Clinical Drug Therapy
RATIONALES FOR NURSING PRACTICE

Clinical Drug Therapy
RATIONALES FOR NURSING PRACTICE

Anne Collins Abrams, RN, MSN
Associate Professor, Emeritus
Department of Baccalaureate and Graduate Nursing
College of Health Sciences
Eastern Kentucky University
Richmond, Kentucky
Chapters 1-6, 13-15, 34-42, 57, 58, 63-65

Carol Barnett Lammon, RN, PhD
Associate Professor
Capstone College of Nursing
University of Alabama
Tuscaloosa, Alabama
Chapters 7-10, 12, 16-20, 26, 29-33, 56, 59-62

Sandra Smith Pennington, RN, PhD
Professor, Emeritus
Department of Nursing
Berea College
Berea, Kentucky;
Academic Dean and Graduate Program Director, RN to MSN Program
Rocky Mountain University of Health Professions
Provo, Utah
Chapters 11, 21-25, 27, 28, 43-55

Consultant
Tracey L. Goldsmith, PharmD
Independent Legal and Healthcare Consultant
Magnolia, Texas

EDITION
9

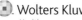 Wolters Kluwer | Lippincott Williams & Wilkins
Health
Philadelphia · Baltimore · New York · London
Buenos Aires · Hong Kong · Sydney · Tokyo

Acquisitions Editor: Hilarie Surrena
Managing Editor: Michelle Clarke
Senior Production Editor: Marian A. Bellus
Director of Nursing Production: Helen Ewan
Senior Managing Editor / Production: Erika Kors
Art Director, Design: Joan Wendt
Art Director, Illustration: Brett MacNaughton
Manufacturing Coordinator: Karin Duffield
Indexer: Michael Ferreira
Compositor: Spearhead

Ninth Edition

9 8 7 6 5 4 3

Printed in China

Library of Congress Cataloging-in-Publication Data

Abrams, Anne Collins.
  Clinical drug therapy: rationales for nursing practice/Anne Collins Abrams, Carol Barnett Lammon, Sandra Smith Pennington; consultant, Tracey L. Goldsmith.—9th ed.
    p. ; cm.
  Includes bibliographical references and index.
  ISBN 978-0-7817-7769-8
  1. Chemotherapy. 2. Drugs. 3. Nursing. I. Lammon, Carol Barnett. II. Pennington, Sandra Smith. III. Title.
  [DNLM: 1. Pharmaceutical Preparations—Nurses' Instruction. 2. Drug Therapy—Nurses' Instruction. QV 55 A161c 2009]
  RM262.A27 2009
  615.5'8—dc22

                                                                      2008032208

RRS1003

Contributors

Susan J. Appel, Ph.D., APRN, ACNP, FNP, BC, CCRN
Associate Professor
University of Alabama at Birmingham
Birmingham, Alabama
Chapter 26

Jennifer Binggeli, PharmD, MBA
Clinical Pharmacist
St. Petersburg, Florida
Chapters 29-33

Kathleen E. Jenks, BSN, MSEd, RN
Associate Professor
Mercy College of Northwest Ohio
Toledo, Ohio
Applying Your Knowledge Features

Marthe Moseley, PhD, RN, CCRN, CCNS
Clinical Nurse Specialist for Critical Care
South Texas Veterans Health Care System
Audie Murphy Hospital
San Antonio, Texas.
Chapters 49 and 51

Mary Annette Wright, RN, MSN, CRNP
Instructor
University of Alabama at Birmingham
Birmingham, Alabama
Chapter 26

Patricia B. Wolff, MSN, ACNS-BC, AOCNS
Clinical Nurse Specialist
Medical Oncology
South Texas Veterans Health Care System
Audie L. Murphy Memorial Veterans Hospital
   Division
San Antonio, Texas
Chapter 42

Susan Alix, RN, MS
Nursing Faculty Instructor
School of Nursing
Worcester State College
Worcester, Massachusetts

Debby Antonella, MSN, RN
Professor
College of Nursing
University of Southern Nevada
Las Vegas, Nevada

April Bigelow, MS, ANP-BC
Assistant Professor
Eastern Michigan University
School of Nursing
Ypsilanti, Michigan

Jean Forsha Byrd, RN, MSN, CNE
Assistant Professor
Community College of Philadelphia
Philadelphia, Pennsylvania

Patricia W. Campbell, RN, MSN
Nursing Faculty
Carolinas College of Health Sciences
Charlotte, North Carolina

Wendy Clark, RN, MSN
Assistant Professor of Nursing
University of Saint Francis
Fort Wayne, Indiana

John F. Conklin, MSN, RN
Nursing Department Chair
Assistant Professor of Nursing
State University of New York Canton

Ellen Cram, PhD, RN
Associate Professor, Clinical
College of Nursing
University of Iowa
Iowa City, Iowa

Angela J. Daniel, MSN, MBA, RN
PhD Candidate School of Nursing
Emory University
Atlanta, Georgia

Jennifer Duhon, RN, MS
Assistant Professor of Nursing
Illinois Central College
East Peoria, Illinois

Susan Ellis-Hermansen, RN, MS
Instructor and Director of Learning Resource Center
University of Maine
Orono, Maine

Brenda L. Haile, RN, DrPH, ACRN
Associate Professor
College of Nursing
Texas Woman's University College of Nursing Houston
    Campus
Houston, Texas

Nancy Hartel, MS, RN, CNE
Associate Professor
St. Joseph's College of Nursing
Syracuse, New York

Karen Hecomovich, MS, RN, BC
Nursing Faculty
Arapahoe Community College.
Littleton, Colorado

Kevin D. Hite, RN, MSN
Assistant Professor of Nursing
Fairmont State University
Fairmont, West Virginia

Jaime Huffman RN, MSN
Instructor of Nursing
Saginaw Valley State University
University Center, Michigan

Immaculata Igbo, MS, PhD
Associate Professor
Prairie View A&M University
Houston, Texas

Michalene A. King, RN, BSN, MSEd, MSN, OhD
Assistant Professor
College of Nursing
University of Akron
Akron, Ohio

Kathie L Kochanowsky, MSN, RN, ANP-C
Nurse practitioner
SpineCare Consultants
Humble, Texas

Judy LaBonte M.S.N., APRN, FNP, BC
Assistant Professor
Baptist College of Health Sciences
Memphis, Tennessee

Melissa Lambert, MSN, RN
Assistant Professor of Nursing
St. Mary's Center for Education
Huntington, West Virginia

John J. Leddy, Ph.D. (Pharmacology)
Assistant Professor
Department of Cellular and Molecular Medicine
University of Ottawa
Ottawa, ON Canada

Adrianne D. Linton, PhD, RN
Chair and Professor, Department of Chronic Nursing Care
School of Nursing Professorship in Aging
University of Texas at San Antonio HSC School of Nursing
San Antonio, Texas

Janet G. Marshall, PhD, RN
Associate Professor
Florida A&M University School of Nursing
Tallahassee, Florida

Kim H McAlister, MSN, RN
Instructor, Clinical
Department of Chronic Nursing Care
UTHSCSA School of Nursing
University of Texas Health Science Center at San Antonio
San Antonio, Texas

Linda McIntosh Liptok, RN, MSN, APRN-BC
Assistant Professor
Kent State University Tuscarawas
New Philadelphia, Ohio

Edna R. Michel-Moyer, CRNP, CS
Professor of Nursing
The Community College of Baltimore County
Catonsville, Maryland

Jane Mighton, RN, BSN, MSN
Nursing Instructor, Term 4
Langara College
Vancouver, British Columbia
Canada

Luke H. Mortensen, PhD, FAHA
Assistant Dean & Professor of Pharmacology and Physiology
Des Moines University
Des Moines, Iowa

Diane E. Mosqueda, RNc, MSN, FNP-C
Nursing Faculty
Houston Community College
Houston, Texas

Sharon Ronaldson, RN, BSN, MEd, PhD
Nursing Instructor
Langara College
Vancouver, BC, Canada

Helene Seibert, RN, MS
Nursing Education Faculty
Southwestern Illinois College
Belleville, Illinois

Patty Shanaberger, RN, MSN, FNP-C
Associate Professor
School of Nursing
El Paso Community College
El Paso, Texas

Cordia A. Starling, RN, EdD
Professor/Dean, School of Nursing
Dalton State College
Dalton, Georgia

Lori Stephens, MN, RN
Nursing Faculty
Skagit Valley College Nursing Department
Mount Vernon, Washington

Judith Swanson, RN, MSN
Assistant Professor of Nursing
Minot State University
Minot, North Dakota

Linda M. Tenofsky, PhD, RN, ANP-BC
Professor/Coordinator Traditional Baccalaureate Program
Department of Nursing
Curry College
Milton, Massachusetts

Charlotte Thayer Wood, PhD
Professor
Mississippi College
School of Nursing
Clinton, Mississippi

Melinda Wang, MSN, WHNP-BC, RN
Assistant Professor of Nursing
Roane State Community College
Harriman, Tennessee

Thomas Worms, MSN, RN
Professor of Nursing
Truman College
Chicago, Illinois

Purpose

The basic precepts underlying previous editions of *Clinical Drug Therapy* also guided the writing of this ninth edition. The overall purpose is to promote safe, effective, and rational drug therapy by

- Providing information that accurately reflects current practices in drug therapy
- Facilitating the acquisition, comprehension, and application of knowledge related to drug therapy. Application requires knowledge about the drug and the patient receiving it.
- Identifying knowledge and skills the nurse can use to smooth the interface between a drug and the patient receiving it

Goals and Responsibilities of Nursing Care Related to Drug Therapy

- Preventing the need for drug therapy, when possible, by promoting health and preventing conditions that require drug therapy
- Using appropriate and effective nonpharmacologic interventions instead of, or in conjunction with, drug therapy when indicated. When used with drug therapy, such interventions may promote lower drug dosage, less frequent administration, and fewer adverse effects.
- Enhancing therapeutic effects by administering drugs accurately and considering patient characteristics that influence responses to drug therapy
- Preventing or minimizing adverse drug effects by knowing the major adverse effects associated with particular drugs, identifying and monitoring patients with characteristics that may increase their risks of experiencing adverse effects, and actively monitoring for the occurrence of adverse effects. When adverse effects occur, early recognition allows interventions to minimize their severity. Because all drugs may cause adverse effects, nurses must maintain a high index of suspicion that signs and symptoms, especially new ones, may be drug induced.
- Teaching patients and caregivers about the role and importance of their medications in treating particular illnesses, accurate administration of medications, nonpharmacologic treatments to use with or instead of pharmacologic treatments, and when to contact a health care provider

Organizational Framework

The content of Clinical Drug Therapy is organized into ten sections, primarily by therapeutic drug groups and their effects on particular body systems. This approach helps students make logical connections between major drug groups and the conditions for which they are used. It also provides a foundation for learning about new drugs, most of which fit into known groups.

The first section contains the basic information required to learn, understand, and apply drug knowledge. The chapters in this section include information about drug names, classifications, prototypes, costs, laws and standards, schedules of controlled substances, drug approval processes, and learning strategies (Chapter 1); cellular physiology, drug transport, pharmacokinetic processes, the receptor theory of drug action, types of drug interactions, and factors that influence drug effects on body tissues (Chapter 2); dosage forms and routes and methods of accurate drug administration (Chapter 3); and guidelines for using the nursing process in drug therapy and general principles of drug therapy (Chapter 4).

Most drug sections include an initial chapter that reviews the physiology of a body system, followed by several chapters that discuss drug groups used to treat disorders of that body system. The seven physiology review chapters are designed to facilitate understanding of drug effects on a body system. These include the central nervous system; the autonomic nervous system; and the endocrine, hematopoietic and immune, respiratory, cardiovascular, and digestive systems. Other chapters within each section emphasize therapeutic classes of drugs and prototypical or commonly used individual drugs, those used to treat common disorders, and those likely to be encountered in clinical nursing practice. Drug chapter content includes a description of a condition (or conditions) for which a drug group is used; a general description of a drug group, including mechanism(s) of action, indications for use, and contraindications; and descriptions and tables of individual drugs, with recommended dosage ranges and routes of administration.

Additional clinically relevant information is presented under the headings of **Nursing Process, Principles of Therapy,** and **Nursing Actions.**

Nursing Process sections emphasize the importance of the nursing process in drug therapy, including assessment of the patient's condition in relation to the drug group, nursing diagnoses, expected outcomes, needed interventions, and evaluation of the patient's progress toward expected outcomes. **Patient Teaching Guidelines** are displayed separately from other interventions to emphasize their importance and for easy student reference.

Principles of Therapy sections present guidelines for maximizing benefits and minimizing adverse effects of drug therapy in various circumstances and populations, including middle-aged and older adults, children and adolescents, and patients with impaired kidney or liver function. General principles are included in Chapter 4; specific principles related to drug groups are included in the chapters where those drug groups are discussed. This approach, rather than separate chapters on pediatric and geriatric pharmacology, for example, was chosen because knowledge about a drug is required before that knowledge can be applied to a specific population with distinctive characteristics and needs in relation to drug therapy.

Each drug chapter includes a **Nursing Actions** display that provides specific nursing responsibilities related to drug administration and patient observation.

Other drug sections include products used to treat infectious, ophthalmic, and dermatologic disorders plus drugs used during pregnancy, labor and delivery, and lactation.

New to This Edition

This thoroughly updated edition includes new content and features:

■ **Updated Drug Information.** Many new drugs have been added: some are additions to well-known drug groups; others represent advances in the drug therapy of some disease processes. In addition, continuing trends in drug dosage formulations are reflected in the increased numbers of fixed-dose combination drug products, long-acting preparations (i.e., 24 hours or longer), and dermatologic (skin patch) products.

■ **Major Revision of Many Chapters.** Chapter revisions reflect current practices in drug therapy, integrate new drugs, and explain the major characteristics of new drug groups. The revisions also reflect a concerted effort to emphasize commonly-used drugs that are likely to be encountered in clinical practice. To this end, approximately 140 drugs were deleted from the chapters.

■ **Evidence-based Practice Displays.** In a landmark report, Crossing the Quality Chasm: A New Health System for the 21st Century (2001), the Institute of Medicine urged health care providers to base care on the best scientific evidence available. In this revision, care has been taken to promote evidence-based practice in pharmacotherapeutics in the text as well as in the evidence-based practice displays.

■ **Black Box Warnings.** A Black Box Warning appearing on the package insert or drug label for a prescription drug identifies a drug with a significant risk of serious or life threatening adverse effects. It is the strongest warning required by the Food and Drug Administration. Throughout this revision, **BLACK BOX WARNINGS** are identified, alerting the nurse to the risk of serious adverse effects.

■ **Applying Your Knowledge.** These threaded case studies provide real-world examples and lend significance to conceptual content. Each drug chapter opens with a patient scenario, which builds throughout the chapter. Case-based questions test students' critical thinking, and special "How Do You Avoid This Medication Error?" questions promote safe and accurate drug administration. The answers to these questions can be found at the end of the book.

■ **Key Terms.** Terms that are key to understanding each chapter's content.

■ **Key Concepts.** These concepts provide the most salient content for the student and appear at the end of each chapter.

■ **Glossary.** Contains definitions of all of the key terms.

Special Features

■ **Readability.** Since the first edition of Clinical Drug Therapy, many students and faculty have commented about the book's clear presentation style.

■ **Organizational Framework.** The book's organizational framework allows it to be used effectively as both a textbook and as a reference. Used as a textbook, students can read chapters in their entirety to learn the characteristics of major drug classes, their prototypical drugs or commonly used representatives, their uses and effects in prevention or treatment of disease processes, and their implications for nursing practice. Used as a reference book, students can readily review selected topics for classroom use or clinical application. Facilitating such uses are a consistent format and frequent headings that allow readers to identify topics at a glance.

■ **Chapter Objectives.** Learning objectives at the beginning of each chapter focus students' attention on important chapter content.

■ **Drugs at a Glance Tables.** These tables highlight and summarize pertinent drug information, including drug names, dosage ranges, and other related facts.

■ **Boxed Displays.** These include information to promote understanding of drug therapy for selected conditions.

■ **Herbal and Dietary Supplements.** Commonly used products are introduced in Chapter 4 and included in selected later chapters. Safety aspects are emphasized.

■ **Patient Teaching Guidelines.** This feature is designed to meet several goals. One is to highlight the importance of teaching patients and caregivers how to manage drug therapy at home, where most medications are taken. This is done by separating teaching from other nursing interventions. Another goal is to promote active and knowledgeable patient participation in drug therapy regimens, which helps to maximize therapeutic effects and minimize adverse effects. In addition, written guidelines allow patients and caregivers to have a source of reference when questions arise in the home setting. A third goal is to make patient teaching easier and less time consuming. Using the guidelines as a foundation, the nurse can simply add or delete information according to a patient's individual needs. To assist both the nurse and patient further, the guidelines contain minimal medical jargon.

■ **Principles of Therapy.** This unique section describes important drug- and patient-related characteristics that need to be considered in drug therapy regimens. Such considerations can greatly increase safety and therapeutic effects, and all health care providers associated with drug therapy should be aware of them. Most chapters contain principles with the headings of **Use in Children, Use in Older Adults, Use in Patients with Renal Impairment, Use in Patients with Hepatic Impairment,** and **Use in Home Care** to denote differences related to age, developmental level, pathophysiology, and setting. Some chapters include principles related to these headings as well: **Genetic and Ethnic Considerations, Use in Critical Illness,** and **Management of Drug Toxicity or Drug Withdrawal.**

■ **Nursing Actions Displays.** These displays emphasize nursing interventions during drug therapy within the following categories: Administer accurately, Observe for therapeutic effects, Observe for adverse effects, and Observe for drug interactions. The inclusion of rationales for interventions provides a strong knowledge base and scientific foundation for clinical practice and critical thinking.

■ **Review and Application Exercises.** Located at the end of each chapter, these exercises include two types of questions. Short Answer questions encourage students to rehearse clinical application strategies in a nonclinical, nonstressful, nondistracting environment. They also promote self-testing in chapter content and can be used to promote classroom discussion. NCLEX-style questions help students prepare for the licensing examination. Answers and rationales for these exercises can be found on the Instructor's Resource CD-ROM.

■ **Appendices.** These include the International System of Units, therapeutic serum drug concentrations for selected drugs, anesthetics, and drugs for erectile dysfunction.

■ **Extensive Index.** Listings of generic and trade names of drugs, nursing process, and other topics provide rapid access to desired information.

Teaching–Learning Package

Nursing students must develop skills in critical thinking, information processing, decision making, collaboration, and problem solving. How can a nurse educator assist students to develop these skills in relation to drug therapy? The ancillary package assists both students and teachers in this development.

The **Study Guide** engages students' interest and active participation by providing a variety of learning exercises and opportunities to practice cognitive skills. Assessing Your Understanding promotes the learning of concepts, principles, and characteristics and uses of major drug groups and can be completed independently or by small groups as in-class learning activities. Applying Your Knowledge scenarios promote appropriate data collection, critical analysis of both drug- and patient-related data, and application of the data in patient care. Practicing for NCLEX, which provides NCLEX-style review questions to help students apply and retain the key information from each chapter.

The companion Web site, http://thepoint.lww.com, provides online updates for faculty and students, links to newly approved drugs, and more.

The free **Student Resource CD-ROM** is an invaluable learning tool that provides 3-D animated demonstrations of pharmacology concepts, medication administration video, and monographs of the most commonly prescribed drugs.

Resources for Instructors:

A set of tools to assist you in teaching your course is available on thePoint at http://thepoint.lww.com. ThePoint is a web-based system that allows you to manage your course and content and provides every resource instructors need in one easy-to-use site.

If, as an instructor, you want help structuring your lessons…

We've provided Guided Lecture Notes that are built on the learning objectives of each chapter. They consist of brief talking points and suggestions for how to present the material in the chapter and are supported by PowerPoint slides, which condense the material into bulleted lists, figures, and tables.

If you need suggestions, aside from straight lecturing, for engaging your students in the material…

We've provided Assignments for each chapter. These cover group assignments, written assignments, clinical assignments, and web-based assignments, so that you can capture the diverse learning styles of your students and be sure they approach the material from a variety of perspectives.

If you want to encourage your students to read the assigned chapter thoroughly before coming to class…

We've provided Pre-Lecture Quizzes (and answers), which are simple multiple-choice and true/false quizzes designed to test whether the student has read and grasped the material before the lecture or other classroom activities begin.

If you'd like your students to start applying what they've learned….

We've provided Discussion Topics and suggested answers to get students talking constructively about how their nursing knowledge works in real-world scenarios. As an added bonus, these discussions can take place online, adding a valuable technologic component to your teaching. We've also provided Case Studies and suggested answers, which encourage students to apply their new knowledge to the types of patient cases they'll likely encounter in practice.

If you're concerned about preparing your students for the NCLEX exams…

We've provided a Test Generator and a set of Student Review Questions, both of which include unique questions for each chapter. These questions are presented in traditional and in alternate-form NCLEX style, so students will become familiar with the format of the exams.

These varied materials allow each instructor to choose or adapt them relevant to his or her circumstances. The authors and publisher hope these resources are truly helpful in easing the day-to-day rigors of teaching pharmacology and invite comments from instructors regarding the materials.

Anne Collins Abrams, RN, MSN
Carol Barnett Lammon, RN, PhD
Sandra Smith Pennington, RN, PhD

Drugs at a Glance tables give students characteristics as well as routes and dosage ranges in an easy-to-read format. Prototype drugs are highlighted in the tables and in the text.

Learning Objectives let students know what they're going to learn in each and every chapter.

Table 24-2	Drugs at a Glance: **Drugs for Hypothyroidism and Hyperthyroidism**	
	ROUTES AND DOSAGE RANGES	
Generic/Trade name	**Adults**	**Children**
Drugs for Hypothyroidism		
P Levothyroxine (Synthroid, Levothroid)	PO 0.05 mg/d initially, increased by 0.025 mg every 2–3 wk until desired response obtained; usual maintenance dose, 0.1–0.2 mg/d (100–200 mcg/d) Myxedema coma, IV 0.4 mg in a single dose; then 0.1–0.2 mg daily Thyroid-stimulating hormone (TSH) suppression in thyroid cancer, nodules, and euthyroid goiters, PO 2.6 mcg/kg/d for 7–10 d *Older adults, patients with cardiac disorders, and patients with hypothyroidism of long duration:* PO 0.0125–0.025 mg/d for 6 wk, then dose is doubled every 6–8 wk until the desired response is obtained Myxedema coma, same as adult dosage	Congenital hypothyroidism, PO as follows: *>12 y:* >150 mcg/d (or 2–3 mcg/kg/d) *6–12 y:* 100–150 mcg/d (or 4–5 mcg/kg/d) *1–5 y:* 75–100 mcg/d (or 5–6 mcg/kg/d) *6–12 mo:* 50–75 mcg/d (or 6–8 mcg/kg/d) *Birth–6 mo:* 25–50 mcg/d (or 8–10 mcg/kg/d)
	PO 300–400 mg/d in divided doses q8h, until the patient is euthyroid; then 100–150 mg/d in 3 divided doses, for maintenance	>10 y: PO 150–300 mg/d in divided doses q8h; usual maintenance dose, 100–300 mg/d in 2 divided doses, q12h 6–10 y: 50–150 mg/d in divided doses q8h
	PO 15–60 mg/d initially, in divided doses q8h until the patient is euthyroid; maintenance, 5–15 mg/d in 2 or 3 doses	PO 0.4 mg/kg/d initially, in divided doses q8h; maintenance dose, one half initial dose
Strong iodine solution (Lugol's solution)	PO 2–6 drops 3 times per day for 10 d before thyroidectomy	PO 2–6 drops 3 times per day for 10 d before thyroidectomy
Saturated solution of	PO 5 drops 3 times per day for 10 d before thyroidectomy	PO 5 drops 3 times per day for 10 d before thyroidectomy
	PO, IV, dosage as calculated by a radiologist trained in nuclear medicine	PO, IV, dosage as calculated by a radiologist trained in nuclear medicine
	PO 40–160 mg/d in divided doses	

Applying Your Knowledge

Jose Rojas is a 24-year-old man who has suffered a head injury while riding his motorcycle without a helmet. He has been admitted for observation, with multiple abrasions and a blow to the head. Mr. Rojas begins to produce massive amounts of clear, pale-yellow urine. The physician diagnoses him with diabetes insipidus and orders desmopressin 0.2 mL in two divided doses intranasally.

 Applying Your Knowledge 22-1

How Can You Avoid This Medication Error?
The nurse prepares Mr. Rojas' medication and administers 0.2 mL of desmopressin intranasally.

Applying Your Knowledge features help students apply concepts to patient care. Most chapters open with a patient scenario, which is then carried through the chapter. Applying Your Knowledge questions require students to take the content they have learned and apply it to the patient in the case study, and special "How Do You Avoid This Medication Error?" questions reinforce safe drug administration. Answers are provided at the end of the book, allowing students to monitor their progress.

LEARNING OBJECTIVES

After studying this chapter, you will be able to:

1. Identify clinical uses of selected hormones.
2. Differentiate characteristics and functions of anterior and posterior pituitary hormones.
3. Recognize the limitations of hypothalamic and pituitary hormones as therapeutic agents.
4. Identify major nursing considerations in the care of patients receiving specific hypothalamic and pituitary hormones.

Nursing Process

Assessment

- Assess for signs and symptoms of thyroid disorders (see Table 24-1). During the course of treatment with thyroid or antithyroid drugs, the patient's blood level of thyroid hormone may range from low to normal to high. At either end of the continuum, signs and symptoms may be dramatic and obvious. As blood levels change toward normal as a result of treatment, signs and symptoms become less obvious. If presenting signs and symptoms are treated too aggressively, they may change toward the opposite end of the continuum and indicate adverse drug effects. Thus, *each patient receiving a drug that alters thyroid function must be assessed for indicators of hypothyroidism, euthyroidism, and hyperthyroidism.*

nursing process continues on page 1060

Nursing Process material helps students think about drug therapy in terms of the nursing process.

Patient Teaching Guidelines give students specific information they may need to educate patients.

Patient Teaching Guidelines · Oral Fluoroquinolones

General Considerations

- Avoid exposure to sunlight during and for several days after taking one of these drugs. Stop taking the drug and notify the prescribing physician if skin burning, redness, swelling, rash, or itching occurs. Sunscreen lotions do not prevent photosensitivity reactions.
- Be very careful if driving or doing other tasks requiring alertness or physical coordination. These drugs may cause dizziness or lightheadedness.

Self-Administration

- Take norfloxacin (Noroxin) levofloxacin solution and ofloxacin (Floxin) 1 hour before or 2 hours after meals on an empty stomach. Ciprofloxacin (Cipro) may be taken with food to decrease GI upset. Gatifloxacin (Teguin), gemifloxacin (Factive), levofloxacin tabs, and moxifloxacin (Avelox) can be taken with or without regard to meals.
- Drink 2 to 3 quarts of fluid daily if able. This helps to prevent kidney problems.
- Do not take antacids containing magnesium or aluminum (e.g., Mylanta or Maalox); any products containing iron, magnesium, calcium (e.g., Tums), or zinc (e.g., multivitamins); sucralfate; or buffered didanosine preparations at the same time, or for several hours before or after a dose of the fluoroquinolone. (Consult product-specific information for individual drug recommendations.)

Evidence-based Practice Boxes give students information they need to —→ improve the quality of care provided to patients.

Black Box Warnings —→ alert nursing students to the risk of serious or life threatening adverse effects associated with a drug.

Pramlintide is given by subcutaneous injection before meals. Opened vials of pramlintide may be stored in a refrigerator or at room temperature for up to 28 days. It cannot be mixed in the same injection with mealtime insulin. Reduction in insulin dosages by 50% is required with initiation of pramlintide therapy to reduce the incidence of hypoglycemia. A **BLACK BOX WARNING** alerts nurses to the danger of severe insulin-induced hypoglycemia with pramlintide therapy, especially in type 1 diabetics. Nausea, another frequent adverse effect of pramlintide, tends to decrease with time and may be reduced with careful titration of the dosage to the therapeutic level. Pramlintide may delay the absorption of concurrently administered oral medications.

Evidence-Based Practice

26-1 Use of Alternative Medicines in Diabetes Mellitus

It is well documented in the literature that a significant number of individuals with diabetes mellitus use complementary and alternative medicine (CAM). CAM includes acupuncture, relaxation techniques, massage, chiropractic, spiritual healing, herbal medicines, and vitamin supplements. Estimates of CAM use by patients with diabetes range as high as 57% in the literature and are comparable with CAM use by nondiabetic individuals. Studies reveal that generally diabetics use the same supplements and alternative remedies as nondiabetic individuals with the exception of increased use of chromium. The literature documents that some patients use CAM to lower blood glucose as well as to treat complications of diabetes; however, the majority of individuals report using CAM for a condition unrelated to diabetes. The use of CAM by diabetics raises several concerns. One obvious concern is the implications of using CAM in replacement of traditional therapies for diabetes such as insulin and oral hypoglycemic drugs; however, one study in the literature suggested that most diabetic patients use CAM in addition to traditional therapies rather than as a replacement for traditional medications. Another study documented that diabetic patients using CAM were more likely to also use preventive care practices such as obtaining a pneumococcal vaccination and visiting their health care provider on a regular basis. A second concern is the potential of CAM to do harm. With regard to herbal and vitamin supplements, harmful effects include potential interactions with traditional drugs as well as increased risk for hepatotoxicity, nephrotoxicity, and poor glycemic control. A third concern is the cost of CAM; one study reported that diabetics using CAM spend as much on the alternative therapies as they do on prescription drugs.

Because the use of CAM is widespread and has the potential for impacting blood glucose levels of diabetic patients, nurses should take careful drug histories, including questions about use of herbal and over-the-counter supplements. Nurses should also educate diabetic patients about the potential impact of complementary therapies on blood glucose levels when this information is available.

Herbal and Dietary Supplements

Increasing numbers of people are choosing alternative medications to complement or, in some cases, to replace prescription medications. With most herbs and dietary supplements, even the commonly used ones (e.g., echinacea, St. John's wort), the effects on blood glucose levels are unknown; well-controlled, long-term studies of effects have not been done; and interactions with antidiabetic drugs are unknown. Thus, anyone with diabetes who wishes to take an herbal or dietary supplement should consult a health care provider, read product labels carefully, seek the most authoritative information available, and monitor blood glucose closely when starting the supplement. Described below are some products that reportedly affect blood sugar and that should be used cautiously, if at all, by patients with diabetes.

←— **Herbal and Dietary Supplement** content is highlighted so students become aware of how these alternative therapies can affect traditional medications.

Nursing Actions Beta-Lactam Antibacterials

NURSING ACTIONS	RATIONALE/EXPLANATION
1. Administer accurately a. With penicillins: (1) Give most oral penicillins on an empty stomach, approximately 1 hour before or 2 hours after a meal. Penicillin V, amoxicillin, and amoxicillin/clavulanate may be given with food.	To decrease binding to foods and inactivation by gastric acid. The latter three drugs are not significantly affected by food.

↑

Nursing Actions give students specific instructions on administration of drugs and observations of patient responses, with rationales for each step.

Review and Application Exercises

Short Answer Exercises

1. Why must aminoglycosides be given parenterally for systemic infections?

2. How are aminoglycosides excreted?

3. What are risk factors for aminoglycoside-induced nephrotoxicity and ototoxicity?

4. How would you assess a patient for nephrotoxicity or ototoxicity?

5. What is the reason for giving an aminoglycoside and an antipseudomonal penicillin in the treatment of serious infections caused by *P. aeruginosa*?

6. Why should an aminoglycoside and an antipseudomonal penicillin not be combined in a syringe or IV fluid for administration?

7. Which laboratory tests need to be monitored regularly for a patient receiving a systemic aminoglycoside?

8. What is the rationale for giving an oral aminoglycoside to treat hepatic coma?

9. What are the main clinical uses of fluoroquinolones?

10. What are adverse effects of fluoroquinolones, and how may they be prevented or minimized?

11. Why is it important to maintain an adequate fluid intake and urine output while taking a fluoroquinolone?

12. Why are fluoroquinolones not preferred drugs for children?

NCLEX-Style Questions

13. A hospitalized patient is scheduled to receive levofloxacin 500 mg PO at 9:00 A.M. The medication administration record also indicates that Maalox 30 mL PO and hydrochlorothiazide 25 mg PO are due at 9:00 A.M. The nurse should
   a. Administer all the medications as scheduled.
   b. Hold the Maalox until 11:00 A.M.
   c. Ask the physician to discontinue hydrochlorothiazide because of increased risk of ototoxicity.
   d. Administer the Maalox and levofloxacin, but hold the hydrochlorothiazide.

14. A critically ill patient is receiving tobramycin 1.5 mg/kg IV every 8 hours. The patient has recently stopped making urine, and the most recent laboratory results indicate that the creatinine level has risen from normal to 3.6 mg/dL. At the next scheduled administration time for tobramycin, the nurse should
   a. Administer half the prescribed dose.
   b. Hold the tobramycin and notify the physician.
   c. Administer tobramycin as prescribed.
   d. Draw a blood sample for testing the tobramycin level before the dose and then administer as prescribed.

15. An outpatient client has just been given a prescription for moxifloxacin 400 mg PO once daily for acute bronchitis. The nurse should teach the patient
   a. not to take moxifloxacin with a meal
   b. to restrict fluid intake to avoid fluid overload
   c. to take moxifloxacin with an antacid (e.g., Tums) to decrease the chance of stomach upset
   d. to avoid prolonged exposure to sunlight

←— **Review and Application Exercises** provide students with the opportunity to review what they just learned. These include both short-answer exercises and NCLEX-style questions.

Acknowledgments

Sincere appreciation is expressed to the following people who assisted in the preparation of this book:

Contributors Susan Appel, Jennifer Binggeli, Kathleen Jenks, Marthe Moseley, and Patricia Wolff, and Mary Annette Wright

Tracey Goldsmith, PharmD, who reviewed all chapters.

Editors and staff at Lippincott Williams and Wilkins

Contents

Chapter Outline

Introduction to Pharmacology

KEY TERMS

- Biotechnology
- Brand or trade name
- Controlled substances
- Drug classifications
- Generic name
- Over-the-counter (OTC) drugs
- Pharmacoeconomics
- Pharmacotherapy
- Placebo
- Prescription drugs
- Prototype
- Systemic effects

LEARNING OBJECTIVES

After studying this chapter, you will be able to:

1. Differentiate between pharmacology and drug therapy.
2. Distinguish between generic and trade names of drugs.
3. Define a prototypical drug.
4. Select authoritative sources of drug information.
5. Discuss major drug laws and standards.
6. Describe the main categories of controlled substances in relation to therapeutic use and potential for abuse.
7. Identify nursing responsibilities in handling controlled substances correctly.
8. Discuss the role of the Food and Drug Administration.
9. Analyze the potential impact of drug costs on drug therapy regimens.
10. Develop personal techniques for learning about drugs and using drug knowledge in patient care.

A Message to Students

You have probably been taking medicines and seeing other people take medicines most of your life. Perhaps you have given medicines to your children, parents, grandparents, or others. Have you ever wondered why it is usually okay to give children Tylenol but not aspirin? Why do a lot of middle-aged and older people take an aspirin a day? Why do people with high blood pressure, heart failure, or diabetes take angiotensin-converting enzyme (ACE) inhibitors, and what are ACE inhibitors? When should an antibiotic NOT be prescribed for an infection?

You are embarking on an exciting journey of discovery as you begin or continue your study of pharmacology. Much of what you learn will be useful in your personal and family life as well as in your professional life as a nurse. The purpose of this book is to help you learn about medications and why, how, when, and where they are used in daily life. Bon voyage!!

Pharmacology and Drug Therapy

Pharmacology is the study of drugs (chemicals) that alter functions of living organisms. Drug therapy, also called *pharmacotherapy*, is the use of drugs to prevent, diagnose, or treat signs, symptoms, and disease processes. When prevention or cure is not a reasonable goal, relief of symptoms can greatly improve a patient's quality of life and ability to function in activities of daily living. Drugs given for therapeutic purposes are called medications.

Medications may be given for local or *systemic effects*. Drugs with local effects, such as sunscreen lotions and local anesthetics, act mainly at the site of application. Those with systemic effects are taken into the body, circulated through the bloodstream to their sites of action in various body tissues, and eventually eliminated from the body. *Most drugs are given for their systemic effects.* Drugs may also be given for acute disorders, such as pain or infection, or to relieve signs and symptoms of long-term disease processes, such as hypertension or diabetes.

Drug Sources

Where do medications come from? Historically, drugs were derived from plants, animals, and minerals. Now, most drugs are synthetic compounds manufactured in laboratories. Chemists, for example, often create a useful new drug by altering the chemical structure of an existing drug. Such techniques and other technologic advances have enabled the production of new drugs as well as synthetic versions of many drugs originally derived from plants and animals. Synthetic drugs are more standardized in their chemical characteristics, more consistent in their effects, and less likely to produce allergic reactions. Semisynthetic drugs (e.g., many antibiotics) are naturally occurring substances that have been chemically modified.

Biotechnology is also an important source of drugs. This process involves manipulating deoxyribonucleic acid (DNA) and ribonucleic acid (RNA) and recombining genes into hybrid molecules that can be inserted into living organisms (*Escherichia coli* bacteria are often used) and repeatedly reproduced. Each hybrid molecule produces a genetically identical molecule, called a clone. Cloning makes it possible to identify the DNA sequence in a gene and to produce the protein product encoded by a gene, such as insulin. Cloning also allows production of adequate amounts of the drug for therapeutic or research purposes. Biotechnology drugs constitute an increasing percentage of drugs now undergoing development, and this trend is expected to continue into the foreseeable future.

Drug Classifications and Prototypes

Drugs are classified according to their effects on particular body systems, their therapeutic uses, and their chemical characteristics. For example, morphine can be classified as a central nervous system depressant and a narcotic or opioid analgesic. The names of therapeutic classifications usually reflect the conditions for which the drugs are used (e.g., antidepressants, antihypertensives). However, the names of many drug groups reflect their chemical characteristics rather than their therapeutic uses (e.g., adrenergics, benzodiazepines). Many drugs fit into multiple groups because they have wide-ranging effects on the human body.

Individual drugs that represent groups of drugs are called *prototypes*. **P Prototypes**, often the first drug of a particular group to be developed, are usually the standard with which newer, similar drugs are compared. For example, morphine is the prototype of opioid analgesics; penicillin is the prototype of antibacterial drugs.

Drug classifications and prototypes are quite stable, and most new drugs can be assigned to a group and compared with an established prototype. However, some groups lack a universally accepted prototype, and some prototypes are replaced over time by newer, more commonly used drugs.

Drug Names

Individual drugs may have several different names, but the two that are most commonly used are the generic name and the trade or brand name. The *generic name* (e.g., amoxicillin) is related to the chemical or official name and is independent of the manufacturer. *The generic name often indicates the drug group* (e.g., *drugs with generic names ending in "cillin" are penicillins*). The *trade or brand name* is designated and patented by the manufacturer. For example, amoxicillin is manufactured by several pharmaceutical companies, some of which assign a specific trade name (e.g., Amoxil, Trimox) and several of which use only the generic name. In drug literature, trade names are capitalized and generic names are presented in lowercase unless in a list or at the beginning of a sentence. Drugs may be prescribed and dispensed by generic or trade name.

Drug Marketing

A new drug is protected by patent for several years, during which time only the pharmaceutical manufacturer that developed it can market it. This is seen as a return on the company's investment in developing a drug, which may require years of work and millions of dollars, and as an incentive for developing other drugs. Other pharmaceutical companies cannot manufacture and market the drug until the patent expires. However, for new drugs that are popular and widely used, other companies often produce similar drugs, with different generic and trade names. Generic drugs are required to be therapeutically equivalent and are less expensive than trade-name drugs.

Pharmacoeconomics

Pharmacoeconomics involves the costs of drug therapy, including costs of purchasing, dispensing (i.e., salaries of pharmacists, pharmacy technicians), storage, administration (i.e., salaries of nurses, costs of supplies), laboratory and other tests used to monitor patient responses, and losses due to expiration. Length of illness or hospitalization is also considered. The goal of most pharmacoeconomic research is to identify drug therapy regimens that provide the desired benefits at the least cost.

Prescription and Nonprescription Drugs

Legally, American consumers have two routes of access to therapeutic drugs. One route is by *prescription* from a licensed health care provider, such as a physician, dentist, or nurse practitioner. The other route is by over-the-counter (OTC) purchase of drugs that do not require a prescription. These routes are regulated by various drug laws. Acquiring and using prescription drugs for nontherapeutic purposes by persons who are not authorized to have the drugs or for whom they are not prescribed is illegal.

American Drug Laws and Standards

Current drug laws and standards have evolved over many years. Their main goal is to protect the public by ensuring that drugs marketed for therapeutic purposes are safe and effective. Their main provisions are further described below and summarized in Table 1-1.

The Food, Drug, and Cosmetic Act of 1938 and its amendments regulate the manufacture, distribution, advertising, and labeling of drugs. The law also requires that official drugs (i.e., those listed in the United States Pharmacopeia and

designated USP) must meet standards of purity and strength as determined by chemical analysis or by animal response to specified doses (bioassay). The Durham-Humphrey Amendment designates drugs that must be prescribed by a licensed physician or nurse practitioner and dispensed by a pharmacist. The Food and Drug Administration (FDA) is charged with enforcing the law. In addition, the Public Health Service regulates vaccines and other biologic products, and the Federal Trade Commission can suppress misleading advertisements of nonprescription drugs.

The Comprehensive Drug Abuse Prevention and Control Act was passed in 1970. Title II of this law, called the Controlled Substances Act, regulates the manufacture and distribution of narcotics, stimulants, depressants, hallucinogens, and anabolic steroids. These drugs are categorized according to therapeutic usefulness and potential for abuse (Box 1-1) and are labeled as *controlled substances* (e.g., morphine is a C-II or Schedule II drug).

Table 1-1	American Drug Laws and Amendments	
YEAR	**NAME**	**MAIN PROVISION(S)**
1906	Pure Food and Drug Act	■ Established official standards and requirements for accurate labeling of drug products ■ Established the forerunner of FDA
1912	Sherley Amendment	Prohibited fraudulent claims of drug effectiveness
1914	Harrison Narcotic Act	Restricted the importation, manufacture, sale, and use of opium, cocaine, marijuana, and other drugs that the Act defined as narcotics
1938	Food, Drug, and Cosmetic Act	■ Revised and broadened FDA powers and responsibilities; gave the FDA control over drug safety ■ Required proof of safety from the manufacturer before a new drug could be marketed ■ Authorized factory inspections ■ Established penalties for fraudulent claims and misleading labels
1945	Amendment	Required governmental certification of biologic products, such as insulin and antibiotics
1952	Durham-Humphrey Amendment	Designated drugs that must be prescribed by a physician and dispensed by a pharmacist (e.g., controlled substances, drugs considered unsafe for use except under supervision by a health care provider, and drugs limited to prescription use under a manufacturer's new drug application)
1962	Kefauver-Harris Amendment	■ Required a manufacturer to provide evidence (from well-controlled research studies) that a drug was effective for claims and conditions identified in the product's labeling ■ Gave the federal government the authority to standardize drug names
1970	Comprehensive Drug Abuse Prevention and Control Act; Title II, Controlled Substances Act	■ Regulated distribution of narcotics and other drugs of abuse ■ Categorized these drugs according to therapeutic usefulness and potential for abuse ■ Updated or replaced all previous laws re: narcotics and other dangerous drugs
1978	Drug Regulation Reform Act	■ Established guidelines for research studies and data to be submitted to the FDA by manufacturers ■ Shortened the time required to develop and market new drugs

YEAR	NAME	MAIN PROVISION(S)
1983	Orphan Drug Act	■ Decreased taxes and competition for manufacturers who would produce drugs to treat selected serious disorders affecting relatively few people
1987		■ Established new regulations designed to speed up the approval process for high-priority medications
1992	Prescription Drug User Fee Act	■ Allowed the FDA to collect user fees from pharmaceutical companies, with each new drug application, to shorten the review time (e.g., by hiring more staff) ■ Specified a review time of 12 months for standard drugs and 6 months for priority drugs
1993	NIH Revitalization Act	Requires inclusion of women and minorities in NIH-funded research studies, including Phase III clinical drug trials
1997	FDA Modernization Act	■ Updated regulation of biologic products ■ Increased patient access to experimental drugs and medical devices ■ Accelerated review of important new drugs ■ Allowed drug companies to disseminate information about off-label (non–FDA-approved) uses and costs of drugs ■ Extended user fees
2002	Best Pharmaceuticals for Children Act	■ Encouraged pharmaceutical companies to conduct studies and label drugs for use in children ■ Provided funds for 5 years for pediatric drug studies

The Drug Enforcement Administration (DEA) enforces the Controlled Substances Act. Individuals and companies legally empowered to handle controlled substances must be registered with the DEA, keep accurate records of all transactions, and provide for secure storage. Prescribers are assigned a number by the DEA and must include the number on all prescriptions they write for a controlled substance. Prescriptions for Schedule II drugs cannot be refilled; a new prescription is required. Nurses are responsible for storing controlled substances in locked containers, administering them only to people for whom they are prescribed, recording each dose given on agency narcotic sheets and on the patient's medication administration record, maintaining an accurate inventory, and reporting discrepancies to the proper authorities.

Historically, drug research was done mainly with young, white males. In 1993, Congress passed the National Institutes

---

Box 1-1	**Categories of Controlled Substances**

Schedule I

Drugs that are not approved for medical use and have high abuse potentials: flunitrazepam (Rohypnol) gamma hydroxybutyric acid (GHB), heroin, lysergic acid diethylamide (LSD), marijuana, 3,4-methylenedioxy-methamphetamine (MDMA or ecstasy), mescaline, peyote, tetrahydrocannabinol.

Schedule II

Drugs that are used medically and have high abuse potentials: opioid analgesics (e.g., codeine, hydromorphone, methadone, meperidine, morphine, oxycodone, oxymorphone), central nervous system (CNS) stimulants (e.g., cocaine, methamphetamine, methylphenidate), and barbiturate sedative-hypnotics (amobarbital, pentobarbital, secobarbital).

Schedule III

Drugs with less potential for abuse than those in Schedules I and II, but abuse may lead to psychological or physical dependence: androgens and anabolic steroids, ketamine, some CNS stimulants (e.g., benzphetamine), and mixtures containing small amounts of controlled substances (e.g., codeine, barbiturates not listed in other schedules).

Schedule IV

Drugs with some potential for abuse: benzodiazepines (e.g., diazepam, lorazepam, temazepam), other sedative-hypnotics (e.g., phenobarbital, chloral hydrate), and some prescription appetite suppressants (e.g., mazindol, phentermine).

Schedule V

Products containing moderate amounts of controlled substances. They may be dispensed by the pharmacist without a physician's prescription but with some restrictions regarding amount, record keeping, and other safeguards. Included are antidiarrheal drugs, such as diphenoxylate and atropine (Lomotil).

of Health (NIH) Revitalization Act, which formalized a policy of the NIH that women and minorities be included in human subject research studies funded by the NIH and that women and minorities be included in clinical drug trials. Now, major drug trials must recruit female subjects and include outcome data on women. In addition, all newly developed drugs must include gender-related effectiveness and safety information in the initial FDA application. Despite these regulations, however, there is still relatively little information about drug effects in women because many commonly used drugs were developed before enactment of these regulations.

In addition to federal laws, state laws also regulate the sale and distribution of controlled drugs. These laws may be more stringent than federal laws; if so, the stricter laws usually apply.

Drug Approval Processes

The FDA is responsible for ensuring that new drugs are safe and effective before approving the drugs and allowing them to be marketed. The FDA reviews research studies (usually conducted or sponsored by pharmaceutical companies) about proposed new drugs; the organization does not test the drugs.

Since 1962, newly developed drugs are extensively tested before being marketed for general use. Initially, drugs are tested in animals and the FDA reviews the test results. Next, clinical trials in humans are done, usually with a randomized, controlled experimental design that involves selection of subjects according to established criteria, random assignment of subjects to experimental groups, and administration of the test drug to one group and a control substance to another group.

Testing proceeds through several phases if there is continuing evidence of drug safety and effectiveness. In Phase I, a few doses are given to a certain number of healthy volunteers to determine safe dosages, routes of administration, absorption, metabolism, excretion, and toxicity. In Phase II, a few doses are given to a certain number of subjects with the disease or symptom for which the drug is being studied, and responses are compared with those of healthy subjects. In Phase III, the drug is given to a larger and more representative group of subjects. In double-blind, placebo-controlled designs, half of the subjects receive the new drug and half receive a *placebo* (an inactive substance similar in appearance to the actual drug), with neither subjects nor researchers knowing who receives which formulation. In crossover studies, subjects serve as their own control; each subject receives the experimental drug during half of the study and a placebo during the other half. Other research methods include control studies in which some patients receive a known drug rather than a placebo; in subject matching, patients are paired with others of similar characteristics. Phase III studies help to determine whether the potential benefits of the drug outweigh the risks. Testing may be stopped during any of the early phases if inadequate effectiveness or excessive toxicity becomes evident. In Phase IV, the FDA evaluates the data from the first three phases for drug safety and effectiveness, allows the drug to be marketed for general use, and requires manufacturers to continue monitoring the drug's effects.

Some approved and marketed drugs (e.g., Vioxx) are later withdrawn, usually because of serious adverse effects that become evident only when the drugs are used in a large, diverse population. In addition, in recent years the FDA has issued warnings about several drugs that can cause serious adverse effects (e.g., antidepressants, nonsteroidal anti-inflammatory drugs [NSAIDs] such as aspirin and ibuprofen, and oseltamivir [Tamiflu], an antiflu drug). As a result, the FDA has been criticized for approving these and other drugs and allowing them to be marketed in the first place. Some authorities are urging major reforms in the drug approval process, the methods of reporting adverse drug effects, and postmarketing surveillance procedures.

Food and Drug Administration Approval

The FDA approves many new drugs annually. New drugs are categorized according to their review priority and therapeutic potential. A status of "1P" indicates a new drug reviewed on a priority (accelerated) basis and with some therapeutic advantages over drugs already available; a status of "1S" indicates standard review and drugs with few, if any, therapeutic advantages (i.e., the new drug is similar to one or more older drugs currently on the market). Most new drugs are "1S" prescription drugs.

The FDA also approves drugs for OTC availability, including the transfer of drugs from prescription to OTC status, and may require additional clinical trials to determine the safety and effectiveness of OTC use. For prescription drugs taken orally, transfer to OTC status may mean different indications for use and lower doses. FDA approval of a drug for OTC availability involves evaluation of evidence that the consumer can use the drug safely, using information on the product label, and shifts primary responsibility for safe and effective drug therapy from health care professionals to consumers. With prescription drugs, a health care professional diagnoses the condition, often with the help of laboratory and other diagnostic tests, and determines a need for the drug. With OTC drugs, the patient must make these decisions, with or without consultation with a health care provider.

Having drugs available OTC has potential advantages and disadvantages for consumers. Advantages include greater autonomy, faster and more convenient access to effective treatment, possibly earlier resumption of usual activities of daily living, fewer visits to a health care provider, and possibly increased efforts by consumers to learn about their symptoms/conditions and recommended treatments. Disadvantages include inaccurate self-diagnoses and potential risks of choosing a wrong or contraindicated drug, delaying treatment by a health care professional, and developing adverse drug reactions and interactions. When a drug is switched from prescription to OTC status, pharmaceutical companies' sales and profits increase and insurance companies' costs decrease. Costs to consumers increase because health insurance policies do not cover OTC drugs.

Sources of Drug Information

There are many sources of drug data, including pharmacology and other textbooks, drug reference books, journal articles, and Internet sites. For the beginning student of pharmacology, a textbook is the best source of information because it describes groups of drugs in relation to therapeutic uses. Drug reference books are most helpful in relation to individual drugs. Two authoritative sources are the *American Hospital Formulary Service* and *Drug Facts and Comparisons*. The former is published by the American Society of Health-System Pharmacists and updated periodically. The latter is published by the Facts and Comparisons division of Lippincott Williams & Wilkins and is updated monthly (loose-leaf edition) or annually (hardbound edition). A less authoritative source is the *Physicians' Desk Reference* (PDR), published yearly, which compiles manufacturers' package inserts for selected drugs.

Numerous drug handbooks (e.g., *Lippincott's Nursing Drug Guide*, published annually) and pharmacologic, medical, and nursing journals also contain information about drugs. Textbook chapters and journal articles often present information about drug therapy for patient's with specific disease processes and may thereby facilitate application of drug knowledge in clinical practice.

Strategies for Studying Pharmacology

- Concentrate on therapeutic classifications and their prototypes. For example, morphine is the prototype of opioid analgesics (see Chap. 6). Understanding morphine makes learning about other opioid analgesics easier because they are compared with morphine.

- Compare a newly encountered drug with a prototype or similar drug when possible. Relating the unknown to the known aids learning and retention of knowledge.

- Try to understand how the drug acts in the body. This understanding allows you to predict therapeutic effects and to predict, prevent, or minimize adverse effects by early detection and treatment.

- Concentrate study efforts on major characteristics. Such characteristics include the main indications for use, common and potentially serious adverse effects, conditions in which the drug is contraindicated or must be used cautiously, and related nursing care needs.

- Keep an authoritative, up-to-date drug reference readily available. A drug reference is a more reliable source of drug information than memory, especially for dosage ranges. Use the reference freely whenever you encounter an unfamiliar drug or when a question arises about a familiar one. In some health care settings, nurses have access to computerized databases of drug information, and these should be consulted for any unfamiliar or infrequently administered drug.

- Use your own words when taking notes or writing drug information cards. Also, write notes, answers to review questions, definitions of new terms, and trade names of drugs encountered in clinical practice settings directly into your pharmacology textbook. The mental processing required for these activities helps in both initial learning and later retention and application of knowledge.

- Rehearse applying drug knowledge in nursing care by asking yourself, "What if I have a patient who is receiving this drug? What must I do to safely administer the drug? For what must I assess the patient before giving the drug and for what must I observe in the patient after drug administration? What if my patient is an elderly person or a child?"

Key Concepts

- Drug therapy or pharmacotherapy is the use of drugs to prevent, diagnose, or treat signs, symptoms, and disease processes.

- Drugs given for therapeutic purposes are called medications.

- Drugs may be given for local or systemic effects; most are given for systemic effects.

- A prototype is an example of a group of drugs, often the first one of the group to be developed.

- Trade names of drugs are determined by manufacturers; generic names are independent of manufacturers.

- Controlled drugs are categorized according to therapeutic usefulness and potential for abuse.

Review and Application Exercises

Short Answer Exercises

1. What is the difference between local and systemic effects of drugs?
2. Can a patient experience systemic effects of local drugs and local effects of systemic drugs? Why or why not?
3. Why is it helpful for nurses to know the generic names of commonly used medications?
4. Why is it helpful to study prototypes of drug groups?
5. List at least three strategies for studying pharmacology.
6. List at least three authoritative sources of drug information.

NCLEX-Style Questions

7. You are caring for a patient who has strong beliefs about not putting anything "un-natural" into her body. Your best response is to tell her that most modern medications are
   a. natural products derived from plants
   b. natural products derived from minerals
   c. synthetic products manufactured in laboratories
   d. synthetic modifications of natural products

8. You are taking care of a patient who is confused about the different medications she is prescribed, and she has noted that some of the names have changed over the course of time she has been on these medications. In your counseling to her it is most important that you keep in mind the following true statement:
   a. A drug can belong to only one group or classification.
   b. A prototype drug is the standard by which similar drugs are compared.
   c. Drug groups and prototypes change frequently and knowledge about a prototype cannot guide knowledge about other drugs in the same class.
   d. The generic name of a drug changes among manufacturers.

9. In understanding the use of controlled substances for your clients, it is important that you know that controlled drugs are
   a. categorized according to prescription or nonprescription status
   b. regulated by state and local laws more than federal laws
   c. those that must demonstrate high standards of safety
   d. scheduled according to medical use and potential for abuse

10. You have a patient who is asking what the difference is between a prescription for 800 mg of a medication that can be purchased over-the-counter in 200 mg per tablet formulations. To answer her, it is important that you know that *over-the-counter drugs*
    a. are considered safe for any consumers to use
    b. are not available for treatment of most commonly occurring symptoms
    c. often differ in indications for use and recommended dosages from their prescription versions
    d. are paid for by most insurance policies

11. A patient is very upset with a drug recall of a medication he has been on for a long time. He states that he feels like he can no longer trust anyone to protect him. In response to his questions about the process of drug development, it is important that you know that with a new drug, the Food and Drug Administration is responsible for
    a. testing the drug with animals
    b. testing the drug with healthy people
    c. marketing the drug to health care providers
    d. evaluating the drug for safety and effectiveness

Selected References

Furberg, C. D., Levin, A. A., Gross, P. A, Shapiro, R. S., & Strom, B. L. (2006). The FDA and drug safety: A proposal for sweeping changes. *Archives of Internal Medicine, 166,* 1938–1942.

Spencer, A. P., & Wingate, S. (2005). Cardiovascular drug therapy in women. *Journal of Cardiovascular Nursing, 20,* 410–419.

Stergachis, A., & Hazlet, T. K. (2005). Pharmacoepidemiology. In J. T. DiPiro, R. L. Talbert, G. C. Yee, G. R. Matzke, B. G. Wells, &

L. M. Posey (Eds.), *Pharmacotherapy: A pathophysiologic approach* (6th ed., pp. 115–123). New York: McGraw-Hill.

U.S. Food and Drug Administration. *Frequently asked questions.* Retrieved June 6, 2005, from http://www.fda.gov/opacom/faqs/faqs.html

Basic Concepts and Processes

LEARNING OBJECTIVES

After studying this chapter, you will be able to:

1. Discuss cellular physiology in relation to drug therapy.
2. Describe the main pathways and mechanisms by which drugs cross biologic membranes and move through the body.
3. Explain each process of pharmacokinetics.
4. Discuss the clinical usefulness of measuring serum drug levels.
5. Describe major characteristics of the receptor theory of drug action.
6. Differentiate between agonist drugs and antagonist drugs.
7. List drug-related and patient-related variables that affect drug actions.
8. Discuss mechanisms and potential effects of drug–drug interactions.
9. Identify signs and symptoms that may occur with adverse drug effects on major body systems.
10. Discuss general management of drug overdose and toxicity.
11. Discuss selected drug antidotes.

Applying Your Knowledge

Mrs. Green, an 89-year-old widow, has recently switched to a new antihypertension medica-tion. She prides herself on being independent and able to manage on her own, despite failing memory and failing health. When you visit as a home health nurse, you assess therapeutic and adverse effects of her medications and compliance to the medical regimen prescribed.

Introduction

All body functions, disease processes, and most drug actions occur at the cellular level. Drugs are chemicals that alter basic processes in body cells. They can stimulate or inhibit normal cellular functions; they cannot add functions. To act on body cells, drugs given for systemic effects must reach adequate concentrations in the blood and other tissue fluids surrounding the cells. Thus, they must enter the body and be circulated to their sites of action (target cells). After they act on cells, they must be eliminated from the body.

How do systemic drugs reach, interact with, and leave body cells? How do people respond to drug actions? The answers to these questions are derived from cellular physiology, pathways and mechanisms of drug transport, pharmacokinetics, pharmacodynamics, and other basic con-cepts and processes that form the foundation of rational drug therapy and the content of this chapter.

Cellular Physiology

Cells are dynamic, busy "factories" (Box 2-1, Fig. 2-1) that take in raw materials, manufacture products required to maintain bodily functions, and deliver those products to their appropriate destinations in the body. Although cells differ from one tissue to another, their common characteristics include the ability to

■ Exchange materials with their immediate environment

■ Obtain energy from nutrients

■ Synthesize hormones, neurotransmitters, enzymes, structural proteins, and other complex molecules

■ Duplicate themselves (reproduce)

■ Communicate with one another via various biologic chemicals, such as neurotransmitters and hormones

Drug Transport Through Cell Membranes

Drugs must reach and interact with or cross the cell membrane to stimulate or inhibit cellular function. Most drugs are given for effects on body cells that are distant from the sites of administration (i.e., systemic effects). To move through the body and reach their sites of action, metabolism, and excretion (Fig. 2-2), drug molecules must cross numerous cell membranes. For example, molecules of most oral drugs must cross

| **Box 2-1** | **Cell Structures and Functions** |

Protoplasm, which comprises the internal environment of body cells, is composed of water, electrolytes (potassium, magnesium, phosphate, sulfate, bicarbonate), proteins, lipids, and carbohydrates. **Water** makes up 70% to 85% of most cells; cellular enzymes, electrolytes, and other chemicals are dissolved or suspended in the water. **Electrolytes** provide chemicals for cellular reactions and are required for some processes (e.g., transmission of electrochemical impulses in nerve and muscle cells). **Proteins** consist of "physical" proteins that form the structure of cells and "chemical" proteins that function mainly as enzymes within the cell. **Lipids**, mainly phospholipids and cholesterol, form the membranes that separate structures inside the cell and the cell itself from surrounding cells and body fluids. **Carbohydrates** play a major role in cell nutrition. Glucose is present in extracellular fluid and is readily available to supply the cell's need for energy. In addition, a small amount of carbohydrate is stored within the cell as glycogen, which can be rapidly converted back to glucose when needed.

The **nucleus** regulates the types and amounts of proteins, enzymes, and other substances to be produced. The **cytoplasm** surrounds the nucleus and contains the working units of the cell. The **cytosol**, the clear fluid portion of the cytoplasm, contains dissolved proteins, electrolytes, and glucose. The **endoplasmic reticulum (ER)** contains ribosomes, which synthesize proteins, including enzymes that synthesize glycogen, triglycerides, and steroids and those that metabolize drugs and other chemicals. The ER is also important in the production of hormones by glandular cells and the production of plasma proteins by liver cells. Most proteins produced by the ribosomes are released into the cytosol where they act as enzymes or structural proteins of the cell. The **Golgi complex** stores the substances produced by the ER. It also packages these substances into secretory granules, which then move out of the Golgi complex into the cytoplasm and, after a stimulus, are released from the cell. **Mitochondria** generate energy for cellular activities and require oxygen. **Lysosomes** are membrane-enclosed vesicles that contain enzymes capable of digesting nutrients (proteins, carbohydrates, fats), damaged cellular structures, foreign substances (e.g., bacteria), and the cell

itself. When a cell becomes worn out or damaged, the membrane around the lysosome breaks and the enzymes (hydrolases) are released. However, lysosomal contents also are released into extracellular spaces and may destroy surrounding cells. Normally, the enzymes are inactivated by enzyme inhibitors and excessive tissue destruction is prevented.

The **cell membrane**, a complex structure of phospholipids, proteins, cholesterol, and carbohydrates, separates intracellular contents from the extracellular environment; provides receptors for hormones and other biologically active substances; participates in electrical events that occur in nerve and muscle cells; and helps regulate growth and proliferation.

The cell membrane covers the entire surface of the cell and consists of a thin, double layer of lipids interspersed with proteins. The lipid layer is composed of phospholipid (fatty acid and phosphate) molecules. The proteins are usually combined with a carbohydrate and called glycoproteins. Some proteins provide structural pores through which water and water-soluble substances (e.g., sodium, potassium, and calcium ions) can diffuse between extracellular and intracellular fluids. Other proteins act as carriers to transport substances through the cell membrane. Still others act to regulate intracellular function or as enzymes to catalyze chemical reactions within the cell.

Cell membrane carbohydrates occur mainly in combination with proteins (glycoproteins) or lipids (glycolipids). Glycoproteins (composed of carbohydrate around a small, inner core of protein and called proteoglycans) often are attached to and cover the entire outside surface of the cell. As a result, the carbohydrate molecules are free to interact with extracellular substances and perform several important functions. First, many have a negative electrical charge that repels other negatively charged substances. Second, the "carbohydrate coat" of some cells attaches to the carbohydrate coat of other cells and thereby connects cells to each other. Third, many of the carbohydrates act as receptor molecules for binding hormones (e.g., insulin). The receptor–hormone combination then activates the attached inner core of protein to perform its enzymatic or other functions in the cell.

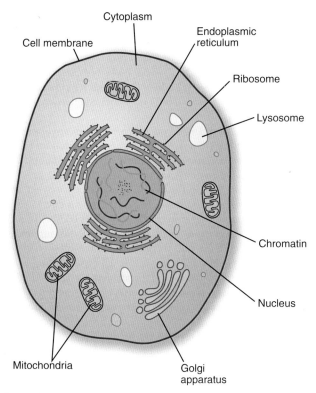

Figure 2-1 ▪ Cytoplasmic organelles of the cell.

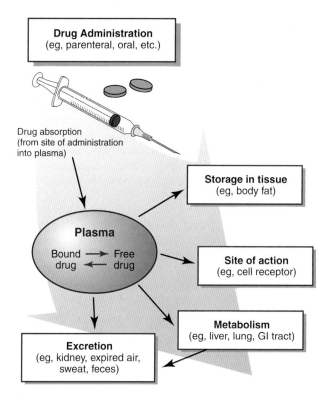

Figure 2-2 ▪ Entry and movement of drug molecules through the body to sites of action, metabolism, and excretion.

the membranes of cells in the gastrointestinal tract, liver, and capillaries to reach the bloodstream, circulate to their target cells, leave the bloodstream and attach to receptors on cells, perform their action, return to the bloodstream, circulate to the liver, reach drug-metabolizing enzymes in liver cells, re-enter the bloodstream (usually as metabolites), circulate to the kidneys, and be excreted in urine. Transport pathways and mechanisms used to move drug molecules through the body are described in Box 2-2 and Figure 2-3.

Pharmacokinetics

Pharmacokinetics involves drug movement through the body (i.e., "what the body does to the drug") to reach sites of action, metabolism, and excretion. Specific processes are absorption, distribution, metabolism (*biotransformation*), and excretion. Metabolism and excretion are often grouped together as drug elimination or clearance mechanisms. Overall, these processes largely determine serum drug levels; onset, peak, and duration of drug actions; therapeutic and adverse effects; and other important aspects of drug therapy.

Absorption

Absorption is the process that occurs from the time a drug enters the body to the time it enters the bloodstream to be circulated. Onset of drug action is largely determined by the rate of absorption; intensity is determined by the extent of absorp-

tion. Numerous factors affect the rate and extent of drug absorption, including dosage form, route of administration, blood flow to the site of administration, gastrointestinal function, the presence of food or other drugs, and other variables. Dosage form is a major determinant of a drug's *bioavailability* (the portion of a dose that reaches the systemic circulation and is available to act on body cells). An intravenous drug is virtually 100% bioavailable; an oral drug is virtually always less than 100% bioavailable because some of it is not absorbed from the gastrointestinal tract and some goes to the liver and is partially metabolized before reaching the systemic circulation.

Most oral drugs must be swallowed, dissolved in gastric fluid, and delivered to the small intestine (which has a large surface area for absorption of nutrients and drugs) before they are absorbed. Liquid medications are absorbed faster than tablets or capsules because they need not be dissolved. Rapid movement through the stomach and small intestine may increase drug absorption by promoting contact with absorptive mucous membrane; it also may decrease absorption because some drugs may move through the small intestine too rapidly to be absorbed. For many drugs, the presence of food in the stomach slows the rate of absorption and may decrease the amount of drug absorbed.

Drugs injected into subcutaneous (Sub-Q) or intramuscular (IM) tissues are usually absorbed more rapidly than oral drugs because they move directly from the injection site to the bloodstream. Absorption is rapid from IM sites because muscle tissue has an abundant blood supply. Drugs injected

| Box 2-2 | Drug Transport Pathways and Mechanisms |

Pathways

There are three main pathways of drug movement across cell membranes. The most common pathway is *direct penetration* of the membrane by lipid-soluble drugs, which are able to dissolve in the lipid layer of the cell membrane. Most systemic drugs are formulated to be lipid soluble so they can move through cell membranes, even oral tablets and capsules that must be sufficiently water soluble to dissolve in the aqueous fluids of the stomach and small intestine.

A second pathway involves passage through *protein channels* that go all the way through the cell membrane. Only a few drugs are able to use this pathway because most drug molecules are too large to pass through the small channels. Small ions (e.g., sodium and potassium) use this pathway, but their movement is regulated by specific channels with a gating mechanism (a flap of protein that opens briefly to allow ion movement and then closes).

The third pathway involves *carrier proteins* that transport molecules from one side of the cell membrane to the other. All of the carrier proteins are selective in the substances they transport; a drug's chemical structure determines which carrier will transport it.

Mechanisms

Once absorbed into the body, drugs are transported to and from target cells by passive diffusion, facilitated diffusion, and active transport.

Passive diffusion, the most common mechanism, involves movement of a drug from an area of higher concentration to one of lower concentration. For example, after oral administration, the initial concentration of a drug is higher in the gastrointestinal tract than in the blood. This promotes movement of the drug into the bloodstream. When the drug is circulated, the concentration is higher in the blood than in body cells, so that the drug moves (from capillaries) into the fluids surrounding the cells or into the cells themselves. Passive diffusion continues until a state of equilibrium is reached between the amount of drug in the tissues and the amount in the blood.

Facilitated diffusion is a similar process, except that drug molecules combine with a carrier substance, such as an enzyme or other protein.

In *active transport*, drug molecules are moved from an area of lower concentration to one of higher concentration. This process requires a carrier substance and the release of cellular energy.

---

intravenously (IV) do not need to be absorbed because they are placed directly into the bloodstream.

Other absorptive sites include the skin, mucous membranes, and lungs. Most drugs applied to the skin are given for local effects (e.g., sunscreens). Systemic absorption is minimal from intact skin but may be considerable when the skin is inflamed or damaged. Also, some drugs are formulated in adhesive skin patches for absorption through the skin (e.g., clonidine, fentanyl, nitroglycerin). Some drugs applied to mucous membranes also are given for local effects. However, systemic absorption occurs from the mucosa of the oral cavity, nose, eye, vagina, and rectum. Drugs absorbed through mucous membranes pass directly into the bloodstream. The lungs have a large surface area for absorption of anesthetic gases and a few other drugs.

Distribution

Distribution involves the transport of drug molecules within the body. After a drug is injected or absorbed into the bloodstream, it is carried by the blood and tissue fluids to its sites of action, metabolism, and excretion. Most drug molecules enter and leave the bloodstream at the capillary level, through gaps between the cells that form capillary walls. Distribution depends largely on the adequacy of blood circulation. Drugs are distributed rapidly to organs receiving a large blood supply, such as the heart, liver, and kidneys. Distribution to other internal organs, muscle, fat, and skin is usually slower.

Protein binding is an important factor in drug distribution (Fig. 2-4). Most drugs form a compound with plasma proteins, mainly albumin, which act as carriers. Drug molecules bound to plasma proteins are pharmacologically inactive because the large size of the complex prevents their leaving the bloodstream through the small openings in capillary walls and reaching their sites of action, metabolism, and excretion. Only the

Lipid-soluble drugs dissolve in the lipid layer of the cell membrane and diffuse into or out of the cell.

Cell membrane

Na^{2+}

Gated channels regulate movement of ions.

K$^+$

Nucleus

Cytoplasm

Carrier proteins attach to drug molecules and move them across cell membranes.

Figure 2-3 ■ Drug transport pathways. Drug molecules cross cell membranes to move into and out of body cells by directly penetrating the lipid layer, diffusing through open or gated channels, or attaching to carrier proteins.

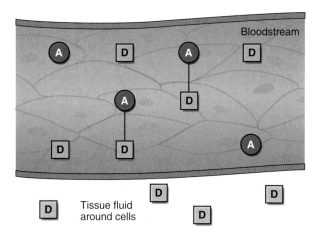

Figure 2-4 ▪ Plasma proteins, mainly albumin (A), act as carriers for drug molecules (D). Bound drug (A–D) stays in the bloodstream and is pharmacologically inactive. Free drug (D) can leave the bloodstream and act on body cells.

free or unbound portion of a drug acts on body cells. As the free drug acts on cells, the decrease in plasma drug levels causes some of the bound drug to be released.

Protein binding allows part of a drug dose to be stored and released as needed. Some drugs also are stored in muscle, fat, or other body tissues and released gradually when plasma drug levels fall. These storage mechanisms maintain lower, more consistent blood levels and reduce the risk of toxicity. Drugs that are highly bound to plasma proteins or stored extensively in other tissues have a long duration of action.

Drug distribution into the central nervous system (CNS) is limited because the blood–brain barrier, which is composed of capillaries with tight walls, limits movement of drug molecules into brain tissue. This barrier usually acts as a selectively permeable membrane to protect the CNS. However, it also can make drug therapy for CNS disorders more difficult because drugs must pass through cells of the capillary wall rather than between cells. As a result, only drugs that are lipid soluble or have a transport system can cross the blood–brain barrier and reach therapeutic concentrations in brain tissue.

Drug distribution during pregnancy and lactation is also unique (see Chap. 65). During pregnancy, most drugs cross the placenta and may affect the fetus. During lactation, many drugs enter breast milk and may affect the nursing infant.

Metabolism

Metabolism is the method by which drugs are inactivated or biotransformed by the body. Most often, an active drug is changed into inactive metabolites, which are then excreted. Some active drugs yield metabolites that are also active and that continue to exert their effects on body cells until they are metabolized further or excreted. Other drugs (called *prodrugs*) are initially inactive and exert no pharmacologic effects until they are metabolized. Most drugs are lipid soluble, a characteristic that aids their movement across cell membranes. However, the kidneys can excrete only water-soluble substances.

Therefore, one function of metabolism is to convert fat-soluble drugs into water-soluble metabolites. Hepatic drug metabolism or clearance is a major mechanism for terminating drug action and eliminating drug molecules from the body.

Most drugs are metabolized by cytochrome P450 (CYP) enzymes in the liver; red blood cells, plasma, kidneys, lungs, and gastrointestinal mucosa also contain drug-metabolizing enzymes. The CYP system consists of several groups of enzymes, some of which metabolize endogenous substances and some of which metabolize drugs. The drug-metabolizing groups are labeled CYP1, CYP2, and CYP3. Individual members of the groups usually metabolize specific drugs; more than one enzyme participates in the metabolism of some drugs. In terms of importance in drug metabolism, the CYP3A4 enzymes are thought to metabolize about 50% of drugs, CYP2D6 enzymes about 25%, CYP2C8/9 about 15%, and CYP1A2, 2C19, 2A6, and 2E1 in decreasing order for the remaining 10%.

CYP enzymes are complex proteins with binding sites for drug molecules (and endogenous substances). They catalyze the chemical reactions of oxidation, reduction, hydrolysis, and conjugation with endogenous substances, such as glucuronic acid or sulfate. With chronic administration, some drugs stimulate liver cells to produce larger amounts of drug-metabolizing enzymes (called *enzyme induction*). Enzyme induction accelerates drug metabolism because larger amounts of the enzymes (and more binding sites) allow larger amounts of a drug to be metabolized during a given time. As a result, larger doses of the rapidly metabolized drug may be required to produce or maintain therapeutic effects. Rapid metabolism may also increase the production of toxic metabolites with some drugs (e.g., acetaminophen). Drugs that induce enzyme production also may increase the rate of metabolism for endogenous steroidal hormones (e.g., cortisol, estrogens, testosterone, vitamin D). However, *enzyme induction does not occur for 1 to 3 weeks after an inducing agent is started*, because new enzyme proteins must be synthesized.

Metabolism also can be decreased or delayed in a process called *enzyme inhibition*, which most often occurs with concurrent administration of two or more drugs that compete for the same metabolizing enzymes. In this case, smaller doses of the slowly metabolized drug may be needed to avoid adverse effects and toxicity from drug accumulation. *Enzyme inhibition occurs within hours or days of starting an inhibiting agent.* Cimetidine, a gastric acid suppressor, inhibits several CYP enzymes (e.g., 1A, 2C, 2D, 3A) and can greatly decrease drug metabolism. The rate of drug metabolism also is reduced in infants (their hepatic enzyme system is immature), in people with impaired blood flow to the liver or severe hepatic or cardiovascular disease, and in people who are malnourished or on low-protein diets.

When drugs are given orally, they are absorbed from the gastrointestinal tract and carried to the liver through the portal circulation. Some drugs are extensively metabolized in the liver, with only part of a drug dose reaching the systemic circulation for distribution to sites of action. This is called the *first-pass effect* or presystemic metabolism.

Excretion

Excretion refers to elimination of a drug from the body. Effective excretion requires adequate functioning of the circulatory system and of the organs of excretion (kidneys, bowel, lungs, and skin). Most drugs are excreted by the kidneys and eliminated (unchanged or as metabolites) in the urine. Some drugs or metabolites are excreted in bile and then eliminated in feces; others are excreted in bile, reabsorbed from the small intestine, returned to the liver (called *enterohepatic recirculation*), metabolized, and eventually excreted in urine. Some oral drugs are not absorbed and are excreted in the feces. The lungs mainly remove volatile substances, such as anesthetic gases. The skin has minimal excretory function. Factors impairing excretion, especially severe renal disease, lead to accumulation of numerous drugs and may cause severe adverse effects if dosage is not reduced.

Serum Drug Levels

A *serum drug level* is a laboratory measurement of the amount of a drug in the blood at a particular time (Fig. 2-5). It reflects dosage, absorption, bioavailability, half-life, and the rates of metabolism and excretion. A minimum effective concentration (MEC) must be present before a drug exerts its pharmacologic action on body cells; this is largely determined by the drug dose and how well it is absorbed into the bloodstream. A toxic concentration is an excessive level at which toxicity occurs. Toxic concentrations may stem from a single large dose, repeated small doses, or slow metabolism that allows the drug to accumulate in the body. Between these low and high concentrations is the therapeutic range, which is the goal of drug therapy—that is, enough drug to be beneficial but not enough to be toxic.

For most drugs, serum levels indicate the onset, peak, and duration of drug action. When a single dose of a drug is given, onset of action occurs when the drug level reaches the MEC. The drug level continues to climb as more of the drug is absorbed, until it reaches its highest concentration and peak drug action occurs. Then, drug levels decline as the drug is eliminated (i.e., metabolized and excreted) from the body. Although there may still be numerous drug molecules in the body, drug action stops when drug levels fall below the MEC. The duration of action is the time during which serum drug levels are at or above the MEC. When multiple doses of a drug are given (e.g., for chronic conditions), the goal is usually to give sufficient doses often enough to maintain serum drug levels in the therapeutic range and avoid the toxic range.

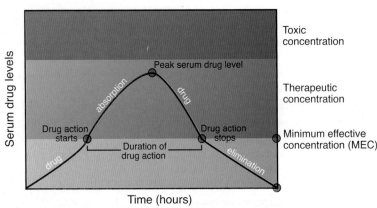

Drug action in relation to serum drug levels and time after a single dose.

A

B Drug action in relation to serum drug levels with repeated doses.

Figure 2-5 ■ Serum drug levels with single (A) and multiple (B) oral drug doses. Drug action starts when enough drug is absorbed to reach the minimum effective concentration (MEC), continues as long as the serum level is above the MEC, wanes as drug molecules are metabolized and excreted (if no more doses are given), and stops when the serum level drops below the MEC. The goal of drug therapy is to maintain serum drug levels in the therapeutic range.

In clinical practice, measuring serum drug levels is useful in several circumstances:

- When drugs with a narrow margin of safety are given, because their therapeutic doses are close to their toxic doses (e.g., digoxin, aminoglycoside antibiotics, lithium)
- To document the serum drug levels associated with particular drug dosages, therapeutic effects, or possible adverse effects
- To monitor unexpected responses to a drug dose such as decreased therapeutic effects or increased adverse effects
- When a drug overdose is suspected

Serum Half-Life

Serum half-life, also called elimination half-life, is the time required for the serum concentration of a drug to decrease by 50%. It is determined primarily by the drug's rates of metabolism and excretion. A drug with a short half-life requires more frequent administration than one with a long half-life.

When a drug is given at a stable dose, four or five half-lives are required to achieve steady-state concentrations and to develop equilibrium between tissue and serum concentrations. Because maximal therapeutic effects do not occur until equilibrium is established, some drugs are not fully effective for days or weeks. To maintain steady-state conditions, the amount of drug given must equal the amount eliminated from the body. When a drug dose is changed, an additional four to five half-lives are required to re-establish equilibrium; when a drug is discontinued, it is eliminated gradually over several half-lives.

Pharmacodynamics

Pharmacodynamics involves drug actions on target cells and the resulting alterations in cellular biochemical reactions and functions (i.e., "what the drug does to the body").

Receptor Theory of Drug Action

Like the physiologic substances (e.g., hormones, neurotransmitters) that normally regulate cell functions, most drugs exert their effects by chemically binding with receptors at the cellular level (Fig. 2-6). Most receptors are proteins located on the surfaces of cell membranes or within cells. Specific receptors include enzymes involved in essential metabolic or regulatory processes (e.g., dihydrofolate reductase, acetylcholinesterase); proteins involved in transport (e.g., sodium–potassium adenosine triphosphatase) or structural processes (e.g., tubulin); and nucleic acids (e.g., DNA) involved in cellular protein synthesis, reproduction, and other metabolic activities.

When drug molecules bind with receptor molecules, the resulting drug–receptor complex initiates physiochemical reactions that stimulate or inhibit normal cellular functions. One type of reaction involves activation, inactivation, or other alterations of intracellular enzymes. Because enzymes catalyze almost all cellular functions, drug-induced changes can markedly increase or decrease the rate of cellular metabolism.

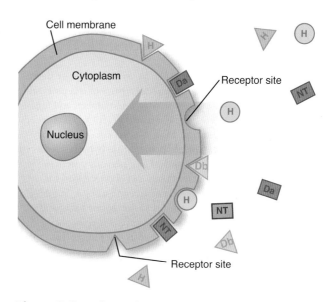

Figure 2-6 ■ Cell membrane contains receptors for physiologic substances such as hormones (H) and neurotransmitters (NT). These substances stimulate or inhibit cellular function. Drug molecules (Da and Db) also interact with receptors to stimulate or inhibit cellular function.

For example, an epinephrine–receptor complex increases the activity of the intracellular enzyme adenyl cyclase, which then causes the formation of cyclic adenosine monophosphate (cAMP). cAMP, in turn, can initiate any one of many different intracellular actions, the exact effect depending on the type of cell.

A second type of reaction involves changes in the permeability of cell membranes to one or more ions. The receptor protein is a structural component of the cell membrane, and its binding to a drug molecule may open or close ion channels. In nerve cells, for example, sodium or calcium ion channels may open and allow movement of ions into the cell. This movement usually causes the cell membrane to depolarize and excite the cell. At other times, potassium channels may open and allow movement of potassium ions out of the cell. This action inhibits neuronal excitability and function. In muscle cells, movement of the ions into the cells may alter intracellular functions, such as the direct effect of calcium ions in stimulating muscle contraction.

A third reaction may modify the synthesis, release, or inactivation of the neurohormones (e.g., acetylcholine, norepinephrine, serotonin) that regulate many physiologic processes. Refer to Box 2-3 for additional elements and characteristics of the receptor theory.

Nonreceptor Drug Actions

Relatively few drugs act by mechanisms other than combination with receptor sites on cells. Drugs that do not act on receptor sites include the following:

- Antacids act chemically to neutralize the hydrochloric acid produced by gastric parietal cells and thereby raise the pH of gastric fluid.

| Box 2-3 | Additional Elements of the Receptor Theory of Drug Action |

- The site and extent of drug action on body cells are determined primarily by specific characteristics of receptors and drugs. Receptors vary in type, location, number, and functional capacity. For example, many different types of receptors have been identified. Most types occur in most body tissues, such as receptors for epinephrine (whether received from stimulation of the sympathetic nervous system or administration of drug formulations) and receptors for growth hormone, thyroid hormone, and insulin. Some occur in fewer body tissues, such as receptors for opioids in the brain and subgroups of receptors for epinephrine in the heart (beta$_1$-adrenergic receptors) and lungs (beta$_2$-adrenergic receptors). Receptor type and location influence drug action. *The receptor is often described as a lock into which the drug molecule fits as a key, and only those drugs able to bond chemically to the receptors in a particular body tissue can exert pharmacologic effects on that tissue.* Thus, all body cells do not respond to all drugs, even though virtually all cell receptors are exposed to any drug molecules circulating in the bloodstream.

  The number of receptor sites available to interact with drug molecules also affects the extent of drug action. Drug molecules must occupy a minimal number of receptors to produce pharmacologic effects. Thus, if many receptors are available but only a few are occupied by drug molecules, few drug effects occur. In this instance, increasing the drug dosage increases the pharmacologic effects. Conversely, if only a few receptors are available for many drug molecules, receptors may be saturated. In this instance, if most receptor sites are occupied, increasing the drug dosage produces no additional pharmacologic effect.

  Drugs vary even more widely than receptors. Because all drugs are chemical substances, chemical characteristics determine drug actions and pharmacologic effects. For example, a drug's chemical structure affects its ability to reach tissue fluids around a cell and bind with its cell receptors. Minor changes in drug structure may produce major changes in pharmacologic effects. Another major factor is the concentration of drug molecules that reach receptor sites in body tissues. Drug- and patient-related variables that affect drug actions are further described later in this chapter.

- When drug molecules chemically bind with cell receptors, pharmacologic effects result from agonism or antagonism. *Agonists* are drugs that produce effects similar to those produced by naturally occurring hormones, neurotransmitters, and other substances. Agonists may accelerate or slow normal cellular processes, depending on the type of receptor activated. For example, epinephrine-like drugs act on the heart to increase the heart rate, and acetylcholine-like drugs act on the heart to slow the heart rate; both are agonists. *Antagonists* are drugs that inhibit cell function by occupying receptor sites. This strategy prevents natural body substances or other drugs from occupying the receptor sites and activating cell functions. After drug action occurs, drug molecules may detach from receptor molecules (i.e., the chemical binding is reversible), return to the bloodstream, and circulate to the liver for metabolism and the kidneys for excretion.

- Receptors are dynamic cellular components that can be synthesized by body cells and altered by endogenous substances and exogenous drugs. For example, prolonged stimulation of body cells with an excitatory agonist usually reduces the number or sensitivity of receptors. As a result, the cell becomes less responsive to the agonist (a process called receptor desensitization or down-regulation). Prolonged inhibition of normal cellular functions with an antagonist may increase receptor number or sensitivity. If the antagonist is suddenly reduced or stopped, the cell becomes excessively responsive to an agonist (a process called receptor up-regulation). These changes in receptors may explain why some drugs must be tapered in dosage and discontinued gradually if withdrawal symptoms are to be avoided.

- Osmotic diuretics (e.g., mannitol) increase the osmolarity of plasma and pull water out of tissues into the bloodstream.

- Drugs that are structurally similar to nutrients required by body cells (e.g., purines, pyrimidines) and that can be incorporated into cellular constituents, such as nucleic acids, interfere with normal cell functioning. Several anticancer drugs act by this mechanism.

- Metal chelating agents combine with toxic metals to form a complex that can be more readily excreted.

Variables That Affect Drug Actions

Historically, expected responses to drugs were based on those occurring when a particular drug was given to healthy adult men (18 to 65 years of age) of average weight (150 lb [70 kg]). However, other groups (e.g., women, children, older adults, different ethnic or racial groups, patients with diseases or symptoms that the drugs are designed to treat) receive drugs and respond differently from healthy adult men. As a result, newer clinical trials include more representatives of these groups. In any patient, however, responses may be altered by both drug- and patient-related variables.

Drug-Related Variables

Dosage

Dosage refers to the frequency, size, and number of doses; it is a major determinant of drug actions and responses, both therapeutic and adverse. If the amount is too small or administered infrequently, no pharmacologic action occurs because the drug does not reach an adequate concentration at target cells. If the amount is too large or administered too often, toxicity (poisoning) may occur. Overdosage may occur with a single large dose or with chronic ingestion of smaller doses.

Dosages recommended in drug literature are usually those that produce particular responses in 50% of the people tested. These dosages usually produce a mixture of therapeutic and adverse effects. The dosage of a particular drug depends on many characteristics of the drug (reason for use, potency, pharmacokinetics, route of administration, dosage form, and others) and of the recipient (age, weight, state of health, and function of cardiovascular, renal, and hepatic systems). Thus, recommended dosages are intended only as guidelines for individualizing dosages.

Route of Administration

Routes of administration affect drug actions and patient responses largely by influencing absorption and distribution. For rapid drug action and response, the IV route is most effective because the drug is injected directly into the bloodstream. For some drugs, the IM route also produces drug action within a few minutes because muscles have a large blood supply. The oral route usually produces slower drug action than parenteral routes. Absorption and action of topical drugs vary according to the drug formulation, whether the drug is applied to skin or mucous membranes, and other factors.

Drug–Diet Interactions

A few drugs are used therapeutically to decrease food absorption in the intestinal tract. For example, orlistat (Xenical) decreases absorption of fats from food and is given to promote weight loss; ezetimibe (Zetia) decreases absorption of cholesterol from food and is given to lower serum cholesterol levels. However, most drug–diet interactions are undesirable because food often slows absorption of oral drugs by slowing gastric emptying time and altering gastrointestinal secretions and motility. Giving medications 1 hour before or 2 hours after a meal can minimize interactions that decrease drug absorption.

In addition, some foods contain certain substances that react with certain drugs. One such interaction occurs between tyramine-containing foods and monoamine oxidase (MAO) inhibitor drugs. Tyramine causes the release of norepinephrine, a strong vasoconstrictive agent, from the adrenal medulla and sympathetic neurons. Normally, norepinephrine is quickly inactivated by MAO. However, because MAO inhibitor drugs prevent inactivation of norepinephrine, ingesting tyramine-containing foods with an MAO inhibitor may produce severe hypertension or intracranial hemorrhage. MAO inhibitors include the antidepressants isocarboxazid and phenelzine and the antiparkinson drugs rasagiline and selegiline. Tyramine-rich foods to be avoided by patients taking MAO inhibitors include aged cheeses, sauerkraut, soy sauce, tap or draft beers, and red wines.

Another interaction may occur between warfarin (Coumadin), an oral anticoagulant, and foods containing vitamin K. Because vitamin K antagonizes the action of warfarin, large amounts of spinach and other green leafy vegetables may offset the anticoagulant effects and predispose the person to thromboembolic disorders.

A third interaction occurs between tetracycline, an antibiotic, and dairy products, such as milk and cheese. The drug combines with the calcium in milk products to form a nonabsorbable compound that is excreted in the feces.

Still another interaction involves grapefruit. Grapefruit contains a substance that strongly inhibits the metabolism of drugs normally metabolized by the CYP3A4 enzyme. This effect greatly increases the blood levels of some drugs (e.g., the widely used "statin" group of cholesterol-lowering drugs) and the effect lasts for several days. Patients who take medications metabolized by the 3A4 enzyme should be advised against eating grapefruit or drinking grapefruit juice.

Drug–Drug Interactions

The action of a drug may be increased or decreased by its interaction with another drug in the body. Most interactions occur whenever the interacting drugs are present in the body; some, especially those affecting the absorption of oral drugs, occur when the interacting drugs are taken at or near the same time. The basic cause of many drug–drug interactions is altered drug metabolism. For example, drugs metabolized by the same enzymes compete for enzyme binding sites and there may not be enough binding sites for two or more drugs. Also, some drugs induce or inhibit the metabolism of other drugs. Protein binding is also the basis for some important drug–drug interactions.

Interactions that can increase the therapeutic or adverse effects of drugs include the following:

- *Additive effects* occur when two drugs with similar pharmacologic actions are taken (e.g., ethanol + sedative drug increases sedative effects).

- *Synergism* occurs when two drugs with different sites or mechanisms of action produce greater effects when taken together (e.g., acetaminophen [nonopioid analgesic] + codeine [opioid analgesic] increases analgesic effects).

- *Interference* by one drug with the metabolism of a second drug may result in intensified effects of the second drug. For example, cimetidine inhibits CYP1A, 2C, and 3A drug-metabolizing enzymes in the liver and therefore interferes with the metabolism of many drugs (e.g., benzodiazepine antianxiety and hypnotic drugs, several cardiovascular drugs). When these drugs are given concurrently with cimetidine, they are likely to cause adverse and toxic effects because blood levels of the drugs are higher. The overall effect is the same as taking a larger dose of the drug whose metabolism is inhibited or slowed.

- *Displacement* (i.e., a drug with a strong attraction to protein-binding sites may displace a less tightly bound drug) of one drug from plasma protein-binding sites by a second drug increases the effects of the displaced drug. This increase occurs because the displaced drug, freed from its bound form, becomes pharmacologically active. The overall effect is the same as taking a larger dose of the displaced drug. For example, aspirin displaces warfarin and increases the drug's anticoagulant effects.

Interactions in which drug effects are decreased include the following:

- An *antidote* drug can be given to antagonize the toxic effects of another drug. For example, naloxone is commonly used to relieve respiratory depression caused by morphine and related drugs. Naloxone molecules displace morphine molecules from their receptor sites on nerve cells in the brain so that the morphine molecules cannot continue to exert their depressant effects.

- Decreased intestinal absorption of oral drugs occurs when drugs combine to produce nonabsorbable compounds. For example, drugs containing aluminum, calcium, or magnesium bind with oral tetracycline (if taken at the same time) to decrease its absorption and therefore its antibiotic effect.

- Activation of drug-metabolizing enzymes in the liver increases the metabolism rate of any drug metabolized mainly by that group of enzymes and therefore decreases the drug's effects. Several drugs (e.g., phenytoin, rifampin) and cigarette smoking are known enzyme inducers.

Patient-Related Variables

Age

The effects of age on drug action are especially important in neonates, infants, and older adults. In children, drug action depends largely on age and developmental stage.

During pregnancy, drugs cross the placenta and may harm the fetus. Fetuses have no effective mechanisms for eliminating drugs because their liver and kidney functions are immature. Newborn infants (birth to 1 month) also handle drugs inefficiently. Drug distribution, metabolism, and excretion differ markedly in neonates, especially premature infants, because their organ systems are not fully developed. Older infants (1 month to 1 year) reach approximately adult levels of protein binding and kidney function, but liver function and the blood–brain barrier are still immature.

Children (1 to 12 years) have a period of increased activity of drug-metabolizing enzymes so that some drugs are rapidly metabolized and eliminated. Although the onset and duration of this period are unclear, a few studies have been done with particular drugs. Theophylline, for example, is eliminated much faster in a 7-year-old child than in a neonate or adult (18 to 65 years). After about 12 years of age, healthy children handle drugs similarly to healthy adults.

In older adults (65 years and older), physiologic changes may alter all pharmacokinetic processes. Changes in the gastrointestinal tract include decreased gastric acidity, decreased blood flow, and decreased motility. Despite these changes, however, there is little difference in drug absorption. Changes in the cardiovascular system include decreased cardiac output and therefore slower distribution of drug molecules to their sites of action, metabolism, and excretion. In the liver, blood flow and metabolizing enzymes are decreased. Thus, many drugs are metabolized more slowly, have a longer action, and are more likely to accumulate with chronic administration. In the kidneys, there is decreased blood flow, decreased glomerular filtration rate, and decreased tubular secretion of drugs. All these changes tend to slow excretion and promote accumulation of drugs in the body. Impaired kidney and liver function greatly increase the risks of adverse drug effects. In addition, older adults are more likely to have acute and chronic illnesses that require the use of multiple drugs or long-term drug therapy. Thus, possibilities for interactions among drugs and between drugs and diseased organs are greatly multiplied.

Body Weight

Body weight affects drug action mainly in relation to dose. The ratio between the amount of drug given and body weight influences drug distribution and concentration at sites of action. In general, people heavier than average may need larger doses, provided that their renal, hepatic, and cardiovascular functions are adequate. Recommended doses for many drugs are listed in terms of grams or milligrams per kilogram of body weight.

Genetic and Ethnic Characteristics

Drugs are given to cause particular effects in recipients. However, when given the same drug in the same dose, by the same route, and in the same time interval, some people experience inadequate therapeutic effects and others experience unusual or exaggerated effects, including increased toxicity. These variations in drug response are often attributed to genetic or ethnic differences in drug metabolism.

Genetics

Genes determine the types and amounts of proteins produced in body cells and thereby control both the physical and chemical functions of the cells. When most drugs enter the body, they interact with proteins (e.g., in plasma, tissues, cell membranes, drug receptor sites) to reach their sites of action, and they interact with other proteins (e.g., drug-metabolizing enzymes in the liver and other organs) to be biotransformed and eliminated from the body. Genetic characteristics that alter any of these proteins can alter drug responses. For example, metabolism of isoniazid, an antitubercular drug, requires the enzyme acetyltransferase. People may metabolize isoniazid rapidly or slowly, depending largely on genetic differences in acetyltransferase activity. Clinically, rapid metabolizers may need larger-than-usual doses to achieve therapeutic effects, and slow metabolizers may need smaller-than-usual doses to avoid toxic effects.

In addition, several genetic variations (called polymorphisms) of the cytochrome P450 drug-metabolizing enzymes have been identified. Specific variations may influence any of the chemical processes by which drugs are metabolized. For example, CYP2D6 metabolizes several antidepressant, antipsychotic, and beta-blocker drugs. Some Caucasians (about 7%) metabolize these drugs poorly and are at increased risk of drug accumulation and adverse effects. CYP2C19 metabolizes diazepam, omeprazole, and some antidepressants. As many as 15% to 30% of Asians may metabolize these drugs poorly and develop adverse effects if dosage is not reduced.

Still another example of genetic variation in drug metabolism is that some people are deficient in glucose-6-phosphate dehydrogenase, an enzyme normally found in red blood cells and other body tissues. These people may have hemolytic anemia when given antimalarial drugs, sulfonamides, analgesics, antipyretics, and other drugs.

Genetic testing to determine a person's reaction to drug therapy is increasing, but clinical use is limited. Much research is being done in this area, especially related to cardiovascular and anticancer drugs (see Pharmacogenetics, below).

Ethnicity

Most drug information has been derived from clinical drug trials using white men. Interethnic variations became evident when drugs and dosages developed for Caucasians produced unexpected responses, including toxicity, when given to individuals from other ethnic groups. One common variation is that African Americans respond differently to some cardiovascular drugs. For example, for African Americans with hypertension, angiotensin-converting enzyme (ACE) inhibitors and beta-adrenergic blocking drugs are less effective and diuretics and calcium channel blockers are more effective. Also, African Americans with heart failure seem to respond better to a combination of hydralazine and isosorbide than do Caucasian patients with heart failure.

Another variation is that Asians usually require much smaller doses of some commonly used drugs, including beta blockers and several psychotropic drugs (e.g., alprazolam, an antianxiety agent, and haloperidol, an antipsychotic). Some documented interethnic variations are included in later chapters.

Pharmacogenetics

Pharmacogenetics involves the study of genetic variations (e.g., gene mutations that produce changes in structure and function of drug-metabolizing enzymes) that result in interindividual differences in drug response. Research has increased with awareness that genetic and ethnic characteristics are important factors and that diverse groups must be included in clinical trials. There is also increased awareness that *each person is genetically unique and must be treated as an individual* rather than as a member of a particular ethnic group. Research is ongoing toward improving drug safety and "personalized medicine," in which prescribers can use a person's genetic characteristics to design a drug therapy regimen to produce the best therapeutic effects and the least adverse effects.

Gender

Most drug-related research has involved men, and the results have been extrapolated to women, sometimes with adjustment of dosage based on the usually smaller size and weight of women. Historically, gender was considered a minor influence on drug action except during pregnancy and lactation. Now, differences between men and women in responses to drug therapy are being increasingly identified, and since 1993, regulations require that major clinical drug trials include women. Data on drug therapy in women are still limited, however. Some identified differences include the following:

- Women who are depressed are more likely to respond to the selective serotonin reuptake inhibitors (SSRIs), such as

fluoxetine (Prozac), than to the tricyclic antidepressants (TCAs), such as amitriptyline (Elavil).
- Women with anxiety disorders may respond less well than men to some antianxiety medications.
- Women with schizophrenia seem to need smaller doses of antipsychotic medications than men. If given the higher doses required by men, women are likely to have adverse drug reactions.
- Women may obtain more pain relief from opioid analgesics (e.g., morphine) and less relief from nonopioid analgesics (e.g., acetaminophen, ibuprofen), compared to men.

Different responses in women are usually attributed to anatomic and physiologic differences. In addition to smaller size and weight, for example, women usually have a higher percentage of body fat, less muscle tissue, smaller blood volume, and other characteristics that may influence responses to drugs. In addition, women have hormonal fluctuations during the menstrual cycle. Altered responses have been demonstrated in some women taking clonidine, an antihypertensive; lithium, a mood-stabilizing agent; phenytoin, an anticonvulsant; propranolol, a beta-adrenergic blocking drug used in the management of hypertension, angina pectoris, and migraine; and antidepressants. In addition, a significant percentage of women with arthritis, asthma, depression, diabetes mellitus, epilepsy, and migraine experience increased symptoms premenstrually. The increased symptoms may indicate a need for adjustments in their drug therapy regimens. Women with clinical depression, for example, may need higher doses of antidepressant medications premenstrually, if symptoms exacerbate, and lower doses during the rest of the menstrual cycle.

There may also be differences in pharmacokinetic processes, although few studies have been done. With absorption, it has been noted that women absorb a larger percentage of an oral dose of two cardiovascular medications compared to men (25% more verapamil and 40% more aspirin). With distribution, women may have higher blood levels of medications that distribute into body fluids (because of the smaller amount of water in which the medication can disperse) and lower blood levels of medications that are deposited in fatty tissues (because of the generally higher percentage of body fat). With metabolism, the CYP3A4 enzyme metabolizes more medications than other enzymes, and women are thought to metabolize the drugs processed by this enzyme 20% to 40% faster than men (and therefore may have lower blood levels than men of similar weight given the same doses). The CYP1A2 enzyme is less active in women so that women who take the cardiovascular drugs clopidogrel or propranolol may have higher blood levels than men (and possibly greater risks of adverse effects if given the same doses as men). With excretion, renally excreted medications may reach higher blood levels because a major mechanism of drug elimination, glomerular filtration, is approximately 20% lower in women.

In general, women given equal dosages or equal weight-based dosages are thought to be exposed to higher concentrations of medications compared to men. Although available data are limited, the main reasons postulated for the gender differences are that women have a lower volume of distribution, lower glomerular filtration, and lower hepatic enzyme activity (except for the medications metabolized by the CYP3A4 enzyme system, which is more active in women). As a result, all women should be monitored closely during drug therapy because they are more likely to experience adverse drug effects than are men.

Pathologic Conditions

Various pathologic conditions may alter some or all pharmacokinetic (PK) processes and lead to decreased therapeutic effects or increased risks of adverse effects. Examples include the following:

- *Cardiovascular disorders* (e.g., myocardial infarction, heart failure, hypotension) may interfere with all PK processes, mainly by decreasing blood flow to sites of drug administration, action, metabolism (liver), and excretion (kidneys).

- *Gastrointestinal disorders* (e.g., vomiting, diarrhea, inflammatory bowel disease, trauma or surgery of the gastrointestinal tract) may interfere with absorption of oral drugs.

- *Hepatic disorders* (e.g., hepatitis, cirrhosis, decreased liver function) mainly interfere with metabolism. Severe liver disease or cirrhosis may interfere with all PK processes.

- *Renal disorders* (e.g., acute or chronic renal failure) mainly interfere with excretion. Severe kidney disease may interfere with all PK processes.

- *Thyroid disorders* mainly affect metabolism. Hypothyroidism slows metabolism, which prolongs drug action and slows elimination. Hyperthyroidism accelerates metabolism, which shortens drug action and hastens elimination.

Psychological Considerations

Psychological considerations influence individual responses to drug administration, although specific mechanisms are unknown. An example is the placebo response. A placebo is a pharmacologically inactive substance. Placebos are used in clinical drug trials to compare the medication being tested with a "dummy" medication. Recipients often report both therapeutic and adverse effects from placebos.

Attitudes and expectations related to drugs in general, a particular drug, or a placebo influence patient response. They also influence compliance or the willingness to carry out the prescribed drug regimen, especially with long-term drug therapy.

Tolerance and Cross-Tolerance

Drug *tolerance* occurs when the body becomes accustomed to a particular drug over time so that larger doses must be given to produce the same effects. *Tolerance* may be acquired to the pharmacologic action of many drugs, especially opioid analgesics, alcohol, and other CNS depressants. Tolerance to pharmacologically related drugs is called *cross-tolerance*. For example, a person who regularly drinks large amounts of alcohol becomes able to ingest even larger amounts before becoming intoxicated—this is tolerance to alcohol. If the person is then given sedative-type drugs or a general anesthetic, larger-than-usual doses are required to produce a pharmacologic effect—this is cross-tolerance.

Tolerance and cross-tolerance are usually attributed to activation of drug-metabolizing enzymes in the liver, which accelerates drug metabolism and excretion. They also are attributed to decreased sensitivity or numbers of receptor sites.

Adverse Effects of Drugs

As used in this book, the term *adverse effects* refer to any undesired responses to drug administration, as opposed to therapeutic effects, which are desired responses. Most drugs produce a mixture of therapeutic and adverse effects; all drugs can produce adverse effects. Adverse effects may produce essentially any symptom or disease process and may involve any body system or tissue. They may be common or rare, mild or severe, localized or widespread—depending on the drug and the recipient. Some adverse effects occur with usual therapeutic doses of drugs (often called side effects); most are more likely to occur and to be more severe with high doses. Common or serious adverse effects are described in Box 2-4. Although adverse effects may occur in anyone who takes medications, they are especially likely to occur with some drugs (e.g., insulin, warfarin) and in older adults, who often take multiple drugs.

For some drug groups and individual drugs that may cause serious or life-threatening adverse effects, the Food and Drug Administration (FDA) requires drug manufacturers to place a **BLACK BOX WARNING (BBW)** on the label of a prescription drug or in the literature describing it. A **BBW** is usually added after a significant number of serious adverse effects have occurred, often several years after a drug is marketed and after it is used in large numbers of people. The **BBW** is the strongest warning from the FDA and often includes prescribing or monitoring information intended to improve the safety of using the particular drug or drug group. In recent years, **BBW**s have been added to antidepressant drugs, nonopioid analgesics, and the antiflu drug oseltamivir (Tamiflu).

⊘ Applying Your Knowledge 2-1

How Can You Avoid This Medication Error?

Mrs. Green is taking a number of medications, including three medications to control her hypertension. During your most recent visit (3 days ago), you instructed Mrs. Green to take her medication with a large glass of water and set up a daily pill calendar. You also checked her vital signs; her blood pressure was 148/70.

Today, you recheck her vital signs and her blood pressure is 96/60. You ask Mrs. Green about her medication and she tells you she has been taking it according to the calendar three times a day.

Box 2-4	Common or Serious Adverse Drug Effects

Central Nervous System (CNS) Effects

CNS effects may result from CNS stimulation (e.g., agitation, confusion, disorientation, hallucinations, psychosis, seizures) or CNS depression (e.g., impaired level of consciousness, sedation, coma, impaired respiration and circulation). CNS effects may occur with many drugs, including most therapeutic groups, substances of abuse, and over-the-counter preparations.

Gastrointestinal (GI) Effects

GI effects (e.g., nausea, vomiting, constipation, diarrhea) commonly occur. Nausea and vomiting occur with many drugs as a result of local irritation of the GI tract or stimulation of the vomiting center in the brain. Diarrhea occurs with drugs that cause local irritation or increase peristalsis. More serious effects include bleeding or ulceration (most often with nonsteroidal anti-inflammatory agents such as ibuprofen) and severe diarrhea/colitis (most often with antibiotics).

Hematologic Effects

Hematologic effects (excessive bleeding, clot formation [thrombosis], bone marrow depression, anemias, *leukopenia*, agranulocytosis, thrombocytopenia) are relatively common and potentially life threatening. Excessive bleeding is often associated with anticoagulants and thrombolytics; bone marrow depression is associated with anticancer drugs.

Hepatic Effects

Hepatic effects (hepatitis, liver dysfunction or failure, biliary tract disorders) are potentially life threatening. The liver is especially susceptible to drug-induced injury because most drugs are circulated to the liver for metabolism and some drugs are toxic to liver cells. Hepatotoxic drugs include acetaminophen (Tylenol), isoniazid (INH), methotrexate (Trexall), phenytoin (Dilantin), and aspirin and other salicylates. In the presence of drug- or disease-induced liver damage, the metabolism of many drugs is impaired. Besides hepatotoxicity, many drugs produce abnormal values in liver function tests without producing clinical signs of liver dysfunction.

Nephrotoxicity

Nephrotoxicity (nephritis, renal insufficiency or failure) occurs with several antimicrobial agents (e.g., gentamicin and other aminoglycosides), nonsteroidal anti-inflammatory agents (e.g., ibuprofen and related drugs), and others. It is potentially serious because it may interfere with drug excretion, thereby causing drug accumulation and increased adverse effects.

Hypersensitivity

Hypersensitivity or allergy may occur with almost any drug in susceptible patients. It is largely unpredictable and unrelated to dose. It occurs in those who have previously been exposed to the drug or a similar substance (antigen) and who have

developed antibodies. When readministered, the drug reacts with the antibodies to cause cell damage and the release of histamine and other substances. These substances produce reactions ranging from mild skin rashes to anaphylactic shock. Anaphylactic shock is a life-threatening hypersensitivity reaction characterized by respiratory distress and cardiovascular collapse. It occurs within a few minutes after drug administration and requires emergency treatment with epinephrine. Some allergic reactions (e.g., serum sickness) occur 1 to 2 weeks after the drug is given.

Drug Fever

Drugs can cause fever by several mechanisms, including allergic reactions, damaging body tissues, interfering with dissipation of body heat, or acting on the temperature-regulating center in the brain. The most common mechanism is an allergic reaction. Fever may occur alone or with other allergic manifestations (e.g., skin rash, hives, joint and muscle pain, enlarged lymph glands, eosinophilia). It may begin within hours after the first dose if the patient has taken the drug before or within about 10 days of continued administration if the drug is new to the patient. If the causative drug is discontinued, fever usually subsides within 48 to 72 hours unless drug excretion is delayed or significant tissue damage has occurred (e.g., hepatitis). Many drugs have been implicated as causes of drug fever, including most antimicrobials

Idiosyncrasy

Idiosyncrasy refers to an unexpected reaction to a drug that occurs the first time it is given. These reactions are usually attributed to genetic characteristics that alter the person's drug-metabolizing enzymes.

Drug Dependence

Drug dependence may occur with mind-altering drugs, such as opioid analgesics, sedative-hypnotic agents, antianxiety agents, and CNS stimulants. Dependence may be physiologic or psychological. Physiologic dependence produces unpleasant physical symptoms when the dose is reduced or the drug is withdrawn. Psychological dependence leads to excessive preoccupation with drugs and drug-seeking behavior.

Carcinogenicity

Carcinogenicity is the ability of a substance to cause cancer. Several drugs are carcinogens, including some hormones and anticancer drugs. Carcinogenicity apparently results from drug-induced alterations in cellular DNA.

Teratogenicity

Teratogenicity is the ability of a substance to cause abnormal fetal development when taken by pregnant women. Drug groups considered teratogenic include antiepileptic drugs and "statin" cholesterol-lowering drugs.

Toxicology: Drug Overdose

Drug toxicity (also called poisoning or overdose) results from excessive amounts of a drug and may damage body tissues. It is a common problem in both adult and pediatric populations. It may result from a single large dose or prolonged ingestion of smaller doses and may involve alcohol or prescription, over-the-counter, or illicit drugs. Clinical manifestations are often nonspecific and may indicate other disease processes. Because of the variable presentation of drug intoxication, health care providers must have a high index of suspicion so that toxicity can be rapidly recognized and treated.

When toxicity occurs in a home or outpatient setting and the victim is collapsed or not breathing, call 911 for emergency aid. If the victim is responsive, someone needs to contact the National Poison Control Center by phone at 1-800-222-1222 or by computer at *www.1-800-222-1222.info*. The caller is connected to a local Poison Control Center and, if possible, needs to tell the responding pharmacist or physician the name of the drug that was taken, the amount, and when. The poison control consultant may recommend treatment measures over the phone or that the victim be taken to a hospital emergency department.

When toxicity occurs in a hospitalized patient or when an outpatient is taken to a hospital, the patient or someone else may know the toxic agent (e.g., accidental overdose of a therapeutic drug, use of an illicit drug, a suicide attempt). Often, however, multiple drugs have been ingested, the causative drugs are unknown, and the circumstances may involve traumatic injury or impaired mental status that make the patient unable to provide useful information. The main goals of treatment are starting treatment as soon as possible after drug ingestion, supporting and stabilizing vital functions, preventing further damage from the toxic agent by reducing absorption or increasing elimination, and administering antidotes when available and indicated. General aspects of care are described in Box 2-5, selected antidotes are listed in Table 2-1, and specific aspects of care are described in relevant chapters.

Box 2-5	General Management of Toxicity

- The first priority is support of vital functions, as indicated by rapid assessment of vital signs and level of consciousness. In serious poisonings, an electrocardiogram is indicated and findings of severe toxicity (e.g., dysrhythmias, ischemia) justify aggressive treatment. Standard cardiopulmonary resuscitation (CPR) measures may be needed to maintain breathing and circulation. An intravenous (IV) line is usually needed to administer fluids and drugs, and invasive treatment or monitoring devices may be inserted.

    Endotracheal intubation and mechanical ventilation are often required to maintain breathing (in unconscious patients), correct hypoxemia, and protect the airway. Hypoxemia must be corrected quickly to avoid brain injury, myocardial ischemia, and cardiac dysrhythmias.

    Serious cardiovascular manifestations often require drug therapy. Hypotension and hypoperfusion may be treated with inotropic and vasopressor drugs to increase cardiac output and raise blood pressure. Dysrhythmias are treated according to Advanced Cardiac Life Support (ACLS) protocols.

    Recurring seizures or status epilepticus requires treatment with anticonvulsant drugs.

- For unconscious patients, as soon as an IV line is established, some authorities recommend a dose of naloxone (2 mg IV) for possible narcotic overdose and thiamine (100 mg IV) for possible brain dysfunction due to thiamine deficiency. In addition, a fingerstick blood glucose test should be done, and if hypoglycemia is indicated, a 50% dextrose solution (50 mL IV) should be given.

- After the patient is out of immediate danger, a thorough physical examination and efforts to determine the drug(s), the amounts, and the time lapse since exposure are needed. If the patient is unable to supply needed information, interview anyone else who may be able to do so. Ask about the use of prescription and over-the-counter drugs, alcohol, and illicit substances.

- There are no standard laboratory tests for poisoned patients, but baseline tests of liver and kidney function are usually indicated. Screening tests for toxic substances are not very helpful because test results may be delayed, many substances are not detected, and the results rarely affect initial treatment. Specimens of blood, urine, or gastric fluids may be obtained for laboratory analysis. Serum drug levels are needed when acetaminophen, alcohol, aspirin, digoxin, lithium, or theophylline is known to be an ingested drug, to assist with treatment.

- For most orally ingested drugs, the initial and major treatment is a single dose of activated charcoal. Sometimes called the "universal antidote," it is useful in many poisonings because it adsorbs many toxins and rarely causes complications. When given within 30 minutes of drug ingestion, it decreases absorption of the toxic drug by about 90%; when given an hour after ingestion, it decreases absorption by about 37%. Activated charcoal (1 g/kg of body weight or 50–100 g) is usually mixed with 240 mL of water (25–50 g in 120 mL of water for children) to make a slurry, which is gritty and unpleasant to swallow. It is often given by nasogastric tube. The charcoal blackens subsequent bowel movements. If used with whole bowel irrigation (WBI; see below), activated charcoal should be given before the WBI solution is started. If given during WBI, the binding capacity of the charcoal is decreased. Activated charcoal does not significantly decrease absorption of some drugs (e.g., ethanol, iron, lithium, metals).

    Multiple doses of activated charcoal may be given in some instances (e.g., ingestion of sustained-release drugs). One regimen is an initial dose of 50 to 100 grams, then 12.5 grams every 1, 2, or 4–6 hours for a few doses.

Adverse effects of activated charcoal include pulmonary aspiration and bowel obstruction from impaction of the charcoal–drug complex. To prevent these effects, unconscious patients should not receive the drug until the airway is secure against aspiration, and many patients are given a laxative (e.g., sorbitol) to aid removal of the charcoal–drug complex.

Ipecac-induced vomiting and gastric lavage are no longer routinely used because of minimal effectiveness and potential complications. Ipecac is no longer recommended to treat poisonings in children in home settings; parents should call a poison control center or a health care provider. Gastric lavage may be beneficial in serious overdoses if performed within an hour of drug ingestion. If the ingested agent delays gastric emptying (e.g., drugs with anticholinergic effects), the time limit may be extended. When used after ingestion of pills or capsules, the tube lumen should be large enough to allow removal of pill fragments.

■ Whole bowel irrigation (WBI) with a polyethylene glycol solution (e.g., Colyte) may be used to remove toxic ingestions of long-acting, sustained-release drugs (e.g., many beta blockers, calcium channel blockers, and theophylline preparations); enteric-coated drugs; and toxins that do not bind well with activated charcoal (e.g., iron, lithium). It may also be helpful in removing packets of illicit drugs, such as cocaine or heroin. When used, 500–2000 mL per hour are given orally or by nasogastric tube until bowel contents are clear. Vomiting is the most common adverse effect. WBI is contraindicated in patients with serious bowel disorders (e.g., obstruction, perforation, ileus), hemodynamic instability, or respiratory impairment (unless intubated).

■ Urinary elimination of some drugs and toxic metabolites can be accelerated by changing the pH of urine (e.g., alkalinizing with IV sodium bicarbonate for salicylate overdose), diuresis, or hemodialysis. Hemodialysis is the treatment of choice in severe lithium and aspirin (salicylate) poisoning.

■ Specific antidotes can be administered when available and as indicated by the patient's clinical condition. Available antidotes vary widely in effectiveness. Some are very effective and rapidly reverse toxic manifestations (e.g., naloxone for opioids, specific Fab fragments for digoxin).

When an antidote is used, its half-life relative to the toxin's half-life must be considered. For example, the half-life of naloxone, a narcotic antagonist, is relatively short compared with the half-life of the longer-acting opioids such as methadone, and repeated doses may be needed to prevent recurrence of the toxic state.

Table 2-1	Antidotes for Overdoses of Selected Therapeutic Drugs		
OVERDOSED DRUG (POISON)	**ANTIDOTE**	**ROUTE AND DOSAGE RANGES**	**COMMENTS**
Acetaminophen (see Chap. 7)	Acetylcysteine (Mucomyst 10% or 20% oral solution, Acetadote 20% [200 mg/mL] injection solution)	PO 140 mg/kg initially, then 70 mg/kg q4h for 17 doses. IV (Acetadote only) Loading dose: 150 mg/kg, diluted in 200 mL 5% dextrose, infused over 15 min. Maintenance dose one: 50 mg/kg, diluted in 500 mL 5% dextrose, infused over 4 h. Maintenance dose two: 100 mg/kg, diluted in 1000 mL 5% dextrose, infused over 16 h	Dilute oral solution to a 5% solution with a cola or other soft drink for oral administration. Follow instructions carefully and note that doses, amounts of diluent, and infusion times are different for the three total IV infusions.
Anticholinergics (atropine; see Chap. 20)	Physostigmine	IV, IM 2 mg; give IV slowly, over at least 2 min	Infrequently used because of its toxicity. Should not be given to patients with a seizure disorder, overdose of unknown drugs, or overdose of drugs known to cause seizures in overdose (e.g., cocaine, lithium). In such circumstances, the risks of seizures outweigh drug benefits.
Benzodiazepines (see Chap. 8)	Flumazenil	IV 0.2 mg over 30 sec; if no response, may give additional 0.3 mg over 30 sec. Additional doses of 0.5 mg may be given at 1-min intervals up to a total amount of 3 mg	Should not be given to patients with overdose of unknown drugs or drugs known to cause seizures in overdose (e.g., cocaine, lithium)

(continued on page 24)

Table 2-1	Antidotes for Overdoses of Selected Therapeutic Drugs (continued)		
OVERDOSED DRUG (POISON)	**ANTIDOTE**	**ROUTE AND DOSAGE RANGES**	**COMMENTS**
Beta blockers (see Chap. 18)	Glucagon	IV 50–150 mcg/kg (5–10 mg for adults) over 1 min initially, then 2–5 mg/h by continuous infusion as needed	Glucagon increases myocardial contractility and raises blood pressure. It does not act on beta-adrenergic receptors and is therefore not affected by beta-blocking drugs.
Calcium channel blockers (see Chaps. 50, 52)	Calcium gluconate 10%	IV 1 g over 5 min; may be repeated	Increases myocardial contractility
Cholinergics (see Chap. 19)	Atropine	Adults: IV 2 mg, repeated as needed Children: IV 0.05 mg/kg, up to 2 mg	If poisoning is due to organophosphates (e.g., insecticides), pralidoxime may be given with the atropine.
Digoxin (see Chap. 48)	Digoxin immune Fab (Digibind)	IV 40 mg (1 vial) for each 0.6 mg of digoxin ingested Reconstitute each vial with 4 mL Water for Injection, then dilute with sterile isotonic saline to a convenient volume and give over 30 min, through a 0.22-micron filter. If cardiac arrest seems imminent, may give the dose as a bolus injection.	Recommended for severe toxicity; reverses cardiac and extracardiac symptoms in a few minutes *Note:* Serum digoxin levels increase after antidote administration, but the drug is bound and therefore inactive.
Heparin (see Chap. 54)	Protamine sulfate	IV 1 mg/100 units of heparin, slowly, over at least 10 min; a single dose should not exceed 50 mg	
Iron (see Chap. 57)	Deferoxamine	IM 1 g q8h PRN IV 15 mg/kg/h if hypotensive	Indicated for serum iron levels >500 mg/dL or serum levels >350 mg/dL with GI or cardiovascular symptoms Can bind and remove a portion of an ingested dose; urine becomes red as iron is excreted
Isoniazid (INH)	Pyridoxine	IV 1 g per gram of INH ingested, at rate of 1 g q2–3 min. If amount of INH unknown, give 5 g; may be repeated.	Indicated for management of seizures and correction of acidosis
Lead	Succimer (Chemet)	Children: PO 10 mg/kg q8h for 5 days	
Opioid analgesics (Chap. 6)	Naloxone (Narcan)	Adults: IV 0.4–2 mg PRN Children: IV 0.1 mg/kg per dose	Can also be given IM, Sub-Q, or by endotracheal tube
Phenothiazine antipsychotic agents (see Chap. 9)	Diphenhydramine (Benadryl)	Adults: IV 50 mg Children: IV 1–2 mg/kg, up to a total of 50 mg	Given to relieve extrapyramidal symptoms (movement disorders)
Thrombolytics (see Chap. 54)	Aminocaproic acid (Amicar)	PO, IV infusion, 5 g initially, then 1–1.25 g/h for 8 h or until bleeding is controlled; maximum dose, 30 g/24h	
Tricyclic antidepressants (see Chap. 10)	Sodium bicarbonate	IV 1–2 mEq/kg initially, then continuous IV drip to maintain serum pH of 7.5	To treat cardiac dysrhythmias, conduction disturbances, and hypotension
Warfarin (see Chap. 54)	Vitamin K_1	PO 5–10 mg daily IV (severe overdose) continuous infusion at rate no faster than 1 mg/min	

Most overdosed patients are treated in emergency rooms and discharged to their homes. A few are admitted to intensive care units (ICUs), often because of unconsciousness and the need for endotracheal intubation and mechanical ventilation. Unconsciousness is a major toxic effect of several commonly ingested substances such as benzodiazepine antianxiety and sedative agents, tricyclic antidepressants, ethanol, and opioid analgesics. Serious cardiovascular effects (e.g., cardiac arrest, dysrhythmias, circulatory impairment) are also common and warrant admission to an ICU.

Key Concepts

■ Drugs can stimulate or inhibit normal cellular activities but cannot add new functions.

■ Most drugs exert their effects by chemically combining with receptors at the cellular level.

■ Receptor proteins can be altered by endogenous substances and exogenous drugs.

■ Pharmacokinetic processes involve absorption, distribution, metabolism, and excretion.

■ Serum drug levels reflect dosage, absorption, bioavailability, elimination half-life, and the rate of elimination.

■ Drug-related variables that affect drug action include dosage, route, drug-diet and drug-drug interactions.

■ Patient-related variables that affect drug action include age, body weight, genetic and ethnic characteristics, gender, pathologic conditions, and psychological status.

■ All drugs can produce adverse effects; adverse effects may produce essentially any symptom or disease process and may involve any body system.

■ Drug toxicity results from excessive amounts of a drug, whether received in a single large dose or multiple smaller doses.

■ Activated charcoal is considered the "universal: antidote; most drugs do not have specific antidotes for overdoses.

Review and Application Exercises

Short Answer Exercises

1. Why do nurses need to understand cellular physiology in relation to drug therapy?

2. What are some factors that decrease absorption of an oral drug?

3. Drug dosage is a major determinant of both therapeutic and adverse drug effects. How can you use this knowledge in monitoring a patient's response to drug therapy?

4. Does protein binding speed or slow drug distribution to sites of action? Why?

5. Are drugs equally distributed throughout the body? Why or why not?

6. What are the implications of hepatic enzyme induction and inhibition in terms of drug metabolism and elimination from the body?

7. For a drug in which biotransformation produces active metabolites, is drug action shortened or lengthened? What difference does this make in patient care?

8. Which pharmacokinetic processes are likely to be impaired with severe cardiovascular disease and with severe renal disease?

9. What are the main elements of the receptor theory of drug action?

10. When drug–drug interactions occur, are drug actions increased or decreased?

11. What are some reasons for individual differences in responses to drugs?

NCLEX-Style Questions

12. You are reading a research report about use of a medication that describes the pharmacokinetics of a particular medication that your patient is on. You know that pharmacokinetics involves
    a. drug effects on human cells
    b. drug binding with receptors
    c. drug absorption, distribution, metabolism, and elimination
    d. drug stimulation of normal cell functions

13. The nurse practitioner has just changed your patient's medication from an oral form to a patch formulation to avoid the "first-pass effect." The NP has explained it to the patient, but the patient still has questions and asks you to explain again what is meant by the first-pass effect. You would be most correct in explaining that this has to do with how
    a. drugs initially bind to plasma proteins
    b. initial renal function is involved in drug excretion
    c. the way drugs first reach their target cells
    d. initial metabolism of an oral drug occurs before it reaches the systemic circulation

14. You are caring for a patient who has worsening liver disease. In monitoring his medication it is important that you know that a patient with liver disease may have impaired
    a. absorption
    b. distribution
    c. metabolism
    d. excretion

15. A patient with an overdose of an oral drug usually receives
    a. a specific antidote
    b. activated charcoal
    c. syrup of ipecac
    d. a strong laxative

16. You are looking up information about the effects of a drug on different receptors. You know that characteristics of receptors include which of the following?
    a. They are carbohydrates located in cell membranes or inside cells.
    b. They are constantly synthesized and degraded in the body.
    c. They bind with molecules of any drug circulating in the bloodstream.
    d. They regulate the actions of all drugs.

Selected References

Bamshad, M. (2005). Genetic influences on health: Does race matter? *Journal of the American Medical Association, 294,* 937–946.

Bauer, L. A. (2005). Clinical pharmacokinetics and pharmacodynamics. In J. T. DiPiro, R. L. Talbert, G. C. Yee, G. R. Matzke, B. G. Wells, & L. M. Posey (Eds.), *Pharmacotherapy: A pathophysiologic approach* (6th ed., pp. 51–73). New York: McGraw-Hill.

Cavallari, L. H., & Lam, Y. W. F. (2005). Pharmacogenetics. In J. T. DiPiro, R. L. Talbert, G. C. Yee, G. R. Matzke, B. G. Wells, & L. M. Posey (Eds.), *Pharmacotherapy: A pathophysiologic approach* (6th ed., pp. 75–90). New York: McGraw-Hill.

Chyka, P. A. (2005). Clinical toxicology. In J. T. DiPiro, R. L. Talbert, G. C. Yee, G. R. Matzke, B. G. Wells, & L. M. Posey (Eds.), *Pharmacotherapy: A pathophysiologic approach* (6th ed., pp. 125–148). New York: McGraw-Hill.

Drug facts and comparisons. (Updated monthly). St. Louis, MO: Facts and Comparisons.

Guyton, A. C., & Hall, J. E. (2006). *Textbook of medical physiology* (11th ed.). Philadelphia: Elsevier.

Lacy, C. F., Armstrong, L. L., Goldman, M. P., & Lance, L. L. (2006). *Drug information handbook* (14th ed.). Hudson, OH: Lexi-Comp.

Manno, M. S. (2006). Preventing adverse drug events. *Nursing, 36,* 56–61.

Munoz, C., & Hilgenberg, C. (2005). Ethnopharmacology. *American Journal of Nursing, 105,* 40–48.

Olson, K. R. (2007). Poisoning. In S. J. McPhee, M. A. Papadakis, & L. M. Tierney, Jr. (Eds.), *Current medical diagnosis & treatment 2007* (46th ed., pp. 1639–1669). New York: McGraw-Hill.

Ries, N. L., & Dart, R. C. (2005). New developments in antidotes. *Medical Clinics of North America, 89,* 1379–1397.

Smeltzer, S. C., & Bare, B. G. (2008). *Brunner & Suddarth's textbook of medical-surgical nursing* (11th ed.). Philadelphia: Lippincott Williams & Wilkins.

Spencer, A. P., & Wingate, S. (2005). Cardiovascular drug therapy in women. *Journal of Cardiovascular Nursing, 20,* 410–419.

Administering Medications

KEY TERMS

- Dosage forms
- Enteric-coated
- "Five rights"
- Parenteral
- Sustained release
- Topical
- Transdermal

LEARNING OBJECTIVES

After studying this chapter, you will be able to:

1. List the "rights" of drug administration.
2. Discuss knowledge and skills needed to implement the "rights" of drug administration.
3. List requirements of a complete drug order or prescription.
4. Accurately interpret drug orders containing common abbreviations.
5. Differentiate drug dosage forms for various routes and purposes of administration.
6. Discuss advantages and disadvantages of oral, parenteral, and topical routes of drug administration.
7. Identify supplies, techniques, and observations needed for safe and accurate administration of drugs by different routes.

Applying Your Knowledge

Juan Sanchez is transferred to your rehabilitation facility after a cerebral vascular accident (stroke) 2 weeks ago. When you review his chart, it indicates he has right-sided hemiparesis and memory deficits.

Introduction

Drugs given for therapeutic purposes are called *medications*. Giving medications to patients is an important nursing responsibility in many health care settings, including ambulatory care, hospitals, long-term care facilities, and patients' homes. The basic requirements for accurate drug administration are often called the *"five rights"*:

1. Right *drug*
2. Right *dose*
3. Right *patient*
4. Right *route*
5. Right *time*

Some people add a sixth "right": documentation. These "rights" require knowledge of the drugs to be given and the patients who are to receive them as well as specific nursing skills and interventions. When one of these "rights" is violated, medication errors can occur. Nurses need to recognize circumstances in which errors are likely to occur and intervene to prevent errors and protect patients. This chapter is concerned with safe and accurate medication administration.

General Principles of Accurate Drug Administration

The following principles should be followed:

- Follow the "rights" consistently.

- Learn essential information about each drug to be given (e.g., indications for use, contraindications, therapeutic effects, adverse effects, any specific instructions about administration).

- Interpret the prescriber's order accurately (i.e., drug name, dose, frequency of administration). Question the prescriber if any information is unclear or if the drug seems inappropriate for the patient's condition.

- Read labels of drug containers for the drug name and concentration (usually in milligrams per tablet, capsule, or milliliter of solution). Many medications are available in different dosage forms and concentrations, and it is extremely important that the correct ones are used.

- Minimize the use of abbreviations for drug names, doses, routes of administration, and times of administration. This promotes safer administration and reduces errors. When abbreviations are used by prescribers or others, interpret them accurately or question the writers about intended meanings.

- Calculate doses accurately. Current nursing practice requires few dosage calculations (most are done by pharmacists). However, when they are needed, accuracy is essential. For medications with a narrow safety margin or potentially serious adverse effects, ask a pharmacist or a colleague to do the calculation also and compare the results. This is especially important when calculating children's dosages.

- Measure doses accurately. Ask a colleague to double-check measurements of insulin and heparin, unusual doses (i.e., large or small), and any drugs to be given intravenously.

- Use the correct procedures and techniques for all routes of administration. For example, use appropriate anatomic landmarks to identify sites for intramuscular (IM) injections, follow the manufacturers' instructions for preparation and administration of intravenous (IV) medications, and use sterile materials and techniques for injectable and eye medications.

- Seek information about the patient's medical diagnoses and condition in relation to drug administration (e.g., ability to swallow oral medications; allergies or contraindications to ordered drugs; new signs or symptoms that may indicate adverse effects of administered drugs; heart, liver, or kidney disorders that may interfere with the patient's ability to eliminate drugs).

- Verify the identity of all patients before administering medications; check identification bands on patients who have them (e.g., in hospitals or long-term care facilities).

- Omit or delay doses as indicated by the patient's condition and report or record omissions appropriately.

- Be especially vigilant when giving medications to children, because there is a high risk of medication errors. One reason is children's great diversity in age, from birth to 18 years, and in weight, from 2 to 3 kilograms to 100 kilograms or more. Another reason is that most drugs have not been tested in children. A third reason is that many drugs are marketed in dosage forms and concentrations suitable for adults. This often requires dilution, calculation, preparation, and administration of very small doses. A fourth reason is that children have limited sites for administration of IV drugs, and several may be given through the same site. In many cases, the need for small volumes of fluid limits flushing between drugs (which may produce undesirable interactions with other drugs and IV solutions).

Legal Responsibilities

Registered and licensed practical nurses are legally empowered, under state nurse practice acts, to give medications ordered by licensed physicians and dentists. In some states, nurse practitioners may prescribe medications.

When giving medications, the nurse is legally responsible for safe and accurate administration. This means that the nurse may be held liable for not giving a drug or for giving a wrong drug or a wrong dose. In addition, the nurse is expected to have sufficient drug knowledge to recognize and question erroneous orders. If, after questioning the prescriber and seeking information from other authoritative sources, the nurse considers that giving a drug is unsafe, the nurse must refuse to give the drug. The fact that a physician wrote an erroneous order does not excuse the nurse from legal liability if he or she carries out that order.

The nurse also is legally responsible for actions delegated to people who are inadequately prepared for or legally barred from administering medications (e.g., nursing assistants). However, certified medical assistants (CMAs) may administer medications in physicians' offices, and certified medication aides (nursing assistants with a short course of training, also called CMAs) often administer medications in long-term care facilities.

The nurse who consistently follows safe practices in giving medications does not need to be excessively concerned about legal liability. The basic techniques and guidelines described in this chapter are aimed at safe and accurate preparation and administration. Most errors result when these practices are not followed.

Legal responsibilities in other aspects of drug therapy are less clear-cut. However, in general, nurses are expected to monitor patients' responses to drug therapy (e.g., therapeutic and adverse effects) and to teach patients safe and effective self-administration of drugs when indicated. These aspects are described more fully in Chapter 4.

Medication Errors

Medication errors continue to receive increasing attention from numerous health care organizations and agencies. Much of this interest stems from a 1999 report of the Institute of Medicine, which estimated that 44,000 to 98,000 deaths occur each year in the United States because of medical errors, including medication errors. Potential adverse patient outcomes of medication and other errors include serious illness, conditions that prolong hospitalization or require additional treatment, and death. Medication errors commonly reported include giving an incorrect dose, not giving an ordered drug, and giving an unordered drug. Specific drugs often associated with errors and adverse drug events (ADEs) include insulin, heparin, and warfarin. The risk of ADEs increases with the number of drugs a patient uses.

Medication errors may occur at any step in the drug distribution process, from the manufacturer to the patient, including prescribing, transcribing, dispensing, and administration. Many steps and numerous people are involved in giving the correct dose of a medication to the intended patient; each step or person has a potential for contributing to a medication error or preventing a medication error. All health care providers involved in drug therapy need to recognize risky situations, intervene to prevent errors when possible, and be extremely vigilant in all phases of drug administration. Recommendations for prevention of medication errors have been developed by several organizations, including the Institute of Medicine (IOM), the Agency for Healthcare Research and Quality (AHRQ), the Joint Commission on Accreditation of Healthcare Organizations (JCAHO), the Institute for Safe Medication Practices (ISMP), and the National Coordinating Council for Medication Error Reporting and Prevention (NCCMERP). Some sources of medication errors and recommendations to prevent them are summarized in Table 3-1.

Table 3-1	Medication Errors: Sources and Prevention Strategies

SOURCES OF ERRORS	RECOMMENDATIONS TO PREVENT ERRORS
Drug manufacturers	
Drugs may have similar names that can lead to erroneous prescribing, dispensing, or administration. For example, the antiseizure drug Lamictal (generic name, lamotrigine) has been confused with Lamisil, an antifungal drug, lamivudine, an antiviral drug, and others. The FDA estimates that about 10% of all reported medication errors result from drug name confusion.	▪ FDA evaluation of proposed trade names in manufacturers' new drug applications in seeking FDA approval for marketing. ▪ When choosing a trade name for a new drug, avoid names that are similar to drugs already on the market. ▪ Design packaging so that all drugs from an individual manufacturer don't look alike in terms of color, appearance, etc. ▪ Clearly designate long-acting drug formulations. ▪ Use Tall Man lettering on drug labels to distinguish between generic drugs with similar names (e.g., NICARdipine, NIFEdipine; vinBLAstine, vinCristine).
In addition to similar names, many drugs, especially those produced by the same manufacturer, have similar packaging. This can lead to errors if container labels are not read carefully, especially if the products are shelved or stored next to each other.	
Long-acting oral dosage forms with various, sometimes unclear indicators (e.g., LA, XL, XR), may be crushed, chewed, or otherwise broken so that the long-acting feature is destroyed. This can cause an overdose.	
Health care agencies	
Prescribers, pharmacists, and nurses may have a heavy workload, with resultant rushing of prescribing, dispensing, and administering medications. They may also experience distractions by interruptions, noise, and other events in the work environment that make it difficult to pay needed attention to the medication-related task.	▪ Provide prescribers with computerized order entry (CPOE) technology and standardized drug order sheets; discourage handwritten drug orders; minimize verbal orders and state procedures to follow when verbal orders are necessary. ▪ Provide computerized technology (e.g., bar coding for patients; handheld scanning devices for nursing staff) to verify the drug, the dose, and the patient identity before administration of a dose and to record administration after a dose. ▪ Provide sufficient pharmacy staff to dispense medications. ▪ Provide sufficient nursing staff to administer medications. ▪ Try to provide a quiet and orderly work environment, with limited human traffic, telephones, and other distractions. ▪ Provide adequate equipment for the required medication-related tasks. For pharmacies, this includes an adequate computer system for accessing databases of drug information and for detecting risks for adverse drug effects and drug–drug interactions.

(continued on page 30)

Table 3-1	Medication Errors: Sources and Prevention Strategies (continued)

SOURCES OF ERRORS	RECOMMENDATIONS TO PREVENT ERRORS
	■ Standardize drug administration materials and equipment (e.g., infusion pumps) throughout the agency. ■ Be sure that all professional staff members know and follow safety standards and medication reconciliation processes mandated by the Joint Commission on Accreditation of Healthcare Organizations (JCAHO).
Prescribers may write orders illegibly; order a drug that is not indicated by the patient's condition; fail to order a drug that is indicated; fail to consider the patient's age, size, kidney function, liver function, and disease process when selecting a drug or dosage; fail to consider other medications the patient is taking, including prescription, over-the-counter, and herbal drugs; lack sufficient knowledge about the drug; fail to monitor for, or instruct others to monitor for, effects of administered drugs; and fail to discontinue drugs appropriately.	■ Use computerized order entry when available. ■ Be sure that any handwritten drug order is legible (e.g., printed in block letters if necessary), clear, and unambiguous. ■ Avoid or minimize the use of abbreviations. ■ Use generic names of medications rather than brand names and include the purpose of the drug. ■ Avoid verbal orders when possible. If a verbal order is necessary, have the person taking the order write the order and read it back, spelling drug names, dosages, routes, and so forth when indicated. ■ Review the patient's health status and other drugs being taken before ordering any new drug. Also, discontinue drugs appropriately when no longer needed. ■ Maintain a current knowledge base about new drugs and changes in uses of drugs for the relevant area of clinical practice.
Pharmacists may not know the patient's condition or recognize an inappropriate or erroneous physician's order. They may dispense incorrect medications, mislabel containers, or fail to determine other drugs being taken.	■ Promote and assist with computerized drug order systems and bar-coding technology, when possible. ■ Verify or request clarification of unclear drug orders. ■ Check the compatibility of newly ordered drugs with available information about a patient's health status and medications already being taken. ■ Verify patient weight and recalculate any dosages based on weight or body surface area, especially for children. ■ Review the original order before dispensing a medication, except in emergency situations. ■ Prepare drugs in a work area with minimal distractions and interruptions. ■ Separate look-alike and sound-alike medications on pharmacy shelves; do not store them next to each other. ■ When possible, dispense medications in a single unit-dose, ready-to-administer form. ■ Maintain current information about sound-alike and look-alike drugs; drugs often associated with medication errors and adverse effects (e.g., insulin, heparin, warfarin); drugs associated with high risks of serious drug–drug interactions; and drug dosage forms that should not be chewed or crushed, tablets that may and may not be split, and capsules that may or may not be opened. ■ For large agencies with many drug orders, encourage specialization in certain areas (e.g., neonatal/pediatric drug therapy; oncology drugs and treatment regimens for various types of cancer). ■ Encourage all health care providers to report medication errors, so that preventive interventions can be developed.
Nurses may have inadequate knowledge about a drug or about the patient receiving the drug; not follow the "five rights"; and fail to question the medication order when indicated.	■ Be aware of agency policies and procedures about medication use, storage, administration, and recording. ■ Maintain an up-to-date knowledge base about drugs and their administration. ■ Make a diligent effort to learn about patients' health status and the drugs they're receiving. ■ Question or clarify any unclear drug orders.

SOURCES OF ERRORS	RECOMMENDATIONS TO PREVENT ERRORS
	▪ Verify medication calculations with another nurse or a pharmacist, especially for children. ▪ Recheck a single dose any time the amount seems unusually large or small. ▪ Verify settings on drug infusion pumps with another nurse, when indicated. ▪ Follow the "five rights" consistently. ▪ Recheck the original drug order when a patient questions whether a particular drug dose should be taken. ▪ Report errors, so that preventive efforts can be designed. ▪ Discuss patients' medications during change-of-shift reports, including new and discontinued drugs, patients' responses to their medications, patient teaching about medications, and medications given 1 to 2 h before report or scheduled to be given 1–2 h in a 1- to 2-h window after each report.
Patients/consumers Outpatients may take drugs from several prescribers; fail to inform one prescriber about drugs prescribed by another health care provider; get prescriptions filled at more than one pharmacy; fail to get prescriptions filled or refilled; underuse or overuse an appropriately prescribed drug; take drugs left over from a previous illness or prescribed for someone else; fail to follow instructions for drug administration or storage; fail to keep appointments for follow-up care; and fail to ask for information when needed.	▪ Inform all health care providers about health status, any drug allergies, and all medications being taken (e.g., prescription, over-the-counter, herbal, and dietary supplements). ▪ Ask prescribers to include the purpose of a drug on the label of all prescription medications. ▪ If able, know names, strengths, doses, and the reason for use of all medications. ▪ Follow instructions about when and how to take medications; do not increase amount or frequency of any medication without checking with a health care provider. Ask questions or request written instructions if needed. ▪ If unable to take medications or if problems occur, discuss with a health care provider. Do not stop taking prescribed medications. ▪ Maintain a current list of all medications being taken. Take the list or the medications to each visit to a health care provider. ▪ Keep all medications in their original containers. ▪ Read labels of medication containers every time a dose is taken. ▪ Do not chew, crush, or break any tablets or capsules unless a health care provider says it is okay to do so.

Medication Systems

Each health care facility has a system for distributing drugs. The unit-dose system, in which most drugs are dispensed in single-dose containers for individual patients, is widely used. In this system, drug orders are checked by a pharmacist or pharmacy technician, who then places the indicated number of doses in the patient's medication drawer at scheduled intervals. When a dose is due to be taken, the nurse removes the medication and gives it to the patient. Unit-dose wrappings of oral drugs should be left in place until the nurse is in the presence of the patient and ready to give the medication. Each dose of a drug must be recorded on the patient's medication administration record (MAR) as soon as possible after administration.

Increasingly, institutions are using automated, computerized, locked cabinets for which each nurse on a unit has a password or code for accessing the cabinet and obtaining a drug dose. An inventory is maintained, and drugs are restocked as needed.

Controlled drugs, such as opioid analgesics, are usually kept as a stock supply in a locked drawer or automated cabinet and replaced as needed. Each dose is signed for and recorded on the patient's MAR. Each nurse must comply with legal regulations and institutional policies for dispensing and recording controlled drugs.

Changes to Prevent Medication Errors

Changes in medication systems are being increasingly implemented, largely in efforts to decrease medication errors and improve patient safety. These include the following:

▪ Computerized provider order entry (CPOE). In this system, a prescriber types a medication order directly into a computer. This decreases errors associated with illegible handwriting and erroneous transcription or dispensing. CPOE, which is already used in many health care facilities, is widely recommended as the preferred alternative to error-prone handwritten orders.

- Bar coding. In 2004, the Food and Drug Administration (FDA) passed a regulation requiring drug manufacturers to put bar codes on current prescription medications and non-prescription medications that are commonly used in hospitals. New drugs must have bar codes within 60 days of their approval. In hospitals, bar codes operate with other agency computer systems and databases that contain a patient's medication orders and medication administration record (MAR). The bar code on the drug label contains the identification number, strength, and dosage form of the drug, and the bar code on the patient's identification band contains the MAR, which can be displayed when a nurse uses a handheld scanning device. When administering medications, the nurse scans the bar code on the drug label, on the patient's identification band, and on the nurse's personal identification badge. A wireless computer network processes the scanned information; gives an error message on the scanner or sounds an alarm if the nurse is about to give the wrong drug or the right drug at the wrong time; and automatically records the time, drug, and dose given on the MAR. The FDA estimates that it will take about 20 years for all U.S. hospitals to implement this system of bar codes for medication administration.

  - For nurses, implementing the bar-coding technology increases the time requirements and interferes with their ability to individualize patient care in relation to medications. Such a system works well with routine medications, but nonroutine situations (e.g., variable doses or times of administration) may pose problems. In addition, in long-term care facilities, it may be difficult to maintain legible bar codes on patient identification bands. Despite some drawbacks, bar coding increases patient safety and therefore should be supported by nurses as it continues to develop.

- Limiting use of abbreviations. The ISMP has long maintained a list of abbreviations that are often associated with medication errors, and the JCAHO now requires accredited organizations to maintain a "Do not use" list (e.g., u or U for units, IU for international units, qd for daily, qod for every other day) that applies to all prescribers and transcribers of medication orders. Other abbreviations are not recommended, as well. In general, it is safer to write out drug names, routes of administration, and so forth and to minimize the use of abbreviations, symbols, and numbers that are often misinterpreted, especially when handwritten.

- Medication reconciliation. This is a process designed to avoid medication errors such as omissions, duplications, dosing errors, or drug interactions that occur when a patient is admitted to a health care agency, transferred from one department or unit to another within the agency, or discharged home from the agency. It involves obtaining an accurate medication history about the prescription, over-the-counter, vitamins, and herbal medications taken at home, including dose and frequency of administration, upon entry into the health care agency. The list of medications developed from the medication history is compared to newly ordered medications and identified discrepancies are resolved. The list is placed in the medical record so that it is accessible to all health care providers, including the prescriber who writes the patient's admission drug orders. When the patient is transferred, the updated list must be communicated to the next health care provider. When a patient is discharged, an updated list should be given to the next provider and to the patient. The patient should be encouraged to keep the list up-to-date when changes are made in the medication regimen and to share the list with future health care providers.

Medication Orders

Medication orders should include the full name of the patient; the name of the drug (preferably the generic name); the dose, route, and frequency of administration; and the date, time, and signature of the prescriber.

Orders in a health care facility may be typed into a computer (the preferred method) or handwritten on an order sheet in the patient's medical record. Occasionally, verbal or telephone orders are acceptable. When taken, they should be written on the patient's order sheet, signed by the person taking the order, and later countersigned by the prescriber. After the order is written, a copy is sent to the pharmacy, where the order is recorded and the drug is dispensed to the appropriate patient care unit. In many facilities, pharmacy staff prepares a computer-generated MAR for each 24-hour period.

For patients in ambulatory care settings, the procedure is essentially the same for drugs to be given immediately. For drugs to be taken at home, written prescriptions are given. In addition to the previous information, a prescription should include instructions for taking the drug (e.g., dose, frequency) and whether the prescription can be refilled. Prescriptions for Schedule II controlled drugs cannot be refilled.

To interpret medication orders accurately, the nurse must know commonly used abbreviations for routes, dosages, and times of drug administration (Table 3-2). Because of medication errors occurring with incorrect or misinterpreted abbreviations, many abbreviations that were formerly commonly used are now banned or no longer recommended by the Joint Commission on Accreditation of Healthcare Organizations (JCAHO), the Institute for Safe Medication Practices (ISMP), and other organizations concerned with increasing patient safety. Thus, it is safer practice to write out such words as "daily" or "three times daily," "at bedtime," "ounce," "teaspoon" or "tablespoon," or "right," "left," or "both eyes" rather

Table 3-2	Common Abbreviations

ROUTES OF DRUG ADMINISTRATION

IM	intramuscular
IV	intravenous
PO	by mouth, oral
SL	sublingual
Sub-Q	subcutaneous

DRUG DOSAGES

cc	cubic centimeter
g	gram
mg	milligram
mcg	microgram
mL	milliliter
oz	ounce
tbsp	tablespoon
tsp	teaspoon

TIMES OF DRUG ADMINISTRATION

ad lib	as desired
PRN	as needed
q4h	every 4 hours
stat	immediately

than using abbreviations, in both medication orders and in transcribing orders to the patient's MAR. If the nurse cannot read the physician's order or if the order seems erroneous, he or she must question the order before giving the drug.

 Applying Your Knowledge 3-1

How Can You Avoid This Medication Error?
You are administering 6 A.M. medications to a patient on a busy medical unit. You enter Mr. Gonzales's room, gently shake him awake, and call him by name. He slowly awakens and appears groggy. You explain that you have his medications, which he takes and then quickly falls back to sleep. On exiting the room, you look at the room number and realize that you just gave medications to Mr. Sanchez.

Drug Preparations and Dosage Forms

Drug preparations and dosage forms vary according to the drug's chemical characteristics, reason for use, and route of adminis-

tration. Some drugs are available in only one dosage form, and others are available in several forms. Characteristics of various dosage forms are described as follows and in Table 3-3.

Dosage forms of systemic drugs include liquids, tablets, capsules, suppositories, and transdermal and pump delivery systems. Systemic liquids are given orally, or PO (Latin *per os*, "by mouth"), or by injection. Those given by injection must be sterile.

Tablets and capsules are given PO. Tablets contain active drug plus binders, colorants, preservatives, and other substances. Capsules contain active drug enclosed in a gelatin capsule. Most tablets and capsules dissolve in the acidic fluids of the stomach and are absorbed in the alkaline fluids of the upper small intestine. *Enteric-coated* tablets and capsules are coated with a substance that is insoluble in stomach acid. This delays dissolution until the medication reaches the intestine, usually to avoid gastric irritation or to keep the drug from being destroyed by gastric acid. Tablets for sublingual (under the tongue) or buccal (held in cheek) administration must be specifically formulated for such use.

Several controlled-release dosage forms and drug delivery systems are available, and more continue to be developed. These formulations maintain more consistent serum drug levels and allow less frequent administration, which is more convenient for patients. Controlled-release oral tablets and capsules are called by a variety of names (e.g., timed release, *sustained release*, extended release), and their names usually include CR, SR, XL, or other indications that they are long-acting formulations. Most of these formulations are given once or twice daily. Some drugs (e.g., alendronate for osteoporosis, fluoxetine for major depression) are available in formulations that deliver a full week's dosage in one oral tablet. Because controlled-release tablets and capsules contain high amounts of drug intended to be absorbed slowly and act over a prolonged period of time, they should never be broken, opened, crushed, or chewed. Such an action allows the full dose to be absorbed immediately and constitutes an overdose, with potential organ damage or death. *Transdermal* (skin patch) formulations include systemically absorbed clonidine, estrogen, fentanyl, and nitroglycerin. These medications are slowly absorbed from the skin patches over varying periods of time (e.g., 1 week for clonidine and estrogen). Pump delivery systems may be external or implanted under the skin and refillable or long acting without refills. Pumps are used to administer insulin, opioid analgesics, antineoplastics, and other drugs.

Solutions, ointments, creams, and suppositories are applied topically to skin or mucous membranes. They are formulated for the intended route of administration. For example, several drugs are available in solutions for nasal or oral inhalation; they are usually self-administered as a spray into the nose or mouth.

Many combination products containing fixed doses of two or more drugs are also available. Commonly used combinations include analgesics, antihypertensive drugs, and cold remedies. Most are oral tablets, capsules, or solutions.

Table 3-3	Drug Dosage Forms

DOSAGE FORMS AND THEIR ROUTES OF ADMINISTRATION	CHARACTERISTICS	CONSIDERATIONS/PRECAUTIONS
Tablets *Regular:* PO, GI tube (crushed and mixed with water)	▪ Contain active drug plus binders, dyes, preservatives ▪ Dissolve in gastric fluids	8 oz of water recommended, to promote dissolution and absorption
Chewable: PO	▪ Colored and flavored, mainly for young children	Children may think tablets are candy; keep out of reach to avoid accidental overdose
Enteric coated: PO	▪ Dissolve in small intestine; mainly used for medications that cause gastric irritation	Do not crush; instruct patients not to chew or crush.
Extended release (XL) (also called sustained release (SR), long acting (LA) and other names: PO	▪ Slowly absorbed; effects prolonged, usually 12–24 h ▪ Contain relatively large amounts of active drug	**Warning:** Crushing to give orally or through a GI tube administers an overdose, with potentially serious adverse effects or death!! *Never crush*; instruct patients not to chew or crush.
Sublingual: Under the tongue *Buccal:* Held in cheek	▪ Dissolve quickly ▪ Medication absorbed directly into the bloodstream and exerts rapid systemic effects	Few medications formulated for administration by SL or buccal routes
Capsules *Regular:* PO	▪ Contain active drug, fillers, and preservatives ▪ Gelatin capsules dissolve in gastric fluid and release medication.	8 oz of fluid recommended to promote dissolution and absorption
Extended release (XL); *sustained release* (SR); *long-acting* (LA): PO	▪ Slowly absorbed; effects prolonged, usually 12–24 h ▪ Contain relatively large amounts of active drug	**Warning:** Emptying a capsule to give the medication orally or through a GI tube administers an overdose, with potentially serious adverse effects or death!! Instruct patients not to bite, chew, or empty these capsules.
Solutions *Oral:* PO, GI tube	▪ Absorbed rapidly because they do not need to be dissolved	Use of appropriate measuring devices and accurate measurement is extremely important.
Parenteral: IV, IM, Sub-Q, intradermal	▪ Medications and all administration devices must be sterile. ▪ IV produces rapid effects; Sub-Q is used mainly for insulin and heparin; IM is used for only a few drugs; intradermal is used mainly to inject skin-test material.	Use of appropriate equipment and accurate measurement is extremely important. Insulin syringes should always be used for insulin, and tuberculin syringes are recommended for measuring small amounts of other drugs.
Suspensions PO, Sub-Q (e.g., NPH, Lente insulins)	▪ Particles of active drug are suspended in a liquid; the liquid must be rotated or shaken before measuring a dose.	Drug particles settle to the bottom on standing. If not remixed, the liquid vehicle is given rather than the drug dose.
Dermatologic Creams, Lotions, Ointments Topically to skin	▪ Most are minimally absorbed through skin and exert local effects at the site of application; some (e.g., skin patches) are absorbed and exert systemic effects.	Formulations vary with intended uses and are not interchangeable. When removed from the patient, skin patches must be disposed of properly to prevent someone else from being exposed to the active drug remaining in the patch.

DOSAGE FORMS AND THEIR ROUTES OF ADMINISTRATION	CHARACTERISTICS	CONSIDERATIONS/PRECAUTIONS
Solutions and Powders for Oral or Nasal Inhalation, Including Metered Dose Inhalers (MDIs)	▪ Oral inhalations are used mainly for asthma; nasal sprays for nasal allergies (allergic rhinitis). ▪ Effective with less systemic effect than oral drugs ▪ Deliver a specified dose per inhalation	Several research studies indicate that patients often do not use MDIs correctly; correct use is essential to obtaining therapeutic effects and avoiding adverse effects.
Eye Solutions and Ointments	▪ Should be sterile ▪ Packaged in small amounts for individual use	Can be systemically absorbed and cause systemic adverse effects
Throat Lozenges	▪ Used for cough and sore throat	
Ear Solutions	▪ Used mainly for ear infections	
Vaginal Creams and Suppositories	▪ Used to treat vaginal infections	
Rectal Suppositories and Enemas	▪ Suppositories may be used to administer sedatives, analgesics, laxatives. ▪ Medicated enemas may be used for constipation or inflammatory bowel diseases.	Effects somewhat unpredictable because absorption is erratic

Calculating Drug Dosages

When calculating drug dosages, the importance of accuracy cannot be overemphasized. Accuracy requires basic skills in mathematics, knowledge of common units of measurement, and methods of using data in performing calculations.

Systems of Measurement

The most commonly used system of measurement is the metric system, in which the meter is used for linear measure, the gram for weight, and the liter for volume. One milliliter (mL) equals 1 cubic centimeter (cc), and both equal 1 gram (g) of water. The household system, with units of drops, teaspoons, tablespoons, and cups, is infrequently used in health care agencies but may be used at home. Table 3-4 lists some commonly used equivalent measurements.

A few drugs are ordered and measured in terms of units or milliequivalents (mEq). Units express biologic activity in animal tests (i.e., the amount of drug required to produce a particular response). Units are unique for each drug. For example, concentrations of insulin and heparin are both expressed in units, but there is no relation between a unit of insulin and a unit of heparin. These drugs are usually ordered in the number of units per dose (e.g., NPH insulin 30 units subcutaneously [Sub-Q] every morning, or heparin 5000 units Sub-Q q12h) and labeled in number of units per milliliter (U 100 insulin contains 100 units/mL; heparin may have 1000, 5000, or 10,000 units/mL). Milliequivalents express the ionic activity of a drug. Drugs such as potassium chloride are ordered and labeled in the number of milliequivalents per dose, tablet, or milliliter.

Mathematical Calculations

Most drug orders and labels are expressed in metric units of measurement. If the amount specified in the order is the same as that on the drug label, no calculations are required, and preparing the right dose is a simple matter. For example, if the order reads "ibuprofen 400 mg PO" and the drug label reads "ibuprofen 400 mg per tablet," it is clear that one tablet is to be given.

Table 3-4	Selected Equivalent Measurements

METRIC	HOUSEHOLD
Weights	
1000 mcg = 1 mg	
1000 mg = 1 g	
30 g	1 oz
454 g	1 lb
1000 g = 1 kg	2.2 lb
Liquids	
1 mL = 1 cc	
5 mL	1 tsp
30 mL	2 tbsp or 1 oz
250 mL	1 cup or 8 oz
500 mL	1 pint
1000 mL = 1 L	1 quart

What happens if the order calls for a 400-mg dose and 200-mg tablets are available? The question is, "How many 200-mg tablets are needed to give a dose of 400 mg?" In this case, the answer can be readily calculated mentally to indicate two tablets. This is a simple example that also can be used to illustrate mathematical calculations. This problem can be solved by several acceptable methods; the following formula is presented because of its relative simplicity for students lacking a more familiar method.

$$\frac{D}{H} = \frac{X}{V}$$

D = desired dose (dose ordered, often in milligrams)
H = on-hand or available dose (dose on the drug label; often in mg per tablet, capsule, or milliliter)
X = unknown (number of tablets, in this example)
V = volume or unit (one tablet, in this example)

$$\frac{400 \text{ mg}}{200 \text{ mg}} = \frac{X \text{ tablet}}{1 \text{ tablet}}$$

Cross multiply:

$$200X = 400$$

$$X = \frac{400}{200} = 2 \text{ tablets}$$

What happens if the order and the label are written in different units? For example, the order may read "amoxicillin 0.5 g" and the label may read "amoxicillin 500 mg/capsule." To calculate the number of capsules needed for the dose, the first step is to convert 0.5 g to the equivalent number of milligrams, or convert 500 mg to the equivalent number of grams. *The desired or ordered dose and the available or label dose must be in the same units of measurement.* Using the equivalents (i.e., 1 g = 1000 mg) listed in Table 3-3, an equation can be set up as follows:

$$\frac{1 \text{ g}}{1000 \text{ mg}} = \frac{0.5 \text{ g}}{X \text{ mg}}$$

$$X = 0.5 \times 1000 = 500 \text{ mg}$$

The next step is to use the new information in the formula, which then becomes

$$\frac{D}{H} = \frac{X}{V}$$

$$\frac{500 \text{ mg}}{500 \text{ mg}} = \frac{X \text{ capsules}}{1 \text{ capsule}}$$

$$500X = 500$$

$$X = \frac{500}{500} = 1 \text{ capsule}$$

The same procedure and formula can be used to calculate portions of tablets or doses of liquids. These are illustrated in the following problems:

1. Order: 25 mg PO
   Label: 50-mg tablet

$$\frac{25 \text{ mg}}{50 \text{ mg}} = \frac{X \text{ tablet}}{1 \text{ tablet}}$$

$$50X = 25$$

$$X = \frac{25}{50} = 0.5 \text{ tablet}$$

2. Order: 25 mg IM
   Label: 50 mg in 1 cc

$$\frac{25 \text{ mg}}{50 \text{ mg}} = \frac{X \text{ cc}}{1 \text{ cc}}$$

$$50X = 25$$

$$X = \frac{25}{50} = 0.5 \text{ cc}$$

3. Order: 4 mg IV
   Label: 10 mg/mL

$$\frac{4 \text{mg}}{10 \text{mg}} = \frac{X \text{ mL}}{1 \text{ mL}}$$

$$10X = 4$$

$$X = \frac{4}{10} = 0.4 \text{ mL}$$

Routes of Administration

Routes of administration depend on drug characteristics, patient characteristics, and desired responses. The major routes are oral (by mouth), *parenteral* (injected), and *topical* (applied to skin or mucous membrane). Each has advantages, disadvantages, indications for use, and specific techniques of administration (Table 3-5). Common parenteral routes are subcutaneous (Sub-Q), intramuscular (IM), and intravenous (IV) injections. Injections require special drug preparations, equipment, and techniques. General characteristics are described below; specific considerations for the IV route are described in Box 3-1.

Drugs for Injection

Injectable drugs must be prepared, packaged, and administered in ways to maintain sterility. Vials are closed containers with rubber stoppers through which a sterile needle can be inserted for withdrawing medication. Single-dose vials usually do not contain a preservative and must be discarded after a dose is withdrawn. Multiple-dose vials contain a preservative and may be reused if aseptic technique is maintained.

Ampules are sealed glass containers, the tops of which must be broken off to allow insertion of a needle and withdrawal of the medication. Broken ampules and any remaining medication are discarded. When vials or ampules contain a powder form of the drug, a sterile solution of water or 0.9% sodium chloride must be added and the drug dissolved before withdrawal. When available, a filter needle is used to withdraw the medication from an ampule or vial because broken glass or rubber fragments may need to be removed from the drug solution. The filter needle is replaced with a regular needle before injecting the patient.

Table 3-5	Routes of Drug Administration

ROUTE AND DESCRIPTION	ADVANTAGES	DISADVANTAGES	COMMENTS
Oral	■ Simple and can be used by most people ■ Convenient; does not require complex equipment ■ Relatively inexpensive	■ Dosage is unknown because some drug is not absorbed and some is metabolized in the liver before reaching the bloodstream. ■ Slow drug action ■ Irritation of gastrointestinal mucosa by some drugs	The oral route should generally be used when possible, considering the patient's condition and ability to take or tolerate oral drugs.
Gastrointestinal (GI) tubes (e.g., nasogastric, gastrostomy)	■ Allows use of GI tract in patients who cannot take oral drugs ■ Can be used over long periods of time, if necessary ■ May avoid or decrease injections	■ With nasogastric tubes, medications may be aspirated into the lungs ■ Small-bore tubes often become clogged ■ Requires special precautions to give correctly and avoid complications	■ Liquid preparations are preferred over crushed tablets and emptied capsules, when available. ■ Tube should be rinsed before and after instilling medication.
Subcutaneous (Sub-Q) injection—injection of drugs under the skin, into the underlying fatty tissue	■ Relatively painless ■ Very small needles can be used ■ Insulin and heparin, commonly used medications, can be given Sub-Q	■ Only a small amount of drug (up to 1 mL) can be given ■ Drug absorption is relatively slow ■ Only a few drugs can be given Sub-Q	The Sub-Q route is commonly used for only a few drugs because many drugs are irritating to Sub-Q tissues. Such drugs may cause pain, necrosis, and abscess formation if injected Sub-Q.
Intramuscular (IM) injection—injection of drugs into selected muscles	■ May be used for several drugs ■ Drug absorption is rapid because muscle tissue has an abundant blood supply	■ A relatively small amount of drug (up to 3 mL) can be given ■ Risks of damage to blood vessels or nerves if needle is not positioned correctly	It is very important to use anatomic landmarks when selecting IM injection sites.
Intravenous (IV) injection— injection of a drug into the bloodstream	■ Allows medications to be given to a patient who cannot take fluids or drugs by GI tract ■ Bypasses barriers to drug absorption that occur with other routes ■ Rapid drug action ■ Larger amounts can be given than by Sub-Q and IM routes ■ Allows slow administration when indicated	■ Time and skill required for venipuncture and maintaining an IV line ■ After it is injected, drug cannot be retrieved if adverse effects or overdoses occur ■ High potential for adverse reactions due to rapid drug action and possible complications of IV therapy (i.e., bleeding, infection, fluid overload, extravasation) ■ Phlebitis and thrombosis may occur and cause discomfort or pain, take days or weeks to subside, and limit the veins available for future therapy	■ The nurse should wear latex gloves to start IV infusions, for protection against exposure to blood-borne pathogens. ■ Phlebitis and thrombosis result from injury to the endothelial cells that form the inner lining (intima) of veins and may be caused by repeated venipunctures, the IV catheter, hypertonic IV fluid, or irritating drugs.

(continued on page 38)

Table 3-5	Routes of Drug Administration (continued)			
ROUTE AND DESCRIPTION	**ADVANTAGES**	**DISADVANTAGES**		**COMMENTS**
Topical administration—application to skin or mucous membranes. Application to mucous membranes includes drugs given by nasal or oral inhalation; by instillation into the lungs, eyes, or nose; and by insertion under the tongue (sublingual), into the cheek (buccal), and into the vagina or rectum.	■ With application to intact skin, most medications act at the site of application, with little systemic absorption or systemic adverse effects. ■ Some drugs are given topically for systemic effects (e.g., medicated skin patches). Effects may last several days, and the patches are usually convenient for patients. ■ With application to mucous membranes, most drugs are well and rapidly absorbed	■ Some drugs irritate skin or mucous membranes and cause itching, rash, or discomfort ■ With inflamed, abraded, or damaged skin, drug absorption is increased and systemic adverse effects may occur ■ Application to mucous membranes may cause systemic adverse effects (e.g., beta blocker eye drops, used to treat glaucoma, can cause bradycardia just as oral beta blockers can)	■ Specific drug preparations must be used for application to skin, eyes, sublingual, buccal, vaginal, and rectal sites.	When available and effective, topical drugs are often preferred over oral or injected drugs, because of fewer and/or less severe systemic adverse effects.

Box 3-1	Principles and Techniques With Intravenous Drug Therapy

Methods

Intravenous (IV) injection or **IV** push is the direct injection of a medication into the vein. The drug may be injected through an injection site on IV tubing or an intermittent infusion device. Most IV push medications should be injected slowly. The time depends on the particular drug, but is often 2 minutes or longer for a dose. Rapid injection should generally be avoided because the drug produces high blood levels and is quickly circulated to the heart and brain, where it may cause adverse or toxic effects. Although IV push may be useful with a few drugs or in emergency situations, slower infusion of more dilute drugs is usually preferred.

Intermittent infusion is administration of intermittent doses, often diluted in 50–100 mL of fluid and infused over 30– 60 minutes. The drug dose is usually prepared in a pharmacy and connected to an IV administration set that controls the amount and flow rate. Intermittent infusions are often connected to an injection port on a primary IV line, through which IV fluids are infusing continuously. The purpose of the primary IV line may be to provide fluids to the patient or to keep the vein open for periodic administration of medications. The IV fluids are usually stopped for the medication infusion, then restarted. Drug doses may also be infused through an intermittent infusion device (e.g., a heparin lock) to conserve veins and allow freedom of motion between drug doses. The devices decrease the amount of IV fluids given to patients who do not need them (i.e., those who are able to ingest adequate amounts of oral fluids) and those who are at risk of fluid overload, especially children and older adults.

An intermittent infusion device may be part of an initial IV line or used to adapt a continuous IV for intermittent use. The devices include a heparin lock or a resealable adapter added to a peripheral or central IV catheter. These devices must be flushed routinely to maintain patency. If the IV catheter has more than one lumen, all must be flushed, whether being used or not. Saline is probably the most commonly used flushing solution; heparin may also be used if recommended by the device's manufacturer or required by institutional policy.

Continuous infusion indicates medications mixed in a large volume of IV fluid and infused continuously, over several hours. For example, vitamins and minerals (e.g., potassium chloride) are usually added to liters of IV fluids. Greater dilution of the drug and administration over a longer time decreases risks of accumulation and toxicity, as well as venous irritation and thrombophlebitis.

Equipment

Equipment varies considerably from one health care agency to another. Nurses must become familiar with the equipment available in their work setting, including IV catheters, types of IV tubing, needles and needleless systems, types of volume control devices, and electronic infusion devices (IV pumps).

Catheters vary in size (both gauge and length), design, and composition (e.g., polyvinyl chloride, polyurethane, silicone). The most common design type is over the needle; the needle is used to start the IV, then it is removed. When choosing a catheter to start an IV, one that is much smaller than the lumen of the vein is recommended. This allows good blood flow and rapidly dilutes drug solutions as they enter the vein. This, in turn, prevents high drug concentrations and risks of toxicity. Also, after a catheter is inserted, it is very important to tape it securely so that it does not move around. Movement of the catheter increases venous irritation and risks of thrombophlebitis and infection. If signs of venous irritation and inflammation develop, the catheter should be removed and a new one inserted at another site. Additional recommendations include application of a topical antibiotic or antiseptic ointment at the IV site after catheter insertion, a sterile occlusive dressing over the site, and limiting the duration of placement to a few days.

Many medications are administered through peripherally inserted central catheters (PICC lines) or central venous catheters, in which the catheter tips are inserted into the superior vena cava, next to the right atrium of the heart. Central venous catheters may have single, double, or triple lumens. Other products, which are especially useful for long-term IV drug therapy, include a variety of implanted ports, pumps, and reservoirs.

If a catheter becomes clogged, do not irrigate it. Doing so may push a clot into the circulation and result in a pulmonary embolus, myocardial infarction, or stroke. It may also cause septicemia, if the clot is infected.

Needleless systems are products with a blunt-tipped plastic insertion device and an injection port that opens. These systems greatly decrease needle-stick injuries and exposure to bloodborne pathogens.

Electronic infusion devices allow amounts and flow rates of IV drug solutions to be set and controlled by a computer. Although the devices save nursing time because the nurse does not need to continually adjust flow rates, the biggest advantage is the steady rate of drug administration. The devices are used in most settings where IV drugs and IV fluids are administered, but they are especially valuable in pediatrics, where very small amounts of medication and IV fluid are needed, and in intensive care units, where strong drugs and varying amounts of IV fluid are usually required. Several types of pumps are available, even within the same health care agency. It is extremely important that nurses become familiar with the devices used in their work setting, so that they can program them accurately and determine whether or not they are functioning properly (i.e., delivering medications as ordered).

Site Selection

IV needles are usually inserted into a vein on the hand or forearm; IV catheters may be inserted in a peripheral site or centrally. In general, recommendations are

- Start at the most distal location. This conserves more proximal veins for later use, if needed. Veins on the back of the hand and on the forearm are often used to provide more comfort and freedom of movement for patients.
- Use veins with a large blood volume flowing through them when possible. Many drugs cause irritation and phlebitis in small veins.
- When possible, avoid the antecubital vein on the inner surface of the elbow, veins over or close to joints, and

veins on the inner aspect of the wrists. Reasons include the difficulty of stabilizing and maintaining an IV line at these sites and inner wrist venipunctures are very painful. *Do not perform venipuncture in foot or leg veins.* The risks of serious or fatal complications are too high.

- Rotate sites when long-term use (more than a few days) of IV fluid or drug therapy is required. Venous irritation occurs with longer duration of site use and with the administration of irritating drugs or fluids. When it is necessary to change an IV site, use the opposite arm if possible.

Drug Preparation

Most IV drugs are prepared for administration in pharmacies and this is the safest practice. When a nurse must prepare a medication, considerations include the following.

- Only drug formulations manufactured for IV use should be given IV. Other formulations contain various substances that are not sterile, pure enough, or soluble enough to be injected into the bloodstream. *In recent years, there have been numerous reports of medication errors resulting from IV administration of drug preparations intended for oral use!!* Such errors can and should be prevented. For example, when liquid medications intended for oral use are measured or dispensed in a syringe (as they often are for children, adults with difficulty in swallowing tablets and capsules, or for administration through a gastrointestinal [GI] tube), the syringe should have a blunt tip that will not connect to or penetrate IV tubing injection sites.
- Use sterile technique during all phases of IV drug preparation.
- Follow the manufacturer's instructions for mixing and diluting IV medications. Some liquid IV medications need to be diluted prior to IV administration, and powdered medications must be reconstituted with the recommended diluent. The diluent recommended by the drug's manufacturer should be used because different drugs require different diluents. In addition, be sure any reconstituted drug is completely dissolved to avoid particles that may be injected into the systemic circulation and lead to thrombus formation or embolism. A filtered aspiration needle should be used when withdrawing medication from a vial or ampule, to remove any particles in the solution. The filter needle should then be discarded, to prevent filtered particles from being injected when the medication is added to the IV fluid. Filters added to IV tubing also help to remove particles.
- Check the expiration date on all IV medications. Many drugs have a limited period of stability after they are reconstituted or diluted for IV administration.
- IV medications should be compatible with the infusing IV fluids. Most are compatible with 5% dextrose in water or saline solutions.
- If adding a medication to a container of IV fluid, invert the container to be sure the additive is well mixed with the solution.
- For any IV medication that is prepared or added to an IV bag, label the medication vial or IV bag with the name of the patient, drug, dosage, date, time of mixing, expiration date, and the preparer's signature.

(continued on page 40)

Box 3-1	Principles and Techniques With Intravenous Drug Therapy (continued)

Drug Administration

■ Most IV medications are injected into a self-sealing site in any of several IV set-ups, including a scalp–vein needle and tubing; a plastic catheter connected to a heparin lock or other intermittent infusion device; or IV tubing and a plastic bag containing IV fluid.

■ Before injecting any IV medication, be sure the IV line is open and functioning properly (e.g., catheter not clotted, IV fluid not leaking into surrounding tissues, phlebitis not present). If leakage occurs, some drugs are very irritating to subcutaneous tissues and may cause tissue necrosis.

■ Maintain sterility of all IV fluids, tubings, injection sites, drug solutions, and equipment coming into contact with the IV system. Because medications and fluids are injected directly into the bloodstream, breaks in sterile technique can lead to serious systemic infection (septicemia) and death.

■ When two or more medications are to be given one after the other, flush the IV tubing and catheter (with the infusing IV fluid or with sterile 0.9% sodium chloride injection) so that the drugs do not come into contact with each other.

■ In general, administer slowly to allow greater dilution of the drug in the bloodstream. Most drugs given by IV push (direct injection) can be given over 2–5 minutes and most drugs diluted in 50–100 mL of IV fluid can be infused in 30–60 minutes.

■ When injecting or infusing medications into IV solutions that contain other additives (e.g., vitamins, insulin, minerals such as potassium or magnesium), be sure the medications are compatible with the other substances. Consult compatibility charts (usually available on nursing units) or pharmacists when indicated.

■ IV flow rates are usually calculated in mL/hour and drops per minute.

Many injectable drugs (e.g., morphine, heparin) are available in prefilled syringes with attached needles. These units are inserted into specially designed holders and used like other needle–syringe units. *Note that many such units, especially those from the same manufacturer, are similar and their use may lead to medication errors if the label is not read carefully.*

Equipment for Injections

Sterile needles and syringes are used to measure and administer parenteral medications; they may be packaged together or separately. Needles are available in various gauges and lengths. The term *gauge* refers to lumen size, with larger numbers indicating smaller lumen sizes. For example, a 25-gauge needle is smaller than an 18-gauge needle. Choice of needle gauge and length depends on the route of administration, the viscosity (thickness) of the solution to be given, and the size of the patient. Usually, a 25-gauge, 5/8- inch needle is used for Sub-Q injections and a 22- or 20-gauge, 1 1/2-inch needle is used for IM injections. Other needle sizes are available for special uses, such as for insulin or intradermal injections. When needles are used, avoid recapping them and dispose of them in appropriate containers. Such containers are designed to prevent accidental needle-stick injuries to health care and housekeeping personnel.

In many settings, needleless systems are used. These systems involve a plastic tip on the syringe that can be used to enter vials and injection sites on IV tubing. Openings created by the tip reseal themselves. Needleless systems were developed because of the risk of injury and spread of bloodborne pathogens, such as the viruses that cause acquired immunodeficiency syndrome and hepatitis B.

Syringes also are available in various sizes. The 3-milliliter size is often used. It is usually plastic and is available with or without an attached needle. Syringes are calibrated so that drug doses can be measured accurately. However, the calibrations vary according to the size and type of syringe.

Insulin and tuberculin syringes are used for specific purposes. Insulin syringes are calibrated to measure up to 100 units of insulin. Safe practice requires that *only* insulin syringes be used to measure insulin and that they be used for no other drugs. Tuberculin syringes have a capacity of 1 milliliter. They should be used for small doses of any drug because measurements are more accurate than with larger syringes.

Sites for Injections

Common sites for Sub-Q injections are the upper arms, abdomen, back, and thighs (Fig. 3-1). Sites for IM injections are the deltoid, dorsogluteal, ventrogluteal, and vastus lateralis muscles. These sites must be selected by first identifying anatomic landmarks (Fig. 3-2). Common sites for IV injections are the veins on the back of the hands and on the forearms (Fig. 3-3). Less common sites include intradermal (into layers of the skin), intra-arterial (into arteries), intra-articular (into joints), and intrathecal (into spinal fluid). Nurses may perform intradermal and intra-arterial injections (if an established arterial line is present); physicians perform intra-articular and intrathecal injections.

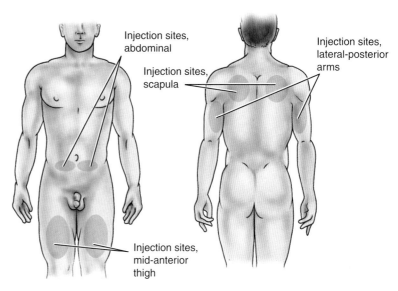

Figure 3-1 ■ Subcutaneous injection sites.

Figure 3-2 ■ Anatomic landmarks and intramuscular (IM) injection sites: (A) ventrogluteal muscle, (B) deltoid muscle, (C) vastus lateralis and rectus femoris muscle, and (D) dorsogluteal muscle.

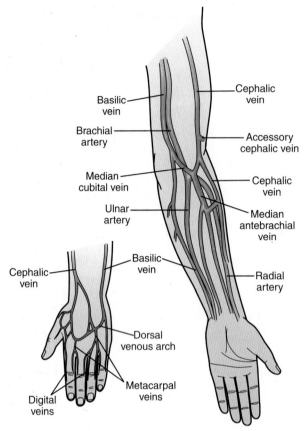

Figure 3-3 ■ Veins of the hand and forearm that may be used to administer intravenous fluids and medications.

Nursing Actions | Drug Administration

NURSING ACTIONS	RATIONALE/EXPLANATION
1. Follow general rules for administering medications safely and effectively.	
a. Prepare and give drugs in well-lighted areas, as free of interruptions and distractions as possible.	To prevent errors in selecting ordered drugs, calculating dosages, and identifying patients
b. Perform hand hygiene before preparing medications and, if needed, during administration.	To prevent infection and cross-contamination
c. Use sterile technique in preparing and administering injections.	To prevent infection. Sterile technique involves using sterile needles, syringes, drug solutions, and cleansing injection sites with an antiseptic.
d. Read the medication administration record (MAR) carefully. Read the label on the drug container, and compare with the MAR in terms of drug, dosage or concentration, and route of administration. Scan bar codes, if available.	For accurate drug administration. Most nursing texts instruct the nurse to read a drug label three times: when removing the container, while measuring the dose, and before returning the container.
e. Do not leave medications unattended.	To prevent ingestion by anyone other than the intended person and to prevent contamination or spilling of medications.
f. Identify the patient by comparing the identification wristband to the medication sheet. Scan barcodes if available.	This is the best way to verify identity. Calling by name, relying on the name on a door or bed, and asking someone else are unreliable methods, although they must be used occasionally when the patient lacks a name band.
g. Identify yourself, if indicated, and state your reason for approaching the patient. For example, "I'm ... I have your medication for you."	Explaining actions helps to decrease patient anxiety and increase cooperation in taking prescribed medication.

NURSING ACTIONS	RATIONALE/EXPLANATION
h. Position the patient appropriately for the intended route of administration.	To prevent complications, such as aspiration of oral drugs into the lungs
i. Provide water or other supplies as needed.	To promote comfort of the patient and to ensure drug administration
j. Do not leave medications at the bedside as a general rule. Common exceptions are nitroglycerin tablets and eye medications.	To prevent omitting or losing the drug or hoarding of the drug by the patient
k. Do not give a drug when signs and symptoms of toxicity are present. Notify the prescriber, and record that the drug was omitted and why.	Additional doses of a drug increase toxicity. However, drugs are not omitted without a careful assessment of the patient's condition and a valid reason.
l. Record drug administration (or omission) as soon as possible and according to agency policies.	To maintain an accurate record of drugs received by the patient
m. Evaluate whether missed scheduled doses should be given at a later time or omitted. Generally, give drugs ordered once or twice daily at a later time. For others, omit the one dose, and give the drug at the next scheduled time.	Patients may be unable to take the drug at the scheduled time because of diagnostic tests or many other reasons. A temporary change in the time of administration—usually for one dose only—may be necessary to maintain therapeutic effects.
n. For medications ordered as needed (PRN), assess the patient's condition; check the physician's orders or MAR for the name, dose, and frequency of administration; and determine the time of the most recently administered dose.	Administration of PRN medications requires nursing assessment and decision making. Analgesics, antiemetics, and antipyretics are often ordered PRN.
o. For narcotics and other controlled substances, sign drugs out on separate narcotic records according to agency policies.	To meet legal requirements for dispensing controlled substances
p. If, at any time during drug preparation or administration, any question arises regarding the drug, the dose, or whether the patient is supposed to receive it, check the original prescriber's order. If the order is not clear, call the prescriber for clarification before giving the drug.	To promote safety and prevent errors. The same procedure applies when the patient questions drug orders at the bedside. For example, the patient may state he has been receiving different drugs or different doses.
2. For oral medications:	
a. With adults	
(1) To give tablets or capsules, open the unit-dose wrapper, place medication in a medicine cup, and give the cup to the patient. For solutions, hold the cup at eye level, and measure the dosage at the bottom of the meniscus. For suspensions, shake or invert containers to mix the medication before measuring the dose.	To maintain clean technique and measure doses accurately. Suspensions settle on standing, and if not mixed, diluent may be given rather than the active drug.
(2) Have the patient in a sitting position when not contraindicated.	To decrease risks of aspirating medication into lungs. Aspiration may lead to difficulty in breathing and aspiration pneumonia.
(3) Give before, with, or after meals as indicated by the specific drug.	Food in the stomach usually delays drug absorption and action. It also decreases gastric irritation, a common side effect of oral drugs.
(4) Give most oral drugs with a full glass (8 oz) of water or other fluid.	To promote dissolution and absorption of tablets and capsules. Also, to decrease gastric irritation by diluting drug concentration.
b. With young children, liquids or chewable tablets are usually given.	Children under 5 years of age are often unable to swallow tablets or capsules.
(1) Measure and give liquids to infants with a dropper or syringe, placing medication on the tongue or buccal mucosa and giving slowly.	For accurate measurement and administration. Giving slowly decreases risks of aspiration.
(2) Medications are often mixed with juice, applesauce, or other vehicle.	To increase the child's ability and willingness to take the medication. If this is done, use a small amount, and be sure the child takes all of it.
c. Do not give oral drugs if the patient is:	
(1) NPO (receiving nothing by mouth)	Oral drugs and fluids may interfere with diagnostic tests or be otherwise contraindicated. Most drugs can be given after diagnostic tests are completed. If the patient is having surgery, preoperative drug orders are cancelled. New orders are written postoperatively.
(2) Vomiting	Oral drugs and fluids increase vomiting. Fluid and electrolyte problems may result from loss of gastric acid.
(3) Excessively sedated or unconscious	To avoid aspiration of drugs into the lungs

(continued on page 44)

Nursing Actions · Drug Administration (continued)

NURSING ACTIONS	RATIONALE/EXPLANATION
3. For medications given by nasogastric or gastrostomy tube: a. Use a liquid preparation when possible. If necessary, crush a tablet or empty a capsule into about 30 mL of water and mix well. Do not crush enteric-coated or sustained-release products, and do not empty sustained-release capsules.	Particles of tablets or powders from capsules may obstruct the tube lumen. Altering sustained-release products increases risks of overdosage and adverse effects.
b. Use a clean bulb syringe or other catheter-tipped syringe.	The syringe allows aspiration and serves as a funnel for instillation of medication and fluids into the stomach. To be sure the tube is in the stomach
c. Before instilling medication, aspirate gastric fluid and check pH or use another method to check tube placement.	
d. Rinse the tube, instill medication by gravity flow, and rinse the tube again with at least 50 mL of water. Do not allow the syringe to empty completely between additions.	Gravity flow is safer than applying pressure. Water "pushes" the drug into the stomach and rinses the tube, thereby maintaining tube patency. Additional water or other fluids may be given according to fluid needs of the patient. Add fluids to avoid instilling air into the stomach unnecessarily.
e. Clamp off the tube from suction or drainage for at least 30 minutes.	To avoid removing the medication from the stomach
4. For subcutaneous (Sub-Q) injections: a. Use only sterile drug preparations labeled or commonly used for Sub-Q injections.	Many parenteral drugs are too irritating to subcutaneous tissue for use by this route.
b. Use a 25-gauge, ⅝-inch needle for most Sub-Q injections.	This size needle is effective for most patients and drugs.
c. Select an appropriate injection site, based on patient preferences, drug characteristics, and visual inspection of possible sites. In long-term therapy, such as with insulin, rotate injection sites. Avoid areas with lumps, bruises, or other lesions.	These techniques allow the patient to participate in his or her care; avoid tissue damage and unpredictable absorption, which occur with repeated injections in the same location; and increase patient comfort and cooperation
d. Cleanse the site with an alcohol sponge.	To prevent infection
e. Tighten the skin or pinch a fold of skin and tissue between thumb and fingers.	Either is acceptable for most patients. If the patient is obese, tightening the skin may be easier. If the patient is very thin, the tissue fold may keep the needle from hitting bone.
f. Hold the syringe like a pencil, and insert the needle quickly at a 45- or 90-degree angle. Use enough force to penetrate the skin and subcutaneous tissue in one smooth movement.	To give the drug correctly with minimal patient discomfort
g. Release the skin so that both hands are free to manipulate the syringe. Pull back gently on the plunger (aspirate). If no blood enters the syringe, inject the drug. If blood is aspirated into the syringe, remove the needle, and reprepare the medication.	To prevent accidental injection into the bloodstream. Blood return in the syringe is an uncommon occurrence. Aspiration is not recommended with heparin injections and possibly not needed with insulin injections.
h. Remove the needle quickly and apply gentle pressure for a few seconds.	To prevent bleeding
5. For intramuscular (IM) injections: a. Use only drug preparations labeled or commonly used for IM injections. Check label instructions for mixing drugs in powder form.	Some parenteral drug preparations cannot be given safely by the IM route.
b. Use a 1½-inch needle for most adults and a ⅝- to 1½-inch needle for children, depending on the size of the patient.	A long needle is necessary to reach muscle tissue, which underlies subcutaneous fat.
c. Use the smallest-gauge needle that will accommodate the medication. A 22-gauge is satisfactory for most drugs; a 20-gauge may be used for viscous medications.	To decrease tissue damage and patient discomfort
d. Select an appropriate injection site, based on patient preferences, drug characteristics, anatomic landmarks, and visual inspection of possible sites. Rotate sites if frequent injections are being given, and avoid areas with lumps, bruises, or other lesions.	To increase patient comfort and participation and to avoid tissue damage. Identification of anatomic landmarks is mandatory for safe administration of IM drugs.

NURSING ACTIONS	RATIONALE/EXPLANATION
e. Cleanse the site with an alcohol sponge.	To prevent infection
f. Tighten the skin, hold the syringe like a pencil, and insert the needle quickly at a 90-degree angle. Use enough force to penetrate the skin and subcutaneous tissue into the muscle in one smooth motion.	To give the drug correctly with minimal patient discomfort
g. Aspirate (see 4g, Sub-Q injections).	
h. Remove the needle quickly and apply pressure for several seconds.	To prevent bleeding

6. For intravenous (IV) injections:

a. Use only drug preparations that are labeled for IV use.	Others are not pure enough for safe injection into the bloodstream or are not compatible with the blood pH (7.35–7.45).
b. Check label instructions for the type and amount of fluid to use for dissolving or diluting the drug.	Some drugs require special preparation techniques to maintain solubility or pharmacologic activity. Most drugs in powder form can be dissolved in sterile water or sodium chloride for injection. Most drug solutions can be given with dextrose or dextrose and sodium chloride IV solutions.
c. Prepare drugs just before use, as a general rule. Also, add drugs to IV fluids just before use.	Some drugs are unstable in solution. In most agencies, drugs are mixed and added to IV fluids in the pharmacy. This is the preferred method because sterility can be better maintained.
d. For venipuncture and direct injection into a vein, apply a tourniquet, select a site in the arm, cleanse the skin with an antiseptic (e.g., povidone-iodine or alcohol), insert the needle, and aspirate a small amount of blood into the syringe to be sure that the needle is in the vein. Remove the tourniquet, and inject the drug slowly. Remove the needle and apply pressure until there is no evidence of bleeding.	For safe and accurate drug administration with minimal risk to the patient. The length of time required to give the drug depends on the specific drug and the amount. Slow administration, over several minutes, allows immediate discontinuation if adverse effects occur.
e. For administration by an established IV line:	
(1) Check the infusion for patency and flow rate. Check the venipuncture site for signs of infiltration and phlebitis before each drug dose.	The solution must be flowing freely for accurate drug administration. If infiltration or phlebitis is present, do not give the drug until a new IV line is begun.
(2) For direct injection, cleanse an injection site on the IV tubing, insert the needle, and inject the drug slowly.	Most tubings have injection sites to facilitate drug administration.
(3) To use a volume-control set, fill it with 50–100 mL of IV fluid, and clamp it so that no further fluid enters the chamber and dilutes the drug. Inject the drug into an injection site after cleansing the site with an alcohol sponge and infuse, usually in 1 hour or less. After the drug is infused, add solution to maintain the infusion.	This method is used for administration of antibiotics on an intermittent schedule. Dilution of the drug decreases adverse effects.
(4) To use a "piggyback" method, add the drug to 50–100 mL of IV solution in a separate container. Attach the IV tubing and a needle. Insert the needle in an injection site on the main IV tubing after cleansing the site. Infuse the drug over 15–60 minutes, depending on the drug.	This method is also used for intermittent administration of antibiotics and other drugs. Whether a volume-control or piggyback apparatus is used depends on agency policy and equipment available.
f. When more than one drug is to be given, flush the line between drugs. Do not mix drugs in syringes or in IV fluids unless the drug literature states that the drugs are compatible.	Physical and chemical interactions between the drugs may occur and cause precipitation, inactivation, or increased toxicity. Most nursing units have charts depicting drug compatibility, or information may be obtained from the pharmacy.

7. For application to skin:

a. Use drug preparations labeled for dermatologic use. Cleanse the skin, remove any previously applied medication, and apply the drug in a thin layer. For broken skin or open lesions, use sterile gloves, tongue blade, or cotton-tipped applicator to apply the drug.	To promote therapeutic effects and minimize adverse effects

(continued on page 46)

Nursing Actions — Drug Administration (continued)

NURSING ACTIONS	RATIONALE/EXPLANATION
8. For instillation of eye drops: a. Use drug preparations labeled for ophthalmic use. Wash hands, open the eye to expose the conjunctival sac, and drop the medication into the sac, without touching the dropper tip to anything. Provide a tissue for blotting any excess drug. If two or more eye drops are scheduled at the same time, wait 1–5 minutes between instillations. With children, prepare the medication, place the child in a head-lowered position, steady the hand holding the medication on the child's head, gently retract the lower lid, and instill the medication into the conjunctival sac.	Ophthalmic preparations must be sterile to avoid infection. Blot any excess drug from the inner canthus near the nose to decrease systemic absorption of the drug. Careful positioning and restraint to avoid sudden movements are necessary to decrease risks of injury to the eye.
9. For instillation of nose drops and nasal sprays: a. Have the patient hold his or her head back, and drop the medication into the nostrils. Give only as ordered With children, place in a supine position with the head lowered, instill the medication, and maintain the position for 2–3 minutes. Then, place the child in a prone position.	When nose drops are used for rhinitis and nasal congestion accompanying the common cold, overuse results in a rebound congestion that may be worse than the original symptom.
10. For instillation of ear medications: a. Open the ear canal by pulling the ear up and back for adults, down and back for children, and drop the medication on the side of the canal.	To straighten the canal and promote maximal contact between medication and tissue
11. For rectal suppositories: a. Lubricate the end with a water-soluble lubricant, wear a glove or finger cot, and insert into the rectum the length of the finger. Place the suppository next to the mucosal wall. b. If the patient prefers and is able, provide supplies for self-administration.	To promote absorption. Allowing self-administration may prevent embarrassment to the patient. Be sure the patient knows the correct procedure.
12. For vaginal medications: a. Use gloves or an applicator for insertion. If an applicator is used, wash thoroughly with soap and water after each use. b. If the patient prefers and is able, provide supplies for self-administration.	Some women may be embarrassed and prefer self-administration. Be sure the patient knows the correct procedure.

Key Concepts

◾ The "five rights" of safe and accurate drug administration are right drug, right dose, right patient, right route, and right time.

◾ Basic knowledge and techniques for accurate drug administration include knowledge of the drug, knowledge of the patient, interpretation of prescriber orders and labels of drug containers, calculations and measurements of doses, and correct techniques for all dosage forms and routes of administration.

◾ Each health care facility has a system for distributing drugs; each nurse in an agency must follow legal and agency policies related to drug administration.

◾ When dosage calculations are required, they *must* be accurate to avoid medication errors and harm to patients.

◾ Question and clarify any unclear drug orders.

◾ Document medication administration according to agency policies.

◾ Identify potential sources of medication errors and intervene to prevent errors when possible.

Review and Application Exercises

Short Answer Exercises

1. When giving an oral medication, what are some interventions to aid absorption and hasten therapeutic effects?

2. What are the advantages and disadvantages of the PO route and the IV route of drug administration?

3. For a patient who receives all medications through a nasogastric feeding tube, which dosage forms are acceptable? Which are unacceptable, and why?

4. What are some legal factors that influence a nurse's administration of medications?

5. When administering medications, what safety precautions are needed with various routes?

6. What safety precautions must the nurse practice consistently to avoid self-injury and exposure to bloodborne pathogens?

7. With a patient who refuses an important medication, what approaches or interventions might persuade the patient to take the medication? Would the same approach be indicated if the medication were a vitamin supplement or a laxative?

NCLEX-Style Questions

8. An important safety measure in drug administration is
   a. calling the patient by name
   b. using appropriate techniques for the ordered route of administration
   c. asking a coworker about an ordered drug
   d. leaving medications at the bedside

9. You are caring for a patient who has been taking his medications with only a small sip of water. You counsel him to drink an 8-oz glass of water with his tablets or capsules, because you know that it aids in which of the following pharmacokinetic processes?
   a. absorption
   b. distribution
   c. biotransformation
   d. excretion

10. When administering medications by nasogastric tube, which of the following nursing actions is indicated?
    a. Verify the position of the tube before giving the drugs.
    b. Aspirate and discard stomach contents.
    c. Mix medications with tube-feeding formulas.
    d. Have the patient sit in a chair.

11. Maintaining sterile technique is necessary while administering which of the following types of medication?
    a. oral suspensions
    b. vaginal suppositories
    c. nasal inhalation products
    d. injections

12. Anatomic landmarks are very important in which of the following routes of drug administration?
    a. oral
    b. inhalation
    c. intramuscular
    d. topical (to skin)

Selected References

Berwick, D. M., Calkins, D. R., McCannot, C. J., & Hackbarth, A. D. (2006). The 100 000 lives campaign: Setting a goal and a deadline for improving health care quality. *Journal of the American Medical Association, 295*, 324–327.

Blank, D. (2006). Bedside bar-coding still lagging in hospitals. *Drug Topics*, May 22, p. 12.

Bootman, J. L., & Cronenwett, L. R. (2007). Medication errors: Prevention strategies. In *Preventing medication errors* (pp. 409–440). Washington, DC: Institute of Medicine, National Academies Press.

Drug facts and comparisons. (Updated monthly). St. Louis, MO: Facts and Comparisons.

Horack, C. L., & Taylor, R. M. (2006). Medication reconciliation: Keeping our patients safe. *Nursing 2006 Critical Care, 1*, 26–33.

Hughes, R. G., & Edgerton, E. A. (2005). Reducing pediatric medication errors. *American Journal of Nursing, 105*, 79–90.

Ketchum, K., Grass, C. A., & Padwojski, A. (2005). Medication reconciliation. *American Journal of Nursing, 105*, 78–85.

Kumpf, V. J., & Chessman, K. H. (2005). Enteral nutrition. In J. T. DiPiro, R. L. Talbert, G. C. Yee, G. R. Matzke, B. G. Wells, & L. M. Posey (Eds.), *Pharmacotherapy: A pathophysiologic approach* (6th ed., pp. 2615–2634). New York: McGraw-Hill.

Manno, M. S. (2006). Preventing adverse drug events. *Nursing, 36*, 56–61.

Manno, M. S., & Hayes, D. D. (2006). Best-practice interventions: How medication reconciliation saves lives. *Nursing, 36*, 63–64.

Paparella, S. (2006). Medication reconciliation: Doing what's right for safe patient care. *Journal of Emergency Nursing, 32*, 516–520.

Smeltzer, S. C., Bare, B. G., Hinkle, J. L., & Cheever, K. H. (2008). *Brunner & Suddarth's textbook of medical-surgical nursing* (11th ed.). Philadelphia: Lippincott Williams & Wilkins.

St. Onge, E. L., Dea, M., & Rose, R. L. (2006). Medication errors and strategies to improve patient safety. *Drug Topics*, May 8, 2006, pp. 36–43.

Stucky, E. R. (2003). Prevention of medication errors in the pediatric inpatient setting. *Pediatrics, 112*, 431–436. (Note: This is a clinical practice guideline from the American Academy of Pediatrics, available online at *www.guideline.gov*)

Tuohy, N., & Paparella, S. (2005). Look-alike and sound-alike drugs: Errors just waiting to happen. *Journal of Emergency Nursing, 31*, 569–571.

Nursing Process in Drug Therapy

LEARNING OBJECTIVES

After studying this chapter, you will be able to:

1. Assess patients for conditions and factors that are likely to influence drug effects, including age, weight, health status, and lifestyle.
2. Obtain a medication history about the patient's use of prescription, over-the-counter (OTC), and social drugs as well as herbal and dietary supplements.
3. Identify nondrug interventions to prevent or decrease the need for drug therapy.
4. Discuss interventions to increase therapeutic effects and decrease adverse effects of drug therapy.
5. Discuss guidelines for rational choices of drugs, dosages, routes, and times of administration.
6. Observe patients for therapeutic and adverse responses to drug therapy.
7. Teach patients and family members how to use prescription and OTC drugs safely and effectively.
8. When indicated, teach patients about the potential effects of herbal and dietary supplements.
9. For patients who use herbal and dietary supplements, provide—or assist them in obtaining—reliable information.
10. Describe major considerations in drug therapy for children, adults, and patients with impaired renal or hepatic function or critical illness.
11. Discuss application of the nursing process in home care settings.
12. Apply evidence-based data about patients and therapeutic drugs in all steps of the nursing process.

Applying Your Knowledge

You are making the first home visit for Robert Walker, an 80-year-old patient with arthritis and hypertension. Upon reading his file, you learn that Mr. Walker lives alone but has a daughter who lives in the area. She visits him once a week and runs his errands. You note he is taking the following medications: Ibuprofen 400 mg every 4 hours, furosemide 20 mg once daily, captopril 25 mg twice a day, and famotidine 20 mg at bedtime.

Introduction

Drug therapy involves the use of drugs to prevent or treat disease processes and manifestations. It may save lives, improve the quality of life, and otherwise benefit recipients. It also may cause adverse effects. Adverse effects and failure to achieve therapeutic effects may occur with correct use, but they are more likely to occur with incorrect use. Prescribers (e.g., physicians, dentists, and nurse practitioners), pharmacists, patients, and nurses all have important roles to play in the safe and effective use of drugs.

For most nurses, drug therapy is one of many responsibilities in patient care. To fulfill this responsibility, the nurse must be knowledgeable about pharmacology (drugs and their effects on the body), physiology (normal body functions), and pathophysiology (alterations in mental and physical functions due to disease processes) and must be adept at using all steps of the nursing process.

Chapter 1 included general information about drugs and suggested strategies for studying pharmacology. Chapter 2 described cellular physiology, concepts, and processes essential to understanding drug effects in humans and general management of drug toxicity. Chapter 3 emphasized drug administration. Although the importance of safe and accurate administration cannot be overemphasized, this is only one aspect of the nursing process in drug therapy. The nurse also must monitor patient responses to drug therapy, both therapeutic and adverse, and teach patients about drugs, both prescribed and OTC. To help the nurse continue to acquire knowledge and skills related to drug therapy, this chapter includes nursing process guidelines, general principles of drug therapy, and general nursing actions. Guidelines, principles, and actions related to specific drugs are included in chapters throughout this text.

Nursing Process in Drug Therapy

The nursing process is a systematic way of gathering and using information to plan and provide individualized patient care and to evaluate the outcomes of care. It involves both cognitive and psychomotor skills. Knowledge of, and skill in, the nursing process are required for drug therapy as in other aspects of patient care. The five steps of the nursing process are assessment, nursing diagnosis, planning and establishing goals for nursing care, interventions, and evaluation. Assessment and interventions are "action" phases, whereas analysis of assessment data, establishing nursing diagnoses and goals, and evaluation are "thinking" phases. However, knowledge and informed, rational thinking should underlie all data collection, decision making, and interventions.

Assessment

Assessment involves collecting data about patient characteristics known to affect drug therapy. This includes observing and interviewing the patient, interviewing family members or others involved in patient care, completing a physical assessment, reviewing medical records for pertinent laboratory and diagnostic test reports, and other methods. Initially (before drug therapy is started or on first contact), assess age, weight, vital signs, health status, pathologic conditions, and ability to function in usual activities of daily living. The effects of these patient-related factors on drug therapy are discussed in Chapter 2. In addition, assess for previous and current use of prescription, nonprescription, and nontherapeutic (e.g., alcohol, caffeine, nicotine, cocaine, marijuana) drugs. A *medication history* (Box 4-1) is useful, or the information can be incorporated into any data collection tool. Specific questions and areas of assessment include the following:

■ What are current drug orders?

■ What does the patient know about current drugs? Is teaching needed?

■ What drugs has the patient taken before? Include any drugs taken regularly, such as those for hypertension, diabetes mellitus, or other chronic conditions. Ask patient about over-the-counter drugs for colds, headaches, or indigestion, because some people do not think of these preparations as drugs.

■ Has the patient ever had an allergic reaction to a drug? If so, what signs and symptoms occurred and how were they managed?

■ Is the patient able to communicate verbally; can he or she swallow oral medications?

■ Does the patient have pathologic conditions that influence drug therapy? For example, all seriously ill patients should be assessed for impaired function of vital organs.

■ Assess for current use of herbal or dietary supplements (e.g., echinacea, glucosamine/chondroitin, vitamins). If so, ask for names, how much is taken and how often, for how long, their reason for use, and perceived benefits or adverse effects.

In addition to nursing assessment data, use progress notes (of any other health care providers), laboratory reports, and other sources to obtain baseline data for monitoring therapeutic or adverse drug effects. Laboratory tests of liver, kidney, and bone marrow function are often helpful because some drugs may damage these organs. Also, if liver or kidney damage exists, drug metabolism or excretion may be altered. Consult authoritative sources for information about the patient's disease processes and ordered drugs, if needed.

After assessment data are obtained, they need to be analyzed to determine the patient's nursing care needs. Although listed as the first step in the nursing process for discussion purposes, assessment is a component of all steps and occurs with every contact with the patient. Ongoing assessment of a patient's health status and response to treatment is needed to determine whether nursing care requirements have changed. In general, nurses must provide care based on available information while knowing that assessment data are always relatively incomplete.

Applying Your Knowledge 4-1

Review Mr. Walker's current medication regimen. Look up the medications, and note the drug class for each. Why do you think this patient is taking them? Are the dosages appropriate for an 80-year-old?

Box 4-1	Medication History

Name_____ Age_____
Health problems, acute and chronic
Are you allergic to any medications?
If yes, describe specific effects or symptoms.

Part 1: Prescription Medications
1. Do you take any prescription medications on a regular basis?
2. If yes, ask the following about each medication.

Name	Dose
Frequency	Specific times
How long taken	Reason for use

3. Do you have any difficulty in taking your medicines? If yes, ask to specify problem areas.
4. Have you had any symptoms or problems that you think are caused by your medicines? If yes, ask to specify.
5. Do you need help from another person to take your medicines?
6. Do you take any prescription medications on an irregular basis? If yes, ask the following about each medication.

Name	Dose
Frequency	Reason
How long taken	

Part 2: Nonprescription Medications
Do you take over-the-counter medications?

		Medication		
Problem	Yes/No	Name	Amount	Frequency
Pain				
Headache				
Sleep				
Cold				
Indigestion				
Heartburn				
Diarrhea				
Constipation				
Other				

Part 3: Social Drugs

	Yes/No	Amount/day
Coffee		
Tea		
Cola drinks		
Alcohol		
Tobacco		

Part 4: Herbal or Dietary Supplements

Do you take any herbal or dietary supplements (e.g., gingko, glucosamine/chondroitin,)? If so, ask for names, how much and how often taken, reason for use, perceived effectiveness, any adverse effects.

Nursing Diagnoses

These statements, as developed by the North American Nursing Diagnosis Association, describe patient problems or needs and are based on assessment data. They should be individualized according to the patient's condition and the drugs prescribed. Thus, the nursing diagnoses needed to adequately reflect the patient's condition vary considerably. Because almost any nursing diagnosis may apply in specific circumstances, this text emphasizes those diagnoses that generally apply to drug therapy.

■ Deficient Knowledge: Drug therapy regimen (e.g., drug ordered; reason for use; expected effects; monitoring of response by health care providers, including diagnostic tests and office visits)

- Deficient Knowledge: Safe and effective self-administration (when appropriate)
- Risk for Injury related to adverse drug effects
- Noncompliance: Overuse
- Noncompliance: Underuse

Planning/Goals

This step involves the expected outcomes of prescribed drug therapy. As a general rule, *goals should be stated in terms of patient behavior, not nurse behavior.* For example, the patient will

- Receive or take drugs as prescribed
- Experience relief of signs and symptoms
- Avoid preventable adverse drug effects
- Self-administer drugs safely and accurately
- Verbalize essential drug information
- Keep appointments for monitoring and follow-up
- Use any herbal and dietary supplements with caution and report such use to health care providers

Interventions

This step involves implementing planned activities and includes any task performed directly with a patient or indirectly on a patient's behalf. Areas of intervention are broad and may include assessment, promoting compliance with prescribed drug therapy, and solving problems related to drug therapy, among others.

General interventions related to drug therapy include promoting health, preventing or decreasing the need for drug therapy, using nondrug measures to enhance therapeutic effects or decrease adverse effects, teaching, individualizing care, administering drugs, and observing patient responses. Some examples include

- Promoting healthful lifestyles in terms of nutrition, fluids, exercise, rest, and sleep
- Performing hand hygiene and other measures to prevent infection
- Ambulating, positioning, and exercising
- Assisting to cough and deep breathe
- Applying heat or cold
- Increasing or decreasing sensory stimulation
- Scheduling activities to promote rest or sleep
- Recording vital signs, fluid intake, urine output, and other assessment data

The intervention of teaching patients and caregivers about drug therapy is essential because most medications are self-administered and patients need information and assistance to use therapeutic drugs safely and effectively. Adequate knowledge, skill, and preparation are required to fulfill teaching responsibilities. Teaching aids to assist the nurse in this endeavor include Box 4-2: Preparing to Teach a Patient or Caregiver; Patient Teaching Guidelines: Safe and Effective Use of Prescription Medications; and Patient Teaching Guidelines: Safe and Effective Use of Over-the-Counter (OTC) Medications. Later drug-related chapters contain more specific patient teaching guidelines for the drugs discussed in those particular chapters.

This chapter includes general principles or guidelines; later drug chapters include those related to particular drug groups. Using established guidelines to individualize nursing care can increase one's knowledge base about safe, effective, and rational drug therapy. These interventions, which reflect integration of knowledge about drugs and the patients receiving them, are presented under the heading of "Principles of Therapy."

Interventions, presented as a separate feature entitled "Nursing Actions," provide specific guidelines related to administering drugs accurately, assessing patients for therapeutic and adverse effects, and observing for drug interactions. Rationales for the interventions are included. This chapter includes general interventions or actions; later drug chapters include those related to particular drug groups.

Evaluation

This step involves evaluating the patient's status in relation to stated goals and expected outcomes. Some outcomes can be evaluated within a few minutes of drug administration (e.g., relief of acute pain after administration of an analgesic), but most require longer periods of time. Over time, the patient is likely to experience brief contacts with many health care providers, which increases the difficulty of evaluating outcomes of drug therapy. However, difficulties can be managed by using appropriate techniques and criteria of evaluation.

General techniques include directly observing the patient's status; interviewing the patient or others about the patient's response to drug therapy; and checking appropriate medical records, including medication records and diagnostic test reports.

General criteria include progress toward stated outcomes, such as relief of symptoms, accurate administration, avoidance of preventable adverse effects, and compliance with instructions for follow-up monitoring by a health care provider. Specific criteria indicate the parameters that must be measured to evaluate responses to particular drugs (e.g., blood sugar with antidiabetic drugs, blood pressure with antihypertensive drugs).

Applying Your Knowledge 4-2

Consider the case of Mr. Walker. When you look at his medication assessment, can you identify possible nursing diagnoses?

Box 4-2	Preparing to Teach a Patient or Caregiver

- Assess learning needs, especially when new drugs are added or new conditions are being treated. This includes finding out what the person already knows about a particular drug. Do not assume that teaching is unneeded, even if the patient has been taking a drug for a while.
- Assess ability to manage a drug therapy regimen (i.e., read printed instructions and drug labels, remember dosage schedules, self-administer medications by ordered routes). A medication history (see Box 4-1) helps to assess the patient's knowledge about drug therapy.
- From assessment data, develop an individualized teaching plan. This saves time for both nurse and patient by avoiding repetition of known material. It also promotes compliance with prescribed drug therapy.
- Try to decrease anxiety. Patients and caregivers may feel overwhelmed by complicated medication regimens. Provide positive reinforcement for effort.
- Choose an appropriate time (e.g., when the patient is mentally alert and not in acute distress from pain or other symptoms) and a place with minimal noise and distractions, when possible.
- Proceed slowly, in small steps; emphasize essential information; and provide opportunities to express concerns or ask questions.
- Provide a combination of verbal and written instructions, which is more effective than either alone. Minimize medical jargon and be aware that patients may have difficulty understanding and retaining the material being taught because of the stress of the illness.
- When explaining a drug to a hospitalized patient, describe the name (preferably both the generic and a trade name), purpose, expected effects, and so on. The purpose can usually be stated in terms of symptoms to be relieved or other expected benefits. In many instances, the drug is familiar

and can be described from personal knowledge. If the drug is unfamiliar, use available resources (e.g., drug reference books, computer drug databases, pharmacists) to learn about the drug and provide accurate information to the patient.
- When teaching a patient about medications to be taken at home, provide specific information and instructions about each drug, including how to take them and how to observe for beneficial and adverse effects. If adverse effects occur, teach them how to manage minor ones and which ones to report to a health care provider. In addition, discuss ways to develop a convenient routine for taking medications, so that usual activities of daily living are minimally disrupted. Allow time for questions and try to ensure that the patient understands how, when, and why to take the medications.
- When teaching a patient about potential adverse drug effects, the goal is to provide needed information without causing unnecessary anxiety. Most drugs produce undesirable effects; some are minor, some are potentially serious. Many people stop taking a drug rather than report adverse reactions. If reactions are reported, it may be possible to continue the drug by reducing dosage, changing the time of administration, or other measures. If severe reactions occur, the drug should be stopped and the prescriber should be notified.
- Emphasize the importance of taking medications as prescribed throughout the teaching session and perhaps at times of other contacts. Common patient errors include taking incorrect doses, taking doses at the wrong times, omitting doses, and stopping a medication too soon. Treatment failure can often be directly traced to these errors.
- Reassess learning needs when medication orders are changed (e.g., when medications are added because of a new illness or stopped).

Patient Teaching Guidelines	Safe and Effective Use of Prescription Medications

General Considerations

- Use drugs cautiously and only when necessary because all drugs affect body functions and may cause adverse effects.
- Use nondrug measures, when possible, to prevent the need for drug therapy or to enhance beneficial effects and decrease adverse effects of drugs.
- Do not take drugs left over from a previous illness or prescribed for someone else, and do not share prescription drugs with anyone else. The likelihood of having the right drug in the right dose is remote, and the risk of adverse effects is high in such circumstances.
- Keep all health care providers informed about all the drugs being taken, including over-the-counter (OTC) products and herbal or dietary supplements.

- Take drugs as prescribed and for the length of time prescribed; notify a health care provider if unable to take a medication. Therapeutic effects greatly depend on taking medications correctly. Altering the dose or time may cause underdosage or overdosage. Stopping a medication may cause a recurrence of the problem for which it was given or withdrawal symptoms. Some medications need to be tapered in dosage and gradually discontinued. If problems occur with taking a drug, report them to a health care provider. An adjustment in dosage or other aspect of administration may solve the problem.
- Follow instructions for follow-up care (e.g., office visits, laboratory or other diagnostic tests that monitor therapeutic or adverse effects of drugs). Some drugs require more frequent monitoring than others. However, safety requires

periodic checks with essentially all medications. With long-term use of a medication, responses may change over time with aging, changes in kidney function, and so on.

- Take drugs in current use (or an up-to-date list) to appointments with a health care provider.
- Get all prescriptions filled at the same pharmacy, when possible. This is an important safety factor in helping to avoid multiple prescriptions of the same or similar drugs and to minimize undesirable interactions of newly prescribed drugs with those already in use.
- Report any drug allergies to all health care providers, and wear a medical identification emblem that lists allergens.
- Ask questions (and write down the answers) about newly prescribed medications, such as:
  - What is the medicine's name?
  - What is it supposed to do (i.e., what symptoms or problems will it relieve)?
  - How and when do I take it, and for how long?
  - Should it be taken with food or on an empty stomach?
- While taking this medicine, should I avoid certain foods, beverages, other medications, certain activities? (For example, alcoholic beverages and driving a car should be avoided with medications that cause drowsiness or decrease alertness.)
  - What side effects are likely and what do I do if they occur?
  - Will the medication affect my ability to sleep or work?
  - What should I do if I miss a dose?
  - Is there a drug information sheet I can have?
- Store medications out of reach of children and, to prevent accidental ingestion, never refer to medications as "candy."
- When taking prescription medications, talk to a doctor, pharmacist, or nurse before starting an OTC medication or herbal or dietary supplement. This is a safety factor to avoid undesirable drug interactions.
- Inform health care providers if you have diabetes or kidney or liver disease. These conditions require special precautions with drug therapy.
- If pregnant, consult your obstetrician before taking any medications prescribed by another physician.
- If breast-feeding, consult your obstetrician or pediatrician before taking any medications prescribed by another health care provider.

Self-Administration

- Develop a routine for taking medications (e.g., at the same time and place each day). A schedule that minimally disrupts usual activities is more convenient and more likely to be followed accurately.

- Take medications in a well-lighted area and read labels of containers to ensure taking the intended drug. Do not take medications if you are not alert or cannot see clearly.
- Most tablets and capsules should be taken whole. If unable to take them whole, ask a health care provider before splitting, chewing, or crushing tablets or taking the medication out of capsules. Some long-acting preparations are dangerous if altered so that the entire dose is absorbed at the same time.
- As a general rule, take oral medications with 6–8 oz of water, in a sitting or standing position. The water helps tablets and capsules dissolve in the stomach, "dilutes" the drug so that it is less likely to upset the stomach, and promotes absorption of the drug into the bloodstream.
- Take most oral drugs at evenly spaced intervals around the clock. For example, if ordered once daily, take about the same time every day. If ordered twice daily or morning and evening, take about 12 hours apart.
- Follow instructions about taking a medication with food, on an empty stomach, or with other medications.
- If a dose is missed, most authorities recommend taking the dose if remembered soon after the scheduled time and omitting the dose if it is not remembered for several hours. If a dose is omitted, the next dose should be taken at the next scheduled time. Do not double the dose.
- If taking a liquid medication (or giving one to a child), measure with a calibrated medication cup or measuring spoon. A dose cannot be measured accurately with household teaspoons or tablespoons because they are different sizes and deliver varying amounts of medication. If the liquid medication is packaged with a measuring cup that shows teaspoons or tablespoons, that should be used to measure doses, for adults or children.
- Use oral or nasal inhalers, eye drops, and skin medications according to instructions. If not clear how a medication is to be used, be sure to ask a health care provider. Correct use is essential for therapeutic effects.
- Report problems or new symptoms to a health care provider.
- Store medications safely, in a cool, dry place. Do not store them in a bathroom; heat, light, and moisture may cause them to decompose. Do not store them near a dangerous substance, which could be taken by mistake. Keep medications in the container in which they were dispensed by the pharmacy, where the label identifies it and gives directions. Do not mix different medications in a single container.
- Discard outdated medications; do not keep drugs for long periods. Drugs are chemicals that may deteriorate over time, especially if exposed to heat and moisture.

Patient Teaching Guidelines — Safe and Effective Use of Over-the-Counter (OTC) Medications

- Read product labels carefully. The labels contain essential information about the name, ingredients, indications for use, usual dosage, when to stop using the medication or when to see a health care provider, possible adverse effects, and expiration dates.
- Use a magnifying glass, if necessary, to read the fine print. If you do not understand the information on labels, ask a physician, pharmacist, or nurse.
- Do not take OTC medications longer or in higher doses than recommended.
- Note that all OTC medications are not safe for everyone. Many OTC medications warn against use with certain illnesses (e.g., hypertension). Consult a health care provider before taking the product if you have a contraindicated condition. If taking any prescription medications, consult a health care provider before taking any OTC drugs to avoid undesirable drug interactions and adverse effects. Some specific precautions include the following:
  - Avoid alcohol if taking sedating antihistamines, cough or cold remedies containing dextromethorphan, or sleeping pills. Because all these drugs cause drowsiness alone, combining any of them with alcohol may result in excessive and potentially dangerous sedation.
  - Avoid OTC sleeping aids if you are taking a prescription sedative-type drug (e.g., for anxiety or nervousness).
  - Ask a health care provider before taking products containing aspirin if you are taking an anticoagulant (e.g., Coumadin).
  - Ask a health care provider before taking other products containing aspirin if you are already taking a regular dose of aspirin to prevent blood clots, heart attack, or

stroke. Aspirin is commonly used for this purpose, often in doses of 81 mg (a child's dose) or 325 mg.
  - Do not take a laxative if you have stomach pain, nausea, or vomiting, to avoid worsening the problem.
  - Do not take a nasal decongestant (e.g., Sudafed), a multisymptom cold remedy containing phenylephrine products, i.e., formulated to remove pseudoephedrine (e.g., Actifed), or an antihistamine-decongestant combination (e.g., Claritin D) if you are taking a prescription medication for high blood pressure. Such products can raise blood pressure and decrease or cancel the blood pressure–lowering effect of the prescription drug. This could lead to severe hypertension and stroke.
- Store OTC drugs in a cool, dry place, in their original containers; check expiration dates periodically and discard those that have expired.
- If pregnant, consult your obstetrician before taking any OTC medications.
- If breast-feeding, consult your pediatrician or family doctor before taking any OTC medications.
- For children, follow any age limits on the label.
- Measure liquid OTC medications with the measuring device that comes with the product (some have a dropper or plastic cup calibrated in milliliters, teaspoons, or tablespoons). If such a device is not available, use a measuring spoon. It is not safe to use household teaspoons or tablespoons because they are different sizes and deliver varying amounts of medication.
- Do not assume continued safety of an OTC medication you have taken for years. Older people are more likely to have adverse drug reactions and interactions because of changes in the heart, kidneys, and other organs that occur with aging and various disease processes.

Integrating Clinical Pathways with Nursing Process

Within a health care agency, nursing responsibilities related to drug therapy may be designated in *clinical pathways*, which are guidelines for the care of patients with particular conditions. Major components include a medical diagnosis, aspects of care related to the medical diagnosis, desired patient outcomes, and time frames (usually days) for achieving the desired outcomes during the expected length of stay.

Medical diagnoses for which clinical pathways are developed are those often encountered in an agency and those that often result in complications or prolonged lengths of stay (e.g., patients having coronary artery bypass grafts or myocardial infarction). Development and implementation of the clinical pathways should be an interdisciplinary, collaborative effort. Thus, all health care professionals involved in the care of a patient should be represented. For patients, a comprehensive pathway extending from illness onset through treatment and recovery could promote continuity of care among agencies and health care providers. In hospital settings, case managers, who

may be non-nurses, usually assess patients' conditions daily to evaluate progress toward the desired outcomes.

Depending on the medical diagnoses, many clinical pathways have specific guidelines related to drug therapy. These guidelines may include any step of the nursing process. With assessment, for example, the clinical pathway may state, "Assess for bleeding if on anticoagulant."

Integrating Evidence-Based Practice with Nursing Process

Evidence-based nursing practice requires a conscientious and continuing effort to provide high-quality care to patients by obtaining and analyzing the best available scientific evidence from research. Then, the scientific evidence is integrated with the nurse's clinical expertise and the patient's preferences and values to yield "best practices" for a patient with a particular disease process or health problem. Evidence-based practice is further described below, and selected elements are described in Box 4-3.

Evidence-based practice (EBP) may include any step of the nursing process, and it does not accept tradition or "that's the way we've always done it" as sufficient rationale for any aspect of nursing care. Requirements for implementing evidence-based practice include

- Using research. Although professional nurses have always been encouraged to use research, EBP structures and formalizes the process. The nurse must use computer skills to search for the best evidence in making decisions about patient care. The search needs to be systematic; obtained data need to be critically analyzed for quality and relevance to the clinical situation.

- Keeping up-to-date in regard to research studies related to one's area of clinical practice. This includes reading research reports and analyzing them to determine their applicability.

- Considering levels of evidence to support clinical decision making. Level A is the strongest level.

- Interpreting research evidence in relation to one's clinical expertise and patient choices to provide a scientific rationale for one's clinical decisions.

- Applying the available information to improve nursing care of an individual or group of patients.

- Evaluating the effectiveness of application—did the intervention improve the patient's condition?

In this text, EBP is presented in boxed features in some chapters and in various sections of some chapters. An example is the use of a particular drug or drugs to treat certain health problems. Although most nurses do not prescribe and therefore do not choose a patient's drug therapy regimen, it is still important for a nurse to know why a drug is used. This knowledge helps in monitoring patients' responses and in teaching patients and may help patients adhere to the prescribed regimen.

Herbal and Dietary Supplements

Herbal and dietary supplements are commonly used, and patients who take them are likely to be encountered in any clinical practice setting. Herbal medicines, also called *botanicals*,

---

| Box 4-3 | Selected Elements of Evidence-based Practice |

Types of Research Studies (Evidence)

Meta-analysis involves a rigorous process of analyzing, comparing, and summarizing multiple studies (e.g., well-designed randomized controlled trials, if available) on a particular topic and combining the results statistically as if they were from one large study.

Systematic reviews usually focus on a clinical topic and answer a specific question. An extensive literature search is conducted to identify all studies with well-designed methodology. The studies are analyzed, critically evaluated, and summarized according to predetermined criteria. For a systematic review, experts follow a rigorous and well-defined process to identify, critically evaluate, synthesize, and summarize the evidence on a particular topic. (The *Cochrane Database of Systematic Reviews* is a highly-respected source of systematic reviews).

Randomized controlled trials (RCTs) study the effect of a treatment (e.g., a drug) on real patients. Such studies include randomizing (a hallmark of high quality research) and blinding (so that neither researcher nor patient knows who is receiving the treatment or intervention) to reduce the likelihood of biasing the results. They also allow comparison between intervention groups and control groups (no intervention). Because RCTs with a large numbers of subjects produce more reliable results than smaller studies, many RCTs are conducted at multiple clinical sites and in multiple countries.

Cohort studies involve large groups of patients who have a specific condition or who receive a particular treatment. These patients are compared with another group who does not have

the condition or does not receive the treatment being studied. Cohort studies are observational and not as reliable as RCTs.

Case control studies compare patients with a specific condition to people who do not have the condition. They are less reliable than RCTs and cohort studies because they collect mainly retrospective data from medical records and patient interviews.

Case series and **case reports** collect reports on the treatment of individual patients or a report on a single patient. Because they are reports of cases and use no control groups with which to compare outcomes, they have no statistical validity.

Levels of Evidence

Although a number of hierarchies or levels of evidence are described in the literature about evidence-based practice, the following levels are used in this text.

Level A indicates that data are derived from multiple randomized clinical trials, meta-analysis, or systematic reviews and provides the strongest evidence or support for clinical decision making and practice. There are also evidence-based clinical practice guidelines. Such guidelines delineate a plan of care for patients with particular health problems (e.g., acute myocardial infarction, asthma). Evidence-based guidelines are based on rigorous scientific evidence (i.e., systematic reviews or RCTs). In many instances, however, when systematic reviews and RCTs are not available, guidelines based on consensus opinions of a group of experts may be the "best

(continued on page 56)

Box 4-3	Selected Elements of Evidence-based Practice (continued)

available evidence" and can assist in clinical decision making. Guidelines on numerous health problems are available from the National Guidelines Clearinghouse (NGC). The NGC is maintained by the Agency for Healthcare Quality and Research, a division of the U.S. Department of Health and Human Services. However, each guideline contains a disclaimer statement that the NGC "does not develop, produce, approve, or endorse the guidelines" and that the guidelines summarized and distributed by NGC are "produced under the auspices of medical specialty societies, relevant professional associations, public or private organizations, other government agencies, health care organizations or plans, and similar entities." Readers with questions about guideline content should contact the guideline developer.

Level B usually indicates that data are derived from a randomized controlled trial, the next strongest evidence for changing or improving practice, after systematic reviews.

Level C indicates that data are derived from consensus opinions of experts, case studies, or standard-of-care recommendations.

Level D or **U** may be used to indicate that data are insufficient, unreliable, or fail to support one or more clinical practices.

Electronic Resources

High-quality Web sites are sponsored by the National Library of Medicine, university health science libraries, hospital libraries, and health care associations and organizations. Most of these resources offer free access to information about patient care. Others require paid subscriptions (e.g., Cochrane reports, most journals). Nurses need to check to see whether their health care or educational organization has an institutional subscription and, if so, how to access the databases. Most of the following Web sites were derived from Dee (2005). The article describes the sites and provides tips for searching them.

Centers for Disease Control and Prevention (CDC)
   www.cdc.gov
Cochrane Database of Systematic Reviews www.cochrane.org
Cumulative Index to Nursing and Allied Health Literature
   (CINAHL) database *www.cinahl.com*
Directory of Information Resources Online (DIRLINE)
   http:dirline.nlm.nih.gov
Healthfinder *www.healthfinder.gov*
Mayo Clinic *www.mayoclinic.com*
MedlinePlus *http://MedlinePlus.gov*
The Merck Manual of Diagnosis and Therapy
   www.merck.com/pubs/mmanual
NLM Gateway *http://gateway.nlm.nih.gov/gw/Cmd*
National Cancer Institute (NCI) *www.cancer.gov*
National Guidelines Clearinghouse *www.guideline.gov*
PubMed *www.ncbi.nlm.nih.gov/PubMed*

---

phytochemicals, and *nutraceuticals,* are derived from plants; other dietary supplements may be derived from a variety of sources. The 1994 Dietary Supplement Health and Education Act (DSHEA) defined a dietary supplement as "a vitamin, a mineral, an herb or other botanical used to supplement the diet." Under this law, herbs can be labeled according to their possible effects on the human body, but the products cannot claim to diagnose, prevent, relieve, or cure specific human diseases unless approved by the Food and Drug Administration (FDA).

It has become evident that nurses need to know about their patient's use of herbal and dietary supplements to provide safe care. An additional impetus came from the Institute of Medicine of the National Academies, which released a report on complementary and alternative medicine (CAM) in 2005 in which they recommended that "health profession schools incorporate sufficient information about … CAM into the standard curriculum at all levels to enable licensed professionals to competently advise their patients about CAM" (cited in Hughes, Jacobs, & Berman., 2007).

More specifically, there are five major concerns associated with the nursing role in relation to herbal products and drug therapy, as follows:

1. Many of the products may not be safe because active ingredients and effects on humans are often unknown. Some contain heavy metals (e.g., lead) and other contaminants (e.g., pesticides); some contain prescription or nonprescription drugs. In addition, ingredients are not standardized and often differ from those listed on the product label.

2. Use of supplements may keep the patient from seeking treatment from a health care provider when indicated. This may allow disease processes to worsen and be more difficult to treat.

3. The products may interact with prescription drugs to decrease therapeutic effects or increase adverse effects. Dangerous interactions have been identified with St. John's wort and some herbs that affect blood clotting mechanisms.

4. Most products have not been studied sufficiently to evaluate their safety or effectiveness. In many studies, the products have not been standardized in terms of types or amounts of active ingredients. In addition, most reported studies have been short-term and with few subjects.

5. Many patients who use supplements do not tell their health care providers. This omission can lead to dangerous interactions when the supplements are combined with prescription or OTC drugs.

In general, nurses need to have an adequate knowledge base to assess and assist patients who use herbal products to do so safely. To develop and maintain a knowledge base, nurses (and patients) need to seek information from authoritative, objective sources rather than product labels, advertisements, or personal testimonials from family members, friends, or celebrities. Some resources are listed below:

■ Table 4-1 describes some commonly used supplements. In later chapters, selected supplements with some scientific support for their use are described in more detail. For example, in Chapter 7 some products reported to be useful in relieving pain, fever, inflammation, or migraines are described.

■ Patient Teaching Guidelines. In this chapter, general information is provided (see Patient Teaching Guidelines: General Information About Herbal and Dietary Supplements). In later chapters, guidelines may emphasize avoidance or caution in using supplements thought to interact adversely with prescribed drugs or particular patient conditions.

■ Assessment guidelines. In this chapter, general information about the use or nonuse of supplements is assessed. In later chapters, specific supplements that may interact with particular drug group(s) are discussed. For example, some supplements are known to increase blood pressure (see Chap. 52) or risk of excessive bleeding (see Chap. 54).

■ End-of-chapter references.

■ A good source of information is the National Center for Complementary and Alternative Medicine (NCCAM) at the National Institutes of Health:

NCCAM Clearinghouse

PO Box 8218

Silver Spring, MD 20907-8218

Tel: 1-888-644-6226

Web site: http://nccam.nih.gov

Table 4-1	Herbal and Dietary Supplements	
NAME/USES	**CHARACTERISTICS**	**REMARKS**
Black Cohosh ■ Most often used to relieve symptoms of menopause (e.g., flushes, vaginal dryness, irritability) ■ May also relieve premenstrual syndrome (PMS) and dysmenorrhea	■ Well tolerated; in overdose may cause nausea, vomiting, dizziness, visual disturbances, and reduced pulse rate ■ Most clinical trials done with Remifemin, in small numbers of women; other trade names include Estroven and Femtrol	■ Did not relieve hot flashes in a 12-month, randomized, double-blind, placebo-controlled NIH* study of 351 menopausal or peri-menopausal women aged 45–55, reported in *Annals of Internal Medicine* (2006) by Newton et al. ■ Not recommended for use longer than 6 months
Capsaicin (Chap. 6) ■ Used to treat pain associated with neuralgia, neuropathy, and osteoarthritis ■ Self-defense as the active ingredient in "pepper spray"	■ A topical analgesic that may inhibit the synthesis, transport, and release of substance P, a pain transmitter ■ Derived from cayenne pepper ■ Adverse effects include skin irritation, itching, redness, and stinging	Applied topically
Chamomile Used mainly for antispasmodic effects in the gastrointestinal (GI) tract; may relieve abdominal cramping	■ Usually ingested as a tea; may delay absorption of oral medications ■ May cause contact dermatitis and severe hypersensitivity reactions, including anaphylaxis, in people allergic to ragweed, asters, and chrysanthemums ■ May increase risks of bleeding	Few studies and little data to support use and effectiveness in GI disorders
Chondroitin (Chap. 7) Arthritis	■ Derived from the trachea cartilage of slaughtered cattle ■ Usually taken with glucosamine ■ Adverse effects may include GI upset, nausea, and headache	Several studies support use

(continued on page 58)

Table 4-1	Herbal and Dietary Supplements (continued)

NAME/USES	CHARACTERISTICS	REMARKS
Creatine Athletes take creatine supplements to gain extra energy, to train longer and harder, and to improve performance	■ An amino acid produced in the liver and kidneys and stored in muscles ■ Causes weight gain, usually within 2 weeks of starting use ■ Legal and available in health food stores as a powder to be mixed with water or juice, as a liquid, and as tablets and capsules	■ Not recommended for use by children because studies have not been done and effects are unknown ■ Nurses and parents need to actively discourage children and adolescents from using creatine supplements.
Echinacea Most often used for the common cold, but also advertised for many other uses (immune system stimulant, anti-infective)	■ Many species, but E. *purpurea* most often used medicinally ■ Effects on immune system include stimulation of phagocytes and monocytes ■ Contraindicated in persons with immune system disorders ■ Hepatotoxic with long-term use	■ Hard to interpret validity of claims because various species and preparations used in reported studies ■ Some evidence (Level B) to support use in patients with the common cold, with possibly shorter durations and less severe symptoms
Feverfew (Chap. 7) Migraines, menstrual irregularities, arthritis	■ May increase risk of bleeding ■ May cause hypersensitivity reactions in people allergic to ragweed, asters, daisies, or chrysanthemums ■ May cause a withdrawal syndrome if use is stopped abruptly	Some studies support use in patients with migraine
Garlic Used to lower serum cholesterol and for other uses	■ Active ingredient thought to be allicin ■ Has antiplatelet activity and may increase risk of bleeding ■ Adverse effects include allergic reactions (asthma, dermatitis), dizziness, nausea, vomiting	Some evidence that garlic has a small cholesterol-lowering effect; no reliable evidence to support other uses
Ginger Used mainly to treat nausea, including motion sickness and postoperative nausea	■ Inhibits platelet aggregation; may increase clotting time ■ Gastroprotective effects in animal studies	Should not be used for morning sickness associated with pregnancy—may increase risk of miscarriage
Ginkgo Biloba Used mainly to improve memory and cognitive function in people with Alzheimer's disease; may be useful in treating peripheral arterial disease	■ May increase blood flow to the brain and legs, improve memory, and decrease intermittent claudication (leg pain with walking) ■ Inhibits platelet aggregation; may increase risks of bleeding with any drug that has antiplatelet effects (e.g., aspirin) ■ Adverse effects include GI upset, headache, bleeding, allergic skin reaction	■ Good evidence (Level A) for small effects in treating dementia and claudication. ■ NIH* is conducting a clinical trial with more than 3,000 volunteers to see if ginkgo prevents the onset of dementia (specifically, Alzheimer's disease), slows cognitive decline and functional disability, and reduces the incidence of cardiovascular disease

NAME/USES	CHARACTERISTICS	REMARKS
Ginseng Used to increase stamina, strength, endurance, and mental acuity	▪ Has various pharmacologic effects that vary with dose and duration of use ▪ Adverse effects include hypertension, nervousness, depression, insomnia, skin rashes, epistaxis, palpitations, vomiting ▪ May increase risks of bleeding with any drug that has antiplatelet effects (e.g., aspirin) ▪ Increases risk of hypoglycemic reactions if taken with antidiabetic drugs ▪ Should not be taken with other herbs or drugs that inhibit monoamine oxidase (e.g., St. John's wort, selegiline); headache, mania, and tremors may occur	▪ Insufficient evidence to support use for any indication ▪ A ginseng abuse syndrome, with insomnia, hypotonia, and edema, has been reported. Caution patients to avoid ingesting excessive amounts. ▪ Instruct patients with cardiovascular disease, diabetes mellitus, or hypertension to check with their health care provider before taking ginseng. ▪ Instruct any patient taking ginseng to avoid long-term use. Siberian ginseng should not be used longer than 3 weeks.
Glucosamine (Chap. 7) Osteoarthritis	▪ Usually used with chondroitin ▪ Has beneficial effects on cartilage ▪ Adverse effects mild, may include GI upset, drowsiness	Several studies support use
Melatonin (Chap. 8) Used mainly for treatment of insomnia and prevention and treatment of jet lag	▪ Several studies of effects on sleep, energy level, fatigue, mental alertness, and mood indicate some improvement, compared with placebo ▪ Contraindicated in persons with hepatic insufficiency or a history of cerebrovascular disease, depression, or neurologic disorders ▪ Adverse effects include altered sleep patterns, confusion, headache, sedation, tachycardia	Patients with renal impairment should use cautiously.
St. John's Wort (Chap. 10) Used for treatment of depression, advertised as an "herbal Prozac"	▪ Active component may be hypericin or hyperforin ▪ Adverse effects include confusion, dizziness, GI upset, photosensitivity ▪ Interacts with many drugs; can decrease effectiveness of birth control pills, anticancer drugs, antivirals used to treat acquired immunodeficiency syndrome (AIDS), and organ transplant drugs (e.g., cyclosporine)	▪ Good evidence (Level A) for improvement in mild to moderate depression; not effective in major or serious depression ▪ Should not be combined with monoamine oxidase inhibitors (MAOI) or selective serotonin reuptake inhibitor (SSRI) antidepressants ▪ Use has declined since serious herb–drug interactions reported.
Saw Palmetto Used to prevent and treat urinary symptoms in men with benign prostatic hyperplasia (BPH)	▪ May have antiandrogenic effects ▪ Adverse effects may include GI upset, headache; diarrhea may occur with high doses.	▪ Some evidence (Level B) of small beneficial effects with doses of 320 mg/day
Valerian (Chap. 8) Used mainly to promote sleep and allay anxiety and nervousness; also has muscle relaxant effects	▪ Adverse effects with acute overdose or chronic use include blurred vision, drowsiness, dizziness, excitability, hypersensitivity reactions, insomnia; also, risk of liver damage from combination products containing valerian and from overdoses averaging 2.5 g ▪ Additive sedation if taken with other CNS depressants	▪ Should not be combined with sedative drugs and should not be used regularly ▪ Many extract products contain 40%–60% alcohol. ▪ Insufficient evidence to support use for treatment of insomnia

GI, gastrointestinal; NIH, National Institutes of Health.

Patient Teaching Guidelines — General Information About Herbal and Dietary Supplements

- Herbal and dietary products are chemicals that have drug-like effects in people. Unfortunately, their effects are largely unknown and may be dangerous for some people because there is little reliable information about them. For most products, little research has been done to determine either their benefits or their adverse effects.

- The safety and effectiveness of these products are not regulated by laws designed to protect consumers, as are pharmaceutical drugs. As a result, the types and amounts of ingredients may not be identified on the product label. In fact, most products contain several active ingredients and it is often not known which ingredient, if any, has the desired pharmacologic effect. In addition, components of plants can vary considerably, depending on the soil, water, and climate where the plants are grown. Quality is also a concern, as heavy metals (e.g., lead), pesticides, and other contaminants have been found in some products.

- These products can be used more safely if they are manufactured by a reputable company that states the ingredients are standardized (meaning that the dose of medicine in each tablet or capsule is the same).

- The product label should also state specific percentages, amounts, and strengths of active ingredients. With herbal medicines especially, different brands of the same herb vary in the amounts of active ingredients per recommended dose. Dosing is also difficult because a particular herb may be available in several different dosage forms (e.g., tablet, capsule, tea, extract) with different amounts of active ingredients.

- These products are often advertised as "natural." Many people interpret this to mean the products are safe and better than synthetic products. This is not true; "natural" does not mean safe, especially when taken concurrently with other herbals, dietary supplements, or drugs.

- When taking herbal or dietary supplements, follow the instructions on the product label. Inappropriate use or taking excessive amounts may cause dangerous side effects.

- Inform health care providers when taking any kind of herbal or dietary supplement to reduce risks of severe adverse effects or drug–supplement interactions.

- Most herbal and dietary supplements should be avoided during pregnancy or lactation and in young children.

- The American Society of Anesthesiologists recommends that all herbal products be discontinued 2–3 weeks before any surgical procedure. Some products (e.g., echinacea, feverfew, garlic, ginkgo, ginseng, valerian, and St. John's wort) can interfere with or increase the effects of some drugs, affect blood pressure or heart rhythm, or increase risks of bleeding; some have unknown effects when combined with anesthetics, other perioperative medications, and surgical procedures.

- Store herbal and dietary supplements out of the reach of children.

General Principles of Drug Therapy

Goals and Guidelines

The goals of drug therapy are to maximize beneficial effects and to minimize adverse effects. To help meet these goals, general guidelines include the following:

- Expected benefits should outweigh potential adverse effects. Thus, drugs usually should not be prescribed for trivial problems or problems for which nondrug measures are effective.

- Drug therapy should be individualized. Many variables influence a drug's effects on the human body. Failure to consider these variables may decrease therapeutic effects or increase risks of adverse effects.

- Drug effects on quality of life should be considered in designing a drug therapy regimen. Quality-of-life issues are also being emphasized in research studies, with expectations of measurable improvement as a result of drug therapy.

Drug Selection and Dosage

Numerous factors must be considered when choosing a drug and dosage range for a particular patient, including the following:

- Minimizing the number of drugs and the frequency of administration increases patient compliance with the prescribed drug regimen and decreases risks of serious adverse effects, including hazardous drug–drug interactions. Notable exceptions to this basic rule are that multiple drugs are commonly used to treat asthma, hypertension, and serious infections.

- Fixed-dose combination drugs, rather then individual drugs that allow greater flexibility of dosage, are commonly used, mainly because patients are more likely to take them. Many of the combination products can be taken once daily, which also promotes compliance.

- The least amount of the least potent drug that yields therapeutic benefit should be given to decrease adverse reactions. For example, if a mild nonopioid and a strong opioid analgesic are both ordered, give the nonopioid drug *if it is effective in relieving pain.*

- In drug literature, recommended dosages are listed in amounts likely to be effective for most people. However, they are only guidelines to be interpreted according to the patient's condition. For example, patients with serious illnesses may require larger doses of some drugs than patients with milder illnesses; patients with severe kidney disease need much smaller doses of renally excreted drugs.

▪ A drug can be started rapidly or slowly. If it has a long half-life and optimal therapeutic effects do not usually occur for several days or weeks, the prescriber may order a limited number of relatively large (*loading*) doses followed by a regular schedule of smaller (*maintenance*) doses. When drug actions are not urgent, therapy may be initiated with a maintenance dose.

Drug Therapy in Special Populations

Drug Therapy in Children

Drug therapy in neonates (birth to 1 month), infants (1 month to 1 year), and children (1 to 12 years) requires special consideration because of the child's changing size, developmental level, and organ function. Physiologic differences alter drug pharmacokinetics (Table 4-2), and drug therapy is less predictable than in adults. Neonates are especially vulnerable to adverse drug effects because of their immature liver and kidney function; neonatal therapeutics are discussed further in Chapter 65.

For many drugs, manufacturers' literature states "safety and effectiveness for use in children have not been established." Still, most drugs given to adults also are given to children, and general principles, techniques of drug administration, and nursing process guidelines apply. Additional principles and guidelines include the following:

▪ **All aspects of pediatric drug therapy must be guided by the child's age, weight, and level of growth and development.**

▪ Safe therapeutic dosage ranges are less well defined for children than for adults. Some drugs are not recommended for use in children, and therefore dosages have not been established. For many drugs, doses for children are extrapolated

Table 4-2	Neonates, Infants, and Children: Physiologic Characteristics and Pharmacokinetic Consequences
PHYSIOLOGIC CHARACTERISTICS	**PHARMACOKINETIC CONSEQUENCES**
Increased thinness and permeability of skin in neonates and infants	Increased absorption of topical drugs (e.g., corticosteroids may be absorbed sufficiently to suppress adrenocortical function)
Immature blood–brain barrier in neonates and infants	Increased distribution of drugs into the central nervous system because myelinization (which creates the blood–brain barrier to the passage of drugs) is not mature until approximately 2 years of age
Increased percentage of body water (70%–80% in neonates and infants, compared with 50%–60% in children older than 2 years of age and adults)	Usually increased volume of distribution in infants and young children, compared with adults. This would seem to indicate a need for larger doses. However, prolonged drug half-life and decreased rate of drug clearance may offset. The net effect is often a need for decreased dosage.
Altered protein binding until approximately 1 year of age, when it reaches adult levels	The amount and binding capacity of plasma proteins may be reduced. This may result in a greater proportion of unbound or pharmacologically active drug and greater risks of adverse drug effects. Dosage requirements may be decreased or modified by other factors. Drugs with decreased protein binding in neonates, compared with older children and adults, include ampicillin (Principen, others), diazepam (Valium), digoxin (Lanoxin), lidocaine (Xylocaine), nafcillin, phenobarbital, phenytoin (Dilantin), salicylates (e.g., aspirin), and theophylline (Theolair).
Decreased glomerular filtration rate in neonates and infants, compared with older children and adults. Kidney function develops progressively during the first few months of life and is fairly mature by 1 year of age.	In neonates and infants, slowed excretion of drugs eliminated by the kidneys. Dosage of these drugs may need to be decreased, depending on the infant's age and level of growth and development.
Decreased activity of liver drug-metabolizing enzyme systems in neonates and infants	Decreased capacity for biotransformation of drugs. This results in slowed metabolism and elimination, with increased risks of drug accumulation and adverse effects.
Increased activity of liver drug-metabolizing enzyme systems in children	Increased capacity for biotransformation of some drugs. This results in a rapid rate of metabolism and elimination. For example, theophylline is cleared about 30% faster in a 7-year-old child than in an adult and approximately four times faster than in a neonate.

from those established for adults. *When pediatric dosage ranges are listed in drug literature, these should be used.* Often, however, dosages are expressed as the amount of drug to be given per kilogram of body weight or square meter of body surface area, and the amount needed for a specific dose must be calculated as a fraction of the adult dose. Body surface area (BSA) is based on height and weight and can be estimated using a nomogram (Fig. 4-1). Use the estimated BSA in the following formula to calculate the child's dose:

$$\frac{\text{Body surface area (in square meters)}}{1.73 \text{ square meters (m}^2)} \times \text{adult dose} = \text{child's dose}$$

■ Dosages obtained from calculations can be used initially and then increased or decreased according to the child's response.

■ Use the oral route of drug administration when possible. Try to obtain the child's cooperation; never force oral medications because forcing may lead to aspiration.

■ Site selection for intramuscular injections depends on age and size. In infants, use thigh muscles because the deltoid muscles are small and the gluteal muscles do not develop until the child is walking. In children older than 18 months of age, use deltoid muscles; injections are considered less painful than in thigh muscles. In children older than 3 years of age, ventrogluteal injections are considered less painful than those in anterior thigh or dorsogluteal areas.

■ Children are fearful of injections. With an immunization schedule that calls for 20 or more injections during childhood plus procedures required by illnesses, interventions are needed to decrease the pain and fear associated with injections, venipunctures, and other "shots." One technique is the application of EMLA (eutectic mixture of lidocaine and

Figure 4-1 ■ Body surface nomograms. To determine the surface area of the patient, draw a straight line between the point representing his or her height on the left vertical scale to the point representing weight on the right vertical scale. The point at which this line intersects the middle vertical scale represents the patient's surface area in square meters (courtesy of Abbott Laboratories).

prilocaine local anesthetics). A disadvantage is that EMLA must be applied an hour before the painful injection. Having parents present and using distraction techniques may also be helpful.

- For safety, keep all medications in childproof containers, out of reach of children, and do not refer to medications as "candy."

Drug Therapy in Older Adults

Aging is a continuum; precisely when a person becomes an "older adult" is not clearly established, but in this book, the term *older adult* refers to people 65 years of age and older. In this population, general nursing process guidelines and principles of drug therapy apply. In addition, adverse effects are likely because of physiologic changes associated with aging (Table 4-3), pathologic changes due to disease processes, multiple drugs for acute and chronic disorders, impaired memory and cognition, and difficulty in complying with drug orders. Overall, the goal of drug therapy may be "care" rather than "cure," with efforts to prevent or control symptoms and to maintain the patient's ability to function in usual activities of daily living. Additional principles include the following:

- Although age in years is important, older adults are quite heterogeneous in their responses to drug therapy and responses differ widely within the same age group. Responses also differ in the same person over time. Physiologic age (i.e., organ function) is more important than chronologic age.

- It may be difficult to separate the effects of aging from the effects of disease processes or drug therapy, particularly long-term drug therapy. Symptoms attributed to aging or disease may be caused by medications. This occurs because older adults are usually less able to metabolize and excrete drugs efficiently. As a result, drugs are more likely to accumulate. *When a patient develops new symptoms or becomes less capable of functioning in usual activities of daily living, consider the possibility of adverse drug effects.* Because new signs and symptoms are often attributed to aging or disease, they may be ignored or treated by prescribing a new drug, when stopping or reducing the dose of an "old" drug is the needed intervention.

- Use nondrug interventions to decrease the need for drugs and to increase their effectiveness or decrease their adverse effects. For example, insomnia is a common complaint among older adults. Preventing it (e.g., by avoiding excessive caffeine and napping) is much safer than taking sedative-hypnotic drugs.

- Medications—both prescription and OTC—should be taken only when necessary. When drug therapy is required, the choice of drug should be based on available drug information regarding effects in older adults.

- Any prescriber should review current medications, including nonprescription drugs and herbal remedies, before prescribing new drugs.

- The basic principle of giving the smallest effective number of drugs applies especially to older adults. A regimen of several drugs increases the risks of adverse drug reactions and interactions. In addition, many older adults are unable to correctly self-administer more than three or four drugs.

- All drugs should be given for the shortest effective time. This interval is not established for most drugs, and many are continued for years. Health care providers must reassess drug regimens periodically to see whether drugs, dosages, or other aspects need to be revised. This is especially important when a serious illness or significant changes in health status have occurred.

- The smallest number of effective doses should be prescribed. This allows less disruption of usual activities and promotes compliance with the prescribed regimen.

- When any drug is started, the dosage should usually be smaller than for younger adults. The dosage can then be increased or decreased according to response. If increased dosage is indicated, increments should be smaller and made at longer intervals in older adults. This conservative, safe approach is often called "start low, go slow."

- For older adults receiving long-term drug therapy at home, assist them to take drugs safely and effectively:

    - If vision is impaired, label drug containers with large lettering for easier readability. A magnifying glass also may be useful.

    - Be sure the patient can open drug containers. For example, avoid childproof containers for an older adult with arthritic hands.

    - Use appropriate devices to schedule drug doses and decrease risks of omitting or repeating doses. Helpful devices include written schedules, calendars, charts, and drug containers with each dose prepared and clearly labeled as to the day and time it is to be taken. With the latter system, the patient can tell at a glance whether a dose has been taken.

    - Enlist family members or friends when necessary.

Applying Your Knowledge 4-3

Given Mr. Walker's age and his drug regimen, what factors related to medication administration should the nurse consider to ensure safe, accurate, and effective drug administration?

Drug Therapy in Patients With Renal Impairment

Many patients have or are at risk for impaired renal function. Patients with disease processes such as diabetes or hypertension may have renal insufficiency on first contact, and this may be worsened by illness, major surgery or trauma, or administration of nephrotoxic drugs. In patients with initially normal renal

Table 4-3	Older Adults: Physiologic Characteristics and Pharmacokinetic Consequences

PHYSIOLOGIC CHARACTERISTICS	PHARMACOKINETIC CONSEQUENCES
Decreased gastrointestinal secretions and motility	Minimal effects on absorption of most oral drugs; effects on extended-release formulations are unknown
Decreased cardiac output	■ Slower absorption from some sites of administration (e.g., gastrointestinal tract, subcutaneous or muscle tissue); effects on absorption from skin and mucous membranes are unknown ■ Decreased distribution to sites of action in tissues, with potential for delaying the onset and reducing the extent of therapeutic effects
Decreased blood flow to the liver and kidneys	Delayed metabolism and excretion, which may lead to drug accumulation and increased risks of adverse or toxic effects
Decreased total body water and lean body mass per kg of weight; increased body fat	Water-soluble drugs (e.g., ethanol, lithium) are distributed into a smaller area, with resultant higher plasma concentrations and higher risks of toxicity with a given dose. Fat-soluble drugs (e.g., diazepam) are distributed to a larger area, accumulate in fat, and have a longer duration of action in the body.
Decreased serum albumin	Decreased availability of protein for binding and transporting drug molecules. This increases serum concentration of free, pharmacologically active drug, especially for those that are normally highly protein bound (e.g., aspirin, warfarin). This may increase risks of adverse effects. However, the drug also may be metabolized and excreted more rapidly, thereby offsetting at least some of the risks. In addition, drug interactions occur with co-administration of multiple drugs that are highly protein bound. The drugs compete for protein-binding sites and are more likely to cause adverse effects with decreased levels of serum albumin. As above, the result is larger concentrations of free drug.
Decreased blood flow to the liver; decreased size of the liver; decreased number and activity of the cytochrome P450 (CYP) oxidative drug-metabolizing enzymes	Slowed metabolism and detoxification of many drugs, with increased risks of drug accumulation and toxic effects. (Numerous drugs metabolized by the CYP enzymes are often prescribed for older adults, including beta blockers, calcium channel blockers, antimicrobials, the statin cholesterol-lowering drugs, and antiulcer drugs. Metabolism of drugs metabolized by conjugative reactions [e.g., acetaminophen, diazepam, morphine, steroids] does not change significantly with aging).
Decreased blood flow to the kidneys; decreased number of functioning nephrons; decreased glomerular filtration rate; and decreased tubular secretion	■ Impaired drug excretion, prolonged half-life, and increased risks of toxicity ■ Age-related alterations in renal function are consistent and well described. When renal blood flow is decreased, less drug is delivered to the kidney for elimination. Renal mass is also decreased and older adults may be more sensitive to drugs that further impair renal function (e.g., nonsteroidal anti-inflammatory drugs such as ibuprofen, which older adults often take for pain or arthritis).

function, renal failure may develop from depletion of intravascular fluid volume, shock due to sepsis or blood loss, seriously impaired cardiovascular function, major surgery, nephrotoxic drugs, or other conditions. Acute renal failure (ARF) may occur in any illness in which renal blood flow or function is impaired. Chronic renal failure (CRF) usually results from disease processes that destroy renal tissue.

With ARF, renal function may recover if the impairment is recognized promptly, contributing factors are eliminated or treated effectively, and medication dosages are adjusted according to the extent of renal impairment. With CRF, effective treatment can help to conserve functioning nephrons and delay progression to end-stage renal disease (ESRD). If ESRD develops, dialysis or transplantation is required.

In relation to drug therapy, the major concern is that the kidneys are unable or less able to excrete drugs and drug metabolites. Guidelines have been established for the use of many drugs; health care providers need to use these recommendations to maximize the safety and effectiveness of drug therapy. Some general guidelines are discussed here; specific guidelines for particular drug groups are included in the appropriate chapters.

Drug therapy must be used very cautiously because of the high risks of drug accumulation and adverse effects. When possible, nephrologists should design drug therapy regimens. However, all health care providers need to be knowledgeable about risk factors for development of renal impairment, illnesses and their physiologic changes (e.g., hemodynamic, renal, hepatic, and metabolic alterations) that affect renal function, and the effects of commonly used drugs on renal function.

Renal status should be monitored in any patient with renal insufficiency or risk factors for developing renal insufficiency. Signs and symptoms of ARF include decreased urine output (less than 600 mL/24 hours), increased blood urea nitrogen, or increased serum creatinine (over 2 mg/dL or an increase of 0.5 mg/dL or more over a baseline value of less than 3.0 mg/dL). In addition, an adequate fluid intake is required to excrete drugs by the kidneys. Any factors that deplete extracellular fluid volume (e.g., inadequate fluid intake; diuretic drugs; loss of body fluids with blood loss, vomiting, or diarrhea) increase the risk of worsening renal impairment in patients with impairment or of causing impairment in those with previously normal function.

Patients with renal impairment may respond to a drug dose or serum concentration differently from patients with normal renal function because of physiologic and biochemical changes. Thus, drug therapy must be individualized according to the extent of renal impairment. This individualization is usually determined by measuring serum creatinine, which is then used to calculate creatinine clearance. Estimations of creatinine clearance are more accurate for patients with stable renal function and average muscle mass (for their age, weight, and height). Estimations are less accurate for emaciated and obese patients and for those with changing renal function, as often occurs in acute illness. If a patient is oliguric (less than 400 mL urine/24 hours), for example, the creatinine clearance should be estimated to be less than 10 mL/min, regardless of the serum creatinine concentration. Also, in elderly patients, serum creatinine is an unreliable indicator of renal function because these patients usually have diminished muscle mass. As a result, they may have a normal serum level of creatinine even if their renal function is markedly reduced.

Some medications can increase serum creatinine levels and create a false impression of renal failure. These drugs, which include cimetidine and trimethoprim, interfere with secretion of creatinine into kidney tubules. As a result, serum creatinine levels are increased without an associated decrease in renal function.

Drug selection should be guided by baseline renal function and the known effects of drugs on renal function, when possible. Many commonly used drugs may adversely affect renal function, including nonsteroidal anti-inflammatory drugs such as ibuprofen (e.g., Advil). Some drugs are excreted exclusively (e.g., aminoglycoside antibiotics, lithium), and most are excreted, to some extent, by the kidneys. Some drugs are contraindicated in renal impairment (e.g., tetracyclines, except doxycycline); others can be used if safety guidelines are followed (e.g., reducing dosage, monitoring serum drug levels and renal function tests, avoiding dehydration). Drugs known to be nephrotoxic should be avoided when possible. In some instances, however, there are no effective substitutes and nephrotoxic drugs must be given. Some commonly used nephrotoxic drugs include aminoglycoside antibiotics, amphotericin B (an antifungal drug), and cisplatin (an anticancer drug).

Dosage of many drugs needs to be decreased in patients with renal failure, including dosage of aminoglycoside antibiotics, most cephalosporin antibiotics, fluoroquinolones, and digoxin. In general, the most effective dosage adjustments are based on the patient's clinical responses and serum drug levels.

Drug Therapy in Patients With Hepatic Impairment

Most drugs are eliminated from the body by hepatic metabolism, renal excretion, or both. Hepatic metabolism depends mainly on blood flow and enzyme activity in the liver and protein binding in the plasma. Patients at risk for impaired liver function include those with primary liver disease (e.g., hepatitis, cirrhosis) and those with disease processes that impair blood flow to the liver (e.g., heart failure, major surgery, trauma) or hepatic enzyme production. An additional factor is hepatotoxic drugs. Fortunately, although the liver is often damaged, it has a great capacity for cell repair and may be able to function with as little as 10% of undamaged hepatic cells.

In relation to drug therapy, acute liver impairment may interfere with drug metabolism and elimination, whereas chronic cirrhosis or severe liver impairment may affect all pharmacokinetic processes. It is difficult to predict the effects of drug therapy because of wide variations in liver function and few helpful diagnostic tests. In addition, with severe hepatic impairment, extrahepatic sites of drug metabolism (e.g., intestine, kidneys, lungs) may become more important in eliminating drugs from the body. Thus, guidelines for drug selection, dosage, and duration of use are not well established. Some general guidelines for increasing drug safety and effectiveness are discussed here; known guidelines for particular drug groups are included in the appropriate chapters.

During drug therapy, patients with impaired liver function require close monitoring for signs and symptoms (e.g., nausea, vomiting, jaundice, liver enlargement) and abnormal results of laboratory tests of liver function. Liver function tests should be monitored in patients with or at risk for liver impairment, especially when patients are receiving potentially hepatotoxic drugs. Indicators of hepatic impairment include serum bilirubin levels above 4 to 5 mg/dL, a prothrombin time greater than 1.5 times control, a serum albumin below 2.0 g/dL, and elevated serum alanine (ALT) and aspartate (AST) aminotransferases. In some patients, abnormal liver function test results may occur without indicating severe liver damage and are often reversible.

Drug selection should be based on knowledge of drug effects on hepatic function. Hepatotoxic drugs should be avoided when possible. If they cannot be avoided, they should be used in the smallest effective doses, for the shortest effective time. Commonly used hepatotoxic drugs include acetaminophen, isoniazid, and cholesterol-lowering statins. Alcohol is toxic to the liver by itself and increases the risks of hepatotoxicity with other drugs.

In addition to hepatotoxic drugs, many other drugs can cause or aggravate liver impairment by decreasing hepatic blood flow and drug-metabolizing capacity. For example, epinephrine and related drugs may cause vasoconstriction in the hepatic artery and portal vein, the two main sources of the liver's blood supply. Beta-adrenergic blocking agents (e.g., propranolol) decrease hepatic blood flow by decreasing cardiac output. Several drugs (e.g., cimetidine, fluoxetine) inhibit hepatic metabolism of many co-administered drugs. The consequence may be toxicity from the inhibited drugs if the dose is not decreased.

Dosage should be reduced for drugs that are extensively metabolized in the liver, because if doses are not reduced, serum drug levels are higher, elimination is slower, and toxicity is more likely to occur in a patient with hepatic disease. For example, some oral drugs are normally extensively metabolized during their "first pass" through the liver, so that a relatively small portion of an oral dose reaches the systemic circulation. In patients with cirrhosis, the blood carrying the drug molecules is shunted around the liver so that oral drugs go directly into the systemic circulation. Some drugs whose dosages should be decreased in patients with hepatic failure include cefoperazone, cimetidine, clindamycin, diazepam, labetalol, lorazepam, morphine, phenytoin, ranitidine, theophylline, and verapamil.

Drug Therapy in Patients With Critical Illness

The term *critical illness*, as used here, denotes patients who are experiencing acute, serious, or life-threatening illness. Critically ill patients are at risk for multiple organ dysfunction, including cardiovascular, renal, and hepatic impairments, that influence all aspects of drug therapy. Drug elimination is often impaired because of decreased blood flow and decreased function of the liver and kidneys.

Although much of critical care nursing is performed in an intensive care unit (ICU), nurses in other settings also care for these patients. For example, nurses in emergency departments often initiate and maintain treatment for several hours; nurses on other hospital units care for patients who are transferred to or from ICUs; and patients formerly cared for in an ICU are on medical-surgical hospital units, in long-term care facilities, or even at home. Moreover, many nursing students are introduced to critical care during their educational programs, many new graduates seek employment in critical care settings, and experienced nurses may transfer to an ICU. Thus, all nurses need to know about drug therapy in critically ill patients. Some general guidelines are discussed here; more specific guidelines related to particular drugs are included in the appropriate chapters.

Drug therapy in critically ill patients is often more complex, more problematic, and less predictable than in most other populations. One reason is that patients often have multiple organ impairments that alter drug effects and increase the risks of adverse drug reactions. Another reason is that patients often require aggressive treatment with large numbers, large doses, and combinations of highly potent drugs that the patient's body may be unable to process effectively.

In this at-risk population, safe and effective drug therapy requires that all involved health care providers be knowledgeable about common critical illnesses, the physiologic changes (e.g., hemodynamic, renal, hepatic, and metabolic alterations) that can be caused by the illnesses, and the drugs used to treat the illnesses. Nurses need to be especially diligent in administering drugs and vigilant in observing patient responses.

Drugs used in patients with critical illness represent most drug classifications and are also discussed in other chapters. Commonly used drugs include analgesics, antimicrobials, cardiovascular agents, gastric acid suppressants, neuromuscular blocking agents, and sedatives. In many instances, the main goals of drug therapy are to support vital functions and relieve life-threatening symptoms.

Drug selection should be guided by the patient's clinical status (e.g., symptoms, severity of illness) and organ function, especially cardiovascular, renal, and hepatic functions.

Route of administration should also be guided by the patient's clinical status. Most drugs are given intravenously (IV) because critically ill patients are often unable to take oral medications and require many drugs, rapid drug action, and relatively large doses. In addition, the IV route achieves more reliable and measurable blood levels

Dosage requirements may vary among patients and within the same patient at different times during an illness. A standard dose may be therapeutic, subtherapeutic, or toxic. Thus, it is especially important that initial dosages are individualized according to the severity of the condition being treated and the patient's characteristics (e.g., age, weight, organ function) and that maintenance dosages are titrated according to patient responses and changes in organ function (e.g., as indicated by symptoms or laboratory tests). In general, to maintain consistent serum drug levels, once-daily drug doses should be given about the same time each day and multiple daily doses should be given at even intervals around the clock.

Laboratory tests are often needed before and during drug therapy to assess the patient's condition (e.g., cardiovascular, renal, and hepatic functions; fluid and electrolyte balance) and response to treatment. For example, serum protein levels should be monitored because drug binding may be significantly altered. Serum albumin, which binds acidic drugs (e.g., phenytoin, diazepam), is often decreased during critical illness. If there is not enough albumin to bind a drug, blood levels of the drug are higher and may cause adverse effects. Also, unbound molecules are metabolized and excreted more readily so that therapeutic effects may be decreased. Alpha$_1$-acid glycoprotein binds basic drugs, and its synthesis may increase during critical illness. As a result, the bound portion of a dose increases for some drugs (e.g., propranolol) and therapeutic blood levels may not be achieved unless higher doses are given. In addition, these drugs are eliminated more slowly than usual.

Drug Therapy in Home Care

As a result of increased outpatient care and brief hospitalizations, patients often recover from illness or surgery at their homes. Skilled nursing care (e.g., managing medication regimens) is often required. Most general principles and nursing responsibilities related to drug therapy apply in home care as in other health care settings. Additional considerations include the following:

▪ In most instances, the role of the nurse is to teach the patient or caregiver to administer medications and monitor their effects.

▪ In a patient's home, the nurse is a guest and must work within the environment to establish rapport, elicit cooperation, and provide nursing care. The initial contact is usually by telephone, and one purpose is to schedule a home visit, preferably at a convenient time for the patient and caregiver. In addition, state the main purpose and approximate length of the visit. Establish a method for contact in case the appointment must be canceled by either party.

▪ Assess the patient's attitude toward the prescribed medication regimen and his or her ability to provide self-care. If the patient is unable to provide self-care, ask who will administer medications and observe for medication effects. Determine the learning needs of the patient or caregiver in relation to the medication regimen.

▪ Ask to see all prescribed and OTC medications that the patient takes, and ask how and when the patient takes each one. With this information, the nurse may be able to reinforce the patient's compliance or identify potential problem areas (e.g., differences between instructions and patient usage of medications, drugs with opposing or duplicate effects, continued use of medications that were supposed to be discontinued, drugs discontinued because of adverse effects).

▪ Ask if the patient takes any herbal medicines or dietary supplements. If so, try to determine the amount, frequency, duration of use, reasons for use, and perceived beneficial or adverse effects. Explain that you need this information because some herbal and dietary supplements may cause various health problems or react adversely with prescription or OTC medications.

▪ Assess the environment for potential safety hazards (e.g., risk of infection with corticosteroids and other immunosuppressants, risk of falls and other injuries with opioid analgesics and other drugs with sedating effects). In addition, assess the patient's ability to obtain medications and keep appointments for follow-up visits to health care providers.

▪ Provide whatever information and assistance is needed for home management of the drug therapy regimen.

  ▪ Most people are accustomed to taking oral drugs, but they may need information about timing in relation to food intake, whether a tablet can be crushed, when to omit a drug, and other aspects.

  ▪ With other routes, the nurse may initially need to demonstrate administration or coach the patient or caregiver through each step.

▪ Demonstrating and having the patient or caregiver do a return demonstration is a good way to teach psychomotor skills (e.g., giving a medication through a GI tube, preparing and administering an injection, or manipulating an IV infusion pump). A written instruction sheet is also helpful. Studies indicate that a combination of verbal and written instructions is more effective than either alone.

▪ In addition to safe and accurate administration, teach the patient and caregiver to observe for beneficial and adverse effects. If adverse effects occur, teach them how to manage minor ones and which ones to report to a health care provider.

▪ Between home visits, maintain contact with patients and caregivers to monitor progress, answer questions, identify problems, and provide reassurance. Patients and caregivers should be given a telephone number to call with questions about medications, adverse effects, and so forth. The nurse may wish to schedule a daily time for receiving and making nonemergency calls. For patients and nurses with computers and Internet access, e-mail may be a convenient and efficient method of communication.

Nursing Actions   Monitoring Drug Therapy

NURSING ACTIONS	RATIONALE/EXPLANATION
1. Prepare medications for administration.	If giving medications to a group of patients, start preparing about 30 minutes before the scheduled administration time when possible, to avoid rushing and increasing the risk of errors.
a. Assemble appropriate supplies and equipment.	Medications and supplies are usually kept on a medication cart in a hospital or long-term care facility.
b. Calculate doses when indicated.	Except for very simple calculations, use pencil and paper to decrease the risk of errors. If unsure about the results, ask a colleague or a pharmacist to do the calculation. Compare results. Accuracy is vital.

(continued on page 68)

Nursing Actions | Monitoring Drug Therapy (continued)

NURSING ACTIONS	RATIONALE/EXPLANATION
c. Check vital signs when indicated.	Check blood pressure (recent recordings) before giving antihypertensive drugs. Check temperature before giving an antipyretic.
d. Check laboratory reports when indicated.	Commonly needed reports include serum potassium levels before giving diuretics; prothrombin time or international normalized ratio (INR) before giving Coumadin; culture and susceptibility reports before giving an antibiotic.
e. Check drug references when indicated.	This is often needed to look up new or unfamiliar drugs; other uses include assessing a drug in relation to a particular patient (e.g., Is it contraindicated? Is it likely to interact with other drugs the patient is taking? Does the patient's ordered dose fit within the dosage range listed in the drug reference? Can a tablet be crushed or a capsule opened without decreasing therapeutic effects or increasing adverse effects?)
2. Administer drugs accurately (see Chap. 3). a. Practice the five rights of drug administration (right drug, right patient, right dose, right route, and right time).	These rights are ensured if the techniques described in Chapter 3 are consistently followed. The time may vary by approximately 30 minutes. For example, a drug ordered for 9 A.M. can be usually given between 8:30 A.M. and 9:30 A.M. No variation is allowed in the other rights.
b. Use correct techniques for different routes of administration.	For example, sterile equipment and techniques are required for injection of any drug.
c. Follow label instructions regarding mixing or other aspects of giving specific drugs.	Some drugs require specific techniques of preparation and administration.
d. In general, do not give antacids with any other oral drugs. When both are ordered, administer at least 2 hours apart.	Antacids decrease absorption of many oral drugs.
3. Observe for therapeutic effects. a. Look for improvement in signs and symptoms, laboratory or other diagnostic test reports, or ability to function.	In general, the nurse should know the expected effects and when they are likely to occur.
b. Ask questions to determine whether the patient is feeling better.	Specific observations depend on the specific drug or drugs being given.
4. Observe for adverse effects. a. Look for signs and symptoms of new problems or worsening of previous disorders. If noted, compare the patient's symptoms with your knowledge base about adverse effects associated with the drugs or consult a drug reference.	All drugs are potentially harmful, although the incidence and severity of adverse reactions vary among drugs and patients. People most likely to have adverse reactions are those with severe liver or kidney disease, those who are very young or very old, those taking several drugs, and those receiving large doses of any drug. Specific adverse effects for which to observe depend on the drugs being given.
b. Check laboratory (e.g., complete blood count [CBC], electrolytes, blood urea nitrogen and serum creatinine, liver function tests) and other diagnostic test reports for abnormal values.	
c. Assess for decreasing ability to function at previous levels.	
d. Ask questions to determine how the patient is feeling and whether he or she is having difficulties that may be associated with drug therapy.	
5. Observe for drug interactions. a. Consider a possible interaction when a patient does not experience expected therapeutic effects or develops adverse effects.	Interactions may occur whenever the patient is receiving two or more drugs concurrently and the number of possible interactions is very large. Although no one can be expected to know or recognize all potential or actual interactions, it is helpful to build a knowledge base about important interactions with commonly used drugs (e.g., warfarin, sedatives, cardiovascular drugs).
b. Look for signs and symptoms of new problems or worsening of previous ones. If noted, compare the patient's symptoms with your knowledge base about interactions associated with the drugs or consult a drug reference to validate your observations.	

Key Concepts

- Nurses must be knowledgeable about drugs and the patients receiving them.
- Nurses need to apply the nursing process in drug therapy as in other aspects of care.
- Children, older adults, people with renal or hepatic dysfunction, and those with critical illness require special consideration in relation to safe and effective drug therapy.

- Nurses are responsible for safe and effective administration of medications and observation of responses in patients of various ages and in a variety of health care settings.
- Teaching patients and caregivers about medications is a necessary and important role.
- Evidence-based nursing practice requires continued searching for and using "best practice" interventions, as based on research and other authoritative evidence.

Review and Application Exercises

Short Answer Exercises

1. Why do nurses need to know the therapeutic and adverse effects of the drugs they give?
2. Given a newly assigned patient, what information is needed about present and previous medications or herbal and dietary supplements?
3. With children, what are some potential difficulties with drug administration, and how can they be prevented or minimized?
4. With older adults, what are some potential difficulties with drug administration, and how can they be prevented or minimized?
5. For older adults, explain what is meant by "start low, go slow" and why it is a good approach to drug therapy.
6. Why is patient teaching about drug therapy needed, and what information should usually be included?
7. Describe at least three important nursing considerations for patients who have renal or hepatic impairment or critical illness.
8. For the home care nurse assisting with a medication regimen, what are some likely differences between the nursing care needed by a child and an adult?
9. For a patient who reports using particular herbal or dietary supplements, how can the nurse evaluate whether they are safe or unsafe in view of the patient's condition and drug therapy regimen?

NCLEX-Style Questions

10. During an initial nursing assessment, the patient reports that he is allergic to a particular medicine. The nurse should
    a. ask what symptoms occurred with the allergic reaction
    b. conduct a detailed medical history and physical examination
    c. disregard the information as unimportant
    d. suspect that the patient overdosed on the drug

11. Interventions to increase safety and effectiveness of drug therapy include
    a. avoiding the use of nondrug measures during drug therapy
    b. using multiple drugs to relieve most symptoms or problems
    c. teaching patients about their drug therapy regimens
    d. avoiding instructions to alter usual activities of daily living

12. When evaluating a patient's response to drug therapy, the nurse should keep in mind that
    a. few drugs cause adverse effects.
    b. drugs may cause virtually any symptom or problem.
    c. patients usually report adverse drug effects without being asked.
    d. therapeutic effects are more important than adverse effects.

13. Considerations in individualizing drug therapy for a child include
    a. age and development
    b. equivalent drug selection and dosage for adults
    c. length of illness
    d. the child's usual diet

14. In teaching a patient about adverse effects of a newly ordered drug, which of the following should be included?
    a. a detailed list of all potential adverse effects
    b. percentages of particular adverse effects that occurred during clinical trials of the drug
    c. adverse effects that the patient is likely to see or feel
    d. research data about rare adverse effects

Selected References

Dee, C. (2005). Making the most of nursing's electronic resources: Accessing evidence-based web sites. *American Journal of Nursing, 105,* 79–85.

Gundling, K. (2005). Update on common dietary supplements. *Emergency Medicine, 37,* 18–28.

Hughes, E. F., Jacobs, B. P., & Berman, B. M. (2007). Complementary and alternative medicine. In S.J . McPhee, M. A. Papadakis, & L. M. Tierney, Jr. (Eds.), *Current medical diagnosis and treatment 2007* (pp. 1743–1766). New York: McGraw-Hill.

Johnston, C. B., Harper, G. M., & Landefeld, C. S. (2007). Geriatric medicine. In S. J. McPhee, M. A. Papadakis, & L. M. Tierney, Jr. (Eds.), *Current medical diagnosis and treatment 2007* (pp. 51–67). New York: McGraw-Hill.

Lindblad, C. I., Gray, S. L., Guay, D. R. P., et al. (2005). Geriatrics. In J. T. DiPiro, R. L. Talbert, G. C. Yee, G. R. Matzke, B. G. Wells, & L. M. Posey (Eds.), *Pharmacotherapy: A pathophysiologic approach* (6th ed., pp. 103–113). New York: McGraw-Hill.

Melnyk, B. M., & Finout-Overholt, E. (2005). *Evidence-based practice in nursing & healthcare.* Philadelphia: Lippincott Williams & Wilkins.

Nahata, M. C., & Taketomo, C. (2005). Pediatrics. In J. T. DiPiro, R. L. Talbert, G. C. Yee, G. R. Matzke, B. G. Wells, & L. M. Posey (Eds.), *Pharmacotherapy: A pathophysiologic approach* (6th ed., pp. 91–101). New York: McGraw-Hill.

Pravikoff, D. S., Tanner, A. B., & Pierce, S. T. (2005). Readiness of U.S. nurses for evidence-based practice. *American Journal of Nursing, 105,* 40–51.

Smeltzer, S. C., Bare, B. G., Hinkle, J. H., & Cheever, K. H. (2008). *Brunner & Suddarth's textbook of medical-surgical nursing* (11th ed., pp. 4–14). Philadelphia: Lippincott Williams & Wilkins.

Stevens, K. R., & Staley, J. M. (2006). The *Quality Chasm* reports, evidence-based practice, and nursing's response to improve healthcare. *Nursing Outlook, 54,* 94–101.

Chapter Outline

Physiology of the Central Nervous System

LEARNING OBJECTIVES

After studying this chapter, you will be able to:

1. Describe the process of neurotransmission.
2. Describe major neurotransmitters and their roles in central nervous system (CNS) functioning.
3. Discuss signs and symptoms of CNS depression.
4. Discuss general types and characteristics of CNS depressant drugs.

Introduction

The central nervous system (CNS), which is composed of the brain and spinal cord, acts as the control center for regulating physical and mental body processes. Afferent or sensory neurons carry messages to the CNS, and efferent or motor neurons carry messages away from the CNS. More specifically, the CNS constantly receives information about blood levels of oxygen and carbon dioxide, body temperature, and sensory stimuli and sends messages to effector organs to adjust the environment toward homeostasis. It is also concerned with higher intellectual functions (e.g., thought, learning, reasoning, problem solving, and memory) and with muscle function, both skeletal and smooth.

The CNS carries out its functions by transmitting electrical and chemical signals among components of the CNS and between the CNS and other parts of the body. Structural components and functions of the CNS are described in Box 5-1; more specific characteristics of neurons and neurotransmission are described below. These characteristics are reviewed to aid in the understanding of drugs that act by altering CNS functions.

Neurons

The CNS is composed of two types of cells: The *neuron* is the basic functional unit, and the *glia* protect, support, and nourish the neuron. Most neurons are composed of a cell body, a dendrite, and an axon. A dendrite has a branching structure with many synapses or sites for receiving stimuli or messages, which are then conducted toward the cell body. An axon is a finger-like projection that carries impulses away from the cell body. The end of the axon branches into presynaptic fibers that end with small, knob-like structures called vesicles. These structures project into the synapse and contain the granules where neurotransmitters are stored. Many axons are covered by myelin, which protects and insulates the axon. An axon together with its myelin sheath is called a nerve fiber. Nerve fibers that transmit the same type of impulses (e.g., pain signals) are found together in a common pathway or tract.

Box 5-1	CNS Structures and Functions

Cerebral Cortex

The cerebral cortex is involved in all conscious processes (e.g., learning, memory, reasoning, verbalization, and voluntary body movements). Some parts receive incoming nerve impulses and are called sensory areas. Other parts send impulses to peripheral structures and are called motor areas. Around the sensory and motor areas are the "association" areas, which occupy the greater portion of the cortex. These areas analyze the information received by the sensory areas and decide on the appropriate response (e.g., stimulation of motor centers to produce movement or speech).

Thalamus

The thalamus receives impulses carrying sensations such as heat, cold, pain, and muscle position sense. These sensations produce a crude awareness in the thalamus; they are relayed to the cerebral cortex, where they are interpreted regarding location, quality, intensity, and significance. The thalamus also relays motor impulses from the cortex to the spinal cord.

Hypothalamus

The hypothalamus has extensive neurologic and endocrine functions. In the CNS, it is connected with the thalamus, medulla oblongata, spinal cord, reticular activating system, and limbic system. In the autonomic nervous system, it is the center for motor control. In the endocrine system, it controls the secretion of all pituitary hormones, is anatomically connected to the posterior pituitary gland, and regulates the activity of the anterior pituitary. The hypothalamus helps maintain homeostasis by constantly adjusting water balance, temperature, hormone levels, blood pressure, and other body functions. It is stimulated or inhibited by nerve impulses from different portions of the nervous system and by concentrations of nutrients, electrolytes, water, and hormones in the blood.

Specific neuroendocrine functions of the hypothalamus include the following:

- Producing oxytocin and antidiuretic hormone (ADH), which are stored in the posterior pituitary gland and released in response to nerve impulses from the hypothalamus. Oxytocin initiates uterine contractions to begin labor and delivery and helps release milk from breast glands during breast-feeding. ADH helps maintain fluid balance by controlling water excretion.
- Regulating body temperature. When body temperature is elevated, sweating and dilation of blood vessels in the skin increase heat loss and lower the temperature. When body temperature is low, sweating stops and vasoconstriction occurs to decrease heat loss and raise the temperature.
- Assisting in regulation of blood pressure by its effects on the vasomotor center located in the medulla oblongata and pons. This center maintains a state of partial contraction in blood vessels (vasomotor tone or vasoconstriction). When nerve impulses from the hypothalamus excite the vasomotor center, vasomotor tone is increased, and blood pressure

is raised. When the impulses inhibit the vasomotor center, vasomotor tone is decreased, with the overall effect of relative vasodilation and lowering of blood pressure.
- Regulating anterior pituitary hormones, including thyroid-stimulating hormone, ACTH, and growth hormone. The hypothalamus secretes a "releasing factor" for each anterior pituitary hormone.
- Regulating food and water intake by the hypothalamic thirst, appetite, hunger, and satiety centers.
- Regulating the physical changes associated with emotions (e.g., increased blood pressure and heart rate). The hypothalamus, thalamus, and cerebral cortex interact to produce the feelings associated with emotions.

Medulla Oblongata

The medulla contains groups of neurons that form the vital cardiac, respiratory, and vasomotor centers. For example, if the respiratory center is stimulated, respiratory rate and depth are increased. If the respiratory center is depressed, respiratory rate and depth are decreased. The medulla also contains reflex centers for coughing, vomiting, sneezing, swallowing, and salivating. The medulla and pons varolii also contain groups of neurons from which cranial nerves 5 through 12 originate.

Reticular Activating System

The reticular activating system is a network of neurons that extends from the spinal cord through the medulla and pons to the thalamus and hypothalamus. It receives impulses from all parts of the body, evaluates the significance of the impulses, and decides which impulses to transmit to the cerebral cortex. It also excites or inhibits motor nerves that control both reflex and voluntary movement. Stimulation of these neurons produces wakefulness and mental alertness, and depression causes sedation and loss of consciousness.

Limbic System

The limbic system borders and interconnects with the thalamus, hypothalamus, basal ganglia, hippocampus, amygdala, and septum. It participates in regulation of feeding behavior, the sleep–wake cycle, emotions (e.g., pleasure, fear, anger, sadness), and behavior (e.g., aggression, laughing, crying). Many nerve impulses from the limbic system are transmitted through the hypothalamus; thus, physiologic changes in blood pressure, heart rate, respiration, and hormone secretion occur in response to emotions.

Cerebellum

The cerebellum, which is connected with motor centers in the cerebral cortex and basal ganglia, coordinates muscle activity. For example, when several skeletal muscles are involved, some are contracted and some are relaxed for smooth, purposeful movements. It also helps maintain balance and posture by receiving nerve impulses from the inner ear that produce appropriate reflex responses.

(continued on page 74)

Box 5-1	CNS Structures and Functions (continued)

Basal Ganglia

The basal ganglia are concerned with skeletal muscle tone and orderly activity. Normal function is influenced by dopamine. Degenerative changes in one of these areas, the substantia nigra, cause dopamine to be released in decreased amounts. This process is a factor in the development of Parkinson's disease.

Pyramidal and Extrapyramidal Systems

The pyramidal and extrapyramidal systems are pathways out of the cerebral cortex that intermingle in the spinal cord. Disease processes affecting higher levels of the CNS involve both tracts. In the pyramidal tract, nerve fibers originate in the cerebral cortex, go down the brain stem to the medulla, where the fibers cross, and continue down the spinal cord, where they end at various levels. Impulses are then carried from the spinal cord to skeletal muscle. Because the fibers cross in the medulla, impulses from the right side of the cerebral cortex control skeletal muscle movements of the left side of the body and impulses from the left control muscle movements of the right side. In the extrapyramidal system, fibers originate mainly in the premotor area of the cerebral cortex and travel to the basal ganglia and brain stem. The fibers are called extrapyramidal because they do not enter the medullary pyramids and cross over.

Brain Metabolism

To function properly, the brain must have an adequate and continuous supply of oxygen, glucose, and thiamine. *Oxygen* is carried to the brain by the carotid and vertebral arteries. The brain requires more oxygen than any other organ. Cerebral cortex cells are very sensitive to lack of oxygen (hypoxia), and interruption of blood supply causes immediate loss of consciousness. Brain stem cells are less sensitive to hypoxia. *Glucose* is required as an energy source for brain cell metabolism. Hypoglycemia (low blood sugar) may cause mental confusion, dizziness, convulsions, loss of consciousness, and permanent damage to the cerebral cortex. *Thiamine* is required for production and use of glucose. Thiamine deficiency can reduce the use of glucose by nerve cells and can cause degeneration of the myelin sheath. Such degeneration in central neurons leads to a form of brain damage known as Wernicke-Korsakoff encephalopathy. Degeneration in peripheral nerves leads to polyneuritis and muscle atrophy, weakness, and paralysis.

Spinal Cord

The spinal cord is continuous with the medulla and extends down through the vertebral column to the sacral area. It consists of 31 segments, each of which is the point of origin for a pair of spinal nerves. The cord is a pathway between the brain and the peripheral nervous system. It carries impulses to and from the brain, along sensory and motor nerve fibers, and is a center for reflex actions. Reflexes are involuntary responses to certain nerve impulses received by the spinal cord (e.g., knee-jerk and pupillary reflexes).

Elements of Neurotransmission

Neurons must be able to communicate with other neurons and body tissues. This communication involves a complex network of electrical and chemical signals that receive, interpret, modify, and send messages. Characteristics that allow neurons to communicate with other body cells include excitability (the ability to produce an action potential or be stimulated) and conductivity (the ability to convey electrical impulses). Specific components of the communication network include neurotransmitters, synapses, and receptors.

Neurotransmitters

Neurotransmitters are chemical substances that carry messages from one neuron to another or from a neuron to other body tissues, such as cardiac or skeletal muscle. They are synthesized and stored in presynaptic nerve terminals and released in response to an electrical impulse (action potential) arriving at the end of the first neuron (presynaptic fiber). The basis for the action potential is the transient opening of ion channels. The entry of calcium ions is required for neurotransmitter release from storage sites in small sacs called synaptic vesicles.

When released from the synaptic vesicles, molecules of neurotransmitter cross the synapse, bind to receptors in the cell membrane of the postsynaptic neuron (Fig. 5-1), and excite or inhibit postsynaptic neurons. Free neurotransmitter molecules (i.e., those not bound to receptors) are rapidly removed from the synapse by three mechanisms: transportation back into the presynaptic nerve terminal (reuptake) for reuse, diffusion into surrounding body fluids, or destruction by enzymes.

The main types of neurotransmitters are amines, amino acids, and peptides, which are derived from body proteins. Most acute CNS responses are caused by fast-acting neurotransmitters (e.g., acetylcholine, dopamine, norepinephrine, serotonin) and amino acids (aspartate, gamma-aminobutyric acid [GABA], glutamate, and glycine). Most prolonged CNS responses are caused by slow-acting neurotransmitters (e.g., adrenocorticotropic hormone [ACTH or corticotropin] and antidiuretic hormone [ADH]).

Several factors affect the availability and function of neurotransmitters, including the following:

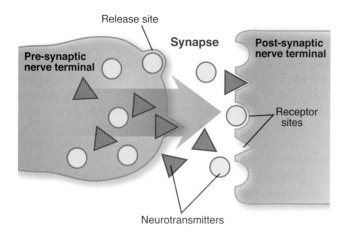

Figure 5-1 ▪ Neurotransmission in the central nervous system. Neurotransmitter molecules (e.g., norepinephrine, acetylcholine), released by the presynaptic nerve, cross the synapse and bind with receptor proteins in the cell membrane of the postsynaptic nerve.

- The availability of precursor proteins and enzymes required to synthesize particular neurotransmitters

- The number and binding capacity of receptors in the cell membranes of presynaptic and postsynaptic nerve endings

- Acid–base imbalances (acidosis decreases and alkalosis increases synaptic transmission)

- Hypoxia, which causes CNS depression (coma occurs within seconds without oxygen)

- Drugs, which may alter neurotransmitter synthesis, release, degradation, or binding to receptors to cause either CNS stimulation or depression

Synapses

Neurons in a chain are separated by a microscopic gap called a *synapse*. Synapses may be electrical, in which sodium and potassium ions conduct an electrical impulse from one neuron to another, or chemical, in which a neurotransmitter conducts the message to the next neuron. The chemical synapse is more commonly used to communicate with other neurons or target cells. Neurotransmitter release and removal occur in the synapses.

Receptors

Receptors are proteins embedded in the cell membranes of neurons. In the CNS, most receptors are on postsynaptic neurons; a few are on presynaptic nerve terminals. A neurotransmitter must bind to receptors to exert an effect on the next neuron in the chain. Some receptors act rapidly to open ion channels, and others interact with intracellular proteins to initiate a second messenger system. For example, when norepinephrine binds with adrenergic receptors, intracellular events include activation of the enzyme adenyl cyclase and the production of cyclic adenosine monophosphate (cAMP). In this case, the

cAMP is a second messenger that activates cellular functions and the physiologic responses controlled by the adrenergic receptors. A neurotransmitter–receptor complex may have an excitatory or inhibitory effect on the postsynaptic neuron.

Receptors are constantly being synthesized and degraded. They increase in number and activity (up-regulation) when there is underactivity at the synapse. They decrease in number and activity (down-regulation) when there is overactivity. Overall, receptors work with other control mechanisms of the nervous system to readjust abnormally stimulated or depressed nerve function toward normal.

Neurotransmission Systems

Neurotransmitters, synapses, and receptors work together to produce communication networks that may be called *neurotransmission* systems. It is the interactions between and among these systems that promote order or disorder in the body's physical and mental processes. Major neurotransmission systems are the cholinergic, dopaminergic, GABA-ergic, noradrenergic, and serotonergic.

The **cholinergic system** uses *acetylcholine* as its neurotransmitter. Acetylcholine is located in many areas of the brain, with high concentrations in the motor cortex and basal ganglia. It is also a neurotransmitter in the autonomic nervous system and at peripheral neuromuscular junctions. Acetylcholine exerts excitatory effects at synapses and nerve–muscle junctions and inhibitory effects at some peripheral sites, such as organs supplied by the vagus nerve. In the CNS, acetylcholine is associated with level of arousal, memory, motor function, and speech.

The **dopaminergic system** uses *dopamine* as its neurotransmitter. Dopamine is found in the substantia nigra, the midbrain, and the hypothalamus. It also is found outside the brain, in renal and mesenteric blood vessels.

In the CNS, dopamine is inhibitory in the basal ganglia but may be excitatory in other areas. Repeated stimulation of dopamine receptors decreases their numbers (down-regulation) and their sensitivity to dopamine (desensitization). Prolonged blockade of dopamine receptors increases their numbers and sensitivity to dopamine. Some receptors (called autoreceptors) occur on the presynaptic nerve terminal. When released, dopamine stimulates these receptors and a negative feedback system is initiated that inhibits further dopamine synthesis and release.

Two groups of dopamine receptors have been identified. They are differentiated by the intracellular events that follow dopamine–receptor binding. One group includes D1 and D5 receptors, which activate adenyl cyclase to produce cAMP. The other group includes D2, D3, and D4 receptors. D2 receptors are thought to inhibit activation of adenyl cyclase and subsequent production of cAMP, suppress calcium ion currents, and activate potassium ion currents. The functions of D3 and D4 receptors have not been delineated. Overall, dopamine actions at the cellular level depend on the subtype of receptor to which it binds and the simultaneous effects of other neurotransmitters at the same target neurons.

The **GABA-ergic system** uses GABA as its neurotransmitter. *Gamma-aminobutyric acid (GABA)* is abundant in the brain and spinal cord. It is the major inhibitory neurotransmitter in the CNS, with a role in many neuronal circuits (estimated at nearly one third of CNS synapses). GABA receptors have been divided into two main types, A and B. The GABA$_A$ receptor is a chloride ion channel that opens when GABA is released from presynaptic neurons. The GABA$_B$ receptor is associated with potassium conductance. There is evidence of multiple subtypes of GABA receptors and important functional differences among them.

The **noradrenergic system** uses *norepinephrine* as its neurotransmitter. Norepinephrine is a catecholamine that is found in relatively large amounts in the hypothalamus and the limbic system and in smaller amounts in most areas of the brain, including the reticular formation. Norepinephrine is mainly an excitatory neurotransmitter that stimulates the brain to generalized increased activity. However, it is inhibitory in a few areas because of inhibitory receptors at some nerve synapses.

Norepinephrine receptors in the CNS are divided into alpha- and beta-adrenergic receptors and their subtypes. Activation of alpha$_1$, beta$_1$, and beta$_2$ receptors stimulates activity of intracellular adenyl cyclase and the production of cAMP. Activation of alpha$_2$ receptors inhibits adenyl cyclase activity and decreases production of cAMP. In addition, alpha$_2$ receptors on the presynaptic nerve ending regulate norepinephrine release (e.g., when high levels of extracellular norepinephrine act on presynaptic alpha$_2$ receptors, the effect is similar to that of a negative feedback system that inhibits the release of norepinephrine). Overall, the noradrenergic system is associated with mood, motor activity, regulation of arousal, and reward. It is thought to play an important role in producing rapid eye movement (REM) sleep, during which dreaming occurs.

The **serotonergic system** uses *serotonin* as its neurotransmitter. Serotonin-synthesizing neurons are widely distributed in the CNS. Because serotonin is synthesized from the amino acid tryptophan, the amount of tryptophan intake in the diet and the enzyme tryptophan hydroxylase control the rate of serotonin production. CNS serotonin is usually an inhibitory neurotransmitter and is associated with mood, the sleep–wake cycle, habituation, and sensory perceptions, including inhibition of pain pathways in the spinal cord. Serotonin is thought to produce sleep by inhibiting CNS activity and arousal. Serotonin receptors are associated with mood, anxiety, and temperature regulation. Activation of some receptors leads to hyperpolarization and neuronal inhibition. Several subtypes of serotonin receptors have been identified.

Serotonin is also found outside the CNS, mainly in mast cells of the lungs and platelets. It plays a major role in the blood coagulation process, during which it is released from platelets and causes vasoconstriction. It may also be involved in the vascular spasm associated with some pulmonary allergic reactions (during which it is released from mast cells) and migraine headaches. However, peripheral serotonin cannot cross the blood–brain barrier.

The **amino acid system** includes several amino acids that may serve as both structural components for protein synthesis and neurotransmitters. *Aspartate* is an excitatory neurotransmitter found in high concentrations in the brain. *Glycine* is an inhibitory neurotransmitter found in the brain stem and spinal cord. Glycine receptors are similar to GABA$_A$ receptors; subtypes have been identified but their functions are unknown.

Glutamate, the most important excitatory neurotransmitter, occurs in high concentrations in most areas of the CNS. Several subtypes of glutamate receptors have been identified, each with a unique distribution in the CNS. The functions of these receptor subtypes have not been established, but research suggests that the N-methyl D-aspartate (NMDA) glutamate receptor subtype plays a role in memory. Some glutamate is needed for normal neurotransmission, but high concentrations can lead to neuronal cell death. Events leading to neuronal death are triggered by excessive activation of NMDA receptors and movement of calcium ions into the neurons. This process may be similar to the neurotoxicity associated with brain injury (e.g., from ischemia, hypoglycemia, or hypoxia), where increased release and impaired reuptake of glutamate lead to excessive stimulation of glutamate receptors and subsequent cell death. Altered glutamate metabolism may also lead to the formation of free radicals, which are implicated in neuronal cell death associated with some neurodegenerative diseases and toxic chemicals, including some drugs of abuse.

Neurotransmission Systems in Selected Central Nervous System Disorders

Abnormalities in neurotransmission systems (e.g., dysfunction or destruction of the neurons that normally produce neurotransmitters; altered receptor response to neurotransmitters) are implicated in many CNS disorders. For example, decreased acetylcholine is a characteristic of Alzheimer's disease; dopamine abnormalities occur in psychosis and Parkinson's disease; GABA abnormalities occur in anxiety, hyperarousal states, and seizure disorders; glutamate has been implicated in the pathogenesis of epilepsy, schizophrenia, stroke, and Huntington's disease; and serotonin abnormalities are thought to be involved in mental depression and sleep disorders.

Although most research has focused on single neurotransmitters and their respective receptors, CNS function in both health and disease is largely determined by interactions among neurotransmission systems. In health, for example, complex mechanisms regulate the amounts and binding capacities of neurotransmitters and receptors, as well as the balance between excitatory and inhibitory forces. When abnormalities occur in any of these elements, the resulting dysregulation and imbalances lead to signs and symptoms of CNS disorders. Overall, then, neurotransmission systems function interdependently; one system may increase, decrease, or otherwise modify the effects of another system.

Except for mental depression, most psychiatric symptoms result from CNS stimulation and usually involve physical and mental hyperactivity. Such hyperactivity reflects observable behaviors and nonobservable thoughts and feelings. In most people, manifestations may include pleasant feelings of mild euphoria and high levels of enthusiasm, energy, and productivity. In people with severe anxiety or psychosis, manifestations include unpleasant feelings of tension, psychomotor agitation, nervousness, and decreased ability to rest and sleep. Many psychiatric disorders, therapeutic drugs, and drugs of abuse may cause varying degrees of CNS stimulation. In general, the pathogenesis of excessive CNS stimulation may involve one or more of the following mechanisms:

▪ Excessive amounts of excitatory neurotransmitters (e.g., norepinephrine, glutamate)

▪ Increased numbers or sensitivity of excitatory receptors

▪ Insufficient amounts of inhibitory neurotransmitters (e.g., GABA)

▪ Decreased numbers or sensitivity of inhibitory receptors

Drugs That Affect the Central Nervous System

Drugs that affect the CNS, sometimes called centrally active drugs, are broadly classified as depressants or stimulants.

CNS depressants (e.g., antipsychotics, opioid analgesics, sedative-hypnotics) produce a general depression of the CNS when given in sufficient dosages. Mild CNS depression is characterized by lack of interest in surroundings and inability to focus on a topic (short attention span). Moderate CNS depression is characterized by drowsiness or sleep; decreased muscle tone; decreased ability to move; and decreased perception of sensations such as pain, heat, and cold. Severe CNS depression is characterized by unconsciousness or coma, loss of reflexes, respiratory failure, and death.

Central nervous system stimulants produce a variety of effects. Mild stimulation is characterized by wakefulness, mental alertness, and decreased fatigue. Increasing stimulation produces hyperactivity, excessive talking, nervousness, and insomnia. Excessive stimulation can cause convulsions, cardiac dysrhythmias, and death.

Key Concepts

▪ The CNS regulates physical and mental body processes through complex communication systems between and among CNS structures.

▪ Afferent neurons carry messages to the CNS; efferent neurons carry messages from the CNS to other body tissues.

▪ Messages are transmitted by the interaction of neurotransmitters and receptors across the synapse.

▪ Major neurotransmitters are acetylcholine, dopamine, GABA, glutamate, norepinephrine, and serotonin. Some excite and some inhibit CNS functions.

▪ Each neurotransmitter has its specific receptors.

▪ CNS depressant drugs are more often used to treat CNS disorders than CNS stimulants.

Review and Application Exercises

Short Answer Exercises

1. Where are neurotransmitters synthesized and stored?
2. What events occur at the synapse between two neurons?
3. After a neurotransmitter is released and acts on receptors, how are the remaining molecules inactivated?
4. What are the main functions of acetylcholine, dopamine, GABA, norepinephrine, and serotonin?
5. What part of the brain is concerned mainly with thoughts, reasoning, and learning?
6. What part of the brain contains vital respiratory and cardiovascular centers?
7. How would you expect a person with CNS depression to look and behave?
8. How would you expect a person with excessive CNS stimulation to look and behave?

NCLEX-Style Questions

9. Up-regulation of receptors occurs when
   a. receptors are degraded faster than they are synthesized.
   b. receptors increase in number and activity.
   c. there is a decrease in both the number and activity of the receptors.
   d. addictive drugs are supplied to patients in diminished amount.

10. A patient has Parkinson's disease. In caring for him and administering medications, the nurse understands his symptoms and his drug regimen as being related to
    a. an increase in the neurotransmitter serotonin
    b. a decrease in the neurotransmitter serotonin
    c. an increase in the neurotransmitter dopamine
    d. a decrease in the neurotransmitter dopamine

11. The neurotransmitter system most associated with rapid eye movement (REM) sleep is
    a. the cholinergic system
    b. the GABA-ergic system
    c. the noradrenergic system
    d. the serotonergic system

12. When caring for a patient with serious sleep disorders that are linked to an imbalance in neurotransmitters, the nurse knows that this patient is most likely to have an abnormal level of
    a. serotonin
    b. GABA
    c. acetylcholine
    d. dopamine

13. A patient is being admitted to a unit with a diagnosis of Wernicke-Korsakoff syndrome. The nurse knows that this condition is triggered by a deficiency in
    a. acetylcholine
    b. calcium
    c. thiamine
    d. insulin

Selected References

Carroll, E. W., & Curtis, R. L. (2005). Organization and control of neural function. In C. M. Porth (Ed.), *Pathophysiology: Concepts of altered health states* (7th ed., pp. 1113–1157). Philadelphia: Lippincott Williams & Wilkins.

Guyton, A. C., & Hall, J. E. (2006). *Textbook of medical physiology* (11th ed.). Philadelphia: Elsevier Saunders.

Smeltzer, S. C., Bare, B. G., Hinkle, J. L., & Cheever, K. H. (2008). *Brunner & Suddarth's textbook of medical-surgical nursing* (11th ed., pp. 2128–2159). Philadelphia: Lippincott Williams & Wilkins.

Opioid Analgesics and Pain Management

LEARNING OBJECTIVES

After studying this chapter, you will be able to:

1. Discuss major types and characteristics of pain.
2. Discuss the nurse's role in assessing and managing patients' pain.
3. List characteristics of opioid analgesics in terms of mechanism of action, indications for use, and major adverse effects.
4. Describe morphine as the prototype of opioid analgesics.
5. Differentiate between ceiling and nonceiling opioids.
6. Explain why higher doses of opioid analgesics are needed when the drugs are given orally.
7. Contrast the use of opioid analgesics in opioid-naive and opioid-tolerant patients.
8. Assess level of consciousness and respiratory status before and after administering opioids.
9. Teach patients about safe, effective use of opioid analgesics.
10. Describe characteristics and treatment of opioid toxicity.
11. Discuss principles of therapy for using opioid analgesics in special populations.
12. Discuss nonopioid drugs used in pain management.

Applying Your Knowledge

Moe Harris is a 53-year-old man who had a lumbar laminectomy with spinal fusion today.

Mr. Harris has experienced chronic low back pain for more than 10 years. During this time, he has been treated with a number of over-the-counter (OTC) and prescription medications for his pain. These drugs have included ibuprofen and hydrocodone with acetaminophen. He is a construction worker, married with three children, a nonsmoker, and drinks beer regularly.

Mr. Harris returns from the postanesthesia recovery room to your care at 10:00 A.M. His vital signs are stable on initial assessment. To treat his pain, the physician has ordered the following:

Morphine 4–8 mg IV, every 2–4 hours as needed, to be given over 5 minutes

After 24 hours, oxycodone 5 mg with acetaminophen 500 mg PO every 4–6 hours, PRN, not to exceed six doses in 24 hours

Introduction

Pain is the most common symptom prompting people to seek health care. This unpleasant, uncomfortable sensation usually indicates tissue damage and impels a person to remove the cause of the damage or seek relief from the pain. When not managed effectively, pain may greatly impair quality of life and ability to perform activities of daily living. The Joint Commission on the Accreditation of Healthcare Organizations (JCAHO) includes assessment and management of pain for all patients in the standards by which it evaluates health care organizations. Opioid (narcotic) analgesics are drugs that relieve moderate to severe pain. To aid understanding of drug actions, selected characteristics of pain and endogenous pain-relieving substances are described.

Physiology of Pain

Pain occurs when tissue damage activates the free nerve endings (pain receptors or nociceptors) of peripheral nerves. *Nociceptors* are abundant in arterial walls, joint surfaces, muscle fascia, periosteum, skin, and soft tissues; they are scarce in most internal organs. Causes of tissue damage may be physical (e.g., heat, cold, pressure, stretch, spasm, ischemia) or chemical (e.g., pain-producing substances are released into the extracellular fluid surrounding the nerve fibers that carry the pain signal). These pain-producing substances activate pain receptors, increase the sensitivity of pain receptors, or stimulate the release of inflammatory substances.

For a person to feel pain, the signal from the nociceptors in peripheral tissues must be transmitted to the spinal cord, then to the hypothalamus and cerebral cortex in the brain. The signal is carried to the spinal cord by two types of nerve cells, A-delta fibers and C fibers. A-delta fibers, which are myelinated and found mainly in skin and muscle, transmit fast, sharp, well-localized pain signals. These fibers release glutamate and aspartate (excitatory amino acid neurotransmitters) at synapses in the spinal cord. C fibers, which are unmyelinated and found in muscle, abdominal viscera, and periosteum,

conduct the pain signal slowly and produce a poorly localized, dull, or burning type of pain. Tissue damage resulting from an acute injury often produces an initial sharp pain transmitted by A-delta fibers followed by a dull ache or burning sensation transmitted by C fibers. C fibers release somatostatin and substance P at synapses in the spinal cord. Glutamate, aspartate, substance P, and perhaps other chemical mediators enhance transmission of the pain signal.

The dorsal horn of the spinal cord is the control center or relay station for information from the A-delta and C nerve fibers, for local modulation of the pain impulse, and for descending influences from higher centers in the central nervous system (CNS; e.g., attention, emotion, memory). Here, nociceptive nerve fibers synapse with non-nociceptive nerve fibers (neurons that carry information other than pain signals). The brain also contains descending pathways that inhibit nociceptive input. Some brain nuclei are serotonergic and project to the dorsal horn of the spinal cord, where they suppress nociceptive transmission. Another inhibitory pathway is noradrenergic and originates in the pons. Thus, increasing the concentration of norepinephrine and serotonin in the synapse inhibits transmission of nerve impulses that carry pain signals to the brain and spinal cord.

In the brain, the thalamus is a relay station for incoming sensory stimuli, including pain. Perception of pain is a primitive awareness in the thalamus, and sensation is not well localized. From the thalamus, pain messages are relayed to the cerebral cortex, where they are perceived more specifically and analyzed to determine actions needed.

Pain may be classified according to origin in body structures (e.g., somatic, visceral, *neuropathic*), duration (e.g., acute, chronic), or cause (e.g., cancer). These types of pain are described in Box 6-1.

| Box 6-1 | Types and Characteristics of Pain |

Acute pain may be caused by injury, trauma, spasm, disease processes, and treatment or diagnostic procedures that damage body tissues. It is often described as sharp or cutting. The intensity of the pain is usually proportional to the amount of tissue damage and the pain serves as a warning system by demanding the sufferer's attention and compelling behavior to withdraw from or avoid the pain-producing stimulus.

Acute pain is called fast pain because it is felt quickly after a pain stimulus is applied. It is aroused by mechanical and thermal stimuli and conducted to the spinal cord by A-delta fibers in the peripheral nerves. Glutamate is the neurotransmitter secreted in the spinal cord at the A-delta nerve fiber endings.

Acute pain is often accompanied by anxiety and objective signs of discomfort (e.g., facial expressions of distress; moaning or crying; positioning to protect the affected part; tenderness, edema, and skin color or temperature changes in the affected part; and either restlessness and excessive movement or limited movement, if movement increases pain). It usually responds to treatment with analgesic drugs and resolves as tissue repair mechanisms heal the damaged area.

Chronic pain (i.e., lasting 3 months or longer) demands attention less urgently, may not be characterized by visible signs, and is often accompanied by emotional stress, increased irritability, depression, social withdrawal, financial distress, loss of libido, disturbed sleep patterns, diminished appetite, weight loss, and decreased ability to perform usual activities of daily living. It may occur with or without evidence of tissue damage and may include acute pain that persists beyond the typical recovery time for the precipitating tissue injury, pain related to a chronic disease, pain without an identifiable cause, and pain associated with cancer. It may arise from essentially any part of the body. It may be continuous or episodic or a combination of both.

Chronic pain may also be called slow pain. It can be elicited by mechanical, thermal, and chemical stimuli and is described as burning, aching, or throbbing. Slow, chronic pain is transmitted by C nerve fibers to the spinal cord and brain. Substance P is the neurotransmitter at C nerve fiber endings; it is released slowly and accumulates over seconds or minutes.

Cancer pain has characteristics of both acute and chronic pain and it may be constant or intermittent. Chronic cancer pain is often caused by tumor spread into pain-sensitive tissues and the resulting tissue destruction. It usually progresses as the disease advances and can be severe and debilitating. Acute pain is often associated with diagnostic procedures or treatment measures (e.g., surgery, chemotherapy). It may also occur with disease progression, with activity, or with the development of drug tolerance.

Somatic pain results from stimulation of nociceptors in skin, bone, muscle, and soft tissue. It is usually well localized and described as sharp, burning, gnawing, throbbing, or cramping. It may be intermittent or constant and acute or chronic. Sprains and other traumatic injuries are examples of acute somatic pain; the bone and joint pain of arthritis is an example of chronic somatic pain, although acute exacerbations may also occur. Somatic pain of low to moderate intensity may stimulate the sympathetic nervous system and produce increased blood pressure, pulse, and respiration; dilated pupils; and increased skeletal muscle tension, such as rigid posture or clenched fists.

Visceral pain, which is diffuse and not well localized, results when nociceptors are stimulated in abdominal or thoracic organs and their surrounding tissues. It includes pain associated with cholecystitis, pancreatitis, uterine disorders,

and liver disease and is often described as deep, dull, aching, or cramping. It may be referred to a different part of the body (e.g., pain from the liver can be referred to the right shoulder area; ischemic pain from the heart can be referred to the left arm or neck area). Severe visceral pain stimulates the parasympathetic nervous system and produces decreased blood pressure and pulse, nausea and vomiting, weakness, syncope, and possibly loss of consciousness.

Neuropathic pain is caused by lesions or physiologic changes that injure peripheral pain receptors, nerves, or the CNS. It is characterized by excessive excitability in the damaged area or surrounding normal tissues, so that nerve cells discharge more easily. As a result, pain may arise spontaneously or from a normally nonpainful stimulus such as a light touch. It is a relatively common cause of chronic pain and is usually described as severe, shooting, burning, or stabbing. It occurs with peripheral neuropathies associated with diabetes mellitus (diabetic neuropathy), herpes zoster infections (postherpetic neuralgia), traumatic nerve injuries, and some types of cancer or cancer treatments. It is difficult to treat because standard analgesics (e.g., nonsteroidal anti inflammatory drugs and opioids) are less effective in neuropathic pain than in other types of pain. Antidepressants and anticonvulsants are often used along with analgesics.

Endogenous Analgesia System

The CNS has its own system for relieving pain by suppressing the transmission of pain signals from peripheral nerves. The system can be activated by nerve signals entering the brain or by morphine-like drugs. Important elements include opioid receptors and endogenous peptides with actions similar to those of morphine. *Opioid receptors* are highly concentrated in some regions of the CNS, including the ascending and descending pain pathways and portions of the brain essential to the *endogenous analgesia system.* The opioid peptides (i.e., *endorphins,* enkephalins, dynorphins) interact with opioid receptors to inhibit perception and transmission of pain signals. Endorphin release can be triggered by excitement, stress, or aerobic exercise. Enkephalins are believed to interrupt the transmission of pain signals at the spinal cord level by inhibiting the release of substance P from C nerve fibers. The

endogenous analgesia system may also inhibit pain signals at other points in the pain pathway.

Drug Therapy for Pain Management

Opioid analgesics are used to prevent or relieve moderate to severe pain. Nonopioid drugs are also used, and a combination of drugs that act by different mechanisms is often the most effective regimen for pain management. Nonopioid drugs belong to several classifications and either have analgesic effects themselves or modify disease processes in a way that reduces pain. Nonopioid analgesics are used in the management of both acute and chronic pain; other nonopioids are used mainly for chronic neuropathic pain or bone pain. In either case, the drugs are often used concurrently with opioids to provide more effective pain relief. Nonopioid drugs used in pain management are listed in Box 6-2 and

| Box 6-2 | Nonopioid Drugs Used to Manage Pain |

Nonopioid analgesics and other drugs are commonly used to prevent or relieve acute and chronic pain. These drugs may be given in combination or concurrently with opioid analgesics for severe pain. They are called adjuvants, co-analgesics, or pain-modifying drugs.

Nonopioid Analgesics

These drugs are mainly acetaminophen and nonsteroidal anti-inflammatory drugs (NSAIDs). Acetaminophen acts on

the parts of the brain that receive pain signals and is one of the safest analgesics for management of mild pain or as a supplement in management of more intense pain. It is especially useful in nonspecific musculoskeletal pain or pain associated with osteoarthritis. The maximum daily dose of acetaminophen is 4000 milligrams, and the drug should be avoided or dosage reduced in patients with renal insufficiency or liver failure. NSAIDs (e.g., ibuprofen) reduce the production of prostaglandins, which in turn reduces inflammatory chemicals

(continued on page 82)

Box 6-2	Nonopioid Drugs Used to Manage Pain (continued)

that cause, increase, or maintain pain signals. NSAIDs are useful in treating many pain conditions that are caused or aggravated by inflammation. They may be used for moderate to severe pain alone or with opioids. Adverse effects include GI bleeding. In patients who require the drugs for long-term treatment of pain, a proton pump inhibitor such as omeprazole (Prilosec) can be given to decrease the risk of GI bleeding.

Antiepileptic Drugs (AEDs)

These drugs are mainly used to treat neuropathic pain, in which they decrease the irritability of overexcited nerve cells that occurs in both epilepsy and neuropathic pain. Decreasing neuronal irritability means the nerve cells carrying pain signals are less likely to discharge spontaneously or in response to stimuli. Gabapentin is commonly used for peripheral neuropathy and postherpetic neuralgia; lamotrigine is beneficial in pain associated with diabetes, human immunodeficiency virus (HIV) infection, and stroke, but dosage must be titrated slowly because of potentially severe adverse effects; and pregabalin is approved for treatment of diabetic neuropathy.

Antidepressants

Tricyclic antidepressants (TCAs) have long been used to relieve neuropathic pain. They inhibit the reuptake of norepinephrine and serotonin in nerve synapses, thereby making these neurotransmitters more available to inhibit pain signals. The drugs cause numerous adverse effects, especially in older adults, but their ability to promote sleep and relieve depression (which often accompanies chronic pain) may be beneficial enough to outweigh their disadvantages.

Venlafaxine and duloxetine are newer antidepressants that also inhibit the reuptake of serotonin and norepinephrine. Duloxetine is FDA approved to treat diabetic neuropathy.

Bisphosphonates

Bisphosphonates (e.g., alendronate, risedronate), drugs most often used to prevent or treat osteoporosis, can relieve pain related to metastatic bone cancer and multiple myeloma.

Corticosteroids

These drugs can reduce inflammation, irritability, and spontaneous discharge in injured nerves and other tissues. They are used to treat neuropathic, visceral, and bone pain. In cancer treatment, they may be given for pain associated with brain metastases and spinal cord compression. Dexamethasone is often used.

Local Anesthetics

Several lidocaine preparations are available to prevent or relieve pain. An oral preparation can be given to relieve mouth and throat pain but is not recommended for long-term use. A transdermal gel and patch (Lidoderm) may be used to relieve the pain of postherpetic neuralgia. Epidural or intrathecal lidocaine (or bupivacaine) can be given with an opioid to reduce neuropathic pain. A mixture of local anesthetics (e.g., eutectic mixture of local anesthetics [EMLA]) may be applied topically in children to decrease the pain of injections and other procedures.

---

discussed mainly in other chapters; opioid analgesics are discussed below.

General Characteristics of Opioid Analgesics

Opioid analgesics relieve moderate to severe pain by inhibiting the transmission of pain signals from peripheral tissues to the brain, reducing the perception of pain sensation in the brain, producing sedation, and decreasing the emotional upsets often associated with pain. They also inhibit the production of pain and inflammation by prostaglandins and leukotrienes in peripheral tissues. Most of these drugs are Schedule II drugs under federal narcotic laws and may lead to drug abuse and dependence. These drugs are called opioids because they act like morphine in the body.

Opioids are well absorbed with oral, intramuscular, or subcutaneous administration. Oral drugs undergo significant first-pass metabolism in the liver, which means that oral doses must be larger than injected doses to have equivalent therapeutic effects. The drugs are extensively metabolized in the liver, and metabolites are excreted in urine. Morphine and meperidine

form pharmacologically active metabolites. Thus, liver impairment can interfere with metabolism, and kidney impairment can interfere with excretion. Drug accumulation and increased adverse effects may occur if dosage is not reduced.

Opioids exert widespread pharmacologic effects, especially in the CNS and the gastrointestinal (GI) system. These effects occur with usual doses and may be therapeutic or adverse, depending on the reason for use. CNS effects include *analgesia*; CNS depression, ranging from drowsiness to sleep to unconsciousness; decreased mental and physical activity; respiratory depression; nausea and vomiting; and pupil constriction. Sedation and respiratory depression are major adverse effects and are potentially life threatening. Newer opioids were developed in an effort to find drugs as effective as morphine in relieving pain while causing less sedation, respiratory depression, and dependence. However, this effort has not been successful: equianalgesic doses of these drugs produce sedative and respiratory depressant effects comparable with those of morphine. In the GI tract, opioids slow motility and may cause constipation and smooth muscle spasms in the bowel and biliary tract.

Because of the potentially fatal adverse effects and risks of drug abuse and dependence, all opioid analgesics have

BLACK BOX WARNINGS. Specific comments and precautions include the following:

- Fentanyl, hydromorphone, methadone, morphine, oxycodone, and oxymorphone have the highest risk of fatal overdoses because of respiratory depression and the highest potential for abuse.

- Most of these drugs are available under generic names and multiple brand names. They also are available in several different dosage formulations, each of which must be used appropriately, for safety and effectiveness. For example, morphine, oxycodone, and oxymorphone are available in both immediate-release and extended-release tablets or capsules. Health care providers and patients must be cautioned to avoid crushing or chewing the tablets or opening capsules, because immediate release of the drug constitutes an overdose. Two exceptions are the Avinza and Kadian capsule formulations of morphine. These capsules contain beads or pellets that can be released from the capsule and sprinkled over applesauce for administration in patients who cannot swallow pills or capsules. However, the beads and pellets should not be crushed or chewed.

- With fentanyl, Actiq and Fentora formulations are indicated only for breakthrough pain in patients who are also taking long-term opioids for chronic pain such as cancer. Duragesic skin patches are indicated only for opioid-tolerant patients who require an opioid analgesic. Ionsys is indicated only for postoperative pain. These formulations require special techniques of administration.

- Prescribed opioids should be kept locked up, even in home settings, to decrease use or theft of the drugs by people other than the patient for whom they are prescribed (e.g., drug abusers and dealers).

Mechanism of Action

Opioids relieve pain by binding to opioid receptors in the brain, spinal cord, and peripheral tissues. When bound to an opioid drug, opioid receptors function like gates that close and thereby block or decrease transmission of pain impulses from one nerve cell to the next. Opioid receptors also activate the endogenous analgesia system. The major types of receptors are mu, kappa, and delta. Most opioid effects (analgesia; CNS depression, with respiratory depression and sedation; euphoria; decreased GI motility; and physical dependence) are attributed to activation of the mu receptors. Analgesia, sedation, and decreased GI motility also occur with activation of kappa receptors. Delta receptors are important in the endogenous analgesia system but may not bind with opioid drugs.

Indications for Use

The main indication for the use of opioid analgesics is to prevent or relieve acute or chronic pain. Specific conditions in which opioids are used include acute myocardial infarction, biliary colic, renal colic, burns and other traumatic injuries, postoperative states, and cancer. These drugs are usually given for chronic pain only when other measures and milder drugs are ineffective, as in terminal cancer. Other clinical uses include

- Before and during surgery to promote sedation, decrease anxiety, facilitate induction of anesthesia, and decrease the amount of anesthesia required
- Before and during invasive diagnostic procedures, such as angiograms and endoscopic examinations
- During labor and delivery (obstetric analgesia)
- Treatment of GI disorders, such as abdominal cramping and diarrhea
- Treatment of acute pulmonary edema (morphine is used)
- Treatment of severe, unproductive cough (codeine may be used)

Contraindications to Use

Opioid analgesics are contraindicated or must be used very cautiously in people with respiratory depression, chronic lung disease, liver or kidney disease, prostatic hypertrophy, increased intracranial pressure, or hypersensitivity reactions to opioids and related drugs.

Subgroups and Individual Drugs

The two main subgroups of opioid analgesics are agonists and agonists/antagonists. The larger group of agonists includes morphine and morphine-like drugs. These agents have activity at mu and kappa opioid receptors and thus produce prototypical opioid effects. As their name indicates, the agonists/antagonists have both agonist and antagonist activity. In addition, numerous combinations of an opioid and acetaminophen or ibuprofen, nonopioid analgesics (see Chap. 7), are available and commonly used in most health care settings. Opioid antagonists are antidote drugs that reverse the effects of opioid agonists. Individual drugs are described in the following sections; trade names and dosages are listed in Table 6-1.

Opioid Agonists

P Morphine, the prototype, is an opium alkaloid that is used mainly to relieve moderate to severe pain. It is a Schedule II controlled drug most often given orally and parenterally. Patient response depends on route of administration and dosage. After IV injection, maximal analgesia and respiratory depression usually occur within 10 to 20 minutes. After IM injection, these effects occur in about 30 minutes. With Sub-Q injection, effects may be delayed up to 60 to 90 minutes. With oral administration of fast-acting (e.g., immediate-release) formulations, peak activity occurs in about 60 minutes. The duration of action is 5 to 7 hours. Long-acting tablets or capsules are given once or twice daily, with the goal of providing pain relief around the clock.

Morphine is about 30% bound to plasma proteins, and its half-life is 2 to 4 hours. It is metabolized in the liver and conjugated to an active metabolite that is excreted by the kidneys. Morphine and its metabolite accumulate in patients with impaired liver or kidney function and may cause prolonged sedation if dosage is not reduced.

Table 6-1	Drugs at a Glance: Opioid Analgesics	

	ROUTES AND DOSAGE RANGES	
Generic/Trade Name	**Adults**	**Children**
Agonists		
Codeine	Pain: PO, Sub-Q, IM 15–60 mg q4–6h PRN; usual dose 30 mg; maximum, 360 mg/24 h Cough: PO 10–20 mg q4h PRN; maximum, 120 mg/24 h	1 y or older, Pain: PO, Sub-Q, IM 0.5 mg/kg q4–6h PRN 2–6 y, Cough: PO 2.5–5 mg q4–6h; maximum, 30 mg/24 h 6–12 y, Cough: PO 5–10 mg q4–6h; maximum, 60 mg/24 h
Fentanyl (Actiq, Duragesic, Fentora, Ionsys, Sublimaze) Note: Actiq, Fentora, and Ionsys are special preparations for specific uses. Check manufacturers' instructions for dosage and administration instructions.	Preanesthetic sedation, IM 0.05–0.1 mg 30–60 min before surgery Analgesic adjunct to general anesthesia, IV total dose of 0.002–0.05 mg/kg, depending on the surgical procedure Adjunct to regional anesthesia, IM or slow IV (over 1–2 min) 0.05–0.1 mg PRN Postoperative analgesia, IM 0.05–0.1 mg, repeat in 1–2 h if needed General anesthesia, IV 0.05–0.1 mg/kg with oxygen and a muscle relaxant (maximum dose 0.15 mg/kg with open heart surgery, other major surgeries, and complicated neurologic or orthopedic procedures) Chronic pain, Duragesic transdermal system 2.5–10 mg every 72 h	Weight at least 10 kg: Conscious sedation or preanesthetic sedation, 5–15 mcg/kg of body weight (100–400 mcg), depending on weight, type of procedure, and other factors. Maximum dose, 400 mcg, regardless of age and weight. 2–12 y: General anesthesia induction and maintenance, IV 2–3 mcg/kg
Hydromorphone (Dilaudid)	PO 2–4 mg q4–6h PRN IM, Sub-Q, IV 1–2 mg q4–6h PRN (may be increased to 4 mg for severe pain) Rectal suppository 3 mg q6–8h	Dosage not established
Meperidine (Demerol)	IM, IV, Sub-Q, PO 50–100 mg q2–4h Obstetric analgesia, IM, Sub-Q 50–100 mg q2–4h for three or four doses	IM, Sub-Q, PO 1.1–1.75 mg/kg, up to adult dose, q3–4h
Methadone (Dolophine)	IM, Sub-Q, PO 2.5–10 mg q3–4h PRN	Not recommended
P Morphine (prototype) (MS Contin, Roxanol, others)	PO immediate-release, 5–30 mg q4h PRN PO controlled-release, 30 mg or more q8–12h IM, Sub-Q 5–20 mg/70 kg q4h PRN IV injection, 2–10 mg/70 kg, diluted in 5 mL water for injection and injected slowly, over 5 min, PRN IV continuous infusion, 0.1–1 mg/mL in 5% dextrose in water solution, by controlled infusion pump Epidurally, 2–5 mg/24 h; intrathecally, 0.2–1 mg/24 h Rectal, 10–20 mg q4h	IM, Sub-Q 0.05–0.2 mg/kg (up to 15 mg) q4h
Oxycodone (OxyContin, Roxicodone, others)	PO, immediate release, 5 mg q6h PRN (OxyIR, Oxydose, OxyFAST); 10–30 mg q4h PRN for other formulations PO, controlled release, 10 mg q12h, increased if necessary	Not recommended for children less than 12 years of age

	ROUTES AND DOSAGE RANGES	
Generic/Trade Name	Adults	Children
Agonists		
Oxymorphone (Numorphan, Opana)	PO (Opana), 10–20 mg q4–6h PO, extended release (Opana ER), 5 mg q12h, increased by 5–10 mg q12h every 3–7 days until pain relieved IM, Sub-Q 1–1.5 mg q4–6h PRN IV 0.5 mg q4–6h PRN Rectal, 5 mg q4–6h PRN Obstetric analgesia, IM 0.5–1 mg	Dosage not established
Propoxyphene (Darvon)	Propoxyphene hydrochloride PO 65 mg q4h PRN (maximal daily dose, 390 mg) Propoxyphene napsylate PO 100 mg q4h PRN (maximal daily dose, 600 mg)	Not recommended Not recommended
Tramadol (Ultram)	PO 50–100 mg q4–6h PRN (maximum, 400 mg/d) Renal impairment (Crcl under 30 mL/min): PO 50–100 mg q12h (maximum dose, 200 mg/d) Hepatic impairment (cirrhosis): PO 50 mg q12h Older adults (65–75 y): Same as adults, unless they also have renal or hepatic impairment Older adults (over 75 y): less than 300mg daily, in divided doses	Dosage not established
Agonists/Antagonists		
Butorphanol (Stadol)	IM, IV 1–4 mg q3–4h PRN Nasal spray 1 mg (one spray in one nostril) q3–4h PRN Older adults IM 1–2 mg q6–8h PRN Renal or hepatic impairment IM 1–2 mg q6–8h	Not recommended for children less than 18 years of age
Nalbuphine (Nubain)	IM, IV, Sub-Q 10 mg/70 kg q3–6h PRN	Not recommended
Opioid antagonist Naloxone (Narcan)	Overdose, IV 0.4–2 mg, repeat every 2–3 minutes if needed. Give IM or Sub-Q if unable to give IV. Postoperative reversal, IV 0.1–0.2 mg q2–3 minutes until desired level of reversal is attained	Birth to 5 y or weight less than 20 kg: 0.1 mg/kg; may repeat every 2–3 minutes if needed Age over 5 y or weight 20 kg or more: 2 mg/dose; may repeat every 2–3 minutes if needed

Crcl, creatinine clearance, PRN, as needed.

Oral administration of morphine is common for chronic pain associated with cancer. When given orally, relatively high doses are required, because part of each dose is metabolized in the liver and never reaches the systemic circulation. Concentrated solutions (e.g., Roxanol) and controlled-release tablets (e.g., MS Contin) have been developed for oral administration of these high doses.

In some cases of severe pain that cannot be controlled by other methods, morphine is administered as a continuous IV infusion. Other routes of administration include epidural, in which the drug is instilled through a catheter placed in the epidural space and slowly diffuses into the spinal cord, and intrathecal, in which the drug is injected directly into the spinal cord. Epidural and intrathecal morphine provide pain relief with very small doses, once or twice daily. When patients cannot take oral medications and injections are undesirable, rectal suppositories can be given.

Codeine is an opium alkaloid and Schedule II drug used for analgesic and antitussive effects. Codeine produces weaker analgesic and antitussive effects and milder adverse effects than morphine. Compared with other opioid analgesics, codeine is more effective when given orally and is less likely to lead to abuse and dependence. The injected drug is more effective than the oral drug in relieving pain, but onset (15 to 30 minutes), peak (30 to 60 minutes), and duration of action (4 to 6 hours) are about the same. Half-life is about 3 hours. Larger doses are required for analgesic than for antitussive effects. Codeine is often given with acetaminophen for additive analgesic effects.

Codeine is metabolized to morphine, which is responsible for its analgesic effects, by the cytochrome P450 2D6 family of enzymes. As many as 10% of whites, Asians, and African Americans have inadequate amounts or activity of the 2D6 enzymes and may therefore receive less pain relief with usual therapeutic doses.

Fentanyl (Sublimaze, others) is a potent opioid agonist that is widely used for preanesthetic medication, postoperative analgesia, and chronic pain that requires an opioid analgesic. Fentanyl is commonly given IV and may also be given IM. In addition, other formulations have been developed for other routes administration. **These formulations are not interchangeable—each must be used appropriately**.

Two transdermal formulations are available. One (Ionsys) is for short-term treatment of acute postoperative pain in hospitalized adults who require opioid analgesics. It is an adhesive skin patch that uses a tiny electric current to deliver a dose of fentanyl through intact skin and into the bloodstream. The patch, which has a button the patient can press for a preset dose of 40 micrograms, is placed on the patient's upper arm or chest and should be activated **only** by the patient (to avoid overdosing). When the Ionsys patch is removed, serum drug levels decline gradually. The other skin patch (Duragesic) is used in the treatment of chronic pain. The active drug is deposited in the skin and slowly absorbed systemically. Duragesic has a slow onset of action (12 to 24 hours), but it lasts about 72 hours. When a Duragesic patch is removed, the drug continues to be absorbed from the skin deposits for 24 hours or longer. With both transdermal formulations, patients should have a fast-acting formulation available for acute pain. An oral lozenge on a stick (Actiq) and a buccal tablet (Fentora) are approved to treat acute (breakthrough) pain in people who have been receiving opioids and have become opioid-tolerant. Because of a risk of respiratory depression, recommended dosages must not be exceeded with any formulation.

Hydrocodone, a Schedule III drug, is similar to codeine in its analgesic and antitussive effects. It is available in oral combination products for cough and with acetaminophen or ibuprofen for pain. Its half-life is about 4 hours, and its duration of action is 4 to 6 hours. Hydrocodone is metabolized to hydromorphone by the cytochrome P450 2D6 enzymes.

Hydromorphone (Dilaudid) is a semisynthetic derivative of morphine that has the same actions, uses, contraindications, and adverse effects as morphine. It is more potent on a milligram basis and more effective orally than morphine. Effects occur in 15 to 30 minutes, peak in 30 to 90 minutes, and last 4 to 5 hours. Hydromorphone is metabolized in the liver to inactive metabolites that are excreted through the kidneys.

Meperidine (Demerol) is a synthetic drug similar to morphine in action and adverse effects. After injection, analgesia occurs in 10 to 20 minutes, peaks in 1 hour, and lasts 2 to 4 hours. After an oral dose, about half is metabolized in the liver and never reaches the systemic circulation. Meperidine is infrequently used for therapeutic purposes, mainly because it produces a neurotoxic metabolite (normeperidine). Normeperidine accumulates with chronic use, large doses, or renal failure and produces CNS stimulation characterized by agitation, hallucinations, and seizures. The half-life of normeperidine is 15 to 30 hours, depending on renal function, and the effects of normeperidine are not reversible with opioid antagonist drugs.

Methadone (Dolophine) is a synthetic drug similar to morphine but with a longer duration of action. It is usually given orally, with which onset and peak of action occur in 30 to 60 minutes. Effects last 4 to 6 hours initially and longer with repeated use. Half-life is 15 to 30 hours, which also lengthens with repeated use. Methadone is used for severe pain and in the detoxification and maintenance treatment of opiate addicts. In 2006, the Food and Drug Administration (FDA) issued an alert about serious adverse effects (e.g., death, overdose, and serious cardiac dysrhythmias) reported in patients taking methadone. The FDA recommended that methadone dosage for pain should be carefully selected and titrated and that patients should be taught not to exceed prescribed dosage or frequency of administration.

Oxycodone (Roxicodone, others) is a derivative of codeine used to relieve moderate pain; its pharmacologic actions are similar to those of other opioid analgesics. It is a Schedule II drug of abuse. With oral administration, action starts in 15 to 30 minutes, peaks in 60 minutes, and lasts 4 to 6 hours. Its half-life is unknown. It is metabolized by the cytochrome P450 2D6 enzymes and excreted through the kidneys.

Oxycodone has been widely used for years, alone or in combination with acetaminophen. Several years ago, controlled-release tablets (OxyContin) in 10-, 20-, 40-, and 80-milligram sizes were marketed for extended treatment of moderate to severe pain (the 80-milligram tablets should be used only by patients who have developed drug tolerance through long-term use of lesser doses). When given every 12 hours, the tablets relieve pain around-the-clock. These effects are advantageous to patients with terminal cancer or other chronic pain conditions. However, OxyContin soon became a popular drug of abuse, leading to many deaths and much criminal activity. Most deaths have resulted from inappropriate use (i.e., not legally prescribed for the user) and by chewing, crushing and snorting through the nose, or crushing and injecting the drug. Chewing or crushing destroys the long-acting feature and constitutes an overdose. Subsequently, the manufacturer and the FDA have issued precautions for prescribing OxyContin and warnings not to crush the product.

Oxymorphone (Numorphan, Opana) is a derivative of morphine with actions, uses, and adverse effects similar to those of morphine. It was formerly available as a solution for injection and as a rectal suppository but was infrequently used. In 2006, oral tablets (immediate-release and extended-release Opana) were approved by the FDA.

Propoxyphene (Darvon) is a synthetic, Schedule IV drug that is chemically related to methadone. It is used for mild to moderate pain but is no more effective than aspirin or acetaminophen, with which it is usually given. Propoxyphene is abused (alone and with alcohol or other CNS depressant drugs), and deaths have occurred from overdoses. In addition, its metabolism produces an active metabolite, norpropoxyphene, which is eliminated in urine. Norpropoxyphene is not an opioid, but it has a long half-life and accumulates with repeated use of propoxyphene. Accumulation is associated with dysrhythmias and pulmonary edema; there have also been reports of apnea, cardiac arrest, and death. Norpropoxyphene cannot be removed by hemodialysis, and naloxone, an opioid antagonist, does not reverse its effects. As a result of these characteristics, propoxyphene has a **BLACK BOX WARNING** that it should not be prescribed for patients at risk for suicide or addiction, that it should be used with caution by patients who take tranquilizers or antidepressant drugs or who use alcohol to excess, and that patients should not exceed recommended dosage and should limit alcohol intake. The drug should be avoided by older adults and should not be used long term. Despite these dangers and warnings, the drug continues to be prescribed.

Tramadol (Ultram) is an oral, synthetic, centrally active analgesic for moderate to severe pain. It is effective and well tolerated in older adults and in people with acute or chronic pain, back pain, fibromyalgia, osteoarthritis, and neuropathic pain. Because it has a low potential for producing tolerance and abuse, it may be used long term for the management of chronic pain. It is not chemically related to opioids and is not a controlled drug. Its mechanism of action includes binding to mu opioid receptors and inhibiting reuptake of norepinephrine and serotonin in the brain, actions that interfere with transmission of pain signals. Analgesia occurs within 1 hour of administration and peaks in 2 to 3 hours with immediate-release tablets. Tramadol causes significantly less respiratory depression than morphine but may cause other morphine-like adverse effects (e.g., drowsiness, nausea, constipation, orthostatic hypotension).

Tramadol is well absorbed after oral administration, even if taken with food. It is minimally bound to plasma proteins, and its half-life is 6 to 7 hours. It is metabolized by the cytochrome P450 3A4 and 2D6 enzymes and forms an active metabolite. About 30% of a dose is excreted unchanged in the urine, and 60% is excreted as metabolites. Dosage should be reduced in people with renal or hepatic impairment. Tramadol is available in oral immediate-release tablets alone and in combination with acetaminophen (Ultracet) as well as an extended-release tablet (Ultram ER) that can be given once daily.

Opioid Agonists/Antagonists

These agents have agonist activity at some receptors and antagonist activity at others. Because of their agonist activity, they are potent analgesics with a lower abuse potential than pure agonists. However, they are considered second-line drugs for treatment of moderate to severe pain. Because of their antagonist activity, they should not be given to people who have been receiving opioid analgesics, and they may produce withdrawal symptoms in people with opioid dependence.

Butorphanol (Stadol) is a synthetic, Schedule IV agonist similar to morphine in analgesic effects and ability to cause respiratory depression. It is used for moderate to severe pain and is given parenterally or topically to nasal mucosa by a metered spray (Stadol NS). After IM or IV administration, analgesia peaks in 30 to 60 minutes. After nasal application, analgesia peaks within 1 to 2 hours. Adverse effects include drowsiness and nausea and vomiting. Butorphanol is not recommended for use in children younger than 18 years of age.

Nalbuphine (Nubain) is a synthetic analgesic used for moderate to severe pain. It is not a controlled drug. It is given IV, IM, or Sub-Q. After IV injection, action starts in 2 to 3 minutes, peaks in 15 to 20 minutes, and lasts for 3 to 6 hours. After IM or Sub-Q injection, action begins in less than 15 minutes, peaks in 30 to 60 minutes, and lasts for 3 to 6 hours. Half-life is 5 hours. The most common adverse effect is sedation; others are minimal at recommended doses.

Opioid Antagonist

An opioid antagonist (antidote) reverses analgesia and the CNS and respiratory depression caused by opioid agonists. It competes with opioids for opioid receptor sites in the brain and thereby prevents opioid binding with receptors or displaces opioids already occupying receptor sites. When an opioid cannot bind to receptor sites, it is "neutralized" and cannot exert its effects on body cells. An opioid antagonist does not relieve the depressant effects of other drugs, such as sedative-hypnotic, antianxiety, and antipsychotic agents. The chief clinical use of an opioid antagonist is to relieve CNS and respiratory depression induced by an opioid.

Naloxone (Narcan) has long been the drug of choice to treat respiratory depression caused by an opioid. Therapeutic effects occur within minutes after IV, IM, or Sub-Q injection and last 1 to 2 hours. Naloxone has a shorter duration of action than opioids, and repeated injections are usually needed. For a long-acting drug such as methadone, injections may be needed for 2 to 3 days. Naloxone produces few adverse effects, and repeated injections can be given safely. This drug should be readily available in all health care settings in which opioids are given. Dosages are listed in Table 6-1.

Applying Your Knowledge 6-1

At 12:00 P.M., you check on Mr. Harris. He complains of postoperative pain. He rates his pain as an 8 on a 10-point scale. Which pain medication will you give, and how much will you administer?

Applying Your Knowledge 6-2

At 1:00 P.M., you visit Mr. Harris's room. You note he is difficult to arouse and has a respiratory rate of 10 breaths per minute. What should be your nursing response?

Table 6-2	Selected Combination Opioid–Nonopioid Products	
OPIOID–NONOPIOID	**STRENGTH (mg)/SELECTED NAMES**	**ADULT DOSAGE RANGES**
Codeine/acetaminophen	30/300 (generic, Tylenol #3)	0.5–2 tabs q4h
Hydrocodone/acetaminophen	5/325 (generic)	1–2 tabs q4–6h, up to 12 tabs/d
	5/500 (generic, Hydrocet, Lorcet HD, Lortab, Vicodin)	1–2 tabs q4–6h, up to 8 tabs/d
	7.5/750 (generic, Vicodin ES)	1 tab q4–6h, up to 5 tabs/d
	10/500 (generic, Lorcet HD, Lortab 10/500)	1 tab q4–6h, up to 6 tabs/d
Hydrocodone/ibuprofen	7.5/200 (Vicoprofen)	1 tab q4–6 h, up to 5 tabs/d
Oxycodone/acetaminophen	5/325 (Percocet, Roxicet)	1 tab q6h
	5/500 (Roxicet 5/500, Tylox)	1 cap q6h
Oxycodone/ibuprofen	5/400 (Combunox)	1 tab, up to 4 tabs/d, not to exceed 7 d
Tramadol/acetaminophen	37.5/325 (generic, Ultracet)	2 tabs q4–6h

Note: Maximum recommended dosage for acetaminophen is 4000 mg/d and for ibuprofen, 2400 mg/d.

 ## Herbal and Dietary Supplement

Capsaicin (Zostrix), a product derived from cayenne chili peppers, is applied topically to the skin to relieve pain associated with osteoarthritis, rheumatoid arthritis, postherpetic neuralgia after a herpes zoster infection (shingles), diabetic neuropathy, postsurgical pain (including pain after mastectomy and amputation), and other complex pain syndromes. It may be most effective in relieving arthritic pain in joints close to skin surfaces (e.g., fingers, elbows, knees). Its analgesic effects are attributed to depletion of substance P in nerve cells. Substance P enhances transmission of painful stimuli from peripheral tissues to the spinal cord. An additional analgesic effect may result from interference with production of prostaglandins and leukotrienes.

Capsaicin is available in a gel, creams, and lotions, in concentrations ranging from 0.025% to 0.25%. It is most effective when applied three or four times daily; effects last 4 to 5 hours. The main adverse effects are itching and stinging. Capsaicin also is the active ingredient in a pepper spray used for self-defense.

⊘ Applying Your Knowledge 6-3

How Can You Avoid This Medication Error?
On the night after his surgery, Mr. Harris requests medication for pain. You note on his chart that the physician has ordered oral pain medication 24 hours after surgery. When Mr. Harris requests medication for pain, you administer Lortab 5/500.

Nursing Process

Assessment

Pain is a subjective experience (whatever the person says it is), and humans display a wide variety of responses. Although pain thresholds (the point at which a tissue-damaging stimulus produces a sensation of pain) are similar, people differ in their perceptions, behaviors, and tolerance of pain. Differences in pain perception may result from psychological components. Stressors such as anxiety, depression, fatigue, anger, and fear tend to increase pain; rest, mood elevation, and diversionary activities tend to decrease pain. Differences in behaviors may or may not indicate pain to observers, and overt signs and symptoms are not reliable indicators of the presence or extent of pain. Especially with chronic pain, overt signs and symptoms may be absent. Differences in the amount or duration of pain a person is willing to suffer before seeking relief often reflect the person's concern about the meaning of the pain and the type or intensity of the painful stimulus. Thus, pain is a complex physiologic, psychological, and sociocultural phenomenon that must be thoroughly assessed if it is to be managed effectively.

The nurse must assess every patient in relation to pain, initially to determine appropriate interventions and later to determine whether the interventions were effective in preventing or relieving pain. Although the patient is usually the best source of data, other people may be questioned about the patient's words and behaviors that indicate pain. This is especially important with young children. During assessment, keep in mind that acute pain may coexist with or be superimposed on chronic pain. Specific assessment data include

- Location. Determining the location may assist in relieving the pain or identifying its underlying cause. Ask the patient to show you where it hurts, if possible, and whether the pain stays in one place or radiates to other parts of the body. The term *referred pain* is used when pain arising from tissue damage in one area of the body is felt in another area. Patterns of referred pain may be helpful in diagnosis. For example, pain of cardiac origin may radiate to the neck, shoulders, chest muscles, and down the arms, often on the left side. This type of pain usually results from myocardial ischemia due to atherosclerotic plaque in coronary arteries. Stomach pain is usually referred to the epigastrium and may indicate gastritis or peptic ulcer. Gallbladder and bile duct pain is often localized in the right upper quadrant of the abdomen. Uterine pain is usually felt as abdominal cramping or low back pain. Deep or chronic pain is more difficult to localize than superficial or acute pain.

- Intensity or severity. Because pain is a subjective experience and cannot be objectively measured, assessment of severity is based on the patient's description and the nurse's observations. Various scales have been developed to measure and quantify pain. These include verbal descriptor scales in which the patient is asked to rate pain as mild, moderate, or severe; numeric scales, with 0 representing no pain and 10 representing severe pain; and visual analog scales, in which the patient chooses the location indicating the level of pain on a continuum.

- Relation to time, activities, and other signs and symptoms. Specific questions include
  - When did the pain start?
  - What activities were occurring when the pain started?
  - Does the pain occur with exercise or when at rest?
  - Do other signs and symptoms occur before, during, or after the pain?
  - Is this the first episode or a recurrent pain?
  - How long does the pain last?
  - What, if anything, decreases or relieves the pain?
  - What, if anything, aggravates the pain?

- Other data. For example, do not assume that postoperative pain is due to the incision and requires opioid analgesics for relief. A person who has had abdominal surgery may have headache, musculoskeletal discomfort, or "gas pains." Also, restlessness may be caused by hypoxia or anxiety rather than pain.

- With patients on opioid analgesics for more than a few days, assess periodically for drug tolerance and the need for higher doses or more frequent administration. Do not assume that increased requests for pain medication indicate inappropriate drug-seeking behavior associated with drug dependence.

Nursing Diagnoses

- Acute Pain
- Chronic Pain
- Impaired Gas Exchange related to sedation and decreased mobility
- Risk for Injury related to sedation and decreased mobility
- Constipation related to slowed peristalsis
- Deficient Knowledge: Effects and appropriate use of opioid analgesics
- Noncompliance: Drug dependence related to overuse

Planning/Goals

The patient will

- Avoid or be relieved of pain.
- Use opioid analgesics appropriately.
- Avoid preventable adverse effects.
- Be monitored for excessive sedation and respiratory depression.
- Be able to communicate and perform other activities of daily living when feasible.

Interventions

Use measures to prevent, relieve, or decrease pain when possible. General measures include those that promote optimal body functioning and those that prevent trauma, inflammation, infection, and other sources of painful stimuli. Specific interventions include the following:

- Encourage pulmonary hygiene techniques (e.g., coughing, deep breathing, ambulation) to promote respiration and prevent pulmonary complications, such as pneumonia and atelectasis.
- Use sterile technique when caring for wounds, urinary catheters, or IV lines.
- Use exercises, ambulation, and position changes to promote circulation and musculoskeletal function.
  - Rub or massage the painful area (e.g., knee pain with osteoarthritis) if feasible and helpful. This intervention is thought to stimulate other nerve fibers that block the nerve fibers carrying pain signals from entering the spinal cord.
- Handle any injured tissue gently, to avoid further trauma.
- Prevent bowel or bladder distention.
- Apply heat or cold.
- Use relaxation or distraction techniques.
- If a patient is in pain on initial contact, try to relieve the pain as soon as possible. After pain is controlled, plan with the patient to avoid or manage future episodes.
- If a patient is not in pain initially but anticipates surgery or an uncomfortable diagnostic procedure, plan with the patient ways to minimize and manage discomfort.

Nursing Process continues on page 90

Evaluation

- Ask patients about their levels of comfort or relief from pain.
- Observe behaviors that indicate the presence or absence of pain.
- Observe participation and ability to function in usual activities of daily living.
- Observe for presence or absence of sedation and respiratory depression.
- Observe for inappropriate drug-seeking behavior (possibly indicating dependence).

Principles of Therapy

Goals of Therapy

The goals of therapy are to relieve pain and discomfort, promote rest and relaxation, allow performance of usual activities of daily living, as health status permits, and minimize the anxiety, depression, and other emotional upsets that develop when pain is not managed effectively. Studies indicate that health care providers often fail to meet these goals with patients experiencing pain. Concerns about respiratory depression, excessive sedation, and drug dependence often contribute to reluctance and delay in administering opioid analgesics. Much of the difficulty has been attributed to inadequate or improper use of opioid analgesics (e.g., prescribing the wrong drug, inadequate dosage, or too-long intervals between doses). Even when opioid analgesics are ordered appropriately, nurses or patients and family members may not administer the drugs effectively. Basic tenets of a more humane approach to pain management are that no person should suffer pain needlessly, that pain occurs when the patient says it does, and that pain should be relieved by whatever means are required, including pharmacologic and nonpharmacologic treatments; that doses of opioids should be titrated to achieve maximal effectiveness; and that dependence rarely results from drugs taken for physical pain. Proponents of this view emphasize the need to assess and monitor all patients receiving opioid analgesics.

Patient Teaching Guidelines Opioid (Narcotic) Analgesics

General Considerations

- Use nonpharmacologic treatments of pain (e.g., exercise, heat and cold applications) instead of or along with analgesics, when effective.
- For pain that is not relieved by nondrug treatments, a non-narcotic analgesic (e.g., acetaminophen or ibuprofen) may be taken.
- For pain that is not relieved by a non-narcotic analgesic, a narcotic may be alternated with a non-narcotic analgesic or a combination product containing a narcotic and non-narcotic may be effective. Use of a narcotic analgesic for acute pain is acceptable and unlikely to lead to addiction.
- Most combination products (e.g., Lorcet, Lortab, Percocet, Vicodin, Tylenol No. 3) contain acetaminophen and there is a risk of liver failure from high doses of acetaminophen or from lower doses in people who already have liver damage (e.g., alcohol abusers). The maximum recommended dose within 24 hours, whether taken alone or in a combination product, is 4000 milligrams (e.g., 8 tablets or capsules containing 500 mg each). If unsure whether a combination product contains acetaminophen, ask a health care provider. In addition to pain relievers, many cold and flu over-the-counter products also contain acetaminophen. The maximum amount of 4000 milligrams should include all sources of acetaminophen. Acetaminophen use leading to liver failure is often implicated in patients requiring a liver transplant.
- For acute episodes of pain that occur at irregular intervals, most opioids may be taken as needed; for acute pain that occurs daily and for chronic pain, the drugs should be taken on a regular schedule, around-the-clock.
- When a choice of pain-relieving medication is available, use the least amount of the mildest drug that is likely to be effective in a particular situation.

- Take only as prescribed. If desired effects are not achieved, report to your health care provider. Do not increase the dose and do not take medication more often than prescribed. Although these principles apply to all medications, they are especially important with opioid analgesics because of potentially serious adverse effects and because analgesics may mask pain for which medical attention is needed.
- Do not drink alcohol or take other drugs that cause drowsiness (e.g., some antihistamines, sedative-type drugs for nervousness or anxiety, sleeping pills) while taking opioids for pain. Combining drugs with similar effects may lead to excessive sedation and difficulty in breathing.
- Do not smoke, cook, drive a car, or operate machinery when drowsy or dizzy or when vision is blurred from medication.
- Sit or lie down at least 30–60 minutes after receiving an opioid by injection. Injected drugs may cause dizziness, drowsiness, and falls when walking around. If it is necessary to get up, ask someone for assistance.
- When hospitalized, ask a health care provider about methods of pain management. For example, if anticipating surgery, ask how postoperative pain will be managed, how you need to report pain and request pain medication, and so on. It is better to take adequate medication and be able to cough, deep breathe, and walk around than to avoid or minimize pain medication and be unable to perform activities that promote recovery and healing. Do not object to having bedrails up or asking for assistance when receiving a strong narcotic analgesic. These are safety measures to prevent falls or other injuries because these drugs may cause drowsiness, weakness, unsteady gait, and blurred vision.

■ Constipation is a common adverse effect of opioid analgesics. It may be prevented or managed by eating high-fiber foods, such as whole-grain cereals, fruits, and vegetables; drinking 2–3 quarts of fluid daily; and being as active as tolerated. If you take these medicines for more than a few days, or if you're the caregiver for someone who takes them, ask a health care provider about a bowel program to prevent constipation. A possible regimen is a daily stool softener (e.g., docusate) and a daily or every other day laxative (e.g., bisacodyl), preferably started at the same time as the narcotic. Docusate and bisacodyl are available over-the-counter.

Self-Administration

■ Take oral narcotic analgesics with 6–8 oz of water, with or after food to reduce nausea.
■ Do not crush or chew long-acting tablets (e.g., MS Contin, OxyContin). The tablets are formulated to release the active drug slowly, over several hours. Crushing or chewing causes immediate release of the drug, with a high risk of overdose and adverse effects, and shortens the duration of pain-relieving effects.
■ Omit one or more doses if severe adverse effects occur (e.g., excessive drowsiness, difficulty in breathing, severe nausea, vomiting, or constipation), and report to a health care provider.

Drug Selection

Prescribers have a wide choice of drugs to use in pain management and several factors should be considered, including the type of pain. Most prescribers use acetaminophen or nonsteroidal anti-inflammatory analgesics (e.g., ibuprofen) for mild pain; continue one of these and add an opioid (e.g., codeine, hydrocodone, or tramadol) for moderate pain; and give a strong opioid (e.g., morphine, fentanyl, hydromorphone) alone for acute, severe pain or combined with nonopioid drugs for chronic severe pain (e.g., cancer or neuropathic pain). Because it is often difficult to control severe pain with a single analgesic, a combination of drugs with different mechanisms of action may be more effective. Combinations may also be effective with lower doses and limit the adverse effects that occur with higher doses. More specific considerations are described below.

Morphine is often the opioid of choice for moderate to severe pain because it is effective, available in several dosage strengths, can be given by several routes, is useful on a short- or long-term basis, and its adverse effects are well known. In addition, it is a "nonceiling" drug (meaning that there is no upper limit to the dosage that can be given to patients who have developed tolerance to previous dosages). This characteristic is especially valuable in patients with severe cancer-related pain, because drug dosage can be increased and titrated to relieve pain when pain increases or *tolerance* develops. Thus, some patients have safely received extremely large doses. Other nonceiling drugs are hydromorphone and methadone. Several opioids are available in long-acting formulations, including fentanyl (Duragesic skin patch), hydromorphone (Palladone extended-release capsules), morphine (MS Contin, Oramorph SR, Avinza, Kadian), oxycodone (OxyContin controlled-release tablets), and tramadol (Ultram ER), which may be an important factor in drug selection. For patients receiving long-acting opioids, a fast-acting opioid also needs to be available for breakthrough pain.

When more than one analgesic is ordered, the least potent drug that is effective in relieving pain should be used. For example, a nonopioid analgesic, such as acetaminophen, rather than an opioid analgesic, should be given when feasible.

Nonopioid analgesics may be alternated or given concurrently with opioid analgesics, especially in chronic pain. This strategy increases patient comfort, reduces the likelihood of drug abuse and dependence, and decreases tolerance to the pain-relieving effects of the opioid analgesics.

Numerous fixed-dose combinations of acetaminophen or ibuprofen and an opioid are available and widely used (see Table 6-2). Prescribers need to assess patients for the use of other products containing an opioid or acetaminophen before prescribing one of these combinations because overuse of these products can result in serious adverse effects.

Route Selection

Opioid analgesics can be given by several routes, either noninvasively (orally, rectally, or transdermally) or invasively (Sub-Q, IM, IV, or by spinal infusion). *When the route is changed (e.g., from oral to injection or vice versa), the dose must also be changed to prevent over dosage or under dosage.* Oral drugs are preferred when feasible, and most patients achieve relief with short-acting or sustained-release oral preparations.

Some drugs can be given by IM or Sub-Q injections for rapid relief of acute pain, but IV injection is usually preferred. Small, frequent IV doses are often effective in relieving pain with minimal risk of serious adverse effects. This is especially advantageous during a serious illness or after surgery. Continuous IV infusion may be used to treat severe pain. A technique called *patient-controlled analgesia* (PCA) allows self-administration. Devices consist of a container of diluted drug connected to an IV line and infusion pump or a specially designed IV bag and special tubing. These devices deliver a dose when the patient pushes a button. Some PCA pumps can also deliver a basic amount of analgesic by continuous infusion, with the patient injecting additional doses when needed. The amount of drug delivered with each dose and the intervals between doses are preset and limited. PCA requires an alert, cooperative patient who can press a button when pain occurs. Studies indicate that analgesia is more effective, patient satisfaction is high, and smaller amounts of drug are used than with as needed administration. PCA is especially useful for patients with postoperative pain or high opioid requirements.

Three other routes may be used to manage acute pain. One is the fentanyl skin patch (Ionsys) described earlier. It is indicated only for short-term treatment of hospitalized, postoperative patients and is the only noninvasive route available for PCA.

Another route involves injection of morphine or fentanyl directly into the CNS through a catheter placed into the epidural or intrathecal space by an anesthesiologist or other physician. This method provides effective analgesia while minimizing depressant effects. The epidural route can be used to administer PCA, and less opioid is required for pain relief than with the IV route. The third route involves the injection of a local anesthetic to provide local or regional analgesia, alone or combined with an opioid. These routes require special administration and monitoring procedures for safe use.

For patients with chronic pain and contraindications to oral or injected medications, some opioids are available in rectal suppositories or skin patches. Morphine, oxymorphone, and hydromorphone can be given rectally with similar potencies and half-lives as when given orally. For patients who cannot take oral medications and whose opioid requirement is too large for rectal administration, the transdermal route is preferred over IV, IM, or Sub-Q injections. A fentanyl skin patch (Duragesic) is commonly used. When first applied, pain relief is delayed about 12 hours (as the drug is gradually absorbed). Because of the delayed effects, doses of a short-acting opioid should be ordered and given as needed during the first 48 hours after the patch is applied. With continued use, the old patch is removed and a new one applied every 72 hours. Opioid overdose can occur with fentanyl patches if the patient has fever (hastens drug absorption) or liver impairment (slows drug metabolism). Analgesics given by a combination of routes may be the most effective regimen.

Drug Dosage

Dosages of opioids should be sufficient to relieve pain without causing unacceptable adverse effects. Thus, dosages should be individualized according to the type and severity of pain; the patient's age, size, and health status; whether the patient is opiate naive (has not received sufficient opioids for development of tolerance) or opiate tolerant (has previously taken opioids and drug tolerance has developed, so that larger-than-usual doses are needed to relieve pain); whether the patient has worsening disease; and other characteristics that influence responses to pain. Additional guidelines include the following:

▪ Small to moderate doses relieve constant, dull pain, and moderate to large doses relieve intermittent, sharp pain caused by trauma or conditions affecting the viscera.

▪ When an opioid is ordered in variable amounts, the smaller amount should be given as long as it is effective in relieving pain.

▪ Dosages of opioids should be reduced for patients who also are receiving other CNS depressants (e.g., antianxiety, antidepressant, antihistaminic, antipsychotic, or other drugs that cause sedation).

▪ Dosages often differ according to the route of administration. Oral doses undergo extensive metabolism on their first pass through the liver, so oral doses are usually much larger than injected doses.

▪ Dosages change when patients are switched from one opioid to another (usually because the first opioid loses its effectiveness, produces unacceptable adverse effects, or is not available in a suitable dosage form for a different route of administration).

Frequency of Administration

Opioid analgesics may be given as needed, within designated time limits, or on a regular schedule. Traditionally, the drugs were often scheduled every 4 to 6 hours as needed (PRN). Numerous studies indicate that such a schedule is often ineffective in managing patients' pain. Because opioids are used for moderate to severe pain, they should in general be scheduled to provide effective and consistent pain relief.

When analgesics are ordered PRN, have a clear-cut system by which the patient requests medication. The patient should know that an analgesic is available and will be given promptly when needed. If a drug cannot be given, explain the reasons to the patient. In addition, offer or give the drug when indicated by the patient's condition rather than waiting for the patient to request medication.

For acute pain, opioids are most effective when given parenterally and at the onset of pain. In chronic, severe pain, opioids are most effective when given on a regular schedule, around the clock.

When feasible, give an analgesic prior to activities known to be uncomfortable or painful (e.g., coughing and deep-breathing exercises, dressing changes, other therapeutic and diagnostic procedures). Allow adequate time for the pain medication to take effect.

Opioids are not recommended for prolonged periods except for advanced cancer. Health care facilities usually have an automatic "stop order" for opioids after 48 to 72 hours; this means that the drug is discontinued when the time limit expires if it is not reordered.

Drug Use in Specific Situations

Cancer

It is important for health care providers to remember that patients with cancer may experience both acute pain (e.g., pain associated with diagnostic tests, surgery or other treatments, disease progression, development of tolerance to opioids) and chronic pain. When opioids are required by patients with chronic pain, the main consideration is patient comfort, not preventing drug addiction. Effective treatment requires that pain be relieved and prevented from recurring; titration of opioid dosage is usually the best approach. With disease progression and the development of drug tolerance, extremely large doses and frequent administration (of *nonceiling opioids*) may be required. Additional guidelines include the following:

▪ Analgesics should be given on a regular schedule, around-the-clock. Patients should be awakened, if necessary, to prevent pain recurrence.

- Oral, rectal, and transdermal routes of administration are generally preferred over injections.

- A nonopioid analgesic (e.g., acetaminophen, ibuprofen) may be used alone for mild pain.

- Oxycodone or codeine can be used for moderate pain, often with a nonopioid analgesic. A combination of the two types of drugs produces additive analgesic effects and may allow smaller doses of the opioid.

- Morphine or another strong opioid (e.g., hydromorphone, fentanyl, oxycodone, methadone) is given for severe pain. Although the dose of morphine can be titrated upward for adequate analgesia, unacceptable adverse effects (e.g., excessive sedation, respiratory depression, nausea and vomiting) may limit the dose. Oral administration is preferred; the initial oral dosage of morphine is usually 10 to 20 mg every 3 to 4 hours.

- When long-acting forms of opioids are given on a regular schedule, fast-acting forms also need to be available for *breakthrough pain* (acute pain that occurs spontaneously or with activity). If supplemental or "rescue" doses are needed frequently, the baseline dose of long-acting medication may need to be increased.

- In addition to analgesics, other drugs may be used to increase patient comfort. For example, some antidepressants and anticonvulsants decrease neuropathic pain. Antiemetics may be given for nausea and vomiting; stool softeners and laxatives are usually needed on a regular schedule to manage constipation. Tolerance does not develop to the constipating effects of opioids.

Biliary, Renal, or Ureteral Colic

When opioids are used to relieve the acute, severe, pain associated with colic, an antispasmodic drug such as atropine may be needed as well. Opioids may increase smooth muscle tone and cause spasm. Atropine does not have strong antispasmodic properties of its own in usual doses, but it reduces the spasm-producing effects of opioids.

Postoperative Use

When opioids are used postoperatively, the goal is to relieve pain without excessive sedation so that patients can do deep-breathing exercises, cough, ambulate, and participate in other activities to promote recovery. Strong opioids are usually given parenterally for a few days. Then, oral opioids or nonopioid analgesics are given.

Burns

In severely burned patients, opioids should be used cautiously. A common cause of respiratory arrest in burned patients is excessive administration of analgesics. Agitation in a burned person may indicate hypoxia or hypovolemia rather than pain. When opioids are necessary, they are usually given IV in small doses. Drugs given by other routes are absorbed erratically in the presence of shock and hypovolemia and may not relieve pain. In addition, unabsorbed drugs may be rapidly absorbed when circulation improves, with the potential for excessive dosage and toxic effects.

Opioid Toxicity: Recognition and Management

Acute toxicity or opioid overdose can occur from therapeutic use or from abuse by drug-dependent people. Overdose may produce severe respiratory depression and coma. The main goal of treatment is to restore and maintain adequate respiratory function. This can be accomplished by inserting an endotracheal tube and starting mechanical ventilation or by giving an opioid antagonist, such as naloxone. Thus, emergency supplies should be readily available in any setting where opioids are used.

Opioid Withdrawal: Prevention and Management

Abstinence from opioids after chronic use produces a withdrawal syndrome characterized by anxiety; restlessness; insomnia; perspiration; pupil dilation; piloerection (goose flesh); anorexia, nausea, and vomiting; diarrhea; elevation of body temperature, respiratory rate, and systolic blood pressure; muscle cramps; and dehydration. Although all opioids produce similar withdrawal syndromes, the onset, severity, and duration vary. With morphine, symptoms begin within a few hours of the last dose, reach peak intensity in 36 to 72 hours, and subside over 8 to 10 days. With methadone, symptoms begin in 1 to 2 days, peak in about 3 days, and subside over several weeks. Heroin, meperidine, methadone, morphine, oxycodone, and oxymorphone are associated with more severe withdrawal symptoms than other opioids. If an opioid antagonist such as naloxone (Narcan) is given, withdrawal symptoms occur rapidly and are more intense but of shorter duration. Despite the discomfort that occurs, withdrawal from opioids is rarely life threatening unless other problems are present. An exception is opioid withdrawal in neonates, which has a high mortality rate if not treated effectively. Signs and symptoms in neonates include tremor, jitteriness, increased muscle tone, screaming, fever, sweating, tachycardia, vomiting, diarrhea, respiratory distress, and possibly seizures.

Recognition and treatment of early, mild symptoms of withdrawal can prevent progression to severe symptoms. Both opioids and nonopioids are used for treatment. Opioids may be used in two ways to provide a safe, therapeutic withdrawal. One technique is to give the opioid from which the person is withdrawing, which immediately reverses the signs and symptoms of withdrawal. Then, dosage is gradually reduced over several days. Another technique is to substitute a long-acting opioid (e.g., methadone) for a short-acting opioid. Methadone is usually given in an adequate dose to control symptoms, once or twice daily, and then is gradually tapered over 5 to 10 days. In neonates undergoing opioid withdrawal, methadone or paregoric may be used.

Clonidine, an antihypertensive drug, is a nonopioid that may be used to treat opioid withdrawal. Clonidine reduces the release of norepinephrine in the brain and thus reduces symptoms associated with excessive stimulation of the sympathetic nervous system (e.g., anxiety, restlessness, insomnia). Blood pressure must be closely monitored during clonidine therapy. Other medications (nonopioid analgesics, antiemetics, antidiarrheals) are often required to treat other symptoms.

Use in Special Populations

Use in Opioid-Tolerant Patients

Whether opioid tolerance results from the use of prescribed therapeutic drugs or the abuse of street drugs, there are two main considerations in using opioid analgesics in this population. First, larger-than-usual doses are required to treat pain. Second, signs and symptoms of withdrawal occur if adequate dosage is not maintained or if opioid antagonists are given.

Use in Children

In general, there is little understanding of the physiology, pathology, assessment, and management of pain in children. Many authorities indicate that children's pain is often ignored or under treated, including children having surgical and other painful procedures for which adults routinely receive an anesthetic, a strong analgesic, or both. This is especially true in preterm and full-term neonates. One reason for inadequate prevention and management of pain in newborns was a common belief that they did not experience pain because of immature nervous systems. However, research indicates that neonates have abundant C fibers and that A-delta fibers are developing during the first few months of life. These are the nerve fibers that carry pain signals from peripheral tissues to the spinal cord. In addition, brain pain centers and the endogenous analgesia system are developed and functional. Endogenous opioids are released at birth and in response to fetal and neonatal distress such as asphyxia or other difficulty associated with the birth process.

Older infants and children may experience pain even when analgesics are readily available. For example, children may fear injections or may be unable to communicate their discomfort. Health care providers or parents may fear adverse effects of opioid analgesics, including excessive sedation, respiratory depression, and addiction.

Other than reduced dosage, there have been few guidelines about the use of opioids in children. With increased knowledge about pain mechanisms, nurses who work with children should be able to manage pain effectively. Specific considerations include the following:

■ Opioids administered during labor and delivery may depress fetal and neonatal respiration. The drugs cross the blood–brain barrier of the infant more readily than that of the mother. Therefore, doses that do not depress maternal respiration may profoundly depress the infant's respiration. Respiration should be monitored closely in neonates, and the opioid antagonist naloxone should be readily available.

■ Expressions of pain may differ according to age and developmental level. Infants may cry and have muscular rigidity and thrashing behavior. Preschoolers may behave aggressively or complain verbally of discomfort. Young school-aged children may express pain verbally or behaviorally, often with regression to behaviors used at younger ages. Adolescents may be reluctant to admit they are uncomfortable or need help. With chronic pain, children of all ages tend to withdraw and regress to an earlier stage of development.

■ It is recommended that opioids be given by routes (e.g., PO, IV, epidurally) other than IM injections, because IM injections are painful and frightening for children. For any child receiving parenteral opioids, vital signs and level of consciousness must be assessed regularly.

■ Opioid formulations for children are not generally available. When children's doses are calculated based on adult doses, the fractions and decimals that often result greatly increase the risk of a dosage error. It is advisable to have two people do the calculations independently and compare results.

■ Opioid rectal suppositories are used more often in children than in adults. Although useful when oral or parenteral routes are not indicated, the dose of medication received by the child is unknown because drug absorption is erratic and because adult suppositories are sometimes cut in half or otherwise altered.

■ Opioid effects in children may differ from those expected in adults because of physiologic and pharmacokinetic differences. Assess regularly and be alert for unusual signs and symptoms.

■ Hydromorphone, methadone, oxycodone, and oxymorphone are not recommended for use in children because safety, efficacy, and dosages have not been established.

■ Like adults, children seem more able to cope with pain when they are informed about what is happening to them and are assisted in developing coping strategies. Age-appropriate doll play, a favorite videotape/DVD, diversionary activities, and other techniques can be used effectively. However, such techniques should be used in conjunction with adequate analgesia, not as a substitute for pain medication.

Use in Older Adults

Opioids should be used cautiously in older adults, especially if they are debilitated; have hepatic, renal, or respiratory impairment; or are receiving other drugs that depress the CNS. Older adults are especially sensitive to respiratory depression, excessive sedation, confusion, and other adverse effects. However, they should receive adequate analgesia, along with vigilant monitoring. Specific recommendations include the following:

■ Use nondrug measures (e.g., heat or cold applications, exercise) and nonopioid analgesics to relieve pain, when effective.

■ When opioids are needed, use those with short half-lives (e.g., oxycodone, hydromorphone) because they are less likely to accumulate.

■ Start with low doses and increase doses gradually, if necessary.

■ Give the drugs less often than for younger adults because the duration of action may be longer.

■ Monitor carefully for sedation or confusion. Also, monitor voiding and urine output because acute urinary retention is more likely to occur in older adults.

■ Assess older adults for ability to self-administer opioids safely. Those with short-term memory loss (common in this population) may require assistance and supervision.

Use in Clients With Renal Impairment

Most opioids are extensively metabolized in the liver to metabolites that are then excreted in urine. In patients with renal impairment, the drugs should be given in minimal doses, for the shortest effective time, because usual doses may produce profound sedation and a prolonged duration of action. Morphine, for example, produces an active metabolite that may accumulate in patients with renal impairment. Meperidine should not be used because a toxic metabolite, normeperidine, may accumulate. Normeperidine is pharmacologically active and a CNS stimulant that may cause muscle spasms, seizures, and psychosis. These effects are not reversed by an opioid antagonist such as naloxone.

Use in Clients With Hepatic Impairment

Because opioid analgesics and related drugs are extensively metabolized by the liver, they may accumulate and cause increased adverse effects in the presence of hepatic impairment. Dosages may need to be reduced, especially with chronic use.

Use in Clients With Critical Illness

Opioids are commonly used to manage pain associated with disease processes and invasive diagnostic and therapeutic procedures. In intensive care units, they are also used concurrently with sedatives and neuromuscular blocking agents, which increases the risks of adverse drug reactions and interactions. In patients with critical illness, opioids are usually given by IV bolus injection or continuous infusion. Guidelines include the following:

■ Assume that all critically ill patients are in pain or at high risk for development of pain.

■ When pain is thought to be present, identify and treat the underlying cause when possible.

■ Assess for pain on a regular schedule around the clock (e.g., every 1 to 2 hours). Use a consistent method for assessing severity, such as a visual analog or numeric scale. If the patient is able to communicate, ask about the location, severity, and so forth. If the patient is unable to communicate needs for pain relief, as is often the case during critical illnesses, the nurse must evaluate posture, body language, risk factors, and other possible indicators of pain.

■ Prevent pain when possible. Interventions include being very gentle when performing nursing care to avoid tissue trauma and positioning patients to prevent ischemia, edema, and misalignment. In addition, give analgesics before painful procedures, when indicated.

■ When pain occurs, manage it to provide relief and prevent its recurrence. In general, opioids should be given continuously or on a regular schedule of intermittent doses, with supplemental or bolus doses when needed for breakthrough pain. When starting a continuous IV infusion of pain medication, a loading dose should be given to attain therapeutic blood levels quickly.

■ Opioids are often given by IV infusion over a prolonged period in patients with trauma and other critical illnesses. They may also be given orally, by transdermal patch, or by epidural infusion, depending on the patient's condition.

■ Opioid agonist drugs are preferred; morphine and fentanyl are commonly used. Mixed agonist–antagonist opioids are not recommended for use in critically ill patients. They may cause opioid withdrawal in those who have been receiving chronic opioid therapy and may also cause psychotomimetic effects.

■ Consult specialists in pain management (e.g., anesthesiologists, clinical pharmacists, physician) when pain is inadequately controlled with the usual measures.

Use in Home Care

Opioids are widely used in the home for both acute and chronic pain. With acute pain, such as in postoperative recovery, the use of an opioid is often limited to a short period and patients self-administer their medications. The need for strong pain medication recedes as healing occurs. The home care nurse may teach patients and caregivers safe usage of the drugs (e.g., that the drugs decrease mental alertness and physical agility, so potentially hazardous activities should be avoided), nonpharmacologic methods of managing pain, and ways to prevent adverse effects of opioids (e.g., constipation). Physical dependence is uncommon with short-term use of opioids for acute pain.

With some types of chronic pain, such as those occurring with low back pain or osteoarthritis, opioids are not indicated for long-term use. Treatment involves nonopioid medications, physical therapy, and other measures. The home care nurse may need to explain the reasons for not using opioids on a long-term basis and to help patients and caregivers learn alternative methods of relieving discomfort.

With cancer pain, as previously discussed, the goal of treatment is to prevent or relieve pain and keep patients comfortable, without concern about addiction. Thus, the home care nurse must assist patients and caregivers in understanding the appropriate use of opioids in cancer care, including administration on a regular schedule, storing the drugs to avoid use by persons other than the patient, and avoiding theft and diversion to street use. The nurse also must be proficient in using and teaching various routes of drug administration and in arranging regimens with potentially very large doses and various combinations of drugs. In addition, an active effort is needed to prevent or manage adverse effects, such as a bowel program to prevent constipation.

Nursing Actions | Opioid Analgesics

NURSING ACTIONS	RATIONALE/EXPLANATION
1. Administer accurately	
a. Check the rate, depth, and rhythm of respirations before each dose. If the rate is fewer than 12 per minute, delay or omit the dose and report to the physician.	Respiratory depression is a major adverse effect of strong analgesics. Assessing respirations before each dose can help prevent or minimize potentially life-threatening respiratory depression.
b. Have the patient lie down to receive injections of opioid analgesics and for at least a few minutes afterward.	Prevents or minimizes hypotension, nausea, and vomiting. These effects are more likely to occur in ambulatory patients. Also, patients may be sedated enough to increase risk of falls or other injuries if they try to ambulate.
c. When injecting opioid analgesics intravenously, give small doses; inject slowly over several minutes; and have opioid antagonist drugs, artificial airways, and equipment for artificial ventilation readily available.	Large doses or rapid intravenous injection may cause severe respiratory depression and hypotension.
d. Put side rails up; instruct the patient not to smoke or try to ambulate without help. Keep the call light within reach.	To prevent falls or other injuries
e. When giving controlled-release tablets, do NOT crush them, and instruct the patient not to chew them.	Crushing or chewing causes immediate release of the drug, with a high risk of overdose and toxicity.
f. Follow the manufacturer's instructions re: administration of alternative formulations of fentanyl (e.g., Actiq, Duragesic, Fentora, and Ionsys).	These formulations have specific indications and require special techniques and precautions. Actiq and Fentora are given orally for transmucosal absorption; Duragesic and Ionsys are applied to the skin for transdermal absorption.
2. Observe for therapeutic effects	
a. A verbal statement of pain relief	Therapeutic effects depend on the reason for use, usually for analgesic effects but sometimes for antitussive or antidiarrheal effects.
b. Decreased behavioral manifestations of pain or discomfort	
c. Sleeping	
d. Increased participation in usual activities of daily living, including interactions with other people in the environment	
e. Fewer and shorter episodes of nonproductive coughing when used for antitussive effects	Opioids relieve cough by depressing the cough center in the medulla oblongata.
f. Lowered blood pressure, decreased pulse rate, slower and deeper respirations, and less dyspnea when morphine is given for pulmonary edema	Morphine may relieve pulmonary edema by causing vasodilation, which in turn decreases venous return to the heart and decreases cardiac work.
g. Decreased diarrhea when given for constipating effects	These drugs slow secretions and motility of the GI tract. Constipation is usually an adverse effect. However, in severe diarrhea or with ileostomy, the drugs decrease the number of bowel movements and make the consistency more paste-like than liquid.
3. Observe for adverse effects	
a. Respiratory depression—hypoxemia, restlessness, dyspnea, slow, shallow breathing, changes in blood pressure and pulse, decreased ability to cough	Respiratory depression is a major adverse effect of opioids and results from depression of the respiratory center in the medulla oblongata. It occurs with usual therapeutic doses and increases in incidence and severity with large doses or frequent administration. *It is especially likely to occur when an opioid is first started and when dosage is increased.*
b. Hypotension	Hypotension stems from drug effects on the vasomotor center in the medulla oblongata that cause peripheral vasodilation and lowering of blood pressure. This is a therapeutic effect with pulmonary edema.
c. Excessive sedation—drowsiness, slurred speech, impaired mobility and coordination, stupor, coma	This is caused by depression of the central nervous system (CNS) and is potentially life threatening.
d. Nausea and vomiting	Opioids stimulate the chemoreceptor trigger zone in the brain. Thus, nausea and vomiting may occur with various routes of administration. They are more likely to occur with ambulation than with recumbency.
e. Constipation	This is caused by the drug's slowing effects on the GI tract. Constipation may be prevented or treated by increased activity, adequate intake of fluid and fiber, and regular administration of stool softeners (e.g., docusate) and stimulant laxatives (e.g., bisacodyl).

NURSING ACTIONS	RATIONALE/EXPLANATION
4. Observe for drug interactions a. Drugs that *increase* effects of opioids: (1) CNS depressants—alcohol, general anesthetics, benzodiazepine antianxiety and hypnotic agents, tricyclic antidepressants, sedating antihistamines, antipsychotic agents, barbiturates, and other drugs that cause sedation	All these drugs alone, as well as the opioids, produce CNS depression. When combined, additive CNS depression results. If dosage of one or more interacting drugs is high, severe respiratory depression, coma, and death may ensue.
(2) Anticholinergics—atropine and other drugs with anticholinergic effects (e.g., antihistamines, tricyclic antidepressants, phenothiazine antipsychotic drugs)	Increased constipation and urinary retention
(3) Antihypertensive drugs	Orthostatic hypotension, an adverse effect of both strong analgesics and antihypertensive drugs, may be increased if the two drug groups are given concurrently.
(4) Monoamine oxidase (MAO) inhibitors	These drugs interfere with detoxification of some opioid analgesics, especially meperidine. They may cause additive CNS depression with hypotension and respiratory depression or CNS stimulation with hyperexcitability and convulsions. If an MAO inhibitor is necessary, dosage should be reduced because the combination is potentially life threatening.
(5) Protease inhibitors—ritonavir, saquinavir, others	May increase CNS and respiratory depression
(6) Cimetidine (Tagamet)	May increase CNS and respiratory depression by inhibiting the cytochrome P450 enzymes that normally metabolize opioids.
b. Drugs that *decrease* effects of opioids: (1) Opioid antagonist (Narcan)	Narcan reverses respiratory depression produced by opioids; it does not reverse respiratory depression caused by other CNS depressants.
(2) Butorphanol, nalbuphine	These analgesics are weak antagonists of opioid analgesics, and they may cause withdrawal symptoms in people who have been receiving opiates or who are physically dependent on opioids.

Key Concepts

- All patients should be assessed for pain. Acute pain may be manifested verbally or by behavior that indicates discomfort; chronic pain may not be characterized by visible signs and is often accompanied by anxiety and depression. If present, pain should be managed effectively, often with a combination of strategies that may include nonpharmacologic treatments, nonopioid analgesics, opioid analgesics, and adjuvant drugs.

- Pain occurs when tissue damage activates free nerve endings (nociceptors) of peripheral nerves. Pain signals are carried from the site of tissue damage to the spinal cord by A-delta and C nerve fibers, then are relayed to the brain where they are perceived as pain.

- Endorphins and enkephalins react with opioid receptors in the CNS to inhibit transmission of pain signals.

- Opioid analgesics react with opioid receptors in the CNS and peripheral tissues to inhibit transmission of pain signals, to reduce the perception of pain, and to reduce the emotional upsets often associated with pain.

- Most opioid analgesics are Schedule II controlled drugs and may cause serious adverse effects (respiratory depression, sedation) and physical dependence. As a result, they all have **BLACK BOX WARNINGS** regarding safe and appropriate use.

- Opioid agonist drugs stimulate opioid receptors; agonists/antagonists have agonist activity at some receptors and antagonist activity at others; antagonists reverse or block the effects of agonists.

- Opioid selection, dosage, and route of administration should be individualized according to the patient's condition.

- For most acute and chronic pain, analgesics are more effective if given on a regular schedule around the clock. When acute pain has subsided or occurs at irregular intervals and when breakthrough pain occurs in patients receiving long-term analgesic therapy for chronic pain, analgesics can be given as needed.

■ For patients who require large doses of opioids to relieve their pain, additional medications and interventions are often needed to manage adverse effects (e.g., nausea, constipation).

■ Pain-relieving interventions must be documented in patient's records and patients must be assessed to determine whether the interventions were effective.

Review and Application Exercises

Short Answer Exercises

1. When assessing a patient for pain, what are the major considerations?

2. What are some nonpharmacologic interventions for pain, and why should they be used instead of or along with analgesics?

3. What are the major adverse effects of opioid analgesics? How do opioid antagonists counteract adverse effects?

4. For a patient who has had major surgery during the previous 24 to 72 hours, what type of analgesic is indicated? Why?

5. What are the potential differences in dosage between short-term (a few days) and long-term (weeks or months) administration of morphine?

6. Explain the rationale for using both opioid analgesics and nonopioid analgesics in the treatment of pain.

7. For a patient with chronic cancer pain, what are the advantages and disadvantages of using opioid analgesics?

8. For a patient with chronic cancer pain, should opioid analgesics be given as needed or on a regular schedule? Why?

9. For a patient who is receiving large doses of an opioid analgesic, what signs and symptoms may indicate drug toxicity or overdose? What interventions are needed for suspected toxicity?

10. For a patient who has been taking an opioid analgesic for a long time, what signs and symptoms would make you suspect opioid withdrawal? What interventions are needed for suspected withdrawal?

NCLEX-Style Questions

11. In administering opioid analgesics to a patient, it is most important that the nurse know that opioid analgesics act mainly by
    a. causing sleep
    b. binding with opioid receptors in the brain and spinal cord
    c. increasing transmission of pain impulses between nerve cells
    d. decreasing the amount of norepinephrine and serotonin in synapses in the brain

12. When caring for a patient who is receiving morphine, it is most important that the nurse regularly assess for which of the following?
    a. respiratory depression
    b. hyperactive bowel sounds
    c. frequent urination
    d. insomnia

13. The nurse is caring for a patient with terminal cancer, who requires significant pain relief. Her family is concerned about addiction. The nurse is most correct in explaining that long-term administration of an opioid under medical supervision does not result in addiction but does result in
    a. tolerance
    b. overdose
    c. withdrawal
    d. hepatotoxicity

14. A postoperative surgical patient is prescribed patient-controlled analgesia, but his family questions why his pain medication is being given in this manner. The nurse is most correct in explaining that the main advantage of patient-controlled analgesia systems is that they
    a. require less nursing time
    b. cause fewer adverse effects
    c. relieve pain more effectively
    d. can be used long term

15. The nurse is caring for a patient with severe cancer pain. The family is questioning when analgesics should be given. The nurse is correct in explaining that in cases of severe pain, analgesics should be given
    a. when the patient asks for them
    b. if a family member or friend asks that they be given
    c. when a patient is restless
    d. on a regular schedule, around-the-clock

Selected References

Baumann, T. J. (2005). Pain management. In J. T. DiPiro, R. L. Talbert, G. C. Yee, G. R. Matzke, B. G. Wells, & L. M. Posey (Eds.), *Pharmacotherapy: A pathophysiologic approach* (6th ed., pp. 1089–1104). New York: McGraw-Hill.

Caulfield, J. S. (2006). Management of chronic nonmalignant pain. *Drug Topics*, 39–46.

Devine, E. C. (2005). Somatosensory function, pain, and headache. In C. M. Porth (Ed.), *Pathophysiology: Concepts of altered health states* (7th ed., pp. 1159–1191). Philadelphia: Lippincott Williams & Wilkins.

Drug facts and comparisons. (Updated monthly). St. Louis, MO: Facts and Comparisons.

Guyton, A. C., & Hall, J. E. (2006). *Textbook of medical physiology* (11th ed., pp 598–609). Philadelphia: Elsevier Saunders.

Joint Commission on Accreditation of Healthcare Organizations. (2005). *2005 Hospital accreditation standards*. Oakbrook Terrace, IL: JCAHO.

Lacy, C. F., Armstrong, L. L., Goldman, M. P., & Lance, L. L. (2006). *Drug information handbook* (14th ed.). Hudson, OH: Lexi-Comp, Inc.

Lausten, G., Gilbert, M., & Wimett, L. (2006). A look back at the most influential drug approvals of 2005. *Nurse Practitioner, 31*, 26–41.

Plaisance, L. (2005). Is your patient's cancer pain under control? *Nursing 2005, 35*, 52–55.

Swegle, J. M., & Logemann, C. (2006). Management of common opioid-induced adverse effects. *American Family Physician, 74*, 1347–1354.

Willens, J. S. (2008). Pain management. In S. C. Smeltzer, B. G. Bare, J. L. Hinkle, & K. H. Cheever (Eds.), *Brunner & Suddarth's textbook of medical-surgical nursing* (11th ed., pp. 258–299). Philadelphia: Lippincott Williams & Wilkins.

Analgesic–Antipyretic–Anti-Inflammatory and Related Drugs

LEARNING OBJECTIVES

After studying this chapter, you will be able to:

1. Discuss the role of prostaglandins in the etiology of pain, fever, and inflammation.
2. Discuss aspirin and other nonsteroidal anti-inflammatory drugs (NSAIDs) in terms of mechanism of action, indications for use, contraindications to use, nursing process, and principles of therapy.
3. Compare and contrast aspirin, other NSAIDs, and acetaminophen in terms of indications for use and adverse effects.
4. Differentiate among antiplatelet, analgesic, and anti-inflammatory doses of aspirin.
5. Differentiate between nonselective NSAIDs and the cyclooxygenase-2 inhibitor, celecoxib.
6. Teach patients interventions to prevent or decrease adverse effects of aspirin, other NSAIDs, and acetaminophen.
7. Identify factors influencing the use of aspirin, NSAIDs, and acetaminophen in special populations.
8. Discuss recognition and management of acetaminophen toxicity.
9. Discuss the use of NSAIDs and antigout drugs.
10. Discuss the use of NSAIDs, triptans, and ergot antimigraine drugs.

Applying Your Knowledge

Julie McKay is a 32-year-old woman who has chronic headache pain. Her first headaches began at age 18 as a combination of migraine type and tension headaches. For acute pain, she uses a combination of Excedrin Migraine (acetaminophen 250 mg, ASA 250 mg, and caffeine 65 mg per tablet), extra-strength acetaminophen (500 mg per tablet), and naproxen sodium (550 mg per tablet). For a typical headache, Julie takes two naproxen sodium tablets at the onset of her pain, followed by two tablets of the acetaminophen every 4 hours and two Excedrin Migraine tablets every 4 hours, starting 2 hours after the acetaminophen. If the pain is not relieved, she takes one naproxen sodium tablet in 12 hours and continues with the Excedrin Migraine and acetaminophen. The headache may last from 3 to 5 days.

Introduction

The analgesic–antipyretic–anti-inflammatory drug group includes chemically and pharmacologically diverse drugs that share the ability to relieve pain, fever, and/or inflammation, symptoms associated with many injuries and illnesses. Drugs discussed in this chapter include

▪ **P Aspirin** (acetylsalicylic acid [ASA]) (the prototype NSAID)

▪ Other *nonsteroidal anti-inflammatory drugs (NSAIDs)*

▪ Acetaminophen

▪ Drugs used to prevent or treat gout and migraine

Aspirin, NSAIDs, and acetaminophen can also be called *antiprostaglandin drugs*, because they inhibit the synthesis of *prostaglandins*. Prostaglandins are chemical mediators found in most body tissues; they help regulate many cell functions and participate in the inflammatory response. They are formed when cellular injury occurs and phospholipids in cell membranes release *arachidonic acid*. Arachidonic acid is then metabolized by *cyclooxygenase (COX)* enzymes to produce prostaglandins, which act briefly in the area where they are produced and are then inactivated. Prostaglandins exert various and opposing effects in different body tissues (Table 7-1). The role of prostaglandins in mediating pain, fever, and inflammation are described in the following sections.

Pain

Pain is the sensation of discomfort, hurt, or distress. It is a common human ailment and may occur with tissue injury and inflammation. Prostaglandins sensitize pain receptors and increase the pain associated with other chemical mediators of inflammation and immunity, such as bradykinin, histamine, and leukotrienes (Box 7-1).

Fever

Fever is an elevation of body temperature above the normal range. Body temperature is controlled by a regulating center in the hypothalamus. Normally, there is a balance between heat production and heat loss so that a constant body temperature is maintained. When there is excessive heat production, mechanisms to increase heat loss are activated. As a result, blood vessels dilate, more blood flows through the skin, sweating occurs, and body temperature usually stays within normal range.

Fever occurs when the set point of the hypothalamus is raised in response to the presence of *pyrogens* (fever-producing agents). Endogenous pyrogenes include cytokines such as interleukin-1, interleukin-6, and tumor necrosis factor (Box 7-1). Exogenous pyrogens include bacteria and their toxins or other byproducts. The upward adjustment of the hypothalamic set point in response to the presence of a pyrogen is mediated by prostaglandin E_2 (see Table 7-1). The body responds to the higher hypothalamic set point by vasoconstriction of blood vessels and shivering, raising the core body temperature to the higher set point. Fever may accompany conditions such as dehydration, inflammation, infectious processes, some drugs, brain injury, or diseases involving the hypothalamus.

Inflammation

Inflammation is the normal body response to tissue damage from any source, and it may occur in any tissue or organ. It is an attempt by the body to remove the damaging agent and repair the damaged tissue. The signs and symptoms of inflammation are the work of a variety of chemical mediators (Box 7-1). Prostaglandin E_2 and others induce inflammation and also enhance the effects of other mediators of the inflammatory response. Local manifestations are redness, heat, edema, and pain. Redness and heat result from vasodilation and increased blood supply. Edema results from leakage of blood plasma into the area. Pain occurs when pain receptors on nerve endings are stimulated by heat, edema, and pressure; chemicals released by

Table 7-1	Prostaglandins	
PROSTAGLANDIN	**LOCATIONS**	**EFFECTS**
PGD_2	Airways, brain, mast cells	▪ Bronchoconstriction
PGE_2	Brain, kidneys, vascular smooth muscle, platelets	▪ Bronchodilation ▪ Gastroprotection ▪ Increased activity of GI smooth muscle ▪ Increased sensitivity to pain ▪ Increased body temperature ▪ Vasodilation
PGF_2	Airways, eyes, uterus, vascular smooth muscle	▪ Bronchoconstriction ▪ Increased activity of GI smooth muscle ▪ Increased uterine contraction (e.g., menstrual cramps)
PGI_2 (Prostacyclin)	Brain, endothelium, kidneys, platelets	▪ Decreased platelet aggregation ▪ Gastroprotection ▪ Vasodilation
PGA_2 (Thromboxane A_2)	Kidneys, macrophages, platelets, vascular smooth muscle	▪ Increased platelet aggregation ▪ Vasoconstriction

GI, gastrointestinal.

Box 7-1	Chemical Mediators of Inflammation and Immunity

Bradykinin is a kinin in body fluids that becomes physiologically active with tissue injury. When tissue cells are damaged, white blood cells (WBCs) increase in the area and ingest damaged cells to remove them from the area. When the WBCs die, they release enzymes that activate kinins. The activated kinins increase and prolong the vasodilation and increased vascular permeability caused by histamine. They also cause pain by stimulating nerve endings for pain in the area. Thus, bradykinin may aggravate and prolong the erythema, heat, and pain of local inflammatory reactions. It also increases mucous gland secretion.

Complement is a group of plasma proteins essential to normal inflammatory and immunologic processes. More specifically, complement destroys cell membranes of body cells (e.g., red blood cells, lymphocytes, platelets) and pathogenic microorganisms (e.g., bacteria, viruses). The system is initiated by an antigen–antibody reaction or by tissue injury. Components of the system (called C1 through C9) are activated in a cascade type of reaction in which each component becomes a proteolytic enzyme that splits the next component in the series. Activation yields products with profound inflammatory effects. C3a and C5a, also called *anaphylatoxins*, act mainly by liberating histamine from mast cells and platelets, and their effects are therefore similar to those of histamine. C3a causes or increases smooth muscle contraction, vasodilation, vascular permeability, degranulation of mast cells and basophils, and secretion of lysosomal enzymes by leukocytes. C5a performs the same functions as C3a and also promotes movement of WBCs into the injured area (chemotaxis). In addition, it activates the lipoxygenase pathway of arachidonic acid metabolism in neutrophils and macrophages, thereby inducing formation of leukotrienes and other substances that increase vascular permeability and chemotaxis.

In the immune response, the complement system breaks down antigen–antibody complexes, especially those in which the antigen is a microbial agent. It enables the body to produce inflammation and localize an infective agent. More specific reactions include increased vascular permeability, chemotaxis, and opsonization (coating a microbe or other antigen so it can be more readily phagocytized).

Cytokines may act on the cells that produce them, on surrounding cells, or on distant cells if sufficient amounts reach the bloodstream. Thus, cytokines act locally and systemically to produce inflammatory and immune responses, including increased vascular permeability and chemotaxis of macrophages, neutrophils, and basophils. Two major types of cytokines are interleukins (produced by leukocytes) and interferons (produced by T lymphocytes or fibroblasts). Interleukin-1 (IL-1) mediates several inflammatory responses, including fever; and IL-2 (also called T-cell growth factor) is required for the growth and function of T lymphocytes. Interferons are cytokines that protect nearby cells from invasion by intracellular microorganisms, such as viruses and rickettsiae. They also limit the growth of some cancer cells.

Histamine is formed (from the amino acid histidine) and stored in most body tissue, with high concentrations in mast cells, basophils, and platelets. Mast cells, which are abundant in skin and connective tissue, release histamine into the vascular system in response to stimuli (e.g., antigen–antibody reaction, tissue injury, and some drugs). After it is released, histamine is highly vasoactive, causing vasodilation (increasing blood flow to the area and producing hypotension) and increasing permeability of capillaries and venules (producing edema). Other effects include contracting smooth muscles in the bronchi (producing bronchoconstriction and respiratory distress), gastrointestinal (GI) tract, and uterus; stimulating salivary, gastric, bronchial, and intestinal secretions; stimulating sensory nerve endings to cause pain and itching; and stimulating movement of eosinophils into injured tissue. Histamine is the first chemical mediator released in the inflammatory response and immediate hypersensitivity reactions (anaphylaxis).

When histamine is released from mast cells and basophils, it diffuses rapidly into other tissues. It then acts on target tissues through both histamine-1 (H_1) and histamine-2 (H_2) receptors. H_1 receptors are located mainly on smooth muscle cells in blood vessels and the respiratory and GI tracts. When histamine binds with these receptors, resulting events include contraction of smooth muscle, increased vascular permeability, production of nasal mucus, stimulation of sensory nerves, pruritus, and dilation of capillaries in the skin. H_2 receptors are also located in the airways, GI tract, and other tissues. When histamine binds to these receptors, there is increased secretion of gastric acid by parietal cells in the stomach mucosal lining, increased mucus secretion and bronchodilation in the airways, contraction of esophageal muscles, tachycardia, inhibition of lymphocyte function, and degranulation of basophils (with additional release of histamine and other mediators) in the bloodstream. In allergic reactions, both types of receptors mediate hypotension (in anaphylaxis), skin flushing, and headache. The peak effects of histamine occur within 1 to 2 minutes of its release and may last as long as 10 minutes, after which it is inactivated by histaminase (produced by eosinophils) or N-methyltransferase.

Leukotrienes, like prostaglandins, are derived from arachidonic acid metabolism. Leukotrienes, identified as LTB_4, LTC_4, LTD_4, and LTE_4, mediate inflammation and immune responses. LTB_4 plays a role in chemotaxis, mediating the aggregation of leukocytes at sites of injury. LTC_4, LTD_4, and LTE_4 produce smooth muscle contractility, bronchospasm, and increased vascular permeability.

Nitric oxide (NO) is synthesized by a variety of cells by the enzyme NO synthase from the amino acid arginine. It readily diffuses across cell membranes, where it reacts with a wide variety of molecules and is inactivated. NO inhibits aggregation of platelets, preventing formation of blood clots. NO relaxes smooth muscles in blood vessels, producing vasodilation. It inhibits inflammation in the walls of blood vessels. NO also plays a role in protecting against invading microbes. Helper T lymphocytes, active in the inflammatory response, secrete NO. NO also enhances the killing of phagocytized microbes within the lysosomes of cells.

Platelet-activating factor (PAF), like prostaglandins and leukotrienes, is derived from arachidonic acid metabolism and has multiple inflammatory activities. It is produced by mast cells, neutrophils, monocytes, and platelets. Because these cells are widely distributed, PAF effects can occur in virtually every organ and tissue. Besides causing platelet aggregation, PAF activates neutrophils, attracts eosinophils, increases vascular permeability, causes vasodilation, and causes IL-1 and tumor necrosis factor–alpha (TNF-alpha) to be released. PAF, IL-1, and TNF-alpha can induce each other's release.

the damaged cells; and prostaglandins. Systemic manifestations include leukocytosis, increased erythrocyte sedimentation rate, fever, headache, loss of appetite, lethargy or malaise, and weakness. Both local and systemic manifestations vary according to the cause and extent of tissue damage. In addition, inflammation may be acute or chronic.

Inflammation may be a component of virtually any illness. Inflammatory conditions affecting organs or systems are often named by adding the suffix "itis" to the involved organ or system (e.g., hepatitis). Current research findings suggest that inflammation may be important in the pathology of disorders (not previously identified as inflammatory conditions) such as heart disease and Alzheimer's disease. *Anti-inflammatory* drugs are indicated when the inflammatory response is inappropriate, abnormal or persistent, or destroys tissue.

General Characteristics of Analgesic–Antipyretic–Anti-Inflammatory and Related Drugs

Mechanism of Action

Aspirin and other NSAIDs inhibit prostaglandin synthesis in both the central nervous system (CNS) and the peripheral nervous system. The action of acetaminophen on prostaglandin inhibition is limited to the CNS. This selective action may explain the inability of acetaminophen to reduce inflammation and the absence of adverse effects in the gastrointestinal (GI) tract, kidneys, and platelets. Aspirin, other NSAIDs, and acetaminophen inhibit the COX enzymes, which are required for prostaglandin formation (Fig. 7-1). Two forms of cyclooxygenase, COX-1 and COX-2, have been identified. Aspirin and other nonselective NSAIDs inhibit both COX-1 and COX-2. The COX-2 inhibitor, celecoxib, is more selective for the COX-2 enzyme. The exact mechanism of action of acetaminophen is unclear.

COX-1 is normally synthesized continuously and is present in all tissues and cell types, especially platelets, endothelial cells, the GI tract, and the kidneys. Prostaglandins produced by COX-1 are important in numerous homeostatic functions and are associated with protective effects on the stomach and kidneys. In the stomach, prostaglandins decrease gastric acid secretion, increase mucus secretion, and regulate blood circulation. In the kidneys, they help maintain adequate blood flow and function. In the cardiovascular system, they help regulate vascular tone (i.e., vasoconstriction and vasodilation) and

platelet function. Drug-induced inhibition of these prostaglandins results in the adverse effects associated with aspirin and related nonselective NSAIDs, especially gastric irritation, ulceration, and bleeding. Inhibition of COX-1 activity in platelets may be more responsible for GI bleeding than inhibition in gastric mucosa.

COX-2 is also normally present in several tissues (e.g., brain, bone, kidneys, GI tract, female reproductive system). However, it is thought to occur in small amounts or to be inactive until stimulated by pain and inflammation. In inflamed tissues, COX-2 is induced by inflammatory chemical mediators such as interleukin-1 and tumor necrosis factor–alpha. In the GI tract, COX-2 is also induced by trauma and *Helicobacter pylori* infection, a common cause of peptic ulcer disease. Overall, prostaglandins produced by COX-2 are associated with pain and other signs of inflammation. Inhibition of COX-2 results in the therapeutic effects of analgesia and anti-inflammatory activity. The COX-2 inhibitor drugs are NSAIDs designed to selectively inhibit COX-2 and relieve pain and inflammation with fewer adverse effects, especially stomach damage; however, with long-term use, adverse effects still occur in the GI, renal, and cardiovascular systems.

Aspirin relieves pain by acting both centrally and peripherally to block the transmission of pain impulses. Related drugs act peripherally to prevent sensitization of pain receptors to various chemical substances released by damaged cells. To relieve fever, the drugs act on the hypothalamus to decrease its response to pyrogens and reset the "thermostat" at a lower level. For inflammation, the drugs prevent prostaglandins from increasing the pain and edema produced by other substances released by damaged cells. Although these drugs relieve symptoms and contribute greatly to the patient's comfort and quality of life, they do not cure the underlying disorders that cause the symptoms.

Aspirin and nonselective NSAIDs also have antiplatelet effects that differ in mechanism and extent. When aspirin is absorbed into the bloodstream, the acetyl portion dissociates and then binds irreversibly to platelet COX-1. This action prevents synthesis of thromboxane A_2, a prostaglandin derivative, thereby inhibiting platelet aggregation. A small single dose (325 mg) irreversibly acetylates circulating platelets within a few minutes, and effects last for the lifespan of the platelets (7 to 10 days). Most other NSAIDs bind reversibly with platelet COX-1 so that antiplatelet effects occur only while the drug is present in the blood. Thus, aspirin has greater effects, but all the drugs except acetaminophen and the COX-2 inhibitors inhibit platelet aggregation, interfere with blood coagulation, and increase the risk of bleeding.

Figure 7-1 ▪ Arachidonic acid metabolic pathways result in production of physiologic and pathologic (i.e., inflammatory) prostaglandins. Nonselective and selective NSAIDs inhibit production of prostaglandins by inhibiting steps in the arachidonic acid pathway.

Indications for Use

Despite many similarities, aspirin, other NSAIDs, and acetaminophen differ in their approved uses.

To Treat Inflammatory Disorders

Aspirin and other NSAIDs are widely used to prevent and treat mild to moderate pain and inflammation associated with musculoskeletal disorders (e.g., degenerative joint disease, rheumatoid arthritis, bursitis). Acetaminophen lacks anti-inflammatory effects but may be useful as an analgesic.

Degenerative joint disease (DJD), also known as osteoarthritis (OA), is a disease that affects the articular cartilage, subchondral bone, and synovium of weight-bearing joints. The joints of the fingers may also be affected by OA. Signs and symptoms of OA include pain, stiffness, and functional impairment. As joint cartilage deteriorates, over time there is less padding and lubricating fluid, underlying bone is exposed, and friction and abrasion lead to inflammation of the synovial membrane lining of the joint. Deformity of the joint occurs as the disease advances.

Rheumatoid arthritis (RA) is a chronic, painful, inflammatory disorder that affects the synovial tissue of hinge-like joints, tissues around these joints, and eventually other body organs are involved (systemic effects). It is an autoimmune disorder characterized by an inflammatory and immune reaction against the body's own tissues. Juvenile rheumatoid arthritis is a chronic, inflammatory, systemic disease that may cause joint or connective tissue damage and visceral lesions throughout the body. Onset may occur before 16 years of age.

Bursitis is an inflammation of the bursa (a cavity in connective tissue that contains synovial fluid; the fluid reduces friction between tendons and bones or ligaments). Common forms include acute painful shoulder, "tennis elbow," "housemaid's knee," and bunions.

To Relieve Pain

Aspirin, other NSAIDs, and acetaminophen are effective in treating mild to moderate pain associated with conditions such as headache, minor trauma (e.g., athletic injuries such as sprains), minor surgery (e.g., dental extraction, episiotomy), and other acute and chronic conditions. These drugs are not recommended to treat pain arising from a visceral origin. Ketorolac (Toradol) is a nonselective NSAID that is used only as an analgesic. Aspirin and other NSAIDs are also effective in relieving *dysmenorrhea* (pain associated with menstruation) since these drugs inhibit prostaglandin-mediated uterine contractions.

To Reduce Fever

Aspirin, other NSAIDs (i.e., ibuprofen), and acetaminophen are all effective in reducing fever in adults. Due to the risk of Reye's syndrome (see contraindications below), aspirin should not be used to treat fever in children.

To Suppress Platelet Aggregation

Low-dose aspirin is indicated for patients that have experienced an ischemic stroke, transient ischemic attack, angina, acute MI, or previous MI, reducing the risk of death and/or recurrent event (Level A). This indication stems from its antiplatelet activity and resultant effects on blood coagulation (i.e., decreased clot formation). Low-dose aspirin can also be used for primary prevention of MI or stroke in healthy adults. Studies such as the Women's Health Study (Ridker, 2005) reveal benefits of this application vary by age, gender, and condition. In this study, aspirin was effective in reducing risk of first MI in men of all ages and women older than 65 years. Aspirin did not afford protection from first MI in women from 40 to 60 years of age. Aspirin reduced risk of first stroke in women of all ages, but no reduction in risk was observed in men. Aspirin was effective in reducing second MI or stroke in both genders, and this effect was not age dependent. In some individuals, aspirin may fail to reduce platelet aggregation, resulting in increased risk for adverse vascular events. Aspirin resistance is described further in Evidence-Based Practice Box 7-1.

Low-dose aspirin (150 mg/day preoperatively and continued for 35 days), unless contraindicated, is also effective for prophylaxis of asymptomatic and symptomatic venous thromboembolism (VTE) in surgical patients (Level A). Additional guidelines for thromboembolism prophylaxis include use of a single dose of aspirin (150 mg) before long distance travel for individuals at high risk for VTE if not contraindicated by other conditions (Level D)

Other Indications

Several studies suggest that use of aspirin and other NSAIDs may protect against development of Alzheimer's disease and a variety of cancers (e.g., colorectal, breast, ovarian, and prostate). These possible benefits are only evident with long-term use and at high doses. The benefits versus risk of side effects such as GI bleeding are unclear at this time. No studies demonstrated any protective benefits from low-dose aspirin therapy. Celecoxib (Celebrex), a COX-2 inhibitor, is used to

treat familial adenomatous polyposis, in which the drug reduces the number of polyps and may decrease risks of colon cancer. Several NSAIDs are formulated as eye drops for use in treating eye disorders (see Chap. 63).

Contraindications to Use

The Food and Drug Administration (FDA) has issued a **BLACK BOX WARNING** regarding increased risk of serious GI adverse events including bleeding, ulceration, and perforation of the stomach and intestines with use of nonselective NSAIDs as well as the selective COX-2 inhibitor, celecoxib. Although celecoxib was formulated to have fewer adverse effects in the GI tract and renal system, long-term use and/or high dosages can result in GI bleeding and renal impairment. Consequently, all NSAIDs and aspirin are contraindicated in the presence of peptic ulcer disease, GI or other bleeding disorders, and impaired renal function. In addition, celecoxib is contraindicated in patients who are allergic to sulfonamides.

Evidence-Based Practice

7-1 Aspirin Resistance

Aspirin resistance can be operationally defined as the failure of aspirin to reduce platelet aggregation resulting in an adverse vascular event such as an MI or stroke. The reported frequency of aspirin resistance is highly variable, ranging from 5.2% up to 60%. Measuring the frequency of aspirin resistance with accuracy is difficult due to the lack of a reliable test to measure the effect of aspirin on platelets. The etiology of aspirin resistance, and even its existence, is hotly debated in the literature; the mechanism of aspirin resistance is unclear. Proposed reasons for aspirin resistance include increased sensitivity of the platelets to the platelet-aggregating effects of collagen; genetic variations in glycoprotein IIA (part of the fibrinogen receptor on platelets); altered drug targets such as a COX-1 polymorphism; poor patient compliance; interactions with nonselective NSAIDs such as ibuprofen, which may compete for COX-1 binding sites; and poor gastrointestinal absorption. Some studies have suggested that aspirin resistance may actually be a dose-related phenomenon, proposing that aspirin-resistant patients might have achieved inhibition of platelet aggregation at higher aspirin doses. Studies have also suggested that aspirin resistance changes over time and may be related to daily variations in platelet activity.

Low-dose aspirin therapy is a Level A recommendation in the evidence-based practice guidelines for prevention of serious vascular events in healthy individuals as well as those at high risk for thrombotic events. An estimated 26 million patients in the United States take ASA therapy to prevent myocardial infarctions and strokes. An aspirin resistance rate of 15% would translate into almost 4 million individuals at risk of a serious vascular event due to treatment failure. The clinical impact of this issue is immense.

References: Martin, C. P., & Talbert, R. L. (2005). Aspirin resistance: An evaluation of current evidence and measurement methods. *Pharmacotherapy, 25*, 942–953.

Patrono, C., & Rocca, B. (2007). Drug insight: Aspirin resistance—Fact or fashion? *National Clinical Practitioner Cardiovascular Medicine, 4*, 42–50.

In people who have demonstrated hypersensitivity to aspirin, all nonaspirin NSAIDs are also contraindicated because cross-hypersensitivity reactions may occur with any drugs that inhibit prostaglandin synthesis. Over-the-counter (OTC) products containing acetaminophen or aspirin/ NSAIDs are contraindicated for chronic alcohol abusers because of possible liver damage (acetaminophen) or stomach bleeding (aspirin and other NSAIDs). The FDA requires an alcohol warning label on all OTC pain relievers and fever reducers. This warning states that people who drink three or more alcoholic drinks daily should ask their health care provider before taking the products.

In children and adolescents, aspirin is contraindicated in the presence of viral infections such as influenza or chickenpox because of its association with *Reye's syndrome*. In pregnancy, aspirin is categorized as Pregnancy Risk Category D. Risks to the pregnant woman include anemia from GI blood loss and postpartum hemorrhage. Potential risks to the fetus include low birth weight, premature closure of the ductus arteriosus, renal toxicity, intracranial hemorrhage, and stillbirth. Furthermore, the safety of most nonselective NSAIDs during pregnancy has not been established.

Ketorolac, an injectable NSAID often used for pain, is contraindicated in patients at risk of excessive bleeding. Thus, ketorolac should not be administered during labor and delivery, before or during any major surgery, with suspected or confirmed cerebrovascular bleeding, or to patients who are currently taking aspirin or other NSAIDs.

The FDA has issued a **BLACK BOX WARNING** regarding increased risk of serious cardiovascular thrombotic events, myocardial infarction, and stroke with use of selective and nonselective NSAIDs. This risk may be increased with long-term use or in patients with history of cardiovascular disease or risk factors for cardiovascular disease. Three COX-2 inhibitors have been marketed in the United States: celecoxib (Celebrex), rofecoxib (Vioxx), and valdecoxib (Bextra). Only celecoxib remains available for prescription at this time. Rofecoxib was voluntarily withdrawn from the market amid concerns resulting from evidence gathered in the Adenomatous Polyp Prevention on Vioxx (APPROVe) study, which showed a significant increase in myocardial infarctions and strokes in subjects receiving rofecoxib versus a placebo. Subsequent review of data from prevention studies involving celecoxib (National Cancer Institute's Adenoma Prevention with Celecoxib trial, or APC trial) and short-term studies of valdecoxib after coronary artery bypass grafting (CABG) surgery indicated that these drugs may also be associated with an increased risk of myocardial infarctions and strokes when used for long periods of time or in high-risk clinical situations such as immediately after heart surgery. In April 2005, valdecoxib was withdrawn from the U.S. market based on data suggesting increased potential for adverse cardiovascular events as well as an increased risk of serious skin reactions such as toxic epidermal necrolysis, Stevens-Johnson syndrome, and erythema multiforme. Although data from long-term clinical trials suggest that nonselective NSAIDs may also be associated with increased cardiovascular risk, short-term use of low doses of NSAIDs for pain relief does not appear to increase the risk of adverse cardiovascular events (with the exception of valdecoxib in post-CABG patients).

A closer look at the function of two contrasting prostaglandin products of the COX enzymes (in vitro) may suggest a possible mechanism for the occurrence of adverse cardiovascular events with long-term use of COX-2 inhibitors. Prostaglandin I_2, a prostaglandin product of COX-2, has been shown to be responsible for inhibition of platelet aggregation, vasodilation, and prevention of proliferation of vascular smooth muscle cells. Thromboxane A_2, a prostaglandin product of COX-1, causes platelet aggregation, vasoconstriction, and vascular proliferation. Aspirin and older nonselective NSAIDs inhibit both prostaglandin I_2 and thromboxane A_2 formation, though the COX-2 inhibitor medications inhibit only prostaglandin I_2 formation, leaving thromboxane A_2 unopposed. It has been proposed that this imbalance may lead to an increased risk of thrombotic events, elevated blood pressure, and accelerated atherogenesis and ultimately an increased risk of cardiovascular events such as myocardial infarction and thrombotic stroke. Although this proposed mechanism is possible, the increased risk of adverse cardiovascular events with long-term use of some nonselective NSAIDs, which inhibit both COX-1 and COX-2 enzymes, cannot be fully explained by this mechanism. Research is ongoing to identify the mechanisms underlying cardiovascular risks associated with selective COX-2 inhibitors.

COX-2 inhibitors may be appropriate for patients at high risk of GI bleeding or for those individuals with intolerance to the nonselective NSAIDs; however, prescribers should carefully evaluate the patient's risk for cardiovascular events before prescribing these drugs. Further FDA review of studies involving NSAIDs and cardiovascular risk is ongoing and may result in additional recommendations in the future.

Classifications and Individual Drugs

Subgroups and selected individual drugs are described below. Indications for use, trade names, and dosage ranges of individual drugs are listed in Table 7-2.

Aspirin and Other Salicylates

P **Aspirin** is the prototype of the analgesic–antipyretic– anti-inflammatory drugs and the most commonly used salicylate. Because it is a nonprescription drug and is widely available, people tend to underestimate its usefulness. It can be purchased in plain, chewable, enteric-coated, and effervescent tablets and rectal suppositories. It is not marketed in liquid form because it is unstable in solution.

Regular aspirin tablets are well absorbed after oral administration; their action starts within 15 to 30 minutes, peaks in 1 to 2 hours, and lasts 4 to 6 hours. Taking aspirin with food

Table 7-2 **Drugs at a Glance:** Analgesic, Antipyretic, Anti-Inflammatory Drugs

Generic/Trade Name	Indications for Use	ROUTES AND DOSAGE RANGES		
		Adults	Children	Comments
Acetaminophen (Tylenol, others)	Pain Fever	PO 325–650 mg q4–6h, or 1000 mg three or four times per day; maximum 4 g/d	PO 10 mg/kg or according to age as follows: 0–3 mo, 40 mg; 4–11 mo, 80 mg; 1–2 y, 120 mg; 2–3 y, 160 mg; 4–5 y, 240 mg; 6–8 y, 320 mg; 9–10 y, 400 mg; 11 y, 480 mg. Doses may be given q4–6h to a maximum of 5 doses in 24 h.	**Warning:** Overdoses may cause fatal liver damage. Maximum recommended dose for adults is 4 g/d, from all sources. Parents and caregivers should ask pediatricians about the amounts of acetaminophen children may take safely.
		Rectal suppository 650 mg q4–6h, maximum of 6 in 24 h	Rectal suppository: age under 3 y, consult physician; age 3–6 y, 120 mg q4–6h, maximum, 720 mg in 24 h; age 6–12 y, 325 mg q4–6h, maximum 2.6 g in 24 h	
P Aspirin	Pain, fever Osteoarthritis (OA), Rheumatoid Arthritis (RA) Prophylaxis of myocardial infarction (MI), transient ischemic attacks (TIAs), and stroke in men Rheumatic fever	*Pain, fever:* PO 325– 650 mg q4h PRN; usual single dose, 650 mg *OA, RA:* PO 2–6 g/d in divided doses *Prophylaxis of MI, TIA, and stroke:* PO 81–325 mg/d *Acute rheumatic fever:* PO 5–8 g/d, in divided doses *TIAs;* PO 1300 mg/d in divided doses (650 mg twice a day or 325 mg four times a day)	*Pain, fever:* PO 10–15 mg/kg q4h, up to 60– 80 mg/kg/d *Recommended doses for weight:* 24–35 lb (10.6–15.9 kg), 162 mg; 36–47 lb (16–21.4 kg), 243 mg; 48–59 lb (21.5–26.8 kg), 324 mg; 60–71 lb (26.9–32.3 kg), 405 mg; 72–95 lb (32.4–43.2 kg), 486 mg; 96 lb or above (43.3 kg or above), 648 mg *Juvenile RA:* PO 60–110 mg/kg/d in divided doses q6–8h *Acute rheumatic fever;* PO 100 mg/kg/d, in divided doses, for 2 wk, then 75 mg/kg/d for 4–6 wk	Therapeutic serum level of salicylate is 100–300 mcg/mL for treatment of arthritis and rheumatic fever; toxicity occurs at levels above 300 mcg/mL.
Celecoxib (Celebrex)	OA RA Familial adenomatous polyposis (FAP)	OA: PO 100 mg twice daily or 200 mg once daily RA: PO 100–200 mg twice daily FAP: PO 200 mg twice daily	Dosage not established	200-mg doses should be taken with food.

(continued on page 108)

| Table 7-2 | **Drugs at a Glance:** Analgesic, Antipyretic, Anti-Inflammatory Drugs (continued) |

| Generic/Trade Name | Indications for Use | ROUTES AND DOSAGE RANGES | | |
		Adults	Children	Comments
Diclofenac potassium (Cataflam) **Diclofenac sodium** (Voltaren, Voltaren XR)	OA RA Ankylosing spondylitis (AS) Pain, dysmenorrhea	OA: PO 100–150 mg/d in divided doses (e.g., 50 mg two or three times or 75 mg twice or 100 mg once daily) RA: PO 150–200 mg/d in two, three, or four divided doses AS: PO 100–125 mg/d in four or five divided doses (e.g., 25 mg four or five times daily) *Pain, dysmenorrhea:* (diclofenac potassium only) PO 50 mg three times daily	Dosage not established	Diclofenac potassium is available only in 50-mg, *immediate-release* tablets. It may be used for all indications. Diclofenac sodium is available in 25-, 50-, and 75-mg *delayed-release* tablets and a 100-mg *extended-release* (XR) tablet. It is not recommended for acute pain or dysmenorrhea.
Diflunisal	OA RA Pain	OA, RA: PO 500–1000 mg/d, in two divided doses, increased to a maximum of 1500 mg/d if necessary *Pain:* PO 500–1000 mg initially, then 250–500 mg q8–12h	Not recommended for use in children <12 years of age	
Etodolac	OA RA Pain	OA, RA: PO 600–1200 mg/d in two to four divided doses *Pain:* PO 200–400 mg q6–8h *Maximum according to weight:* 1200 mg/d for 60 kg (132 lbs) or more; 20 mg/kg/d for <60 kg	Dosage not established	Available in *immediate-release* and *extended-release* (XR) tablets of various strengths. The immediate-release forms should be used to treat acute pain.
Flurbiprofen (Ansaid)	OA RA	OA, RA: PO 200–300 mg/d in two, three, or four divided doses	Dosage not established	
Ibuprofen (Advil, Motrin, PediaCare Fever)	OA RA Pain, dysmenorrhea Fever	OA, RA: PO 300–600 mg 3 or 4 times per day; maximum, 2400 mg/d *Pain, dysmenorrhea:* PO 400 mg q4–6h PRN; maximum, 3200 mg/d	1–12 y: Fever, initial temperature 39.2°C (102.5°F) or less, PO 5 mg/kg q6–8h; initial temperature above 39.2°C (102.5°F), PO 10 mg/kg q6–8h; maximum dose, 40 mg/kg/d *Juvenile arthritis:* PO 20–40 mg/kg/d, in three or four divided doses	Available in numerous dosage forms and concentrations, including regular tablets; chewable tablets; capsules; oral suspensions (of 100 mg/5 mL); and oral drops (of 40 mg/mL, for infants)

Generic/Trade Name	Indications for Use	ROUTES AND DOSAGE RANGES		
		Adults	Children	Comments
Indomethacin (Indocin, Indocin SR)	OA RA AS Tendinitis Bursitis Acute painful shoulder Acute gout Closure of patent ductus arteriosus (IV only)	PO, rectal suppository; 75 mg/d initially, increased by 25 mg/d at weekly intervals to a maximum of 150–200 mg/d, if necessary *Acute gouty arthritis, acute painful shoulder;* PO 75–150 mg/d in three or four divided doses until pain and inflammation are controlled (e.g., 3–5 d for gout; 7–14 d for painful shoulder), then discontinued	*Premature infants with patent ductus arteriosus;* IV 0.2–0.3 mg/kg q12h for a total of three doses	The sustained-release form is not recommended for acute gouty arthritis.
Ketoprofen (Oruvail)	Pain Dysmenorrhea OA RA	*Pain, dysmenorrhea:* PO 25–50 mg q6–8h PRN OA, RA: PO 150–300 mg/d in three or four divided doses Extended-release; 200 mg once daily Maximum; 300 mg/d for regular formulation; 200 mg/d for extended release; 100–150 mg/d for clients with impaired renal function	Do not give to children <16 years unless directed by a physician.	Extended-release capsules are available as generic ketoprofen and Oruvail. Note that the names do not contain any letters (e.g., SR, XL) that indicate long-acting dosage forms.
Ketorolac (Toradol)	Moderately severe, acute pain, for short-term (up to 5 days) treatment	IV, IM 30 mg q6h PRN to a maximum of 120 mg/d PO 10 mg q4–6h to a maximum of 40 mg/d Older adults (>65 y), those with renal impairment, those with weight < 50 kg (110 lbs); IV, IM 15 mg q6h to a maximum of 60 mg/d	Dosage not established	Treatment is started with one or more injected doses, followed by oral doses when the client is able to take them. Maximum duration of both injected and oral doses, 5 days
Meloxicam (Mobic)	OA	PO 7.5 mg once daily; increased to 15 mg once daily if necessary	Dosage not established	May be taken without regard to meals
Nabumetone	OA RA	PO 1000–2000 mg/day in one or two doses	Dosage not established	Available in 500-mg and 750-mg tablets

(continued on page 110)

Table 7-2		Drugs at a Glance: Analgesic, Antipyretic, Anti-Inflammatory Drugs (continued)

| Generic/Trade Name | Indications For Use | ROUTES AND DOSAGE RANGES | | |
		Adults	Children	Comments
Naproxen (Naprosyn) **Naproxen sodium** (Aleve, Anaprox, Naprelan)	OA RA Juvenile arthritis AS Pain Dysmenorrhea Bursitis Tendinitis Acute gout	*Naproxen:* PO 250–500 mg twice daily *Gout:* PO 750 mg initially, then 250 mg q8h until symptoms subside Maximum, 1250 mg/d *Naproxen sodium: Pain, dysmenorrhea, acute tendinitis, bursitis:* PO 550 mg q12h or 275 mg q6–8h Maximum, 1375 mg/d *OA, RA, AS:* PO 275–550 mg twice a day *Acute gout:* PO 825 mg initially, then 275 mg q8h until symptoms subside Controlled-release (Naprelan); 750– 1000 mg once daily	*Juvenile arthritis (naproxen only):* PO 10 mg/kg/d in two divided doses. Oral suspension (125 mg/5 mL) twice daily according to weight: 13 kg (29 lb), 2.5 mL; 25 kg (55 lb), 5 mL; 39 kg (84 lb), 7.5 mL OTC preparation not recommended for children < 12 y	Available in several dosage strength tablets, in a suspension, and in immediate- and delayed-release formulations
Oxaprozin (Daypro)	OA RA	PO 600–1200 mg once daily Maximum; 1800 mg/d or 26 mg/kg/d, whichever is lower, in divided doses	Dosage not established	Lower doses recommended for patients with low body weight or milder disease
Piroxicam (Feldene)	OA RA	PO 20 mg/d or 10 mg twice daily	Dosage not established	
Salsalate (Disalcid, others)	Pain, fever Rheumatic fever OA RA	PO 3000 mg/d in divided doses	Dosage not established	May be taken with food to decrease GI effects. Administer with full glass of water to prevent tablet or capsule from lodging in esophagus
Sulindac (Clinoril)	OA RA Ankylosing spondylitis Bursitis Tendinitis Acute painful shoulder Acute gout	PO 150–200 mg twice a day; maximum, 400 mg/d *Acute gout, acute painful shoulder:* PO 200 mg twice a day until pain and inflammation subside (e.g., 7–14 d), then reduce dosage or discontinue	Dosage not established	

GI, gastrointestinal; PRN, as needed.

slows absorption but also decreases gastric irritation. Absorption of enteric-coated aspirin and rectal suppositories is slower and less complete.

Aspirin is distributed to all body tissues and fluids, including fetal tissues, breast milk, and the CNS. The highest concentrations are found in the plasma, liver, heart, and lungs. In plasma, aspirin binds to albumin (75% to 90%). Aspirin has a short half-life of 15 to 20 minutes because it is rapidly converted to salicylic acid, an active metabolite. Salicylic acid has a half-life of 2 to 3 hours at low doses and 6 to 12 hours at therapeutic anti-inflammatory doses. It undergoes oxidation and conjugation in the liver, and its metabolites are excreted through the kidneys. In alkaline urine (e.g., pH of 8), renal excretion of salicylate is greatly increased.

Diflunisal is a salicylic acid derivative that differs chemically from aspirin. It is reportedly equal or superior to aspirin in mild to moderate pain, RA, and OA. Compared with aspirin, it has less *antipyretic* effect, causes less gastric irritation, and has a longer duration of action.

Salsalate (Disalcid) is a salicylate with antipyretic, analgesic, antirheumatic, and anti-inflammatory properties. It is indicated for relief of pain and fever as well as treatment of rheumatic fever, RA, and OA. It is absorbed in the small intestine rather than in the stomach and is reported to cause fewer GI adverse effects than aspirin. Onset, peak, and duration of action are similar to aspirin. The drug is metabolized in the liver and excreted in the urine.

NSAIDs

Propionic acid derivatives include flurbiprofen (Ansaid), ibuprofen (Motrin, Advil), ketoprofen (Oruvail), naproxen (Naprosyn), and oxaprozin (Daypro). In addition to their use as anti-inflammatory agents, some are used as analgesics and antipyretics. Ibuprofen, ketoprofen, and naproxen are available OTC, with recommended doses smaller and durations of use shorter than those for prescription formulations. Although these drugs are usually better tolerated than aspirin, they are much more expensive and may cause all the adverse effects associated with aspirin and other prostaglandin inhibitors.

Ibuprofen, a commonly used drug, is well absorbed with oral administration. Its action starts in about 30 minutes, peaks in 1 to 2 hours, and lasts 4 to 6 hours. The drug is highly bound (about 99%) to plasma proteins and has a half-life of about 2 hours. It is metabolized in the liver and excreted by the kidneys. It is available by prescription and OTC; in tablets, chewable tablets, capsules, oral suspension, and oral drops; and for use by adults and children.

Acetic acid derivatives include indomethacin (Indocin) and sulindac (Clinoril). These drugs have strong anti-inflammatory effects and more severe adverse effects than the propionic acid derivatives. Potentially serious adverse effects include GI ulceration, bone marrow depression, hemolytic anemia, mental confusion, depression, and psychosis. These effects are especially associated with indomethacin; sulindac was developed in an effort to find equally effective but less toxic derivatives. Adverse reactions occur less often with sulindac but are still common.

In addition to other uses, intravenous (IV) indomethacin is approved for treatment of patent ductus arteriosus in premature infants. The ductus arteriosus joins the pulmonary artery to the aorta in the fetal circulation. When it fails to close at time of birth (i.e., patent ductus arteriosus), blood is shunted from the aorta to the pulmonary artery, causing severe cardiopulmonary problems.

Related drugs are **etodolac, ketorolac** (Toradol), and **nabumetone** (Relafen). Etodolac reportedly causes less gastric irritation, especially in older adults at high risk of GI bleeding. Ketorolac is used only for pain, and although it can be given

orally, its unique characteristic is that it can be given by injection. Parenteral ketorolac reportedly compares with morphine and other opioids in analgesic effectiveness for moderate or severe pain. However, its use is limited to 5 days because it increases the risk of bleeding. Hematomas and wound bleeding have been reported with postoperative use. An intranasal form of ketorolac is currently in phase III drug testing trials and shows promise in relieving postsurgical pain and in reducing the amount of other analgesics (e.g., morphine) required in the postoperative period.

Oxicam drugs include meloxicam (Mobic) and piroxicam (Feldene). Meloxicam has a serum half-life of 15 to 20 hours and is excreted about equally in urine and feces. Piroxicam has a half-life of about 50 hours. The long half-lives allow the drugs to be given once daily, but optimal efficacy may not occur for 1 to 2 weeks.

Diclofenac sodium (Voltaren) is chemically different from but pharmacologically similar to other NSAIDs. Formulations are delayed or extended-release and onset of action is therefore delayed. Peak action occurs in about 2 hours and effects last 12 to 15 hours. The formulation of diclofenac potassium (Cataflam) is immediate-release; action starts quickly, peaks in about 20 minutes to 2 hours, and also lasts 12 to 15 hours. As a result, the potassium salt may be given for rapid relief of pain and primary dysmenorrhea. Diclofenac has a serum half-life of about 2 hours and is excreted mainly in the urine.

Only one COX-2 inhibitor, **celecoxib,** is currently marketed in the United States; however, several other COX-2 inhibitors (e.g., lumiracoxib, parecoxib, and etoricoxib) are currently under review by the FDA. COX-2 inhibitors were designed to selectively block production of prostaglandins associated with pain and inflammation without blocking those associated with protective effects on gastric mucosa, renal function, and platelet aggregation. Thus, they produce less gastric irritation and renal impairment than aspirin and other NSAIDs. However, with prolonged use or high dosages, GI bleeding, renal impairment, and associated hypertension and edema are still risks. COX-2 inhibitors are not associated with increased risk of bleeding because they do not have the antiplatelet effects of aspirin and other NSAIDs.

Celecoxib (Celebrex) is well absorbed with oral administration; peak plasma levels and peak action occur approximately 3 hours after an oral dose. It is highly protein bound (97%) and its serum half-life is about 11 hours. It is metabolized by the cytochrome P450 enzymes in the liver to inactive metabolites that are then excreted in the urine. A small amount is excreted unchanged in the urine.

Applying Your Knowledge 7-1

Review Julie's medications. What would be the most likely adverse reaction to this medication regimen, considering the total amount of medication that Julie may take for her headaches?

Acetaminophen

Acetaminophen (also called APAP, an abbreviation of *N*-acetyl-*p*-aminophenol) is a nonprescription drug commonly used as an aspirin substitute because it does not cause nausea, vomiting, or GI bleeding, and it does not interfere with blood clotting. It is equal to aspirin in analgesic and antipyretic effects, but it lacks anti-inflammatory activity.

Acetaminophen is well absorbed with oral administration, and peak plasma concentrations are reached within 30 to 120 minutes. Duration of action is 3 to 4 hours.

Acetaminophen is metabolized in the liver (Fig. 7-2); approximately 94% is excreted in the urine as nontoxic glucuronate and sulfate conjugates and 2% is excreted unchanged. The remaining 4% is metabolized by cytochrome P450 enzymes to a toxic metabolite, which is normally inactivated by conjugation with glutathione and excreted in urine. With usual therapeutic doses, a sufficient amount of glutathione is available in the liver to detoxify acetaminophen. However, in acute or chronic overdose situations, the supply of glutathione may become depleted. In the absence of glutathione, the toxic metabolite combines with liver cells and causes damage or fatal liver necrosis. In people who abuse alcohol, usual therapeutic doses may cause or increase liver damage. The probable mechanism for increased risk of hepatotoxicity in this population is that ethanol induces drug-metabolizing cytochrome P450 enzymes in the liver and reduces the available supply of glutathione. The resulting rapid metabolism of acetaminophen produces enough toxic metabolite to exceed the available glutathione and results in hepatotoxicity.

Acetaminophen is available in tablet, liquid, and rectal suppository forms and is found in numerous combination products marketed as analgesics and cold remedies. It is often prescribed with codeine, hydrocodone, or oxycodone for added analgesic effects.

Applying Your Knowledge 7-2

How Can You Avoid This Medication Error?
Julie comes down with a cold and calls the office. You advise her to take Sinutab (acetaminophen 325 mg and pseudoephedrine hydrochloride 30 mg per tablet) for relief of her symptoms in addition to her usual treatment of headache.

Drugs Used to Treat Gout and Hyperuricemia

Uric acid is a waste product resulting from protein metabolism. Elevated serum levels (*hyperuricemia*) may result from a genetic defect in purine metabolism resulting in an inability to metabolize uric acid (a waste product of protein metabolism). These individuals are sometimes called "overproducers" of uric acid. Hyperuricemia may also result from an inability to excrete uric acid, and these individuals are termed "under-excreters." Hyperuricemia may be asymptomatic or may lead to urate deposits in various tissues. In the musculoskeletal system, often in the feet, urate deposits produce periodic episodes of severe pain, edema, and inflammation (gouty arthritis). In the kidneys, urate deposits may form renal calculi or cause other damage. Secondary hyperuricemia may occur in conditions characterized by high cell destruction or turnover (e.g., leukemia, multiple myeloma, cancer chemotherapy), producing gout.

Individual drugs used to treat gout and hyperuricemia are described below; dosages are listed in Table 7-3.

Allopurinol (Zyloprim) is used to prevent or treat hyperuricemia, which occurs with gout and with antineoplastic drug therapy. Uric acid is formed by purine metabolism and an enzyme called xanthine oxidase. Allopurinol prevents

Figure 7-2 ■ Acetaminophen metabolic pathway.

Table 7-3	**Drugs at a Glance:** Drugs Used in Gout	

	ROUTES AND DOSAGE RANGES	
Generic/Trade Name	**Adults**	**Children**
Allopurinol (Zyloprim)	Mild gout, PO 200–400 mg/d Severe gout, PO 400–600 mg/d Hyperuricemia in clients with renal insufficiency, PO 100–200 mg/d Secondary hyperuricemia from anticancer drugs, PO 100–200 mg/d; maximum 800 mg/d	Secondary hyperuricemia from anticancer drugs: <6 y, PO 150 mg/d; 6–10 y, PO 300 mg/d
Colchicine	Acute attacks, PO 1.2 mg initially followed by 0.6 mg q1h or 1.2 mg q2 h until pain is relieved or diarrhea ensues.*The total amount to control pain and inflammation is usually 4–8 mg. IV 1–2 mg initially, then 0.5 mg q3–6h until response is obtained; maximum total dose 4 mg Prophylaxis, PO 0.6–1.2 mg/d	Dosage not established
Probenecid (Benemid)	PO 250 mg twice a day for 1 wk, then 500 mg twice a day	>2 y, PO 40 mg/kg/d in divided doses
Sulfinpyrazone (Anturane)	PO 100–200 mg twice a day, gradually increased over 1 wk to a maximum of 400–800 mg/d	Dosage not established

Recommended dosage varies, and some authorities do not recommend dosing until diarrhea occurs.

formation of uric acid by inhibiting xanthine oxidase. It is especially useful in treating chronic gout characterized by *tophi* (deposits of uric acid crystals in the joints, kidneys, and soft tissues) and impaired renal function. The drug promotes resorption of urate deposits and prevents their further development. Acute attacks of gout may result when urate deposits are mobilized. These may be prevented by concomitant administration of colchicine until serum uric acid levels are lowered.

Colchicine is an anti-inflammatory drug used to prevent or treat acute attacks of gout. In acute attacks, colchicine may be used for relieving inflammation, joint pain, and edema. Colchicine is no longer considered a first line medication to treat gout due to drug toxicities, and an NSAID (e.g., indomethacin) that is equally effective in treating gout is often preferentially prescribed. Colchicine decreases inflammation by decreasing the movement of leukocytes into body tissues containing urate crystals. It has no direct analgesic or antipyretic effects. In patients unable to tolerate the severe GI side effects of oral colchicine (i.e., nausea, vomiting, severe diarrhea, and abdominal pain) colchicine may be given intravenously; however, it is important to note that oral and intravenous dosages of colchicine are not the same to avoid making a dangerous drug error. Colchicine causes severe local irritation to tissues and therefore should never be administered intramuscularly or subcutaneously. Because colchicine is toxic to the bone marrow, it is limited to only 7 days of therapy. Reduced dosages are required in the presence of diminished renal or liver function, and colchicine should not be used in individuals with combined renal and hepatic insufficiency.

Probenecid (Benemid) increases the urinary excretion of uric acid. This *uricosuric* action is used therapeutically to treat hyperuricemia and gout. It is not effective in acute attacks of gouty arthritis but prevents hyperuricemia and tophi associated with chronic gout. Probenecid may cause acute gout until serum uric acid levels are within the normal range; concomitant administration of colchicine prevents this effect. (Probenecid also is used with penicillin, most often in treating sexually transmitted diseases. It increases blood levels and prolongs the action of penicillin by decreasing the rate of urinary excretion.)

Sulfinpyrazone (Anturane) is a uricosuric agent similar to probenecid. It is not effective in acute gout but prevents or decreases tissue changes of chronic gout. Colchicine is usually given during initial sulfinpyrazone therapy to prevent acute gout.

Drugs Used to Treat Migraine

Migraine headaches are characterized by periodic attacks of pain, nausea, and increased sensitivity to light and sound. Migraines demonstrate a familial pattern and are thought to be inherited as an autosomal dominant trait with incomplete penetrance. During childhood, migraine headaches are evenly distributed between genders; however, in adulthood migraines affect females three times more often than males. Migraine headaches are believed to result from periods of neural hyperexcitability, resulting in vasodilation. Vasodilation leads to pain and further neural hyperexcitability, specifically activation of the trigeminal nerve. Activation of the trigeminal nerve results in release of neuropeptides that trigger an inflammatory response within the meningeal blood vessels. Hormones, especially estrogen, are also thought to play a role in the pattern of migraine headaches. This is supported by the observation that many women experience migraine headaches at the time of their menstrual cycle. Finally, "trigger chemicals" found in foods such as monosodium glutamate (MSG), chocolate, aged cheese, and wine are associated with migraine headaches.

Drugs used to treat migraine headaches can be divided into two categories: medications used to treat acute pain and medications used to prevent migraine headaches from occurring. Drugs used for migraine prophylaxis are different in their classification and mechanism of action from medications useful in treating the acute pain of a migraine headache. Prophylactic drugs include beta blockers such as propranolol (see Chap. 18), calcium channel blockers such as nifedipine (see Chap. 50), tricyclic antidepressants such as imipramine (see Chap. 10), and anticonvulsants such as valproic acid (see Chap. 11).

Drugs used for relieving the acute pain of migraine headaches include aspirin, other NSAIDs, and acetaminophen. In most studies, aspirin, ibuprofen, naproxen, tolfenamic acid, and the combination of aspirin, acetaminophen, and caffeine seem to be the most effective in treating migraine pain. Aspirin may be combined with metoclopramide to enhance absorption and treat migraine associated nausea. Aspirin may also be combined with caffeine to speed absorption. Acetaminophen is usually combined with another analgesic such as aspirin or an opioid, rather than taken alone, when used to treat migraine pain. For severe migraine pain, opioid analgesics (see Chap. 6) may be prescribed.

Serotonin receptor (5-HT$_{1B}$ and 5-HT$_{1D}$) agonists (also known as triptans) and ergot alkaloids are prescription medications indicated for aborting acute migraine headaches. The triptans and ergot alkaloids are discussed in this section. Individual drugs are described below. Dosages are given in Table 7-4.

Almotriptan (Axert), **eletriptan** (Relpax), **frovatriptan** (Frova), **naratriptan** (Amerge), **rizatriptan** (Maxalt), **sumatriptan** (Imitrex), and **zolmitriptan** (Zomig), called "triptans," were developed specifically for the treatment of moderate or severe migraines. They are called selective serotonin 5-HT$_{1B}$ and 5-HT$_{1D}$ receptor agonists because they act on a specific serotonin (5-hydroxytryptamine, or 5-HT) receptor subtypes in the brain. Binding to serotonin receptors in the intracranial blood vessels results in vasoconstriction. Binding to serotonin receptors within the trigeminal nervous system suppresses the release of inflammatory neuropeptides, reducing inflammation in meningeal blood vessels. By constricting blood vessels and reducing vascular inflammation, triptans are effective in aborting acute migraine headaches. The drugs vary in onset of action, with subcutaneous sumatriptan acting the most rapidly and starting to relieve migraine headache within 10 minutes. Most patients obtain relief within 1 to 2 hours with all of the oral drugs. The drugs are metabolized in the liver by monoamine oxidase or cytochrome P450 enzymes; metabolism of eletriptan, rizatriptan, and zolmitriptan produces active

metabolites. Subcutaneous sumatriptan produces more adverse effects than the oral drugs, which have similar adverse effects (e.g., pain, paresthesias, nausea, dizziness, drowsiness). These drugs are considered safer than ergot alkaloids.

Because of their vasoconstrictive properties, triptans are contraindicated in patients with a history of angina pectoris, myocardial infarction, or uncontrolled hypertension. Use caution with the concurrent use of antidepressants (e.g., SSRIs, SNRIs, and MAOIs), meperidine, and dextromethorphan with triptans since all of these medications have the potential to increase serotonin levels in the brain. Serotonin syndrome, a potentially fatal reaction, may occur when two drugs that raise the serotonin levels in the brain are taken concurrently, resulting in restlessness, hallucinations, loss of coordination, tachycardia, rapid changes in blood pressure, fever, hyperactive reflexes, nausea, vomiting, and diarrhea. Serotonin syndrome occurs most frequently when a medication is initially started or the dosage is increased. Serotonin syndrome is treated by withdrawing the medications that caused this reaction and administering IV fluids and supportive medications such as cyproheptadine (Periactin) to block serotonin production and benzodiazepines to relax muscles and decrease agitation

Ergotamine tartrate (Ergomar) is an ergot alkaloid used only in the treatment of migraine. Ergot preparations relieve migraine by activating 5-HT$_{1D}$ receptors on intracranial blood vessels, resulting in vasoconstriction. Ergotamine is most effective when given sublingually or by inhalation at the onset of headache. When given orally, ergotamine is erratically absorbed, and therapeutic effects may be delayed for 20 to 30 minutes. Ergotamine is contraindicated during pregnancy and in the presence of severe hypertension, peripheral vascular disease, coronary artery disease, renal or hepatic disease, and severe infections. **Ergotamine tartrate and caffeine** (Cafergot) is a commonly used antimigraine preparation. Caffeine reportedly increases the absorption and vasoconstrictive effects of ergotamine.

Dihydroergotamine mesylate (DHE 45) is a semisynthetic derivative of ergotamine with similar mechanism of action and contraindications. The FDA has issued a **BLACK BOX WARNING** advising against concurrent therapy of dihydroergotamine with CYP 3A4 inhibitors (e.g., protease inhibitors, macrolide antibiotics, ketoconazole, grapefruit juice, and others) because the resulting increased serum levels of dihydroergotamine have been reported to result in serious or life-threatening peripheral and cerebral ischemia.

Herbal and Dietary Supplements

In addition to the drugs described above, many herbal medicines are used to relieve pain and/or inflammation. For most of these (e.g., comfrey, marigold, peppermint, primrose, ginger), such usage is anecdotal and unsupported by clinical studies. For a few supplements, there is some evidence of effectiveness with few adverse effects.

Table 7-4	Drugs at a Glance: Drugs Used in Migraine

GENERIC/TRADE NAME	ROUTES AND DOSAGE RANGES
Serotonin Agonists (Triptans)	
Almotriptan (Axert)	PO 6.25 mg, repeat after 2 h if necessary. Maximum, 12.5 mg/24h
Eletriptan (Relpax)	PO 20–40 mg as a single dose, repeat after 2 h if necessary. Maximum dose, 80 mg/d
Frovatriptan (Frova)	PO 2.5 mg; repeat after 2 h if necessary. Maximum dose, 7.5 mg
Naratriptan (Amerge)	PO 1–2.5 mg as a single dose; repeat in 4 h if necessary. Maximum, 5 mg/d
Rizatriptan (Maxalt)	PO 5–10 mg as a single dose; repeat after 2 h if necessary. Maximum dose, 30 mg/d
Sumatriptan (Imitrex)	PO 25–100 mg as a single dose. Maximum dose, 300 mg/d
	Sub-Q 6 mg as a single dose. Maximum, 12 mg/d
	Nasal spray 5, 10, or 20 mg by unit-dose spray device. Maximum, 40 mg/d
Zolmitriptan (Zomig)	PO 1.25–2.5 mg as a single dose; may repeat after 2 h if necessary. Maximum dose, 10 mg/d
	Nasal spray 0.5, 1, 2.5, or 5 mg by unit-dose spray device. Maximum, 10 mg/d
	Orally disintegrating tablets (Zomig-ZMT) 2.5–5 mg as a single dose; may repeat after 2 h if necessary. Maximum dose, 10 mg/d
Ergot Preparations	
Dihydroergotamine mesylate (DHE 45)	IM 1 mg at onset of migraine, may be repeated hourly, if necessary, to a total of 3 mg
	IV 1 mg, repeated, if necessary, after 1 h; maximum dose 2 mg. Do not exceed 6 mg/wk.
Ergotamine tartrate (Ergomar)	PO, sublingually, 1–2 mg at onset of migraine, then 2 mg q30 min, if necessary, to a maximum of 6 mg/24 h or 10 mg/wk
	Inhalation, 0.36 mg (one inhalation) at onset of migraine, repeat in 5 min, if necessary, to a maximum of 6 inhalations/24 h
Ergotamine tartrate and caffeine (Cafergot)	*Adults:* PO 2 tablets at onset of migraine, then 1 tablet q30 min, if necessary, up to 6 tablets per attack or 10 tablets/wk
	Rectal suppository 0.5–1 suppository at onset of migraine, repeat in 1 h, if necessary, up to two suppositories per attack or five suppositories/wk
	Children: PO 0.5–1 tablet initially, then 0.5 tablet q30 min, if necessary, to a maximum of three tablets

Feverfew is an herbal medicine with some evidence of effectiveness in migraine, especially in reducing incidence and severity. Its main active ingredient is thought to be parthenolide. Feverfew is thought to inhibit platelet aggregation, prostaglandin synthesis, and the release of inflammatory mediators such as histamine, but its exact mechanism in migraine prophylaxis is unknown. It is contraindicated in pregnant and lactating women.

In general, patients should be encouraged to try standard methods of preventing and treating migraine before taking products with uncertain benefits and risks. For example, commercial preparations of feverfew are not standardized and may contain different amounts of parthenolide. The usual recommended dose is 25 to 50 milligrams daily with food, but more studies are needed.

Adverse effects include hypersensitivity reactions in people who are allergic to ragweed, asters, chrysanthemums, or daisies, and stopping the preparation abruptly can result in withdrawal symptoms of pain and stiffness. No interactions with OTC or prescription drugs have been reported, but there is a potential for increasing risks of bleeding in patients taking an antiplatelet drug (e.g., aspirin) or an anticoagulant (e.g., warfarin).

Chondroitin and glucosamine can each be used alone but are more often taken in combination to relieve the pain of osteoarthritis. Chondroitin sulfate (CS), a supplement extracted from animal cartilage or manufactured synthetically and used to treat arthritis, is thought to delay the breakdown of joint cartilage (by inhibiting elastase, a proteolytic enzyme found in synovial membranes), to stimulate synthesis of new cartilage (by stimulating chondrocytes to produce collagen and proteoglycan), and to promote the "shock-absorbing" quality of cartilage (by retaining water).

Chondroitin is a normal component of joint cartilage, which also contains water (65% to 80%), collagen, proteoglycans, and chondrocytes that produce new collagen and proteoglycans. CS was first used as a dietary supplement because studies suggested that it would promote healing of cartilage damaged by inflammation or injury. The daily dose of CS is based on weight: less than 120 pounds, 800 milligrams; 120 to 200 pounds, 1200 milligrams; more than 200 pounds, 1600 milligrams. CS is usually taken with food, in two to four divided doses.

Proponents of CS cite clinical trials that indicate beneficial effects and low incidence of adverse effects. In 2003, a meta-analysis of 15 high-quality, randomized, double-blind controlled trials comparing chondroitin and glucosamine to placebo or active control concluded that oral CS significantly improved symptoms, including joint mobility, in patients with OA. Adverse effects were found to be statistically similar to placebo in all studies. The main adverse effect of CS is reportedly minor stomach upset. In addition, there is a theoretical risk of bleeding because of the drug's structural similarity to heparin, but there have been no reports of bleeding from the use of CS.

Opponents question whether CS is absorbed systemically, because of its large molecular size, and whether it is able to reach cartilage cells. They also state that little is known about long-term toxicity of the compound.

Glucosamine, a synthetic supplement, is also taken for arthritis. Glucosamine is an essential structural component of joint connective tissue. With OA, glucosamine production is decreased, synovial fluid becomes thin and less effective in lubricating the joint, and joint cartilage deteriorates. The rationale for taking supplementary glucosamine is to reduce cartilage breakdown and improve cartilage production and repair.

Some studies indicate that glucosamine may decrease mild to moderate pain caused by OA in some patients, possibly as well as NSAIDs. Other studies indicate little or no benefit when glucosamine is compared with placebo. There is controversy about the ability of glucosamine to affect cartilage structure and delay joint deterioration. Most studies are criticized as being too small, of too short a duration, and of having flawed designs. A study of 212 patients with knee OA indicated that long-term use of glucosamine improves symptoms and prevents changes in joint structure. These patients took 1500 milligrams of glucosamine sulfate or placebo once a day for 3 years. Radiographs of the knees were taken before starting glucosamine and after 1 and 3 years of treatment. The researchers concluded that significant improvement of symptoms and less joint deterioration occurred in patients receiving glucosamine. Critics of this study said the pain relief was minor and the radiographic changes were insignificant and did not indicate improvement in disease progression.

The previously mentioned 2003 meta-analysis, which compared chondroitin and glucosamine with placebo or con-

trols, concluded that structural improvement as measured by joint space narrowing was significantly demonstrated in patients receiving glucosamine. Glucosamine significantly improved joint structure and symptoms in patients with OA of the knee.

Glucosamine is available as a hydrochloride salt and as a sulfate salt. Most studies have been performed with glucosamine sulfate (GS), which is the preferred form. Dosage of GS is based on weight: less than 120 pounds, 1000 milligrams; 120 to 200 pounds, 1500 milligrams; more than 200 pounds, 2000 milligrams. GS is usually taken with food, in two to four divided doses.

There are no known contraindications to the use of glucosamine, but it should be avoided during pregnancy and lactation and in children, because effects are unknown. Adverse effects include GI upset (e.g., epigastric pain, heartburn, nausea, constipation, diarrhea), drowsiness, headache, and skin rash. No interactions with OTC or prescription drugs have been reported.

In an effort to clarify the efficacy of glucosamine and chondroitin, the Glucosamine/Chondroitin Arthritis Intervention Trial (GAIT), funded by the National Institutes of Health, was conducted at 16 rheumatology centers around the United States. The results of this study, published in 2006, suggest the benefit of glucosamine and chondroitin depends on pain severity. In people with moderate-to-severe knee OA pain, glucosamine was more effective in relieving pain than celecoxib, either supplement alone, or a placebo. In subjects with mild OA knee pain, glucosamine and chondroitin did not show effectiveness over a placebo. Based on the GAIT results, the Arthritis Foundation issued a statement supportive of the potential benefits of using glucosamine and chondroitin as part of the overall treatment plan in individuals with moderate to severe knee OA (Level A). Because benefits of glucosamine and chondroitin may be delayed, some physicians suggest taking the supplements for 3 months (glucosamine 500 mg and chondroitin 400 mg three times a day) and then evaluating for clinical improvement (e.g., less pain, improved ability to walk).

A Cochrane review of studies including 13 herbal medicines proposed for relief of back pain was completed in 2006. Three herbal medicines seemed to reduce low back pain more than a placebo. The review reported moderate evidence that 50 to 100 milligrams of *Harpagophytum procumbens* (Devil's claw) and 120 to 240 milligrams of *Salix alba* (White willow bark) are useful in the short-term treatment of acute nonspecific low back pain and limited evidence that the topical application of *Capsicum frutescens* (Cayenne) is beneficial. Devil's claw is proposed to have anti-inflammatory actions; however, this effect is not due to arachidonic acid metabolism. Devil's claw is contraindicated in patients with ulcers or in pregnant women because the drug may stimulate uterine contractions. Chemical components of Devil's claw are reported to affect chronotropic (heart rate) and inotropic (force of contraction) cardiac function and lower blood glucose. Consequently, individuals with cardiac disorders, dysrhythmias, and diabetes should exercise caution in using Devil's claw. White willow bark contains salicylate-like chemical compounds and shares similar adverse reactions, contraindications, and drug interactions with other salicylates (i.e., aspirin). Capsicum is thought to reduce pain by depleting substance P, a mediator in the transmission of pain impulses from peripheral receptors to the central nervous system. Capsicum should not be used by pregnant women. Simultaneous use of heat treatments with capsicum should be avoided to prevent possible skin irritation.

Many herbal medications have the potential to interact with aspirin, other NSAIDs, and acetaminophen. Ginkgo, garlic, ginger, bilberry, dong quai, feverfew, ginseng, tumeric, meadowsweet, and willow possess antiplatelet actions and may interact with aspirin and other NSAIDs, increasing the risk of bleeding. Camomile, motherworth, horse chestnut, fenugreek, and red clover possess coumarin-like activity and may increase the risk of bleeding when taken with ASA or other NSAIDs. Ginkgo (and possibly some of the previously mentioned herbs) may also increase the risk of bleeding when used with acetaminophen. Echinacea and kava are potentially hepatotoxic and may increase the risk of liver damage when used concurrently with acetaminophen. Willow and meadowsweet may increase the risk of nephrotoxicity when taken concurrently with acetaminophen.

Nursing Process

Assessment

- Assess for signs and symptoms of pain, such as location, severity, duration, and factors that cause or relieve the pain (see Chap. 6).
- Assess for fever (thermometer readings above 99.6°F [37.3°C] are usually considered fever). Hot, dry skin; flushed face; reduced urine output; and concentrated urine may accompany fever if the person also is dehydrated.
- Assess for inflammation. Local signs are redness, heat, edema, and pain or tenderness; systemic signs include fever, elevated white blood cell count (leukocytosis), and weakness.
- With arthritis or other musculoskeletal disorders, assess for pain and limitations in activity and mobility.
- Ask about use of OTC analgesic, antipyretic, or anti-inflammatory drugs and herbal or dietary supplements.
- Ask about allergic reactions to aspirin or NSAIDs.
- Assess for history of peptic ulcer disease, GI bleeding, liver, or kidney disorders.
- With migraine, assess severity and patterns of occurrences.

Nursing Diagnoses

- Acute Pain
- Chronic Pain

- Activity Intolerance related to pain
- Risk for Poisoning: Acetaminophen overdose
- Risk for Injury related to adverse drug effects (GI bleeding, renal insufficiency, liver damage)
- Deficient Knowledge: Therapeutic and adverse effects of commonly used drugs
- Deficient Knowledge: Correct use of OTC drugs for pain, fever, and inflammation

Planning/Goals

The patient will

- Experience relief of discomfort with minimal adverse drug effects
- Experience increased mobility and activity tolerance
- Inform health care providers if taking aspirin, an NSAID or acetaminophen regularly.
- Self-administer the drugs safely
- Avoid overuse of the drugs
- Use measures to prevent accidental ingestion or overdose, especially in children
- Experience fewer and less severe attacks of migraine

Interventions

Implement measures to prevent or minimize pain, fever, and inflammation.

- Treat the disease processes (e.g., infection, arthritis) or circumstances (e.g., impaired blood supply, lack of physical activity, poor positioning or body alignment) thought to be causing pain, fever, or inflammation.
- Treat pain as soon as possible; early treatment may prevent severe pain and anxiety and allow the use of milder analgesic drugs. Use distraction, relaxation techniques, or other nonpharmacologic techniques along with drug therapy, when appropriate.
- With acute musculoskeletal injuries (e.g., sprains) think *RICE: Rest, Ice, Compression, Elevation* to decrease pain, swelling, and inflammation. Cold therapy should be applied for 20 minutes every 3 to 4 hours for 48 hours.
- Assist patients with migraine to identify and avoid "triggers."
- Assist patients to drink 2 to 3 liters of fluid daily when taking an NSAID regularly. This strategy decreases gastric irritation and helps to maintain good kidney function. With long-term use of aspirin, fluids help to prevent precipitation of salicylate crystals in the urinary tract. With antigout drugs, fluids help to prevent precipitation of urate crystals and formation of urate kidney stones. Fluid intake is especially important initially when serum uric acid levels are high and large amounts of uric acid are being excreted.
- Provide appropriate teaching for any drug therapy (see accompanying displays).

Evaluation

- Interview and observe regarding relief of symptoms.
- Interview and observe regarding mobility and activity levels.
- Interview and observe regarding safe, effective use of the drugs.
- Select drugs appropriately.

Applying Your Knowledge 7-3

Given Julie's medication regimen, what nursing measures should be implemented to decrease the probability of GI bleeding?

Principles of Therapy

Use of Aspirin

When pain, fever, or inflammation is present, aspirin is effective across a wide range of clinical conditions. Like any other drug, aspirin must be used appropriately to maximize therapeutic benefits and minimize adverse reactions.

For pain, aspirin is useful alone when the discomfort is of low to moderate intensity. For more severe pain, aspirin may be combined with an oral opioid (e.g., codeine) or given between opioid doses. Aspirin and opioid analgesics act by different mechanisms, so such use is rational. For acute pain, aspirin is taken when the pain occurs and is often effective within a few minutes. For chronic pain, a regular schedule of administration, such as every 4 to 6 hours, is more effective.

For fever, aspirin is effective if drug therapy is indicated. However, aspirin is contraindicated in children because of its association with Reye's syndrome.

For inflammation, aspirin is useful in both short- and long-term therapy of conditions characterized by pain and inflammation, such as RA or OA. Although effective, the high doses and frequent administration required for anti-inflammatory effects increase the risks of GI upset, ulceration, and bleeding.

For acute pain or fever, plain aspirin tablets are preferred. For chronic pain, long-term use in arthritis, and daily use for antiplatelet effects, enteric-coated tablets may be better tolerated. Rectal suppositories are sometimes used when oral administration is contraindicated.

Drug Dosage

The dose of aspirin given depends mainly on the condition being treated. Low doses (325 mg initially and 80 mg daily) are used for antiplatelet effects in preventing arterial thrombotic disorders such as myocardial infarction or stroke. Because aspirin is highly protein bound, lower-than-average doses are needed for patients with low serum albumin levels, because a larger proportion of each dose is free to exert pharmacologic activity. Larger doses are needed for anti-inflammatory effects (maximum daily dosage of 8000 mg) than for analgesic and antipyretic effects (325 to 650 mg every 4 hours). In general, patients taking low-dose aspirin to prevent myocardial infarction or stroke should continue to take the aspirin if prescribed a COX-2 inhibitor NSAID because the COX-2 inhibitors have little effect on platelet function.

Toxicity: Recognition and Management

Salicylate intoxication (*salicylism*) may occur with an acute overdose or with chronic use of therapeutic doses, especially the higher doses taken for anti-inflammatory effects. Chronic ingestion of large doses saturates a major metabolic pathway, thereby slowing drug elimination, prolonging the serum half-life, and causing drug accumulation.

Prevention

To decrease risks of toxicity, plasma salicylate levels should be measured when an acute overdose is suspected and periodically when large doses of aspirin are taken long term. Therapeutic levels are 150 to 300 micrograms per milliliter. Signs of salicylate toxicity occur at serum levels greater than 200; severe toxic effects may occur at levels greater than 400.

Signs and Symptoms

Manifestations of salicylism include nausea, vomiting, fever, fluid and electrolyte deficiencies, tinnitus, decreased hearing, visual changes, drowsiness, confusion, hyperventilation, and others. Severe CNS dysfunction (e.g., delirium, stupor, coma, seizures) indicates life-threatening toxicity.

Treatment

In mild salicylism, stopping the drug or reducing the dose is usually sufficient. In severe salicylate overdose, treatment is symptomatic and aimed at preventing further absorption from the GI tract; increasing urinary excretion; and correcting fluid, electrolyte, and acid–base imbalances. When the drug may still be in the GI tract, gastric lavage and activated charcoal help reduce absorption. IV sodium bicarbonate produces an alkaline urine in which salicylates are more rapidly excreted, and hemodialysis effectively removes salicylates from the blood. IV fluids are indicated when high fever or dehydration is present. The specific content of IV fluids depends on the serum electrolyte and acid–base status.

Use of NSAIDs

Nonaspirin NSAIDs are widely used and preferred by many people because of less gastric irritation and GI upset compared with aspirin. Many NSAIDs are prescription drugs used primarily for analgesia and anti-inflammatory effects in arthritis and other musculoskeletal disorders. However, several are approved for more general use as an analgesic or antipyretic. Ibuprofen, ketoprofen, and naproxen are available by prescription and OTC. Patients must be instructed to avoid combined use of prescription and nonprescription NSAIDs because of the high risk of adverse effects. NSAIDs commonly cause gastric mucosal damage, and prolonged use may lead to gastric ulceration and

Patient Teaching Guidelines | Drugs Used in Migraine

General Considerations

■ Try to identify and avoid situations known to precipitate acute attacks of migraine.

■ For mild or infrequent migraine attacks, acetaminophen, aspirin, or another nonsteroidal anti-inflammatory drug may be effective.

■ For moderate-to-severe migraine attacks, the drug of first choice is probably sumatriptan (Imitrex) or a related drug, if not contraindicated (e.g., by heart disease or hypertension). However, one of these drugs should not be taken if an ergot preparation has been taken within the previous 24 hours.

■ If you have frequent or severe migraine attacks, consult a physician about medications to prevent or reduce the frequency of acute attacks.

■ Never take an antimigraine medication prescribed for someone else or allow someone else to take yours. The medications used to relieve acute migraine can constrict blood vessels, raise blood pressure, and cause serious adverse effects.

■ Chronic overuse of analgesics, preparations containing sedatives or caffeine, triptans, opioids, or ergotamine may play a role in causing rebound headaches.

Self-Administration

■ Take medication at onset of pain, when possible, to prevent development of more severe symptoms.

■ With triptans, take oral drugs (except for rizatriptan and zolmitriptan orally disintegrating tablets) with fluids. If symptoms recur, a second dose may be taken. However, do not take a second dose of almotriptan, eletriptan, frovatriptan, rizatriptan, or zolmitriptan sooner than 2 hours after the first dose, or a second dose of naratriptan sooner

than 4 hours after the first dose. Do not take more than 12.5 mg of almotriptan, 80 mg of eletriptan, 7.5 mg of frovatriptan, 5 mg of naratriptan, 30 mg of rizatriptan, or 10 mg of zolmitriptan in any 24-hour period.

■ Rizatriptan and zolmitriptan are available in a regular tablet, which can be taken with fluids, and in an orally disintegrating tablet, which can be dissolved on the tongue and swallowed without fluids. The tablet should be removed from its package with dry hands and placed on the tongue immediately. Zolmitriptan is also available as a nasal spray. The usual dose is one spray into one nostril, not to exceed 10 mg/d (2 doses).

■ Sumatriptan can be taken by mouth, injection, or nasal spray. Instructions should be strictly followed for the prescribed method of administration. For the nasal spray, the usual dose is one spray into one nostril. If symptoms return, a second spray may be taken 2 hours or longer after the first spray. Do not take more than 40 mg of nasal spray or 200 mg orally or by injection in any 24-hour period. If self-administering injectable sumatriptan, be sure to give in fatty tissue under the skin. This drug must not be taken intravenously; serious, potentially fatal reactions may occur.

■ If symptoms of an allergic reaction (e.g., shortness of breath, wheezing, heart pounding, swelling of eyelids, face or lips, skin rash, or hives) occur after taking a triptan drug, tell your prescribing physician immediately and do not take any additional doses without specific instructions to do so.

■ With ergot preparations, report signs of poor blood circulation, such as tingling sensations or coldness, numbness, or weakness of the arms and legs. These are symptoms of ergot toxicity. To avoid potentially serious adverse effects, do not exceed recommended doses.

Patient Teaching Guidelines | Acetaminophen, Aspirin, and Other NSAIDs

General Considerations

■ Aspirin and other anti-inflammatory drugs such as ibuprofen are used to relieve pain, fever, and inflammation. Aspirin is as effective as the more costly medications but at typical doses is more likely to cause stomach irritation and bleeding problems.

■ Many prescription and OTC medications for pain, fever, and colds/flu/sinusitis contain acetaminophen, aspirin, or other NSAIDs. There is a risk of overdosing when taking different products containing the same or similar medications. Read all drug labels carefully and do not exceed the *total* recommended dosage for any medication.

■ It is generally safe to take an occasional dose of aspirin or an NSAID for pain or fever if taking low-dose aspirin to prevent heart attack or stroke.

■ Improvement of symptoms with NSAIDs depends on the reason for use. When taken for pain, the drugs usually act within 30 to 60 minutes; when taken for inflammatory disorders, improvement may occur within 24 to 48 hours with aspirin and 1 to 2 weeks with other NSAIDs.

■ Taking a medication for fever is not usually recommended unless the fever is high or is accompanied by other symptoms. Fever is one way the body fights infection.

■ Do not take OTC ibuprofen more than 3 days for fever or 10 days for pain. If these symptoms persist or worsen, or if new symptoms develop, contact a health care provider.

■ Avoid aspirin for approximately 2 weeks before and after major surgery or dental work to decrease the risk of excessive bleeding. If pregnant, do not take aspirin for approximately 2 weeks before the estimated delivery date.

■ Inform any health care provider if taking acetaminophen, aspirin, ibuprofen, or any other NSAID regularly.

■ Inform health care providers if you have ever had an allergic reaction (e.g., asthma, difficulty in breathing, hives), severe GI symptoms (e.g., ulcer, bleeding), or rash or other skin disorder after taking aspirin, ibuprofen, or similar drugs.

■ Avoid or minimize alcoholic beverages because alcohol increases gastric irritation and risks of bleeding. The Food and Drug Administration requires an alcohol warning on

(continued on page 120)

Patient Teaching Guidelines — Acetaminophen, Aspirin, and Other NSAIDs (continued)

the labels of OTC pain and fever relievers and urges people who drink three or more alcoholic drinks every day to ask their doctors before using the products.

■ To avoid accidental ingestion and aspirin poisoning, store aspirin in a closed childproof container and keep out of children's reach.

Self-Administration

■ Take aspirin and other NSAIDs with a full glass of liquid and food to decrease stomach irritation. Meloxicam (Mobic) may be taken without regard to food.

■ Swallow enteric-coated aspirin whole; do not chew or crush. The coating is applied to decrease stomach irritation by making the tablet dissolve in the intestine. Also do not take with an antacid, which can cause the tablet to dissolve in the stomach.

■ Swallow any long-acting pills or capsules whole; do not chew or crush. If you are unsure whether the medication you are taking is long acting, ask your health care provider.

■ Drink 2 to 3 quarts of fluid daily when taking an NSAID regularly. This decreases gastric irritation and helps to maintain good kidney function.

■ Report signs of bleeding (e.g., nose bleed, vomiting blood, bruising, blood in urine or stools), difficulty breathing, skin rash or hives, ringing in ears, dizziness, severe stomach upset, or swelling and weight gain.

Acetaminophen

■ Acetaminophen is often the initial drug of choice for relieving mild to moderate pain and fever because it

does not cause gastric irritation or bleeding. It may be taken on an empty stomach.

■ Acetaminophen is an effective aspirin substitute for pain or fever but not for inflammation or prevention of heart attack or stroke.

■ Do not exceed recommended doses of acetaminophen due to risk of life-threatening liver damage. People with liver disorders such as hepatitis or those who ingest alcoholic beverages frequently should use extreme caution.

■ Do not exceed recommended duration of use (longer than 5 days in children, 10 days in adults, or 3 days for fever in adults and children) without consulting a physician.

■ Avoid or minimize alcoholic beverages because alcohol increases risk of liver damage. People who ingest three or more alcoholic drinks every day should ask their doctors before taking products containing acetaminophen.

Antigout Drugs

■ When colchicine is taken for acute gout, pain is usually relieved in 4 to 12 hours with IV administration and in 24 to 48 hours with oral administration. Inflammation and edema may not decrease for several days.

■ With colchicine for chronic gout, carry the drug and take as directed when pain begins until relief is obtained or nausea, vomiting, and diarrhea occur.

■ Drink 2 to 3 quarts of fluid daily with antigout drugs. An adequate fluid intake helps prevent formation of uric acid kidney stones. Fluid intake is especially important initially, when uric acid levels in the blood are high and large amounts or uric acid are being excreted in the urine.

■ When allopurinol is taken, blood levels of uric acid usually decrease to normal range within 1 to 3 weeks.

bleeding even in the absence of prior warning signs. Because NSAIDs lead to renal impairment in some patients, blood urea nitrogen and serum creatinine should be checked approximately 2 weeks after starting any of the agents.

NSAIDs inhibit platelet activity only while drug molecules are in the bloodstream, not for the life of the platelet (approximately 1 week) as aspirin does. Thus, they are not prescribed therapeutically for antiplatelet effects.

Effects of NSAIDs on Other Drugs

NSAIDs decrease effects of certain drugs. With angiotensin-converting enzyme (ACE) inhibitors, decreased antihypertensive effects are probably caused by sodium and water retention. With beta blockers, decreased antihypertensive effects are attributed to NSAID inhibition of renal prostaglandin synthesis, which allows unopposed pressor systems to produce hypertension. With diuretics, decreased effects on hypertension and edema are attributed to retention of sodium and water. Chronic use of NSAIDs, particularly ibuprofen, has been shown to inhibit the cardioprotective effects of low-dose aspirin by competing with aspirin for COX-1 inhibition.

NSAIDs increase effects of other drugs. With anticoagulants, prothrombin time may be prolonged, and risks of bleed-

ing are increased by NSAID-induced gastric irritation and antiplatelet effects. With cyclosporine, nephrotoxicity associated with both drugs may be increased. With digoxin, ibuprofen and indomethacin may increase serum levels. With phenytoin, serum drug levels and pharmacologic effects, including adverse or toxic effects, may be increased. With lithium, serum drug levels and risk of toxicity may be increased (except with sulindac, which has no effect or may decrease serum lithium levels). With methotrexate (MTX), risks of toxicity (e.g., stomatitis, bone marrow suppression, nephrotoxicity) may be increased. Celecoxib and meloxicam apparently do not increase MTX toxicity.

Use of Acetaminophen

Acetaminophen is effective and widely used for the treatment of pain and fever. It has two major advantages over aspirin: acetaminophen does not cause gastric irritation or increase the risk of bleeding. It is the drug of choice for children with febrile illness (because of the association of aspirin with Reye's syndrome), elderly adults with impaired renal function (because aspirin and NSAIDs may cause further impairment), and pregnant women (because aspirin is associated with several maternal and fetal disorders, including bleeding).

Despite the high degree of safety of acetaminophen when used appropriately, it is not the drug of choice for people with hepatitis or other liver disorders or for those who drink substantial amounts of alcoholic beverages. The major drawback to acetaminophen use is potentially fatal liver damage with overdose. The kidneys and myocardium may also be damaged.

Toxicity: Recognition and Management

Acetaminophen poisoning may occur with a single large dose (possibly as little as 6 g, but usually 10–15 g) or with chronic ingestion of excessive doses (5–8 g/day for several weeks or 3–4 g/day for 1 year). Potentially fatal hepatotoxicity is the main concern and is most likely to occur with doses of 20 grams or more. Metabolism of acetaminophen produces a toxic metabolite that is normally inactivated by combining with glutathione. In overdose situations, the supply of glutathione is depleted and the toxic metabolite accumulates and directly damages liver cells (see Fig. 7-2). Acute renal failure may also occur.

Prevention

The recommended maximum daily dose is 4 grams for adults; additional amounts constitute an overdose. Ingestion of an overdose may be accidental or intentional. One contributing factor may be that some people think the drug is so safe that they can take any amount without harm. Another may be that people take the drug in several formulations without calculating or realizing that they are taking potentially harmful amounts. For example, numerous brand names of acetaminophen are available OTC, and acetaminophen is an ingredient in many prescription and OTC combination products (e.g., Percocet; OTC cold, flu, headache, and sinus remedies). For chronic alcohol abusers, short-term ingestion of usual therapeutic doses may cause hepatotoxicity, and it is recommended that these persons ingest no more than 2 grams daily. The FDA has issued a warning advising individuals who ingest three or more alcoholic drinks daily to avoid acetaminophen or to ask a physician before using even small doses. Another recommendation is to limit duration of use (5 days or less in children, 10 days or less in adults, and 3 days in both adults and children when used to reduce fever) unless directed by a physician.

Because of multiple reports of liver damage from acetaminophen poisoning, the FDA has strengthened the warning on products containing acetaminophen and emphasized that the maximum adult dose of 4 grams daily, from all sources, should not be exceeded.

Signs and Symptoms

Early symptoms (12–24 hours after ingestion) are nonspecific (e.g., anorexia, nausea, vomiting, diaphoresis) and may not be considered serious or important enough to report or seek treatment. At 24 to 48 hours symptoms may subside, but tests of liver function (e.g., aspartate aminotransferase, alanine aminotransferase, bilirubin, prothrombin time) begin to show increased levels. Later manifestations may include jaundice, vomiting, and CNS stimulation with excitement and delirium, followed by vascular collapse, coma, and death. Peak hepato-

toxicity occurs in 3 to 4 days; recovery in nonfatal overdoses occurs in 7 to 8 days.

Plasma acetaminophen levels should be obtained when an overdose is known or suspected, preferably within 4 hours after ingestion and every 24 hours for several days. Minimal hepatotoxicity is associated with plasma levels of less than 120 micrograms per milliliter at 4 hours after ingestion or less than 30 micrograms per milliliter at 12 hours after ingestion. With blood levels greater than 300 micrograms per milliliter at 4 hours after ingestion, about 90% of patients develop liver damage.

Treatment

Gastric lavage is recommended if overdose is detected within 4 hours after ingestion, and activated charcoal can be given to inhibit absorption. In addition, the specific antidote is acetylcysteine (Mucomyst), a mucolytic agent given by inhalation in respiratory disorders. For acetaminophen poisoning, acetylcysteine (Mucomyst) may be given orally or intravenously (Acetadote) (dosages are listed with other antidotes in Chap. 2). The drug provides cysteine, a precursor substance required for the synthesis of glutathione. The synthesized glutathione combines with a toxic metabolite and decreases hepatotoxicity. Acetylcysteine is most beneficial if given within 8 to 10 hours of acetaminophen ingestion but may be helpful within 36 hours. It does not reverse damage that has already occurred.

Applying Your Knowledge 7-4

How much acetaminophen is Julie possibly consuming in a 24-hour time period, and what danger does this present?

Treatment of Specific Disorders

Arthritis

The primary goals of treatment are to control pain and inflammation and to minimize immobilization and disability. Rest, exercise, physical therapy, and drugs are used to attain these goals. Few of these measures prevent or slow joint destruction.

Osteoarthritis (OA)

The main goal of drug therapy is relief of pain. Acetaminophen (4 g/day) is the initial drug of choice unless contraindicated by liver disease or hypersensitivity (Level A). Aspirin and other NSAIDs are also effective in reducing pain and inflammation (Level A); an antacid, H_2 blocker, or proton pump inhibitor may be added to the treatment regime for gastroprotection (Level A). Ibuprofen and other propionic acid derivatives are often used, although available NSAIDs have comparable effectiveness. A drug may be given for 2 or 3 weeks on a trial basis. If therapeutic benefits occur, the drug may be continued; if no benefits seem evident or toxicity occurs, another drug may be tried. A COX-2 inhibitor may be preferred for patients at high risk of GI ulceration and bleeding; however, caution must be used for individuals with cardiovascular risk factors or renal dysfunction (Level B). NSAIDs are usually given in analgesic doses for OA, rather than the larger anti-inflammatory doses given for RA.

Additional treatments for knee OA include topical capsaicin, oral chondroitin and glucosamine, and intra-articular injections of corticosteroids (see Chap. 23) or hyaluronic acid (e.g., Synvisc, a product that helps restore the "shock-absorbing" ability of joint structures). Patients who continue to have severe pain and functional impairment despite medical treatment may need knee replacement surgery.

Rheumatoid Arthritis (RA)

Acetaminophen may be useful to relieve pain (Level A); however, aspirin or another NSAID may be preferred because these drugs offer relieve pain as well as anti-inflammatory effects (Level B). Aspirin is effective, but many people are unable to tolerate the adverse effects associated with anti-inflammatory doses. When aspirin is used, dosage usually ranges between 2 and 6 grams daily but should be individualized to relieve symptoms, maintain therapeutic salicylate blood levels, and minimize adverse effects. For people who cannot take aspirin, another NSAID may be given. For those who cannot take aspirin or a nonselective NSAID because of GI irritation, peptic ulcer disease, bleeding disorders, or other contraindications, the selective COX-2 inhibitor NSAID, celecoxib, may be preferred. NSAIDs are usually given in larger, anti-inflammatory doses for RA, rather than the smaller, analgesic doses given for OA. Corticosteroids such as prednisone are also useful in slowing joint damage due to inflammation.

Disease-modifying antirheumatic drugs (DMARDs) include a variety of medications used to relieve symptoms and slow joint destruction (so called disease-modifying effects). DMARDs are the drugs of choice to treat active rheumatoid arthritis (Level B-C). DMARDs, as well as corticosteroids, may cause serious adverse effects, including greatly increased susceptibility to infection. Methotrexate (MTX), which is also used in cancer chemotherapy, is an example of a DMARD given in smaller doses for RA. About 75% of patients have a beneficial response, with improvement usually evident within 4 to 8 weeks (i.e., less morning stiffness, pain, joint edema, and fatigue). Biologic response modifiers, a type of DMARD, include drugs such as adalimumab (Humira), etanercept (Enbrel), infliximab (Remicade), and leflunomide (Arava), which modify the immune system by inhibiting cytokines, which mediate inflammation (see Chap. 41). Clinical improvement usually occurs within a few weeks. According to the Arthritis Foundation, a biologic response modifier given along with MTX may be the most effective and aggressive treatment for individuals with severe RA.

Hyperuricemia and Gout

Opinions differ regarding treatment of asymptomatic hyperuricemia. Some authorities do not believe that drug therapy is indicated, and others believe that lowering serum uric acid levels may prevent joint inflammation and renal calculi. Allopurinol, probenecid, or sulfinpyrazone may be given for this purpose. Colchicine also should be given for several weeks to prevent acute attacks of gout while serum uric acid levels are being lowered. During initial administration of these drugs, a high fluid intake (to produce approximately 2000 mL of urine per day) and alkaline urine are recommended to prevent renal calculi. Urate crystals are more likely to precipitate in acid urine.

Acute Migraine

Evidence-based guidelines for treating acute migraine headache as reported by the American Academy of Neurology include the following recommendations for adults: aspirin and other oral NSAIDs including combination products containing caffeine are effective first line treatment for mild to moderate migraine headaches (Level A). Acetaminophen is not usually used as monotherapy for migraine pain (Level B). Preparations containing sedatives such as butalbital should be limited due to the possibility of overuse headaches and withdrawal issues (Level C). Because nausea and vomiting often accompany migraine pain, oral or parenteral antiemetics may be prescribed (Level B-C depending on the antiemetic drug). Parenteral metoclopramide may also be used as monotherapy to treat migraine headaches (Level B). For moderate to severe migraine attacks, sumatriptan and related drugs are effective (Level A). They cause fewer adverse effects than ergot preparations and are usually well tolerated. However, because they are strong vasoconstrictors, they should not be taken by people with coronary artery disease or hypertension. They are also expensive compared with other antimigraine drugs. When nausea and vomiting accompany migraine headache and a triptan is indicated, sumatriptan may be given intranasal or subcutaneously (Level C).

Ergot alkaloids such as ergotamine and ergotamine-caffeine combination are effective treatment for moderate to severe migraine headaches (Level B). Dihydroergotamine (DHE 45) IM/Sub-Q may be used for patients with moderate to severe migraine pain (Level B). DHE 45 nasal spray is safe and effective for treating acute migraines (Grade A) and may be considered when migraine pain is accompanied by nausea and vomiting (Level C). If an ergot preparation is used, it should be given at the onset of headache, and the patient should lie down in a quiet, darkened room. For further information regarding best migraine practices for adults, the student is referred to the American Academy of Neurology Web site, www.neurology.org.

Evidence-based guidelines for acute treatment of migraine headache as reported by the American Academy of Neurology (endorsed by the Academy of Pediatrics and the American Headache Society) include the following recommendations for children. Ibuprofen is effective for treating acute migraine headaches in children (Level A), and acetaminophen is probably effective and also can be considered for treating migraine pain (Level B). Aspirin is not recommended for children under the age of 15 due to the risk of Reye's syndrome. Several triptans were evaluated for acute migraine pain in children and adolescents. Rizatriptan and zolmitriptan were not superior to placebos for treating acute migraine pain in children, but sumatriptan nasal spray is effective for the treatment of acute migraine pain in adolescents (Level A). There are no data for the use of oral sumatriptan in children or adolescents and limited data on the efficacy of subcutaneous sumatriptan (Level U). For further evidence-based practice guidelines for treating and preventing migraine headaches in children and adolescents, the student is referred to the American Academy of Neurology Web site, www.neurology.org

Both categories of migraine abortive drugs (e.g., ergot alkaloids and serotonin agonists) exert powerful vasoconstrictive effects and have the potential to raise blood pressure. For this reason, ergot alkaloids and serotonin agonists should not be used within 24 hours of each other when treating migraine headaches.

Excessive use of simple analgesics, analgesics containing sedatives (e.g., butalbital) or caffeine, triptans, opioids, or ergotamine are believed to play a role in triggering overuse headaches, also called "rebound headaches." The most common clinical approach to management of overuse headaches involves tapering and/or cessation of the overused medication accompanied by temporary treatment of the rebound headache. Patients must be educated about the risks of chronic use of analgesics and encouraged to limit use of abortive and prophylactic migraine drugs appropriately. Use of nonpharmacologic therapies such as psychotherapy, biofeedback, and relaxation training may also be useful.

Perioperative

Aspirin should generally be avoided for 1 to 2 weeks before and after surgery because it increases the risk of bleeding. Most other NSAIDs should be discontinued approximately 3 days before surgery; nabumetone and piroxicam have long half-lives and must be discontinued approximately 1 week before surgery. NSAIDs, administered intraoperatively, have been shown to reduce postoperative pain and use of opioids after abdominal surgery. After surgery, especially after relatively minor procedures, such as dental extractions and episiotomies, an NSAID may be used to relieve pain. Caution is needed because of increased risk of bleeding, and the drug should not be given if there are other risk factors for bleeding. In addition, ketorolac, the only injectable NSAID, has been used to relieve postoperative pain. This drug has several advantages over opioid analgesics, but bleeding and hematomas may occur.

Cancer

Cancer often produces chronic pain from tumor invasion of tissues or complications of treatment (chemotherapy, surgery, or radiation). As with acute pain, acetaminophen, aspirin, or other NSAIDs prevent sensitization of peripheral pain receptors by inhibiting prostaglandin formation. NSAIDs are especially effective for pain associated with bone metastases. For mild pain, acetaminophen or an NSAID may be used alone; for moderate to severe pain, these drugs may be continued and an opioid analgesic added. Nonopioid and opioid analgesics may be given together or alternated; a combination of analgesics is often needed to provide optimal pain relief. Aspirin is contraindicated for the patient receiving chemotherapy that depresses the bone marrow because of the high risk of thrombocytopenia and bleeding.

Use in Special Populations

Use in Children

Acetaminophen is usually the drug of choice for pain or fever in children. Children seem less susceptible to liver toxicity than adults, apparently because they form less of the toxic metabolite during metabolism of acetaminophen. However, there is a risk of overdose and hepatotoxicity because acetaminophen is a very common ingredient in OTC cold, flu, fever, and pain remedies. An overdose can occur with large doses of one product or smaller amounts of several different products. In addition, toxicity has occurred when parents or caregivers have given the liquid concentration intended for children to infants. The concentrations are different and cannot be given interchangeably. Infants' doses are measured with a dropper, and children's doses are measured by teaspoon. Caution parents and caregivers to ask pediatricians for written instructions on giving acetaminophen to their children, to read the labels of all drug products very carefully, and to avoid giving children acetaminophen from multiple sources. Ibuprofen also may be given for fever. Alternating acetaminophen and ibuprofen every 4 hours over a 3-day period to control fever in young children (ages 6–36 months) has been shown to be more effective than monotherapy with either agent. Ibuprofen is preferred over acetaminophen when treating acute migraine headache pain in children and adolescents.

Aspirin is not recommended because of its association with Reye's syndrome, a life-threatening illness characterized by encephalopathy, hepatic damage, and other serious problems. Reye's syndrome usually occurs after a viral infection, such as influenza or chickenpox, during which aspirin was given for fever. A rare, but serious, adverse effect of ibuprofen and NSAIDs in children is the occurrence of severe skin reactions, such as Stevens-Johnson syndrome or toxic epidermal necrolysis. For children with juvenile RA, aspirin, ibuprofen, or naproxen may be given. Pediatric indications for use and dosages have not been established for most of the other drugs.

When an NSAID is given during late pregnancy to prevent premature labor, it may adversely affect the kidneys of the fetus. When an NSAID is given shortly after birth to close a patent ductus arteriosus, it may adversely affect the kidneys of the neonate.

Use in Older Adults

The American Geriatric Society recommends acetaminophen be the initial consideration for treatment of middle to moderate pain of musculoskeletal origin (Level B). Acetaminophen is usually safe in recommended doses unless liver damage is present or the person is a chronic alcohol abuser. Aspirin is usually safe in the low doses prescribed for prevention of myocardial infarction and stroke (antiplatelet effects). Aspirin and other NSAIDs are probably safe in therapeutic doses for occasional use as an analgesic or antipyretic. The incidence of musculoskeletal disorders (e.g., OA) is higher in older adults, and aspirin or another NSAID is often prescribed. Older patients on long-term NSAIDs should be evaluated for GI blood loss, renal dysfunction, edema, hypertension, and drug–

drug or drug–disease interactions (Level A). Use of gastroprotective agents is recommended for individuals at risk of upper GI bleeding events (Level B). A COX-2 inhibitor may be preferred in older adults because they are less likely to cause gastric ulceration and bleeding; however, this benefit must be weighed against the increased risk of cardiovascular events.

Use in Patients With Renal Impairment

Acetaminophen, aspirin, and other NSAIDs can cause or aggravate renal impairment even though they are eliminated mainly by hepatic metabolism. Acetaminophen is normally metabolized in the liver to metabolites that are excreted through the kidneys; these metabolites may accumulate in patients with renal failure. In addition, acetaminophen is nephrotoxic in overdose because it forms a metabolite that attacks kidney cells and may cause necrosis. Aspirin is nephrotoxic in high doses, and protein binding of aspirin is reduced in patients with renal failure so that blood levels of active drug are higher. In addition, aspirin and other NSAIDs can decrease blood flow in the kidneys by inhibiting synthesis of prostaglandins that dilate renal blood vessels. When renal blood flow is normal, these prostaglandins have limited activity. However, when renal blood flow is decreased, synthesis of these prostaglandins is increased, and they protect the kidneys from ischemia and hypoxia by antagonizing the vasoconstrictive effects of angiotensin II, norepinephrine, and other substances. Thus, in patients who depend on prostaglandins to maintain an adequate renal blood flow, the prostaglandin-blocking effects of aspirin and NSAIDs result in constriction of renal arteries and arterioles, decreased renal blood flow, decreased glomerular filtration rate, and retention of salt and water. NSAIDs can also cause kidney damage by other mechanisms, including a hypersensitivity reaction that leads to acute renal failure, manifested by proteinuria, hematuria, or pyuria. Biopsy reports usually indicate inflammatory reactions such as glomerulonephritis or interstitial nephritis.

People at highest risk from the use of these drugs are those with pre-existing renal impairment; those older than 50 years of age; those taking diuretics; and those with hypertension, diabetes, or heart failure. Measures to prevent or minimize renal damage include avoiding nephrotoxic drugs when possible, treating the disorders that increase risk of renal damage, stopping the NSAID if renal impairment occurs, monitoring renal function, reducing dosage, and maintaining hydration.

The role of COX-2 inhibitor NSAIDs in renal impairment is not clear. Although it was hoped that these drugs would have protective effects on the kidneys, studies indicate that their effects on the kidneys are similar to those of the older nonselective NSAIDs.

Use in Patients With Hepatic Impairment

Except for acetaminophen, the effects of NSAIDs on liver function and the effects of hepatic impairment on most NSAIDs are largely unknown. Because the drugs are metabolized in the liver, they should be used with caution and in lower doses in people with impaired hepatic function or a history of liver disease. For example, some authorities recommend a maximum daily dose of 2 grams for people with hepatitis (compared with a maximum daily dose of 4 grams for people who do not have impaired liver function).

Acetaminophen can cause fatal liver necrosis in overdose because it forms a metabolite that can destroy liver cells. The hepatotoxic metabolite is formed more rapidly when drug-metabolizing enzymes in the liver have been stimulated by ingestion of alcohol, cigarette smoking, and drugs such as anticonvulsants and others. Thus, alcoholics are at high risk of hepatotoxicity with usual therapeutic doses.

In cirrhotic liver disease, naproxen and sulindac may be metabolized more slowly and aggravate hepatic impairment if dosage is not reduced. In liver impairment, blood levels of oral sumatriptan and related antimigraine drugs may be high because less of the drug is metabolized on its first pass through the liver and a higher proportion of a dose reaches the systemic circulation. Thus, the drugs should be used cautiously, possibly in reduced dosage.

Use in Patients With Critical Illness

Acetaminophen, aspirin, and other NSAIDs are infrequently used during critical illness, partly because they are usually given orally and many patients are unable to take oral medications. Pain is more likely to be treated with injectable opioid analgesics in this population. Acetaminophen may be given by rectal suppository for pain or fever in patients who are unable to take oral drugs.

These drugs may be risk factors for renal or hepatic impairment or bleeding disorders. For example, if a patient has a history of taking aspirin, including the low doses prescribed for antithrombotic effects, there is a risk of bleeding from common therapeutic (e.g., intramuscular injections, venipuncture, inserting urinary catheters or GI tubes) or diagnostic (e.g., drawing blood, angiography) procedures. If a patient has been taking an NSAID regularly, he or she may be more likely to experience renal failure if the critical illness causes dehydration or requires treatment with one or more nephrotoxic drugs. If a patient presents with acute renal failure, NSAID ingestion must be considered as a possible cause. If a patient is known to drink alcoholic beverages and take acetaminophen, he or she may be more likely to experience impaired liver function.

Use in Home Care

Home use of acetaminophen, NSAIDs, and other analgesic drugs is extremely widespread. Many people are aware of the beneficial effects of these drugs in relieving pain, but they may not be adequately informed about potential problems associated with use of the drugs. Thus, the home care nurse may need to assist patients in perceiving a need for additional information and provide that information. Specific suggestions include reading and following instructions on labels of OTC analgesics, not exceeding recommended dosages without consulting a health care provider, and avoiding multiple sources of acetaminophen or NSAIDs (e.g., multiple OTC NSAIDs or an OTC and a prescription NSAID). In addition, adverse drug effects should be reviewed with patients, and patients should be assessed for characteristics (e.g., older age group, renal impairment, overuse of the drugs) that increase the risks of adverse effects.

Nursing Actions Analgesic–Antipyretic–Anti-Inflammatory, and Related Drugs

NURSING ACTIONS	RATIONALE/EXPLANATION
1. Administer accurately	
a. Give aspirin and other nonsteroidal anti-inflammatory drugs (NSAIDs) with a full glass of water or other fluid and with or just after food.	To decrease gastric irritation. Even though food delays absorption and decreases peak plasma levels of some of the drugs, it is probably safer to give them with food. Meloxicam may be given without regard to food.
b. Do not crush tablets or open capsules of long-acting dosage forms and instruct patients not to crush or chew the products. Examples include: (1) Enteric-coated aspirin (e.g., Ecotrin) (2) Diclofenac sodium (Voltaren or Voltaren XR) (3) Diflunisal (Dolobid) (4) Etodolac (Lodine XL) (5) Indomethacin or Indocin SR (6) Ketoprofen or Oruvail extended-release capsules (7) Naproxen delayed-release (EC-Naprosyn) or naproxen sodium controlled-release (Naprelan)	Breaking the tablets or capsules allows faster absorption, destroys the long-acting feature, and increases risks of adverse effects and toxicity from overdose.
c. Give antimigraine preparations at the onset of headache.	To prevent development of more severe symptoms
d. Give rapidly disintegrating tablets for migraine relief by placing tablet on the tongue. Do not give with water.	Allows drug to dissolve and be absorbed
2. Observe for therapeutic effects	
a. When drugs are given for pain, observe for decreased or absent manifestations of pain.	Pain relief is usually evident within 30–60 minutes.
b. When drugs are given for fever, record temperature every 2–4 hours, and observe for a decrease.	
c. When drugs are given for arthritis and other inflammatory disorders, observe for decreased pain, edema, redness, heat, and stiffness of joints. Also observe for increased joint mobility and exercise tolerance.	With aspirin, improvement is usually noted within 24–48 hours. With most of the NSAIDs, 1–2 weeks may be required before beneficial effects become evident.
d. When colchicine is given for acute gouty arthritis, observe for decreased pain and inflammation in involved joints.	Therapeutic effects occur within 4–12 hours after intravenous colchicine administration and 24–48 hours after oral administration. Edema may not decrease for several days.
e. When allopurinol, probenecid, or sulfinpyrazone is given for hyperuricemia, observe for normal serum uric acid level (approximately 2–8 mg/100 mL).	Serum uric acid levels usually decrease to normal range within 1–3 weeks.
f. When allopurinol, probenecid, or sulfinpyrazone is given for chronic gout, observe for decreased size of tophi, absence of new tophi, decreased joint pain and increased joint mobility, and normal serum uric acid levels.	
g. When triptans or ergot preparations are given to treat migraine headache, observe for relief of symptoms.	Therapeutic effects are usually evident within 15–30 minutes.
3. Observe for adverse effects	
a. With analgesic–antipyretic–anti-inflammatory and antigout agents, observe for:	
(1) Gastrointestinal problems—anorexia, nausea, vomiting, diarrhea, bleeding, ulceration	These are common reactions, more likely with aspirin, indomethacin, piroxicam, sulindac, colchicine, and sulfinpyrazone and less likely with acetaminophen, celecoxib, diflunisal, etodolac, ibuprofen, and naproxen.
(2) Hematologic problems—petechiae, bruises, hematuria, melena, epistaxis, and bone marrow depression (leukopenia, thrombocytopenia, anemia)	Bone marrow depression is more likely to occur with colchicine.
(3) Central nervous system effects—headache, dizziness, fainting, ataxia, insomnia, confusion, drowsiness	These effects are relatively common with indomethacin and may occur with most of the other drugs, especially with high dosages.
(4) Skin rashes, dermatitis	Rare but serious skin reactions, such as Stevens-Johnson syndrome or toxic epidermal necrolysis, are possible.
(5) Hypersensitivity reactions with dyspnea, bronchospasm, skin rashes	These effects may simulate asthma in people who are allergic to aspirin and aspirin-like drugs; most likely to occur in patients with a history of nasal polyps.

(continued on page 126)

Nursing Actions — Analgesic–Antipyretic–Anti-Inflammatory, and Related Drugs (continued)

NURSING ACTIONS	RATIONALE/EXPLANATION
(6) Tinnitus, blurred vision	Tinnitus (ringing or roaring in the ears) is a classic sign of aspirin overdose (salicylate intoxication). It occurs with NSAIDs as well.
(7) Nephrotoxicity—decreased urine output; increased blood urea nitrogen (BUN); increased serum creatinine; hyperkalemia; retention of sodium and water with resultant edema	More likely to occur in people with pre-existing renal impairment
(8) Cardiovascular effects—increased hypertension, edema. With long-term use, increased risk of myocardial infarction or stroke.	NSAIDs can cause sodium and water retention. Mechanism of adverse cardiovascular events is not fully understood; however, they may be partially explained by inhibition of prostaglandin I_2 formation, which increases risk of thromboembolic events.
(9) Hepatotoxicity—liver damage or failure	Occurs mainly with acetaminophen, in overdose or in people with underlying liver disease
b. With triptan antimigraine drugs, observe for:	
(1) Chest tightness or pain, hypertension, drowsiness, dizziness, nausea, fatigue, paresthesias	Most adverse effects are mild and transient. However, because of their vasoconstrictive effects, they may cause or aggravate angina pectoris and hypertension.
c. With ergot antimigraine drugs, observe for:	
(1) Nausea, vomiting, diarrhea	These drugs have a direct effect on the vomiting center of the brain and stimulate contraction of gastrointestinal smooth muscle.
(2) Symptoms of ergot poisoning (ergotism)—coolness, numbness, and tingling of the extremities; headache; vomiting; dizziness; thirst; convulsions; weak pulse; confusion; angina-like chest pain; transient tachycardia or bradycardia; muscle weakness and pain; cyanosis; gangrene of the extremities	The ergot alkaloids are highly toxic; poisoning may be acute or chronic. Acute poisoning is rare; chronic poisoning is usually a result of overdosage. Circulatory impairments may result from vasoconstriction and vascular insufficiency. Large doses also damage capillary endothelium and may cause thrombosis and occlusion. Gangrene of extremities rarely occurs with usual doses unless peripheral vascular disease or other contraindications are also present.
(3) Hypertension	Blood pressure may rise as a result of generalized vasoconstriction induced by the ergot preparation.
(4) Hypersensitivity reactions—local edema and pruritus, anaphylactic shock	Allergic reactions are relatively uncommon.
4. Observe for drug interactions	
a. Drugs that *increase* effects of aspirin and other NSAIDs:	
(1) Acidifying agents (e.g., ascorbic acid)	Acidify urine and thereby decrease the urinary excretion rate of salicylates
(2) Alcohol	Increases gastric irritation and occult blood loss
(3) Anticoagulants, oral	Increase risk of bleeding substantially. People taking anticoagulants should avoid aspirin and aspirin-containing products.
(4) Codeine, hydrocodone, oxycodone	Additive analgesic effects because of different mechanisms of action. Aspirin or an NSAID can often be used with these drugs to provide adequate pain relief without excessive doses and sedation.
(5) Corticosteroids (e.g., prednisone)	Additive gastric irritation and possible ulcerogenic effects
b. Drug that *increases* effects of celecoxib:	
(1) Fluconazole (and possibly other azole antifungal drugs)	Inhibits liver enzymes that normally metabolize celecoxib; increases serum celecoxib levels
c. Drugs that *decrease* effects of aspirin and other NSAIDs:	
(1) Alkalinizing agents (e.g., sodium bicarbonate)	Increase rate of renal excretion
(2) Misoprostol (Cytotec)	This drug, a prostaglandin, was developed specifically to prevent aspirin and NSAID-induced gastric ulcers.
(3) Ibuprofen may negate the cardioprotective benefits of low-dose aspirin	Ibuprofen competes with aspirin for COX-1 Inhibition.
d. Drugs that *increase* effects of indomethacin:	
(1) Anticoagulants, oral	Increase risk of gastrointestinal bleeding. Indomethacin causes gastric irritation and is considered an ulcerogenic drug.
(2) Corticosteroids	Increase ulcerogenic effect

NURSING ACTIONS	RATIONALE/EXPLANATION
(3) Salicylates	Increase ulcerogenic effect
(4) Heparin	Increases risk of bleeding. These drugs should not be used concurrently.
e. Drugs that *decrease* effects of indomethacin:	
(1) Antacids	Delay absorption from the gastrointestinal tract
f. Drugs that *decrease* effects of allopurinol, probenecid, and sulfinpyrazone:	
(1) Alkalinizing agents (e.g., sodium bicarbonate)	Decrease risks of renal calculi from precipitation of uric acid crystals. Alkalinizing agents are recommended until serum uric acid levels return to normal.
(2) Colchicine	Decreases attacks of acute gout. Recommended for concurrent use until serum uric acid levels return to normal.
(3) Diuretics	Decrease uricosuric effects
(4) Salicylates	Mainly at salicylate doses of less than 2 grams per day, decrease uricosuric effects of probenecid and sulfinpyrazone but do not interfere with the action of allopurinol. Salicylates are uricosuric at doses greater than 5 grams per day.
g. Drugs that *increase* effects of ergot preparations:	
(1) Vasoconstrictors (e.g., ephedrine, epinephrine, phenylephrine)	Additive vasoconstriction with risks of severe, persistent hypertension and intracranial hemorrhage
(2) Any drug that inhibits CYP3A4 enzyme metabolism (protease inhibitors, macrolide antibiotics, ketoconazole, grapefruit juice, others)	CYP3A4 enzyme inhibition increases the amount of ergot preparation that remains in the body, resulting in life-threatening peripheral and cerebral vasoconstriction and ischemia.
h. Drugs that *increase* effects of triptan antimigraine drugs:	
(1) Antidepressants (SSRIs, SNRIs, MAOIs)	Serotonin syndrome, a potentially life-threatening reaction, may occur when two drugs that affect serotonin levels in the body are taken concurrently. Symptoms of serotonin syndrome include restlessness, hallucinations, fever, loss of coordination, tachycardia, rapid changes in blood pressure, hyperactive reflexes, nausea, vomiting, and diarrhea.
(2) MAOIs	Increase serum levels of triptans and may cause serious adverse effects, including cardiac dysrhythmias and myocardial infarction
	Triptans and MAOIs must not be taken concurrently; a triptan should be taken for at least 2 weeks after an MAOI is discontinued.
(3) Ergot preparations	**Triptans and ergot preparations should not be taken concurrently or within 24 hours of each other, because severe hypertension and stroke may occur.**
i. Drugs that *increase* effects of eletriptan (Relplax)	
(1) Any drug that inhibits CYP3A4 enzyme metabolism. Examples include protease inhibitors, macrolide antibiotics, ketoconazole, grapefruit juice, others.	Inhibition of CYP3A4 enzymes increases the amount of eletriptan that remains in the body, resulting in toxicity.

Key Concepts

▪ Aspirin, other NSAIDs, and acetaminophen inhibit COX enzymes, which are required for prostaglandin formation.

▪ Aspirin and other nonselective NSAIDs inhibit both COX-1 and COX-2. The COX-2 inhibitor, celecoxib, is more selective for the COX-2 enzyme. The exact mechanism of action of acetaminophen is unclear.

▪ Prostaglandins produced by COX-1 are important in regulating homeostasis and are associated with platelet aggregation and protective effects on the stomach and kidneys.

Drug-induced inhibition results in gastric ulceration, renal dysfunction, and diminished blood clotting.

▪ Prostaglandins produced by COX-2 are associated with pain and inflammation. Drug-induced inhibition results in therapeutic effects of analgesia and anti-inflammatory activity.

▪ Individuals with hypersensitivity to aspirin should not take NSAIDs due to the risk of cross-sensitivity to other antiprostaglandin drugs.

■ The use of gastroprotective drugs such as antacids, H_2 blockers, and proton pump inhibitors may be indicated to prevent upper gastrointestinal bleeding with chronic use of aspirin and other nonselective NSAIDs.

■ In children and adolescents, aspirin is contraindicated in the presence of viral infections due to the risk of Reye's syndrome. Acetaminophen is the drug of choice for fever in children. Acetaminophen and ibuprofen may be alternated in the treatment of children with fever.

■ The major drawback of acetaminophen use is the potentially fatal liver damage with overdose. Acetylcysteine is the specific antidote to acetaminophen overdose.

■ Allopurinol, which inhibits the synthesis of uric acid, is the drug of choice for individuals with gout due to "overproduction" of uric acid.

■ Colchicine is the only antigout drug with anti-inflammatory effects; it is useful for treating acute attacks.

■ Probenecid and sulfinpyrazone are uricosuric drugs effective in treating individuals with gout who "under-excrete" uric acid.

■ During treatment for gout, encourage individuals to increase fluid intake to 2000 milliliters per day to prevent renal calculi.

■ Aspirin, other NSAIDs, and acetaminophen may be useful in the treatment of mild infrequent migraine pain.

■ Serotonin receptor agonists and ergot alkaloids are effective in aborting acute migraine headaches. These medicines are powerful vasoconstrictors and may raise blood pressure. They should not be used within 24 hours of each other when treating migraine headaches.

■ Overuse of all types of analgesics may lead to overuse or rebound headaches.

Review and Application Exercises

Short Answer Exercises

1. How do aspirin and other NSAIDs produce analgesic, antipyretic, anti-inflammatory, and antiplatelet effects?

2. What adverse effects occur with aspirin and other NSAIDs, especially with daily ingestion?

3. Compare and contrast the uses and effects of aspirin, ibuprofen, and acetaminophen.

4. For a 6-year-old child with fever, would aspirin or acetaminophen be preferred? Why?

5. For a 50-year-old adult with RA, would aspirin, another NSAID, or acetaminophen be preferred? Why?

6. For a 75-year-old adult with OA and a long history of "stomach trouble," would aspirin, another NSAID, or acetaminophen be preferred? Why?

7. What are some nursing interventions to decrease the adverse effects of aspirin, other NSAIDs, and acetaminophen?

8. When teaching a patient about home use of aspirin, other NSAIDs, and acetaminophen, what information must be included?

9. What is the rationale for using acetylcysteine in the treatment of acetaminophen toxicity?

10. What is the rationale for combining opioid and nonopioid analgesics in the treatment of moderate pain?

11. If you were a patient, what information do you think would be most helpful in home management of migraine?

NCLEX-Style Questions

12. The nurse would question the pain medication order for which of the following patients?
    a. acetaminophen for OA in a 60-year-old man with peptic ulcer disease
    b. celecoxib for RA in a 48-year-old woman taking warfarin
    c. acetaminophen for a headache in a 55-year-old man scheduled for surgery in the morning
    d. aspirin for a feverish 12-year-old child with influenza

13. The most important laboratory tests the nurse should evaluate for a patient who takes an overdose of acetaminophen are
    a. plasma salicylate
    b. aspartate aminotransferase and alanine aminotransferase, bilirubin, and prothrombin time
    c. blood urea nitrogen and creatinine
    d. hemoglobin, hematocrit, and complete blood count

14. Which of the following nursing interventions is most important when allopurinol is prescribed for the treatment of gout?
    a. Monitor stools for occult blood.
    b. Encourage an acid ash diet to acidify the urine.
    c. Encourage fluid intake of at least 3000 mL of fluid per day.
    d. Encourage the use of aspirin when an OTC analgesic is necessary.

15. Prior to administering sumatriptan for migraine headaches, the nurse should assess for
    a. bradycardia
    b. elevated blood glucose level
    c. adequate urine output
    d. use of ergot preparations in past 24 hours

Selected References

Abebe, W. (2002). Herbal medication: Potential for adverse interactions with analgesic drugs. *Journal of Clinical Pharmacy and Therapeutics, 27,* 391–401.

American Geriatric Society, Panel on Persistent Pain in Older Persons. (2002, June). *The management of persistent pain in older persons.* Retrieved January 30, 2007, from http://www.guidelines.gov/summary/summary.aspx?doc_id=3365&nbr=002591&string=N

American Pain Society. (2002). *Pain in osteoarthritis, rheumatoid arthritis, and juvenile chronic arthritis.* Retrieved January 30, 2007, from http://www.guidelines.gov/summary/summary.aspx?doc_id=3691&nbr=002917&string=g

Center for Drug Evaluation and Research. (2006, July 19). *FDA Public Health Advisory: Combined use of 5-hydroxytryptamine receptor agonists (triptans), selective serotonin reuptake inhibitors (SSRIs) or selective serotonin/norepinephrine reuptake inhibitors (SNRIs) may result in life-threatening serotonin syndrome.* Rockville, MD: Center for Drug Evaluation and Research.

Clegg, D. O., Reda, D. J., Harris, C. L., Klein, M. A., O'Dell, J. R., Hooper, M. M., Bradley, J. D., Bingham, C. O., Weisman, M. H., Jackson, C. G., Lane, N. E., Cush, J. J., Moreland, L. W., Schumacher, H. R., Oddis, C. V., Wolfe, F., Molitor, J. A., Yocum, D. E., Schnitzer, T. J., Furst, D. E., Sawitzke, A. D., Shi, H., Brandt, K. D., Moskowitz, R. W., & Williams, H. J. (2006). Glucosamine, chondroitin sulfate and the two in combination for painful knee osteoarthritis. *New England Journal of Medicine, 354,* 795–808.

Cook, N. R., Lee, I., Gaziano, J. M., Gordon, D., Ridker, P. M., Manson, J. E., Hennekens, C. H., & Buring, J. E. (2005). Low-dose aspirin in the primary prevention of cancer. *Journal of the American Medical Association, 294,* 47–55.

Devine, E. C. (2005). Somatosensory function, pain and headache. In C. M. Porth (Ed.), *Pathophysiology: Concepts of altered health states* (7th ed., pp. 1159–1191). Philadelphia: Lippincott Williams & Wilkins.

Drug facts and comparisons. (Updated monthly). St. Louis, MO: Facts and Comparisons.

Fetrow, C. W., & Avila, J. R. (2003). *Professional's handbook of complementary and alternative medicines* (3rd ed.). Philadelphia: Lippincott Williams & Wilkins.

Gagnier, J. J., van Tulder, M. W., Berman, B., & Bombardier, C. (2007). Herbal medicine for low back pain: A Cochrane review. *Spine, 32,* 82–92.

Grassi, L., Andrasid, F., D'Amico, D., Usai, S., Rigamonti, A., Leone, M., & Bussone, G. (2003). Treatment of chronic daily headache with medication overuse. *Neurological Sciences, 24,* S125–S127.

Hansen, K. E., & Elliott, M. E. (2005). Osteoarthritis. In J. T. DiPiro, R. L. Talbert, G. C. Yee, G. R. Matzke, B. G. Wells, & L. M. Posey (Eds.), *Pharmacotherapy: A pathophysiologic approach* (6th ed., pp. 1685–1703). New York: McGraw-Hill.

Hawkins, D. W., & Rahn, D. W. (2005). Gout and hyperuricemia. In J. T. DiPiro, R. L. Talbert, G. C. Yee, G. R. Matzke, B. G. Wells, & L. M. Posey (Eds.), *Pharmacotherapy: A pathophysiologic approach* (6th ed., pp. 1705–1711). New York: McGraw-Hill.

King, D. S., & Herndon, K. C. (2005). Headache disorders. In J. T. DiPiro, R. L. Talbert, G. C. Yee, G. R. Matzke, B. G. Wells, & L. M.

Posey (Eds.), *Pharmacotherapy: A pathophysiologic approach* (6th ed., pp. 1105–1120). New York: McGraw-Hill.

Kunert, M. P. (2005). Alterations in temperature regulation. In C. M. Porth (Ed.), *Pathophysiology: Concepts of altered health states* (7th ed., pp. 201–215). Philadelphia: Lippincott Williams & Wilkins.

Lewis, D., Ahwal, S., Hershey, A., Hirtz, D., Yonker, M., & Silberstein, S. (2005). Pharmacological treatment of migraine headache in children and adolescents. Report of the American Academy of Neurology Quality Standards Subcommittee and the Practice Committee of the Child Neurology Society [Electronic version]. *Pediatrics, 115,* 1107. Retrieved on January 30, 2007, from http://pediatrics.org/cgi/content/full/115/4/1107

Martin, C. P., & Talbert, R. L. (2005). Aspirin resistance: An evaluation of current evidence and measurement methods. *Pharmacotherapy, 25,* 942–953.

Michigan Quality Improvement Consortium. (2003, August). *Medical management of adults with osteoarthritis.* Retrieved January 30, 2007, from http://www.guidelines.gov/summary/summary.aspx?doc_id=8164&nbr=004551&string=n

Patrono, C., & Rocca, B. (2007). Drug insight: Aspirin resistance—Fact or fashion? *National Clinical Practitioner Cardiovascular Medicine, 4,* 42–50.

Porth, C. M. (2005). Inflammation and healing. In C. M. Porth (Ed.), *Pathophysiology: Concepts of altered health states* (7th ed., pp. 387–402). Philadelphia: Lippincott Williams & Wilkins.

Richy, F., Bruyere, O., Cucherat, M., Henrotin, Y., & Reginster, J. Y. (2003). Structural and symptomatic efficacy of glucosamine and chondroitin in knee osteoarthritis, a comprehensive meta-analysis. *Archives of Internal Medicine, 163,* 1514–1522.

Ridker, P. M., Cook, N. R., Lee, I., Gordon, D., Gaziano, J. M., Manson, J. E., Hennekens, C. H., & Buring, J. E. (2005). A randomized trial of low-dose aspirin in the primary prevention of cardiovascular disease in women. *New England Journal of Medicine, 352,* 1293–1304.

Rizzo, D. B. (2005). Disorders of skeletal function: Rheumatic disorders. In C. M. Porth (Ed.), *Pathophysiology: Concepts of altered health states* (7th ed., pp. 1417–1440). Philadelphia: Lippincott Williams & Wilkins.

Sarrell, E. M., Wielunsky, E., & Cohen, H. A. (2006). Antipyretic treatment in young children with fever. *Archives of Pediatrics and Adolescent Medicine, 160,* 197–202.

Schuna, A. A. (2005). Rheumatoid arthritis. In J. T. DiPiro, R. L. Talbert, G. C. Yee, G. R. Matzke, B. G. Wells, & L. M. Posey (Eds.), *Pharmacotherapy: A pathophysiologic approach* (6th ed., pp. 1671–1683). New York: McGraw-Hill.

Scottish Intercollegiate Guidelines Network. (2002, October). Prophylaxis of venous thromboembolism. Retrieved February 7, 2007, from http://www.guidelines.gov/summary/summary.aspx?doc_id=3485&nbr=002711&string=low

Silberstein, S. D. (2000). Practice parameter: Evidence-based guidelines for migraine (an evidence-based review). *Neurology, 55,* 754–762.

Smeltzer, S. C., Bare, B. G., Hinkle J. L., & Cheever, K. H. (2008). *Brunner & Suddarth's textbook of medical-surgical nursing* (11th ed.). Philadelphia: Lippincott Williams & Wilkins.

Zarraga, I. G. E., & Schwarz, E. R. (2007). Coxibs and heart disease: What we have learned and what else we need to know. *Journal of the American College of Cardiology, 49,* 1–14.

Antianxiety and Sedative-Hypnotic Drugs

LEARNING OBJECTIVES

After studying this chapter, you will be able to:

1. Discuss characteristics, sources, and signs and symptoms of anxiety.
2. Discuss functions of sleep and consequences of sleep deprivation.
3. Describe nondrug interventions to decrease anxiety and insomnia.
4. List characteristics of benzodiazepine antianxiety and hypnotic drugs in terms of mechanism of action, indications for use, nursing process implications, and potential for abuse and dependence.
5. Describe strategies for preventing, recognizing, or treating benzodiazepine withdrawal reactions.
6. Contrast characteristics of selected nonbenzodiazepines and benzodiazepines.
7. Teach patients guidelines for rational, safe use of antianxiety and sedative-hypnotic drugs.
8. Discuss the use of flumazenil and other treatment measures for overdose of benzodiazepines.

Applying Your Knowledge

Gertrude Portman is an 88-year-old woman who has been admitted for observation due to a syncopal episode. She is in the early stages of Alzheimer's disease and appears very anxious and agitated. Mrs. Portman has the following medical orders for sedation:

Alprazolam (Xanax) 0.25–0.5 mg 2–4 times daily for anxiety; Venlafaxine (Effexor XR) 75 mg daily; and Zolpidem (Ambien) 5 mg PO at half strength (HS) for sleep.

Introduction

Antianxiety and sedative-hypnotic agents are central nervous system (CNS) depressants that have similar effects. Antianxiety drugs (also known as *anxiolytics*) and *sedatives* promote relaxation, and hypnotics produce sleep. The difference between the effects depends largely on dosage. Large doses of antianxiety and sedative agents produce sleep, and small doses of *hypnotics* produce antianxiety or sedative effects. In addition, therapeutic doses of hypnotics taken at bedtime may have residual sedative effects ("morning hangover") the following day. Because these drugs produce varying degrees of CNS depression, some are also used as anticonvulsants and anesthetics.

The main drugs used to treat insomnia are the benzodiazepines and the nonbenzodiazepine hypnotics. Benzodiazepines are also used to treat short-term symptoms of acute anxiety in response to stressful situations. Antidepressants (i.e., selective serotonin reuptake inhibitors [SSRIs], tricyclics [TCAs], and newer miscellaneous drugs) are preferred as first line drugs for long-term treatment of most chronic anxiety disorders, with benzodiazepines considered second line drugs (see Evidence-Based Practice Box 8-1). Antidepressant medications are discussed in more detail in Chapter 10. The barbiturates, a historically important group of CNS depressants, are obsolete for most uses, including treatment of anxiety and insomnia. A few may be used as intravenous general anesthetics (see Appendix C), phenobarbital may be used to treat seizure disorders (see Chap. 11), and some are abused (see Chap. 14).

To promote understanding of the uses and effects of both benzodiazepines and nonbenzodiazepines, anxiety and insomnia are described in the following sections. The clinical manifestations of these disorders are similar and overlapping; that is, daytime anxiety may be manifested as nighttime difficulty in sleeping because the person cannot "turn off" worries, and difficulty in sleeping may be manifested as anxiety, fatigue, and decreased ability to function during usual waking hours.

Evidence-Based Practice

8-1 Treatment of Generalized Anxiety Disorder: Antidepressants Versus Anxiolytics

Historically, the benzodiazepine and nonbenzodiazepine antianxiety drugs have been the drugs of choice for treatment of generalized anxiety disorder. More recently, the antidepressants have been increasingly prescribed to treat generalized anxiety disorder.

A Cochrane Review (2002) of 15 clinical trials was conducted to determine the efficacy of antidepressants for treating generalized anxiety disorder. Antidepressants (i.e., imipramine, venlafaxine, and paroxetine) were found to be effective in the treatment of generalized anxiety disorder and were generally well tolerated by patients with anxiety. There was no evidence to determine that one class of antidepressants is more effective than another in treating adults with generalized anxiety disorder. In children with generalized anxiety disorder, one study showed Sertraline to be efficacious.

For the purposes of this review, only studies including subjects with generalized depression as a sole diagnosis were included; however, anxiety disorders are often comorbid with depression. The comorbidity rate for general anxiety disorder and depression is estimated to be as high as 62%. Studies of twins suggest a shared genetic basis for generalized anxiety disorder and depression. This comorbidity often results in worse treatment outcomes, increased risk for suicidality, greater recurrence of symptoms, and greater utilization of health care resources.

When generalized anxiety disorder is comorbid with depression, antidepressants may have a therapeutic advantage in that one drug can be beneficial for treating both conditions. However, antidepressants may result in an initial increase in agitation and anxiety resulting in just enough clinical improvement to allow the depressed and suicidal patient the energy to carry out suicidal plans. The nurse must be vigilant in monitoring patients with comorbid anxiety and depression for treatment-induced suicidality.

Kapczinski, F., Lima, M. S., Souza, J. S., Cunha, A., & Schmitt, R. (2002). Antidepressants for generalized anxiety disorder. Cochrane Database Systematic Reviews, 2, CD003592.

Anxiety

Anxiety is a common disorder that may be referred to as nervousness, tension, worry, or other terms that denote an unpleasant feeling. It occurs when a person perceives a situation as threatening to physical, emotional, social, or economic well-being. Anxiety may occur in association with everyday events related to home, work, school, social activities, and chronic illness, or it may occur episodically, in association with acute illness, death, divorce, losing a job, starting a new job, or taking a test. Situational anxiety is a normal response to a stressful situation. It may be beneficial when it motivates the person toward constructive, problem-solving, coping activities. Symptoms may be quite severe, but they usually last only 2 to 3 weeks.

Although there is no clear boundary between normal and abnormal anxiety, when anxiety is severe or prolonged and impairs the ability to function in usual activities of daily living, it is called an *anxiety disorder*. The American Psychiatric Association delineates anxiety disorders as medical diagnoses in the *Diagnostic and Statistical Manual of Mental Disorders, 4th edition, Text Revision (DSM-IV-TR)*. This classification includes several types of anxiety disorders (Box 8-1). Generalized anxiety disorder (GAD) is emphasized in this chapter.

The pathophysiology of anxiety disorders is unknown, but there is evidence of a biologic basis and possible imbalances among several neurotransmission systems. A simplistic view involves an excess of excitatory neurotransmitters (e.g., norepinephrine) or a deficiency of inhibitory neurotransmitters (e.g., gamma-aminobutyric acid [GABA]).

The noradrenergic system is associated with the hyperarousal state experienced by patients with anxiety (i.e., feelings of panic, restlessness, tremulousness, palpitations, hyperventilation), which is attributed to excessive norepinephrine. Norepinephrine is released from the locus ceruleus (LC) in response to an actual or a perceived threat. The LC is a brain stem nucleus that contains many noradrenergic neurons and has extensive projections to the limbic system, cerebral cortex, and cerebellum. The involvement of the noradrenergic system in anxiety is supported by the observations that drugs that stimulate activity in the LC (e.g., caffeine) may cause symptoms of anxiety, and drugs used to treat anxiety (e.g., benzodiazepines) decrease neuronal firing and norepinephrine release in the LC.

Neuroendocrine factors also play a role in anxiety disorders. Perceived threat or stress activates the hypothalamic–pituitary–adrenal axis and corticotropin-releasing factor (CRF), one of its components. CRF activates the LC, which then releases norepinephrine and generates anxiety. Overall, CRF is considered important in integrating the endocrine, autonomic, and behavioral responses to stress.

GABA is the major inhibitory neurotransmitter in the brain and spinal cord. $GABA_A$ receptors are attached to chloride channels in nerve cell membranes. When GABA interacts with $GABA_A$ receptors, chloride channels open, chloride ions move into the neuron, and the nerve cell is less able to be excited (i.e., generate an electrical impulse).

Box 8-1	Anxiety Disorders

Generalized Anxiety Disorder (GAD)

Major diagnostic criteria for GAD include worry about two or more circumstances and multiple symptoms for 6 months or longer, and elimination of disease processes or drugs as possible causes. The frequency, duration, or intensity of the worry is exaggerated or out of proportion to the actual situation. Symptoms are related to motor tension (e.g., muscle tension, restlessness, trembling, fatigue), overactivity of the autonomic nervous system (e.g., dyspnea, palpitations, tachycardia, sweating, dry mouth, dizziness, nausea, diarrhea), and increased vigilance (feeling fearful, nervous, or keyed up; difficulty concentrating; irritability; insomnia).

Symptoms of anxiety occur with numerous disease processes, including medical disorders (e.g., hyperthyroidism, cardiovascular disease, cancer) and psychiatric disorders (e.g., mood disorders, schizophrenia, substance use disorders). They also frequently occur with drugs that affect the central nervous system (CNS). With CNS stimulants (e.g., nasal decongestants, antiasthma drugs, nicotine, caffeine), symptoms occur with drug administration; with CNS depressants (e.g., alcohol, benzodiazepines), symptoms are more likely to occur when the drug is stopped, especially if stopped abruptly.

When the symptoms are secondary to medical illness, they may decrease as the illness improves. However, most persons with GAD experience little relief when one stressful situation or problem is resolved. Instead, they quickly move on to another worry. Additional characteristics of GAD include its chronicity, although the severity of symptoms fluctuates over time; its frequent association with somatic symptoms (e.g., headache, gastrointestinal complaints, including irritable bowel syndrome); and its frequent coexistence with depression, other anxiety disorders, and substance abuse or dependence.

Obsessive-Compulsive Disorder (OCD)

An obsession involves an uncontrollable desire to dwell on a thought or a feeling; a compulsion involves repeated performance of some act to relieve the fear and anxiety associated with an obsession. OCD is characterized by obsessions or compulsions that are severe enough to be time consuming (e.g., take more than an hour per day), cause marked distress, or impair the person's ability to function in usual activities or relationships. The compulsive behavior provides some relief from anxiety but is not pleasurable. The person recognizes that the obsessions or compulsions are excessive or unreasonable and attempts to resist them. When patients resist or are prevented from performing the compulsive behavior, they experience increasing anxiety and often abuse alcohol or antianxiety, sedative-type drugs in the attempt to relieve anxiety.

Panic Disorder

Panic disorder involves acute, sudden, recurrent attacks of anxiety, with feelings of intense fear, terror, or impending doom. It may be accompanied by such symptoms as palpitations, sweating, trembling, shortness of breath or a feeling of smothering, chest pain, nausea, or dizziness. Symptoms usually build to a peak over about 10 minutes and may require medication to be relieved. Afterward, the person is usually preoccupied and worried about future attacks.

A significant number (50–65%) of patients with panic disorder are thought to also have major depression. In addition, some patients with panic disorder also develop agoraphobia, a fear of having a panic attack in a place or situation where one cannot escape or get help. Combined panic disorder and agoraphobia often involves a chronic, relapsing pattern of significant functional impairment and may require lifetime treatment.

Post-Traumatic Stress Disorder (PTSD)

PTSD develops after seeing or being involved in highly stressful events that involve actual or threatened death or serious injury (e.g., natural disasters, military combat, violent acts such as rape or murder, explosions or bombings, serious automobile accidents). The person responds to such an event with thoughts and feelings of intense fear, helplessness, or horror and develops symptoms such as hyperarousal, irritability, outbursts of anger, difficulty sleeping, difficulty concentrating, and an exaggerated startle response. These thoughts, feelings, and symptoms persist as the traumatic event is relived through recurring thoughts, images, nightmares, or flashbacks in which the actual event seems to be occurring. The intense psychic discomfort leads people to avoid situations that remind them of the event; become detached from other people; have less interest in activities they formerly enjoyed; and develop other disorders (e.g., anxiety disorders, major depression, alcohol or other substance abuse).

The response to stress is highly individualized and the same event or type of event might precipitate PTSD in one person and have little effect in another. Thus, most people experience major stresses and traumatic events during their lifetimes, but many do not develop PTSD. This point needs emphasis because many people seem to assume that PTSD is the normal response to a tragic event and that intensive counseling is needed. For example, counselors converge upon schools in response to events that are perceived to be tragic or stressful. Some authorities take the opposing view, however, that talking about and reliving a traumatic event may increase anxiety in some people and thereby increase the likelihood that PTSD will occur.

Social Anxiety Disorder (SAD)

This disorder involves excessive concern about scrutiny by others, which may start in childhood and be lifelong. Affected persons are afraid they will say or do something that will embarrass or humiliate them. As a result, they try to avoid certain situations (e.g., public speaking) or experience considerable distress if they cannot avoid them. They are often uncomfortable around other people or experience anxiety in many social situations. SAD may be inherited; there is a threefold increase in the occurance of SAD in related family members.

The serotonin system, although not as well understood, is also thought to play a role in anxiety. Both serotonin reuptake inhibitors and serotonin receptor agonists are now used to treat anxiety disorders. Research has suggested two possible roles for the serotonin receptor HT_{1A}. During embryonic development, stimulation of HT_{1A} receptors by serotonin is thought to play a role in development of normal brain circuitry necessary for normal anxiety responses. However, during adulthood, SSRIs act through HT_{1A} receptors to reduce anxiety responses.

Additional causes of anxiety disorders include medical conditions (anxiety disorder due to a general medical condition according to the *DSM-IV-TR*), psychiatric disorders, and substance abuse. Almost all major psychiatric illnesses may be associated with symptoms of anxiety (e.g., dementia, major depression, mania, schizophrenia). Anxiety related to substance abuse is categorized in the *DSM-IV-TR* as substance-induced anxiety disorder.

Sleep and Insomnia

Sleep is a recurrent period of decreased mental and physical activity during which a person is relatively unresponsive to sensory and environmental stimuli. Normal sleep allows rest, renewal of energy for performing activities of daily living, and alertness on awakening.

When a person retires for sleep, there is an initial period of drowsiness or sleep latency, which lasts about 30 minutes. After the person is asleep, cycles occur approximately every 90 minutes during the sleep period. During each cycle, the sleeper progresses from drowsiness (stage I) to deep sleep (stages III and IV). These stages are characterized by depressed body functions, non–rapid eye movement (non-REM), and non-dreaming, and they are thought to be physically restorative. Activities that occur during these stages include increased tissue repair, synthesis of skeletal muscle protein, and secretion of growth hormone. At the same time, there is decreased body temperature, metabolic rate, glucose consumption, and production of catabolic hormones. Stage IV is followed by a period of 5 to 20 minutes of REM, dreaming, and increased physiologic activity.

REM sleep is thought to be mentally and emotionally restorative; REM deprivation can lead to serious psychological problems, including psychosis. It is estimated that a person spends about 75% of sleeping hours in non-REM sleep and about 25% in REM sleep. However, older adults often have a different pattern, with less deep sleep, more light sleep, more frequent awakenings, and generally more disruptions.

Insomnia, prolonged difficulty in going to sleep or staying asleep long enough to feel rested, is the most common sleep disorder. Insomnia has many causes, including such stressors as pain, anxiety, illness, changes in lifestyle or environment, and various drugs. Occasional sleeplessness is a normal response to many stimuli and is not usually harmful. Insomnia is said to be chronic when it lasts longer than 1 month. As in anxiety, several neurotransmission systems are apparently involved in regulating sleep–wake cycles and producing insomnia.

General Characteristics of Benzodiazepines

Benzodiazepines are widely used for anxiety and insomnia and are also used for several other indications. They have a wide margin of safety between therapeutic and toxic doses and are rarely fatal, even in overdose, unless combined with other CNS depressant drugs, such as alcohol. They are Schedule IV drugs under the Controlled Substances Act. They are drugs of abuse and may cause physiologic dependence; therefore, withdrawal symptoms occur if the drugs are stopped abruptly. To avoid withdrawal symptoms, benzodiazepines should be gradually tapered and discontinued. They do not induce drug-metabolizing enzymes or suppress REM sleep. They may cause characteristic effects of CNS depression, including excessive sedation, impairment of physical and mental activities, and respiratory depression. They are not recommended for long-term use.

Benzodiazepines differ mainly in their plasma half-lives, production of active metabolites, and clinical uses. Drugs with half-lives longer than 24 hours (e.g., chlordiazepoxide, diazepam, clorazepate, flurazepam) form active metabolites that also have long half-lives and tend to accumulate, especially in older adults and people with impaired liver function. These drugs require 5 to 7 days to reach steady-state serum levels. Therapeutic effects (e.g., decreased anxiety or insomnia) and adverse effects (e.g., sedation, ataxia) are more likely to occur after 2 or 3 days of therapy than initially. Such effects accumulate with chronic usage and persist for several days after the drugs are discontinued. Drugs with half-lives shorter than 24 hours (e.g., alprazolam, lorazepam, midazolam, oxazepam, temazepam, triazolam) do not have active metabolites and do not accumulate. Although the drugs produce similar effects, they differ in clinical uses mainly because their manufacturers developed and promoted them for particular purposes. All benzodiazepines are effective sedative-hypnotics, but only flurazepam, temazepam, and triazolam are marketed for the treatment of insomnia.

Mechanism of Action

Benzodiazepines bind with benzodiazepine receptors in nerve cells of the brain; this receptor complex also has binding sites for GABA, an inhibitory neurotransmitter. This GABA–benzodiazepine receptor complex regulates the entry of chloride ions into the cell. When GABA binds to the receptor complex, chloride ions enter the cell and hyperpolarize the cell membrane, making the cell membrane more stable and less responsive to excitatory neurotransmitters, such as norepinephrine. Benzodiazepines bind at a different site on the receptor complex and enhance the inhibitory effect of GABA to relieve anxiety, tension, and nervousness and to produce sleep. The decreased neuronal excitability also accounts for the usefulness of benzodiazepines as muscle relaxants, hypnotics, and anticonvulsants.

At least two benzodiazepine receptors, called BZ1 and BZ2, have been identified in the brain. BZ1 is thought to be

Table 8-1	Pharmacokinetics of Benzodiazepines

Generic Name	Protein Binding (%)	Half-Life (H)	Metabolite(S)	ACTION Onset	ACTION Peak	ACTION Duration
Alprazolam	80	7–15	Inactive	30 min	1–2 h	4–6 h
Chlordiazepoxide	96	5–30	Active	10–15 min	1–4 h	2–3 d
Clonazepam	97	20–50	Inactive	varies	1–4 h	weeks
Clorazepate	97	40–50	Active	rapid	1–2 h	days
Diazepam	98	20–80	Active	PO 30–60 min IV 1–5 min	1–2 h 30 min	3 h 15–60 min
Flurazepam	97	2–3	Active	15–45 min	30–60 min	6–8 h
Lorazepam	85	10–20	Inactive	PO 1–30 min IM 15–30 min IV 5–20 min	2–4 h 60–90 min 30 min	12–24 h 12–24 h 4 h
Midazolam		1–2	Active	15 min		30–60 min
Oxazepam	87	5–20	Inactive	slow	2–4 h	2–4 h
Temazepam	96	9–12	Inactive	30–60 min	2–3 h	6–8 h
Triazolam	78–89	2–5	Inactive	15–30 min	1–2 h	4–6 h

concerned with sleep mechanisms. BZ2 is associated with memory, motor, sensory, and cognitive functions.

Pharmacokinetics

Benzodiazepines are well absorbed with oral administration, and most are given orally. A few (e.g., diazepam, lorazepam) are given both orally and parenterally. They are highly lipid soluble, widely distributed in body tissues, and highly bound to plasma proteins (85% to 98%). The high lipid solubility allows the drugs to easily enter the CNS and perform their actions. Then, the drugs are redistributed to peripheral tissues, from which they are slowly eliminated. Diazepam, for example, is an extremely lipid-soluble drug that enters the CNS and acts within 1 to 5 minutes after intravenous (IV) injection. However, the duration of action of a single IV dose is short (30 to 100 minutes) because the drug rapidly leaves the CNS and distributes peripherally. Thus, the pharmacodynamic effects (e.g., sedation) do not correlate with plasma drug levels because the drugs move in and out of the CNS rapidly. This redistribution allows a patient to awaken even though the drug may remain in the blood and other peripheral tissues for days or weeks before it is completely eliminated. The pharmacokinetic profile of some benzodiazepines is given in Table 8-1.

Benzodiazepines are mainly metabolized in the liver by the cytochrome P450 enzymes (3A4 subgroup) and glucuronide conjugation. Some (e.g., midazolam) are also metabolized by CYP3A4 enzymes in the intestine. Most benzodiazepines are oxidized by the enzymes to metabolites that are then conjugated. For example, diazepam is converted to *N*-desmethyl-diazepam (N-DMDZ), an active metabolite with a

long elimination half-life (up to 200 hours). N-DMDZ is further oxidized to oxazepam and then conjugated and excreted. With repeated drug doses, N-DMDZ accumulates and may contribute to both long-lasting antianxiety effects and to adverse effects. If oxidation is impaired (e.g., in older adults, in individuals with liver disease, with concurrent use of drugs that inhibit oxidation), higher blood levels of both the parent drugs and metabolites increase the risks of adverse drug effects. In contrast, lorazepam, oxazepam, and temazepam are conjugated only, so their elimination is not impaired by the above factors. Drug metabolites are excreted through the kidneys.

Indications for Use

Major clinical uses of the benzodiazepines are as antianxiety, hypnotic, and anticonvulsant agents. They also are given for preoperative sedation, prevention of agitation and delirium tremens in acute alcohol withdrawal, and treatment of anxiety symptoms associated with depression, acute psychosis, or mania. Thus, they are often given concurrently with antidepressants, antipsychotics, and mood stabilizers.

Not all benzodiazepines are approved for all uses; Table 8-2 lists indications for the individual benzodiazepines. Diazepam has been extensively studied and has more approved uses than others.

Contraindications to Use

Contraindications to benzodiazepines include severe respiratory disorders, severe liver or kidney disease, hypersensitivity reactions, and a history of alcohol or other drug abuse. The drugs must be used very cautiously when taken concurrently with any other CNS depressant drugs.

Individual Drugs

Benzodiazepines

P **Diazepam** (Valium) is the prototype benzodiazepine. High-potency benzodiazepines such as **alprazolam** (Xanax), **lorazepam** (Ativan), and **clonazepam** (Klonopin) may be more commonly prescribed due to their greater therapeutic effects and rapid onset of action. The trade names, indications for use,

and dosage ranges of individual benzodiazepines are listed in Table 8-2.

Other Antianxiety and Sedative-Hypnotic Drugs

Several nonbenzodiazepine drugs of varied characteristics are also used as antianxiety and sedative-hypnotic agents. These include many antidepressants, buspirone, clomipramine, and hydroxyzine as antianxiety agents and chloral hydrate,

Table 8-2 Drugs at a Glance: Benzodiazepines

Generic/Trade Name	Clinical Indications	ROUTES AND DOSAGE RANGES	
		Adults	**Children**
Alprazolam (Xanax, Xanax XR)	Anxiety Panic disorder	*Anxiety:* PO 0.25–0.5 mg 3 times daily; maximum, 4 mg daily in divided doses *Older or debilitated adults:* PO 0.25 mg 2–3 times daily, increased gradually if necessary *Panic disorder:* PO 0.5 mg 3 times daily initially, gradually increase to 4–10 mg daily Xanax XR: PO 0.5–1 mg daily; gradually increase PRN to maximum dose of 3–6 mg daily	Dosage not established
Chlordiazepoxide (Librium)	Anxiety Acute alcohol withdrawal	PO 15–100 mg daily, once at bedtime or in 3–4 divided doses IM, IV 50–100 mg; maximum, 300 mg daily *Older or debilitated adults:* PO 5 mg 2–4 times daily; IM, IV 25–50 mg	>6 y: PO 5–10 mg 2–4 times daily <6 y: Not recommended
Clonazepam (Klonopin, Klonopin wafers)	Seizure disorders Panic disorder	*Seizure disorders:* PO 0.5 mg 3 times daily, increased by 0.5–1 mg every 3 days until seizures are controlled or adverse effects occur; maximum, 20 mg daily *Panic disorder:* PO 0.25 mg 2 times daily, increasing to 1 mg daily after 3 days	*Up to 10 y or 30 kg:* 0.01–0.03 mg/kg/d initially; not to exceed 0.05 mg/kg/d, in 2 or 3 divided doses; increase by 0.25–0.5 mg every third day until a daily dose of 0.1–0.2 mg/kg is reached
Clorazepate (Tranxene)	Anxiety Seizure disorders	PO 7.5 mg 3 times daily, increased by no more than 7.5 mg/wk; maximum, 90 mg daily	9–12 y: PO 7.5 mg 2 times daily, increased by no more than 7.5 mg/wk; maximum, 60 mg daily <9 y: Not recommended
P **Diazepam** (Valium)	Anxiety Seizure disorders Acute alcohol withdrawal Muscle spasm Preoperative sedation	PO 2–10 mg 2–4 times daily IM, IV 5–10 mg, repeated in 3–4 hours if necessary; give IV slowly, no faster than 5 mg (1 mL) per minute Older or debilitated adults: PO 2–5 mg once or twice daily, increased gradually if needed and tolerated	PO 1–2.5 mg 3–4 times daily, increased gradually if needed and tolerated *>30 d and <5 y of age:* Seizures, IM, IV 0.2–0.5 mg/2–5 min to a maximum of 5 mg *5 y or older:* Seizures, IM, IV 1 mg/2–5 min to a maximum of 10 mg

(continued on page 136)

Table 8-2		Drugs at a Glance: Benzodiazepines (continued)	
		ROUTES AND DOSAGE RANGES	
Generic/Trade Name	**Clinical Indications**	**Adults**	**Children**
Flurazepam (Dalmane)	Insomnia	PO 15–30 mg	Not for use in children <15 years of age
Lorazepam (Ativan)	Anxiety Preoperative sedation	PO 2–6 mg/d in 2–3 divided doses IM 0.05 mg/kg to a maximum of 4 mg IV 2 mg, diluted with 2 mL of sterile water, sodium chloride, or 5% dextrose injection; do not exceed 2 mg/min *Older or debilitated adults:* PO 1–2 mg/d in divided doses	
Midazolam (Versed)	Preoperative sedation Sedation before short diagnostic tests and endoscopic examinations Induction of general anesthesia Supplementation of nitrous oxide/oxygen anesthesia for short surgical procedures	*Preoperative sedation:* IM 0.05–0.08 mg/kg approximately 1 h before surgery *Prediagnostic test sedation:* IV 0.1–0.15 mg/kg or up to 0.2 mg/kg initially; maintenance dose, approximately 25% of initial dose; reduce dose by 25%–30% if an opioid analgesic is also given *Induction of anesthesia:* IV 0.3–0.35 mg/kg initially, then reduce dose as above for maintenance; reduce initial dose to 0.15–0.3 mg/kg if a narcotic is also given	Preoperative or preprocedure sedation, induction of anesthesia: PO syrup 0.25–1 mg/kg (maximum dose, 20 mg) as a single dose
Oxazepam (Serax)	Anxiety Acute alcohol withdrawal	PO 10–30 mg 3–4 times daily *Older or debilitated adults:* PO 10 mg 3 times daily, gradually increased to 15 mg 3 times daily if necessary	
Temazepam (Restoril)	Insomnia	PO 15–30 mg	Not for use in children <18 years of age
Triazolam (Halcion)	Insomnia	PO 0.125–0.25 mg	Not for use in children <18 years of age

eszopiclone, ramelteon, zaleplon, and zolpidem as sedative-hypnotics. Miscellaneous nonbenzodiazepines are listed in Table 8-3.

Buspirone (BuSpar) differs chemically and pharmacologically from other antianxiety drugs. Its mechanism of action is unclear, but it apparently interacts with serotonin and dopamine receptors in the brain. Compared with the benzodiazepines, buspirone lacks muscle relaxant and anticonvulsant effects, does not cause sedation or physical or psychological dependence, does not increase the CNS depression of alcohol and other drugs, and is not a controlled substance. Adverse effects include nervousness and excitement. Thus, patients wanting and accustomed to sedative effects may not like the drug or comply with instructions for its use. Its only clinical indication for use is the short-term treatment of anxiety. Although some beneficial effects may occur within 7 to 10 days, optimal effects may require 3 to 4 weeks. Because therapeutic effects may be delayed, buspirone is not considered

beneficial for immediate effects or occasional (as needed, or PRN) use. Buspirone is rapidly absorbed after oral administration. Peak plasma levels occur within 45 to 90 minutes. It is metabolized by the liver to inactive metabolites, which are then excreted in the urine and feces. Its elimination half-life is 2 to 3 hours.

Chloral hydrate (Noctec, Aquachloral), the oldest sedative-hypnotic drug, is relatively safe, effective, and inexpensive in usual therapeutic doses. It reportedly does not suppress REM sleep. Tolerance develops after approximately 2 weeks of continual use. It is a drug of abuse and may cause physical dependence.

Clomipramine (Anafranil), **escitalopram** (Lexapro), **fluoxetine** (Prozac, Sarafem), **paroxetine** (Paxil), **sertraline** (Zoloft), and **venlafaxine** (Effexor, extended release only) are antidepressants generally prescribed for depression (see Chap. 10); however, they are also considered to be first line treatment for anxiety disorders. The Food and Drug Administration

| Table 8-3 | | Drugs at a Glance: Miscellaneous Antianxiety and Sedative-Hypnotic Agents | |

Generic/ Trade Name	Major Clinical Use	ROUTES AND DOSAGE RANGES	
		Adults	Children
Antianxiety Agents			
Buspirone (BuSpar)	Anxiety	PO 5 mg 3 times daily, increased by 5 mg/d at 2- to 3-day intervals if necessary. Usual maintenance dose 20–30 mg/d in divided doses; maximum dose 60 mg/d.	Not recommended
Clomipramine (Anafranil)	Obsessive-compulsive disorder (OCD)	PO 25 mg/d initially; increase to 100 mg/d during the first 2 wk and to a maximum dose of 250 mg/d over several weeks if necessary.	PO 25 mg/d initially, gradually increased over 2 wk to a maximum of 3 mg/kg/d or 100 mg, whichever is smaller. Then increase to 3 mg/kg/d or 200 mg per day if necessary.
Escitalopram (Lexapro)	Generalized anxiety disorder (GAD)	PO 10 mg once daily, may increase after 1 wk, maximum dose 20 mg/d	Not recommended
Hydroxyzine (Vistaril)	Anxiety, sedative, pruritus	PO 75–400 mg/d in 3 or 4 divided doses Pre- and postoperative and pre- and postpartum sedation, IM 25–100 mg in a single dose	PO 2 mg/kg per day in 4 divided doses. Pre- and postoperative sedation, IM 1 mg/kg in a single dose.
Paroxetine (Paxil, Paxil CR)	Generalized anxiety disorder (GAD) Obsessive-compulsive disorder (OCD) Post-traumatic stress disorder (PTSD)	PO 20 mg/d, may increase by 10 mg/d every week to maximum dose 50 mg/d. In elderly, 10 mg/d, may increase to maximum dose 40 mg/d.	FOR OCD: 10–60 mg/d Not recommended for GAD or PTSD
	Panic disorders	PO 10 mg/d, increase by 10 mg/d every week to maximum dose 60 mg/d; maximum dose in elderly 40 mg/d.	Not recommended
	Social anxiety disorder (SAD)	PO 20 mg/d, may increase by 10 mg/d every week to maximum dose of 60 mg/d. In elderly, PO 10 mg/d may increase to maximum dose of 40 mg/d	Not recommended
Sertraline (Zoloft)	Obsessive-compulsive disorder (OCD) Panic disorder Post-traumatic stress disorder (PTSD) Social anxiety disorder (SAD)	OCD, PO 50 mg once daily Panic disorder and PTSD, PO 25 mg once daily initially, increased after 1 wk to 50 mg once daily SAD: PO 25 mg daily initially, increasing after 1 week to 50 mg; maximum dose 200 mg daily	OCD, 6–12 y: PO 25 mg once daily; 13–17 y, PO 50 mg once daily
Venlafaxine extended release (Effexor XR)	Generalized anxiety disorder (GAD) Panic disorder Social anxiety disorder (SAD)	PO 37.5–75 mg once daily initially, increased up to 225 mg daily if necessary PO 75 mg once daily	Dosage not established
Sedative-Hypnotic Agents			
Chloral hydrate (Aquachloral, Noctec)	Sedative, hypnotic	*Sedative:* PO, rectal suppository 250 mg 3 times per day Hypnotic: PO, rectal suppository 500–1000 mg at bedtime; maximum dose, 2 g/d	*Sedative:* PO, rectal suppository 25 mg/kg per day, in 3 or 4 divided doses *Hypnotic:* PO, rectal suppository 50 mg/kg at bedtime; maximum single dose, 1 g

(continued on page 138)

| Table 8-3 | | Drugs at a Glance: Miscellaneous Antianxiety and Sedative-Hypnotic Agents (continued) | |

Generic/ Trade Name	Major Clinical Use	ROUTES AND DOSAGE RANGES	
		Adults	**Children**
Sedative Hypnotic Agents			
Eszopiclone (Lunesta)	Hypnotic	PO 2 mg at bedtime; may be increased to 3 mg if needed. For elderly, debilitated patients, and those with hepatic impairment, 1 mg PO at bedtime; may be increased to 2 mg if needed.	Not recommended
Ramelteon (Rozerem)	Hypnotic	PO 8 mg at bedtime	Not recommended
Zaleplon (Sonata)	Hypnotic	PO 10 mg at bedtime; 5 mg for adults who are elderly, of low weight, or have mild to moderate hepatic impairment	Dosage not established
Zolpidem (Ambien)	Hypnotic	PO 10 mg at bedtime; 5 mg for older adults and those with hepatic impairment	Not recommended

(FDA) has issued a **BLACK BOX WARNING** about the risk of suicidality (suicidal thinking or behavior) in young adults being treated with antidepressant medications. The nurse should observe the patient carefully for signs of clinical worsening, unusual behavior changes, or suicidality when administering antidepressant medications to adults.

Eszopiclone (Lunesta) is the first oral nonbenzodiazepine hypnotic to be approved for long-term use (≤12 months). During drug testing, tolerance to the hypnotic benefits of eszopiclone was not observed over a 6-month period. Eszopiclone increases total sleep time and reduces the amount of time needed to fall asleep. Studies show the drug does not reduce nighttime awakenings. Eszopiclone is classified as a Schedule IV controlled substance by the Controlled Substance Act.

The hypnotic effect of eszopiclone is believed to be due to interaction with the GABA$_A$ receptor at location close to or coupled with the benzodiazepine receptors. Eszopiclone is rapidly absorbed after oral administration, reaching peak plasma levels 1 hour after administration. Onset of action may be delayed by approximately 1 hour if the drug is taken with a high-fat or heavy meal. Eszopiclone has a half-life of 6 hours. It is metabolized in the liver by CYP3A4 and CYP2E1 enzyme systems via oxidation and demethylation processes, producing metabolites that are much less reactive with GABA$_A$ receptors than the parent drug. Eszopiclone is eliminated primarily by the renal system.

The drug is contraindicated in patients with hypersensitivity reactions, and it should be used cautiously during pregnancy and lactation and in people who are depressed or have impaired hepatic or respiratory function. Adverse reactions include behavior changes such as reduced inhibition,

aggression or bizarre behavior, worsening depression and suicidal ideation, hallucinations, and *anterograde amnesia* (short-term memory loss). A commonly reported reaction to eszopiclone is an unpleasant taste. Elderly patients, those with hepatic impairment or debilitating conditions, and those taking drugs that inhibit CYP3A4 enzymes (e.g., antidepressants, antifungals, erythromycin, grapefruit, protease inhibitors, others) require lower dosages to reduce adverse effects. Eszopiclone should not be taken with alcohol or other CNS depressants to avoid additive effects.

Hydroxyzine (Vistaril) is an antihistamine with sedative and antiemetic properties. Clinical indications for use include anxiety, preoperative sedation, nausea and vomiting associated with surgery or motion sickness, and pruritus and urticaria associated with allergic dermatoses.

Ramelteon (Rozerem) is the newest oral nonbenzodiazepine hypnotic, approved for the long-term treatment of insomnia characterized by difficulty with sleep onset. Unlike other nonbenzodiazepine hypnotics, which bind to GABA$_A$ receptors, ramelteon binds to melatonin receptors in the central nervous system. Stimulation of melatonin receptors by ramelteon, like endogenous melatonin, is thought to play a role in the maintenance of the circadian rhythm, which helps regulate the normal sleep–wake cycle. Ramelteon does not appear to cause rebound insomnia post-treatment. Because it does not produce physical dependence, ramelteon is not classified as a controlled substance.

Ramelteon is rapidly absorbed orally, reaching peak plasma levels in about 45 minutes. Ramelteon is moderately protein bound (82%) and undergoes rapid hepatic first pass metabolism by CYP1A2 and to a lesser degree CYP2C and CYP3A4 enzyme systems. Ramelteon is excreted primarily in the urine and does not accumulate in the body with daily dosing due to the short half-life of the drug (1 to 2.6 hours). Patients should avoid taking ramelteon with a high fatty meal because onset of action may be delayed by the presence of food.

Ramelteon is contraindicated in patients with severe hepatic impairment or in those patients taking fluvoxamine, a strong CYP1A2 inhibitor. The drug should be used with caution in those with depression or impaired respiratory function. Ramelteon may affect the endocrine hormones, resulting in decreased testosterone levels, increased prolactin levels, and decreased cortisol levels. Common adverse reactions to ramelteon include headache, fatigue, dizziness, nausea, diarrhea, arthralgia/myalgia, and taste changes. Like other hypnotics, ramelteon should not be taken with alcohol because of excessive sedation and respiratory depression.

Zaleplon (Sonata) is an oral, nonbenzodiazepine hypnotic approved for the short-term treatment (7 to 10 days) of insomnia. It binds to the benzodiazepine BZ1 receptor and apparently enhances the inhibitory effects of GABA, as do the benzodiazepines. It is a Schedule IV controlled substance; a few studies indicate abuse potential similar to that associated with benzodiazepines.

Zaleplon is well absorbed, but bioavailability is only about 30% because of extensive presystemic or "first-pass" hepatic metabolism. Action onset is rapid and peaks in 1 hour. A high-fat, heavy meal slows absorption and may reduce the drug's effectiveness in inducing sleep. It is 60% bound to plasma proteins, and its half-life is 1 hour. The drug is metabolized mainly by aldehyde oxidase and slightly by the cytochrome P450 3A4 enzymes to inactive metabolites. The metabolites and a small amount of unchanged drug are excreted in the urine.

The drug is contraindicated in patients with hypersensitivity reactions and during lactation, and it should be used cautiously during pregnancy and in people who are depressed or have impaired hepatic or respiratory function. Adverse effects include depression, drowsiness, nausea, dizziness, headache, hypersensitivity, impaired coordination, and short-term memory impairment. To decrease risks of adverse effects, dosage should be reduced in patients with mild to moderate hepatic impairment and should be avoided in those with severe hepatic impairment. No dosage adjustment is needed with mild to moderate renal impairment; drug effects with severe renal impairment have not been studied. Dosage should also be reduced in older adults. Drug safety and effectiveness in children have not been established. Japanese patients may be at higher-than-average risk of adverse effects because these subjects had higher peak plasma levels and longer durations of action in clinical trials. These effects were attributed to differences in body weight or drug-metabolizing enzymes resulting from dietary, environmental, or other factors.

Zaleplon should not be taken concurrently with alcohol or other CNS depressant drugs because of the increased risk of excessive sedation and respiratory depression. There is also a risk of increased serum zaleplon levels if the drug is taken concurrently with cimetidine (see Chap. 59). Cimetidine inhibits both the aldehyde oxidase and cytochrome P450 3A4 enzymes that metabolize zaleplon. If cimetidine is taken, zaleplon dosage should be reduced to 5 milligrams. It is very important that patients taking zaleplon be taught about this interaction because cimetidine is available without prescription, and the patient may not inform the health care provider who prescribes zaleplon about taking cimetidine.

Overall, zaleplon is effective in helping a person get to sleep and has several advantages as a hypnotic, including the rapid onset, absence of active metabolites, absence of clinically significant cytochrome P450 drug interactions, rapid clearance from the body, and absence of major memory impairments. However, it may not increase total sleep time or decrease the number of awakenings during sleeping hours.

Zolpidem (Ambien and Ambien CR), like zaleplon and eszopiclone, is a nonbenzodiazepine hypnotic. It differs structurally from the benzodiazepines but produces similar effects. Zolpidem is a Schedule IV drug approved for short-term treatment (7 to 10 days) of insomnia. Zolpidem should be given with caution to patients with signs and symptoms of major depression because of increased risk of intentional overdose.

Zolpidem is well absorbed with oral administration and has a rapid onset of action, usually within 20 to 30 minutes. Its half-life is 2.5 hours, and its hypnotic effects last 6 to 8 hours. A newer controlled release form of zolpidem (Ambien CR) contains a rapid releasing layer of medication which aids a person in falling asleep and a second layer which is released more slowly to promote sleep all night. Zolpidem is 90% bound to plasma proteins. Bioavailability, peak plasma concentration, and half-life are increased in older adults and in patients with impaired hepatic function. Dosage should be reduced for these groups. Zolpidem is metabolized to inactive metabolites that are then eliminated by renal excretion. Dosage reductions are not required for patients with renal impairment, but these patients should be closely monitored.

Adverse effects include daytime drowsiness, dizziness, nausea, diarrhea, and anterograde amnesia. Rebound insomnia may occur for a night or two after stopping the drug, and withdrawal symptoms may occur if it is stopped abruptly after approximately a week of regular use. Zolpidem should not be taken concurrently with alcohol or other CNS depressant drugs because of the increased risk of excessive sedation and respiratory depression.

Herbal and Dietary Supplements

Numerous preparations have been used to relieve anxiety and insomnia. None has been adequately studied regarding dosage; effects; or interactions with prescribed drugs, over-the-counter drugs, or other supplements. Three products are commonly used.

Kava is derived from a shrub found in many South Pacific islands. It is claimed to be useful in numerous disorders, including anxiety, depression, insomnia, asthma, pain, rheumatism, muscle spasms, and seizures. It suppresses emotional excitability and may produce a mild euphoria. Effects include analgesia, sedation, diminished reflexes, impaired gait, and pupil dilation. Kava has been used or studied most often for treatment of anxiety, stress, and restlessness. It is thought to act similarly to the benzodiazepines by interacting with $GABA_A$ receptors on nerve cell membranes. This action and limited evidence from a few small clinical trials may support use of the herb in the treatment of anxiety, insomnia, and seizure disorders. However, additional studies are needed to delineate therapeutic and adverse effects, dosing recommendations, and drug interactions when used for these conditions.

Adverse effects include impaired thinking, judgment, motor reflexes, and vision. Serious adverse effects may occur with long-term, heavy use, including decreased plasma proteins, decreased platelet and lymphocyte counts, dyspnea, and pulmonary hypertension. Kava should not be taken concurrently with other CNS depressant drugs (e.g., benzodiazepines, ethanol), antiplatelet drugs, or levodopa (increases Parkinson symptoms). In addition, it should not be taken by women who are pregnant or lactating or by children under 12 years of age. Finally, it should be used cautiously by patients with renal disease, thrombocytopenia, or neutropenia. In 2002, the Food and Drug Administration (FDA) issued a warning that products containing kava have been implicated in at least 25 cases of severe liver toxicity (e.g., hepatitis, cirrhosis, liver failure).

Melatonin is a hormone produced by the pineal gland, an endocrine gland in the brain. Endogenous melatonin is derived from the amino acid tryptophan, which is converted to serotonin, which is then enzymatically converted to melatonin in the pineal gland. Exogenous preparations are produced synthetically and may contain other ingredients. Melatonin products are widely available. Recommended doses on product labels usually range from 0.3 to 5 milligrams.

Melatonin influences sleep–wake cycles; it is released during sleep, and serum levels are very low during waking hours. Prolonged intake of exogenous melatonin can reset the sleep–wake cycle. As a result, it is widely promoted for prevention and treatment of jet lag (considered a circadian rhythm disorder) and treatment of insomnia. It is thought to act similarly to the benzodiazepines in inducing sleep. In several studies of patients with sleep disturbances, those taking melatonin experienced modest improvement compared with those taking a placebo. Other studies suggest that melatonin supplements improve sleep in older adults with melatonin deficiency and decrease weight loss in people with cancer. Large, controlled studies are needed to determine the effects of long-term use and the most effective regimen when used for jet lag.

Melatonin supplements are contraindicated in patients with hepatic insufficiency because of reduced clearance. They are also contraindicated in people with a history of cerebrovascular disease, depression, or neurologic disorders. They should be used cautiously by people with renal impairment and those taking benzodiazepines or other CNS depressant

drugs. Adverse effects include altered sleep patterns, confusion, headache, hypothermia, pruritus, sedation, and tachycardia.

Valerian is an herb used mainly as a sedative-hypnotic. It apparently increases the amount of GABA in the brain, probably by inhibiting the transaminase enzyme that normally metabolizes GABA. Increasing GABA, an inhibitory neurotransmitter, results in calming, sedative effects.

There are differences of opinion about the clinical usefulness of valerian; some practitioners say that studies indicate the herb's effectiveness as a sleep aid and mild antianxiety agent, whereas other practitioners say that these studies were flawed by small samples, short durations, and poor definitions of patient populations. An expert panel convened by the U.S. Pharmacopeia and a recent Cochrane Review (2006) concluded that there is insufficient evidence to support the use of valerian for treating insomnia (Level U).

Adverse effects with acute overdose or chronic use include blurred vision, cardiac disturbance, excitability, headache, hypersensitivity reactions, insomnia, and nausea. There is a risk of hepatotoxicity from overdosage and from using combination herbal products containing valerian. Valerian should not be taken by people with hepatic impairment (risk of increased liver damage) or by pregnant or breast-feeding women (effects are unknown). The herb should not be taken concurrently with any other sedatives, hypnotics, alcohol, or CNS depressants because of the potential for additive CNS depression.

Applying Your Knowledge 8-1

Legal/Ethical Dilemma

Mrs. Portman's daughter questions you about the medication her mother is receiving. She feels that her mother is too sedated and does not want her to receive any more medication. Without the medications, Mrs. Portman wanders away and is at risk to hurt herself. What would you do?

Nursing Process

Assessment

Assess the patient's need for antianxiety or sedative-hypnotic drugs, including intensity and duration of symptoms. Manifestations are more obvious with moderate to severe anxiety or insomnia. Some guidelines for assessment include the following:

■ What is the patient's statement of the problem? Does the problem interfere with usual activities of daily living? If so, how much and for how long?

■ Try to identify factors that precipitate anxiety or insomnia in the patient. Some common precursors are physical symptoms; feeling worried, tense, or nervous; factors such as illness, death of a friend or family member, divorce, or job stress; and excessive CNS stimulation from caffeine-containing beverages or drugs such as bronchodilators and nasal decongestants. In addition, excessive daytime sleep and too little exercise and activity may cause insomnia, especially in older patients.

■ Observe for behavioral manifestations of anxiety, such as psychomotor agitation, facial grimaces, tense posture, and others.

■ Observe for physiologic manifestations of anxiety. These signs may include increased blood pressure and pulse rate, increased rate and depth of respiration, increased muscle tension, and pale, cool skin.

■ If behavioral or physiologic manifestations seem to indicate anxiety, try to determine whether this is actually the case. Because similar manifestations may indicate pain or other problems rather than anxiety, the observer's perceptions must be validated by the patient before appropriate action can be taken.

■ If insomnia is reported, observe for signs of sleep deprivation such as drowsiness, slow movements or speech, and difficulty concentrating or focusing attention.

■ Obtain a careful drug history, including the use of alcohol and sedative-hypnotic drugs, and assess the likelihood of drug abuse and dependence. People who abuse other drugs, including alcohol, are likely to abuse antianxiety and sedative-hypnotic drugs. Also, assess for use of CNS stimulant drugs (e.g., appetite suppressants, bronchodilators, nasal decongestants, caffeine, cocaine) and herbs (e.g., ephedra).

■ Identify coping mechanisms used in managing previous situations of stress, anxiety, and insomnia. These are very individualized. Reading, watching television, listening to music, or talking to a friend are examples. Some people are quiet and inactive; others participate in strenuous activity. Some prefer to be alone; others prefer being with a friend, family member, or group.

■ After drug therapy for anxiety or insomnia is begun, assess the patient's level of consciousness and functional ability before each dose so that excessive sedation can be avoided.

Nursing Diagnoses

■ Ineffective Individual Coping related to need for antianxiety or sedative-hypnotic drug

■ Deficient Knowledge: Appropriate uses and effects of antianxiety or sedative-hypnotic drugs

■ Deficient Knowledge: Nondrug measures for relieving anxiety and insomnia

■ Noncompliance: Overuse

■ Risk for Injury related to sedation, respiratory depression, impaired mobility, and other adverse effects

■ Sleep Pattern Disturbance: Insomnia related to one or more causes (e.g., anxiety, daytime sleep)

Planning/Goals

The patient will

■ Feel more calm, relaxed, and comfortable with anxiety; experience improved quantity and quality of sleep with insomnia

■ Be monitored for excessive sedation and impaired mobility to prevent falls or other injuries (in health care settings)

■ Verbalize and demonstrate nondrug activities to reduce or manage anxiety or insomnia

■ Demonstrate safe, accurate drug usage

■ Notify a health care provider if he or she wants to stop taking a benzodiazepine; agree to not stop taking a benzodiazepine abruptly

■ Avoid preventable adverse effects, including abuse and dependence

Interventions

Use nondrug measures to relieve anxiety or to enhance the effectiveness of antianxiety drugs.

■ Assist patients to identify and avoid or decrease situations that cause anxiety and insomnia, when possible. In addition, help them to understand that medications do not solve underlying problems.

■ Support the patient's usual coping mechanisms when feasible. Provide the opportunity for reading, exercising, listening to music, or watching television; promote contact with significant others; or simply allow the patient to be alone and uninterrupted for a while.

■ Use interpersonal and communication techniques to help the patient manage anxiety. The degree of anxiety and the clinical situation largely determine which techniques are appropriate. For example, staying with the patient, showing interest, listening, and allowing him or her to verbalize concerns may be beneficial.

■ Providing information may be a therapeutic technique when anxiety is related to medical conditions. People vary in the amount and kind of information they want, but usually the following topics should be included:

  ■ The overall treatment plan, including medical or surgical treatment, choice of outpatient care or hospitalization, expected length of treatment, and expected outcomes in terms of health and ability to function in activities of daily living

  ■ Specific diagnostic tests, including preparation; aftereffects, if any; and how the patient will be informed of results

  ■ Specific medication and treatment measures, including expected therapeutic results

  ■ What the patient must do to carry out the plan of treatment

Nursing Process continues on page 142

- When offering information and explanations, keep in mind that anxiety interferes with intellectual functioning. Thus, communication should be brief, clear, and repeated as necessary, because patients may misunderstand or forget what is said.
- Modify the environment to decrease anxiety-provoking stimuli. Modifications may involve altering temperature, light, and noise levels.
- Use measures to increase physical comfort. These may include a wide variety of activities, such as positioning, helping the patient bathe or ambulate, giving back rubs, or providing fluids of the patient's choice.
- Consult with other services and departments on the patient's behalf. For example, if financial problems were identified as a cause of anxiety, social services may be able to help.
- When a benzodiazepine is used with diagnostic tests or minor surgery, provide instructions for postprocedure care to the patient or to family members, preferably in written form.

Implement measures to decrease the need for or increase the effectiveness of sedative-hypnotic drugs, such as the following:

- Modify the environment to promote rest and sleep (e.g., reduce noise and light).
- Plan care to allow uninterrupted periods of rest and sleep, when possible.
- Relieve symptoms that interfere with rest and sleep. Drugs such as analgesics for pain or antitussives for cough are usually safer and more effective than sedative-hypnotic drugs. Nondrug measures, such as positioning, exercise, and back rubs, may be helpful in relieving muscle tension and other discomforts. Allowing the patient to verbalize concerns, providing information so that he or she knows what to expect, or consulting other personnel (e.g., social worker, chaplain) may be useful in decreasing anxiety.
- Help the patient modify lifestyle habits to promote rest and sleep (e.g., limiting intake of caffeine-containing beverages, limiting intake of fluids during evening hours if nocturia interferes with sleep, avoiding daytime naps, having a regular schedule of rest and sleep periods, increasing physical activity, not trying to sleep unless tired or drowsy).

In addition, patient guidelines for antianxiety and sedative-hypnotic drugs are presented in the accompanying display.

Evaluation

- Decreased symptoms of anxiety or insomnia and increased rest and sleep are reported or observed.
- Excessive sedation and motor impairment are not observed.
- The patient reports no serious adverse effects.
- Monitoring of prescriptions (e.g., "pill counts") does not indicate excessive use.

Principles of Therapy

Drug Dosage

With benzodiazepines, dosage must be individualized and carefully titrated because requirements vary widely among patients. With antianxiety agents, the goal is to find the lowest effective dose that does not cause excessive daytime drowsiness or impaired mobility. In general, start with the smallest dose likely to be effective (e.g., diazepam 2 mg three times daily or equivalent doses of others). Then, according to patient response, doses can be titrated upward to relieve symptoms of anxiety and avoid adverse drug effects. The maximum daily dose of diazepam is 40 milligrams per day or (equivalent doses of other drugs). With hypnotics, the lowest effective doses should be taken on an intermittent basis, not every night. Additional guidelines include the following:

- Smaller-than-usual doses may be indicated in patients receiving cimetidine or other drugs that decrease the hepatic metabolism of benzodiazepines, in older adults, and in debilitated patients. With alprazolam, the most commonly prescribed benzodiazepine, the dose should be reduced by 50% if given concurrently with the antidepressant fluvoxamine.
- In older adults, most benzodiazepines are metabolized more slowly, and half-lives are longer than in younger adults. Exceptions are lorazepam and oxazepam, whose half-lives and dosages are the same for older adults as for younger ones. The recommended initial dose of zaleplon and zolpidem is 5 milligrams, one half of that recommended for younger adults. Dosages of eszopiclone should also be reduced for older adults, beginning with 1 milligram initially, not to exceed 2 milligrams at bedtime.
- Larger-than-usual doses may be needed for patients who are severely anxious or agitated. Also, large doses are usually required to relax skeletal muscle; control muscle spasm; control seizures; and provide sedation before surgery, cardioversion, endoscopy, and angiography.
- When benzodiazepines are used with opioid analgesics, the analgesic dose should be reduced initially and increased gradually to avoid excessive CNS depression.

Applying Your Knowledge 8-2

Mrs. Portman is given 0.5 mg of alprazolam at 2:00 P.M. You assess her at 6:00 P.M. and prepare her for her dinner. Mrs. Portman is very drowsy and has difficulty feeding herself. After dinner, Mrs. Portman begins to experience mild anxiety and you prepare to administer an appropriate dose of medication. What would you prepare and why?

Patient Teaching Guidelines | Antianxiety and Sedative-Hypnotic Drugs

General Considerations

▪ "Nerve pills" and "sleeping pills" can relieve symptoms temporarily, but they do not cure or solve the underlying problems. With rare exceptions, these drugs are recommended only for short-term use. For long-term relief, counseling or psychotherapy may be more beneficial because it can help you learn other ways to decrease your nervousness and difficulty in sleeping.

▪ Use nondrug measures to promote relaxation, rest, and sleep when possible. Physical exercise, reading, craft work, stress management, and relaxation techniques are safer than any drug.

▪ Try to identify and avoid factors that cause nervousness or insomnia, such as caffeine-containing beverages and stimulant drugs. This may prevent or decrease the severity of nervousness or insomnia so that sedative-type drugs are not needed. If the drugs are used, these factors can cancel or decrease the drugs' effects. Stimulant drugs include asthma and cold remedies and appetite suppressants.

▪ Most "nerve pills" and "sleeping pills" belong to the same chemical group and have similar effects, including the ability to decrease nervousness, cause drowsiness, and cause dependence. Thus, there is no logical reason to take a combination of the drugs for anxiety, or to take one drug for daytime sedation and another for sleep. Ativan, Xanax, Valium, and Restoril are commonly used examples of this group, but there are several others as well.

▪ Inform all health care providers when taking a sedative-type medication, preferably by the generic and trade names. This helps avoid multiple prescriptions of drugs with similar effects and reduces the risk of serious adverse effects from overdose.

▪ Do not perform tasks that require alertness if drowsy from medication. The drugs often impair mental and physical functioning, especially during the first several days of use, and thereby make routine activities potentially hazardous. Avoid smoking, ambulating without help, driving a car, operating machinery, and other potentially hazardous tasks. These activities may lead to falls or other injuries if undertaken while alertness is impaired.

▪ Avoid alcohol and other depressant drugs (e.g., over-the-counter [OTC] antihistamines and sleeping pills, narcotic analgesics, sedating herbs such as kava and valerian, and the dietary supplement melatonin) while taking any antianxiety or sedative-hypnotic drugs (except buspirone). An antihistamine that causes drowsiness is the active ingredient in OTC sleep aids (e.g., Compoz, Nytol, Sominex, Unisom) and in many pain reliever products with "PM" as part of their names (e.g., Tylenol PM). Because these drugs depress brain functioning when taken alone, combining them produces additive depression and may lead to

excessive drowsiness, difficulty breathing, traumatic injuries, and other potentially serious adverse drug effects.

▪ Store drugs safely, out of reach of children and adults who are confused or less than alert. Accidental or intentional ingestion may lead to serious adverse effects. Also, do not keep the drug container at the bedside, because a person sedated by a previous dose may take additional doses.

▪ Do not share these drugs with anyone else. These mind-altering, brain-depressant drugs should be taken only by those people for whom they are prescribed.

▪ Do not stop taking a Valium-related drug abruptly. Withdrawal symptoms can occur. When being discontinued, dosage should be gradually reduced, as directed by and with the supervision of a health care provider.

▪ Do not take most "sleeping pills" every night. Many sleeping pills lose their effectiveness in 2–4 weeks if taken nightly, and cause sleep disturbances when stopped. If longer drug therapy for insomnia is needed, eszopiclone (Lunesta) and ramelteon (Rozerem) are approved for long-term use.

▪ Alprazolam (Xanax) is sometimes confused with ranitidine (Zantac), a drug for heartburn and peptic ulcers.

Self-Administration

▪ Follow instructions carefully about how much, how often, and how long to take the drugs. These drugs produce more beneficial effects and fewer adverse reactions when used in the smallest effective doses and for the shortest duration feasible in particular circumstances. All of the Valium-related drugs, eszopiclone (Lunesta), zaleplon (Sonata), and zolpidem (Ambien) can cause physical dependence, which may eventually cause worse problems than the original anxiety or insomnia.

▪ Take sleeping pills just before going to bed so that you are lying down when the expected drowsiness occurs.

▪ Omit one or more doses if excessive drowsiness occurs to avoid difficulty breathing, falls, and other adverse drug effects.

▪ Take oral benzodiazepines with a glass of water; they may be taken with food if stomach upset occurs.

▪ Take buspirone on a daily schedule. It is not fully effective until after 3–4 weeks of regular use; it is ineffective for occasional use.

▪ Take nonbenzodiazepine hypnotics on an empty stomach, at bedtime, because fatty heavy meals delay onset of action.

▪ Take Xanax XR once daily, preferably in the morning. Take the tablet intact; do not crush, chew, or break it.

▪ Take Klonopin wafers (orally disintegrating tablets) by carefully peeling open the foil packaging and placing the tablet in the mouth. Disintegration quickly occurs in saliva, and the tablet can be swallowed with or without water.

Drug Administration

Frequency of Administration

The antianxiety benzodiazepines are often given in three or four daily doses. This is necessary for the short-acting agents, but there is no pharmacologic basis for multiple daily doses of the long-acting drugs. Because of their prolonged actions, all or

most of the daily dose can be given at bedtime. This schedule promotes sleep, and there is usually enough residual sedation to maintain antianxiety effects throughout the next day. If necessary, one or two small supplemental doses may be given during the day. Although the hypnotic benzodiazepines vary in their onset of action, they should be taken at bedtime because it is safer for patients to be recumbent when drowsiness occurs.

Eszopiclone, ramelteon, zaleplon, and zolpidem also should be taken at bedtime because of their rapid onset of action.

Duration of Therapy

Benzodiazepines should be given for the shortest effective period to decrease the likelihood of drug abuse and physiologic and psychological dependence. Few problems develop with short-term use unless an overdose is taken or other CNS depressant drugs (e.g., alcohol) are taken concurrently. Most problems occur with long-term use, especially of larger-than-usual doses. In general, an antianxiety benzodiazepine should not be taken for longer than 4 months and a hypnotic benzodiazepine should not be taken more than three or four nights a week for approximately 3 weeks.

For buspirone, recommendations for duration of therapy have not been established. For zaleplon and zolpidem, the recommended duration is no longer than 10 days. Eszopiclone is approved for long-term treatment of insomnia and may be taken up to 12 months. Ramelteon, the only non-controlled substance scheduled hypnotic, is approved for long-term use.

Benzodiazepine Withdrawal: Prevention and Management

Physical dependence on benzodiazepines, which is associated with longer use and higher doses, is indicated by withdrawal symptoms when the drugs are stopped. Mild symptoms occur in approximately half the patients taking therapeutic doses for 6 to 12 weeks; severe symptoms are most likely to occur when high doses are taken regularly for more than 4 months and then abruptly discontinued. Although the drugs have not been proven effective for more than 4 months of regular use, this period is probably exceeded quite often in clinical practice.

Withdrawal symptoms may be caused by the abrupt separation of benzodiazepine molecules from their receptor sites and the resulting acute decrease in GABA neurotransmission. Because GABA is an inhibitory neurotransmitter, less GABA may produce a less inhibited CNS and therefore symptoms of hyperarousal or CNS stimulation. Common manifestations include increased anxiety, psychomotor agitation, insomnia, irritability, headache, tremor, and palpitations. Less common but more serious manifestations include confusion, abnormal perception of movement, depersonalization, psychosis, and seizures.

Severe symptoms are most likely to occur with short-acting drugs (e.g., alprazolam, lorazepam, triazolam) unless they are discontinued very gradually. Symptoms may occur within 24 hours of stopping a short-acting drug, but they usually occur 4 to 5 days after stopping a long-acting drug such as diazepam. Symptoms can be relieved by administration of a benzodiazepine.

To prevent withdrawal symptoms, the drug should be tapered in dose and gradually discontinued. Reducing the dose by 10% to 25% every 1 or 2 weeks over 4 to 16 weeks usually is effective. However, the rate may need to be even slower with high doses or long-term use. After the drug is discontinued, the patient should be monitored for a few weeks for symptoms of withdrawal or recurrence of symptoms for which the drug was originally prescribed.

Benzodiazepine Toxicity: Recognition and Management

Toxic effects of benzodiazepines include excessive sedation, respiratory depression, and coma. **Flumazenil** (Romazicon) is a specific antidote that competes with benzodiazepines for benzodiazepine receptors and reverses toxicity. Clinical indications for use include benzodiazepine overdose and reversal of sedation after diagnostic or therapeutic procedures. The degree of sedation reversal depends on the plasma concentration of the ingested benzodiazepine and the flumazenil dose and frequency of administration. The drug acts rapidly, with onset within 2 minutes and peak effects within 6 to 10 minutes. However, the duration of action is short (serum half-life is 60 to 90 minutes) compared with that of most benzodiazepines, so repeated doses are usually required. Adverse effects include precipitation of acute benzodiazepine withdrawal symptoms, agitation, confusion, and seizures. Re-sedation and hypoventilation may occur if flumazenil is not given long enough to coincide with the duration of action of the benzodiazepine.

The drug should be injected into a freely flowing IV line in a large vein. Dosage recommendations vary with use. For reversal of conscious sedation or general anesthesia, the initial dose is 0.2 milligrams over 15 seconds, then 0.2 milligrams every 60 seconds, if necessary, to a maximum of 1.0 milligrams (total of five doses). For overdose, the initial dose is 0.2 milligrams over 30 seconds, wait 30 seconds, then 0.3 milligrams over 30 seconds, then 0.5 milligrams every 60 seconds up to a total dose of 3 milligrams, if necessary, for the patient to reach the desired level of consciousness. Slow administration and repeated doses are recommended to awaken the patient gradually and decrease the risks of causing acute withdrawal symptoms. A patient who does not respond within 5 minutes of administering the total recommended dose should be reassessed for other causes of sedation.

Mrs. Portman continues to receive her medication for a few days and then is no longer given the alprazolam. She begins to experience anxiety, agitation, and irritability. What is the possible explanation for these symptoms?

Drug Therapy for Anxiety

Antianxiety drugs are not recommended for treating everyday stress and anxiety. Some authorities believe such use promotes reliance on drugs and decreases development of healthier coping mechanisms. For severe anxiety associated with a temporary stressful situation, an anxiolytic drug may be beneficial for short-term use as needed; prolonged therapy is not recommended. These drugs are most clearly indicated when anxiety causes disability and interferes with job performance, interpersonal relationships, and other activities of daily living. Because anxiety often accompanies pain, antianxiety agents are sometimes used to treat pain. However, in the management of chronic pain, antianxiety drugs have not demonstrated a definite benefit and in some cases may actually heighten the pain awareness. Anxiety about recurrence of pain is better controlled by adequate analgesia than by antianxiety drugs.

Because benzodiazepines are equally effective in relieving acute anxiety, other factors may assist the prescriber in choosing a particular drug for a particular patient. For example, alprazolam, clorazepate, and diazepam decrease anxiety within 30 to 60 minutes. Thus, one of these drugs may be preferred when rapid onset of drug action is desired. Lorazepam and oxazepam have a slower onset of action and thus are not recommended for acute symptoms of anxiety. Because they have short half-lives and their elimination does not depend on the cytochrome P450 oxidizing enzymes in the liver, lorazepam and oxazepam are the drugs of choice for patients who are elderly, have liver disease, or are taking drugs that interfere with hepatic drug-metabolizing enzymes.

For chronic anxiety disorders, prescribers must consider the type of anxiety disorder before prescribing treatment. Antidepressants are considered first line drugs for the treatment of most anxiety disorders; however, benzodiazepines may be prescribed as second line drugs for some anxiety disorders. Although benzodiazepines are effective anxiolytics, long-term use is associated with concerns over tolerance, dependency, withdrawal, lack of efficacy for treating the depression that often accompanies anxiety disorders, and the need for multiple daily dosing with some benzodiazepines. In studies comparing the effects of antidepressants and benzodiazepines for treating generalized anxiety disorder (GAD), it was concluded that benzodiazepines work faster (within a few days) but that antidepressants are more effective after 4 to 6 weeks. Some clinicians prescribe a combination of a benzodiazepine and an antidepressant. The benzodiazepine provides relief during the 2 to 3 weeks required for antidepressant effects, and then it is tapered and discontinued while the antidepressant is continued. Antidepressants do not cause cognitive impairment or dependence, as do benzodiazepines. In addition, patients with GAD often have depression as well. Thus, an antidepressant can relieve both anxiety and depression, but a benzodiazepine is not effective for treating depression.

One factor to consider in the use of antidepressants is that these drugs can increase the agitation and hyperarousal already present in the patient with GAD. To minimize stimulation, initial doses of antidepressants should be about 50% less than the doses for depression. Then, the dose can be increased over 1 to 2 weeks. The optimal maintenance dose of an antidepressant for GAD is usually the same as for depression. Another factor is that patients may not be willing to take antidepressants long term because of the sexual dysfunction and weight gain associated with the drugs.

Buspirone is an alternative antianxiety agent, especially for patients with conditions (e.g., chronic obstructive lung disease) that may be aggravated by the sedative and respiratory depressant effects of benzodiazepines. A Cochrane Review (2006) found BuSpar to be useful in the treatment of GAD, especially those that had not previously been taking a benzodiazepine; however, it may not be superior to benzodiazepines. Longer term studies are needed to answer this question. BuSpar has a delayed onset of action for up to 2 to 4 weeks. Thus, buspirone is not useful for acute episodes of anxiety, and it may be difficult to persuade some patients to take the drug long enough to be effective. Adverse effects are usually mild and can include nausea and dizziness. Buspirone should not be taken in combination with monoamine oxidase inhibitors; otherwise, buspirone has few drug–drug interactions. When used to treat GAD, some clinicians recommend relatively high doses of 30 to 60 milligrams daily (in two or three divided doses).

Overall, a combination of drug therapy and psychotherapy may be the most effective treatment for GAD. Antidepressants, buspirone, and benzodiazepines are the drugs of choice; cognitive behavioral therapy (CBT) is probably the nonpharmacologic treatment of choice. Drug therapy can relieve the symptoms; CBT can help patients learn to manage their anxiety and decrease their negative thinking. After anxiety is under control, some clinicians recommend continuing drug therapy for at least a year.

Although selective serotonin reuptake inhibitors are preferred for the treatment of panic disorders because they are effective and well tolerated, benzodiazepines continue to be the most commonly prescribed medication for treatment of panic disorders. Longer acting benzodiazepines such as clonazepam and alprazolam XR are useful in treating breakthrough panic symptoms that may occur at the end of therapy with shorter acting medications. Selective serotonin reuptake inhibitors and venlafaxine are first line therapy for social anxiety disorder; however, benzodiazepines may be prescribed in children after failure to respond to all other types of drug therapy. Benzodiazepines are not generally prescribed for obsessive-compulsive disorder; selective serotonin reuptake inhibitors and clomipramine are preferred therapy for this condition. Although benzodiazepines may be useful in reducing acute anxiety associated with post-traumatic stress syndrome (PTSD), they are not considered effective in the long-term management of PTSD.

Drug Therapy for Insomnia

In general, sedative-hypnotic drugs should be used only when insomnia causes significant distress and resists management by nonpharmacologic means; they should not be used for occasional sleeplessness. The goal of treatment is to relieve anxiety or sleeplessness without permitting sensory perception, responsiveness to the environment, or alertness to drop below safe levels. The drugs of choice for most patients are the benzodiazepines and the nonbenzodiazepine hypnotics, eszopiclone, ramelteon, zaleplon, and zolpidem. However, for patients with insomnia associated with major depression, antidepressants are preferred.

Sedative-hypnotic drugs should not be taken every night unless necessary. Intermittent administration helps maintain drug effectiveness and decreases the risks of drug abuse and dependence. It also decreases disturbances of normal sleep patterns. For chronic insomnia, only eszopiclone is recommended for long-term treatment (≤12 months). Most benzodiazepine hypnotics lose their effectiveness in producing sleep after 4 weeks of daily use; triazolam loses effectiveness in 2 weeks. It is not helpful to switch from one drug to another because cross-tolerance develops. To restore the sleep-producing effect, administration of the hypnotic drug must be interrupted for 1 to 2 weeks.

When sedative-hypnotic drugs are prescribed for outpatients, the prescription should limit the number of doses dispensed and the number of refills. This is one way of decreasing the risk of abuse and suicide.

As with the antianxiety benzodiazepines, most hypnotic benzodiazepines are oxidized in the liver by the cytochrome P450 enzymes to metabolites that are then conjugated and excreted through the kidneys. An exception is **temazepam** (Restoril), which is eliminated only by conjugation with glucuronide. Thus, temazepam is the drug of choice for patients who are elderly, have liver disease, or are taking drugs that interfere with hepatic drug-metabolizing enzymes.

Use in Special Populations

Use in Children

Anxiety is a common disorder among children and adolescents. When given antianxiety and sedative-hypnotic drugs, they may have unanticipated or variable responses, including paradoxical CNS stimulation and excitement rather than CNS depression and calming. Few studies have been done in children. Thus, much clinical usage of these drugs is empiric, not approved by the FDA, and not supported by data. As with other populations, benzodiazepines should be given to children only when clearly indicated, in the lowest effective dose, and for the shortest effective time.

Drug pharmacodynamics and pharmacokinetics are likely to be different in children than in adults. Pharmacodynamic differences may stem from changes in neurotransmission systems in the brain as the child grows. Pharmacokinetic differences may stem from changes in distribution or metabolism of drugs; absorption seems similar to that in adults. In relation to distribution, children usually have a lesser percentage of body fat than adults. Thus, antianxiety and sedative-hypnotic drugs, which are usually highly lipid soluble, cannot be as readily stored in fat as they are in adults. This often leads to shorter half-lives and the need for more frequent administration. In relation to metabolism, young children (e.g., preschoolers) usually have a faster rate than adults and may therefore require relatively high doses for their size and weight. In relation to excretion, renal function is usually similar to that of adults and most of the drugs are largely inactive. Thus, with normal renal function, excretion probably has little effect on blood levels of active drug or the child's response to the drug.

Oral and parenteral diazepam has been used extensively in children, in all age groups older than 6 months. Other benzodiazepines are not recommended for particular age groups (see Table 8-2). The effects of buspirone, eszopiclone, zaleplon, and zolpidem in children are unknown, and these drugs are not recommended for use in children. Because there are reproductive concerns over the use of ramelteon in children due to decreased testosterone levels and increased prolactin levels, ramelteon is not recommended for use in children and adolescents.

The FDA has issued **BLACK BOX WARNINGS** for the use of most antidepressants (including the SSRIs) in children and adolescents. SSRIs may increase suicidality in children and adolescents with major depressive or other psychiatric disorders, especially during the first months of treatment. Although these drugs are generally prescribed for depression, they are also indicated for treatment of some anxiety disorders in children (see Table 8-3). The benefit versus risk must be carefully weighed before administering these medications to children or adolescents. The nurse should observe the patient carefully for signs of clinical worsening, unusual behavior changes, or suicidality.

Use in Older Adults

Most antianxiety and sedative-hypnotic drugs are metabolized and excreted more slowly in older adults, so the effects of a given dose last longer. In addition, several of the benzodiazepines produce pharmacologically active metabolites, which prolong drug actions. Thus, the drugs may accumulate and increase adverse effects if dosages are not reduced. The initial dose of any antianxiety or sedative-hypnotic drug should be small, and any incremental increases should be made gradually to decrease the risks of adverse effects. Adverse effects include oversedation, dizziness, confusion, hypotension, and impaired mobility, which may contribute to falls and other injuries unless patients are carefully monitored and safeguarded. Benzodiazepines may produce paradoxical excitement and aggression in adults older than 50 years of age who have a history of psychosis. SSRIs are considered by some clinicians to be first line interventions for anxiety in older patients because of their efficacy and relatively low incidence of side effects.

Benzodiazepines should be tapered rather than discontinued abruptly in older adults, as in other populations. Withdrawal symptoms may occur within 24 hours after abruptly stopping a short-acting drug but may not occur for several days after stopping a long-acting agent.

For anxiety, short-acting benzodiazepines, such as alprazolam or lorazepam, are preferred over long-acting agents, such as diazepam. Buspirone may be preferred over a benzodiazepine because it does not cause sedation, psychomotor impairment, or increased risk of falls. However, it must be taken on a regular schedule and is not effective for PRN use.

For insomnia, sedative-hypnotic drugs should usually be avoided or their use minimized in older adults. Finding and treating the causes and using nondrug measures to aid sleep are much safer. If a sedative-hypnotic is used, shorter-acting benzodiazepines are preferred because they are eliminated more rapidly and are therefore less likely to accumulate and cause adverse effects. In addition, dosages should be smaller than for younger adults, the drugs should not be used every night or for longer than a few days, and older adults should be monitored closely for adverse effects. If zaleplon or zolpidem is used, the recommended dose for older adults is half that of younger adults (5 mg). With eszopiclone, reduced dosing recommendations begin at 1 milligram with a maximum dosage of 2 milligrams at night. No dosage changes are required for elderly patients using ramelteon.

Use in Patients With Hypoalbuminemia

Patients with hypoalbuminemia (e.g., from malnutrition or liver disease) are at risk of adverse effects if they take drugs that are highly bound to plasma proteins, such as the benzodiazepines, buspirone, and zolpidem. If a benzodiazepine is given to patients with low serum albumin levels, alprazolam or lorazepam is preferred because these drugs are less extensively bound to plasma proteins and less likely to cause adverse effects. If buspirone or zolpidem is given, dosage may need to be reduced.

Use in Patients With Renal Impairment

Patients with renal impairment are often given sedatives to relieve anxiety and depression, and excessive sedation is the major adverse effect. It may be difficult to assess the patient for excessive sedation because drowsiness, lethargy, and mental status changes are also common symptoms of uremia.

All benzodiazepines undergo hepatic metabolism and then elimination in urine. Several of the drugs produce active metabolites that are normally excreted by the kidneys. If renal excretion is impaired, the active metabolites may accumulate and cause excessive sedation and respiratory depression.

Buspirone is contraindicated in patients with severe renal impairment. Eszopiclone, ramelteon, zaleplon, and zolpidem may be used by these patients and do not require dosage reduction.

Use in Patients With Hepatic Impairment

Benzodiazepines undergo hepatic metabolism and then elimination in urine. In the presence of liver disease (e.g., cirrhosis, hepatitis), the metabolism of most benzodiazepines is slowed, with resultant accumulation and increased risk of adverse effects. If a benzodiazepine is needed, lorazepam and oxazepam are preferred antianxiety agents, and temazepam is the preferred hypnotic. These drugs require only conjugation with glucuronide for elimination, and liver disease does not significantly affect this process. If other benzodiazepines are given to patients with advanced liver disease, small initial doses and slow, gradual increases are indicated. Buspirone is metabolized in the liver and should not be used by patients with severe hepatic impairment. Eszopiclone, ramelteon, zaleplon, and zolpidem are metabolized more slowly in patients with liver impairment, and reduced dosages are recommended for patients with mild to moderate liver dysfunction (see Table 8-3). Ramelteon, eszopiclone, and zaleplon should not be used by patients with severe liver impairment.

Use in Patients With Critical Illness

Antianxiety and sedative-hypnotic drugs are often used in critically ill patients to relieve stress, anxiety, and agitation. By their calming effects, they may also decrease cardiac workload (e.g., heart rate, blood pressure, force of myocardial contraction, myocardial oxygen consumption) and respiratory effort. Additional benefits include improving tolerance of treatment measures (e.g., mechanical ventilation); keeping confused patients from harming themselves by pulling out IV catheters, feeding or drainage tubes, wound drains, and other treatment devices; and allowing more rest or sleep. Dosage of sedative drugs can be titrated to some extent by assessing patients according to a sedation scale. For example, the Ramsay scale rates levels of sedation numerically, with 1 indicating a wide-awake and agitated patient and 6 indicating an unresponsive patient. The desirable level is usually 2 or 3, levels which indicate that the patient is calm, drowsy, but easily aroused and responsive to commands. In addition to sedation, the drugs often induce amnesia, which may be a desirable effect in the critically ill.

Benzodiazepines are commonly used sedatives in critical care units. The drugs may be given orally or by gastrointestinal tube when the patient is able to take medications enterally, needs a fairly stable sedative dose, and is expected to need prolonged sedation (e.g., patients receiving mechanical ventilation). However, most patients receive IV sedatives, often in conjunction with opioid analgesics for pain control. IV drugs are usually given by infusion, sometimes by intermittent bolus injection. The infusions may be given on a short-term (e.g., a few days) or long-term (e.g., weeks) basis. Response to the benzodiazepines is somewhat unpredictable because most drug data were derived from short-term administration of the drugs to non–critically ill adults and may differ significantly with long-term infusions and administration to critically ill patients.

Lorazepam (Ativan) is probably the benzodiazepine of first choice. It has a slow onset of action (5 to 20 minutes) because of delayed brain penetration but an intermediate to prolonged duration. In addition, there is little accumulation and its elimination is not significantly affected by hepatic or renal disease. Because of the slow onset of action of lorazepam, an IV injection of diazepam or midazolam (Versed) is usually given to achieve rapid sedative effects. Midazolam is short acting when given in a single IV injection or for a short time to patients with normal hepatic, renal, and cardiac function. However, in the critical care setting, it is usually given by continuous IV infusion and both midazolam and an active metabolite may accumulate. Overall, drug effects are less predictable in these patients because changes in protein binding, hepatic metabolism, and other factors lead to wide variations in drug elimination and duration of action. Some people (e.g., those being mechanically ventilated, those who have had cardiac surgery, those with septic shock or acute renal failure) have continued to be sedated for days or hours after the drug is discontinued. In patients with renal failure, active metabolites may accumulate to high levels. For these reasons, plus its high cost, some clinicians recommend using midazolam for IV bolus dosing before starting lorazepam and for short-term periods of less than 48 hours.

Diazepam also may be given to patients who require rapid sedation (e.g., those with extreme agitation). It acts within 1 to 5 minutes after IV injection and lasts about 30 to 100 minutes. However, diazepam should not be given long term because its metabolism forms an active metabolite with an extremely long half-life, which accumulates and may cause excessive sedation and respiratory depression.

Although the risk of adverse effects with a benzodiazepine is high in critically ill patients, routine use of flumazenil, the benzodiazepine antidote, is generally not recommended because it may cause seizures or cardiac arrest. These effects are most likely to occur in people with a history of seizures, cardiac arrest, head injury, cerebral hypoxia, or chronic benzodiazepine use.

Use in Home Care

Although antianxiety and sedative-hypnotic drugs are not recommended for long-term use, they are often used at home. Previously described precautions and teaching needs related to safe use of the drugs apply in home care just as they do in other settings. The home care nurse should encourage patients to use nondrug methods of reducing anxiety and insomnia and should review the risks of injuries if mental and physical responses are slowed by the drugs. In addition, assess patients for signs and symptoms of overuse; withdrawal; and use of other sedating drugs, including alcohol, sedating antihistamines, and other prescription drugs. Although the home care nurse is more likely to encounter these drugs as legal prescriptions, they are also commonly abused street drugs.

Nursing Actions   Antianxiety and Sedative-Hypnotic Drugs

NURSING ACTIONS	RATIONALE/EXPLANATION
1. Administer accurately	To avoid excessive sedation and other adverse effects
a. If a patient appears excessively sedated when a dose of an antianxiety or sedative-hypnotic drug is due, omit the dose and record the reason.	
b. For oral sedative-hypnotics:	
(1) Prepare the patient for sleep before giving hypnotic doses of any drug.	Most of the drugs cause drowsiness within 15–30 minutes. The patient should be in bed when he or she becomes drowsy to increase the therapeutic effectiveness of the drug and to decrease the likelihood of falls or other injuries.
(2) Give with a glass of water or other fluid. Avoid taking with or immediately after a fatty or heavy meal.	The fluid enhances dissolution and absorption of the drug for a quicker onset of action. Fatty foods delay onset of action.
(3) Raise bedrails and instruct the patient to stay in bed or to ask for help if necessary to get out of bed.	To avoid falls and other injuries related to sedation and impaired mobility
c. For benzodiazepines:	
(1) Give orally, when feasible.	These drugs are well absorbed from the gastrointestinal (GI) tract, and onset of action occurs within a few minutes. Diazepam is better absorbed orally than intramuscularly (IM). When given IM, the drug crystallizes in tissue and is absorbed very slowly.
(2) Do not mix injectable diazepam with any other drug in a syringe or add to intravenous (IV) fluids.	Diazepam is physically incompatible with other drugs and solutions.
(3) Give IM benzodiazepines undiluted, deeply, into large muscle masses, such as the gluteus muscle of the hip.	These drugs are irritating to tissues and may cause pain at injection sites.
(4) With IV benzodiazepines, be very careful to avoid intra-arterial injection or extravasation into surrounding tissues. Have equipment available for respiratory assistance.	These drugs are very irritating to tissues and may cause venous thrombosis, phlebitis, local irritation, edema, and vascular impairment. They may also cause respiratory depression and apnea.
(5) Give IV **diazepam** slowly, over at least 1 minute for 5 mg (1 mL); into large veins (not hand or wrist veins); by direct injection into the vein or into IV infusion tubing as close as possible to the venipuncture site.	To avoid apnea and tissue irritation
(6) Give IV **lorazepam** slowly, over at least 1 minute for 2 mg, by direct injection into the vein or into IV infusion tubing. Immediately before injection, dilute with an equal volume of sterile water for injection, 0.9% sodium chloride injection, or 5% dextrose in water.	To avoid apnea, hypotension, and tissue irritation

NURSING ACTIONS	RATIONALE/EXPLANATION
(7) Give IV **midazolam** slowly, over approximately 2 minutes, after diluting the dose with 0.9% sodium chloride injection or 5% dextrose in water.	Rapid IV injection may cause severe respiratory depression and apnea; dilution facilitates slow injection.
(8) Midazolam may be mixed in the same syringe with morphine sulfate, and atropine sulfate.	No apparent chemical or physical incompatibilities occur with these substances.
(9) Do not crush, break, or allow patient to chew extended-release forms of **alprazolam**.	Increased drug absorption may lead to toxicity.
(10) Carefully peel open packaging of orally disintegrating tablets of **clonazepam** and place in the mouth. Be sure your hands are dry when handling tablets.	Tablets rapidly dissolve when moistened and can be swallowed with or without water.
d. Give **hydroxyzine** orally or deep IM only. When given IM for preoperative sedation, it can be mixed in the same syringe with atropine, and most opioid analgesics likely to be ordered at the same time.	IM hydroxyzine is very irritating to tissues.
e. Give **clomipramine** in divided doses, with meals, initially; after titration to a stable dose, give the total daily dose at bedtime.	Giving with meals decreases adverse effects on the GI tract; giving the total dose once daily at bedtime decreases daytime sedation.

2. Observe for therapeutic effects

a. When a drug is given for antianxiety effects, observe for:

(1) An appearance of being relaxed, perhaps drowsy, but easily aroused

(2) Verbal statements such as "less worried," "more relaxed," "resting better"

(3) Decrease in or absence of manifestations of anxiety, such as rigid posture, facial grimaces, crying, elevated blood pressure and heart rate

(4) Less time spent in worrying or compulsive behaviors

b. When a drug is given for hypnotic effects, drowsiness should be evident within approximately 30 minutes, and the patient usually sleeps for several hours.

c. When diazepam or lorazepam is given IV for control of acute convulsive disorders, seizure activity should decrease or stop almost immediately. When a drug is given for chronic anticonvulsant effects, lack of seizure activity is a therapeutic effect.

d. When hydroxyzine is given for nausea and vomiting, absence of vomiting and verbal statements of relief indicate therapeutic effects.

e. When hydroxyzine is given for antihistaminic effects in skin disorders, observe for decreased itching and fewer statements of discomfort.

Therapeutic effects depend largely on the reason for use. With benzodiazepines, decreased anxiety and drowsiness may appear within a few minutes.

With buspirone, antianxiety effects may occur within 7–10 days of regular use, with optimal effects in 3–4 weeks.

3. Observe for adverse effects

a. Excessive sedation—drowsiness, stupor, difficult to arouse, impaired mental processes, impaired mobility, respiratory depression, confusion

b. Hypotension

c. Pain and induration at injection sites

d. Paradoxical excitement, anger, aggression, and hallucinations

Most adverse effects are caused by central nervous system (CNS) depression.

These effects are more likely to occur with large doses or if the recipient is elderly, debilitated, or has liver disease that slows drug metabolism. Respiratory depression and apnea stem from depression of the respiratory center in the medulla oblongata; they are most likely to occur with large doses or rapid IV administration of diazepam, lorazepam, or midazolam. Excessive drowsiness is more likely to occur when drug therapy is begun, and it usually decreases within a week.

Hypotension probably results from depression of the vasomotor center in the brain and is more likely to occur with large doses or rapid IV administration of diazepam, lorazepam, or midazolam.

Parenteral solutions are irritating to tissues.

(continued on page 150)

Nursing Actions — Antianxiety and Sedative-Hypnotic Drugs (continued)

NURSING ACTIONS	RATIONALE/EXPLANATION
e. Chronic intoxication—sedation, confusion, emotional lability, muscular incoordination, impaired mental processes including anterograde amnesia, mental depression, GI problems, weight loss	These signs and symptoms may occur with benzodiazepines and are similar to those occurring with chronic alcohol abuse (see Chap. 14).
f. Withdrawal or abstinence syndrome—anxiety, insomnia, restlessness, irritability, tremors, postural hypotension, seizures	These signs and symptoms may occur when benzodiazepines are discontinued abruptly, especially after high doses or long-term use.
g. With buspirone, the most common adverse effects are headache, dizziness, nausea, nervousness, fatigue, and excitement. Less frequent effects include dry mouth, chest pain, tachycardia, palpitations, drowsiness, confusion, and depression.	
h. With nonbenzodiazepine hypnotics, common adverse effects include daytime drowsiness, dizziness, headache, nausea and diarrhea. Less frequent effects include ataxia, confusion, paradoxical excitation.	

4. Observe for drug interactions

NURSING ACTIONS	RATIONALE/EXPLANATION
a. Drugs that *increase* effects of antianxiety and sedative-hypnotic drugs:	
(1) CNS depressants—alcohol, opioid analgesics, tricyclic antidepressants, sedating antihistamines, phenothiazine and other antipsychotic agents	All these drugs produce CNS depression when given alone. Any combination increases CNS depression, sedation, and respiratory depression. Combinations of these drugs are hazardous and should be avoided. Ingesting alcohol with antianxiety or sedative-hypnotic drugs may cause respiratory depression, coma, and convulsions. Although buspirone does not appear to cause additive CNS depression, concurrent use with other CNS depressants is best avoided.
(2) Amprenavir, clarithromycin, cimetidine, diltiazem, erythromycin, fluoxetine, fluvoxamine, itraconazole, ketoconazole, metoprolol, nefazodone, omeprazole, oral contraceptives, propranolol, ritonavir, valproic acid	These drugs inhibit cytochrome P450 3A4 enzymes that metabolize most benzodiazepines and many nonbenzodiazepine sedative hypnotics. Midazolam should be avoided in patients receiving a CYP3A4 inhibitor drug; lorazepam or propofol may be used for sedation. These drugs do not affect elimination of lorazepam or temazepam.
b. Drugs that *decrease* effects of antianxiety and sedative-hypnotic agents:	
(1) CNS stimulants—antiasthma drugs, appetite suppressants, bronchodilators (e.g., albuterol, theophylline), nasal decongestants (e.g., phenylephrine, pseudoephedrine), and lifestyle drugs (e.g., caffeine, nicotine)	Phenylephrine and pseudoephedrine are available alone or in multisymptom cold remedies.
(2) Enzyme inducers (e.g., carbamazepine, isoniazid, phenytoin, rifampin)	With chronic use, these drugs antagonize their own actions and the actions of other drugs metabolized by the same enzymes in the liver. They increase the rate of drug metabolism and elimination from the body.
c. Drug that *increases* effects of zaleplon:	
(1) Cimetidine	Inhibits both aldehyde oxidase and CYP3A4 enzymes that metabolize zaleplon, thereby greatly increasing serum levels and risks of toxicity
d. Drug that *increases* effects of zolpidem:	
(1) Ritonavir	Inhibits hepatic metabolism of zolpidem and may cause severe sedation and respiratory depression. These drugs should not be given concurrently.

Key Concepts

- Anxiety is a common disorder that occurs when a person perceives a situation as threatening to physical, emotional, social, or economic well-being.

- When anxiety is severe or prolonged and impairs the ability to function in usual activities of daily living, it is called an anxiety disorder. The American Psychiatric Association delineates anxiety disorders as medical diagnosis in the *Diagnostic and Statistical Manual of Mental Disorders, 4th edition, Text Revision*.

- Examples of anxiety disorders include generalized anxiety disorder, obsessive-compulsive disorder, panic disorder, post-traumatic stress disorder, and social anxiety disorder.

- Insomnia is a prolonged difficulty in going to sleep or staying asleep long enough to feel rested.

- Benzodiazepines are indicated as sedatives-hypnotics, antianxiety agents, muscle relaxants, and anticonvulsants.

- Benzodiazepines and some nonbenzodiazepine hypnotics are Schedule IV drugs under the Controlled Substance Act and can cause physical dependence and withdrawal syndromes.

- The choice of benzodiazepine for a particular purpose and patient depends on the pharmacokinetics of the drug. Benzodiazepines differ in their plasma half-live, production of active metabolites, and metabolism.

- Benzodiazepine and most nonbenzodiazepine hypnotics are indicated for short-term use only; tolerance develops after approximately 2 weeks. Eszopiclone, a nonbenzodiazepine hypnotic, is approved for use up to 12 months.

- Contraindications to most antianxiety and sedative-hypnotics include severe respiratory disorders, severe liver or kidney disease, hypersensitivity reaction, and a history of drug or alcohol abuse.

- Concurrent use of antianxiety or sedative-hypnotic drugs with other CNS depressants should be avoided to prevent respiratory depression and excessive sedation.

- The specific antidote to benzodiazepine overdose is flumazenil. Flumazenil has a shorter half-life than many benzodiazepines, and repeated dosages may be needed to avoid re-sedation and hypoventilation.

- Ramelteon binds to melatonin receptors to produce sleep. It is not a controlled substance and is approved for long-term use.

- Antidepressants, such as the selective serotonin reuptake inhibitors, are considered first line treatment for anxiety; benzodiazepines are considered second line drugs.

- There is an increased risk for suicidality in children, adolescents, and adults treated with antidepressant medications.

- Buspirone is indicated for short-term treatment of anxiety; however, it may take up to 3 to 4 weeks to achieve optimal effects.

- Generally, in older adults dosages of antianxiety and sedative-hypnotic drugs should be decreased.

Review and Application Exercises

Short Answer Exercises

1. What is anxiety, and how may it be manifested?

2. How do benzodiazepines act to relieve anxiety?

3. What are some nonpharmacologic interventions to decrease anxiety?

4. When assessing a patient before giving an antianxiety benzodiazepine, what assessment data would cause the nurse to omit the dose?

5. Why is sleep necessary? What functions does sleep fulfill?

6. Why are nonpharmacologic interventions to promote relaxation and sleep usually preferred over the use of sedative-hypnotic drugs?

7. What is the main difference between sedatives and hypnotics?

8. In terms of nursing care, what difference does it make whether a benzodiazepine is metabolized to active or inactive metabolites?

9. What are drug dependence, tolerance, and withdrawal symptoms in relation to the benzodiazepines?

10. What are some special precautions for using sedatives and hypnotics in older adults and those with renal or hepatic impairment or critical illness?

11. For an ambulatory patient beginning a prescription for a benzodiazepine antianxiety or hypnotic agent, what instructions must be emphasized for safe, effective, and rational drug use?

12. When assisting in home care of a patient taking a benzodiazepine, what kinds of data would the nurse collect to evaluate whether the patient is using the drug appropriately or abusing it?

NCLEX-Style Questions

13. When using flumazenil (Romazicon) as an antidote for benzodiazepine overdose, the nurse should
    a. Administer the antidote IM into a large muscle.
    b. Inject the antidote IV push over 5 seconds.
    c. Observe for re-sedation after administration of the antidote.
    d. Administer the antidote one time only.

14. When administering benzodiazepines to patients with malnutrition or liver disease, the nurse should monitor carefully for
    a. toxicity
    b. withdrawal
    c. paradoxical excitation
    d. seizures

15. Which statement would indicate to the nurse the need for further patient teaching?
    a. "I only use my medication when I really need it."
    b. "I avoid smoking after taking my sleeping pill."
    c. "I skip my evening glass of wine when I take my sleeping pill."
    d. "My sister often has a sleep problem similar to mine."

Selected References

Aina, Y. I., & Susman, J. L. (2006). Understanding comorbidity with depression and anxiety disorders. *Journal of American Osteopath Association, 106*(Suppl. 2), S9–S14.

American Psychiatric Association. (2000). *Diagnostic and statistical manual of mental disorders* (4th ed., text revision). Washington, DC: American Psychiatric Association.

American Psychiatric Association. (2004, November). *Practice guideline for the treatment of patients with acute stress disorder and posttraumatic stress disorder.* Retrieved February 19, 2007, from http://www.guideline.gov/summary/summary.aspx?doc_id=5954&nbr=003920&string=an

Chessick, C. A., Allen, M. H., Thase, M. E., & Batista Miralha Souza, J. J. S. S. (2006). Azapirones for generalized anxiety disorder. *Cochrane Database Systematic Reviews, 3*, CD006115.

Drug facts and comparisons. (Updated monthly). St. Louis, MO: Facts and Comparisons.

Fetrow, C. W., & Avila, J. R. (2003). *Professional's handbook of complementary and alternative medicines* (3rd ed.). Philadelphia: Lippincott Williams & Wilkins.

Jackson, C. W., & Curtis, J. L. (2005). Sleep disorders. In J. T. DiPiro, R. L. Talbert, G. C. Yee, G. R. Matzke, B. G. Wells, & L. M. Posey (Eds.), *Pharmacotherapy: A pathophysiologic approach* (6th ed., pp. 1685–1703). New York: McGraw-Hill.

Kapczinski, F., Lima, M. S., Souza, J. S., Cunha, A., & Schmitt, R. (2007). Antidepressants for generalized anxiety disorder *Cochrane Database Systematic Reviews, 2*, CD003592.

Kirkwood, C. K., Makela, E. H., & Wells, B. G. (2005). Anxiety disorders II: Posttraumatic stress disorder and obsessive-compulsive disorder. In J. T. DiPiro, R. L. Talbert, G. C. Yee, G. R. Matzke, B. G. Wells, & L. M. Posey (Eds.), *Pharmacotherapy: A pathophysiologic approach* (6th ed., pp. 1685–1703). New York: McGraw-Hill.

Kirkwood, C. K., & Melton, S. T. (2005). Anxiety disorders I: Generalized anxiety, panic, and social anxiety disorders. In J. T. DiPiro, R. L. Talbert, G. C. Yee, G. R. Matzke, B. G. Wells, & L. M. Posey (Eds.), *Pharmacotherapy: A pathophysiologic approach* (6th ed., pp. 1685–1703). New York: McGraw-Hill.

Middeldorp, C. M., Cath, D. C., Dyck, R. V., & Boomsma, D. I. (2005). The co-morbidity of anxiety and depression in the perspective of genetic epidemiology. A review of twin and family studies. *Psychological Medicine, 35*, 611–624.

Miyasaka, L. S., Atallah, A. N., & Soares, B. G. O. (2006). Valerian for anxiety disorders *Cochrane Database Systematic Reviews, 4*, CD004515.

Nichols, J., Alper, C., & Milkin, T. (2007). Strategies for the management of insomnia: An update on pharmacologic therapies [electronic version]. *Formulary, 42*, 86–98.

Porth, C. M. (2005). Sleep disorders. In C. M. Porth (Ed.), *Pathophysiology: Concepts of altered health states* (7th ed.). Philadelphia: Lippincott Williams & Wilkins.

Antipsychotic Drugs

KEY TERMS

- Akathisia
- Anhedonia
- Choreoathetoid
- Delusions
- Dystonia
- Extrapyramidal effects
- Hallucinations
- Neuroleptic
- Neuroleptic malignant syndrome
- Paranoia
- Psychosis
- Schizophrenia
- Tardive dyskinesia

LEARNING OBJECTIVES

After studying this chapter, you will be able to:

1. Discuss common manifestations of psychotic disorders, including schizophrenia.
2. Discuss characteristics of phenothiazines and related antipsychotics.
3. Compare characteristics of "atypical" antipsychotic drugs with those of "typical" phenothiazines and related antipsychotic drugs.
4. Describe the main elements of acute and long-term treatment of psychotic disorders.
5. State interventions to decrease adverse effects of antipsychotic drugs.
6. State interventions to promote compliance with outpatient use of antipsychotic drugs.

Applying Your Knowledge

Caroline Jones is brought to the mental health clinic by a friend. The friend says that Caroline has been seeing things that are not there and has become more withdrawn. Caroline has not taken care of her personal hygiene for some time. She is diagnosed with acute psychosis and is treated with psychotherapy and the medications haloperidol and risperidone.

Introduction

Psychosis

Antipsychotic drugs are used mainly for the treatment of *psychosis*, a severe mental disorder characterized by disordered thought processes (disorganized and often bizarre thinking); blunted or inappropriate emotional responses; bizarre behavior ranging from hypoactivity to hyperactivity with agitation, aggressiveness, hostility, and combativeness; social withdrawal in which a person pays less-than-normal attention to the environment and other people; deterioration from previous levels of occupational and social functioning (poor self-care and interpersonal skills); hallucinations; and paranoid delusions. *Hallucinations* are sensory perceptions of people or objects that are not present in the external environment. More specifically, people see, hear, or feel stimuli that are not visible to external observers, and they cannot distinguish between these false perceptions and reality. Hallucinations occur in delirium, dementias, schizophrenia, and other psychotic states. In schizophrenia or bipolar affective disorder, they are usually auditory; in delirium, they are usually visual or tactile; and in dementia, they are usually visual. *Delusions* are false beliefs that persist in the absence of reason or evidence. Deluded people often believe that other people control their thoughts, feelings, and behaviors or seek to harm them (*paranoia*). Delusions indicate severe mental illness. Although they are commonly associated with schizophrenia, delusions also occur with delirium, dementias, and other psychotic disorders.

Psychosis may be acute or chronic. Acute episodes, also called confusion or delirium, have a sudden onset over hours to days and may be precipitated by physical disorders (e.g., brain damage related to cerebrovascular disease or head injury, metabolic disorders, infections); drug intoxication with adrenergics, antidepressants, some anticonvulsants, amphetamines, cocaine, and others; and drug withdrawal after chronic use (e.g., alcohol, benzodiazepine antianxiety or sedative-hypnotic agents). In addition, acute psychotic episodes may be superimposed on chronic dementias and psychoses, such as schizophrenia. This chapter focuses primarily on schizophrenia as a chronic psychosis.

Schizophrenia

Although *schizophrenia* is often referred to as a single disease, it includes a variety of related disorders. The lifetime prevalence of schizophrenia in the United States is approximately 1%. Males and females are equally affected; however, the disorder manifests itself earlier in males (early twenties for males as compared with late twenties to early thirties for females).

The etiology of schizophrenia is unknown. The neurodevelopmental model proposes that schizophrenia results when abnormal brain synapses are formed in response to an intrauterine insult during the second trimester of pregnancy when neuronal migration is normally taking place. Intrauterine events such as upper respiratory infection, obstetric complications, and neonatal hypoxia have been associated with schizophrenia. The emergence of psychosis in response to the formation of these abnormal circuits in adolescence or early adulthood corresponds to the time period of neuronal maturation. Some studies of patients with schizophrenia have shown early neurologic abnormalities in infancy and early childhood, such as abnormal movements or motor developmental delays in infancy and psychological abnormalities as early as 4 years of age. This early onset of abnormalities coupled with emergence of schizophrenia in young adulthood suggests a neurodegenerative etiology for schizophrenia as well.

Genetics is strongly suspected to play a role in the development of schizophrenia. Family studies identify increased risk if a first degree relative has the illness (10%), if a second degree relative has the illness (3%), if both parents have the illness (40%), and if a monozygotic twin has the illness (48%). Adoption studies of twins suggest that heredity rather than environment is a key factor in the development of schizophrenia.

Many genetic studies are underway to identify the gene or genes responsible for schizophrenia. Possible genes linked to schizophrenia include mutations in *WKL1* on chromosome 22, which is thought to play a role in catatonic schizophrenia; mutations in *DISC1*, which causes delays in migration of brain neurons in mouse models; and mutation in the gene responsible for the glutamate receptor, which regulates the amount of glutamine in synapses.

Symptoms may begin gradually or suddenly, usually during adolescence or early adulthood. According to the American Psychiatric Association's *Diagnostic and Statistical Manual of Mental Disorders, 4th edition, Text Revision (DSM-IV-TR)* characteristic psychotic symptoms must have been present during a 1-month period with presence of some overt psychotic symptoms for at least 6 months before schizophrenia can be diagnosed. Behavioral manifestations of schizophrenia are categorized as positive and negative symptoms. Positive symptoms are characterized by central nervous system (CNS) stimulation and include agitation, behavioral disturbances, delusions, disorganized speech, hallucinations, insomnia, and paranoia. Negative symptoms are characterized by lack of pleasure (*anhedonia*), lack of motivation, blunted affect, poor grooming and hygiene, poor social skills, poverty of speech, and social withdrawal. Antipsychotic drugs are generally more effective in treating positive symptoms than negative symptoms. A recent Cochrane Review looked at the efficacy of antidepressants for treating the negative symptoms of schizophrenia (see Evidence-Based Practice Box 9-1).

Evidence-Based Practice

9-1 Are Antidepressant Medications Effective for the Treatment of Negative Symptoms of Schizophrenia?

Traditional antipsychotic medications are more efficacious for the treatment of positive symptoms of schizophrenia than negative symptoms. Newer atypical antipsychotics are reported to be marginally more efficacious; however, they often do not usually achieve satisfactory reduction of negative symptoms, resulting in a condition known as residual schizophrenia. Antidepressants are sometimes added to the therapeutic regime for patients with residual schizophrenia due to their stimulating or activating effect on symptoms of depression such as mood and affect. Only five studies were available for the Cochrane Review (2007) to determine the safety and efficacy of the addition of an antidepressant to antipsychotic drug therapy for treatment of negative symptoms of schizophrenia. In these studies, patients treated with an antidepressant plus an antipsychotic drug showed more clinically significant improvement in negative symptoms of schizophrenia compared with those given an antipsychotic plus a placebo. There were no statistically significant differences in adverse effects between the two groups. The review concluded that the combination of antidepressants and antipsychotics may be effective in treating negative symptoms of schizophrenia; however, more studies are needed to provide information about long-term outcomes of this treatment such as compliance rates, relapse rates, recurrence of negative symptoms, and ability to function cognitively and socially.

An important nursing implication to consider: Some antidepressants can inhibit the metabolism of antipsychotic drugs, increasing the risk of toxicity and adverse effects.

Rummel, C., Kissling, W., & Leucht, S. (2006). Antidepressants for the negative symptoms of schizophrenia (*Cochrane Datatbase of Systematic Reviews*, 6, CD005581.)

There is evidence of abnormal neurotransmission systems in the schizophrenic brain, especially in the dopaminergic, serotonergic, and glutamatergic systems. There is also evidence of extensive interactions among neurotransmission systems. In addition, illnesses or drugs that alter neurotransmission in one system are likely to alter neurotransmission in other systems. The dopaminergic, serotoninergic, and glutamatergic systems have been studied most.

The dopaminergic system has been more extensively studied than other systems, because schizophrenia has historically been attributed to increased dopamine activity in the brain. Stimulation of dopamine can initiate psychotic symptoms or exacerbate an existing psychotic disorder. The importance of dopamine is further supported by two findings: (1) antipsychotic drugs exert their therapeutic effects by decreasing dopamine activity (i.e., blocking dopamine receptors), and (2) drugs that increase dopamine levels in the brain (e.g., bromocriptine, cocaine, levodopa) can cause signs and symptoms of psychosis.

In addition to the increased amount of dopamine, dopamine receptor subtypes and their location are also involved. In general, over-activity of dopamine$_2$ (D$_2$) receptors in the basal ganglia, hypothalamus, limbic system, brain stem, and medulla is thought to account for the positive symptoms of schizophrenia, and under-activity of dopamine$_1$ (D$_1$) receptors in the prefrontal cortex is thought to account for the negative symptoms.

The serotonergic system, which is widespread in the brain, is mainly inhibitory in nature. In schizophrenia, serotonin apparently decreases dopamine activity in the part of the brain associated with negative symptoms, causing or aggravating these symptoms.

The glutamatergic neurotransmission system involves glutamate, the major excitatory neurotransmitter in the CNS. Glutamate receptors are widespread and possibly located on every neuron in the brain. They are also diverse, and their functions may vary according to subtypes and their locations in particular parts of the brain. When glutamate binds to its receptors, the resulting neuronal depolarization activates signaling molecules (e.g., calcium, nitric oxide) within and between brain cells. Thus, glutamatergic transmission may affect every CNS neuron and is considered essential for all mental, sensory, motor, and affective functions. Dysfunction of glutamatergic neurotransmission has been implicated in the development of psychosis.

In addition, the glutamatergic system interacts with the dopaminergic and gamma-aminobutyric acid (GABA) systems and possibly other neurotransmission systems. In people with schizophrenia, evidence indicates the presence of abnormalities in the number, density, composition, and function of glutamate receptors. In addition, glutamate receptors are genetically encoded and can interact with environmental factors (e.g., stress, alcohol and other drugs) during brain development. Thus, glutamatergic dysfunction may account for the roles of genetic and environmental risk factors in the development of schizophrenia as well as the cognitive impairments and negative symptoms associated with the disorder.

General Characteristics of Antipsychotic Drugs

Antipsychotic drugs (neuroleptics) are derived from several chemical groups. These drugs may be broadly categorized as first-generation or "typical" agents and second-generation or "atypical" agents. First-generation drugs include the phenothiazines and *older* nonphenothiazines, such as haloperidol (Haldol) and thiothixene (Navane), which share similar pharmacologic actions, clinical uses, and adverse effects. Second-generation agents or *newer* nonphenothiazines include clozapine, risperidone, paliperidone, olanzapine, quetiapine, ziprasidone, and aripiprazole.

Mechanism of Action

Most antipsychotic drugs bind to D$_2$ dopamine receptors and block the action of dopamine (Fig. 9-1). However, drug binding to the receptors does not account for antipsychotic effects because binding occurs within a few hours after a drug dose, and antipsychotic effects may not occur until the drugs have been given for a few weeks. Manifestations of hyperarousal (e.g., anxiety, agitation, hyperactivity, insomnia, aggressive or combative behavior) are relieved more quickly than hallucinations, delusions, and thought disorders. One view of the delayed effects is that the blockade of dopamine receptors leads to changes in the receptors and postreceptor effects on cell

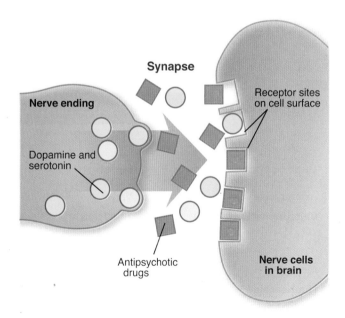

Figure 9-1 ▪ Antipsychotic drugs prevent dopamine and serotonin from occupying receptor sites on neuronal cell membranes and exerting their effects on cellular functions. This action leads to changes in receptors and cell functions that account for therapeutic effects (i.e., relief of psychotic symptoms). Other neurotransmitters and receptors may also be involved.

metabolism and function. With chronic drug administration (i.e., chronic blockade of dopamine receptors), dopamine receptors up-regulate, increasing the number of receptors on postsynaptic and possibly presynaptic nerve cell membranes. Clozapine (Clozaril) and other atypical agents block dopamine receptors as well as serotonin and glutamate receptors. Overall, the drugs "re-regulate" the abnormal neurotransmission systems associated with psychosis.

Indications for Use

The major clinical indication for use of antipsychotic drugs is schizophrenia. The drugs also are used to treat psychotic symptoms associated with brain impairment induced by head injury, tumor, stroke, alcohol withdrawal, overdoses of CNS stimulant drugs, and other disorders. They may be useful in the manic phase of bipolar affective disorder to control manic behavior until lithium, the drug of choice, becomes effective.

The phenothiazines are also used for clinical indications not associated with psychiatric illness. These include treatment of nausea, vomiting, and intractable hiccups. The drugs relieve nausea and vomiting by blocking dopamine receptors in the chemoreceptor trigger zone, a group of neurons in the medulla oblongata that causes nausea and vomiting when activated by physical or psychological stimuli. The mechanism by which the drugs relieve hiccups is unclear. **Promethazine** (Phenergan) is not used for antipsychotic effects but is often used for antiemetic, sedative, and antihistaminic effects.

Contraindications to Use

Because of their wide-ranging adverse effects, antipsychotic drugs may cause or aggravate a number of conditions. They are contraindicated in patients with liver damage, coronary artery disease, cerebrovascular disease, parkinsonism, bone marrow depression, severe hypotension or hypertension, coma, or severely depressed states. They should be used cautiously in people with seizure disorders, diabetes mellitus, glaucoma, prostatic hypertrophy, peptic ulcer disease, and chronic respiratory disorders.

Individual Drugs

Phenothiazines and first-generation "typical" nonphenothiazines are similar in ability to relieve symptoms of psychosis; however, they differ in potency and adverse effects produced. Second-generation "atypical" nonphenothiazines are equally effective in relieving symptoms of psychosis; however, they have a more favorable adverse effect profile. For this reason they are considered first-line therapy for schizophrenia.

Phenothiazines

These drugs are historically important because **P chlorpromazine** (Thorazine), the first drug to effectively treat psychotic disorders, belongs to this group. These drugs have been used since the 1950s, but their usage and clinical importance have waned in recent years.

The phenothiazines are well absorbed after oral and parenteral administration. They are distributed to most body tissues and reach high concentrations in the brain. They are metabolized in the liver by the cytochrome P450 enzyme system; several produce pharmacologically active metabolites. Metabolites are excreted in urine. These drugs do not cause psychological dependence, but they may cause physical dependence manifested by withdrawal symptoms (e.g., lethargy, difficulty sleeping) if they are abruptly discontinued. Pharmacokinetics of various antipsychotics are presented in Table 9-1.

| Table 9-1 | Pharmacokinetics of Antipsychotic Drugs |

Generic Name	Route	ACTION				Half-Life (Hours)
		Onset	Peak	Duration		
Aripiprazole	PO	Varies	3–5 h	24 h		75–146
Chlorpromazine	PO	30–60 min	2–4 h	4–6 h (10–12 h for extended release)		3–40
	IM	Unknown	2–3 h	4–18 h		3–40
Clozapine	PO	Unknown	1–6 h	4–12 h		9–17
Fluphenazine decanoate	IM	24–72 h	24 h	1–3 wks		7–10 days
Fluphenazine hydrochloride	PO	60 min	3–5 h	6–8 h		5–15
Haloperidol	PO	2 h	2–6 h	8–12 h		21–24
	IM	20–30 min	30–45 min	4–8 h		
Haloperidol decanoate	IM	3–9 days	Unknown	1 month		3 wk

		ACTION			
Generic Name	**Route**	**Onset**	**Peak**	**Duration**	**Half-Life (Hours)**
Olanzapine	PO	Varies	4–5 h	weeks	20–27
Paliperidone	PO	Varies	24 h	Unknown	23 h
Perphenazine	PO	Varies	Unknown	Unknown	Unknown
	IM/IV	5–10 min	1–2 h	6 h	
Quetiapine	PO	Varies	2–4 h	8–10 h	6
Risperidone	PO	1–2 h	3–17 h	weeks	20–30
Thiothixene	PO	Slow	1–3 h	12 h	3–4
Trifluoperazine	PO	Varies	2–4 h	<12 h	3–40
	IM	Rapid	1–2 h	<12 h	3–40
Ziprasidone	PO	Varies	1 h	6–8 h	3
Ziprasidone mesylate	IM	Unknown	1 h	Unknown	2–5

Phenothiazines have many effects, including CNS depression, autonomic nervous system depression (antiadrenergic and anticholinergic effects), antiemetic effects, lowering of body temperature, and hypersensitivity reactions. Additional adverse effects include increased prolactin levels, producing gynecomastia and galactorrhea; sexual dysfunction, including decreased libido, impaired ability to reach orgasm, and erectile/ejaculatory dysfunction; reduced seizure threshold, especially in those with seizure disorders; dysrhythmias due to prolongation of the QT interval; and weight gain. *Neuroleptic malignant syndrome*, a rare but potentially fatal adverse effect, is characterized by rigidity, severe hyperthermia, agitation, confusion, delirium, dyspnea, tachycardia, respiratory failure, and acute renal failure. Supportive treatments for neuroleptic malignant syndrome include hydration, cooling measures and antipyretics to reduce fever, benzodiazepines to reduce agitation, dantrolene to directly relax muscles, and bromocriptine or amantadine (dopamine agonists) to reduce CNS depression.

Phenothiazines differ mainly in potency and adverse effects. Low-potency phenothiazines include chlorpromazine and thioridazine. Perphenazine is an example of a medium-potency phenothiazine. High-potency phenothiazines include trifluoperazine and fluphenazine. With low-potency drugs, higher dosages are required to achieve the same antipsychotic effect as smaller dosages of high-potency drugs. High-potency antipsychotic drugs are more likely to produce early extrapyramidal side effects (e.g., acute dystonia, parkinsonism, and akathisia) than low-potency drugs; however, the risk for late extrapyramidal effects (e.g., tardive dyskinesia) occurs with all phenothiazines. High-potency drugs also carry increased risk for neuroleptic malignant syndrome when compared with lower potency drugs. Anticholinergic side effects (e.g., blurred vision, constipation, dry mouth, photophobia, tachycardia, and urinary hesitancy), antiadrenergic effects such as orthostatic hypotension, and CNS depression (sedation) occur more frequently with low-potency drugs than with high-potency drugs.

Information about administration, dosage, and other characteristics of individual phenothiazine drugs are listed in Table 9-2.

Nonphenothiazines

Nonphenothiazines include first-generation "typical" antipsychotics, which share many similarities to phenothiazines, and second-generation "atypical" antipsychotics, which vary in relation to typical drugs and to each other. Details about administration, dosage, and other characteristics of selected nonphenothiazines are listed in Table 9-3.

First-Generation "Typical" Antipsychotics

Haloperidol (Haldol) is a butyrophenone used in psychiatric disorders. A related drug, droperidol, is used in anesthesia and as an antiemetic. Haloperidol is a frequently used, long-acting drug. It is well absorbed after oral or intramuscular (IM) administration, is metabolized in the liver, and is excreted in urine and bile. It may cause adverse effects similar to those of the phenothiazines. Haloperidol is a high-potency drug, producing a relatively low incidence of orthostatic hypotension and sedation and a high incidence of extrapyramidal effects.

Haloperidol may be used as the initial drug for treating psychotic disorders or as a substitute in patients who are hypersensitive or refractory to the phenothiazines. It also is used to treat some conditions in which other antipsychotic drugs are not used, including mental retardation with hyperkinesia (abnormally increased motor activity), Tourette's syndrome (a rare disorder characterized by involuntary movements and vocalizations), and Huntington's disease (a rare genetic disorder that involves progressive psychiatric symptoms and involuntary movements). For patients who are unable or unwilling to take the oral drug as prescribed, a slowly absorbed, long-acting formulation (haloperidol decanoate) may be given IM, once monthly.

Thiothixene (Navane), another high-potency drug, is used only for antipsychotic effects. Compared with haloperi-

Table 9-2 **Drugs at a Glance:** Phenothiazine Antipsychotic Drugs

Generic/Trade Name	Routes of Administration and Dosage Ranges	MAJOR SIDE EFFECTS (INCIDENCE)		
		Sedation	Extrapyramidal Reactions	Hypotension
P Chlorpromazine (Thorazine)	*Adults:* PO 200–600 mg daily in divided doses. Dose may be increased by 100 mg daily q2–3 days until symptoms are controlled, adverse effects occur, or a maximum daily dose of 2 g is reached. IM 25–100 mg initially for acute psychotic symptoms, repeated in 1–4 hours PRN until control is achieved. *Elderly or debilitated adults:* PO one third to one half usual adult dose, increased by 25 mg daily q2–3 days if necessary. IM 10 mg q6–8h until acute symptoms are controlled. *Children:* PO, IM 0.5 mg/kg q4–8h. Maximum IM dose, 40 mg daily in children under 5 y of age and 75 mg for older children.	High	Moderate	Moderate to high
Fluphenazine decanoate (Prolixin Decanoate)	*Adults under 50 y:* IM; Sub-Q 12.5 mg initially followed by 25 mg every 2 weeks. Dosage requirements rarely exceed 100 mg q2–6 wk. *Adults over 50 y, debilitated clients, or clients with a history of extrapyramidal reactions:* 2.5 mg initially followed by 2.5–5 mg q10–14 days *Children:* No dosage established	Low to moderate	High	Low
Fluphenazine hydrochloride (Prolixin, Permitil)	*Adults:* PO 2.5–10 mg initially, gradually reduced to maintenance dose of 1–5 mg (doses above 3 mg are rarely necessary). Acute psychosis: 1.25 mg initially, increased gradually to 2.5–10 mg daily in 3–4 divided doses. *Elderly or debilitated adults:* PO 1–2.5 mg daily; IM one third to one half the usual adult dose *Children:* PO 0.75–10 mg daily in children 5 to 12 y. IM no dosage established.	Low to moderate	High	Low
Perphenazine (Trilafon)	*Adults:* PO 16–64 mg daily in divided doses. Acute psychoses: IM 5–10 mg initially, then 5 mg q6h if necessary. Maximum daily dose, 15 mg for ambulatory clients and 30 mg for hospitalized clients. *Elderly or debilitated adults:* PO, IM one third to one half usual adult dose *Children:* PO dosages not established, but the following amounts have been given in divided doses: ages 1–6 y, 4–6 mg daily; 6–12 y, 6 mg daily; over 12 y, 6–12 mg daily	Low to moderate	High	Low

Generic/Trade Name	Routes of Administration and Dosage Ranges	MAJOR SIDE EFFECTS (INCIDENCE)		
		Sedation	Extrapyramidal Reactions	Hypotension
Prochlorperazine (Compazine)	*Adults:* PO 10 mg 3–4 times daily, increased gradually (usual daily dose, 100–150 mg). IM 10–20 mg; may be repeated in 2–4 h. Switch to oral form as soon as possible. *Children over 2 y:* PO, rectal 2.5 mg 2–3 times daily; IM 0.06 mg/lb	Moderate	High	Low
Trifluoperazine (Stelazine)	*Adults:* Outpatients PO 2–4 mg daily in divided doses. Hospitalized clients, PO 4–10 mg daily in divided doses. Acute psychoses: IM 1–2 mg q4–5h, maximum of 10 mg daily. *Elderly or debilitated adults:* PO, IM one third to one half usual adult dose. If given IM, give at less frequent intervals than above. *Children 6 y and over:* PO, IM 1–2 mg daily, maximum daily dose 15 mg *Children under 6 y:* no dosage established	Moderate	High	Low

dol, thiothixene is more likely to produce orthostatic hypotension. Thiothixene can be given orally or parenterally.

Second-Generation "Atypical" Antipsychotics

In recent years, the "atypical" or newer nonphenothiazines have become the drugs of first choice. They have virtually replaced phenothiazines and related drugs except in patients doing well on older drugs and in the treatment of acute psychotic episodes. The atypical drugs have both similarities and differences when compared with other antipsychotic drugs and with each other. The main similarity is their effectiveness in treating the positive symptoms of psychosis; the main differences are greater effectiveness in relieving negative symptoms of schizophrenia and fewer resulting movement disorders (i.e., extrapyramidal symptoms such as acute dystonia, parkinsonism, akathisia, and tardive dyskinesia). Although adverse effects are generally milder and more tolerable than with older drugs, clozapine may cause life-threatening agranulocytosis, and some of these drugs have been associated with weight gain, hyperglycemia, diabetes, and neuroleptic malignant syndrome.

All second-generation or atypical antipsychotics share a **BLACK BOX WARNING** for elderly patients with dementia-related psychosis. For these patients, the second-generation antipsychotics are associated with increased mortality risk primarily due to cardiovascular disorders or infections.

P Clozapine (Clozaril), the prototype of the atypical agents, is chemically different from the older antipsychotic drugs. It blocks both dopamine and serotonin receptors in the brain. Clozapine is restricted to patients with treatment-resistant schizophrenia and those patients who have exhibited recurrent suicidal behavior.

Advantages of clozapine include improvement of negative symptoms, without causing the extrapyramidal effects associated with older antipsychotic drugs. However, despite these advantages, it is a second-line drug, recommended only for patients who have not responded to treatment with at least two other antipsychotic drugs or who exhibit recurrent suicidal behavior. The reason for the second-line status of clozapine is its association with agranulocytosis, a life-threatening decrease in white blood cells (WBCs), which usually occurs during the first 3 months of therapy. A **BLACK BOX WARNING** alerts health practitioners to this dangerous side effect. Weekly WBC counts are required during the first 6 months of therapy; if acceptable WBC counts are maintained, then WBC counts can be monitored every 2 weeks. Nurses should also be aware of a **BLACK BOX WARNING** for dose-related increased risk for seizures in individuals with prior history or predisposing factors. Additional **BLACK BOX WARNINGS** for clozapine (especially in the first months of treatment) include increased risk for fatal myocarditis, orthostatic hypotension with or without syncope, and rarely cardiopulmonary arrest. Clozapine is also more likely to cause constipation, drowsiness, and weight gain than other atypical drugs. Clozapine is metabolized primarily by CYP1A2 enzymes and to a lesser degree by CYP2D6 and CYP3A4 enzymes.

Olanzapine (Zyprexa) is indicated for treatment of schizophrenia and the acute phase of bipolar disorder. It has therapeutic effects similar to those of clozapine, but adverse effects may differ. Compared with clozapine, olanzapine is more likely

Table 9-3	Drugs at a Glance: Nonphenothiazine Antipsychotic Drugs

	ROUTES AND DOSAGE RANGES	
Generic/Trade Name	**Adults**	**Children**
First-Generation, "Typical" Drugs		
Haloperidol (Haldol)	Acute psychosis, PO 1–15 mg/d initially in divided doses, gradually increased to 100 mg/d, if necessary; usual maintenance dose, 2–8 mg daily; IM 2–10 mg q1–8h until symptoms are controlled (usually within 72 h) Chronic schizophrenia, PO 6–15 mg/d; maximum 100 mg/d; dosage is reduced for maintenance, usually 15–20 mg/d Haloperidol decanoate IM, initial dose up to 100 mg, depending on the previous dose of oral drug, then titrated according to response. Usually given every 4 weeks. Tourette's syndrome, PO 6–15 mg/d; maximum 100 mg/d; usual maintenance dose, 9 mg/d Mental retardation with hyperkinesia, PO 80–120 mg/d, gradually reduced to a maintenance dose of approximately 60 mg/d; IM 20 mg/d in divided doses, gradually increased to 60 mg/d if necessary. Oral administration should be substituted after symptoms are controlled. *Elderly or debilitated adults:* Same as for children <12 y	12 y and older: Acute psychosis, chronic refractory schizophrenia, Tourette's syndrome, mental retardation with hyperkinesia: same as for adults <12 y: Acute psychosis, PO 0.5–1.5 mg/d initially, gradually increased in increments of 0.5 mg; usual maintenance dose, 2–4 mg/d. IM dosage not established. Chronic refractory schizophrenia, dosage not established Tourette's syndrome, PO 1.5–6 mg/d initially in divided doses; usual maintenance dose, 1.5 mg/d Mental retardation with hyperkinesia, PO 1.5 mg/d initially, in divided doses, gradually increased to a maximum of 15 mg/d, if necessary. When symptoms are controlled, dosage is gradually reduced to the minimum effective level. IM dosage not established.
Thiothixene (Navane)	PO 6–10 mg/d in divided doses; maximum 60 mg/d Acute psychosis, IM 8–16 mg/d in divided doses; maximum 30 mg/d *Elderly or debilitated adults:* PO, IM one third to one half the usual adult dosage	12 y and older: Same as adults <12 y: Dosage not established
Second-Generation, "Atypical" Drugs		
Aripiprazole (Abilify) (Abilify Discmelt)	PO 10–15 mg once daily; maximum dose 30 mg/d	Dosage not established
Olanzapine (Zyprexa) (Zyprexa ODT)	PO 5–10 mg/d initially; given once daily at bedtime; increased over several weeks to 20 mg/d, if necessary	Dosage not established
Paliperidone (Invega)	PO 6 mg daily in the morning, may be increased over several weeks to maximum of 12 mg/d	Dosage not established
P Clozapine (Clozaril) (FazoClo ODT)	PO 12.5 mg once or twice daily. Increase by 25–50 mg/d every 3–7 days up to a maximum dose of 900 mg/d	Dosage not establisheds
Quetiapine (Seroquel)	PO 25 mg bid initially; increased by 25–50 mg two or three times daily on second and third days, as tolerated, to 300–400 mg, in two or three divided doses on the fourth day	Dosage not established

ROUTES AND DOSAGE RANGES

Generic/Trade Name	Adults	Children
	Additional increments or decrements can be made at 2-day intervals; maximum dose 800 mg/d *Elderly or debilitated adults:* Use lower initial doses and increase more gradually, to a lower target dose than for other adults. *Hepatic impairment:* PO, same as for elderly or debilitated adults	
Risperidone (Risperdal)	PO, initially 1 mg twice daily (2 mg/d); increase to 2 mg twice daily on the second day (4 mg/d); increase to 3 mg twice daily on the third day (6 mg/d), if necessary. Usual maintenance dose, 4 to 8 mg/d. After initial titration, dosage increases or decreases should be made at a rate of 1 mg/wk. *Elderly or debilitated adults:* PO, initially 0.5 mg twice daily (1 mg/d); increase in 0.5-mg increments to 1.5 mg twice daily (3 mg/d) *Renal or hepatic impairment:* PO, same as for elderly or debilitated adults	13–17 y: PO, initially 0.5 mg/d. Increase 1–2 mg/d for a target dose of 3 mg/d. Dosage range is 1–6 mg/d.
(Risperdal Consta)	IM 25 mg every 2 wk; maximum dose not to exceed 50 mg/2 wk. Oral Risperdal should be continued for first 3 weeks of therapy to ensure adequate blood levels are maintained.	< 18 y: Dosage not established
Ziprasidone (Geodon)	PO 20 mg twice daily with food, initially; gradually increased up to 80 mg twice daily, if necessary	
Ziprasidone mesylate	IM 10–20 mg every 4 h up to a maximum of 40 mg/d, not to exceed 3 days for treatment of acute agitation in schizophrenia	Not recommended

to cause extrapyramidal effects and less likely to cause agranulocytosis. Compared with the typical antipsychotics, olanzapine reportedly causes less sedation, extrapyramidal symptoms, anticholinergic effects, and orthostatic hypotension. However, it has been associated with weight gain, hyperglycemia, and initiation or aggravation of diabetes mellitus.

The drug is well absorbed after oral administration; its absorption is not affected by food. A steady-state concentration is reached after approximately 1 week of once-daily administration. Olanzapine is metabolized in the liver by the CYP1A2 and to a lesser degree CYP2D6 and CYP2C19 enzymes. It is excreted in urine and feces.

Quetiapine (Seroquel), like the other atypical agents, blocks both dopamine and serotonin receptors and relieves both positive and negative symptoms of psychosis and is also indicated for the acute manic phase of bipolar disorder. After oral administration, quetiapine is well absorbed and may be taken without regard to meals. It is extensively metabolized in the liver by CYP3A4 enzymes. Clinically significant drug interactions may occur with drugs that induce or inhibit the liver enzymes, and dosage of quetiapine may need to be increased in patients taking enzyme inducers (e.g., carbamazepine, phenytoin, rifampin) or decreased in patients taking enzyme inhibitors (e.g., cimetidine, erythromycin). Common adverse effects include drowsiness, headache, orthostatic hypotension, and weight gain.

Risperidone (Risperdal) also blocks both dopamine and serotonin receptors and relieves both positive and negative symptoms of psychosis as well as the acute manic phase of bipolar disorder. It is a frequently prescribed, first-choice agent that is usually well tolerated. A Cochrane Review (2005) compared risperidone and olanzapine and concluded that both drugs were effective in treating schizophrenia. The main difference noted between the two drugs was in adverse effects; patients taking risperidone experienced significantly less weight gain than with olanzapine.

Risperidone is well absorbed with oral administration. Peak blood levels occur in 1 to 2 hours, but therapeutic effects are delayed for 1 to 2 weeks. Risperidone is metabolized mainly in the liver by the CYP2D6 enzymes and produces an active metabolite. Effects are attributed approximately equally to risperidone and the metabolite. Slow metabolizers of risperidone require lower doses to avoid toxicity. Most (70%) of the drug is excreted in urine and some (14%) in feces. Adverse effects include agitation, anxiety, headache, insomnia, dizziness, and hypotension. Risperidone may also cause parkinsonism and other movement disorders, especially at higher doses, but is less likely to do so than the typical antipsychotic drugs.

Paliperidone (Invega), an active metabolite of risperidone, blocks both dopamine and serotonin receptors. It is effective in treating both positive and negative symptoms. Paliperidone is administered orally in an extended-release tablet and reaches peak blood levels 24 hours after administration. The half-life of paliperidone is 23 hours. The cytochrome P450 system plays a very limited role in the metabolism of paliperidone, resulting in fewer drug interactions with other antipsychotics. The drug is eliminated by the renal system. Adverse effects include akathisia, extrapyramidal effects, QT prolongation, orthostatic hypotension, syncope, hyperprolactinemia, and hyperglycemia.

Ziprasidone (Geodon) is another atypical agent used to treat schizophrenia and the acute manic phase of bipolar disorder. It may be given orally or intramuscularly. It is effective in suppressing many of the negative symptoms such as blunted affect, lack of motivation, and social withdrawal. Additional benefits include a decrease in weight and improvement in cholesterol and triglyceride levels. Ziprasidone is contraindicated in people who are allergic to the drug, who are pregnant or lactating, who have a prolonged QT interval on electrocardiogram (ECG), or who have a history of severe heart disease. It must be used cautiously in people with impaired renal or hepatic function and cardiovascular disease. Because it may prolong the QT interval and cause torsades de pointes, a potentially fatal type of ventricular tachycardia, ziprasidone is probably not a drug of first choice.

Ziprasidone is metabolized in the liver by CYP3A4 enzymes and excreted in urine. Adverse effects include cardiac dysrhythmias, drowsiness, headache, and nausea; weight gain is less likely than with other antipsychotic drugs.

Aripiprazole (Abilify) is approved for the treatment of schizophrenia and acute mania associated with bipolar disorder. It is the first in a new category of drugs called partial dopamine agonists. A partial agonist is a drug that has the ability to block a receptor if it is overstimulated and to stimulate a receptor if it is understimulated. The beneficial effect of aripiprazole in patients with schizophrenia is proposed to involve a combination of partial agonist activity at D_2 and serotonin $5\text{-}HT_{1A}$ receptors and antagonist activity at serotonin $5\text{-}HT_{2A}$ receptors. Aripiprazole also blocks $alpha_1$ adrenergic receptors, increasing the risk for orthostatic hypotension, and exerts an antihistamine effect by H_1 blockade. Aripiprazole may also cause neuroleptic malignant syndrome, tardive dyskinesia, weight gain, hyperglycemia, and diabetes mellitus.

Aripiprazole is well absorbed orally, with or without food. It is 99% protein bound. It is metabolized in the liver by the CYP3A4 and CYP2D6 enzyme systems and has an active metabolite. Generally, no dosage adjustment for aripiprazole is

required on the basis of hepatic or renal impairment. Slow metabolizers of aripiprazole require significantly lower doses to avoid drug toxicity.

Applying Your Knowledge 9-1

After 6 weeks of therapy, Ms. Jones has far fewer symptoms; however, she has been observed to have a gradual loss of muscle movement. What adverse reaction is likely to be occurring?

Nursing Process

Assessment

Assess the patient's mental health status, need for antipsychotic drugs, and response to drug therapy. There is a wide variation in response to drug therapy. Close observation of physical and behavioral reactions is necessary to evaluate effectiveness and to individualize dosage schedules. Accurate assessment is especially important when starting drug therapy and when increasing or decreasing dosage. Some assessment factors include the following:

■ Interview the patient and family members. Attempts to interview an acutely psychotic person yield little useful information because of the patient's distorted perception of reality. The nurse may be able to assess the patient's level of orientation and delusional and hallucinatory activity. If possible, try to determine from family members or others what the patient was doing or experiencing when the acute episode began (i.e., predisposing factors, such as increased environmental stress or alcohol or drug ingestion); whether this is a first or a repeated episode of psychotic behavior; whether the person has physical illnesses, takes any drugs, or uses alcohol; whether the patient seems to be a hazard to self or others; and some description of pre-illness personality traits, level of social interaction, and ability to function in usual activities of daily living.

■ Observe the patient for the presence or absence of psychotic symptoms such as agitation, hyperactivity, combativeness, and bizarre behavior.

■ Obtain baseline data to help monitor the patient's response to drug therapy. Some authorities advocate initial and periodic laboratory tests of liver, kidney, and blood functions, as well as electrocardiograms. Such tests may assist in early detection and treatment of adverse drug effects. Baseline blood pressure readings also may be helpful.

■ Continue assessing the patient's response to drug therapy and his or her ability to function in activities of daily living, whether the patient is hospitalized or receiving outpatient treatment.

Nursing Diagnoses

- Altered Thought Processes related to psychosis
- Self-Care Deficit related to the disease process or drug-induced sedation
- Impaired Physical Mobility related to sedation
- Altered Tissue Perfusion related to hypotension
- Risk for Injury related to excessive sedation and movement disorders (extrapyramidal effects)
- Risk for Violence: Self-Directed or Directed at Others
- Noncompliance related to underuse of prescribed drugs

Planing/Goals

The patient will

- Become less agitated within a few hours of the start of drug therapy, and less psychotic within 1–3 weeks
- Be kept safe while sedated from drug therapy
- Be cared for by staff in areas of nutrition, hygiene, exercise, and social interactions when unable to provide self-care
- Improve in ability to participate in self-care activities
- Avoid preventable adverse drug effects, especially those that impair safety
- Be helped to take medications as prescribed and return for follow-up appointments with health care providers

Interventions

Use nondrug measures when appropriate to increase the effectiveness of drug therapy and to decrease adverse reactions.

- Drug therapy is ineffective if the patient does not receive sufficient medication; many people are unable or unwilling to take medications as prescribed. Any nursing action aimed toward more accurate drug administration increases the effectiveness of drug therapy.

    Specific nursing actions must be individualized to the patient and/or caregiver. Some general nursing actions that may be helpful include emphasizing the therapeutic benefits expected from drug therapy; answering questions or providing information about drug therapy and other aspects of the treatment plan; devising a schedule of administration times that is as convenient as possible for the patient; and assisting the patient or caregiver in preventing or managing adverse drug effects (see accompanying patient teaching guidelines). Most adverse effects are less likely to occur or be severe with the newer atypical drugs than with phenothiazines and other older drugs.

- Supervise ambulation to prevent falls or other injuries if the patient is drowsy or elderly or has postural hypotension.

- Several measures can help prevent or minimize hypotension, such as having the patient lie down for approximately an hour after a large oral dose or an injection of antipsy-

chotic medication; applying elastic stockings; and instructing the patient to change positions gradually, elevate legs when sitting, avoid standing for prolonged periods, and avoid hot baths (hot baths cause vasodilation and increase the incidence of hypotension). In addition, the daily dose can be decreased or divided into smaller amounts.

- Dry mouth and oral infections can be decreased by frequently brushing the teeth; rinsing the mouth with water; chewing sugarless gum or candy; and ensuring an adequate fluid intake. Excessive water intake should be discouraged because it may lead to serum electrolyte deficiencies.

- The usual measures of increasing fluid intake, dietary fiber, and exercise can help prevent constipation.

- Support caregivers in efforts to maintain contact with inpatients and provide care for outpatients. One way is to provide caregivers with telephone numbers of health care providers and to make periodic telephone calls to caregivers.

- Provide patient teaching regarding drug therapy (see accompanying display).

Evaluation

- Interview the patient to determine the presence and extent of hallucinations and delusions.
- Observe the patient for decreased signs and symptoms.
- Document abilities and limitations in self-care.
- Note whether any injuries have occurred during drug therapy.
- Interview the caregiver about the patient's behavior and medication response (i.e., during a home visit or telephone call).

Applying Your Knowledge 9-2

Ms. Jones says she is dizzy when she gets up. What nursing measures can be implemented to prevent injury?

Principles of Therapy

Goals of Therapy

Overall, the goal of treatment is to relieve symptoms with minimal or tolerable adverse drug effects. In patients with acute psychosis, the goal during the first week of treatment is to decrease symptoms (e.g., aggression, agitation, combativeness, hostility) and normalize patterns of sleeping and eating. The next goals may be increased ability for self-care and increased socialization. Therapeutic effects usually occur gradually, over 1 to 2 months. Long-term goals include increasing the patient's ability to cope with the environment, promoting optimal functioning in self-care and activities of daily living, and preventing acute episodes and hospitalizations. With drug therapy,

Patient Teaching Guidelines | Antipsychotic Drugs

Antipsychotic drugs are given to patients with schizophrenia, a chronic mental illness. Because of the nature of the disease, a responsible adult caregiver is needed to prompt a patient about taking particular doses and to manage other aspects of the drug therapy regimen, as follows.

General Considerations

■ Ask about the planned drug therapy regimen, including the desired results, when results can be expected, and the tentative length of drug therapy.

■ Maintain an adequate supply of medication to ensure regular administration. Consistent blood levels are necessary to control symptoms and to prevent recurring episodes of acute illness and hospitalization.

■ Do not allow the patient to drive a car, operate machinery, or perform activities that require alertness when drowsy from medication. Drowsiness, slowed thinking, and impaired muscle coordination are especially likely during the first 2 weeks of drug therapy but tend to decrease with time.

■ Report unusual side effects and all physical illnesses, because changes in drug therapy may be indicated.

■ Try to prevent the patient from taking unprescribed medications, including those available without prescription or those prescribed for another person, to prevent undesirable drug interactions. Alcohol and sleeping pills should be avoided because they may cause excessive drowsiness and decreased awareness of safety hazards in the environment.

■ Keep all physicians informed about all the medications being taken by the patient, to decrease risks of undesirable drug interactions.

■ These drugs should be tapered in dosage and discontinued gradually; they should not be stopped abruptly.

■ Notify your physician if you become pregnant or intend to become pregnant

Medication Administration

Assist or prompt the patient to:

■ Take medications in the correct doses and at the correct times, to maintain blood levels and beneficial effects.

■ Avoid taking these medications with antacids. If an antacid is needed (e.g., for heartburn), it should be taken 1 hour before or 2 hours after the antipsychotic drug. Antacids decrease absorption of these drugs from the intestine.

■ Lie down for approximately an hour after receiving medication, if dizziness and faintness occur.

■ Take the medication at bedtime, if able, so that drowsiness aids sleep and is minimized during waking hours.

■ Practice good oral hygiene, including dental checkups, thorough and frequent toothbrushing, drinking fluids, and frequent mouth rinsing. Mouth dryness is a common side effect of the drugs. Although it is usually not serious, dry mouth can lead to mouth infections and dental cavities.

■ Minimize exposure to sunlight, wear protective clothing, and use sunscreen lotions. Sensitivity to sunlight occurs with some of the drugs and may produce a sunburn type of skin reaction.

■ Avoid exposure to excessive heat. Some of these medications may cause fever and heat prostration with high environmental temperatures. In hot weather or climates, keep the client indoors and use air conditioning or fans during the hours of highest heat levels.

---

patients often can participate in psychotherapy, group therapy, or other treatment modalities; return to community settings; and return to their pre-illness level of functioning.

Drug Selection

The physician caring for a patient with psychosis has a greater choice of drugs than ever before. Some general factors to consider include the patient's age and physical condition, the severity and duration of illness, the frequency and severity of adverse effects produced by each drug, the patient's use of and response to antipsychotic drugs in the past, the supervision available, and the physician's experience with a particular drug.

The atypical drugs are the drugs of choice, especially for patients who are newly diagnosed with schizophrenia, because these drugs may be more effective in relieving some symptoms, they usually produce milder adverse effects, and patients seem to take them more consistently. The ability of the atypical antipsychotics to reduce adverse effects is seen as a significant advantage, because patients are more likely to take the drugs. Better compliance with drug therapy helps prevent acute episodes of psychosis and repeated hospitalizations, thereby reducing the overall cost of care, according to studies. A major drawback is the high cost of these drugs, which may preclude their use in some patients.

An additional drawback and concern is weight gain and abnormal glucose metabolism. Most of the drugs in the atypical group have been associated with weight gain, especially with the chronic use required for treatment of schizophrenia. Recent reports also associate clozapine, olanzapine, paliperidone, risperidone, quetiapine, and aripiprazole with changes in blood glucose levels, including hyperglycemia and diabetes mellitus. In some extreme cases, ketoacidosis, hyperosmolar coma, and death have been reported. A causal relationship between use of these drugs and onset of diabetes has not been established. However, before starting one of the drugs, patients should be assessed for diabetes or risk factors related to the development of diabetes (e.g., obesity; personal or family history of diabetes; symptoms of diabetes such as polyuria, polydipsia, or polyphagia). If symptoms or risk factors are identified, blood glucose levels should be checked before starting the drug and periodically during treatment.

When compared with atypical antipsychotic drugs, traditional or typical antipsychotic drugs are apparently equally effective, but some patients who do not respond well to one of them may respond to another. Because the typical drugs are similarly effective, some physicians base their choice on a drug's adverse effects. In addition, some physicians use a phenothiazine first and prescribe a nonphenothiazine as a second-line drug for patients with chronic schizophrenia whose symptoms have not been controlled by the phenothiazines and for patients with hypersensitivity reactions to the phenothiazines. Thioridazine (Mellaril), formerly a commonly used drug, is now indicated only when other drugs are ineffective because of its association with serious cardiac dysrhythmias.

Patients who are unable or unwilling to take daily doses of a maintenance antipsychotic drug may be given periodic injections of a long-acting form of fluphenazine, haloperidol, or risperidone. Extrapyramidal symptoms may be more problematic with depot injections of antipsychotic drugs.

Any person who has had an allergic or hypersensitivity reaction to an antipsychotic drug usually should not be given that drug (or any drug in the same chemical group) again. Cross-sensitivity occurs, and the likelihood of another allergic reaction is high.

There is no logical basis for giving more than one antipsychotic drug at a time. There is no therapeutic advantage, and the risk of serious adverse reactions is increased.

Dosage and Administration

Dosage and route of administration must be individualized according to the patient's condition and response; in some cases prescribers may exceed the recommended maximum dosage approved by the Food and Drug Administration (FDA). Oral drugs undergo extensive first-pass metabolism in the liver so that a significant portion of a dose does not reach the systemic circulation and low serum drug levels are produced. In contrast, IM doses avoid first-pass metabolism and produce serum drug levels approximately double those of oral doses. Thus, usual IM doses are approximately half the oral doses.

Initial drug therapy for acute psychotic episodes may require IM administration and hospitalization; symptoms are usually controlled within 48 to 72 hours, after which oral drugs can be given. When treatment is initiated with oral drugs, divided daily doses are recommended. Oral concentrates are better absorbed than pills and can be similar to IM administration in the time to reach peak serum concentrations. For maintenance therapy, once-daily dosing is usually preferred. A single bedtime dose is effective for most patients. This schedule increases compliance with prescribed drug therapy, allows better nighttime sleep, and decreases hypotension and daytime sedation. Effective maintenance therapy requires close supervision and contact with the patient and family members.

Duration of Therapy

In schizophrenia, antipsychotic drugs are usually given for years because there is a high rate of relapse (acute psychotic episodes) when drug therapy is discontinued, most often by patients who become unwilling or unable to continue their medication regimen. Drug therapy usually is indicated for at least 1 year after an initial psychotic episode and for at least 5 years, perhaps for life, after multiple episodes. Several studies indicate that low-dose, continuous maintenance therapy is effective in long-term prevention of recurrent psychosis. With wider use of maintenance therapy and the newer, better-

tolerated antipsychotic drugs, patients may experience fewer psychotic episodes and hospitalizations.

Drug Withdrawal: Recognition and Treatment

Antipsychotic drugs can cause symptoms of withdrawal when suddenly or rapidly discontinued. Specific symptoms are related to drug potency, extent of dopaminergic blockade, and anticholinergic effects. Low-potency drugs (e.g., chlorpromazine), for example, have strong anticholinergic effects, and sudden withdrawal can cause cholinergic effects such as diarrhea, drooling, and insomnia. To prevent withdrawal symptoms, drugs should be tapered in dosage and gradually discontinued over several weeks.

Treatment of Extrapyramidal Symptoms

Extrapyramidal effects (i.e., abnormal movements) are more likely to occur with usage of older high-potency antipsychotic drugs than with the newer atypical agents. Such neuromuscular symptoms appear in fewer than half of the patients taking traditional antipsychotic drugs and are better handled by reducing dosage, if this does not cause recurrence of psychotic symptoms. Acute *dystonia* (manifested by severe spasms of muscles of the face, neck, tongue, or back) typically occurs early in treatment and constitutes an emergency. Severe manifestations of acute dystonia include oculogyric crisis (severe involuntary upward rotation of the eyes) and opisthotonus (severe spasm of back muscles, causing head, and heals to bend backward and the body to bow forward). Acute dystonia is treated with intramuscular or intravenous administration of anticholinergic medications such as benztropine or diphenhydramine. *Akathisia* (manifested by motor restlessness and inability to be still) usually occurs in the first few months of treatment with antipsychotics. Switching to a second-generation atypical medication may be indicated to treat akathisia.

Anticholinergics, benzodiazepines, and beta blockers may also be prescribed to control the urge to move. Parkinsonism (manifested by resting tremor, bradykinesia, rigidity, and postural instability) may occur in the first month of therapy with antipsychotics due to dopamine receptor blockade. Centrally acting anticholinergic drugs such as benztropine, diphenhydramine, and amantadine are useful in treating drug-induced parkinsonism. Levodopa and direct dopamine agonists (e.g., bromocriptine) should not be used to treat antipsychotic-induced parkinsonism because these drugs can counteract the effectiveness of the antipsychotic drug and may result in a recurrence of psychotic symptoms. *Tardive dyskinesia* (*choreoathetoid* or twisting worm-like movements of the face and tongue) is an irreversible late extrapyramidal effect of antipsychotic drugs. Often, the slow worm-like tongue movements are the earliest sign that tardive dyskinesia is developing. These abnormal movements of the face and tongue may interfere with eating and speech. Over time, abnormal movements may appear in other parts of the body. There is no curative treatment for tardive dyskinesia; anticholinergic drugs, dosage reduction, or use of an alternative second-generation drug may be helpful. Because prevention is the best treatment for tardive dyskinesia, the nurse should be alert to early signs of this movement disorder.

Perioperative Use

A major concern about giving traditional antipsychotic drugs perioperatively is their potential for adverse interactions with other drugs. For example, the drugs potentiate the effects of general anesthetics and other CNS depressants that are often used before, during, and after surgery. As a result, risks of hypotension and excessive sedation are increased unless doses of other drugs are reduced. If hypotension occurs and requires vasopressor drugs, phenylephrine or norepinephrine should be used rather than epinephrine because antipsychotic drugs inhibit the vasoconstrictive (blood pressure–raising) effects of epinephrine. Guidelines for perioperative use of the newer, atypical drugs have not been developed. Cautious use is indicated because they may also cause hypotension, sedation, and other adverse effects.

Use in Special Populations

Use in Children

Antipsychotic drugs are used mainly for childhood schizophrenia, which is often characterized by more severe symptoms and a more chronic course than adult schizophrenia. Drug therapy is largely empiric, because few studies have been conducted in children and adolescents. Guidelines for the use of antipsychotic drugs have been published by the American Academy of Child and Adolescent Psychiatry. Major recommendations are listed in Box 9-1.

It is not clear which antipsychotics are safest and most effective in children and adolescents. Drug pharmacodynamics and pharmacokinetics are likely to be different in children compared with adults. Pharmacodynamic differences may stem from changes in neurotransmission systems in the brain as children grow. Pharmacokinetic differences may stem from changes in distribution or metabolism of drugs; absorption seems similar to that of adults. In relation to distribution, children usually have a lesser percentage of body fat than adults. Thus, antipsychotic drugs, which are highly lipid soluble, cannot be as readily stored in fat as they are in adults. This often leads to shorter half-lives and the need for more frequent administration. In relation to metabolism, children usually have a faster rate than adults and may therefore require relatively high doses for their size and weight. In relation to excretion, children's renal function is usually similar to that of adults, and most of the drugs are largely inactivated by liver metabolism. Thus, with normal renal function, excretion probably has little effect on blood levels of active drug or a child's response to the drug.

Although the newer drugs are being used, children's dosages have not been established for most of these drugs, and long-term effects are unknown. Risperdal has recently been approved by the FDA as the first atypical antipsychotic drug for the treatment of schizophrenia in adolescents, ages 13 to

---

Box 9-1	Guidelines for the Use of Antipsychotic Drugs by the American Academy of Child and Adolescent Psychiatry

- Give a thorough psychiatric and physical examination before starting drug therapy.
- Choose a medication based on potency, adverse effects, and the client's medication response history, if available. A newer, atypical drug is probably the drug of first choice.
- Give the chosen drug at least 4–6 weeks before evaluating its effectiveness. If an inadequate response is then evident, a new antipsychotic drug should be tried.
- After an adequate response is obtained, continue drug therapy for at least several months. For newly diagnosed children who are symptom free for 6–12 months, it may be feasible to stop the drug for a trial period to reassess condition and drug dosage. In general, the lowest effective dose is recommended.
- Use psychosocial and psychotherapeutic interventions along with antipsychotic drugs.
- Have the physician or another health care provider maintain contact with the child and his or her parents or guardian and monitor responses to the medication. For example, weight charts and calculations of body mass index should be maintained with the atypical drugs because most are associated with weight gain and some are associated with the development of diabetes.
- Conduct more controlled studies of drug effects in children and adolescents.

From the American Academy of Child and Adolescent Psychiatry's Practice Parameter for the Assessment and Treatment of Children and Adolescents with Schizophrenia.

---

17. Quetiapine, although not recommended for use in children, has a **BLACK BOX WARNING** for increased risk of suicidality in children and adolescents with major depressive or other psychiatric disorder, especially in the first months of treatment. Traditional drugs are not usually recommended for children younger than 12 years of age. However, prochlorperazine (Compazine), trifluoperazine (Stelazine), and haloperidol (Haldol) may be used in children aged 2 to 12 years.

Dosage regulation is difficult because children may require lower plasma levels for therapeutic effects, but they also metabolize antipsychotic drugs more rapidly than adults. A conservative approach is to begin with a low dose and increase it gradually (no more than once or twice a week), if necessary. Divided doses may be useful initially, with later conversion to once daily at bedtime. Older adolescents may require doses comparable with those of adults.

Adverse effects may be different in children. For example, extrapyramidal symptoms with conventional drugs are more likely to occur in children than in adults. If they do occur, dosage reduction is more effective in alleviating them than are

| Box 9-2 | Considerations Regarding Use of Antipsychotic Drugs in Older Adults |

Drug Selection

With traditional antipsychotic drugs, haloperidol and fluphenazine may be better tolerated, but they cause a high incidence of extrapyramidal symptoms. With atypical drugs, clozapine is a second-line agent because it produces many adverse effects. Olanzapine, quetiapine, risperidone, ziprasidone, or aripiprazole may be useful, but little information is available about their use in older adults. Ziprasidone should not be used in older adults with cardiac dysrhythmias or severe cardiovascular disease. All second-generation atypical antipsychotics carry a **BLACK BOX WARNING** for elderly patients with dementia-related psychosis due to increased mortality associated with cardiovascular events and infections.

Dosage

When the drugs are required, the recommended starting dosage is 25%–33% of the dosage recommended for younger adults. Dosage should also be increased more gradually, if necessary, and according to clinical response. The basic principle of "start low, go slow" is especially applicable. After symptoms are controlled, dosage should be reduced to the lowest effective level. Some specific drugs and dosage ranges include haloperidol 0.25–1.5 mg qd to qid; clozapine 6.25 mg qd, initially; risperidone 0.5 mg qd, initially; quetiapine, a lower initial dose, slower dose titration, and a lower target dose in older

adults. No reduction of dosage is required based on age for aripiprazole.

As in other populations, antipsychotic drugs should be tapered in dosage and discontinued gradually rather than discontinued abruptly.

Adverse Effects

Older adults are at high risk of adverse effects because metabolism and excretion are usually slower or more likely to be impaired than in younger adults. With traditional antipsychotic drugs, anticholinergic effects (e.g., confusion, memory impairment, hallucinations, urinary retention, constipation, heat stroke) may be especially problematic. In addition, cardiovascular effects (e.g., hypotension, dysrhythmias) may be especially dangerous in older adults, who often have underlying cardiovascular diseases. Tardive dyskinesia, which may occur with long-term use of the typical antipsychotic drugs, may develop more rapidly and at lower drug dosages in older adults than in younger clients. There is also a risk of neuroleptic malignant syndrome, a rare but serious disorder characterized by confusion, dizziness, fever, and rigidity. Other adverse effects include oversedation, dizziness, confusion, and impaired mobility, which may contribute to falls and other injuries unless clients are carefully monitored and safeguarded. With atypical drugs, many of these adverse effects are less likely to occur, especially at the reduced dosages recommended for older adults.

the anticholinergic antiparkinson drugs commonly used in adults. In addition, hypotension is more likely to develop in children. Blood pressure should be closely monitored during initial dosage titration.

Use in Older Adults

Antipsychotic drugs should be used cautiously in older adults. Before they are started, a thorough assessment is necessary, because psychiatric symptoms are often caused by organic disease or other drugs. If this is the case, treating the disease or stopping the offending drug may eliminate the need for an antipsychotic drug. In addition, older adults are more likely to have problems for which the drugs are contraindicated (e.g., severe cardiovascular disease, liver damage, Parkinson's disease) or must be used very cautiously (diabetes mellitus, glaucoma, prostatic hypertrophy, peptic ulcer disease, chronic respiratory disorders).

If antipsychotic drugs are used to control acute agitation in older adults, they should be used in the lowest effective dose for the shortest effective duration. If the drugs are used to treat dementia, they may relieve some symptoms (e.g., agitation, hallucinations, hostility, suspiciousness, uncooperativeness), but they do not improve memory loss and may further impair cognitive functioning. All second-generation or atypical antipsychotics share a **BLACK BOX WARNING** for elderly patients with dementia-related psychosis. For these patients, the second-

generation antipsychotics are associated with increased mortality risk primarily due to cardiovascular disorders or infections.

For older adults in long-term care facilities, there is concern that antipsychotic drugs may be overused to control agitated or disruptive behavior caused by nonpsychotic disorders and for which other treatments are preferable. For example, patients with dementia may become agitated because of environmental or medical problems. Alleviating such causes, when possible, is safer and more effective than administering antipsychotic drugs. Inappropriate use of antipsychotic drugs exposes patients to adverse drug effects and does not resolve underlying problems.

Because of the many implications for patient safety and welfare, federal regulations have been established for the use of antipsychotics in facilities receiving Medicare and Medicaid funds. These regulations include appropriate (e.g., psychotic disorders, delusions, schizophrenia, dementia and delirium that meet certain criteria) and inappropriate (e.g., agitation not thought to indicate potential harm to the resident or others, anxiety, depression, uncooperativeness, wandering) indications. When antipsychotics are required in older adults, several issues should be considered (Box 9-2).

Use in Various Ethnic Groups

Most antipsychotic drugs are metabolized in the liver by enzymes in the cytochrome P450 system. The ability of an individual to produce these enzymes and metabolize drugs efficiently is dependent on genetics, which is influenced by ethnic/racial makeup; however, subgroups within a racial or ethnic category often exhibit genetic variations and therefore different clinical responses to medications. Individuals with strong enzyme activity are known as fast metabolizers, whereas those with slower rates of enzyme activity are slow metabolizers. Fast metabolizers eliminate drugs rapidly and may need a larger-than-usual dose to achieve therapeutic effects, and slow metabolizers eliminate drugs slowly and therefore are at risk of drug accumulation and adverse effects. For example, in fast metabolizers, risperidone has a half-life of 3 hours and its active metabolite has a half-life of 21 hours. In slow metabolizers, risperidone has a half-life of 20 hours and its active metabolite has a half-life of 30 hours. About 6% to 8% of Caucasians are thought to be slow metabolizers. Furthermore, due to the possibility of genetic variation in one enzyme in the cytochrome P450 system and not another, it is possible for a person to be a fast metabolizer of one antipsychotic drug and a slow metabolizer of another. Although much more research is needed, especially with the atypical drugs and with other factors that may be involved, several studies documented differences in antipsychotic drug effects in non-Caucasian populations. Some studies have suggested that atypical antipsychotics may be preferable for treating ethnic minorities because they have fewer extrapyramidal and other adverse effects.

African Americans tend to respond more rapidly; experience a higher incidence of adverse effects, including tardive dyskinesia; and metabolize antipsychotic drugs more slowly than whites. When compared with haloperidol, olanzapine has been associated with fewer extrapyramidal reactions in African Americans.

In addition, compared with Caucasians with psychotic disorders, African Americans may be given higher doses and more frequent injections of long-acting antipsychotic drugs, both of which may increase the incidence and severity of adverse effects.

Asians generally metabolize antipsychotic drugs slowly and therefore have higher plasma drug levels for a given dose than Caucasians. Most studies have been done with haloperidol and in a limited number of Asian subgroups. Thus, it cannot be assumed that all antipsychotic drugs and all people of Asian heritage respond in the same way. To avoid drug toxicity, initial doses should be approximately half the usual doses given to Caucasians and later doses should be titrated according to clinical response and serum drug levels.

A few studies have noted that Hispanics metabolize antipsychotic drugs slowly, requiring lower doses than Caucasians.

Use in Patients With Renal Impairment

Because most antipsychotic drugs are extensively metabolized in the liver and the metabolites are excreted through the kidneys, the drugs should be used cautiously in patients with impaired renal function. Renal function should be monitored periodically during long-term therapy. If renal function test results (e.g., blood urea nitrogen) become abnormal, the drug

may need to be lowered in dosage or discontinued. Because risperidone is metabolized to an active metabolite, recommended dosage reductions and titrations for patients with renal impairment are the same as those for older adults.

With highly sedating antipsychotic drugs, it may be difficult to assess the patient for excessive sedation because drowsiness, lethargy, and mental status changes may also occur with renal impairment.

Use in Patients With Hepatic Impairment

Antipsychotic drugs undergo extensive hepatic metabolism and then elimination in urine. In the presence of liver disease (e.g., cirrhosis, hepatitis), metabolism may be slowed and drug elimination half-lives prolonged, with resultant accumulation and increased risk of adverse effects. Thus, the drugs should be used cautiously in patients with hepatic impairment.

Jaundice has been associated with phenothiazines, usually after 2 to 4 weeks of therapy. It is considered a hypersensitivity reaction, and patients should not be re-exposed to a phenothiazine. If antipsychotic drug therapy is required in these patients, a drug from a different chemical group should be given. Overall, there is no conclusive evidence that pre-existing liver impairment increases the risk of jaundice, and patients with alcoholic cirrhosis have been treated without complications. With risperidone, recommended dosage reductions and titrations for patients with hepatic impairment are the same as those for older adults. With quetiapine, higher plasma levels occur in patients with hepatic impairment and a slower rate of dose titration and a lower target dose are recommended.

Periodic liver function tests (e.g., gamma-glutamyl transpeptidase, alkaline phosphatase, bilirubin) are probably indicated, especially with long-term therapy or the use of clozapine, haloperidol, thiothixene, or a phenothiazine.

Use in Patients With Critical Illness

Antipsychotic drugs are infrequently used in patients who are critically ill. Some patients become acutely agitated or delirious and need sedation to prevent injuring themselves by thrashing about, removing tubes and intravenous (IV) catheters, and so forth. Some physicians prefer a benzodiazepine-type of sedative, whereas others may use haloperidol. Before giving either drug, causes of delirium (e.g., drug intoxication or withdrawal) should be identified and eliminated if possible.

If haloperidol is used, it is usually given IV, by bolus injection. The initial dose is 0.5 to 10 milligrams, depending on the severity of the agitation. It should be injected at a rate no faster than 5 milligrams per minute; the dose can be repeated every 30 to 60 minutes, up to a total amount of 30 milligrams, if necessary. Haloperidol has relatively weak sedative effects and does not cause respiratory depression. However, it can cause hypotension in patients who are volume depleted or receiving antihypertensive drugs. It can also cause cardiac dysrhythmias, including life-threatening torsades de pointes, in patients who are receiving large doses (>50 mg/day) or who have abnormal serum electrolyte levels (e.g., calcium, potassium, magnesium). Patients should be on a cardiac monitor and the ECG should be checked for a prolonged QT interval.

For patients with chronic schizophrenia who are stabilized on an antipsychotic drug when they experience a critical illness, either continuing or stopping the drug may cause difficulties. Continuing the drug may worsen signs and symptoms of the critical illness (e.g., hypotension). Stopping it may cause symptoms of withdrawal.

Little information is available about the newer drugs. If quetiapine is used, very low doses are recommended in older adults, patients with hepatic impairment, debilitated patients, and those predisposed to hypotension. A critically ill patient could have all of these conditions.

Use in Home Care

Chronically mentally ill patients, such as those with schizophrenia, are among the most challenging in the caseload of the home care nurse. Major recurring problems include failure to take antipsychotic medications as prescribed and the concurrent use of alcohol and other drugs of abuse. Either problem is likely to lead to acute psychotic episodes and hospitalizations. The home care nurse must assist and support caregivers' efforts to maintain medications and manage adverse drug effects, other aspects of daily care, and follow-up psychiatric care. In addition, the home care nurse may need to coordinate the efforts of several health and social service agencies or providers.

Applying Your Knowledge 9-3

When making a home visit to Ms. Jones, the nurse observes that the patient is confused, is experiencing muscle twitching, and has a fever. What is the most likely explanation for these symptoms?

Nursing Actions — Antipsychotic Drugs

NURSING ACTIONS	RATIONALE/EXPLANATION
1. Administer accurately	
a. Check doses carefully, especially when starting or stopping an antipsychotic drug, or substituting one for another.	Doses are often changed. When a drug is started, initial doses are usually titrated upward over days or weeks, then reduced for maintenance; when the drug is stopped, doses are gradually reduced; when substituting, dosage of one may be increased while dosage of the other is decreased.
b. With older, typical drugs:	
(1) Give once daily, 1–2 hours before bedtime, when feasible.	Peak sedation occurs in about 2 hours and aids sleep. Also, adverse effects such as dry mouth and hypotension are less bothersome.
(2) When preparing solutions, try to avoid skin contact. If contact is made, wash the area immediately.	These solutions are irritating to the skin and many cause contact dermatitis.
(3) Mix liquid concentrates with at least 60 mL of fruit juice or water just before administration.	To mask the taste. If the patient does not like juice or water, check the package insert for other diluents. Some of the drugs may be mixed with coffee, tea, milk, or carbonated beverages.
(4) For intramuscular injections, give only those preparations labeled for IM use; do not mix with any other drugs in a syringe; change the needle after filling the syringe; inject slowly and deeply into gluteal muscles; and have the patients lie down for 30–60 minutes after the injection.	These drugs are physically incompatible with many other drugs, and a precipitate may occur; parenteral solutions are irritating to body tissues and changing needles helps protect the tissues of the injection tract from unnecessary contact with the drug; injecting into a large muscle mass decreases tissue irritation; lying down helps to prevent orthostatic hypotension.
(5) With parenteral fluphenazine, give the hydrochloride salt IM only; give the decanoate and enanthate salts IM or subcutaneously (Sub-Q).	To decrease tissue irritation
c. With newer, atypical drugs:	
(1) Give aripiprazole and paliperidone once daily, without regard to meals.	Manufacturer's recommendation
(2) Give olanzapine once daily, without regard to meals; with oral disintegrating tablets, peel back foil covering, transfer tablet to dry cup or fingers, and place the tablet into the mouth.	Manufacturer's recommendation. The disintegrating tablet does not require fluid.
(3) Give quetiapine in 2 or 3 daily doses.	
(4) Give risperidone twice daily; mix the oral solution with 3–4 oz of water, coffee, orange juice, or low-fat milk; do not mix with cola drinks or tea.	Manufacturer's recommendation
(5) Give Risperdal Consta deep IM into gluteal muscles.	Manufacturer's recommendation
(6) Give ziprasidone twice daily with food.	Manufacturer's recommendation

(continued on page 170)

Nursing Actions Antipsychotic Drugs (continued)

NURSING ACTIONS	RATIONALE/EXPLANATION
2. Observe for therapeutic effects a. When the drug is given for acute psychotic episodes, observe for decreased agitation, combativeness, and psychomotor activity.	The sedative effects of antipsychotic drugs are exerted within 48–72 hours. Sedation that occurs with treatment of acute psychotic episodes is a therapeutic effect. Sedation that occurs with treatment of nonacute psychotic disorders, or excessive sedation at any time, is an adverse reaction. These therapeutic effects may not be evident for 3–6 weeks after drug therapy is begun.

2. Observe for therapeutic effects

  a. When the drug is given for acute psychotic episodes, observe for decreased agitation, combativeness, and psychomotor activity.

  b. When the drug is given for acute or chronic psychosis, observe for decreased psychotic behavior, such as:

    (1) Decreased auditory and visual hallucinations

    (2) Decreased delusions

    (3) Continued decrease in or absence of agitation, hostility, hyperactivity, and other behavior associated with acute psychosis

    (4) Increased socialization

    (5) Increased ability in self-care activities

    (6) Increased ability to participate in other therapeutic modalities along with drug therapy.

  c. When the drug is given for antiemetic effects, observe for decreased or absent nausea or vomiting.

3. Observe for adverse effects

  a. With phenothiazines and related drugs, observe for:

    (1) Excessive sedation—drowsiness, lethargy, fatigue, slurred speech, impaired mobility, and impaired mental processes

Excessive sedation is most likely to occur during the first few days of treatment of an acute psychotic episode, when large doses are usually given. Psychotic clients also seem sedated because the drug lets them catch up on psychosis-induced sleep deprivation. Sedation is more likely to occur in elderly or debilitated people. Tolerance to the drugs' sedative effects develops, and sedation tends to decrease with continued drug therapy.

    (2) Extrapyramidal reactions

      Akathisia—compulsive, involuntary restlessness and body movements

Akathisia is the most common extrapyramidal reaction, and it may occur about 5–60 days after the start of antipsychotic drug therapy. The motor restlessness may be erroneously interpreted as psychotic agitation necessitating increased drug dosage. This condition can sometimes be controlled by substituting an antipsychotic drug that is less likely to cause extrapyramidal effects or by giving an anticholinergic antiparkinson drug.

      Parkinsonism—loss of muscle movement (akinesia), muscular rigidity and tremors, shuffling gait, postural abnormalities, mask-like facial expression, hypersalivation, and drooling

These symptoms are the same as those occurring with idiopathic Parkinson's disease. They can be controlled with anticholinergic antiparkinson drugs, given along with the antipsychotic drug for about 3 months, then discontinued. This reaction may occur about 5–30 days after antipsychotic drug therapy is begun.

      Dyskinesias (involuntary, rhythmic body movements) and dystonias (uncoordinated, bizarre movements of the neck, face, eyes, tongue, trunk, or extremities)

These are less common extrapyramidal reactions, but they may occur suddenly, approximately 1–5 days after drug therapy is started, and be very frightening to the patients and health care personnel. The movements are caused by muscle spasms and result in exaggerated posture and facial distortions. These symptoms are sometimes misinterpreted as seizures, hysteria, or other disorders. Antiparkinson drugs are given parenterally during acute dystonic reactions, but continued administration is not usually required. These reactions occur most often in younger people.

      Tardive dyskinesia—hyperkinetic movements of the face (sucking and smacking of lips, tongue protrusion, and facial grimaces) and choreiform movements of the trunk and limbs

This syndrome occurs after months or years of high-dose antipsychotic drug therapy. The drugs may mask the symptoms so that the syndrome is more likely to be diagnosed when dosage is decreased or the drug is discontinued for a few days. It occurs gradually and at any age but is more common in older people, women, and people with organic brain disorders. The condition is usually irreversible, and there is no effective treatment. Symptoms are not controlled and may be worsened by antiparkinson drugs. Low dosage and short-term use of antipsychotic drugs help prevent tardive dyskinesia; drug-free periods may aid early detection.

NURSING ACTIONS	RATIONALE/EXPLANATION
(3) Antiadrenergic effects—hypotension, tachycardia, dizziness, faintness, fatigue	Hypotension is potentially one of the most serious adverse reactions to the antipsychotic drugs. It is most likely to occur when the patient assumes an upright position after sitting or lying down (orthostatic or postural hypotension), but it does occur in the recumbent position. It is caused by peripheral vasodilation. Orthostatic hypotension can be assessed by comparing blood pressure readings taken with the patient in supine and standing positions. Tachycardia occurs as a compensatory mechanism in response to hypotension and as an anticholinergic effect in which the normal vagus nerve action of slowing the heart rate is blocked.
(4) Anticholinergic effects—dry mouth, dental caries, blurred vision, constipation, paralytic ileus, urinary retention	These atropine-like effects are common with therapeutic doses and are increased with large doses of phenothiazines.
(5) Respiratory depression—slow, shallow breathing and decreased ability to breathe deeply, cough, and remove secretions from the respiratory tract	This stems from general central nervous system (CNS) depression, which causes drowsiness and decreased movement. It may cause pneumonia or other respiratory problems, especially in people with hypercarbia and chronic lung disease.
(6) Endocrine effects—menstrual irregularities, possibly impotence and decreased libido in the male client, weight gain	These apparently result from drug-induced changes in pituitary and hypothalamic functions.
(7) Hypothermia or hyperthermia	Antipsychotic drugs may impair the temperature-regulating center in the hypothalamus. Hypothermia is more likely to occur. Hyperthermia occurs with high doses and warm environmental temperatures.
(8) Hypersensitivity reactions: *Cholestatic hepatitis*—may begin with fever and influenza-like symptoms followed in approximately 1 week by jaundice	Cholestatic hepatitis results from drug-induced edema of the bile ducts and obstruction of the bile flow. It occurs most often in women and after 2–4 weeks of receiving the drug. It is usually reversible if the drug is discontinued.
Blood dyscrasias—leukopenia, agranulocytosis (fever, sore throat, weakness)	Some degree of leukopenia occurs rather often and does not seem to be serious. Agranulocytosis, on the other hand, occurs rarely but is life threatening. Agranulocytosis is most likely to occur during the first 4–10 weeks of drug therapy, in women, and in older people.
Skin reactions—photosensitivity, dermatoses	Skin pigmentation and discoloration may occur with exposure to sunlight.
(9) Electrocardiogram (ECG) changes, cardiac dysrhythmias	ECG changes may portend dysrhythmias, especially in people with underlying heart disease. Ziprasidone may prolong the QT/QTc interval, an ECG change associated with torsades de pointes, a life-threatening dysrhythmia.
(10) Neuroleptic malignant syndrome—fever (may be confused with heat stroke), muscle rigidity, agitation, confusion, delirium, dyspnea, tachycardia, respiratory failure, acute renal failure	A rare but potentially fatal reaction that may occur hours to months after initial drug use. Symptoms usually develop rapidly over 24–72 hours. Treatment includes stopping the antipsychotic drug, giving supportive care related to fever and other symptoms, and drug therapy (dantrolene, a skeletal muscle relaxant, and amantadine or bromocriptine, dopamine-stimulating drugs).

b. With aripiprazole, observe for:
  (1) CNS effects—anxiety, headache, somnolence, blurred vision, akathisia, tardive dyskinesia, neuroleptic malignant syndrome
  (2) GI effects—nausea, vomiting, constipation, dysphagia
  (3) Cardiovascular effects—orthostatic hypotension
  (4) Other—weight gain, hyperglycemia
c. With clozapine, observe for:
  (1) CNS effects—drowsiness, dizziness, headache, seizures
  (2) Gastrointestinal (GI) effects—nausea, vomiting, constipation
  (3) Cardiovascular effects—hypotension, tachycardia

(continued on page 172)

Nursing Actions Antipsychotic Drugs (continued)

NURSING ACTIONS	RATIONALE/EXPLANATION
(4) Hematologic effects—agranulocytosis	This is the most life-threatening adverse effect of clozapine. Patients' white blood cell (WBC) counts must be checked before starting clozapine, every week during the first six months of therapy, then every 2 weeks as long as WBC counts are satisfactory. WBC levels should be monitored weekly for 4 weeks after the drug is discontinued.

d. With olanzapine, observe for:
  (1) CNS effects—drowsiness, dizziness, akathisia, tardive dyskinesia, neuroleptic malignant syndrome
  (2) GI effects—constipation
  (3) Cardiovascular effects—hypotension, tachycardia
  (4) Other—weight gain, hyperglycemia, diabetes, hyperlipidemia

e. With quetiapine, observe for:
  (1) CNS effects—drowsiness, dizziness, headache, tardive dyskinesia, neuroleptic malignant syndrome
  (2) GI effects—anorexia, nausea, vomiting
  (3) Cardiovascular effects—orthostatic hypotension, tachycardia
  (4) Other—weight gain, hyperglycemia, diabetes

f. With paliperidone, observe for:
  (1) CNS effects — akathisia, extrapyramidal effects, syncope
  (2) GI effects — possible obstruction in patients with known GI narrowing
  (3) Cardiovascular effects — QT prolongation, arrythmias, orthostatic hypotension
  (4) Other — hyperglycemia, hyperprolactinemia

g. With risperidone, observe for:
  (1) CNS effects—agitation, anxiety, drowsiness, dizziness, headache, insomnia, tardive dyskinesia, neuroleptic malignant syndrome
  (2) GI effects—nausea, vomiting, constipation
  (3) Cardiovascular effects—orthostatic hypotension, dysrhythmias
  (4) Other—photosensitivity

h. With ziprasidone, observe for:
  (1) CNS effects—drowsiness, headache, extrapyramidal reactions
  (2) GI effects—nausea, constipation
  (3) Cardiovascular effects—dysrhythmias, hypotension, ECG changes
  (4) Other—fever

4. Observe for drug interactions

NURSING ACTIONS	RATIONALE/EXPLANATION
a. Drugs that *increase* effects of antipsychotic drugs:	
(1) Anticholinergics (e.g., atropine)	Additive anticholinergic effects
(2) Antidepressants, tricyclic	Potentiation of sedative and anticholinergic effects. Additive CNS depression, sedation, orthostatic hypotension, urinary retention, and glaucoma may occur unless dosages are decreased. Apparently these two drug groups inhibit the metabolism of each other, thus prolonging the actions of both groups if they are given concurrently.
(3) Antihistamines	Additive CNS depression and sedation
(4) CNS depressants—alcohol, opioid analgesics, antianxiety agents, sedative-hypnotics	Additive CNS depression. Also, severe hypotension, urinary retention, seizures, severe atropine-like reactions, and other adverse effects may occur, depending on which group of CNS depressant drugs is given.
(5) Propranolol	Additive hypotensive and ECG effects
(6) Thiazide diuretics, such as hydrochlorothiazide	Additive hypotension
(7) Lithium	Acute encephalopathy, including irreversible brain damage and dyskinesias, has been reported.

NURSING ACTIONS	RATIONALE/EXPLANATION
b. Drugs that *decrease* effects of antipsychotic drugs: (1) Antacids	Oral antacids, especially aluminum hydroxide and magnesium trisilicate, may inhibit gastrointestinal absorption of antipsychotic drugs.
(2) Norepinephrine, phenylephrine	Antagonize the hypotensive effects of antipsychotic drugs
c. Drugs that alter effects of antipsychotics by altering hepatic metabolism: (1) Cimetidine, ketaconazole, nefazodone, grapefruit juice, erythromycin, fluoxetine increase the effects of clozapine, quetiapine, and ziprasidone.	CYP3A4 enzyme inhibition slows the metabolism of drugs dependent on this enzyme system.
(2) Carbamazepine, phenytoin, rifampin, and St. John's wort may decrease the effects of clozapine, quetiapine, and ziprasidone.	CYP3A4 enzyme induction speeds the metabolism of drugs dependent on this enzyme system.
(3) Cimetidine, fluvoxamine, and fluoroquinolone antibiotics increase the effects of clozapine, haloperidol, olanzapine, thioridazine, and thiothixene.	CYP1A2 enzyme inhibition slows the metabolism of drugs dependent on this enzyme system.
(4) Carbamazepine and cigarette smoke may decrease effects of clozapine, haloperidol, olanzapine, thioridazine, and thiothixene.	CYP1A2 enzyme induction speeds the metabolism of drugs dependent on this enzyme system.
(5) Fluoxetine, paroxetine, and quinidine may increase the effects of phenothiazines, risperidone, and aripiprazole.	CYP2D6 enzyme inhibition slows the metabolism of drugs dependent on this enzyme system.
(6) Carbamazepine may decrease the effects of phenothiazines, risperidone, and aripirazole.	CYP2D6 enzyme induction speeds the metabolism of drugs dependent on this enzyme system.

Key Concepts

∎ First-generation antipsychotics, or "typical antipsychotics," include the phenothiazines and older nonphenothiazines such as haloperidol and thiothixene.

∎ Second-generation antipsychotics, or "atypical antipsychotics," include newer nonphenothiazine drugs. They are also considered first choice therapy for schizophrenia because they have a more favorable side effect profile, producing fewer extrapyramidal movement disorders.

∎ The mechanism of action of first-generation antipsychotic drugs is blockade of D_2 receptors.

∎ The mechanism of action of second-generation antipsychotics is blockade of dopamine and serotonin receptors.

∎ Antipsychotic drugs are indicated to treat psychosis, including disorders such as schizophrenia and the manic phase of bipolar disorder.

∎ Positive symptoms of schizophrenia respond to drug therapy more readily than negative symptoms. The second-generation "atypical" nonphenothiazine drugs may be slightly more effective in treating negative symptoms of schizophrenia.

∎ Therapeutic effects to antipsychotics may take several weeks to achieve maximum therapeutic effect.

∎ All first-generation antipsychotics are considered equal in ability to relieve symptoms of psychosis; however, they differ in potency and side effects.

∎ Adverse effects occurring more frequently in low-potency drugs as compared with high-potency drugs include anticholinergic effects, antiadrenergic effects (orthostatic hypotension), and CNS depression (sedation).

∎ Adverse effects more common to high-potency drugs as compared with low-potency drugs include early extrapyramidal effects (acute dystonia, akathisia, parkinsonism).

∎ Early extrapyramidal effects are treated by reducing dosage, changing to a second-generation antipsychotic, or use of anticholinergic medications. Akathisia may also be treated with benzodiazepines and beta blockers to reduce the urge to move.

∎ Tardive dyskinesia, a late extrapyramidal effect, may occur with all phenothiazine and typical nonphenothiazine drugs and is generally considered to be irreversible. It may be treated by reducing dosages or switching to a second-generation antipsychotic. Prevention through early detection is key.

∎ Neuroleptic malignant syndrome (a potentially fatal adverse effect characterized by rigidity, severe hyperthermia, agitation, confusion, delirium, dyspnea, tachycardia, respiratory failure, and acute renal failure) is treated with hydration, cooling measures and antipyretics to reduce fever, benzodiazepines to reduce agitation, dantrolene to directly relax muscles, and bromocriptine or amantadine (dopamine agonists) to reduce CNS depression.

Review and Application Exercises

Short Answer Exercises

1. How do antipsychotic drugs act to relieve psychotic symptoms?

2. What are some uses of antipsychotic drugs other than the treatment of schizophrenia?

3. What are major adverse effects of older antipsychotic drugs?

4. When instructing a patient to rise slowly from a sitting or lying position, which adverse effect of an antipsychotic drug is the nurse trying to prevent?

5. In a patient receiving an antipsychotic drug, what appearances or behaviors would lead the nurse to suspect an extrapyramidal reaction?

6. Are antipsychotic drugs likely to be overused and abused? Why or why not?

7. In an older patient taking an antipsychotic drug, what special safety measures are needed? Why?

8. How do clozapine, olanzapine, quetiapine, risperidone, ziprasidone, and aripiprazole compare with older antipsychotic drugs in terms of therapeutic and adverse effects?

9. What can the home care nurse do to prevent acute psychotic episodes and hospitalization of chronically mentally ill patients?

NCLEX-Style Questions

10. For patients taking clozapine, the nurse should assess which of the following laboratory values weekly?
    a. complete blood count (CBC)
    b. hemoglobin and hematocrit
    c. blood urea nitrogen and creatinine
    d. liver enzyme studies

11. Patients taking ziprasidone (Geodon) may have prolonged QT intervals, placing them at risk for which of the following?
    a. atrial fibrillation
    b. torsades de pointes
    c. complete heart block
    d. atrial tachycardia

12. The nurse should administer long-acting injections of antipsychotic drugs in which of the following ways?
    a. intramuscularly into the deltoid muscle
    b. subcutaneously into the abdomen
    c. intramuscularly into the gluteal muscle
    d. intravenously into a large vein

13. When administering atypical antipsychotics, the nurse should be alert to possible
    a. renal failure
    b. liver failure
    c. diabetes mellitus
    d. hypertension

14. In monitoring the status of a patient on a long-term course of a phenothiazine antipsychotic, the nurse needs to be most aware that an adverse effect of long-term use of phenothiazine antipsychotics is the development of which of the following?
    a. glaucoma
    b. tardive dyskinesia
    c. hypertension
    d. diabetes

Selected References

Alexopoulos, G., Streim, J., Carpenter, D., & Docherty, J. (2004). Expert consensus panel for using antipsychotic drugs in older patients. *Journal of Clinical Psychiatry, 65,* 5–99, 100–102.

American Academy of Child and Adolescent Psychiatry, Work Group on Quality Issues. (2001). The practice parameter for the assessment and treatment of children and adolescents with schizophrenia. *Journal of the American Academy of Child & Adolescent Psychiatry, 40,* 4S–23S.

American Psychiatric Association. (2000). *Diagnostic and statistical manual of mental disorders* (4th ed., text revision). Washington, DC: American Psychiatric Association.

American Psychiatric Association, Work Group on Schizophrenia. (2004). *Practice guideline for the treatment of patients with schizophrenia* (2nd ed.). Retrieved April 19, 2007, from www.psych.org

Correll, C., Leucht, S., & Kane, J. (2004). Lower risk for tardive dyskinesia associated with second-generation antipsychotics: A systematic review of 1-year studies. *American Journal of Psychiatry, 161,* 414–425.

Crismon, M. L., & Buckley, P. F. (2005). Schizophrenia. In J. T. DiPiro, R. L. Talbert, G. C. Yee, G. R. Matzke, B. G. Wells, & L. M. Posey (Eds.), *Pharmacotherapy: A pathophysiologic approach* (6th ed., pp. 1109–1233). New York: McGraw-Hill.

Drug facts and comparisons. (Updated monthly). St. Louis, MO: Facts and Comparisons.

Jayaram, M. B., & Stroup, S. (2005). Risperidone versus olanzapine for schizophrenia *Cochrane Database of Systematic Reviews, 2,* CD005237.

Munoz, C., & Hilgenberg, E. (2005). Ethnopharmacology. *American Journal of Nursing, 105,* 40–48.

Rummel, C., Kissling, W., & Leucht, S. (2007). Antidepressants for the negative symptoms of schizophrenia *Cochrane Database of Systematic Reviews, 6,* CD005581.

Antidepressants and Mood Stabilizers

LEARNING OBJECTIVES

After studying this chapter, you will be able to:

1. Describe major features of depression and bipolar disorder.
2. Discuss characteristics of antidepressants in terms of mechanism of action, indications for use, adverse effects, principles of therapy, and nursing process implications.
3. Compare and contrast the different categories of antidepressants: selective serotonin reuptake inhibitors (SSRIs), tricyclic antidepressants (TCAs), mixed serotonin-norepinephrine reuptake inhibitors (SNRIs), monoamine oxidase (MAO) inhibitors, and other atypical antidepressants.
4. Discuss selected characteristics of atypical antidepressants.
5. Describe the use of lithium in bipolar disorder.
6. Describe the use of atypical antipsychotics in the manic phase of bipolar disorder.
7. Discuss interventions to increase safety of lithium therapy.
8. Describe the nursing role in preventing, recognizing, and treating overdoses of antidepressant drugs and lithium.
9. Analyze important factors in using antidepressant drugs and lithium in special populations.

Applying Your Knowledge

While in the hospital, Carl Mehring, age 70, is diagnosed with chronic depression secondary to his chronic heart failure, hypertension, diabetes mellitus, and renal insufficiency. As Mr. Mehring's health has declined, so has his interest in his family, friends, and hobbies. His physician prescribes sertraline 50 mg PO at bedtime.

Introduction

Mood disorders include depression, *dysthymia*, bipolar disorder, and *cyclothymia* (Box 10-1). It is difficult to determine the prevalence of depression in the United States; however, major depressive disorder is relatively common in adults and is increasingly being diagnosed in children and adolescents. The National Comorbidity Survey Replication Study (2003) revealed that 16.2% of study participants had experienced a major depressive disorder in their lifetime. Major depression occurs more often in women than in men and shows familial tendencies with increased risk for depression in individuals with an affected twin or first degree relative. *Postnatal depression* is a major depressive episode occurring after the birth of a child (see Evidence-Based Practice Box 10-1). Major

Box 10-1	Types of Mood Disorders

Depression

Depression, often described as the most common mental illness, is characterized by depressed mood, feelings of sadness, or emotional upset, and it occurs in all age groups. Mild depression occurs in everyone as a normal response to life stresses and losses and usually does not require treatment; severe or major depression is a psychiatric illness and requires treatment. Major depression also is categorized as unipolar, in which people of usually normal moods experience recurrent episodes of depression.

Major Depression

The American Psychiatric Association's *Diagnostic and Statistical Manual of Mental Disorders*, 4th edition, lists criteria for a major depressive episode as a depressed mood plus at least five of the following symptoms for at least 2 weeks:

Loss of energy, fatigue
Indecisiveness
Difficulty thinking and concentrating
Loss of interest in appearance, work, and leisure and sexual activities
Inappropriate feelings of guilt and worthlessness
Loss of appetite and weight loss, or excessive eating and weight gain
Sleep disorders (hypersomnia or insomnia)
Somatic symptoms (e.g., constipation, headache, atypical pain)
Obsession with death, thoughts of suicide
Psychotic symptoms, such as hallucinations and delusions

Dysthymia

Dysthymia involves a chronically depressed mood and at least two other symptoms (e.g., anorexia, overeating, insomnia, hypersomnia, low energy, low self-esteem, poor concentration, feelings of hopelessness) for 2 years. Although the symptoms may cause significant social and work-related impairments, they are not severe enough to meet the criteria for major depression.

Bipolar Disorder

Bipolar disorder involves episodes of depression alternating with episodes of mania. *Mania* is characterized by excessive CNS stimulation with physical and mental hyperactivity (e.g., agitation, constant talking, constant movement, grandiose ideas, impulsiveness, inflated self-esteem, little need for sleep, poor concentration, racing thoughts, short attention span) for at least 1 week. Symptoms are similar to those of acute psychosis or schizophrenia. *Hypomania* involves the same symptoms, but they are less severe, indicate less CNS stimulation and hyperactivity, and last 3 or 4 days.

Cyclothymia

Cyclothymia is a mild type of bipolar disorder that involves periods of hypomania and depression that do not meet the criteria for mania and major depression. Symptoms must be present for at least 2 years. It does not usually require drug therapy.

---

depression is associated with impaired ability to function in usual activities and relationships. The average depressive episode lasts about 5 months, and having one episode is a risk factor for developing another episode.

Bipolar disorder is divided into subtypes that are defined by the presentation of the mood disorder. Bipolar disorder type I is characterized by a episodes of major depression plus mania and occurs equally in men and women. Bipolar disorder type II is characterized by episodes of major depression plus hypomanic episodes and occurs more frequently in women. Bipolar spectrum disorder broadens the definition of bipolar disorder to include conditions such as cyclothymia and dysthymia. The prevalence of bipolar disorders is estimated to range up to 5% of the adult population.

Depression and antidepressant drug therapy are emphasized in this chapter. Bipolar disorder and mood-stabilizing drugs are also discussed.

Etiology of Depression

Despite extensive study and identification of numerous potential contributory factors, the etiology of depression is unclear. It is likely that depression results from interactions among several complex factors. Two of the major theories of depression pathogenesis are described in the following sections.

Monoamine Neurotransmitter Dysfunction

Depression is thought to result from a deficiency of norepinephrine and/or serotonin. Recent studies suggest that deficiencies of dopamine may also play a role in depression. This hypothesis stemmed from studies demonstrating that antidepressant drugs increase the amounts of norepinephrine and/or serotonin in the central nervous system (CNS) synapse by inhibiting their reuptake into the presynaptic neuron. Serotonin received increased attention after the selective serotonin reuptake inhibitor (SSRI) antidepressants were marketed. Serotonin helps regulate several behaviors that are disturbed in depression, such as mood, sleep, appetite, energy level, and cognitive and psychomotor functions.

Emphasis shifted toward receptors because the neurotransmitter view did not explain why the amounts of neurotransmitter increased within hours after single doses of a drug, but relief of depression occurred only after weeks of drug therapy. Researchers identified changes in norepinephrine and serotonin receptors with chronic antidepressant drug therapy. Studies demonstrated that chronic drug administration results in

Evidence-Based Practice

10-1 Antidepressants and Postnatal Depression

Postnatal depression is defined as a depressive episode that meets the DSM-IV criteria for major depression and occurs within 4 weeks of childbirth. Many clinicians extend this time criteria for the diagnosis of postnatal depression up to 6 months after delivery. The Edinburgh Postnatal Depression Scale, which elicits responses to a series of 10 statements about the mother's feelings during the past week, is commonly used by health care providers to screen for postnatal depression. Postnatal depression is common, affecting 12% to 15% of new mothers. For women with a history of postnatal depression the risk of recurrence is 33%, and suicide is the main cause of maternal death within the first year of childbirth. Postnatal depression may resolve without treatment within 3 to 6 months; however, 25% of affected mothers will still be depressed 1 year after delivery. Treatment generally involves the use of psychotherapy and/or antidepressants; however, there is limited information available to guide the selection of the most efficacious antidepressants for treatment of postnatal depression. One random controlled trial evaluated the use of cognitive behavior therapy and fluoxetine and found that both were effective in treating postnatal depression. Sertraline, paroxetine, venlafaxine, and nortriptyline have been reported to be safe for use by nursing mothers of healthy infants; however, fluoxetine is not recommended because it can cause irritability, sleep disturbances, and poor feeding in exposed breast-feeding infants. Third trimester intrauterine exposure to fluoxetine and other SSRIs may result in a *neonatal withdrawal syndrome*, which shares some similarity to a mild serotonin syndrome. Common symptoms include irritability, prolonged crying, respiratory distress, rigidity, and possibly seizures. Care for neonatal withdrawal syndrome is supportive; symptoms usually abate within a few days.

A Cochrane Review investigated the use of antidepressants in women with a past history of postnatal depression and concluded that there was no clear evidence to recommend antidepressant prophylaxis. Given the limited evidence available on the treatment of postnatal depression, further research is needed.

It seems apparent that long-term administration of antidepressant drugs produces complex changes in the sensitivities of both presynaptic and postsynaptic receptor sites.

Overall, there is increasing awareness that balance, integration, and interactions among norepinephrine, serotonin, and possibly other neurotransmission systems (e.g., dopamine, acetylcholine) are probably more important etiologic factors than single neurotransmitter or receptor alterations. For example, animal studies indicate that serotonin is required for optimal functioning of the neurons that produce norepinephrine. Changes in neurons may also play a major role.

Neuroendocrine Factors

In addition to monoamine neurotransmission systems, researchers have identified nonmonoamine systems that influence neurotransmission and are significantly altered in depression. A major nonmonoamine is corticotropin-releasing factor or hormone (CRF or CRH), whose secretion is increased in people with depression. CRF-secreting neurons are widespread in the CNS, and CRF apparently functions as a neurotransmitter and mediator of the endocrine, autonomic, immune, and behavioral responses to stress as well as a releasing factor for corticotropin. Hypothalamic CRF is part of the hypothalamic–pituitary–adrenal (HPA) axis, which becomes hyperactive in depression. As a result, there is increased secretion of CRF by the hypothalamus, adrenocorticotropic hormone (ACTH) by the anterior pituitary, and cortisol by the adrenal cortex. The increased cortisol (part of the normal physiologic response to stress) is thought to decrease the numbers or sensitivity of cortisol receptors (down-regulation) and lead to depression. This view is supported by animal studies indicating that antidepressant drugs restore the ability of cortisol receptors to bind with cortisol. This alteration of cortisol receptors takes about 2 weeks, the approximate time interval required for the drugs to improve symptoms of depression. Extrahypothalamic CRF is also increased in depression. Secretion of both hypothalamic and extrahypothalamic CRF apparently returns to normal with recovery from depression.

Other neuroendocrine factors in patients with depression are thought to include abnormalities in the secretion and function of thyroid and growth hormones.

Additional Factors

Additional factors thought to play a role in the etiology of depression include the immune system, genetic factors, and environmental factors.

Immune cells (e.g., T lymphocytes, B lymphocytes) produce cytokines (e.g., interleukins, interferons, tumor necrosis factor), which affect neurotransmission. Possible mechanisms of cytokine-induced depression include increased CRF and activation of the HPA axis, alteration of monoamine neurotransmitters in several areas of the brain, or cytokines functioning as neurotransmitters and exerting direct effects on brain function.

Genetic factors are considered important mainly because close relatives of a depressed person are more likely to experience depression.

fewer and less sensitive receptors on the postsynaptic membrane. This down-regulation or desensitization of receptors, first noted with beta-adrenergic receptors and later with norepinephrine and serotonin receptors, corresponds with therapeutic drug effects. All known treatments for depression lead to the down-regulation of beta receptors, which coincides with the behavioral changes associated with antidepressant drug therapy.

Alpha$_2$-adrenergic receptors (called autoreceptors), located on presynaptic nerve terminals, may also play a role. When these receptors are stimulated, they inhibit the release of norepinephrine. There is evidence that alpha$_2$ receptors are also down-regulated by antidepressant drugs, thus allowing increased norepinephrine release. With serotonin receptors, available antidepressants may increase the sensitivity of postsynaptic receptors and decrease the sensitivity of presynaptic receptors.

Physiologically, presynaptic receptors regulate the release and reuptake of neurotransmitters; postsynaptic receptors participate in the transmission of nerve impulses to target tissues.

Environmental factors include stressful life events, which apparently change brain structure and function and contribute to the development of depression in some people. Changes have been identified in CRF, the HPA axis, and the noradrenergic neurotransmission system, all of which are activated as part of the stress response. These changes are thought to cause a hypersensitive or exaggerated response to later stressful events, including mild stress or daily life events. Most studies have involved early life trauma such as physical or sexual abuse in childhood.

Etiology of Bipolar Disorder

Like depression, *mania* and *hypomania* have historically been associated with abnormal functioning of neurotransmitters or receptors, such as a relative excess of excitatory neurotransmitters (e.g., norepinephrine) or a relative deficiency of inhibitory neurotransmitters (e.g., gamma-aminobutyric acid [GABA]). Another more recent proposed etiology for bipolar disorder is alteration in neuronal growth and survival in areas of the brain (e.g., subgenual precortex, hippocampus) involved with mood and memory. Mood-stabilizing drugs such as lithium have been shown to stimulate neuronal growth and reduce brain atrophy in individuals with long-standing mood disorders. Secondary causes of manic and hypomanic behavior include drugs that stimulate the CNS, CNS diseases and infections, and electrolyte or endocrine disorders.

General Characteristics of Antidepressant Drugs

Drugs used in the pharmacologic management of depressive disorders are derived from several chemical groups. Older antidepressants include the tricyclic antidepressants (TCAs) and the *monoamine oxidase (MAO) inhibitors*. Newer drugs include the *selective serotonin reuptake inhibitors (SSRIs)*, the mixed serotonin-norepinephrine reuptake inhibitors (SNRIs), and several atypical antidepressant drugs that differ from TCAs, MAO inhibitors, SSRIs, and SNRIs. General characteristics of antidepressants include the following:

- All are effective in relieving depression, but they differ in their adverse effects.

- All must be taken for 2 to 4 weeks before depressive symptoms improve.

- They are given orally, absorbed from the small bowel, enter the portal circulation, and circulate through the liver, where they undergo extensive first-pass metabolism before reaching the systemic circulation.

- They are metabolized by the cytochrome P450 enzymes in the liver. Many antidepressants and other drugs are metabolized by the 2D6 or 3A4 subgroup of the enzymes. Thus, antidepressants may interact with each other and with a wide variety of drugs that are normally metabolized by the same subgroups of enzymes.

Mechanisms of Action

Although the actions of antidepressant drugs are still being studied in relation to newer information about brain function and the etiology of mood disorders, these drugs apparently normalize abnormal neurotransmission systems in the brain by altering the amounts of neurotransmitters and the number or sensitivity of receptors. They may also modify interactions among neurotransmission systems and affect endocrine function (e.g., the HPA axis and cortisol activity).

After neurotransmitters are released from presynaptic nerve endings, the molecules that are not bound to receptors are normally inactivated by reuptake into the presynaptic nerve fibers that released them or metabolized by MAO. Most antidepressants prevent the reuptake of multiple neurotransmitters; SSRIs selectively inhibit the reuptake of serotonin, and MAO inhibitors prevent the metabolism of neurotransmitter molecules. These mechanisms thereby increase the amount of neurotransmitter available to bind to receptors.

With chronic drug administration, receptors adapt to the presence of increased neurotransmitter by decreasing their number or sensitivity to the neurotransmitter. More specifically, norepinephrine receptors, especially postsynaptic beta receptors and presynaptic alpha$_2$ receptors, are down-regulated. The serotonin receptor 5-HT$_2$, a postsynaptic receptor, and cortisol (glucocorticoid) receptors may also be down-regulated.

Thus, antidepressant effects are attributed to changes in receptors rather than changes in neurotransmitters. Although some of the drugs act more selectively on one neurotransmission system than another initially, this selectivity seems to be lost with chronic administration.

With lithium, the exact mechanism of action is unknown. However, it is known to affect the synthesis, release, and reuptake of several neurotransmitters in the brain, including acetylcholine, dopamine, GABA, and norepinephrine. It also stabilizes postsynaptic receptor sensitivity to neurotransmitters, probably by competing with calcium, magnesium, potassium, and sodium ions for binding sites. Long-term administration of lithium may also stimulate neuronal growth, exerting a neuroprotective effect on areas of the brain involved with mood.

Indications for Use

Antidepressant therapy may be indicated if depressive symptoms persist at least 2 weeks, impair social relationships or work performance, and occur independently of life events. In addition, antidepressants are increasingly being used for treatment of anxiety disorders. TCAs may be used in children and adolescents in the management of enuresis (bedwetting or involuntary urination resulting from a physical or psychological disorder). In this setting, TCAs may be given after physical causes (e.g., urethral irritation, excessive intake of fluids) have been ruled out. TCAs and duloxetine (an SNRI) are also commonly used in the treatment of neuropathic pain. MAO inhibitors are considered third-line drugs, largely because of their potential for serious interactions with certain foods and other drugs.

Contraindications to Use

Antidepressants are contraindicated or must be used with caution in patients with acute schizophrenia; mixed mania and depression; suicidal tendencies; severe renal, hepatic, or cardiovascular disease; narrow-angle glaucoma; and seizure disorders. A **BLACK BOX WARNING** alerts health care providers to the increased risk of suicidal ideation in children, adolescents, and young adults 18 to 24 years of age when taking antidepressant medications. Health care providers should be aware that worsening symptoms could be a result of underlying disease or drug therapy. Symptoms of concern include anxiety, agitation, panic attacks, insomnia, irritability, hostility, impulsivity, akathisia, hypomania, and mania. The presence of these symptoms, especially if new (i.e., not part of the patient's presenting symptoms), severe, or abrupt in onset, should prompt evaluation of drug therapy and possible discontinuation of medications. If the decision is made to discontinue antidepressant therapy, it is important that medications be tapered rather than abruptly discontinued.

 Applying Your Knowledge 10-1

How Can You Avoid This Medication Error?

Mr. Mehring is talking with his pastor when you arrive to administer his medication. He asks you to just leave the medication and he will take it when he finishes his visit. You leave the medication with Mr. Mehring and chart it as given.

Types of Antidepressants and Individual Drugs

Additional characteristics of antidepressants and lithium are described in the following sections. Names, indications for use, and dosage ranges of individual drugs are listed in Table 10-1.

Table 10-1	**Drugs at a Glance:** Antidepressant Agents	
GENERIC/TRADE NAME	**CLINICAL INDICATIONS**	**ROUTES AND DOSAGE RANGES**
Tricyclic Antidepressants **Amitriptyline** (Elavil)	Depression	PO 50–100 mg once daily at bedtime, gradually increased to 150 mg daily if necessary; IM 80–120 mg daily in 4 divided doses *Adolescents and older adults:* PO 10 mg 3 times daily and 20 mg at bedtime
Clomipramine (Anafranil)	Obsessive-compulsive disorder (OCD)	PO 25 mg daily, increased to 100 mg daily by end of 2 wk, in divided doses, with meals. Give maintenance dose in a single dose at bedtime. Maximum dose, 250 mg daily. *Children and adolescents:* PO 25 mg daily, increased to 3 mg/kg or 100 mg, whichever is smaller, over 2 wk. Give maintenance dose in a single dose at bedtime. Maximum dose, 3 mg/kg or 200 mg, whichever is smaller.
Desipramine (Norpramin)	Depression	PO 100–200 mg daily in divided doses or as a single daily dose. Give maintenance dose once daily. Maximum dose, 300 mg/d. *Adolescents and older adults:* PO 25–100 mg daily in divided doses or as a single daily dose. Maximum dose, 150 mg/d.
Doxepin (Sinequan)	Depression	PO 75–150 mg daily, in divided doses or a single dose at bedtime. Maximum dose, 300 mg/d.
P Imipramine (Tofranil)	Depression Childhood enuresis	PO 75 mg daily in 3 divided doses, gradually increased to 200 mg daily if necessary. Maintenance dose, 75–150 mg daily. *Adolescents and older adults:* PO 30–40 mg daily in divided doses, increased to 100 mg daily if necessary. *Children >6 y:* Enuresis, PO 25–50 mg 1 h before bedtime
Nortriptyline (Aventyl, Pamelor)	Depression	PO 25 mg 3 or 4 times daily or in a single dose (75–100 mg) at bedtime. Maximum dose, 150 mg/d. *Adolescents and older adults:* 30–50 mg/d, in divided doses or a single dose once daily.

(continued on page 180)

Table 10-1 Drugs at a Glance: Antidepressant Agents (continued)

GENERIC/TRADE NAME	CLINICAL INDICATIONS	ROUTES AND DOSAGE RANGES
Selective Serotonin Reuptake Inhibitors (SSRIs)		
Citalopram (Celexa)	Depression	PO 20 mg once daily, morning or evening, increased to 40 mg daily in 1 wk, if necessary *Elderly/hepatic impairment:* PO 20 mg daily
Escitalopram (Lexapro)	Depression Generalized anxiety disorder (GAD)	PO 10 mg once daily. May increase to maximum dose of 20 mg after minimum of 1 wk of therapy
Fluoxetine (Prozac, Prozac Weekly, Sarafem)	Depression OCD Bulimia nervosa Premenstrual dysphoric disorder (Sarafem)	PO 20 mg once daily in the morning, increased after several weeks if necessary. Give doses larger than 20 mg once in the morning or in 2 divided doses, morning and noon; maximum daily dose 80 mg. Prozac Weekly (delayed-release capsules), PO 90 mg once each wk, starting 7 days after the last 20-mg dose *Children and adolescents 8–17 y for depression:* PO 10 mg/d. May increase to 20 mg/d if necessary.
Paroxetine (Paxil, Paxil CR)	Depression GAD OCD Panic disorder Social anxiety disorder	PO 20 mg once daily in the morning, increased at 1 wk or longer intervals, if necessary; usual range, 20–50 mg/d; maximum dose, 60 mg/d. Controlled-release (CR) tablets, PO 25 mg once daily in the morning, increased up to 62.5 mg/d if necessary *Elderly or debilitated adults:* PO 10 mg once daily, increased if necessary. Maximum dose, 40 mg. *Severe renal or hepatic impairment:* Same as for older adults
Sertraline (Zoloft)	Depression OCD Panic disorder Post-traumatic stress disorder (PTSD)	Depression, OCD, PO 50 mg once daily morning or evening, increased at 1-wk or longer intervals to a maximum daily dose of 200 mg Panic, PTSD, PO 25 mg once daily, increased after 1 wk to 50 mg once daily *Children:* OCD, 6–12 y, 25 mg once daily; 13–17 y, 50 mg once daily
Serotonin-Norepinephrine Reuptake Inhibitors (SNRIs)		
Duloxetine (Cymbalta)	Depression GAD	PO 30–60 mg/d, increase by 30-mg increments every week up to a maximum daily dose of 120 mg/d. Contraindicated for hepatic impairment, lower doses for renal impairment.
Venlafaxine (Effexor, Effexor XR)	Depression GAD (XR form)	Immediate-release tablets, PO initially 75 mg/d in 2 or 3 divided doses with food. Increase by 75 mg/d (4 d or longer between increments) up to 225 mg/d if necessary. Extended-release (XR) capsules, PO initially 37.5 or 75 mg/d in a single dose morning or evening. Increase by 75 mg/d (4 d or longer between increments) up to 225 mg/d if necessary. *Hepatic or renal impairment:* Reduce dose by 50% and increase very slowly.
Monoamine Oxidase (MAO) Inhibitors		
Phenelzine (Nardil)	Depression	PO 15 mg 3 times daily
Tranylcypromine (Parnate)	Depression	PO 30 mg daily in divided doses
Other Atypical Antidepressants		
Bupropion (Wellbutrin, Wellbutrin SR, Wellbutrin XL, Zyban)	Depression (Wellbutrin) Smoking cessation (Zyban)	Immediate-release tablets, PO 100 mg twice daily, increased to 100 mg 3 times daily (at least 6 h apart) if necessary. Maximum single dose, 150 mg.

GENERIC/TRADE NAME	CLINICAL INDICATIONS	ROUTES AND DOSAGE RANGES
		Sustained-release (SR) tablets, PO 150 mg once daily in the morning, increased to 150 mg twice daily (at least 8 h apart). Maximum single dose, 150 mg.
		Wellbutrin XL: PO 150 mg once daily in the morning. May increase to target dose of 300 mg on or after fourth day of therapy. Maximum single dose, 450 mg.
Mirtazapine (Remeron)	Depression	PO 15 mg/d
Trazodone (Desyrel)	Depression	PO 100–300 mg daily, increased to a maximum dose of 600 mg daily if necessary
Mood-Stabilizing Agents		
Lithium carbonate (Eskalith, Lithobid)	Bipolar disorder (mania)	PO 600 mg 3 times daily or 900 mg twice daily (slow-release forms)
		Maintenance dose, PO 300 mg 3 or 4 times daily to maintain a serum lithium level of 0.6–1.2 mEq/L
Aripiprazole (Abilify)	Bipolar disorder (acute mania)	PO 30 mg/d
Olanzapine (Zyprexa)	Bipolar disorder (acute mania)	PO 10–15 mg/d initially; may increase by 5 mg qd PRN to maximum dose of 20 mg/d.
		Elderly or debilitated adults: PO 5 mg/d
Quetiapine (Seroquel)	Bipolar disorder (acute mania)	PO 50 mg twice daily on day 1
		PO 100 mg twice daily on day 2
		PO 150 mg twice daily on day 3
		PO 200 mg twice daily on day 4
		If needed, may continue to increase maximum dose 800 mg/d.
	Bipolar disorder (depressive episodes)	PO 50 mg at bedtime. May increase by 50 mg/d to maximum dose 600 mg at bedtime.
Olanzapine/fluoxetine (Symbyax)	Bipolar disorder (depressive episodes)	PO 6/25 mg at bedtime. May increase to maximum 18/75 mg/d.
Risperidone (Risperdal)	Bipolar disorder (acute mania)	PO 2–3 mg/d initially. May increase 1 mg/d to maximum dose of 6 mg/d.
		Elderly or debilitated adults: PO 0.5mg/d, may increase by 0.5 mg/d to 3 mg/d, then may increase by 1 mg/wk to maximum dose of 6 mg/d.
		Adolescents 10–17 y: 0.5 mg/d initially. Titrate 0.5–1 daily to a target dose of 2.5 mg/d. Dosage range 0.5–6 mg/d.
Ziprasidone (Goeden)	Bipolar disorder (acute mania)	PO 40 mg twice daily. May increase to maximum dose 80 mg twice daily.
Carbamazepine (Tegretol)	Bipolar disorder	PO 100–200 mg initially. May increase to maximum 1600 mg/d.
Lamotrigine (Lamictal)	Bipolar disorder (maintenance)	PO 50 mg/d initially; may increase to maximum of 200 mg/d.
Valproic acid (Depakene)	Bipolar disorder (acute mania)	PO 250 mg/d; may increase rapidly to lowest effective dose. Maximum dose 60 mg/kg/d.

Tricyclic Antidepressants

TCAs, of which **P** imipramine is the prototype, are similar drugs that produce a high incidence of adverse effects such as sedation, orthostatic hypotension, cardiac dysrhythmias, anti-cholinergic effects (e.g., blurred vision, dry mouth, constipation, urinary retention), and weight gain. They are well absorbed after oral administration, but first-pass metabolism by the liver results in blood level variations of 10- to 30-fold among people given identical doses. After they are absorbed, these drugs are widely distributed in body tissues and metabolized in the liver by CYP2D6 enzymes in the liver to active and inactive metabolites. Because of adverse effects on the heart, especially in overdose, baseline and follow-up electrocardiograms (ECGs) are recommended for all patients. **Amitriptyline** (Elavil) is a commonly used TCA.

Selective Serotonin Reuptake Inhibitors

SSRIs, of which P **fluoxetine** (Prozac, Sarafem) is the prototype, produce fewer serious adverse effects than the TCAs. They are well absorbed with oral administration, undergo extensive first-pass metabolism in the liver, are highly protein bound (56%–95%), and have a half-life of 24 to 72 hours, which may lead to accumulation with chronic administration. Fluoxetine also forms an active metabolite with a half-life of 7 to 9 days. Thus, steady-state blood levels are achieved slowly, over several weeks, and drug effects decrease slowly (over 2 to 3 months) when fluoxetine is discontinued. Sertraline (Zoloft) and citalopram (Celexa) also have active metabolites, but fluoxetine and paroxetine (Paxil) are more likely to accumulate. Escitalopram (Lexapro), paroxetine, and sertraline reach steady-state concentrations in 1 to 2 weeks. SSRIs are usually given once daily.

Because SSRIs are highly bound to plasma proteins, they compete with endogenous compounds and other medications for binding sites, resulting in drug interactions. Because the drugs are highly lipid soluble, they accumulate in the CNS and other adipose-rich tissue. Metabolism of most SSRIs is accomplished by CYP2D6 enzymes, with the exception of citalopram and escitalopram, which are metabolized by CYP3A4 and CYP2C19.

Adverse effects include a high incidence of gastrointestinal (GI) symptoms (e.g., nausea, diarrhea, and weight loss) and sexual dysfunction (e.g., delayed ejaculation in men, impaired orgasmic ability in women). Most SSRIs also cause some degree of CNS stimulation (e.g., anxiety, nervousness, insomnia), which is most prominent with fluoxetine. Because serotonin release from platelets is essential for hemostasis and psychotropic drugs interfere with serotonin reuptake, these agents are associated with increased risk of GI bleeding. Concomitant use of nonsteroidal anti-inflammatory drugs (NSAIDS), aspirin, or warfarin increases this risk.

Serotonin syndrome, a serious and sometimes fatal reaction characterized by hypertensive crisis, hyperpyrexia, extreme agitation progressing to delirium and coma, muscle rigidity, and seizures, may occur due to combined therapy with an SSRI and an MAO inhibitor or other drugs that potentiate serotonin neurotransmission. An SSRI or SNRI and an MAO inhibitor should not be given concurrently or within 2 weeks of each other. In most cases, if a patient taking an SSRI is to be transferred to an MAO inhibitor, the SSRI should be discontinued at least 14 days before starting the MAO inhibitor. However, due to the prolonged half-life, fluoxetine should be discontinued at least 5 weeks before starting an MAO inhibitor.

On his return visit to the physician 2 weeks later, Mr. Mehring's wife complains that she sees no improvement in her husband's mood and that he is taking too much medication. How would you respond?

Mixed Serotonin-Norepinephrine Reuptake Inhibitors (SNRIs)

Venlafaxine (Effexor) and **duloxetine** (Cymbalta) inhibit the neuronal uptake of serotonin and norepinephrine, increasing the activity of these neurotransmitters in the brain. Venlafaxine is also a weak inhibitor of dopamine neuronal reuptake. These drugs are similar to SSRIs in terms of therapeutic effects but exhibit more anticholinergic, CNS sedation, and cardiac conduction abnormalities than most of the SSRIs.

Venlafaxine crosses the placenta and may enter breast milk. It is metabolized in the liver and excreted in urine. It is contraindicated during pregnancy, and women should use effective birth control methods while taking this drug. Adverse effects include CNS (anxiety, dizziness, dreams, insomnia, nervousness, somnolence, tremors), GI (anorexia, nausea, vomiting, constipation, diarrhea), cardiovascular (hypertension, tachycardia, vasodilation), genitourinary (abnormal ejaculation, impotence, urinary frequency), and dermatologic (sweating, rash, pruritus) symptoms. Venlafaxine does not interact with drugs metabolized by the cytochrome P450 system, but it should not be taken concurrently with MAO inhibitors because of increased serum levels and risks of serotonin syndrome. If a patient taking venlafaxine is to be transferred to an MAO inhibitor, the venlafaxine should be discontinued at least 7 days before starting the MAO inhibitor. If a patient taking an MAO inhibitor is to be transferred to venlafaxine, the MAO inhibitor should be discontinued at least 14 days before starting venlafaxine.

Duloxetine (Cymbalta) is highly protein bound, extensively metabolized by CYP 2D6 and CYP1A2 enzymes in the liver, and excreted by the kidneys. It is not recommended for use in patients with severe renal or any degree of liver impairment. In addition to sharing similar adverse effects as venlafaxine, duloxetine is also associated with hepatic toxicity, leading to increased liver transaminases and bilirubin. Use of alcohol increases the risk of liver damage, and duloxetine is not recommended for patients with significant alcohol use. Duloxetine, like venlafaxine, should not be given concurrently with an MAO inhibitor. Allow at least 5 days after duloxetine is discontinued before switching to therapy with a MAO inhibitor and allow at least 14 days after discontinuation of an MAO inhibitor before initiating treatment with duloxetine.

Duloxetine crosses the placenta and exposed infants, especially in the third trimester, have demonstrated symptoms consistent with drug discontinuation syndrome and serotonin syndrome, requiring prolonged hospitalization. The drug may be excreted in the breast milk as well. During pregnancy, duloxetine should only be used if benefit outweighs risk, and tapering of the medication during the third trimester may be appropriate.

Monoamine Oxidase Inhibitors

MAO inhibitors are rarely used in clinical practice today, mainly because they may interact with some foods and drugs to produce severe hypertension and possible heart attack or stroke. Foods that interact contain tyramine, a monoamine precursor of norepinephrine. Normally, tyramine is deactivated in the GI tract and liver so that large amounts do not reach the systemic circulation. When deactivation is blocked by MAO inhibitors, tyramine is absorbed systemically and transported to adrenergic nerve terminals, where it causes a sudden release of large amounts of norepinephrine. Foods that should be avoided include aged cheeses and meats, concentrated yeast extracts, sauerkraut, and fava beans. Drugs that should be avoided include CNS stimulants (e.g., amphetamines, cocaine), adrenergics (e.g., pseudoephedrine), antidepressants (SSRIs, SNRIs), buspirone, levodopa, and meperidine.

Atypical Antidepressants

Bupropion (Wellbutrin, Zyban) inhibits the reuptake of dopamine, norepinephrine, and serotonin. It was marketed with warnings related to seizure activity. Seizures are most likely to occur with doses above 450 milligrams per day and in patients known to have a seizure disorder.

After an oral dose, peak plasma levels are reached in about 2 hours. The average drug half-life is about 14 hours. The drug is metabolized in the liver by CYP2B6 among other enzymes and excreted primarily in the urine. Several metabolites are pharmacologically active. Dosage should be reduced in patients with impaired hepatic or renal function. Acute episodes of depression usually require several months of drug therapy. Bupropion is also effective as a long-term smoking cessation aid.

Bupropion has few adverse effects on cardiac function and does not cause orthostatic hypotension or sexual dysfunction. However, in addition to seizures, the drug has CNS stimulant effects (agitation, anxiety, excitement, increased motor activity, insomnia, restlessness) that may require a sedative during the first few days of administration. These effects may increase the risk of abuse. Other common adverse effects include dry mouth, headache, nausea and vomiting, and constipation.

Mirtazapine (Remeron) blocks presynaptic alpha$_2$-adrenergic receptors (which increase the release of norepinephrine), serotonin receptors, and histamine H$_1$ receptors. Consequently, the drug decreases anxiety, agitation, insomnia, and migraine headaches as well as depression.

Mirtazapine is well absorbed after oral administration, and peak plasma levels occur within 2 hours after an oral dose. It is metabolized in the liver, mainly to inactive metabolites. Common adverse effects include drowsiness (with accompanying cognitive and motor impairment), increased appetite, weight gain, dizziness, dry mouth, and constipation. It does not cause sexual dysfunction.

Mirtazapine should not be taken concurrently with other CNS depressants (e.g., alcohol, benzodiazepine antianxiety or hypnotic agents) because of additive sedation. In addition, it should not be taken concurrently with an MAO inhibitor or for 14 days after an MAO inhibitor is stopped. An MAO inhibitor should not be started until at least 14 days after mirtazapine is stopped.

Trazodone (Desyrel) is used more often for sedation and sleep than for depression because high doses (>300 mg/day) are required for antidepressant effects, and these amounts cause excessive sedation in many patients. The drug is often given concurrently with a stimulating antidepressant, such as bupropion, fluoxetine, sertraline, or venlafaxine.

Trazodone is well absorbed with oral administration, and peak plasma concentrations are obtained within 30 minutes to 2 hours. It is metabolized by CYP3A4 in the liver and excreted primarily by the kidneys. Adverse effects include sedation, dizziness, edema, cardiac dysrhythmias, and priapism (prolonged and painful penile erection).

Mood-Stabilizing Agents

Lithium carbonate (Eskalith) is a naturally occurring metallic salt that is used in patients with bipolar disorder, mainly to treat and prevent manic episodes. It is well absorbed after oral administration, with peak serum levels in 1 to 3 hours after a dose and steady-state concentrations in 5 to 7 days. Serum lithium concentrations should be monitored frequently because they vary widely among patients taking similar doses and because of the narrow range between therapeutic and toxic levels.

Lithium is not metabolized by the body; it is entirely excreted by the kidneys, so adequate renal function is a prerequisite for lithium therapy. Approximately 80% of a lithium dose is reabsorbed in the proximal renal tubules. The amount of reabsorption depends on the concentration of sodium in the proximal renal tubules. A sodium deficit causes more lithium to be reabsorbed and increases the risk of lithium toxicity. A sodium excess causes more lithium to be excreted (i.e., lithium diuresis) and may lower serum lithium levels to nontherapeutic ranges.

Before lithium therapy is begun, baseline studies of renal, cardiac, and thyroid status should be obtained because adverse drug effects involve these organ systems. Baseline electrolyte studies are also necessary.

Anticonvulsants (see Chap. 11) are also used as mood-stabilizing agents in bipolar disorder because they modify nerve cell function. Carbamazepine (Tegretol), lamotrigine (Lamictal), and valproate (Depakene) are currently approved by the Food and Drug Administration (FDA) for treating bipolar disorder. Other anticonvulsants (e.g., gabapentin, topiramate, oxcarbazepine) are being used and studied regarding their effects in bipolar disorder but are not approved by the FDA for this purpose.

Both typical and atypical **antipsychotics** (see Chap. 9) are used to decrease dopamine activity in the treatment of the mania phase of bipolar disorder. Both have similar efficacy in reducing acute mania, psychomotor agitation, and psychosis; however, the atypical antipsychotics are associated with fewer adverse effects. Currently, aripiprazole, quetiapine, risperidone, olanzapine (monotherapy or combination with fluoxetine), and ziprasidone are approved by the FDA for this indication.

 ## Herbal Supplement

St. John's wort (*Hypericum perforatum*) is an herb that is widely self-prescribed for depression. Several studies, most of which used about 900 milligrams per day of a standardized extract, indicate its usefulness in mild to moderate depression, with fewer adverse effects than antidepressant drugs. A 3-year, multicenter study by the National Institutes of Health concluded that the herb is not effective in major depression.

Antidepressant effects are attributed mainly to hypericin, although several other active components have also been identified. The mechanism of action is unknown, but the herb is thought to act similarly to antidepressant drugs. Some herbalists refer to St. John's wort as "natural Prozac."

Adverse effects, which are usually infrequent and mild, include constipation, dizziness, dry mouth, fatigue, GI distress, nausea, photosensitivity, restlessness, skin rash, and sleep disturbances. These symptoms are relieved by stopping the herb.

Drug interactions may be extensive. St. John's wort may reduce effectiveness of cyclosporine, HIV protease inhibitors, oral contraceptives, digoxin, warfarin, and theophylline through interactions mediated by CYP3A4, CYP2C9, CYP1A2, and CYP2C19 enzyme systems as well as other mechanisms. St. John's wort should not be combined with alcohol, antidepressant drugs (e.g., MAO inhibitors, SSRIs, TCAs), nasal decongestants or other over-the-counter cold and flu medications, bronchodilators, opioid analgesics, or amino acid supplements containing phenylalanine and tyrosine. All of these interactions may result in hypertension, possibly severe.

Most authorities agree that there is insufficient evidence to support the use of St. John's wort for mild to moderate depression and that more studies are needed to confirm the safety and effectiveness of this herb. Most of the previous studies were considered flawed.

Overall, both consumers and health care professionals seem to underestimate the risks of taking this herbal supplement. For patients who report use of St. John's wort, teach them to purchase products from reputable sources because the amount and type of herbal content may vary among manufacturers; to avoid taking antidepressant drugs, alcohol, and cold and flu medications while taking St. John's wort; to avoid the herb during pregnancy because effects are unknown; and to use sunscreen lotions and clothing to protect themselves from sun exposure.

Nursing Process

Assessment

Assess the patient's condition in relation to depressive disorders.

- Identify patients at risk for current or potential depression. Areas to assess include health status, family and social relationship, and work status. Severe or prolonged illness, impaired interpersonal relationships, inability to work, and job dissatisfaction may precipitate depression. Depression also occurs without an identifiable cause.

- Observe for signs and symptoms of depression. Clinical manifestations are nonspecific and vary in severity. For example, fatigue and insomnia may be caused by a variety of disorders and range from mild to severe. When symptoms are present, try to determine their frequency, duration, and severity.

- When a patient appears depressed or has a history of depression, assess for suicidal thoughts and behaviors. Statements indicating a detailed plan, accompanied by the intent, ability, and method for carrying out the plan, place the patient at high risk for suicide.

- Identify the patient's usual coping mechanisms for stressful situations. Coping mechanisms vary widely, and behavior that may be helpful to one patient may not be helpful to another. For example, one person may prefer being alone or having decreased contact with family and friends, whereas another may find increased contact desirable.

Nursing Diagnoses

- Dysfunctional Grieving related to loss (of health, ability to perform usual tasks, job, significant other, and so forth)
- Self-Care Deficit related to fatigue and self-esteem disturbance with depression or sedation with antidepressant drugs
- Sleep Pattern Disturbance related to mood disorder or drug therapy
- Risk for Injury related to adverse drug effects
- Risk for Violence: Self-Directed or Directed at Others
- Deficient Knowledge: Effects and appropriate use of antidepressant and mood-stabilizing drugs

Planning/Goals

The patient will

- Experience improvement of mood and depressive state
- Receive or self-administer the drugs correctly
- Be kept safe while sedated during therapy with the TCAs and related drugs
- Be assessed regularly for suicidal tendencies. If present, caretakers will implement safety measures.

- Be cared for by staff in areas of nutrition, hygiene, exercise, and social interactions when unable to provide self-care
- Resume self-care and other usual activities
- Avoid preventable adverse drug effects

Interventions

Use measures to prevent or decrease the severity of depression. General measures include supportive psychotherapy and reduction of environmental stress. Specific measures include the following:

- Support the patient's usual mechanisms for handling stressful situations, when feasible. Helpful actions may involve relieving pain or insomnia, scheduling rest periods, and increasing or decreasing socialization.
- Call the patient by name, encourage self-care activities, allow him or her to participate in setting goals and making decisions, and praise efforts to accomplish tasks. These actions promote a positive self-image.
- When signs and symptoms of depression are observed, initiate treatment before depression becomes severe. Institute suicide precautions for patients at risk. These usually involve close observation, often on a one-to-one basis, and removal of potential weapons from the environment. For patients hospitalized on medical-surgical units, transfer to a psychiatric unit may be needed.
- Provide patient teaching regarding drug therapy (see accompanying display).

Evaluation

- Observe for behaviors indicating lessened depression.
- Interview regarding feelings and mood.
- Observe and interview regarding adverse drug effects.
- Observe and interview regarding suicidal thoughts and behaviors.

Principles of Therapy

Drug Selection

Because the available drugs have similar efficacy in treating depression, the choice of an antidepressant depends on the patient's age; medical conditions; previous history of drug response, if any; and the specific drug's adverse effects. Cost also needs to be considered. Although the newer drugs are much more expensive than the TCAs, they may be more cost effective overall because TCAs are more likely to cause serious adverse effects, they require monitoring of plasma drug levels and ECGs, and patients are more likely to stop taking them. The SSRIs are the drugs of first choice. These drugs are effective and usually produce fewer and milder adverse effects than

other drugs. Guidelines for choosing one SSRI over another have not been established.

TCAs are second-line drugs for the treatment of depression. Initial selection of TCAs may be based on the patient's previous response or susceptibility to adverse effects. For example, if a patient (or a close family member) responded well to a particular drug in the past, that is probably the drug of choice for repeated episodes of depression. The response of family members to individual drugs may be significant because there is a strong genetic component to depression and drug response. If therapeutic effects do not occur within 4 weeks, the TCA probably should be discontinued or changed, because some patients tolerate or respond better to one TCA than to another. For potentially suicidal patients, an SSRI or another newer drug is preferred over a TCA because the TCAs are much more toxic in overdoses.

MAO inhibitors are third-line drugs for the treatment of depression because of their potential interactions with other drugs and certain foods. An MAO inhibitor is most likely to be prescribed when the patient does not respond to other antidepressant drugs or when electroconvulsive therapy is refused or contraindicated.

Criteria for choosing bupropion, mirtazapine, duloxetine, and venlafaxine are not clearly defined. Bupropion does not cause orthostatic hypotension or sexual dysfunction. Mirtazapine decreases anxiety, agitation, migraines, and insomnia, as well as depression. In addition, it does not cause sexual dysfunction or clinically significant drug–drug interactions. Duloxetine relieves painful physical symptoms (overall pain, backache, shoulder pain, etc.) associated with depression, thereby reducing remission rates, and reduces depression-associated anxiety. However, duloxetine has CNS stimulant effects and can produce hepatotoxicity. Venlafaxine has stimulant effects, increases blood pressure, and causes sexual dysfunction, but it does not cause significant drug–drug interactions.

For patients with certain concurrent medical conditions, antidepressants may have adverse effects. For patients with cardiovascular disorders, most antidepressants can cause hypotension, but the SSRIs, bupropion, and venlafaxine are rarely associated with cardiac dysrhythmias. Duloxetine, venlafaxine, and MAO inhibitors can increase blood pressure. For patients with seizure disorders, bupropion, clomipramine, and duloxetine should be avoided. SSRIs, MAO inhibitors, and desipramine are less likely to cause seizures. For patients with diabetes mellitus, SSRIs may have a hypoglycemic effect. Duloxetine may slightly increase fasting glucose levels, and bupropion and venlafaxine have little effect on blood sugar levels. Duloxetine can cause mydriasis, increasing intraocular pressure in patients with narrow-angle glaucoma.

Lithium is the drug of choice for patients with bipolar disorder. When used therapeutically, lithium is effective in controlling mania in 65% to 80% of patients. When used prophylactically, the drug decreases the frequency and intensity of manic cycles. Carbamazepine (Tegretol), lamotrigine (Lamictal), and valproate (Depakene) are anticonvulsants

Patient Teaching Guidelines | Antidepressants and Lithium

General Considerations

■ Take antidepressants as directed to maximize therapeutic benefits and minimize adverse effects. Do not alter doses when symptoms subside. Antidepressants are usually given for several months, perhaps years. Lithium therapy may be lifelong.

■ Therapeutic effects (relief of symptoms) may not occur for 2–4 weeks after drug therapy is started. As a result, it is very important not to think the drug is ineffective and stop taking it prematurely.

■ Do not take other prescription or over-the-counter drugs without consulting a health care provider, including over-the-counter cold remedies. Potentially serious drug interactions may occur.

■ Do not take the herbal supplement St. John's wort while taking a prescription antidepressant drug. Serious interactions may occur.

■ Inform any physician, surgeon, dentist, or nurse practitioner about the antidepressant drugs being taken. Potentially serious adverse effects or drug interactions may occur if certain other drugs are prescribed.

■ Avoid activities that require alertness and physical coordination (e.g., driving a car, operating other machinery) until reasonably sure the medication does not make you drowsy or impair your ability to perform the activities safely.

■ Avoid alcohol and other central nervous system depressants (e.g., any drugs that cause drowsiness). Excessive drowsiness, dizziness, difficulty breathing, and low blood pressure may occur, with potentially serious consequences.

■ Learn the name and type of a prescribed antidepressant drug to help avoid undesirable interactions with other drugs or a physician prescribing other drugs with similar effects. There are several different types of antidepressant drugs, with different characteristics and precautions for safe and effective usage.

■ Escitalopram (Lexapro) is a derivative of citalopram (Celexa), and the two medications should not be taken concomitantly.

■ Bupropion is a unique drug prescribed for depression (brand name Wellbutrin) and for smoking cessation (brand name Zyban). It is extremely important not to increase the dose or take the two brand names at the same time (as might happen with different physicians or filling prescriptions at different pharmacies). Overdoses may cause seizures, as well as other adverse effects. When used for smoking cessation, Zyban is recommended for up to 12 weeks if progress is being made. If significant progress is not made by approximately 7 weeks, it is considered unlikely that longer drug use will be helpful.

■ Do not stop taking any antidepressant drug without discussing it with a health care provider. If a problem occurs, the type of drug, the dose, or other aspects may be changed to solve the problem and allow continued use of the medication.

■ Counseling, support groups, relaxation techniques, and other nonmedication treatments are recommended along with drug therapy.

■ Notify your physician if you become pregnant or intend to become pregnant during therapy with antidepressant drugs.

Self-Administration

■ With a selective serotonin reuptake inhibitor (e.g., Celexa, Lexapro, Paxil, Prozac, Zoloft), take in the morning because the drug may interfere with sleep if taken at bedtime. In addition, notify a health care provider if a skin rash or other allergic reaction occurs. Allergic reactions are uncommon but may require that the drug be discontinued.

■ With a tricyclic antidepressant (e.g., amitriptyline), take at bedtime to aid sleep and decrease adverse effects. Also, report urinary retention, fainting, irregular heartbeat, seizures, restlessness, and mental confusion. These are potentially serious adverse drug effects.

■ With venlafaxine (Effexor), take as directed or ask for instructions. This drug is often taken twice daily. Notify a health care provider if a skin rash or other allergic reaction occurs. An allergic reaction may require that the drug be discontinued.

■ With duloxetine (Cymbalta), swallow the medication whole, do not crush, chew, or sprinkle capsule contents on food.

■ There are short-, intermediate-, and long-acting forms of bupropion that are taken 3 times, 2 times, or 1 time per day, respectively. Be sure to take your medication as prescribed by your physician.

■ With lithium, several precautions are needed for safe use:
  1. Take with food or milk or soon after a meal to decrease stomach upset.
  2. Do not alter dietary salt intake. Decreased salt intake (e.g., low-salt diet) increases risk of adverse effects from lithium. Increased intake may decrease therapeutic effects.
  3. Drink 8–12 glasses of fluids daily; avoid excessive intake of caffeine-containing beverages. Caffeine has a diuretic effect and dehydration increases lithium toxicity.
  4. Do not take diuretic medications without consulting a health care provider. Diuretics cause loss of sodium and water, which increases lithium toxicity.
  5. Minimize activities that cause excessive perspiration, such as sweating during heavy exercise, sauna use, or outdoor activities during hot summer days. Loss of salt in sweat increases the risk of adverse effects from lithium.
  6. Report for measurements of lithium blood levels as instructed, and do not take the morning dose of lithium until the blood sample has been obtained. Regular measurements of blood lithium levels are necessary for safe and effective lithium therapy. Accurate measurement of serum drug levels requires that blood be drawn approximately 12 hours after the previous dose of lithium.
  7. If signs of overdose occur (e.g., vomiting, diarrhea, unsteady walking, tremor, drowsiness, muscle weakness), stop taking lithium and contact the prescribing physician or other health care provider.

with mood-stabilizing properties that may be used for patients who do not respond to lithium.

Drug Dosage and Administration

Dosage of antidepressant drugs should be individualized according to clinical response. Antidepressant drug therapy is usually initiated with small, divided doses that are gradually increased until therapeutic or adverse effects occur.

With SSRIs and venlafaxine, therapy is begun with once-daily oral administration of the manufacturer's recommended dosage. Dosage may be increased after 3 or 4 weeks if depression is not relieved. As with most other drugs, smaller doses may be indicated in older adults and in patients taking multiple medications. Duloxetine is initiated with twice-a-day oral administration without regard to food.

Applying Your Knowledge 10-3

Mr. Mehring reports he is having difficulty sleeping. What measures should be initiated?

With TCAs, therapy is begun with small doses, which are increased to the desired dose over 1 to 2 weeks. Minimal effective doses are approximately 150 milligrams per day of imipramine (Tofranil) or its equivalent. TCAs can be administered once or twice daily because they have long elimination half-lives. After dosage is established, TCAs are often given once daily at bedtime. This regimen is effective and well tolerated by most patients. Elderly patients may experience fewer adverse reactions if divided doses are continued. With TCAs, measurement of plasma levels is helpful in adjusting dosages.

With bupropion, seizures are more likely to occur with large single doses, large total doses, and large or abrupt increases in dosage. Recommendations to avoid these risk factors are as follows:

- Give bupropion in equally divided doses, three times daily (at least 6 hours apart) for immediate-release tablets, twice daily for sustained-release tablets, and once a day for extended-release forms of bupropion XL.

- The maximal single dose of immediate-release tablets is 150 milligrams (sustained-release, 200 mg; XL, 450 mg).

- The recommended initial dose is 200 milligrams, gradually increased to 300 milligrams. If no clinical improvement occurs after several weeks of 300 milligrams per day, the dosage may be increased to 450 milligrams, the maximal daily dose for immediate-release tablets (sustained-release, 400 mg; XL, 450 mg).

- The recommended maintenance dose is the lowest amount that maintains remission.

With lithium, dosage should be based on serum lithium levels, control of symptoms, and occurrence of adverse effects. Measurements of serum levels are required because therapeutic doses are only slightly lower than toxic doses and because

patients vary widely in rates of lithium absorption and excretion. Thus, a dose that is therapeutic in one patient may be toxic in another. Lower doses are indicated for older adults and for patients with conditions that impair lithium excretion (e.g., diuretic drug therapy, dehydration, low-salt diet, renal impairment, decreased cardiac output).

When lithium therapy is being initiated, the serum drug concentration should be measured two or three times weekly in the morning, 12 hours after the last dose of lithium. For most patients, the therapeutic range of serum drug levels is 0.5 to 1.2 milliequivalents per liter (SI units, 0.5 to 1.2 mmol/L). Serum lithium levels should not exceed 1.5 milliequivalents per liter, because the risk of serious toxicity is increased at higher levels.

After symptoms of mania are controlled, lithium doses should be lowered. Serum lithium levels should be measured at least every 3 months during long-term maintenance therapy.

Duration of Drug Therapy

Guidelines for the duration of antidepressant drug therapy are not well established, and there are differences of opinion. Some authorities recommend 9 months of treatment after symptoms subside for a first episode of depression, 5 years after symptoms subside for a second episode, and long-term therapy after a third episode. Recent studies support the use of long-term maintenance therapy for patients at high risk of recurrent depression at antidepressant dosages that helped the patient achieve remission.

With lithium, long-term therapy is the usual practice because of a high recurrence rate if the drug is discontinued. When lithium is discontinued, most often because of adverse effects or the patient's lack of adherence to the prescribed regimen, gradually tapering the dose over 2 to 4 weeks delays recurrence of symptoms.

Effects of Antidepressants on Other Drugs

The SSRIs are strong inhibitors of the cytochrome P450 enzyme system, which metabolizes many drugs, especially those metabolized by the 1A2, 2D6, and 3A4 groups of enzymes. Inhibiting the enzymes that normally metabolize or inactivate a drug produces the same effect as an excessive dose of the inhibited drug. As a result, serum drug levels and risks of adverse effects are greatly increased. Specific interactions include the following:

- Fluoxetine, paroxetine, and sertraline inhibit 2D6 enzymes and slow metabolism of bupropion, codeine, desipramine, dextromethorphan, flecainide, metoprolol, nortriptyline, phenothiazines, propranolol, risperidone, and timolol.

- TCAs are metabolized by 2D6 enzymes and may inhibit the metabolism of other drugs metabolized by the 2D6 group (other antidepressants, phenothiazines, carbamazepine, flecainide, propafenone). Lower-than-usual doses of both the TCA and the other drug may be needed.

- Mirtazapine and venlafaxine are not thought to have clinically significant effects on cytochrome P450 enzymes, but few studies have been done and effects are unknown.

- Duloxetine competes with other drugs metabolized by the CYP2D6 enzymes (flecainide, phenothiazines, propafenone, TCAs, and thioridazine), increasing risk of toxicity. Because of increased risk of ventricular arrhythmias and sudden death, duloxetine should not be given with thioridazine.

Toxicity: Recognition and Management

Some antidepressant drugs are highly toxic and potentially lethal when taken in large doses. Toxicity is most likely to occur in depressed patients who intentionally ingest large amounts of drug in suicide attempts and in young children who accidentally gain access to medication containers. Measures to prevent acute poisoning from drug overdose include dispensing only a few days' supply (i.e., 5 to 7 days) to patients with suicidal tendencies and storing the drugs in places inaccessible to young children. General measures to treat acute poisoning include early detection of signs and symptoms, stopping the drug, and instituting treatment if indicated. Specific symptoms and signs of overdose and treatment measures for selected antidepressants are discussed below.

SSRIs and SNRIs

Symptoms of overdose include nausea, vomiting, agitation, restlessness, hypomania, and other signs of CNS stimulation. Management includes symptomatic and supportive treatment, such as maintaining an adequate airway and ventilation, monitoring cardiac rhythm, and administering activated charcoal.

TCAs

Overdose symptoms occur 1 to 4 hours after drug ingestion and consist primarily of CNS depression and cardiovascular effects (e.g., nystagmus, tremor, restlessness, seizures, hypotension, dysrhythmias, myocardial depression). Death usually results from cardiac, respiratory, and circulatory failure. Management of TCA toxicity consists of performing gastric lavage and giving activated charcoal to reduce drug absorption, establishing and maintaining a patent airway, performing continuous ECG monitoring of comatose patients or those with respiratory insufficiency or wide QRS intervals, giving intravenous fluids and vasopressors for severe hypotension, and giving intravenous phenytoin (Dilantin) or fosphenytoin (Cerebyx) or a parenteral benzodiazepine (e.g., lorazepam) if seizures occur.

MAO inhibitors

Symptoms of overdose occur 12 hours or more after drug ingestion and consist primarily of adrenergic effects (e.g., tachycardia, increased rate of respiration, agitation, tremors, convulsive seizures, sweating, heart block, hypotension, delirium, coma). Management consists of diuresis, acidification of urine, or hemodialysis to remove the drug from the body.

Atypical Antidepressants

Symptoms of bupropion overdose include agitation and other mental status changes, nausea and vomiting, and seizures. General treatment measures include hospitalization, decreasing absorption (e.g., giving activated charcoal to conscious patients), and supporting vital functions. If seizures occur, an intravenous benzodiazepine (e.g., lorazepam) is the drug of first choice.

Mood-Stabilizing Agents

Toxic manifestations of lithium overdosage occur at serum lithium levels greater than 2.5 milliequivalents per liter and include nystagmus, tremors, oliguria, confusion, impaired consciousness, visual or tactile hallucinations, choreiform movements, convulsions, coma, and death. Treatment involves supportive care to maintain vital functions, including correction of fluid and electrolyte imbalances. With severe overdoses, hemodialysis is preferred because it removes lithium from the body.

Antidepressant Discontinuation Syndrome: Prevention and Management

Antidepressant discontinuation syndrome has been reported with sudden termination of most antidepressant drugs. In general, symptoms occur more rapidly and may be more intense with drugs that have a short half-life and/or with long-term antidepressant therapy. As with other psychotropic drugs, these antidepressant drugs should be tapered in dosage and discontinued gradually unless severe drug toxicity, anaphylactic reactions, or other life-threatening conditions are present. Tapering of most antidepressants may take 6 to 8 weeks to avoid antidepressant discontinuation syndrome. Lower dosages may require less tapering time, and more tapering time may be needed to discontinue long-term maintenance therapy. The occurrence of withdrawal symptoms may indicate that the patient has omitted doses or stopped taking the drug.

The most clearly defined withdrawal syndromes are associated with SSRIs and TCAs. With SSRIs, withdrawal symptoms include dizziness, gastrointestinal upset, lethargy or anxiety/hyperarousal, dysphoria, sleep problems, and headache which can last from several days to several weeks. More serious symptoms may include aggression, hypomania, mood disturbances, and suicidal tendencies. Fluoxetine has a long half-life and has not been associated with withdrawal symptoms. Other SSRIs and SNRIs have short half-lives and may cause withdrawal reactions if stopped abruptly. Paroxetine, which has a half-life of approximately 24 hours and does not produce active metabolites, may be associated with relatively severe withdrawal symptoms even when discontinued gradually, over 7 to 10 days. Symptoms may include a flu-like syndrome with nausea, vomiting, fatigue, muscle aches, dizziness, headache, and insomnia. The short-acting SSRIs and SNRIs should be tapered in dosage and gradually discontinued to prevent or minimize withdrawal reactions.

TCAs have strong anticholinergic effects. When TCAs are abruptly discontinued cholinergic rebound may occur. Symptoms of excessive cholinergic activity include hypersalivation, diarrhea, urinary urgency, abdominal cramping, and sweating. The patient may benefit from short-term use of an anticholinergic agent such as atropine or benztropine to alleviate symptoms of cholinergic rebound. TCA tapering should be gradual and may take up to 3 months.

Perioperative Use

Antidepressants must be used very cautiously, if at all, perioperatively because of the risk of serious adverse effects and adverse interactions with anesthetics and other commonly used drugs. It is usually recommended that antidepressants be tapered in dosage and gradually discontinued. MAO inhibitors are contraindicated and should be discontinued at least 10 days before elective surgery. TCAs should be discontinued several days before elective surgery and resumed several days after surgery. SSRIs and other antidepressants have not been studied in relation to perioperative use; however, it seems reasonable to discontinue the drugs when feasible because of potential adverse effects, especially on the cardiovascular system and CNS.

Lithium should be stopped 1 to 2 days before surgery and resumed when full oral intake of food and fluids is allowed. Lithium may prolong the effects of anesthetics and neuromuscular blocking drugs.

Use in Special Populations

Use in Various Ethnic Groups

Antidepressant drug therapy for nonwhite populations in the United States is based primarily on dosage recommendations, pharmacokinetic data, and adverse effects derived from white recipients. However, several studies document differences in drug effects in nonwhite populations. The differences are mainly attributed to genetic or ethnic variations in drug-metabolizing enzymes in the liver. Although all ethnic groups are genetically heterogeneous and individual members may respond differently, health care providers must consider potential differences in responses to drug therapy.

African Americans tend to have higher plasma drug levels for a given dose, respond more rapidly, experience a higher incidence of adverse effects, and metabolize TCAs more slowly than whites. To decrease adverse effects, initial doses may need to be lower than those given to whites, and later doses should be titrated according to clinical response and serum drug levels. In addition, baseline and periodic ECGs are recommended to detect adverse drug effects on the heart. Studies have not been done with newer antidepressants. With lithium, African Americans report more adverse reactions than whites and may need smaller doses.

Asians tend to metabolize antidepressant drugs slowly and therefore have higher plasma drug levels for a given dose than whites. Most studies have been done with TCAs and a limited number of Asian subgroups. Thus, it cannot be assumed that all antidepressant drugs and all people of Asian heritage respond the same. To avoid drug toxicity, initial doses should be approximately half the usual doses given to whites, and later doses should be titrated according to clinical response and serum drug levels. This recommendation is supported by a survey from several Asian countries that reported the use of much smaller doses of TCAs than in the United States. In addition, baseline and periodic ECGs are also recommended for Asian patients to detect adverse drug effects on the heart. Studies have not been done with newer antidepressants. With lithium, there are no apparent differences between effects in Asians and whites.

Information regarding the reaction of the Hispanic population to antidepressant drugs is largely unknown. Few studies have been performed; some report a need for lower doses of TCAs and greater susceptibility to adverse effects, whereas others report no differences between Hispanics and whites.

Use in Children

Between 3% and 5% of children and adolescents in the United States are affected by major depression; the risk for depression increases after puberty. Antidepressant drugs are widely prescribed in children and adolescents, in whom depression commonly occurs. However, only a few drugs are actually FDA approved for use in the pediatric population, and the FDA warns against the use of paroxetine in children and adolescents. TCAs are not efficacious for depression in children and adolescents (Level A). There is only limited evidence in support of SSRIs for treating depression in children and adolescents, and these medications should be reserved for treatment of severe depression (Level B). Because of the increased risk of suicidality, children and adolescents taking all antidepressants must be closely monitored (Level C).

For most children and adolescents, it is probably best to reserve drug therapy for those who do not respond to nonpharmacologic treatments such as cognitive behavior therapy (Level A) and those whose depression is persistent or severe enough to impair function in usual activities of daily living. The long-term effects of antidepressant drugs on the developing brain are unknown. FDA-approved SSRIs are considered first-line antidepressants and safer than TCAs and MAO inhibitors for children with depression. Fluoxetine is approved for treatment of pediatric major depression. (In addition, fluoxetine, sertraline, and fluvoxamine are approved for treatment of obsessive-compulsive disorder in children.) Common adverse effects include sedation and activation; it is often difficult to distinguish therapeutic effects (improvement of mood, increased energy and motivation) from the adverse effects of behavioral activation (agitation, hypomania, restlessness).

Safety and effectiveness have not been established for MAO inhibitors in children younger than 16 years of age or for bupropion, duloxetine, mirtazapine, and venlafaxine in children younger than 18 years of age.

TCAs are not recommended for use in children younger than 12 years of age except for short-term treatment of enuresis in children older than 6 years of age. Amitriptyline, desipramine, imipramine, and nortriptyline are the TCAs most commonly prescribed to treat depression in children older than 12 years of age. Because of potentially serious adverse effects, blood pressure, ECGs, and plasma drug levels should be monitored. There is evidence that children metabolize TCAs faster than adults, and withdrawal symptoms (e.g., increased GI motility, malaise, and headache) are more common in children than in adults. Several TCAs are approved for treatment of depression in adolescents. (Clomipramine is approved for treatment of obsessive-compulsive disorder in children, and imipramine is also approved for treating childhood enuresis in children older than 6 years of age.)

Divided doses may be better tolerated and minimize withdrawal symptoms. When a TCA is used for enuresis, effectiveness may decrease over time, and no residual benefits continue after the drug is stopped. Common adverse effects include sedation, fatigue, nervousness, and sleep disorders. A TCA probably is not a drug of first choice for adolescents because TCAs are more toxic in overdose than other antidepressants, and suicide is a leading cause of death in adolescents.

For adolescents, it may be important to discuss sexual effects because the SSRIs and SNRIs cause a high incidence of sexual dysfunction (e.g., anorgasmia, decreased libido, erectile dysfunction). Bupropion and mirtazapine are unlikely to cause sexual dysfunction.

Lithium is not approved for use in children younger than 12 years of age, but it has been used to treat bipolar disorder and aggressiveness. Children normally excrete lithium more rapidly than adults. As with adults, initial doses should be relatively low and gradually increased according to regular measurements of serum drug levels. Risperidone has recently been approved by the FDA for use in adolescents aged 10 to 17 years with type I bipolar disorder. It can be used alone or in combination with lithium or valproate for the treatment of acute mania or mixed episodes.

Use in Older Adults

SSRIs are the drugs of choice in older adults as in younger ones because they produce fewer sedative, anticholinergic, cardiotoxic, and psychomotor adverse effects than the TCAs and related antidepressants. These drugs produce similar adverse effects in older adults as in younger adults. Although their effects in older adults are not well delineated, SSRIs may be eliminated more slowly, and smaller or less frequent doses may be prudent. SNRIs may also be used in older adults, with smaller initial doses and increments recommended. The weight loss often associated with SSRIs and SNRIs may be undesirable in older adults. Use of maintenance antidepressant therapy is beneficial to prevent recurrence of depression in older adults.

TCAs may cause or aggravate conditions that are common in older adults (e.g., cardiac conduction abnormalities, urinary retention, narrow-angle glaucoma). In addition, impaired compensatory mechanisms make older adults more likely to experience anticholinergic effects, confusion, hypotension, and sedation. If a TCA is chosen for an older adult, nortriptyline or desipramine is preferred. In addition, any TCA should be given in small doses initially and gradually increased over several weeks, if necessary, to achieve therapeutic effects. Initial and maintenance doses should be small

because the drugs are metabolized and excreted more slowly than in younger adults. Initial dosage should be decreased by 30% to 50% to avoid serious adverse reactions; increments should be small. Vital signs, serum drug levels, and ECGs should be monitored regularly.

MAO inhibitors may be more likely to cause hypertensive crises in older adults because cardiovascular, renal, and hepatic functions are often diminished.

With lithium, initial doses should be low and increased gradually, according to regular measurements of serum drug levels.

Use in Patients With Renal Impairment

Antidepressants should be used cautiously in the presence of severe renal impairment. Mild or moderate impairment contributes to few adverse effects, but severe impairment may increase plasma drug levels and adverse effects of virtually all antidepressants. Thus, small initial doses, slow increases, and less frequent dosing are indicated.

Lithium is eliminated only by the kidneys, and it has a very narrow therapeutic range. If given to a patient with renal impairment or unstable renal function, the dose must be markedly reduced and plasma lithium levels must be closely monitored.

Use in Patients With Hepatic Impairment

Hepatic impairment leads to reduced first-pass metabolism of most antidepressant drugs, resulting in higher plasma levels. The drugs should be used cautiously in patients with severe liver impairment. Cautious use means lower doses, longer intervals between doses, and slower dose increases than usual. Duloxetine is not recommended for use in patients with any hepatic insufficiency.

Fluoxetine and sertraline are less readily metabolized to their active metabolites in patients with hepatic impairment. For example, in patients with cirrhosis, the average half-life of fluoxetine may increase from 2 to 3 days to more than 7 days and that of norfluoxetine, the active metabolite, from 7 to 9 days to 12 days. Clearance of sertraline is also decreased in patients with cirrhosis. Paroxetine has a short half-life and no active metabolites, but increased plasma levels can occur with severe hepatic impairment.

TCAs are also less readily metabolized in people with severe hepatic impairment (e.g., severe cirrhosis). This increases the risk of adverse effects such as sedation and hypotension.

Use in Patients With Critical Illness

Critically ill patients may be receiving an antidepressant when the critical illness develops or may need a drug to combat the depression that often develops with major illness. The decision to continue or start an antidepressant should be based on a thorough assessment of the patient's condition, other drugs being given, potential adverse drug effects, and other factors. If an antidepressant is given, its use must be cautious and slow and the patient's responses carefully monitored because critically ill patients are often frail and unstable, with multiple organ dysfunctions.

Use in Home Care

Whatever the primary problem for which a home care nurse is visiting a patient, he or she must be vigilant for signs and symptoms of major depression. Depression often accompanies any serious physical illness and may occur in many other circumstances as well. The main role of the nurse may be recognizing depressive states and referring patients for treatment. If an antidepressant medication was recently started, the nurse may need to remind the patient that it usually takes 2 to 4 weeks to take effect. The nurse should encourage the patient to continue taking the medication. In addition, the nurse should observe the patient's response and assess for suicidal thoughts or plans, especially at the beginning of therapy or when dosages are increased or decreased. The family should be taught to report any change in the patient's behavior, especially anxiety, agitation, panic attacks, insomnia, irritability, hostility, impulsivity, akathisia, hypomania, and mania. A patient who has one or more of these symptoms may be at greater risk for worsening depression or suicidality.

Nursing Actions   Antidepressants

NURSING ACTIONS	RATIONALE/EXPLANATION
1. Administer accurately	
a. Give most selective serotonin reuptake inhibitors (SSRIs) once daily in the morning; citalopram, escitalopram, and sertraline may be given morning or evening.	To prevent insomnia
b. Mix sertraline oral concentrate (20 mg/mL) in 4 oz of water, ginger ale, lemon/lime soda, lemonade, or orange juice only; give immediately after mixing.	Manufacturer's recommendations
c. Give tricyclic antidepressants (TCAs) and mirtazapine at bedtime.	To aid sleep and decrease daytime sedation
d. Give venlafaxine and lithium with food.	To decrease gastrointestinal (GI) effects (e.g., nausea and vomiting)
2. Observe for therapeutic effects	
a. With antidepressants for depression, observe for statements of feeling better or less depressed; increased appetite, physical activity, and interest in surroundings; improved sleep patterns; improved appearance; decreased anxiety; decreased somatic complaints.	Therapeutic effects occur 2–4 weeks after drug therapy is started.
b. With antidepressants for anxiety disorders, observe for decreased symptoms of the disorders (see Chap. 8).	
c. With lithium, observe for decreases in manic behavior and mood swings.	Therapeutic effects do not occur until approximately 7–10 days after therapeutic serum drug levels (1–1.5 mEq/L with acute mania; 0.6–1.2 mEq/L for maintenance therapy) are attained. In mania, a benzodiazepine or an antipsychotic drug is usually given to reduce agitation and control behavior until the lithium takes effect.
3. Observe for adverse effects	
a. With SSRIs and SNRIs, observe for dizziness, headache, nervousness, insomnia, nausea, diarrhea, dizziness, dry mouth, sedation, skin rash, sexual dysfunction.	GI upset and diarrhea are common with SSRIs; GI upset, diarrhea, agitation, and insomnia are common with venlafaxine. Although numerous adverse effects may occur, they are usually less serious than those occurring with most other antidepressants. Compared with the TCAs, SSRIs and other newer drugs are less likely to cause significant sedation, hypotension, and cardiac dysrhythmias, but they are more likely to cause nausea, nervousness, and insomnia.
b. With TCAs, observe for:	Most adverse effects result from anticholinergic or antiadrenergic activity. Cardiovascular effects are most serious in overdose.
(1) Central nervous system (CNS) effects—drowsiness, dizziness, confusion, poor memory	
(2) GI effects—nausea, dry mouth, constipation	
(3) Cardiovascular effects—cardiac dysrhythmias, tachycardia, orthostatic hypotension	
(4) Other effects—blurred vision, urinary retention, sexual dysfunction, weight gain or loss	
c. With monoamine oxidase (MAO) inhibitors, observe for blurred vision, constipation, dizziness, dry mouth, hypotension, urinary retention, hypoglycemia.	Anticholinergic effects are common. Hypoglycemia results from a drug-induced reduction in blood sugar.

(continued on page 192)

Nursing Actions Antidepressants (continued)

NURSING ACTIONS	RATIONALE/EXPLANATION
d. With bupropion, observe for seizure activity, CNS stimulation (agitation, insomnia, hyperactivity, hallucinations, delusions), headache, nausea and vomiting, weight loss.	Adverse effects are most likely to occur if recommended doses are exceeded. Note that bupropion has few, if any, effects on cardiac conduction and does not cause orthostatic hypotension.
e. With mirtazapine, observe for sedation, confusion, dry mouth, constipation, nausea and vomiting, hypotension, tachycardia, urinary retention, photosensitivity, skin rash, weight gain.	· Common effects are drowsiness, dizziness, and weight gain. Has CNS depressant and anticholinergic effects.
f. With lithium, observe for:	Most patients who take lithium experience adverse effects.
(1) Metallic taste, hand tremors, nausea, polyuria, polydipsia, diarrhea, muscular weakness, fatigue, edema, weight gain	Symptoms listed in (1) are common, occur at therapeutic serum drug levels (0.6–1.2 mEq/L), and usually subside during the first few weeks of drug therapy. Symptoms listed in (2) occur at higher serum drug levels (1.5–2.5 mEq/L). Nausea may be decreased by giving lithium with meals. Propranolol (Inderal), 20–120 mg daily, may be given to control tremors.
(2) More severe nausea and diarrhea, vomiting, ataxia, incoordination, dizziness, slurred speech, blurred vision, tinnitus, muscle twitching and tremors, increased muscle tone	Severe adverse effects may be managed by decreasing lithium dosage, omitting a few doses, or discontinuing the drug temporarily. Toxic symptoms occur at serum drug levels above 2.5 mEq/L.
(3) Leukocytosis	Lithium mobilizes white blood cells (WBCs) from bone marrow to the bloodstream. Maximum increase in WBCs occurs in 7–10 days.
4. Observe for drug interactions	
a. Drugs that *increase* effects of SSRIs:	Drug interactions with the SSRIs vary with individual drugs.
(1) Cimetidine	May increase serum drug levels of SSRIs by slowing their metabolism
(2) MAO inhibitors	**SSRIs and MAO inhibitors should not be given concurrently or close together because serious and fatal reactions have occurred.** The reaction, attributed to excess serotonin and called the serotonin syndrome, may cause hyperthermia, muscle spasm, agitation, delirium, and coma. To avoid this reaction, an SSRI should not be started for at least 2 weeks after an MAO inhibitor is discontinued, and an MAO inhibitor should not be started for at least 2 weeks after an SSRI has been discontinued (5 weeks with fluoxetine, because of its long half-life).
(3) Linezolid	The antibiotic linezolid is a reversible nonselective MAO inhibitor (see above).
(4) Sumatriptan	Postmarketing studies report concomitant use of SSRIs and sumatriptan may result in weakness, hyperreflexia, and incoordination.
(5) Nonsteroidal anti-inflammatory drugs (NSAIDs), aspirin, warfarin	Serotonin release by platelets plays a role in hemostasis, and SSRIs may interfere with this release, resulting in an increased incidence of GI bleeding. Concomitant use of NSAIDs, aspirin, or warfarin potentiates this risk.
(6) Metoclopramide, sibutramine tramadol	Increased risk of serotonin syndrome
b. Drugs that *decrease* effects of SSRIs:	
(1) Carbamazepine, phenytoin, rifampin	These drugs induce liver enzymes that accelerate the metabolism of the SSRIs.
(2) Cyproheptadine	This is an antihistamine with antiserotonin effects.
c. Drugs that *increase* effects of mirtazapine and venlafaxine:	
(1) MAO inhibitors	See SSRIs, above. **These drugs and MAO inhibitors should not be given concurrently or close together because serious and fatal reactions have occurred.** Mirtazapine should be stopped at least 14 days and venlafaxine at least 7 days before starting an MAO inhibitor, and an MAO inhibitor should be stopped at least 14 days before starting mirtazapine or venlafaxine.

NURSING ACTIONS	RATIONALE/EXPLANATION
d. Drugs that *increase* the effects of duloxetine:	
(1) CYP1A2 inhibitors (fluvoxamine, quinolone antibiotics)	These drugs prevent metabolism of duloxetine, increasing serum levels.
(2) CYP2D6 inhibitors (fluoxetine, quinidine, paroxetine)	These drugs prevent metabolism of duloxetine, increasing serum levels.
(3) MAO inhibitors (MAOIs)	**Duloxetine and MAOIs should not be given concurrently or close together because serious and fatal reactions have occurred.** Duloxetine should not be given within 14 days of stopping an MAOI, and an MAOI should not be given within 5 days of stopping duloxetine.
e. Drugs that *increase* effects of TCAs:	
(1) Antidysrhythmics (e.g., quinidine, disopyramide, procainamide)	Additive effects on cardiac conduction, increasing risk of heart block
(2) Antihistamines, atropine, and other drugs with anticholinergic effects	Additive anticholinergic effects (e.g., dry mouth, blurred vision, urinary retention, constipation)
(3) Antihypertensives	Additive hypotension
(4) Cimetidine	Increases risks of toxicity by decreasing hepatic metabolism and increasing blood levels of TCAs
(5) CNS depressants (e.g., alcohol, benzodiazepine antianxiety and hypnotic agents, opioid analgesics)	Additive sedation and CNS depression
(6) MAO inhibitors	**TCAs should not be given with MAO inhibitors or within 2 weeks after an MAO inhibitor drug;** hyperpyrexia, convulsions, and death have occurred with concurrent use.
(7) SSRIs	Inhibit metabolism of TCAs
f. Drugs that *decrease* effects of TCAs:	
(1) Carbamazepine, phenytoin, rifampin, nicotine (cigarette smoking)	These drugs induce drug-metabolizing enzymes in the liver, which increases the rate of TCA metabolism and elimination from the body.
g. Drugs that *increase* effects of MAO inhibitors:	
(1) Anticholinergic drugs (e.g., atropine, antipsychotic agents, TCAs)	Additive anticholinergic effects
(2) Adrenergic agents (e.g., epinephrine, phenylephrine), alcohol (some beers and wines), levodopa, meperidine	Hypertensive crisis and stroke may occur.
h. Drugs that *increase* effects of lithium:	
(1) Angiotensin-converting enzyme inhibitors (e.g., captopril)	Decrease renal clearance of lithium and thus increase serum lithium levels and risks of toxicity.
(2) Diuretics (e.g., furosemide, hydrochlorothiazide)	Increase neurotoxicity and cardiotoxicity of lithium by increasing excretion of sodium and potassium and thereby decreasing excretion of lithium.
(3) NSAIDs	Decrease renal clearance of lithium and thus increase serum levels and risks of lithium toxicity.
(4) Phenothiazines	Increased risk of hyperglycemia
(5) TCAs	May increase effects of lithium and are sometimes combined with lithium for this purpose. These drugs also may precipitate a manic episode and increase risks of hypothyroidism.
i. Drugs that *decrease* effects of lithium:	
(1) Acetazolamide, sodium chloride (in excessive amounts), drugs with a high sodium content (e.g., ticarcillin), theophylline	Increase excretion of lithium

Key Concepts

- Major depression is associated with impaired ability to function in usual activities and relationships.

- Postnatal depression is a major depressive episode occurring after the birth of a child.

- Bipolar disorder type I is characterized by episodes of major depression plus mania and occurs equally in men and women.

- Bipolar disorder type II is characterized by episodes of major depression plus hypomanic episodes and occurs more frequently in women.

- Antidepressants must be taken for 2 to 4 weeks before depressive symptoms improve.

- A **BLACK BOX WARNING** alerts health care providers to the increased risk of suicidal ideation in children, adolescents, and young adults 18 to 24 years of age when taking antidepressant medications.

- SSRIs are considered to be first-line medications in the treatment of depression because they have a more favorable side effect profile (e.g., GI symptoms, sexual dysfunction, CNS stimulation, and increased risk of GI bleeding).

- TCAs, second-line medications in the treatment of depression, produce a high incidence of adverse effects (e.g., sedation, orthostatic hypotension, cardiac dysrhythmias, anticholinergic effects, and weight gain).

- MAO inhibitors are considered third-line medications in the treatment of depression because of a high incidence of food and drug interactions which potentially lead to hypertensive crisis.

- Serotonin syndrome, a serious and sometimes fatal reaction characterized by hypertensive crisis, hyperpyrexia, extreme agitation progressing to delirium and coma, muscle rigidity, and seizures, may occur due to combined therapy with an SSRI or SNRI and an MAO inhibitor or other drug that potentiates serotonin neurotransmission. An SSRI or SNRI and an MAO inhibitor should not be given concurrently or within 2 weeks of each other. Fluoxetine, because of a long half-life, must be discontinued at least 5 weeks before starting an MAO inhibitor.

- SNRIs are similar to SSRIs in terms of therapeutic effects but exhibit more anticholinergic, CNS sedation, and cardiac conduction abnormalities.

- Some antidepressant drugs are highly toxic and potentially lethal when taken in large doses.

- Antidepressant discontinuation syndrome has been reported with sudden termination of most antidepressant drugs.

- SSRIs are the drugs of choice in older adults with depression.

- Moist antidepressants should be used cautiously in the presence of renal or hepatic impairment.

- Lithium is the drug of choice to treat bipolar disorder. Lithium has a narrow therapeutic index, and dosage is determined by serum lithium levels, control of symptoms, and occurrence of adverse effects. Therapeutic range for serum lithium level is 0.5 to 1.2 milliequivalents per liter.

- Anticonvulsants (e.g., carbamazepine, lamotrigine, and valorous acid) are also used to treat bipolar disorder.

- Atypical antipsychotics are useful in the treatment of the acute mania phase of bipolar disorder.

- Most authorities agree that there is insufficient evidence to support the use of St John's wort for treatment of depression.

Review and Application Exercises

Short Answer Exercises

1. During the initial assessment of any patient, what kinds of appearances or behaviors may indicate depression?

2. Is antidepressant drug therapy indicated for most episodes of temporary sadness? Why or why not?

3. What are the major groups of antidepressant drugs?

4. How do the drugs act to relieve depression?

5. When a patient begins antidepressant drug therapy, why is it important to explain that relief of depression may not occur for a few weeks?

6. What are common adverse effects of TCAs, and how may they be minimized?

7. What is the advantage of giving a TCA at bedtime rather than in the morning?

8. For a patient taking an MAO inhibitor, what information would you provide for preventing a hypertensive crisis?

9. How do the SSRIs differ from TCAs?

10. How do the newer drugs, including mirtazapine and venlafaxine, compare with the SSRIs in terms of adverse effects and adverse drug–drug interactions?

11. List the main elements of treatment of antidepressant overdoses.

12. What are common adverse effects of lithium, and how may they be minimized?

13. What is the nurse's role in assessing and managing depression in special populations? In the home setting?

NCLEX-Style Questions

14. A nurse is teaching the importance of proper diet to a patient taking tranylcypromine (Parnate), an MAO inhibitor, for depression. Which of the following food selections by the patient indicates that further teaching is needed?
    a. a tossed salad and a bowl of vegetable soup
    b. a sandwich with salami and Swiss cheese
    c. a hamburger and french fries
    d. a cold plate with cottage cheese, chicken salad, and grapes

15. A patient taking lithium is having problems with coordination and unstable gait. The patient's lithium level is 2.3 milliequivalents per liter. The nurse should do which of the following?
    a. Continue to administer the lithium three times per day.
    b. Skip a dose of lithium and then resume the regular medication schedule.
    c. Administer an extra dose of lithium.
    d. Withhold the lithium and notify the prescriber of the lithium level.

16. Today your patient begins a new drug regimen of escitalopram (Lexapro) for depression. Before administering this medication, you should assess for which of the following?
    a. prior recent use of MAO inhibitor antidepressants
    b. prior diet high in tyramine-containing foods
    c. history of cigarette use
    d. history of seizure disorders

17. Your patient has been taking imipramine (Tofranil) for 1 week for depression. He tells you he is going to stop taking this medication because it isn't working. Your best response is which of the following?
    a. "Contact your prescriber about taking a different antidepressant medication."
    b. "It may take up to 4 weeks before this medication makes you feel better."
    c. "You should slowly taper rather than suddenly discontinue this medication."
    d. "You should take an extra dose today to build up your blood level and get faster results."

Selected References

American Psychiatric Association. (2000). *Diagnostic and statistical manual of mental disorders* (4th ed., text revision). Washington, DC: American Psychiatric Association.

Bhatia, S. K., & Bhatia, S. C. (2007). Childhood and adolescent depression. *American Family Physician, 75*. Retrieved May, 8, 2007, from http://www.aaafp.org/afp/20070101/73.html

Blier, P., Keller, M. B., Pollack, M. H., Thase, M. E., Zajecka, J. M., & Dunner, D. L. (2007). Preventing recurrent depression: Long-term treatment for major depressive disorder. *Journal of Clinical Psychiatry, 68*, e06.

Burgess, S., Geddes, J., Hawton, K., Townsend, E., Jamison, K., & Goodwin, G. (2007) Lithium for maintenance treatment of mood disorders *Cochrane Database of Systematic Reviews, 3*, CD003013.

Cipriani, A., Brambilla, P., Furukawa, T., Geddes, J., Gregis, M., Hotopf, M., Malvini, L., & Barbui, C. (2007). Fluoxetine versus other types of pharmacotherapy for depression. *Cochrane Database of Systematic Reviews, 4*, CD004195.

Drug facts and comparisons. (Updated monthly). St. Louis, MO: Facts and Comparisons.

Fava, M., Mallinckrodt, C. H., Detke, M. J., Watkin, J. G., & Wohlreich, N. M. (2004). The effect of duloxetine on painful physical symptoms in depressed patients: Do improvements in these symptoms result in higher remission rates? *Journal of Clinical Psychiatry, 65*, 521–530.

Fetrow, C. W., & Avila, J. R. (2003). *Professional's handbook of complementary and alternative medicines* (3rd ed.). Philadelphia: Lippincott Williams & Wilkins.

Fochtmann, L. J., & Gelenberg, A. J. (2005). *Guideline watch: Practice guideline for the treatment of patients with major depressive disorder* (2nd ed.). Arlington, VA: American Psychiatric Association.

Frankhauser, M. P., & Freeman, M. P. (2005). Bipolar disorder. In J. T. DiPiro, R. L. Talbert, G. C. Yee, G. R. Matzke, B. G. Wells, & L. M. Posey (Eds.), *Pharmacotherapy: A pathophysiologic approach* (6th ed., pp. 1257–1284). New York: McGraw-Hill.

Hirschfeld, R. M. A. (2005). *Guideline watch: Practice guideline for the treatment of patients with bipolar disorder* (2nd ed.). Arlington: VA: American Psychiatric Association.

Howard, L. (2005). Clinical evidence concise: Postnatal depression. A publication of BMJ Publishing Group. Reprinted in *American Family Physician*. Retrieved May 22, 2007, from http://www.aaafp.org/afp/20051001/bmj.html

Howard, L. M., Hoffbrand, S., Henshaw, C., Boath, L., & Bradley, E. (2006) Antidepressant prevention of postnatal depression. *Cochrane Database of Systematic Reviews, 2*, CD004363.

Kando, J. C., Wells, B. G., & Hayes, P. E. (2005). Depressive disorders. In J. T. DiPiro, R. L. Talbert, G. C. Yee, G. R. Matzke, B. G. Wells, & L. M. Posey (Eds.), *Pharmacotherapy: A pathophysiologic approach* (6th ed., pp. 1235–1255). New York: McGraw-Hill.

Kessler, R.C., Berglundy P., Demler, O., Jin, R., Koretz., D., Merikangas, K.R., Rush, J., Walters, E. E., Wang, P.S. (2003). The epidemiology of major depressive disorder: Results from the National Comorbidity Survey Replication CNCS-R. *JAMA, 289*, 3095–3105.

Mottram, P., Wilson, K., & Strobl, J. (2007) Antidepressants for depressed elderly (Cochrane Review). *Cochrane Database of Systematic Reviews, 1*, CD003491.

Munoz, C., & Hilgenberg, C. (2005) Ethnopharmacology. *American Journal of Nursing, 105*, 40–48.

Warner, C. H., Bobo, W., Warner, C., Reid, S., & Rachal, J. (2006) Antidepressant discontinuation syndrome. *American Family Physician, 74*. Retrieved May 22, 2007, from http://www.aaafp.org/afp/20060801/449.html

Antiseizure Drugs

KEY TERMS

- Anticonvulsant
- Convulsion
- Epilepsy
- Gingival hyperplasia
- Monotherapy
- Seizure
- Seizure threshold
- Status epilepticus
- Tonic-clonic

LEARNING OBJECTIVES

After studying this chapter, you will be able to:

1. Identify types and potential causes of seizures.
2. Discuss major factors that influence choice of an antiseizure drug for a patient with a seizure disorder.
3. Recognize characteristics and effects of commonly used antiseizure drugs.
4. Differentiate between older and more recent antiseizure drugs.
5. Compare advantages and disadvantages between monotherapy and combination drug therapy for seizure disorders.
6. Apply the nursing process with patients receiving antiseizure drugs.
7. Describe strategies for prevention and treatment of status epilepticus.
8. Discuss the use of antiseizure drugs in special populations.

Applying Your Knowledge

Frank DeLaney is an 18-year-old college freshman who has been diagnosed with generalized and partial seizures. He has experienced at least three tonic-clonic seizures in the past 6 months and was started on phenytoin 1 month ago. The phenytoin has decreased the number of seizures but has not been successful in controlling the seizures to the degree the patient would like. The prescriber at the student health center has added carbamazepine to the antiseizure regimen. You are working in the student health center and are counseling Frank about his disease process and medical regimen.

Introduction

Seizure Disorders

The terms *seizure* and *convulsion* are often used interchangeably, although they are not the same. A seizure involves a brief episode of abnormal electrical activity in nerve cells of the brain that may or may not be accompanied by visible changes in appearance or behavior. A convulsion is a tonic-clonic type of seizure characterized by spasmodic contractions of involuntary muscles.

Seizures may occur as single events in response to hypoglycemia, fever, electrolyte imbalances, overdoses of numerous drugs (e.g., amphetamine, cocaine, isoniazid, lidocaine, lithium, methylphenidate, antipsychotics, theophylline), and withdrawal of alcohol or sedative-hypnotic drugs. Treatment of the underlying problem or temporary use of an antiseizure drug may relieve the seizures. An antiseizure drug is also called an antiepileptic drug (AED) or an *anticonvulsant*.

Epilepsy

When seizures occur in a chronic, recurrent pattern, they characterize a disorder known as *epilepsy*, which usually requires long-term drug therapy. Epilepsy is characterized by sudden, abnormal, hypersynchronous firing of neurons diagnosed by clinical signs and symptoms of seizure activity and by the presence of abnormal brain wave patterns on the electroencephalogram. Epilepsy can be classified as idiopathic or attributable to a secondary cause. Secondary causes in infancy include developmental defects, metabolic disease, or birth injury. Fever is a common cause during late infancy and early childhood, and inherited forms usually begin in childhood or adolescence. When epilepsy begins in adulthood, it is often caused by an acquired neurologic disorder (e.g., head injury, stroke, brain tumor) or alcohol and other drug effects. The incidence of epilepsy is higher in young children and older adults than in other age groups.

Seizures are broadly classified as partial or generalized. Partial seizures begin in a specific area of the brain and often indicate a localized brain lesion such as birth injury, trauma, stroke, or tumor. They produce symptoms ranging from simple motor and sensory manifestations to more complex abnormal movements and bizarre behavior. Movements are usually automatic, repetitive, and inappropriate to the situation, such as chewing, swallowing, or aversive movements (automatisms). In simple partial seizures, consciousness is not impaired; in complex partial seizures, the level of consciousness is decreased.

Generalized seizures are bilateral and symmetric and have no discernible point of origin in the brain. The most common type is the *tonic-clonic* or major motor seizure. The tonic phase involves sustained contraction of skeletal muscles; abnormal postures, such as opisthotonos; and absence of respiration, during which the person becomes cyanotic. The clonic phase is characterized by rapid rhythmic and symmetric jerking movements of the body. Tonic-clonic seizures are sometimes preceded by an aura—a brief warning, such as a flash of light or a specific sound or smell. In children, febrile seizures (i.e., tonic-clonic seizures that occur with fever in the absence of other identifiable causes) are the most common form of epilepsy.

Another type of generalized seizure is the absence seizure, characterized by abrupt alterations in consciousness that last only a few seconds. Other types of generalized seizures include the myoclonic type (contraction of a muscle or group of muscles) and the akinetic type (absence of movement). Some people are subject to mixed seizures.

Status epilepticus is a life-threatening emergency characterized by generalized tonic-clonic convulsions lasting for several minutes or occurring at close intervals during which the patient does not regain consciousness. Hypotension, hypoxia, and cardiac dysrhythmias may also occur. There is a high risk of permanent brain damage and death unless prompt, appropriate treatment is instituted. In a person taking medications for a diagnosed seizure disorder, the most common cause of status epilepticus is abruptly stopping AEDs. In other patients, regardless of whether they have a diagnosed seizure disorder, causes of status epilepticus include brain trauma or tumors, systemic or central nervous system (CNS) infections, alcohol withdrawal, and overdoses of drugs (e.g., cocaine, theophylline).

General Characteristics of Antiseizure Drugs

Antiseizure drugs can usually control seizure activity but do not cure the underlying disorder. Numerous difficulties, for both clinicians and patients, have been associated with AED therapy, including trials of different drugs; consideration of monotherapy versus combination therapy using two or more drugs; the need to titrate dosage over time; lack of seizure control while drugs are being selected and dosages adjusted; social stigma and adverse drug effects, often leading to poor patient compliance; and undesirable drug interactions among AEDs and between AEDs and other medications. Attempts to overcome these difficulties have led to the development of several new drugs in recent years.

Drug therapy for epilepsy is rapidly evolving as older, more toxic drugs are being replaced by newer drugs with better adverse effect profiles that maintain better control of seizures. In this chapter, older drugs that are still commonly used (phenytoin, carbamazepine, ethosuximide, phenobarbital, valproate) as well as newer drugs (gabapentin, lamotrigine, levetiracetam, oxcarbazepine, tiagabine, topiramate, zonisamide) are discussed.

Mechanism of Action

Although the exact mechanism of action of most AEDs is unknown, the drugs are thought to suppress seizures in one of the following ways: by decreasing movement of ions into nerve cells, by altering the activity of neurotransmitters (e.g., gamma-aminobutyric acid [GABA], glutamate), or by a combination of these mechanisms. Because movement of sodium and calcium ions is required for normal conduction of nerve impulses, blocking these ions decreases responsiveness to stimuli and results in stabilized, less excitable cell membranes. Increasing the activity of GABA, the major inhibitory neurotransmitter in the brain, and decreasing the activity of glutamate, the major excitatory neurotransmitter, also decrease nerve cell excitability. The actions of both sodium channel blockers (e.g., phenytoin, oxcarbazepine) and GABA enhancers (e.g., benzodiazepines, most of the newer AEDs) increase the amount of stimulation required to produce a seizure (called the *seizure threshold*). Overall, the AEDs are thought to stabilize neuronal membranes and decrease neuronal firing in response to stimuli. Some seem able to suppress abnormal neuronal firing without suppressing normal neurotransmission.

Indications for Use

The major clinical indication for AEDs is the prevention or treatment of seizures, especially the chronic recurring seizures of epilepsy. Indications for particular drugs depend on the types and severity of seizures involved. For example, most of the newer drugs are indicated for use with one or two other AEDs to treat more severe seizure disorders that do not respond to a single drug. However, oxcarbazepine is approved for monotherapy, and studies indicate that most of the other newer drugs may also be effective as monotherapy in some types of seizures.

In addition to maintenance treatment of epilepsy, AEDs are used to stop acute, tonic-clonic convulsions and status epilepticus. The drug of choice is an intravenous (IV) benzodiazepine, usually lorazepam. A systematic review of trials in both adult and pediatric patients concluded lorazepam was significantly better than diazepam or phenytoin for the immediate control of status epilepticus (Level A). After acute seizure activity is controlled, a longer-acting drug, such as phenytoin or fosphenytoin, is given to prevent recurrence. AEDs also are used prophylactically in patients with brain trauma from injury or surgery.

In addition to seizure disorders, AEDs are used to treat bipolar disorder (e.g., carbamazepine, valproate). The Food and Drug Administration (FDA) has recently approved valproate for the treatment of acute mania. Carbamazepine has also been found useful, especially in more refractory bipolar episodes. Often these medications are combined with lithium for maximum effect. Both drugs are also used in the management of chronic neuropathic pain. Carbamazepine is approved for treatment of the pain associated with trigeminal neuralgia.

Gabapentin is the first oral medication approved by the FDA for the management of postherpetic neuralgia. Studies indicate that patients receiving gabapentin experienced significant pain relief, improvement in sleep, and improved overall quality of life. Some of the other, newer AEDs are being tested for effectiveness in relation to bipolar, neuropathic pain, and other disorders. Because the drugs are being used for other indi-

cations than seizure disorders, some people suggest they be called neuromodulators or neurostabilizers rather than AEDs or anticonvulsants.

Contraindications to Use

AEDs are contraindicated or must be used with caution in patients with CNS depression. Phenytoin, carbamazepine, gabapentin, lamotrigine, levetiracetam, oxcarbazepine, tiagabine, topiramate, and valproate are contraindicated in patients who have experienced a hypersensitivity reaction to the particular drug (usually manifested by a skin rash, arthralgia, and other symptoms). Phenytoin, carbamazepine, ethosuximide, lamotrigine, topiramate, and zonisamide are contraindicated or must be used cautiously in patients with hepatic or renal impairment. Additional contraindications include phenytoin in patients with sinus bradycardia or heart block, carbamazepine in those with bone marrow depression (e.g., leukopenia, agranulocytosis), and tiagabine and valproic acid in people with liver disease. All of the drugs must be used cautiously during pregnancy because they are teratogenic in animals.

Individual Drugs

Most AEDs are well absorbed with oral administration and are usually given by this route. Most are metabolized in the liver, and a few are eliminated mainly through the kidneys. The large majority commonly produce adverse effects such as ataxia (impaired muscular coordination such as a staggering gait when trying to walk), confusion, dizziness, and drowsiness. Some may cause serious or life-threatening adverse effects such as cardiac dysrhythmias, bone marrow depression, or pancreatitis. Because AEDs are so diverse, they cannot be adequately discussed as groups. Consequently, the drugs are described indi-

Table 11-1		**Drugs at a Glance:** Antiseizure Drugs		
		ROUTES AND DOSAGE RANGES		
Generic/Trade Name	**Types of Seizures Used to Treat**	**Adults**	**Children**	**Remarks**
Carbamazepine (Tegretol)	Partial, generalized tonic-clonic, and mixed seizures	Epilepsy, PO 200 mg twice daily, increased gradually to 600–1200 mg daily if needed, in 3 or 4 divided doses Trigeminal neuralgia, PO 200 mg daily, increased gradually to 1200 mg if necessary Bipolar disorder, PO 400 mg in 2 divided doses, increased gradually to 1600 mg if necessary	>12 y: PO 200 mg twice daily; may increase to 1000 mg daily for children 12–15 years and 1200 mg for children over 15 y, if necessary 6–12 y: PO 100 mg twice daily (tablet) or 50 mg 4 times daily (suspension), increase to 1000 mg daily if necessary, in 3 or 4 divided doses	■ Available in oral and chewable tablets, extended-release tablets and capsules, and a suspension of 100 mg/5 mL ■ The suspension is absorbed more rapidly and produces higher peak drug levels than tablets. ■ Therapeutic serum drug level is 4 to 12 mcg/mL (SI units, 17–51 µmol/L).

		ROUTES AND DOSAGE RANGES		
Generic/Trade Name	**Types of Seizures Used to Treat**	**Adults**	**Children**	**Remarks**
Clonazepam (Klonopin)	Myoclonic or akinetic seizures, alone or with other AEDs; possibly effective in generalized tonic-clonic and psychomotor seizures	PO 1.5 mg/d, increased by 0.5 mg/d every 3–7 d if necessary; maximum dose, 20 mg/d	PO 0.01–0.03 mg/kg/d, increased by 0.25–0.5 mg/d every 3–7 days if necessary; maximum dose, 0.2 mg/kg/d	Schedule IV drug
Clorazepate (Tranxene)	Partial seizures, with other AEDs	PO maximal initial dose 7.5 mg 3 times daily; increased by 7.5 mg every week, if necessary; maximum dose, 90 mg/d	>12 y: PO same as adults 9–12 y: PO maximal initial dose 7.5 mg two times daily; increased by 7.5 mg every week, if necessary; maximum dose, 60 mg/d	Schedule IV drug
Diazepam (Valium)	Acute convulsive seizures, status epilepticus	IV 5–10 mg no faster than 2 mg/min; repeat every 5–10 min if needed; maximum dose, 30 mg. Repeat in 2–4 h if necessary; maximum dose, 100 mg/24 h	>30 d and <5 y of age: IV 0.2–0.5 mg over 2–3 min, every 2–5 min up to a maximum of 5 mg 5 y and older: IV 1 mg every 2–5 min up to a maximum of 10 mg. Repeat in 2–4 h if necessary.	Schedule IV drug
Ethosuximide (Zarontin)	Absence seizures; also may be effective in myoclonic and akinetic epilepsy	PO initially 500 mg/d, increased by 250 mg weekly until seizures are controlled or toxicity occurs; maximum dose, 1500 mg/d	PO initially 250 mg/d, increased at weekly intervals until seizures are controlled or toxicity occurs; maximum dose, approximately 750–1000 mg/d	Available in oral capsules and syrup Therapeutic serum drug level is 40–80 mcg/mL.
Fosphenytoin (Cerebyx)	Status epilepticus and short-term use in clients who cannot take oral phenytoin	Nonemergent seizures, IV, IM loading dose 10–20 mg PE/kg; maintenance dose 4–6 mg PE/kg/d; status epilepticus, IV 15–20 mg PE/kg, at a rate of 100–150 mg PE/min	<12 y: Loading dose (if not pervious phenytoin): 10–20 mg PE/kg IV no faster than 3 mg PE/kg/min (no >150 mg/min) Maintenance dose, 4–6 mg PE/kg/d divided into 2 or more doses	Much easier to give IV than phenytoin; can also be given IM
Gabapentin (Neurontin)	Partial seizures, with other AEDs	PO 900 mg daily, in 3 divided doses; increased up to 1800 mg/d if necessary. Intervals between doses should not exceed 12 h. Renal impairment: Crcl >60 mL/min, 400 mg 3 times daily (1200 mg/d); Crcl 30–60 mL/min, 300 mg 2 times daily (600 mg/d); Crcl 15–30 mL/min, 300 mg once daily; Crcl <15 mL/min, 300 mg every other day. For patients on hemodialysis, 200–300 mg after each 4 h of hemodialysis.	>12 y: PO 900–1800 mg/d, in 3 divided doses (same as adults) 3–12 y: 10–15 mg/kg/d, in 3 divided doses, increased if necessary. Intervals between doses should not exceed 12 h.	Does not cause significant drug–drug interactions Clinical trial data indicate that monitoring serum levels is not necessary for safe use.

(continued on page 200)

| Table 11-1 | **Drugs at a Glance:** Antiseizure Drugs (continued) |

Generic/Trade Name	Types of Seizures Used To Treat	ROUTES AND DOSAGE RANGES		
		Adults	**Children**	**Remarks**
Lamotrigine (Lamictal)	Partial seizures, with other AEDs Lennox-Gastaut syndrome, with other AEDs	With AEDs other than valproic acid: PO 50 mg once daily for 2 wk, then 50 mg twice daily (100 mg/d) for 2 wk, then increase by 100 mg/d at weekly intervals to a maintenance dose. Usual maintenance dose, 300–500 mg/d in 2 divided doses. With AEDs including valproic acid: PO 25 mg every other day for 2 wk, then 25 mg once daily for 2 wk, then increase by 25 to 50 mg/d every 1–2 wk to a maintenance dose. Usual maintenance dose, 100–150 mg/d in 2 divided doses.	2–12 y: With enzyme-inducing AEDs, initially, PO 0.15 mg/kg/d in 1 or 2 doses for 2 wk. If calculated dose is 2.5–5 mg, give 5 mg on alternate days for 2 wk, then 0.3 mg/kg/d in 1 or 2 doses, rounded to nearest 5 mg, for 2 wk. Maintenance dose, PO 5–15 mg/kg/d in 2 divided doses >12 y: With enzyme-inducing AEDs, initially, PO 25 mg every other day for 2 wk, then 25 mg daily for 2 wk Maintenance dose, PO 100–400 mg daily in 1 or 2 divided doses With valproic acid, PO 50 mg daily for 2 wk, then 100 mg daily in 2 divided doses for 2 wk Maintenance dose, PO 300–500 mg daily in 1 or 2 doses	Valproic acid slows lamotrigine's metabolism by approximately 50%. If lamotrigine is combined with other AEDs plus valproic acid, dosage must be substantially reduced.
Levetiracetam (Keppra)	Partial seizures, with other AEDs	PO 500 mg twice daily initially, increased by 1000 mg/d every 2 wk, if necessary. Maximum dose, 3000 mg daily. *Renal Impairment:* Crcl >80, 500–1500 mg; Crcl 50–80, 500–1000 mg; Crcl 30–50, 250–750 mg; Crcl <30, 250–500 mg End-stage renal disease, on hemodialysis, 500–1000 mg, with a supplemental dose of half the total daily dose (250–500 mg)	For adjunctive treatment of partial seizures or refractory seizures: 4-5 y: 10 mg/kg PO twice daily, can increase the daily dose every 2 wk by increments of 20 mg/kg to recommended dose of 30 mg/kg twice daily (60 mg/kg/d).	Tablets should be swallowed whole; should not crush or chew tablets
Lorazepam (Ativan)	Acute convulsive seizures, status epilepticus	IV 2–10 mg, diluted in an equal amount of sterile water for injection, 0.9% sodium chloride injection, or 5% dextrose in water, and injected over 2 min	0.1 mg/kg IV over 2–5 min for status. A second dose of 0.05 mg/kg IV may be repeated in 10–15 min if needed.	Schedule IV drug

ROUTES AND DOSAGE RANGES

Generic/Trade Name	Types of Seizures Used To Treat	Adults	Children	Remarks
Oxcarbazepine (Trileptal)	Partial seizures, as monotherapy or with other AEDs in adults, with other AEDs in children 4–16 years old	PO 600 mg twice daily (1200 mg/d); maximum dose, 2400 mg/d Severe renal impairment (Crcl <30 mL/min), PO 300 mg twice daily (600 mg/d) and increased slowly until response achieved	With other AEDs, PO 8–10 mg/kg/d, not to exceed 600 mg twice daily. Titrate to reach target dose over 2 wk.	▪ Available in 150-, 300-, and 600-mg scored tablets and a 60 mg/mL fruit-flavored suspension
Phenobarbital	Generalized tonic-clonic and partial seizures	PO 100–300 mg daily in 2–3 divided doses	PO 5 mg/kg per day in 2–3 divided doses	Serum drug levels of 10–25 mcg/mL are in the therapeutic range.
P **Phenytoin** (Dilantin)	Generalized tonic-clonic and some partial seizures Prevention and treatment of seizures occurring during or after neurosurgery	PO 100 mg three times daily initially; 300 mg (long-acting) once daily as maintenance IV 100 mg q6–8h; maximum 50 mg/min	PO 4–7 mg/kg/d in divided doses. Dosing children is highly variable; dosage adjustment based on serum concentrations.	▪ Available in chewable tablets, oral suspension, immediate-release and extended-release capsules, and solution for injection ▪ Therapeutic serum level is 5–20 mcg/mL (SI units 40–80 μmol/L). Concentrations at or above the upper therapeutic level may be associated with toxicity.
Tiagabine (Gabitril)	Partial seizures, with other AEDs	PO 4 mg daily for 1 wk, increased by 4–8 mg/wk until desired effect; maximum dose 56 mg/d in 2–4 divided doses.	12–18 y: PO 4 mg daily for 1 wk, increased to 8 mg/d in 2 divided doses for 1 wk; then increased by 4–8 mg/wk up to a maximum of 32 mg/d in 2 to 4 divided doses <12 y: not recommended.	Most experience obtained in patients receiving at least one concomitant enzymeinducing AED. Use in noninduced patients (e.g., those receiving valproate monotherapy) may require lower doses or a slower dose titration.
Topiramate (Topamax)	Partial seizures, with other AEDs	PO 25–50 mg daily, increased by 25–50 mg per week until response. Usual dose, 400 mg daily in 2 divided doses.	2–16 y: PO wk 1, 25 mg every P.M., increase by 1–3 mg/kg/d at 1- or 2-wk intervals until response. Usual dose 5–9 mg/kg/d, in 2 divided doses.	

(continued on page 202)

Table 11-1	Drugs at a Glance: Antiseizure Drugs (continued)

		ROUTES AND DOSAGE RANGES		
Generic/Trade Name	**Types of Seizures Used To Treat**	**Adults**	**Children**	**Remarks**
Valproic acid (Depakene capsules); **Sodium valproate** (Depakene syrup, Depacon injection); **Divalproex sodium** (Depakote enteric-coated tablets)	Absence, mixed, and complex partial seizures	PO 10–15 mg/kg/d, increase weekly by 5–10 mg/kg/d, until seizures controlled, adverse effects occur, or the maximum dose (60 mg/kg/d) is reached. Give amounts >250 mg/d in divided doses. Usual daily dose, 1000–1600 mg, in divided doses. IV client's usual dose, diluted in 5% dextrose or 0.9% sodium chloride injection	PO 15–30 mg/kg/d	■ Therapeutic serum levels are 50–100 mcg/mL (SI units 350–700 µmol/L) ■ Note: Dosage ranges are the same for the different formulations; doses are in valproic acid equivalents. ■ Do not give IV >14 d; switch to oral product when possible. Several formulations of valproic acid are available in the United States. These products may contain valproic acid as the acid, as the sodium salt (sodium valproate), or a combination of the two (divalproex sodium).
Zonisamide (Zonegran)	Partial seizures, with other AEDs	PO 100–200 mg daily as a single dose or as 2–3 divided doses; increase by 100 mg/d every 1–2 wk if necessary; maximum dose, 600 mg daily	<16 y: 1–2 mg/kg PO given once daily or in divided doses twice daily; increase by 1–2 mg/kg/d only every 1–2 wk. Target range is 4–8 mg/kg/d.	Individuals allergic to sulfonamide should not take zonisamide.

AED, antiepileptic drug; Crcl, creatinine clearance; µmol/L, micromol/L; PE, phenytoin equivalent.

vidually. Types of seizures for which the drugs are used and specific dosages are listed in Table 11-1.

P **Phenytoin** (Dilantin), the prototype, is one of the oldest and most widely used AEDs. It is often the initial drug of choice, especially in adults. In addition to treatment of seizure disorders, it is sometimes used to treat cardiac dysrhythmias.

With oral phenytoin, the rate and extent of absorption vary with the drug formulation. Peak plasma drug levels occur in 2 to 3 hours with prompt-acting forms and in about 12 hours in long-acting forms. Intramuscular (IM) phenytoin is poorly absorbed and not recommended. The drug is metabolized in the liver to inactive metabolites that are excreted in the urine.

Phenytoin is highly bound (90%) to plasma proteins, and only the free drug (the fraction not bound to plasma albumin) is therapeutically active. For most people, dosage is calculated on the basis of the total phenytoin value. The recognized therapeutic range, assuming a normal plasma albumin level, reflects the amount of phenytoin that is bound to albumin along with the unbound (free) portion. Monitoring the free phenytoin serum level (normal levels 0.8 to 2.0 mcg/mL) should be done in patients with altered albumin levels (elderly persons or those with cirrhosis, burns, malnutrition, cachexia, or nephrotic syndrome) and with factors that may decrease the affinity of phenytoin for albumin or cause displacement of the drug (e.g., renal failure, interacting drugs [warfarin, salicylate, valproate], or increased bilirubin). Conditions or factors that decrease binding increase the available free portion of the drug and therefore these patients require lower-than-normal total plasma levels to achieve the normal therapeutic effects.

The most common adverse effects of phenytoin affect the CNS (e.g., ataxia, drowsiness, lethargy) and gastrointestinal (GI) tract (e.g., nausea, vomiting). *Gingival hyperplasia*, an overgrowth of gum tissue, is also common, especially in children. Long-term use may lead to an increased risk of osteoporosis because of its effect on vitamin D metabolism. Serious reactions are uncommon but may include allergic reactions, hepatitis, nephritis, bone marrow depression, and mental confusion.

Phenytoin may interact with many other drugs, mainly because it induces drug-metabolizing enzymes in the liver. Thus, it can increase the metabolism of itself and many other drugs, both AEDs and non-AEDs. In addition, many other drugs can affect phenytoin metabolism and protein binding.

Phenytoin is available as a capsule (generic and brand name), chewable tablet, oral suspension, and injectable solution. The injectable solution is highly irritating to tissues, and special techniques are required when the drug is given IV. Patients should not switch between generic and trade name formulations of phenytoin because of differences in absorption and bioavailability. If a patient is stabilized on a generic formulation and switches to Dilantin, there is a risk of higher serum phenytoin levels and toxicity. If a patient takes Dilantin and switches to a generic form, there is a risk of lower serum phenytoin levels, loss of therapeutic effectiveness, and seizures. There may also be differences in bioavailability among generic formulations manufactured by different companies.

Applying Your Knowledge 11-1

How do you determine if Frank is receiving an adequate dosage of phenytoin?

Fosphenytoin (Cerebyx) is a water-soluble prodrug formulation that is rapidly hydrolyzed to phenytoin after IV or IM injection. It is approved for treatment of status epilepticus and for short-term use in patients who cannot take oral phenytoin. In contrast to other preparations of injectable phenytoin, fosphenytoin causes minimal tissue irritation, can be diluted with 5% dextrose or 0.9% sodium chloride solution, and can be given IV more rapidly. Dose, concentration in dosing solutions, and infusion rate of IV fosphenytoin is expressed as phenytoin sodium equivalents (PE) to prevent the need for calculating molecular weight–based adjustments when converting between fosphenytoin and phenytoin sodium doses. Fosphenytoin is available in 2-mL and 10-mL vials with 50 mg PE/mL (fosphenytoin 50 mg PE = phenytoin 50 mg). For IV administration, fosphenytoin can be diluted to a concentration of 1.5 to 25 mg PE/mL, and infused at a maximal rate of 150 mg PE/minute.

Carbamazepine (Tegretol) is used to treat seizure disorders as well as trigeminal neuralgia and bipolar disorder. It is given orally, and peak blood levels are reached in about 1.5 hours with the liquid suspension, in 4 to 5 hours with conventional tablets, and in 3 to 12 hours with extended-release forms (tablets and capsules). Carbamazepine is metabolized in the

liver to an active metabolite. Because it induces its own metabolism, its half-life shortens with chronic administration. It is contraindicated in patients with previous bone marrow depression or hypersensitivity to carbamazepine and in those taking monoamine oxidase (MAO) inhibitors. MAO inhibitors should be discontinued at least 14 days before carbamazepine is started. Different brands may not be bioequivalent and should not be used interchangeably without evaluating serum blood levels. The drug has a narrow therapeutic index and the FDA has issued a **BLACK BOX WARNING** regarding the development of an aplastic anemia and agranulocytosis with use of carbamazepine.

Applying Your Knowledge 11-2

Even though Frank has not indicated a history of a psychiatric disorder, what question should you ask before Frank begins treatment with the carbamazepine?

Clonazepam (Klonopin), **clorazepate** (Tranxene), **diazepam** (Valium), and **lorazepam** (Ativan) are benzodiazepines (see Chap. 8) used in seizure disorders. Clonazepam and clorazepate are used in long-term treatment of seizure disorders, alone or with other AEDs. Tolerance to antiseizure effects develops with long-term use. Clonazepam has a long half-life and may require weeks of continued administration to achieve therapeutic serum blood levels. As with other benzodiazepines, clonazepam produces physical dependence and withdrawal symptoms. Because of clonazepam's long half-life, withdrawal symptoms may appear several days after administration is stopped. Abrupt withdrawal may precipitate seizure activity or status epilepticus.

Diazepam and lorazepam are used to terminate acute convulsive seizures, especially the life-threatening seizures of status epilepticus. Diazepam has a short duration of action and must be given in repeated doses. Lorazepam has become the drug of choice to treat status epilepticus because its effects last longer than those of diazepam.

Ethosuximide (Zarontin) is the AED of choice for absence seizures and may be used with other AEDs for treatment of mixed types of seizures. It is well absorbed after oral administration and reaches peak serum levels in 3 to 7 hours; a steady-state serum concentration is reached in about 5 days. It is eliminated mainly by hepatic metabolism to inactive metabolites, and about 20% is excreted unchanged through the kidneys. Its elimination half-life is approximately 30 hours in children and 60 hours in adults.

Gabapentin (Neurontin) is used with other AEDs for treatment of partial seizures. In addition, it is commonly used to treat postherpetic neuralgia and other conditions such as chronic pain syndromes, including neuropathies (i.e., diabetic and others). Gabapentin is 60% absorbed with usual doses, circulates largely in a free state because of minimal binding to plasma proteins, is not appreciably metabolized, and is eliminated by the kidneys as unchanged drug. Its elimination half-life is 5 to 7 hours in patients with normal renal function and as much as 50 hours in patients with impaired renal function, depending on creatinine clearance.

Adverse effects of gabapentin include dizziness, drowsiness, fatigue, loss of muscle coordination, tremor, nausea, vomiting, abnormal vision, gingivitis, and pruritus. Most adverse effects subside spontaneously or with dosage reduction. However, the first dose of gabapentin should be administered at bedtime, because the drug can cause significant somnolence and dizziness with the first dose. Gabapentin reportedly does not cause significant drug–drug interactions. Because the drug is eliminated only by the kidneys, dosage must be reduced in patients with renal impairment. Although it is structurally related to GABA, the drug does not interact with GABA receptors in the brain; its mechanism of action is unknown.

Lamotrigine (Lamictal) is used with other AEDs for treatment of partial seizures. It is thought to reduce the release of glutamate, an excitatory neurotransmitter, in the brain. It is well absorbed after oral administration, with peak plasma levels reached in 1.5 to 4.5 hours. Lamotrigine is about 55% bound to plasma proteins. It is metabolized in the liver to an inactive metabolite and eliminated mainly in the urine.

Adverse effects of lamotrigine include dizziness, drowsiness, headache, ataxia, blurred or double vision, nausea and vomiting, and weakness. The FDA has issued a **BLACK BOX WARNING** related to the potential development of serious dermatologic reactions. Because a serious skin rash may occur, especially in children, lamotrigine should not be given to children younger than 16 years of age and should be discontinued at the first sign of skin rash in an adult. Skin rash is more likely to occur with concomitant valproic acid therapy, high lamotrigine starting dose, and rapid titration rate. It may resolve if lamotrigine is discontinued, but it progresses in some patients to more severe forms, such as Stevens-Johnson syndrome or toxic epidermal necrosis.

Lamotrigine has little effect on the metabolism of other AEDs, but other AEDs affect its metabolism. Phenytoin, carbamazepine, and phenobarbital induce drug-metabolizing enzymes in the liver and accelerate its metabolism. Valproic acid inhibits those enzymes and thereby slows its metabolism by approximately 50%. If lamotrigine is combined with other AEDs plus valproic acid, dosage must be substantially reduced. To discontinue, dosage should be tapered over at least 2 weeks.

Levetiracetam (Keppra) is a newer drug approved for treatment of partial seizures, in combination with other AEDs. It is chemically unrelated to other AEDs, and its mechanism of action is unknown. It inhibits abnormal neuronal firing but does not affect normal neuronal excitability or function.

Levetiracetam is well and rapidly absorbed with oral administration; peak plasma levels occur in about 1 hour. Food reduces peak plasma levels by 20%, and these levels do not occur until 1.5 hours; however, this does not affect the extent of drug absorption. The drug is minimally bound (10%) to plasma proteins and reaches steady-state plasma concentrations after 2 days of twice-daily administration. This rapid attainment of therapeutic effects is especially useful for patients with frequent or severe seizures. The majority of a dose (66%) is eliminated by the kidneys as unchanged drug, and the dose must be reduced in patients with impaired renal function. The drug is not metabolized by the liver and does not affect the hepatic metabolism of other drugs. Thus, it has a low potential for drug interactions.

Levetiracetam was well tolerated in clinical trials, and the incidence of adverse events was similar to that of placebo. Common adverse effects include drowsiness, dizziness, and fatigue. Others include decreases in red and white blood cell counts, double vision, amnesia, anxiety, ataxia, emotional lability, hostility, nervousness, paresthesia, pharyngitis, and rhinitis.

Overall, levetiracetam has pharmacokinetic and other characteristics that may make it especially useful in patients who require combination AED therapy, who take drugs with increased potential for drug interactions, or who have impaired liver function.

Oxcarbazepine (Trileptal) is a newer drug that is structurally related to carbamazepine. It is approved for both monotherapy and adjunctive (with other AEDs) therapy in adults with partial seizures and for adjunctive therapy only in children. For patients receiving carbamazepine or oxcarbazepine, either drug may be substituted for the other without tapering the dose of one or gradually increasing the dose of the other. However, the equivalent dosage of oxcarbazepine is 50% higher than the carbamazepine dosage. In older adults, the recommended equivalent oxcarbazepine dosage is 20% higher than the carbamazepine dosage.

Oxcarbazepine is well absorbed after oral administration, with peak plasma levels occurring in about 5 hours. Most effects are attributed to an active metabolite produced during first-pass metabolism in the liver; the metabolite is 40% protein bound. The elimination half-life is 2 hours for oxcarbazepine and 9 hours for the metabolite. The metabolite is conjugated with glucuronic acid in the liver and excreted in the urine, along with a small amount of unchanged drug. Dosage must be reduced in patients with severe renal impairment (i.e., creatinine clearance < 30 mL/min).

Adverse effects are similar in adult and pediatric patients and when oxcarbazepine is used alone or with other AEDs. They include cardiac dysrhythmias, drowsiness, dizziness, hypotension, nausea, vomiting, skin rash, and hyponatremia. A Cochrane systematic review indicated that oxcarbazepine added to other AEDs was significantly more effective than placebo in decreasing seizure frequency in adults and children with drug-resistant partial epilepsy (Level A). Because of the risk of hyponatremia, oxcarbazepine should be used with caution in patients taking other drugs that decrease serum sodium levels, and serum sodium levels should be monitored periodically during maintenance therapy. Some studies indicate that skin reactions occur less often with oxcarbazepine than with carbamazepine.

Several drug–drug interactions may occur with oxcarbazepine. The drug inhibits cytochrome P450 2C19 enzymes and induces 3A4 enzymes to influence the metabolism of other drugs metabolized by these enzymes. For example, oxcarbazepine increases metabolism of estrogens and may decrease the effectiveness of oral contraceptives and postmenopausal estrogen replacement therapy. In addition, other drugs that induce cytochrome P450 enzymes, including phenytoin, may reduce plasma levels of the active metabolite by about one third. Drugs that inhibit these enzymes (e.g., cimetidine, erythromycin) do not significantly affect the elimination of oxcarbazepine or its metabolite.

Phenobarbital is a long-acting barbiturate that is used alone or with another AED (most often phenytoin). Its use has declined with the advent of other AEDs that cause less sedation and cognitive impairment. CNS depression and other adverse effects associated with barbiturates may occur, but drug dependence and barbiturate intoxication are unlikely with usual antiepileptic doses. Because phenobarbital has a long half-life (50 to 140 hours), it takes 2 to 3 weeks to reach therapeutic serum levels and 3 to 4 weeks to reach a steady-state concentration. It is metabolized in the liver; about 25% is eliminated unchanged in the urine. It induces drug-metabolizing enzymes in the liver and thereby accelerates the metabolism of most AEDs when given with them. Effects on other drugs begin 1 or 2 weeks after phenobarbital therapy is started.

Tiagabine (Gabitril), which may increase GABA levels in the brain, is used with other AEDs in patients with partial seizures. After oral administration, tiagabine is well absorbed; peak plasma levels occur in about 45 minutes if taken on an empty stomach and 2.5 hours if taken with food. It is highly protein bound (96%) and is extensively metabolized in the liver by the cytochrome P450 3A family of enzymes. Only 1% of the drug is excreted unchanged in the urine, and the metabolites are excreted in urine and feces. The elimination half-life is 4 to 7 hours in patients receiving enzyme-inducing AEDs (e.g., phenytoin, carbamazepine). Patients with impaired liver function may need smaller doses because the drug is cleared more slowly. CNS effects (e.g., confusion, drowsiness, impaired concentration or speech) are the most common adverse effects. GI upset and a serious skin rash may also occur.

Topiramate (Topamax), which has a broad spectrum of antiseizure activity, may act by increasing the effects of GABA and other mechanisms. It is rapidly absorbed and produces peak plasma levels about 2 hours after oral administration. The average elimination half-life is about 21 hours, and steady-state concentrations are reached in about 4 days with normal renal function. It is 20% bound to plasma proteins. Topiramate is not extensively metabolized and is primarily eliminated unchanged through the kidneys. For patients with a creatinine clearance below 70 milliliters per minute, dosage should be reduced by one half.

The most common adverse effects are ataxia, drowsiness, dizziness, and nausea. Renal stones may also occur. Interventions to help prevent renal stones include maintaining an adequate fluid intake, avoiding concurrent use of topiramate with other drugs associated with renal stone formation or increased urinary pH (e.g., triamterene, zonisamide), and avoiding topiramate in people with conditions requiring fluid restriction (e.g., heart failure) or a history of renal stones. Additive CNS depression may occur with alcohol and other CNS depressant drugs.

Valproic acid preparations (Depakene, Depakote, Depacon) are chemically unrelated to other AEDs. They are thought to enhance the effects of GABA in the brain and are also used to treat manic reactions in bipolar disorder and to prevent migraine headache. Valproic acid preparations are well absorbed after oral administration and produce peak plasma levels in 1 to 4 hours (15 minutes to 2 hours with the syrup). They are highly bound (90%) to plasma proteins. They are primarily metabolized in the liver, and metabolites are excreted through the kidneys. Valproic acid (Depakene) is available in capsules, and sodium valproate is a syrup formulation. Divalproex sodium (Depakote) contains equal parts of valproic acid and sodium valproate and is available as delayed-release tablets and sprinkle capsules. Depacon is an injectable formulation of valproate. Dosages of all formulations are expressed in valproic acid equivalents. The FDA has issued a **BLACK BOX WARNING** as hepatic failure and life-threatening pancreatitis have been reported in both children and adults receiving valproate. In addition, valproate can produce teratogenic effects such as neural tube defects if taken during pregnancy.

Depakene, Depakote, and Depacon all produce less sedation and cognitive impairment than phenytoin and phenobarbital. Potentially serious adverse effects, although uncommon, include hepatotoxicity and pancreatitis. The drugs are contraindicated in people who have had hypersensitivity reactions to any of the preparations and people with hepatic disease or impaired hepatic function.

Zonisamide (Zonegran) is chemically a sulfonamide. (It is contraindicated for use in patients who are allergic to sulfonamides.) It is approved for adjunctive treatment of partial seizures and may also be effective for monotherapy and generalized seizures. It is thought to act by inhibiting the entry of sodium and calcium ions into nerve cells.

Zonisamide is well absorbed with oral administration and produces peak plasma levels in 2 to 6 hours. It is 40% bound to plasma proteins and also binds extensively to red blood cells. Its elimination half-life is about 63 hours in plasma and more than 100 hours in red blood cells. It is metabolized by the cytochrome P450 3A enzymes and perhaps other pathways. It is excreted in the urine as unchanged drug (35%) and metabolites (65%). Patients with impaired renal function may require lower doses or a slower titration schedule.

Adverse effects of zonisamide include drowsiness, dizziness, ataxia, confusion, abnormal thinking, nervousness, and fatigue, which can be reduced by increasing the dosage gradually, over several weeks. There is also a risk of kidney stones, which is higher in patients with an inadequate fluid intake or who also take topiramate or triamterene. Skin rash, including the life-threatening Stevens-Johnson syndrome, has been observed.

Drugs that induce the cytochrome P450 enzymes (e.g., carbamazepine, phenytoin) increase the metabolism of zonisamide and reduce its half-life. However, administration with cimetidine, which inhibits the cytochrome P450 enzymes, does not seem to inhibit zonisamide metabolism or increase its half-life.

Zonisamide apparently does not induce or inhibit cytochrome P450 enzymes and therefore has little effect on the metabolism of other drugs.

Nursing Process

Assessment

Assess patient status in relation to seizure activity and other factors:

- If the patient has a known seizure disorder and is taking antiseizure drugs, helpful assessment data can be obtained by interviewing the client. Some questions and guidelines include the following:

  - How long has the patient had the seizure disorder?

  - How long has it been since seizure activity occurred, or what is the frequency of seizures?

  - Does any particular situation or activity precipitate a seizure?

  - How does the seizure affect the patient? For example, what parts of the body are involved? Does he or she lose consciousness? Is he or she drowsy and tired afterward?

  - Which antiseizure drugs are taken? How do they affect the patient? How long has the patient taken the drugs? Is the currently ordered dosage the same as what the patient has been taking? Does the patient usually take the drugs as prescribed, or does he or she find it difficult to do so?

  - What other drugs are taken? This includes both prescription and nonprescription drugs, as well as those taken regularly or periodically. This information is necessary because many drugs interact with antiseizure drugs to decrease seizure control or increase drug toxicity.

  - What is the patient's attitude toward the seizure disorder? Clues to attitude may include terminology, willingness or reluctance to discuss the seizure disorder, compliance or rejection of drug therapy, and others.

- Check reports of serum drug levels for abnormal values.

- Identify risk factors for seizure disorders. In people without previous seizure activity, seizure disorders may develop with brain surgery, head injury, hypoxia, hypoglycemia, drug overdosage (CNS stimulants, such as amphetamines or cocaine, or local anesthetics, such as lidocaine), and withdrawal from CNS depressants, such as alcohol and barbiturates.

- To observe and record seizure activity accurately, note the location (localized or generalized); specific characteristics of abnormal movements or behavior; duration; concomi-

tant events, such as loss of consciousness and loss of bowel or bladder control; and postseizure behavior.

- Assess for risk of status epilepticus. Risk factors include recent changes in antiseizure drug therapy, chronic alcohol ingestion, use of drugs known to cause seizures, and infection.

Nursing Diagnoses

- Ineffective Coping related to denial of the disease process and need for long-term drug therapy
- Deficient Knowledge: Disease process
- Deficient Knowledge: Drug effects
- Risk for Injury: Trauma related to ataxia, dizziness, confusion
- Risk for Injury: Seizure activity or drug toxicity
- Ineffective Management of Therapeutic Regimen: Individual: Underuse of Medications

Planning/Goals

The patient will

- Take medications as prescribed
- Experience control of seizures
- Avoid serious adverse drug effects
- Verbalize knowledge of the disease process and treatment regimen
- Avoid discontinuing antiseizure medications abruptly
- Keep follow-up appointments with health care providers

Interventions

Use measures to minimize seizure activity. Guidelines include the following:

- Help the patient identify conditions under which seizures are likely to occur. These precipitating factors, to be avoided or decreased when possible, may include ingestion of alcoholic beverages or stimulant drugs; fever; severe physical or emotional stress; and sensory stimuli, such as flashing lights and loud noises. Identification of precipitating factors is important because lifestyle changes (e.g., reducing stress, reducing alcohol and caffeine intake, increasing exercise, improving sleep and diet) and treatment of existing disorders can reduce the frequency of seizures.

- Assist the patient in planning how to get enough rest and exercise and eat a balanced diet, if needed.

- Discuss the seizure disorder, the plan for treatment, and the importance of complying with prescribed drug therapy with the patient and family members (see accompanying patient teaching display).

- Involve the patient in decision making when possible.

- Inform the patient and family that seizure control is not gained immediately when drug therapy is started. The goal is to avoid unrealistic expectations and excessive frustration while drugs and dosages are being changed in an effort to determine the best regimen for the patient.

- Discuss social and economic factors that promote or prevent compliance.
- Protect a patient experiencing a generalized tonic-clonic seizure by
  - Placing a small pillow or piece of clothing under the head if injury could be sustained from the ground or floor
  - Not restraining the patient's movements; fractures may result
  - Loosening tight clothing, especially around the neck and chest, to promote respiration
  - Turning the patient to one side so that accumulated secretions can drain from the mouth and throat when convulsive movements stop. The cyanosis, abnormal movements, and loss of consciousness that characterize a generalized tonic-clonic seizure can be quite alarming to witnesses. Most of these seizures, however, subside within 3 or 4 minutes, and the person starts responding and regaining normal skin color. If the person has one seizure after another (status epilepticus), has trouble breathing or continued cyanosis, or has sustained an injury, further care is needed, and a physician should be notified immediately.
- When risk factors for seizures, especially status epilepticus, are identified, try to prevent or minimize their occurrence.

Evaluation

- Interview and observe for decrease in or absence of seizure activity.
- Interview and observe for avoidance of adverse drug effects, especially those that impair safety.
- When available, check laboratory reports of serum drug levels for therapeutic ranges or evidence of underdosing or overdosing.

Principles of Therapy

Goal of Therapy

Drug therapy is the main treatment of epilepsy for patients of all ages. The goal is to control seizure activity with minimal adverse drug effects. To meet this goal, therapy must be individualized. In most patients, treatment with a single AED is sufficient to meet this goal. However, in 20% to 30% of patients, two or more AEDs are required. In general, combination therapy is associated with more severe adverse effects, interactions among AEDs, poor compliance, and higher costs.

Drug Selection

Several factors should be considered when developing a therapeutic regimen using one or more AEDs.

Seizure Type

Type of seizure is a major factor in drug selection. Therefore, an accurate diagnosis is essential before drug therapy is started. In general, for activity against both partial and generalized seizures, the AEDs lamotrigine, levetiracetam, topiramate, valproic acid, and zonisamide are used. For partial seizures, carbamazepine, gabapentin, oxcarbazepine, phenobarbital, phenytoin, and tiagabine are considered most useful. For absence seizures, ethosuximide is the drug of choice, and clonazepam and valproate are also effective. For mixed seizures, a combination of drugs is usually necessary.

Guidelines for newer drugs are evolving as research studies are performed and clinical experience with their use increases. Most of these agents are approved for combination therapy with other AEDs in patients whose seizures are not adequately controlled with a single drug. However, oxcarbazepine is approved for monotherapy of partial seizures, and some other drugs are also thought to be effective as monotherapy (e.g., lamotrigine, valproate).

Adverse Effects

Adverse effects may be the deciding factor in choosing an AED because most types of seizures can be treated effectively by a variety of drugs. The use of carbamazepine and valproic acid increased largely because they cause less sedation and cognitive and psychomotor impairment than phenobarbital and phenytoin. Most of the newer AEDs reportedly cause fewer adverse effects and are better tolerated than the older drugs, even though these newer drugs may also cause potentially serious adverse effects. Fewer and milder adverse effects may greatly increase a patient's willingness to comply with the prescribed regimen and attain seizure control.

Monotherapy Versus Combination Therapy

A single drug (*monotherapy*) is recommended when possible. If effective in controlling seizures, monotherapy has the advantages of fewer adverse drug effects, fewer drug–drug interactions, lower cost, and usually greater patient compliance. If the first drug, in adequate dosage, fails to control seizures or causes unacceptable adverse effects, then another agent should be tried as monotherapy. Most practitioners recommend sequential trials of two to three agents as monotherapy before considering combination therapy.

When substituting one AED for another, the second drug should be added and allowed to reach therapeutic blood levels before the first drug is gradually decreased in dosage and discontinued. This is not necessary when substituting oxcarbazepine for carbamazepine or vice versa, because the drugs are similar.

When monotherapy is ineffective, a second, and sometimes a third, drug may be added. If combination therapy is

Patient Teaching Guidelines | Antiseizure Medications

General Considerations

- Take the medications as prescribed. This is extremely important. These drugs must be taken regularly to maintain blood levels adequate to control seizure activity. At the same time, additional doses must not be taken because of increased risks of serious adverse reactions.

- Do not suddenly stop taking any antiseizure medication. Severe, even life-threatening, seizures may occur if the drugs are stopped abruptly.

- Discuss any problems (e.g., seizure activity, excessive drowsiness, other adverse effects) associated with an antiseizure medication with the prescribing clinician or other health care professional. Adjusting dose or time of administration may relieve the problems.

- Do not drive a car, operate machinery, or perform other activities requiring physical and mental alertness when drowsy from antiseizure medications. Excessive drowsiness, decreased physical coordination, and decreased mental alertness increase the likelihood of injury.

- Do not take other drugs without the physician's knowledge and inform any other physician or dentist about taking antiseizure medications. There are many potential drug interactions in which the effects of the antiseizure drug or other drugs may be altered when drugs are given concomitantly.

- Do not take any other drugs that cause drowsiness, including over-the-counter antihistamines and sleep aids.

- Carry identification, such as a MedicAlert device, with the name and dose of the medication being taken. This is necessary for rapid and appropriate treatment in the event of a seizure, accidental injury, or other emergency situation.

- Notify your clinician if you become pregnant or intend to become pregnant during therapy. Oxcarbazepine (Trileptal) decreases the effectiveness of oral contraceptive drugs. Many antiseizure medications are tetragenic.

- Notify your clinician if you are breast-feeding or intend to breast-feed during therapy.

Self-Administration

- Take most antiseizure medications with food or a full glass of fluid. This will prevent or decrease nausea, vomiting, and gastric distress, which are adverse reactions to most of these drugs. Levetiracetam (Keppra), oxcarbazepine (Trileptal), topiramate (Topamax), and zonisamide (Zonegran) may be taken with or without food.

- When taking generic phenytoin or the Dilantin brand of phenytoin:

1. Do not switch from a generic to Dilantin, or vice versa, without discussing with the prescribing clinician. There are differences in formulations that may upset seizure control and cause adverse effects.

2. Ask your clinician if you should take (or give a child) supplements of folic acid, calcium, vitamin D, or vitamin K. These supplements may help to prevent some adverse effects of phenytoin.

3. Brush and floss your teeth and have regular dental care to prevent or delay a gum disorder called *gingival hyperplasia.*

4. If you have diabetes, you may need to check your blood sugar more often or take a higher dose of your antidiabetic medication. Phenytoin may inhibit the release of insulin and increase blood sugar.

5. Notify your clinician or another health care professional if you develop a skin rash, severe nausea and vomiting, swollen glands, bleeding, swollen or tender gums, yellowish skin or eyes, joint pain, unexplained fever, sore throat, unusual bleeding or bruising, persistent headache, or any indication of infection or bleeding, and if you become pregnant.

6. If you are taking phenytoin liquid suspension or giving it to a child, mix it thoroughly immediately before use and measure it with a calibrated medicine cup or a measuring teaspoon. Do not use regular teaspoons because they hold varying amounts of medication.

- If you are taking oxcarbazepine liquid suspension or giving it to a child, mix it thoroughly immediately before use. Measure it with the syringe supplied by the manufacturer and squirt the medication directly into the mouth. Store the suspension at room temperature and use the bottle within 7 weeks or discard the amount remaining. It is helpful to write the date opened and the expiration date on the container.

- With valproic acid, the regular capsule should not be opened and the tablet should not be crushed for administration. The sprinkle capsule may be opened and the contents sprinkled on soft food for administration. The syrup formulation may be diluted in water or milk but should not be mixed in carbonated beverages.

- Swallow tablets or capsules of valproic acid (Depakene or Depakote) whole; chewing or crushing may cause irritation of the mouth and throat.

- Taking valproic acid at bedtime may reduce dizziness and drowsiness.

- Lamotrigine may cause photosensitivity. When outdoors, wear protective clothing and sunscreen.

- If taking lamotrigine, notify the clinician immediately if a skin rash or decreased seizure control develops.

---

ineffective, the clinician may need to reassess the patient for type of seizure, medical conditions or drug–drug interactions that aggravate the seizure disorder or decrease the effectiveness of AEDs, and compliance with the prescribed drug therapy regimen.

Dosage Form

Dosage forms may increase seizure control, patient convenience, and compliance. For example, extended-release or long-acting dosage forms can maintain more consistent serum drug levels and decrease frequency of administration. Most of the AEDs are available in oral tablets or capsules, and a few are available as oral liquids or injectable solutions.

Cost

Cost should be considered because it may be a major factor in patient compliance. Although the newer drugs are generally effective and better tolerated than older agents, they are also quite expensive. When possible, clinicians can encourage compliance by choosing drugs that are covered by patients' insurance plans or, for uninsured patients, choosing less expensive drug therapy regimens or facilitating enrollment of the patient in manufacturer or state drug discount programs.

Pregnancy Risk

Sexually active adolescent girls and women of childbearing potential who require an AED must be evaluated and monitored very closely because all of the AEDs are considered teratogenic. In general, infants exposed to one AED have a significantly higher risk of birth defects than those who are not exposed, and infants exposed to two or more AEDs have a significantly higher risk than those exposed to one AED.

Drug Dosage

The dosage of most drugs is determined empirically by observation of seizure control and adverse effects.

- Usually, larger doses are needed for a single drug than for multiple drugs; for patients with a large body mass (assuming normal liver and kidney function); and in cases of trauma, surgery, and emotional stress.

- Smaller doses are usually required for patients who have liver disease or who are taking multiple drugs. Smaller doses of gabapentin, levetiracetam, and topiramate must be given in the presence of renal impairment, and smaller doses of lamotrigine must be given when combined with valproic acid and another AED.

- For most drugs, initial doses are relatively low and gradually increased until seizures are controlled or adverse effects occur. Then doses may be lowered to the minimum effective level, to decrease adverse effects. Adverse effects are more likely to occur during initiation of treatment. If treatment is started too aggressively, patients may be unwilling to continue a particular medication even if doses are reduced in amount or frequency of administration.

- When one AED is being substituted for another, dosage of the one being added is gradually increased while the one being discontinued is gradually decreased. The first drug is usually stopped when therapeutic effects or therapeutic serum drug levels of the second drug are attained.

- When an AED is being discontinued, its dosage should always be tapered gradually, usually over 1 to 3 months. Abruptly stopping an AED may exacerbate seizures or cause status epilepticus.

- When fosphenytoin is substituted for oral phenytoin, the same total daily dosage (in phenytoin equivalents) may be given IV or IM.

- For patients receiving carbamazepine or oxcarbazepine, either agent may be substituted for the other without gradual reduction or titration of the dose. For most patients, the equivalent oxcarbazepine dosage is 50% higher than the carbamazepine dosage. When switching between agents in older adults, the recommended equivalent oxcar-

bazepine dosage is 20% higher than the carbamazepine dosage.

Monitoring Antiepileptic Drug Therapy

The effectiveness of drug therapy is evaluated primarily by patient response in terms of therapeutic or adverse effects. Periodic measurements of serum drug levels are recommended, especially when multiple AEDs are being given. This strategy helps to

- Document blood levels associated with particular drug dosages, seizure control, or adverse drug effects

- Assess and document therapeutic failures

- Assess for drug malabsorption or patient noncompliance

- Guide dosage adjustments

- Evaluate possible drug-related adverse effects

To be useful, serum drug levels must be interpreted in relation to clinical responses, because there are wide variations among patients receiving similar doses, probably due to differences in hepatic metabolism. In other words, doses should not be increased or decreased solely to maintain a certain serum drug level. In addition, the timing of collection of blood samples in relation to drug administration is important. For routine monitoring, blood samples should generally be obtained in the morning, before the first daily dose of an AED.

Several antiseizure drugs have the potential to cause blood, liver, or kidney disorders. For this reason, it is usually recommended that baseline blood studies (e.g., complete blood count, platelet count) and liver function tests (e.g., bilirubin, serum protein, aspartate aminotransferase) be performed before drug therapy starts and periodically thereafter.

When drug therapy fails to control seizures, there are several possible causes. A common one is the patient's failure to take the antiseizure drug as prescribed. Other causes include incorrect diagnosis of the type of seizure, use of the wrong drug for the type of seizure, inadequate drug dosage, and too-frequent changes or premature withdrawal of drugs. Additional causes may include drug overdoses (e.g., theophylline), severe electrolyte imbalances (e.g., hyponatremia), or use of alcohol or recreational drugs.

Duration and Discontinuation of Therapy

Antiseizure drug therapy may be discontinued for some patients, usually after a seizure-free period of at least 2 years. Although opinions differ about whether, when, and how the drugs should be discontinued, studies indicate that medications can be stopped in approximately two thirds of patients whose epilepsy is completely controlled with drug therapy. Advantages of discontinuation include avoiding adverse drug effects and decreasing costs; disadvantages include recurrence of seizures, with possible status epilepticus. Even if drugs cannot be stopped completely, periodic attempts to decrease the number or dosage of drugs are probably desirable to minimize adverse reactions. Discontinuing drugs, changing drugs, or changing dosage must be done gradually over 2 to 3 months for each drug and with close medical supervision because sudden withdrawal or dosage decreases may cause status epilepticus. Only one drug should be reduced in dosage or gradually discontinued at a time.

Toxicity: Recognition and Management

Signs and symptoms of overdose and toxicity are usually extensions of known adverse effects. Severe overdoses disturb vital functions (e.g., CNS depression with confusion, impaired consciousness and possible coma, respiratory depression; cardiovascular problems such as dysrhythmias and hypotension) and are life threatening. Fatalities have been reported with most antiseizure drugs.

If toxicity is suspected, serum drug levels should be assessed in patients taking those drugs with established therapeutic ranges. There are no specific antidotes, and treatment is symptomatic and supportive. For example, gastric lavage and activated charcoal may be indicated to prevent absorption of additional drug; an endotracheal tube should be inserted prior to lavage, to prevent aspiration. (Activated charcoal is not effective in adsorbing topiramate and is not recommended for topiramate overdose.) Hemodialysis is effective in removing drugs that are poorly bound to plasma proteins and that are excreted mainly or partly by the kidneys (e.g., gabapentin, levetiracetam, topiramate, valproate). Vital signs, electrocardiogram, level of consciousness, pupillary reflexes, and urine output should be monitored.

Effects of Antiepileptic Drugs on Nonantiepileptic Drugs

Interactions between AEDs and many non-AEDs may be clinically significant. Because AEDs depress the CNS and cause drowsiness, their combination with any other CNS depressants may cause excessive sedation and other adverse CNS effects. AEDs may also decrease the effects of numerous other drugs, mainly by inducing drug-metabolizing enzymes in the liver. Enzyme induction means that the affected drugs are metabolized and eliminated more quickly. In some cases, larger doses of the affected drugs are needed to achieve therapeutic effects.

The older AEDs produce more effects on non-AEDs than newer agents. Phenytoin reduces the effects of cardiovascular drugs (e.g., amiodarone, digoxin, disopyramide, dopamine, mexiletine, quinidine), female sex hormones (i.e., estrogens, oral contraceptives, levonorgestrel), adrenal corticosteroids, antipsychotic drugs (e.g., phenothiazines, haloperidol), oral antidiabetic agents (e.g., sulfonylureas), doxycycline, furosemide, levodopa, methadone, and theophylline. The consequence of increasing metabolism of oral contraceptives may be unintended pregnancy. The consequence of decreasing the effects of sulfonylureas may be greater difficulty in controlling blood sugar levels in diabetic patients who require both drugs. Phenytoin decreases the therapeutic effects of acetaminophen

but may increase the risk of hepatotoxicity by accelerating production of the metabolite that damages the liver. Carbamazepine reduces the effects of tricyclic antidepressants, oral anticoagulants, oral contraceptives, bupropion, cyclosporine, doxycycline, felodipine, and haloperidol. Carbamazepine has the same effects on acetaminophen as phenytoin.

Few interactions have been reported with the newer drugs. Topiramate decreases effects of digoxin and oral contraceptives. Levetiracetam does not induce or inhibit hepatic metabolism of drugs, and risks of interactions are minimal. Oxcarbazepine decreases effectiveness of felodipine and oral contraceptives (a barrier type of contraception is recommended during oxcarbazepine therapy). Zonisamide interacts with other AEDs, but no interactions have been reported with non-AEDs. More interactions with these drugs may be observed with longer clinical use.

Treatment of Status Epilepticus

An IV benzodiazepine (e.g., lorazepam 0.1 mg/kg at 2 mg/minute) is the drug of choice for rapid control of tonic-clonic seizures. However, seizures often recur unless the benzodiazepine is repeated or another, longer-acting drug, such as IV phenytoin (20 mg/kg at 50 mg/minute) or fosphenytoin (20 mg/kg phenytoin equivalents at 150 mg/minute), is given. Further treatment is based on the patient's response to these medications. Because there is a risk of significant respiratory depression with IV benzodiazepines, personnel and supplies for emergency resuscitation must be readily available.

Use in Special Populations

Use in Children

Oral drugs are absorbed slowly and inefficiently in newborns. If an antiseizure drug is necessary during the first 7 to 10 days of life, IM phenobarbital is effective. Metabolism and excretion also are delayed during the first 2 weeks of life, but rates become more rapid than those of adults by 2 to 3 months of age. In infants and children, oral drugs are rapidly absorbed and have short half-lives. This produces therapeutic serum drug levels earlier in children than in adults. Rates of metabolism and excretion also are increased. Consequently, children require higher doses per kilogram of body weight than adults.

The rapid rate of drug elimination persists until approximately 6 years of age and then decreases until it stabilizes at around the adult rate by 10 to 14 years of age. AEDs must be used cautiously to avoid excessive sedation and interference with learning and social development.

There is little information about the effects of the newer AEDs in children. Most of the drugs are approved for use in children (i.e., gabapentin, lamotrigine, oxcarbazepine, tiagabine, and topiramate, but not levetiracetam and zonisamide). Oxcarbazepine is metabolized faster in children younger than 8 years of age, and the rate of metabolism is similar to that in adults after 8 years of age. Several studies indicated that oxcarbazepine is effective in monotherapy and combination therapy, with relatively few and mild adverse effects. Reports of behavioral problems, aggression, thought disorders, and hyperkinesias have been reported with the use of gabapentin in children 3 to 12 years of age.

Use in Older Adults

Seizure disorders commonly occur in older adults and require drug therapy. Older adults often have multiple medical conditions, take multiple drugs, and have decreases in protein binding and liver and kidney function. As a result, older adults are at high risk of adverse drug effects and adverse drug–drug interactions with AEDs. For example, reduced levels of serum albumin may increase the active portion of highly protein bound AEDs (e.g., phenytoin, valproic acid) and increase risks for adverse effects even when total serum drug concentrations are normal. Similarly, decreased elimination by the liver and kidneys may lead to drug accumulation, with subsequent risks of dizziness, impaired coordination, and injuries due to falls.

In addition to the ataxia, confusion, dizziness, and drowsiness that may occur with most AEDs, older adults are also more likely to develop some adverse effects associated with specific drugs. For example, with carbamazepine they may develop hyponatremia, especially if they also take sodium-losing diuretics (e.g., furosemide, hydrochlorothiazide), or cardiac dysrhythmias, especially if they have underlying heart disease. Older adults with pre-existing heart disease should have a thorough cardiac evaluation before starting carbamazepine therapy. These effects may also occur with oxcarbazepine. With valproic acid, older adults may develop a tremor that is difficult to diagnose because of its gradual onset and similarity to the tremor occurring with Parkinson's disease. The tremor is often dose-related and reverses when the drug is reduced in dosage or discontinued.

Most of these potential problems can be averted or minimized by using AEDs very cautiously in older adults. In general, small initial doses, slow titration to desired doses, and small maintenance doses are needed. Using controlled-release formulations to minimize peak plasma concentrations may also be helpful. In addition, frequent assessment of patients for adverse effects and periodic monitoring of serum drug levels, liver function, and kidney function are indicated.

Use in Patients With Renal Impairment

Phenytoin is often used to prevent or treat seizure disorders in patients who are seriously ill. With renal impairment, protein binding is decreased and the amount of free, active drug is higher than in patients with normal renal function. Total phenytoin levels are still more commonly obtained in routine clinical practice; however, free levels are more relevant in the setting of renal failure. The use of phenobarbital in patients with severe renal impairment requires markedly reduced dosage, close monitoring of plasma drug levels, and frequent observation for toxic effects. Smaller doses of gabapentin, levetiracetam, oxcarbazepine, topiramate, and zonisamide must be given in the presence of renal impairment because these drugs are eliminated primarily through the kidneys. Dosage of oxcarbazepine should be decreased by 50% in patients with creati-

nine clearance of less than 30 milliliters per minute. Zonisamide should not be given to patients with renal failure and should be discontinued in patients who develop acute renal failure or increased serum creatinine and blood urea nitrogen levels during therapy. Elimination of tiagabine is not significantly affected by renal insufficiency, renal failure, or hemodialysis, and dose adjustment for renal dysfunction is not necessary. Renal stones have been reported with topiramate and zonisamide.

Use in Patients With Hepatic Impairment

Most AEDs are metabolized in the liver and may accumulate in the presence of liver disease or impaired liver function. The drugs should be used cautiously. Tiagabine is cleared more slowly in patients with liver impairment. Increased plasma levels of unbound tiagabine, increased elimination half-life, and increased frequency of neurologic adverse effects (e.g., ataxia, dizziness, drowsiness, tremor) have been observed in patients with mild and moderate hepatic insufficiency. Doses may need to be reduced or given at less frequent intervals. Topiramate may also be cleared more slowly even though it is eliminated mainly through the kidneys and does not undergo significant hepatic metabolism. It should be used with caution in the presence of hepatic impairment.

Valproic acid is a hepatotoxic drug and contraindicated for use in patients with hepatic impairment. No dosage adjustment is indicated with levetiracetam, oxcarbazepine, or zonisamide.

Use in Patients With Critical Illness

Phenytoin is often used to prevent or treat seizure disorders in critically ill patients, including those with head injuries. Phenytoin therapy can best be monitored by measuring free serum phenytoin concentrations, but laboratories usually report the total serum drug concentration. In some patients, a low total phenytoin level may still be therapeutic, and a dosage increase is not indicated. The occurrence of nystagmus (abnormal movements of the eyeball) indicates phenytoin toxicity; the drug should be reduced in dosage or discontinued until serum levels decrease. Because phenytoin is extensively metabolized in the liver, patients with severe illnesses may metabolize the drug more slowly and therefore experience toxicity.

For patients in critical care units for other disorders, a history of long-term antiepileptic therapy may be a risk factor for seizures, including status epilepticus, if the AED is stopped abruptly. At the same time, the use of continuous nasogastric enteral feedings may decrease the absorption of phenytoin administered through the same route, predisposing the patient to the risk of seizure activity. In addition, continuing an AED may complicate drug therapy for other conditions because of adverse effects and potential drug–drug interactions. For example, phenytoin decreases ventricular automaticity and should not be used in critically ill patients with sinus bradycardia or heart block.

Use in Home Care

The home care nurse must work with patients and family members to implement and monitor AED therapy. When an

AED is started, a few weeks may be required to titrate the dosage and determine whether the chosen drug is effective in controlling seizures. The nurse can play an important role in clinical assessment of the patient in three ways: (1) interviewing the family about the occurrence of seizures (a log of date, time, duration, and characteristics of seizures can be very helpful), (2) ensuring that the patient keeps appointments for serum drug level testing and follow-up care, and (3) encouraging compliance with the prescribed regimen. With long-term use of the drugs, the nurse must monitor the patient for therapeutic and adverse drug effects, especially with changes in drugs or dosages. The nurse can also play a role in drawing the blood for levels of anticonvulsants to ensure appropriate dosing. With any evidence that the patient is not taking medica-

tion as directed, the nurse may need to review the potential loss of seizure control and potential for status epilepticus.

 Applying Your Knowledge 11-3

How Can You Avoid This Medication Error?
Frank is scheduled for an outpatient diagnostic test that requires him to be NPO after midnight. So, you advise him not to eat or drink anything after midnight, including medication, the night before his procedure. The next morning, before Frank has his procedure, he experiences a tonic-clonic seizure.

Nursing Actions   Antiseizure Drugs

NURSING ACTIONS	RATIONALE/EXPLANATION
1. Administer accurately a. Give on a regular schedule about the same time each day. b. Give most oral antiseizure drugs after meals or with a full glass of water or other fluid; levetiracetam, oxcarbazepine, topiramate, and zonisamide may be taken with or without food.	To maintain therapeutic blood levels of drugs Most antiseizure drugs cause some gastric irritation, nausea, or vomiting. Taking the drugs with food or fluid helps decrease gastrointestinal side effects.
c. To give phenytoin: (1) Shake oral suspensions of the drug vigorously before pouring and always use the same measuring equipment.	In suspensions, particles of drug are suspended in water or other liquid. On standing, drug particles settle to the bottom of the container. Shaking the container is necessary to distribute drug particles in the liquid vehicle. If the contents are not mixed well every time a dose is given, the liquid vehicle will be given initially, and the concentrated drug will be given later. That is, underdosage will occur at first, and little if any therapeutic benefit will result. Overdosage will follow, and the risks of serious toxicity are greatly increased. Using the same measuring container ensures consistent dosage. Calibrated medication cups or measuring teaspoons or tablespoons are acceptable. Regular household teaspoons and tablespoons used for eating and serving are not acceptable because sizes vary widely.
(2) Do not mix parenteral phenytoin in the same syringe with any other drug.	Phenytoin solution is highly alkaline (pH approximately 12) and physically incompatible with other drugs. A precipitate occurs if mixing is attempted.
(3) Give phenytoin as an undiluted intravenous (IV) bolus injection at a rate not exceeding 50 mg/min, then flush the IV line with normal saline or dilute in 50–100 mL of normal saline (0.9% NaCl) and administer over approximately 30–60 minutes. If piggybacked into a primary IV line, the primary IV solution must be normal saline or the line must be flushed with normal saline before and after administration of phenytoin. An in-line filter is recommended.	Phenytoin cannot be diluted or given in IV fluids other than normal saline because it precipitates within minutes. Slow administration and dilution decrease local venous irritation from the highly alkaline drug solution. Rapid administration must be avoided because it may produce myocardial depression, hypotension, cardiac dysrhythmias, and even cardiac arrest.
d. To give IV fosphenytoin: (1) Check the physician's order and the drug concentration carefully.	The dose is expressed in phenytoin equivalents (PE; fosphenytoin 50 mg PE = phenytoin 50 mg).
(2) Dilute the dose in 5% dextrose or 0.9% sodium chloride solution to a concentration of 1.5 mg PE/mL to 25 mg PE/mL and infuse no faster than 150 mg PE/min.	The drug is preferably diluted in the pharmacy and labeled with the concentration and duration of the infusion. For a 100-mg PE dose, diluting with 4 mL yields the maximum concentration of 25 mg PE/mL; this amount could be infused in about 1 min at the maximal recommended rate. A 1-g loading dose could be added to 50 mL of 0.9% sodium chloride and infused in approximately 10 min at the maximal recommended rate.

NURSING ACTIONS	RATIONALE/EXPLANATION
(3) Consult a pharmacist or the manufacturer's literature if any aspect of the dose or instructions for administration are unclear.	To avoid error
e. To give carbamazepine and phenytoin suspensions by nasogastric (NG) feeding tube, dilute with an equal amount of water, and rinse the NG tube before and after administration.	Absorption is slow and decreased, possibly because of drug adherence to the NG tube. Dilution and tube irrigation decrease such adherence.
f. To give oxcarbazepine suspension, use the 10-mL oral dosing syringe provided by the manufacturer with each bottle. Also check expiration date.	For accurate measurement and a reminder that the suspension is given orally only. The suspension is stored at room temperature and must be used within 7 weeks after opening the bottle.
2. Observe for therapeutic effects	
a. When the drug is given on a long-term basis to prevent seizures, observe for a decrease in or absence of seizure activity.	Therapeutic effects begin later with antiseizure drugs than with most other drug groups because the antiseizure drugs have relatively long half-lives. Optimum therapeutic benefits of phenytoin occur approximately 7–10 days after drug therapy is started.
b. When the drug is given to stop an acute convulsive seizure, seizure activity usually slows or stops within a few minutes.	Intravenous lorazepam is the drug of choice for controlling an acute convulsion.
3. Observe for adverse effects	
a. Central nervous system (CNS) effects—ataxia, dizziness, drowsiness, double vision	These effects are common, especially during the first week or two of drug therapy.
b. Gastrointestinal effects—anorexia, nausea, vomiting	These common effects of oral drugs can be reduced by taking the drugs with food or a full glass of water.
c. Hypersensitivity reactions—often manifested by skin disorders such as rash, urticaria, exfoliative dermatitis, Stevens-Johnson syndrome (a severe reaction accompanied by headache, arthralgia, and other symptoms in addition to skin lesions)	These may occur with almost all the antiseizure drugs. Some are mild; some are potentially serious but rare. These skin reactions are usually sufficient reason to discontinue the drug. About 25%–30% of patients with allergic reactions to carbamazepine are likely to be allergic to oxcarbazepine.
d. Blood dyscrasias—anemia, leukopenia, thrombocytopenia, agranulocytosis	Most antiseizure drugs decrease blood levels of folic acid, which may progress to megaloblastic anemia. The other disorders indicate bone marrow depression and are potentially life threatening. They do not usually occur with phenytoin, but may infrequently occur with most other antiseizure drugs.
e. Respiratory depression	This is not likely to be a significant adverse reaction except when a depressant drug, such as lorazepam, is given IV to control acute seizures, such as status epilepticus. Even then, respiratory depression can be minimized by avoiding overdosage and rapid administration.
f. Liver damage—hepatitis symptoms, jaundice, abnormal liver function test results	Hepatic damage may occur with phenytoin, and fatal hepatotoxicity has been reported with valproic acid.
g. Gingival hyperplasia	Occurs often with phenytoin, especially in children. It may be prevented or delayed by vigorous oral hygiene.
h. Hypocalcemia	May occur when antiseizure drugs are taken in high doses and over long periods
i. Hyponatremia	May occur with carbamazepine and oxcarbazepine, especially if taken concurrently with sodium-losing diuretics (e.g., furosemide, hydrochlorothiazide). Usually transient and levels return to normal with fluid restriction or dose reduction.
j. Lymphadenopathy resembling malignant lymphoma	This reaction has occurred with several antiseizure drugs, most often with phenytoin.
k. Pancreatitis	Life-threatening pancreatitis has occurred after short- and long-term therapy with valproic acid. Patients should be monitored for the development of acute abdominal pain, nausea, and vomiting.
l. Kidney stones	May occur with topiramate and zonisamide. Inadequate fluid intake or concurrent administration of triamterene may increase risk.

(continued on page 214)

Nursing Actions Antipsychotic Drugs (continued)

NURSING ACTIONS	RATIONALE/EXPLANATION
4. Observe for drug interactions	
a. Drugs that *increase* effects of antiseizure drugs:	
(1) CNS depressants—alcohol, sedating antihistamines, benzodiazepines, opioid analgesics, sedatives	Additive CNS depression
(2) Most other antiseizure drugs	Additive or synergistic effects. The drugs are often given in combination, to increase therapeutic effects.
b. Drugs that *decrease* effects of antiseizure drugs:	
(1) Tricyclic antidepressants, antipsychotic drugs	These drugs may lower the seizure threshold and precipitate seizures. Dosage of antiseizure drugs may need to be increased.
(2) Carbemazepine, phenytoin, and other enzyme inducers	These drugs inhibit themselves and other antiseizure drugs by activating liver enzymes and accelerating the rate of drug metabolism.
c. Additional drugs that alter effects of phenytoin and fos-phenytoin:	
(1) Alcohol (acute ingestion), allopurinol, amiodarone, benzodiazepines, chlorpheniramine, cimetidine, fluconazole, fluoxetine, isoniazid, metronidazole, miconazole, omeprazole, paroxetine, sertraline, and trimethoprim increase effects.	These drugs increase phenytoin toxicity by inhibiting hepatic metabolism of phenytoin or by displacing it from plasma protein-binding sites.
(2) Alcohol (chronic ingestion), antacids, antineoplastics, folic acid, pyridoxine, rifampin, sucralfate, and theophylline decrease effects.	These drugs decrease effects of phenytoin by decreasing absorption, accelerating metabolism, or by unknown mechanisms.
(3) Phenobarbital has variable interactions with phenytoin.	Phenytoin and phenobarbital have complex interactions with unpredictable effects. Although phenobarbital induces drug metabolism in the liver and may increase the rate of metabolism of other anticonvulsant drugs, its interaction with phenytoin differs. Phenobarbital apparently decreases serum levels of phenytoin and perhaps its half-life. Still, the anticonvulsant effects of the two drugs together are greater than those of either drug given alone. The interaction apparently varies with dosage, route, time of administration, the degree of liver enzyme induction already present, and other factors. Thus, whether a significant interaction will occur in a client is unpredictable. Probably the most important clinical implication is that close observation of the patient is necessary when either drug is being added or withdrawn.
d. Additional drugs that alter effects of carbamazepine:	
(1) Cimetidine, clarithromycin, diltiazem, erythromycin, haloperidol, isoniazid, valproic acid, and verapamil increase effects.	Most of these drugs inhibit the cytochrome P450 enzymes (1A2, 2C8, and/or 3A4 groups) that normally metabolize carbamazepine, thereby increasing blood levels of carbamazepine. Valproic acid inhibits an epoxide hydrolase enzyme and causes an active metabolite to accumulate. Toxicity may result even if carbamazepine blood levels are at therapeutic concentrations.
(2) Alcohol, phenytoin, and phenobarbital decrease effects.	These drugs increase activity of hepatic drug-metabolizing enzymes, thereby decreasing blood levels of carbamazepine.
e. Drugs that alter the effects of gabapentin:	
(1) Antacids	Reduce absorption of gabapentin. Gabapentin should be given at least 2 hours after a dose of an antacid to decrease interference with absorption.
f. Drugs that alter effects of lamotrigine:	
(1) Valproic acid increases effects.	Valproic acid inhibits the liver enzymes that metabolize lamotrigine, thereby increasing blood levels and slowing metabolism of lamotrigine. As a result, lamotrigine dosage must be substantially reduced when the drug is given in a multidrug regimen that includes valproic acid.
(2) Carbamazepine, phenytoin, and phenobarbital decrease effects.	These drugs induce drug-metabolizing enzymes in the liver and thereby increase the rate of metabolism of themselves and of lamotrigine.

NURSING ACTIONS	RATIONALE/EXPLANATION
g. Drugs that *decrease* effects of oxcarbazepine: (1) Phenobarbital, phenytoin, valproic acid, verapamil	These drugs induce drug-metabolizing enzymes in the liver and thereby increase the metabolism and hasten the elimination of oxcarbazepine.
h. Drug that *increase* effects of phenobarbital: (1) Valproic acid	May increase plasma levels of phenobarbital as much as 40%, probably by inhibiting liver metabolizing enzymes
i. Additional drugs that *increases* effects of valproate: (1) Cimetidine (2) Salicylates	Inhibits drug-metabolizing enzymes, thereby slowing elimination from the body and increasing blood levels of valproic acid Displace valproic acid from binding sites on plasma proteins, thereby increasing the serum level of unbound valproic acid
j. Drugs that *decrease* effects of zonisamide: (1) Carbamazepine, phenytoin, phenobarbital	These drugs induce drug-metabolizing enzymes in the liver and thereby increase the metabolism and hasten the elimination of zonisamide.
k. Interactions with clonazepam, lorazepam, and diazepam	These drugs are benzodiazepines, discussed in Chapter 8.

Key Concepts

- Seizures are classified as idiopathic or secondary (caused by tumors, metabolic disorders, overdoses of numerous drugs, or withdrawal of alcohol or sedative-hypnotic drugs).

- When seizures occur in a chronic, recurrent pattern, they characterize a disorder known as epilepsy, which usually requires long-term drug therapy.

- Types of seizure include generalized (generalized tonic-clonic seizures) and partial and (simple or complex, depending on whether consciousness is altered).

- Status epilepticus is a life-threatening emergency that may result in hypotension, hypoxia, cardiac dysrhythmias, permanent brain damage, and death unless prompt, appropriate treatment is instituted.

- Newer antiepileptic medications have better adverse effect profiles with enhanced seizure control.

- Monotherapy should guide initial management of seizure disorders.

- When an AED is being discontinued, its dosage should always be tapered gradually, usually over 1 to 3 months. Abruptly stopping an AED may exacerbate seizures or cause status epilepticus.

- Serum drug levels monitoring is useful for most AEDs and must be interpreted in relation to clinical responses.

- Adverse effect profiles vary with individual AEDs; potential teratogenic adverse effects, drug interactions, hypersensitivity reactions, and blood dyscrasias have been reported.

- All doses of fosphenytoin should be prescribed in terms of its phenytoin equivalent (PE).

- **BLACK BOX WARNINGS** have been issued by the FDA for the following AEDs: carbamazepine, divalproex sodium, lamotrigine, and valproic acid and its derivatives.

Review and Application Exercises

Short Answer Exercises

1. For a patient with a newly developed seizure disorder, why is it important to verify the type of seizure by electroencephalogram before starting AEDs?

2. What are the indications for use of the major AEDs?

3. What are the major adverse effects of commonly used AEDs, and how can they be minimized?

4. What are the advantages and disadvantages of treatment with a single drug and of treatment with multiple drugs?

5. Which of the benzodiazepines are used as AEDs?

6. What are the advantages of carbamazepine and valproic acid compared with the benzodiazepines, phenytoin, and phenobarbital?

7. How are the newer drugs similar to or different from phenytoin?

8. What is the treatment of choice for an acute convulsion or status epilepticus?

9. Why is it important when teaching patients to emphasize that none of the AEDs should be stopped abruptly?

10. How can a home care nurse monitor AED therapy during a home visit?

NCLEX-Style Questions

11. An 18-year-old patient presents to the clinic with complaints of breast tenderness, nausea, vomiting, and absence of menses for 2 months. She has a history of a seizure disorder that is well controlled with oxcarbazepine (Trileptal). She believes that she has been taking her oral contraceptives as directed but asks if she could be pregnant. The nurse recognizes that the best response to the patient's question is which of the following?
    a. "Oxcarbazepine can decreases the effectiveness of oral contraceptive drugs, so we need to do a pregnancy test."
    b. "You can't be pregnant if you have been taking your pills correctly."
    c. "Don't worry; birth control pills are very effective."
    d. "Taking antiseizure drugs with oral contraceptives significantly decreases your risk of pregnancy."

12. A patient scheduled for her next dose of phenytoin (Dilantin) has a serum plasma phenytoin level of 16 mcg/mL. Based on this information, the nurse should do which of the following?
    a. Administer the drug.
    b. Hold the dose and obtain another plasma drug level before the next dose.
    c. Hold the drug and notify the prescriber.
    d. Administer half of the prescribed dose.

13. A patient taking gabapentin (Neurontin) begins to exhibit tremors, dizziness, and abnormal vision. The nurse should assess the patient for signs of which of the following?
    a. additional adverse effects of gabapentin
    b. liver dysfunction
    c. impending seizure activity
    d. cardiac toxicity and dysrhythmias

14. A patient is started on phenytoin (Dilantin). A teaching plan for the patient should include strategies to minimize which of the following common side effects?
    a. hypoglycemia
    b. photosensitivity
    c. gingival hyperplasia
    d. hyponatremia

15. A patient is brought to the emergency department with ongoing tonic-clonic seizure activity. The health care provider orders lorazepam (Ativan) 4 mg IV. Lorazepam is the drug of choice for which of the following types of seizures?
    a. partial seizures
    b. tonic-clonic seizures
    c. absence seizures
    d. status epilepticus

Selected References

Castillo, S., Schmidt, D. B., & White, S. (2000). Oxcarbazepine add-on for drug-resistant partial epilepsy (Cochrane Review). *Cochrane Database of Systematic Reviews*, Issue 3.

Drug facts and comparisons. (Updated monthly). St. Louis, MO: Facts and Comparisons.

EFNS Task Force. (2005). *EFNS guideline on the diagnosis and management of alcohol-related seizures: Report of an EFNS task force.* Retrieved February 27, 2007, from http://www.guidelines.gov/summary/summary.aspx?doc_id=9648

Gamble, C. L., Williamson, P. R., & Marson, A. G. (2006). Lamotrigine versus carbamazepine monotherapy for epilepsy (Cochrane Review). *Cochrane Database of Systematic Reviews*, Issue 1. Art. no.: CD001031.

Lacy, C. F., Armstrong, L. L., Goldman, M. P., & Lance, L. L. (2007). *Lexi-Comp's drug information handbook* (15th ed.). Hudson, OH: American Pharmaceutical Association.

Muller, M., Marson, A. G., & Williamson, P. R. (2006). Oxcarbazepine versus phenytoin monotherapy for epilepsy (Cochrane Review). *Cochrane Database of Systematic Reviews*, Issue 2. Art. no.: CD003615.

Prasad, K., Al-Roomi, K., Krishnan, P. R., & Sequeira, R. (Cochrane Epilepsy Group) (2005). Anticonvulsant therapy for status epilepticus (Cochrane Review). *Cochrane Database of Systematic Reviews*, Issue 4. Art. no.: CD0037230.

Young, G. B. (2006). Status epilepticus and refractory status epilepticus: introductory and summary statements. *Advances in Neurology, 97,* 183–185.

CHAPTER 12

Antiparkinson Drugs

KEY TERMS

- Akinesia
- Anticholinergic drugs
- Basal ganglia
- Bradykinesia
- Dopaminergic drugs
- Extrapyramidal reactions
- Hypertensive crisis
- "Off-time"
- Parkinson's disease
- Parkinsonism
- Substantia nigra

LEARNING OBJECTIVES

After studying this chapter, you will be able to:

1. Describe major characteristics of Parkinson's disease.
2. Differentiate the types of commonly used antiparkinson drugs.
3. Discuss therapeutic and adverse effects of dopaminergic and anticholinergic drugs.
4. Discuss the use of antiparkinson drugs in selected populations.
5. Apply the nursing process with patients experiencing parkinsonism.

Applying Your Knowledge

Lee Sung is an 81-year-old woman who had been experiencing hand tremors, slow movement, a shuffling gait, and excessive salivation. Her physician diagnosed her with Parkinson's disease and started her on levodopa/carbidopa 25/100 four times a day and benztropine mesylate at bedtime. Following a fall, she is admitted for evaluation.

Introduction

Parkinson's disease (also called *parkinsonism*) is a chronic, progressive, degenerative disorder of the central nervous system (CNS) characterized by resting tremor, bradykinesia, rigidity, and postural instability. Approximately 85% of the 1.5 million Americans with Parkinson's disease are over the age of 50. Parkinson's disease occurs slightly more often in men than in women. The disease occurs more often in Caucasian and Hispanic/Latino individuals than in African Americans. Idiopathic parkinsonism results from progressive destruction of or degenerative changes in dopamine-producing nerve cells in the *substantia nigra* in the *basal ganglia*, the area in the midbrain that controls smooth voluntary movement. The cause of the nerve-cell damage is unknown; age-related degeneration, genetics, and exposure to environmental toxins are possible etiologic factors. A total of nine genetic linkages and four genes have been associated with Parkinson's disease, including mutations of alpha-synuclein and parkin genes. A high incidence of mutation in the parkin-2 gene has been associated with early-onset parkinsonism. Signs and symptoms of Parkinson's disease also may occur with other CNS diseases, brain tumors, and head injuries. Drugs that deplete dopamine stores or block dopamine receptors, including the older antipsychotic drugs (phenothiazines and haloperidol), reserpine, and metoclopramide, can produce movement disorders such as secondary parkinsonism (also known as *extrapyramidal reactions*, see Chap. 9).

The basal ganglia in the brain normally contain substantial amounts of the neurotransmitters dopamine and acetylcholine. The correct balance of dopamine and acetylcholine is important in regulating posture, muscle tone, and voluntary movement. People with Parkinson's disease have an imbalance in these neurotransmitters, resulting in a decrease in inhibitory brain dopamine and a relative increase in excitatory acetylcholine.

217

The first symptom of Parkinson's disease is often a resting tremor that begins in the fingers and thumb of one hand (pill-rolling movements), eventually spreading over one side of the body and progressing to the contralateral limbs. Other common symptoms include slow movement (*bradykinesia*), inability to move (*akinesia*), rigid limbs, shuffling gait, stooped posture, mask-like facial expression, and a soft speaking voice. Less common symptoms may include depression, personality changes, loss of appetite, sleep disturbances, speech impairment, or sexual difficulty. Approximately 15% to 20% of individuals with Parkinson's disease develop dementia. The severity of disease manifestations usually worsen over time. However, disease progression is often quite gradual, and patients may retain near-normal functional abilities for several years.

General Characteristics of Antiparkinson Drugs

Drugs used in Parkinson's disease help correct the neurotransmitter imbalance by increasing levels of dopamine (*dopaminergic drugs*) or inhibiting the actions of acetylcholine in the brain (*anticholinergic drugs*).

Dopaminergic Drugs

Levodopa, carbidopa, amantadine, bromocriptine, entacapone, pramipexole, ropinirole, rotigotine-transdermal, selegiline, tolcapone, and rasagiline increase dopamine concentrations in the brain, exerting dopaminergic activity, directly or indirectly. P **Levodopa** (L-dopa) is the mainstay of drug therapy for idiopathic parkinsonism. Carbidopa is used only in conjunction with levodopa. The other drugs are used as adjunctive agents, usually with levodopa.

Mechanism of Action

Dopaminergic drugs increase the amount of dopamine in the brain by various mechanisms (Fig. 12-1). Amantadine increases dopamine release and decreases dopamine reuptake by presynaptic nerve fibers. Bromocriptine, pramipexole, ropinirole, and rotigotine-transdermal are dopamine agonists that directly stimulate postsynaptic dopamine receptors. Levodopa is a precursor substance that is converted to dopamine. Selegiline selectively blocks one of the enzymes (MAO-B) that normally inactivates dopamine. Rasagiline is an irreversible MAO inhibitor. It is effective in blocking the MAO-B enzyme; however, studies have not yet established whether rasagiline is *selective* for the MAO-B enzyme. Entacapone and tolcapone block another enzyme (COMT) that normally inactivates dopamine and levodopa.

Indications for Use

Amantadine, entacapone, levodopa, pramipexole, rasagiline, ropinirole, rotigotine-transdermal, selegiline, and tolcapone are indicated for the treatment of idiopathic parkinsonism. Amantadine is also therapeutic for secondary parkinsonism (or extrapyramidal reaction). Carbidopa is used only to decrease peripheral breakdown of levodopa and allow more to reach the brain.

Some of the other drugs have additional uses. Bromocriptine is also used in the treatment of acromegaly, amenorrhea, and galactorrhea associated with hyperprolactinemia. Selegiline-transdermal has been approved to treat major depressive disorder. The Food and Drug Administration (FDA) has issued a **BLACK BOX WARNING** regarding an increased risk of suicidality in children and adolescents when treated with antidepressant including selegiline-transdermal. Dopaminergic drugs (e.g., levodopa, cabergoline, pramipexole, ropinirole, and rotigotine-transdermal) may also be prescribed to reduce the symptoms of restless leg syndrome (RLS). Individuals with RLS, also known as Ekbom's syndrome, experience paresthesias of the muscles, particularly in the calf and thighs, creating the urge to move. The paresthesia is relieved by movement, returning when the individual is at rest or trying to sleep. The disorder may result in insomnia, mental distress, and in some cases suicide. Historically, amantadine has been prescribed to prevent or treat influenza A viral infections; however, the Advisory Committee on Immunization Practices (ACIP) of the CDC no longer recommends this practice due to high levels of viral resistance to amantadine.

Contraindications to Use

Levodopa is contraindicated in patients with known hypersensitivity to the drug. Because levodopa can dilate pupils and raise intraocular pressure, it is contraindicated in narrow-angle glaucoma. Levodopa may activate malignant melanoma; therefore, it should not be administered to individuals with suspicious skin lesions or a history of melanoma. Concurrent administration of nonselective MAO inhibitors (used in the treatment of depression) and levodopa can result in extreme elevations in blood pressure or *hypertensive crisis*. To avoid this adverse effect, MAO-A inhibitors should be discontinued 14 days prior to beginning levodopa therapy. In addition, levodopa must be used with caution in patients with severe cardiovascular, pulmonary, renal, hepatic, or endocrine disorders; depression; and peptic ulcer disease. Safe use in pregnancy has not been established. Bromocriptine is an ergot derivative and therefore is contraindicated in people who are hypersensitive to ergot alkaloids or who have uncontrolled hypertension. Entacapone, rasagiline, rotigotine-transdermal, selegiline, and tolcapone are contraindicated in people with hypersensitivity reactions to the drugs. Rasagiline is also contraindicated with foods containing tyramine or sympathomimetic amine–containing medications (e.g., nonprescription cold/cold preparations and anesthetics) due to the risk of hypertensive crisis and with antidepressants (e.g., tricyclics, SSRIs, SNRIs, mirtazapine), meperidine, and dextromethorphan due to the potential for inducing serotonin syndrome. Rotigotine-transdermal is contraindicated in patients with hypersensitivity to sulfites; this may be more common in patients who also have asthma. Tolcapone is also contraindicated in patients with liver disease.

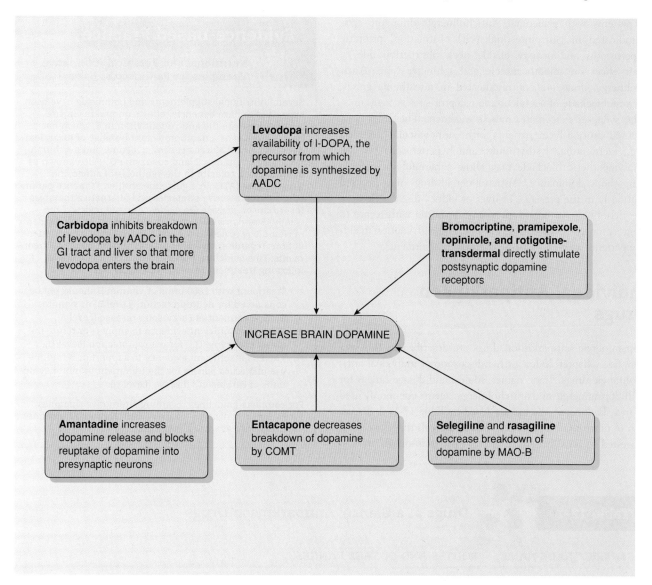

Figure 12-1 ■ Mechanisms by which dopaminergic drugs increase dopamine in the brain. AADC, amino acid decarboxylase; COMT, catechol-O-methyltransferase; MAO-B, monoamine oxidase B.

Anticholinergic Drugs

Anticholinergic drugs are discussed in Chapter 20 and are described here only in relation to their use in the treatment of Parkinson's disease. Only anticholinergic drugs that are centrally active (i.e., those that penetrate the blood–brain barrier) are useful in treating parkinsonism. Atropine and scopolamine are centrally active but are not used because of a high incidence of adverse reactions. In addition to the primary anticholinergic drugs, an antihistamine (diphenhydramine) is used for parkinsonism because of its strong anticholinergic effects.

Mechanism of Action

Anticholinergic drugs decrease the effects of acetylcholine. This decreases the relative excess of acetylcholine in relation to the amount of dopamine that occurs in Parkinson's disease.

Indications for Use

Anticholinergic drugs are used in idiopathic parkinsonism to decrease salivation, spasticity, and tremors. They are used primarily in people who have minimal symptoms or who cannot tolerate levodopa, or in combination with other antiparkinson drugs. Anticholinergic drugs are usually not effective for bradykinesia or other symptoms of Parkinson's disease. Anticholinergic agents also are used to relieve symptoms of secondary parkinsonism (extrapyramidal reaction) that can occur with the use of antipsychotic drugs. If used for this purpose, a course of therapy of approximately 3 months is recommended because symptoms usually subside by then, even if the antipsychotic drug is continued.

Contraindications to Use

Because anticholinergic drugs can increase intraocular pressure, due to mydriasis and cycloplegia, they are contraindicated in patients with glaucoma. Anticholinergic drugs are contraindicated in gastrointestinal (GI) obstruction, prostatic hypertrophy, and urinary bladder-neck obstruction due to their effect on smooth muscle and sphincter tone. Anticholinergic drugs are contraindicated in myasthenia gravis, because blockade of acetylcholine receptor sites at neuromuscular synapses exacerbates muscle weakness. The drugs must be used cautiously in patients with cardiovascular disorders (e.g., tachycardia, dysrhythmias, and hypertension) because parasympathetic blockade may allow a harmful increase in sympathetic dominance. Anticholinergic drugs must be used cautiously in the presence of liver or kidney disease. Because acetylcholine is an important neurotransmitter with regard to memory function, these drugs must be used with caution in elderly patients with pre-existing cognitive impairments.

Individual Antiparkinson Drugs

Dopaminergic antiparkinson drugs are described in this section. See Chapter 20 for further discussion of individual anticholinergic drugs. Trade names, routes, and dosage ranges for both dopaminergic and anticholinergic agents commonly used to treat Parkinson's disease are listed in Table 12-1. A discussion of nutritional supplements and botanicals that have been suggested to have beneficial effects on parkinsonism are dis-

Table 12-1	Drugs at a Glance: Antiparkinson Drugs

GENERIC/TRADE NAME	ROUTES AND DOSAGE RANGES
Dopaminergic Agents	
P Levodopa	PO 0.5–1 g/d initially in 3 or 4 divided doses, increase gradually by no more than 0.75 g/d, every 3–7 d. The rate of dosage increase depends mainly on the client's tolerance of adverse effects, especially nausea and vomiting. Average maintenance dose, 3–6 g/d; maximum dose, 8 g/d. Dosage must be reduced when carbidopa is also given (see carbidopa, below).
Carbidopa (Lodosyn)	PO 70–100 mg/d, depending on dosage of levodopa; maximum dose, 200 mg/d
Levodopa/carbidopa (Sinemet)	*Patients not receiving levodopa:* PO 1 tablet of 25 mg carbidopa/100 mg levodopa 3 times daily or 1 tablet of 10 mg carbidopa/100 mg levodopa 3 or 4 times daily, increased by 1 tablet every day or every other day until a dosage of 8 tablets daily is reached Sinemet CR PO 1 tablet twice daily at least 6 h apart initially, increased up to 8 tablets daily and q4h intervals if necessary *Patients receiving levodopa:* Discontinue levodopa at least 8 h before starting Sinemet. PO 1 tablet of 25 mg carbidopa/250 mg levodopa 3 or 4 times daily for clients taking >1500 mg levodopa or 1 tablet of 25 mg carbidopa/100 mg levodopa for clients taking <1500 mg levodopa
Levodopa/carbidopa/ entacapone (Stalevo)	Patients already taking the drugs separately can be switched to the combination tablet containing an equivalent amount of each drug. For patients taking >600 mg levodopa daily when starting entacapone, dosage should be titrated and stabilized with the individual drugs before using the combination product. Patients taking <600 mg levodopa daily may be started directly on the corresponding dosage of Stalevo, but levodopa dosage may need to be reduced.

GENERIC/TRADE NAME	ROUTES AND DOSAGE RANGES
Amantadine (Symmetrel)	PO 100 mg twice a day
Bromocriptine (Parlodel)	PO 1.25 mg twice a day with meals, increased by 2.5 mg/d every 2–4 wk if necessary for therapeutic benefit. Reduce dose gradually if severe adverse effects occur.
Entacapone (Comtan)	PO 200 mg with each dose of levodopa/carbidopa, up to 8 times (1600 mg) daily
Pramipexole (Mirapex)	PO wk 1, 0.125 mg 3 times daily; wk 2, 0.25 mg 3 times daily; wk 3, 0.5 mg 3 times daily; wk 4, 0.75 mg 3 times daily; wk 5, 1 mg 3 times daily; wk 6, 1.25 mg 3 times daily; wk 7, 1.5 mg 3 times daily
	Renal impairment: Creatinine clearance (Crcl) > 60 mL/min, 0.125 mg 3 times daily initially, up to a maximum of 1.5 mg 3 times daily; Crcl 35–59 mL/min, 0.125 mg 2 times daily initially, up to a maximum of 1.5 mg 2 times daily; Crcl 15–34 mL/min, 0.125 mg once daily, up to a maximum of 1.5 mg once daily
Rasagiline (Azilect)	PO 1 mg/d. When combined with levodopa, the starting dose is 0.5 mg/d and may be increased to 1 mg/d if necessary.
Ropinirole (Requip)	PO wk 1, 0.25 mg 3 times daily; wk 2, 0.5 mg 3 times daily; wk 3, 0.75 mg 3 times daily; wk 4, 1 mg 3 times daily
Rotigotine-transdermal (Neupro)	TDS: 2 mg/24 h initially, increase in weekly increments of 2 mg/24 h up to a maximum dose of 8 mg/24 h.
Selegiline (Eldepryl)	PO 5 mg twice daily, morning and noon
Anticholinergic Agents	
Benztropine (Cogentin)	PO 0.5–1 mg at bedtime initially, gradually increased to 4–6 mg daily if necessary
Diphenhydramine (Benadryl)	PO 25 mg 3 times daily, gradually increased to 50 mg 4 times daily if necessary
	Adults: Drug-induced extrapyramidal reactions, IM, IV 10–50 mg; maximal single dose, 100 mg; maximal daily dose, 400 mg
	Children: Drug-induced extrapyramidal reactions, IM 5 mg/kg per day; maximal daily dose, 300 mg
Trihexyphenidyl (Trihexy)	PO 1–2 mg daily initially, gradually increased to 12–15 mg daily, until therapeutic or adverse effects occur
	Adults: Drug-induced extrapyramidal reactions, PO 1 mg initially, gradually increased to 5–15 mg daily if necessary

TDS, transdermal delivery system.

cussed in Evidence-Based Practice Box 12-1. No supplements are currently recommended by the American Academy of Neurology practice guidelines.

P Levodopa is the most effective drug available for the treatment of Parkinson's disease. It relieves all major symptoms, especially bradykinesia and rigidity. Levodopa does not alter the underlying disease process, but it may improve a patient's quality of life.

Levodopa acts to replace dopamine in the basal ganglia of the brain. Dopamine cannot be used for replacement therapy because it does not penetrate the blood–brain barrier. Levodopa readily penetrates the CNS and is converted to dopamine by the enzyme amino acid decarboxylase (AADC). The dopamine is stored in presynaptic dopaminergic neurons and functions like endogenous dopamine. In advanced stages of Parkinson's disease, there are fewer dopaminergic neurons and thus less storage capacity for dopamine derived from levodopa. As a result, levodopa has a shorter duration of action and drug effects "wear off" between doses or during duration of action ("*off-time*"), resulting in sudden fluctuations in symptoms including severe hypomobility (freezing). Apomorphine

injection is a non-ergot dopamine agonist approved for acute intermittent treatment of these sudden episodic symptoms. Similar to other opioids, apomorphine may cause nausea and vomiting and should be administered concurrently with the antiemetic, trimethobenzamide. Due to the occurrence of hypotension and loss of consciousness, apomorphine should not be given with 5-HT$_3$ antagonists (e.g., ondansetron, granisetron, dolasetron, palonosetron, and alosetron). In peripheral tissues (e.g., GI tract, liver), levodopa is metabolized extensively by AADC and to a lesser extent by COMT. Because most levodopa is metabolized in peripheral tissues, large doses are required to obtain therapeutic levels of dopamine in the brain. These large amounts increase adverse drug effects. To reduce levodopa dosage and decrease adverse effects, carbidopa, an AADC inhibitor, is given to decrease the peripheral metabolism of levodopa. The combination of levodopa and carbidopa greatly increases the amount of available levodopa, so that levodopa dosage can be reduced by approximately 70%. The two drugs are usually given together in a fixed-dose formulation called Sinemet. When carbidopa inhibits the decarboxylase pathway of levodopa metabolism, the COMT pathway becomes more important (see entacapone and tolcapone, COMT inhibitors, below). A newer product, Stalevo, combines levodopa, carbidopa, and entacapone to further decrease metabolism of levodopa.

Levodopa is well absorbed from the small intestine after oral administration, reaches peak serum levels within 30 to 90 minutes, and has a short serum half-life (1–3 hours). Absorption is decreased by delayed gastric emptying, hyperacidity of gastric secretions, and competition with amino acids (from digestion of protein foods) for sites of absorption in the small intestine. Pyridoxine (vitamin B$_6$) promotes the breakdown of levodopa, reducing its effectiveness. Levodopa is metabolized to 30 or more metabolites, some of which are pharmacologically active and probably contribute to drug toxicity; the metabolites are excreted primarily in the urine, usually within 24 hours.

Because of adverse effects and recurrence of parkinsonian symptoms after a few years of levodopa therapy, levodopa is usually reserved for patients with significant symptoms and functional disabilities. In addition to treating Parkinson's disease, levodopa also may be useful in other CNS disorders in which symptoms of parkinsonism occur (e.g., juvenile Huntington's chorea, chronic manganese poisoning). Levodopa relieves only parkinsonian symptoms in these conditions.

Applying Your Knowledge 12-1

Mrs. Sung tells you that she has a friend who takes her medication for Parkinson's disease once a day, and questions you why she must take her medication more than once a day. What is the most appropriate response?

Carbidopa (Lodosyn) inhibits the enzyme AADC. As a result, less levodopa is decarboxylated in peripheral tissues; more levodopa reaches the brain, where it is decarboxylated to dopamine; and much smaller doses of levodopa can be given. Carbidopa does not penetrate the blood–brain barrier. Although carbidopa is available alone, it is most often given in the levodopa/carbidopa fixed-dose combination product, Sinemet.

Amantadine (Symmetrel) increases the release and inhibits the reuptake of dopamine in the brain, thereby increasing dopamine levels. The drug relieves symptoms rapidly, within 1 to 5 days, but it loses efficacy with 6 to 8 weeks of continuous administration. Consequently, it is usually given for 2- to 3-week periods during initiation of drug therapy with longer-acting agents (e.g., levodopa) or when symptoms worsen. Amantadine is often given with levodopa. Compared with other antiparkinson drugs, amantadine is considered less effective than levodopa but more effective than anticholinergic agents.

Amantadine is well absorbed from the GI tract and has a relatively long duration of action. It is excreted unchanged in the urine. Dosage must be reduced with impaired renal function to avoid drug accumulation.

Bromocriptine (Parlodel) is an ergot derivative that directly stimulates dopamine receptors in the brain. It is used in the treatment of idiopathic Parkinson's disease, with levodopa/carbidopa, to prolong effectiveness and allow reduced dosage of levodopa. Cabergoline is a synthetic ergot long-acting dopamine agonist, approved by the FDA for use in hyperprolactinemia. An unlabeled use of this mediation has been to improve motor symptoms of parkinsonism; however, the higher dosage required to treat parkinsonism is associated with increased risk for the development of serious heart valve damage due to fibrosis. Another ergot dopamine agonist, pergolide (Permax), was removed from the market for similar adverse effects on heart valves.

Entacapone (Comtan) and **tolcapone** (Tasmar) are COMT inhibitors. COMT plays a role in brain metabolism of dopamine and metabolizes approximately 10% of peripheral levodopa. By inhibiting COMT, entacapone and tolcapone increase levels of dopamine in the brain and relieve symptoms more effectively and consistently. Although the main mechanism of action seems to be inhibiting the metabolism of levodopa in the bloodstream, the drugs may also inhibit COMT in the brain and prolong the activity of dopamine at the synapse. These drugs are used only in conjunction with levodopa/carbidopa, and dosage of levodopa must be reduced.

Entacapone is well absorbed with oral administration and reaches a peak plasma level in 1 hour. It is highly protein bound (98%), has a half-life of about 2.5 hours, and is metabolized in the liver to an inactive metabolite. Dosage must be reduced by 50% in the presence of impaired liver function. The parent drug and the metabolite are 90% excreted through the biliary tract and feces; 10% is excreted in the urine. Adverse effects include confusion, dizziness, drowsiness, hallucinations, nausea, and vomiting. These can be reduced by lowering the dose of either levodopa or entacapone. Although there were few instances of liver enzyme elevation or hemoglobin decreases during clinical trials, it is recommended that liver enzymes and red blood cell counts be done periodically.

Tolcapone is also well absorbed with oral administration. Its elimination half-life is 2 to 3 hours, and it is metabolized in the liver. During clinical trials, diarrhea was a common adverse effect. Because of several reports of liver damage and deaths from liver failure, the FDA has issued a **BLACK BOX WARNING.** Tolcapone should be used only in patients who do not respond to other drugs. When used, liver aminotransferase enzymes (serum alanine aminotransferase [ALT] and aspartate aminotransferase [AST]) should be monitored every 2 weeks for 1 year, then every 4 weeks for 6 months, then every 2 months. Tolcapone should be discontinued if ALT and AST are elevated, if symptoms of liver failure occur (anorexia, abdominal tenderness, dark urine, jaundice, clay-colored stools), or if parkinsonian symptoms do not improve after 3 weeks of taking tolcapone.

Pramipexole (Mirapex), **ropinirole** (Requip), and **rotigotine-transdermal** (Neupro) stimulate dopamine receptors in the brain. They are approved for both beginning and advanced stages of Parkinson's disease. In early stages, one of these drugs can be used alone to improve motor performance, improve ability to participate in usual activities of daily living, and delay levodopa therapy. In advanced stages, one of these drugs can be used with levodopa and perhaps other antiparkinson drugs to provide more consistent relief of symptoms between doses of levodopa and allow reduced dosage of levodopa. These drugs are not ergot derivatives and may not cause some adverse effects associated with bromocriptine (e.g., pulmonary and peritoneal fibrosis, constriction of coronary arteries).

Pramipexole is rapidly absorbed with oral administration. Peak serum levels are reached in 1 to 3 hours after a dose and steady-state concentrations in about 2 days. It is less than 20% bound to plasma proteins and has an elimination half-life of 8 to 12 hours. Most of the drug is excreted unchanged in the urine; only 10% of the drug is metabolized. As a result, renal failure may cause higher-than-usual plasma levels and possible toxicity, but hepatic disease is unlikely to alter drug effects.

Ropinirole is also well absorbed with oral administration. It reaches peak serum levels in 1 to 2 hours and steady-state concentrations within 2 days. It is 40% bound to plasma proteins and has an elimination half-life of 6 hours. It is metabolized by the cytochrome P450 enzymes in the liver to inactive metabolites, which are excreted through the kidneys. Less than 10% of ropinirole is excreted unchanged in the urine. Thus, liver failure may decrease metabolism, allow drug accumulation, and increase adverse effects. Renal failure does not appear to alter drug effects.

Rotigotine is the first transdermal system to treat early idiopathic Parkinson's disease. The 24-hour duration of the transdermal system offers extended symptom control and significantly decreases the amount of "off-time". Onset of action is 1 to 3 hours after placing the patch, with peak action at 15 to 18 hours. The most common side effects reported include application site reactions, somnolence, nausea and vomiting, and dizziness.

Selegiline (Eldepryl) inhibits metabolism of dopamine by monoamine oxidase (MAO), which exists in two types, MAO-A and MAO-B, both of which are found in the CNS and peripheral tissues. They are differentiated by their relative specificities for individual catecholamines. MAO-A acts more specifically on tyramine, norepinephrine, epinephrine, and serotonin. This enzyme is the main subtype in GI mucosa and in the liver and is responsible for metabolizing dietary tyramine. If MAO-A is inhibited in the intestine, tyramine in various foods is absorbed systemically rather than deactivated. As a result, there is excessive stimulation of the sympathetic nervous system and severe hypertension and stroke can occur. This is sometimes called the "cheese reaction" because aged cheeses are high in tyramine. This life-threatening reaction can also occur with some medications (e.g., sympathomimetics) that are normally metabolized by MAO. MAO-B metabolizes dopamine; in the brain, most MAO activity is due to type B. At oral dosages of 10 milligrams per day or less, selegiline inhibits MAO-B *selectively* and is unlikely to cause severe hypertension and stroke. However, at dosages greater than 10 milligrams per day, selectivity is lost and metabolism of both MAO-A and MAO-B is inhibited. Dosages greater than 10 milligrams per day should be avoided in patients with Parkin-

son's disease. Selegiline inhibition of MAO-B is irreversible, and drug effects persist until more MAO is synthesized in the brain, which may take several months.

In early Parkinson's disease, selegiline may be effective as monotherapy (Level A). In advanced disease, it is given to enhance the effects of levodopa. Its addition aids symptom control and allows the dosage of levodopa/carbidopa to be reduced. Once proposed to have neuroprotective properties, it is now believed that there is insufficient evidence to recommend the use of selegiline to confer neuroprotection in patients with Parkinson's disease (Level U).

Rasagiline is the newest irreversible MAO inhibitor. It is indicated for initial treatment for idiopathic parkinsonism and as an adjunct therapy with levodopa to reduce "off time" when movements are poorly controlled. Because it has not been determined to be selective for MAO-B in humans, care must be taken to avoid tyramine-containing foods as well as sympathomimetic medications to prevent hypertensive crisis. In addition, rasagiline has the potential to increase serotonin neurotransmission. When given with other drugs that enhance stimulation of serotonergic receptors (e.g., antidepressants, St. John's wort, dextromethorphan, and meperidine), serotonin syndrome, a potential fatal CNS toxicity reaction characterized by hyperpyrexia and death, can occur. Rasagiline should be discontinued at least 14 days before beginning treatment with most antidepressants or other MAO inhibitors. Fluoxetine should be discontinued at least 5 weeks before initiating rasagiline, due to its long half-life. Rasagiline is well absorbed orally, metabolized in the liver, and excreted primarily by the kidney.

Nursing Process

Assessment

Assess for signs and symptoms of Parkinson's disease and drug-induced extrapyramidal reactions. These may include the following, depending on the severity and stage of progression.

- Slow movements (bradykinesia) and difficulty in changing positions, assuming an upright position, eating, dressing, and other self-care activities
- Stooped posture
- Accelerating gait with short steps
- Tremor at rest (e.g., "pill rolling" movements of fingers)
- Rigidity of arms, legs, and neck
- Mask-like, immobile facial expression
- Speech problems (e.g., low volume, monotonous tone, rapid, difficult to understand)
- Excessive salivation and drooling
- Dysphagia
- Excessive sweating
- Constipation from decreased intestinal motility
- Mental depression from self-consciousness and embarrassment over physical appearance and activity limitations.

Nursing Process continues on page 224

The intellect is usually intact until the late stages of the disease process.

Nursing Diagnoses

- Bathing/Grooming Self-Care Deficit related to tremors and impaired motor function
- Impaired Physical Mobility related to alterations in balance and coordination
- Deficient Knowledge: Safe usage and effects of antiparkinson drugs
- Imbalanced Nutrition: Less Than Body Requirements related to difficulty in chewing and swallowing food

Planning/Goals

The patient will

- Experience relief of excessive salivation, muscle rigidity, spasticity, and tremors
- Experience improved motor function, mobility, and self-care abilities
- Increase knowledge of the disease process and drug therapy
- Take medications as instructed
- Avoid falls and other injuries from the disease process or drug therapy.

Interventions

Use measures to assist the patient and family in coping with symptoms and maintaining function. These include the following:

- Provide physical therapy for heel-to-toe gait training; widening stance to increase balance and base of support; other exercises.
- Encourage ambulation and frequent changes of position, assisted if necessary.
- Help with active and passive range-of-motion exercises.
- Encourage self-care as much as possible. Cutting meat; opening cartons; giving frequent, small meals; and allowing privacy during mealtime may be helpful. If the client has difficulty chewing or swallowing, chopped or soft foods may be necessary. Hook-and-loop-type fasteners or zippers are easier to handle than buttons. Slip-on shoes are easier to manage than laced ones.
- Spend time with the patient and encourage socialization with other people. Victims of Parkinson's disease tend to become withdrawn, isolated, and depressed.
- Schedule rest periods. Tremor and rigidity are aggravated by fatigue and emotional stress.
- Provide facial tissues if drooling is a problem.
- Provide appropriate patient teaching related to drug therapy (see accompanying display).

Evaluation

- Interview and observe for relief of symptoms.
- Interview and observe for increased mobility and participation in activities of daily living.
- Interview and observe regarding correct usage of medications

Patient Teaching Guidelines   Antiparkinson Drugs

General Considerations

- Beneficial effects of antiparkinson drugs may not occur for a few weeks; do not stop taking the drugs before they have had a chance to work.
- Do not take other drugs without the physician's knowledge and consent. This is necessary to avoid adverse drug interactions. Prescription and nonprescription drugs may interact with antiparkinson drugs to increase or decrease effects.
- Avoid driving an automobile or operating other potentially hazardous machinery if vision is blurred or drowsiness occurs with levodopa.
- Change positions slowly, especially when assuming an upright position, and wear elastic stockings, if needed, to prevent dizziness from a drop in blood pressure.
- Pathologic gambling, increased libido, and hypersexuality have been reported with dopamine agonist medications.

Self- or Caregiver Administration

- Take antiparkinson drugs with or just after food to prevent or reduce anorexia, nausea, and vomiting.
- Do not crush or chew levodopa/carbidopa Sinemet CR. It is formulated to be released slowly; crushing or chewing destroys this feature.

- Take or give selegiline in the morning and at noon. This schedule decreases stimulating effects that may interfere with sleep if the drug is taken in the evening.
- Take or give entacapone with each dose of levodopa/carbidopa, up to 8 times daily.
- Decrease excessive mouth dryness by maintaining an adequate fluid intake (2000–3000 mL daily if not contraindicated) and using sugarless chewing gum and hard candies. Both anticholinergics and levodopa may cause mouth dryness. This is usually a therapeutic effect in Parkinson's disease. However, excessive mouth dryness causes discomfort and dental caries.
- Report adverse effects. Adverse effects can often be reduced by changing drugs or dosages. However, some adverse effects usually must be tolerated for control of disease symptoms.
- With rotigotine-transdermal, apply to clean dry intact-skin on abdomen, thigh, hip, flank, shoulder or upper arm. Rotate sites and do not reuse a site in less than 14 days. If shaving is necessary, wait 3 days to use the site. If the patch comes off, reapply to a fresh site.
- Remove rotigotine-transdermal patch before an MRI or cardioversion to avoid skin burns.

Applying Your Knowledge 12-2

Because Mrs. Sung was admitted following a fall and is experiencing many of the typical symptoms of a person with Parkinson's disease, she may be having ongoing difficulty with ambulation. What referral should you initiate to improve her safety?

Principles of Therapy

Goals of Therapy

Antiparkinson drugs aim to control symptoms, maintain functional ability in activities of daily living, minimize adverse drug effects, and slow disease progression.

Drug Selection

Choices of antiparkinson drugs depend largely on the type of parkinsonism (e.g., idiopathic or drug induced) and the severity of symptoms. In addition, because of difficulties with levodopa therapy (e.g., adverse effects, loss of effectiveness in a few years, possible acceleration of the loss of dopaminergic neurons in the brain), several drug therapy strategies and combinations are used to delay the start of levodopa therapy and, after it is started, to reduce levodopa dosage. Whenever possible, drug selection should be evidence based.

- For secondary parkinsonism, an anticholinergic agent is usually recommended; however, amantadine is also effective.

- For early idiopathic parkinsonism, when symptoms and functional disability are relatively mild, several drugs may be used in monotherapy. Selegiline may be considered as initial symptomatic treatment prior to beginning therapy with other dopaminergic agents (Level A).

- Amantadine may be used with patients with motor fluctuations for reducing dyskinesia (Level C). An anticholinergic agent may also be effective, relieving tremor in approximately 50% of patients.

- Either levodopa or a dopamine agonist may be prescribed as the initial dopaminergic agent in the treatment of Parkinson's disease. Levodopa is a better choice for improving motor disability, but dopamine agonists are better at lessening motor complications (Level A).

- For advanced idiopathic parkinsonism, a combination of medications is used. Two advantages of combination therapy are better control of symptoms and reduced dosage of individual drugs.

- The following recommendations are for reducing "off-time". Entacapone and rasagiline may be prescribed to reduce "off-time" with levodopa therapy (Level A). Pramipexole, ropinirole, and tolcapone can also be considered to reduce "off-time" (Level B); however, tolcapone requires careful monitoring for liver failure. Apomorphine, cabergoline (off-label use), and selegiline may be considered to reduce "off-time" (Level C). Rotigotine has been shown to significantly reduce "off-time" over a sustained 24-hour transdermal delivery of medication. Sustained-release carbidopa/levodopa and bromocriptine may be disregarded to reduce "off-time" (Level C). There is no difference in the rate of motor complications between intermediate-release levodopa and sustained-release levodopa formulations when initiating levodopa therapy (Level B).

- An anticholinergic agent may be given with levodopa alone or with a levodopa/carbidopa combination.

- Amantadine may be given in combination with levodopa or other antiparkinson agents.

- A dopamine agonist is usually given with levodopa/carbidopa. The combination provides more effective relief of symptoms and allows lower dosage of levodopa. Although available dopamine agonists are similarly effective, pramipexole, ropinirole, and rotigotine-transdermal cause less severe adverse effects than ergots such as bromocriptine.

- The levodopa/carbidopa combination is probably the most effective drug when bradykinesia and rigidity become prominent. However, because levodopa becomes less effective after approximately 5 to 7 years, many clinicians use other drugs first and reserve levodopa for use when symptoms become more severe.

- Selegiline may be given with levodopa/carbidopa and with entacapone, because selegiline acts in the brain and entacapone acts peripherally.

- Entacapone is used only with levodopa/carbidopa; simultaneous administration of carbidopa and entacapone significantly increases the plasma half-life of levodopa. (Stalevo is a newer product that combines levodopa, carbidopa, and entacapone.)

- Tolcapone should be used only when other drugs are ineffective, because of its association with liver failure.

- Rasagiline may be used as monotherapy or as an adjunct to levodopa.

- When changes are made in a drug therapy regimen, one change at a time is recommended so that effects of the change are clear.

Drug Dosage

The dosage of antiparkinson drugs is highly individualized. The general rule is to start with low initial dosage and gradually increase it until therapeutic effects, adverse effects, or maximum drug dosage is achieved. Additional guidelines include the following:

- The optimal dose is the lowest one that allows the patient to function adequately. Optimal dosage may not be established for 6 to 8 weeks with levodopa.

- Dosages need to be adjusted as parkinsonism progresses.

- Dosage must be individualized for levodopa and carbidopa. Only 5% to 10% of a dose of levodopa reaches the CNS, even with the addition of carbidopa. When carbidopa is given with levodopa, the dosage of levodopa must be reduced by approximately 75%. A daily dose of approximately 70 to 100 milligrams of carbidopa is required to saturate peripheral AADC. At least 12 hours should elapse between the last dose of levodopa and initiation of carbidopa/levodopa therapy to avoid drug toxicity.

- A levodopa/carbidopa combination is available in three dosage formulations (10 mg carbidopa/100 mg levodopa, 25 mg carbidopa/100 mg levodopa, and 25 mg carbidopa/250 mg levodopa) of immediate-release tablets (Sinemet) and two dosage formulations (25 mg carbidopa/100 mg levodopa, 50 mg carbidopa/200 mg levodopa) of sustained-release tablets (Sinemet CR). Various preparations can be mixed to administer optimal amounts of each ingredient. Sinemet CR is not as well absorbed as the short-acting form, and a patient being transferred to Sinemet CR needs a dosage increase of approximately one third.

- With levodopa, dosage should be gradually increased to the desired therapeutic level. In addition, therapeutic effects may be increased and adverse effects decreased by frequent administration of small doses.

- With pramipexole, ropinirole, and rotigotine-transdermal, dosage is started at low levels and gradually increased over several weeks. When the drugs are discontinued, they should be tapered in dosage over 1 week. With pramipexole, lower doses are indicated in older adults and those with renal impairment; with ropinirole and rotigotine-transdermal lower doses may be needed with hepatic impairment.

- Entacapone (200 mg) should be taken with each dose of levodopa (up to 8 times per day). Each tablet of Stalevo contains 200 milligrams of entacapone along with various amounts of levodopa and carbidopa.

- When combinations of drugs are used, dosage adjustments of individual components are often necessary. When levodopa is added to a regimen of anticholinergic drug therapy, for example, the anticholinergic drug need not be discontinued or reduced in dosage. However, when a dopaminergic drug is added to a regimen containing levodopa/carbidopa, dosage of levodopa/carbidopa must be reduced.

- Rasagiline may be used as monotherapy or as an adjunct with levodopa. When used with levodopa, reduced dosages of both rasagiline and levodopa are indicated. In the presence of mild liver dysfunction or concurrent therapy with ciprofloxacin or other CYP1A2 inhibitors, rasagiline dosage should be reduced by half.

⊘ Applying Your Knowledge 12-3

How Can You Avoid This Medication Error?
The physician writes a drug order for levodopa/carbidopa 25/100. The pharmacy supplies Sinemet CR 25/100 and you administer the medication.

Use in Special Populations

Use in Children
Safety and effectiveness for use in children have not been established for most antiparkinson drugs, including the centrally acting anticholinergics (all ages), levodopa (<12 years), and bromocriptine (<15 years). Because parkinsonism is a degenerative disorder of adults, antiparkinson drugs are most likely to be used in children for other purposes, anticholinergics are sometimes given to children who have drug-induced extrapyramidal reactions.

Use in Older Adults
Dosage of amantadine may need to be reduced because the drug is excreted mainly through the kidneys, and renal function is usually decreased in older adults. Dosage of levodopa/carbidopa may need to be reduced because of an age-related decrease in peripheral AADC, the enzyme that carbidopa inhibits.

Anticholinergic drugs may cause blurred vision, dry mouth, tachycardia, and urinary retention. They also decrease sweating and may cause fever or heatstroke. Fever may occur in any age group, but heatstroke is more likely to occur in older adults, especially with cardiovascular disease, strenuous activity, and high environmental temperatures. When centrally active anticholinergics are given for Parkinson's disease, agitation, mental confusion, hallucinations, and psychosis may occur. Many other drugs in addition to the primary anticholinergics have significant anticholinergic activity, such as some antihistamines in over-the-counter cold remedies and sleep aids, tricyclic antidepressants, and phenothiazine antipsychotic drugs. When anticholinergic drugs are needed in older adults, dosage should be minimized, combinations of drugs with anticholinergic effects should be avoided, and patients should be closely monitored for adverse drug effects.

Older patients are at increased risk of having hallucinations with dopamine agonist drugs. Pramipexole dosage may need to be reduced in older adults with impaired renal function. Changes in the skin of patients over the age of 80 may result in increased absorption and higher blood levels of rotigotine-transdermal.

Use in Patients With Renal Impairment
With amantadine, excretion is primarily via the kidneys, and the drug should be used with caution in patients with renal failure. With pramipexole, clearance is reduced in patients with moderate or severe renal impairment, and lower initial and maintenance doses are recommended. With ropinirole, rotigotine-transdermal, and entacapone, no dosage adjustments are needed for renal impairment.

Use in Patients With Hepatic Impairment
With ropinirole and rasagiline, cautious use in patients with hepatic impairment is warranted, and dosage may need to be reduced. Reduced dosages of rotigotine-transdermal are indicated with severe hepatic impairment. With tolcapone, ele-

vated liver enzymes and deaths from liver failure have been reported, prompting a **BLACK BOX WARNING** by the FDA regarding the potential for acute liver failure. Tolcapone therapy should not be initiated for any individual with liver disease or elevated liver enzymes. Liver transaminase enzymes should be monitored frequently on the schedule previously described. The drug should be withdrawn and not reinstated at the earliest sign of liver dysfunction. With entacapone periodic measurements of liver transaminase enzymes are recommended, although liver failure has not been associated with this drug.

Use in Home Care

The home care nurse can help patients and caregivers understand that the purpose of drug therapy is to control symptoms and that noticeable improvement may not occur for several weeks. Also, the nurse can encourage patients to consult physical therapists, speech therapists, and dietitians to help maintain their ability to perform activities of daily living. In addition, teaching about preventing or managing adverse drug effects may be necessary. Caregivers may need to be informed that most activities (e.g., eating, dressing) take longer and require considerable effort by patients with parkinsonism.

Nursing Actions   Antiparkinson Drugs

NURSING ACTIONS	RATIONALE/EXPLANATION
1. Administer accurately	
a. Give most antiparkinson drugs with or just after food; entacapone can be given without regard to meals.	To prevent or reduce nausea and vomiting
b. Do not crush Sinemet CR and instruct clients not to chew the tablet.	Crushing and chewing destroys the controlled-release feature of the formulation.
c. Do not give levodopa with iron preparations or multivitamin–mineral preparations containing iron.	Iron decreases absorption of levodopa.
d. Give selegiline in the morning and at noon.	To decrease central nervous system (CNS) stimulating effects that may interfere with sleep if the drug is taken in the evening
e. Give entacapone with each dose of levodopa/carbidopa, up to 8 times daily. Apply rotigotine-transdermal system to clean dry intact skin on abdomen, thigh, hip, flank, shoulder, or upper arm. Rotate sites & do not reuse a site in less than 14 days. Wait 3 days to use a site if shaving is necessary.	These measures promote optimal absorption.
2. Observe for therapeutic effects	
a. With anticholinergic agents, observe for decreased tremor, salivation, drooling, and sweating.	Decreased salivation and sweating are therapeutic effects when these drugs are used in Parkinson's disease, but they are adverse effects when the drugs are used in other disorders.
b. With levodopa and dopaminergic agents, observe for improvement in mobility, balance, posture, gait, speech, handwriting, and self-care ability. Drooling and seborrhea may be abolished, and mood may be elevated.	Therapeutic effects are usually evident within 2–3 weeks, as levodopa dosage approaches 2–3 g/d, but may not reach optimum levels for 6 months.
3. Observe for adverse effects	
a. With anticholinergic drugs, observe for atropine-like effects, such as:	
(1) Tachycardia and palpitations	These effects may occur with usual therapeutic doses but are not likely to be serious except in people with underlying heart disease.
(2) Excessive CNS stimulation (tremor, restlessness, confusion, hallucinations, delirium)	This effect is most likely to occur with large doses of trihexyphenidyl (Trihexy) or benztropine (Cogentin). It may occur with levodopa.
(3) Sedation and drowsiness	These are most likely to occur with benztropine. The drug has antihistaminic and anticholinergic properties, and sedation is attributed to the antihistamine effect.
(4) Constipation, impaction, paralytic ileus	These effects result from decreased gastrointestinal motility and muscle tone. They may be severe because decreased intestinal motility and constipation also are characteristics of Parkinson's disease; thus, additive effects may occur.

(continued on page 228)

Nursing Actions Antiparkinson Drugs (continued)

NURSING ACTIONS	RATIONALE/EXPLANATION
(5) Urinary retention	This reaction is caused by loss of muscle tone in the bladder and is most likely to occur in elderly men who have enlarged prostate glands.
(6) Dilated pupils (mydriasis), blurred vision, photophobia	Ocular effects are due to paralysis of accommodation and relaxation of the ciliary muscle and the sphincter muscle of the iris.
b. With levodopa, observe for:	
(1) Anorexia, nausea, and vomiting	These symptoms usually disappear after a few months of drug therapy. They may be minimized by giving levodopa with food, gradually increasing dosage, administering smaller doses more frequently or adding carbidopa so that dosage of levodopa can be reduced.
(2) Orthostatic hypotension—check blood pressure in both sitting and standing positions q4h while the client is awake.	This effect is common during the first few weeks but usually subsides eventually. It can be minimized by arising slowly from supine or sitting positions and by wearing elastic stockings.
(3) Cardiac dysrhythmias (tachycardia, premature ventricular contractions) and increased myocardial contractility	Levodopa and its metabolites stimulate beta-adrenergic receptors in the heart. People with pre-existing coronary artery disease may need a beta-adrenergic blocking agent (e.g., propranolol) to counteract these effects.
(4) Dyskinesia—involuntary movements that may involve only the tongue, mouth, and face or the whole body	Dyskinesia eventually develops in most people who take levodopa. It is related to duration of levodopa therapy rather than dosage. Carbidopa may heighten this adverse effect, and there is no way to prevent it except by decreasing levodopa dosage. Many people prefer dyskinesia to lowering drug dosage and subsequent return of the parkinsonism symptoms.
(5) CNS stimulation—restlessness, agitation, confusion, delirium	This is more likely to occur with levodopa/carbidopa combination drug therapy.
(6) Abrupt swings in motor function (on–off phenomenon)	This fluctuation may indicate progression of the disease process. It often occurs after long-term levodopa use.
c. With amantadine, observe for:	
(1) CNS stimulation—insomnia, hyperexcitability, ataxia, dizziness, slurred speech, mental confusion, hallucinations	Compared with other antiparkinson drugs, amantadine produces few adverse effects. The ones that occur are mild, transient, and reversible. However, adverse effects increase if daily dosage exceeds 200 mg.
(2) Livedo reticularis—patchy, bluish discoloration of skin on the legs	This is a benign but cosmetically unappealing condition. It usually occurs with long-term use of amantadine and disappears when the drug is discontinued.
d. With bromocriptine, observe for:	
(1) Nausea	These symptoms are usually mild and can be minimized by starting with low doses and increasing the dose gradually until the desired effect is achieved. If adverse effects do occur, they usually disappear with a decrease in dosage.
(2) Confusion and hallucinations	
(3) Hypotension	
e. With pramipexole and ropinirole, observe for:	These effects occurred more commonly than others during clinical trials.
(1) Nausea	
(2) Confusion, hallucinations	
(3) Dizziness, drowsiness	
(4) Dyskinesias	
(5) Orthostatic hypotension	
f. With selegiline, observe for:	
(1) CNS effects—agitation, ataxia, bradykinesia, confusion, dizziness, dyskinesias, hallucinations, insomnia	
(2) Nausea, abdominal pain	
g. With rasagiline observe for:	These effects occurred more commonly than others in clinical trials.
(1) Arthralgia	
(2) Dyspepsia	
(3) Depression	
(4) Orthostatic hypotension	
(5) Flu-like syndrome	

NURSING ACTIONS	RATIONALE/EXPLANATION
h. With entacapone and tolcapone, observe for: (1) Anorexia, nausea, vomiting, diarrhea, constipation (2) Dizziness, drowsiness (3) Dyskinesias and dystonias (4) Hallucinations (5) Orthostatic hypotension	These effects occurred more commonly than others during clinical trials.
i. With rotigotine-transdermal observe for: (1) Skin irritation (2) Nausea and vomiting (3) Somnolence (4) Dizziness (5) Orthostatic hypotension	These effects occurred more commonly than others during clinical trials.
4. Observe for drug interactions a. Drugs that *increase* effects of anticholinergic drugs: (1) Antihistamines, disopyramide (Norpace), thiothixene (Navane), phenothiazines, and tricyclic antidepressants	These drugs have anticholinergic properties and produce additive anticholinergic effects.
b. Drugs that *decrease* effects of anticholinergic drugs: (1) Cholinergic agents	These drugs counteract the inhibition of gastrointestinal motility and tone, which is a side effect of anticholinergic drug therapy.
c. Drugs that *increase* effects of levodopa: (1) Amantadine, anticholinergic agents, bromocriptine, carbidopa, entacapone, pramipexole, ropinirole, selegiline, tolcapone, rotigotine-transdermal.	These drugs are often used in combination for treatment of Parkinson's disease.
(2) Tricyclic antidepressants	These drugs potentiate levodopa effects and increase the risk of cardiac arrhythmias in people with heart disease.
(3) Monoamine oxidase type A (MAO-A) inhibitors, including isocarboxazid (Marplan), phenelzine (Nardil), and tranylcypromine (Parnate)	The combination of a catecholamine precursor (levodopa) and MAO-A inhibitors that decrease metabolism of catecholamines can result in excessive amounts of dopamine, epinephrine, and norepinephrine. Heart palpitations, headache, hypertensive crisis, and stroke may occur. Levodopa and MAO-A inhibitors should not be given concurrently. Also, levodopa should not be started within 2 weeks after an MAO-A inhibitor is discontinued. Effects of MAO-A inhibitors persist for 1–2 weeks after their discontinuation. These effects are unlikely to occur with selegiline, an MAO-B inhibitor, which more selectively inhibits the metabolism of dopamine. However, selectivity may be lost at doses higher than the recommended 10 mg/d. Selegiline is used with levodopa. Rasagiline is also indicated for adjunctive therapy with levodopa.
d. Drugs that *decrease* effects of levodopa: (1) Anticholinergics	Although anticholinergics are often given with levodopa for increased antiparkinson effects, they also may decrease effects of levodopa by delaying gastric emptying. This causes more levodopa to be metabolized in the stomach and decreases the amount available for absorption from the intestine.
(2) Alcohol; benzodiazepines (e.g., diazepam [Valium]); antiemetics; antipsychotics such as phenothiazines, haloperidol (Haldol), and thiothixene (Navane)	The mechanisms by which most of these drugs decrease effects of levodopa are not clear. Phenothiazines block dopamine receptors in the basal ganglia.
(3) Oral iron preparations	Iron binds with levodopa and reduces levodopa absorption, possibly by as much as 50%.
(4) Pyridoxine (vitamin B_6)	Pyridoxine stimulates decarboxylase, the enzyme that converts levodopa to dopamine. As a result, more levodopa is metabolized in peripheral tissues, and less reaches the CNS, where antiparkinson effects occur.
e. Drugs that *increase* effects of rasagiline: (1) Ciprofloxacin	Inhibits CYPIA2 enzymes responsible for the metabolism of rasagiline.

(continued on page 230)

Nursing Actions Antiparkinson Drugs (continued)

NURSING ACTIONS	RATIONALE/EXPLANATION
(2) Antidepressants (SSRIs, MAOIs, St. John's wort), Dextromethorphan, Meperidine	Combining drugs that enhance serotonin neurotransmission by different mechanisms can result in excessive serotonin neurotransmission, a potentially fatal condition called serotonin syndrome, characterized by CNS toxicity and hyperpyrexia. Rasagailine should be discontinued 14 days before treatment with any of these drugs. Fluoxetine should be discontinued 5 weeks before treatment with rasagiline due to the long half-life of fluoxetine.
f. Drugs that decrease effects of dopaminergic antiparkinson drugs: (1) Antipsychotic drugs (2) Metoclopramide (Reglan)	These drugs are dopamine antagonists and therefore inhibit the effects of dopamine agonists.

Key Concepts

- Parkinsonism is a progressive neurodegenerative disorder characterized by a deficit of dopamine and a relative excess of acetylcholine.

- Classic symptoms of Parkinson's disease include resting tremor, bradykinesia, rigidity, and postural instability.

- Dopaminergic drugs increase dopamine concentrations in the brain, exerting dopaminergic activity, directly or indirectly.

- Dopamine activity can be increased by increasing dopamine release and reducing neuronal reuptake (amantadine), directly stimulating dopamine receptors (apomorphine, bromocriptine, pramipexole, ropinirole, rotigotine-transdermal), replacement of dopamine or its precursor (levodopa,), or inhibition of metabolism of

dopamine by MAO or COMT enzymes (rasagiline, selegiline, entacapone, tolcapone).

- Carbidopa prevents levodopa breakdown in the periphery, resulting in higher brain concentrations with lower levodopa dosages.

- Anticholinergic drugs (e.g., benztropine, trihexyphenidyl, and diphenhydramine) decrease the effect of acetylcholine in the brain.

- Combinations of antiparkinson drugs are often given to reduce dosages and achieve better control of symptoms.

- Care must be taken to avoid serious food or drug interactions that may diminish treatment effectiveness (levodopa) or be potentially fatal (selegiline and rasagiline).

Review and Application Exercises

Short Answer Exercises

1. Which neurotransmitter is deficient in idiopathic and drug-induced parkinsonism?

2. How do the antiparkinson drugs act to alter the level of the deficient neurotransmitter?

3. What are the advantages and disadvantages of the various drugs used to treat parkinsonism?

4. Why is it desirable to delay the start of levodopa therapy and, after it is started, to reduce dosage as much as possible?

5. What is the rationale for various combinations of antiparkinson drugs?

6. What are the major adverse effects of antiparkinson drugs, and how can they be minimized?

NCLEX-Style Questions

7. A patient's wife has asked the nurse for an explanation of how an imbalance in neurotransmitters in Parkinson's disease affects her husband. The nurse is correct in telling her that the disease is involved in an imbalance of neurotransmitters in which of the following structures?
   a. basal ganglia
   b. cerebral cortex
   c. limbic system
   d. reticular activating system

8. The nurse is able to explain the use of medications for Parkinson's disease, using core knowledge that the main pathophysiology of Parkinson's disease is a decrease in the brain content of which of the following substances?
   a. acetylcholine
   b. serotonin
   c. glutamate
   d. dopamine

9. Periodic assessment of a patient with parkinsonism should include which of the following?
   a. blood tests of liver function
   b. blood tests of kidney function
   c. evaluation of mental status
   d. evaluation of responses to drug therapy

10. The main purpose of combination drug therapy for parkinsonism is to
    a. stop disease progression
    b. relieve adverse effects of other drugs
    c. reduce dosage of levodopa
    d. delay the need for drug therapy

11. The nurse demonstrates understanding of the use of combination therapy for Parkinson's disease by knowing that carbidopa is usually given along with levodopa because it
    a. crosses the blood–brain barrier and acts centrally
    b. inhibits peripheral breakdown of levodopa
    c. directly stimulates dopamine receptors in the brain
    d. decreases adverse effects of anticholinergic antiparkinson drugs

Selected References

Centers for Disease Control and Prevention. (2006, June 28). Prevention and control of influenza. MMWR, 155, 1–41.

Drug facts and comparisons. (Updated monthly). St. Louis, MO: Facts and Comparisons.

Jackson, C. W., & Curtis, J. L. (2005). Sleep disorders. In J. T. DiPiro, R. L. Talbert, G. C. Yee, G. R. Matzke, B. G. Wells, & L. M. Posey (Eds.), *Pharmacotherapy: A pathophysiologic approach* (6th ed., pp. 1329–1330). New York: McGraw-Hill.

Nelson, M. V., Berchou, R. C., & LeWitt, P. A. (2005). Parkinson's disease. In J. T. DiPiro, R. L. Talbert, G. C. Yee, G. R. Matzke, B. G. Wells, & L. M. Posey (Eds.), *Pharmacotherapy: A pathophysiologic approach* (6th ed., pp. 1075–1088). New York: McGraw-Hill.

Porth, C. M., & Curtis, R. L. (2005). Disorders of motor function. In C. M. Porth (Ed.), *Pathophysiology: Concepts of altered health states* (7th ed., pp. 1210–1212). Philadelphia: Lippincott Williams & Wilkins.

Smeltzer, S. C., Bare, B. G., Hinkle, J. L., & Cheever, K. H. (2008). *Brunner & Suddarth's textbook of medical-surgical nursing* (11th ed., pp. 2311–2319). Philadelphia: Lippincott Williams & Wilkins.

Sommers, M. S., Johnson, S. A., & Beery, T. A. (2007). *Diseases and disorders: A nursing therapeutics manual* (3rd ed., pp. 697–701). Philadelphia: F. A. Davis.

Quality Standards Subcommittee of the American Academy of Neurology. (2002, January 8). *Practice parameter: Initiation of treatment for Parkinson's disease (An evidence-based review)*. Retrieved January 17, 2007, from http://www.guidelines.gov/summary.aspx?doc_id=3123

Quality Standards Subcommittee of the American Academy of Neurology. (2006, April 11). *Practice parameter: Treatment of Parkinson disease with motor fluctuations and dyskinesia (An evidence-based review)*. Retrieved January 17, 2007, from http://www.guidelines.gov/summary.aspx?doc_id=9124

Quality Standards Subcommittee of the American Academy of Neurology. (2006, April 11). *Practice parameter: Neuroprotective strategies and alternative therapies for Parkinson's disease (An evidence-based review)*. Retrieved January 17, 2007, from http://www.guidelines.gov/summary.aspx?doc_id=9122

Skeletal Muscle Relaxants

KEY TERMS

- Clonic
- Malignant hyperthermia
- Muscle spasm
- Spasticity
- Tonic

LEARNING OBJECTIVES

After studying this chapter, you will be able to:

1. Discuss common symptoms and disorders for which skeletal muscle relaxants are used.
2. Differentiate uses and effects of selected skeletal muscle relaxants.
3. Describe nonpharmacologic interventions to relieve muscle spasm and spasticity.
4. Apply the nursing process with patients experiencing muscle spasm or spasticity.

Applying Your Knowledge

Annette Milewski, age 52, has had multiple sclerosis since she was 33 years of age. She is prescribed baclofen (Lioresal) 15 mg PO 3 times per day to control spasticity. Her family and a home health aide provide the care she requires. You are the home health nurse visiting for her monthly evaluation.

Introduction

Skeletal muscle relaxants are used to decrease muscle spasm or spasticity that occurs in certain neurologic and musculoskeletal disorders. (Neuromuscular blocking agents used as adjuncts to general anesthesia for surgery are included in Appendix C.)

Muscle Spasm

Muscle spasm or cramp is a sudden, involuntary, painful muscle contraction that occurs with musculoskeletal trauma (e.g., overuse or injury of skeletal muscle, twisting a joint, or tearing a ligament as with a sprain) or inflammation (e.g., bursitis, arthritis). Muscle spasm also occurs with acute or chronic low back pain. Spasms may be *clonic* (alternating contraction and relaxation) or *tonic* (sustained contraction). Muscle spasms commonly occur and may cause significant disability when inflammation, edema, and pain interfere with coordination and mobility.

Spasticity

Spasticity involves increased muscle tone or contraction and stiff, awkward movements. It occurs in neurologic disorders such as multiple sclerosis, spinal cord injury, traumatic brain injury, cerebral palsy, and post-stroke syndrome. Because spasticity is caused by nerve damage in the brain and spinal cord, it is a permanent condition that may be painful and disabling.

In patients with spinal cord injury, spasticity requires treatment when it impairs safety, mobility, and the ability to perform activities of daily living (e.g., self-care in hygiene, eating, dressing, and work or recreational activities). Stimuli that precipitate spasms vary from one individual to another and may include muscle stretching, bladder infections or stones, constipation and bowel distention, or infections. Each person should be assessed for personal precipitating factors, so that these factors can be avoided if possible. Treatment measures include passive range-of-motion and muscle-stretching exercises and antispasmodic medications (e.g., baclofen, dantrolene).

Multiple Sclerosis

Multiple sclerosis (MS), a major cause of neurologic disability among young and middle-aged adults, occurs more often in women than in men and usually has a pattern of exacerbations and remissions. It is considered an autoimmune disorder that occurs in genetically susceptible individuals, and its cause is unknown. MS involves destruction of portions of the myelin sheath that covers nerves in the brain, spinal cord, and optic nerve. Myelin normally insulates the neuron from electrical activity and conducts electrical impulses rapidly along nerve fibers. When myelin is destroyed (a process called demyelination, which probably results from inflammation), fibrotic lesions are formed and nerve conduction is slowed or blocked around the lesions. Lesions in various states of development (e.g., acute, subacute, chronic) often occur at multiple sites in the central nervous system (CNS). Muscle weakness and other symptoms vary according to the location and duration of the myelin damage.

In recent years, researchers have discovered that nerve cells can be repaired (remyelinated) if the process that damaged the myelin is stopped before the oligodendrocytes (the cells that form myelin) are destroyed. Other researchers are trying to develop methods for enhancing nerve conduction velocity in demyelinated nerves.

People with minimal symptoms do not require treatment but should be encouraged to maintain a healthy lifestyle. Those with more extensive symptoms should try to avoid emotional stress, extremes of environmental temperature, infections, and excessive fatigue. Physical therapy may help maintain muscle tone, and occupational therapy may help maintain ability to perform activities of daily living.

Drug therapy for MS may involve various medications for different stages of the disease (see Evidence-Based Practice Box 13-1). Corticosteroids, potent anti-inflammatory drugs, are used to treat acute exacerbations (see Chap. 23); interferon beta, glatiramer, and mitoxantrone suppress the immune system and are given to prevent relapses (see Chap. 41). Other drugs (e.g., antibiotics, antidepressants, anticonvulsants for neuropathic pain) are used to treat symptoms. A skeletal muscle relaxant (e.g., baclofen, tizanidine, or dantrolene) is used to treat the symptom of spasticity. In some cases, decreasing spasticity may not be desirable, because patients with severe leg weakness may require some degree of spasticity to ambulate. In cases of severe spasticity, baclofen may be given intrathecally through an implanted subcutaneous pump.

Evidence-Based Practice

13-1 Drug Therapy for Relapsing, Remitting Multiple Sclerosis

Acute Exacerbations

▪ High-dose methylprednisolone (e.g., 500–1000 mg IV daily for 3–5 days) (Level A)

Disease-Modifying Drugs

▪ Interferon beta-1a (Avonex, Rebif) and interferon beta-1b (Betaseron) (Level A). In 2005, the FDA issued a warning that "Severe hepatic injury, including cases of hepatic failure, has been reported in patients taking Avonex."
▪ Glatiramer (Copaxone) (Level A)
▪ Mitoxantrone (Novantrone) (Level B). In 2005, the FDA issued a warning about risks of cardiotoxicity and secondary acute myelogenous leukemia (AML).

Sources: Information adapted from Goodin et al. (2002) and the National Collaborating Centre for Chronic Conditions (United Kingdom) (2004) (articles obtained from the National Guideline Clearinghouse at www.guideline.gov). Please consult the cited journals or the National Guideline Clearinghouse for additional information regarding drug therapy of MS.

Applying Your Knowledge 13-1

What general teaching points should you emphasize with Mrs. Milewski and her caregivers to prevent exacerbation of symptoms?

General Characteristics of Skeletal Muscle Relaxants

Mechanism of Action

All skeletal muscle relaxants except dantrolene are centrally active drugs. Pharmacologic action is usually attributed to general depression of the CNS but may involve blockage of nerve impulses that cause increased muscle tone and contraction. It is unclear whether relief of pain results from muscle relaxation or sedative effects. In addition, although parenteral administration of some drugs (e.g., diazepam, methocarbamol) relieves pain associated with acute musculoskeletal trauma or inflammation, it is uncertain whether oral administration of usual doses exerts a beneficial effect in acute or chronic disorders.

Baclofen and diazepam increase the effects of gamma-aminobutyric acid, an inhibitory neurotransmitter. Tizanidine inhibits motor neurons in the brain. Dantrolene is the only skeletal muscle relaxant that acts peripherally on the muscle itself; it inhibits the release of calcium in skeletal muscle cells, thereby decreasing the strength of muscle contraction.

Indications for Use

Skeletal muscle relaxants are used primarily as adjuncts to other treatment measures such as physical therapy. Occasionally, parenteral agents are given to facilitate orthopedic procedures and examinations. In spastic disorders, skeletal muscle relaxants are indicated when spasticity causes severe pain or inability to tolerate physical therapy, sit in a wheelchair, or participate in self-care activities of daily living (e.g., eating, dressing). The drugs should not be given if they cause excessive muscle weakness and impair rather than facilitate mobility and function. Dantrolene also is indicated for prevention and treatment of *malignant hyperthermia* (see "Individual Drugs").

Contraindications to Use

Most skeletal muscle relaxants cause CNS depression and have the same contraindications as other CNS depressants. They should be used cautiously in patients with impaired renal or hepatic function or respiratory depression and in patients who must be alert for activities of daily living (e.g., driving a car, operating potentially hazardous machinery). Cyclobenzaprine has high levels of anticholinergic activity and therefore should be used cautiously in patients with glaucoma, urinary retention, cardiac dysrhythmias, or tachycardia.

Applying Your Knowledge 13-2

During your assessment, you note that Mrs. Milewski is having more weakness in her lower extremities during this visit as compared with your visit 1 month ago. You also note that the prescriber has recently increased the dose of baclofen from 10 to 15 mg. How would you respond?

Individual Drugs

Individual skeletal muscle relaxants are described below. Routes and dosage ranges are listed in Table 13-1.

Baclofen (Lioresal) is used mainly to treat spasticity in MS and spinal cord injuries. It is contraindicated in people with hypersensitivity reactions and in those with muscle spasm from rheumatic disorders. It can be given orally and intrathecally through an implanted subcutaneous pump. Check the literature from the pump manufacturer for information about pump implantation and drug infusion techniques.

Oral baclofen begins to act in 1 hour, peaks in 2 hours, and lasts 4 to 8 hours. It is metabolized in the liver and excreted in urine; its half-life is 3 to 4 hours. Dosage must be reduced in patients with impaired renal function. Common adverse effects include drowsiness, dizziness, confusion, constipation, fatigue, headache, hypotension, insomnia, nausea, and weakness. When discontinued, dosage should be tapered and the drug withdrawn over 1 to 2 weeks.

Carisoprodol (Soma) is used to relieve discomfort from acute, painful musculoskeletal disorders. It is not recom-

mended for long-term use. If used long term or in high doses, it can cause physical dependence, and it may cause symptoms of withdrawal if stopped abruptly. The drug is contraindicated in patients with intermittent porphyria, a rare metabolic disorder characterized by acute abdominal pain and neurologic symptoms. Oral drug acts within 30 minutes, peaks in 1 to 2 hours, and lasts 4 to 6 hours. It is metabolized in the liver and has a half-life of 8 hours. Common adverse effects include drowsiness, dizziness, and impaired motor coordination.

Cyclobenzaprine (Flexeril) has the same indication for use as carisoprodol. It is contraindicated in patients with cardiovascular disorders (e.g., recent myocardial infarction, dysrhythmias, heart block) or hyperthyroidism. The oral drug acts in 1 hour, peaks in 4 to 6 hours, and lasts 12 to 24 hours. The half-life is 1 to 3 days. Duration of use should not exceed 3 weeks. Common adverse effects are drowsiness, dizziness, and anticholinergic effects (e.g., dry mouth, constipation, urinary retention, tachycardia).

Dantrolene (Dantrium) acts directly on skeletal muscle to inhibit muscle contraction. It is used to relieve spasticity in neurologic disorders (e.g., MS, spinal cord injury) and to prevent or treat malignant hyperthermia, a rare but life-threatening complication of anesthesia characterized by hypercarbia, metabolic acidosis, skeletal muscle rigidity, fever, and cyanosis. For preoperative prophylaxis in people with previous episodes of malignant hyperthermia, the drug is given orally for 1 to 2 days before surgery. For intraoperative malignant hyperthermia, the drug is given intravenously (IV). After an occurrence during surgery, the drug is given orally for 1 to 3 days to prevent recurrence of symptoms.

Oral dantrolene acts slowly, peaking in 4 to 6 hours and lasting 8 to 10 hours, whereas IV drug acts more quickly and lasts 6 to 8 hours. Common adverse effects include drowsiness, dizziness, diarrhea, and fatigue. The most serious adverse effect is potentially fatal hepatitis, with jaundice and other symptoms that usually occur within 1 month of starting drug therapy. Liver function tests should be monitored periodically in all patients receiving dantrolene. These adverse effects do not occur with short-term use of IV drug for malignant hyperthermia.

Metaxalone (Skelaxin) is used to relieve discomfort from acute, painful musculoskeletal disorders. It is contraindicated in patients with anemias or severe renal or hepatic impairment. Oral drug acts within 60 minutes, peaks in 2 hours, and lasts 4 to 6 hours. It has a half-life of 2 to 3 hours, is metabolized in the liver, and is excreted in urine. Common adverse effects include drowsiness, dizziness, and nausea; hepatotoxicity and hemolytic anemia may also occur. Liver function should be monitored during therapy.

Methocarbamol (Robaxin) is used to relieve discomfort from acute, painful musculoskeletal disorders. It may also be used to treat tetanus. The parenteral form is contraindicated in patients with renal impairment, because the solution contains polyethylene glycol. The oral drug acts within 30 minutes and peaks in 2 hours, and the parenteral drug acts rapidly, but peak and duration of action are unknown. Methocarbamol has a

Table 13-1	Drugs at a Glance: Skeletal Muscle Relaxants	

	ROUTES AND DOSAGE RANGES	
Generic/Trade Name	**Adults**	**Children**
Baclofen (Lioresal)	PO 5 mg 3 times daily for 3 d; 10 mg 3 times daily for 3 d; 15 mg 3 times daily for 3 d; then 20 mg 3 times daily, if necessary Intrathecal via implanted pump: Dosage varies widely; see manufacturer's recommendations.	<12 years: Safety not established
Carisoprodol (Soma)	PO 350 mg 3 or 4 times daily, with the last dose at bedtime	<12 years: Not recommended
Cyclobenzaprine (Flexeril)	PO 10 mg 3 times daily. Maximal recommended duration, 3 weeks; maximal recommended dose, 60 mg daily	<15 years: Safety and effectiveness have not been established.
Dantrolene (Dantrium)	PO 25 mg daily initially, gradually increased weekly (by increments of 50–100 mg/d) to a maximal dose of 400 mg daily in 4 divided doses Preoperative prophylaxis of malignant hyperthermia: PO 4–8 mg/kg/d in 3–4 divided doses for 1 or 2 days before surgery Intraoperative malignant hyperthermia: IV push 1 mg/kg initially, continued until symptoms are relieved or a maximum total dose of 10 mg/kg has been given Postcrisis follow-up treatment: PO 4–8 mg/kg/d in 4 divided doses for 1–3 days	Spasticity: PO 1 mg/kg/d initially, gradually increased to a maximal dose of 3 mg/kg 4 times daily, not to exceed 400 mg daily Malignant hyperthermia: Same as adult
Diazepam (Valium)	PO 2–10 mg 3 or 4 times daily IM, IV 5–10 mg repeated in 3–4 hours if necessary	PO 0.12–0.8 mg/kg/d in 3 or 4 divided doses IM, IV 0.04–0.2 mg/kg in a single dose, not to exceed 0.6 mg/kg within an 8-h period
Metaxalone (Skelaxin)	PO 800 mg 3 or 4 times daily	>12 years: Same as adult <12 years: Safety and effectiveness have not been established.
Methocarbamol (Robaxin)	PO 1.5–2 g 4 times daily for 48–72 hours, reduced to 1 g 4 times daily for maintenance IM 500 mg q8h IV 1–3 g daily at a rate not to exceed 300 mg/min (3 mL of 10% injection). Do not give IV more than 3 days.	Safety and effectiveness have not been established except for treatment of tetanus (IV 15 mg/kg every 6 h as indicated).
Tizanidine (Zanaflex)	PO 4 mg q6–8h initially, increased gradually if needed. Maximum of 3 doses and 36 mg in 24 h	Safety and effectiveness have not been established.

half-life of 1 to 2 hours. It is metabolized in the liver and excreted in urine and feces. Common adverse effects with oral drug include drowsiness, dizziness, nausea, and urticaria; effects with injected drug also include fainting, incoordination, and hypotension. The drug may also give urine a green, brown, or black color. This is considered a harmless effect, but patients should be informed about it.

Tizanidine (Zanaflex) is an alpha$_2$-adrenergic agonist, similar to clonidine, that is used to treat spasticity in patients with MS, spinal cord injury, or brain trauma. It should be used cautiously in patients with renal or hepatic impairment and hypotension. It is given orally, and it begins to act within 30 to 60 minutes, peaks in 1 to 2 hours, and lasts 3 to 4 hours. Its half-life is 3 to 4 hours. It is metabolized in the liver and excreted in urine. Common adverse effects include drowsiness, dizziness, constipation, dry mouth, and hypotension. Hypotension may be significant and occur at usual doses. The drug may also cause psychotic symptoms, including hallucinations.

Nursing Process

Assessment

Assess for muscle spasm and spasticity.

- With muscle spasm, assess for:
  - **Pain.** This is a prominent symptom of muscle spasm and is usually aggravated by movement. Try to determine the location as specifically as possible, as well as the intensity, duration, and precipitating factors (e.g., traumatic injury, strenuous exercise).
  - **Accompanying signs and symptoms,** such as bruises (ecchymoses), edema, or signs of inflammation (redness, heat, edema, tenderness to touch)
- With spasticity, assess for pain and impaired functional ability in self-care (e.g., eating, dressing). In addition, severe spasticity interferes with ambulation and other movement as well as exercises to maintain joint and muscle mobility.

Nursing Diagnoses

- Pain related to muscle spasm
- Impaired Physical Mobility related to spasm and pain
- Bathing/Hygiene Self-Care Deficit related to spasm and pain
- Deficient Knowledge: Nondrug measures to relieve muscle spasm, pain, and spasticity and safe usage of skeletal muscle relaxants
- Risk for Injury: Dizziness, sedation related to CNS depression

Planning/Goals

The patient will

- Experience relief of pain and spasm
- Experience improved motor function
- Increase self-care abilities in activities of daily living
- Take medications as instructed
- Use nondrug measures appropriately
- Be safeguarded when sedated from drug therapy

Interventions

Use adjunctive measures for muscle spasm and spasticity.

- Physical therapy (massage, moist heat, exercises)
- Relaxation techniques
- Correct posture and lifting techniques (e.g., stooping rather than bending to lift objects, holding heavy objects close to the body, *not* lifting excessive amounts of weight)
- Regular exercise and use of warm-up exercises. Strenuous exercise performed on an occasional basis (e.g., weekly or monthly) is more likely to cause acute muscle spasm.

Evaluation

- Interview and observe for relief of symptoms.
- Interview and observe regarding correct usage of medications and nondrug therapeutic measures.

Principles of Therapy

Goals of Therapy

Skeletal muscle relaxants aim to relieve pain, muscle spasm, and muscle spasticity without impairing the ability to perform self-care activities of daily living.

Applying Your Knowledge 13-3

Mrs. Milewski's family gives her all of her morning medications as soon as she wakes up. Mrs. Milewski is complaining about an upset stomach. What should be changed?

Drug Selection

Choice of a skeletal muscle relaxant depends mainly on the disorder being treated.

- For acute muscle spasm and pain, oral or parenteral drugs may be used. These drugs cause sedation and other adverse effects and are recommended for short-term use. Cyclobenzaprine should not be used longer than 3 weeks.
- For orthopedic procedures, parenteral agents are preferred because they have greater sedative and pain-relieving effects.
- For spasticity in people with MS, baclofen (Lioresal) and tizanidine (Zanaflex) are approved. The two drugs are similarly effective, but tizanidine may cause fewer adverse effects.
- None of the skeletal muscle relaxants has been established as safe for use during pregnancy and lactation.
- For children, the drug should be chosen from those with established pediatric dosages.

Use in Special Populations

Use in Children

For most of the skeletal muscle relaxants, safety and effectiveness for use in children 12 years of age and younger have not been established. The drugs should be used only when clearly indicated, for short periods, when close supervision is available for monitoring drug effects (especially sedation), and when mobility and alertness are not required.

Use in Older Adults

Any CNS depressant or sedating drug should be used cautiously in older adults. Risks of falls, mental confusion, and other

Patient Teaching Guidelines | Skeletal Muscle Relaxants

General Considerations

- Use nondrug measures, such as exercises and applications of heat and cold, to decrease muscle spasm and spasticity.
- Avoid activities that require mental alertness or physical coordination (e.g., driving an automobile, operating potentially dangerous machinery) if drowsy from medication.
- Do not take other drugs without the physician's knowledge, including nonprescription drugs. The major risk occurs with concurrent use of alcohol, antihistamines, sleeping aids, or other drugs that cause drowsiness.

- Avoid herbal preparations that cause drowsiness or sleep, including valerian.

Self-Administration

- Take the drugs with milk or food, to avoid nausea and stomach irritation.
- Do not stop drugs abruptly. Dosage should be decreased gradually, especially with baclofen (Lioresal), carisoprodol (Soma), and cyclobenzaprine (Flexeril). Suddenly stopping baclofen may cause hallucinations; stopping the other drugs may cause fatigue, headache, and nausea.

---

adverse effects are higher because of impaired drug metabolism and excretion.

Use in Patients With Renal Impairment

The skeletal muscle relaxants should be used cautiously in patients with renal impairment. Dosage of baclofen must be reduced.

Use in Patients With Hepatic Impairment

Dantrolene may cause potentially fatal hepatitis, with jaundice and other symptoms that usually occur within 1 month of starting drug therapy. Liver function tests should be monitored periodically in all patients receiving dantrolene.

Metaxalone and tizanidine can cause liver damage. Thus, liver function should be assessed before starting either drug and periodically during treatment. If liver damage occurs, the drugs should be stopped. The drugs should not be given to patients with pre-existing liver disease.

Use in Home Care

The home care nurse is likely to be involved with the use of baclofen, dantrolene, or tizanidine in chronic spastic disorders. Patients may need continued assessment of drug effects, monitoring of functional abilities, assistance in arranging blood tests of liver function, and other care. Caregivers may need instruction about nonpharmacologic interventions to help prevent or relieve spasticity.

Nursing Actions | Skeletal Muscle Relaxants

NURSING ACTIONS	RATIONALE/EXPLANATION
1. Administer accurately	
a. Give baclofen and metaxalone with milk or food.	To decrease gastrointestinal distress
b. Do not mix parenteral diazepam in a syringe with any other drugs.	Diazepam is physically incompatible with other drugs.
c. Inject intravenous (IV) diazepam directly into a vein or the injection site nearest the vein (during continuous IV infusions) at a rate of approximately 2 mg/min.	Diazepam may cause a precipitate if diluted. Avoid contact with IV solutions as much as possible. A slow rate of injection minimizes the risks of respiratory depression and apnea.
d. Avoid extravasation with IV diazepam, and inject intramuscular (IM) diazepam deeply into a gluteal muscle.	To prevent or reduce tissue irritation
e. With IV methocarbamol, inject or infuse slowly, no more than 3 mL/min.	Rapid administration may cause bradycardia, hypotension, and dizziness.
f. With IV methocarbamol, have the patient lie down during and at least 15 minutes after administration.	To minimize orthostatic hypotension and other adverse drug effects
g. Avoid extravasation with IV methocarbamol, and give IM methocarbamol deeply into a gluteal muscle (no more than 5mL per site).	Parenteral methocarbamol is a hypertonic solution that is very irritating to tissues. Thrombophlebitis may occur at IV injection sites, and sloughing of tissue may occur at sites of extravasation or IM injections.
2. Observe for therapeutic effects	
a. When the drug is given for acute muscle spasm, observe for: (1) Decreased pain and tenderness (2) Increased mobility (3) Increased ability to participate in activities of daily living	Therapeutic effects usually occur within 30 minutes after IV injection of diazepam or methocarbamol.

(continued on page 238)

Nursing Actions | **Skeletal Muscle Relaxants** (continued)

NURSING ACTIONS	RATIONALE/EXPLANATION
b. When the drug is given for spasticity in chronic neurologic disorders, observe for: (1) Increased ability to maintain posture and balance (2) Increased ability for self-care (e.g., eating and dressing) (3) Increased tolerance for physical therapy and exercises	
3. **Observe for adverse effects** a. With centrally active agents, observe for: (1) Drowsiness and dizziness (2) Blurred vision, lethargy, flushing	These are the most common adverse effects. These effects occur more often with IV administration of drugs. They are usually transient. These effects are most likely to occur with large oral doses.
(3) Nausea, vomiting, abdominal distress, constipation or diarrhea, ataxia, areflexia, flaccid paralysis, respiratory depression, tachycardia, hypotension (4) Hypersensitivity—skin rash, pruritus	The drug should be discontinued if hypersensitivity reactions occur. Serious allergic reactions (e.g., anaphylaxis) are rare. Most likely to occur with long-term use of large doses
(5) Psychological or physical dependence with diazepam and other antianxiety agents b. With a peripherally active agent (dantrolene), observe for: (1) Drowsiness, fatigue, lethargy, weakness, nausea, vomiting	Adverse effects are usually transient. These effects are the most common.
(2) Headache, anorexia, nervousness (3) Hepatotoxicity	Less common effects This potentially serious adverse effect is most likely to occur in people older than 35 years of age who have taken the drug 60 days or longer. Women older than 35 years of age who take estrogens have the highest risk. Hepatotoxicity can be prevented or minimized by administering the lowest effective dose, monitoring liver enzymes (aspartate aminotransferase [AST] and alanine aminotransferase [ALT]) during therapy, and discontinuing the drug if no beneficial effects occur within 45 days.
4. **Observe for drug interactions** a. Drugs that *increase* effects of skeletal muscle relaxants: (1) Central nervous system (CNS) depressants (alcohol, antianxiety agents, antidepressants, antihistamines, antipsychotic drugs, sedative-hypnotics)	Additive CNS depression with increased risks of excessive sedation and respiratory depression or apnea
(2) Monoamine oxidase inhibitors (3) Antihypertensive agents	May potentiate effects by inhibiting metabolism of muscle relaxants Increased hypotension, especially with tizanidine

Key Concepts

- Muscle spasms usually result from trauma to the affected skeletal muscle.
- Spasticity results from damage to nerves in the brain and spinal cord.
- Both muscle spasms and spasticity can cause pain and disability.
- Physical therapy and other nonpharmacologic treatments are useful in treating muscle spasm and spasticity.

- Most muscle relaxant drugs are CNS depressants; only dantrolene acts on the muscle.
- The etiology of multiple sclerosis (MS) is unknown, and there is presently no cure.
- Drugs used to relieve spasticity with MS are baclofen and tizanidine.
- Other drugs used to treat MS include corticosteroids, disease-modifying drugs, and drugs used to treat various symptoms other than spasticity.

Review and Application Exercises

Short Answer Exercises

1. How do skeletal muscle relaxants act to relieve spasm and pain?

2. What are the indications for the use of skeletal muscle relaxants?

3. What are the contraindications to the use of skeletal muscle relaxants?

4. What are the major adverse effects of skeletal muscle relaxants, and how can they be minimized?

5. What are some nonpharmacologic interventions to use instead of, or along with, skeletal muscle relaxants?

NCLEX-Style Questions

6. The nurse who is administering baclofen (Lioresal) knows that the adverse effect she needs to monitor most closely includes which of the following?
   a. muscle spasms
   b. insomnia
   c. nervousness
   d. hypotension

7. Which of the following muscle relaxants is the only one that acts peripherally on muscles?
   a. dantrolene (Dantrium)
   b. baclofen (Lioresal)
   c. methocarbamol (Robaxin)
   d. diazepam (Valium)

8. A patient with MS who has progressive and severe leg weakness has questions about his medications. The provider has discontinued his antispasmodic and he wants to know why this may be the case. The nurse is correct in telling him that
   a. There are no effective medications that reduce spasticity in MS.
   b. Spasticity is not an effect of MS.
   c. He may need some degree of spasticity to ambulate, which may be why the medication was eliminated, but he should ask his provider.
   d. His provider was concerned about serious side effects from the medications.

Selected References

Aminoff, M. J. (2007). Nervous system. In S. J. McPhee, M. A. Papadakis, & L. M. Tierney, Jr. (Eds.), *Current medical diagnosis and treatment 2007* (46th ed., pp. 998–1062). New York: McGraw-Hill.

Bainbridge, J. L. & Corboy, J. R. (2005). Multiple sclerosis. In J. T. DiPiro, R. L. Talbert, G. C. Yee, G. R. Matzke, B. G. Wells, & L. M. Posey (Eds.), *Pharmacotherapy: A pathophysiologic approach* (6th ed., pp. 1007–1021). New York: McGraw-Hill.

Drug facts and comparisons. (Updated monthly). St. Louis, MO: Facts and Comparisons.

Goodin, D. S., Frohman, E. M., Garmany, G. P., Jr., Halper, J., Likosky, W. H., Lublin, F. D., Silberberg, D. H., Stuart, W. H., & van den Noort, S. (2002). Disease modifying therapies in multiple sclerosis: Report of the Therapeutics and Technology Assessment Subcommittee of the American Academy of Neurology and the MS Council for Clinical Practice Guidelines. *Neurology, 58,* 169–178. (Updated in 2005 with FDA-issued warnings about serious adverse effects with Avonex and Novantrone.)

McGinty, L. A. (2008). Management of patients with neurologic infections, autoimmune disorders, and neuropathies. In S. C. Smeltzer, B. G. Bare, J. L. Hinkle, & K. H. Cheever (Eds.), *Brunner & Suddarth's textbook of medical-surgical nursing* (11th ed., pp. 2269–2299). Philadelphia: Lippincott Williams & Wilkins.

National Collaborating Centre for Chronic Conditions. (2004). *Multiple sclerosis. National clinical guideline for diagnosis and management in primary and secondary care.* London (UK): National Institute for Clinical Excellence (NICE).

Porth, C. M., & Curtis, R. L. (2005). Disorders of motor function. In C. M. Porth (Ed.), *Pathophysiology: Concepts of altered health states* (7th ed., pp. 1193–1226). Philadelphia: Lippincott Williams & Wilkins.

Substance Abuse Disorders

KEY TERMS

- Alcohol abuse
- Hallucinogen
- Physical dependence
- Psychological dependence
- Substance abuse
- Tolerance

LEARNING OBJECTIVES

After studying this chapter, you will be able to:

1. Identify risk factors for development of drug dependence.
2. Describe the effects of alcohol, cocaine, marijuana, and nicotine on selected body organs.
3. Compare and contrast characteristics of dependence associated with alcohol, benzodiazepines, cocaine, and opiates.
4. Describe specific antidotes for overdoses of central nervous system (CNS) depressant drugs and the circumstances indicating their use.
5. Outline major elements of treatment for overdoses of commonly abused drugs that do not have antidotes.
6. Describe interventions to prevent or manage withdrawal reactions associated with alcohol, benzodiazepines, cocaine and other CNS stimulants, and opiates.

Applying Your Knowledge

Bryan Wilson is a 24-year-old man who regularly uses marijuana, alcohol, and tobacco. He also occasionally uses cocaine as a recreational drug. He is seen in the ER in acute intoxication. He is admitted for withdrawal and treatment.

Introduction

Substance abuse is a significant health, social, economic, and legal problem. It is often associated with substantial damage to the abuser and society (e.g., crime, child and spouse abuse, traumatic injury, chronic health problems, death). In this chapter, substance abuse is defined as self-administration of a drug for prolonged periods or in excessive amounts to the point of producing physical or psychological dependence, impairing functions of body organs, reducing the ability to function in usual activities of daily living, and decreasing the ability and motivation to function as a productive member of society.

Most drugs of abuse are those that affect the CNS and alter the state of consciousness. Commonly abused drugs include CNS depressants (e.g., alcohol, antianxiety and sedative-hypnotic agents, opioid analgesics), CNS stimulants (e.g., cocaine, methamphetamine, methylphenidate, nicotine), and other mind-altering drugs (e.g., marijuana, "ecstasy"). Although these drugs produce different effects, they are associated with feelings of pleasure, positive reinforcement, and compulsive self-administration. Most are also associated with *tolerance* if used repeatedly. This means that the body adjusts to the drugs so that higher doses are needed to achieve feelings of pleasure ("reward") or stave off withdrawal symptoms ("punishment"). Both reward and punishment serve to reinforce continued substance abuse.

Many drugs of abuse activate the pleasure or reward system in the brain by altering neurotransmission systems. For example, cocaine and methamphetamine increase the availability of the neurotransmitters dopamine and norepinephrine. Prolonged drug abuse damages nerve cells in the brain and alters brain functions. The damage is long lasting.

Drugs of abuse seem to be readily available. Internet Web sites have become an important source of the drugs. In some instances, instructions for manufacturing particular drugs are available. Although patterns of drug abuse vary in particular populations and in geographic areas, continuing trends seem to include increased use of methamphetamine, "club drugs," prescription drugs, and using multiple drugs at the same time.

Dependence

Characteristics of drug dependence include craving a drug, often with unsuccessful attempts to decrease its use; compulsive drug-seeking behavior; physical dependence (withdrawal symptoms if drug use is decreased or stopped); and continuing to take a drug despite adverse consequences (e.g., drug-related illnesses, mental or legal problems, job loss or decreased ability to function in an occupation, impaired family relationships).

Psychological dependence involves feelings of satisfaction and pleasure from taking the drug. These feelings, perceived as extremely desirable by the drug-dependent person, contribute to acute intoxication, development and maintenance of drug-abuse patterns, and return to drug-taking behavior after periods of abstinence.

Physical dependence involves physiologic adaptation to chronic use of a drug so that unpleasant symptoms occur when the drug is stopped, when its action is antagonized by another drug, or when its dosage is decreased. The withdrawal or abstinence syndrome produces specific manifestations according to the type of drug and does not occur as long as adequate dosage is maintained. Attempts to avoid withdrawal symptoms reinforce psychological dependence and promote continuing drug use and relapses to drug-taking behavior. Tolerance is often an element of drug dependence, and increasing doses are therefore required to obtain psychological effects or avoid physical with-

drawal symptoms. A person may be dependent on several drugs; most substance abusers use multiple drugs.

Drug dependence is a complex phenomenon. Although the cause is unknown, one theory is that drugs stimulate or inhibit neurotransmitters in the brain to produce pleasure and euphoria or to decrease unpleasant feelings such as anxiety. For example, dopaminergic neurons in the limbic system are associated with the brain's reward system and are thought to be sites of action of alcohol, amphetamines, cocaine, nicotine, and opiates. These major drugs of abuse increase dopaminergic transmission and the availability of dopamine. For example, amphetamines promote dopamine release and inhibit its reuptake, and cocaine inhibits dopamine reuptake. These actions are believed to stimulate the brain's reward system and lead to compulsive drug administration and abuse.

The noradrenergic neurotransmission system, which uses norepinephrine as its neurotransmitter, is often involved as well as the dopaminergic system. Noradrenergic neurons innervate the limbic system and cerebral cortex and are important in setting mood and affect. Drugs that alter noradrenergic transmission have profound effects on mood and affect. Amphetamines and cocaine increase noradrenergic transmission, as with dopaminergic transmission, by promoting the release of norepinephrine and/or inhibiting its reuptake. Increased norepinephrine leads to mood elevation and euphoria, which promotes continued drug abuse. Increased norepinephrine also leads to major adverse effects of amphetamines and cocaine, including myocardial infarction, severe hypertension, and stroke, as well as profound mood swings from euphoria to depression.

Other factors important in developing drug dependence include the specific drug; the amount, frequency, and route of administration; the person's psychological and physiologic characteristics; and environmental or circumstantial characteristics. Peer pressure is often an important factor in initial and continuing drug ingestion. A genetic factor seems evident in *alcohol abuse*: Studies indicate that children of abusers are at risk of becoming abusers themselves, even if reared away from the abusing parent. See Box 14-1 for additional general characteristics of substance abuse and dependence.

Box 14-1	Characteristics of Substance Abuse and Dependence

- Substance abuse involves all socioeconomic levels and affects all age groups. It is especially prevalent among adolescents and young adults. Patterns of abuse may vary by age group. For example, adolescents and young adults are more likely to use illicit drugs and older adults are more likely to abuse alcohol and prescription drugs. Health care professionals (e.g., physicians, pharmacists, nurses) are also considered at high risk for development of substance abuse disorders, at least partly because of easy access.
- A person who abuses one drug is likely to abuse others.
- Multiple drugs are often abused concurrently. Alcohol, for example, is often used with other drugs of abuse, probably

because it is legal and readily available. In addition, alcohol, marijuana, opioids, and sedatives are often used to combat the anxiety and nervousness induced by cocaine, methamphetamine, and other CNS stimulants.
- Drug effects vary according to the type of substance being abused, the amount, route of administration, duration of use, and phase of substance abuse (e.g., acute intoxication, withdrawal syndromes, organ damage, medical illness). Thus, acute intoxication often produces profound behavioral changes and chronic abuse often leads to serious organ damage and impaired ability to function in work, family, or social settings. Withdrawal symptoms are

(continued on page 242)

Box 14-1	Characteristics of Substance Abuse and Dependence (continued)

characteristic of particular types of drugs and are usually opposite to the effects originally produced. For example, withdrawal symptoms of alcohol and sedative-type drugs are mainly agitation, nervousness, and hyperactivity.

■ Abusers of alcohol and other drugs are not reliable sources of information about the types or amounts of drugs used. Most abusers understate the amount and frequency of substance use; heroin addicts may overstate the amount used in attempts to obtain higher doses of methadone. In addition, those who use illegal street drugs may not know what they have taken because of varying purity, potency, additives, contaminants, names, and substitutions of one drug for another.

■ Substance abusers rarely seek health care unless circumstances force the issue. Thus, most substance abuse comes to the attention of health care professionals when the abuser experiences a complication such as acute intoxication, withdrawal, or serious medical problems resulting from chronic drug overuse, misuse, or abuse.

■ Smoking or inhaling drug vapors is a preferred route of administration for cocaine, marijuana, and nicotine because the drugs are rapidly absorbed from the large surface area of the lungs. Then, they rapidly circulate to the heart and brain without dilution by the systemic circulation or metabolism by enzymes.

■ Substance abusers who inject drugs intravenously (IV) are prey to serious problems because they use impure drugs of unknown potency, contaminated needles, poor hygiene, and other dangerous practices. Specific problems include overdoses, death, and numerous infections (e.g., hepatitis, human immunodeficiency virus infection, endocarditis, phlebitis, cellulitis at injection sites).

Many drugs abused for their mind-altering properties have clinical usefulness and are discussed elsewhere: "Antianxiety and Sedative-Hypnotic Drugs" (Chap. 8), "Opioid Analgesics and Pain Management" (Chap. 6), and "Central Nervous System Stimulants" (Chap. 15). This chapter describes commonly abused substances, characteristics and treatment of substance-related disorders, and drugs used to treat substance-related disorders (Table 14-1).

Table 14-1	Drugs at a Glance: Drugs Used to Treat Substance Abuse Disorders

GENERIC/ TRADE NAME	INDICATIONS FOR USE	ROUTES AND DOSAGE RANGES	COMMENTS
Bupropion (Zyban)	Smoking cessation	PO 150 mg once daily for 3 d, then increase to 150 mg twice daily, at least 8 h apart. Maximum dose, 300 mg/d	
Chlordiazepoxide (Librium)	Alcohol detoxification; benzodiazepine withdrawal	PO 50 mg q6–8h initially, then tapered over 1–2 wk	
Clonidine (Catapres)	Alcohol withdrawal; opiate withdrawal	*Alcohol withdrawal:* PO 0.3–0.6 mg q6h	Unlabeled uses
		Opiate withdrawal: PO 2 mcg/kg 3 times daily for 7–10 d	May cause hypotension
Disulfiram (Antabuse)	Chronic alcohol abuse, to prevent continued alcohol ingestion	PO 125–500 mg daily	Limited effectiveness because many alcoholics will not take the drug; should not be given until at least 12 h after alcohol ingestion
Flumazenil (Romazicon)	Acute intoxication or overdose of benzodiazepine antianxiety or sedative-hypnotic drugs	IV 0.1–0.2 mg/min up to 1 mg	May precipitate acute withdrawal symptoms
Haloperidol (Haldol)	Psychotic symptoms associated with acute intoxication with cocaine and other CNS stimulants	IM 2–5 mg q 30 min–6 h PRN for psychotic behavior	Other antipsychotic agents may also be used.

GENERIC/ TRADE NAME	INDICATIONS FOR USE	ROUTES AND DOSAGE RANGES	COMMENTS
Lorazepam (Ativan)	Excessive CNS stimulation associated with acute intoxication with cocaine and other CNS stimulants, hallucinogens, marijuana, inhalants, and phencyclidine; alcohol withdrawal	*Agitation:* IM q 30 min–6 h PRN; *alcohol withdrawal hallucinations or seizures:* IM 2 mg, repeated if necessary; *benzodiazepine withdrawal:* PO 2 mg q6–8h initially, then tapered over 1–2 wk	1 wk of tapering usually adequate for withdrawal from short-acting benzodiazepines; 2 wk needed for long-acting benzodiazepines
Methadone	Opioid withdrawal; maintenance therapy for heroin addiction	*Withdrawal:* PO 20–80 mg daily initially, reduced by 5–10 mg daily over 7–10 days; *maintenance:* PO 20–80 mg daily	Maintenance doses of 60–80 mg daily more effective than 20–30 mg daily to decrease heroin use
Naloxone (Narcan)	Acute intoxication or overdose of opioids (heroin, morphine, others)	IV 0.4–2 mg q3min	May precipitate acute withdrawal symptoms
Naltrexone (ReVia, Vivitrol)	Opioid dependence; alcohol dependence	PO 50 mg daily IM (Vivitrol) 380 mg once monthly in buttocks	With opiate dependence, should not be started until patient is opioid-free for at least 7 days
Nicotine (Habitrol, Nicoderm CQ, Nicorette, Nicotrol, Nicotrol Inhaler, Nicotrol NS)	Aid smoking cessation by relieving nicotine withdrawal symptoms	*Transdermal patches, Habitrol, Nicoderm:* 21 mg/d for 6 wk; then 14 mg/d for 2 wk; then 7 mg/d for 2 wk *Nicotrol patch:* 15 mg/16 h for 6 wk *Nicotrol chewing gum:* 1 piece every 1–2 h for wk 1–6; 1 piece every 2–4 h for wk 7–9; 1 piece every 4–8 h for wk 10–12 *Nicotrol inhaler:* 6–12 cartridges/d for 3 mo, then gradually taper dosage over 6–12 wk, then discontinue *Nicotrol nasal spray:* 1 spray to each nostril, every 1–2 h, to a maximum of 80 sprays (40 mg) per day for heavy smokers. Taper by using less often or spraying 1 nostril per dose.	Should not be used while continuing to smoke because of high risk of serious adverse effects Used patches contain enough nicotine to be toxic to children and pets; they should be discarded in a safe manner.
Varenicline (Chantix)	Smoking cessation	PO days 1–3, 0.5 mg once daily; days 4–7, 0.5 mg twice daily; day 8 through end of treatment (total of 12–24 wk), 1 mg twice daily	

CNS, Central nervous system

Central Nervous System Depressants

CNS depressants are drugs that slow down or "depress" brain activity. They include alcohol, antianxiety and sedative-hypnotic agents, and opiates.

Alcohol (Ethanol)

Alcohol is commonly abused around the world. It is legal and readily available, and its use is accepted in most societies. Excessive amounts and long-term abuse damages essentially all organ systems of the body. Alcohol is thought to exert its effects on the CNS mainly by enhancing the activity of gamma-aminobutyric acid, an inhibitory neurotransmitter, or by inhibiting the activity of glutamate, an excitatory neurotransmitter. Other neurotransmitters (e.g., dopamine, opioid peptides, serotonin) may also be affected.

When alcohol is ingested orally, a portion is inactivated in the stomach (by the enzyme alcohol dehydrogenase) and not absorbed systemically. Women have less enzyme activity than men and therefore absorb about 30% more alcohol than men when comparable amounts are ingested according to weight and size. As a result, women are especially vulnerable to adverse effects of alcohol, including more rapid intoxication from smaller amounts of alcohol and earlier development of hepatic cirrhosis and other complications of alcohol abuse.

In men and women, alcohol is absorbed partly from the stomach but mostly from the upper small intestine. It is rapidly absorbed when the stomach and small intestine are empty.

Food delays absorption by diluting the alcohol and delaying gastric emptying. After it is absorbed, alcohol is quickly distributed to all body tissues, partly because it is lipid soluble and crosses cell membranes easily. The alcohol concentration in the brain rapidly approaches that in the blood, and CNS effects usually occur within a few minutes. These effects depend on the amount ingested, how rapidly it was ingested, whether the stomach was empty, and other factors. Effects with acute intoxication usually progress from feelings of euphoria and relaxation to impaired mental and motor functions, stupor, and sleep. Excited behavior may occur because of depression of the cerebral cortex, which normally controls behavior. The person may seem more talkative and outgoing or more impulsive and aggressive because inhibitions and self-control are decreased.

The rate of alcohol metabolism largely determines the duration of CNS effects. Most alcohol is oxidized in the liver to acetaldehyde, which can be used for energy or converted to fat and stored. When metabolized to acetaldehyde, alcohol no longer exerts depressant effects on the CNS. Although the rate of metabolism differs with acute ingestion or chronic intake and some other factors, it is approximately 120 milligrams per kilogram of body weight or 10 milliliters per hour. This is the amount of alcohol contained in approximately 2/3 ounce of whiskey, 3 to 4 ounces of wine, or 8 to 12 ounces of beer. *Alcohol is metabolized at the same rate regardless of the amount present in body tissues.*

In older adults, the pharmacokinetics of alcohol are essentially the same as in younger adults. However, equivalent amounts of alcohol produce higher blood levels in older adults because of changes in body composition (e.g., a greater proportion of fatty tissue).

Alcohol may cause significant interactions when used with other drugs. These interactions often differ between acute and chronic ingestion. Acute ingestion inhibits drug-metabolizing enzymes, which slows the metabolism of some drugs, thereby increasing their effects and the likelihood of toxicity. Chronic ingestion induces metabolizing enzymes. This increases the rate of metabolism and decreases drug effects. Long-term ingestion of large amounts of alcohol, however, causes liver damage and impaired ability to metabolize drugs. Because so many variables influence alcohol's interactions with other drugs, it is difficult to predict effects of interactions in particular people. However, some important interactions include those with other CNS depressants, antihypertensive agents, antidiabetic agents, oral anticoagulants, and disulfiram. These are summarized in Box 14-2.

Alcohol Dependence and Its Treatment

Alcohol dependence involves acute or chronic consumption of alcohol in excess of the limits accepted by the person's culture, at times considered inappropriate by that culture, and to the extent that physical health and social relationships are impaired. Psychological dependence, physical dependence, tolerance, and cross-tolerance with other CNS depressants are prominent characteristics.

Acute intoxication impairs thinking, judgment, and psychomotor coordination. These impairments lead to poor work

| Box 14-2 | Alcohol Interactions With Other Drugs |

- With other CNS depressants (e.g., sedative-hypnotics, opioid analgesics, antianxiety agents, antipsychotic agents, general anesthetics, tricyclic antidepressants), alcohol potentiates CNS depression and increases risks of excessive sedation, respiratory depression, and impaired mental and physical functioning. Combining alcohol with these drugs may be lethal and should be avoided.
- With antihypertensive agents, alcohol potentiates vasodilation and hypotensive effects.
- With oral antidiabetic drugs that decrease blood sugar, alcohol potentiates hypoglycemic effects. These drugs include acarbose (Precose), exenatide (Byetta), glipizide (Glucotrol), glyburide (DiaBeta), glimepiride (Amaryl), miglitol (Glyset), nateglinide (Starlix), pioglitazone (Actos), pramlintide (Symlin), repaglinide (Prandin), and rosiglitazone (Avandia). With metformin (Glucophage), alcohol may increase the risk of lactic acidosis.
- With oral anticoagulants (e.g., warfarin), alcohol interactions vary. Acute ingestion increases anticoagulant effects and the risk of bleeding. Chronic ingestion decreases anticoagulant effects by inducing drug-metabolizing enzymes in the liver and increasing the rate of warfarin metabolism. However, if chronic ingestion has caused liver damage, metabolism of warfarin may be slowed. This increases the risk of excessive anticoagulant effect and bleeding.
- With disulfiram (Antabuse), alcohol produces significant distress (flushing, tachycardia, bronchospasm, sweating, nausea and vomiting). This reaction may be used to treat alcohol dependence.
- A disulfiram-like reaction also may occur with other drugs, including the antimicrobial drugs cefoperazone (Cefobid) and metronidazole (Flagyl).

performance, accidents, and disturbed relationships with other people. Conscious control of behavior is lost, and exhibitionism and aggressiveness often result. Chronic ingestion may cause severe organ damage and mental problems.

Signs and symptoms of alcohol withdrawal include agitation, anxiety, tremors, sweating, nausea, tachycardia, fever, hyperreflexia, postural hypotension, and, if severe, convulsions and delirium. Delirium tremens, the most serious form of alcohol withdrawal, is characterized by confusion, disorientation, delusions, visual hallucinations, and other signs of acute psychosis. The intensity of the alcohol withdrawal syndrome varies with the duration and amount of alcohol ingestion. Withdrawal symptoms start within a few hours after a person's last drink and last for several days; moderate to severe withdrawal symptoms often lead to hospitalization in a critical care unit.

Alcohol dependence is a progressive illness, and early recognition and treatment are desirable. The alcohol-dependent person is unlikely to seek treatment for alcohol abuse unless an acute illness or other situation forces the issue. He or she is likely, however, to seek treatment for other disorders, such as nervousness, anxiety, depression, insomnia, and gastroenteritis. Thus, health professionals may recognize alcohol abuse in its early stages if they are aware of indicative assessment data.

If the patient does not admit that alcohol abuse is a problem and agrees to participate in a treatment program, success is unlikely. The patient may fail to make return visits or may seek treatment elsewhere. If the patient agrees to treatment, the three primary approaches are psychological counseling, referral to a self-help group such as Alcoholics Anonymous, and drug therapy.

Applying Your Knowledge 14-1

For Mr. Wilson's treatment to be successful, what are the primary approaches that should be used?

Acute intoxication with alcohol does not usually require treatment. If the patient is hyperactive and combative, a sedative-type drug may be given. The patient must be closely observed because sedatives potentiate alcohol, and excessive CNS depression may occur. If the patient is already sedated and stuporous, he or she can be allowed to sleep off the alcohol effects. If the patient is comatose, supportive measures are indicated. For example, respiratory depression may require insertion of an artificial airway and mechanical ventilation.

Benzodiazepine antianxiety agents are the drugs of choice for treating alcohol withdrawal syndromes. They can help the patient participate in rehabilitation programs and can be gradually reduced in dosage and discontinued. They provide adequate sedation and have a significant anticonvulsant effect. Some physicians prefer a benzodiazepine with a long half-life (e.g., diazepam [Valium] or **chlordiazepoxide** [Librium]), whereas others prefer one with a short half-life (e.g., **lorazepam** [Ativan] or oxazepam). Lorazepam and oxazepam are less likely to accumulate and may be best for older adults or patients with hepatic disease. Alcoholic patients usually require high doses of benzodiazepines because of the drugs' cross-tolerance with alcohol.

Seizures require treatment if they are repeated or continuous. Antiseizure drugs need not be given for more than a few days unless the person has a pre-existing seizure disorder. **Clonidine** (Catapres) may be given to reduce symptoms (e.g., hyperactivity, tremors) associated with excessive stimulation of the sympathetic nervous system. Midazolam or propofol may be useful for treating delirium tremens because their doses can be easily titrated to manage the symptoms.

Applying Your Knowledge 14-2

Although Mr. Wilson's acute intoxication may not require treatment, his chronic abuse of alcohol will result in the need for treatment of alcohol withdrawal symptoms. The physician prescribes a benzodiazepine. Why?

Drug therapy for maintenance of sobriety is limited, mainly because of poor compliance. The drugs approved for this purpose include **disulfiram** (Antabuse) and **naltrexone** (ReVia, Vivitrol). Disulfiram interferes with hepatic metabolism of alcohol and allows accumulation of acetaldehyde. If alcohol is ingested during disulfiram therapy, acetaldehyde causes nausea and vomiting, dyspnea, hypotension, tachycardia, syncope, blurred vision, headache, and confusion. Severe reactions include respiratory depression, cardiovascular collapse, cardiac dysrhythmias, myocardial infarction, congestive heart failure, unconsciousness, convulsions, and death. The reaction lasts as long as alcohol is present in the blood. Ingestion of prescription and over-the-counter medications that contain alcohol may cause a reaction in the disulfiram-treated alcoholic. Disulfiram alone may produce adverse reactions of drowsiness, fatigue, impotence, headache, and dermatitis. Disulfiram also interferes with the metabolism of phenytoin and warfarin, which may increase blood levels of the drugs and increase their toxicity. Because of these reactions, disulfiram must be given only with the patient's full consent, cooperation, and knowledge.

Naltrexone is an opiate antagonist that reduces craving for alcohol and increases abstinence rates when combined with psychosocial treatment. A possible mechanism is blockade of the endogenous opioid system, which is thought to reinforce alcohol craving and consumption. The most common adverse effect is nausea; others include anxiety, dizziness, drowsiness, headache, insomnia, nervousness, and vomiting. Naltrexone is hepatotoxic in high doses and contraindicated in patients with acute hepatitis or liver failure. Formerly an oral tablet that required daily administration, with which adherence is a problem, naltrexone is now available in an extended-release solution (Vivitrol) that can be injected once each month.

In addition to drug therapy to treat withdrawal and maintain sobriety, alcohol abusers often need treatment of coexisting medical illnesses and psychiatric disorders, such as depression. Antidepressant drugs seem to decrease alcohol intake as well as relieve depression in this population.

Applying Your Knowledge 14-3

Preparations are being made for Mr. Wilson's discharge and outpatient therapy. He is prescribed Antabuse. Why is he given this drug, and what will he experience if he consumes alcohol while taking it?

Benzodiazepines

Benzodiazepines are widely used for antianxiety and sedative-hypnotic effects (see Chap. 8) and are also widely abused, mainly by people who also abuse alcohol and/or other drugs. Benzodiazepines rarely cause respiratory depression or death, even in overdose, unless taken with alcohol or other drugs. They may, however, cause oversedation, memory impairment, poor motor coordination, and confusion. Withdrawal reactions can be extremely uncomfortable. Symptoms begin 12 to 24 hours after the last dose of a short-acting drug such as alprazolam (Xanax) and peak at 24 to 72 hours. With long-acting drugs such as diazepam and chlordiazepoxide, symptoms begin 24 to 48 hours after the last dose and peak within 5 to 8 days.

Combining any of these drugs with each other or with alcohol can cause serious depression of vital functions and death. Unfortunately, abusers often combine drugs in their quest for a greater "high" or to relieve the unpleasant effects of CNS stimulants and other street drugs.

Benzodiazepine Dependence and Its Treatment

This type of dependence resembles alcohol dependence in symptoms of intoxication and withdrawal. Other characteristics include physical dependence, psychological dependence, tolerance, and cross-tolerance. Signs and symptoms of withdrawal include anxiety, tremors and muscle twitching, weakness, dizziness, distorted visual perceptions, nausea and vomiting, insomnia, nightmares, tachycardia, weight loss, postural hypotension, generalized tonic-clonic seizures, and delirium that resembles the delirium tremens of alcoholism or a major psychotic episode. Convulsions are more likely to occur during the first 48 hours of withdrawal and delirium after 48 to 72 hours.

Treatment may involve overdose and withdrawal syndromes. Overdose produces intoxication similar to that produced by alcohol. There may be a period of excitement and emotional lability followed by progressively increasing signs of CNS depression (e.g., impaired mental function, muscular incoordination, sedation). Treatment is unnecessary for mild overdose if vital functions are adequate. The patient usually sleeps off the effects of the drug. The rate of recovery depends primarily on the amount of drug ingested and its rate of metabolism. More severe overdoses cause respiratory depression and coma.

Flumazenil (Romazicon) is a specific antidote that can reverse benzodiazepine-induced sedation, coma, and respiratory depression. The drug competes with benzodiazepines for benzodiazepine receptors. It has a short duration of action, and repeated IV injections are usually needed. Recipients must be closely observed because symptoms of overdose may recur when the effects of a dose of flumazenil subside and because the drug may precipitate acute withdrawal symptoms (e.g., agitation, confusion, seizures) in benzodiazepine abusers.

Treatment of withdrawal may involve administration of a benzodiazepine to relieve acute signs and symptoms and then tapering the dose until the drug can be discontinued. Benzodiazepine withdrawal syndromes can be life threatening. The person may experience cardiovascular collapse, generalized tonic-clonic seizures, and acute psychotic episodes. These can be prevented by gradually withdrawing the offending drug. If they do occur, each situation requires specific drug therapy and supportive measures. Withdrawal reactions should be supervised and managed by experienced people, such as health care professionals or staff at detoxification centers.

Opioids

Opioids are potent analgesics and extensively used in pain management (see Chap. 6). They are also commonly abused. Legal opioid analgesics are increasingly being diverted from their appropriate use and bought and sold as street drugs. Because therapeutic opioids are discussed elsewhere, the focus here is heroin, a common drug of abuse. It is a Schedule I drug in the United States and is not used therapeutically.

Heroin produces the same effects as naturally occurring endorphins and other opioid drugs. The drug rapidly enters the brain, where it is converted to morphine. Morphine stimulates opioid receptors in the reward system of the brain, which causes greater amounts of dopamine to be released.

Heroin may be taken by IV injection, smoking, or nasal application (snorting). IV injection produces intense euphoria, which occurs within seconds, lasts a few minutes, and is followed by a period of sedation. Effects diminish over approximately 4 hours, depending on the dose. Addicts may inject several times daily, cycling between desired effects and symptoms of withdrawal. Tolerance to euphoric effects develops rapidly, leading to dosage escalation and continued use to avoid withdrawal. Like other opioids, heroin causes severe respiratory depression with overdose and produces a characteristic abstinence syndrome.

Opioid Dependence and Its Treatment

Opioids produce tolerance and high degrees of psychological and physical dependence. Most other drugs that produce dependence do so with prolonged usage of large doses, but morphine-like drugs produce dependence with repeated administration of small doses. Medical usage of these drugs produces physical dependence and tolerance but rarely leads to use or abuse for mind-altering effects. Thus, "addiction" should not be an issue when the drugs are needed for pain management in patients with cancer or other severe illnesses. Although deaths from overdoses of opioid analgesics (e.g., oxycodone, hydrocodone, methadone, fentanyl) have increased in recent years, these deaths are usually associated with nonmedical use rather than pain management. Also, most overdose deaths involve multiple drugs.

Acute effects of opioid administration vary according to dosage, route of administration, and physical and mental characteristics of the user. They may produce euphoria, sedation, analgesia, respiratory depression, postural hypotension, vasodilation, pupil constriction, and constipation.

Treatment may be needed for overdose or withdrawal syndromes. Overdose may produce severe respiratory depression and coma. Insertion of an endotracheal tube and mechanical ventilation may be required. Drug therapy consists of an opioid antagonist (e.g., naloxone) to reverse opioid effects. Giving an opioid antagonist can precipitate withdrawal symptoms. If there is no response to the opioid antagonist, the symptoms may be caused by depressant drugs other than opioids. In addition to profound respiratory depression, pulmonary edema, hypoglycemia, pneumonia, cellulitis, and other infections often accompany opioid overdose and require specific treatment measures.

Symptoms of opioid withdrawal may resemble severe flu, with rhinorrhea, sneezing, yawning, lacrimation, abdominal cramping, leg cramping, piloerection (gooseflesh), nausea, vomiting, diarrhea, and dilated pupils. Onset and duration of symptoms are determined by the half-life of the abused opioid. For example, symptoms occur within 36 to 72 hours and last about 7 to 10 days with heroin. They occur in 72 to 96 hours and last at least 14 days with methadone.

Signs and symptoms of withdrawal can be reversed immediately by giving the drug producing the dependence. Therapeutic withdrawal involves gradually reducing dosage over several days. Clonidine, a drug used mainly for hypertension, is sometimes used to relieve withdrawal symptoms associated with excessive stimulation of the sympathetic nervous system.

Ideally, the goal of treatment for opioid abuse is abstinence from further opioid usage. Because this goal is rarely met, long-term drug therapy may be used to treat heroin dependence. One method uses opioid substitutes to prevent withdrawal symptoms and improve a lifestyle that revolves around obtaining, using, and recovering from a drug. **Methadone** has long been used for this purpose, usually a single, daily oral dose given in a methadone clinic. Proponents say that methadone blocks euphoria produced by heroin, acts longer, and reduces preoccupation with drug use. This allows a more normal lifestyle for the patient and reduces morbidity and mortality associated with the use of illegal and injected drugs. Also, because methadone is free, the heroin addict does not commit crimes to obtain drugs. Opponents say that methadone maintenance only substitutes one type of drug dependence for another. In addition, a substantial percentage of those receiving methadone maintenance therapy abuse other drugs, including cocaine.

A second treatment option is **naltrexone** (ReVia), an opioid antagonist that prevents opioids from occupying receptor sites and thereby prevents their physiologic effects. Used to maintain opioid-free states in the opioid addict, it is recommended for use in conjunction with psychological counseling to promote patient motivation and compliance. If the patient taking naltrexone has mild or moderate pain, nonopioid analgesics (e.g., acetaminophen or a nonsteroidal anti-inflammatory drug) should be given. If the patient has severe pain and requires an opioid, it should be given in a setting staffed and equipped for cardiopulmonary resuscitation because respiratory depression may be deeper and more prolonged than usual. In addition, patients needing elective surgery and opioid analgesics should be instructed to stop taking naltrexone at least 72 hours before the scheduled procedure.

A third drug therapy option is **buprenorphine** (Buprenex), a Schedule III agonist-antagonist analgesic that is occasionally injected therapeutically to relieve pain and is also a drug of abuse. It is given orally (Subutex, Suboxone) to treat opioid dependence. Suboxone also contains naloxone, a narcotic antagonist, to prevent buprenorphine abuse for mind-altering effects. Physicians who prescribe the drug for outpatient use must meet several restrictions and are required to have 8 hours of special training.

Central Nervous System Stimulants

Amphetamines and Related Drugs

Amphetamines and some related drugs (see Chap. 15) are used therapeutically for narcolepsy and attention deficit-hyperactivity disorder (ADHD). However, amphetamines are more important as drugs of abuse than therapeutic agents. The effects of amphetamines are similar to those of cocaine. The drugs increase the activity of norepinephrine and dopamine by increasing their release, blocking their reuptake, and inhibiting the enzyme (monoamine oxidase) that normally metabolizes catecholamine neurotransmitters.

Methamphetamine is a commonly abused drug that is often manufactured in illegal "meth labs." Purchase and possession of the ingredients for its manufacture are restricted by law. The drug is taken orally, by IV injection, and by inhalation (after chemical treatment to produce crystals, which are then heated and the vapors smoked or inhaled). Inhalation or IV injection produces a pleasurable sensation that lasts only a few minutes.

Methylphenidate (Ritalin, others), a prescription drug used to treat ADHD, is increasingly being used for nonmedical purposes. The drug is obtained by diverting it from legitimate channels (e.g., buying, stealing, sharing among friends). A mild CNS stimulant, methylphenidate tablets are taken orally, crushed and taken intranasally, or dissolved in water and injected. The pattern of abuse is similar to that of other CNS stimulants, with episodes of binge use followed by severe depression and continued use despite serious adverse consequences.

Amphetamine Dependence and Its Treatment

Amphetamines and related drugs produce stimulation and euphoria. Small amounts produce mental alertness, wakefulness, and increased energy for a few hours. Tolerance develops rapidly, so users increase the amount and frequency of administration to regain the state of stimulation, continuing use as long as the drug is available and then "crashing" with profound fatigue and depression. Large amounts and long-term use damages the brain and may cause aggression, hallucinations, memory loss, paranoia, psychosis, and violence as well as serious cardiac dysrhythmias, severe dental disease, and stroke.

Acute ingestion of these drugs masks underlying fatigue or depression; withdrawal allows these conditions to emerge in an exaggerated form. The resulting exhaustion and depression reinforce the compulsion to continue using the drugs. Users may take them alone or to counteract the effects of other drugs. In the latter case, these drugs may be part of a pattern of polydrug use in which CNS depressants such as alcohol or sedative-type drugs ("downers") are alternated with CNS stimulants, such as amphetamines ("uppers").

Treatment is mainly concerned with overdosage because these drugs do not produce physical dependence and withdrawal as alcohol, opioids, and sedative-hypnotic drugs do. The patient is likely to be hyperactive, agitated, and hallucinating (toxic psychosis) and may have tachycardia, fever, and other symptoms. Symptomatic treatment includes sedation, lowering of body temperature, and administration of an antipsychotic drug. Sedative-type drugs must be used with great caution, however, because depression and sleep usually follow amphetamine use, and these after-effects can be aggravated by sedative administration.

Cocaine

Cocaine is a popular drug of abuse. It produces strong CNS stimulation by preventing reuptake of catecholamine neurotransmitters (e.g., dopamine, norepinephrine), which increases and prolongs neurotransmitter effects. The two main drug forms are cocaine hydrochloride powder and "crack." Crack is strong, inexpensive, and extremely addicting. It is prepared by altering cocaine hydrochloride with chemicals and heat to form rock-like formations of cocaine base. The process removes impurities and results in a very potent drug. Cocaine powder is commonly inhaled (snorted) through the nose; "crack" is heated and the vapors inhaled. Both forms are rapidly absorbed; peak blood levels are higher with "crack" than with cocaine powder. The effects of cocaine use are very short. The euphoria from smoking "crack" lasts about 5 to 10 minutes and that from snorting the powder may last 15 to 30 minutes. Cocaine is also metabolized and eliminated rapidly; the half-life is about 1 hour.

In addition to intense euphoria, acute use of cocaine or "crack" produces increased energy and alertness, sexual arousal, tachycardia, increased blood pressure, and restlessness. High doses can cause cardiac dysrhythmias, convulsions, myocardial infarction, respiratory failure, stroke, and death, even in young, healthy adults and even with initial exposure. Cocaine withdrawal begins within hours of stopping drug use and lasts up to several days. Symptoms include depression (which may be profound), drowsiness, fatigue, and sleep disturbances (e.g., nightmares).

When cocaine and alcohol are present in the body at the same time, the drugs are converted to cocaethylene, a substance that has a longer duration of action and is more toxic to the brain than either drug alone. This mixture is the most common two-drug combination that results in drug-related death.

Cocaine Dependence and Its Treatment

Cocaine is not thought to produce physical dependence. However, the euphoria associated with intake and the depression and fatigue associated with stopping intake are believed to induce psychological dependence and compulsive use. Because cocaine effects are very brief, users often ingest the drug every few minutes as long as it is available. Crack cocaine reportedly can cause psychological dependence with one use.

Drug therapy of cocaine dependence is largely symptomatic. Thus, agitation and hyperactivity may be treated with a benzodiazepine antianxiety agent, psychosis may be treated with **haloperidol** (Haldol) or another antipsychotic agent, car-

diac dysrhythmias may be treated with usual antidysrhythmic drugs, myocardial infarction may be treated by standard methods, and so forth. Initial detoxification and long-term treatment are best accomplished in centers or units that specialize in substance-abuse disorders. Long-term treatment of cocaine abuse usually involves psychotherapy, behavioral therapy, and 12-step programs. In addition, many patients also abuse other drugs and need treatment for coexisting psychiatric disorders.

Nicotine

Nicotine, one of many active ingredients in tobacco products, is the ingredient that promotes compulsive use, abuse, and dependence. Inhaling smoke from a cigarette produces CNS stimulation in a few seconds. The average cigarette contains approximately 6 to 8 milligrams of nicotine and delivers approximately 1 milligram of nicotine systemically to the smoker (most is burned or dissipated as "sidestream" smoke). Nicotine obtained from chewing tobacco produces longer-lasting effects because it is more slowly absorbed than inhaled nicotine. Nicotine produces its effects by increasing levels of dopamine and other substances in the brain.

Nicotine is readily absorbed through the lungs, skin, and mucous membranes. It is extensively metabolized, mainly in the liver, and its metabolites are eliminated by the kidneys. It is also excreted in breast milk of nursing mothers. Adverse effects include nausea in new smokers at low blood levels and in experienced smokers at blood levels higher than their accustomed levels. Nicotine poisoning can occur in infants and children from ingestion of tobacco products, skin contact with used nicotine transdermal patches, or chewing nicotine gum. Poisoning may also occur with accidental ingestion of insecticide sprays containing nicotine. Oral ingestion usually causes vomiting, which limits the amount of nicotine absorbed. Toxic effects of a large dose may include hypertension, cardiac dysrhythmias, convulsions, coma, respiratory arrest, and paralysis of skeletal muscle. With chronic tobacco use, nicotine is implicated in the vascular disease and sudden cardiac death associated with smoking. However, the role of nicotine in the etiology of other disorders (e.g., cancer, pulmonary disease) associated with chronic use of tobacco is unknown.

Nicotine Dependence and Its Treatment

Nicotine dependence is characterized by compulsive use and the development of tolerance and physical dependence. Mental depression is also associated with nicotine dependence. Cigarette smokers may smoke to obtain the perceived pleasure of nicotine's effects, avoid the discomfort of nicotine withdrawal, or both. Evidence indicates a compulsion to smoke when blood levels of nicotine become low. Abstinence from smoking leads to signs and symptoms of withdrawal (e.g., anxiety, irritability, difficulty concentrating, restlessness, headache, increased appetite, weight gain, sleep disturbances), which usually begin within 24 hours of the last exposure to nicotine.

Most tobacco users who quit do so on their own. For those who are strongly dependent and unable or unwilling to quit on their own, there are two main methods of treatment. One method is nicotine replacement therapy with drug formulations of nicotine. These products prevent or reduce withdrawal symptoms, but they do not produce the subjective effects or peak blood levels seen with cigarettes.

Nicotine is available in transdermal patches, chewing gum, an oral inhaler, and a nasal spray. The gum, inhaler, and spray are used intermittently during the day; the transdermal patch is applied once daily. Transdermal patches produce a steady blood level of nicotine and patients seem to use them more consistently than they use the other products. The patches and gum are available over-the-counter; the inhaler and nasal spray require a prescription. The products are contraindicated in people with significant cardiovascular disease (angina pectoris, dysrhythmias, or recent myocardial infarction). Adverse effects include soreness of mouth and throat (with gum), nausea, vomiting, dizziness, hypertension, dysrhythmias, confusion, and skin irritation at sites of transdermal patch application. Nicotine products are intended to be used for limited periods of 3 to 6 months, with tapering of dosage and discontinuation. Although they are effective in helping smokers achieve abstinence, many users resume smoking.

Other smoking-cessation drugs for nicotine dependence include bupropion, an antidepressant (see Chap. 10) and **varenicline** (Chantix). The antidepressant formulation of **bupropion** is marketed as Wellbutrin; the smoking-cessation formulation is Zyban, a sustained-release tablet. Varenicline (Chantix) blocks some nicotine receptors and thereby decreases the ability of nicotine to stimulate dopamine activity in the brain (the "reward" system). It also stimulates some other nicotine receptors and thereby decreases symptoms of nicotine withdrawal (the "punishment" system). Both medications are generally well tolerated. The most common adverse effects are insomnia with bupropion and nausea with varencicline.

Overall, treatment regimens that combine counseling and behavioral therapy with drug therapy are more successful than those using drug therapy alone. In addition, a combination of drugs (e.g., Zyban and nicotine transdermal patches) may be more effective than either drug alone.

Marijuana

Marijuana and other cannabis preparations are obtained from *Cannabis sativa*, the hemp plant, which grows in most parts of the world, including the entire United States. Marijuana and hashish are the two cannabis preparations used in the United States. Marijuana is obtained from leaves and stems; hashish, prepared from plant resin, is 5 to 10 times as potent as commonly available marijuana. These cannabis preparations contain several related compounds called cannabinoids. Delta-9-tetrahydrocannabinol (Δ-9-THC) is the main psychoactive ingredient, but metabolites and other constituents also may exert pharmacologic activity. THC binds to and activates cannabinoid receptors in areas of the brain that control memory, thought, concentration, time and depth perception, and coordinated movement. THC decreases activity of the neurons in each of these areas and thereby impairs these functions.

It also stimulates dopamine and the reward system of the brain, thereby producing euphoria, relaxation, and more intense sensations.

Cannabis preparations are difficult to classify. Some people call them depressants; some call them stimulants; and others label them as mind-altering, hallucinogenic, psychotomimetic, or unique in terms of fitting into drug categories. It is also difficult to predict the effects of these drugs. Factors that influence a person's response include dose, route of administration, personality traits, and the amount of active ingredients, which varies with the climate and soil where the plants are grown and with the method of preparation. Reportedly, the THC content of marijuana products is higher now than previously, so that effects may be even more unpredictable.

Marijuana can be taken orally but is more often smoked and inhaled through the lungs. It is more potent and more rapid in its actions when inhaled. After smoking, subjective effects begin in about 10 minutes and last 2 to 3 hours. However, THC accumulates in fatty tissues and has a long half-life, so that impairment of musculoskeletal coordination and other adverse effects may last for more than 24 hours. Low doses are mildly intoxicating and similar to small amounts of alcohol. Large doses can produce panic reactions and hallucinations similar to acute psychosis. Effects wear off as THC is metabolized to inactive products.

Numerous adverse effects have been reported with marijuana use. In addition to CNS effects and impaired ability to perform common tasks of everyday life, THC may cause serious cardiovascular (e.g., hypertension, bradycardia, vasoconstriction; hypotension may occur with high doses), respiratory (e.g., damage to mucosa, chronic bronchitis with cough and wheezing, respiratory infections, possibly increased risk of lung cancer because the amount of some carcinogens is much higher in marijuana than in tobacco smoke), and other physiologic effects, especially with chronic use. In addition, there is a high risk of infection, especially in patients with acquired immunodeficiency syndrome (AIDS) or other immune system impairments, because marijuana products can be contaminated with fecal matter and various microorganisms (e.g., aspergillus, salmonella). Some authorities believe that adverse effects are now more common and serious than previously thought, because of the higher THC content in marijuana preparations.

Except for dronabinol (Marinol), marijuana and other cannabis preparations are illegal and not used therapeutically in most of the United States. Dronabinol, a formulation of Δ-9-THC, is used to treat nausea and vomiting associated with anticancer drugs and to stimulate appetite in patients with AIDS. The risks of abuse are high, and the drug may cause physical and psychological dependence. It is a Schedule III controlled drug. Cannabinoids can also decrease intraocular pressure and may be useful in treating glaucoma. Some people promote legalization of marijuana for medical uses. However, clinicians state that such usage is no more effective than available legal treatments that have less abuse potential.

Marijuana Dependence and Its Treatment

Tolerance and psychological dependence do not usually develop with occasional use but may occur with chronic use; physical dependence rarely occurs. There is no specific treatment other than abstinence.

Hallucinogens

Hallucinogenic drugs include a variety of substances that cause mood changes, anxiety, distorted sensory perceptions, hallucinations, delusions, depersonalization, pupil dilation, elevated body temperature, and elevated blood pressure.

Dextromethorphan

Dextromethorphan is a cough suppressant found in many OTC multisymptom cold and cough remedies. It is a synthetic drug derived from an opioid analgesic. It does not have analgesic or sedative effects. It is a CNS depressant but is usually classified as a *hallucinogen* because of dissociative effects similar to those of phencyclidine (PCP) and ketamine (see below) when it is taken in the high doses characteristic of abuse. (The maximum recommended therapeutic dose is 120 mg in 24 hours, taken in 15- to 30-mg amounts every 4 to 6 hours; abusers may take as much as 360 mg at one time).

Adverse effects include blurred vision, brain damage, confusion, dizziness, drowsiness, excessive sweating, hallucinations, impaired breathing, impaired judgment and mental functioning, loss of consciousness, loss of physical coordination, muscle twitches, nausea and vomiting, paranoia, rapid and irregular heartbeat, seizures, slurred speech, and death. In addition, OTC products contain other ingredients (e.g., acetaminophen, antihistamines, decongestants) that are also toxic in overdose. In 2005, the Food and Drug Administration (FDA) issued a warning against DM abuse after the deaths of five teenagers were associated with the ingestion of DM capsules. Overdose requires emergency treatment and may involve activated charcoal and IV naloxone, a narcotic antagonist.

LSD

LSD (lysergic acid diethylamide) is a synthetic derivative of a compound in ergot and some varieties of morning glory seeds. It is very potent, and small doses can alter normal brain functioning. LSD is usually distributed as a soluble powder and ingested in capsule, tablet, or liquid form. The exact mechanism of action is unknown, and effects cannot be predicted accurately. LSD alters sensory perceptions and thought processes; impairs most intellectual functions, such as memory and problem-solving ability; distorts perception of time and space; and produces sympathomimetic reactions, including increased blood pressure, heart rate, and body temperature, as well as pupil dilation. Adverse reactions include self-injury and possibly suicide, violent behavior, psychotic episodes, "flashbacks" (a phenomenon characterized by psychological effects and hallucinations that may recur days, weeks, or months after the drug is taken), and possible chromosomal damage resulting in birth defects.

Mescaline

Mescaline is an alkaloid of the peyote cactus. It is the least active of the commonly used psychotomimetic agents but produces effects similar to those of LSD. It is usually ingested in the form of a soluble powder or capsule.

Phencyclidine

Phencyclidine (PCP) produces excitement, delirium, hallucinations, and other profound psychological and physiologic effects, including a state of intoxication similar to that produced by alcohol; altered sensory perceptions; impaired thought processes; impaired motor skills; psychotic reactions; sedation and analgesia; nystagmus and diplopia; and pressor effects that can cause hypertensive crisis, cerebral hemorrhage, convulsions, coma, and death. Death from overdose also has occurred as a result of respiratory depression. Bizarre murders, suicides, and self-mutilations have been attributed to the schizophrenic reaction induced by PCP, especially in high doses. The drug also produces flashbacks.

PCP is usually distributed in liquid or crystal form and can be ingested, inhaled, or injected. It is usually sprayed or sprinkled on marijuana or herbs and smoked. Probably because it is cheap, easily synthesized, and readily available, PCP is often sold as LSD, mescaline, cocaine, or THC (the active ingredient in marijuana). It may also be added to marijuana without the user's knowledge. Consequently, the drug user may experience severe and unexpected reactions, including death.

Hallucinogen Dependence and Its Treatment

Tolerance develops, but there is no apparent physical dependence or abstinence syndrome. Psychological dependence probably occurs but is usually not intense. Users may prefer one of these drugs, but they apparently do without or substitute another drug if the one they favor is unavailable. A major danger with these drugs is their ability to impair judgment and insight, which can lead to panic reactions in which users may try to injure themselves (e.g., by running into traffic). There is no specific treatment for hallucinogen dependence. Those who experience severe panic reactions may be kept in a safe, supportive environment until drug effects wear off or may be given a sedative-type drug.

"Club" and "Date-Rape" Drugs

"Ecstasy," flunitrazepam (Rohypnol), gamma-hydroxybutyrate (GHB), and ketamine are reported to be widely used, mainly by adolescents and young adults. The "club drug" designation stems from use at all-night dance parties called "raves"; the "date-rape drug" designation stems from reported use of these drugs in unaware females to facilitate sexual conquest.

Ecstasy

Ecstasy (3,4 methylenedioxy-methamphetamine or MDMA) is an illegal, Schedule I derivative of amphetamine. It is structurally similar to methamphetamine and mescaline and produces stimulant and hallucinogenic effects. MDMA first became popular with adolescents and young adults at "raves," but its use has spread to a variety of settings and age groups. It is usually taken orally, as a tablet, but it may be crushed and snorted or injected. Users report increased energy and perception, euphoria, and feelings of closeness to others. These effects occur within an hour after oral ingestion and last 4 to 6 hours.

Ecstasy is extremely dangerous, and usage is decreasing as users become more aware of serious adverse effects. Adverse effects include acute psychiatric symptoms (e.g., anxiety, panic, depression, paranoid thinking), cardiac dysrhythmias, coma, dehydration, delirium, hypertension, hyperthermia, hyponatremia, rhabdomyolysis, seizures, tachycardia, and death. These effects have occurred with a single use. Another major concern is the drug's neurotoxicity. Early effects include spasmodic jerking, involuntary jaw clenching, and teeth grinding. Long-term or permanent changes may result from damage to the nerve cells in the brain that use serotonin as a neurotransmitter. MDMA increases the release and inhibits reuptake of serotonin. This action floods the brain with high amounts of serotonin, which is important in emotion, mood, and memory. Chronic use of MDMA may deplete serotonin and lead to sadness or depression, insomnia, memory impairment, low energy or passivity, and a decreased ability to feel emotions or pleasure.

In addition to the many adverse effects of MDMA, users also need to be concerned about the actual product they are taking. There have been numerous reports of other drugs (e.g., LSD, methamphetamine, ketamine, PCP) being sold as ecstasy. All of these drugs may have serious adverse effects as well.

MDMA is not thought to cause dependence or withdrawal syndromes. Emergency treatment of MDMA abuse usually involves decreasing the high body temperature, replacing fluids and electrolytes, and monitoring for cardiovascular complications.

Flunitrazepam (Rohypnol)

Flunitrazepam is a benzodiazepine (see Chap. 8) that is manufactured and used in Europe and other parts of the world. It is a Schedule I drug in the United States and has never been approved for any therapeutic use. The drug is usually taken orally, but the tablets are sometimes ground into a powder and snorted. Flunitrazepam is often taken with other drugs, including alcohol, cocaine, heroin, or marijuana. In addition to intentional use, the odorless and colorless drug has reportedly been added to punch and other drinks at fraternity parties and other social events, leading to its designation as a "date-rape" drug.

Even when flunitrazepam is taken alone in relatively low doses, the drug can cause muscle relaxation, general sedative and hypnotic effects, and the appearance of intoxication, with slurred speech, poor coordination, swaying, and bloodshot eyes. These effects begin within 30 minutes, peak within 2 hours, and may last 8 hours or longer, depending on dosage. Other adverse effects include confusion, dizziness, drowsiness, hypotension, memory impairment, and visual disturbances. In high doses, flunitrazepam causes a loss of muscle control, loss of consciousness, and partial amnesia. Combining the drug with alcohol increases its adverse effects.

As with other benzodiazepines, flunitrazepam causes dependence. After dependence has developed, stopping the drug induces withdrawal symptoms such as extreme anxiety, confusion, headache, irritability, muscle pain, and restlessness. Cardiovascular collapse, convulsions, delirium, hallucinations, numbness and tingling of the extremities, and shock also may occur. Withdrawal seizures can occur a week or longer after stopping the drug. The main treatment for flunitrazepam dependence is gradually tapering and discontinuing the drug.

Gamma-Hydroxybutyrate (GHB)

GHB is a Schedule I controlled drug whose only approved use in the United States is for research. It is a CNS depressant that is structurally related to the inhibitory neurotransmitter, gamma-aminobutyric acid (GABA). Usage of GHB has increased in recent years, mainly in the party or dance-club setting, and is increasingly involved in poisonings, overdoses, date rapes, visits to hospital emergency departments, and fatalities. Some users admit they took the drug intentionally; some say the drug was added to their drinks without their knowledge or consent. In addition to its use as a "club" or "date-rape" drug, GHB is sometimes used by body builders for alleged anabolic effects. Formerly sold in health food stores as a nutritional supplement with numerous claims of beneficial effects, the drug became a controlled drug in 2000 after serious illnesses and deaths were reported. However, precursor substances (that are converted to GHB in the body) are reportedly still available in gyms and health food stores as dietary supplements.

GHB is available in an odorless, colorless liquid or as a white powder and is taken orally, often combined with alcohol. Effects include drowsiness, respiratory depression, seizures, unconsciousness, and vomiting. As with other sedative drugs, respiratory depression leading to hypoxia and death is the most serious adverse effect. Treatment of acute toxicity is mainly symptomatic and supportive.

With chronic use, GHB and its precursors (gammabutyrolactone, butanediol) are reported to induce tolerance and produce dependence. Withdrawal symptoms of severe agitation, mental status changes (including symptoms of psychosis), elevated blood pressure, and tachycardia occur within hours of the last dose.

Ketamine

Ketamine is an anesthetic that is chemically related to PCP and used mainly by veterinarians. It has become a "recreational" drug, and its effects are similar to those of PCP and LSD (e.g., distorted senses and perceptions, dissociative reactions). The hallucinations produced by ketamine last about an hour, but the user's senses, judgment, coordination, and self-control may be impaired as long as 24 hours after the initial use of the drug. These effects produce a high risk of injuries. Other effects include respiratory depression, heart rate abnormalities, and a withdrawal syndrome. Ketamine is a Schedule III controlled substance.

Ketamine is usually injected, but it may be taken orally, smoked, or swallowed. It is sometimes added to marijuana cigarettes. Effects include increased blood pressure, tachycardia, respiratory depression, airway obstruction, apnea, hypertonic muscles and movement disorders, and psychosis. With overdoses, seizures, polyneuropathy, increased intracranial pressure, respiratory arrest, and cardiac arrest may occur. With chronic use, flashbacks and other effects may last up to 2 years after stopping the drug. Long-term effects include tolerance and possibly physical and/or psychological dependence.

Inhalants

These drugs include volatile solvents such as acetone, toluene, and gasoline, substances that produce chemical vapors that can be inhaled to induce mind-altering effects. These solvents may be constituents of some types of glues, plastic cements, aerosol sprays, butane lighter, spray paints, degreasers or cleaning fluids, paint thinners and removers, felt-tip marker fluids, and other products. Some general inhalation anesthetics, such as nitrous oxide, have also been abused to the point of dependence. Nitrous oxide may be an ingredient in whipped cream dispensers and products that boost octane levels in racing cars. Volatile solvents are most often abused by preadolescents and adolescents who squeeze glue into a plastic bag, for example, and sniff the fumes. Suffocation sometimes occurs when the sniffer loses consciousness while the bag covers the face.

These substances produce symptoms comparable with those of acute alcohol intoxication, including initial mild euphoria followed by ataxia, confusion, and disorientation. Some substances in gasoline and toluene also may produce symptoms similar to those produced by the hallucinogens, including euphoria, hallucinations, recklessness, and loss of self-control. Large doses may cause convulsions, coma, and death.

Inhalants can harm the brain, liver, heart, kidneys, and lungs, and abuse of any drug during adolescence may interfere with brain development. Substances containing gasoline, benzene, or carbon tetrachloride are especially likely to cause serious damage to the liver, kidneys, and bone marrow. Inhalants can also produce psychological dependence, and some produce tolerance. There is some question about whether physical dependence occurs. If it does occur, it is considered less intense than the physical dependence associated with alcohol and opioids.

Nursing Process

Assessment

Assess patients for signs of alcohol and other drug abuse, including abuse of prescription drugs such as antianxiety agents, opioids, and sedative-hypnotics. Some general screening-type questions are appropriate for any initial nursing assessment. The overall purpose of these questions is to determine whether a current or potential problem exists and whether additional information is needed. Some patients may refuse to answer or give answers that contradict other assessment data. Denial of excessive drinking and of problems resulting from alcohol use is a prominent characteristic of alcoholism; underreporting the extent of drug use is common in other types of drug abuse as well. Useful information includes each specific drug, the amount, the frequency of administration, and the duration of administration. If answers to general questions reveal problem areas, such as long-term use of alcohol or psychotropic drugs, more specific questions can be formulated to assess the scope and depth of the problem. It may be especially difficult to obtain needed information about illegal "street drugs," most of which have numerous, frequently changed names. For nurses who often encounter substance abusers, efforts to keep up with drug names and terminology may be helpful.

▪ Interview the patient regarding alcohol and other drug use to help determine immediate and long-term nursing care needs. For example, information may be obtained that would indicate the likelihood of a withdrawal reaction; the risk of increased or decreased effects of a variety of drugs; and the patient's susceptibility to drug abuse. People who abuse one drug are likely to abuse others, and abuse of multiple drugs is a more common pattern than abuse of a single drug. These and other factors aid effective planning of nursing care.

▪ Assess behavior that may indicate drug abuse, such as alcohol on the breath, altered speech patterns, staggering gait, hyperactivity or hypoactivity, and other signs of excessive CNS depression or stimulation. Impairments in work performance and in interpersonal relationships also may be behavioral clues.

▪ Assess for disorders that may be caused by substance abuse. These disorders may include infections, liver disease, accidental injuries, and psychiatric problems of anxiety or depression. These disorders may be caused by other factors, of course, and are nonspecific.

▪ Check laboratory reports, when available, for abnormal liver function test results, indications of anemia, abnormal white blood cell counts, abnormal electrolytes (hypocalcemia, hypomagnesemia, and acidosis are common in alcoholics), and alcohol and drug levels in the blood.

Nursing Diagnoses

▪ Ineffective Coping related to reliance on alcohol or other drugs

▪ Risk for Injury: Adverse effects of abused drug(s)

▪ Disturbed Thought Processes related to use of psychoactive drugs

▪ Risk for Other- or Self-Directed Violence related to disturbed thought processes, impaired judgment, and impulsive behavior

▪ Imbalanced Nutrition: Less Than Body Requirements related to drug effects and drug-seeking behavior

- Dysfunctional Family Processes: Alcoholism
- Risk for Injury: Infection, hepatitis, or AIDS related to use of contaminated needles and syringes for IV drugs

Planning/Goals

- Safety will be maintained for patients impaired by alcohol and drug abuse.
- Information will be provided regarding drug effects and treatment resources.
- The patient's efforts toward stopping drug usage will be recognized and reinforced.

Interventions

- Administer prescribed drugs correctly during acute intoxication or withdrawal.
- Decrease environmental stimuli for the person undergoing drug withdrawal.
- Record vital signs; cardiovascular, respiratory, and neurologic functions; mental status; and behavior at regular intervals.
- Support use of resources for stopping drug abuse (psychotherapy, treatment programs).
- Request patient referrals to psychiatric/mental health physicians, nurse clinical specialists, or self-help programs when indicated.
- Use therapeutic communication skills to discuss alcohol or other drug-related health problems, health-related benefits of stopping substance use or abuse, and available services or treatment options.
- Teach nondrug techniques for coping with stress and anxiety.
- Provide positive reinforcement for efforts toward quitting substance abuse.
- Inform smokers with young children in the home that cigarette smoke can precipitate or aggravate asthma and upper respiratory disorders in children.
- Inform smokers with nonsmoking spouses or other members of the household that secondhand smoke can increase the risks of cancer and lung disease in the nonsmokers as well as the smoker.
- For smokers who are concerned about weight gain if they quit smoking, emphasize that the health benefits of quitting far outweigh the disadvantages of gaining a few pounds, and discuss ways to control weight without smoking.

Evaluation

- Observe for improved behavior (e.g., less impulsiveness, improved judgment and thought processes, commits no injury to self or others).

- Observe for use or avoidance of nonprescribed drugs while hospitalized.
- Interview to determine the client's insight into personal problems stemming from drug abuse.
- Verify enrollment in a treatment program.
- Observe for appropriate use of drugs to decrease abuse of other drugs.

Principles of Therapy

Prevention of Substance Abuse

Alcohol and other drug abuse have devastating effects on individuals and communities. The losses of worker productivity and the astronomical costs of dealing with associated crime, violence, traumatic injuries, medical illness, and psychiatric disorders are depleting governmental units of resources that could provide more benefit to society if used for education and other purposes. Consequently, all citizens need to be concerned about this modern plague and support efforts to prevent people from starting drug abuse in the first place. Although there are difficulties in trying to prevent conditions for which causes are not known, some of the following community-wide and individual measures may be helpful:

- Decrease the availability of commonly abused drugs. Most efforts at prevention have tried to reduce the supply of drugs. For example, laws designate certain drugs as illegal and provide penalties for possession or use of these drugs; regulate circumstances in which legal drugs, such as opioid analgesics, may be used; and regulate the sale of alcoholic beverages. In recent years, laws to restrict the availability of ingredients used to manufacture methamphetamine and those to increase cigarette taxes and prevent smoking in public places have been passed.

  Despite these efforts, drugs of abuse seem to be widely available, in homes, on the street, and from Internet sources. In many cases, prescription sedatives, analgesics, or methylphenidate preparations are obtained by various means and used for nonmedical purposes. Thus, every individual or family member has a responsibility for safe use and storage of these drugs so they cannot be diverted to illegal, nonmedical use.

- Decrease the demand for drugs. It is a simple axiom that drugs of abuse would not be available if there were no market for them. Because decreasing demand involves changing attitudes, it is very difficult but more effective in the long run. In general, American society has had a permissive attitude toward the use of alcohol and other drugs of abuse. This climate may be changing somewhat as evidenced by public support of laws increasing the costs of tobacco products and banning smoking in public places. Efforts to change attitudes and decrease demand for drugs can be made through education and counseling about such topics as drug effects and nondrug ways to cope with the stresses and problems of daily life. Although community-wide efforts are important and should be supported, each individual must take personal responsibility for drinking alcoholic beverages and taking mind-altering drugs for the purpose of "getting high." Initially, conscious, voluntary choices are made to drink or not to drink, to take a drug or not to take it. This period varies somewhat, but drug dependence develops in most instances only after prolonged use. When mind-altering drugs are prescribed for a legitimate reason, the patient must use them in prescribed doses and preferably for a short time.

■ Drug prescribers can help prevent drug abuse by prescribing drugs appropriately, prescribing mind-altering drugs in limited amounts and for limited periods, using nondrug measures when they are likely to be effective, educating patients about the drugs prescribed for them, participating in drug education programs, and recognizing, as early as possible, patients who are abusing or who are likely to abuse drugs. Some authorities recommend that physicians question all patients about smoking cigarettes and offer cessation treatment when indicated.

■ Nurses can help prevent drug abuse by administering drugs appropriately, using nondrug measures when possible, teaching patients about drugs prescribed for them, and participating in drug education programs. Some resources for information and educational materials are listed in Box 14-3.

| Box 14-3 | Sources of Information About Substance Abuse |

■ The National Institute on Drug Abuse (NIDA) of the National Institutes of Health supports most of the world's research on the health aspects of drug abuse and addiction.
6001 Executive Blvd.
Bethesda, MD 20892-9561
Telephone: (301) 443-1124
www.drugabuse.gov; also www.nida.nih.gov
■ Substance Abuse & Mental Health Services Administration (SAMHSA)
1 Choke Cherry Road
Rockville, MD 20857
Telephone: (240) 276-2130
www.samhsa.org
■ The National Institute on Alcohol Abuse and Alcoholism (NIAAA) conducts and supports research on the causes, consequences, prevention, and treatment of alcohol abuse and disseminates research findings to general, professional, and academic audiences. Publications and research information are available at www.niaaa.nih.gov.
SAMHSA's National Clearinghouse for Alcohol and Drug Information (NCADI) Web site is http://ncadi.samhsa.gov

■ Parents can help prevent drug abuse by talking to their children about the dangers of substance abuse (e.g., brain damage and other serious health problems, as well as traumatic injuries, sexually transmitted diseases, etc.), limiting availability of abused substances in the home (e.g., alcohol; prescription pain relievers such as Percocet, Vicodin, and OxyContin; prescription sedatives such as Xanax; prescription methylphenidate for ADHD; OTC cold and cough remedies containing dextromethorphan; household products that can be abused by inhalation), monitoring the use and amounts of those products that are available, minimizing their own use of drugs, and avoiding heavy cigarette smoking. Children are more likely to use illegal drugs if their parents have a generally permissive attitude about drug taking, if either parent takes mind-altering drugs regularly, and if either parent is a heavy cigarette smoker.

■ Substance abuse often starts during adolescence and is especially hazardous then, because the brain is still developing and especially vulnerable to damage. Teenagers obtain prescription drugs from prescribers (e.g., for ADHD; with tales of anxiety and stress or difficulty sleeping), friends, stealing them from family members, ordering them over the Internet, as well as on the street from dealers (who may be friends or schoolmates). Preteens may also abuse drugs, including alcohol, cough syrup containing dextromethorphan, and inhalants.

■ Pregnant women should avoid alcohol, nicotine, and other drugs of abuse because of potentially harmful effects on the fetus.

Goals of Therapy

The major goals of treatment for substance abuse are detoxification, initiation of abstinence, and prevention of relapse. Patients who are likely to benefit from treatment are those who admit that substance abuse is causing significant problems in their ability to function in activities of daily living. Despite advances in treatment and the many adverse consequences of substance abuse, relapses to drug-taking behavior are common among those who have been detoxified or even abstinent for varying periods of time.

Treatment of Substance Abuse

Treatments for substance abuse are limited but increasing; more treatment facilities are needed. For most health professionals, contact with substance abusers is more likely to occur in acute situations, such as intoxication or overdose, withdrawal syndromes, or various medical-surgical illnesses associated with the substance abuse. In general, treatment depends on the type, extent, and duration of drug-taking behavior and the particular situation for which treatment is needed.

Psychological rehabilitation efforts should be part of any treatment program for a drug-dependent person. Several approaches may be useful, including inpatient and outpatient psychotherapy, voluntary self-help groups (e.g., Alcoholics Anonymous, Narcotics Anonymous), and other types of emotional support and counseling. Substance abusers are assisted and encouraged to develop more healthful coping skills to deal with life stresses and to alter the environment or relationships in which substance abuse occurs. Much of this counseling is done by health care providers who specialize in treatment of drug dependence.

In addition to or along with "talk" therapy (e.g., cognitive behavior therapy), an intervention with some success is contingency management (also called motivational incentives), in which incentives or rewards are given for not using drugs (e.g., as evidenced by drug-free urine tests) with abusers of cocaine, marijuana, and methamphetamine. Rewards include vouchers of some kind that can be used to purchase various products. In one study, patients who remained abstinent for the entire treatment period of 14 weeks received vouchers for $570, which could be exchanged for movie passes, sports or hobby equipment, and other purchases that would not enable or encourage substance abuse.

Drug therapy is limited in treating drug dependence for several reasons. First, specific antidotes are available only for benzodiazepines (flumazenil) and opioid narcotics (naloxone). Second, there is a high risk of substituting one abused drug for another. Third, there are significant drawbacks to giving CNS stimulants to reverse effects of CNS depressants, and vice versa. Fourth, there is often inadequate information about the types and amounts of drugs taken.

Two of the more successful drug therapy regimens are methadone administration for heroin dependence and nicotine replacement or other drug therapy (e.g., bupropion or varenicline) for nicotine dependence. With both treatments, however, a combination of drug therapy and counseling is more effective than either alone.

Despite these drawbacks, however, there are some clinical indications for drug therapy, including treatment of overdose or withdrawal syndromes. Even when drug therapy is indicated, there are few guidelines for optimal use. Doses, for example, must often be estimated initially and then titrated according to response. Drug therapy may be provided by primary care prescribers or prescribers who specialize in treatment of drug dependence.

General care of patients with drug overdose is primarily symptomatic and supportive. The aim of treatment is usually to support vital functions, such as respiration and circulation, until the drug is metabolized and eliminated from the body. For example, respiratory depression from an overdose of a CNS depressant drug may be treated by inserting an artificial airway and mechanical ventilation. Removal of some drugs can be hastened by hemodialysis.

Treatment of substance abuse may be complicated by the presence of other disorders. For example, medical illnesses and other psychiatric disorders are common.

Key Concepts

▪ Drug abuse damages the brain and other body organs.

▪ Health professionals most often encounter substance abusers when they are intoxicated, overdosed, undergoing withdrawal, or have illnesses stemming from substance abuse.

▪ Drug therapy for substance abuse is most effective when combined with counseling and psychotherapy.

▪ Because substance abuse often starts during childhood and adolescence, health professionals, parents, teachers, and others need to teach children about risks of drug abuse and strategies to resist peer pressure to use drugs of abuse, limit access to drugs of abuse, and support programs and activities designed to decrease drug abuse in this population.

Review and Application Exercises

Short Answer Exercises

1. Why is it important to assess each patient in relation to alcohol and other substance abuse?

2. What are the signs and symptoms of overdose with alcohol, benzodiazepine antianxiety or sedative-hypnotic agents, cocaine, and opiates?

3. What are general interventions for treatment of drug overdoses?

4. What are specific antidotes for opioid and benzodiazepine overdoses, and how are they administered?

5. Which commonly abused drugs may produce life-threatening withdrawal reactions if stopped abruptly?

6. How can severe withdrawal syndromes be prevented, minimized, or safely managed?

7. What are the advantages of treating substance abuse disorders in centers established for that purpose?

NCLEX-Style Questions

8. The nurse who is caring for a patient who has been abusing alcohol may expect to see what symptom as the patient enters withdrawal?
   a. sleep
   b. muscle relaxation
   c. euphoria
   d. agitation

9. The nurse taking care of an adolescent with a history of compulsive drug use is questioned by her parents about the reasons behind such drug use. The nurse is most correct when she states that compulsive drug use is attributed mainly to
   a. drug stimulation of the "reward" center in the brain
   b. a belief that the drugs are not harmful
   c. parental pressure to do well in school
   d. a permissive attitude toward taking drugs by parents and society

10. The nurse may expect an order to administer flumazenil (Romazicon) as an antidote for a patient admitted with an overdose of
    a. alcohol
    b. benzodiazepines
    c. opioids
    d. amphetamines

11. The nurse who is caring for a patient admitted with acute overdosage of cocaine knows that this is most likely to cause
    a. severe lung damage
    b. anaphylaxis
    c. life-threatening cardiac dysrhythmias
    d. hypotension

12. Which of the following drug products can be used to aid smoking cessation?
    a. naltrexone (ReVia)
    b. disulfiram (Antabuse)
    c. bupropion (Zyban)
    d. dronabinol (Marinol)

Selected References

Doering, P. L. (2005). Substance-related disorders: Alcohol, nicotine, and caffeine. In J. T. DiPiro, R. L. Talbert, G. C. Yee, G. R. Matzke, B. G. Wells, & L. M. Posey (Eds.), *Pharmacotherapy: A pathophysiologic approach* (6th ed., pp. 1193–1208). New York: McGraw-Hill.

Doering, P. L. (2005). Substance-related disorders: Overview and depressants, stimulants and hallucinogens. In J. T. DiPiro, R. L. Talbert, G. C. Yee, G. R. Matzke, B. G. Wells, & L. M. Posey (Eds.), *Pharmacotherapy: A pathophysiologic approach* (6th ed., pp. 1175–1191). New York: McGraw-Hill.

Donaher, P. A., & Welsh, C. (2006). Managing opioid addiction with buprenorphine. *American Family Physician, 73*, 1573–1578.

Eisendrath, S. J., & Lichtmacher, J. E. (2007). Psychiatric disorders. In S. J. McPhee, M. A. Papadakis, & L. M. Tierney, Jr. (Eds), *Current medical diagnosis and treatment 2007* (46th ed., pp 1063–1122). New York: McGraw-Hill.

Friedman, R. A. (2006). The changing face of teenage drug abuse—The trend toward prescription drugs. *New England Journal of Medicine, 354*, 1448–1450.

Jorenby, D. E., Hays, J. T., & Rigotti, N. A. (2006). Efficacy of varenicline, an alpha₄beta₂ nicotinic acetylcholine receptor partial agonist, vs placebo or sustained-release bupropion for smoking cessation: A randomized controlled trial. *Journal of the American Medical Association, 296*, 56–63.

Kuehn, B. M. (2005). Methadone treatment marks 40 years. *Journal of the American Medical Association, 294*, 887–889.

Molnar, A. (2006). One drink over the line. *Nursing 2006 Critical Care, 1*, 20–33.

Moore, B. A. (2005). Respiratory effects of marijuana and tobacco use in a U.S. sample. *Journal of General Internal Medicine, 20*, 33–37.

O'Connor, P. G. (2005). Methods of detoxification and their role in treating patients with opioid dependence [editorial]. *Journal of the American Medical Association, 94*, 961–963.

Porth, C. M. (2005). *Pathophysiology: Concepts of altered health states* (7th ed.). Philadelphia: Lippincott Williams & Wilkins.

Rollo, K. L., & Ewen, B. (2007). Meth: The crystal that kills. *Nursing 2007 Critical Care, 2*, 54–60.

Smeltzer, S. C., Bare, B. G., Hinkle, J.L., & Cheever, K.H. (2008). *Brunner & Suddarth's textbook of medical-surgical nursing* (11th ed.). Philadelphia: Lippincott Williams & Wilkins.

Central Nervous System Stimulants

LEARNING OBJECTIVES

After studying this chapter, you will be able to:

1. Describe general characteristics of central nervous system (CNS) stimulants.
2. Discuss reasons for decreased use of amphetamines for therapeutic purposes.
3. Discuss the rationale for treating attention deficit-hyperactivity disorder with CNS stimulants.
4. Identify effects and sources of caffeine.
5. Identify nursing interventions to prevent, recognize, and treat stimulant overdose.

Applying Your Knowledge

Kevin Granata was diagnosed with attention deficit-hyperactivity disorder (ADHD) at age 8. He is now 11 years old and a student at the school where you are the school nurse. As a result of taking methylphenidate (Ritalin) 15 mg daily and receiving individual counseling, Kevin's attention span and school performance improved.

Part of the annual school physical examination for all children is to track height and weight. Kevin's height and weight is less than normal for his age group, and he has lost weight since his examination last year. When you talk with his teachers, they report that he is restless in class and has an extremely short attention span. He has had more difficulty getting along with his classmates.

Introduction

Many drugs stimulate the central nervous system (CNS), but only a few are used therapeutically, and their indications for use are limited. Two disorders treated with CNS stimulants are *attention deficit-hyperactivity disorder* (ADHD) and *narcolepsy*.

Attention Deficit-Hyperactivity Disorder (ADHD)

ADHD is the most common psychiatric or neurobehavioral disorder in children. It is usually diagnosed between 3 and 7 years of age and may affect as many as 6% to 7% of school-age children. It is characterized by persistent hyperactivity, a short attention span, difficulty completing assigned tasks or schoolwork, restlessness, and impulsiveness. Such behaviors make it difficult for the child to get along with others (e.g., family members, peer groups, teachers) and to function in situations requiring controlled behavior (e.g., classrooms).

ADHD continues into adolescence and adulthood in approximately 50% of cases and may affect 4% of adults in the United States. In adolescents and adults, hyperactivity is not prominent, but impulsiveness, inattention, and difficulties in structured settings such as school or work may continue. In addition, some studies indicate that children with ADHD are more likely to have learning disabilities, mood disorders, and substance abuse disorders as adolescents and adults. A major criterion for diagnosing later ADHD is a previous diagnosis of ADHD by 7 years of age. Some authorities believe this age limit is too restrictive. The diagnosis of ADHD in adults has greatly increased in recent years, with a concomitant increase in the use of prescribed CNS stimulants for its treatment.

Narcolepsy

Narcolepsy is a sleep disorder characterized by daytime "sleep attacks" in which the person goes to sleep at any place or at any time. Signs and symptoms also include excessive daytime drowsiness, fatigue, muscle weakness and hallucinations at onset of sleep, and disturbances of nighttime sleep patterns. The hazards of drowsiness during normal waking hours and suddenly going to sleep in unsafe environments restrict activities of daily living.

Narcolepsy affects men and women equally and usually begins during the teenage or young adult years. Its cause is unknown, and sleep studies are required for an accurate diagnosis. In addition to drug therapy, prevention of sleep deprivation, regular sleeping and waking times, avoiding shift work, and short naps may be helpful in reducing daytime sleepiness. However, even adequate amounts of nighttime sleep do not produce full alertness.

General Characteristics of Stimulants

CNS stimulants act by facilitating initiation and transmission of nerve impulses that excite other cells. The drugs are somewhat selective in their actions at lower doses but tend to involve the entire CNS at higher doses. In ADHD, the drugs improve academic performance, behavior, and interpersonal relationships. Major groups of stimulants are amphetamines and related drugs and xanthines.

Amphetamines increase the amounts of norepinephrine, dopamine, and possibly serotonin in the brain, thereby producing mood elevation or euphoria, increasing mental alertness and capacity for work, decreasing fatigue and drowsiness, and prolonging wakefulness. However, large doses produce signs of excessive CNS stimulation (e.g., agitation, confusion, hyperactivity, difficulty concentrating on tasks, hyperactivity, nervousness, restlessness) and sympathetic nervous system stimulation (e.g., increased heart rate and blood pressure, pupil dilation, slowed gastrointestinal [GI] motility, and other symptoms). Overdoses can result in psychosis, convulsions, stroke, cardiac arrest, and death.

Amphetamines are Schedule II drugs under the Controlled Substances Act and have a high potential for drug abuse and dependence. These drugs are widely sold on the street and commonly abused (see Chap. 14). Amphetamine-related drugs (methylphenidate and dexmethylphenidate) have essentially the same effects as the amphetamines and are also Schedule II drugs. These drugs have long had **BLACK BOX WARNINGS** about the risk of drug dependence. In recent years, warnings have been added to all drugs used to treat ADHD about the risks of sudden death, serious cardiovascular problems (e.g., heart attack, hypertension), and psychiatric illnesses (e.g., psychosis, aggression, mania).

Xanthines stimulate the cerebral cortex, increasing mental alertness and decreasing drowsiness and fatigue. Other effects include myocardial stimulation with increased cardiac output and heart rate, diuresis, and increased secretion of pepsin and hydrochloric acid. Large doses can impair mental and physical functions by producing agitation, anxiety, cardiac dysrhythmias, gastritis, insomnia, nervousness and restlessness.

Indications for Use

Amphetamines and methylphenidate are used in the treatment of narcolepsy and ADHD. Atomoxetine and dexmethylphenidate are indicated only for ADHD. Caffeine (a xanthine) is an ingredient in nonprescription analgesics and stimulants that promote wakefulness (e.g., NoDoz). A combination of caffeine and sodium benzoate is occasionally used as a respiratory stimulant in neonates. Modafinil is approved only for treatment of narcolepsy.

Contraindications to Use

CNS stimulants also stimulate the cardiovascular system and thus are contraindicated in patients with cardiovascular disorders (e.g., angina, dysrhythmias, hypertension) that are likely to be aggravated by the drugs. They also are contraindicated in patients with anxiety or agitation, glaucoma, or hyperthyroidism. They are usually contraindicated in patients with a history of drug abuse. Caffeine is not recommended for people with cardiac dysrhythmias, a history of stroke, peptic ulcer disease, bipolar mood disorder, and schizophrenia.

Individual Drugs

Individual drugs are described below. Dosages are listed in Table 15-1.

Amphetamines and Related Drugs

P **Amphetamine**, **dextroamphetamine** (Dexedrine), and **methamphetamine** (Desoxyn) are closely related drugs that share characteristics of the amphetamines as a group. Except for the amphetamine/dextroamphetamine mixture of **Adderall**, which is used for treatment of ADHD in children and adults, amphetamines are more important as drugs of abuse than as therapeutic agents. A newer amphetamine, **lisdexamfetamine** (Vyvanse), is approved for treatment of ADHD. The drug reportedly delays the stimulation associated with other amphetamines and may be less prone to abuse.

Methylphenidate (e.g., Ritalin) is chemically related to amphetamines and produces similar actions and adverse effects.

Table 15-1 **Drugs at a Glance:** Central Nervous System Stimulants

Names/Indications for Use	ROUTES AND DOSAGE RANGES	
	Adults	**Children**
Amphetamines		
P Amphetamine ADHD Narcolepsy	Narcolepsy: PO 5–60 mg/d in divided doses	Narcolepsy: *6 y and older:* PO 5 mg/d initially, increased at weekly intervals if necessary ADHD: *3–5 y:* PO 2.5 mg/d initially, increased at weekly intervals if necessary *6 y and older:* PO 5 mg once or twice daily initially, increased at weekly intervals until optimal response or maximum dose of 40 mg/d
Dextroamphetamine (Dexedrine) ADHD Narcolepsy		Narcolepsy: *6 y and older:* PO 5 mg/d initially, increased at weekly intervals to effective dose ADHD: *3–5 y:* PO 2.5 mg/d initially, increased at weekly intervals until response *6 y and older:* PO 5 mg once or twice daily initially, increased at weekly intervals until optimal response or maximum dose of 40 mg/d
Lisdexamfetamine (Vyvanse) ADHD in Children		ADHD: *6–12 y:* PO 30 mg once daily, increased if necessary. Maximum dose, 70 mg/d
Methamphetamine (Desoxyn) ADHD in children		PO 5 mg/d initially, increased if necessary. Usual dose 20–25 mg/d, in 2 divided doses.
Amphetamine mixture (Adderall, Adderall XR) ADHD Narcolepsy	Narcolepsy: PO 10 mg/d initially, increased if necessary ADHD: Extended release, 20 mg/d	ADHD: *3–5 y:* PO 2.5 mg/d, increased if necessary *6 y and older:* PO 5 mg 1–2 times daily, increased if necessary. Maximum dose 40 mg/d in 1–3 divided doses. Extended release: *6 y and older:* PO 5–10 mg/d, increased at weekly intervals if necessary. Maximum dose, 30 mg/d. *13–17 y:* PO 10 mg once daily, increased to 20 mg if necessary
Amphetamine-Related Drugs		
Dexmethylphenidate (Focalin, Focalin XR) ADHD	PO 5–10 mg/d, increased if necessary. Maximum dose, 20 mg/d.	*6 y and older:* PO 2.5–5 mg/d, increased if necessary. Maximum dose 20 mg/d.
Methylphenidate (MPH) (Immediate release[IR]), Generic MPH, Methylin, Ritalin)	ADHD: IR: PO 2.5–5 mg twice daily, before breakfast and lunch; increased by 5–10 mg/d at weekly intervals if necessary. Maximum dose 90 mg/d.	*6 y and older:* ADHD IR: PO 2.5–5 mg twice daily, before breakfast and lunch; increased by 5–10 mg/d at weekly intervals if necessary. Maximum dose 90 mg/d.
(Extended release, Concerta, Metadate CD, Metadate ER, Methylin ER, Ritalin LA, Ritalin SR, Daytrana skin patch) ADHD Narcolepsy	ADHD: Metadate CD, Ritalin LA: PO 20 mg once daily, increased if necessary. Maximum dose, 60 mg/d. Narcolepsy: PO 10 mg 2–3 times daily, up to 60 mg/d	Concerta PO: 18 mg once daily, increased if necessary. Maximum dose 54 mg/d for children 6–12 y, 72 mg/d for children 13–17 y Metadate ER, Methylin ER, Ritalin SR may be substituted once the daily dose is titrated with immediate-release MPH tablets and the 8-hour dose corresponds to the extended release tablet size. Daytrana topical to skin for 9 h/d, 10 mg first week, then increase dose weekly until desired response

(continued on page 260)

Table 15-1	Drugs at a Glance: Central Nervous System Stimulants (continued)	
	ROUTES AND DOSAGE RANGES	
Names/Indications for Use	**Adults**	**Children**
Other Drugs		
Atomoxetine (Strattera) ADHD	PO 40 mg/d initially, increased after 3 d to 80 mg/d; given as a single dose in the morning, or as 2 divided doses in morning and early evening	Weight 70 kg or more: PO 0.5 mg/kg/d, increased after 3 d to approximately 1.2 mg/kg/d; given as a single dose in the morning, or as 2 divided doses in morning and early evening
Modafinil (Provigil) Narcolepsy; shift work disorder; excessive daytime sleepiness	PO 200 mg once daily, in the morning. Dosage should be reduced by 50% with severe hepatic impairment.	Dosage not established for children under 16 years of age.

It is well absorbed after oral administration. In children, peak plasma levels occur in about 2 hours with immediate-release tablets and in about 5 hours with extended-release tablets. The drug is mostly metabolized in the liver and excreted in the urine. Methylphenidate is marketed by generic and various trade names and in several dosage forms, including immediate release and chewable tablets, extended release capsules, and a transdermal patch. These dosage forms are not interchangeable. Methylphenidate has become a drug of abuse and its nonmedical use, alone or with other drugs, has increased emergency department visits by adolescents and young adults.

Dexmethylphenidate (Focalin) is very similar to methylphenidate and the amphetamines. It is well absorbed after oral administration and reaches peak plasma levels in 1 to 1.5 hours. It is metabolized in the liver and excreted in urine.

Xanthines

Caffeine is a frequently consumed CNS stimulant worldwide, and most is obtained from dietary sources (e.g., coffee, tea, soft drinks). The caffeine content of coffee and tea beverages is determined by the particular coffee bean or tea leaf and the method of preparation. Caffeine is added to about 70% of the soft drinks ingested in the United States. In addition, so-called energy drinks are widely used, especially by teenagers and young adults. These products contain large amounts of caffeine and most contain large amounts of sugar.

In low to moderate amounts, caffeine increases alertness, wakefulness, and capacity for work; decreases fatigue; and delays sleep. Large amounts cause anxiety, agitation, diarrhea, hyperactivity, insomnia, irritability, nausea, nervousness, premature ventricular contractions, restlessness, tachycardia, tremors, and vomiting. Toxic amounts may cause delirium and seizures. With large amounts or chronic use, caffeine has been implicated as a causative or aggravating factor in cardiovascular disease (hypertension, dysrhythmias), GI disorders (esophageal reflux, peptic ulcers), reproductive disorders, osteoporosis (may increase loss of calcium in urine), psychiatric disturbances, and drug-abuse liability.

Caffeine produces tolerance to its stimulating effects and physical dependence occurs. Abstinence produces withdrawal symptoms, including drowsiness, fatigue, headache, and irritability, within 18 to 24 hours after stopping caffeine intake.

Caffeine is well absorbed from the GI tract and reaches a peak blood level within 30 to 45 minutes of oral ingestion. It easily crosses the blood–brain barrier and has a half-life of 3.5 to 5 hours. It is extensively metabolized, mainly in the liver, and excreted mainly in urine.

Pharmaceutical preparations of caffeine include an oral drug and a solution for injection. Caffeine is an ingredient in some nonprescription analgesic preparations and may increase analgesia. It is combined with an ergot alkaloid to treat migraine headaches (e.g., Cafergot) and is the active ingredient in nonprescription stimulant (antisleep) preparations. A combination of caffeine and sodium benzoate is used as a respiratory stimulant in neonatal apnea unresponsive to other therapies.

Because of the widespread ingestion of caffeine-containing beverages and the wide availability of over-the-counter products that contain caffeine, toxicity may result from concomitant consumption of caffeine from several sources. Some authorities recommend that normal, healthy, nonpregnant adults consume no more than 250 milligrams of caffeine daily. Common sources and amounts of caffeine are summarized in Table 15-2.

Theophylline preparations are xanthines used in the treatment of respiratory disorders, such as asthma and bronchitis. In these conditions, the desired effect is bronchodilation and improvement of breathing; CNS stimulation is then an adverse effect (see Chap. 44).

Other Drugs

Atomoxetine (Strattera), a second-line drug for the treatment of ADHD in children and adults, has a low risk of abuse and dependence compared with the other drugs used for ADHD. It acts to inhibit reuptake of norepinephrine in nerve synapses. It is not a controlled drug. Atomoxetine is rapidly absorbed with oral administration, with peak plasma levels in 1 to 2 hours. It is highly protein bound (98%), and elimination half-life is

Table 15-2	Sources of Caffeine		
SOURCE	**AMOUNT (oz)**	**CAFFEINE (mg)**	**COMMENTS**
Coffee			
Brewed, regular	5–8	40–180	Caffeine content varies with product and preparation.
Instant	5–8	30–120	
Espresso	2	120	
Starbucks (regular)	12	58–279	
	16	116–372	
Tea			
Brewed, leaf or bag	8	80	Caffeine content varies with product and preparation.
Instant	8	50	
Iced	12	70	
Soft Drinks			
Coke, Diet Coke	12	45	Most other cola drinks contain 35–45 mg/12 oz.
Pepsi, Diet Pepsi	12	38	
Mountain Dew	12	54	
Energy Drinks			
Amp	8.4	75	Sugar 31 g (6 tsp)
Full throttle	16	141	Sugar 58 g (12 tsp)
Monster	16	140	Sugar 54 g (11 tsp)
Red Bull	8	80	Sugar 39 g (8 tsp)
Rockstar	16	160	Sugar 60 g (12 tsp)
SoBe Adrenaline Rush	8.3	79	Sugar 35 g (7 tsp)
SoBe No Fear	16	66	Sugar 66 g (13 tsp)
Tab Energy	10.5	95	Sugar 0 g
OTC Analgesics			
Anacin, Vanquish	1 tablet or caplet	30	
APAP-Plus, Excedrin, Midol	1 tablet, caplet, or geltab	60–65	
OTC Antisleep Products			
Caffedrine, NoDoz, Vivarin	1 tablet or capsule	200	
OTC Diuretic			
Aqua-Ban	1 tablet	100	PO 2 tablets 3 times daily
Prescription Drugs			
Cafergot	1 tablet	100	Also contains ergotamine. PO 2 tablets at onset of migraine, then 1 tablet every hour if needed, up to 6 tablets per attack or 2 suppositories per attack
	1 rectal suppository	100	
Fiorinal	1 capsule	40	Also contains a barbiturate and is a Schedule III controlled drug. PO 1–2 caplets every 4 hours, up to 6 caplets in 24 hours.

about 5 hours. Atomoxetine is metabolized in the liver by cytochrome P450 enzymes 2D6 and 2C19 and is excreted mainly in urine. Dosage should be reduced by 50% with moderate hepatic insufficiency and by 75% with severe hepatic insufficiency. The drug may be taken with or without food. Common adverse effects include abdominal pain, anorexia, cough, dry mouth, headache, insomnia, nausea, and vomiting.

There is a **BLACK BOX WARNING** that suicidal ideation may occur in children and adolescents.

Modafinil (Provigil) is used to treat narcolepsy and to improve wakefulness in other sleep disorders (e.g., obstructive sleep apnea/hypopnea syndrome, shift work sleep disorder). It is also used to decrease the fatigue associated with multiple sclerosis and other disorders.

Modafinil's ability to promote wakefulness is similar to that of amphetamines and methylphenidate, but its mechanism of action is unknown. Like other CNS stimulants, it has psychoactive effects that alter mood, perception, and thinking. It is a Schedule IV controlled drug. It is rapidly absorbed, reaches peak plasma levels in 2 to 4 hours, is 60% bound to plasma proteins, and is 90% metabolized by the liver to metabolites that are then excreted in urine.

Modafinil is not recommended for patients with a history of left ventricular hypertrophy or ischemic changes on electrocardiograms. Adverse effects include anxiety, chest pain, dizziness, dyspnea, dysrhythmias, headache, nausea, palpitations, and nervousness. Dosage should be reduced by 50% in patients with severe hepatic impairment.

Herbal and Dietary Supplements

Guarana is made from the seeds of a South American shrub. The main active ingredient is caffeine, which is present in greater amounts than in coffee beans or dried tea leaves. Guarana is widely used as a source of caffeine by soft drink manufacturers. It is also used as a flavoring agent and is an ingredient in herbal stimulant and weight-loss products, energy drinks, vitamin supplements, candies, and chewing gums. The product, which may also contain theophylline and theobromine, is also available in teas, extracts, elixirs, capsules, and tablets of vari-

ous strengths. In general, the caffeine content of a guarana product is unknown, and guarana may not be listed as an ingredient. As a result, consumers may not know how much caffeine they are ingesting in products containing guarana.

As with caffeine from other sources, guarana may cause excessive nervousness and insomnia. It is contraindicated during pregnancy and lactation and should be used cautiously, if at all, in people who are sensitive to the effects of caffeine or who have cardiovascular disease. Overall, the use of guarana as a CNS stimulant and weight-loss aid is not recommended and should be discouraged.

Nursing Process

Assessment

- Assess use of stimulant and depressant drugs (prescribed, over-the-counter, or street drugs).

- Assess caffeine intake as a possible cause of anxiety, nervousness, insomnia, or tachycardia, alone or in combination with other CNS stimulants. Heavy users of caffeine may also be taking other psychoactive medications, especially CNS depressants such as antianxiety and sedative-hypnotic drugs.

- Try to identify potentially significant sources of caffeine intake.

Patient Teaching Guidelines   Caffeine

General considerations

- There are numerous sources of caffeine, including coffee, cocoa, tea, most soft drinks, and several OTC medications. In addition, "energy drinks" (e.g., Red Bull, Monster, many others) containing high amounts of caffeine and sugar are popular with teenagers and young adult. They are aggressively marketed to this population for weight loss, increased endurance and wakefulness, decreased fatigue, and legal "highs." Parents may think the drinks will help their children in school; coaches may think the drinks will help athletic performance. There is no evidence for these claims, and the risks of excessive caffeine intake are high. There are increasing visits to hospital emergency rooms and calls to poison centers for teens that become ill from excessive caffeine.

    Some of the drinks also contain B vitamins, which can cause rapid heartbeat, heart palpitations, and numbness and tingling in the hands and feet when taken in large doses, and some are being mixed with alcoholic beverages. Two large companies produce "energy beers," and a drink containing a mixture of Red Bull and vodka has been popular for several years. There is a great potential for traumatic injuries and alcohol poisoning with these products.

    In general, authorities recommend no more than 250 milligrams of caffeine per day for healthy adults and little

to none for people with heart disease. Signs and symptoms of excess caffeine intake (e.g., anxiety, agitation, heart palpitations, insomnia, nausea, nervousness, tremors) usually occur with ingestion of 500 milligrams per day or more.

- Prevent nervousness, anxiety, tremors and insomnia from excessive intake by decreasing consumption of caffeinated beverages or by drinking decaffeinated coffee, tea, and cola. Sprite and 7 UP have no caffeine.

- Parents need to supervise and possibly limit their children's intake of caffeinated beverages, especially energy drinks. If children do consume such products, parents need to discuss with them the consequences of drinking too much.

- Parents and health care providers should caution high school and college students that caffeine, in any form, is not a substitute for adequate rest and sleep. Being tired and sleepy are normal and necessary resting mechanisms for the body.

Self-Administration

- Limit intake of caffeinated beverages and read labels of over-the-counter stay-awake products and multi-ingredient pain reliever products so that you do not develop trouble sleeping as well as brain, heart, and stomach problems from excessive caffeine intake.

- Assess for conditions that are aggravated by CNS stimulants.
- For a child with possible ADHD, assess behavior as specifically and thoroughly as possible.
- For any patient receiving amphetamines or methylphenidate, assess behavior for signs of tolerance and abuse.

Nursing Diagnoses

- Sleep Pattern Disturbance related to hyperactivity, nervousness, insomnia
- Risk for Injury: Adverse drug effects (excessive cardiac and CNS stimulation, drug dependence)
- Deficient Knowledge: Drug effects on children and adults
- Noncompliance: Overuse of drug

Planning/Goals

The patient will

- Take CNS stimulants safely and accurately
- Improve attention span and task performance (children and adults with ADHD) and decrease hyperactivity (children with ADHD)
- Have fewer sleep episodes during normal waking hours (for patients with narcolepsy)

Interventions

- For a child receiving a CNS stimulant, assist parents in scheduling drug administration to increase beneficial effects and help prevent drug dependence and stunted growth. In addition, ask parents to control drug distribution and monitor the number of pills or capsules available and the number prescribed. The goals are to prevent overuse by the child for whom the drug is prescribed and to prevent the child from sharing his medication with other children who wish to take the drug for nonmedical purposes.
- Record weight at least weekly.
- Promote nutrition to avoid excessive weight loss.
- Provide information about the condition for which a stimulant drug is being given and the potential consequences of overusing the drug.

Evaluation

- Ask parents and teachers of children with ADHD to report on behavior and academic performance.
- For adolescents and adults with ADHD, ask the patient or family about the patient's ability to function in work, school, or social environments.
- Assess for decreased inappropriate sleep episodes in patients with narcolepsy.

Principles of Therapy

Goals of Therapy

The main goal of therapy with CNS stimulants is to relieve symptoms of the disorders for which they are given. A secondary goal is to have patients use the drugs appropriately. Stimulants are often misused and abused by people who want to combat fatigue and delay sleep, such as long-distance drivers, students, and athletes. College students reportedly use stimulants as study aids. Use of stimulants for these purposes is not justified. These drugs are dangerous for drivers and those involved in similar activities and have no legitimate use in athletics.

Applying Your Knowledge 15-1

A teacher comes to the health office and tells you that he has observed Kevin selling his methylphenidate (Ritalin) to the school's star soccer player. What advice will you give this teacher and what obligation do you have regarding Kevin's personal health information?

Drug Dosage

When a CNS stimulant is prescribed, it is started with a low dose that is then increased as necessary, usually at weekly intervals, until an effective dose (i.e., decreased symptoms) or the maximum daily dose is reached. In addition, the number of doses that can be obtained with one prescription should be limited. This action reduces the likelihood of drug dependence or diversion (use by people for whom the drug is not prescribed).

Toxicity: Recognition and Management

Overdoses may occur with acute or chronic ingestion of large amounts of a single stimulant, combinations of stimulants, or concurrent ingestion of a stimulant and another drug that slows the metabolism of the stimulant. Signs of toxicity may include severe agitation, cardiac dysrhythmias, combativeness, confusion, delirium, hallucinations, high body temperature, hyperactivity, hypertension, insomnia, irritability, nervousness, panic states, restlessness, tremors, seizures, coma, circulatory collapse, and death.

Treatment is largely symptomatic and supportive. In general, place the patient in a cool room, monitor cardiac function and body temperature, and minimize external stimulation. Activated charcoal (1 g/kg of body weight) may be given. With amphetamines, urinary acidification, IV fluids, and IV diuretics (e.g., furosemide, mannitol) hasten drug excretion. IV diazepam or lorazepam may be given to control agitation, hyperactivity, or seizures, and haloperidol may be given to control symptoms of psychosis. If cardiovascular collapse occurs, fluid replacement and vasopressors may be used. If a long-

Patient Teaching Guidelines | CNS Stimulants for ADHD

General Considerations

■ When diagnosed with ADHD and before taking any medication for it, adult patients and parents of children should inform a health care provider about any other stimulant drugs being taken, involvement in strenuous activities of any kind, any heart disease, or any family history of sudden cardiac death. All ADHD drugs stimulate the heart and blood vessels. The effects are usually a faster heartbeat and increased blood pressure, but cardiac arrest, stroke, or sudden death may occur.

■ These drugs may mask symptoms of fatigue, impair physical coordination, and cause dizziness or drowsiness. Use caution while driving or performing other tasks requiring alertness.

■ Notify a health care provider of nervousness, insomnia, heart palpitations, vomiting, fever, or skin rash. These are adverse drug effects and dosage may need to be reduced.

■ Avoid other stimulants, including caffeine.

■ Record weight at least weekly; report excessive losses.

■ The drugs may cause weight loss; caloric intake (of nutritional foods) may need to be increased, especially in children.

■ Take stimulant drugs only as prescribed. These drugs have a high potential for abuse. The risks of serious health problems and drug dependence are lessened if they are

taken correctly. The likelihood of medical problems is greatly increased when ADHD medication is used improperly or in combination with other drugs.

■ Get adequate rest and sleep. Do not take stimulant drugs to delay fatigue and sleep; these are normal, necessary resting mechanisms for the body.

■ Keep these medications away from children, preferably in a locked cabinet. Parents (or a school nurse) need to dispense each dose and to be sure the drug is taken only by the child for whom it was prescribed.

Self-Administration and Administration to Children

■ Take (or give) regular tablets approximately 30 to 45 minutes before meals.

■ Take (or give) the last dose of the day in the afternoon, before 6 P.M., to avoid interference with sleep.

■ Ritalin SR, Concerta, Metadate CD, and Metadate ER are long-acting forms of methylphenidate. They should be swallowed whole, without crushing or chewing.

■ Use the Daytrana skin patch exactly as prescribed. See the manufacturer's instructions for opening, applying, removing, and disposing of the skin patch.

■ If excessive weight loss, nervousness, or insomnia develops, ask the prescribing physician if the dose can be reduced or taken on a different schedule to relieve these adverse effects.

acting form of the stimulant drug has been ingested, saline cathartics may be useful to remove undissolved drug granules.

With caffeine, ingestion of 15 to 30 milligrams per kilogram of body weight (e.g., 1–2 g for a person weighing 70 kg [150 lb]) may cause myocardial irritability, muscle tremors or spasms, and vomiting. Oral doses of 5 grams or more may cause death. Signs of toxicity are correlated with serum levels of caffeine. Several cups of coffee (or beverages that contain similar amounts of caffeine) may produce levels of 5 to 10 micrograms per liter and symptoms of agitation and tremors. Cardiac dysrhythmias and seizures occur at higher levels. Additional manifestations of caffeine toxicity include opisthotonus, decerebrate posturing, muscle hypertonicity, rhabdomyolysis with subsequent renal failure, pulmonary edema, hyperglycemia, hypokalemia, leukocytosis, ketosis, and metabolic acidosis.

Treatment is symptomatic and supportive, with activated charcoal if indicated. IV diazepam or lorazepam may be used to control seizures. Hemodialysis is indicated if the serum caffeine concentration is more than 100 micrograms per microliter or if life-threatening seizures or cardiac dysrhythmias occur.

Applying Your Knowledge 15-2

Kevin comes to the health office complaining that his heart is racing. He is very agitated and has tremors in his hands. What actions should you initiate?

Effects of Central Nervous System Stimulants on Other Drugs

Caffeine may increase adverse effects of clozapine and theophylline by decreasing their metabolism and increasing their blood levels. It may increase effects of aspirin by increasing aspirin absorption. It may decrease effects of lithium by increasing lithium clearance. **Dexmethylphenidate** and **methylphenidate** may increase effects of phenytoin and antidepressants (selective serotonin reuptake inhibitors and tricyclics), and they may decrease effects of antihypertensive drugs. **Modafinil** may increase effects of citalopram, clomipramine, diazepam, phenytoin, propranolol, sertraline, tricyclic antidepressants, and warfarin. It may decrease effects of cyclosporine and oral contraceptives. **Atomoxetine** may increase the effects of drugs that stimulate cardiovascular function (e.g., increase heart rate and blood pressure).

Use in Special Populations

Use in Children

CNS stimulants are not recommended for ADHD in children younger than 3 years of age. When used, parents need to monitor their children's use of ADHD medications, and dosage must be carefully titrated and monitored to avoid excessive CNS stimulation, anorexia, and insomnia. Suppression of weight and height (e.g., less than the estimated average of 2 inches per year) may occur, and growth should be monitored during drug therapy. In children with psychosis or Tourette's syndrome, CNS stimulants may exacerbate symptoms. In children and adolescents with pre-existing heart disease, usual doses of dextroamphetamine may cause sudden death.

In ADHD, careful documentation of baseline symptoms over approximately 1 month is necessary to establish the diagnosis and evaluate outcomes of treatment. This can be done with videotapes of behavior, observations and ratings by clinicians familiar with ADHD, and by interviewing the child, parents, or caretakers. Some authorities believe that this condition is overdiagnosed and that stimulant drugs are prescribed unnecessarily. Guidelines for treatment of ADHD include the following:

■ Counseling and psychotherapy (e.g., parental counseling, family therapy) are recommended along with drug therapy for effective treatment and realistic expectations of outcomes.

■ Young children may not require treatment until starting school. Then, the goal of drug therapy is to control symptoms, facilitate learning, and promote social development.

■ Drug therapy is indicated when symptoms are moderate to severe; are present for several months; and interfere in social, academic, or behavioral functioning).

■ Methylphenidate is commonly prescribed and usually given daily for the first 3 to 4 weeks of treatment to allow caregivers to assess beneficial and adverse effects. Desirable effects may include improvement in behavior, attention span, and quality and quantity of school work and better relationships with other children and family members. Adverse effects include appetite suppression and weight loss, which may be worse during the first 6 months of therapy.

■ A drug holiday (i.e., stopping drug therapy) is recommended at least annually to evaluate the child's treatment regimen. Dosage adjustments are usually needed as the child grows and hepatic metabolism slows. Also, drug holidays decrease weight loss and growth suppression.

Applying Your Knowledge 15-3

What might be a drug-related reason for Kevin's weight loss? How would you instruct Kevin on the appropriate way to take his medicine?

Use in Older Adults

CNS stimulants should be used cautiously in older adults. As with most other drugs, slowed metabolism and excretion increase the risks of accumulation and toxicity. Older adults are likely to experience anxiety, confusion, insomnia, and nervousness from excessive CNS stimulation. In addition, older adults often have cardiovascular disorders (e.g., angina, dysrhythmias, hypertension) that may be aggravated by the cardiac-stimulating effects of the drugs, including dietary caffeine. In general, reduced doses are safer in older adults.

Nursing Actions — Central Nervous System Stimulants

NURSING ACTIONS	RATIONALE/EXPLANATION
1. Administer accurately	
a. Give the first dose of a CNS stimulant drug early in the day or upon awakening; give the last dose at least 6 hours before bedtime.	To avoid interference with sleep. If insomnia occurs, give the last dose of the day at an earlier time or decrease the dose.
b. For children with attention deficit-hyperactivity disorder (ADHD), give immediate-release forms of amphetamines and methylphenidate about 30–45 minutes before meals.	To minimize the drugs' appetite-suppressing effects and risks of interference with nutrition and growth
c. Do not crush or open and instruct patients not to bite or chew long-acting forms of amphetamine mixture (Adderall XR) or methylphenidate (Concerta, Metadate CD, Metadate ER, Ritalin SR).	Breaking the tablets or capsules destroys the extended-release feature and allows the drug to be absorbed faster. An overdose may result.
d. With transdermal methylphenidate (Daytrana), follow instructions exactly for application, timing, removal, and disposal.	Correct use is required for the most beneficial effects and fewest adverse effects. The skin patch should be removed after 9 hours.
e. Give atomoxetine with or without food.	
2. Observe for therapeutic effects	
a. Fewer "sleep attacks" with narcolepsy	Therapeutic effects depend on the reason for use.
b. Improved behavior and performance of cognitive and psychomotor tasks with ADHD	Effects of most ADHD drugs start within approximately 2 hours after drug administration.
c. Increased mental alertness and decreased fatigue	

(continued on page 266)

Nursing Actions — Central Nervous System Stimulants (continued)

NURSING ACTIONS	RATIONALE/EXPLANATION
3. Observe for adverse effects	Adverse effects may occur with acute or chronic ingestion of any CNS stimulant drugs. These reactions are more likely to occur with large doses.
a. Excessive central nervous system (CNS) stimulation—anxiety, hyperactivity, nervousness, insomnia, tremors, convulsions, psychotic behavior	
b. Cardiovascular effects—tachycardia, other dysrhythmias, hypertension	These reactions are caused by the sympathomimetic effects of the drugs.
c. Gastrointestinal effects—anorexia, gastritis, weight loss, nausea, diarrhea, constipation	
d. With the methylphenidate patch (Daytrana), skin irritation at the site of application	Skin irritation can be minimized by correct application and rotating sites.
4. Observe for drug interactions	
a. Drugs that *increase* the effects of CNS stimulants:	
(1) Other CNS stimulant drugs	Such combinations are potentially dangerous and should be avoided or minimized.
(2) Albuterol and related antiasthmatic drugs, pseudoephedrine	These drugs cause additive CNS- and cardiac-stimulating effects.
b. Drugs that *decrease* effects of CNS stimulants:	
(1) CNS depressants	IV diazepam or lorazepam may be used to decrease agitation, hyperactivity, and seizures occurring with stimulant overdose.
c. Drugs that *increase* effects of amphetamines:	
(1) Alkalinizing agents (e.g., antacids)	Drugs that increase the alkalinity of the gastrointestinal tract increase intestinal absorption of amphetamines, and urinary alkalinizers decrease urinary excretion. Increased absorption and decreased excretion serve to potentiate drug effects.
(2) Monoamine oxidase (MAO) inhibitors	Potentiate amphetamines by slowing drug metabolism. These drugs thereby increase the risks of headache, subarachnoid hemorrhage, and other signs of a hypertensive crisis. The combination may cause death and should be avoided.
d. Drugs that *decrease* effects of amphetamines:	
(1) Acidifying agents	Urinary acidifying agents (e.g., ammonium chloride) increase urinary excretion and lower blood levels of amphetamines. Decreased absorption and increased excretion serve to decrease drug effects.
(2) Antipsychotic agents	Decrease or antagonize the excessive CNS stimulation produced by amphetamines. Chlorpromazine (Thorazine) or haloperidol (Haldol) is sometimes used in treating amphetamine overdose.
e. Drugs that *increase* effects of methylphenidate:	
(1) Chlorpromazine, fluoxetine, miconazole, paroxetine, ritonavir, ropinirole	These drugs inhibit the cytochrome P450 2D6 enzymes that normally metabolize methylphenidate
f. Drugs that *decrease* effects of methylphenidate:	
(1) Carbamazepine	
g. Drugs that *increase* effects of modafinil:	
(1) Clarithromycin, diclofenac, doxycycline, erythromycin, imatinib, itraconazole	These drugs inhibit cytochrome P450 3A4 enzymes that partly metabolize modafinil.
h. Drugs that *decrease* effects of modafinil:	
(1) Carbamazepine, phenytoin, rifampin	These drugs induce cytochrome P450 3A4 enzymes that partly metabolize modafinil.
i. Drugs that increase effects of caffeine:	
(1) Fluvoxamine, mexiletine, theophylline	These drugs inhibit the cytochrome P450 1A2 enzymes that participate in the metabolism of caffeine. Decreased metabolism may increase adverse effects.
(2) Cimetidine, oral contraceptives	May impair caffeine metabolism
j. Drugs that *decrease* effects of caffeine:	
(1) Carbamazepine, phenytoin, rifampin	These drugs induce drug-metabolizing enzymes, thereby decreasing blood levels and increasing clearance of caffeine.

Key Concepts

- ADHD is characterized by hyperactivity, impulsivity, and a short attention span.
- ADHD usually starts in childhood and may persist through adulthood.
- CNS stimulants improve behavior and attention in patients with ADHD.
- Narcolepsy is characterized by daytime drowsiness and unpredictable "sleep attacks."
- Prescribed CNS stimulants are also abused and used for nonmedical purposes.
- All of the CNS stimulants, including caffeine, can cause life-threatening health problems with excessive intake.

Review and Application Exercises

Short Answer Exercises

1. What kinds of behaviors may indicate narcolepsy?
2. What kinds of behaviors may indicate ADHD?
3. What is the rationale for treating narcolepsy and ADHD with CNS stimulants?
4. What are the major adverse effects of CNS stimulants, and how may they be minimized?
5. Do you think children taking CNS stimulants for ADHD should have drug-free periods? Justify your answer.

NCLEX-Style Questions

6. The nurse caring for a child with ADHD knows that when a CNS stimulant is used, the following outcomes may be expected:
   a. increased behavioral problems
   b. improved performance in schoolwork
   c. decreased ability to complete a task
   d. increased hyperactivity

7. The nurse caring for a child who is receiving a CNS stimulant for ADHD knows that it is most important to monitor for which of the following?
   a. abnormal liver function
   b. weight loss
   c. fever
   d. seizure activity

8. Caffeine and other CNS stimulants may cause which of the following adverse effects?
   a. increased appetite
   b. respiratory depression
   c. sedation
   d. cardiac dysrhythmias

Selected References

Belden, H. (2006). ADHD therapy to be applied transdermally. *Drug Topics*, p. 14. (May 22).

Doering, P. L. (2005). Substance-related disorders: Alcohol, nicotine, and caffeine. In J. T. DiPiro, R. L. Talbert, G. C. Yee, G. R. Matzke, B. G. Wells, & L. M. Posey (Eds.), *Pharmacotherapy: A pathophysiologic approach* (6th ed., pp. 1193–1208). New York: McGraw-Hill.

Dopheide, J. A., Theesen, K. A., & Malkin, M. (2005). Childhood disorders. In J. T. DiPiro, R. L. Talbert, G. C. Yee, G. R. Matzke, B. G. Wells, & L. M. Posey (Eds.), *Pharmacotherapy: A pathophysiologic approach* (6th ed., pp. 1133–1145). New York: McGraw-Hill.

Drug facts and comparisons. (Updated monthly). St. Louis, MO: Facts and Comparisons.

Eisendrath, S. J., & Lichtmacher, J. E. (2007). Psychiatric disorders. In S. J. McPhee, M. A. Papadakis, & L. M. Tierney, Jr. (Eds.), *Current medical diagnosis and treatment 2007* (46th ed., pp. 1063–1122). New York: McGraw-Hill.

Lacy, C. F., Armstrong, L. L., Goldman, M. P., & Lance, L.L. (2006). *Lexi-Comp's drug information handbook* (14th ed.). Hudson, OH: Lexi-Comp.

Porth, C. M. (2005). Sleep and sleep disorders. In C. M. Porth (Ed.), *Pathophysiology: Concepts of altered health states*, (7th ed., pp. 268–270). Philadelphia: Lippincott Williams & Wilkins.

Smeltzer, S. C., Bare, B. G., Hinkle, J. L., & Cheever, K. H. (2008). *Brunner & Suddarth's textbook of medical-surgical nursing* (11th ed.). Philadelphia: Lippincott Williams & Wilkins.

Wolraich, M. L., McGuinn, L., & Doffing, M. (2007). Treatment of attention deficit hyperactivity disorder in children and adolescents: Safety considerations. *Drug Safety, 30*, 17–26.

Woodard, R. (2006). The diagnosis and medical treatment of ADHD in children and adolescents in primary care: A practical guide. *Pediatric Nursing, 32*, 363–370.

Drugs Affecting the Autonomic Nervous System

Chapter Outline

Physiology of the Autonomic Nervous System

LEARNING OBJECTIVES

After studying this chapter, you will be able to:

1. Identify physiologic effects of the sympathetic nervous system.
2. Differentiate subtypes and functions of sympathetic nervous system receptors.
3. Identify physiologic effects of the parasympathetic nervous system.
4. Differentiate subtypes and functions of parasympathetic nervous system receptors.
5. Describe signal transduction and the intracellular events that occur when receptors of the autonomic nervous system are stimulated.
6. State names and general characteristics of drugs affecting the autonomic nervous system.

Introduction

The nervous system is composed of two main divisions, the central nervous system (CNS) and the peripheral nervous system (PNS) (Fig. 16-1). The CNS includes the brain and spinal cord. It receives and processes incoming sensory information and responds by sending out signals that initiate or modify body processes.

The PNS includes all the neurons and ganglia found outside the CNS. The PNS includes afferent neurons and efferent neurons. Afferent neurons carry sensory input from the periphery to the CNS and modify motor output through the action of reflex arcs. Efferent neurons carry motor signals from the CNS to the peripheral areas of the body.

The efferent portion of the PNS is further subdivided into the somatic nervous system and the *autonomic nervous system (ANS)*. The somatic nervous system innervates skeletal muscles and controls voluntary movement. The ANS, without conscious thought or effort, controls involuntary activities in smooth muscle, secretory glands, and in the visceral organs of the body such as the heart.

The functions of the ANS can be broadly described as activities designed to maintain a constant internal environment (homeostasis), to respond to stress or emergencies, and to repair body tissues. The ANS is regulated by centers in the CNS, including the hypothalamus, brain stem, and spinal cord. It is subdivided into the sympathetic nervous system and the parasympathetic nervous system.

Structure and Function of the Autonomic Nervous System

Nerve impulses are generated and transmitted to body tissues in the *sympathetic nervous system* and the *parasympathetic nervous system*, as they are in the CNS (see Chap. 5). *Preganglionic* nerve

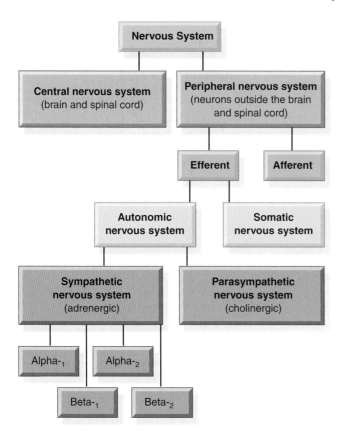

Figure 16-1 ▪ Divisions of the human nervous system.

impulses travel from the CNS along the presynaptic nerves to ganglia. Ganglia are bundles of nerve tissue composed of the terminal end of the presynaptic neuron and clusters of postsynaptic neuron cell bodies. A *neurotransmitter* is released from the terminal end of the presynaptic neuron, allowing the nervous impulse to bridge the synapse between the presynaptic and postsynaptic nerve. The *postganglionic* impulses travel from the ganglia to target or effector tissues of the heart, blood vessels, glands, other visceral organs, and smooth muscle. A neurotransmitter is released from the terminal end of the postsynaptic neuron, allowing the impulse to reach the effector tissue, stimulate a *receptor*, and bring about a response (Fig. 16-2).

The main neurotransmitters of the ANS are acetylcholine and norepinephrine (see Chap. 5). Acetylcholine is synthesized from acetylcoenzyme A and choline. It is released at preganglionic fibers of both the sympathetic nervous system and parasympathetic nervous system and at postganglionic fibers of the parasympathetic nervous system. Acetylcholine is also released from postganglionic sympathetic neurons that innervate the sweat glands and from motor neurons of the somatic nervous system that innervate the skeletal muscles. The nerve fibers that secrete acetylcholine are called cholinergic fibers. Acetylcholine acts on receptors in body organs and tissues to cause parasympathetic effects.

Norepinephrine is synthesized from the amino acid tyrosine by a series of enzymatic conversions that also produce

dopamine and *epinephrine* (i.e., tyrosine → dopamine → norepinephrine → epinephrine). Norepinephrine is the end product of this chemical reaction, except in the adrenal medulla, where most of the norepinephrine is converted to epinephrine. Norepinephrine is released at most postganglionic fibers of the sympathetic nervous system. Nerve fibers secreting norepinephrine are called adrenergic fibers. Norepinephrine acts on receptors in body organs and tissues to cause sympathetic effects.

Neurotransmitters, such as acetylcholine and norepinephrine, as well as medications and hormones that can bind to receptors in the ANS, are collectively called *ligands*. When receptors located on target tissues are stimulated by a ligand, a cascade of intracellular events known as signal transduction is initiated. The ligand that binds the receptor is the *first messenger*. In most cases, this ligand–receptor interaction activates a cell membrane–bound G protein and an effector enzyme, which then activate a molecule inside the cell called a *second messenger*. This second messenger is the link between events that are occurring outside the cell (i.e., receptor activation by the ligand) and resulting events that will occur inside the cell, such as opening ion channels, stimulating other enzymes, and increasing intracellular calcium levels. These intracellular events ultimately produce the physiologic responses to neurotransmitter and hormone release or drug administration. Figure 16-3 illustrates the intracellular events of *signal transduction* that occur when an adrenergic beta receptor is stimulated by epinephrine.

Involuntary organs and tissues in the body are innervated by both divisions of the ANS; however, most organs are predominantly controlled by one system. For example, in the gastrointestinal tract, the parasympathetic nervous system predominates and stimulation of the parasympathetic nervous system regulates the routine activities of digestion and elimination.

The two divisions of the ANS are usually antagonistic in their actions on a particular organ. When the sympathetic system excites a particular organ, the parasympathetic system often inhibits it and vice versa. Stimulation of the ANS causes excitatory effects in some organs but inhibitory effects in others. For example, sympathetic stimulation of the heart causes an increased rate and force of myocardial contraction; parasympathetic stimulation decreases rate and force of contraction, thereby resting the heart. In the gastrointestinal tract, stimulation of the parasympathetic nervous system promotes digestion; sympathetic stimulation decreases blood flow and impairs digestion. Exceptions to this antagonistic action include sweating and regulation of arteriolar blood-vessel diameter, which is controlled by the sympathetic nervous system.

Sympathetic Nervous System

The sympathetic nervous system is stimulated by physical or emotional stress, such as strenuous exercise or work, pain, hemorrhage, intense emotions, and temperature extremes. Increased capacity for vigorous muscle activity in response to a perceived threat, whether real or imaginary, is often called the fight-or-flight reaction. Specific body responses include

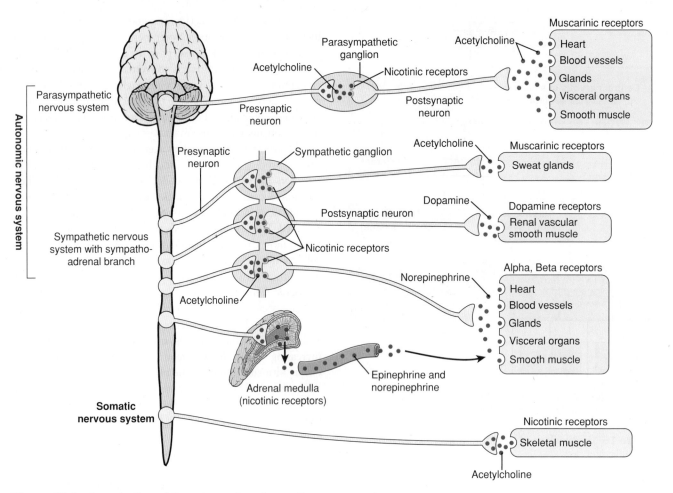

Figure 16-2 ■ Organization of the autonomic and somatic nervous systems.

- Increased arterial blood pressure and cardiac output
- Increased blood flow to the brain, heart, and skeletal muscles; decreased blood flow to viscera, skin, and other organs not needed for fight-or-flight
- Increased rate of cellular metabolism—increased oxygen consumption and carbon dioxide production
- Increased breakdown of muscle glycogen for energy
- Increased blood sugar
- Increased mental activity and ability to think clearly
- Increased muscle strength
- Increased rate of blood coagulation
- Increased rate and depth of respiration
- Pupil dilation to aid vision
- Increased sweating (Note that acetylcholine is the neurotransmitter for this sympathetic response. This is a deviation from the normal postganglionic neurotransmitter, which is norepinephrine.)

These responses are protective mechanisms designed to help the person cope with the stress or get away from it. The intensity and duration of the sympathetic response depends on the amounts of norepinephrine and epinephrine present.

Norepinephrine is synthesized in adrenergic nerve endings and released into the synapse when adrenergic nerve endings are stimulated. It exerts intense but brief effects on presynaptic and postsynaptic adrenergic receptors. The effects of norepinephrine are terminated by reuptake of most of the neurotransmitter back into the nerve endings, where it is packaged into vesicles for reuse as a neurotransmitter. This reuptake and termination process can be inhibited by cocaine and tricyclic antidepressant medications and is responsible for the activation of the sympathetic nervous system seen with these drugs. The remainder of the norepinephrine, which was not taken back into the nerve endings, diffuses into surrounding tissue fluids and blood or it is metabolized by *monoamine oxidase (MAO)* or *catechol-O-methyltransferase (COMT)*.

Norepinephrine also functions as a circulating neurohormone, along with epinephrine. In response to adrenergic nerve stimulation, norepinephrine and epinephrine are secreted into the bloodstream by the adrenal medullae and transported to all body tissues. They are continually present in arterial blood in amounts that vary according to the degree of stress present and the ability of the adrenal medullae to respond to stimuli. The larger proportion of the circulating hormones (approximately 80%) is epinephrine. These catecholamines exert the same effects on target tissues as those caused by direct stimulation of

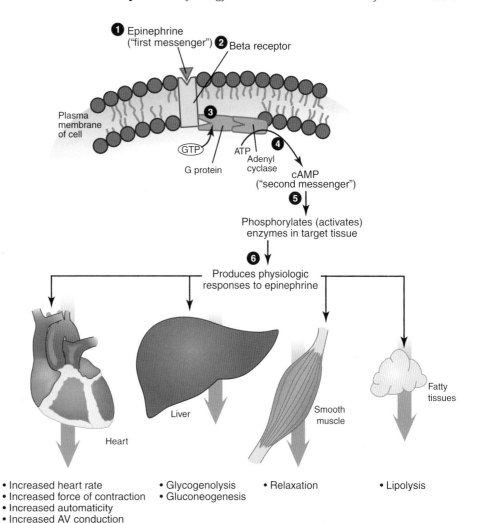

① Epinephrine ("first messenger") ② Beta receptor

Plasma membrane of cell

③ GTP · ATP · Adenyl cyclase

G protein

④ cAMP ("second messenger")

⑤ Phosphorylates (activates) enzymes in target tissue

⑥ Produces physiologic responses to epinephrine

Heart
- Increased heart rate
- Increased force of contraction
- Increased automaticity
- Increased AV conduction

Liver
- Glycogenolysis
- Gluconeogenesis

Smooth muscle
- Relaxation

Fatty tissues
- Lipolysis

Figure 16-3 ■ Signal transduction mechanism for an adrenergic beta receptor. Epinephrine (1), the "first messenger," interacts with a beta receptor (2). This hormone–receptor complex activates a G protein, which reacts with a guanosine triphosphate (GTP) (3). The activated G protein then activates the enzyme adenyl cyclase, which (4) catalyzes the conversion of adenosine triphosphate (ATP) to cyclic adenosine monophosphate (cAMP), the "second messenger." (5) cAMP activates enzymes, which bring about the biologic responses to epinephrine (6).

the sympathetic nervous system. However, the effects last longer because the hormones are removed from the blood more slowly. These hormones are metabolized mainly in the liver by the enzymes MAO and COMT.

Dopamine is also an adrenergic neurotransmitter and catecholamine. In the brain, dopamine is essential for normal function (see Chap. 5). In peripheral tissues, its main effects are on the heart and blood vessels of the renal system and viscera, where it produces vasodilation.

Adrenergic Receptors

When norepinephrine and epinephrine act on body cells that respond to sympathetic nerve or catecholamine stimulation, they interact with two distinct *adrenergic* receptors, alpha and beta. Norepinephrine acts mainly on alpha receptors; epinephrine acts on both alpha and beta receptors. These receptors have been further subdivided into alpha$_1$, alpha$_2$, beta$_1$, and beta$_2$ receptors. A beta$_3$ receptor has been identified, and studies suggest that stimulation of this receptor may augment heat production, produce lipolysis (thermogenesis), and increase energy expenditure. Several compounds are being tested to treat obesity, hyperglycemia, and the problem of insulin resist-

ance in diabetes. Currently, there are no beta$_3$ agonist drugs approved by the Food and Drug Administration for human use.

When dopamine acts on body cells that respond to adrenergic stimulation, it can activate alpha$_1$ and beta$_1$ receptors as well as dopaminergic receptors. Only dopamine can activate dopaminergic receptors. Dopamine receptors are located in the brain, in blood vessels of the kidneys and other viscera, and probably in presynaptic sympathetic nerve terminals. Activation (agonism) of these receptors may result in stimulation or inhibition of cellular function. Like alpha and beta receptors, dopamine receptors are divided into several subtypes (D$_1$ to D$_5$), and specific effects depend on which subtype of receptor is activated. Table 16-1 describes the locations of adrenergic receptors in the body and the response that occurs when each receptor is stimulated.

The intracellular events resulting from signal transduction after stimulation of adrenergic receptors are thought to include the following mechanisms:

■ *Alpha$_1$ receptors:* Activation of alpha$_1$ receptors in smooth muscle cells is thought to open ion channels, allow calcium ions to move into the cell, and produce muscle

Table 16-1	Adrenergic Receptors	
TYPE	**LOCATION**	**EFFECTS OF STIMULATION**
Alpha₁	Blood vessels	Vasoconstriction
	Kidney	Decreased renin secretion
	Intestinal smooth muscle	Relaxation
	Liver	Glycogenolysis, gluconeogenesis
	Genitourinary smooth muscle	Contraction
	Eye (radial muscle)	Blinking, mydriasis
	Pregnant uterus	Uterine contraction
	Male sexual organs	Ejaculation
Alpha₂	Nerve endings	Inhibit release of norepinephrine
	Vascular smooth muscle	Vasoconstriction
	Pancreatic beta cells	Inhibit insulin secretion
	Platelets	Aggregation
Beta₁	Heart	Increased heart rate, force of contraction, automaticity, and rate of atrioventricular conduction
	Kidney	Increased renin release
Beta₂	Bronchioles	Bronchodilation
	Blood vessels	Vasodilation
	Gastrointestinal tract	Decreased motility and tone
	Liver	Glycogenolysis, gluconeogenesis
	Urinary bladder	Relaxed detrusor muscle
	Pregnant uterus	Relaxation
Beta₃	Adipose tissue Gastrointestinal tract	Increased metabolism
Dopamine	Blood vessels of kidney, heart, other viscera	Vasodilation

contraction (e.g., vasoconstriction, gastrointestinal and bladder-sphincter contraction).

■ *Alpha₂ receptors:* In the brain, some of the norepinephrine released into the synaptic cleft between neurons returns to the nerve endings from which it was released and stimulates presynaptic alpha₂ receptors. This negative feedback prevents calcium-mediated release of norepinephrine from storage vesicles into the synapse, resulting in decreased sym-

pathetic outflow and an antiadrenergic effect. Also, cyclic adenosine monophosphate (cAMP) is decreased.

■ *Beta₁, beta₂, and beta₃ receptors:* Activation of these receptors stimulates activity of adenyl cyclase (an enzyme in cell membranes), which stimulates formation of cyclic adenosine monophosphate (cAMP). cAMP serves as a second messenger and can initiate several different intracellular actions, with specific actions depending on the type of cell. cAMP is rapidly degraded by an enzyme called phosphodiesterase to 5' adenosine monophosphate (AMP). Drugs such as theophylline inhibit phosphodiesterase and increase cAMP concentrations, resulting in bronchodilation (see Chap. 44).

■ *Dopaminergic receptors D₁ and D₅:* Activation of these receptors is thought to stimulate the production of cAMP, as does activation of beta₁ and beta₂ receptors.

■ *Dopaminergic receptor D₂:* Activation of this receptor is thought to inhibit formation of cAMP and to alter calcium- and potassium-ion currents. D₃ and D₄ receptors are subgrouped with D₂ receptors, but the effects of their activation have not been clearly delineated.

The number of receptors and the binding activity of receptors to target organs and tissues are dynamic and may be altered. These phenomena are most clearly understood with beta receptors. For example, when chronically exposed to high concentrations of substances that stimulate their function, the beta receptors decrease in number and become less efficient in stimulating adenyl cyclase. The resulting decrease in beta-adrenergic responsiveness is called desensitization or *down-regulation* of receptors. Conversely, when chronically exposed to substances that block their function, the receptors may increase in number and become more efficient in stimulating adenyl cyclase. The resulting increase in beta-adrenergic responsiveness, called hypersensitization or *up-regulation*, may lead to an exaggerated response when the blocking substance is withdrawn.

Parasympathetic Nervous System

Functions stimulated by the parasympathetic nervous system are often described as resting, reparative, or vegetative functions. They include digestion, excretion, cardiac deceleration, anabolism, and near vision.

Approximately 75% of all parasympathetic nerve fibers are in the vagus nerves. These nerves supply the thoracic and abdominal organs; their branches go to the heart, lungs, esophagus, stomach, small intestine, the proximal half of the colon, the liver, gallbladder, pancreas, and the upper portions of the ureters. Other parasympathetic fibers supply pupillary sphincters and circular muscles of the eye; lacrimal, nasal, submaxillary, and parotid glands; descending colon and rectum; lower portions of the ureters and bladder; and genitalia.

Specific body responses to parasympathetic stimulation include

■ Dilation of blood vessels in the skin

■ Decreased heart rate, possibly bradycardia

■ Increased secretion of digestive enzymes and motility of the gastrointestinal tract

■ Constriction of smooth muscle of bronchi

■ Increased secretions from glands in the lungs, stomach, intestines, and skin (sweat glands)

■ Constricted pupils (from contraction of the circular muscle of the iris) and accommodation to near vision (from contraction of the ciliary muscle of the eye)

■ Contraction of smooth muscle in the urinary bladder

■ Contraction of skeletal muscle

■ Release of *nitrous oxide* from the endothelium of blood vessels, resulting in decreased platelet aggregation, decreased inflammation, relaxation of vascular smooth muscle, and dilation of blood vessels

Parasympathetic responses are regulated by acetylcholine, a neurotransmitter in the brain, ANS, and neuromuscular junctions. Acetylcholine is formed in cholinergic nerve endings from choline and acetylcoenzyme A, in a chemical reaction catalyzed by choline acetyltransferase. After its release from the nerve ending, the effect of acetylcholine on receptors of the parasympathetic nervous system is brief and measured in milliseconds. The action of acetylcholine on receptors is terminated due to rapid metabolism by acetylcholinesterase, an enzyme present in the nerve ending and on the surface of the receptor organ. Acetylcholinesterase splits the active acetylcholine into inactive acetate and choline. The choline is taken up again by the presynaptic nerve terminal and reused to form more acetylcholine. Acetylcholine exerts excitatory effects at nerve synapses and neuromuscular junctions and inhibitory effects at some peripheral sites such as the heart.

Cholinergic Receptors

When acetylcholine acts on body cells that respond to parasympathetic nerve stimulation, it interacts with two types of *cholinergic* receptors: *nicotinic* and *muscarinic*. Nicotinic receptors are located in motor nerves and skeletal muscle. When they are activated by acetylcholine, the cell membrane depolarizes and produces muscle contraction. Muscarinic receptors are located in most internal organs, including the cardiovascular, respiratory, gastrointestinal, and genitourinary systems. When muscarinic receptors are activated by acetylcholine, the affected cells may be excited or inhibited in their functions.

Nicotinic and muscarinic receptors have been further subdivided, with two types of nicotinic and five types of muscarinic receptors identified. Although the subtypes of cholinergic receptors have not been as well characterized as those of the adrenergic receptors, the intracellular events resulting from signal transduction after receptor stimulation are thought to include the following mechanisms:

■ *Muscarinic$_1$ receptors:* Muscarinic$_1$ receptors are expressed primarily in the CNS, autonomic ganglia, and the gastric and salivary glands. Activation of these receptors results in a series of processes during which phospholipids in the cell

membrane and inside the cell are broken down. One of the products of phospholipid metabolism is inositol phosphate. Inositol phosphate acts as a second messenger to increase the intracellular concentration of calcium. Calcium also acts as a second messenger and functions to activate several intracellular enzymes, initiate contraction of smooth muscle cells, increase secretions of exocrine glands, increase cognitive function, and decrease dopamine release.

■ *Muscarinic$_2$ receptors:* Receptor activation results in inhibition of adenyl cyclase in the heart, smooth muscle, and brain. As a result, less cAMP is formed to act as a second messenger and stimulate intracellular activity. Receptor stimulation also results in activation of potassium channels in cell membranes of the heart. The overall consequences of M$_2$ activation are inhibition of cardiac function, increased contraction of smooth muscle, and inhibition of neuronal transmission.

■ *Muscarinic$_3$ receptors:* Muscarinic$_3$ receptors are expressed primarily in the CNS, smooth muscle, glands, and heart. Activation apparently causes the same cascade of intracellular processes as with activation of the M$_1$ receptors resulting in decreased dopamine release, increased smooth muscle contraction, and increased glandular secretion. In addition, nitrous oxide is generated from vascular endothelial cells, resulting in dilation of vessels.

■ *Muscarinic$_4$ receptors:* Activation of these receptors in the CNS results in a molecular response similar to M$_2$ receptor activation. Muscarinic$_4$ activation results in inhibition of neurotransmitter release in the CNS and periphery, analgesia, and facilitation of dopamine release.

■ *Muscarinic$_5$ receptors:* Receptor activation results in a molecular response similar to M$_1$ receptor activation. The receptor has been identified in central nervous system tissues (especially the substantia nigra); its activation results in dilation of cerebral arteries and arterioles and facilitation of dopamine release. Muscarinic$_5$ activation also plays a role in augmentation of drug-seeking behavior and reward.

Although five muscarinic receptor subtypes have been identified, currently available drug therapies do not selectively differentiate among the various receptor subtypes.

■ *Nicotinic$_n$ receptors:* These receptors are located on autonomic ganglia and the adrenal medulla. Activation results in enhanced transmission of nerve impulses at all parasympathetic and sympathetic ganglia and release of epinephrine from the adrenal medullae.

■ *Nicotinic$_m$ receptors:* These are located at neuromuscular junctions in skeletal muscle. Their activation causes muscle contraction.

■ *Nicotinic$_{CNS}$ receptors:* These receptors are located on presynaptic nerve fibers in the brain and spinal cord. Their activation promotes the release of acetylcholine in the cerebral cortex.

Nicotinic receptors are composed of five different protein subunits. The protein subunits that make up a nicotinic$_n$ receptor vary from those that make up a nicotinic$_m$ receptor, thus allowing the development of medications that are more selective in their actions. For example, neuromuscular blocking medications such as pancuronium, which act selectively at nicotinic$_m$ receptors, can paralyze skeletal muscles in patients when limiting movement is therapeutic (such as in the ventilated patient or during surgery), without adversely affecting the other functions of the ANS.

Characteristics of Autonomic Drugs

Many drugs are used clinically because of their ability to stimulate or block activity of the sympathetic nervous system or parasympathetic nervous system. Drugs that stimulate activity act like endogenous neurotransmitter substances; drugs that block activity prevent the actions of both endogenous substances and stimulating drugs.

Because ANS receptors are widespread throughout the body, drugs that act on the ANS usually affect the entire body rather than certain organs and tissues. Drug effects depend on which branch of the ANS is involved and whether it is stimulated or inhibited by drug therapy. Thus, knowledge of the physiology of the ANS is required if drug effects are to be understood and predicted. In addition, it is becoming increasingly important to understand receptor activity and the consequences of stimulation or inhibition. More drugs are being developed to stimulate or inhibit particular subtypes of receptors. This is part of the continuing effort to design drugs that act more selectively on particular body tissues and decrease adverse effects on other body tissues. For example, drugs such as terbutaline have been developed to stimulate beta$_2$ receptors in the respiratory tract and produce bronchodilation (a desired effect) with decreased stimulation of beta$_1$ receptors in the heart (an adverse effect).

The terminology used to describe autonomic drugs is often confusing because different terms are used to refer to the same phenomenon. Thus, sympathomimetic, *adrenergic*, and alpha- and beta-adrenergic agonists are used to describe a drug that has the same effects on the human body as stimulation of the sympathetic nervous system. Parasympathomimetic, cholinomimetic, and *cholinergic* are used to describe a drug that has the same effects on the body as stimulation of the parasympathetic nervous system. There are also drugs that oppose or block stimulation of these systems. Sympatholytic, *antiadrenergic*, and alpha- and beta-adrenergic blocking drugs inhibit sympathetic stimulation. Parasympatholytic, *anticholinergic*, and cholinergic blocking drugs inhibit parasympathetic stimulation. This book uses the terms adrenergic, antiadrenergic, cholinergic, and anticholinergic when describing medications.

Key Concepts

- The ANS controls involuntary activities in smooth muscle, secretory glands, and in the visceral organs of the body such as the heart.

- The ANS functions to maintain homeostasis, to respond to stress, and to repair body tissues.

- The ANS is comprised of the sympathetic and parasympathetic nervous system; these two divisions are usually antagonistic in their actions on a particular organ. Exceptions to this antagonism are sweating and regulation of arteriolar diameter, which are controlled by the sympathetic nervous system.

- Release of neurotransmitters allows nerve impulses in the ANS to bridge synapses and travel from presynaptic to postsynaptic nerves, eventually stimulating receptors located on effector organs.

- Stimulation of receptors in the sympathetic nervous system produces adrenergic effects. Blockade of receptors produces antiadrenergic effects.

- Stimulation of receptors in the parasympathetic nervous system produces cholinergic effects. Blockade of receptors produces anticholinergic effects.

- Drugs that activate ANS receptors (function like endogenous neurotransmitters) stimulate the ANS.

- Drugs that block activity of ANS receptors prevent the actions of both endogenous neurotransmitters and ANS agonists.

- Adrenergic receptors include alpha and beta receptors as well as dopamine receptors; there are several subtypes.

- Cholinergic receptors include muscarinic and nicotinic receptors; there are several subtypes.

- The number of receptors in the ANS is dynamic and can be up-regulated or down-regulated as needed.

Review and Application Exercises

Short Answer Exercises

1. What are the major differences between the sympathetic and parasympathetic branches of the ANS?

2. What are the major sympathetic nervous system and parasympathetic nervous system neurotransmitters?

3. What are the locations and functions of sympathetic nervous system receptors?

4. What is meant when drugs are described as adrenergic, sympathomimetic, antiadrenergic, sympatholytic, cholinergic, or anticholinergic?

Selected References

Carroll, E. W., & Curtis, R. L. (2005). Organization and control of neural function. In C. M. Porth (Ed.), *Pathophysiology: Concepts of altered health states* (7th ed., pp. 1149–1157). Philadelphia: Lippincott Williams & Wilkins.

Westfall, T. C., & Westfal, D. P. (2006). Neurotransmission: The autonomic and somatic motor nervous systems. In L. L. Brunton, J. S. Lazo, & K. L. Parker (Eds.), *Goodman & Gilman's the pharmacological basis of therapeutics* (11th ed., pp. 137–180). New York: McGraw-Hill.

Adrenergic Drugs

LEARNING OBJECTIVES

After studying this chapter, you will be able to:

1. Identify effects produced by stimulation of alpha- and beta-adrenergic receptors.
2. List characteristics of adrenergic drugs in terms of effects on body tissues, indications for use, adverse effects, nursing process implications, principles of therapy, and observation of patient responses.
3. Discuss use of epinephrine to treat anaphylactic shock, acute bronchospasm, and cardiac arrest.
4. Identify patients at risk for the adverse effects associated with adrenergic drugs.
5. List commonly used over-the-counter preparations and herbal preparations that contain adrenergic drugs.
6. Discuss principles of therapy and nursing process for using adrenergic drugs in special populations.
7. Describe signs and symptoms of toxicity due to noncatecholamine adrenergic drugs.
8. Discuss treatment of overdose with noncatecholamine adrenergic drugs.
9. Teach the patient about safe, effective use of adrenergic drugs.

Applying Your Knowledge

Alexsey Sobechenko is a 71-year-old man with chronic obstructive pulmonary disease (COPD). He has had asthma for all of his adult life and is admitted to the hospital with acute respiratory distress secondary to pneumonia. He has a very modest pension and is covered by Medicare, which sometimes makes it difficult for him to pay for all of his medical supplies and medication. Although Mr. Sobechenko has never been a smoker, he did work as a welder for 45 years. Due to his acute bronchospasm, his physician orders epinephrine 1:10,000 IV stat.

Introduction

Adrenergic drugs produce effects similar to those produced by stimulation of the sympathetic nervous system and therefore have widespread effects on body tissues (see Chap. 16). Major therapeutic uses and adverse effects of adrenergic medications derive from drug action on the heart, blood vessels, and lungs. Some adrenergic drugs are exogenous formulations of naturally occurring neurotransmitters and hormones, such as norepinephrine, epinephrine, and dopamine. Other adrenergic medications, such as phenylephrine, pseudoephedrine, and isoproterenol, are synthetic chemical relatives of naturally occurring neurotransmitters and hormones.

Specific effects of adrenergic medications depend mainly on the type of *adrenergic receptor* activated by the drug. The drugs discussed in this chapter (epinephrine, ephedrine, pseudoephedrine, isoproterenol, and phenylephrine) affect multiple adrenergic receptors and have many clinical uses. Other adrenergic drugs are more selective for specific adrenergic receptors or are given topically to produce more localized therapeutic effects and fewer systemic adverse effects. These drugs have relatively restricted clinical indications and are discussed more extensively elsewhere ("Drugs Used in Hypotension and Shock," Chap. 51; "Drugs for Asthma and Other Bronchoconstrictive Disorders," Chap. 44; "Nasal Decongestants, Antitussives, and Cold Remedies," Chap. 46; and "Drugs Used in Ophthalmic Conditions," Chap. 63). Table 17-1 groups commonly used adrenergic drugs by adrenergic receptor activity and gives their clinical use.

General Characteristics of Adrenergic Drugs

Mechanisms of Action

Adrenergic drugs have three mechanisms of action. For the most part, adrenergic drugs interact directly with postsynaptic $alpha_1$- or beta-adrenergic receptors on the surface membrane of target organs and tissues (Fig. 17-1). The drug–receptor complex then alters the permeability of the cell membrane to ions or extracellular enzymes. The influx of these molecules stimulates intracellular metabolism and production of other enzymes, structural proteins, energy, and other products required for cell function and reproduction. Epinephrine, isoproterenol, norepinephrine, and phenylephrine are examples of direct-acting adrenergic drugs.

Some adrenergic drugs exert indirect effects on *postsynaptic* adrenergic receptors. Indirect adrenergic effects may be produced by drugs such as amphetamines, which increase the amount of norepinephrine released into the synapse from storage sites in nerve endings (Fig. 17-2A). Norepinephrine then stimulates the alpha and beta receptors, producing sympathetic effects in the body. Inhibition of norepinephrine reuptake from the synapse is another mechanism that produces indirect adrenergic effects. Remember that norepinephrine reuptake is the major way that sympathetic nerve transmission is terminated. Drugs such as tricyclic antidepressants and cocaine block norepinephrine reuptake, resulting in stimulation of alpha- and beta-adrenergic receptors (Fig. 17-2B).

The third mechanism of adrenergic drug action is called mixed acting and is a combination of direct and indirect receptor stimulation. Mixed-acting drugs directly stimulate adrenergic receptors by binding to them and indirectly stimulate adrenergic receptors by increasing the release of norepineph-

Table 17-1	Commonly Used Adrenergic Drugs
GENERIC/TRADE NAME	**MAJOR CLINICAL USES**
Alpha and Beta Activity	
Dopamine	Hypotension and shock
Epinephrine (Adrenalin)	Allergic reactions, cardiac arrest, hypotension and shock, local vasoconstriction, bronchodilation, cardiac stimulation, ophthalmic conditions
Ephedrine	Bronchodilation, cardiac stimulation, nasal decongestion
Pseudoephedrine (Sudafed)	Nasal decongestion
Norepinephrine (Levophed)	Hypotension and shock
Alpha Activity	
Naphazoline hydrochloride (Privine)	Nasal decongestion
Oxymetazoline hydrochloride (Afrin)	Nasal decongestion
Phenylephrine (Neo-Synephrine)	Hypotension and shock, nasal decongestion, ophthalmic conditions
Tetrahydrozoline hydrochloride (Tyzine, Visine)	Nasal decongestion, local vasoconstriction in the eye
Beta Activity	
Albuterol (Proventil)	Bronchodilation
Arformoterol (Brovana)	Bronchodilation
Dobutamine (Dobutrex)	Cardiac stimulation
Formoterol (Foradil)	Bronchodilation
Isoproterenol (Isuprel)	Bronchodilation, cardiac stimulation
Metaproterenol (Alupent)	Bronchodilation
Pirbuterol (Maxair)	Bronchodilation
Salmeterol (Serevent)	Bronchodilation
Terbutaline (Brethine)	Bronchodilation, preterm labor inhibition

rine into synapses. Ephedrine and pseudoephedrine are examples of mixed-acting adrenergic drugs.

Because many body tissues have both alpha and beta receptors, the effect produced by an adrenergic drug depends on the type of receptor activated and the number of affected receptors in a particular body tissue. Some adrenergic drugs are nonselective, acting on both alpha and beta receptors. Other medications are more selective, acting only on certain subtypes of receptors (see Table 17-1).

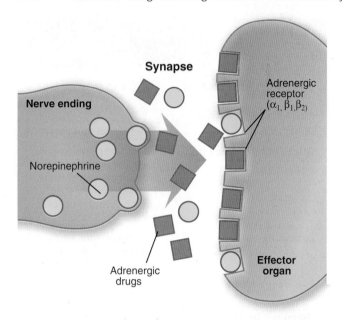

Figure 17-1 ■ Mechanism of direct adrenergic drug action. Adrenergic drugs interact directly with postsynaptic alpha₁ and beta receptors on target effector organs, activating the organ in a similar fashion as the neurotransmitter norepinephrine.

The predominant effect in response to activation of alpha₁ receptors by an adrenergic drug is vasoconstriction of blood vessels, which increases the blood pressure. This is sometimes referred to as a *pressor* (or *vasopressor*) effect. Alpha₁-activated vasoconstriction of blood vessels in nasal mucous membranes decreases nasal congestion, resulting in a *decongestant* effect. Other adrenergic effects resulting from alpha₁ activation include mydriasis, contraction of gastrointestinal (GI) and genitourinary sphincters, and elevated blood glucose.

The predominant effect in response to activation of beta₁ receptors in the heart is cardiac stimulation. Beta₁ activation results in increased force of myocardial contraction, or a positive inotropic effect; increased heart rate, or a positive chronotropic effect; and increased speed of electrical conduction in the heart, or a positive dromotropic effect. Another adrenergic effect resulting from beta₁ activation is increased renin secretion from the kidneys.

The predominant clinical effect in response to activation of beta₂ receptors is bronchodilation. Activation of beta₂ receptors in blood vessels results in vasodilation and increased blood flow to the heart, brain, and skeletal muscles, tissues needed for the "fight-or-flight" sympathetic response. Beta₂ activation also results in hepatic glycogenolysis and gluconeogenesis and decreased pancreatic insulin secretion, resulting in hyperglycemia. Other adrenergic effects resulting from beta₂ activation include relaxation of smooth muscle in the uterus, urinary bladder, and GI tract.

Activation of beta₃-adrenergic receptors produces lipolysis and increased release of free fatty acids into the blood.

It is interesting to note that drugs that activate *alpha₂* receptors on *presynaptic* nerve fibers do not produce a sympathetic effect. These drugs inhibit the release of the *neurotransmitter* norepinephrine into synapses of the sympathetic nervous system, thus exerting an antiadrenergic response in the body. Although activation of presynaptic alpha₂ receptors in the periphery is not of clinical significance, activation of these receptors in the central nervous system (CNS) by medications is useful in treating hypertension (see Chaps. 18 and 52).

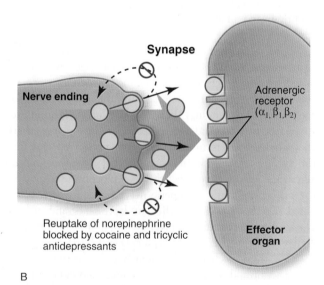

A   B

Figure 17-2 ■ Mechanisms of indirect adrenergic drug action. Stimulation of postsynaptic alpha₁, beta₁, and beta₂ receptors results from adrenergic medications that act indirectly, increasing the release of norepinephrine into the synapse (**A**) or inhibiting the reuptake of norepinephrine from the synapse (**B**).

Indications for Use

Clinical indications for the use of adrenergic drugs stem mainly from their effects on the heart, blood vessels, and bronchi. They are often used as emergency drugs in the treatment of acute cardiovascular, respiratory, and allergic disorders.

In cardiac arrest, Stokes-Adams syndrome (sudden attacks of unconsciousness caused by heart block), and profound bradycardia, they may be used as cardiac stimulants. In hypotension and shock, they may be used to increase blood pressure. In hemorrhagic or hypovolemic shock, the drugs are second-line agents that may be used if adequate fluid volume replacement does not restore sufficient blood pressure and circulation to maintain organ perfusion.

In bronchial asthma and other obstructive pulmonary diseases, the drugs are used as bronchodilators to relieve bronchoconstriction and bronchospasm. In upper respiratory infections, including the common cold and sinusitis, they may be given orally or applied topically to the nasal mucosa to reduce nasal congestion (decongestant effect).

Adrenergic drugs are useful in treating a variety of symptoms of allergic disorders. Severe allergic reactions are characterized by hypotension, bronchoconstriction, and laryngoedema. As vasoconstrictors, the drugs are useful in correcting the hypotension that often accompanies severe allergic reactions. The drug-induced vasoconstriction of blood vessels in mucous membranes produces a decongestant effect to relieve edema in the respiratory tract, skin, and other tissues. As bronchodilators, the drugs also help relieve the bronchospasm of severe allergic reactions. Adrenergic drugs may be used to treat allergic rhinitis, acute hypersensitivity (anaphylactoid reactions to drugs, animal serums, insect stings, and other allergens), serum sickness, urticaria, and angioneurotic edema.

Other clinical uses of adrenergic drugs include relaxation of uterine musculature and inhibition of uterine contractions in preterm labor. They also may be added to local anesthetics for their vasoconstrictive effect, thus preventing unwanted systemic absorption of the anesthetic; prolonging anesthesia; and reducing bleeding. Topical uses include application to skin and mucous membranes for vasoconstriction and hemostatic effects and to the eyes for vasoconstriction and mydriasis.

Contraindications to Use

Contraindications to using adrenergic drugs include cardiac dysrhythmias, angina pectoris, hypertension, hyperthyroidism, and cerebrovascular disease; stimulation of the sympathetic nervous system worsens these conditions. Narrow-angle glaucoma is a contraindication, because the drugs result in mydriasis, closure of the filtration angle of the eye, and increased intraocular pressure. Hypersensitivity to an adrenergic drug or any component is also a contraindication. For example, some adrenergic preparations contain sulfites, to which some people are allergic.

Adrenergic drugs are contraindicated with local anesthesia of distal areas with a single blood supply (e.g., fingers, toes, nose, ears) because of potential tissue damage and sloughing from vasoconstriction. They should not be given during the second stage of labor because they may delay progression. They should be used with caution in patients with anxiety, insomnia, and psychiatric disorders because of their stimulant effects on the CNS and in older adults because of their cardiac- and CNS-stimulating effects.

Individual Drugs

Adrenergic drugs are described in this section. Generic and trade names, routes, and dosages are listed in Table 17-2.

Epinephrine and Other Adrenergic Drugs

P Epinephrine (Adrenalin) is the prototype of the adrenergic drugs. When it is given systemically, the effects may be therapeutic or adverse, depending on the reason for use, dosage, and route of administration. Epinephrine stimulates alpha$_1$ and all beta receptors. At usual doses, beta-adrenergic effects on the heart and vascular and other smooth muscles predominate. However, at high doses, alpha$_1$-adrenergic effects (e.g., vasoconstriction) predominate. Numerous epinephrine solutions are available for various routes of administration (Table 17-3). Solutions vary widely in the amount of drug they contain. They must be used correctly to avoid potentially serious hazards.

The effects and clinical indications for epinephrine are the same as for most adrenergic drugs. Epinephrine is the adrenergic drug of choice for relieving the acute bronchospasm and laryngeal edema of anaphylactic shock, the most serious allergic reaction. It is used in cardiac arrest for its cardiac stimulant and peripheral vasoconstrictive effects. Peripheral vasoconstriction allows shunting of blood to the heart and brain, with increased perfusion pressure in the coronary and cerebral circulations. This action is thought to be the main beneficial effect in cardiac arrest and cardiopulmonary resuscitation (CPR). Epinephrine is also added to local anesthetics for vasoconstrictive effects, which include prolonging the action of the local anesthetic drug, preventing systemic absorption, and minimizing bleeding.

Epinephrine is not given orally, because enzymes in the GI tract and liver destroy it. It may be given by inhalation, injection, or topical application. Epinephrine crosses the placenta but not the blood–brain barrier. When given by injection, it acts rapidly but has a short duration of action. Intravenous (IV) epinephrine acts almost immediately to produce an increase in blood pressure; a positive inotropic and positive chronotropic effect on the myocardium; hyperglycemia; bronchodilation; and vasoconstriction of arterioles in the skin, mucosa, and most viscera. For acute asthma attacks, subcutaneous (Sub-Q) administration usually produces bronchodilation within 5 to 10 minutes; maximal effects may occur within 20 minutes. Parenteral epinephrine should be used with caution in infants and children, because syncope has occurred with use in asthmatic children. Most epinephrine is rapidly metabolized in the liver to inactive metabolites, which are

Table 17-2 Drugs at a Glance: Selected Adrenergic Drugs

| Generic/Trade Name | Use | PREPARATIONS, ROUTES, AND DOSAGE RANGES | |
		Adults	Children
Epinephrine (Adrenalin)	Bronchodilator	**Aqueous epinephrine (1:1000 [1 mg/mL]):** Sub-Q/IM 0.1–0.25 mg q 20 min to 4 h PRN. Max dose 1 mg. **IV injection (1:10,000 [0.1 mg/mL]):** IV 0.1–0.25 mg injected slowly **Epinephrine 1% solution for inhalation (1:100):** Instill no more than 10 drops into nebulizer reservoir. Administer 1–3 inhalations 4–6 times/day. **Metered-dose inhaler (160–250 mcg/ puff):** 1 puff at onset of bronchospasm. Repeat if needed after 1–5 min. Dose is individualized to patients' needs.	**Aqueous epinephrine (1:1000 sol [1 mg/mL]):** Sub-Q/IM 0.01 mg/kg q 20 min to 4 h PRN. Max dose 0.5 mg. **Epinephrine 1% solution for inhalation (1:100):** Instill no more than 10 drops into nebulizer reservoir. Administer 1–3 inhalations 4–6 times/day.
	Profound bradycardia/ hypotension	**Continuous IV infusion:** 2–10 mcg/min	**IV/IO injection (1:10,000 [0.1 mg/mL]):** IV 0.01 mg/kg q 3–5 min PRN
	Cardiac arrest	**Aqueous epinephrine (1:1000 [1 mg/mL]):** IV 0.5 mg diluted to 10 mL with NS Or **IV/IO injection (1:10,000 [0.1 mg/mL]):** IV 0.5–1 mg q 3–5 min PRN **Endotracheally (1:10,000 [0.1 mg/mL]):** ETT 2–2.5 mg q 3–5 min PRN	**IV/IO injection (1:10,000 [0.1 mg/mL]):** IV 0.01 mg/kg q 3–5 min PRN for infants and children (maximum dosage 1 mg). IV 0.03 mg/kg q 3–5 min PRN for neonates (maximum dosage 1 mg). **Endotracheally (1:1000 [1 mg/mL]):** ETT up to 0.1 mg/kg q 3–5 min PRN (maximum dosage 10 mg for infants and children).
	Allergic reaction/ anaphylaxis	**Aqueous epinephrine (1:1000 [1 mg/mL]):** Sub-Q/IM 0.1–0.5 mg q 5–15 min. Max dose 1 mg. **IV injection (1:10,000 [0.1 mg/mL]):** IV 0.1–0.25 mg over 5–10 min q 5–15 min PRN, THEN 1–4 mcg/min continuous infusion if severe anaphylactic shock. **EpiPen Autoinjector:** IM 0.3 mg; may repeat	**Aqueous epinephrine (1:1000 [1 mg/mL]):** Sub-Q/IM 0.01 mg/kg q 20 min–4 h PRN. Max dose 0.5 mg. **IV injection (1:100,000 [0.01 mg/mL]):** IV 0.1 mg over 5–10 min once, THEN 0.1–1.5 mcg/ kg/min continuous infusion **EpiPen Jr. Autoinjector:** IM 0.15 mg; may repeat
	Ophthalmic agent	**Epinephrine HCl 0.1%, 0.5%, 1%, and 2%:** 1–2 drops in eyes once or twice daily	

Generic/Trade Name	Use	PREPARATIONS, ROUTES, AND DOSAGE RANGES	
		Adults	Children
	Nasal agent for hemostasis	**Epinephrine nasal solution 0.1% (1:1000):** 1–2 drops per nostril q 4–6 h	
Ephedrine	Asthma	PO: 12.5–25 mg q4h. Do not exceed 150 mg/24h	6–12 y: PO 6.25–12.5 mg q4–6h. 2–6 y: PO 0.3–0.5 mg/kg q4–6h
	Hypotension	IM, Sub-Q: 25–50 mg IV push: 5–25 mg/dose slowly, repeated q 5–10 min as needed then q3–4h. Do not exceed 150 mg/24h.	
	Nasal congestion	PO: 25–50 mg q4h 0.25% nasal spray or 1% nasal jelly	
Pseudoephedrine (Sudafed)	Nasal congestion	Give 30–60 mg PO q4–6h or 120 mg sustained-release formula q12h. Do not exceed 240 mg/24h.	6–12 y: PO 30 mg q6h. Do not exceed 120 mg/24h. 2–5 y: PO 15 mg q6h. Do not exceed 60 mg/24h.
Isoproterenol (Isuprel)	Cardiac dysrhythmias	IV 20–60 mcg (1–3 mL) bolus initially, followed by IV infusion. Can use 1:50,000 solution for IV bolus undiluted. For IV bolus using 1:5000 solution, dilute 0.2 mg to 10 mL with sodium chloride or 5% dextrose injection and give 1–3 mL. For IV infusion, dilute 2 mg of 1:5000 solution in 500 mL 5% dextrose injection. Dosage depends on type of dysrhythmia and ranges from 2–20 mcg/min. Titrate to patient's response.	
	Shock	IV infusion, Dilute 1 mg of 1:5000 solution in 500 mL 5% dextrose injection. Dosage ranges from 0.5–5 mcg/ min. Titrate to patient's response.	
Phenylephrine (Neo-Synephrine, others)	Hypotension/shock	**IM, Sub-Q:** 2–5 mg q1–2h. Initial dose not to exceed 5 mg. Repeat no more often than every 10–15 min. **IV bolus:** 0.1 – 0.5 mg, diluted in NaCl injection, given slowly q 10–15 min as needed. Initial dose not to exceed 0.5 mg. **IV infusion:** 10 mg in 500 mL D5W or NS. Infuse at 100–180 mcg/min initially. When BP stable, reduce to maintenance rate of 40–60 mcg/min.	
	Nasal congestion	**Nasal decongestants:** 0.25%, 0.5%, 1.0% solutions 2–3 drops or sprays q4h. Therapy should not exceed 3 days.	
	Ophthalmic agent/ mydriatic agent	**Ophthalmic preparations:** 2.5% or 10% solutions. Instill one drop. May be repeated in 10–60 min.	

IO, intraosseous, BP, blood pressure, D5W, dextrose 5% in water; NS, 0.9% sodium chloride.

then excreted in the urine. The remaining epinephrine is deactivated by reuptake at synaptic receptor sites. Epinephrine is excreted in breast milk.

Epinephrine is the active ingredient in many over-the-counter (OTC) inhalation products for asthma (e.g., MicroNe-frin, Primatene Mist, others), producing bronchodilation. Treatment guidelines for asthma recommend use of anti-inflammatory medications (e.g., corticosteroids) and prescription bronchodilators (e.g., beta$_2$-adrenergic agonists) for the optimal treatment of asthma. OTC epinephrine preparations

Table 17-3	Epinephrine Concentrations and Administration Routes

FINAL CONCENTRATION	ROUTE
1% (1:100)	Inhalation
0.5% (1:200)	Subcutaneous
0.1% (1:1000)	Subcutaneous
	Intramuscular
0.01% (1:10,000)	Intravenous
0.001% (1:100,000)	Intradermal (in combination with local anesthetics)

have a short duration of action, which promotes frequent and excessive use. Prolonged use may cause adverse effects and result in the development of tolerance to the therapeutic effects of the drug. There is also concern by some health professionals that reliance on OTC medications may delay the asthmatic patient from seeking medical care. Another area of concern is the ozone-depleting propellants used in OTC inhalation products such as Primatene Mist. At this time, however, these medications have "essential use designation" by the Food and Drug Administration (FDA) because they constitute the only OTC inhalation products available to individuals with asthma. Supporters site that OTC bronchodilators are much less costly than prescription medications and are an affordable "rescue treatment" option for patients who do not have insurance coverage for prescription medications. People who have heart disease or are elderly should not use these products on a regular basis.

Ephedrine is a mixed-acting adrenergic drug that acts by stimulating alpha$_1$ and beta receptors and causing release of norepinephrine from presynaptic terminals. Its actions are less potent but longer lasting than those of epinephrine. Ephedrine produces more CNS stimulation than other adrenergic drugs. It may be used in the treatment of bronchial asthma to prevent bronchospasm, but it is less effective than epinephrine for acute bronchospasm and respiratory distress.

Ephedrine can be given orally or parenterally. When given orally, therapeutic effects occur within 1 hour and last 3 to 5 hours. When given Sub-Q, it acts in approximately 20 minutes, and its effects last approximately 60 minutes. When given intramuscularly, it acts in approximately 10 to 20 minutes, and its effects last less than 60 minutes. Ephedrine is excreted unchanged in the urine. Acidic urine increases the rate of drug elimination.

Ephedrine is a common ingredient in OTC antiasthma tablets (e.g., Bronkaid, Primatene, others). The tablets contain 12.5 to 25 milligrams of ephedrine and 100 to 130 milligrams of theophylline, a xanthine bronchodilator. Other clinical uses include shock associated with spinal or epidural anesthesia, Stokes-Adams syndrome, allergic disorders, nasal congestion, and eye disorders.

The nurse reviews the drug order. Why did the physician order this medication IV instead of PO?

Pseudoephedrine (Sudafed) is a related drug, stimulating alpha$_1$ and beta receptors. It is used as a bronchodilator and nasal decongestant. Pseudoephedrine is given orally and is available OTC alone and as an ingredient in several multi-ingredient sinus, allergy, and cold remedies. Pseudoephedrine is eliminated primarily in the urine. Its elimination may be slowed by alkaline urine, which promotes drug reabsorption in the renal tubules. Pseudoephedrine and ephedrine are ingredients used in making methamphetamine, a highly addictive and illegal drug of abuse. The Combat Methamphetamine Epidemic Act (part of the U.S. Patriot Act) requires drug stores to control OTC access to these drugs by placing these medications behind the counter and documenting each purchase by the customer.

Isoproterenol (Isuprel) is a synthetic catecholamine that acts on beta$_1$- and beta$_2$-adrenergic receptors. Its main actions are to stimulate the heart, dilate blood vessels in skeletal muscle, and relax bronchial smooth muscle. Compared with epinephrine, isoproterenol has similar cardiac stimulant effects, but it does not affect alpha receptors and therefore does not cause vasoconstriction. It is well absorbed when given by injection or as an aerosol. However, absorption is unreliable with sublingual and oral preparations, so their use is not recommended. It is metabolized more slowly than epinephrine by the enzyme catechol-O-methyltransferase (COMT). It is not well metabolized by monoamine oxidase (MAO), which may account for its slightly longer duration of action than epinephrine.

Isoproterenol may be used as a cardiac stimulant in heart block and cardiogenic shock and as a bronchodilator in respiratory conditions characterized by bronchospasm. However, beta$_2$-selective agonists (e.g., albuterol, others) are preferred for bronchodilating effects because they cause less cardiac stimulation. Too-frequent use of inhaled isoproterenol may lead to tolerance and decreased bronchodilating effects.

Phenylephrine (e.g., Neo-Synephrine, others) is a synthetic drug that acts on alpha-adrenergic receptors to produce vasoconstriction. Vasoconstriction decreases cardiac output and renal perfusion and increases peripheral vascular resistance and blood pressure. There is little cardiac stimulation because phenylephrine does not activate beta$_1$ receptors in the heart or beta$_2$ receptors in blood vessels.

Phenylephrine may be given to increase blood pressure in hypotension and shock. Compared with epinephrine, phenylephrine produces longer lasting elevation of blood pressure (20–50 minutes with injection). When given systemically, phenylephrine produces a reflex bradycardia. This effect may be used therapeutically to relieve paroxysmal atrial tachycardia. However, other medications such as calcium channel blockers (see Chaps. 49 and 50) are more likely to be used for this purpose. A **BLACK BOX WARNING** for parenteral use of Neo-Synephrine alerts prescribers to be familiar with complete prescribing information before use. Other uses of phenylephrine include local application for nasal decongestant and mydriatic effects. Phenylephrine is often an ingredient in prescription and nonprescription cold and allergy remedies. However, a recent systematic review and meta-analysis of oral phenylephrine demonstrated that the OTC 10-milligram dose is ineffective for treatment of nasal congestion. The low bioavailability of phenylephrine (38%) may contribute to this lack of efficacy at lower doses. Dosages of 25 milligrams or higher did demonstrate some effectiveness in reducing nasal congestion; however, this dosage exceeds the OTC recommended dose, potentially increasing the incidence of adverse effects. The reviewers recommended that OTC phenylephrine be classified as Category III (data are insufficient to classify as safe and effective, and further testing is required). Phenylephrine is excreted primarily in the urine.

Herbal and Dietary Supplements

Ephedra (ma huang) is an OTC dietary supplement used for weight control, boosting sports performance, and increasing energy levels. Ephedra is a plant source of ephedrine alkaloids, including ephedrine and pseudoephedrine. The OTC use of ephedra has been linked to increased risk of hypertension, heart attack, stroke, and death. The Dietary Supplement Health and Education Act of 1994 grants the FDA the authority to remove a dietary supplement from the market if it "presents a significant or unreasonable risk of illness or injury when used according to its labeling or under ordinary conditions of use." In 2004, using this law, the FDA prohibited the sale of any dietary supplements containing ephedrine alkaloids (i.e., ephedra).

Nursing Process

Assessment

Assess the patient's status in relation to the following conditions.

- **Allergic disorders.** It is standard procedure to question a patient about allergies on initial contact or admission to a health care agency. If the patient reports a previous allergic reaction, try to determine what caused it and what specific symptoms occurred. It may be helpful to ask if swelling, breathing difficulty, or hives (urticaria) occurred. With anaphylactic reactions, severe respiratory distress (from bronchospasm and laryngeal edema) and profound hypotension (from vasodilation) may occur.
- **Asthma.** If the patient is known to have asthma, assess the frequency of attacks, the specific signs and symptoms experienced, the precipitating factors, the actions taken to obtain relief, and the use of bronchodilators or other med-

ications on a long-term basis. With acute bronchospasm, respiratory distress is clearly evidenced by loud, rapid, gasping, wheezing respirations. Acute asthma attacks may be precipitated by exposure to allergens or respiratory infections. When available, check arterial blood gas reports for the adequacy of oxygen–carbon dioxide gas exchange. Hypoxemia ($\downarrow Po_2$), hypercarbia ($\uparrow Pco_2$), and acidosis ($\downarrow pH$) may occur with acute bronchospasm.

- **Chronic obstructive pulmonary disorders.** Emphysema and chronic bronchitis are characterized by bronchoconstriction and dyspnea with exercise or at rest. Check arterial blood gas reports when available. Hypoxemia, hypercarbia, and acidosis are likely with chronic bronchoconstriction. Acute bronchospasm may be superimposed on the chronic bronchoconstrictive disorder, especially with a respiratory infection.
- **Cardiovascular status.** Assess for conditions that are caused or aggravated by adrenergic drugs (e.g., angina, hypertension, tachydysrhythmias).

Nursing Diagnoses

- Impaired Gas Exchange related to bronchoconstriction
- Ineffective Tissue Perfusion related to hypotension and shock or vasoconstriction with drug therapy
- Imbalanced Nutrition: Less than Body Requirements related to anorexia
- Disturbed Sleep Pattern: Insomnia, nervousness
- Noncompliance: Overuse
- Risk for Injury related to cardiac stimulation (dysrhythmias, hypertension)
- Deficient Knowledge: Drug effects and safe usage

Planning/Goals

The patient will

- Receive or self-administer drugs accurately
- Experience relief of symptoms for which adrenergic drugs are given
- Comply with instructions for safe drug use
- Demonstrate knowledge of adverse drug effects to be reported
- Avoid preventable adverse drug effects
- Avoid combinations of adrenergic drugs

Interventions

Use measures to prevent or minimize conditions for which adrenergic drugs are required.

- Decrease exposure to allergens. Allergens include cigarette smoke, foods, drugs, air pollutants, plant pollens, insect venoms, and animal dander. Specific allergens must be determined for each person.

Nursing Process continues on page 286

■ For patients with chronic lung disease, use measures to prevent respiratory infections. These include interventions to aid removal of respiratory secretions, such as adequate hydration, ambulation, deep-breathing and coughing exercises, and chest physiotherapy. Immunizations with pneumococcal pneumonia vaccine and annual influenza vaccine are also strongly recommended.

■ When administering substances known to produce hypersensitivity reactions (penicillin and other antibiotics, allergy extracts, vaccines, local anesthetics), observe the recipient carefully for at least 30 minutes after administration. Have adrenergic and other emergency drugs and equipment readily available in case a reaction occurs.

■ Use noninvasive interventions in addition to adrenergic medications when treating shock and hypotension. These include applying external pressure over a bleeding site to control hemorrhage and placing the patient in a recumbent position to improve venous return and blood pressure.

Provide appropriate teaching for drug therapy (see accompanying patient teaching display).

Evaluation

■ Observe for increased blood pressure and improved tissue perfusion when a drug is given for hypotension and shock or anaphylaxis.

■ Interview and observe for improved breathing and arterial blood gas reports when a drug is given for bronchoconstriction or anaphylaxis.

■ Interview and observe for decreased nasal congestion.

Principles of Therapy

Drug Selection and Administration

The choice of drug, dosage, and route of administration depends largely on the reason for use (see Table 17-1). Adrenergic drugs are given IV only for emergencies, such as cardiac

---

Patient Teaching Guidelines | Adrenergic Drugs

General Considerations

■ Take no other medications without the physician's knowledge and approval. Many over-the-counter (OTC) cold remedies and appetite suppressants contain adrenergic drugs. Use of these along with prescribed adrenergic drugs can result in overdose and serious cardiovascular or central nervous system problems. In addition, adrenergic drugs interact with numerous other drugs to increase or decrease effects; some of these interactions may be life threatening.

■ Herbal preparations of ephedra or ma huang contain derivatives of ephedrine and should not be taken with other adrenergic medications. Excessive central nervous system and cardiovascular stimulation may result. (Sale of supplements containing ephedra was banned by the FDA in 2003.)

■ Tell your health care provider if you are pregnant, breast-feeding, taking any other prescription or OTC drugs, or if you are allergic to sulfite preservatives.

■ Use these drugs only as directed. The potential for abuse is high, especially for the patient with asthma or other chronic lung disease who is seeking relief from labored breathing. Some of these drugs are prescribed for long-term use, but excessive use does not increase therapeutic effects. Instead, it causes tolerance and decreased benefit from usual doses and increases the incidence and severity of adverse reactions.

■ Frequent cardiac monitoring and checks of flow rate, blood pressure, and urine output are necessary if you are receiving intravenous adrenergic drugs to stimulate your heart or raise your blood pressure. These measures increase the safety and benefits of drug therapy rather than indicate the presence of a critical condition. Ask your nurse if you have concerns about your condition.

■ You may feel anxious or tense; have difficulty sleeping; and experience palpitations, blurred vision, headache, tremor, dizziness, and pallor. These are effects of the medication. Use of relaxation techniques to promote rest and decrease muscle tension may be helpful.

■ Use caution when driving or performing activities requiring alertness, dexterity, and good vision.

■ Report adverse reactions such as fast pulse, palpitations, and chest pain so that drug dosage can be re-evaluated and therapy changed if needed.

Self-Administration

■ Do not use topical decongestants longer than 3 to 5 days. Long-term use may be habit forming. Burning on use and rebound congestion after the dose wears off are common. Stop using the medication gradually.

■ Stinging may occur when using ophthalmic preparations. Do not let the tip of the applicator touch your eye or anything else during administration of the medication, to avoid contamination. Do not wear soft contact lenses while using ophthalmic adrenergic drugs; discoloration of the lenses may occur. Report blurred vision, headache, palpitations, and muscle tremors to your health care provider.

■ Follow guidelines for use of your inhaler. Do not increase the dosage or frequency; tolerance may occur. Report chest pain, dizziness, or failure to obtain relief of symptoms. Saliva and sputum may be discolored pink with isoproterenol.

■ Learn to self-administer an injection of epinephrine if you have severe allergies. Always carry your injection kit with you. Seek immediate medical care after self-injection of epinephrine.

■ If you are diabetic, monitor your glucose levels carefully because adrenergic medications may elevate them.

arrest, severe arterial hypotension, circulatory shock, and anaphylactic shock. IV or Sub-Q epinephrine is the drug of choice in anaphylactic shock. No standard doses of individual adrenergic drugs are always effective; the dose must be individualized or titrated to the patient's response. This is especially true in emergencies, but it also applies to long-term use.

 Applying Your Knowledge 17-2

How Can You Avoid This Medication Error?
Epinephrine 1 mg is ordered to be given in a 1:10,000 dilution. You add 1 mL of normal saline and administer the drug.

Treatment of Specific Disorders

Because adrenergic drugs are often used in crises, they must be readily available in all health care settings (e.g., hospitals, long-term care facilities, physicians' offices). All health care personnel should know where emergency drugs are stored.

Anaphylaxis

Anaphylactic shock or *anaphylaxis* is a type I immunoglobulin E-mediated allergic reaction to a foreign substance (*antigen*) that has entered the body. Some typical antigens include foods (e.g., shellfish, peanuts, eggs), medications (e.g., penicillin, vaccinations, enzymes, iodine contrast media), and insect bites/stings (e.g., bees, ants). During an anaphylactic reaction, mast cells release chemical mediators such as histamine, serotonin, platelet-activating factor, prostaglandins, and leukotrienes. The resulting increased capillary permeability and smooth muscle contraction lead to edema, bronchospasm, and airway obstruction. Vasodilation results in hypotension and shock. Anaphylactic reactions occur on second or subsequent exposure to an antigen. Symptoms develop rapidly; typical symptom onset ranges from 30 minutes to 2 hours after exposure to the antigen.

Epinephrine is the drug of choice for the treatment of anaphylaxis (Level A). It relieves bronchospasm, laryngeal edema, and hypotension. In conjunction with its alpha (vasoconstriction) and beta (cardiac stimulation, bronchodilation) effects, epinephrine acts as a physiologic antagonist of histamine and other bronchoconstricting and vasodilating substances released during anaphylactic reactions. People susceptible to severe allergic responses should carry a syringe of epinephrine at all times. EpiPen and EpiPen Jr. are prefilled, autoinjection syringes for intramuscular self-administration of epinephrine in emergency situations (Figure 17-3). The thigh is the preferred site for autoinjection, providing more rapid absorption and higher blood levels of epinephrine that the arm in children and adults for either intramuscular or subcutaneous administration. Victims of anaphylaxis who have been taking beta-adrenergic blocking drugs (e.g., propranolol [Inderal]) do not respond as readily to epinephrine as those not taking beta blockers. Larger doses of epinephrine and large amounts of IV fluids may be required.

Adjunct medications that may be useful in treating severe cases of anaphylaxis include corticosteroids, norepinephrine, and aminophylline. Antihistamines are considered second-line treatment; their usefulness is limited because histamine plays a minor role in causing anaphylaxis compared with leukotrienes and other inflammatory mediators. Antihista-

Figure 17-3 ■ To use the EpiPen Autoinjector, grasp the unit in your fist with the black tip pointing down. When ready to inject, activate the unit by removing the gray activation cap with your other hand. Firmly thrust the device into the outer thigh at a 90-degree angle and hold in place for several seconds. After removing the autoinjector, massage the injection site to enhance absorption. (Note: The injection can be made through clothing.)

mines should never be used alone in the treatment of anaphylaxis. Diphenhydramine is often used as a second-line adjunctive treatment; however, studies show that a combination of ranitidine and diphenhydramine is more efficacious than diphenhydramine alone.

Applying Your Knowledge 17-3

The physician orders piperacillin/tazobactam, a beta-lactam antibiotic, to treat Mr. Sobechenko's pneumonia. Within 15 minutes of the start of the antibiotic infusion, the patient has an anaphylactic reaction. He is agitated and flushed and complains of palpitations. He is having severe difficulty breathing due to bronchospasm. The physician orders epinephrine. What are the nursing implications for Mr. Sobechenko's reaction to the antibiotic, and what assessment is needed relative to the adverse effects of epinephrine?

Cardiopulmonary Resuscitation

Epinephrine is often administered during CPR. The most important action of epinephrine during cardiac arrest is constriction of peripheral blood vessels, which shunts blood to the central circulation and increases blood flow to the heart and brain. This beneficial effect comes at the expense of increased oxygen consumption by the myocardium, ventricular dysrhythmias, and myocardial dysfunction after resuscitation. Epinephrine was once considered the drug of choice in the treatment of all types of cardiac arrest. The most recent Advanced Cardiac Life Support (ACLS) guidelines for health professionals (2005) continue to support epinephrine for first use in pulseless sudden cardiac arrest, classifying it as class indeterminate for the treatment of defibrillation-resistant ventricular tachycardia and ventricular fibrillation during cardiac arrest. Class indeterminate refers to a promising treatment that lacks research evidence of benefit. Vasopressin may also be used as an alternative pressor to epinephrine during sudden pulseless cardiac arrest situations due to ventricular tachycardia or ventricular fibrillation (see Evidence-Based Practice Box 17-1). Epinephrine is still considered the drug of choice for the treatment of cardiac arrest in cases of nonventricular tachycardia/fibrillation such as asystole or pulseless electrical activity. Epinephrine is beneficial in these situations because it stimulates electrical and mechanical activity and produces myocardial contraction.

The specific effects of epinephrine depend largely on the dose and route of administration. The optimal dose in CPR has not been established. ACLS guidelines recommend epinephrine 1 milligram intravenously every 3 to 5 minutes. If this fails, higher doses of epinephrine may be given but are not recommended. Research has shown that high doses of epinephrine may produce significantly higher rates of resuscitation but no improvement on long-term survival or neurologic outcome. In addition, there is growing evidence that higher doses of epinephrine may be harmful to both adults and children.

Evidence-Based Practice

17-1 Epinephrine Versus Vasopressin for Cardiac Arrest

There is ongoing debate and research regarding the pharmacologic approach to cardiac arrest that will produce the highest rate of restoration of spontaneous circulation and the highest neurologically intact survival rates post-resuscitation. Historically, epinephrine has been the drug of choice in cardiac arrest situations; however, the American Heart Association (AHA) guidelines (2000) recommended vasopressin as an alternate pressor, classifying it Class IIb (usefulness of the drug is supported by fair to good research).

In the most recent AHA guidelines (2005), changes were made with regard to the use of epinephrine versus vasopressin for cardiac arrest management. Epinephrine is still the recommended pressor in cardiac arrest due to asystole and pulseless electrical activity. Epinephrine is also recommended in pulseless sudden cardiac arrest due to ventricular tachycardia or ventricular fibrillation (Class IIb recommendation). However, the 2005 AHA guidelines state that one dose of vasopressin may replace either the first or second dose of epinephrine in all cardiac arrest algorithms, including asystole and pulseless electrical activity. Vasopressin has been reclassified in the 2005 AHA guidelines from Class IIb (AHA 2000 guidelines) to class indeterminate (promising treatment that lacks research evidence of benefit).

When used during resuscitation efforts, vasopressin is given as a single dose of 40 units intravenously or intraosseously and onset of action may take up to 20 minutes (see Chap. 22). An advantage of vasopressin over epinephrine is the ability of vasopressin to increase coronary blood flow and the availability of oxygen to the myocardium during resuscitation efforts.

Both epinephrine and vasopressin have been shown to positively influence restoration of spontaneous circulation; however, no vasopressor has been shown to improve the rate of survival to discharge with an intact neurologic status after cardiac arrest. Further research is needed to determine the most effective treatment for cardiac arrest. It is imperative that nurses in critical care areas maintain current Advanced Cardiac Life Support (ACLS) certification and stay alert to research findings that may influence ACLS protocols for resuscitation in the future.

Hypotension and Shock

In hypotension and shock, initial efforts involve identifying and treating the cause when possible. Such treatments include placing the patient in the recumbent position, blood transfusions, fluid and electrolyte replacement, treatment of infection, and use of positive inotropic drugs and other medications to treat heart failure. If these measures are ineffective in raising the blood pressure enough to maintain perfusion to vital organs such as the brain, kidneys, and heart, vasopressor drugs may be used. The usual goal of vasopressor drug therapy is to maintain tissue perfusion and a mean arterial pressure of at least 80 to 100 mm Hg.

Nasal Congestion

Adrenergic drugs are given topically and systemically to constrict blood vessels in nasal mucosa and decrease the nasal congestion associated with the common cold, allergic rhinitis, and sinusitis. Topical agents are effective, undergo little systemic absorption, are available OTC, and are widely used. However, overuse leads to decreased effectiveness (tolerance), irritation and ischemic changes in the nasal mucosa, and rebound congestion. These effects can be minimized by using small doses only when necessary and for no longer than 3 to 5 days.

Oral drugs have a slower onset of action than topical ones but may last longer. They also may cause more adverse effects, which may occur with usual therapeutic doses and are especially likely with high doses. The most problematic adverse effects are cardiac and CNS stimulation; the risks for hypertension and cerebral hemorrhage are greater in hypertensive people. Commonly used oral agents are pseudoephedrine and ephedrine.

Toxicity of Adrenergics: Recognition and Management

Unlike catecholamines, which are quickly cleared from the body, excessive use of noncatecholamine adrenergic drugs (phenylephrine, ephedrine, and pseudoephedrine) can lead to overdose and toxicity. These drugs are an ingredient in OTC products such as nasal decongestants, cold preparations, and appetite suppressants. Phenylephrine and ephedrine have a narrow therapeutic index; toxic doses are only two to three times greater than the therapeutic dose. Pseudoephedrine toxicity occurs with doses four to five times greater than the normal therapeutic dose. Ephedrine and ephedra-containing herbal preparations (e.g., ma huang, herbal ecstasy) are often abused as an alternative to amphetamines. These substances were banned in the United States in 2003.

The primary clinical manifestation of noncatecholamine adrenergic drug toxicity is severe hypertension, which may lead to headache, confusion, seizures, and intracranial hemorrhage. Reflex bradycardia and atrioventricular block also have been associated with phenylephrine toxicity.

Treatment involves maintaining an airway and assisting with ventilation if needed. Activated charcoal may be administered early in treatment. Hypertension is aggressively treated with vasodilators such as phentolamine or nitroprusside. Beta blockers are not used alone to treat hypertension without first administering a vasodilator, to avoid a paradoxical increase in blood pressure. Dialysis and hemoperfusion are not effective in clearing these drugs from the body. Urinary acidification may enhance elimination of ephedrine and pseudoephedrine; however, this technique is not routinely used because of the risk of renal damage from myoglobin deposition in the kidney.

Use in Special Populations

Use in Children

Adrenergic agents are used to treat asthma, hypotension, shock, cardiac arrest, and anaphylaxis in children. However, guidelines for safe and effective use of adrenergic drugs in children are not well established. Children are very sensitive to drug effects, including cardiac and CNS stimulation, and recommended doses usually should not be exceeded.

Epinephrine is mainly used in children for treatment of bronchospasm due to asthma or allergic reactions. Parenteral epinephrine may cause syncope when given to asthmatic children. Isoproterenol is rarely given parenterally to children, but

if it is, the first dose should be approximately half the adult dose, and later doses should be based on the response to the first dose. There is little reason to use the inhalation route, because in children, as in adults, selective beta$_2$ agonists such as albuterol are preferred for bronchodilation in asthma.

Phenylephrine is most often used to relieve congestion of the upper respiratory tract and may be given topically, as nose drops. Doses must be carefully measured. Rebound nasal congestion occurs with overuse.

Use in Older Adults

Adrenergic agents are used to treat asthma, hypotension, shock, cardiac arrest, and anaphylaxis in older adults. These drugs stimulate the heart to increase rate and force of contraction and blood pressure. Because older adults often have chronic cardiovascular conditions (e.g., angina, dysrhythmias, congestive heart failure, coronary artery disease, hypertension, peripheral vascular disease) that are aggravated by adrenergic drugs, careful monitoring by the nurse is required.

Adrenergic drugs are often prescribed as bronchodilators and decongestants in older adults. Therapeutic doses increase the workload of the heart and may cause symptoms of impaired cardiovascular function. Overdoses may cause severe cardiovascular dysfunction, including life-threatening dysrhythmias. The drugs also cause CNS stimulation. With therapeutic doses, anxiety, restlessness, nervousness, and insomnia often occur in older adults. Overdoses may cause hallucinations, convulsions, CNS depression, and death.

Adrenergics are ingredients in OTC asthma remedies, cold remedies, nasal decongestants, and appetite suppressants. Cautious use of these preparations is required in older adults. The drugs should not be taken concurrently with prescription adrenergic drugs because of the high risk of overdose and toxicity.

Ophthalmic preparations of adrenergic drugs also should be used cautiously. For example, phenylephrine is used as a vasoconstrictor and mydriatic. Applying larger-than-recommended doses to the normal eye or usual doses to the traumatized, inflamed, or diseased eye may result in sufficient systemic absorption of the drug to cause increased blood pressure and other adverse effects.

Use in Patients With Renal Impairment

Adrenergic drugs exert effects on the renal system that may cause problems for patients with renal impairment. For example, adrenergic drugs with alpha$_1$ activity cause constriction of renal arteries, thereby diminishing renal blood flow and urine production. These drugs also constrict urinary sphincters, causing urinary retention and painful urination, especially in men with prostatic hyperplasia.

Many adrenergic drugs and their metabolites are eliminated by the renal system. In the presence of renal disease, these compounds may accumulate and cause increased adverse effects.

Use in Patients With Hepatic Impairment

The liver is rich in the enzymes MAO and COMT, which are responsible for metabolism of circulating epinephrine and other adrenergic drugs (e.g., norepinephrine, dopamine, isoproterenol). However, other tissues in the body also possess these enzymes and are capable of metabolizing natural and synthetic catecholamines. Any unchanged drug can be excreted in the urine. Many noncatecholamine adrenergic drugs are excreted largely unchanged in the urine. Therefore, liver disease is not usually considered a contraindication to administering adrenergic drugs.

Use in Patients With Critical Illness

Adrenergic drugs are important emergency drugs. They are essential for treating hypotension, shock, asystole and other dysrhythmias, acute bronchospasm, and anaphylaxis. Although they may save the life of a critically ill patient, use of adrenergic drugs may result in secondary health problems that require monitoring and intervention. These health problems include

- Potential for the vasopressor action of adrenergic drugs to result in diminished renal perfusion and decreased urine output
- Potential for adrenergic drugs with $beta_1$ activity to induce irritable cardiac dysrhythmias
- Potential for adrenergic drugs with $beta_1$ activity to increase myocardial oxygen requirement
- Potential for adrenergic drugs with vasopressor action to decrease perfusion to the liver, with subsequent liver damage
- Hyperglycemia, hypokalemia, and hypophosphatemia due to $beta_1$-adrenergic effects
- Severe hypertension and reflex bradycardia
- Tissue necrosis after extravasation
- Limb ischemia due to profound vasoconstriction

Nursing Actions   Adrenergic Drugs

NURSING ACTIONS	RATIONALE/EXPLANATION
1. Administer accurately	
a. Check package inserts or other references if not absolutely sure about the preparation, concentration, or method of administration for an adrenergic drug.	The many different preparations and concentrations available for various routes of administration increase the risk of medication error unless extreme caution is used. Preparations for intravenous (IV), subcutaneous, inhalation, ophthalmic, or nasal routes must be used by the designated route only.
b. To give epinephrine subcutaneously, use a tuberculin syringe, aspirate, and massage the injection site.	The tuberculin syringe is necessary for accurate measurement of the small doses usually given (often less than 0.5 mL). Aspiration is necessary to avoid inadvertent IV administration of the larger, undiluted amount of drug intended for subcutaneous use. Massaging the injection site accelerates drug absorption and thus relief of symptoms.
c. For inhalation, be sure to use the correct drug concentration, and use the nebulizing device properly.	Inhalation medications are often administered by patients themselves or by respiratory therapists if intermittent positive-pressure breathing is used. The nurse may need to demonstrate and supervise self-administration initially.
d. Do not give epinephrine and isoproterenol at the same time or within 4 hours of each other.	Both of these drugs are potent cardiac stimulants, and the combination could cause serious cardiac dysrhythmias. However, they have synergistic bronchodilating effects, and doses can be alternated and given safely if the drugs are given no more closely together than 4 hours.
e. Follow package insert guidelines carefully when diluting epinephrine for IV injection or IV infusion. Administer in an intensive care unit, when possible, using an infusion pump and a central IV line. Use parenteral solutions of epinephrine only if clear. Epinephrine is unstable in alkaline solutions.	Dilution increases safety of administration. A solution that is brown or contains a precipitate should not be used. Discoloration indicates chemical deterioration of epinephrine. Do not administer at the same time that sodium bicarbonate is being administered.
f. For IV infusion of isoproterenol and phenylephrine: (1) Administer in an intensive care unit when possible.	These drugs are given IV in emergencies, during which the patient's condition must be carefully monitored. Frequent recording of blood pressure and pulse and continuous electrocardiographic monitoring are needed.
(2) Use only clear drug solutions.	A brownish color or precipitate indicates deterioration, and such solutions should not be used.
(3) Dilute isoproterenol in 5% dextrose injection. Phenylephrine can be diluted in 5% dextrose injection or 0.9% sodium chloride solution. Do not add the drug until ready to use.	Mixing solutions when ready for use helps to ensure drug stability. Note that drug concentration varies with the amount of drug and the amount of IV solution to which it is added.

NURSING ACTIONS	RATIONALE/EXPLANATION
(4) Use an infusion device to regulate flow rate accurately.	Flow rate usually requires frequent adjustment according to blood pressure measurements. An infusion device helps to regulate drug administration, so wide fluctuations in blood pressure are avoided.
(5) Use a "piggyback" IV apparatus.	Only one bottle contains an adrenergic drug, and it can be regulated or discontinued without disruption of the primary IV line.
(6) Start the adrenergic drug solution slowly and increase flow rate according to the patient's response (e.g., blood pressure, color, mental status). Slow or discontinue the solution gradually as well.	To avoid abrupt changes in circulation and blood pressure
g. When giving adrenergic drugs as eye drops or nose drops, do not touch the dropper to the eye or nose.	Contaminated droppers can be a source of bacterial infection.
2. Observe for therapeutic effects	These depend on the reason for use.
a. When the drug is used as a bronchodilator, observe for absence or reduction of wheezing, less labored breathing, and decreased rate of respirations.	Indicates prevention or relief of bronchospasm. Acute bronchospasm is usually relieved within 5 minutes by injected or inhaled epinephrine or inhaled isoproterenol.
b. When epinephrine is given in anaphylactic shock, observe for decreased tissue edema and improved breathing and circulation.	Epinephrine injection usually relieves laryngeal edema and bronchospasm within 5 minutes and lasts for approximately 20 minutes.
c. When isoproterenol or phenylephrine is given in hypotension and shock, observe for increased blood pressure, stronger pulse, and improved urine output, level of consciousness, and color.	These are indicators of improved circulation.
d. When a drug is given nasally for decongestant effects, observe for decreased nasal congestion and ability to breathe through the nose.	The drugs act as vasoconstrictors to reduce engorgement of nasal mucosa.
e. When given as eye drops for vasoconstrictor effects, observe for decreased redness. When giving for mydriatic effects, observe for pupil dilation.	
3. Observe for adverse effects	Adverse effects depend to some extent on the reason for use. For example, cardiovascular effects are considered adverse reactions when the drugs are given for bronchodilation. Adverse effects occur with usual therapeutic doses and are more likely to occur with higher doses.
a. Cardiovascular effects—cardiac dysrhythmias, hypertension	Tachycardia and hypertension are common; if severe or prolonged, myocardial ischemia or heart failure may occur. Premature ventricular contractions and other serious dysrhythmias may occur. Propranolol (Inderal) or another beta blocker may be given to decrease heart rate and hypertension resulting from overdosage of adrenergic drugs. Phentolamine may be used to decrease severe hypertension.
b. Excessive central nervous system (CNS) stimulation— nervousness, anxiety, tremor, insomnia	These effects are more likely to occur with ephedrine or high doses of other adrenergic drugs. Sometimes, a sedative-type drug is given concomitantly to offset these effects.
c. Rebound nasal congestion, rhinitis, possible ulceration of nasal mucosa	These effects occur with excessive use of nasal decongestant drugs.
4. Observe for drug interactions	
a. Drugs that *increase* effects of adrenergic drugs:	Most of these drugs increase incidence or severity of adverse reactions.
(1) Anesthetics, general (e.g., halothane)	Increased risk of cardiac dysrhythmias. Potentially hazardous.
(2) Anticholinergics (e.g., atropine)	Increased bronchial relaxation. Also increased mydriasis and therefore contraindicated with narrow-angle glaucoma.
(3) Antidepressants, tricyclic (e.g., amitriptyline [Elavil])	Increased pressor response with IV epinephrine
(4) Antihistamines	May increase pressor effects
(5) Cocaine	Increases pressor and mydriatic effects by inhibiting uptake of norepinephrine by nerve endings. Cardiac dysrhythmias, convulsions, and acute glaucoma may occur.
(6) Digoxin	Sympathomimetics, especially beta-adrenergics like epinephrine and isoproterenol, increase the likelihood of cardiac dysrhythmias due to ectopic pacemaker activity.

(continued on page 292)

Nursing Actions   Adrenergic Drugs (continued)

NURSING ACTIONS	RATIONALE/EXPLANATION
(7) Doxapram (Dopram)	Increased pressor effect
(8) Ergot alkaloids	Increased vasoconstriction. Extremely high blood pressure may occur. There also may be decreased perfusion of fingers and toes.
(9) Monoamine oxidase (MAO) inhibitors (e.g., isocarboxazid [Marplan])	**CONTRAINDICATED. THE COMBINATION MAY CAUSE DEATH.** When these drugs are given concurrently with adrenergic drugs, there is danger of cardiac dysrhythmias, respiratory depression, and acute hypertensive crisis with possible intracranial hemorrhage, convulsions, coma, and death. Effects of a MAO inhibitor may not occur for several weeks after treatment is started and may last up to 3 weeks after the drug is stopped. Every patient taking a MAO inhibitor should be warned against taking any other medication without the advice of a physician or pharmacist.
(10) Methylphenidate (Ritalin)	Increased pressor and mydriatic effects. The combination may be hazardous in glaucoma.
(11) Thyroid preparations (e.g., Synthroid)	Increased adrenergic effects, resulting in increased likelihood of dysrhythmias
(12) Xanthines (in caffeine-containing substances, such as coffee, tea, cola drinks; theophylline)	Synergistic bronchodilating effect. Sympathomimetics with CNS-stimulating properties (e.g., ephedrine, isoproterenol) may produce excessive CNS stimulation with cardiac dysrhythmias, emotional disturbances, and insomnia.
(13) Beta-adrenergic blocking agents (e.g., propranolol [Inderal])	May augment hypertensive response to epinephrine (see also b[4] below)
b. Drugs that *decrease* effects of adrenergics drugs:	
(1) Anticholinesterases (e.g., neostigmine [Prostigmin], pyridostigmine [Mestinon]) and other cholinergic drugs	Decrease mydriatic effects of adrenergics; thus, the two groups should not be given concurrently in ophthalmic conditions.
(2) Antihypertensives (e.g., methyldopa)	Generally antagonize pressor effects of adrenergics, which act to increase blood pressure while antihypertensives act to lower it.
(3) Antipsychotic drugs (e.g., haloperidol [Haldol])	Block the vasopressor action of epinephrine. Therefore, epinephrine should not be used to treat hypotension induced by these drugs.
(4) Beta-adrenergic blocking agents (e.g., propranolol [Inderal])	Decrease bronchodilating effects of adrenergics and may exacerbate asthma. Contraindicated with asthma.
(5) Phentolamine	Antagonizes vasopressor effects of adrenergics

Occurrence of any of these adverse effects may complicate the already complex care of critically ill patients. Careful assessment and prompt nursing intervention are essential.

Use in Home Care

Adrenergic drugs are often used in the home setting. Frequently prescribed drugs include bronchodilators and nasal decongestants. OTC drugs with the same effects are also commonly used to treat asthma, allergic rhinitis, cold symptoms, and appetite suppression for weight control. A major function of the home care nurse is to teach patients to use the drugs correctly (especially metered-dose inhalers), to report excessive CNS or cardiac stimulation to a health care provider, and to not take OTC drugs or herbal preparations with the same or similar ingredients as prescription drugs.

Excessive adverse effects are probably most likely to occur in children and older adults. Older adults often have other illnesses that may be aggravated by adrenergic drugs or they may take other drugs whose effects may be altered by concomitant use of adrenergics.

Key Concepts

■ Adrenergic drugs produce effects similar to those produced by stimulation of the sympathetic nervous system.

■ Specific effects of adrenergic medications depend mainly on the type of adrenergic receptor activated by the drug.

■ Adrenergic drugs have three mechanisms of action: direct interaction with adrenergic receptors, indirect stimulation of adrenergic receptors by the neurotransmitter norepinephrine, or mixed acting, which is a combination of direct and indirect receptor stimulation.

- Because many body tissues have both alpha and beta receptors, the effect produced by an adrenergic drug depends on the type of receptor activated and the number of affected receptors in a particular body tissue.

- The *predominant* effect in response to activation of alpha₁ receptors by an adrenergic drug is vasoconstriction of blood vessels, increasing blood pressure. This is called a vasopressor or pressor effect.

- The *predominant* effect in response to activation of beta₁ receptors by an adrenergic drug is cardiac stimulation.

- The *predominant* effect in response to activation of beta₂ receptors is bronchodilation.

- The *predominant* effect in response to activation of beta₃ receptors is lipolysis and increased release of free fatty acids into the blood.

- Drugs that stimulate presynaptic alpha₂ receptors inhibit the release of norepinephrine into SNS synapses, thus exerting an *antiadrenergic response* in the body. Drugs that stimulate presynaptic alpha₂ receptors in the central nervous system are useful in treating hypertension.

- Adrenergic drugs are used as cardiac stimulants, vasopressors, bronchodilators, nasal decongestants, uterine relaxants, adjuncts to local anesthetics, and for hemostatic (topical) and mydriatic effects (topical).

- Epinephrine is the drug of choice to treat anaphylaxis.

- Individuals susceptible to severe allergic reactions should carry epinephrine in the form of an autoinjector such as EpiPen or EpiPen Jr for self-administration in emergency situations. Allergic individuals should also wear a medic alert tag or carry documentation of severe allergies.

- Use of beta-adrenergic blocking drugs (e.g., propanolol and others) may decrease the effectiveness of epinephrine in cases of anaphylaxis. Higher doses of epinephrine and use of intravenous fluids may be required to maintain a patent airway and restore blood pressure.

- Epinephrine is recommended as a vasopressor in cardiac arrest situations; however, current ACLS guidelines state vasopressin may replace either the first or second dose of epinephrine in all cardiac arrest algorithms. A benefit of epinephrine in arrest situations due to asystole or pulseless electrical activity is the added ability to stimulate electrical and mechanical activity and produce myocardial contraction.

- Contraindications to adrenergic drugs include cardiac dysrhythmias, angina, hypertension, hyperthyroidism, cerebrovascular disease, narrow-angle glaucoma, and hypersensitivity to sulfites. Local anesthetics containing adrenergics should not be used in any area of the body with a single blood supply (e.g., fingers, toes, nose, and ears).

- Epinephrine stimulates alpha₁ and beta receptors.

- Ephedrine stimulates alpha₁ and beta receptors

- Pseudoephedrine stimulates alpha₁ and beta receptors.

- Isoproterenol stimulates beta₁ and beta₂ receptors.

- Phenylephrine stimulates alpha₁ receptors.

- Dietary supplements containing ephedrine alkaloids (ephedra) are prohibited in the United States.

Review and Application Exercises

Short Answer Exercises

1. How do adrenergic drugs act to relieve symptoms of acute bronchospasm, anaphylaxis, cardiac arrest, hypotension and shock, and nasal congestion?

2. Which adrenergic receptors are stimulated by administration of epinephrine?

3. Why is it important to have epinephrine and other adrenergic drugs readily available in all health care settings?

4. Which adrenergic drug is the drug of choice to treat acute anaphylactic reactions?

5. Why is inhaled epinephrine not a drug of choice for long-term treatment of asthma and other bronchoconstrictive disorders?

6. What are the major adverse effects of adrenergic drugs?

7. Why are patients with cardiac dysrhythmias, angina pectoris, hypertension, or diabetes mellitus especially likely to experience adverse reactions to adrenergic drugs?

8. For a patient who reports frequent use of OTC asthma remedies and cold remedies, what teaching is needed to increase patient safety?

9. Mentally rehearse nursing interventions for various emergency situations (anaphylaxis, acute respiratory distress, cardiac arrest) in terms of medications and equipment needed and how to obtain them promptly.

10. What signs and symptoms occur with overdose of noncatecholamine adrenergic drugs? What interventions are needed to treat the toxicity?

NCLEX-Style Questions

11. You are caring for a patient with nasal congestion. His medical history includes depression. Which of the following medications would contraindicate the use of pseudoephedrine (Sudafed) to treat his nasal congestion?
    a. fluoxetine (Prozac)
    b. amitriptyline (Elavil)
    c. isocarboxazid (Marplan)
    d. lithium (Lithotab)

12. When giving a drug with beta₂ agonist activity, you know that the main therapeutic benefit is
    a. vasoconstriction and elevation of the blood pressure
    b. relaxation of bronchial smooth muscle and bronchodilation
    c. elevated heart rate and improved force of myocardial contraction
    d. uterine contraction and induction of labor

13. A patient with asthma tells the nurse he is using his metered-dose inhaler of epinephrine more frequently than prescribed to control wheezing. The nurse is concerned because this behavior may result in
    a. drug tolerance
    b. heart failure
    c. drug toxicity
    d. diabetes mellitus

14. The nurse teaches the diabetic patient using adrenergic medications to anticipate
    a. no change in blood glucose levels
    b. a decrease in blood glucose levels
    c. an increase in blood glucose levels
    d. more fluctuation in blood glucose levels

15. When the nurse responds to hypotension due to hypovolemic shock, which of the following should be administered first?
    a. epinephrine (Adrenalin)
    b. isoproterenol (Isuprel)
    c. normal saline IV
    d. ephedrine

16. Which of the following drugs is first administered by the nurse to treat an anaphylactic reaction to penicillin?
    a. diphenhydramine (Benadryl)
    b. epinephrine (Adrenalin)
    c. isoproterenol (Isuprel)
    d. dexamethasone (Decadron)

Selected References

American Heart Association. (2005). Guidelines for cardiopulmonary resuscitation and emergency cardiovascular care. *Circulation, 112,* IV58–IV66.

Barletta, J. F. (2005). Cardiopulmonary resuscitation. In J. T. DiPiro, R. L. Talbert, G. C. Yee, G. R. Matzke, B. G. Wells, & L. M. Posey (Eds.), *Pharmacotherapy: A pathophysiologic approach* (6th ed., pp. 171–183). New York: McGraw-Hill.

DiPiro, J. T., & Ownby, D. R. (2005). Allergic and pseudoallergic drug reactions. In J. T. DiPiro, R. L. Talbert, G. C. Yee, G. R. Matzke, B. G. Wells, & L. M. Posey (Eds.), *Pharmacotherapy: A pathophysiologic approach* (6th ed., pp. 1599–1611). New York: McGraw-Hill.

Drug facts and comparisons. (Updated monthly). St. Louis, MO: Facts and Comparisons.

Fetrow, C. W., & Avila, J. R. (2004). *Professional's handbook of complementary and alternative medicines* (3rd ed.). Springhouse, PA: Springhouse.

Hatton, R. C., Winterstein, A. G., McKelvey, R. P., Shuster, J., & Hendeles, L. (2007). Efficacy and safety of oral phenylephrine: A systemic review and meta-analysis. *Annuals of Pharmacotherapy, 41,* 381–390

Joint Task Force of Practice Parameters; American Academy of Allergy, Asthma and Immunology; American College of Allergy, Asthma and Immunology; & Joint Council of Allergy, Asthma and Immunology. (2005). The diagnosis and management of anaphylaxis: An updated practice parameter. *Journal of Allergy and Clinical Immunology, 115*(Suppl. 2), S483–S523.

Miano, T. A., & Crouch, M. A. (2006). Evolving role of vasopressin in the treatment of cardiac arrest. *Pharmacotherapy, 26*(6), 828–839.

Porth, C. M., & Curtis, R. L. (2005). Heart failure and circulatory shock. In C. M. Porth (Ed.), *Pathophysiology: Concepts of altered health states* (7th ed., pp. 603–330). Philadelphia: Lippincott Williams & Wilkins.

Smeltzer, S. C., Bare, B. G., Hinkle, J. L., & Cheever, K. H. (2008). Shock and multisystem failure. *Brunner & Suddarth's textbook of medical-surgical nursing* (11th ed., pp. 355–379). Philadelphia: Lippincott Williams & Wilkins.

Wenzel, V., Kismer, A., Arntz, R., Sitter, H., Stadlbauer, K. H., & Lindner, K H.., European Resuscitation Council During Cardiopulmonary Resuscitation Study Group. (2004). A comparison of vasopressin and epinephrine for out-of-hospital cardiopulmonary resuscitation. *New England Journal of Medicine, 350*(2), 105–113.

Antiadrenergic Drugs

LEARNING OBJECTIVES

After studying this chapter, you will be able to:

1. List characteristics of antiadrenergic drugs in terms of effects on body tissues, indications for use, nursing process implications, principles of therapy, and observation of patient response.
2. Discuss alpha$_1$-adrenergic blocking drugs and alpha$_2$-adrenergic agonists in terms of indications for use, adverse effects, and other selected characteristics.
3. Compare and contrast beta-adrenergic blocking drugs in terms of cardioselectivity, indications for use, adverse effects, and other selected characteristics.
4. Teach patients about safe, effective use of antiadrenergic drugs.
5. Discuss principles of therapy and nursing process for using antiadrenergic drugs in special populations.

Applying Your Knowledge

William Jones is a 58-year-old Caucasian man with a long history of hypertension. He has hyperlipidemia, type 2 diabetes mellitus, and coronary artery disease with a history of a myocardial infarction (MI) and triple coronary artery bypass graft. He is prescribed Lopressor 100 mg daily and clonidine transdermal patch every 7 days.

Introduction

Antiadrenergic drugs decrease or block the effects of sympathetic nerve stimulation, endogenous catecholamines (e.g., epinephrine), and adrenergic drugs. The drugs are chemically diverse and have a wide spectrum of pharmacologic activity. Specific effects depend mainly on the patient's health status when a drug is given and the drug's binding with particular adrenergic receptors. Included in this chapter are centrally active antiadrenergic drugs such as clonidine, which are used primarily in the treatment of hypertension, and peripherally active alpha- and beta-adrenergic blocking agents, which are used to treat various cardiovascular and other disorders. A few uncommonly used antiadrenergic drugs for hypertension are included in Chapter 52.

A basal level of sympathetic tone is necessary to maintain normal body functioning, including regulation of blood pressure, blood glucose levels, and stress response. Therefore the goal of antiadrenergic drug therapy is to suppress pathologic stimulation—not the normal physiologic response to activity, stress, and other stimuli.

General Characteristics of Antiadrenergic Drugs

Mechanisms of Action

Antiadrenergic effects can occur either when alpha$_1$ or beta receptors are blocked by adrenergic antagonists or when presynaptic alpha$_2$ receptors are stimulated by agonist drugs. Most antiadrenergic drugs have *antagonist* or blocking effects when they bind with alpha$_1$, beta$_1$, beta$_2$, or a combination of receptors in peripheral tissues, thus preventing adrenergic effects. Antiadrenergic drugs may be nonselective, exerting antiadrenergic effects on several adrenergic receptors simultaneously; or they may act selectively, blocking only one adrenergic receptor.

Clonidine and related drugs have *agonist* effects at presynaptic alpha$_2$ receptors in the brain. As stated in Chapter 17, this agonist effect results in a negative feedback type of mechanism that decreases the release of additional norepinephrine. Thus the overall effect is decreased sympathetic outflow from the brain and decreased activation of alpha and beta receptors by norepinephrine throughout the body.

Alpha-Adrenergic Agonists and Blocking Drugs

Alpha$_2$-adrenergic agonists such as clonidine (Catapres) inhibit the release of norepinephrine in the brain, thereby decreasing the effects of sympathetic nervous system stimulation throughout the body. A major clinical effect is decreased blood pressure. Although clinical effects are attributed mainly to drug action at presynaptic alpha$_2$ receptors in the brain, postsynaptic alpha$_2$ receptors in the brain and peripheral tissues (e.g., vascular smooth muscle) may also be involved. Activation of alpha$_2$ receptors in the pancreatic islets suppresses insulin secretion.

Some *alpha-adrenergic blocking drugs* may be selective for alpha$_1$ receptors in peripheral tissues such as smooth muscles and glands innervated by sympathetic nerve fibers. These drugs act primarily in the skin, mucosa, intestines, lungs, and kidneys to block or prevent alpha-mediated vasoconstriction. Specific effects of alpha$_1$-adrenergic blocking drugs include dilation of arterioles and veins, increased local blood flow, decreased blood pressure, constriction of pupils, and increased motility of the gastrointestinal (GI) tract. Alpha-adrenergic antagonists often activate reflexes that oppose the decrease in blood pressure by increasing heart rate and cardiac output and by causing fluid retention.

Alpha$_1$-adrenergic blocking drugs such as tamsulosin also can prevent alpha-mediated contraction of smooth muscle in nonvascular tissues. This action makes these drugs useful in the treatment of benign prostatic hyperplasia (BPH), a condition characterized by obstructed urine flow as the enlarged prostate gland presses on the urethra. Alpha$_1$-blocking agents can decrease urinary retention and improve urine flow by relaxing muscles in the prostate and urinary bladder. Patients diagnosed with BPH should be evaluated for prostatic cancer before starting drug therapy because the signs and symptoms of BPH and prostatic cancer are similar. The two conditions may also coexist.

Nonselective alpha-adrenergic blocking drugs such as phentolamine occupy peripheral alpha$_1$ receptors, causing vasodilation, and presynaptic alpha$_2$ receptors, causing cardiac stimulation. Consequently, decreased blood pressure is accompanied by tachycardia and perhaps other dysrhythmias.

Beta-Adrenergic Blocking Drugs

Beta-adrenergic blocking agents occupy beta-adrenergic receptor sites and prevent the receptors from responding to sympathetic nerve impulses, circulating catecholamines, and beta-adrenergic drugs (Fig. 18-1).

Beta$_1$ receptor blockade has an inhibitory effect on the cardiovascular system, resulting in decreased heart rate (negative *chronotropy*), decreased force of myocardial contraction (negative *inotropy*), slowed conduction through the atrioventricular (AV) node (negative *dromotropy*), decreased automaticity of ectopic pacemakers, decreased cardiac output at rest and with exercise, and decreased blood pressure in supine and standing positions, especially in people with hypertension. Chronic use of beta blockers is associated with increased very–low-density lipoprotein (VLDL) and decreased high-density lipoprotein (HDL) cholesterol. These changes pose a potential risk for patients with cardiovascular disease. Beta$_1$ receptor blockade also results in decreased renin secretion from the kidneys, decreased production of aqueous humor in

Figure 18-1 ■ Beta-adrenergic blocking agents prevent epinephrine and norepinephrine from occupying receptor sites on cell membranes. This action alters cell functions normally stimulated by epinephrine and norepinephrine, according to the number of receptor sites occupied by the beta-blocking drugs. (Adapted by J. Harley from *Encyclopedia Britannica Medical and Health Annual*. [1983]. Chicago: Encyclopedia Britannica.)

the eye, and diminished portal vein pressure in patients with cirrhosis.

Beta$_2$ receptor blockade produces bronchoconstriction of the smooth muscles in the respiratory tract, especially in people with asthma or other chronic lung diseases. Beta$_2$ receptor blockade also results in less effective metabolism of glucose (decreased glycogenolysis) when needed by the body, especially in people taking beta-blocking agents along with antidiabetic drugs. These diabetic patients may experience more severe and prolonged hypoglycemia. In addition, tachycardia, the early warning symptom of hypoglycemia, may be blocked by the medication, thereby delaying recognition and treatment. Beta$_2$ receptor blockade also increases the tone of smooth muscles in the GI tract, urinary bladder, and uterus.

Indications for Use

Alpha-Adrenergic Agonists and Blocking Drugs

Alpha$_2$ agonists are used in the treatment of hypertension. Clonidine, administered by the epidural route, is also approved for the relief of severe pain in cancer patients. A **BLACK BOX WARNING** alerts health care professionals that epidural administration of clonidine is not recommended for obstetrical, postpartum, or peri-operative pain management due to the risk for adverse effects resulting from hypotension and bradycardia. Investigational uses of clonidine include the treatment of tic disorders, postmenopausal hot flashes, migraine, attention deficit-hyperactivity disorder, drug-induced akathisia, and alcohol withdrawal and opioid dependence, as well as use as adjunct medication during anesthesia. Clonidine has not received approval by the U.S. Food and Drug Administration (FDA) for these purposes.

Selective alpha$_1$-adrenergic blocking drugs are used in the treatment of hypertension, BPH, and vasospastic disorders. The use of selective alpha$_1$-adrenergic blockers for the treatment of BPH was evaluated by an expert panel of the American Urological Association (AUA). The resulting clinical guidelines recommend alfuzosin, doxazosin, tamsulosin, and terazosin as equally effective in relieving the lower urinary tract symptoms of BPH, with only slight variations noted in the adverse effects profile of the individual alpha$_1$-adrenergic blockers. The AUA guidelines note insufficient data to support a recommendation for the use of prazosin for treatment of lower urinary tract symptoms secondary to BPH.

Nonselective alpha-blocking drugs are used as antihypertensive drugs only when hypertension is caused by excessive catecholamines. Excessive catecholamines may result from overdoses of adrenergic drugs or from pheochromocytoma, a rare tumor of the adrenal medulla that secretes epinephrine and norepinephrine and causes hypertension, tachycardia, and cardiac dysrhythmias. Although the treatment of choice for pheochromocytoma is surgical excision, alpha-adrenergic blocking drugs are useful adjuncts. They are given before and during surgery, usually in conjunction with beta blockers

to block the sympathetic effect of excessive catecholamine secretion.

Nonselective alpha blockers also are used in vascular diseases characterized by vasospasm, such as Raynaud's disease and frostbite, in which they improve blood flow. Phentolamine also can be used to prevent tissue necrosis due to extravasation of potent vasoconstrictors such as norepinephrine and dopamine into subcutaneous tissues.

Beta-Adrenergic Blocking Drugs

Clinical indications for use of beta-blocking agents are mainly cardiovascular disorders (e.g., angina pectoris, cardiac tachydysrhythmias, hypertension, myocardial infarction [MI], heart failure [HF]) and glaucoma.

In angina, beta blockers decrease myocardial contractility, cardiac output, heart rate, and blood pressure. These effects decrease myocardial oxygen demand (cardiac workload), especially in response to activity, exercise, and stress. In dysrhythmias, the drugs slow the sinus rate and prolong conduction through the AV node, thereby slowing the ventricular response rate to supraventricular tachydysrhythmias. In hypertension, the actions of beta blockers are unclear. Possible mechanisms include reduced cardiac output, inhibition of renin, and inhibition of sympathetic nervous system stimulation in the brain. However, the drugs effective in hypertension do not consistently demonstrate these effects; for example, a drug may lower blood pressure without reducing cardiac output or inhibiting renin.

After acute MI, beta blockers help protect the heart from reinfarction and decrease mortality rates over several years. Possible mechanisms include reduction in cardiac workload and prevention or reduction in the incidence of catecholamine-induced dysrhythmias. In HF, beta blockers play an important role but require careful monitoring on the part of the physician and the nurse. Administration of beta blockers may potentially worsen the condition of people with HF by blocking the sympathetic stimulation that helps maintain cardiac output. However, in many patients with HF, even those of advanced age and with advanced disease, the drugs are beneficial. For these patients, beta blockers decrease the risk of sudden cardiac death and may reduce ventricular remodeling that accompanies HF and leads to further deterioration of cardiac function.

In glaucoma, the drugs reduce intraocular pressure by binding to beta-adrenergic receptors in the ciliary body of the eye and decreasing formation of aqueous humor.

Contraindications to Use

Alpha$_2$ agonists are contraindicated in patients with hypersensitivity to the drugs, and methyldopa is also contraindicated in patients with active liver disease. Alpha-adrenergic blocking agents are contraindicated in angina pectoris, MI, HF, and stroke.

Beta-adrenergic blocking agents are contraindicated in bradycardia and heart block. Nonselective beta blockers are contraindicated with asthma and other allergic or pulmonary conditions characterized by bronchoconstriction; however, the selective beta$_1$ blockers may be used in people with these disorders. Research has shown that beta blockers can be beneficial in selected patients with mild to moderate chronic HF; however, the drugs have not been proven safe for people older than 80 years of age or those with severe HF.

Individual Drugs

Selected antiadrenergic medications are described in the following sections. Trade names, clinical indications, and dosage ranges are presented in Table 18-1 for alpha-adrenergic

agonists and blocking drugs and in Table 18-2 for beta-adrenergic blocking drugs.

Alpha-Adrenergic Agonists and Blocking Drugs

Alpha$_2$-adrenergic agonists include clonidine and methyldopa. These drugs produce similar therapeutic and adverse effects but differ in their pharmacokinetics and frequency of administration. Oral **clonidine** (Catapres) reduces blood pressure within 1 hour, reaches peak plasma levels in 3 to 5 hours, and has a plasma half-life of approximately 12 to 16 hours (longer with

Table 18-1	**Drugs at a Glance:** Alpha-Adrenergic Agonists and Blocking Drugs	

GENERIC/TRADE NAME	CLINICAL INDICATIONS	ROUTES AND DOSAGE RANGES
Alpha$_2$ Agonists		
Clonidine (Catapres)	Hypertension	PO 0.1 mg 2 times daily initially, gradually increased if necessary. Average maintenance dose, 0.2–0.8 mg/d. Transdermal 0.1-mg patch every 7 d initially; increase every 7–14 d to 0.2 mg or 0.3 mg if necessary. Maximum dose, two 0.3-mg patches every 7 d
Methyldopa	Hypertension	*Adults:* PO 250 mg 2 or 3 times daily initially, increased gradually at intervals of not less than 2 d until blood pressure is controlled or a daily dose of 3 g is reached
		Children: PO 10 mg/kg/d in 2 to 4 divided doses initially, increased or decreased according to response. Maximal dose, 65 mg/kg/d or 3 g daily, whichever is less
Selective Alpha$_1$-Blocking Drugs		
Alfuzosin (UroXatral)	BPH	PO 10 mg daily after same meal each day
Doxazosin (Cardura)	Hypertension BPH	PO 1 mg once daily initially, increased to 2 mg, then to 4, 8, and 16 mg if necessary
Prazosin (Minipress)	Hypertension BPH	PO 1 mg 2 to 3 times daily initially, increased if necessary to a total daily dose of 20 mg in divided doses. Average maintenance dose, 6–15 mg/d
Tamsulosin HCl (Flomax)	BPH	PO 0.4 mg/d after same meal each day. Dose may be increased if needed after 2–4 wk trial period.
Terazosin (Hytrin)	Hypertension	PO 1 mg at bedtime initially, increased gradually to maintenance dose, usually 1–5 mg once daily
	BPH	1–5 mg once daily
Nonselective Alpha-Blocking Drugs		
Phentolamine	Hypertension caused by pheochromocytoma	*Before and during surgery for pheochromocytoma:* IV, IM 5–20 mg as needed to control blood pressure
	Prevention of tissue necrosis from extravasation of vasoconstrictive drugs	*Prevention of tissue necrosis:* IV 10 mg in each liter of IV solution containing a potent vasoconstrictor
		Treatment of extravasation: Sub-Q 5–10 mg in 10 mL saline, infiltrated into the area within 12 h

BPH, benign prostatic hyperplasia.

Table 18-2	Drugs at a Glance: Beta-Adrenergic Blocking Agents

GENERIC/TRADE NAME	CLINICAL INDICATIONS	ROUTES AND DOSAGE RANGES
Nonselective Blocking Agents		
Levobunolol (Betagan)	Glaucoma	Topically to affected eye, 1 drop twice daily
Metipranolol (OptiPranolol)	Glaucoma	Topically to each eye, 1 drop once or twice daily
Propranolol (Inderal)	Hypertension	PO 40 mg twice daily initially, may be increased to 120–240 mg daily in divided doses Sustained-release capsules, PO 80 mg once daily, may be increased to 120–160 mg once daily Maximal daily dose, 640 mg
	Angina pectoris	PO 80–320 mg in 2–4 divided doses Sustained release, PO 80–160 mg once daily Maximal daily dose, 320 mg
	Dysrhythmias	PO 10–30 mg, q6–8h Life-threatening dysrhythmias, IV 1–3 mg at a rate not to exceed 1 mg/min with electrocardiographic and blood-pressure monitoring
	Myocardial infarction	PO 180–240 mg daily in 3 or 4 divided doses Maximal daily dose, 240 mg
	Hypertrophic subaortic stenosis	PO 20–40 mg daily in 3 or 4 divided doses Sustained release, PO 80–160 mg once daily
	Migraine prophylaxis	PO 80–240 mg daily in divided doses Sustained release, PO 80 mg once daily
Pindolol (Visken)*	Hypertension	PO 5 mg twice daily initially, increased by 10 mg every 3–4 wk, to a maximal daily dose of 60 mg if necessary
Nadolol (Corgard)	Hypertension Angina pectoris	Hypertension, PO 40 mg once daily initially, gradually increased. Usual daily maintenance dose, 80–320 mg Angina, PO 40 mg once daily initially, increased by 40–80 mg at 3- to 7-d intervals. Usual daily maintenance dose, 80–240 mg
Sotalol (Betapace, Betapace AF)	Cardiac dysrhythmias	PO 80–160 mg twice daily
Timolol (Blocadren, Timoptic)	Hypertension Myocardial infarction Glaucoma	Hypertension, PO 10 mg twice daily initially, increased at 7-d intervals to a maximum of 60 mg/d in 2 divided doses; usual maintenance dose, 20–40 mg daily Myocardial infarction, PO 10 mg twice daily Glaucoma, topically to eye, 1 drop of 0.25% or 0.5% solution (Timoptic) in each eye twice daily
Cardioselective Blocking Agents		
Acebutolol (Sectral)*	Hypertension Ventricular dysrhythmias	Hypertension, PO 400 mg daily in 1 or 2 doses; usual maintenance dose, 400–800 mg daily Dysrhythmias, PO 400 mg daily in 2 divided doses; usual maintenance dose, 600–1200 mg daily

(continued on page 300)

Table 18-2	Drugs at a Glance: Beta-Adrenergic Blocking Agents (continued)	
GENERIC/TRADE NAME	**CLINICAL INDICATIONS**	**ROUTES AND DOSAGE RANGES**
Atenolol (Tenormin)	Hypertension Angina pectoris Myocardial infarction	Hypertension, PO 50–100 mg daily Angina, PO 50–100 mg daily, increased to 200 mg daily if necessary Myocardial infarction, IV 5 mg over 5 min, then 5 mg 10 min later, then 50 mg PO 10 min later, then 50 mg 12 h later. Thereafter, PO 100 mg daily, in 1 or 2 doses, for 6–9 d or until discharge from hospital
Betaxolol (Betoptic, Kerlone)	Glaucoma Hypertension	Topically to each eye, 1 drop twice daily Hypertension, PO 10–20 mg daily
Bisoprolol (Zebeta)	Hypertension	PO 5–20 mg once daily
Esmolol (Brevibloc)	Supraventricular tach-yarrhythmias	IV 50–200 mcg/kg/min; average dose, 100 mcg/kg/min, titrated to effect with close monitoring of client's condition
Metoprolol (Lopressor)	Hypertension Myocardial infarction	Hypertension, PO 100 mg daily in single or divided doses, increased at 7-d or longer intervals; usual maintenance dose, 100–450 mg/d Myocardial infarction, early treatment, IV 5 mg every 2 min for total of 3 doses (15 mg), then 50 mg PO q6h for 48 h, then 100 mg PO twice daily. Myocardial infarction, late treatment, PO 100 mg twice daily, for at least 3 months, up to 1–3 y
Alpha–Beta-Blocking Agents **Carvedilol** (Coreg)*	Hypertension Congestive heart failure	PO 6.25 mg twice daily for 7–14 d, then increase to 12.5 mg twice daily if necessary for 7–14 d, then increase to 25 mg twice daily if necessary (maximum dose)
Labetalol (Trandate, Normodyne)	Hypertension, including hypertensive emergencies	PO 100 mg twice daily IV 20 mg over 2 min then 40–80 mg every 10 min until desired blood pressure achieved or 300 mg given IV infusion 2 mg/min (e.g., add 200 mg of drug to 250 mL 5% dextrose solution for a 2 mg/3 mL concentration)

* These drugs also have intrinsic sympathomimetic activity (ISA).

renal impairment). Approximately half the oral dose is metabolized in the liver, and the remainder is excreted unchanged in urine. When transdermal clonidine is given, therapeutic plasma levels are reached in 2 to 3 days and last 1 week.

Methyldopa (Aldomet) is an older drug with low to moderate absorption. With oral drug, peak plasma levels are reached in 2 to 4 hours, and peak antihypertensive effects occur in approximately 2 days. When discontinued, blood pressure increases in approximately 2 days. Intravenous (IV) administration reduces blood pressure in 4 to 6 hours and lasts 10 to 16 hours. Methyldopa is metabolized to some extent in the liver but is largely excreted in urine. In patients with renal impair-

ment, blood pressure–lowering effects may be pronounced and prolonged because of slower excretion. In addition to the adverse effects that occur with all these drugs, methyldopa also may cause hemolytic anemia and hepatotoxicity (e.g., jaundice, hepatitis).

Alpha$_1$-adrenergic antagonists include alfuzosin, doxazosin, prazosin, terazosin, and tamsulosin. **P** **Prazosin** (Minipress), the prototype, is well absorbed after oral administration and reaches peak plasma concentrations in 1 to 3 hours; action lasts approximately 4 to 6 hours. The drug is highly bound to plasma proteins, and the plasma half-life is approximately 2 to 3 hours. It is extensively metabolized in the liver, and its metabolites are excreted by the kidneys. **Doxazosin** (Cardura) and **terazosin** (Hytrin) are similar to prazosin but have longer half-lives (doxazosin, 10–20 hours; terazosin, approximately 12 hours) and durations of action (doxazosin, up to 36 hours; terazosin, 18 hours or longer). Prazosin must be taken in multiple doses. Doxazosin and terazosin may usually be taken once daily to control hypertension or symptoms of BPH.

Tamsulosin (Flomax) is the first alpha$_1$ antagonist designed specifically to treat BPH. Tamsulosin blocks alpha$_1$ receptors in the male genitourinary system, producing smooth-muscle relaxation in the prostate gland and urinary bladder neck. Urinary flow rate is improved, and symptoms of BPH are reduced. Because of the specificity of tamsulosin for receptors in the genitourinary system, this drug causes less orthostatic hypotension than other alpha$_1$ antagonists.

After oral administration, more than 90% of tamsulosin is absorbed. Administration with food decreases bioavailability by 30%. Tamsulosin is highly protein bound and is metabolized by the liver. Approximately 10% of the drug is excreted unchanged in the urine. An advantage of tamsulosin is the ability to start the drug at the recommended dosage. Most of the alpha$_1$ antagonists must be gradually increased to the recommended dosage. Common adverse effects include abnormal ejaculation and dizziness.

Alfuzosin (UroXatral) is another alpha$_1$-blocking drug specifically indicated for BPH. This moderately protein bound, extended-release medication is similar to prazosin but has the advantage of once-a-day dosing. It has a half-life of 10 hours and a duration of action of 24 hours. Alfuzosin should be taken after meals to promote absorption. It is metabolized extensively in the liver by cytochrome P450 3A4 enzymes and should not be given with potent inhibitors of this enzyme such as ketoconazole, itraconazole, or ritonavir or in the presence of moderate to severe liver insufficiency, because drug toxicity will occur. In addition, alfuzosin can prolong the Q–T interval and therefore should be used with caution in people with congenital or acquired Q–T prolongation. Common adverse effects include dizziness, headache, fatigue, and increased incidence of upper respiratory infections.

Of the alpha-adrenergic blocking drugs, **phenoxybenzamine** (Dibenzyline) is an old drug that exerts its action by binding permanently to alpha receptors and producing drug effects until the body builds new receptors. Therefore the drug action of phenoxybenzamine is long acting, persisting for 3 to 4 days. **Phentolamine** (Regitine) is similar to phenoxybenzamine but more useful clinically. Phentolamine acts competitively at alpha receptors and is therefore short acting; effects last only a few hours and can be reversed by an alpha-adrenergic stimulant drug such as norepinephrine.

Beta-Adrenergic Blocking Drugs

Numerous beta-blocking drugs are marketed in the United States. Although they produce similar effects, they differ from the prototype **P** **propranolol** (Inderal) with respect to several properties.

Clinical Indications

Propranolol is the oldest and most extensively studied beta blocker. In addition to its use in the treatment of hypertension, dysrhythmias, angina pectoris, and MI, propranolol is used to treat a wide variety of other conditions. In hypertrophic obstructive cardiomyopathy, it is used to improve exercise tolerance by increasing stroke volume. In pheochromocytoma, it is used in conjunction with an alpha-blocking drug to counter the effect of excessive catecholamine secretion, thereby preventing tachycardia and dysrhythmias. In dissecting aortic aneurysms, it is used to decrease systolic blood pressure. In hyperthyroidism, it decreases heart rate, cardiac output, and tremor.

Propranolol is also useful, by an unknown mechanism, for the prevention of migraine headache. However, it is not helpful in acute attacks of migraine headache. It also relieves palpitation and tremor associated with anxiety and stage fright, but it is not approved for clinical use as an antianxiety drug. Some people experiencing alcohol withdrawal may also benefit from administration of propranolol.

Research indicates that propranolol may be useful in treating cirrhosis of the liver. The drug may decrease the incidence of the initial episode of bleeding esophageal varices, prevent rebleeding episodes, and decrease the mortality rate due to hemorrhage.

Most beta blockers are approved for the treatment of hypertension. A beta blocker may be used alone or with another antihypertensive drug, such as a diuretic. **Labetalol** (Trandate, Normodyne) is also approved for treatment of hypertensive emergencies. **Atenolol** (Tenormin), metoprolol (Lopressor), **nadolol** (Corgard), and **propranolol** are approved as antianginal agents. **Betaxolol** (Betoptic, Kerlone) and **timolol** are used for hypertension and glaucoma. **Levobunolol** (Betagan) and **metipranolol** (OptiPranolol) are used only for glaucoma.

Acebutolol (Sectral), **esmolol** (Brevibloc), **propranolol**, and **sotalol** (Betapace and Betapace AF) are approved as antidysrhythmic agents. **Atenolol, metoprolol, propranolol,** and **timolol** (Blocadren, Timoptic) are used to prevent MI or reinfarction.

A growing number of studies demonstrate that **carvedilol** (Coreg), a *cardioselective* alpha–beta blocker, is useful not only in treating mild to moderate cases of chronic HF but also in reducing the risk of sudden death. Carvedilol has been shown to reduce risk of death or hospitalization in patients with mild to moderate HF by 38%. Despite concern that people who have severe HF or are more advanced in age would not be able to tolerate beta blockers, carvedilol appears to be well tolerated, even if the HF is advanced. Exactly how beta blockers benefit patients with HF is unclear. Possible mechanisms of action include blockade of the damaging effects of sympathetic stimulation on the heart, beta receptor up-regulation, decreased sympathetic stimulation due to decreased plasma norepinephrine and antidysrhythmic effects, and improved diastolic function by lengthening diastolic filling time. Research has shown that carvedilol demonstrates antioxidant activity. The clinical significance of this finding for patients with HF is not yet clear. **Metoprolol**, a cardioselective beta blocker, is also indicated for the treatment of stable heart failure along with an ACE inhibitor, a diuretic, and digoxin. Studies show metoprolol reduces hospitalizations for exacerbation of heart failure and reduces cardiovascular mortality.

Applying Your Knowledge 18-1

What is the potential benefit of using Lopressor for Mr. Jones' hypertension and his coronary history?

Receptor Selectivity

Levobunolol, metipranolol, penbutolol, nadolol, pindolol, propranolol, sotalol, and timolol are nonselective beta blockers. The term *nonselective* means that the drugs block both beta$_1$ (cardiac) and beta$_2$ (mainly smooth muscle in the bronchi and blood vessels) receptors. Blockade of beta$_2$ receptors is associated with adverse effects such as bronchoconstriction, peripheral vasoconstriction, and interference with glycogenolysis.

Acebutolol, atenolol, betaxolol, bisoprolol, esmolol, and metoprolol are cardioselective agents, which means they have more effect on beta$_1$ receptors than on beta$_2$ receptors. As a result, they may cause less bronchospasm, less impairment of glucose metabolism, and less peripheral vascular insufficiency. These drugs are preferred when beta blockers are needed by patients with diabetes mellitus, peripheral vascular disorders, or asthma or other bronchospastic pulmonary disorders (see Evidence-Based Practice Box 18-1). However, cardioselectivity is lost at higher doses because most organs have both beta$_1$ and beta$_2$ receptors rather than one or the other exclusively.

Labetalol and carvedilol block alpha$_1$ receptors to cause vasodilation and beta$_1$ and beta$_2$ receptors to cause all the effects of the nonselective agents. Both alpha- and beta-adrenergic blocking actions contribute to antihypertensive effects, but it is unclear whether these drugs have any definite advantage over other beta blockers. They may cause less bradycardia but more postural hypotension than other beta-blocking agents, and they may cause less reflex tachycardia than other vasodilators.

Intrinsic Sympathomimetic Activity

Drugs with *intrinsic sympathomimetic activity* (ISA) (acebutolol, carvedilol, penbutolol, and pindolol) have a chemical structure similar to that of catecholamines. As a result, they can block some beta receptors and stimulate others. It was once thought that these drugs would produce fewer adverse effects than other beta blockers; however, this has not occurred clinically. The primary use for medications with intrinsic sympathomimetic activity is to treat people who experience bradycardia with other beta blockers. These medications should not be used to prevent recurrent MI because of their potential to increase dysrhythmias and oxygen consumption by the myocardium.

Evidence-Based Practice

18-1 Cardioselective Beta Blockers in Patients With Asthma or Chronic Obstructive Pulmonary Disease

Beta blockers have been shown to benefit patients with hypertension, heart failure, and myocardial infarction. However, they have traditionally been considered contraindicated in patients with obstructive airway disorders because of the bronchoconstrictive effects of beta blockade. This Cochrane review (which included a meta-analysis of 19 randomized, blinded, controlled trials on single-dose treatment with beta blockers and 10 studies on continued treatment with beta blockers) sought to assess the effect of cardioselective beta blockers on respiratory function in patients with asthma or chronic obstructive pulmonary disease (COPD) by assessing the effect of the beta blocker on the forced expiratory volume in 1 second (FEV$_1$). The reviewers divided beta blockers into those with or without ISA for this analysis and looked at the effect of a single dose as well as continued beta$_1$ blocker therapy. Cardioselective beta blockers produced no significant change in FEV$_1$ or respiratory symptoms compared with a placebo when given as a single dose or for longer duration. There was no significant difference in FEV$_1$ with beta-blocker therapy based on presence or absence of ISA properties. In view of this review and the demonstrated benefits of beta blockers in conditions such as heart failure, coronary artery disease, and hypertension, the reviewers concluded that cardioselective beta blockers are safe for short-term use in patients with mild to moderate asthma or COPD. Further research is needed to establish long-term safety.

Membrane-Stabilizing Activity

Several beta blockers have a *membrane-stabilizing effect* that is sometimes described as quinidine-like (i.e., producing myocardial depression). Because the doses required to produce this effect are much higher than those used for therapeutic effects, this characteristic is considered clinically insignificant.

Potassium Channel Blockade

Unique among beta blockers, sotalol exerts an antidysrhythmic effect by blocking potassium channels in cell membranes, thereby prolonging repolarization and the refractory period of the heart. At low doses, beta-blocking effects predominate, and at high doses, antidysrhythmic effects predominate. Sotalol is used to treat life-threatening ventricular dysrhythmias and to maintain normal sinus rhythm in patients who frequently reconvert to atrial fibrillation/flutter (see Chap. 49). A **BLACK BOX WARNING** alerts health care professionals that appropriate use of sotalol (Betapace and Betapace AF) requires continuous ECG monitoring for 3 days after the patient is stabilized on a maintenance dose to minimize risk from drug-induced dysrhythmias. Calculation of creatinine clearance is necessary before initiating sotalol therapy to prevent drug accumulation and toxicity. Furthermore, substitution of Betapace for Betapace AF should be avoided due to significant differences in labeling, including patient package insert, dosing administration, and safety information.

Lipid Solubility

The more lipid-soluble beta blockers were thought to penetrate the central nervous system (CNS) more extensively and cause adverse effects such as confusion, depression, hallucinations, and insomnia. Some clinicians state that this characteristic is important only in terms of drug usage and excretion in certain disease states. Thus a water-soluble, renally excreted beta blocker may be preferred in patients with liver disease and a lipid-soluble, hepatically metabolized drug may be preferred in patients with renal disease.

Routes of Elimination

Most beta-blocking drugs are metabolized in the liver. Atenolol, nadolol, and an active metabolite of acebutolol are excreted by the kidneys; dosage must be reduced in the presence of renal failure.

Routes of Administration

Most beta blockers can be given orally. Atenolol, esmolol, labetalol, metoprolol, and propranolol also can be given IV, and ophthalmic solutions are applied topically to the eye. Betaxolol and timolol are available in oral and ophthalmic forms.

Duration of Action

Acebutolol, atenolol, bisoprolol, penbutolol, and nadolol have long serum half-lives and can usually be given once daily. Carvedilol, labetalol, metoprolol, pindolol, sotalol, and timolol are usually given twice daily. Propranolol required administration several times daily until development of a sustained-release capsule allowed once-daily dosing.

Nursing Process

Assessment

- Assess the patient's condition in relation to disorders in which antiadrenergic drugs are used. Because most of the drugs are used to treat hypertension, assess blood-pressure patterns over time, when possible, including antihypertensive drugs used and the response obtained. With other cardiovascular disorders, check blood pressure for elevation and pulse for tachycardia or dysrhythmia, and determine the presence or absence of chest pain, migraine headache, or hyperthyroidism. If the client reports or medical records indicate one or more of these disorders, assess for specific signs and symptoms. With BPH, assess for signs and symptoms of urinary retention and difficulty voiding.

- Assess for conditions that contraindicate the use of antiadrenergic drugs.

- Assess vital signs to establish a baseline for later comparisons.

- Assess for use of prescription and nonprescription drugs that are likely to increase or decrease effects of antiadrenergic drugs.

- Assess for lifestyle habits that are likely to increase or decrease effects of antiadrenergic drugs (e.g., ingestion of caffeine or nicotine).

Nursing Diagnoses

- Decreased Cardiac Output related to drug-induced postural hypotension (alpha$_2$ agonists, alpha$_1$-blocking agents, nonselective alpha-blocking agents, and beta blockers) and worsening HF (beta blockers)

- Impaired Gas Exchange related to drug-induced bronchoconstriction with beta blockers

- Sexual Dysfunction in men related to impotence and decreased libido

- Fatigue related to decreased cardiac output

- Noncompliance with drug therapy related to adverse drug effects or inadequate understanding of drug regimen

- Risk for Injury related to hypotension, dizziness, sedation

- Deficient Knowledge of drug effects and safe usage

Planning/Goals

The patient will

- Receive or self-administer drugs accurately

- Experience relief of symptoms for which antiadrenergic drugs are given

- Comply with instructions for safe drug usage

- Avoid stopping antiadrenergic drugs abruptly

- Demonstrate knowledge of adverse drug effects to be reported

- Avoid preventable adverse drug effects

- Keep appointments for blood pressure monitoring and other follow-up activities

Interventions

Use measures to prevent or decrease the need for antiadrenergic drugs. Because the sympathetic nervous system is stimulated by physical and emotional stress, efforts to decrease stress may indirectly decrease the need for drugs to antagonize sympathetic effects. Such efforts may include the following:

- Helping the patient stop or decrease cigarette smoking. Nicotine stimulates the CNS and the sympathetic nervous system to cause tremors, tachycardia, and elevated blood pressure.

- Teaching measures to relieve pain, anxiety, and other stresses

- Counseling regarding relaxation techniques

- Helping the patient avoid temperature extremes

- Helping the patient avoid excessive caffeine in coffee or other beverages

- Helping the patient develop a reasonable balance among rest, exercise, work, and recreation

Nursing Process continues on page 304

- Recording vital signs at regular intervals in hospitalized clients to monitor for adverse effects
- Helping with activity or ambulation as needed to prevent injury from dizziness

In addition, teaching guidelines are included in the accompanying display.

Evaluation

- Observe for decreased blood pressure when antiadrenergic drugs are given for hypertension.
- Interview regarding decreased chest pain when beta blockers are given for angina.
- Interview and observe for signs and symptoms of adverse drug effects (e.g., edema, tachycardia with alpha agonists and blocking agents; bradycardia, congestive HF, bronchoconstriction with beta blockers).
- Interview regarding knowledge and use of drugs.

Principles of Therapy

Drug Selection and Administration

Alpha-Adrenergic Agonists and Blocking Drugs

When an alpha$_1$-blocking agent (doxazosin, prazosin, terazosin) is given for hypertension, "first-dose syncope" may occur due to hypotension. This reaction can be prevented or minimized by starting with a low dose, increasing the dose gradually, and giving the first dose at bedtime. The decreased blood pressure also stimulates reflex mechanisms to raise blood pressure

(increase heart rate and cardiac output, fluid retention), and a diuretic may be necessary.

When an alpha$_2$ agonist is given for hypertension, it is very important not to stop the drug abruptly because of the risk of rebound hypertension. For example, to discontinue clonidine, the dosage should be gradually reduced over 2 to 4 days.

Beta-Adrenergic Blocking Drugs

For most people, a nonselective beta blocker that can be taken once or twice daily is acceptable. For others, the choice of a beta blocker depends largely on the patient's condition and response to the drugs. For example, cardioselective drugs are preferred for patients who have pulmonary disorders and diabetes mellitus, and drugs with intrinsic sympathomimetic activity may be preferred for those who experience significant bradycardia with beta blockers lacking this property.

Dosage of beta blockers must be individualized because of wide variations in plasma levels from comparable doses. Variations are attributed to the initial metabolism in the liver, the extent of binding to plasma proteins, and the degree of beta-adrenergic stimulation that the drugs must overcome. In general, low doses should be used initially and increased gradually until therapeutic or adverse effects occur. Adequacy of dosage or extent of beta blockade can be assessed by determining whether the heart rate increases in response to exercise.

Metoprolol and carvedilol are indicated for treatment of HF. Treatment should begin with a low dose of the beta blocker, often administered concurrently with an angiotensin-converting enzyme (ACE) inhibitor, a diuretic, and digoxin. The purpose of the ACE inhibitor is to counteract any initial aggravation of the HF symptoms due to the beta blocker.

Patient Teaching Guidelines — Alpha$_2$ Agonists and Alpha-Blocking Drugs

General Considerations

- Have your blood pressure checked regularly. Report high or low values to your health care provider.
- The adverse reactions of palpitations, weakness, and dizziness usually disappear with continued use. However, they may recur with conditions promoting vasodilation (dosage increase, exercise, high environmental temperatures, ingesting alcohol or a large meal).
- To prevent falls and injuries, if the above reactions occur, sit down or lie down immediately and flex arms and legs. Change positions slowly, especially from supine to standing.
- Do not drive a car or operate machinery if drowsy or dizzy from medication.
- Do not stop the drugs abruptly. Hypertension, possibly severe, may develop.
- With methyldopa, report any signs of abdominal pain, nausea, vomiting, diarrhea, or jaundice to your health

care provider. Regular blood tests are needed to make sure the medication is working as it should.
- Do not take over-the-counter or other medications without the physician's knowledge. Many drugs interact to increase or decrease the effects of antiadrenergic drugs.

Self-Administration

- Sedation and first-dose syncope may be minimized by taking all or most of the prescribed dose at bedtime.
- When using the clonidine transdermal patch, select a hairless area on the upper arm or torso for the application. The patch is changed once a week.
- Avoid alcohol use with these medications because excessive drowsiness may occur.
- With extended-release medications such as alfuzosin (UroXatral), do not crush, split, or chew the tablets, because overdose may occur.
- Take alfuzosin (UroXatral) and tamsulosin (Flomax) after a meal.

Patient Teaching Guidelines   Beta-Blocking Drugs

General Considerations

■ Count your pulse daily and report to a health care provider if under 50 for several days in succession. This information helps to determine if the drug therapy needs to be altered to avoid more serious adverse effects.

■ Report weight gain (more than 2 lb within a week), ankle edema, shortness of breath, or excessive fatigue. These are signs of heart failure. If they occur, the drug may be stopped.

■ Report fainting spells, excessive weakness, or difficulty in breathing. Beta-blocking drugs decrease the usual adaptive responses to exercise or stress. Syncope may result from hypotension, bradycardia, or heart block; its occur-

rence probably indicates stopping or decreasing the dose of the drug.

■ Do not stop taking the drugs abruptly. Stopping the drugs suddenly may cause or aggravate chest pain (angina).

■ Do not take over-the-counter or other medications without the physician's knowledge. Many drugs interact to increase or decrease the effects of beta-blocking agents.

Self-Administration

■ Consistently take the drug at the same time each day with or without food. This maintains consistent therapeutic blood levels.

■ Do not crush or chew long-acting forms of these medications.

The purpose of the diuretic is to manage fluid retention. The purpose of digoxin is to improve cardiac output. The patient should be closely monitored for adverse effects such as worsening HF.

Current evidence based practice guidelines by the American Heart Association and the American College of Cardiology recommend early use of an oral beta blocker with or without reperfusion therapy after an acute MI along with oxygen, aspirin, nitroglycerin, and an anticoagulant (heparin or low-molecular weight heparin). Adjunctive medications may include clopidogrel and a glycoprotein IIb/IIIa receptor blocker. Intravenous beta-blocker therapy is appropriate for patients with acute MI accompanied by tachyarrhythmias or high blood pressures; however, there is a higher risk of early cardiogenic shock in more hemodynamically at-risk patients. Patients with acute MI that have documented heart failure or high risk for shock may not be candidates for early beta-blocker treatment; it is important to individualize treatment in these cases. Beta-blocker therapy should be continued for at least 2 years post-MI. (A beta blocker with intrinsic sympathomimetic activity should not be used for this purpose.) Studies have shown that such use of a beta blocker may reduce mortality by as much as 25%. Accompanying post-MI beta-blocker therapy, most patients will also receive aspirin and an angiotensin-converting enzyme inhibitor for secondary prevention of death stroke and recurrent MI. Adjunctive medications may include statins for hyperlipidemia and anticoagulation with warfarin.

A **BLACK BOX WARNING** alerts health care providers that beta blockers should not be discontinued abruptly. Long-term blockade of beta-adrenergic receptors increases the receptors' sensitivity to epinephrine and norepinephrine when the drugs are discontinued. There is a risk of severe hypertension, angina, dysrhythmias, and MI from the increased or excessive sympathetic nervous system stimulation. Thus the dosage should be tapered and gradually discontinued to allow beta-adrenergic receptors to return to predrug density and sensitivity. An optimal tapering period has not been defined.

Some authorities recommend 1 to 2 weeks, and others recommend reducing the dosage over approximately 10 days to 30 milligrams per day of propranolol (or an equivalent amount of other drugs) and continuing this amount at least 2 weeks before the drug is stopped completely. Treatment with beta blockers should be restarted if angina worsens or acute coronary insufficiency develops during the tapering process.

Beta blockers are indicated to reduce hemodynamic complications during the perioperative period. Esmolol is often the beta blocker of choice in this situation because it is cardioselective, can be given IV, and has a rapid onset of action. Cardiac output may be an important factor in determining the amount of IV anesthetic needed for induction, and esmolol is known to reduce cardiac output. A recent study found that propofol requirements for induction were reduced by 25% after pretreatment with esmolol. During the intraoperative and postoperative periods, esmolol is useful for controlling tachycardia and hypertension. With some types of anesthesia such as desflurane, intraoperative administration of esmolol promotes more rapid awakening after anesthesia and reduced need for opioid analgesics. Postoperatively, esmolol may also be useful in preventing myocardial ischemia.

Various drugs may be used to treat adverse effects of beta blockers. Atropine can be given for bradycardia, digoxin and diuretics for HF, vasopressors for hypotension, and bronchodilator drugs for bronchoconstriction.

It is important to note that bronchodilation does not occur in a patient taking beta blockers when given epinephrine to treat an allergic reaction to an allergen or during allergy testing. This absence of the normal response to epinephrine is due to drug-induced beta$_2$ blockade.

Applying Your Knowledge 18-2

What explanation do you give Mr. Jones when he asks what the patch does for his condition?

Use in Special Populations

Use in Children

Most alpha-adrenergic agonists and blocking agents have not been established as safe and effective in children.

Beta-adrenergic blocking drugs are used in children for disorders similar to those in adults. However, safety and effectiveness have not been established, and manufacturers of most of the drugs do not recommend pediatric use or suggest dosages. The drugs are probably contraindicated in young children with resting heart rates of less than 60 beats per minute.

When beta blockers are given, general guidelines include the following:

■ Adjust dosage for body weight.

■ Monitor responses closely. Children are more sensitive to adverse drug effects than adults.

■ Remember that if beta blockers are given to infants (up to 1 year of age) with immature liver function, blood levels may be higher and accumulation is more likely even when doses are based on weight.

■ When monitoring responses, remember that heart rate and blood pressure vary among children according to age and level of growth and development. They also differ from those of adults.

■ Recall that children are more likely to have asthma than adults. Thus they may be at greater risk of drug-induced bronchoconstriction.

Propranolol is probably the most frequently used beta blocker in children. The drug is given orally for hypertension, and dosage should be individualized. The usual dosage range is 2 to 4 milligrams per kilogram of body weight per day, in two equal doses. Calculation of the dosage on the basis of body surface area is not recommended because of possible excessive blood levels of drug and greater risk of toxicity. As with adults, the drug should not be stopped abruptly and should be tapered gradually over 1 to 3 weeks.

Use in Older Adults

Alpha$_2$-adrenergic agonists may be used to treat hypertension in older adults, and alpha$_1$-adrenergic antagonists may be used to treat hypertension and BPH. Dosage of these drugs should be reduced because older adults are more likely to experience adverse drug effects, especially with impaired renal or hepatic function. As with other populations, these drugs should not be stopped suddenly. Instead, they should be tapered in dosage and discontinued gradually, over 1 to 2 weeks.

Older adults undergoing cataract surgery are at risk of a surgical complication, intraoperative *floppy iris syndrome*, if they are taking selective alpha$_1$-blockers for BPH or hypertension. Pupil dilation is necessary for cataract surgery. Alpha$_1$ blockers may cause the pupil to constrict and the iris to relax, complicating the surgical procedure. It is important for individuals to alert eye surgeons of alpha$_1$ blockers therapy so

special precautions during surgery can be implemented to reduce potential complications.

Beta-adrenergic blocking drugs are commonly used in older adults for angina, dysrhythmias, hypertension, HF, prevention of recurrent MI, and glaucoma. Several recent clinical trials and research studies demonstrated that older adults can tolerate and benefit from use of beta blockers in the treatment of HF. In hypertension, beta blockers are not recommended for monotherapy because older adults may be less responsive than younger adults. Thus the drugs are probably most useful as second drugs (with diuretics) in patients who require multidrug therapy and patients who also have angina pectoris or another disorder for which a beta blocker is indicated.

Whatever the indications for beta blockers in older adults, the drugs should be used cautiously and patients' responses should be monitored closely. Older adults are likely to have disorders that put them at higher risk of adverse drug effects, such as HF and other cardiovascular conditions, renal or hepatic impairment, and chronic pulmonary disease. Thus they may experience bradycardia, bronchoconstriction, and hypotension to a greater degree than younger adults. Dosage usually should be reduced because of decreased hepatic blood flow and subsequent slowing of drug metabolism. As in other populations, beta blockers should be tapered in dosage and discontinued over 1 to 3 weeks to avoid myocardial ischemia and other potentially serious adverse cardiovascular effects.

⊘ **Applying Your Knowledge 18-3**

How Can You Avoid This Medication Error?
You are preparing medication for Mr. Jones. The pharmacy has substituted Lopressor with a generic drug. Mr. Jones informs you that he cannot take another form of the drug, so you hold the dose and do not administer today's metoprolol.

Use in Various Ethnic Groups

Most studies involve adults with hypertension and compare drug therapy responses between African Americans and Caucasians. Findings indicate that monotherapy with alpha$_1$ blockers and combination therapy with alpha and beta blockers is equally effective in the two groups. However, monotherapy with beta blockers is less effective in African Americans than in Caucasians. When beta blockers are used in African Americans, they should usually be part of a multidrug treatment regimen, and higher doses may be required. In addition, labetalol, an alpha and beta blocker, has been shown to be more effective in the African-American population than propranolol, timolol, or metoprolol. According to the U.S. Carvedilol Heart Failure Trials Program and the COPERNICUS trials, African Americans with HF responded favorably to a combination of carvedilol plus ACE inhibitors, even when their condition was advanced.

Several studies indicate that Asians achieve higher blood levels of beta blockers with given doses and, in general, need much smaller doses than Caucasians. This increased sensitivity to the drugs may result from slower metabolism and excretion.

Use in Patients With Renal Impairment

Centrally acting alpha$_2$ agonists such as clonidine and methyldopa are eliminated by a combination of liver metabolism and renal excretion. Renal impairment may result in slower excretion of these medications, with subsequent accumulation and increased adverse effects.

Alpha$_1$-adrenergic antagonists such as prazosin, terazosin, alfuzosin, doxazosin, and tamsulosin are eliminated primarily by liver metabolism and biliary excretion. Therefore renal impairment is not a contraindication to use of these medications. However, the kidneys excrete tolazoline, and reduced dosage should be considered in the presence of renal impairment.

Many beta blockers are eliminated primarily in the urine and pose potentially serious problems for patients with renal failure. In renal failure, dosage of acebutolol, atenolol, and nadolol must be reduced because they are eliminated mainly through the kidneys. The dosage of acebutolol and nadolol should be reduced if creatinine clearance is less than 50 milliliters per minute, and the dosage of atenolol should be reduced if the creatinine clearance is less than 35 milliliters per minute.

Use in Patients With Liver Impairment

Caution must be used when administering centrally acting alpha$_2$-adrenergic agonists such as clonidine and methyldopa to patients with liver impairment. These medications rely on hepatic metabolism as well as renal elimination to clear the body. Furthermore, methyldopa has been associated with liver disorders such as hepatitis and hepatic necrosis.

Alpha$_1$-adrenergic medications such as prazosin, alfuzosin, terazosin, doxazosin, and tamsulosin rely heavily on liver metabolism and biliary excretion to clear the body. Liver impairment may result in increased drug levels and adverse effects.

In the presence of hepatic disease (e.g., cirrhosis) or impaired blood flow to the liver (e.g., reduced cardiac output from any cause), dosage of some beta blockers such as propranolol, metoprolol, and timolol should be substantially reduced because these drugs are extensively metabolized in the liver. The use of atenolol or nadolol is preferred in liver disease because both are eliminated primarily by the kidneys.

Use in Patients With Critical Illness

Antiadrenergic drugs are one of several families of medications that may be used to treat urgent or malignant hypertension. An alpha$_2$ agonist such as clonidine might be prescribed under such conditions. A loading dose of clonidine 0.2 milligrams,

followed by 0.1 milligram per hour until the diastolic pressure falls below 110 mm Hg, may be administered. A dose of 0.7 milligrams should not be exceeded when using clonidine to treat malignant hypertension.

Beta blockers may be used in the treatment of acute MI. Early administration of a beta blocker after an acute MI results in a lower incidence of reinfarction, ventricular dysrhythmias, and mortality. These results have been demonstrated with several different agents; however, those with intrinsic sympathomimetic activity are not prescribed for this purpose. Patients must be carefully monitored for hypotension and HF when receiving beta blockers after an MI.

Use in Home Care

Antiadrenergic drugs are commonly used in the home setting, mainly to treat chronic disorders in adults. With alpha$_1$-adrenergic blocking drugs, the home care nurse may need to teach patients ways to avoid orthostatic hypotension. Most patients probably take these medications for hypertension. However, some older men with BPH take one of these drugs to aid urinary elimination. For an older man taking one of these drugs, the home care nurse must assess the reason for use to teach the patient and monitor for drug effects.

With beta-adrenergic blocking drugs, the home care nurse may need to assist patients and caregivers in assessing for therapeutic and adverse drug effects. It is helpful to have the patient or someone else in the household count and record the radial pulse daily, preferably about the same time interval before or after taking a beta blocker. Several days of a slow pulse should probably be reported to the health care provider who prescribed the beta blocker, especially if the patient also has excessive fatigue or signs of HF.

If wheezing respirations (indicating bronchoconstriction) develop in a patient taking a nonselective beta blocker, the patient or the home care nurse must consult the prescribing physician about changing to a cardioselective beta blocker. If a patient has diabetes mellitus, the home care nurse must interview and observe the patient for alterations in blood sugar control, especially increased episodes of hypoglycemia. If a patient has hypertension, the home care nurse must teach the patient to avoid over-the-counter (OTC) asthma and cold remedies, decongestants, appetite suppressants, and herbal preparations such as ma huang, black cohosh, and St. John's wort because these drugs act to increase blood pressure and may reduce the benefits of antiadrenergic medications. In addition, OTC analgesics such as ibuprofen, ketoprofen, and naproxen may raise blood pressure by causing retention of sodium and water.

Applying Your Knowledge 18-4

Mr. Jones has diabetes and is therefore at increased risk of what complication from Lopressor?

Nursing Actions | Antiadrenergic Drugs

NURSING ACTIONS	RATIONALE/EXPLANATION
1. Administer accurately	
a. With alpha$_2$ agonists:	
(1) Give all or most of a dose at bedtime, when possible.	To minimize daytime drowsiness and sedation
(2) Apply the clonidine skin patch to a hairless, intact area on the upper arm or torso; then apply adhesive overlay securely. Do not cut or alter the patch. Remove a used patch and fold its adhesive edges together before discarding. Apply a new patch in a new site.	To promote effectiveness and safe usage
b. With alpha$_1$-blocking drugs:	
(1) Give the first dose of doxazosin, prazosin, or terazosin at bedtime.	To prevent fainting from severe orthostatic hypotension
(2) Give alfuzosin and tamsulosin after the same meal each day.	Drug absorption is delayed in fasting conditions.
c. With beta-adrenergic blocking drugs:	
(1) Check blood pressure and pulse frequently, especially when dosage is being increased.	To monitor therapeutic effects and the occurrence of adverse reactions. Some patients with heart rates between 50 and 60 beats per minute may be continued on a beta blocker if hypotension or escape dysrhythmias do not develop.
(2) See Table 18–2 and manufacturers' literature regarding intravenous (IV) administration.	Specific instructions vary with individual drugs.
2. Observe for therapeutic effects	
a. With alpha$_2$ agonists and alpha-blocking drugs:	
(1) With hypertension, observe for decreased blood pressure.	With most of the drugs, blood pressure decreases within a few hours. However, antihypertensive effects with clonidine skin patches occur 2–3 days after initial application (overlap with oral clonidine or other antihypertensive drugs may be needed) and persist 2–3 days when discontinued.
(2) With benign prostatic hyperplasia, observe for improved urination.	The patient may report a larger stream, less nocturnal voiding, and more complete emptying of the bladder.
(3) In pheochromocytoma, observe for decreased pulse rate, blood pressure, sweating, palpitations, and blood sugar.	Because symptoms of pheochromocytoma are caused by excessive sympathetic nervous system stimulation, blocking stimulation with these drugs produces a decrease or absence of symptoms.
(4) In Raynaud's disease or frostbite, observe affected areas for improvement in skin color and temperature and in the quality of peripheral pulses.	These conditions are characterized by vasospasm, which diminishes blood flow to the affected part. The drugs improve blood flow by vasodilation.
b. With beta-blocking drugs:	
(1) With hypertension, observe for decreasing blood pressure.	Blood pressure is lowered when sympathetic nervous system activity is inhibited.
(2) With angina, observe for absence of chest pain, nausea, vomiting, sweating, and anxiety.	Angina is characterized by inadequate blood flow and oxygenation to the myocardium. The drugs reduce cardiac workload and therefore reduce oxygen demand.
(3) With dysrhythmias, observe for regular pulse and signs of adequate cardiac output.	Rhythm disturbances decrease cardiac output.
3. Observe for adverse effects	Adverse effects are usually extensions of therapeutic effects.
a. With alpha$_2$ agonists and alpha-blocking drugs:	
(1) Hypotension	Hypotension may range from transient postural hypotension to a more severe hypotensive state resembling shock. "First-dose syncope" may occur with prazosin and related drugs.
(2) Sedation, drowsiness	Sedation can be minimized by increasing dosage slowly and giving all or most of the daily dose at bedtime.
(3) Tachycardia	Tachycardia occurs as a reflex mechanism to increase blood supply to body tissues in hypotensive states.
(4) Edema	These drugs promote retention of sodium and water. Concomitant diuretic therapy may be needed to maintain antihypertensive effects with long-term use.
(5) Impaired ejaculation	Blockade of the sympathetic nervous system impedes efferent nerve conduction to the seminal vesicles.

NURSING ACTIONS	RATIONALE/EXPLANATION
(6) Prolonged Q–T interval and dysrhythmias with alfuzosin	Prolongation of the Q–T interval increases the risk of ventricular dysrhythmias such as torsades de pointes.
b. With beta-blocking drugs:	
(1) Bradycardia and heart block	These are extensions of the therapeutic effects, which slow conduction of electrical impulses through the atrioventricular node, particularly in patients with compromised cardiac function.
(2) Congestive heart failure—edema, dyspnea, fatigue	Caused by reduced force of myocardial contraction
(3) Bronchospasm—dyspnea, wheezing	Caused by drug-induced constriction of bronchi and bronchioles. It is more likely to occur in people with bronchial asthma or other obstructive lung disease.
(4) Fatigue and dizziness, especially with activity or exercise	These symptoms occur because the usual sympathetic nervous system stimulation in response to activity or stress is blocked by drug action.
(5) Central nervous system (CNS) effects—depression, insomnia, vivid dreams, and hallucinations	The mechanism by which these effects are produced is unknown.

4. Observe for drug interactions

a. Drugs that *increase* effects of alpha-antiadrenergic drugs:	
(1) Other antihypertensive drugs	Additive antihypertensive effects
(2) CNS depressants	Additive sedation and drowsiness
(3) Nonsteroidal anti-inflammatory drugs	Additive sodium and water retention, possible edema
(4) Epinephrine	Epinephrine increases the hypotensive effects of phentolamine and should not be given to treat shock caused by these drugs. Because epinephrine stimulates both alpha- and beta-adrenergic receptors, the net effect is vasodilation and a further drop in blood pressure.
(5) Ketoconazole, itraconazole, and ritonavir (with alfuzosin)	These drugs inhibit the enzyme CYP3A4, which is responsible for the metabolism of alfuzosin.
b. Drugs that *decrease* effects of alpha-antiadrenergic drugs:	
(1) Alpha adrenergics (e.g., norepinephrine)	Norepinephrine is a strong vasoconstricting agent and is the drug of choice for treating shock caused by overdosage of, or hypersensitivity to, phentolamine or phentalamine.
(2) Estrogens, oral contraceptives, nonsteroidal anti-inflammatory drugs	These drugs may cause sodium and fluid retention and thereby decrease antihypertensive effects of alpha-antiadrenergic drugs.
c. Drugs that *increase* effects of beta-adrenergic blocking drugs (e.g., propranolol):	
(1) Other antihypertensives	Synergistic antihypertensive effects. Patients who do not respond to beta blockers or vasodilators alone may respond well to the combination. Also, beta blockers prevent reflex tachycardia, which usually occurs with vasodilator antihypertensive drugs.
(2) Phentolamine	Synergistic effects to prevent excessive hypertension before and during surgical excision of pheochromocytoma
(3) Cimetidine, furosemide	Increase plasma levels by slowing hepatic metabolism
(4) Digoxin	Additive bradycardia, heart block
(5) Phenytoin	Potentiates cardiac depressant effects of propranolol
(6) Quinidine	The combination may be synergistic in treating cardiac arrhythmias. However, additive cardiac depressant effects also may occur (bradycardia, decreased force of myocardial contraction [negative inotropy], decreased cardiac output).
(7) Verapamil, IV	IV verapamil and IV propranolol should never be used in combination because of additive bradycardia and hypotension.
d. Drugs that *decrease* effects of beta-adrenergic blocking drugs:	
(1) Antacids	Decrease absorption of several oral beta blockers
(2) Atropine	Increases heart rate and may be used to counteract excessive bradycardia caused by beta blockers
(3) Isoproterenol	Stimulates beta-adrenergic receptors and therefore antagonizes effects of beta-blocking agents. Isoproterenol also can be used to counteract excessive bradycardia.
(4) Cocaine	May reduce or cancel the effects of beta-blocking drugs

Key Concepts

■ Antiadrenergic drugs decrease or block the effects of sympathetic nerve stimulation, endogenous catecholamines (e.g., epinephrine), and adrenergic drugs.

■ Antiadrenergic effects can occur either when alpha$_1$ or beta receptors are blocked by adrenergic antagonists or when presynaptic alpha$_2$ receptors are stimulated by agonist drugs.

■ Most antiadrenergic drugs have antagonist or blocking effects when they bind with alpha$_1$, beta$_1$, beta$_2$, or a combination of receptors in peripheral tissues, thus preventing adrenergic effects.

■ Alpha$_2$-adrenergic agonists such as clonidine (Catapres) inhibit the release of norepinephrine in the brain, thereby decreasing the effects of sympathetic nervous system stimulation throughout the body.

■ Alpha$_2$ agonists are used in the treatment of hypertension

■ Selective alpha$_1$-adrenergic blocking drugs are used in the treatment of hypertension, BPH, and vasospastic disorders.

■ Clinical indications for beta-blocking agents are mainly cardiovascular disorders (e.g., angina pectoris, cardiac tachydysrhythmias, hypertension, myocardial infarction [MI], heart failure [HF]) and glaucoma.

■ Antiadrenergic drugs should not be abruptly discontinued.

Review and Application Exercises

Short Answer Exercises

1. How do alpha$_2$ agonists and alpha$_1$-blocking drugs decrease blood pressure?

2. What are safety factors in administering and monitoring the effects of alpha$_2$ agonists and alpha$_1$-blocking drugs?

3. Why should a patient be cautioned against stopping alpha$_2$ agonists and alpha$_1$-blocking drugs abruptly?

4. What are the main mechanisms by which beta blockers relieve angina pectoris?

5. How are beta blockers thought to be "cardioprotective" in preventing repeat MIs?

6. What are some noncardiovascular indications for the use of propranolol?

7. What are the main differences between cardioselective and nonselective beta blockers?

8. Why are cardioselective beta blockers preferred for patients with asthma or diabetes mellitus?

9. List at least five adverse effects of beta blockers.

10. Explain the drug effects that contribute to each adverse reaction.

11. What signs, symptoms, or behaviors would lead you to suspect adverse drug effects?

12. Do the same adverse effects occur with beta-blocker eye drops that occur with systemic drugs? If so, how may they be prevented or minimized?

13. What information needs to be included in teaching patients about beta-blocker therapy?

14. What is the risk of abruptly stopping a beta-blocker drug rather than tapering the dose and gradually discontinuing the drug, as recommended?

15. How can beta blockers be both therapeutic and nontherapeutic for HF?

NCLEX-Style Questions

16. A patient with a history of emphysema is prescribed propanolol (Inderal) to treat hypertension. In this situation, the nurse should assess for the presence of
a. hyperglycemia
b. tachycardia
c. bronchoconstriction
d. respiratory depression

17. Your diabetic patient requires a beta blocker to treat a tachydysrhythmia. Due to the beta-blocker therapy, you should teach this patient not to rely on which of the following signs of developing hypoglycemia?
a. increased thirst
b. irritability
c. tachycardia
d. hunger

18. A patient is taking clonidine (Catapres), an alpha$_2$ blocker, for hypertension. It is important for the nurse to give this patient which of the following instructions?
a. Change from lying to standing positions slowly.
b. Rest often to avoid exercise intolerance.
c. Promptly report episodes of wheezing and difficulty breathing.
d. Take the medication in the morning to avoid insomnia.

19. You are taking care of a patient receiving intravenous dopamine (Intropin), a vasoconstrictor. What must you be prepared to administer if extravasation occurs?
    a. phentolamine (Regitine)
    b. propranolol (Inderal)
    c. esmolol (Brevibloc)
    d. tamsulosin (Flomax)

20. The nurse should monitor which of the following tests in a hypertensive patient taking methyldopa (Aldomet)?
    a. prostate-specific antigen
    b. serum electrolytes
    c. blood glucose
    d. liver studies

21. Which of the following instructions should be given to the patient with benign prostatic hyperplasia before taking his first dose of prazosin (Minipress)?
    a. Take your medication in the morning after meals.
    b. Take your medication at bedtime.
    c. Take your medication on an empty stomach.
    d. Take your medication with a glass of milk.

Selected References

American Urological Association. (2003, updated 2006). *Guideline on the management of benign prostatic hyperplasia (BPH)*. Retrieved August 15, 2005, from http://www.auanet.org/guidelines/main_reports/bph_management/preface_toc.pdf

Chang, D. F., & Campbell, J. R. (2005). Intraoperative floppy iris syndrome associated with tamsulosin. *Journal of Cataract Refractive Surgery, 31,* 664–673.

Drug facts and comparisons. (Updated monthly). St. Louis, MO: Facts and Comparisons.

Fetrow, C. W., & Avila, J. R. (2004). *Complementary and alternative medicines* (3rd ed.). Springhouse, PA: Springhouse.

Hospital Interventions Quality Improvement Organization Support Center. (2006, August). Facts you can work with. Early beta-blocker therapy for acute myocardial infarction. Retrieved from www.acc.org/qualityandscience/clinical/practice_advisory/pdfs/committBetaBlockerFACTSheet.pdf

Lee, M. (2005). Management of benign prostatic hyperplasia. In J. T. DiPiro, R. L. Talbert, G. C. Yee, G. R. Matzke, B. G. Wells, & L. M. Posey (Eds.), *Pharmacotherapy: A pathophysiologic approach* (6th ed., pp. 1535–1546). New York: McGraw-Hill.

Measures FACT Sheet. Beta-blockers for acute myocardial infarction. (April, 2005). Retrieved from www.ahrq.gov/clinic/commitfact.htm

Salpeter, S., Ormiston, T., Salpeter, E., & Wood-Baker, R. (2002). Cardioselective beta-blockers for reversible airway disease. *Cochrane Database of Systematic Reviews, Issue 4*. Retrieved July 23, 2007, from http://www.cochrane.org/reviews/en/ab002992.html

Spinler, S., & deDenus, S. (2005). Acute coronary syndromes. In J. T. DiPiro, R. L. Talbert, G. C. Yee, G. R. Matzke, B. G. Wells, & L. M. Posey (Eds.), *Pharmacotherapy: A pathophysiologic approach* (6th ed., pp. 291–319). New York: McGraw-Hill.

Cholinergic Drugs

KEY TERMS

- Acetyl-cholinesterase
- Alzheimer's disease
- Anticholinesterase
- Cholinergic
- Myasthenia gravis

LEARNING OBJECTIVES

After studying this chapter, you will be able to:

1. Describe effects and indications for use of selected cholinergic drugs.
2. Discuss drug therapy for myasthenia gravis.
3. Discuss the use of cholinergic drug therapy for paralytic ileus and urinary retention.
4. Discuss drug therapy for Alzheimer's disease.
5. Describe major nursing care needs of patients receiving cholinergic drugs.
6. Describe signs, symptoms, and treatment of overdose with cholinergic drugs.
7. Discuss atropine and pralidoxime as antidotes for cholinergic drugs.
8. Discuss principles of therapy for using cholinergic drugs in special populations.
9. Teach patients about safe, effective use of cholinergic drugs.

Applying Your Knowledge

Betty Humbarger is a 39-year-old woman who has myasthenia gravis. The use of neostigmine 30 mg three to four times a day has controlled her symptoms.

Introduction

Cholinergic drugs stimulate the parasympathetic nervous system in the same manner as acetylcholine (see Chap. 16). Some drugs act directly to stimulate cholinergic receptors; others act indirectly by inhibiting the enzyme *acetylcholinesterase*, thereby slowing acetylcholine metabolism at autonomic nerve synapses. Selected drugs are discussed here in relation to their use in *myasthenia gravis*, *Alzheimer's disease*, and atony of the smooth muscle of the gastrointestinal (GI) and urinary systems, which results in paralytic ileus and urinary retention, respectively.

In normal neuromuscular function, acetylcholine is released from nerve endings and binds to nicotinic receptors on cell membranes of muscle cells to cause muscle contraction. Myasthenia gravis is an autoimmune disorder in which autoantibodies are thought to destroy nicotinic receptors for acetylcholine on skeletal muscle. As a result, acetylcholine is less able to stimulate muscle contraction, and muscle weakness occurs.

In normal brain function, acetylcholine is an essential neurotransmitter and plays an important role in cognitive functions, including memory storage and retrieval. Alzheimer's disease, the most common type of dementia in adults, is characterized by abnormalities in the cholinergic, serotonergic, noradrenergic, and glutamatergic neurotransmission systems (see Chap. 5). In the cholinergic system, there is a substantial loss of neurons that secrete acetylcholine in the brain and decreased activity of choline acetyltransferase, the enzyme required for synthesis of acetylcholine.

Acetylcholine stimulates cholinergic receptors in the gut to promote normal secretory and motor activity. Cholinergic stimulation results in increased peristalsis and relaxation of the smooth muscle in sphincters to facilitate movement of flatus and feces. The secretory functions of the salivary and gastric glands are also stimulated.

Acetylcholine stimulates cholinergic receptors in the urinary system to promote normal urination. Cholinergic stimulation results in contraction of the detrusor muscle and relaxation of the urinary sphincter to facilitate emptying the urinary bladder.

General Characteristics of Cholinergic Drugs

Mechanisms of Action and Effects

Direct-acting cholinergic drugs are synthetic derivatives of choline. Most direct-acting cholinergic drugs are quaternary amines, carry a positive charge, and are lipid insoluble. They do not readily enter the central nervous system; thus their effects occur primarily in the periphery. Direct-acting cholinergic drugs are highly resistant to metabolism by acetylcholinesterase, the enzyme that normally metabolizes acetylcholine. This allows the drugs to have a longer duration of action than acetylcholine would produce. Direct-acting cholinergic drugs have widespread systemic effects when they activate muscarinic receptors in cardiac muscle, smooth muscle, exocrine glands, and the eye (Fig. 19-1).

Specific effects of direct-acting cholinergic drugs include

- Decreased heart rate, vasodilation, and unpredictable changes in blood pressure
- Increased tone and contractility in GI smooth muscle, relaxation of sphincters, and increased salivary-gland and GI secretions
- Increased tone and contractility of smooth muscle (detrusor) in the urinary bladder and relaxation of the sphincter
- Increased tone and contractility of bronchial smooth muscle
- Increased respiratory secretions
- Constriction of pupils (miosis) and contraction of ciliary muscle, resulting in accommodation for near vision

Indirect-acting cholinergic, or *anticholinesterase*, drugs decrease the inactivation of acetylcholine in the synapse by the enzyme acetylcholinesterase. Acetylcholine can then accumulate in the synapse and enhance the activation of postsynaptic muscarinic as well as nicotinic receptors (Fig. 19-2). In addition to the cholinergic drug effects described above, the added effect of indirect-acting cholinergic drugs on nicotinic

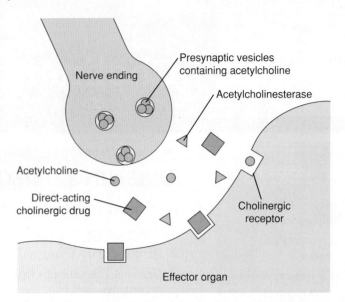

Figure 19-1 ■ Mechanism of direct cholinergic drug action. Direct-acting cholinergic drugs interact with postsynaptic cholinergic receptors on target effector organs, activating the organ in a similar fashion as the neurotransmitter acetylcholine.

receptors in skeletal muscles results in improved skeletal muscle tone and strength. Indirect-acting cholinergic medications for Alzheimer's disease are widely distributed, including to the central nervous system. Thus indirect-acting cholinergic drugs are able to improve cholinergic neurotransmission in the brain.

Anticholinesterase drugs are classified as either reversible or irreversible inhibitors of acetylcholinesterase. The reversible inhibitors exhibit a moderate duration of action and have several therapeutic uses, such as for Alzheimer's disease and myasthenia gravis, as described later. The irreversible inhibitors produce prolonged effects and are highly toxic. These agents are used primarily as poisons (i.e., insecticides and nerve gases); management of the toxicity caused by these agents is discussed later in this chapter. The only therapeutic use of these drugs is in the treatment of glaucoma (see Chap. 63).

Indications for Use

Cholinergic drugs have limited but varied uses. A direct-acting drug, bethanechol, is used to treat urinary retention due to urinary bladder atony and postoperative abdominal distention due to paralytic ileus. The anticholinesterase agents are used in the diagnosis and treatment of myasthenia gravis. They are also used to reverse the action of nondepolarizing neuromuscular blocking agents, such as tubocurarine, used in surgery (see Appendix C). Anticholinesterase agents do not reverse the neuromuscular blockade produced by depolarizing neuromuscular blocking agents, such as succinylcholine. In addition, donepezil, rivastigmine, and galantamine are anticholinesterase agents approved for treatment of Alzheimer's disease. Rivastigmine is also approved for treatment of mild to moderate dementia due to Parkinson's disease. Cholinergic drugs may also be used to treat glaucoma (see Chap. 63).

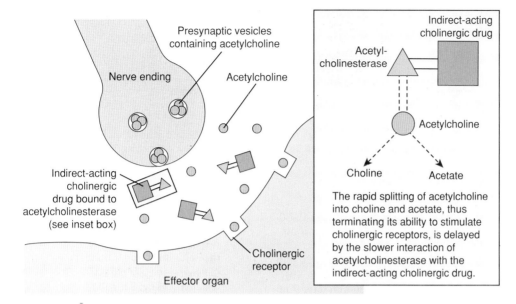

Figure 19-2 ▪ Mechanism of indirect cholinergic drug action. Indirect-acting cholinergic drugs prevent the enzymatic breakdown of the neurotransmitter acetylcholine. The acetylcholine remains in the synapse and continues to interact with cholinergic receptors on target effector organs, producing a cholinergic response.

Labels in figure:
- Presynaptic vesicles containing acetylcholine
- Nerve ending
- Acetylcholine
- Indirect-acting cholinergic drug bound to acetylcholinesterase (see inset box)
- Cholinergic receptor
- Effector organ
- Indirect-acting cholinergic drug
- Acetylcholinesterase
- Acetylcholine
- Choline
- Acetate

The rapid splitting of acetylcholine into choline and acetate, thus terminating its ability to stimulate cholinergic receptors, is delayed by the slower interaction of acetylcholinesterase with the indirect-acting cholinergic drug.

Contraindications to Use

Cholinergic drugs are contraindicated in urinary or GI tract obstruction because they increase the contractility of smooth muscle in the urinary and GI systems and may result in injury to structures proximal to the obstruction. Cholinergic drugs are contraindicated in individuals with asthma because they may cause bronchoconstriction and increased respiratory secretions. Individuals with peptic ulcer disease should not use cholinergic drugs because they increase gastric acid secretion. These drugs are also contraindicated in patients with inflammatory abdominal conditions and recent bowel surgery, because the drugs cause increased tone and motility of the intestinal smooth muscle and may lead to rupture of the bowel. Individuals with coronary artery disease should not take cholinergics because they can result in bradycardia, vasodilation, and hypotension.

Patients with hyperthyroidism should avoid cholinergic drugs. In the individual with hyperthyroidism, the initial response to cholinergic medications (bradycardia and hypotension) triggers the baroreceptor reflex. As this reflex attempts to resolve the hypotension, norepinephrine is secreted from sympathetic nerves regulating the heart. Norepinephrine may trigger reflex tachycardia and other cardiac dysrhythmias.

Pregnant women should not take cholinergic medications.

Individual Drugs

Cholinergic drugs are described in the following sections. Trade names, clinical indications, and dosage ranges are listed in Table 19-1.

Direct-Acting Cholinergics

Bethanechol (Urecholine) is a synthetic derivative of choline. Because the drug produces smooth-muscle contractions, it

should not be used in obstructive conditions of the urinary or GI tracts.

Reversible Indirect-Acting Cholinergics (Anticholinesterases)

P **Neostigmine** (Prostigmin) is the prototype anticholinesterase agent. It is used for long-term treatment of myasthenia gravis and as an antidote for tubocurarine and other nondepolarizing skeletal muscle relaxants used in surgery. Neostigmine, like bethanecol, is a quaternary amine and carries a positive charge. This reduces its lipid solubility and results in poor absorption from the GI tract. Consequently, oral doses are much larger than parenteral doses. When it is used for long-term treatment of myasthenia gravis, resistance to its action may occur and larger doses may be required.

Edrophonium (Tensilon) is a short-acting cholinergic drug used to diagnose myasthenia gravis, to differentiate between myasthenic crisis and cholinergic crisis, and to reverse the neuromuscular blockade produced by nondepolarizing skeletal muscle relaxants. It is given IM or IV by a physician who remains in attendance. Atropine, an antidote, and life-support equipment, such as ventilators and endotracheal tubes, must be available when the drug is given.

Physostigmine salicylate (Antilirium) is the only anticholinesterase capable of crossing the blood–brain barrier. Unlike other drugs in this group, physostigmine is not a quaternary amine, does not carry a positive charge, and therefore is more lipid soluble. It is sometimes used as an antidote for overdosage of anticholinergic drugs, including atropine, antihistamines, tricyclic antidepressants, and phenothiazine antipsychotics. However, its potential for causing serious adverse effects limits its usefulness. Some preparations of physostigmine are also used in the treatment of glaucoma (see Chap. 63).

Pyridostigmine (Mestinon) is similar to neostigmine in actions and uses and in adverse effects. It may have a longer

Table 19-1	Drugs at a Glance: Selected Cholinergic Drugs	

	ROUTES AND DOSAGE RANGES	
Generic/Trade Name	**Adults**	**Children**
Direct-Acting Cholinergics		
Bethanechol (Urecholine)	PO 10–50 mg 2 to 4 times daily, maximum single dose not to exceed 50 mg	Safety and efficacy not established <8 y. PO: 0.6 mg/kg 3 to 4 times daily.
Indirect-Acting Cholinergics (Anticholinesterase Drugs)		
Edrophonium (Tensilon)	*Diagnosis of myasthenia gravis:* *IV route preferred:* 2 mg IV over 15–30 sec; 8 mg IV given 45 sec later if no response. Test dose may be repeated in 30 min. *IM route:* 10 mg; may follow up with an additional 2 mg 30 min later if no response. *Differentiation of myasthenic crisis from cholinergic crisis:* 2 mg IV, observe response for 60 sec. May repeat with subsequent doses of 3 mg and 5 mg if no response to initial dose. BE PREPARED to intubate.	*Diagnosis of myasthenia gravis:* *Infants:* 0.5 mg IV. <34 kg: 1 mg IV; may titrate up to 5 mg if no response. >34 kg: 2 mg IV; may titrate up to 10 mg if no response. *Children <34 kg:* 2 mg IM. *Children >34 kg:* 5 mg, IM
Neostigmine (Prostigmin)	*Prevention/treatment of postoperative distention and urinary retention:* 0.25–0.5 mg IM or Sub-Q q 4–6 h for 2–3 d. *Treatment of myasthenia gravis:* Dosage individualized to patient needs. PO 15–375 mg/day in 3 or 4 divided doses. Sub-Q, IV, or IM 0.5 mg initially. Individualize subsequent doses. *Diagnosis of myasthenia gravis:* 0.022 mg/kg IM *Antidote for nondepolarizing neuromuscular blockers:* Give atropine sulfate 0.6–1.2 mg IV several min before slow IV injection of neostigmine 0.5–2 mg. Repeat as needed; total dose not to exceed 5 mg	*Prevention/treatment of postoperative distention and urinary retention* Safety and efficacy not established *Treatment of myasthenia gravis:* PO 0.3–0.6 mg/kg q3–4h Sub-Q, IV, IM 0.01–0.04 mg/kg/dose q2–3h as needed *Diagnosis of myasthenia gravis:* 0.04 mg/kg IM *Antidote for nondepolarizing neuromuscular blockers* Give 0.008–0.025 mg/kg atropine sulfate IV several min before slow IV injection of neostigmine 0.07–0.08 mg/kg.
Physostigmine (Antilirium)	IM, IV 0.5–2 mg. Give IV slowly, no faster than 1 mg/min to avoid adverse effects of bradycardia, respiratory distress, and seizures.	
Pyridostigmine (Mestinon)	PO 60 mg 3 times daily initially; individualize dose to control symptoms. Average dose in 24 h: 600 mg. Range in 24 h: 60–1500 mg. IM, IV slowly: 1/30th the oral dose	PO 7 mg/kg/d divided into 5 or 6 doses *Neonates of mothers with myasthenia gravis, who have difficulty with sucking/breathing/swallowing:* 0.05–0.15 mg/kg IM. Change to syrup as soon as possible.
Indirect-Acting Cholinergics for Alzheimer's Disease (Anticholinesterase Drugs)		
Donepezil (Aricept)	PO 5 mg daily at bedtime for 4–6 wk, then increase to 10 mg daily if needed.	

| | ROUTES AND DOSAGE RANGES | |
Generic/Trade Name	Adults	Children
Galantamine (Razadyne, Razadyne ER).	PO 8 mg/d initially, with food; increase to 16 mg/d after 4 wks if needed. May continue to increase q 4 wk up to maximum dose of 24 mg/d.	
Rivastigmine (Exelon), (Exelon Patch)	PO 1.5 mg twice daily with food initially. May titrate to higher doses at 1.5-mg intervals q 2 wk to a maximum dose of 12 mg/d. TDS initially 4–6 mg/24 h patch. Increase to 9.5 mg/24 h patch after 4 weeks. Maximum dose 9.5 mg/ 24 h patch.	
Tacrine (Cognex)	PO 40 mg/d (10 mg 4 times daily) for 6 wk. If aminotransferase levels are satisfactory after weekly monitoring, may increase the dose to 80 mg/d (20 mg 4 times daily). If liver function remains normal, may increase daily dose by 10 mg q 6 wk to a total of 120–160 mg/d.	

TDS, transdermal delivery system.

duration of action and lower incidence of side effects than neostigmine, and it is the maintenance drug of choice for patients with myasthenia gravis. An added advantage is the availability of a slow-release form, which is effective for 8 to 12 hours. When this form is taken at bedtime, the patient does not have to take other medications during the night and does not awaken too weak to swallow.

Reversible Indirect-Acting Cholinergics (Anticholinesterases) for Alzheimer's Disease

Donepezil (Aricept) is used to treat mild to moderate Alzheimer's disease. In long-term studies, donepezil delayed the progression of the disease for up to 55 weeks. Donepezil increases acetylcholine in the brain by inhibiting its metabolism. Donepezil is well absorbed after oral administration, and absorption is unaffected by food. The drug is highly bound (96%) to plasma proteins. It is metabolized in the liver to several metabolites, some of which are pharmacologically active; metabolites and some unchanged drug are excreted mainly in urine. Adverse effects include nausea, vomiting, diarrhea, bradycardia, and possible aggravation of asthma, peptic ulcer disease, and chronic obstructive pulmonary disease.

Galantamine (Razadyne) is a newer long-acting anticholinesterase agent approved by the U.S. Food and Drug Administration (FDA) for the treatment of Alzheimer's disease. Its pharmacokinetics and adverse-effect profile are similar to donepezil and rivastigmine.

Rivastigmine (Exelon) is a long-acting central anticholinesterase agent approved for the treatment of mild to moderate dementia due to Alzheimer's disease and Parkinson's disease. Oral rivastigmine lasts 12 hours, making twice-a-day dosing possible. Rivastigmine transdermal is applied as a patch once a day. Like other drugs in this class, it is not a cure for Alzheimer's disease but does slow the progression of symptoms. Rivastigmine is metabolized by the liver and excreted in the feces. It has an adverse-effect profile similar to donepezil. Dosages are typically increased slowly untill therapeutic dosage is reached to minimize certain side effects (e.g., nausea, vomiting, loss if appetite). It may be taken with food to decrease GI distress.

Nursing Process

Assessment

Assess the patient's condition in relation to disorders for which cholinergic drugs are used.

- In patients known to have myasthenia gravis, assess for muscle weakness. This may be manifested by ptosis (drooping) of the upper eyelid and diplopia (double vision) caused by weakness of the eye muscles. More severe disease may be indicated by difficulty in chewing, swallowing, and speaking; accumulation of oral secretions,

Nursing Process continues on page 318

which the patient may be unable to expectorate or swallow; decreased skeletal muscle activity, including impaired chest expansion; and eventual respiratory failure.

- In patients with possible urinary retention, assess for bladder distention, time and amount of previous urination, and fluid intake.

- In patients with possible paralytic ileus, assess for presence of bowel sounds, abdominal distention, and elimination pattern.

- In patients with Alzheimer's disease, assess for abilities and limitations in relation to memory, cognitive functioning, self-care activities, and pre-existing conditions that may be aggravated by a cholinergic drug.

Nursing Diagnoses

- Impaired Gas Exchange related to increased respiratory secretions, bronchospasm, and/or respiratory paralysis

- Ineffective Breathing Pattern related to bronchoconstriction

- Ineffective Airway Clearance related to increased respiratory secretions

- Self-Care Deficit related to muscle weakness, cognitive impairment, or diplopia

- Deficient Knowledge: Drug administration and effects

Planning/Goals

The patient will

- Verbalize or demonstrate correct drug administration

- Improve in self-care abilities

- Regain usual patterns of urinary and bowel elimination

- Maintain effective oxygenation of tissues

- Report adverse drug effects

- For patients with myasthenia gravis, at least one family member will verbalize or demonstrate correct drug administration, symptoms of too much or too little drug, and emergency care procedures.

- For patients with dementia, a caregiver will verbalize or demonstrate correct drug administration and knowledge of adverse effects to be reported to a health care provider.

Interventions

- Use measures to prevent or decrease the need for cholinergic drugs. Ambulation, adequate fluid intake, and judicious use of opioid analgesics or other sedative-type drugs help prevent postoperative urinary retention. In myasthenia gravis, muscle weakness is aggravated by exercise and improved by rest. Therefore, scheduling activities to avoid excessive fatigue and to allow adequate rest periods may be beneficial.

- With drug therapy for Alzheimer's disease, assist and teach caregivers to:

- Maintain a quiet, stable environment and daily routines to decrease confusion (e.g., verbal or written reminders, simple directions, adequate lighting, calendars, personal objects within view and reach).

- Avoid altering dosage or stopping the drug without consulting the prescribing physician.

- Be sure that the patient keeps appointments for supervision and blood tests.

- Report signs and symptoms (i.e., skin rash, jaundice, light-colored stools) that may indicate hepatotoxicity for patients taking tacrine.

- Notify surgeons about tacrine therapy. Exaggerated muscle relaxation may occur if succinylcholine-type drugs are given.

- Do not give cholinergic drugs for bladder atony and urinary retention or for paralytic ileus in the presence of an obstruction.

- For long-term use, assist patients and families to establish a schedule of drug administration that best meets the patient's needs.

- With myasthenia gravis, recommend that one or more family members be trained in cardiopulmonary resuscitation.

In addition, teaching guidelines are given in the accompanying display.

Evaluation

- Observe and interview about the adequacy of urinary elimination.

- Observe abilities and limitations in self-care.

- Question the patient and at least one family member of the patient with myasthenia gravis about correct drug usage, symptoms of underdosage and overdosage, and emergency care procedures.

- Question caregivers of patients with dementia about the patient's level of functioning and response to medication.

Principles of Therapy

Use in Myasthenia Gravis

Guidelines for the use of anticholinesterase drugs in myasthenia gravis include the following:

- Drug dosage should be increased gradually until maximal benefit is obtained. Larger doses are often required with increased physical activity, emotional stress, infections, and sometimes premenstrually.

- Some patients with myasthenia gravis cannot tolerate optimal doses of anticholinesterase drugs unless atropine is given to decrease the severity of adverse reactions due to muscarinic activation. However, atropine should be given only if necessary because it may mask the sudden increase of adverse effects. Such an increase is the first sign of overdose.

▪ Drug dosage in excess of the amount needed to maintain muscle strength and function can produce a cholinergic crisis. A cholinergic crisis is characterized by excessive stimulation of the parasympathetic nervous system. If early symptoms are not treated, hypotension and respiratory failure may occur. At high doses, anticholinesterase drugs weaken rather than strengthen skeletal muscle contraction because excessive amounts of acetylcholine accumulate at motor endplates and reduce nerve impulse transmission to muscle tissue.

▪ Some people acquire partial or total resistance to anticholinesterase drugs after taking them for months or years. Therefore do not assume that drug therapy that is effective initially will continue to be effective over the long-term course of the disease.

▪ All anticholinesterase drugs should be taken with food or milk to decrease the risk of gastric distress and ulceration.

Applying Your Knowledge 19-1

Ms. Humbarger tells you that she usually increases the dose of her medication according to her symptoms and that she usually requires less medication when she is in the hospital. What is your most appropriate action/response?

Cholinergic vs. Myasthenic Crisis: Recognition and Management

Differentiating myasthenic crisis from cholinergic crisis may be difficult because both are characterized by respiratory difficulty or failure. It is necessary to differentiate between them, however, because they require opposite treatment measures. Myasthenic crisis is an exacerbation of the disease process

Patient Teaching Guidelines ▸ Cholinergic Drugs

General Considerations

▪ Because cholinergic drugs used for urinary retention usually act within 60 minutes after administration, be sure bathroom facilities are available.

▪ Wear a medical alert identification device if taking long-term cholinergic drug therapy for myasthenia gravis, hypotonic bladder, or Alzheimer's disease.

▪ Atropine 0.6 mg IV may be administered for overdose of cholinergic drugs.

▪ Record symptoms of myasthenia gravis and effects of drug therapy, especially when drug therapy is initiated and medication doses are being titrated. The amount of medication required to control symptoms of myasthenia gravis varies greatly and the physician needs this information to adjust the dosage correctly.

▪ Do not overexert yourself if you have myasthenia gravis. Rest between activities. Although the dose of medication may be increased during periods of increased activity, it is desirable to space activities to obtain optimal benefit from the drug, at the lowest possible dose, with the fewest adverse effects.

▪ Report increased muscle weakness, difficulty breathing, or recurrence of myasthenic symptoms to the physician. These are signs of drug underdosage (myasthenic crisis) and indicate a need to increase or change drug therapy.

▪ Report adverse reactions, including abdominal cramps, diarrhea, excessive oral secretions, difficulty in breathing, and muscle weakness. These are signs of drug overdosage (cholinergic crisis) and require immediate discontinuation of drugs and treatment by the physician. Respiratory failure can result if this condition is not recognized and treated properly.

▪ Patients taking tacrine need weekly monitoring of liver aminotransferase levels for 18 weeks when initiating

therapy and weekly monitoring for 6 weeks after any increase in dose. Caregivers should report any signs or symptoms of adverse drug reactions such as nausea, vomiting, diarrhea, rash, jaundice, or change in the color of stools. The drug should not be suddenly discontinued.

▪ If dizziness or syncope occurs when taking tacrine, donepezil, or other anticholinesterase drugs, ambulation should be supervised to avoid injury.

▪ Caregivers should record observed effects of anticholinesterase medications given to treat Alzheimer's disease. These medications are often titrated upward to improve cognitive function and delay symptom progression, and this information will be helpful to the prescriber.

Self- or Caregiver Administration

▪ Take drugs as directed on a regular schedule to maintain consistent blood levels and control of symptoms.

▪ Do not chew or crush sustained-release medications.

▪ Take oral cholinergics on an empty stomach to lessen nausea and vomiting. Also, food decreases absorption of tacrine by up to 40%.

▪ Ensure adequate fluid intake if vomiting or diarrhea occurs as a side effect of cholinergic medications.

▪ Avoid taking St. John's wort because concurrent use may reduce blood levels of donepezil.

▪ Remove Exelon Patch from sealed pouch immediately before application. Apply Exelon Patch to clean dry infact skin on upper or lower back, upper arm, or chest. Select a new site with each patch application and do not re-use a site within 14 days. Do not cut or tear patch. Remove the patch after 24 hours. You may bath, swim, or shower while wearing the patch.

and its clinical manifestations, requiring more anticholinesterase drug. Cholinergic crisis is a drug-induced overstimulation of the parasympathetic nervous system, requiring discontinuation of any anticholinesterase drug that the patient has been receiving.

An accurate diagnosis may be determined from signs and symptoms and their timing in relation to medication; that is, signs and symptoms having their onset within approximately 1 hour after a dose of anticholinesterase drug are more likely to be caused by cholinergic crisis (too much drug). Signs and symptoms beginning 3 hours or more after a drug dose are more likely to be caused by myasthenic crisis (too little drug).

If the differential diagnosis cannot be made on the basis of signs and symptoms, the patient can be intubated, mechanically ventilated, and observed closely until a diagnosis is possible. Still another way to differentiate between the two conditions is for the physician to inject a small dose of IV edrophonium (Tensilon). The ideal test dose of edrophonium has not been determined. An incremental dosing schedule begins with 2 milligrams IV, followed by a 60-second period of time during which the response of the individual is observed. Subsequent doses of 3 and 5 milligrams may be given if indicated by a lack of response. If the edrophonium test causes a dramatic improvement in breathing, the test is considered positive and the diagnosis is myasthenic crisis. If the edrophonium test makes the patient even weaker, the diagnosis is cholinergic crisis. Edrophonium or any other diagnostic pharmacologic agent should be administered only after endotracheal intubation and controlled ventilation have been instituted.

Treatment for cholinergic crisis includes withdrawal of anticholinesterase drugs; administration of atropine, an anticholinergic drug (see Chap. 20); and measures to maintain respiration. It is important to understand that atropine reverses only the muscarinic effects of cholinergic crisis, having no effect on reversing nicotinic receptor–mediated skeletal muscle weakness. Endotracheal intubation and mechanical ventilation may be necessary due to this profound skeletal muscle weakness, including muscles of respiration.

Treatment for myasthenic crisis includes administration of additional anticholinesterase medications and measures to maintain respirations until the medications are effective in improving muscle strength.

Use in Alzheimer's Disease

The goal of drug therapy for Alzheimer's disease is to slow the loss of memory and cognition, thus preserving the independence of the individual for as long as possible. Practice guidelines developed by the American Academy of Neurology (2001, reviewed 2003) recommend early diagnosis and treatment of Alzheimer's disease with cholinesterase inhibitors for all patients with mild to moderate symptoms. Although these drugs do not cure Alzheimer's disease, they do delay the onset of the disease somewhat and bring about a slight improvement in cognition and function. Additional medications that may be beneficial in slowing the progression of

Evidence-Based Practice

19-1 The Role of Inflammation and NSAIDs in Alzheimer's Disease

There is research evidence that brain inflammation may contribute to the changes in the brain associated with Alzheimer's disease. Some studies have indicated that the long-term use of nonsteroidal anti-inflammatory drugs (NSAIDs), such as ibuprofen, naproxen, and aspirin, before the onset of symptoms of Alzheimer's disease may help prevent the disorder. Other researchers have suggested that NSAIDs may help slow the progression of the disease. A clinical trial tested two NSAIDs, rofecoxib (Vioxx) and naproxen (Aleve), and found these drugs did not delay the progression of Alzheimer's disease in those previously diagnosed with the disorder. The Alzheimer's Disease Anti-inflammatory Prevention Trial (ADAPT) was designed to test celecoxib (Celebrex) and naproxen to determine if NSAIDs are beneficial in preventing Alzheimer's disease in healthy older people. However, the ADAPT study was suspended because of concerns over increased adverse cardiovascular events associated with the use of NSAIDS (see Chap. 7). At this time, NSAIDs are not recommended for the prevention or treatment of Alzheimer's disease.

Alzheimer's disease include high-dose vitamin E therapy, selegiline, and memantine (Namenda), an N-methyl D-aspartate (NMDA) antagonist. Estrogen is not recommended as a treatment for Alzheimer's disease. Although some studies suggest that inflammation may play a role in Alzheimer's disease, anti-inflammatory drugs such as prednisone or NSAIDs are not recommended for treatment at this time (see Evidence-Based Practice Box 19-1).

Toxicity of Cholinergic Drugs: Recognition and Management

Atropine, an anticholinergic, antimuscarinic drug, is a specific antidote to cholinergic agents. The drug and equipment for its injection should be readily available whenever cholinergic drugs are given. It is important to note that atropine reverses only the muscarinic effects of cholinergic drugs, primarily in the heart, smooth muscle, and glands. Atropine does not interact with nicotinic receptors and therefore cannot reverse the nicotinic effects of skeletal-muscle weakness or paralysis due to overdose of the indirect cholinergic drugs.

Management of Mushroom Poisoning

Muscarinic receptors in the parasympathetic nervous system were given their name because they can be stimulated by muscarine, an alkaloid that is found in small quantities in the *Amanita muscaria* mushroom. Some mushrooms found in North America, such as the Clitocybe and Inocybe mushrooms, however, contain much larger quantities of muscarine. Accidental or intentional ingestion of these mushrooms results in intense cholinergic stimulation (cholinergic crisis) and is potentially fatal. Atropine is the specific antidote for mushroom poisoning.

Toxicity of Irreversible Anticholinesterase Agents: Recognition and Management

Most irreversible anticholinesterase agents are highly lipid soluble and can enter the body by a variety of routes, including the eye, skin, respiratory system, and GI tract. Because they readily cross the blood–brain barrier, their effects are seen peripherally as well as centrally.

Exposure to toxic doses of irreversible anticholinesterase agents, such as organophosphate insecticides (malathion, parathion) or nerve gases (sarin, tabun, soman), produces a cholinergic crisis characterized by excessive cholinergic (muscarinic) stimulation and neuromuscular blockade. This cholinergic crisis occurs because the irreversible anticholinesterase poison binds to the enzyme acetylcholinesterase and inactivates it. Consequently, acetylcholine remains in cholinergic synapses and causes excessive stimulation of muscarinic and nicotinic receptors.

Emergency treatment includes decontamination procedures such as removing contaminated clothing, flushing the poison from skin and eyes, and using activated charcoal and lavage to remove ingested poison from the GI tract. Pharmacologic treatment includes administering atropine to counteract the muscarinic effects of the poison (e.g., salivation, urination, defecation, bronchial secretions, laryngospasm, bronchospasm).

To relieve the neuromuscular blockade produced by nicotinic effects of the poison, a second drug, pralidoxime, is needed. Pralidoxime (Protopam), a cholinesterase reactivator, is a specific antidote for overdose with irreversible anticholinesterase agents. Pralidoxime treats toxicity by causing the anticholinesterase poison to release the enzyme acetylcholinesterase. The reactivated acetylcholinesterase can then degrade excess acetylcholine at the cholinergic synapses, including the neuromuscular junction. Because pralidoxime cannot cross the blood–brain barrier, it is effective only in the peripheral areas of the body. Pralidoxime must be given as soon after the poisoning as possible. If too much time passes, the bond between the irreversible anticholinesterase agent and acetylcholinesterase becomes stronger and pralidoxime is unable to release the enzyme from the poison.

Treatment of anticholinesterase overdose may also require diazepam or lorazepam to control seizures. Mechanical ventilation may be necessary to treat respiratory paralysis.

Use in Special Populations

Use in Children

Bethanechol is occasionally used to treat urinary retention and paralytic ileus, but safety and effectiveness for children younger than 8 years of age have not been established. Neostigmine is used to treat myasthenia gravis and to reverse neuromuscular blockade after general anesthesia but is not recommended for urinary retention. Pyridostigmine may be used in the neonate of a mother with myasthenia gravis to treat difficulties with sucking, swallowing, and breathing.

Although galantamine and donepezil are approved only for the treatment of Alzheimer's disease, these medications are currently under investigation to treat attention deficit-hyperactivity disorder (ADHD). Some studies have shown that these medications may be useful in treating the child with ADHD by improving cognition relative to executive functioning, including planning, time-management, and organizational skills.

Precautions and adverse effects for cholinergic drugs are the same for children as for adults.

Use in Older Adults

Indirect-acting cholinergic drugs may be used in patients with myasthenia gravis or Alzheimer's disease or to treat overdoses of atropine and other centrally acting anticholinergic drugs (e.g., those used for parkinsonism). Older adults are more likely to experience adverse drug effects because of age-related physiologic changes and superimposed pathologic conditions.

Use in Patients With Renal Impairment

Because bethanechol and other cholinergic drugs increase pressure in the urinary tract by stimulating detrusor muscle contraction and relaxation of urinary sphincters, they are contraindicated for patients with urinary tract obstructions or weaknesses in the bladder wall. Administering a cholinergic drug to these people might result in rupture of the bladder.

Some aspects of the pharmacokinetics of cholinergic drugs are unknown. Many of the drugs are degraded enzymatically by cholinesterases. However, a few (e.g., neostigmine, pyridostigmine) undergo hepatic metabolism and tubular excretion in the kidneys. Renal impairment may result in accumulation and increased adverse effects, especially with chronic use.

Use in Patients With Hepatic Impairment

The hepatic metabolism of neostigmine and pyridostigmine may be impaired by liver disease, resulting in increased adverse effects.

Use in Critical Illness

Cholinergic drugs have several specific uses in critical illness:

- Neostigmine, pyridostigmine, and edrophonium to reverse neuromuscular blockade (skeletal muscle paralysis) caused by nondepolarizing muscle relaxants

- Anticholinesterase drugs to treat myasthenic crisis and improve muscle strength

- Physostigmine in severe cases as an antidote to anticholinergic poisoning with drugs such as atropine or tricyclic antidepressants

Use in Home Care

Medications to treat long-term conditions such as myasthenia gravis or Alzheimer's disease are often administered in the home setting. The person using the drugs may have difficulty with self-administration. The patient with myasthenia gravis may have diplopia or diminished muscle strength that makes it difficult to self-administer medications. Strict adherence to timely medication administration promotes optimal blood levels of drugs and optimal symptom control. The patient with Alzheimer's disease may have problems with remembering to take medications and may easily underdose or overdose him- or herself. It is important to work with responsible family members in such cases to ensure accurate drug administration.

 Applying Your Knowledge 19-2

How Can You Avoid This Medication Error?
After administering her medication, you leave Ms. Humbarger's room to tend to other patients. When you return 4 hours later, Ms. Humbarger complains that she is having increased difficulty breathing. You recognize this as a cholinergic crisis and prepare to administer the antidote atropine.

Nursing Actions Cholinergic Drugs

NURSING ACTIONS	RATIONALE/EXPLANATION
1. Administer accurately	
a. Give oral bethanechol before meals.	If these drugs are given after meals, nausea and vomiting may occur because the drug stimulates contraction of muscles in the gastrointestinal (GI) tract.
b. With pyridostigmine and other drugs for myasthenia gravis, give at regularly scheduled intervals with food or milk.	For consistent blood levels and control of symptoms. These drugs increase the risk of GI distress and ulceration.
c. Give tacrine on an empty stomach, 1 hour before or 2 hours after a meal, if possible, at regular intervals around the clock (e.g., q6h). Give with meals if GI upset occurs.	Food decreases absorption and decreases serum drug levels by 30% or more. Regular intervals increase therapeutic effects and decrease adverse effects.
d. Give donepezil at bedtime.	Manufacturer's recommendation
e. Give galantamine and rivastigmine with food.	To decrease GI distress
2. Observe for therapeutic effects	
a. When the drug is given for postoperative hypoperistalsis, observe for bowel sounds, passage of flatus through the rectum, or a bowel movement.	These are indicators of increased GI muscle tone and motility.
b. When bethanechol or neostigmine is given for urinary retention, micturition usually occurs within approximately 60 minutes. If it does not, urinary catheterization may be necessary.	
c. When the drug is given to clients with myasthenia gravis, observe for increased muscle strength as shown by:	
(1) Decreased or absent ptosis of eyelids	With neostigmine, onset of action is 2–4 hours after oral administration and 10–30 minutes after injection. Duration is approximately 3–4 hours. With pyridostigmine, onset of action is approximately 30–45 minutes after oral use, 15 minutes after IM injection, and 2–5 minutes after IV injection. Duration is approximately 4–6 hours. The long-acting form of pyridostigmine lasts 8–12 hours.
(2) Decreased difficulty with chewing, swallowing, and speech	
(3) Increased skeletal muscle strength, increased tolerance of activity, less fatigue	
d. With cholinergic drugs to treat Alzheimer's disease (tacrine, donepezil, galantamine, and rivastigmine) observe for improvement in memory and cognitive functioning in activities of daily living.	Improved functioning is most likely to occur in patients with mild to moderate dementia.
3. Observe for adverse effects	Adverse effects occur with usual therapeutic doses but are more likely with large doses. They are caused by stimulation of the parasympathetic nervous system.
a. Central nervous system effects—convulsions, dizziness, drowsiness, headache, loss of consciousness	
b. Respiratory effects—increased secretions, bronchospasm, laryngospasm, respiratory failure	
c. Cardiovascular effects—dysrhythmias (bradycardia, tachycardia, atrioventricular block), cardiac arrest, hypotension, syncope	These may be detected early by regular assessment of blood pressure and heart rate. Bradycardia is probably the most likely dysrhythmia to occur. GI effects commonly occur. Tacrine may be hepatotoxic.

NURSING ACTIONS	RATIONALE/EXPLANATION
d. GI effects—nausea and vomiting, diarrhea, increased peristalsis, abdominal cramping, increased secretions (i.e., saliva, gastric and intestinal secretions). With tacrine, observe for signs of hepatotoxicity (e.g., jaundice, elevated liver enzymes).	
e. Other effects—increased frequency and urgency of urination, increased sweating, miosis, skin rash	Skin rashes are most likely to occur from formulations of neostigmine or pyridostigmine that contain bromide.
4. Observe for drug interactions	
a. Drugs that *increase* effects of direct-acting cholinergics such as bethanechol:	
(1) Other cholinergic drugs	Have additive cholinergic effect
(2) Cholinesterase inhibitors	Prevent degradation of cholinesterase and prolong cholinergic response
b. Drugs that *decrease* effects of cholinergic agents:	
(1) Anticholinergic drugs (e.g., atropine)	Antagonize effects of cholinergic drugs (miosis; increased tone and motility in smooth muscle of GI tract, bronchi, and urinary bladder; bradycardia). Atropine is the specific antidote for overdosage with cholinergic drugs.
(2) Antihistamines	Most antihistamines have anticholinergic properties that antagonize effects of cholinergic drugs.
c. Drugs that *decrease* effects of anticholinesterase agents:	
(1) Corticosteroids	May antagonize anticholinesterase agents and increase muscle weakness in myasthenia gravis. However, corticosteroids are often prescribed for their anti-immune effect.
(2) Aminoglycoside antibiotics (e.g., gentamicin)	Can produce neuromuscular blockade that antagonizes effects of anticholinesterase drugs and causes muscle weakness in myasthenia gravis
(3) Succinylcholine	Increased and prolonged neuromuscular blockade occurs when indirect-acting cholinergics and succinylcholine are given concurrently.
d. Drug that *increases* effects of tacrine:	
(1) Cimetidine	Slows metabolism of tacrine in the liver, thereby increasing risks of accumulation and adverse effects

Key Concepts

- Cholinergic drugs stimulate the parasympathetic nervous system directly by stimulating cholinergic receptors or indirectly by inhibiting the enzymatic metabolism of acetylcholine in synapses.

- Both direct-acting cholinergic drugs and indirect-acting cholinergic drugs (or anticholinesterase drugs) have widespread parasympathetic effects when they activate muscarinic receptors in cardiac muscle, smooth muscle, exocrine glands, and the eye.

- Indirect-acting cholinergic drugs also stimulate nicotinic receptors in skeletal muscles, resulting in improved skeletal muscle tone and strength.

- The direct-acting cholinergic drug, bethanechol, is used to treat urinary retention due to urinary bladder atony and postoperative abdominal distention due to paralytic ileus.

- Indirect-acting cholinergic or anticholinesterase drugs are indicated to treat myasthenia gravis and Alzheimer's disease.

- Edrophonium is used to differentiate between myasthenic crisis (too little cholinergic medication) and cholinergic crisis (too much cholinergic medication).

- Atropine reverses muscarinic effects due to overdose of cholinergic drugs but does not reverse the nicotinic effects of skeletal-muscle weakness or paralysis due to overdose of indirect cholinergic drugs.

- Pralidoxime, a cholinesterase reactivator, is the specific treatment for neuromuscular blockade due to overdose with irreversible indirect cholinergic drugs.

Review and Application Exercises

Short Answer Exercises

1. What are the actions of cholinergic drugs?

2. Which neurotransmitter is involved in cholinergic (parasympathetic) stimulation?

3. When a cholinergic drug is given to treat myasthenia gravis, what is the expected effect?

4. What is the difference between cholinergic crisis and myasthenic crisis? How are they treated?

5. When indirect-acting cholinergic drugs are used to treat Alzheimer's disease, what is the desired effect?

6. Is a cholinergic drug the usual treatment of choice for urinary bladder atony? Why or why not?

7. What are the adverse effects of cholinergic drugs?

8. How are overdoses of cholinergic drugs treated?

NCLEX-Style Questions

9. A patient with myasthenia gravis is admitted to the emergency department with complaints of muscle weakness and respiratory distress. You give an ordered "test dose" of edrophonium (Tensilon) and the patient ceases to breathe, requiring mechanical ventilation. The results of this test dose indicate
   a. The patient is underdosed on his medications and is in myasthenic crisis.
   b. The patient is allergic to edrophonium and is having an anaphylactic reaction.
   c. The patient is overdosed on his medications and is in cholinergic crisis.
   d. The patient's condition is not due to myasthenia gravis because edrophonium did not improve the symptoms.

10. A 65-year-old patient has been admitted with a diagnosis of benign prostatic hyperplasia. How should the nurse respond to an order for bethanechol (Urecholine) to treat urinary retention in this situation?
    a. Give the medication as ordered.
    b. Insert a Foley catheter before administering the medication.
    c. Provide a urinal because urinary frequency will increase after drug administration.
    d. Question this order because the patient's urinary retention is due to an obstructive process.

11. The nurse should be prepared to administer which of the following drugs as an antidote to cholinergic drug overdose?
    a. epinephrine (Adrenalin)
    b. diphenhydramine (Benadryl)
    c. atropine (AtroPen)
    d. propanolol (Inderal)

12. You are teaching family members how to administer galantamine for Alzheimer's disease. Your instructions should include which of the following?
    a. Take this medication with food.
    b. Take this medication on an empty stomach.
    c. Take this medication at bedtime.
    d. Take this medication at the start of each day.

13. When treating a patient in cholinergic crisis due to exposure to an organophosphate insecticide, the nurse must be prepared to administer which drug to relieve neuromuscular blockade?
    a. atropine (AtroPen)
    b. pralidoxime (Protopam)
    c. epinephrine (Adrenalin)
    d. physostigmine (Antilirium)

Selected References

Doody, R. S., Stevens, J. C., Beck, C., Dubinsky, R. M., Kaye, J. A., Gwyther, L., Mohs, R. C., Thal, L. J., Whitehouse, P. J., DeKosky, S. T., & Cummings, J. L. (2001, reviewed 2003). Report of the Quality Standards Subcommittee of the American Academy of Neurology Practice parameter: Management of dementia (an evidence-based review). *Neurology, 56,* 1154–1166.

Drug facts and comparisons. (Updated monthly). St. Louis, MO: Facts and Comparisons.

Faulkner, J. D., Bartlet, J., & Hicks, P. (2005). Alzheimer's disease. In J. T. DiPiro, R. L. Talbert, G. C. Yee, G. R. Matzke, B. G. Wells, & L. M. Posey (Eds.), *Pharmacotherapy: A pathophysiologic approach* (6th ed., pp. 1157–1173). New York: McGraw-Hill.

Myasthenia Gravis Foundation of America, Inc. (2006, Sept. 30). *Health care professionals: Clinical overview of myasthenia gravis.* Retrieved August 29, 2007, from http://www.myasthenia.org/hp_clinicaloverview.cfm

National Institute on Aging. (2006, Dec. 14). *Treatment for Alzheimer's disease: Alzheimer's Disease Education & Referral Center.* Retrieved August 29, 2007, from http://www.nia.nih.gov/Alzheimers/AlzheimersInformation/Treatment/

Smeltzer, S. C., Bare, B. G., Hinkle, J. L., & Cheever, K. H. (2008). *Brunner & Suddarth's textbook of medical-surgical nursing* (11th ed., pp. 2285–2288). Philadelphia: Lippincott Williams & Wilkins.

Anticholinergic Drugs

LEARNING OBJECTIVES

After studying this chapter, you will be able to:

1. List characteristics of anticholinergic drugs in terms of effects on body tissues, indications for use, nursing process implications, observation of patient response, and teaching patients.
2. Discuss atropine as the prototype of anticholinergic drugs.
3. Discuss clinical disorders or symptoms for which anticholinergic drugs are used.
4. Describe the mechanism by which atropine relieves bradycardia.
5. Review anticholinergic effects of antipsychotics, tricyclic antidepressants, and antihistamines.
6. Discuss principles of therapy and nursing process for using anticholinergic drugs in special populations.
7. Describe the signs and symptoms of atropine or anticholinergic drug overdose and its treatment.
8. Teach patients about the safe, effective use of anticholinergic drugs.

Applying Your Knowledge

J. E. Smoot is a 77-year-old man who has chronic obstructive pulmonary disease and experiences a syncopal episode. He is admitted to your unit with stable vital signs. The physician orders ipratropium two puffs four times a day and places Mr. Smoot on a cardiac monitor.

Introduction

Anticholinergic drugs block the action of acetylcholine on the parasympathetic nervous system. Most anticholinergic drugs interact with muscarinic cholinergic receptors in the brain, secretory glands, heart, and smooth muscle and are sometimes called *antimuscarinic drugs*. When given at high doses, a few anticholinergic drugs are also able to block *nicotinic receptors* in autonomic ganglia and skeletal muscles. Glycopyrrolate is an example of such a medication. This drug class includes belladonna alkaloids and their derivatives, such as atropine, and many synthetic substitutes.

Most anticholinergic medications are either *tertiary amines* or *quaternary amines* (Table 20-1). Tertiary amines are uncharged lipid-soluble molecules. Atropine and scopolamine are tertiary amines and therefore are able to cross cell membranes readily. They are well absorbed from the gastrointestinal (GI) tract and conjunctiva, and they cross the blood–brain barrier. Tertiary amines are excreted in the urine.

Some belladonna derivatives and synthetic anticholinergics are quaternary amines. These drugs carry a positive charge and are lipid insoluble. Consequently, they do not readily cross cell

Table 20-1	Common Tertiary Amine and Quaternary Amine Anticholinergic Drugs

TERTIARY AMINES	QUATERNARY AMINES
Atropine	Glycopyrrolate (Robinul)
Benztropine (Cogentin)	Ipratropium (Atrovent)
Darifenacin hydrobromide (Enablex)	
Dicyclomine hydrochloride (Bentyl)	Methscopolamine (Pamine)
Flavoxate (Urispas)	
l-Hyoscyamine (Anaspaz)	
Oxybutynin (Ditropan)	Tiotropium (Spiriva)
Scopolamine	Trospium chloride (Sanctura)
Solifenacin succinate (Vesicare)	
Tolterodine (Detrol, Detrol LA, and Oxytrol)	
Trihexyphenidyl (Trihexy)	

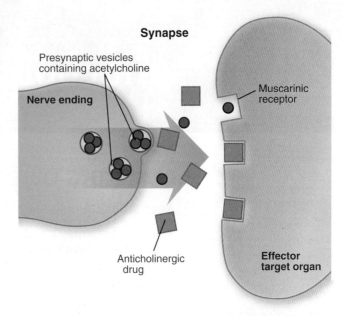

Figure 20-1 ■ Mechanism of action of anticholinergic drugs. Anticholinergic (antimuscarinic) drugs prevent acetylcholine from interacting with muscarinic receptors on target effector organs, thus blocking or decreasing a parasympathetic response in these organs.

membranes. They are poorly absorbed from the GI tract and do not cross the blood–brain barrier. Quaternary amines are excreted largely in the feces.

General Characteristics of Anticholinergic Drugs

Mechanism of Action and Effects

These drugs act by occupying receptor sites on target organs innervated by the parasympathetic nervous system, thereby leaving fewer receptor sites free to respond to acetylcholine (Fig. 20-1). Parasympathetic response is absent or decreased, depending on the number of receptors blocked by anticholinergic drugs and the underlying degree of parasympathetic activity. Because cholinergic *muscarinic receptors* are widely distributed in the body, anticholinergic drugs produce effects in a variety of locations, including the central nervous system (CNS), heart, smooth muscle, glands, and the eye.

Specific effects on body tissues and organs include the following:

- CNS stimulation followed by depression, which may result in coma and death. This is most likely to occur with large doses of anticholinergic drugs that cross the blood–brain barrier (atropine, scopolamine, and antiparkinson agents).

- Decreased cardiovascular response to parasympathetic (vagal) stimulation that slows heart rate. Atropine is the anticholinergic drug most often used for its cardiovascular effects. According to Advanced Cardiac Life Support (ACLS) protocol, atropine is the drug of choice to treat symptomatic sinus bradycardia. Low doses (<0.5 mg) may

produce a slight and temporary decrease in heart rate; however, moderate to large doses (0.5–1 mg) increase heart rate by blocking parasympathetic vagal stimulation. Although the increase in heart rate may be therapeutic in bradycardia, it can be an adverse effect in patients with other types of heart disease because atropine increases the myocardial oxygen demand. Atropine usually has little or no effect on blood pressure. Large doses cause facial flushing because of dilation of blood vessels in the neck.

- Bronchodilation and decreased respiratory tract secretions. Anticholinergics block the action of acetylcholine in bronchial smooth muscle when given by inhalation. This action reduces intracellular GMP, a bronchoconstrictive substance. When anticholinergic drugs are given systemically, respiratory secretions decrease and may become viscous, resulting in mucous plugging of small respiratory passages. Administering the medications by inhalation decreases this effect while preserving the beneficial bronchodilation effect.

- Antispasmodic effects in the GI tract due to decreased muscle tone and motility. The drugs have little inhibitory effect on gastric acid secretion with usual doses and insignificant effects on pancreatic and intestinal secretions.

- *Mydriasis* and *cycloplegia* in the eye. Normally, anticholinergics do not change intraocular pressure, but with narrow-angle glaucoma, they may increase intraocular pressure and precipitate an episode of acute glaucoma. When the pupil is fully dilated, photophobia may be uncomfortable, and reflexes to light and accommodation may disappear.

▪ Miscellaneous effects include decreased secretions from salivary and sweat glands; relaxation of ureters, urinary bladder, and the detrusor muscle; and relaxation of smooth muscle in the gallbladder and bile ducts.

The clinical usefulness of anticholinergic drugs is limited by their widespread effects. Consequently, several synthetic drugs have been developed in an effort to increase selectivity of action on particular body tissues, especially to retain the antispasmodic and antisecretory effects of atropine while eliminating its adverse effects. This effort has been less than successful—all the synthetic drugs produce atropine-like adverse effects when given in sufficient dosage.

Some synthetic drugs are used for antispasmodic effects in GI disorders and overactive urinary bladder. Another group of synthetic drugs includes centrally active anticholinergics used in the treatment of Parkinson's disease (see Chap. 12). They balance the relative cholinergic dominance that causes the movement disorders associated with parkinsonism.

Indications for Use

Anticholinergic drugs are used for disorders in many body systems. Clinical indications include the following.

GI Disorders. Anticholinergics have been used for peptic ulcer disease, gastritis, pylorospasm, and diverticulitis. These conditions are often characterized by excessive gastric acid and abdominal pain because of increased motility and spasm of GI smooth muscle. However, anticholinergics are weak inhibitors of gastric acid secretion, even in maximal doses that usually produce intolerable adverse effects, making them a second choice for treatment of peptic ulcers. Although the drugs do not heal peptic ulcers, they may relieve abdominal pain by relaxing GI smooth muscle. In addition, anticholinergics may be helpful in reducing the frequency of bowel movements and abdominal discomfort associated with irritable colon or colitis. Anticholinergics are not usually prescribed for chronic inflammatory disorders (e.g., diverticulitis, ulcerative colitis) or acute intestinal infections (e.g., bacterial, viral, amebic). Other drugs are more useful in treating the diarrhea and increased intestinal motility that occurs in these conditions.

Genitourinary Disorders. Anticholinergic drugs are the drugs of choice for their antispasmodic effects on smooth muscle to relieve the symptoms of urinary incontinence and frequency that accompany an overactive bladder. In infections such as cystitis, urethritis, and prostatitis, the drugs decrease the frequency and pain of urination. The drugs are also given to increase bladder capacity in enuresis, paraplegia, or neurogenic bladder.

Ophthalmology. Anticholinergic drugs are applied topically for mydriatic and cycloplegic effects to aid examination or surgery. They are also used to treat some inflammatory disorders. Anticholinergic preparations used in ophthalmology are discussed further in Chapter 63.

Respiratory Disorders. Anticholinergic drugs are used for respiratory disorders characterized by bronchoconstriction (i.e., asthma, chronic bronchitis). Ipratropium or tiotropium bromide may be given by inhalation for bronchodilating effects (see Chap. 44).

Cardiac Disorders. Atropine may be given to increase heart rate in bradycardia and heart block characterized by hypotension and shock.

Parkinson's Disease. Anticholinergic drugs are given for their central effects in decreasing salivation, spasticity, and tremors. They are used mainly in patients who have minimal symptoms, who do not respond to levodopa, or who cannot tolerate levodopa because of adverse reactions or contraindications. An additional use of anticholinergic drugs is to relieve Parkinson-like symptoms that occur with older antipsychotic drugs.

Preoperative Use. Anticholinergics are given to prevent vagal stimulation and potential bradycardia, hypotension, and cardiac arrest. They are also given to reduce respiratory tract secretions, especially in head and neck surgery and bronchoscopy.

Toxicity and Poisoning. Anticholinergics are used treat anticholinesterase toxicity, mushroom poisoning, or organophosphate pesticide poisoning (see Chap. 19). Atropine is given to treat excessive cholinergic stimulation.

Contraindications to Use

Contraindications to the use of anticholinergic drugs include any condition characterized by symptoms that would be aggravated by the drugs. Some of these are prostatic hypertrophy, myasthenia gravis, hyperthyroidism, glaucoma, tachydysrhythmia, myocardial infarction, and heart failure unless bradycardia is present. Anticholinergic drugs should not be given in hiatal hernia or other conditions contributing to reflux esophagitis because the drugs delay gastric emptying, relax the cardioesophageal sphincter, and increase esophageal reflux.

Individual Drugs

The therapeutic uses, dosages, and routes of administration for selected anticholinergic drugs are presented in Table 20-2.

Belladonna Alkaloids and Derivatives

P **Atropine**, the prototype of anticholinergic drugs, is a naturally occurring belladonna alkaloid that can be extracted from the belladonna plant or prepared synthetically. It is usually prepared as atropine sulfate, a salt that is very soluble in water. It is well absorbed from the GI tract and distributed throughout the body. It crosses the blood–brain barrier to enter the CNS, where large doses produce stimulant effects and toxic doses produce depressant effects. Atropine is also absorbed systemically when applied locally to mucous membranes. The drug is rapidly excreted in the urine. Pharmacologic effects are of short duration except for ocular effects, which may last for several days.

Table 20-2	Drugs at a Glance: Selected Anticholinergic Drugs		

		ROUTES AND DOSAGE RANGES	
Generic/TradeName	**Use**	**Adults**	**Children**
Belladonna Alkaloids and Derivatives			
Atropine	Systemic use	PO, IM, Sub-Q, IV 0.4–0.6 mg	PO, IM, Sub-Q, IV: 7–16 lb: 0.1 mg 16–24 lb: 0.15 mg 24–40 lb: 0.2 mg 40–65 lb: 0.3 mg 65–90 lb: 0.4 mg under 90 lb: 0.4–0.6 mg
	Surgery	IM, Sub-Q, or IV 0.4–0.6 mg prior to induction. Use 0.4-mg dose with cyclopropane anesthesia.	0.1 mg (newborn) to 0.6 mg (12 y) given Sub-Q 30 min prior to surgery
	Bradyarrhythmias	IV 0.5 mg (up to 3 mg) q 3–5 min PRN	
	Antidote for cholinergic poisoning	IV Titrate large doses of 2–3 mg as needed until signs of atropine toxicity appear and cholinergic crisis is controlled.	
Ophthalmic atropine (Isopto-Atropine)	Mydriatic/cycloplegia/ inflammation of uveal tract	*For refraction:* Instill 1 or 2 drops of 1% solution into eye(s) 1 h before refraction. *For uveitis:* Instill 1–2 drops of 1% solution into eye(s) 4 times daily.	*For refraction:* Instill 1–2 drops of 0.5% solution twice daily for 1–3 d before procedure.
Homatropine (Isopto-Homatropine)	Mydriatic/cycloplegia/ inflammation of uveal tract	*For refraction:* Instill 1–2 drops of 2% solution or 1 drop of 5% solution into eye before procedure. May repeat at 5–10 min intervals as needed. *For uveitis:* Instill 1 or 2 drops of 2% or 5% solution 2–4 times daily or every 3–4 h as needed.	*For refraction:* Instill 1 drop of 2% solution into eye before procedure. May repeat q 10 min as needed. *For uveitis:* Instill 1 drop of 2% solution 2–4 times daily
Hyoscyamine (Anaspaz)	Antispasmodic/antisecretory for gastrointestinal (GI) and genitourinary (GU) disorders	PO, SL 0.125–0.25 mg 3 or 4 times daily before meals and at bedtime. PO (timed- release formula): 0.375–0.75mg q12h. IM, IV, Sub-Q: 0.25–0.5 mg q6h	*Children 2–10 y:* PO 0.062–0.125 mg q 6–8h. *Children under 2 y:* half of the previous dose
Ipratropium (Atrovent)	Bronchodilation	2 puffs (36 mcg) of aerosol 4 times daily. Additional inhalations may be needed. Do not exceed 12 puffs/24h. Solution for inhalation: 500 mcg, 3 or 4 times daily.	
	Nasal spray for rhinorrhea	2 sprays/nostril of 0.03% spray 2 or 3 times daily. 2 sprays/nostril of 0.06% spray 3–4 times daily.	2 sprays/nostril of 0.03% spray 2 or 3 times daily
Scopolamine	Systemic use	PO 0.4–0.8 mg daily. Sub-Q, IM 0.32–0.65 mg IV 0.32–0.65 mg diluted in sterile water for injection	Not approved for PO use under 6 y *Parenteral:* 0.006 mg/kg *Maximum dose:* 0.3 mg

		ROUTES AND DOSAGE RANGES	
Generic/TradeName	**Use**	**Adults**	**Children**
	Antiemetic	*Transdermal:* Apply disk 4 h before antiemetic effect is needed. Replace q3d.	Not approved in children
	Mydriatic/cycloplegia/ inflammation of uveal tract	*For refraction:* Instill 1 or 2 drops into eye 1 h before refracting. *For uveitis:* Instill 1 or 2 drops into eye(s) up to 3 times daily.	Same as adult dose
Tiotropium bromide (Spiriva)	Bronchodilation	Inhalation of contents of one capsule (18 mcg) daily using the HandiHaler inhalation device	Safety and efficacy not established
Antisecretory/Antispasmodic Anticholinergics for Gastrointestinal Disorders			
Dicyclomine hydrochloride (Bentyl)	Antisecretory/antispasmodic	PO 20–40 mg before meals and at bedtime IM 20 mg before meals and at bedtime	
Glycopyrrolate (Robinul)	Antisecretory/antispasmodic Preanesthetic	PO 1–2 mg 2 or 3 times daily IM, IV 0.1–0.2 mg IM 0.004 mg/kg 30–60 min before anesthesia	*under 12 y:* Not recommended *under 2 y:* 0.004 mg/lb IM 30–60 min before anesthesia *2–12 y:* 0.002–0.004 mg/lb IM 30–60 min before anesthesia
Anticholinergics Used in Parkinson's Disease			
Benztropine (Cogentin)	Parkinsonism	PO, IM, IV 0.5–1 mg at bedtime. May increase up to 6 mg given at bedtime or in 2–4 divided doses.	
	Drug-induced extrapyramidal symptoms	*For acute dystonia:* IM, IV 1–2 mg. May repeat if needed. For prevention: PO 1–2 mg.	
Trihexyphenidyl (Trihexy)	Parkinsonism	PO 1–2 mg. Increase by 2-mg increments at 3- to 5-d intervals until a total of 6–10 mg is given daily in divided doses 3–4 times daily at mealtimes and bedtimes.	
	Drug-induced extrapyramidal symptoms	PO 1 mg initially. Increase as needed to control symptoms.	
Urinary Antispasmodics			
Darifenacin hydrobromide (Enablex)	Overactive bladder	PO 7.5 mg once daily. May increase to 15 mg if needed to control symptoms.	Safety and efficacy not established
Flavoxate (Urispas)	Overactive bladder	PO 100–200 mg 3 or 4 times daily. Reduce when symptoms improve.	*under 12 y:* Safety and efficacy not established
Oxybutynin (Ditropan and Ditropan XL, Oxytrol transdermal system)	Overactive bladder	PO 5 mg 2 or 3 times daily. Maximum dose 5 mg 4 times daily. *Extended-release* 5 mg PO daily up to 30 mg/daily. TDS: Apply TDS every 3–4 days.	*older than 5 y:* 5 mg PO twice daily. Maximum dose 5 mg 3 times daily

(continued on page 330)

| Table 20-2 | Drugs at a Glance: Selected Anticholinergic Drugs (continued) | | |

		ROUTES AND DOSAGE RANGES	
Generic/TradeName	Use	Adults	Children
Solifenacin succinate (VESIcare)	Overactive bladder	PO 5 mg once daily. May increase to 10 mg once daily if needed to control symptoms.	Safety and efficacy not established
Tolterodine (Detrol and Detrol LA)	Overactive bladder	PO 2 mg twice daily. May decrease to 1 mg when symptoms improve. Reduce doses to 1 mg PO twice daily in presence of hepatic impairment.	Safety and efficacy not established
Trospium chloride (Sanctura)	Overactive bladder	PO 20 mg twice daily at least 1 h before meals or on an empty stomach	Safety and efficacy not established

PRN, *as needed*; SL, *sublingual*; TDS, *transdermal system.*

Belladonna tincture is a mixture of alkaloids in an aqueous–alcohol solution. It is most often used in GI disorders because of its antispasmodic effect. It is an ingredient in several drug mixtures.

Homatropine hydrobromide is a semisynthetic derivative of atropine used as eye drops to produce mydriasis and cycloplegia. Compared with atropine, homatropine may be preferable, because ocular effects do not last as long.

Hyoscyamine (Anaspaz) is a belladonna alkaloid used in GI and genitourinary disorders characterized by spasm, increased secretion, and increased motility. It has the same effects as other atropine-like drugs.

Ipratropium (Atrovent) is an anticholinergic drug chemically related to atropine. When given as a nasal spray, it is useful in treating rhinorrhea due to allergy or the common cold. When given as an inhalation treatment or aerosol to patients with chronic obstructive pulmonary disease (COPD), it is beneficial as a bronchodilator. An advantage of administration of anticholinergic drugs by the respiratory route over the systemic route is less thickening of respiratory secretions and therefore a reduced incidence of mucous-plugged airways.

Scopolamine is similar to atropine in terms of uses, adverse effects, and peripheral effects but different in central effects. When it is given parenterally, scopolamine depresses the CNS and causes amnesia, drowsiness, euphoria, relaxation, and sleep. Effects of the drug appear more quickly and disappear more readily than those of atropine. Scopolamine also is used in motion sickness. It is available as oral tablets and as a transdermal adhesive disk that is placed behind the ear. The disk (Transderm-V) protects against motion sickness for 72 hours.

Tiotropium bromide (Spiriva HandiHaler) is a dry powder in capsule form intended for oral inhalation with the Handi-Haler inhalation device. This long-acting, antimuscarinic, anticholinergic, quaternary ammonium compound inhibits M_3 receptors in smooth muscle, resulting in bronchodilation. Tiotropium is indicated for daily maintenance treatment of bronchospasm associated with COPD. It is not indicated for acute episodes of bronchospasm (i.e., rescue therapy). Tiotropium is eliminated via the renal system, and patients with moderate to severe renal dysfunction should be carefully monitored for drug toxicity. No dosage adjustments are required for older patients or patients with hepatic impairment or mild renal impairment.

Antisecretory/Antispasmodic Anticholinergics Used in Gastrointestinal Disorders

Dicyclomine and **glycopyrrolate** are older medications, previously commonly used to treat peptic ulcer disease. With the introduction of medications such as proton pump inhibitors and other drugs that more effectively treat hyperacidity with fewer adverse effects (see Chap. 59), anticholinergics are infrequently prescribed today. Dicyclomine is also useful as an antispasmodic agent for treatment of irritable bowel syndrome.

Centrally Acting Anticholinergics Used in Parkinson's Disease

Older anticholinergic drugs such as atropine are rarely used to treat Parkinson's disease because of their undesirable peripheral effects (e.g., dry mouth, blurred vision, photophobia, constipation, urinary retention, tachycardia). Newer, centrally acting synthetic anticholinergic drugs are more selective for muscarinic receptors in the CNS and are designed to produce fewer adverse effects.

Trihexyphenidyl (Trihexy) is used in the treatment of parkinsonism and extrapyramidal reactions caused by some antipsychotic drugs. Trihexyphenidyl relieves smooth muscle spasm by a direct action on the muscle and by inhibiting the parasympathetic nervous system. The drug supposedly has fewer adverse effects than atropine, but approximately half the recipients report mouth dryness, blurring of vision, and other adverse effects common to anticholinergic drugs. Trihexyphenidyl requires the same precautions as other anticholinergic drugs and is contraindicated in glaucoma.

Benztropine (Cogentin) is a synthetic drug with both anticholinergic and antihistaminic effects. Its anticholinergic activity approximates that of atropine. A major clinical use is to treat acute dystonic reactions caused by antipsychotic drugs and to prevent their recurrence in patients receiving long-term antipsychotic drug therapy. It also may be given in small doses to supplement other antiparkinson drugs. In full dosage, adverse reactions are common.

Urinary Antispasmodics

Darifenacin (Enablex) is a competitive, antimuscarinic, anticholinergic agent with selective affinity for M_3 receptors involved in contraction of the urinary bladder. Darifenacin is indicated for the treatment of overactive bladder, reducing symptoms of urge incontinence, urgency, and frequency. After oral administration, darifenacin is 98% protein bound and extensively metabolized in the liver by CYP3A4 and CYP2D6 enzymes. A small group of individuals (approximately 7% Caucasian and 2% African American) are poor metabolizers of the drug and may require reduced dosages to avoid adverse effects. Dosage should also be reduced in individuals with moderate liver dysfunction and avoided in those individuals with severe liver impairment.

Flavoxate (Urispas) was developed specifically to counteract spasm in smooth muscle tissue of the urinary tract. It has anticholinergic, local anesthetic, and analgesic effects. Thus, the drug relieves dysuria, urgency, frequency, and pain with genitourinary infections, such as cystitis and prostatitis.

Oxybutynin (Ditropan, Ditropan XL, and Oxytrol transdermal system) has direct antispasmodic effects on smooth muscle and anticholinergic effects. It increases bladder capacity and decreases frequency of voiding in patients with neurogenic bladder. Oxybutynin is available in an extended-release form for once-daily dosing and a transdermal system that can be administered every 3 to 4 days.

Solifenacin (VESIcare) is a competitive, antimuscarinic, anticholinergic agent indicated for the treatment of overactive bladder with symptoms of urgency, urge incontinence, and frequency. Solifenacin is well absorbed after oral administration, 98% bound to plasma proteins, and extensively metabolized in the liver by CYP3A4 enzymes. Dosages should be reduced in individuals with moderate renal or liver impairment, and solifenacin is not recommended for those with severe liver impairment. Solifenacin may prolong QT intervals, especially at higher dosages, potentially resulting in dysrhythmias.

Tolterodine (Detrol and Detrol LA) is a competitive antimuscarinic, anticholinergic agent that inhibits bladder contraction, decreases detrusor muscle pressure, and delays the urge to void. It is used to treat urinary frequency, urgency, and urge incontinence. Tolterodine is more selective for muscarinic receptors in the urinary bladder than in other areas of the body, such as the salivary glands, and therefore anticholinergic adverse effects are less marked. Reduced doses (1 mg) are recommended for patients with hepatic dysfunction. Tolterodine is also available in an extended-release form.

Trospium chloride (Sanctura) is an antimuscarinic, anticholinergic drug for treatment of urgency, urge incontinence, and urinary frequency associated with overactive bladder. Trospium reduces the tone of smooth muscle in the bladder, exerting an antispasmodic effect. Because of its quaternary structure, less than 10% of an orally administered dose is absorbed, and food further delays absorption. Therefore, it is recommended that the medication be taken at least 1 hour before meals or on an empty stomach. Absorbed trospium is eliminated by a combination of glomerular filtration and active tubular secretion. Trospium has the potential for interaction with other drugs that are eliminated by active tubular secretion (e.g., digoxin, procainamide, pancuronium, morphine, vancomycin, metformin, tenofovir), resulting in increased serum concentration of either trospium or the co-administered drug because of competition for the urinary tubular pump. Reduced dosages of trospium are recommended for patients with renal insufficiency and those older than 75 years of age who may be less able to tolerate the adverse effects of anticholinergic drugs.

Nursing Process

Assessment

- Assess the patient's condition in relation to disorders for which anticholinergic drugs are used (i.e., check for bradycardia or heart block, diarrhea, dysuria, abdominal pain, and other disorders). If the patient reports or medical records indicate a specific disorder, assess for signs and symptoms of that disorder (e.g., Parkinson's disease).
- Assess for disorders in which anticholinergic drugs are contraindicated (e.g., glaucoma, prostatic hypertrophy, reflux esophagitis, myasthenia gravis, hyperthyroidism).
- Assess use of other drugs with anticholinergic effects, such as antihistamines (histamine$_1$ receptor antagonists [see Chap. 45]), antipsychotic agents, and tricyclic antidepressants.

Nursing Diagnoses

- Impaired Urinary Elimination: Decreased bladder tone and urine retention
- Constipation related to slowed GI function
- Disturbed Thought Processes: Confusion, disorientation, especially in older adults
- Deficient Knowledge: Drug effects and accurate usage
- Risk for Injury related to drug-induced blurred vision and photophobia
- Risk for Noncompliance related to adverse drug effects
- Risk for Altered Body Temperature: Hyperthermia

Planning/Goals

The patient will

- Receive or self-administer the drugs correctly
- Experience relief of symptoms for which anticholinergic drugs are given

Nursing Process continues on page 332

■ Be assisted to avoid or cope with adverse drug effects on vision, thought processes, bowel and bladder elimination, and heat dissipation

Interventions

Use measures to decrease the need for anticholinergic drugs. For example, with peptic ulcer disease, teach the client to avoid factors known to increase gastric secretion and GI motility (alcohol; cigarette smoking; caffeine-containing beverages, such as coffee, tea, and cola drinks; ulcerogenic drugs, such as aspirin). Late evening snacks also should be avoided because increased gastric acid secretion occurs approximately 90 minutes after eating and may cause pain and awakening from sleep. Although milk was previously considered an "ulcer food," it contains protein and calcium, which promote acid secretion, and is a poor buffer of gastric acid. Thus, drinking large amounts of milk should be avoided.

Patient Guidelines for Anticholinergic Drugs are presented in the accompanying display.

Evaluation

■ Interview and observe in relation to safe, accurate drug administration.

■ Interview and observe for relief of symptoms for which the drugs are given.

■ Interview and observe for adverse drug effects.

Applying Your Knowledge 20-1

Mr. Smoot experiences symptomatic bradycardia, with a heart rate in the range of 40 to 50 beats per minute. The standing order is to give atropine 1 mg IV. You administer the medication. What response is expected?

Principles of Therapy

Treatment of Specific Disorders

Renal or Biliary Colic

Atropine is sometimes given with morphine or meperidine to relieve the severe pain of renal or biliary colic. It acts mainly to decrease the spasm-producing effects of the opioid analgesics. It has little antispasmodic effect on the involved muscles and is not used alone for this purpose.

Overactive Urinary Bladder

Urinary antispasmodics are useful in relieving the urgency, frequency, and urge incontinence associated with overactive bladder. Although these medications are formulated to be more selective for the muscarinic receptors in the smooth muscle of the urinary bladder, unwanted anticholinergic effects such as dry mouth, constipation, and mydriasis may occur.

Preoperative Use in Patients With Glaucoma

Glaucoma is usually listed as a contraindication to anticholinergic drugs because the drugs impair outflow of aqueous humor and may cause an acute attack of glaucoma (increased intraocular pressure). However, anticholinergic drugs can be given safely before surgery to patients with open-angle glaucoma (80% of patients with primary glaucoma) if they are receiving miotic drugs such as pilocarpine. If anticholinergic preoperative medication is needed in patients predisposed to angle closure, the hazard of causing acute glaucoma can be minimized by also giving pilocarpine eye drops and acetazolamide.

Gastrointestinal Disorders

In peptic ulcer disease, more effective drugs have been developed, and anticholinergics are rarely used. When anticholinergic drugs are given for GI disorders, larger doses may be given at bedtime to prevent pain and awakening during sleep.

Parkinson's Disease

When anticholinergic drugs are used in parkinsonism, small doses are given initially and gradually increased. This regimen decreases adverse reactions.

Extrapyramidal Reactions

When anticholinergic drugs are used in drug-induced extrapyramidal reactions (Parkinson-like symptoms), they should be prescribed only if symptoms occur. They should not be used routinely to prevent extrapyramidal reactions, because fewer than half of patients taking antipsychotic drugs experience such reactions. Most drug-induced reactions last approximately 3 months and do not recur if anticholinergic drugs are discontinued at that time. (An exception is tardive dyskinesia, which does not respond to anticholinergic drugs and may be aggravated by them.)

Muscarinic Agonist Poisoning

Atropine is the antidote for poisoning by cholinergic (muscarinic) agonists such as certain species of mushrooms, cholinergic agonist drugs, cholinesterase inhibitor drugs, and insecticides containing organophosphates. Symptoms of muscarinic poisoning include salivation, lacrimation, visual disturbances, bronchospasm, diarrhea, bradycardia, and hypotension. Atropine prevents the poison from interacting with the muscarinic receptor, thus reversing the toxic effects.

Asthma and Other Chronic Obstructive Lung Diseases

Oral anticholinergics are not used to treat asthma and other COPDs because of the possibility of thickened respiratory secretions and formation of mucous plugs in airways. Administration of ipratropium or tiotropium by inhalation causes the beneficial bronchodilating effect.

Toxicity of Anticholinergics: Recognition and Management

Overdose of atropine or other anticholinergic drugs produces the usual pharmacologic effects in a severe and exaggerated

Patient Teaching Guidelines | Anticholinergic Drugs

General Considerations

■ Do not take other drugs without the physician's knowledge. In addition to some prescribed antiparkinson drugs, antidepressants, antihistamines, and antipsychotic drugs with anticholinergic properties, over-the-counter sleeping pills and antihistamines have anticholinergic effects. Taking any of these concurrently could cause overdosage or excessive anticholinergic effects.

■ Use measures to minimize risks of heat exhaustion and heat stroke:
   ■ Wear light, cool clothing in warm climates or environments.
   ■ Maintain fluid and salt intake if not contraindicated.
   ■ Limit exposure to direct sunlight.
   ■ Limit physical activity.
   ■ Take frequent cool baths.
   ■ Ensure adequate ventilation, with fans or air conditioners if necessary.
   ■ Avoid alcoholic beverages.

■ Use sugarless chewing gum and hard candy, if not contraindicated, to relieve mouth dryness.

■ Carry out good dental hygiene practices (e.g., regular brushing of teeth) to prevent dental caries and loss of teeth that may result from drug-induced xerostomia (dry mouth from decreased saliva production). This is more likely to occur with long-term use of these drugs.

■ To prevent injury due to blurring of vision or drowsiness, avoid potentially hazardous activities (e.g., driving or operating machinery).

■ To reduce sensitivity to light (photophobia), dark glasses can be worn outdoors in strong light.

■ If you wear contact lenses and experience dry eyes, use an ophthalmic lubricating solution.

■ When using anticholinergic ophthalmic preparations, if eye pain occurs, stop using the medication and contact your physician or health care provider. This may be a warning sign of undiagnosed glaucoma.

■ Notify your physician or health care provider if urinary retention or constipation occurs.

■ Tell your physician or health care provider if you are pregnant or breast-feeding or allergic to sulfite preservatives or any other atropine compound.

Self-Administration

■ Take anticholinergic drugs for gastrointestinal disorders 30 minutes before meals and at bedtime.

■ Safeguard anticholinergic medications from children because they are especially sensitive to atropine poisoning.

■ To prevent constipation, eat a diet high in fiber. Include whole grains, fruits, and vegetables in your daily menu. Also, drink 2 to 3 quarts of fluid a day and exercise regularly.

■ Take trospium at least 1 hour before meals or on an empty stomach.

■ To take tiotropium, follow the manufacturer's guidelines for using the HandiHaler to self-administer the drug by inhalation. Place a capsule into the center of the Handi-Haler inhalation device. Pierce the capsule by pressing and releasing the button on the side of the inhalation device. Inhale through the mouthpiece to disperse the drug. **Do not** swallow tiotropium capsules. Avoid allowing tiotropium powder to enter the eyes.

■ Rotate sites on the hips, abdomen, or buttocks and apply Oxytrol transdermal system to clean, dry skin.

■ Do not crush or chew extended-release anticholinergic medications. Swallow whole with liquid.

---

form. The anticholinergic overdose syndrome is characterized by hyperthermia; hot, dry, flushed skin; dry mouth; mydriasis; delirium; tachycardia; paralytic ileus; and urinary retention. Myoclonic movements and choreoathetosis may be seen. Seizures, coma, and respiratory arrest may also occur. Treatment involves use of activated charcoal to absorb ingested poison. Hemodialysis, hemoperfusion, peritoneal dialysis, and repeated doses of charcoal are not effective.

Physostigmine salicylate (Antilirium), an acetylcholinesterase inhibitor, is a specific antidote for overdose of anticholinergics. It is usually given intravenously (IV) at a slow rate of injection, because rapid administration may cause bradycardia, hypersalivation (with subsequent respiratory distress), and seizures. The adult dose is 2 milligrams (no more than 1 mg/min), and the pediatric dose is 0.5 to 1 milligrams (no more than 0.5 mg/min). Repeated doses may be given if life-threatening dysrhythmias, convulsions, or coma occur with anticholinergic overdose. However, the benefit of repeat dosing must be balanced against the risk of physostigmine overdose. Excessive administration of physostigmine can precipitate a cholinergic crisis, leading to seizures and dysrhythmias. Atropine is the antidote for physostigmine overdose.

Diazepam or a similar drug may be given for excessive CNS stimulation (e.g., delirium, excitement) that accompanies anticholinergic toxicity. Ice bags, cooling blankets, and tepid sponge baths may help reduce fever. Artificial ventilation and cardiopulmonary resuscitative measures are used if excessive depression of the CNS causes coma and respiratory failure. Infants, children, and the elderly are especially susceptible to the toxic effects of anticholinergic drugs.

Anticholinergic drugs have potential intoxicating effects. Abuse of these drugs may produce euphoria, disorientation, hallucinations, and paranoia in addition to the classic anticholinergic adverse reactions.

Use in Special Populations
Use in Children

Systemic anticholinergics, including atropine, glycopyrrolate, and scopolamine, are given to children of all ages for essentially the same effects as for adults. Most of the antisecretory, antispasmodic drugs for GI disorders are not recommended for children. With the urinary antispasmodics, flavoxate is not recommended for children younger than 12 years of age; oxybutynin is not recommended for children younger than 5 years of age; and the safety and efficacy of darifenacin, solifenacin, tolterodine, and trospium are not established in children. Similarly, the safety and efficacy of ipratropium and tiotropium, which are used for bronchodilation in chronic lung disorders, are not established in children.

Anticholinergic drugs cause the same adverse effects in children as in adults. However, the effects may be more severe in children, who are especially sensitive to these drugs. Facial flushing is common, and skin rashes may occur.

Ophthalmic anticholinergic drugs should be used only with close medical supervision. Cyclopentolate and tropicamide have been associated with behavioral disturbances and psychotic reactions in children. Tropicamide also has been associated with cardiopulmonary collapse.

Use in Older Adults

Anticholinergic drugs are given in older adults for the same purposes as in younger adults. In addition to the primary anticholinergic drugs, many others are commonly prescribed for older adults have high anticholinergic activity, including many antihistamines (histamine$_1$ receptor antagonists), tricyclic antidepressants, and antipsychotic drugs.

Older adults are especially likely to have significant adverse reactions because of slowed drug metabolism and the frequent presence of several disease processes. Some common adverse effects, with suggestions for reducing their impact, are

- Blurred vision. Patients may need help with ambulation, especially with stairs or in other potentially hazardous environments. Remove obstacles and hazards when possible.

- Confusion. Provide whatever assistance is needed to prevent falls and other injuries.

- Heat stroke. Help avoid precipitating factors, such as strenuous activity and high environmental temperatures.

- Constipation. Encourage or assist with an adequate intake of high-fiber foods and fluids and adequate exercise when feasible.

- Urinary retention. Encourage adequate fluid intake and avoid high doses of the drugs. Men should be examined for prostatic hypertrophy.

- Hallucinations and other psychotic symptoms. These are most likely to occur with the centrally active anticholinergics given for Parkinson's disease or drug-induced extrapyramidal effects, such as trihexyphenidyl or benztropine. Regulate and supervise dosage of these drugs carefully.

Applying Your Knowledge 20-2

Mr. Smoot complains about being unable to move his bowels and is having difficulty with urination. How should the nurse respond?

Use in Patients With Renal Impairment

Anticholinergic drugs that have a tertiary amine structure, such as atropine, are eliminated by a combination of hepatic metabolism and renal excretion. In the presence of renal impairment, they may accumulate and cause increased adverse effects. Quaternary amines are eliminated largely in the feces and are less affected by renal impairment.

Use in Patients With Hepatic Impairment

Some anticholinergic drugs are metabolized by the liver. Therefore, in the presence of hepatic impairment, they may accumulate and cause adverse effects. Darifenacin, solifenacin, and tolterodine are examples of such medications. Dosages should be reduced and/or given less frequently in the presence of liver impairment.

Use in Patients With Critical Illness

Atropine is an important drug in the emergency drug box. According to ACLS guidelines, atropine is the first drug to be administered in the emergency treatment of bradydysrhythmias. Atropine 0.5 milligrams should be administered IV every 3 to 5 minutes and may be repeated up to 3 milligrams (0.03–0.04 mg/kg total dose). For patients with asystole, 1 milligram of atropine is administered IV or IO and repeated every 3 to 5 minutes if asystole persists, up to 0.04 milligrams per kilogram of body weight. Administration of atropine in doses less than 0.5 milligrams should be avoided, because this may result in a paradoxical bradycardia. Atropine may be administered by endotracheal tube in patients without IV access. The recommended dose is 2 to 3 milligrams diluted in 10 milliliters of normal saline.

Use in Home Care

Anticholinergic drugs are commonly used in home care with children and adults. Children and older adults are probably most likely to experience adverse effects of these drugs and should be monitored carefully. With older patients, the home care nurse needs to assess medication regimens for combinations of drugs with anticholinergic effects, especially if mental confusion develops or worsens. The home care nurse may also need to teach older patients or caregivers that the drugs prevent sweating and heat loss and increase risks of heat stroke if precautions to avoid overheating are not taken.

 Applying Your Knowledge 20-3

How Can You Avoid This Medication Error?

Mr. Bing is another patient of yours on the unit. He is a 50-year-old man with a medical history of cholelithiasis, glaucoma, and hypertension. He has had surgery today to remove his gallbladder. You assess Mr. Bing and find that he is experiencing nausea. The resident on call orders a scopolamine patch. You follow the order and apply the patch.

Nursing Actions Anticholinergic Drugs

NURSING ACTIONS	RATIONALE/EXPLANATION
1. Administer accurately	
a. For gastrointestinal disorders, give most oral anticholinergic drugs approximately 30 min before meals and at bedtime.	To allow the drugs to reach peak antisecretory effects by the time ingested food is stimulating gastric acid secretion. Bedtime administration helps prevent awakening with abdominal pain.
b. When given before surgery, parenteral preparations of atropine can be mixed in the same syringe with several other common preoperative medications, such as meperidine (Demerol), morphine, oxymorphone (Numorphan), and promethazine (Phenergan).	The primary reason for mixing medications in the same syringe is to decrease the number of injections and thus decrease patient discomfort. Note, however, that extra caution is required when mixing drugs to be sure that the dosage of each drug is accurate. Also, if any question exists regarding compatibility with another drug, it is safer not to mix the drugs, even if two or three injections are required.
c. When applying topical atropine solutions or ointment to the eye, be sure to use the correct concentration and blot any excess from the inner canthus.	Atropine ophthalmic preparations are available in several concentrations (usually 1%, 2%, and 3%). Excess medication should be removed so the drug will not enter the naso-lacrimal (tear) ducts and be absorbed systemically through the mucous membrane of the nasopharynx or be carried to the throat and swallowed.
d. Parenteral glycopyrrolate can be given through the tubing of a running intravenous infusion of physiologic saline or lactated Ringer's solution.	
e. Do not crush extended-release or long-acting forms of anticholinergic drugs such as Detrol LA, Ditropan XL, VESIcare, and Enablex.	Crushing long-acting medications may result in high blood levels of the medication and increased adverse effects.
f. Take trospium (Sanctura) on an empty stomach.	Food interferes with absorption.
g. Follow the manufacturer's guidelines for administration of tiotropium using the HandiHaler inhalation device. Use the drug immediately after opening. Do not allow the powder to enter the eyes.	This ensures proper dosage and prevents reduced effectiveness. Drug powder in the eyes may cause blurred vision and pupil dilation.
2. Observe for therapeutic effects	
	Therapeutic effects depend primarily on the reason for use. Thus, a therapeutic effect in one condition may be an adverse effect in another condition.
a. When a drug is given for *peptic ulcer disease* or other gastrointestinal disorders, observe for decreased abdominal pain.	Relief of abdominal pain is due to the smooth muscle relaxant or antispasmodic effect of the drug.
b. When the drug is given for *diagnosing* or *treating eye disorders,* observe for pupil dilation (mydriasis) and blurring of vision (cycloplegia).	Note that these ocular effects are considered adverse effects when the drugs are given for problems not related to the eyes.
c. When the drug is given for *symptomatic bradycardia,* observe for increased pulse rate.	These drugs increase heart rate by blocking action of the vagus nerve.
d. When the drug is given for *urinary-tract disorders,* such as cystitis or enuresis, observe for decreased frequency of urination. When the drug is given for *renal colic due to stones,* observe for decreased pain. When the drug is given for *overactive bladder,* observe for fewer symptoms of urgency, urge incontinence, and frequency.	Anticholinergic drugs decrease muscle tone and spasm in the smooth muscle of the ureters and urinary bladder.
e. When the centrally acting anticholinergics are given for *Parkinson's disease,* observe for decrease in tremor, salivation, and drooling.	Decreased salivation is a therapeutic effect with parkinsonism but an adverse reaction in most other conditions.
3. Observe for adverse effects	
a. Tachycardia	These depend on reasons for use and are dose related. Tachycardia may occur with usual therapeutic doses because anticholinergic drugs block vagal action, which normally slows heart rate. Tachycardia is not likely to be serious except in patients with underlying heart disease. For example, in patients with angina pectoris, prolonged or severe tachycardia may increase myocardial ischemia to the point of causing an acute attack of angina (chest pain) or even myocardial infarction. In patients with congestive heart failure, severe or prolonged tachycardia can increase the workload of the heart to the point of causing acute heart failure or pulmonary edema.

(continued on page 336)

Nursing Actions | Anticholinergic Drugs (continued)

NURSING ACTIONS	RATIONALE/EXPLANATION
b. Excessive central nervous system (CNS) stimulation (tremor, restlessness, confusion, hallucinations, delirium) followed by excessive CNS depression (coma, respiratory depression)	These effects are more likely to occur with large doses of atropine because atropine crosses the blood-brain barrier. Large doses of trihexyphenidyl (Trihexy) also may cause CNS stimulation.
c. Sedation and amnesia with scopolamine or benztropine (Cogentin)	This may be a therapeutic effect but becomes an adverse reaction if severe or if the drug is given for another purpose. Benztropine has anticholinergic and antihistaminic properties. Apparently, drowsiness and sedation are caused by the antihistaminic component.
d. Constipation or paralytic ileus	These effects are the result of decreased gastrointestinal motility and muscle tone. Constipation is more likely with large doses or parenteral administration. Paralytic ileus is not likely unless the drugs are given to patients who already have decreased gastrointestinal motility.
e. Decreased oral and respiratory tract secretions, which cause mouth dryness and thick respiratory secretions	Mouth dryness is more annoying than serious in most cases and is caused by decreased salivation. However, patients with chronic lung disease, who usually have excessive secretions, tend to retain them with the consequence of frequent respiratory tract infections.
f. Paradoxical bronchospasm	This effect is detrimental and requires that the drug be discontinued.
g. Urinary retention	This reaction is caused by loss of bladder tone and is most likely to occur in elderly men with enlarged prostate glands. Thus, the drugs are usually contraindicated with prostatic hypertrophy.
h. Hot, dry skin; fever; heat stroke	These effects are due to decreased sweating and impairment of the normal heat-loss mechanism. Fever may occur with any age group. Heat stroke is more likely to occur with cardiovascular disease, strenuous physical activity, and high environmental temperatures, especially in older people.
i. Ocular effects—mydriasis, blurred vision, photophobia	These are adverse effects when anticholinergic drugs are given for conditions not related to the eyes.
j. Angioedema with tiotropium	This effect requires that the drug be discontinued.
4. Observe for drug interactions	
a. Drugs that *increase* effects of anticholinergic drugs: antihistamines, disopyramide, phenothiazines, thioxanthene agents, tricyclic antidepressants, amantadine	These drugs have anticholinergic properties and produce additive anticholinergic effects.
b. Drugs that *decrease* effects of anticholinergic drugs: cholinergic drugs	These drugs counteract the inhibition of gastrointestinal motility and tone induced by atropine. They are sometimes used in atropine overdose.
c. For trospium, use caution when administering concurrently with drugs that are eliminated by active tubular secretion (e.g., digoxin, metformin, morphine, pancuronium, procainamide, tenofovir, vancomycin).	As these drugs compete for urinary tubular pumps, increased serum concentration of trospium or the co-administered drug may occur.
d. For solifenacin and darifenacin: ketaconazole and other inhibitors of CYP3A4 enzymes increase the effect of anticholinergic drugs.	Ketaconazole inhibits the metabolism of solifenacin and darifenacin, increasing effects.

Key Concepts

- Anticholinergic drugs block the action of acetylcholine on the parasympathetic nervous system.

- Most anticholinergic drugs interact with muscarinic cholinergic receptors in the brain, secretory glands, heart, and smooth muscle and are sometimes called antimuscarinic drugs.

- Cholinergic (muscarinic) receptors are widespread throughout the body, producing effects in a variety of locations including the central nervous system, heart, smooth muscle, glands, and the eye.

- Synthetic anticholinergics were developed to exert more selective effects on particular body tissues.

- Anticholinergic drugs (e.g., dicyclomine or glycopyrrolate) are indicated for antispasmodic effects in GI disorders. Historically, they have also been used to treat peptic ulcer disease; however, they are weak inhibitors of gastric acid secretion and have been largely replaced other more effective medications (e.g., proton pump inhibitors)

- Urinary antispasmodic anticholinergic drugs are the drugs of choice for treatment of symptoms of overactive bladder.

- Ophthalmic anticholinergic preparations are indicated for mydriatic and cycloplegic effects to aid in eye examination and surgery.

- Ipratropium and tiotropium are anticholinergic medications given by inhalation for bronchodilation effects in the treatment of asthma and chronic bronchitis.

- Atropine is the drug of choice to treat bradycardia.

- Anticholinergic medications are indicated in the relief of central nervous system symptoms of Parkinson's disease or extrapyramidal symptoms associated with some antipsychotic drugs.

- Anticholinergic drugs are given preoperatively to prevent anesthesia-associated complications such as bradycardia, excessive respiratory secretions, and hypotension.

- Anticholinergic drugs are contraindicated for patients with benign prostatic hypertrophy, myasthenia gravis, hyperthyroidism, narrow-angle glaucoma, tachydysrhythmias, myocardial infarction, heart failure, or conditions associated with esophageal reflux.

- Anticholinergic overdose is characterized by hyperthermia; hot, dry, flushed skin; dry mouth; mydriasis; delirium; tachycardia; paralytic ileus; urinary retention; myoclonic movements; seizures; coma; and respiratory arrest. Physostigmine is the specific antidote for anticholinergic overdose.

- Atropine is the antidote for muscarinic agonist poisoning.

Review and Application Exercises

Short Answer Exercises

1. How do anticholinergic drugs exert their therapeutic effects?

2. What are the indications and contraindications for use of anticholinergic drugs?

3. What is the effect of anticholinergic drugs on heart rate, and what is the mechanism for this effect?

4. Under what circumstances is it desirable to administer atropine before surgery, and why?

5. What are adverse effects of anticholinergic drugs?

6. What treatment measures are indicated for a patient with an overdose of a drug with anticholinergic effects?

7. Name two other commonly used drug groups that have anticholinergic effects.

8. What nursing observations and interventions are needed to increase patient safety and comfort during anticholinergic drug therapy?

NCLEX-Style Questions

9. Your 62-year-old patient has a sinus bradycardia with a rate of 48 beats per minute. He is confused, and his skin is cool and clammy. What is the drug of choice in this situation?
   a. atropine sulfate
   b. epinephrine (Adrenalin)
   c. isoproterenol (Isuprel)
   d. dopamine (Intropin)

10. Your patient is taking an anticholinergic medication. Which of the following instructions would be appropriate for this patient?
   a. Limit oral intake because these medications cause fluid retention.
   b. Be sure a bathroom is near because these medications may cause diarrhea.
   c. Avoid overheating and wear cool, loose clothing because these medications impair sweating.
   d. Change positions slowly because these medications may cause orthostatic hypotension.

11. Shortly after administration of the first dose of atropine, your patient complains of acute eye pain. The nurse should
    a. Administer a PRN (as needed) dose of analgesic, such as acetaminophen.
    b. Place a cool, damp cloth over the patient's eyes for comfort.
    c. Hold further doses of atropine and notify the physician immediately.
    d. Prepare to treat an allergic reaction to atropine with epinephrine (Adrenalin).

12. Your patient with chronic lung disease is in respiratory distress due to acute bronchospasm. Which of the following orders for treatment of this condition would you question?
    a. epinephrine (Adrenalin)
    b. albuterol (Ventolin)
    c. aminophylline (Truphylline)
    d. tiotropium (Spiriva)

Selected References

American Heart Association. (2005). Guidelines for cardiopulmonary resuscitation and emergency cardiovascular care. *Circulation, 112,* IV58–IV66.

Barletta, J. F. (2005). Cardiopulmonary resuscitation. In J. T. DiPiro, R. L. Talbert, G. C. Yee, G. R. Matzke, B. G. Wells, & L. M. Posey (Eds.), *Pharmacotherapy: A pathophysiologic approach* (6th ed., pp. 171–183). New York: McGraw-Hill.

Drug facts and comparisons. (Updated monthly). St. Louis, MO: Facts and Comparisons.

Nelson, M. V., Berchou, R. C., & LeWitt, P. A. (2005). Parkinson's disease. In J. T. DiPiro, R. L. Talbert, G. C. Yee, G. R. Matzke, B. G. Wells, & L. M. Posey (Eds.), *Pharmacotherapy: A pathophysiologic approach* (6th ed., pp. 1075–1088). New York: McGraw-Hill.

Rovner, E., Wyman, J., Lackner, T., & Guay, D. (2005). Urinary incontinence. In J. T. DiPiro, R. L. Talbert, G. C. Yee, G. R. Matzke, B. G. Wells, & L. M. Posey (Eds.), *Pharmacotherapy: A pathophysiologic approach* (6th ed., pp. 1547–1563). New York: McGraw-Hill.

SECTION 4

Drugs Affecting the Endocrine System

Chapter Outline

LEARNING OBJECTIVES

After studying this chapter, you will be able to:

1. Examine the relationship between the endocrine system and the central nervous system.
2. Describe general characteristics and functions of hormones.
3. Compare steroid and protein hormones in relation to site of action and pharmacokinetics.
4. Examine hormonal action at the cellular level.
5. Describe the second-messenger roles of cyclic adenosine monophosphate and calcium within body cells.
6. Differentiate between physiologic and pharmacologic doses of hormonal drugs.

Introduction

The endocrine system participates in the regulation of essentially all body activities, including metabolism of nutrients and water, reproduction, growth and development, and adapting to changes in internal and external environments. The major elements of the endocrine system are the *hypothalamus*, pituitary gland, thyroid gland, parathyroid glands, pancreas, adrenal glands, ovaries, and testes. These tissues function through *hormones*, substances that are synthesized and secreted into body fluids by one group of cells and have physiologic effects on other body cells. Hormones act as chemical messengers to transmit information between body cells and organs. Most hormones from the traditional endocrine glands are secreted into the bloodstream and act on distant organs.

In addition to the major endocrine organs, other tissues also produce hormones. These endocrine-like cells intermingle with nonendocrine cells in various organs. Their hormones are secreted into tissue fluids and act locally on nearby cells, as in the following examples:

- The gastrointestinal mucosa produces hormones that are important in the digestive process (e.g., gastrin, enterogastrone, secretin, cholecystokinin).
- The kidneys produce erythropoietin, a hormone that stimulates the bone marrow to produce red blood cells.
- White blood cells produce cytokines that function as messengers among leukocytes in inflammatory and immune processes.
- Many body tissues produce prostaglandins and leukotrienes, which have a variety of physiologic effects.

Neoplasms also may produce hormones. In endocrine tissues, neoplasms may be an added source of the hormone normally produced by the organ. In nonendocrine tissues, various hormones may be produced. For example, lung tumors may produce corticotropin (adrenocorticotropic hormone [ACTH]), antidiuretic hormone, or parathyroid hormone; kidney tumors may produce parathyroid hormone. The usual effects are those of excess hormone secretion.

This chapter focuses on the traditional endocrine organs and their hormones. Specific organs are discussed in the following chapters; general characteristics of the endocrine system and hormones are described in the following sections and in Box 21-1.

Endocrine System–Nervous System Interactions

The endocrine and nervous systems are closely connected, anatomically and physiologically, and work in harmony to integrate and regulate body functions. In general, the nervous system regulates rapid muscular and sensory activities by secreting substances that act as neurotransmitters, circulating hormones, and local hormones (e.g., norepinephrine, epinephrine). The endocrine system regulates slow metabolic activities by secreting hormones that control cellular metabolism, transport of substances across cell membranes, and other functions (e.g., reproduction, growth and development, secretion).

The main connecting link between the nervous system and the endocrine system is the hypothalamus, which responds to nervous system stimulation by producing hormones. Secretion of almost all hormones from the pituitary gland is controlled by the hypothalamus. Special nerve fibers originating in the hypothalamus and ending in the posterior pituitary gland control secretions of the posterior pituitary. The hypothalamus secretes hormones, called releasing and inhibitory factors, that regulate functions of the anterior pituitary. The anterior pituitary, in turn, secretes hormones that act on target tissues, usually to stimulate production of other hormones. For example, hypothalamic corticotropin-releasing hormone stimulates the anterior pituitary to produce corticotropin, and corticotropin, in turn, stimulates the adrenal cortex to produce cortisol. This complex interrelationship is often referred to as the *hypothalamic–pituitary–adrenocortical (HPA) axis*. It functions by *a negative feedback system*, in which hormone secretion is stimulated when hormones are needed and inhibited when they are not needed. The hypothalamic–pituitary–thyroid axis also functions by a negative feedback mechanism.

Box 21-1	Major Hormones and Their General Functions

Anterior pituitary hormones are growth hormone (also called somatotropin), corticotropin, thyroid-stimulating hormone, follicle-stimulating hormone, luteinizing hormone, and prolactin. Most of these hormones function by stimulating secretion of other hormones.

Posterior pituitary hormones are antidiuretic hormone (ADH or vasopressin) and oxytocin. ADH helps maintain fluid balance; oxytocin stimulates uterine contractions during childbirth.

Adrenal cortex hormones, commonly called corticosteroids, include the glucocorticoids, such as cortisol, and the mineralocorticoids, such as aldosterone. Glucocorticoids influence carbohydrate storage, exert anti-inflammatory effects, suppress corticotropin secretion, and increase protein catabolism. Mineralocorticoids help regulate electrolyte balance, mainly by promoting sodium retention and potassium loss. The adrenal cortex also produces sex hormones. The adrenal medulla hormones are epinephrine and norepinephrine (see Chap. 17).

Thyroid hormones include triiodothyronine (T_3 or liothyronine) and tetraiodothyronine (T_4 or thyroxine). These hormones regulate the metabolic rate of the body and greatly influence growth and development.

Parathyroid hormone, also called parathormone or PTH, regulates calcium and phosphate metabolism.

Pancreatic hormones are insulin and glucagon, which regulate the metabolism of glucose, lipids, and proteins.

Ovarian hormones (female sex hormones) are estrogens and progesterone. Estrogens promote growth of specific body cells and development of most female secondary sexual characteristics. Progesterone helps prepare the uterus for pregnancy and the mammary glands for lactation.

Testicular hormone (male sex hormone) is testosterone, which regulates development of masculine characteristics.

Placental hormones are chorionic gonadotropin, estrogen, progesterone, and human placental lactogen, all of which are concerned with reproductive functions.

General Characteristics of Hormones

Hormones are extremely important in regulating body activities. Their normal secretion and function help to maintain the internal environment and determine response and adaptation to the external environment. Hormones participate in complex interactions with other hormones and nonhormone chemical substances in the body to influence every aspect of life. Although hormones are usually studied individually, virtually all endocrine functions are complex processes that are influenced by more than one hormone.

Although hormones circulating in the bloodstream reach essentially all body cells, some (e.g., growth hormone, thyroid hormone) affect almost all cells, whereas others affect specific "target" tissues (e.g., corticotropin stimulates the adrenal cortex). In addition, one hormone can affect different tissues (e.g., ovarian estrogen can act on ovarian follicles to promote their maturation, on the endometrial lining of the uterus to stimulate its growth and cyclic changes, on breast tissue to stimulate growth of milk ducts, and on the hypothalamic–pituitary system to regulate its own secretion), or several hormones can affect a single tissue or function (e.g., catecholamines, glucagon, secretin, and prolactin regulate lipolysis [release of fatty acids from adipose tissue]).

Several hormones are secreted in cyclic patterns. For example, ACTH, cortisol, and growth hormone are secreted in 24-hour (circadian) cycles, whereas estrogen and progestin secretion are related to the 28-day menstrual cycle.

Hormone Pharmacokinetics

Protein-derived hormones (amines, amino acids, peptides, and polypeptides) are synthesized, stored, and released into the bloodstream in response to a stimulus. The steroid hormones, which are synthesized in the adrenal cortex and gonads from cholesterol, are released as they are synthesized. Most hormones are constantly present in the blood; plasma concentrations vary according to body needs, the rate of synthesis and release, and the rate of metabolism and excretion.

Protein-derived hormones usually circulate in an unbound, active form. Steroid and thyroid hormones are transported by specific carrier proteins synthesized in the liver. (Some drugs may compete with a hormone for binding sites on the carrier protein. If this occurs, hormone effects are enhanced because more unbound, active molecules are available to act on body cells.)

Hormones must be continuously inactivated to prevent their accumulation and excessive effects. Several mechanisms operate to eliminate hormones from the body. The water-soluble, protein-derived hormones have a short duration of action and are inactivated by enzymes mainly in the liver and kidneys. The lipid-soluble steroid and thyroid hormones have a longer duration of action because they are bound to plasma proteins. After they are released by the plasma proteins, these hormones are conjugated in the liver to inactive forms and then excreted in bile or urine. A third, less common mechanism is inactivation by enzymes at receptor sites on target cells.

Hormone Action at the Cellular Level

Hormones modify rather than initiate cellular reactions and functions. After hormone molecules reach a responsive cell, they bind with receptors in the cell membrane (e.g., catecholamines and protein hormones) or inside the cell (e.g., steroid and thyroid hormones). The number of hormone receptors and the affinity of the receptors for the hormone are the major determinants of target-cell response to hormone action.

The main target organs for a given hormone contain large numbers of receptors. However, the number of receptors may be altered by various conditions. For example, receptors may be increased (called *up-regulation*) when there are low levels of hormone. This allows the cell to obtain more of the needed hormone than it can obtain with fewer receptors. Receptors may be decreased (called *down-regulation*) when there are excessive amounts of hormone. This mechanism protects the cell by making it less responsive to excessive hormone levels. Receptor up-regulation and down-regulation occur with chronic exposure to abnormal levels of hormones. In addition, receptor proteins may be decreased by inadequate formation or antibodies that destroy them. Thus, receptors are constantly being synthesized and degraded, so the number of receptors may change within hours. Receptor affinity for binding with hormone molecules probably changes as well.

After binding occurs, the resulting hormone–receptor complex initiates intracellular biochemical reactions, depending on the particular hormone and the type of cell. Many hormones act as a "first messenger" to the cell, and the hormone–receptor complex activates a "second messenger." The second messenger then activates intracellular structures to produce characteristic cellular functions and products. Steroid hormones from the adrenal cortex, ovaries, and testes stimulate target cells to synthesize various proteins (e.g., enzymes, transport and structural proteins) needed for normal cellular function.

Second-Messenger System

Three major *second-messenger systems*, cyclic adenosine monophosphate (cAMP), calcium–calmodulin, and phospholipid products, are described in this section.

Cyclic AMP is the second messenger for many hormones, including corticotropin, catecholamines, glucagon, thyroid-stimulating hormone, follicle-stimulating hormone, luteinizing hormone, parathyroid hormone, secretin, and antidiuretic hormone. It is formed by the action of the enzyme adenyl cyclase on adenosine triphosphate, a component of all cells and the main source of energy for cellular metabolism. After it is formed, cAMP activates a series of enzyme reactions that alter cell function. The amount of intracellular cAMP is increased by hormones that activate adenyl cyclase (e.g., the pituitary hormones, calcitonin, glucagon, parathyroid hormone) and is decreased by hormones that inactivate adenyl cyclase (e.g., angiotensin, somatostatin). Cyclic AMP is inactivated by phosphodiesterase enzymes.

Calcium is the second messenger for angiotensin II, a strong vasoconstrictor that participates in control of arterial blood pressure, and for gonadotropin-releasing hormone. The postulated sequence of events is that hormone binding to receptors increases intracellular calcium. The calcium binds with an intracellular regulatory protein called calmodulin. The calcium–calmodulin complex activates protein kinases, which then regulate contractile structures of the cell, cell membrane permeability, and intracellular enzyme activity. Specific effects include contraction of smooth muscle, changes in the secretions produced by secreting cells, and changes in ciliary action in the lungs.

Phospholipid products are mainly involved with local hormones. *Phospholipids* are major components of the cell membrane portion of all body cells. Some local hormones activate cell membrane receptors and transform them into phospholipase C, an enzyme that causes some of the phospholipids in cell membranes to split into smaller molecules (e.g., inositol triphosphate and diacylglycerol). These products then act as second messengers to intracellular structures. Inositol triphosphate mobilizes intracellular calcium ions and the calcium ions then fulfill their functions as second messengers, as described previously. Diacylglycerol activates protein kinase C, an enzyme important in cell reproduction. Also, the lipid component of diacylglycerol is arachidonic acid, the precursor for prostaglandins, leukotrienes, and other local hormones with extensive effects.

Steroid Stimulation of Protein Synthesis

Steroid hormones are lipid soluble and therefore cross cell membranes easily. Inside the cell cytoplasm, the hormone molecules bind with specific receptor proteins. The hormone–receptor complex then enters the nucleus of the cell, where it activates nucleic acids (DNA and RNA) and the genetic code to synthesize new proteins.

Hormonal Disorders

Abnormal secretion and function of hormones, even minor alterations, can impair physical and mental health. Malfunction of an endocrine organ is usually associated with hyposecretion, hypersecretion, or inappropriate secretion of its hormones. Any malfunction can produce serious disease or death.

Glandular Hypofunction

Hypofunction may be associated with a variety of circumstances, including the following:

1. A congenital defect may result in the absence of an endocrine gland, the presence of an abnormally developed gland, or the absence of an enzyme required for glandular synthesis of its specific hormone.

2. The endocrine gland may be damaged or destroyed by impaired blood flow, infection or inflammation, autoimmune disorders, or neoplasms.

3. The endocrine gland may atrophy and become less able to produce its hormone because of aging, drug therapy, disease, or unknown reasons.

4. The endocrine gland may produce adequate hormone, but the hormone may not be able to function normally because of receptor defects (not enough receptors or the receptors present are unable to bind with the hormone).

5. Even if there is adequate hormone and adequate binding to receptors, intracellular metabolic processes (e.g., enzyme function, protein synthesis, energy production) may not respond appropriately.

Glandular Hyperfunction

Hyperfunction is usually characterized by excessive hormone production. Excessive amounts of hormone may occur from excessive stimulation and enlargement of the endocrine gland, from a hormone-producing tumor of the gland, or from a hormone-producing tumor of nonendocrine tissues (e.g., some primary lung tumors produce antidiuretic hormone and ACTH).

Use of Hormonal Drugs

Hormonal drugs are powerful drugs that produce widespread therapeutic and adverse effects. Hormones given for therapeutic purposes may be natural hormones from human or animal sources or synthetic. Many of the most important hormones have been synthesized, and synthetic preparations may have more potent and prolonged effects than naturally occurring hormones. Administration of one hormone may alter effects of other hormones through complex hormone interactions.

Hormones are given for physiologic or pharmacologic effects and are more often given for disorders resulting from endocrine gland hypofunction than for those related to hyperfunction. Physiologic use involves giving small doses as a replacement or substitute for the amount secreted by a normally functioning endocrine gland. Such use is indicated only when a gland cannot secrete an adequate amount of hormone. Examples of physiologic use include insulin administration in diabetes mellitus and adrenal corticosteroid administration in Addison's disease. Pharmacologic use involves relatively large doses for effects greater than physiologic effects. For example, adrenal corticosteroids are widely used for anti-inflammatory effects in endocrine and nonendocrine disorders.

Key Concepts

- The endocrine system is comprised of the hypothalamus of the brain, pituitary gland, thyroid gland, parathyroid glands, pancreas, adrenal glands, ovaries, and testes.

- Endocrine tissues function through hormones, which act as chemical messengers to transmit information between body cells and organs.

- Water-soluble, protein-derived hormones have a short duration of action and are inactivated by enzymes mainly in the liver and kidneys.

- Lipid-soluble steroid and thyroid hormones have a longer

- duration of action because they are bound to plasma proteins.

- Secretion of almost all hormones from the pituitary gland is controlled by the hypothalamus.

- The endocrine and nervous systems are closely connected, anatomically and physiologically, and work in harmony to integrate and regulate body functions.

- ACTH, cortisol, and growth hormone are secreted in 24-hour (circadian) cycles, whereas estrogen and progestin secretion are related to the 28-day menstrual cycle.

■ Many hormones act as a "first messenger" to the cell, and the hormone–receptor complex activates a "second messenger," which activates intracellular structures to produce characteristic cellular functions and products.

■ Receptors are capable of increasing (up-regulation) or decreasing (down-regulation) with chronic exposure to abnormal levels of hormones.

Review and Application Exercises

Short Answer Exercises

1. How do hormones function in maintaining homeostasis?

2. What is the connection between the nervous system and the endocrine system?

3. What is meant by a negative feedback system?

4. Because classic hormones are secreted into blood and circulated to essentially all body cells, why do they not affect all body cells?

5. What are the functions and characteristics of the pituitary gland?

Selected References

Corwin, E. J. (2006). *Handbook of Pathophysiology* (3rd ed.). Philadelphia: Lippincott Williams & Wilkins.

Guyton, A. C., & Hall, J. E. (2006). *Textbook of medical physiology* (11th ed.). Philadelphia: W. B. Saunders.

Huether, S. E. (2006). Mechanisms of hormonal regulation. In K. L. McCance and S. E. Huether (Eds.), *Pathophysiology: The biologic basis for disease in adults and children* (5th ed., pp. 655–681). Philadelphia: Elsevier Mosby.

Hypothalamic and Pituitary Hormones

LEARNING OBJECTIVES

After studying this chapter, you will be able to:

1. Identify clinical uses of selected hormones.
2. Differentiate characteristics and functions of anterior and posterior pituitary hormones.
3. Recognize the limitations of hypothalamic and pituitary hormones as therapeutic agents.
4. Identify major nursing considerations in the care of patients receiving specific hypothalamic and pituitary hormones.

Applying Your Knowledge

Jose Rojas is a 24-year-old man who has suffered a head injury while riding his motorcycle without a helmet. He has been admitted for observation, with multiple abrasions and a blow to the head. Mr. Rojas begins to produce massive amounts of clear, pale-yellow urine. The physician diagnoses him with diabetes insipidus and orders desmopressin 0.2 mL in two divided doses intranasally.

Introduction

The hypothalamus of the brain and the pituitary gland interact to control most metabolic functions of the body and to maintain homeostasis (Fig. 22-1). They are anatomically connected by the funnel-shaped hypophyseal stalk. The hypothalamus controls secretions of the pituitary gland. The pituitary gland, in turn, regulates secretions or functions of other body tissues, called target tissues. The pituitary gland is actually two glands, each with different structures and functions. The anterior pituitary is composed of different types of glandular cells that synthesize and secrete different hormones. The posterior pituitary is anatomically an extension of the hypothalamus and is composed mainly of nerve fibers. Although it does not manufacture any hormones itself, it stores and releases hormones synthesized in the hypothalamus.

Types of Hormones

Hypothalamic Hormones

Hormones are chemical messenger with specific regulatory effect on the cells that control various bodily functions. The hypothalamus produces a *releasing hormone* to accelerate the secretion of a given hormone or an *inhibiting hormone* that decreases hormone secretion that corresponds to each of the major hormones of the anterior pituitary gland.

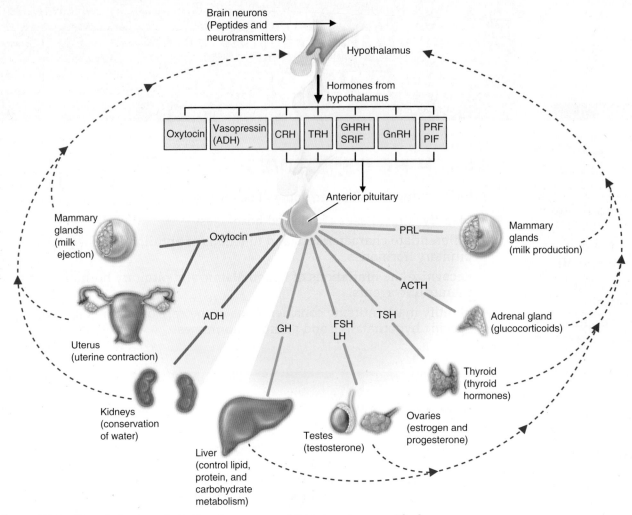

Figure 22-1 ■ Hypothalamic and pituitary hormones and their target organs. The hypothalamus produces hormones that act on the anterior pituitary or are stored in the posterior pituitary. The anterior pituitary produces hormones that act on various body tissues and stimulate production of other hormones. T_3, triiodothyronine; T_4, thyroxine; TRH, thyrotropin-releasing hormone; TSH, thyroid-stimulating hormone.

Corticotropin-releasing hormone or **factor** (CRH or CRF) causes release of *corticotropin* (also called *adrenocorticotropic hormone [ACTH]*) in response to stress and threatening stimuli. CRH is secreted most often during sleep, and its secretion is influenced by several neurotransmitters. Acetylcholine and serotonin stimulate secretion, and gamma-aminobutyric acid (GABA) and norepinephrine inhibit secretion. The ability of CRH to stimulate corticotropin secretion is increased by vasopressin and decreased or prevented by somatostatin and elevated levels of glucocorticoids. CRH can be used in the diagnosis of Cushing's disease, a disorder characterized by excess cortisol.

Growth hormone–releasing hormone (GHRH) causes release of *growth hormone* (GH) in response to low blood levels of GH. Secretion of hypothalamic GHRH is stimulated by dopamine, norepinephrine, epinephrine, GABA, acetylcholine, and serotonin. The stimulatory effect of GHRH on secretion of GH is blocked by somatostatin. GHRH may

be used to test pituitary function and to stimulate growth in children with GHRH deficiency.

Growth hormone release–inhibiting hormone (somatostatin) inhibits release of GH and is distributed throughout the brain and spinal cord, where it functions as a neurotransmitter. It is also found in the intestines and the pancreas, where it regulates secretion of insulin and glucagon. Somatostatin secretion is increased by several neurotransmitters, including acetylcholine, dopamine, epinephrine, GABA, and norepinephrine.

Somatostatin also inhibits other functions, including secretion of corticotropin, *thyroid-stimulating hormone* (*TSH* or *thyrotropin*), prolactin, pancreatic secretions (e.g., insulin, glucagon), and gastrointestinal (GI) secretions (gastrin, cholecystokinin, secretin, vasoactive intestinal peptide) as well as GI motility, bile flow, and mesenteric blood flow. Hypothalamic somatostatin blocks the action of GHRH and decreases thyrotropin-releasing hormone (TRH)–induced release of

TSH. GH stimulates secretion of somatostatin, and the effects of somatostatin on TSH may contribute to TSH deficiency in children being treated with GH. A long-acting somatostatin analog, octreotide (Sandostatin), may be used to treat acromegaly, carcinoid tumors, and vasoactive intestinal peptide tumors (VIPomas).

Thyrotropin-releasing hormone (TRH) causes release of TSH in response to stress, such as exposure to cold. TRH may be used in diagnostic tests of pituitary function and hyperthyroidism.

Gonadotropin-releasing hormone (GnRH) causes release of follicle-stimulating hormone (FSH) and luteinizing hormone (LH). Several synthetic equivalents of GnRH are used clinically.

Prolactin-releasing factor is active during lactation after childbirth. **Prolactin-inhibitory factor** (PIF) is active at times other than during lactation.

Anterior Pituitary Hormones

The anterior pituitary gland produces seven hormones. Two of these, GH and prolactin, act directly on their target tissues; the other five act indirectly by stimulating target tissues to produce other hormones.

Corticotropin, also called ACTH, stimulates the adrenal cortex to produce corticosteroids. Secretion is controlled by the hypothalamus and by plasma levels of cortisol, the major corticosteroid. A negative feedback mechanism inhibits the release of cortisol when plasma levels are adequate for body needs. Corticotropin is less predictable and less convenient than glucocorticoids and therefore has no apparent advantages.

GH, also called *somatotropin*, stimulates growth of body tissues. It regulates cell division and protein synthesis required for normal growth and promotes an increase in cell size and number, including growth of muscle cells and lengthening of bone. These effects occur mainly via altered metabolism of carbohydrate, protein, and fat by direct and indirect effects. GH is often considered an insulin antagonist because it suppresses the abilities of insulin to stimulate uptake of glucose in peripheral tissues and enhance glucose synthesis in the liver. Paradoxically, administration of GH produces hyperinsulinemia by stimulating insulin secretion. In addition, GH stimulates protein anabolism in many tissues. The hormone also enhances fat utilization by stimulating triglyceride breakdown and oxidation in fat-storing cells.

Levels of GH rise rapidly during adolescence, peak in the 20s, and then start to decline. Deficient GH in children produces *dwarfism*, a condition marked by severely decreased linear growth and, frequently, severely delayed mental, emotional, dental, and sexual growth as well. If untreated, excessive GH in preadolescents produces gigantism, resulting in heights of eight or nine feet.

In adults, deficient GH (less than expected for age) can cause increased fat, reduced skeletal and heart muscle mass, reduced strength, reduced ability to exercise, and worsened cholesterol levels (i.e., increased low-density lipoprotein cho-

lesterol and decreased high-density lipoprotein cholesterol), which increase risk factors for cardiovascular disease. Excessive GH in adults produces *acromegaly*, a chronic disease characterized by an abnormal pattern of bone and connective-tissue growth associated with an increased incidence of diabetes mellitus and hypertension.

Thyrotropin (also called TSH) regulates secretion of thyroid hormones. Thyrotropin secretion is controlled by a negative feedback mechanism in proportion to metabolic needs. Thus, increased thyroid hormones in body fluids inhibit secretion of thyrotropin by the anterior pituitary and of TRH by the hypothalamus.

FSH, one of the gonadotropins, stimulates functions of sex glands. FSH is produced by the anterior pituitary gland of both sexes, beginning at puberty. It acts on the ovaries in a cyclical fashion during the reproductive years, stimulating growth of ovarian follicles. These follicles then produce estrogen, which prepares the endometrium for implantation of a fertilized ovum. FSH acts on the testes to stimulate the production and growth of sperm (spermatogenesis), but it does not stimulate secretion of male sex hormones.

LH (also called interstitial cell-stimulating hormone) is another gonadotropin that stimulates hormone production by the gonads of both sexes. In women, LH is important in the maturation and rupture of the ovarian follicle (ovulation). After ovulation, LH acts on the cells of the collapsed follicular sac to produce the corpus luteum, which then produces progesterone during the last half of the menstrual cycle. When blood progesterone levels rise, a negative feedback effect is exerted on hypothalamic and anterior pituitary secretion of gonadotropins. Decreased pituitary secretion of LH causes the corpus luteum to die and stop producing progesterone. Lack of progesterone causes slough and discharge of the endometrial lining as menstrual flow. (Of course, if the ovum has been fertilized and attached to the endometrium, menstruation does not occur.) In men, LH stimulates the Leydig's cells in the spaces between the seminiferous tubules to secrete androgens, mainly testosterone.

Prolactin plays a part in milk production by nursing mothers. It is not usually secreted in nonpregnant women because of the hypothalamic hormone PIF. During late pregnancy and lactation, various stimuli, including suckling, inhibit the production of PIF, and thus prolactin is synthesized and released.

Melanocyte-stimulating hormone (MSH) plays a role in skin pigmentation and has recently been found to play important roles in feeding and energy metabolism as well as in inflammation. Recently, MSH, particularly gamma-MSH, has been linked to cardiovascular regulation and sodium metabolism.

Posterior Pituitary Hormones

The posterior pituitary gland stores and releases two hormones that are synthesized by nerve cells in the hypothalamus.

Antidiuretic hormone (ADH), also called vasopressin, functions to regulate water balance. When ADH is secreted, it makes renal tubules more permeable to water. This allows water in renal tubules to be reabsorbed into the plasma and so conserves body water. In the absence of ADH, little water is reabsorbed, and large amounts are lost in the urine.

ADH is secreted when body fluids become concentrated (high amounts of electrolytes in proportion to the amount of water) and when blood volume is low. In the first instance, ADH causes reabsorption of water, dilution of extracellular fluids, and restoration of normal osmotic pressure. In the second instance, ADH raises blood volume and arterial blood pressure toward homeostatic levels.

Oxytocin functions in childbirth and lactation. It initiates uterine contractions at the end of gestation to induce childbirth, and it causes milk to move from breast glands to nipples so the infant can obtain the milk by suckling.

Individual Drugs

Although hypothalamic hormones and pituitary hormones have few therapeutic uses, they have important functions when used in certain circumstances, and drug formulations of most hormones have been synthesized. Selected drugs are described below. Indications for use, routes, and dosage ranges are listed in Table 22-1.

Hypothalamic Hormones

Goserelin (Zoladex), **histrelin** (Vantas), **leuprolide** (Lupron), **nafarelin** (Synarel), and **triptorelin** (Trelstar) are equivalent

to GnRH. After initial stimulation of LH and FSH secretion, chronic administration of therapeutic doses inhibits gonadotropin secretion. This action results in decreased production of testosterone and estrogen, which is reversible when administration is stopped. In males, testosterone is reduced to castrate levels. In premenopausal females, estrogens are reduced to postmenopausal levels. These effects occur within 2 to 4 weeks after drug therapy is begun. In children with central precocious puberty, gonadotropins (testosterone in males; estrogen in females) are reduced to prepubertal levels.

These GnRH equivalents cannot be given orally, because they would be destroyed by enzymes in the GI tract. Most are given by injection and are available in depot preparations that can be given once monthly or less often. Adverse effects are basically those of testosterone or estrogen deficiency. When given for prostate cancer, the drugs may cause increased bone pain and increased difficulty in urinating during the first few weeks of treatment. The drugs may also cause or aggravate depression.

Octreotide (Sandostatin) has pharmacologic actions similar to those of somatostatin. Indications for use include acromegaly, in which the drug reduces blood levels of GH and insulin-like growth factor-1 (IGF-1); carcinoid tumors, in which it inhibits diarrhea and flushing; and vasoactive intestinal peptide tumors, in which it relieves diarrhea (by decreasing GI secretions and motility). It is also used to treat diarrhea in acquired immunodeficiency syndrome (AIDS) and other

Table 22-1	**Drugs at a Glance:** Hypothalamic and Pituitary Drugs		
		ROUTES AND DOSAGE RANGES	
Generic/Trade name	**Indications for use**	**Adults**	**Children**
Hypothalamic Hormones			
Goserelin (Zoladex)	Endometriosis Metastatic breast cancer Prostate cancer	Sub-Q implant into upper abdominal wall, 3.6 mg every 28 days or 10.8 mg every 3 mo	
Histrelin (Vantas; Supprelin LA)	Palliative treatment of advanced prostate cancer (Vantas) CPR (Supprelin LA) in children	1 implant Sub-Q q 12 mo	*Supprelin LA,* Implant Sub-Q q 12 mo
Leuprolide (Lupron)	Advanced prostatic cancer CPP in children Endometriosis Uterine fibroid tumors	Endometriosis, uterine fibroids, IM depot injection, 3.75 mg every mo or 11.25 mg every 3 mo for 6 mo Prostate cancer, Sub-Q 1 mg daily; IM depot 7.5 mg every mo, 22.5 mg every 3 mo, or 30 mg every 4 mo; implant (Viadur) one (72 mg) every 12 mo	CPP, Sub-Q 50 mcg/kg/d; IM Depot-Ped, weight 25 kg or less, 7.5 mg; more than 25 to 37.5 kg, 11.25 mg; more than 37.5 kg, 15 mg every mo

		ROUTES AND DOSAGE RANGES	
Generic/Trade name	Indications for use	Adults	Children
Nafarelin (Synarel)	Endometriosis CPP in children	1 spray (200 mcg) in one nostril in the morning and 1 spray in the other nostril in the evening (400 mcg/d), starting between the 2nd and 4th days of the menstrual cycle	2 sprays (400 mcg) in each nostril morning and evening (1600 mcg/d), until resumption of puberty is desired
Octreotide (Sandostatin; LAR Depot [long-acting])	Acromegaly Carcinoid tumors Vasoactive intestinal peptide tumors Diarrhea	Acromegaly, Sub-Q 50–100 mcg 3 times daily; long-acting: 100–200 mcg 3 times daily, may be adjusted up to 500 mcg 3 times daily Carcinoid tumors, Sub-Q 100–600 mcg daily (average 300 mcg) in 2–4 divided doses Intestinal tumors, Sub-Q 200–300 mcg daily in 2–4 divided doses Diarrhea, IV, Sub-Q 50 mcg 2 or 3 times daily initially, then adjusted according to response	Dosage not established but 1–10 mcg/kg reportedly well tolerated in young clients
Triptorelin (Trelstar)	Advanced prostatic cancer	3.75 mg depot injection IM	
Anterior Pituitary Hormones			
Corticotropin (Acthrel; HP Acthar Gel)	Stimulate synthesis of hormones by the adrenal cortex Diagnostic test of adrenal function Treatment of acute exacerbation of multiple sclerosis	Diagnostic use, IM Sub-Q up to 80 units as a single injection. HP Acthar Gel, IM or Sub-Q 40–80 units q24–72 IM 80–120 units daily for 2–3 wk	
Cosyntropin (Cortrosyn)	Diagnostic test in suspected adrenal insufficiency	IM, IV 0.25 mg (equivalent to 25 units ACTH)	*older than 2 y:* same as adult dose *under 2 y:* IM, IV 0.125 mg
Growth hormone: **Somatrem** **Somatropin** (Genotropin, Humatrope, Norditropin, Nutropin, Serostim)	Promote growth in children whose growth is impaired by a deficiency of endogenous growth hormone		*Somatrem,* IM up to 0.1 mg/kg 3 times per wk *Somatropin,* IM up to 0.06 mg/kg 3 times per wk
HCG (Chorex, Choron, Pregnyl)	Cryptorchidism Induce ovulation in the treatment of infertility	Cryptorchidism and male hypogonadism, IM 500–4000 units 2–3 times per wk for several wk To induce ovulation, IM 5000–10,000 units in 1 dose, 1 d after treatment with menotropins	*Preadolescent boys:* Cryptorchidism and hypogonadism, IM 500–4000 units 2–3 times per wk for several wk
Choriogonadotropin alpha (Ovidrel)	Induce ovulation in the treatment of infertility	250 mcg Sub-Q in 1 dose, 1 d after treatment with menotropins	
Follitropin alfa (Gonal-F, Gonal-F RFF pen)	Stimulate ovulation	Sub-Q 75 IU of FSH to maximum daily dose of 300 IU Prefilled pen: 300–900 IU IV of FSH as individualized dosage	

(continued on page 350)

Table 22-1   Drugs at a Glance: Hypothalamic and Pituitary Drugs (continued)

| Generic/Trade name | Indications for use | ROUTES AND DOSAGE RANGES | |
		Adults	Children
Follitropin beta (Follistim)	Stimulate ovulation	Sub-Q 75 IU of FSH to maximum daily dose of 300 IU	
Menotropins (Pergonal)	Combined with HCG to induce ovulation in treatment of infertility caused by lack of pituitary gonadotropins	IM 1 ampule (75 units FSH and 75 units LH) daily for 9–12 d, followed by HCG to induce ovulation	
Pegvisomant (Somavert)	Acromegaly unresponsive to other management strategies	Load: 40 mg Sub-Q Maintenance: 10 mg Sub-Q; titrate by 5 mg increments q4–6 wk according to IGF-1 levels to maximum of 30 mg/d	
Thyrotropin alfa (Thyrogen)	Diagnostic test of thyroid function	IM 0.9 mg every 24 h for 2 doses or every 72 h for 3 doses	*under 16 y:* Dosage not established
Urofollitropin (Bravelle)	Stimulate ovulation	Sub-Q 150 IU of FSH daily for the first 5 d to maximum daily dose of 450 IU	
Posterior Pituitary Hormones			
Desmopressin (DDAVP, Stimate)	Neurogenic diabetes insipidus Hemostasis (parenteral only) in spontaneous, trauma-induced, and perioperative bleeding	Diabetes insipidus, intranasally 0.1–0.4 mL/d, usually in 2 divided doses Hemophilia A, von Willebrand's disease, IV 0.3 mcg/kg in 50 mL sterile saline, infused over 15–30 min	*3 mo–2 y:* Diabetes insipidus, intranasally 0.05–0.3 mL/d in 1–2 doses *Weight more than 10 kg:* Hemophilia A, von Willebrand's disease, same as adult dosage *Weight 10 kg or less:* Hemophilia A, von Willebrand's disease, IV 0.3 mcg/kg in 10 mL of sterile saline
Vasopressin (Pitressin)	Diabetes insipidus	IM, Sub-Q, intranasally on cotton pledgets, 0.25–0.5 mL (5–10 units) 2–3 times daily	IM, Sub-Q, intranasally on cotton pledgets, 0.125–0.5 mL (2.5–10 units) 3–4 times daily
Oxytocin (Pitocin)	Induce labor Control postpartum bleeding	Induction of labor, IV 1-mL ampule (10 units) in 1000 mL of 5% dextrose injection (10 units/1000 mL = 10 milliunits/mL), infused at 0.2–2 milliunits/min initially, then regulated according to frequency and strength of uterine contractions Prevention or treatment of postpartum bleeding, IV 10–40 units in 1000 mL of 5% dextrose injection, infused at 125 mL/h (40 milliunits/min) or 0.6–1.8 units (0.06–0.18 mL) diluted in 3–5 mL sodium chloride injection and injected slowly; IM 0.3–1 mL (3–10 units)	

ACTH, adrenocorticotropic hormone; CPP, central precocious puberty; FSH, follicle-stimulating hormone; HCG, human chorionic gonadotropin; IGF-1, insulin-like growth factor-1; LH, luteinizing hormone.

conditions. The drug is most often given subcutaneously and may be self-administered. The long-acting formulation (Sandostatin LAR Depot) must be given intramuscularly in a gluteal muscle. Dosage should be reduced for older adults.

Anterior Pituitary Hormones

Corticotropin (ACTH, Acthar Gel), which is obtained from animal pituitary glands, is mainly of historical interest. For therapeutic purposes, it has been replaced by adrenal corticosteroids. It may be used occasionally as a diagnostic test to differentiate primary adrenal insufficiency (Addison's disease, which is associated with atrophy of the adrenal gland) from secondary adrenal insufficiency caused by inadequate pituitary secretion of corticotropin. However, **cosyntropin** (Cortrosyn), a synthetic formulation, is more commonly used to test for suspected adrenal insufficiency.

Growth hormone is synthesized from bacteria by recombinant DNA technology. **Somatropin** (e.g., Humatrope) is therapeutically equivalent to endogenous GH produced by the pituitary gland. The main clinical use of GH is for children whose growth is impaired by a deficiency of endogenous hormone. The drugs are ineffective when impaired growth results from other causes or after puberty, when epiphyses of the long bones have closed. GH is also used to treat short stature in children that is associated with chronic renal failure or Turner's syndrome (a genetic disorder that occurs in girls). In adults, the drugs may be used to treat deficiency states (e.g., those caused by disease, surgery, or radiation of the pituitary gland) or the tissue wasting associated with AIDS. In general, dosage should be individualized according to response. Excessive administration can cause gigantism.

Human chorionic gonadotropin (HCG; e.g., Chorex) produces physiologic effects similar to those of naturally occurring LH. In males, it is used to evaluate the ability of Leydig's cells to produce testosterone, to treat hypogonadism due to pituitary deficiency, and to treat cryptorchidism (undescended testicle) in preadolescent boys. In women, recombinant HCG **choriogonadotropin alpha** (Ovidrel) is used in combination with menotropins to induce ovulation in the treatment of infertility. Excessive doses or prolonged administration can lead to sexual precocity, edema, and breast enlargement caused by oversecretion of testosterone and estrogen.

Menotropins (Pergonal), a gonadotropin preparation obtained from the urine of postmenopausal women, contains both FSH and LH. It is usually combined with HCG to induce ovulation in the treatment of infertility caused by lack of pituitary gonadotropins.

Pegvisomant (Somavert) is a GH receptor antagonist used in the treatment of acromegaly in adults who are unable to tolerate or are resistant to other management strategies. The drug selectively binds to GH receptors, blocking the binding of endogenous GH. In general, dosage should be individualized according to response. Dosage reduction of hypoglycemic agents may be required because the drug may increase glucose

tolerance. Increased dosages of pegvisomant may be necessary when administered with narcotics. The drug should be used with caution in the elderly and in people with renal or hepatic disease.

Thyrotropin alfa (Thyrogen) is a synthetic formulation of TSH used as a diagnostic adjunct for serum thyroglobin (Tg) testing in individuals with well-differentiated thyroid cancer. The testing can be performed with or without radioiodine imaging. Because there is a risk of missing the diagnosis of thyroid cancer or predicting the extent of the disease, thyroid hormone withdrawal Tg testing radioactive imaging is the standard test for evaluating the presence, extent, and location of thyroid cancer. Thyrotropin alfa must be used cautiously in patients with coronary artery disease and with a large amount of residual thyroid tissue as the drug produces a temporary rise of thyroid hormone concentration in the blood.

Urofollitropin (Bravelle), **follitropin alfa** (Gonal-F), and **follitropin beta** (Follistim) are drug preparations of FSH. These drugs are used to stimulate ovarian function in the treatment of infertility and are used sequentially with HCG. Urofollitropin is extracted from the urine of postmenopausal women and acts directly on the ovaries to stimulate follicular ovulation. The development of follitropin alfa and follitropin beta as recombinant products advances the treatment of infertility, appears to be well tolerated, and has similar efficacy. A new liquid formulation of follitropin alfa (Gonal-F RFF Pen) is available in a prefilled and ready-to-use multidose FSH injection.

Posterior Pituitary Hormones

Desmopressin (DDAVP, Stimate) and vasopressin (Pitressin) are synthetic equivalents of ADH. A major clinical use is the treatment of neurogenic diabetes insipidus, a disorder characterized by a deficiency of ADH and the excretion of large amounts of dilute urine. Diabetes insipidus may be idiopathic, hereditary, or acquired as a result of trauma, surgery, tumor, infection, or other conditions that impair the function of the hypothalamus or posterior pituitary.

Parenteral desmopressin is also used as a hemostatic in patients with hemophilia A or mild to moderate von Willebrand's disease (type 1). The drug is effective in controlling spontaneous or trauma-induced bleeding and intraoperative and postoperative bleeding when given 30 minutes before the procedure. Vasopressin is also used in the treatment of bleeding esophageal varices because of its vasoconstrictive effects. Desmopressin may be inhaled intranasally; vasopressin must be injected.

Oxytocin (Pitocin) is a synthetic drug that exerts the same physiologic effects as the posterior pituitary hormone. Thus, it promotes uterine contractility and is used clinically to induce labor and in the postpartum period to control bleeding. Oxytocin must be used only when clearly indicated and when the recipient can be supervised by well-trained personnel, as in a hospital.

Applying Your Knowledge 22-1

How Can You Avoid This Medication Error?

The nurse prepares Mr. Rojas' medication and administers 0.2 mL of desmopressin intranasally.

Nursing Process

Assessment

Assess for disorders for which hypothalamic and pituitary hormones are given.

- For children with impaired growth, assess height and weight (actual and compared with growth charts) and diagnostic radiographic reports of bone age.

- For patients with diabetes insipidus, assess baseline blood pressure, weight, ratio of fluid intake to urine output, urine specific gravity, and laboratory reports of serum electrolytes.

- For patients with diarrhea, assess the number and consistency of stools per day as well as hydration status.

- For patients with infertility, assess drug-specific adverse effects (dizziness, nausea, headache and abdominal cramps, hot flashes/flushes, ovarian enlargement, blurring of vision and other visual symptoms).

Nursing Diagnoses

- Deficient Knowledge: Drug administration and effects
- Altered Growth and Development
- Anxiety related to multiple injections
- Risk for Injury: Adverse drug effects
- Ineffective Coping related to frustration with difficulty with conception

Planning/Goals

The patient will

- Experience relief of symptoms without serious adverse effects

- Take or receive the drug accurately

- Comply with procedures for monitoring and follow-up

- Cope effectively and acknowledge feelings of grief, disappointment, and failure

Interventions

- For children receiving GH, help the family set reasonable goals for increased height and weight and comply with accurate drug administration and follow-up procedures (e.g., periodic radiographs to determine bone growth and progress toward epiphyseal closure; recording

height and weight at least weekly). Patient Guidelines for Growth Hormone are given in the accompanying display.

- For patients with diabetes insipidus, help them develop a daily routine to monitor their response to drug therapy (e.g., weigh themselves; monitor fluid intake and urine output for approximately equal amounts; check urine specific gravity [should be at least 1.015] and replace fluids accordingly).

- For patients with infertility, reinforce teaching about potential risks and benefits of drug therapy and about proper self-administration techniques of preparation, injection, and disposal of medication and supplies. Educate about evaluating basal body temperature patterns and continuing medical supervision as long as the drugs are being taken, and alert the couple about the risk of multiple births. Refer to local support groups, and acknowledge feelings of grief, disappointment, and failure. Patient Guidelines for Fertility Drugs are given in the accompanying display.

Evaluation

- Interview and observe for compliance with instructions for taking the drug(s).

- Observe for relief of symptoms for which pituitary hormones were prescribed.

- Observe for effective coping with the underlying condition and the effects of treatment.

Applying Your Knowledge 22-2

What nursing measures should be implemented to appropriately monitor Mr. Rojas?

Principles of Therapy

Hypothalamic hormones and pituitary hormones have few therapeutic uses. Most hypothalamic hormones are used to diagnose pituitary insufficiency. Pituitary hormones are not used extensively because most conditions in which they are indicated are uncommon, other effective agents are available for some uses, and deficiencies of target-gland hormones (e.g., corticosteroids, thyroid hormones, male or female sex hormones) are usually more effectively treated with those hormones than with anterior pituitary hormones that stimulate their secretion. However, the hormones perform important functions when used in particular circumstances, and drug formulations of most hormones have been synthesized for these purposes.

Because the hormones are proteins, they must be given by injection or nasal inhalation. If taken orally, the hormones would be destroyed by the proteolytic enzymes in the GI tract.

Hypothalamic Hormones

Hypothalamic hormones are rarely used in most clinical practice settings. The drugs should be prescribed by health care providers who are knowledgeable about endocrinology and should be administered according to the manufacturers' literature.

Applying Your Knowledge 22-3

The nurse returns to Mr. Rojas' room to assess the patient. Mr. Rojas has an elevated blood pressure of 190/100. His sodium level is low, at 117 mEq/L, and his urine osmolality is below normal. How do you respond?

Pituitary Hormones

Most drug therapy with pituitary hormones is given to replace or supplement naturally occurring hormones in situations involving inadequate function of the pituitary gland (hypopituitarism). Conditions resulting from excessive amounts of pituitary hormones (hyperpituitarism) are more often treated with surgery or radiation. Diagnosis of suspected pituitary disorders should be thorough to promote more effective treatment, including drug therapy. Dosage of all pituitary hormones must be individualized, because the responsiveness of affected tissues varies.

Toxicity: Abuse of Growth Hormone

Inappropriate use of GH is an increasing concern. Young athletes may use the drug for bodybuilding and to enhance athletic performance. If so, they are likely to use relatively high doses. In addition, the highest levels of physiologic hormone are secreted during adolescence. The combination of high pharmacologic and high physiologic amounts increases risks of health problems from excessive hormone. Also, there is little evidence that hormone use increases muscle mass or strength beyond that achieved with exercise alone.

Middle-aged and older adults may use GH to combat the effects of aging, such as decreased energy, weaker muscles and joints, and wrinkled skin. One source of the product is apparently "anti-aging" clinics. Although it is not illegal for health care providers to prescribe GH for these populations, such use is unproven in safety and effectiveness. Endocrinologists emphasize that optimal adult levels of GH are unknown, and use of GH to slow aging is unproven and potentially dangerous because the long-term effects are unknown.

Possible adverse effects associated with GH, especially with high doses or chronic use, include acromegaly, diabetes, hypertension, and increased risk of serious cardiovascular disease (e.g., heart failure). There is also concern about a possible link between GH, which stimulates tumor growth, and cancer. GH stimulates the release of IGF-1 (also called somatomedin), a substance that circulates in the blood and stimulates cell division. Most tumor cells have receptors that recognize IGF-1, bind it, and allow it to enter the cell, where it could trigger uncontrolled cell division. This concern may be greater for middle-aged and older adults, because malignancies are more common in these groups than in adolescents and young adults.

Applying Your Knowledge 22-4

Legal/Ethical Dilemma

During his stay, Mr. Rojas' family comes to visit him often. You meet his mother and his two younger brothers. After one of their visits, Mr. Rojas confides that Juan, age 13, is taking GH because he is in the 35th height percentile for his age. His other brother, Miguel, age 15, plays basketball and wants to be taller. Miguel has convinced his brother Juan to share his drug with him. What action should you take and why?

Patient Teaching Guidelines ▪ Growth Hormone

General Considerations

- Growth hormone (GH) is taken to normalize growth and development in children with a GH deficiency, not for people merely desiring an increase in stature. The drugs are contraindicated in children after epiphyseal closure occurs.
- GH is taken until a satisfactory height has been achieved, epiphyseal closure occurs, or until no further stimulation of growth occurs.
- Periodic tests of growth curve, bone age, serum glucose levels, thyroid function, and somatomedin levels are necessary, as well as funduscopic eye examinations.
- Children who have GH deficiency may develop slipped capital femoral epiphysis more frequently, and those with scoliosis may see a progression of the condition.

Self-Administration

- Take GH only if prescribed and as prescribed.
- Continue with medical supervision as long as GH is being taken.
- Ask a health care provider if you are uncertain about how to administer GH.
- Report severe hip or knee pain or the development of a limp to the prescriber immediately, because this may indicate slipped capital femoral epiphysis. In addition, report any signs of severe headache or acute visual changes, because they may indicate the complication of increased intracranial pressure.

Patient Teaching Guidelines | Fertility Drugs

General Considerations

- Fertility drugs stimulate ovulation and fertility. Pregnancy typically may occur within 4–6 weeks of therapy.
- These drugs are contraindicated in pregnant women. If pregnancy is suspected, the drugs should be discontinued, and the physician who prescribed them should be notified.
- These drugs should not be used by women who are breast-feeding or by children.
- In many cases, couples who are infertile experience feelings of grief, disappointment, and failure. Often they can benefit from participation in local support groups.

Self-Administration

- Take fertility drugs only if prescribed and as prescribed.
- Continue with medical supervision as long as the drugs are being taken.

- Ask the health care provider if you are uncertain about how the drug is administered; proper use of infusion devices; and how to monitor basal body temperature patterns.
- Monitor ovulation and discontinue the drug, if instructed, when ovulation is suspected.
- Recognize that the risk of multiple births is increased with the use of these drugs.
- Report adverse effects, such as dizziness, nausea, headache and abdominal cramps, hot flashes/flushes, and blurring of vision and other visual symptoms.
- For maximum desired response, have intercourse daily beginning the day before human chorionic gonadotropin therapy until ovulation occurs.

Nursing Actions | Hypothalamic and Pituitary Hormones

NURSING ACTIONS	RATIONALE/EXPLANATION
1. Administer accurately a. Read the manufacturer's instructions and drug labels carefully before drug preparation and administration.	These hormone preparations are given infrequently and often require special techniques of administration.
2. Observe for therapeutic effects	Therapeutic effects vary widely, depending on the particular pituitary hormone given and the reason for use.
a. With goserelin and related drugs, observe for ovulation or decreased symptoms of endometriosis and absence of menstruation.	Therapeutic effects depend on the reason for use. Note that different formulations are used to stimulate ovulation and treat endometriosis.
b. With corticotropin, therapeutic effects stem largely from increased secretion of adrenal cortex hormones, especially the glucocorticoids, and include anti-inflammatory effects (see Chap. 23).	Corticotropin is usually not recommended for the numerous nonendocrine inflammatory disorders that respond to glucocorticoids. Administration of glucocorticoids is more convenient and effective than administration of corticotropin.
c. With chorionic gonadotropin, menotropins, follitropin alpha, and follitropin beta given in cases of female infertility, ovulation and conception are therapeutic effects.	
d. With chorionic gonadotropin given in cryptorchidism, the therapeutic effect is descent of the testicles from the abdomen to the scrotum.	
e. With growth hormone, observe for increased skeletal growth and development.	Indicated by appropriate increases in height and weight
f. With antidiuretics (desmopressin and vasopressin), observe for decreased urine output, increased urine specific gravity, decreased signs of dehydration, decreased thirst.	These effects indicate control of diabetes insipidus.
g. With oxytocin given to induce labor, observe for the beginning or the intensifying of uterine contractions.	
h. With oxytocin given to control postpartum bleeding, observe for a firm uterine fundus and decreased vaginal bleeding.	
i. With octreotide given for diarrhea, observe for decreased number and fluidity of stools.	Octreotide is often used to control diarrhea associated with a number of conditions.
3. Observe for adverse effects a. With goserelin, observe for headache, nausea, lightheadedness, and local edema, pain, and pruritus after subcutaneous injections.	Systemic reactions occur infrequently.

NURSING ACTIONS	RATIONALE/EXPLANATION
b. With corticotropin, observe for sodium and fluid retention, edema, hypokalemia, hyperglycemia, osteoporosis, increased susceptibility to infection, myopathy, behavioral changes.	These adverse reactions are in general the same as those produced by adrenal cortex hormones. Severity of adverse reactions tends to increase with dosage and duration of corticotropin administration.
c. With human chorionic gonadotropin given to preadolescent boys, observe for sexual precocity, breast enlargement, and edema.	Sexual precocity results from stimulation of excessive testosterone secretion at an early age.
d. With growth hormone, observe for mild edema, headache, localized muscle pain, weakness, and hyperglycemia.	Adverse effects are not common. Another adverse effect may be development of antibodies to the drug, but this does not prevent its growth-stimulating effects.
e. With menotropins, observe for symptoms of ovarian hyperstimulation, such as abdominal discomfort, weight gain, ascites, pleural effusion, oliguria, and hypotension.	Adverse effects can be minimized by frequent pelvic examinations to check for ovarian enlargement and by laboratory measurement of estrogen levels. Multiple gestation (mostly twins) is a possibility and is related to ovarian overstimulation.
f. With desmopressin, observe for headache, nasal congestion, nausea, and increased blood pressure. A more serious adverse reaction is water retention and hyponatremia.	Adverse reactions usually occur only with high dosages and tend to be relatively mild. Water intoxication (headache, nausea, vomiting, confusion, lethargy, coma, convulsions) may occur with any antidiuretic therapy if excessive fluids are ingested.
g. With pegvisomant, observe for pain, injection site reaction, nausea, flu syndrome, and diarrhea.	Adverse effects are usually mild or occur infrequently.
h. With vasopressin, observe for water intoxication; chest pain, myocardial infarction, increased blood pressure; abdominal cramps, nausea, and diarrhea.	With high doses, vasopressin constricts blood vessels, especially coronary arteries, and stimulates smooth muscle of the gastrointestinal tract. Special caution is necessary in clients with heart disease, asthma, or epilepsy.
i. With oxytocin, observe for excessive stimulation or contractility of the uterus, uterine rupture, and cervical and perineal lacerations.	Severe adverse reactions are most likely to occur when oxytocin is given to induce labor and delivery.
j. With octreotide, observe for dysrhythmias, bradycardia, diarrhea, headache, hyperglycemia, injection-site pain, and symptoms of gallstones.	These are more common effects, especially in those receiving octreotide for acromegaly.
k. With triptorelin, observe for hot flushes, skeletal pain, impotence, headache, and hypertension.	Adverse reactions due to decreased levels of LH and FSH
4. Observe for drug interactions	
a. Drugs that *increase* effects of vasopressin: (1) General anesthetics, chlorpropamide (Diabinese)	Potentiate vasopressin
b. Drug that *decreases* effects of vasopressin: (1) Lithium	Inhibits the renal tubular reabsorption of water normally stimulated by vasopressin
c. Drugs that *increase* effects of oxytocin: (1) Estrogens	With adequate estrogen levels, oxytocin increases uterine contractility. When estrogen levels are low, the effect of oxytocin is reduced.
(2) Vasoconstrictors or vasopressors (e.g., ephedrine, epinephrine, norepinephrine)	Severe, persistent hypertension with rupture of cerebral blood vessels may occur because of additive vasoconstrictor effects. This is a potentially lethal interaction and should be avoided.

Key Concepts

■ The hypothalamus and the pituitary gland interact to control most metabolic functions of the body and to maintain homeostasis.

■ The anterior pituitary gland produces seven hormones: 6H, ACTH, TSH, FSH, LH, MSH, and prolactin.

■ The posterior pituitary gland stores and releases two hormones that are synthesized by nerve cells in the hypothalamus: ADH and oxytocin.

■ Antidiuretic hormone (ADH), also called vasopressin, functions to regulate water balance.

Review and Application Exercises

Short Answer Exercises

1. What hormones are secreted by the hypothalamus and pituitary, and what are their functions?

2. What are the functions and clinical uses of ADH and GH?

3. What are adverse effects of the hypothalamic and pituitary hormones used in clinical practice?

NCLEX-Style Questions

4. Because growth hormone (GH) is an insulin antagonist, administration of GH to a person with type 1 diabetes mellitus may result in which of the following?
   a. hyperglycemia
   b. an increase in insulin production
   c. a decreased need for insulin
   d. no significant effect

5. The father of an 11-year-old boy is concerned because his son is shorter than his friends. He asks the nurse whether the boy should be taking GH so that he can be competitive when playing basketball in middle school. Both of the boy's parents are of short stature. Which of the following is the best response on the part of the nurse?
   a. "The treatment is very expensive so we need to check and see if your insurance will cover it."
   b. "Don't worry; many basketball players who are short in stature are successful."
   c. "Short stature is not the only requirement for treatment with GH. Let's spend some time discussing the assessment that is being done to determine your son's need for GH."
   d. "GH will not increase your child's stature, because you and your wife are also very short."

6. Your patient has an IV order for cosyntropin (Cortrosyn) and asks why he is to be given this medication. You explain that it is not a treatment but is commonly used to test for which of the following conditions?
   a. hypothalamic dysfunction
   b. thyroid cancer
   c. pituitary dysfunction
   d. adrenal insufficiency

7. A patient taking high doses of vasopressin has a blood pressure of 188/96 mm Hg and complains of abdominal cramps, nausea, and diarrhea. The nurse contacts the prescribing provider and recognizes that these GI symptoms result from which of the following conditions?
   a. smooth-muscle stimulation of the GI tract
   b. neurologic toxicity
   c. gastroparesis
   d. drug interaction with a nutrient

Selected References

Corwin, E. J. (2006). *Handbook of pathophysiology* (3rd ed.). Philadelphia: Lippincott Williams & Wilkins.

Drug facts and comparisons. (Updated monthly). St. Louis, MO: Facts and Comparisons.

Humphreys, M. H. (2007). Cardiovascular and renal actions of melanocyte-stimulating hormone peptides. *Current Opinion in Nephrology and Hypertension, 16*, 32–38.

Lacy, C. F., Armstrong, L. L., Goldman, M. P., & Lance, L. L. (2007). *Lexi-Comp's drug information handbook* (15th ed.). Hudson, OH: American Pharmaceutical Association.

Porth, C. M. (2005). *Pathophysiology: Concepts of altered health states* (7th ed.). Philadelphia: Lippincott Williams & Wilkins.

Stelmach, R., Patrocínio, M., Nunes, T., Ribeiro, M., & Cukier, A. (2005). Effect of treating allergic rhinitis with corticosteroids in patients with mild-to-moderate persistent asthma. *Chest, 128*, 3140–3147.

Corticosteroids

KEY TERMS

- Addison's disease
- Addisonian crisis
- Adrenocortical insufficiency
- Aldosterone
- Corticosteroids
- Cortisol
- Cushing's disease
- Glucocorticoids
- Immunosuppression
- Mineralocorticoids
- Negative feedback mechanism
- Steroids

LEARNING OBJECTIVES

After studying this chapter, you will be able to:

1. Review physiologic effects of endogenous corticosteroids.
2. Discuss clinical indications for use of exogenous corticosteroids.
3. Differentiate between physiologic and pharmacologic doses of corticosteroids.
4. Differentiate between short-term and long-term corticosteroid therapy.
5. Recognize at least 10 adverse effects of long-term corticosteroid therapy.
6. Explain the pathophysiologic basis of adverse drug effects.
7. Examine the potential benefits for administering corticosteroids topically when possible rather than systemically.
8. Analyze the use other drugs and interventions to decrease the need for corticosteroids.
9. Discuss the use of corticosteroids in selected populations and conditions.
10. Apply the nursing process with a patient receiving long-term systemic corticosteroid therapy, including teaching needs.

Applying Your Knowledge

Sue Hubble is a 70-year-old African-American woman. She is 5 feet 9 inches tall and weighs 275 pounds. She has type 2 diabetes mellitus and, as a result of lifelong smoking, has been diagnosed with chronic obstructive pulmonary disease (COPD). In her home, she uses oxygen. In addition to her respiratory drugs and her drugs for diabetes, she has been taking prednisone 20 mg PO daily for the past month. You are Ms. Hubble's home care nurse.

Introduction

Corticosteroids, also called *glucocorticoids* or *steroids*, are hormones produced by the adrenal cortex, part of the adrenal glands. These hormones affect almost all body organs and are extremely important in maintaining homeostasis when secreted in normal amounts. Disease results from inadequate or excessive secretion. Exogenous corticosteroids are used as drugs in a variety of disorders. Their use must be closely monitored, because they have profound therapeutic and adverse effects. To understand the effects of corticosteroids used as drugs (exogenous corticosteroids), it is necessary to understand the physiologic effects and other characteristics of the endogenous hormones.

Secretion of Endogenous Corticosteroids

Corticosteroid secretion is controlled by the hypothalamus, the anterior pituitary, and adrenal cortex (the hypothalamic–pituitary–adrenal, or HPA, axis). Various stimuli (e.g., low plasma levels of corticosteroids, pain, anxiety, trauma, illness, anesthesia) activate the system. These stimuli cause the hypothalamus of the brain to secrete corticotropin-releasing hormone or factor (CRH or CRF), which stimulates the anterior pituitary gland to secrete corticotropin, and corticotropin then stimulates the adrenal cortex to secrete corticosteroids.

The rate of corticosteroid secretion is usually maintained within relatively narrow limits but changes according to need. When plasma corticosteroid levels rise to an adequate level, secretion of corticosteroids slows or stops. The mechanism by which the hypothalamus and anterior pituitary "learn" that no more corticosteroids are needed is called a *negative feedback mechanism.*

This negative feedback mechanism is normally very important, but it does not work during stress responses. The stress response activates the sympathetic nervous system (SNS) to produce more epinephrine and norepinephrine and the adrenal cortex to produce as much as 10 times the normal amount of cortisol. The synergistic interaction of these hormones increases the person's ability to respond to stress. However, the increased SNS activity continues to stimulate cortisol production (the main glucocorticoids secreted as part of the body's response to stress) and overrules the negative feedback mechanism. Excessive and prolonged corticosteroid secretion damages body tissues.

Corticosteroids are secreted directly into the bloodstream. *Cortisol* is approximately 90% bound to plasma proteins, and this high degree of protein binding slows cortisol movement out of the plasma, so that it has a relatively long plasma half-life of 60 to 90 minutes. The remaining 10% is unbound and biologically active. In contrast, aldosterone is only 60% bound to plasma proteins and has a short half-life of 20 minutes. In general, protein binding functions as a storage area from which the hormones are released as needed. This promotes more consistent blood levels and more uniform distribution to the tissues.

Types of Endogenous Corticosteroids

The adrenal cortex produces approximately 30 steroid hormones, which are divided into glucocorticoids, mineralocorticoids, and adrenal sex hormones. Chemically, all corticosteroids are derived from cholesterol and have similar chemical structures. Despite their similarities, however, slight differences cause them to have different functions.

Glucocorticoids

The term *corticosteroids* actually refers to all secretions of the adrenal cortex, but it is most often used to designate the glucocorticoids, which are important in metabolic, inflammatory, and immune processes. Glucocorticoids include cortisol, corticosterone, and cortisone. Cortisol accounts for at least 95% of glucocorticoid activity; corticosterone and cortisone accounts for a small amount of activity. Glucocorticoids are secreted cyclically, with the largest amount being produced in the early morning and the smallest amount during the evening hours (in people with a normal day–night schedule). At the cellular level, glucocorticoids account for most of the characteristics and physiologic effects of the corticosteroids (Box 23-1).

| **Box 23-1** | **Effects of Glucocorticoids on Body Processes and Systems** |

Carbohydrate Metabolism

- ↑ Formation of glucose (gluconeogenesis) by breaking down protein into amino acids. The amino acids are then transported to the liver, where they are acted on by enzymes that convert them to glucose. The glucose is then returned to the circulation for use by body tissues or storage in the liver as glycogen.
- ↓ Cellular use of glucose, especially in muscle cells. This is attributed to a ↓effect of insulin on the proteins that normally transport glucose into cells and by ↓numbers and functional capacity of insulin receptors.
- Both the ↑production and ↓use of glucose promote higher levels of glucose in the blood (hyperglycemia) and may lead to diabetes mellitus. These actions also increase the amount of glucose stored as glycogen in the liver, skeletal muscles, and other tissues.

Protein Metabolism

- ↑ Breakdown of protein into amino acids (catabolic effect); ↑ rate of amino acid transport to the liver and conversion to glucose

- ↓Rate of new protein formation from dietary and other amino acids (antianabolic effect)
- The combination of ↑breakdown of cell protein and ↓protein synthesis leads to protein depletion in virtually all body cells except those of the liver. Thus, glycogen stores in the body are ↑and protein stores are ↓.

Lipid Metabolism

- ↑Breakdown of adipose tissue into fatty acids; the fatty acids are transported in the plasma and used as a source of energy by body cells.
- ↑Oxidation of fatty acids within body cells

Inflammatory and Immune Responses

- ↓Inflammatory response. Inflammation is the normal bodily response to tissue damage and involves three stages. First, a large amount of plasma-like fluid leaks out of capillaries into the damaged area and becomes clotted. Second, leukocytes migrate into the area. Third, tissue healing occurs, largely by growth of fibrous scar tissue. Normal or physiologic amounts of glucocorticoids probably do not significantly affect inflammation and healing, but large amounts of glucocorticoids inhibit all three stages of the inflammatory process.

More specifically, corticosteroids stabilize lysosomal membranes (and thereby prevent the release of inflammatory proteolytic enzymes); ↓capillary permeability (and thereby↓leakage of fluid and proteins into the damaged tissue); ↓the accumulation of neutrophils and macrophages at sites of inflammation (and thereby impair phagocytosis of pathogenic microorganisms and waste products of cellular metabolism); and ↓production of inflammatory chemicals, such as interleukin-1, prostaglandins, and leukotrienes, by injured cells.

■ ↓Immune response. The immune system normally protects the body from foreign invaders, and several immune responses overlap inflammatory responses, including phagocytosis. In addition, the immune response stimulates the production of antibodies and activated lymphocytes to destroy the foreign substance. Glucocorticoids impair protein synthesis, including the production of antibodies; ↓the numbers of circulating lymphocytes, eosinophils, and macrophages; and ↓amounts of lymphoid tissue. These effects help to account for the immunosuppressive and antiallergic actions of the glucocorticoids.

Cardiovascular System

■ Help to regulate arterial blood pressure by modifying vascular smooth muscle tone, by modifying myocardial contractility, and by stimulating renal mineralocorticoid and glucocorticoid receptors

■ ↑The response of vascular smooth muscle to the pressor effects of catecholamines and other vasoconstrictive agents

↑, *increase/increased;* ↓, *decrease/decreased.*

Nervous System

■ Physiologic amounts help to *maintain normal nerve excitability;* pharmacologic amounts ↓nerve excitability, slow activity in the cerebral cortex, and alter brain wave patterns.

■ ↓Secretion of corticotropin-releasing hormone by the hypothalamus and of corticotropin by the anterior pituitary gland. This results in suppression of further glucocorticoid secretion by the adrenal cortex (negative feedback system).

Musculoskeletal System

■ Maintain muscle strength when present in physiologic amounts but cause muscle atrophy (from protein breakdown) when present in excessive amounts

■ ↓Bone formation and growth and↑bone breakdown. Glucocorticoids also ↓intestinal absorption and ↑renal excretion of calcium. These effects contribute to bone demineralization (osteoporosis) in adults and to ↓linear growth in children.

Respiratory System

■ Maintain open airways. Glucocorticoids do not have direct bronchodilating effects, but help to maintain and restore responsiveness to the bronchodilating effects of endogenous catecholamines, such as epinephrine.

■ Stabilize mast cells and other cells to inhibit the release of bronchoconstrictive and inflammatory substances, such as histamine.

Gastrointestinal System

■ ↓Viscosity of gastric mucus. This effect may ↓protective properties of the mucus and contribute to the development of peptic ulcer disease.

Mineralocorticoids

Mineralocorticoids are a class of steroids that play a vital role in the maintenance of fluid and electrolyte balance through their influence on salt and water metabolism. *Aldosterone* is the main mineralocorticoid and is responsible for approximately 90% of mineralocorticoid activity. Characteristics and physiologic effects of mineralocorticoids are summarized in Box 23-2.

| **Box 23-2** | **Effects of Mineralocorticoids on Body Processes and Systems** |

■ The overall physiologic effects are to conserve sodium and water and eliminate potassium. Aldosterone increases sodium reabsorption from kidney tubules, and water is reabsorbed along with the sodium. When sodium is conserved, another cation must be excreted to maintain electrical neutrality of body fluids; thus, potassium is excreted. This is the only potent mechanism for controlling the concentration of potassium ions in extracellular fluids.

■ Secretion of aldosterone is controlled by several factors, most of which are related to kidney function. In general, secretion is increased when the potassium level of extracellular fluid is high, the sodium level of extracellular fluid is low, the renin–angiotensin system of the kidneys is activated, or the anterior pituitary gland secretes corticotropin.

■ Inadequate secretion of aldosterone causes hyperkalemia, hyponatremia, and extracellular fluid volume deficit (dehydration). Hypotension and shock may result from decreased cardiac output. Absence of mineralocorticoids causes death.

■ Excessive secretion of aldosterone produces hypokalemia, hypernatremia, and extracellular fluid volume excess (water intoxication). Edema and hypertension may result.

Adrenal Sex Hormones

The adrenal cortex secretes male (androgens) and female (estrogens and progesterone) sex hormones. Compared with the effect of hormones produced by the testes and ovaries, the adrenal sex hormones have an insignificant effect on normal body function. Adrenal androgens, secreted continuously in small quantities by both sexes, are responsible for most of the physiologic effects exerted by the adrenal sex hormones. They increase protein synthesis (anabolism), which increases the mass and strength of muscle and bone tissue; they affect development of male secondary sex characteristics; and they increase hair growth and libido in women. Excessive secretion of adrenal androgens in women causes masculinizing effects (e.g., hirsutism, acne, breast atrophy, deepening of the voice, amenorrhea). Female sex hormones are secreted in small amounts and normally exert few physiologic effects. Excessive secretion may produce feminizing effects in men (e.g., breast enlargement, decreased hair growth, voice changes).

Disorders of the Adrenal Cortex

Disorders of the adrenal cortex involve increased or decreased production of corticosteroids, especially cortisol as the primary glucocorticoid and aldosterone as the primary mineralocorticoid. These disorders include the following:

■ **Primary adrenocortical insufficiency** (*Addison's disease*) is associated with destruction of the adrenal cortex by disorders such as tuberculosis, cancer, or hemorrhage; with atrophy of the adrenal cortex caused by autoimmune disease or prolonged administration of exogenous corticosteroids; and with surgical excision of the adrenal glands. In primary adrenocortical insufficiency, there is inadequate production of both cortisol and aldosterone.

■ **Secondary adrenocortical insufficiency**, produced by inadequate secretion of corticotropin, is most often caused by prolonged administration of corticosteroids. This condition is largely a glucocorticoid deficiency; mineralocorticoid secretion is not significantly impaired.

■ **Congenital adrenogenital syndromes and adrenal hyperplasia** result from deficiencies in one or more enzymes required for cortisol production. Low plasma levels of cortisol lead to excessive corticotropin secretion, which then leads to excessive adrenal secretion of androgens and hyperplasia (abnormal increase in number of cells).

■ **Androgen-producing tumors** of the adrenal cortex, which are usually benign, produce masculinizing effects.

■ **Adrenocortical hyperfunction** (*Cushing's disease*) may result from excessive corticotropin or a primary adrenal tumor. Adrenal tumors may be benign or malignant. Benign tumors often produce one corticosteroid normally secreted by the adrenal cortex, but malignant tumors often secrete several corticosteroids.

■ **Hyperaldosteronism** is a rare disorder caused by adenoma (a benign tissue from glandular tissue) or hyperplasia of the adrenal cortex cells that produce aldosterone. It is characterized by hypokalemia, hypernatremia, hypertension, thirst, and polyuria.

General Characteristics of Exogenous Corticosteroids

Mechanisms of Action

Like endogenous glucocorticoids, exogenous drug molecules act at the cellular level by binding to glucocorticoid receptors in target tissues. The drugs are lipid soluble and easily diffuse through the cell membranes of target cells. Inside the cell, they bind with receptors in intracellular cytoplasm. The drug–receptor complex then moves to the cell nucleus, where it interacts with DNA to stimulate or suppress gene transcription.

Glucocorticoids increase or decrease transcription of many genes to alter the synthesis of proteins that regulate their many physiologic effects (e.g., enzymes, transport proteins, structural proteins). Metabolic effects do not occur for at least 45 to 60 minutes because of the time required for protein synthesis. Several hours or days may be needed for full production of proteins.

Because the genes vary in different types of body cells, glucocorticoid effects also vary, depending on the specific cells being targeted. For example, supraphysiologic concentrations of glucocorticoids induce the synthesis of lipolytic and proteolytic enzymes and other specific proteins in various tissues. Overall, corticosteroids have multiple mechanisms of action and effects (Fig. 23-1), including the following:

■ **Inhibiting arachidonic acid metabolism.** Normally, when a body cell is injured or activated by various stimuli, the enzyme phospholipase A_2 causes the phospholipids in cell membranes to release arachidonic acid. Free arachidonic acid is then metabolized to produce proinflammatory prostaglandins (see Chap. 7) and leukotrienes. At sites of tissue injury or inflammation, corticosteroids induce the synthesis of proteins that suppress the activation of phospholipase A_2. This action, in turn, decreases the release of arachidonic acid and the formation of prostaglandins and leukotrienes.

■ **Strengthening or stabilizing biologic membranes.** Two biologic membranes are especially important in inflammatory processes. Stabilization of cell membranes inhibits the release of arachidonic acid and production of prostaglandins and leukotrienes, as described above. Stabilization of lysosomal membranes inhibits release of bradykinin, histamine, enzymes, and perhaps other substances from lysosomes. (Lysosomes are intracellular structures that contain inflammatory chemical mediators and enzymes that destroy cellular debris and phagocytized pathogens.) This reduces capillary permeability and thus prevents leakage of fluid into the injured area and development of edema. It also reduces the chemicals that normally cause vasodilation and tissue irritation.

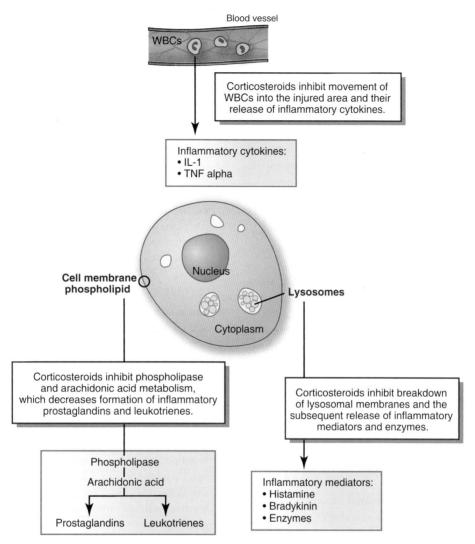

Figure 23-1 ▪ Inflammatory processes and anti-inflammatory actions of corticosteroids. Cellular responses to injury include the following. Phospholipid in the cell membrane is acted on by phospholipase to release arachidonic acid. Metabolism of arachidonic acid produces the inflammatory mediators prostaglandins and leukotrienes. Lysosomal membrane breaks down and releases inflammatory chemicals (e.g., histamine, bradykinin, intracellular digestive enzymes). White blood cells (WBCs) are drawn to the area and release inflammatory cytokines (e.g., interleukin-1 [IL-1], tumor necrosis factor [TNF] alpha). Overall, corticosteroid drugs act to inhibit the release, formation, or activation of various inflammatory mediators.

- **Inhibiting the production of interleukin-1, tumor necrosis factor, and other cytokines.** This action also contributes to the anti-inflammatory and immunosuppressant effects of glucocorticoids.

- **Impairing phagocytosis.** The drugs inhibit the ability of phagocytic cells to leave the bloodstream and move into the injured or inflamed tissue.

- **Impairing lymphocytes.** The drugs inhibit the ability of these immune cells to increase in number and perform their functions.

- **Inhibiting tissue repair.** The drugs inhibit the growth of new capillaries, fibroblasts, and collagen needed for tissue repair.

Indications for Use

Corticosteroids are extensively used to treat many different disorders. Except for replacement therapy in deficiency states, the use of corticosteroids is largely empiric. Because the drugs affect virtually every aspect of inflammatory and immune responses, they are used in the treatment of a broad spectrum of diseases with an inflammatory or immunologic component.

Corticosteroid preparations applied topically in ophthalmic and dermatologic disorders are discussed in Chapters 63 and 64, respectively. The corticosteroids discussed in this chapter are used to treat potentially serious or disabling disorders. These disorders include the following:

■ **Allergic** or hypersensitivity disorders, such as allergic reactions to drugs, serum and blood transfusions, and dermatoses with an allergic component

■ **Collagen** disorders, such as systemic lupus erythematosus, scleroderma, and periarteritis nodosa. Collagen is the basic structural protein of connective tissue, tendons, cartilage, and bone, and it is therefore present in almost all body tissues and organ systems. The collagen disorders are characterized by inflammation of various body tissues. Signs and symptoms depend on which body tissues or organs are affected and the severity of the inflammatory process.

■ **Dermatologic** disorders that may be treated with systemic corticosteroids include acute contact dermatitis, erythema multiforme, herpes zoster (prophylaxis of postherpetic neuralgia), lichen planus, pemphigus, skin rashes caused by drugs, and toxic epidermal necrolysis.

■ **Endocrine** disorders, such as adrenocortical insufficiency and congenital adrenal hyperplasia. Corticosteroids are given to replace or substitute for the natural hormones (both glucocorticoids and mineralocorticoids) in cases of insufficiency and to suppress corticotropin when excess secretion causes adrenal hyperplasia. These conditions are rare and account for a small percentage of corticosteroid usage.

■ **Gastrointestinal** disorders, such as ulcerative colitis and regional enteritis (Crohn's disease)

■ **Hematologic** disorders, such as idiopathic thrombocytopenic purpura or acquired hemolytic anemia

■ **Hepatic** disorders characterized by edema, such as cirrhosis and ascites

■ **Neoplastic disease**, such as acute and chronic leukemias, Hodgkin's disease, other lymphomas, and multiple myeloma. The effectiveness of corticosteroids in these conditions probably stems from their ability to suppress lymphocytes and other lymphoid tissue.

■ **Neurologic** conditions, such as cerebral edema, brain tumor, acute spinal cord injury, and myasthenia gravis

■ **Ophthalmic** disorders, such as optic neuritis, sympathetic ophthalmia, and chorioretinitis

■ **Organ or tissue transplants and grafts** (e.g., kidney, heart, bone marrow). Corticosteroids suppress cellular and humoral immune responses (see Chap. 41) and help prevent rejection of transplanted tissue. Drug therapy is usually continued as long as the transplanted tissue is in place.

■ **Renal** disorders characterized by edema, such as the nephrotic syndrome

■ **Respiratory** disorders, such as asthma, status asthmaticus, chronic obstructive pulmonary disease (COPD), and inflammatory disorders of nasal mucosa (rhinitis). In asthma, corticosteroids increase the number of beta-adrenergic receptors and increase or restore responsiveness of beta receptors to beta-adrenergic bronchodilating drugs. In asthma, COPD, and rhinitis, the drugs decrease mucus secretion and inflammation.

■ **Rheumatic** disorders, such as ankylosing spondylitis, acute and chronic bursitis, acute gouty arthritis, rheumatoid arthritis, and osteoarthritis

■ **Shock.** Corticosteroids are clearly indicated only for shock resulting from *adrenocortical insufficiency* (adrenal or *Addisonian crisis*), which may mimic hypovolemic or septic shock. The use of corticosteroids in septic shock has been highly controversial, and randomized studies and meta-analyses have indicated that corticosteroids are not beneficial in treating septic shock. However, more recent small studies indicate possible clinical usefulness in septic shock, because this form of shock may be associated with relative adrenal insufficiency. In anaphylactic shock resulting from an allergic reaction, corticosteroids may increase or restore cardiovascular responsiveness to adrenergic drugs.

Indications for use, routes, and dosage ranges are given in Table 23-1.

Table 23-1	Drugs at a Glance: Corticosteroids*

	ROUTES AND DOSAGE RANGES	
Generic/Trade Name	**Adults**	**Children**
Glucocorticoids		
Beclamethasone oral inhalation (QVAR)	1–2 inhalations (40–80 mcg) 2 times daily (maximum daily dose 320 mcg)	
Nasal inhalation (Beconase AQ)	1–2 inhalations (42–84 mcg in each nostril) 2 times daily; as maintenance, 1 inhalation each nostril	*older than 6 y:* 1–2 inhalations (42–84 mcg) each nostril daily
Betamethasone (Celestone)	PO 0.6–7.2 mg daily initially, gradually reduced to lowest effective dose	
Betamethasone acetate and sodium phosphate (Celestone Soluspan)	IM 0.5–9 mg daily Intra-articular injection 0.25–2 mL	

ROUTES AND DOSAGE RANGES

Generic/Trade Name	Adults	Children
Budesonide oral inhalation (Pulmicort Terbuhaler, Pulmicort Respules)	Turbuhaler, 200–400 mcg twice daily	Turbuhaler, *older than 6 y*: 200 mcg twice daily Respules, *12 mo–8 y*: 0.5 mg daily in 1 single or 2 divided doses
Nasal inhalation (Rhinocort)	256 mcg daily initially (2 sprays each nostril morning and evening or 4 sprays each nostril every morning). When symptoms are controlled, reduce dosage to lowest effective maintenance dose.	*older than 6 y*: Same as adults
Oral capsule (Entocort EC)	Crohn's disease, PO 9 mg once daily in the morning, for up to 8 wk	
Cortisone	PO 25–300 mg daily, individualized for condition and response	
Dexamethasone (Decadron)	PO 0.75–9 mg daily in 2–4 doses; higher ranges for serious diseases	
Dexamethasone acetate	IM 8–16 mg (1–2 mL) in single dose, repeated every 1–3 wk if necessary	
Dexamethasone sodium phosphate	IM, IV 0.5–9 mg, depending on severity of disease	
Flunisolide oral inhalation (AeroBid)	2 inhalations (500 mcg) twice daily	*6–15 y*: Same as adults
Nasal inhalation (Nasarel)	2 sprays in each nostril twice daily; maximal daily dose 8 sprays in each nostril	*6–14 y*: 1 spray in each nostril 3 times daily or 2 sprays in each nostril 2 times daily; maximal daily dose 4 sprays in each nostril
Fluticasone (Flovent) oral inhalation	2 inhalations (88 mcg) 2 times daily (maximum daily dose 440 mcg inhaled 2 times daily)	*under 12 y*: not recommended
(Flonase) nasal inhalation	200 mcg daily initially (2 sprays each nostril once daily or 1 spray each nostril twice daily). After a few days, reduce dosage to 100 mcg daily (1 spray each nostril once daily) for maintenance therapy.	*12 y and older*: 100 mcg daily (1 spray per nostril once daily)
Hydrocortisone (Cortef)	PO 20–240 mg daily, depending on condition and response	
Hydrocortisone sodium phosphate	IV, IM, Sub-Q 15–240 mg daily in 2 divided doses	
Hydrocortisone sodium succinate	IV, IM 100–400 mg initially, repeated at 2, 4, or 6 hour intervals if necessary	
Hydrocortisone retention enema (Cortenema)	Rectally, one enema (100 mg) nightly for 21 d or until optimal response	
Hydrocortisone acetate intrarectal foam (Cortifoam)	1 applicatorful 1–2 times daily for 2–3 wk, then once every 2–3 d if needed	
Methylprednisolone (Medrol)	PO 4–48 mg daily initially, gradually reduced to lowest effective level	
Methylprednisolone sodium succinate (Solu-Medrol)	IV, IM 10–40 mg initially, adjusted to condition and response	Infants and children: IV, IM not less than 0.5 mg/kg/24 hours
Methylprednisolone acetate (Depo-Medrol)	IM 40–120 mg once daily	

(continued on page 364)

| Table 23-1 | Drugs at a Glance: Corticosteroids* (continued) | |

	ROUTES AND DOSAGE RANGES	
Generic/Trade Name	**Adults**	**Children**
Mometasone (Nasonex)	2 sprays (50 mcg/spray) in each nostril once daily (200 mcg/d)	*older than 12 y:* Same as adults *3–11 y:* 1 spray (50 mcg) in each nostril once daily (100 mcg/d)
Prednisolone	PO 5–60 mg daily initially, adjusted fo maintenance	
Prednisolone acetate	IM 4–60 mg daily initially, adjusted for maintenance	
Prednisone	PO 5–60 mg daily initially, reduced for maintenance	PO: 0.25 - 2mg /kg/dose every 6 h for 48 h, then 1–2 mg/kg/24 h, (maximum 60 mg/24 h)
Triamcinolone	PO 4–48 mg daily initially, reduced for maintenance	
Triamcinolone acetonide (Kenalog-40)	IM 2.5–60 mg daily, depending on the disease. Reduce dosage and start oral therapy when feasible.	
Oral inhalation (Azmacort)	2 inhalations (200 mcg) 3–4 times daily or 4 inhalations (400 mcg) 2 times daily	*6–12 y:* 1–2 inhalations (100–200 mcg) 3–4 times daily or 2–4 inhalations (200–400 mcg) 2 times daily. Maximum daily dose, 12 inhalations (1200 mcg)
Nasal inhalation (Nasacort)	2 sprays (110 mcg) in each nostril once daily (total dose 220 mcg/d). May increase to maximal daily dose of 440 mcg if indicated	*6 y or older:* 2 sprays (110 mcg) in each nostril once daily (220 mcg/d) initially; reduce to 1 spray per nostril once daily (110 mcg/d)
Triamcinolone diacetate (Aristocort Forte)	IM 20–80 mg initially	
Mineralocorticoid **Fludrocortisone** (Florinef)	Chronic adrenocortical insufficiency, PO 0.1 mg daily Salt-losing adrenogenital syndromes, PO 0.1–0.2 mg daily	PO 0.05–0.1 mg daily

Ophthalmic and dermatologic preparations are discussed in Chapters 63 and 64, respectively.

Contraindications to Use

Corticosteroids are contraindicated in systemic fungal infections and in people who are hypersensitive to drug formulations. They should be used with caution in patients at risk for infections (they may decrease resistance), patients with infections (they may mask signs and symptoms so that infections become more severe before they are recognized and treated), diabetes mellitus (they cause or increase hyperglycemia), peptic ulcer disease, inflammatory bowel disorders, hypertension, congestive heart failure, and renal insufficiency.

Applying Your Knowledge 23-1

You arrive at Ms. Hubble's home and begin your assessment of the patient. You notice the appearance of white patches on Ms. Hubble's mouth. What action do you take?

All adrenal corticosteroids are available as drug preparations, as are many synthetic derivatives developed by altering the basic steroid molecule in efforts to increase therapeutic effects while minimizing adverse effects. When corticosteroids are administered from sources outside the body, they are given mainly for replacement or therapeutic purposes. Replacement involves small doses to correct a deficiency state and restore normal function (physiologic effects). Therapeutic purposes require relatively large doses to exert pharmacologic effects. Drug effects involve extension of the physiologic effects of endogenous corticosteroids and new effects that do not occur with small, physiologic doses. The most frequently desired pharmacologic effects are anti-inflammatory, immunosuppressive, antiallergic, and antistress. These are glucocorticoid effects. Mineralocorticoid and androgenic effects are usually considered adverse reactions.

■ The drugs are palliative; they control many symptoms but do not cure underlying disease processes. In chronic disorders, they may enable patients to continue the usual activities of daily living and delay disability. However, the disease may continue to progress, and long-term use of systemic corticosteroids inevitably produces serious adverse effects.

■ Drug effects vary, so a specific effect may be considered therapeutic in one patient but adverse in another. For example, an increased blood sugar level is therapeutic for the patient with adrenocortical insufficiency or an isletcell adenoma of the pancreas but is an adverse reaction for most patients, especially those with diabetes mellitus. In addition, some patients respond more favorably or experience adverse reactions more readily than others taking equivalent doses. This is partly caused by individual differences in the rate at which corticosteroids are metabolized.

■ Administration of exogenous corticosteroids suppresses the HPA axis. This decreases secretion of corticotropin, which, in turn, causes atrophy of the adrenal cortex and decreased production of endogenous adrenal corticosteroids.

■ P **Hydrocortisone**, the exogenous equivalent of endogenous cortisol, is the prototype of corticosteroid drugs. When a new corticosteroid is developed, it is compared with hydrocortisone to determine its potency in producing anti-inflammatory and antiallergic responses, increasing deposition of liver glycogen, and suppressing secretion of corticotropin. Daily administration of physiologic doses (15–20 mg of hydrocortisone or its equivalent) or administration of pharmacologic doses (more than 15–20 mg of hydrocortisone or its equivalent) for approximately 2 weeks suppresses the HPA axis. HPA recovery usually occurs within a few weeks or months after corticosteroids are discontinued but may take 9 to 12 months. During that time, supplemental corticosteroids are usually needed during stressful situations (e.g., fever, illness, surgical procedures) to improve the patient's ability to respond to stress and prevent acute adrenocortical insufficiency.

■ Anti-inflammatory activity of glucocorticoids is approximately equal when the drugs are given in equivalent doses (hydrocortisone 20 mg, prednisone and prednisolone 5 mg, methylprednisolone and triamcinolone 4 mg, dexamethasone 0.75 mg, and betamethasone 0.6 mg). Mineralocorticoid activity is high in cortisone (which is rarely used); intermediate in hydrocortisone, prednisolone, and prednisone; and low in newer agents.

■ Duration of action also varies and is only known for oral drugs. Betamethasone and dexamethasone last 48 hours; methylprednisolone, prednisolone, prednisone, and triamcinolone last 18 to 36 hours; and hydrocortisone lasts 18 hours.

■ Corticosteroids are metabolized in the liver (mainly by cytochrome P450 3A4 enzymes) and conjugated to inactive metabolites. About 25% of the metabolites are excreted in the bile, then in the feces. The other 75% enter the circulation and are excreted by the kidneys. Metabolism is slowed by hepatic disease, and excretion is slowed by renal disease. In these conditions, corticosteroids may accumulate and cause signs and symptoms of hypercorticism.

Applying Your Knowledge 23-2

Ms. Hubble asks you why she has to take the prednisone because it has not made her COPD go away. How should you respond?

Nursing Process

Assessment

Initiation of Corticosteroid Therapy

■ For a patient expected to receive short-term corticosteroid therapy, the major focus of assessment is the extent and severity of symptoms. Such data can then be used to evaluate the effectiveness of drug therapy.

■ For a patient expected to receive long-term, systemic corticosteroid therapy, a thorough assessment is needed. This may include diagnostic tests for diabetes mellitus, tuberculosis, and peptic ulcer disease, because these conditions may develop from or be exacerbated by administration of corticosteroid drugs. If one of these conditions is present, corticosteroid therapy must be altered and other drugs given concomitantly.

■ If acute infection is found on initial assessment, it should be treated with appropriate antibiotics either before corticosteroid drugs are started or concomitantly with corticosteroid therapy. This is necessary because corticosteroids may mask symptoms of infection and impair healing. Thus, even minor infections can become serious if left untreated during corticosteroid therapy. If infection occurs during long-term corticosteroid therapy, appropriate antibiotic therapy (as determined by culture of the causative microorganism and antibiotic sensitivity studies) is again indicated. Also, increased doses of corticosteroids are usually indicated to cope with the added stress of the infection.

Previous or Current Corticosteroid Therapy

Initial assessment of every patient should include information about previous or current treatment with systemic corticosteroids. This can usually be determined by questioning the client or reviewing medical records.

■ If the nurse determines that the patient has taken corticosteroids in the past, additional information is needed about the specific drug and dosage taken, the purpose and length of therapy, and when therapy was stopped. Such information is necessary for planning nursing care. If the patient had an acute illness and received an oral or

Nursing Process continues on page 366

injected corticosteroid for approximately 1 week or received corticosteroids by local injection or application to skin lesions, no special nursing care is likely to be required. However, if the patient took systemic corticosteroids for 2 weeks or longer during the past year, nursing observations must be especially vigilant. Such a patient may be at higher risk for acute adrenocortical insufficiency during stressful situations. If the patient has surgery, corticosteroid therapy is restarted either before or on the day of surgery and continued, in decreasing dosage, for a few days after surgery. In addition to anesthesia and surgery, potentially significant sources of stress include hospitalization, various diagnostic tests, concurrent infection or other illnesses, and family problems.

If the patient is currently taking a systemic corticosteroid drug, again the nurse must identify the drug, the dosage and schedule of administration, the purpose for which the drug is being taken, and the length of time involved. After this basic information is obtained, the nurse can further assess patient status and plan nursing care. Some specific factors include the following:

■ If the patient undergoes anesthesia and surgery, expect that higher doses of corticosteroids will be given for several days. This may be done by changing the drug, the route of administration, and the dosage. Specific regimens vary according to type of anesthesia, surgical procedure, patient condition, prescriber preference, and other variables. A patient having major abdominal surgery may be given 300 to 400 mg of hydrocortisone (or the equivalent dosage of other drugs) on the day of surgery and then be tapered back to maintenance dosage within a few days.

■ Note that additional corticosteroids may be given in other situations as well. One extra dose may be adequate for a short-term stress situation, such as an angiogram or other invasive diagnostic test.

■ Using all available data, assess the likelihood of the patient having acute adrenal insufficiency.

■ Assess for signs and symptoms of adrenocortical excess and adverse drug effects.

■ Assess for signs and symptoms of the disease for which long-term corticosteroid therapy is being given.

Nursing Diagnoses

■ Disturbed Body Image related to cushingoid changes in appearance

■ Imbalanced Nutrition: Less Than Body Requirements related to protein and potassium losses

■ Imbalanced Nutrition: More Than Body Requirements related to sodium and water retention and hyperglycemia

■ Excess Fluid Volume related to sodium and water retention

■ Risk for Injury related to adverse drug effects of impaired wound healing, increased susceptibility to infection, weakening of skin and muscles, osteoporosis, gastrointestinal

ulceration, diabetes mellitus, hypertension, and acute adrenocortical insufficiency

■ Ineffective Coping related to chronic illness; long-term drug therapy and drug-induced mood changes, irritability and insomnia

■ Deficient Knowledge related to disease process and corticosteroid drug therapy

Planning/Goals
The patient will

■ Take the drug correctly

■ Practice measures to decrease the need for corticosteroids and minimize adverse effects

■ Be monitored regularly for adverse drug effects

■ Keep appointments for follow-up care

■ Be assisted to cope with body image changes

■ Verbalize or demonstrate essential drug information

Interventions

For patients on long-term, systemic corticosteroid therapy, use supplementary drugs as ordered and nondrug measures to decrease dosage and adverse effects of corticosteroid drugs. Specific measures include the following:

■ Help patients set reasonable goals of drug therapy. For example, partial relief of symptoms may be better than complete relief if the latter requires larger doses or longer periods of treatment with systemic drugs.

■ In patients with bronchial asthma and COPD, other treatment measures should be continued during corticosteroid therapy. With asthma, the corticosteroid needs to be given on a regular schedule; inhaled bronchodilators can usually be taken as needed.

■ In patients with rheumatoid arthritis, rest, physical therapy, and salicylates or other nonsteroid anti-inflammatory drugs are continued. Systemic corticosteroid therapy is reserved for severe, acute exacerbations when possible.

■ Help patients identify stressors and find ways to modify or avoid stressful situations when possible. For example, most patients probably do not think of extreme heat or cold or minor infections as significant stressors. However, they can be for people taking corticosteroids. This assessment of potential stressors must be individualized because a situation viewed as stressful by one patient may not be stressful to another.

■ Encourage activity, if not contraindicated, to slow demineralization of bone (osteoporosis). This is especially important in postmenopausal women who are not taking replacement estrogens, because they are very susceptible to osteoporosis. Walking is preferred if the patient is able. Range-of-motion exercises are indicated in immobilized or bedridden people. Also, bedridden patients taking corticosteroids should have their positions changed frequently because these drugs thin the skin and increase the risk of pressure ulcers. This risk is further increased if edema also is present.

■ Dietary changes may be beneficial in some patients. Salt restriction may help prevent hypernatremia, fluid retention, and edema. Foods high in potassium may help prevent hypokalemia. A diet high in protein, calcium, and vitamin D may help prevent osteoporosis. Increased intake of vitamin C may help decrease bleeding in the skin and soft tissues.

■ Avoid exposing the patient to potential sources of infection by washing hands frequently; using aseptic technique when changing dressings; keeping health care personnel and visitors with colds or other infections away from the patient; and following other appropriate measures. Reverse or protective isolation is sometimes indicated, commonly for those patients who have had organ transplantation and are receiving corticosteroids to help prevent rejection of the transplanted organ.

■ Handle tissues very gently during any procedures (e.g., bathing, assisting out of bed, venipunctures). Because long-term corticosteroid therapy weakens the skin and bones, there are risks of skin damage and fractures with even minor trauma.

Patient Guidelines for Long-Term Corticosteroid Therapy are presented in the accompanying display.

Evaluation

■ Interview and observe for relief of symptoms for which corticosteroids were prescribed.

■ Interview and observe for accurate drug administration.

■ Interview and observe for use of nondrug measures indicated for the condition being treated.

■ Interview and observe for adverse drug effects on a regular basis.

■ Interview regarding drug knowledge and effects to be reported to health care providers.

Applying Your Knowledge 23-3

You test Ms. Hubble's blood glucose level, and it is 345 mg/dL. Why is this patient hyperglycemic, and what action should you take?

Principles of Therapy

Goal of Therapy

The goal of corticosteroid therapy is usually to reduce symptoms to a tolerable level. Total suppression of symptoms may require excessively large doses and produce excessive adverse effects. Because systemic corticosteroids can cause serious adverse reactions, indications for their clinical use should be as clear-cut as possible.

Drug Selection

Choice of corticosteroid drug is influenced by many factors, including the purpose for use, characteristics of specific drugs, desired route of administration, characteristics of individual patients, and expected adverse effects. Some guidelines for rational drug choice include the following:

■ Hydrocortisone and cortisone are usually the drugs of choice in adrenocortical insufficiency, which requires replacement of both glucocorticoids and mineralocorticoids whether caused by Addison's disease, adrenalectomy, or inadequate corticotropin. These drugs have greater mineralocorticoid activity compared with other corticosteroids. If additional mineralocorticoid activity is required, fludrocortisone can be given.

■ Prednisone is often the glucocorticoid of choice in nonendocrine disorders in which anti-inflammatory, antiallergic, antistress, and immunosuppressive effects are desired. A corticosteroid drug with primarily glucocorticoid activity is necessary.

■ Beclomethasone (QVAR, Beconase AQ), budesonide (Pulmicort, Rhinocort), flunisolide (AeroBid), fluticasone (Flonase, Flovent), mometasone (Nasonex), and triamcinolone (Azmacort, Nasacort) are corticosteroids formulated to be given by oral or nasal inhalation in respiratory disorders. Their use replaces, prevents, delays, or decreases use of systemic drugs and thereby decreases risks of serious adverse effects. However, high doses or frequent use may suppress adrenocortical function.

■ Dexamethasone (parenterally or orally) is considered the corticosteroid of choice for cerebral edema associated with brain tumors, craniotomy, or head injury, because dexamethasone is thought to penetrate the blood–brain barrier more readily and achieve higher concentrations in cerebrospinal fluids and tissues. It also has minimal sodium- and water-retaining properties. With brain tumors, the drug is more effective in metastatic lesions and glioblastomas than astrocytomas and meningiomas.

■ Hydrocortisone, dexamethasone, and methylprednisolone are among those drugs that may be given parenterally and are useful in acute, life-threatening situations that require such administration, usually intravenously (IV). This requirement limits the choice of drugs, because not all corticosteroids are available in injectable preparations.

Drug Dosage

Many factors have an effect on drug dosage, such as the specific drug to be given, the desired route of administration, the reason for use, expected adverse effects, and patient characteristics. In general, the smallest effective dose should be given for the shortest effective time. The dosage must be individualized

Patient Teaching Guidelines | Long-Term Corticosteroid Therapy

General Considerations

- In most instances, corticosteroids are used to relieve symptoms; they do not cure the underlying disease process. However, they can improve comfort and quality of life.

- When taking an oral corticosteroid (e.g., prednisone) for longer than 2 weeks, it is extremely important to take the drug as directed. Missing a dose or two, stopping the drug, changing the amount or time of administration, taking extra drug (except as specifically directed during stress situations), or any other alterations may result in complications. Some complications are relatively minor; several are serious, even life threatening. When these drugs are being discontinued, the dosage is gradually reduced over several weeks. They must not be stopped abruptly.

- Wear a special medical alert bracelet or tag or carry an identification card stating the drug being taken; the dosage; the prescriber's name, address, and telephone number; and instructions for emergency treatment. If an accident or emergency situation occurs, health care providers must know about corticosteroid drug therapy to give additional amounts during the stress of the emergency.

- Report to all health care providers consulted that corticosteroid drugs are being taken or have been taken within the past year. Current or previous corticosteroid therapy can influence treatment measures, and such knowledge increases the ability to provide appropriate treatment.

- Maintain regular medical supervision. This is extremely important so that the prescriber can detect adverse reactions, evaluate disease status, and evaluate drug response and indications for dosage change, as well as other responsibilities that can be carried out only with personal contact between the prescriber and the patient. Periodic blood tests, x-ray studies, and other tests may be performed during long-term corticosteroid therapy.

- Take no other drugs, prescription or nonprescription, without notifying the prescriber who is supervising corticosteroid therapy. Corticosteroid drugs influence reactions to other drugs, and some other drugs interact with corticosteroids either to increase or decrease their effects. Thus, taking other drugs can decrease the expected therapeutic benefits or increase the incidence or severity of adverse effects.

- Avoid exposure to infection when possible. Avoid crowds and people known to have an infection. Also, wash hands frequently and thoroughly. These drugs increase the likelihood of infection, so preventive measures are necessary. Also, if infection does occur, healing is likely to be slow.

- Practice safety measures to avoid accidents (e.g., falls and possible fractures due to osteoporosis, cuts or other injuries because of delayed wound healing, soft tissue trauma because of increased tendency to bruise easily).

- Weigh frequently when starting corticosteroid therapy and at least weekly during long-term maintenance. An initial weight gain is likely to occur and is usually attributed to increased appetite. Later weight gains may be caused by fluid retention.

- Ask the prescriber about the amount and kind of activity or exercise needed. As a general rule, being as active as possible helps to prevent or delay osteoporosis, a common

adverse effect. However, increased activity may not be desirable for everyone. A patient with rheumatoid arthritis, for example, may become too active when drug therapy relieves joint pain and increases mobility.

- Follow instructions for other measures used in treatment of the particular condition (e.g., other drugs and physical therapy for rheumatoid arthritis). Such measures may allow smaller doses of corticosteroids and decrease adverse effects.

- Because the corticosteroid impairs the ability to respond to stress, dosage may need to be temporarily increased with illness, surgery, or other stressful situations. Clarify with the prescriber predictable sources of stress and the amount of drug to be taken if the stress cannot be avoided.

- In addition to stressful situations, report sore throat, fever, or other signs of infection; weight gain of 5 pounds or more in a week; or swelling in the ankles or elsewhere. These symptoms may indicate adverse drug effects and changes in corticosteroid therapy may be indicated.

- Muscle weakness and fatigue or disease symptoms may occur when drug dosage is reduced, withdrawn, or omitted (e.g., the nondrug day of alternate-day therapy). Although these symptoms may cause some discomfort, they should be tolerated if possible rather than increasing the corticosteroid dose. If severe, of course, dosage or time of administration may have to be changed.

- Dietary changes may be helpful in reducing some adverse effects of corticosteroid therapy. Decreasing salt intake (e.g., by not adding table salt to foods and avoiding obviously salty foods, such as many snack foods and prepared sandwich meats) may help decrease swelling. Eating high-potassium foods, such as citrus fruits and juices or bananas, may help prevent potassium loss. An adequate intake of calcium, protein, and vitamin D (meat and dairy products are good sources) may help to prevent or delay osteoporosis. Vitamin C (e.g., from citrus fruits) may help to prevent excessive bruising.

- Do not object when your prescriber reduces your dose of oral corticosteroid, with the goal of stopping the drug entirely or continuing with a smaller dose. Long-term therapy should be used only when necessary because of the potential for serious adverse effects, and the lowest effective dose should be given.

- With local applications of corticosteroids, there is usually little systemic absorption and few adverse effects, compared with oral or injected drugs. When effective in relieving symptoms, it is better to use a local than a systemic corticosteroid. In some instances, combined systemic and local application allows administration of a lesser dose of the systemic drug.

  Commonly used local applications are applied topically for skin disorders; by oral inhalation for asthma; and by nasal inhalation for allergic rhinitis. Although long-term use is usually well tolerated, systemic toxicity can occur if excess corticosteroid is inhaled or if occlusive dressings are used over skin lesions. Thus, a corticosteroid for local application must be applied correctly and not overused.

- Corticosteroids are not the same as the steroids often abused by athletes and body builders. Those are anabolic steroids derived from testosterone, the male sex hormone.

Self- or Caregiver Administration

- Take an oral corticosteroid with a meal or snack to decrease gastrointestinal upset.
- If taking the medication once a day or every other day, take before 9 A.M. if taking multiple doses, take at evenly spaced intervals throughout the day.
- Report to the prescriber if unable to take a dose orally because of vomiting or some other problem. In some circumstances, the dose may need to be given by injection.
- If taking an oral corticosteroid in tapering doses, be sure to follow instructions exactly to avoid adverse effects.
- When applying a corticosteroid to skin lesions, do not apply more often than ordered and do not cover with an occlusive dressing unless specifically instructed to do so.
- With an intranasal corticosteroid, use on a regular basis (usually once or twice daily) for the best anti-inflammatory effects.

- With an oral-inhalation corticosteroid, use on a regular schedule for anti-inflammatory effects. The drugs are *not* effective in relieving acute asthma attacks or shortness of breath and should not be used "as needed" for that purpose. Use metered-dose inhalers as follows (unless instructed otherwise by a health care provider):
  1. Shake canister thoroughly.
  2. Place canister between lips (both open and pursed lips have been recommended) or outside lips.
  3. Exhale completely.
  4. Activate canister while taking a slow, deep breath.
  5. Hold breath for 10 seconds or as long as possible.
  6. Wait at least 1 minute before taking additional inhalations.
  7. Rinse mouth after inhalations to decrease the incidence of oral thrush (a fungal infection).
  8. Rinse mouthpiece at least once per day.

according to the severity of the disorder being treated, whether the disease is acute or chronic, and the patient's response to drug therapy. (Dosage for children is calculated according to severity of disease rather than weight.) If life-threatening disease is present, high doses are usually given until acute symptoms subside. Then the dose is gradually reduced until a maintenance dose is determined or the drug is discontinued. If life-threatening disease is not present, relatively high doses may still be given initially and then lowered. Doses should be gradually reduced (tapered) over several days. With long-term corticosteroid therapy, periodic attempts to reduce dosage are desirable to decrease adverse effects. One way is to reduce the dose gradually until symptoms worsen, indicating the minimally effective dose.

Physiologic doses (approximately 15–20 mg of hydrocortisone or its equivalent daily) are given to replace or substitute for endogenous adrenocortical hormone. Pharmacologic doses (supraphysiologic amounts) are usually required for anti-inflammatory, antiallergic, antistress, and immunosuppressive effects.

Compared with hydrocortisone, newer corticosteroids are more potent on a weight basis but are equipotent in anti-inflammatory effects when given in equivalent doses. Statements of equivalency with hydrocortisone are helpful in evaluating new drugs, comparing different drugs, and changing drugs or dosages. However, dosage equivalents apply only to drugs given orally or IV.

Drug Administration

Routes of Administration

Corticosteroids can be given by several different routes, based on the clinical problem, to produce local or systemic effects. If feasible, these drugs should be given locally rather than systemically to prevent or decrease systemic toxicity. In recent years there have been several formulations developed for oral inhalation in the treatment of asthma and for nasal inhalation in the treatment of allergic rhinitis. When these drugs must be given

systemically, the oral route is preferred. Parenteral administration is indicated only for patients who are seriously ill or unable to take oral medications.

For intramuscular or IV injections, sodium phosphate or sodium succinate salts are used because they are most soluble in water. For intra-articular or intralesional injections, acetate salts are used because they have low solubility in water and provide prolonged local action.

Frequency of Administration

Scheduling of drug administration is more important with corticosteroids than with most other drug classes. Most adverse effects occur with long-term administration of high doses. A major adverse reaction is suppression of the HPA axis and subsequent loss of adrenocortical function. Certain schedules are often recommended to prevent or minimize HPA suppression.

Corticosteroids can be given in relatively large, divided doses for approximately 48 to 72 hours in acute situations until the condition has been brought under control. After acute symptoms subside or 48 to 72 hours have passed, the dosage is tapered so that a slightly smaller dose is given each day until the drug can be discontinued completely (total period of use: approximately 1 week). Such a regimen may be useful in allergic reactions, contact dermatitis, exacerbations of chronic conditions (e.g., bronchial asthma), and stressful situations such as surgery.

Daily administration is required in cases of chronic adrenocortical insufficiency. The entire daily dose can be taken each morning, between 6 and 9 A.M. This schedule simulates normal endogenous corticosteroid secretion.

Alternate-day therapy (ADT), in which a double dose is taken every other morning, is usually preferred for other chronic conditions. This schedule allows rest periods so that adverse effects are decreased while anti-inflammatory effects continue. ADT seems to be as effective as more frequent administration in most patients with bronchial asthma, ulcerative colitis, and other conditions for which long-term corticosteroid therapy is prescribed. ADT is used only for maintenance therapy (i.e., clinical signs and symptoms are controlled initially with more frequent drug administration). ADT can be started after symptoms have subsided and stabilized.

Intermediate-acting glucocorticoids (e.g., prednisone, prednisolone, methylprednisolone) are the drugs of choice for ADT. Long-acting drugs (e.g., betamethasone, dexamethasone) are not recommended because of their prolonged suppression of adrenocortical function.

ADT has other advantages. It probably decreases susceptibility to infection and does not retard growth in children, as do other schedules.

ADT is not usually indicated in patients who have previously received corticosteroids on a long-term basis. First, these patients already have maximal HPA suppression, so a major advantage of ADT is lost. Second, if these patients begin ADT, recurrence of symptoms and considerable discomfort may occur on days when drugs are omitted. Patients with severe disease and very painful or disabling symptoms also may experience severe discomfort with ADT.

Stress Dosage Corticosteroid Therapy

Long-term use of pharmacologic doses (e.g., more than 5 mg of prednisone daily) produces adverse reactions. For this reason, long-term corticosteroid therapy should be reserved for life-threatening conditions or severe, disabling symptoms that do not respond to treatment with more benign drugs or other measures. For people receiving chronic corticosteroid therapy, dosage must be increased during periods of stress or illness. Some common sources of stress for most people include surgery and anesthesia, infections, anxiety, and extremes of temperature. Note that events that are stressful for one patient may not be stressful for another. Some guidelines for corticosteroid dosage during stress include the following:

■ During minor or relatively mild illness (e.g., viral upper respiratory infection, any febrile illness, strenuous exercise, gastroenteritis with vomiting and diarrhea, minor surgery), doubling the daily maintenance dose is usually adequate. After the stress period is over, dosage may be reduced abruptly to the usual maintenance dose.

■ During major stress or severe illness, even larger doses are necessary. For example, a patient undergoing abdominal surgery may require 300 to 400 mg of hydrocortisone on the day of surgery. This dose can gradually be reduced to usual maintenance doses within approximately 5 days if postoperative recovery is uncomplicated. As a general rule, it is better to administer excessive doses temporarily than to risk inadequate doses and adrenal insufficiency. The patient also may require sodium chloride and fluid replacement, antibiotic therapy if infection is present, and supportive measures if shock occurs.

■ During acute stress situations of short duration, such as traumatic injury or invasive diagnostic tests (e.g., angiography), a single dose of approximately 100 mg of hydrocortisone immediately after the injury or before the diagnostic test is usually sufficient.

■ Many chronic diseases that require long-term corticosteroid therapy are characterized by exacerbations and remissions. Dosage of corticosteroids usually must be increased during acute flare-ups of disease symptoms but can then be decreased gradually to maintenance levels.

Treatment of Specific Disorders

Allergic Rhinitis

Allergic rhinitis (also called seasonal rhinitis, hay fever, and perennial rhinitis) is a common problem for which corticosteroids are given by nasal spray, once or twice daily. Therapeutic effects usually occur within a few days with regular use. Systemic adverse effects are minimal with recommended doses but may occur with higher doses, including adrenocortical insufficiency from HPA suppression.

Arthritis

Corticosteroids are the most effective drugs for rapid relief of the pain, edema, and restricted mobility associated with acute episodes of joint inflammation. They are usually given on a short-term basis. When inflammation is limited to three or fewer joints, the preferred route of drug administration is by injection directly into the joint. Intra-articular injections relieve symptoms in approximately 2 to 8 weeks, and several formulations are available for this route. However, corticosteroids do not prevent disease progression and joint destruction. As a general rule, a joint should not be injected more often than three times yearly because of risks of infection and damage to intra-articular structures from the injections and from overuse when pain is relieved.

Asthma

Corticosteroids are commonly used in the treatment of asthma because of their anti-inflammatory effects. In addition, corticosteroids increase the effects of adrenergic bronchodilators to prevent or treat bronchoconstriction and bronchospasm. The drugs work by increasing the number and responsiveness of beta-adrenergic receptors and preventing the tolerance usually associated with chronic administration of these bronchodilators. Research studies indicate that responsiveness to beta-adrenergic bronchodilators increases within 2 hours and that numbers of beta receptors increase within 4 hours. A meta-analysis of randomized controlled trials was completed to determine the efficacy of corticosteroids on the outcome in patients with acute exacerbations of COPD. Findings are outlined in Evidence-Based Practice Box 23-1.

In acute asthma or status asthmaticus unrelieved by inhaled beta-adrenergic bronchodilators, high doses of systemic corticosteroids are given orally or IV along with bronchodilators for approximately 5 to 10 days. Although these high doses suppress the HPA axis, the suppression lasts for only 1 to 3 days, and other serious adverse effects are avoided. Thus, systemic corticosteroids are used for short-term therapy, as needed, and not for long-term treatment. People who regularly use inhaled corticosteroids also require high doses of systemic drugs during acute attacks because aerosols are not effective. As soon as acute symptoms subside, the dose should be tapered; the lowest effective maintenance dose should be used, or the drug should be discontinued. In chronic asthma, inhaled corticosteroids are the drugs of first choice. This recommendation evolved from increased knowledge about the importance of inflammation in the pathophysiology of asthma and the development of aerosol corticosteroids that are effective with minimal adverse effects. Inhaled drugs may be given alone or with systemic drugs. In general, inhaled corticosteroids can replace oral drugs when daily dosage of the oral drug has been tapered to 10 to 15 milligrams of prednisone or the equivalent. When a patient is being switched from an oral to an inhaled corticosteroid, the inhaled drug should be started during tapering of the oral drug, approximately 1 or 2 weeks before discontinuing or reaching the lowest anticipated dose of the oral drug. When a patient requires a systemic corticosteroid, co-administration of an aerosol allows smaller doses of the systemic corticosteroid. Although the inhaled drugs can cause suppression of the HPA axis and adrenocortical function, especially at higher doses, they are much less likely to do so than systemic drugs. However, a **BLACK BOX WARNING** has been issued by the Food and Drug Administration (FDA) for individuals who are transferred from systemically active corticosteroids to flunisolide inhaler because deaths have occurred from adrenal insufficiency.

Cancer

Corticosteroids are commonly used in the treatment of lymphomas, lymphocytic leukemias, and multiple myeloma. In these disorders, corticosteroids inhibit cell reproduction and are cytotoxic to lymphocytes. In addition to their anticancer effects in hematologic malignancies, corticosteroids are beneficial in treatment of several signs and symptoms that often accompany cancer, although the mechanisms of action are unknown and drug/dosage regimens vary widely. Cortico-

steroids are used to treat anorexia, nausea and vomiting, cerebral edema and inflammation associated with brain metastases or radiation of the head, spinal cord compression, pain and edema related to pressure on nerves or bone metastases, graft-versus-host disease after bone marrow transplantation, and other disorders that occur in patients with cancer. Patients tend to feel better when taking corticosteroids, although the basic disease process may be unchanged.

Primary Central Nervous System Lymphomas

Formerly considered rare tumors of older adults, central nervous system lymphomas are being diagnosed more frequently in younger patients. They are usually associated with chronic *immunosuppression* caused by immunosuppressant drugs or acquired immunodeficiency syndrome (AIDS). Many of these lymphomas are very sensitive to corticosteroids, and therapy is indicated when the diagnosis is established.

Other Central Nervous System Tumors

Corticosteroid therapy may be useful in both supportive and definitive treatment of brain and spinal cord tumors, and neurologic signs and symptoms often improve dramatically within 24 to 48 hours. Corticosteroids help relieve symptoms by controlling edema around the tumor, at operative sites, and at sites receiving radiation therapy. Some patients no longer require corticosteroids after surgical or radiation therapy, whereas others require continued therapy to manage neurologic symptoms. Adverse effects of long-term corticosteroid therapy may include mental changes ranging from mild agitation to psychosis and steroid myopathy (muscle weakness and atrophy) that may be confused with tumor progression. Mental symptoms usually improve if drug dosage is reduced and resolve if the drug is discontinued; steroid myopathy may persist for weeks or months.

Chemotherapy-Induced Emesis

Corticosteroids have strong antiemetic effects; the mechanism is unknown. One effective regimen is a combination of an oral or IV dose of dexamethasone (10–20 mg) and a serotonin antagonist or metoclopramide given immediately before the chemotherapeutic drug. This regimen is the treatment of choice for chemotherapy with cisplatin, which is a strongly emetic drug.

Chronic Obstructive Pulmonary Disease

Corticosteroids are more helpful in acute exacerbations than in stable COPD. However, oral corticosteroids may improve pulmonary function and symptoms in some patients. For example, for a patient with inadequate relief from a bronchodilator, a trial of a corticosteroid (e.g., prednisone 20–40 mg each morning for 5–7 days) may be justified. Treatment should be continued only if there is significant improvement. As in other conditions, the lowest effective dose is needed to minimize adverse drug effects.

Inhaled corticosteroids can also be tried. They produce minimal adverse effects, but their effectiveness in COPD has not been clearly demonstrated.

Inflammatory Bowel Disease

Crohn's disease and ulcerative colitis often require periodic corticosteroid therapy.

In moderate Crohn's disease, oral prednisone, 40 milligrams daily, is usually given until symptoms subside. With severe disease, patients often require hospitalization, IV fluids for hydration, and parenteral corticosteroids until symptoms subside. An oral form of budesonide (Entocort EC) may be used for Crohn's disease. The capsule dissolves in the small intestine and acts locally before being absorbed into the bloodstream and transported to the liver for metabolism. It has fewer adverse effects than systemic corticosteroids but is also less effective and more expensive.

In ulcerative colitis, corticosteroids are usually used when aminosalicylates (e.g., mesalamine) are not effective or when symptoms are more severe. Initially, hydrocortisone enemas may be effective. If not effective, oral prednisone (20–60 mg daily) may be given until symptoms subside. In severe disease, oral prednisone may be required initially. After remission of symptoms is achieved, the dose can be tapered by 2.5 to 5 milligrams per day each week to a dose of 20 milligrams. Then, tapering may be slowed to 2.5 to 5 milligrams per day every other week. As in Crohn's disease, patients with severe ulcerative colitis often require hospitalization and parenteral corticosteroids. One regimen uses IV hydrocortisone 300 milligrams per day or the equivalent dose of another drug. When the patient's condition improves, oral prednisone can replace the IV corticosteroid.

Spinal Cord Injury

High-dose corticosteroid therapy to treat spinal cord injury is a common practice in clinical settings, although controversy exists regarding its use. Data suggest that methylprednisolone may be effective in acute spinal cord injury when given in high doses within 8 hours of the injury. Methylprednisolone improves neurologic recovery, although it does not improve mortality, and its use is unlikely to result in normal neurologic function. In addition, severe adverse outcomes, including wound and systemic infections, gastrointestinal hemorrhage, and pneumonia, have been reported.

Prevention of Acute Adrenocortical Insufficiency

Suppression of the HPA axis may occur with corticosteroid therapy and may lead to life-threatening inability to increase cortisol secretion when needed to cope with stress. It is most likely to occur with abrupt withdrawal of systemic corticosteroid drugs. The risk of HPA suppression is high with systemic drugs given for more than a few days, although patients vary in degree and duration of suppression with comparable doses, and the minimum dose and duration of therapy that cause suppression are unknown.

When corticosteroids are given for replacement therapy, adrenal insufficiency is lifelong, and drug administration must be continued. When the drugs are given for purposes other than replacement and then discontinued, the HPA axis usually recovers within several weeks to months, but recovery may take a year. Several strategies have been developed to minimize HPA suppression and risks of acute adrenal insufficiency, including

■ Administering a systemic corticosteroid during high-stress situations (e.g., moderate or severe illness, trauma, surgery) to patients who have received pharmacologic doses for 2 weeks within the previous year or who receive long-term systemic therapy (i.e., are steroid dependent)

■ Giving short courses of systemic therapy for acute disorders, such as asthma attacks, then decreasing the dose or stopping the drug within a few days

■ Gradually tapering the dose of any systemic corticosteroid. Although specific guidelines for tapering dosage have not been developed, higher doses and longer durations of administration in general require slower tapering, possibly over several weeks. The goal of tapering may be to stop the drug or to decrease the dosage to the lowest effective amount.

■ Using local rather than systemic therapy when possible, alone or in combination with low doses of systemic drugs. Numerous preparations are available for local application, including aerosols for oral or nasal inhalation; formulations for topical application to the skin, eyes, and ears; and drugs for intra-articular injections.

■ Using ADT, which involves titrating the daily dose to the lowest effective maintenance level, then giving a double dose every other day

Use in Special Populations

Use in Children

Corticosteroids are used for the same conditions in children as in adults; a common indication is for treatment of asthma. With severe asthma, continual corticosteroid therapy may be required. For children with asthma, evidence indicates that with inhaled corticosteroids, starting with a moderate dose of inhaled corticosteroid is comparable with starting with a high dose and titrating down. A concern with children is growth retardation, which can occur short term with small doses and administration by inhalation. Many children have a growth spurt when the corticosteroid is discontinued. Adult stature does not appear to be affected by inhaled corticosteroid therapy during childhood.

Parents and prescribers can monitor drug effects by recording height and weight weekly. ADT is less likely to impair normal growth and development than daily administration. In addition, for both systemic and inhaled corticosteroids, each child's dose should be titrated to the lowest effective amount.

Use in Older Adults

Corticosteroids are used for the same conditions in older adults as in younger ones. Older adults are especially likely to have conditions that are aggravated by the drugs (e.g., congestive heart failure, hypertension, diabetes mellitus, arthritis, osteoporosis, increased susceptibility to infection, concomitant drug therapy that increases risks of gastrointestinal ulceration and bleeding). Consequently, risk–benefit ratios of systemic corticosteroid therapy should be carefully considered, especially for long-term therapy.

When used, lower doses are usually indicated because of decreased muscle mass, plasma volume, hepatic metabolism, and renal excretion in older adults. In addition, therapeutic and adverse responses should be monitored regularly by a health care provider (e.g., blood pressure, serum electrolytes, and blood glucose levels at least every 6 months). As in other populations, adverse effects are less likely to occur with oral or nasal inhalations than with oral drugs.

Use in Patients With Renal Impairment

Systemic corticosteroids should be used with caution because of slowed excretion, with possible accumulation and signs and symptoms of hypercorticism. In renal transplantation, corticosteroids are extensively used, along with other immunosuppressive drugs, to prevent or treat rejection reactions. In these patients, as in others, adverse effects of systemic corticosteroids may include infections, hypertension, glucose intolerance, obesity, cosmetic changes, bone loss, growth retardation in children, cataracts, pancreatitis, peptic ulcerations, and psychiatric disturbances. Doses should be minimized, and eventually the drugs can be withdrawn in some patients.

Use in Patients With Hepatic Impairment

Metabolism of corticosteroids is slowed by severe hepatic disease, and corticosteroids may accumulate and cause signs and symptoms of hypercorticism. In addition, patients with liver disease should be given prednisolone rather than prednisone. Liver metabolism of prednisone is required to convert it to its active form, prednisolone.

Use in Patients With Critical Illness

Corticosteroids have been extensively used in the treatment of serious illness, with much empiric usage.

Adrenal Insufficiency

Adrenal insufficiency is the most clear-cut indication for use of a corticosteroid, and even a slight impairment of the adrenal response during severe illness can be lethal if corticosteroid therapy is not instituted. For example, hypotension is a common symptom in critically ill patients, and hypotension caused by adrenal insufficiency may mimic either hypovolemic or septic shock. If adrenal insufficiency is the cause of the hypotension, administration of corticosteroids can eliminate the need for vasopressor drugs to maintain adequate tissue perfusion.

However, adrenal insufficiency may not be recognized because hypotension and other symptoms also occur with many illnesses. The normal response to critical illness (e.g., pain, hypovolemia) is an increased and prolonged secretion of cortisol. If this does not occur, or if too little cortisol is produced, a state of adrenal insufficiency exists. One way to evaluate a patient for adrenal insufficiency is a test in which a

baseline serum cortisol level is measured, after which corticotropin is given IV to stimulate cortisol production, and the serum cortisol level is measured again in approximately 30 to 60 minutes. Test results are hard to interpret in seriously ill patients, though, because serum cortisol concentrations that would be normal in normal subjects may be low in this population. In addition, a lower-than-expected rise in serum cortisol levels may indicate a normal HPA axis that is already maximally stimulated or interference with the ability of the adrenal cortex to synthesize cortisol. Thus, a critically ill patient may have a limited ability to increase cortisol production in response to stress.

In any patient suspected of having adrenal insufficiency, a single IV dose of corticosteroid seems justified. If the patient does have adrenal insufficiency, the corticosteroid may prevent immediate death and allow time for other diagnostic and therapeutic measures. If the patient does not have adrenal insufficiency, the single dose is not harmful.

Acute Respiratory Failure in Chronic Obstructive Pulmonary Disease

Some studies support the use of IV methylprednisolone. Thus, if other medications do not produce adequate bronchodilation, it seems reasonable to try an IV corticosteroid during the first 72 hours of the illness. However, corticosteroid therapy increases the risks of pulmonary infection.

Adult Respiratory Distress Syndrome

Although corticosteroids have been widely used, several well-controlled studies demonstrate that the drugs are not beneficial in early treatment or in prevention of adult respiratory distress syndrome (ARDS). Thus, corticosteroids should be used in these patients only if there are other specific indications.

Sepsis

Sepsis may be complicated by impaired corticosteroid production. There is sufficient evidence to support that giving a long course of low dose of corticosteroids in patients with septic shock could improved survival without causing harm. However, overall corticosteroids did not impact on mortality

Acquired Immunodeficiency Syndrome

Adrenal insufficiency is being increasingly recognized in patients with AIDS, who should be assessed and treated for it, if indicated. In addition, corticosteroids improve survival and decrease risks of respiratory failure with pneumocystosis, a common cause of death in patients with AIDS. The recommended regimen is prednisone 40 milligrams twice daily for 5 days, then 40 milligrams once daily for 5 days, then 20 milligrams daily until completion of treatment for pneumocystosis. The effect of corticosteroids on risks of other opportunistic infections or neoplasms is unknown.

Use in Home Care

Corticosteroids are extensively used in the home setting, by all age groups, for a wide variety of disorders, and by most routes of administration. Because of potentially serious adverse effects, especially with oral drugs, it is extremely important that these drugs be used as prescribed. A major responsibility of home care nurses is to teach, demonstrate, supervise, monitor, or do whatever is needed to facilitate correct use. In addition, home care nurses must teach patients and caregivers interventions to minimize adverse effects of these drugs.

Nursing Actions · Corticosteroids

NURSING ACTIONS	RATIONALE/EXPLANATION
1. Administer accurately a. Read the drug label carefully to be certain of having the correct preparation for the intended route of administration.	Many corticosteroid drugs are available in several different preparations. For example, hydrocortisone is available in formulations for intravenous (IV) or intramuscular (IM) administration, for intraarticular injection, and for topical application in creams and ointments of several different strengths. These preparations cannot be used interchangeably without causing potentially serious adverse reactions and decreasing therapeutic effects. Some drugs are available for only one use. For example, several preparations are for topical use only; beclomethasone is prepared only for oral and nasal inhalation.
b. With oral corticosteroids: (1) Give single daily doses or alternate day doses between 6 and 9 A.M.	Early-morning administration causes less suppression of hypothalamic–pituitary–adrenal (HPA) function.
(2) Give multiple doses at evenly spaced intervals. (3) If dosage is being tapered, follow the exact schedule. (4) Give with meals or snacks. (5) With oral budesonide (Entocort EC), ask the patient to swallow the drug whole, without biting or chewing.	To avoid adverse effects To decrease gastrointestinal (GI) upset This drug is formulated to dissolve in the intestine and have local anti-inflammatory effects. Biting or chewing allows it to dissolve in the stomach.
(6) Do *not* give these drugs with an antacid containing aluminum or magnesium (e.g., Maalox, Mylanta). c. For IV or IM administration: (1) Shake the medication vial well before withdrawing medication. (2) Give a direct IV injection over at least 1 minute. d. For oral or nasal inhalation of a corticosteroid, check the instruction leaflet that accompanies the inhaler.	The antacids decrease absorption of corticosteroids, with possible reduction of therapeutic effects. Most of the injectable formulations are suspensions, which need to be mixed well for accurate dosage. To increase safety of administration These drugs are given by metered-dose inhalers or nasal sprays, and correct usage of the devices is essential to drug administration and therapeutic effects.
2. Observe for therapeutic effects	The primary objective of corticosteroid therapy is to relieve signs and symptoms, because the drugs are not curative. Therefore, therapeutic effects depend largely on the reason for use.
a. With adrenocortical insufficiency, observe for absence or decrease of weakness, weight loss, anorexia, nausea, vomiting, hyperpigmentation, hypotension, hypoglycemia, hyponatremia, and hyperkalemia.	These signs and symptoms of impaired metabolism do not occur with adequate replacement of corticosteroids.
b. With rheumatoid arthritis, observe for decreased pain and edema in joints, greater capacity for movement, and increased ability to perform usual activities of daily living. c. With asthma and chronic obstructive pulmonary disease, observe for decrease in respiratory distress and increased tolerance of activity. d. With skin lesions, observe for decreasing inflammation. e. When the drug is given to suppress the immune response to organ transplants, therapeutic effect is the absence of signs and symptoms indicating rejection of the transplanted tissue.	

NURSING ACTIONS	RATIONALE/EXPLANATION
3. Observe for adverse effects	These are uncommon with replacement therapy but common with long-term administration of the pharmacologic doses used for many disease processes. Adverse reactions may affect every body tissue and organ.
a. Adrenocortical insufficiency—fainting, weakness, anorexia, nausea, vomiting, hypotension, shock, and if untreated, death	This reaction is likely to occur in patients receiving daily corticosteroid drugs who encounter stressful situations. It is caused by drug-induced suppression of the HPA axis, which makes the patient unable to respond to stress by increasing adrenocortical hormone secretion.
b. Adrenocortical excess (hypercorticism or Cushing's disease)	Most adverse effects result from excessive corticosteroids.
(1) "Moon face," "buffalo hump" contour of shoulders, obese trunk, thin extremities	This appearance is caused by abnormal fat deposits in cheeks, shoulders, breasts, abdomen, and buttocks. These changes are more cosmetic than physiologically significant. However, the alterations in self-image can lead to psychological problems. These changes cannot be prevented, but they may be partially reversed if corticosteroid therapy is discontinued or reduced in dosage.
(2) Diabetes mellitus—glycosuria, hyperglycemia, polyuria, polydipsia, polyphagia, impaired healing, and other signs and symptoms	Corticosteroid drugs can cause hyperglycemia and diabetes mellitus or aggravate pre-existing diabetes mellitus by their effects on carbohydrate metabolism.
(3) Central nervous system effects—euphoria, psychological dependence, nervousness, insomnia, depression, personality and behavioral changes, aggravation of pre-existing psychiatric disorders	Some patients enjoy the drug-induced euphoria so much that they resist attempts to withdraw the drug or decrease its dosage.
(4) Musculoskeletal effects—osteoporosis, pathologic fractures, muscle weakness and atrophy, decreased linear growth in children	Demineralization of bone produces thin, weak bones that fracture easily. Fractures of vertebrae, long bones, and ribs are relatively common, especially in postmenopausal women and immobilized patients. Myopathy results from abnormal protein metabolism. Decreased growth in children results from impaired bone formation and protein metabolism.
(5) Cardiovascular, fluid, and electrolyte effects—fluid retention, edema, hypertension, congestive heart failure, hypernatremia, hypokalemia, metabolic alkalosis	These effects result largely from mineralocorticoid activity, which causes retention of sodium and water. They are more likely to occur with older corticosteroids, such as hydrocortisone and prednisone.
(6) Gastrointestinal effects—nausea, vomiting, possible peptic ulcer disease, increased appetite, obesity	
(7) Increased susceptibility to infection and delayed wound healing	Caused by suppression of normal inflammatory and immune processes and impaired protein metabolism
(8) Menstrual irregularities, acne, excessive facial hair	Caused by excessive sex hormones, primarily androgens
(9) Ocular effects—increased intraocular pressure, glaucoma, cataracts	
(10) Integumentary effects—skin becomes reddened, thinner, has stretch marks, and is easily injured	
4. Observe for drug interactions	
a. Drugs that *increase* effects of corticosteroids:	
(1) Estrogens, oral contraceptives, ketoconazole, macrolide antibiotics (e.g., erythromycin)	These drugs apparently inhibit the enzymes that normally metabolize corticosteroids in the liver.
(2) Diuretics (e.g., furosemide, thiazides)	Increase hypokalemia
b. Drugs that *decrease* effects of corticosteroids:	
(1) Antacids, cholestyramine	Decrease absorption
(2) Carbamazepine, phenytoin, rifampin	These drugs induce microsomal enzymes in the liver and increase the rate at which corticosteroids are metabolized or deactivated.

Key Concepts

■ The most frequently desired pharmacologic effects of exogenous corticosteroids are anti-inflammatory, immunosuppressive, antiallergic, and antistress.

■ Mineralocorticoid and androgenic effects of exogenous corticosteroids are usually considered adverse reactions.

■ Daily administration of corticosteroids and mineralocorticoids is required in cases of chronic adrenocortical insufficiency (Addison's disease).

■ Adrenocortical hyperfunction (Cushing's disease) may result from excessive corticotropin or a primary adrenal tumor.

■ Strategies to minimize HPA suppression and risks of acute adrenal insufficiency, include (1) administering a systemic corticosteroid during high-stress situations to those who receive long-term systemic therapy (i.e., are steroid dependent); (2) giving short courses of systemic therapy for acute disorders; (3) gradually tapering the dose of any systemic corticosteroid; (4) using local rather than systemic therapy when possible, alone or in combination with low doses of systemic drugs; and (5) using ADT.

■ Adverse effects of systemic corticosteroids may include infections, hypertension, glucose intolerance, obesity, cosmetic changes, bone loss, growth retardation in children, cataracts, pancreatitis, peptic ulcerations, and psychiatric disturbances.

■ A **BLACK BOX WARNING** has been issued by the FDA for individuals who are transferred from systemically active corticosteroids to flunisolide inhaler; deaths have been reported from adrenal insufficiency.

Review and Application Exercises

Short Answer Exercises

1. What are the main characteristics and functions of cortisol?

2. What is the difference between glucocorticoid and mineralocorticoid components of corticosteroids?

3. How do glucocorticoids affect body metabolism?

4. What is meant by the HPA axis?

5. What are the mechanisms by which exogenous corticosteroids may cause adrenocortical insufficiency and excess?

6. What adverse effects are associated with chronic use of systemic corticosteroids?

7. What are the main differences between administering corticosteroids in adrenal insufficiency versus in other disorders?

8. When a corticosteroid is given by inhalation to patients with asthma, what is the expected effect?

NCLEX-Style Questions

9. Your patient is being discontinued from long-term systemic corticosteroid therapy. You know that it is important to taper the dose in long-term systemic corticosteroid therapy rather than stopping the drug abruptly, because tapering results in which of the following?
   a. less suppression of hypothalamic–pituitary–adrenal function
   b. increased patient compliance with drug therapy
   c. greater tolerance of adverse effects
   d. significantly increased anti-inflammatory effect

10. A nurse is instructing a patient regarding the correct way follow the order, "prednisone 10 mg PO once daily." The nurse should tell the patient to take
    a. the entire dose once a day at bedtime
    b. the entire dose once a day on arising
    c. half of the dose in the morning and half at bedtime
    d. one third of the dose in the morning and two thirds in the afternoon

11. A patient who has been on long-term corticosteroid therapy begins to gain weight and complains that her rings no longer fit on her hands. She asks the nurse why she is gaining weight. The nurse tells the patient that the most likely cause of later weight gain when undergoing corticosteroid therapy is
    a. increased appetite
    b. hyperglycemia
    c. muscle hypertrophy
    d. fluid retention

12. A patient taking an inhaled steroid should be instructed to rinse her mouth after administration of the drug to avoid development of which of the following conditions?
    a. anorexia
    b. nausea and vomiting
    c. thrush
    d. gingival hyperplasia

13. Patients taking oral or IV glucocorticoids have an increased risk for which of the following conditions?
    a. allergic reaction
    b. hypotension
    c. hypoglycemia
    d. infection

Selected References

Annane, D., Bellissant, E., Bollaert, P. E., Briegel, J., Keh, D., & Kupfer, Y. (2007). Corticosteroids for treating severe sepsis and septic shock. *Cochrane Database of Systematic Reviews*, Issue 2. Art No.: CD002243

Corwin, E. J. (2006). *Handbook of pathophysiology* (3rd ed.). Philadelphia: Lippincott Williams & Wilkins.

Drug facts and comparisons. (Updated monthly). St. Louis, MO: Facts and Comparisons.

Guyton, A. C., & Hall, J. E. (2006). *Textbook of medical physiology* (11th ed.). Philadelphia: W. B. Saunders.

Lacy, C. F., Armstrong, L. L., Goldman, M. P., & Lance, L. L. (2007). *Lexi-Comp's drug information handbook* (15th ed.). Hudson, OH: American Pharmaceutical Association.

Mash, B., Bheekie, A., & Jones, P. W. (2007). Inhaled versus oral steroids for adults with chronic asthma. *Cochrane Database of Systematic Reviews*, Issue 2. Art No.: CD002160.

Matfin, G., Kuenzi, J. A., & Guven, S. (2005). Disorders of endocrine control of growth and metabolism. In C. M. Porth (Ed.), *Pathophysiology: Concepts of altered health states* (7th ed., pp. 961–985). Philadelphia: Lippincott Williams & Wilkins.

McCance, K. L., & Huether, S. E. (2006). *Pathophysiology: The biologic basis for disease in adults and children* (5th ed., pp. 655–681). Philadelphia: Elsevier Mosby.

Wood-Baker, R. R., Gibson, P., Hannay, M., Walters, E. H., & Walters, J. A. E. (2007). Systemic corticosteroids for acute exacerbations of chronic obstructive pulmonary disease. *Cochrane Database of Systematic Reviews*, Issue 1. Art No.: CD0012288.

Thyroid and Antithyroid Drugs

LEARNING OBJECTIVES

After studying this chapter, you will be able to:

1. Recognize physiologic effects of thyroid hormone.
2. Assess subclinical, symptomatic, and severe effects of inadequate or excessive thyroid hormone.
3. Describe characteristics, uses, and effects of thyroid drugs.
4. Identify characteristics, uses, and effects of antithyroid drugs.
5. Evaluate the influence of thyroid and antithyroid drugs on the metabolism of other drugs.
6. Teach patients effective self-care activities related to the use of thyroid and antithyroid drugs.
7. Apply the nursing process with patients receiving thyroid and antithyroid drugs.

Applying Your Knowledge

Brenda Zalewski is a 45-year-old woman who had a goiter as a child and a thyroidectomy at age 12. She has been taking a synthetic thyroid preparation since that time. Ms. Zalewski takes a maintenance dose of Synthroid 0.1 mg PO daily. She is 5 feet 8 inches tall and weighs 215 pounds.

Introduction

Normal serum levels of thyroid hormones and a physiologic state of normal thyroid function (*euthyroid*) require a functioning thyroid gland and feedback mechanism. The thyroid gland produces three hormones: *thyroxine*, triiodothyronine, and calcitonin. Thyroxine (also called T_4) contains four atoms of iodine, and triiodothyronine (also called T_3) contains three atoms of iodine. T_3 is more potent than T_4 and has a more rapid onset but a shorter duration of action. Despite these minor differences, the two hormones produce the same physiologic effects and have the same actions and uses. Calcitonin functions in calcium metabolism and is discussed in Chapter 25.

Production of T_3 and T_4 depends on the presence of iodine and tyrosine in the thyroid gland. In a series of chemical reactions, iodine atoms become attached to tyrosine, an amino acid derived from dietary protein, to form the thyroid hormones T_3 and T_4. After they are formed, the hormones are stored within the chemically inactive thyroglobulin molecule. Tyrosine forms the basic structure of thyroglobulin.

Thyroid hormones are released into the circulation when the thyroid gland is stimulated by thyroid-stimulating hormone (thyrotropin or TSH) from the anterior pituitary gland (Fig. 24-1). The hormones become largely bound to plasma proteins with only the small unbound remaining

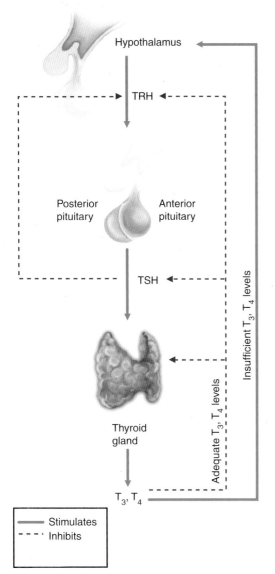

Figure 24-1 ■ Thyroid-releasing hormone (TRH) from the hypothalamus stimulates the anterior pituitary to release thyroid-stimulating hormone (TSH). It also inhibits the hypothalamus from releasing TRH. TSH stimulates the thyroid gland to releases T_3 and T_4. It also inhibits the hypothalamus from releasing TRH and the anterior pituitary from releasing more TSH. The release of T_3 and T_4 from the thyroid gland inhibits TRH release from the hypothalamus, TSH release from the pituitary, and further T_3 and T_4 release from the thyroid gland. Falling T_3 and T_4 levels stimulate the hypothalamus to release TRH, and the process repeatedly continues to maintain effective hormone levels. ACTH, adrenocorticotropic hormone; CRH, corticotropin-releasing hormone; FSH, follicle-stimulating hormone; GH, growth hormone; GHRH, growth hormone–releasing hormone; GnRH, gonadotropin-releasing hormone; LH, luteinizing hormone; PIF, prolactin-inhibiting factor; PRL, prolactin; PRF, prolactin-releasing factor; SRIF, somatotropin release-inhibiting factor.

biologically active. The bound thyroid hormones are released to tissue cells very slowly. In tissue cells, the hormones combine with intracellular proteins so they are again stored. They are released slowly within the cell and used over a period of days or weeks. When they are used by the cells, the thyroid hormones release iodine atoms. Most of the iodine is reabsorbed and used to produce new thyroid hormones; the remainder is excreted in the urine.

Thyroid hormones control the rate of cellular metabolism and thereby influence the functioning of virtually every cell in the body. The heart, skeletal muscle, liver, and kidneys are especially responsive to the stimulating effects of thyroid hormones. The brain, spleen, and gonads are less responsive. Thyroid hormones are required for normal growth and development and are considered especially critical for brain and skeletal development and maturation.

Thyroid hormones also influence linear growth; brain function, including intelligence and memory; neural development; dentition; and bone development. These hormones are thought to act mainly by controlling intracellular protein synthesis. Some specific physiologic effects include

- Increased rate of cellular metabolism and oxygen consumption with a resultant increase in heat production
- Increased heart rate, force of contraction, and cardiac output (increased cardiac workload)
- Increased carbohydrate metabolism
- Increased fat metabolism, including increased lipolytic effects of other hormones and metabolism of cholesterol to bile acids
- Inhibition of pituitary secretion of TSH

Two types of thyroid disorders requiring drug therapy are hypothyroidism and hyperthyroidism. These disorders produce opposing effects on body tissues, depending on the levels of circulating thyroid hormone. Specific effects and clinical manifestations are listed in Table 24-1.

Hypothyroidism

Primary *hypothyroidism* occurs when disease or destruction of thyroid gland tissue causes inadequate production of thyroid hormones. Common causes of primary hypothyroidism include chronic (Hashimoto's) *thyroiditis*, an autoimmune disorder characterized by inflammation of the thyroid gland, and treatment of hyperthyroidism with antithyroid drugs, radiation therapy, or surgery. Other causes include previous radiation to the thyroid area of the neck and treatment with amiodarone, lithium, or iodine preparations. Secondary hypothyroidism occurs when there is decreased TSH from the anterior pituitary gland or decreased thyrotropin-releasing hormone (TRH) secreted from the hypothalamus.

Congenital hypothyroidism (*cretinism*) occurs when a child is born with a poorly functioning or absent thyroid gland. Cretinism is uncommon in the United States but may occur with a lack of iodine in the mother's diet. Symptoms are rarely present at birth but develop gradually during infancy and early childhood, and they include poor growth and development, lethargy and inactivity, feeding problems, slow pulse, subnormal temperature, and constipation. If cretinism is untreated until the child is several months old, permanent mental retardation is likely to result.

Adult hypothyroidism (*myxedema*) may be subclinical or clinical and occurs much more often in women than in men. Subclinical hypothyroidism, the most common thyroid disorder, involves a mildly elevated serum TSH and normal serum thyroxine levels. It is usually asymptomatic. If the thyroid gland cannot secrete enough hormone despite excessive release of TSH, hypothyroidism occurs, and a *goiter* (visible enlargement of the thyroid gland) may occur from the overstimulation. Clinical hypothyroidism produces variable signs and symptoms, depending on the amount of circulating thyroid hormone. Initially, manifestations (see Table 24-1) are mild and vague. They usually increase in incidence and severity over time as the thyroid gland gradually atrophies and functioning glandular tissue is replaced by nonfunctioning fibrous connective tissue.

Myxedema coma is severe, life-threatening hypothyroidism characterized by coma, hypothermia, cardiovascular collapse, hypoventilation, and severe metabolic disorders such as hyponatremia, hypoglycemia, and lactic acidosis. Predisposing factors include exposure to cold, infection, trauma, respiratory disease, and administration of central nervous system depressants (e.g., anesthetics, analgesics, sedatives). A person with severe hypothyroidism cannot metabolize and excrete the drugs.

Table 24-1	Thyroid Disorders and Their Effects on Body Systems
HYPOTHYROIDISM	**HYPERTHYROIDISM**
Cardiovascular Effects	
Increased capillary fragility	Tachycardia
Decreased cardiac output	Increased cardiac output
Decreased blood pressure	Increased blood volume
Decreased heart rate	Increased systolic blood pressure
Cardiac enlargement	Decreased diastolic blood pressure
Congestive heart failure	Cardiac dysrhythmias
Anemia	Congestive heart failure
More rapid development of atherosclerosis and its complications (e.g., coronary artery and peripheral vascular disease)	
Central Nervous System Effects	
Apathy and lethargy	Nervousness
Emotional dullness	Emotional instability
Slow speech, perhaps slurring and hoarseness as well	Restlessness
Hypoactive reflexes	Anxiety
Forgetfulness and mental sluggishness	Insomnia
Excessive drowsiness and sleeping	Hyperactive reflexes
Metabolic Effects	
Intolerance of cold	Intolerance of heat
Subnormal temperature	Low-grade fever
Increased serum cholesterol Weight gain	Weight loss despite increased appetite
Gastrointestinal Effects	
Decreased appetite	Increased appetite
Constipation	Abdominal cramps Diarrhea Nausea and vomiting
Muscular Effects	
Weakness	Weakness
Fatigue	Fatigue

HYPOTHYROIDISM	HYPERTHYROIDISM
Vague aches and pains	Muscle atrophy
	Tremors
Integumentary Effects	
Dry, coarse, and thickened skin	Moist, warm, flushed skin due to vasodilation and
Puffy appearance of face and eyelids	increased sweating
Dry and thinned hair	Hair and nails soft
Thick and hard nails	
Reproductive Effects	
Prolonged menstrual periods	Amenorrhea or oligomenorrhea
Infertility or sterility	
Decreased libido	
Miscellaneous Effects	
Increased susceptibility to infection	Dyspnea
Increased sensitivity to narcotics, barbiturates, and anesthetics due to slowed metabolism of these drugs	Polyuria
	Hoarse, rapid speech
	Increased susceptibility to infection
	Excessive perspiration
	Localized edema around the eyeballs, which produces characteristic eye changes, including exophthalmos

Hyperthyroidism

Hyperthyroidism is characterized by excessive secretion of thyroid hormone and usually involves an enlarged thyroid gland that has an increased number of cells and an increased rate of secretion. It may be associated with *Graves' disease*, nodular goiter, thyroiditis, overtreatment with thyroid drugs, functioning thyroid carcinoma, and pituitary adenoma that secretes excessive amounts of TSH. The hyperplastic thyroid gland may secrete 5 to 15 times the normal amount of thyroid hormone. As a result, body metabolism is greatly increased. Specific physiologic effects and clinical manifestations of hyperthyroidism are listed in Table 24-1. These effects vary, depending on the amount of circulating thyroid hormone, and they usually increase in incidence and severity with time if hyperthyroidism is not treated.

Subclinical hyperthyroidism is defined as a reduced TSH (less than 0.1 microunit/L) and normal T_3 and T_4 levels. The most common cause is excess thyroid hormone therapy. Subclinical hyperthyroidism is a risk factor for osteoporosis in postmenopausal women who do not take estrogen replacement therapy, because it leads to reduced bone mineral density. It also greatly increases the risk of atrial fibrillation in patients older than 60 years of age.

Thyroid storm or thyrotoxic crisis is a rare but severe complication characterized by extreme symptoms of hyperthyroidism, such as severe tachycardia, fever, dehydration, heart failure, and coma. It is most likely to occur in patients with hyperthyroidism that has been inadequately treated, especially when stressful situations occur (e.g., trauma, infection, surgery, emotional upset).

It should be noted that iodine is present in foods (especially seafood and kelp) and in radiographic contrast dyes. Reports of iodine-induced hyperthyroidism have been reported after ingestion of dietary sources of iodine.

General Characteristics of Thyroid and Antithyroid Drugs

Mechanism of Action

Thyroid drugs such as the synthetic drug levothyroxine provide an exogenous source of thyroid hormone. Antithyroid drugs act by decreasing production or release of thyroid hormones. The thioamide drugs inhibit synthesis of thyroid hormone. Iodine preparations inhibit the release of thyroid hormones and cause them to be stored within the thyroid gland. Radioactive iodine emits rays that destroy the thyroid gland tissue.

Indications for Use

Thyroid drugs are indicated for primary or secondary hypothyroidism, cretinism, and myxedema. Antithyroid drugs may be necessary for hyperthyroidism associated with Graves' disease, nodular goiter, thyroiditis, overtreatment with thyroid drugs, functioning thyroid carcinoma, and pituitary adenoma that secretes excessive amounts of TSH. Antithyroid drugs may also be indicated for thyroid storm. The Food and Drug Administration (FDA) has issued a **BLACK BOX WARNING** regarding the use of thyroid hormones for the treatment of obesity or for weight loss, either alone or with other therapeutic agents.

Additional administration of thyroid preparations in euthyroid individuals may produce serious or life-threatening manifestations of toxicity; this effect is increased when given in conjunction with sympathomimetic amines, often used for their anorectic effects in weigh loss management.

Contraindications to Use

Iodine preparations and thioamide antithyroid drugs are contraindicated in pregnancy, because they can lead to goiter and hypothyroidism in the fetus or newborn. Radioactive iodine is contraindicated during lactation as well. Because radioactive iodine may cause cancer and chromosome damage in children, it should be used only for hyperthyroidism that cannot be controlled by other drugs or surgery.

Individual Drugs

Thyroid and antithyroid drugs are described in the following section. Dosages are listed in Table 24-2.

Table 24-2	**Drugs at a Glance:** Drugs for Hypothyroidism and Hyperthyroidism	

| | ROUTES AND DOSAGE RANGES | |
Generic/Trade name	Adults	Children
Drugs for Hypothyroidism		
P Levothyroxine (Synthroid, Levothroid)	PO 0.05 mg/d initially, increased by 0.025 mg every 2–3 wk until desired response obtained; usual maintenance dose, 0.1–0.2 mg/d (100–200 mcg/d) Myxedema coma, IV 0.4 mg in a single dose; then 0.1–0.2 mg daily Thyroid-stimulating hormone (TSH) suppression in thyroid cancer, nodules, and euthyroid goiters, PO 2.6 mcg/kg/d for 7–10 d *Older adults, patients with cardiac disorders, and patients with hypothyroidism of long duration:* PO 0.0125–0.025 mg/d for 6 wk, then dose is doubled every 6–8 wk until the desired response is obtained Myxedema coma, same as adult dosage	Congenital hypothyroidism, PO as follows: *older than 12 y:* >150 mcg/d (or 2–3 mcg/kg/d) *6–12 y:* 100–150 mcg/d (or 4–5 mcg/kg/d) *1–5 y:* 75–100 mcg/d (or 5–6 mcg/kg/d) *6–12 mo:* 50–75 mcg/d (or 6–8 mcg/kg/d) *Birth–6 mo:* 25–50 mcg/d (or 8–10 mcg/kg/d)
Drugs for Hyperthyroidism		
P Propylthiouracil	PO 300–400 mg/d in divided doses q8h, until the patient is euthyroid; then 100–150 mg/d in 3 divided doses, for maintenance	*older than 10 y:* PO 150–300 mg/d in divided doses q8h; usual maintenance dose, 100–300 mg/d in 2 divided doses, q12h *6–10 y:* 50–150 mg/d in divided doses q8h
Methimazole (Tapazole)	PO 15–60 mg/d initially, in divided doses q8h until the patient is euthyroid; maintenance, 5–15 mg/d in 2 or 3 doses	PO 0.4 mg/kg/d initially, in divided doses q8h; maintenance dose, one half initial dose
Strong iodine solution (Lugol's solution)	PO 2–6 drops 3 times per day for 10 d before thyroidectomy	PO 2–6 drops 3 times per day for 10 d before thyroidectomy
Saturated solution of potassium iodide (SSKI)	PO 5 drops 3 times per day for 10 d before thyroidectomy	PO 5 drops 3 times per day for 10 d before thyroidectomy
Sodium iodide ^{131}I (Iodotope)	PO, IV, dosage as calculated by a radiologist trained in nuclear medicine	PO, IV, dosage as calculated by a radiologist trained in nuclear medicine
Propranolol (Inderal)	PO 40–160 mg/d in divided doses	

Thyroid Drugs (Used in Hypothyroidism)

P **Levothyroxine** (Synthroid, Levothroid), a synthetic preparation of T_4, is the drug of choice for long-term treatment of hypothyroidism and serves as the prototype. This potent form of T_4 contains a uniform amount of hormone and can be given parenterally. Absorption with oral administration varies from 48% to 79% of the dose administered. Taking the medication on an empty stomach increases absorption; malabsorption syndromes cause excessive fecal loss. Most (99%) of the circulating levothyroxine is bound to serum proteins, including thyroid-binding globulin as well as thyroid-binding prealbumin and albumin. Levothyroxine has a long half-life of about 6 to 7 days in euthyroidism (normal thyroid function) but is prolonged to 9 to 10 days in hypothyroidism and shortened to 3 to 4 days in hyperthyroidism.

Applying Your Knowledge 24-1

While Ms. Zalewski is in the hospital, you are administering her daily medications. Hospital routine is to administer all once-daily medications at 9:00 A.M. When reviewing the medication administration sheets, you note Ms. Zalewski is to receive Synthroid at 9:00 A.M. Breakfast trays are usually served to patients between 8:00 and 8:30 A.M. What action should you take with regard to administration of the Synthroid?

Antithyroid Drugs (Used in Hyperthyroidism)

P **Propylthiouracil** (PTU) is the prototype of the thioamide antithyroid drugs. It can be used alone to treat hyperthyroidism, as part of the preoperative preparation for thyroidectomy, before or after radioactive iodine therapy, and in the treatment of thyroid storm. PTU acts by inhibiting production of thyroid hormones and peripheral conversion of T_4 to the more active T_3. It does not interfere with release of thyroid hormones previously produced and stored. Thus, therapeutic effects do not occur for several days or weeks until the stored hormones have been used.

PTU is well absorbed with oral administration, and peak plasma levels occur within 30 minutes. Plasma half-life is 1 to 2 hours. However, duration of action depends on the half-life within the thyroid gland rather than plasma half-life. Because this time is relatively short, PTU must be given every 8 hours. The drug is metabolized in the liver and excreted in urine.

Methimazole (Tapazole) is similar to PTU in actions, uses, and adverse reactions. It is also well absorbed with oral administration and rapidly reaches peak plasma levels.

Strong iodine solution (Lugol's solution) and **saturated solution of potassium iodide** (SSKI) are iodine preparations sometimes used in short-term treatment of hyperthyroidism.

These drugs inhibit release of thyroid hormones, causing them to accumulate in the thyroid gland. Lugol's solution is usually used to treat thyrotoxic crisis and to decrease the size and vascularity of the thyroid gland before thyroidectomy. SSKI is more often used as an expectorant but may be given as preparation for thyroidectomy. Iodine preparations should not be followed by propylthiouracil, methimazole, or radioactive iodine because the latter drugs cause release of stored thyroid hormone and may precipitate acute hyperthyroidism.

Sodium iodide [131]I (Iodotope) is a radioactive isotope of iodine. The thyroid gland cannot differentiate between regular iodide and radioactive iodide, so it picks up the radioactive iodide from the circulating blood. As a result, small amounts of radioactive iodide can be used as a diagnostic test of thyroid function, and larger doses are used therapeutically to treat hyperthyroidism. Therapeutic doses act by emitting beta and gamma rays, which destroy thyroid tissue and thereby decrease production of thyroid hormones. It is also used to treat thyroid cancer.

Propranolol (Inderal) is an antiadrenergic, not an antithyroid, drug. It does not affect thyroid function, hormone secretion, or hormone metabolism. It is most often used to treat cardiovascular conditions, such as dysrhythmias, angina pectoris, and hypertension. When given to patients with hyperthyroidism, propranolol blocks beta-adrenergic receptors in various organs and thereby controls symptoms of hyperthyroidism resulting from excessive stimulation of the sympathetic nervous system. These symptoms include tachycardia, palpitations, excessive sweating, tremors, and nervousness. Propranolol is useful for controlling symptoms during the delayed response to thioamide drugs and radioactive iodine, before thyroidectomy, and in treating thyrotoxic crisis. When the patient becomes euthyroid and hyperthyroid symptoms are controlled by definitive treatment measures, propranolol should be tapered and discontinued.

Nursing Process

Assessment

■ Assess for signs and symptoms of thyroid disorders (see Table 24-1). During the course of treatment with thyroid or antithyroid drugs, the patient's blood level of thyroid hormone may range from low to normal to high. At either end of the continuum, signs and symptoms may be dramatic and obvious. As blood levels change toward normal as a result of treatment, signs and symptoms become less obvious. If presenting signs and symptoms are treated too aggressively, they may change toward the opposite end of the continuum and indicate adverse drug effects. Thus, *each patients receiving a drug that alters thyroid function must be assessed for indicators of hypothyroidism, euthyroidism, and hyperthyroidism.*

Nursing Process continues on page 384

- Check laboratory reports for serum TSH (normal = 0.5 to 4.2 μU/mL) when available. An elevated serum TSH is the first indication of primary hypothyroidism and commonly occurs in middle-aged women, even in the absence of other signs and symptoms. Serum TSH is used to monitor response to drugs that alter thyroid function.

Nursing Diagnoses

- Decreased Cardiac Output related to disease- or drug-induced thyroid disorders
- Imbalanced Nutrition: Less Than Body Requirements with hyperthyroidism
- Imbalanced Nutrition: More Than Body Requirements with hypothyroidism
- Ineffective Thermoregulation related to changes in metabolism rate and body heat production
- Deficient Knowledge: Disease process and drug therapy

Planning/Goals

The patient will

- Achieve normal blood levels of thyroid hormone
- Receive or take drugs accurately
- Experience relief of symptoms of hypothyroidism or hyperthyroidism
- Be assisted to cope with symptoms until therapy becomes effective
- Avoid preventable adverse drug effects
- Maintain the therapeutic and avoid the adverse effects of drug therapy

Interventions

Use nondrug measures to control symptoms, increase effectiveness of drug therapy, and decrease adverse reactions. Some areas for intervention include the following:

- **Environmental temperature.** Regulate for the patient's comfort, when possible. Patients with *hypothyroidism* are very intolerant of cold, due to their slow metabolism rate. Chilling and shivering should be prevented because of added strain on the heart. Please provide blankets and warm clothes as needed. Patients with *hyperthyroidism* are very intolerant of heat and perspire excessively, due to their rapid metabolism rate. Provide cooling baths and lightweight clothing as needed.

- **Diet.** Despite a poor appetite, *hypothyroid* patients are often overweight because of a slow metabolism rate. Thus, a low-calorie, weight-reduction diet may be indicated. In addition, an increased intake of high-fiber foods is usually needed to prevent constipation as a result of decreased gastrointestinal secretions and motility. Despite a good appetite, *hyperthyroid* patients are often underweight because of a rapid metabolism rate. They often need extra calories and nutrients to prevent tissue breakdown.

These can be provided by extra meals and snacks. The patient may wish to avoid highly seasoned and high-fiber foods because they may increase diarrhea.

- **Fluids.** With *hypothyroidism*, patients need an adequate intake of low-calorie fluids to prevent constipation. With *hyperthyroidism*, patients need large amounts of fluids (3000–4000 mL/day) unless contraindicated by cardiac or renal disease. The fluids are needed to eliminate heat and waste products produced by the hypermetabolic state. Much of the patient's fluid loss is visible as excessive perspiration and urine output.

- **Activity.** With *hypothyroidism*, encourage activity to maintain cardiovascular, respiratory, gastrointestinal, and musculoskeletal function. With *hyperthyroidism*, encourage rest and quiet, nonstrenuous activity. Because patients differ in what they find restful, this must be determined with each patient. A quiet room, reading, and soft music may be helpful. Mild sedatives are often given. The patient is caught in the dilemma of needing rest because of the high metabolic rate but being unable to rest because of nervousness and excitement.

- **Skin care.** *Hypothyroid* patients are likely to have edema and dry skin. When edema is present, inspect pressure points, turn often, and avoid trauma when possible. Edema increases risks of skin breakdown and decubitus ulcer formation. Also, increased capillary fragility increases the likelihood of bruising from seemingly minor trauma. When skin is dry, use soap sparingly and lotions and other lubricants freely.

- **Eye care.** *Hyperthyroid* patients may have exophthalmos. In mild cases, use measures to protect the eye. For example, dark glasses, local lubricants, and patching of the eyes at night may be needed. Diuretic drugs and elevating the head of the bed may help reduce periorbital edema and eyeball protrusion. If the eyelids cannot close, they are sometimes taped shut to avoid corneal abrasion. In severe exophthalmos, the preceding measures are taken and large doses of corticosteroids are usually given.

Patient Guidelines for Levothyroxine and for Propyl-thiouracil or Methimazole are presented in the accompanying displays.

Evaluation

- Interview and observe for compliance with instructions for taking medications.
- Observe for relief of symptoms.
- Check laboratory reports for normal blood levels of TSH or thyroid hormones.
- Interview and observe for adverse drug effects.
- Check appointment records for compliance with follow-up procedures.

Applying Your Knowledge 24-2

You are preparing a teaching plan for Ms. Zalewski. Considering her height and weight, what should you include for this patient?

Principles of Therapy

Goals of Therapy

The goal of treatment with thyroid drugs is to restore the individual to a euthyroid state with normal metabolism. In hypothyroidism, the goal of thyroid replacement therapy is to administer a dosage in sufficient amounts to compensate for the thyroid deficit, so as to resolve symptoms and restore serum TSH and thyroid hormone to normal. In hyperthyroidism, the goals are to reduce thyroid hormone production to relieve symptoms, return serum TSH and thyroid hormone levels to normal, and avoid complete destruction of the thyroid gland.

Applying Your Knowledge 24-3

You are performing the assessment of Ms. Zalewski and observe tachycardia, increased systolic blood pressure, nervousness, insomnia, hunger, and fatigue. What laboratory test should be assessed and what action should you take?

Thyroid Drugs

Drug Selection

Regardless of the cause of hypothyroidism and the age at which it occurs, the specific treatment is replacement of thyroid hormone from an exogenous source. Synthetic levothyroxine is the drug of choice for thyroid hormone replacement because of uniform potency, once-daily dosing, and low cost. In patients with subclinical hypothyroidism, levothyroxine should be given if the serum TSH level is higher than 10 microunits per liter. There is some difference of opinion about treatment for TSH values between 5 and 10 microunits per liter. Arguments for treatment of subclinical hypothyroidism are the high rate of progression to symptomatic hypothyroidism, improvement of cholesterol metabolism (e.g., low-density lipoprotein, or "bad" cholesterol, is reduced with treatment), and improvement in left ventricular function.

In patients with symptomatic hypothyroidism, levothyroxine therapy is definitely indicated. In addition to improvement of metabolism, treatment may also improve cardiac function, energy level, mood, muscle function, and fertility. In myxedema coma, levothyroxine is given intravenously, along with interventions to relieve precipitating factors and to support vital functions until the thyroid hormone becomes effective, often within 24 hours.

Drug Dosage

Dosage is influenced by the choice of drug, the patient's age and general condition, severity and duration of hypothyroidism, and clinical response to drug therapy. The dosage must be individualized to approximate the amount of thyroid

Patient Teaching Guidelines   Levothyroxine

General Considerations
- Thyroid hormone is required for normal body functioning and for life. When a person's thyroid gland is unable to produce enough thyroid hormone, levothyroxine is used as a synthetic substitute. Thus, levothyroxine therapy for hypothyroidism is lifelong; stopping it may lead to life-threatening illness.
- Periodic tests of thyroid function are needed.
- Dosage adjustments are made according to clinical response and results of thyroid function tests.
- Do not switch from one brand name to another; effects may be different.
- Levothyroxine stimulates the central nervous system and the heart; excessive stimulation may occur if it is taken with other stimulating drugs. Thus, you should consult a health care provider before taking over-the-counter drugs that stimulate the heart or cause nervousness

(e.g., asthma remedies, cold remedies, decongestants). In addition, you should probably limit your intake of caffeine-containing beverages to 2 to 3 servings daily.

Self-Administration
- Take every morning, on an empty stomach, for best absorption. Also, do not take the drug with an antacid (e.g., Tums, Maalox), an iron preparation, or sucralfate (Carafate). These drugs decrease absorption of levothyroxine. If it is necessary to take one of these drugs, take levothyroxine 2 hours before or 4 to 6 hours after the other drug.
- Take at about the same time each day for more consistent blood levels and more normal body metabolism.
- Report chest pain, heart palpitations, nervousness, or insomnia. These adverse effects result from excessive stimulation and may indicate that drug dosage or intake of other stimulants needs to be reduced.

Patient Teaching Guidelines | Propylthiouracil or Methimazole

General Considerations

- These drugs are sometimes called *antithyroid drugs* because they are given to decrease the production of thyroid hormone by an overactive thyroid gland.
- These drugs must be taken for 1 year or longer to decrease thyroid hormone levels to normal.
- Periodic tests of thyroid function and drug dosage adjustments are needed.
- Ask the prescribing physician if it is necessary to avoid or restrict amounts of seafood or iodized salt. These sources of iodide may need to be reduced or omitted during antithyroid drug therapy.

Self-Administration

- Take at regular intervals around the clock, usually every 8 hours.
- Report fever, sore throat, unusual bleeding or bruising, headache, skin rash, yellowing of the skin, or vomiting. If these adverse effects occur, drug dosage may need to be reduced or the drug may need to be discontinued.
- Consult a health care provider before taking over-the-counter drugs. Some drugs contain iodide, which can increase the likelihood of goiter and the risk of adverse effects from excessive doses of iodide (e.g., some cough syrups, asthma medications, and multivitamins may contain iodide).

---

hormone needed to make up the deficit in endogenous hormone production. As a general rule, initial dosage is relatively small. Dosage is gradually increased at approximately 2-week intervals until symptoms are relieved and a normal serum TSH level (0.5–4.2 microunits/L) is reestablished. Maintenance dosage for long-term therapy is based on the patient's clinical status and periodic measurement of serum TSH.

Duration of Therapy

Thyroid replacement therapy in the patient with hypothyroidism is lifelong. Medical supervision is needed frequently during early treatment and at least annually after the patient's condition has stabilized and maintenance dosage has been determined.

Hypothyroidism and the Metabolism of Other Drugs

Changes in the rate of body metabolism affect the metabolism of many drugs. Most drugs given to patients with hypothyroidism have a prolonged effect, because drug metabolism in the liver is delayed and the glomerular filtration rate of the kidneys is decreased. Drug absorption from the intestine or a parenteral injection site also may be slowed. As a result, dosage of many other drugs should be reduced, including digoxin and insulin. In addition, people with hypothyroidism are especially likely to experience respiratory depression and myxedema coma with opioid analgesics and other sedating drugs. These drugs should be avoided when possible. However, when necessary, they are given very cautiously and in dosages of approximately one third to one half the usual dose. Even then, patients must be observed very closely for respiratory depression.

After thyroid replacement therapy is started and stabilized, the patient becomes euthyroid (having normal thyroid gland function), has a normal rate of metabolism, and can tolerate usual doses of most drugs if other influencing factors are not present. On the other hand, excessive doses of

thyroid drugs may produce hyperthyroidism and a greatly increased rate of metabolism. In this situation, larger doses of most other drugs are necessary to produce the same effects. However, rather than increasing dosage of other drugs, dosage of thyroid drugs should be reduced so the patient is euthyroid again.

Adrenal Insufficiency

When hypothyroidism and adrenal insufficiency coexist, the adrenal insufficiency should be treated with a corticosteroid drug before starting thyroid replacement. Thyroid hormones increase tissue metabolism and tissue demands for adrenocortical hormones. If adrenal insufficiency is not treated first, administration of thyroid hormone may cause acute adrenocortical insufficiency, a life-threatening condition.

Antithyroid Drugs

Treatment of hyperthyroidism depends on the cause. If the cause is an adenoma or multinodular goiter surgery or radioactive iodine therapy is recommended, especially in older patients. If the cause is excessive doses of levothyroxine (for hypothyroidism), the dose of levothyroxine should be reduced. If the cause is Graves' disease, antithyroid drugs, radioactive iodine, surgery, or a combination of these methods may be warranted. All these methods reduce the amount of thyroid hormones circulating in the bloodstream.

Drug Selection

The antithyroid drugs include the thioamide derivatives (propylthiouracil and methimazole) and iodine preparations (Lugol's solution and SSKI). The thioamide drugs are inexpensive and relatively safe, and they do not damage the thyroid gland. These drugs may be used as the primary treatment (for which they may be given 6 months to 2 years) or to decrease blood levels of thyroid hormone before radioactive iodine therapy or surgery.

Radioactive iodine is a frequently used treatment. It is safe, effective, inexpensive, and convenient. One disadvantage is hypothyroidism, which usually develops within a few months and requires lifelong thyroid hormone replacement therapy. Another disadvantage is the delay in therapeutic benefits. Results may not be apparent for 3 months or longer, during which time severe hyperthyroidism must be brought under control with one of the thioamide antithyroid drugs.

Other iodine preparations are not used in long-term treatment of hyperthyroidism. They are indicated when a rapid clinical response is needed, as in thyroid storm and acute hyperthyroidism, or to prepare a hyperthyroid person for thyroidectomy. A thioamide drug is given to produce a euthyroid state, and an iodine preparation is given to reduce the size and vascularity of the thyroid gland to reduce the risk of excessive bleeding. Maximal effects are reached in approximately 10 to 15 days of continuous therapy, and this is probably the primary advantage. Disadvantages of this combination of drugs include the following:

- They may produce goiter, hyperthyroidism, or both.
- They cannot be used alone. Therapeutic benefits are temporary, and symptoms of hyperthyroidism may reappear and even be intensified if other treatment methods are not also used.
- Radioactive iodine cannot be used effectively for a prolonged period in a patient who has received iodine preparations. Even if the iodine preparation is discontinued, the thyroid gland is saturated with iodine and does not attract enough radioactive iodine for treatment to be effective. Also, if radioactive iodine is given later, acute hyperthyroidism is likely to result because the radioactive iodine causes the stored hormones to be released into the circulation.
- Although giving a thioamide drug followed by an iodine preparation is standard preparation for thyroidectomy, the opposite sequence of administration is unsafe. If the iodine preparation is given first and followed by PTU or methimazole, the patient is likely to experience acute hyperthyroidism because the thioamide causes release of the stored thyroid hormones.

Drug Dosage

Dosage of the thioamide antithyroid drugs is relatively large until a euthyroid state is reached, usually in 6 to 8 weeks. A maintenance dose, in the smallest amount that prevents recurrent symptoms of hyperthyroidism, is then given for 1 year or longer. Dosage should be decreased if the thyroid gland enlarges or signs and symptoms of hypothyroidism occur.

Radioactive iodide is usually given in a single dose to middle-aged and elderly people on an outpatient basis. For most patients, no special radiation precautions are necessary. If a very large dose is given, the patient may be isolated for 8 days, which is the half-life of radioactive iodide.

Duration of Therapy

No clear-cut guidelines exist regarding duration of antithyroid drug therapy because exacerbations and remissions occur. It is usually continued until the patient is euthyroid for 6 to 12 months. Diagnostic tests to evaluate thyroid function or a trial withdrawal then may be implemented to determine whether the patient is likely to remain euthyroid without further drug therapy. If a drug is to be discontinued, this is usually done gradually over weeks or months.

The therapeutic effects of radioactive iodide are delayed for several weeks or as long as 6 months. During this time, symptoms may be controlled with thioamide drugs or propranolol.

Hyperthyroidism and the Metabolism of Other Drugs

Treatment of hyperthyroidism changes the rate of body metabolism, including the rate of metabolism of many drugs. In the hyperthyroid state, drug metabolism may be very rapid, and higher doses of most drugs may be necessary to achieve therapeutic results. When the patient becomes euthyroid, the rate of drug metabolism is decreased. Consequently, doses of all medications should be evaluated and probably reduced to avoid severe adverse effects.

Use in Special Populations

Use in Children

For hypothyroidism, replacement therapy is required because thyroid hormone is essential for normal growth and development. As in adults, levothyroxine is the drug of choice in children and dosage needs may change with growth. For congenital hypothyroidism (cretinism), drug therapy should be started within 6 weeks of birth and continued for life. Initially, the recommended dose is 10 to 15 micrograms per kilogram of body weight per day. Delay in replacement therapy may result in permanent retardation despite resolution of the symptoms that resulted from thyroid deficit. Then, maintenance doses for long-term therapy vary with the child's age and weight, usually decreasing over time to a typical adult dose at 11 to 20 years of age. Infants requiring thyroid hormone replacement need relatively large doses. After thyroid drugs are started, the maintenance dosage is determined by periodic radioimmunoassay of serum thyroxine levels and by periodic radiographs to follow bone development.

To monitor drug effects on growth in children, height and weight should be recorded and compared with growth charts at regular intervals. Children should be monitored closely for adverse drug effects, which are similar to those seen in adults.

For hyperthyroidism, PTU or methimazole is used. Potential risks for adverse effects are similar to those in adults. Radioactive iodine may cause cancer and chromosome damage in children; therefore, this agent should be used only for hyperthyroidism that cannot be controlled by other antithyroid drugs or surgery.

Nursing Actions Thyroid and Antithyroid Drugs

NURSING ACTIONS	RATIONALE/EXPLANATION
1. Administer accurately	
a. With thyroid drugs:	
(1) Administer in a single daily dose, on an empty stomach (e.g., before breakfast).	Fasting increases drug absorption; early administration allows peak activity during daytime hours and is less likely to interfere with sleep.
(2) Check the pulse rate before giving the drug. If the rate is over 100 per minute or if any changes in cardiac rhythm are noted, consult the physician before giving the dose.	Tachycardia or other cardiac dysrhythmias may indicate adverse cardiac effects. Dosage may need to be reduced or the drug stopped temporarily.
(3) To give levothyroxine to an infant or young child, the tablet may be crushed and a small amount of formula or water added. After it is mixed, administer it soon, by spoon or dropper. Do *not* store the liquid very long. The crushed tablet may also be sprinkled on a small amount of food (e.g., cereal, applesauce).	Accurate and consistent administration is vital to promoting normal growth and development.
(4) Do not switch among various brands or generic forms of the drug.	Differences in bioavailability have been identified among products. Changes in preparations may alter dosage and therefore symptom control.
b. With antithyroid and iodine drugs:	
(1) Administer q8h.	All these drugs have rather short half-lives and must be given frequently and regularly to maintain therapeutic blood levels. In addition, if iodine preparations are not given every 8 hours, symptoms of hyperthyroidism may recur.
(2) Dilute iodine solutions in a full glass of fruit juice or milk, if possible, and have the patient drink the medication through a straw.	Dilution of the drug reduces gastric irritation and masks the unpleasant taste. Using a straw prevents staining the teeth.
2. Observe for therapeutic effects	
a. With thyroid drugs, observe for:	
(1) Increased energy and activity level, less lethargy and fatigue	Therapeutic effects result from a return to normal metabolic activities and relief of the symptoms of hypothyroidism. Therapeutic effects may be evident as early as 2 or 3 days after drug therapy is started or delayed up to approximately 2 weeks. All signs and symptoms of myxedema should disappear in approximately 3 to 12 weeks.
(2) Increased alertness and interest in surroundings	
(3) Increased appetite	
(4) Increased pulse rate and temperature	
(5) Decreased constipation	
(6) Reversal of coarseness and other changes in skin and hair	
(7) With cretinism, increased growth rate (record height periodically)	
(8) With myxedema, diuresis, weight loss, and decreased edema	
(9) Decreased serum cholesterol and possibly decreased creatine phosphokinase, lactate dehydrogenase, and aspartate aminotransferase levels	These serum levels are often elevated with myxedema and may return to normal when thyroid replacement therapy is begun.
b. With antithyroid and iodine drugs, observe for:	
(1) Slower pulse rate	With propylthiouracil and methimazole, some therapeutic effects are apparent in 1 or 2 weeks, but euthyroidism may not occur for 6 or 8 weeks.
(2) Slower speech	
(3) More normal activity level (slowing of hyperactivity)	With iodine solutions, therapeutic effects may be apparent within 24 hours. Maximal effects occur in approximately 10 to 15 days. However, therapeutic effects may not be sustained. Symptoms may reappear if the drug is given longer than a few weeks, and they may be more severe than initially.
(4) Decreased nervousness	
(5) Decreased tremors	
(6) Improved ability to sleep and rest	
(7) Weight gain	

NURSING ACTIONS	RATIONALE/EXPLANATION
3. Observe for adverse effects	
a. With thyroid drugs, observe for tachycardia and other cardiac dysrhythmias, angina pectoris, myocardial infarction, congestive heart failure, nervousness, hyperactivity, insomnia, diarrhea, abdominal cramps, nausea and vomiting, weight loss, fever, intolerance to heat.	Most adverse reactions stem from excessive doses, and signs and symptoms produced are the same as those occurring with hyperthyroidism. Excessive thyroid hormones make the heart work very hard and fast in attempting to meet tissue demands for oxygenated blood and nutrients. Symptoms of myocardial ischemia occur when the myocardium does not get an adequate supply of oxygenated blood. Symptoms of congestive heart failure occur when the increased cardiac workload is prolonged. Cardiovascular problems are more likely to occur in patients who are elderly or who already have heart disease.
b. With propylthiouracil and methimazole, observe for:	
(1) Hypothyroidism—bradycardia, congestive heart failure, anemia, coronary artery and peripheral vascular disease, slow speech and movements, emotional and mental dullness, excessive sleeping, weight gain, constipation, skin changes, and others	
(2) Blood disorders—leukopenia, agranulocytosis, hypoprothrombinemia	Leukopenia may be difficult to evaluate because it may occur with hyperthyroidism and with antithyroid drugs. Agranulocytosis occurs rarely but is the most severe adverse reaction; the earliest symptoms are likely to be sore throat and fever. If these occur, report them to the physician immediately.
(3) Integumentary system—skin rash, pruritus, alopecia	
(4) Central nervous system (CNS)—headache, dizziness, loss of sense of taste, drowsiness, paresthesias	
(5) Gastrointestinal system—nausea, vomiting, abdominal discomfort, gastric irritation, cholestatic hepatitis	
(6) Other—lymphadenopathy, edema, joint pain, drug fever	
c. With iodine preparations, observe for:	Adverse effects are uncommon with short-term use.
(1) Iodism—metallic taste, burning in mouth, soreness of gums, excessive salivation, gastric or respiratory irritation, rhinitis, headache, redness of conjunctiva, edema of eyelids	
(2) Hypersensitivity—acneiform skin rash, pruritus, fever, jaundice, angioedema, serum sickness	Allergic reactions rarely occur.
(3) Goiter with hypothyroidism	Uncommon but may occur in adults and newborns whose mothers have taken iodides for long periods
4. Observe for drug interactions	
a. Drugs that *increase* effects of thyroid hormones:	
(1) *Activating antidepressants* (e.g., bupropion, venlafaxine), adrenergic antiasthmatic drugs (e.g., albuterol, epinephrine), nasal decongestants	These drugs may cause CNS and cardiovascular stimulation when taken alone. When combined with thyroid hormones, excessive cardiovascular stimulation may occur and cause myocardial ischemia, cardiac dysrhythmias, hypertension, and other adverse cardiovascular effects. Excessive CNS stimulation may produce anxiety, nervousness, hyperactivity, and insomnia.
b. Drugs that *decrease* effects of thyroid hormones:	
(1) Antacids, cholestyramine, iron, sucralfate	Decrease absorption of levothyroxine; give levothyroxine 2 hours before or 4 to 6 hours after one of these drugs.
(2) Antihypertensives	Decrease cardiac-stimulating effects
(3) Estrogens, including oral contraceptives containing estrogens	Estrogens increase thyroxine-binding globulin, thereby increasing the amount of bound, inactive levothyroxine in patients with hypothyroidism. This decreased effect does not occur in patients with adequate thyroid-hormone secretion because the increased binding is offset by increased T_4 production. Women taking oral contraceptives may need larger doses of thyroid hormone replacement than would otherwise be needed.
(4) Propranolol (Inderal)	This drug decreases cardiac effects of thyroid hormones. It is used in hyperthyroidism to reduce tachycardia and other symptoms of excessive cardiovascular stimulation.
(5) Phenytoin, rifampin	Induce enzymes that metabolize (inactivate) levothyroxine more rapidly
c. Drug that *increases* effects of antithyroid drugs:	
(1) Lithium	Acts synergistically to produce hypothyroidism

Use in Older Adults

Signs and symptoms of thyroid disorders may mimic those of other disorders that often occur in older adults (e.g., congestive heart failure). Therefore, a thorough physical examination and diagnostic tests of thyroid function are necessary before starting any type of treatment.

For hypothyroidism, levothyroxine is given. Thyroid hormone replacement increases the workload of the heart and may cause serious adverse effects in older adults, especially those with cardiovascular disease. Cardiac effects also may be increased in patients receiving bronchodilators or other cardiac stimulants. Patients who are older or who have cardiovascular disease require cautious treatment because of a high risk of adverse effects on the cardiovascular system. Thus, these patients are given smaller initial dosages and smaller increments at longer intervals than younger adults. For example, the drugs should be given in small initial dosages (e.g., 25 mcg/day) and increased by 25 micrograms pre day at monthly intervals until a euthyroid state is attained and a maintenance dose established. Periodic measurements of serum TSH levels are indicated to monitor drug therapy, and doses can be adjusted when indicated.

Blood pressure and pulse should be monitored regularly. As a general rule, the drug should not be given if the resting heart rate is more than 100 beats per minute.

For hyperthyroidism, PTU or methimazole may be used, but radioactive iodine is often preferred because it is associated with fewer adverse effects than other antithyroid drugs or surgery. Patients should be monitored closely for hypothyroidism, which usually develops within a year after receiving treatment for hyperthyroidism.

Use in Patients With Renal Impairment

Some thyroid and antithyroid drugs are excreted by the kidneys, and dosage adjustment may be required in the presence of renal impairment. PTU is an example of such medication.

Most drugs given to patients with hypothyroidism have a prolonged effect, because the glomerular filtration rate of the kidneys is decreased.

Use in Patients With Hepatic Impairment

The liver plays an important role in thyroid hormone metabolism, and euthyroidism is important for normal hepatic function and bilirubin metabolism. Drugs used to treat hypothyroidism and hyperthyroidism are commonly metabolized in the liver. Therefore, in the presence of hepatic impairment, drugs may accumulate and cause adverse effects. Drug metabolism in the liver is delayed in patients with hypothyroidism, so most drugs given to these patients have a prolonged effect. Conversely, individuals who are hyperthyroid metabolize drugs more slowly than in the euthyroid state.

Use in Patients With Critical Illness

Individuals in thyroid storm or thyrotoxic crisis are commonly managed in the critical care unit. Increased rate of cellular metabolism and oxygen consumption occur with a resultant increase in heat production. The hypermetabolic state increases the metabolism of medications, so increased or more frequent dosing may be necessary.

Use in Home Care

The home care nurse may be involved in a wide range of activities, including assessing the patient's response to therapy, teaching about the disease process, managing symptoms, and preventing and managing adverse drug effects.

 Applying Your Knowledge 24-4

How Can You Avoid This Medication Error?

Ms. Zalewski complains about acid indigestion. You notice that alumina and magnesia gel (Maalox) has been ordered for her and give a dose with her morning medication.

Key Concepts

- Propylthiouracil (PTU) is the prototype of the thioamide antithyroid drugs and is used alone to treat hyperthyroidism, as part of the preoperative preparation for thyroidectomy, before or after radioactive iodine therapy, and in the treatment of thyroid storm.

- Patients should be monitored closely for hypothyroidism while taking antithyroid drugs, which may typically develop within a year after receiving treatment for hyperthyroidism.

- Levothyroxine (Synthroid, Levothroid), a synthetic preparation of T_4, is the drug of choice for long-term treatment of hypothyroidism and serves as the prototype.

- Thyroid replacement therapy in the patient with hypothyroidism is lifelong; no clear-cut guidelines exist regarding duration of antithyroid drug therapy because exacerbations and remissions Replacement therapy usually continues until the patient is euthyroid for 6 to 12 months.

- For congenital hypothyroidism (cretinism), drug therapy should be started within 6 weeks of birth and continued for life or mental retardation may result.

▪ Individuals with hypothyroidism are especially likely to experience respiratory depression and myxede a coma with opioid analgesics and other sedating drugs.

▪ The FDA has issued a **BLACK BOX WARNING** regarding the use of thyroid hormones for the treatment of obesity or for weight loss, either alone or with other therapeutic agents. Significant and serious complications may develop in euthyroid individuals taking thyroid hormones.

Review and Application Exercises

Short Answer Exercises

1. Where is TSH produced, and what is its function?

2. What is the role of thyroid hormones in maintaining body functions?

3. What signs and symptoms are associated with hypothyroidism?

4. In primary hypothyroidism, are blood levels of TSH increased or decreased?

5. What are adverse effects of drug therapy for hypothyroidism?

6. What signs and symptoms are associated with hyperthyroidism?

7. Which drugs reduce blood levels of thyroid hormone in hyperthyroidism, and how do they act?

8. What are adverse effects of drug therapy for hyperthyroidism?

9. When propranolol is used in the treatment of hyperthyroidism, what are its expected effects?

10. What is the effect of thyroid disorders on metabolism of other drugs?

NCLEX-Style Questions

11. A male patient asks a nurse when he should take his daily dose of levothyroxine. The nurse recommends that the patient take the drug
    a. before breakfast on an empty stomach
    b. with meals in divided doses
    c. at bedtime with a snack
    d. whenever it is convenient

12. Which of the following agents is the drug of first choice for treatment of hypothyroidism?
    a. propranolol (Inderal)
    b. levothyroxine (Synthroid, Levothroid)
    c. methimazole
    d. propylthiouracil (PTU)

13. Which of the following patients with Graves' disease would be the most appropriate candidate for sodium iodide ^{131}I therapy?
    a. an 8-year-old boy
    b. a 28-year-old breast-feeding mother
    c. a 35-year-old pregnant woman
    d. a 40-year-old man

14. The nurse who is taking care of a patient with hyperthyroidism and receives an order to administer propranolol knows that it is ordered to relieve which of the following symptoms?
    a. heat intolerance
    b. exophthalmos
    c. dry skin
    d. tachycardia

15. Which of the following orders should a nurse question in a patient with hypothyroidism?
    a. psyllium seed (Metamucil)
    b. levothyroxine (Synthroid)
    c. morphine sulfate
    d. albuterol (Ventolin inhaler)

Selected References

Abraham, P., Avenell, A., Watson, W. A., Park, C. M., & Bevan, J. S. (2005). Antithyroid drug regimen for treating Graves' hyperthyroidism. *Cochrane Database of Systematic Reviews*, Issue 2. ART No. CD003420.

Bach-Huynh, T., & Jonklaas, J. (2006). Thyroid medications during pregnancy. *Therapeutic Drug Monitoring, 28*, 431–441.

Corwin, E. J. (2006). *Handbook of pathophysiology* (3rd ed.). Philadelphia: Lippincott Williams & Wilkins.

Drug facts and comparisons. (Updated monthly). St. Louis, MO: Facts and Comparisons.

Guyton, A. C., & Hall, J. E. (2006). *Textbook of medical physiology* (11th ed.). Philadelphia: W. B. Saunders.

Lacy, C. F., Armstrong, L. L., Goldman, M. P., & Lance, L. L. (2007). *Lexi-Comp's drug information handbook* (15th ed.). Hudson, OH: American Pharmaceutical Association.

Matfin, G., Kuenzi, J. A., & Guven, S. (2005). Disorders of endocrine control of growth and metabolism. In C. M. Porth (Ed.), *Pathophysiology: Concepts of altered health states* (7th ed., pp. 961–985). Philadelphia: Lippincott Williams & Wilkins.

Nayak, B., & Hodak, S. P. (2007). Hyperthyroidism. *Endocrinology and Metabolism Clinics of North America, 36,* 617–656.

Walsh, J. P., Ward, L. C., Burke, V., Bhagat, C. I., Shiels, L., Henley, D., Gillett, M. J., Gilbert, R., Tanner, M., & Stuckey, B. G. (2006). Small changes in thyroxine dosage do not produce measurable changes in hypothyroid symptoms, well-being, or quality of life: Results of a double-blind, randomized clinical trial. *Journal of Clinical Endocrinology & Metabolism, 91,* 2624–2630.

Hormones That Regulate Calcium and Bone Metabolism

LEARNING OBJECTIVES

After studying this chapter, you will be able to:

1. Examine the roles of parathyroid hormone, calcitonin, and vitamin D in regulating calcium metabolism.
2. Manage individuals at risk for hypocalcemia.
3. Discuss prevention and treatment of hypocalcemia and osteoporosis.
4. Manage individuals at risk for hypercalcemia.
5. Outline appropriate management strategies of hypercalcemia as a medical emergency.
6. Evaluate the use of calcium and vitamin D supplements, calcitonin, and bisphosphonate drugs in the treatment of osteoporosis.

Applying Your Knowledge

Carolyn Taylor is a 68-year-old retired teacher. She has chronic venous insufficiency and osteoporosis. Ms. Taylor has suffered two fractures from falls in recent years. She has been menopausal for 16 years and has not been on estrogen replacement therapy due to her vascular disease. Her physician prescribes alendronate in the once-weekly dose.

Introduction

Three hormones regulate calcium and bone metabolism, *parathyroid hormone (PTH)*, calcitonin, and vitamin D, which act to maintain normal serum levels of calcium. When serum calcium levels are decreased, hormonal mechanisms are activated to raise them; when they are elevated, mechanisms act to lower them (Fig. 25-1). Overall, the hormones alter absorption of dietary calcium from the gastrointestinal tract, movement of calcium from bone to serum, and excretion of calcium through the kidneys.

Disorders of calcium and bone metabolism include hypocalcemia, hypercalcemia, osteoporosis, Paget's disease, and bone breakdown associated with breast cancer and multiple myeloma. Drugs used to treat these disorders mainly alter serum calcium levels or strengthen bone. This chapter describes the characteristics of the hormones, calcium, phosphorus, and some associated disorders.

Hormones Involved in Calcium Metabolism

Parathyroid Hormone

PTH secretion is stimulated by low serum calcium levels and inhibited by normal or high levels (a negative feedback system). Because phosphate is closely related to calcium in body functions, PTH also regulates phosphate metabolism. In general, when serum calcium levels increase, serum

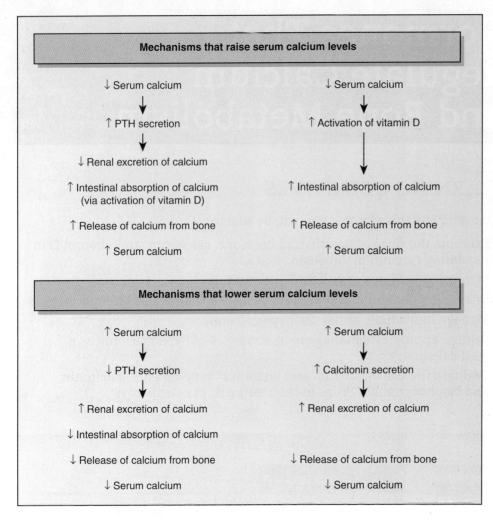

Mechanisms that raise serum calcium levels

↓ Serum calcium

↑ PTH secretion

↓ Renal excretion of calcium

↑ Intestinal absorption of calcium (via activation of vitamin D)

↑ Release of calcium from bone

↑ Serum calcium

↓ Serum calcium

↑ Activation of vitamin D

↑ Intestinal absorption of calcium

↑ Release of calcium from bone

↑ Serum calcium

Mechanisms that lower serum calcium levels

↑ Serum calcium

↓ PTH secretion

↑ Renal excretion of calcium

↓ Intestinal absorption of calcium

↓ Release of calcium from bone

↓ Serum calcium

↑ Serum calcium

↑ Calcitonin secretion

↑ Renal excretion of calcium

↓ Release of calcium from bone

↓ Serum calcium

Figure 25-1 ■ Hormonal regulation of serum calcium levels. When serum calcium levels are low (hypocalcemia), there is increased secretion of parathyroid hormone (PTH) and increased activation of vitamin D. These mechanisms lead to decreased loss of calcium in the urine, increased absorption of calcium from the intestine, and increased resorption of calcium from the bone. These mechanisms work together to raise serum calcium levels to normal.

When serum calcium levels are high (hypercalcemia), there is decreased secretion of PTH and increased secretion of calcitonin. These mechanisms lead to increased loss of calcium from the intestine and decreased resorption of calcium from bone. These mechanisms lower serum calcium levels to normal.

phosphate levels decrease, and vice versa. Thus, an inverse relationship exists between calcium and phosphate.

When the serum calcium level falls below the normal range, PTH raises the level by acting on bone, intestines, and kidneys. In bone, breakdown is increased, so that calcium moves from bone into the serum. In the intestines, there is increased absorption of calcium ingested in food (PTH activates vitamin D, which increases intestinal absorption). In the kidneys, there is increased reabsorption of calcium in the renal tubules and less urinary excretion. The opposite effects occur with phosphate (e.g., PTH decreases serum phosphate and increases urinary phosphate excretion).

Disorders of parathyroid function are related to insufficient production of PTH (hypoparathyroidism) or excessive production of PTH (hyperparathyroidism). *Hypoparathyroidism* is most often caused by removal of or damage to the parathyroid glands during neck surgery. *Hyperparathyroidism* is most often caused by a tumor or hyperplasia of a parathyroid gland. It also may result from ectopic secretion of PTH by malignant tumors (e.g., carcinomas of the lung, pancreas, kidney, ovary, prostate gland, or bladder). Clinical manifestations and treatment of hypoparathyroidism are the same as those of hypocalcemia. Clinical manifestations and treatment of hyperparathyroidism are the same as those of hypercalcemia.

Calcitonin

Calcitonin is a hormone from the thyroid gland whose secretion is controlled by the concentration of ionized calcium in the blood flowing through the thyroid gland. When the serum level of ionized calcium is increased, secretion of calcitonin is increased. The function of calcitonin is to lower serum calcium in the presence of hypercalcemia, which it does by decreasing movement of calcium from bone to serum and increasing urinary excretion of calcium. The action of calcitonin is rapid but of short duration. Thus, this hormone has little effect on long-term calcium metabolism.

Vitamin D (Calciferol)

Vitamin D (Calciferol) is a fat-soluble vitamin that includes both ergocalciferol (obtained from foods) and cholecalciferol (formed by exposure of skin to sunlight). It functions as a hormone and plays an important role in calcium and bone metabolism. The main action of vitamin D is to raise serum calcium levels by increasing intestinal absorption of calcium and mobilizing calcium from bone. It also promotes bone formation by providing adequate serum concentrations of minerals. Vitamin D is not physiologically active in the body. It must be converted to an intermediate metabolite in the liver, then to an active metabolite (1,25-dihydroxyvitamin D or calcitriol) in the kidneys. PTH and adequate hepatic and renal function are required to produce the active metabolite.

Deficiency of vitamin D causes inadequate absorption of calcium and phosphorus. This, in turn, leads to low levels of serum calcium and stimulation of PTH secretion. In children, this sequence of events produces inadequate mineralization of bone (rickets), a rare condition in the United States. In adults, vitamin D deficiency causes osteomalacia, a condition characterized by decreased bone density and strength.

Calcium and Phosphorus

Calcium and phosphorus are discussed together because they are closely related physiologically. These mineral nutrients are found in many of the same foods, from which they are absorbed together. They are regulated by PTH and excreted through the kidneys. They are both required in cellular structure and function and, as calcium phosphate, in formation and maintenance of bones and teeth. Their characteristics and functions are summarized in Box 25-1.

Box 25-1	Characteristics and Functions of Calcium and Phosphorus

Calcium

Calcium is the most abundant cation in the body. Approximately 99% is located in the bones and teeth; the rest is in the extracellular fluid and soft tissues. Approximately half of serum calcium is bound, mostly to serum proteins, and is physiologically inactive. The other half is ionized and physiologically active. Ionized calcium can leave the vascular compartment and enter cells, where it participates in intracellular functions. An adequate amount of free (ionized) calcium is required for normal function of all body cells.

Calcium is obtained from the diet, but only 30% to 50% is absorbed from the small intestine; the rest is lost in feces. Absorption is increased in the presence of vitamin D, lactose, moderate amounts of fat, and high protein intake; increased acidity of gastric secretions; and a physiologic need. Absorption is inhibited by vitamin D deficiency; a high-fat diet; the presence of oxalic acid (from beet greens, chard), which combines with calcium to form insoluble calcium oxalate in the intestine; alkalinity of intestinal secretions, which leads to formation of insoluble calcium phosphate; diarrhea or other conditions of rapid intestinal motility, which do not allow sufficient time for absorption; and immobilization.

Calcium is lost from the body in feces, urine, and sweat. Even when there is deficient intake, approximately 150 mg are lost daily through the intestines (in mucosal and biliary secretions and sloughed intestinal cells). In lactating women, relatively large amounts are lost in breast milk.

Functions

▪ Calcium participates in many metabolic processes, including the regulation of:
  ▪ Cell membrane permeability and function
  ▪ Nerve-cell excitability and transmission of impulses (e.g., it is required for release of neurotransmitters at synapses)
  ▪ Contraction of cardiac, skeletal, and smooth muscle
  ▪ Conduction of electrical impulses in the heart
  ▪ Blood coagulation and platelet adhesion processes
  ▪ Hormone secretion
  ▪ Enzyme activity
  ▪ Catecholamine release from the adrenal medulla
  ▪ Release of chemical mediators (e.g., histamine from mast cells)

▪ Calcium is required for building and maintaining bones and teeth. Bone calcium is composed mainly of calcium phosphate and calcium carbonate. In addition to these bound forms, a small amount of calcium is available for exchange with serum. This acts as a reserve supply of calcium. Calcium is constantly shifting between bone and serum as bone is formed and broken down. When serum calcium levels become low, calcium moves into serum.

Requirements and Sources

The calcium requirement of normal adults is approximately 1000 mg daily. Increased daily amounts are needed by growing children (1200 mg), pregnant or lactating women (1200 mg), and postmenopausal women who do not take replacement estrogens (1500 mg to prevent osteoporosis).

The best sources of calcium are milk and milk products. Three 8-oz glasses of milk daily contain approximately the amount needed by healthy adults. Calcium in milk is readily used by the body because milk also contains lactose and vitamin D, both of which are involved in calcium absorption. Other sources of calcium include vegetables (e.g., broccoli, spinach, kale, mustard greens) and seafood (e.g., clams, oysters).

Phosphorus

Phosphorus is one of the most important elements in normal body function. Most phosphorus is combined with calcium in bones and teeth as calcium phosphate (approximately 80%). The remainder is distributed in every body cell and in extracellular fluid. It is combined with carbohydrates, lipids, proteins, and various other compounds.

Phosphorus is obtained from the diet, and approximately 70% of dietary phosphorus is absorbed from the gastrointestinal (GI) tract. The most efficient absorption occurs when calcium and phosphorus are ingested in approximately equal amounts. Because this equal ratio is present in milk, milk is probably the best source of phosphorus. In general, factors that increase or decrease calcium absorption act the same way on phosphorus absorption. Vitamin D enhances, but is not essential for, phosphorus absorption. Large amounts of calcium or aluminum in the GI tract may combine with phosphate to form insoluble compounds and thereby decrease absorption of phosphorus.

(continued on page 396)

| Box 25-1 | Characteristics and Functions of Calcium and Phosphorus (continued) |

Phosphorus is lost from the body primarily in urine. In people with acute or chronic renal failure, phosphorus intake is restricted because excretion is impaired.

Functions

Phosphorus, most of which is located intracellularly as the phosphate ion, performs many metabolic functions:

- It is an essential component of deoxyribonucleic acid, ribonucleic acid, and other nucleic acids in body cells. Thus, it is required for cell reproduction and body growth.
- It combines with fatty acids to form phospholipids, which are components of all cell membranes in the body. This reaction also prevents buildup of excessive amounts of free fatty acids.
- It forms a phosphate buffer system, which helps to maintain acid–base balance. When excess hydrogen ions are present in kidney tubules, phosphate combines with them and allows their excretion in urine. At the same time,

bicarbonate is retained by the kidneys and contributes to alkalinity of body fluids. Although there are other buffering systems in the body, failure of the phosphate system leads to metabolic acidosis (retained hydrogen ions or acid and lost bicarbonate ions or base).

- It is necessary for cellular use of glucose and production of energy.
- It is necessary for proper function of several B vitamins (i.e., the vitamins function as coenzymes in various chemical reactions only when combined with phosphate).

Requirements and Sources

Daily requirements for phosphorus are approximately 800 mg for normal adults and 1200 mg for growing children and pregnant or lactating women. Phosphorus is widely available in foods. Good sources are milk and other dairy products, meat, poultry, fish, eggs, and nuts. There is little risk of phosphorus deficiency with an adequate intake of calcium and protein.

Calcium Disorders and Bone Metabolism

The calcium disorders are *hypocalcemia* and *hypercalcemia*, either of which can be life threatening. The bone disorders discussed in this chapter are those characterized by increased resorption of calcium and loss of bone mass. These disorders weaken bone and lead to fractures, pain, and disability. Selected calcium and bone disorders are described in Box 25-2.

| Box 25-2 | Calcium and Bone Disorders |

Hypocalcemia

Hypocalcemia is an abnormally low blood calcium level (i.e., <8.5 mg/dL). It may be caused by inadequate intake of calcium and vitamin D, numerous disorders (e.g., diarrhea or malabsorption syndromes that cause inadequate absorption of calcium and vitamin D, hypoparathyroidism, renal failure, severe hypomagnesemia, hypermagnesemia, acute pancreatitis, rhabdomyolysis, tumor lysis syndrome, vitamin D deficiency), and several drugs (e.g., cisplatin, cytosine arabinoside, foscarnet, ketoconazole, pentamidine, agents used to treat hypercalcemia). Calcium deficits caused by inadequate dietary intake affect bone tissue rather than serum calcium levels. Hypocalcemia associated with renal failure is caused by two mechanisms. First, inability to excrete phosphate in urine leads to accumulation of phosphate in the blood (hyperphosphatemia). Because phosphate levels are inversely related to calcium levels, hyperphosphatemia induces hypocalcemia. Second, when kidney function is impaired, vitamin D conversion to its active metabolite is impaired. This results in decreased intestinal absorption of calcium.

Clinical manifestations are characterized by increased neuromuscular irritability, which may progress to tetany. Tetany is characterized by numbness and tingling of the lips, fingers, and toes; twitching of facial muscles; spasms of skeletal muscle;

carpopedal spasm; laryngospasm; and convulsions. In young children, hypocalcemia may be manifested by convulsions rather than tetany and erroneously diagnosed as epilepsy. This may be a serious error because anticonvulsant drugs used for epilepsy may further decrease serum calcium levels. Severe hypocalcemia may cause lethargy or confusion.

Hypercalcemia

Hypercalcemia is an abnormally high blood calcium level (i.e., >10.5 mg/dL). It may be caused by hyperparathyroidism, hyperthyroidism, malignant neoplasms, vitamin D or vitamin A intoxication, aluminum intoxication, prolonged immobilization, adrenocortical insufficiency, and ingestion of thiazide diuretics, estrogens, and lithium. Cancer is a common cause, especially carcinomas (of the breast, lung, head and neck, or kidney) and multiple myeloma. Cancer stimulates bone breakdown, which increases serum calcium levels. Increased urine output leads to fluid volume deficit. This leads, in turn, to increased reabsorption of calcium in renal tubules and decreased renal excretion of calcium. Decreased renal excretion potentiates hypercalcemia. Patients at risk for hypercalcemia should be monitored for early signs and symptoms so treatment can be started before severe hypercalcemia develops.

Clinical manifestations are caused by the decreased ability of nerves to respond to stimuli and the decreased ability of muscles to contract and relax. Hypercalcemia has a depressant effect on nerve and muscle function. Gastrointestinal problems with hypercalcemia include anorexia, nausea, vomiting, constipation, and abdominal pain. Central nervous system problems include apathy, depression, poor memory, headache, and drowsiness. Severe hypercalcemia may produce lethargy, syncope, disorientation, hallucinations, coma, and death. Other signs and symptoms include weakness and decreased tone in skeletal and smooth muscle, dysphagia, polyuria, polyphagia, and cardiac dysrhythmias. In addition, calcium may be deposited in various tissues, such as the conjunctiva, cornea, and kidneys. Calcium deposits in the kidneys (renal calculi) may lead to irreversible damage and impairment of function.

Osteoporosis

Osteoporosis is characterized by decreased bone density (osteopenia) and weak, fragile bones that often lead to fractures, pain, and disability. Although any bones may be affected, common fracture sites are the vertebrae of the lower dorsal and lumbar spines, wrists, and hips. Risk factors include female sex, advanced age, small stature, lean body mass, white or Asian race, positive family history, low calcium intake, menopause, sedentary lifestyle, nulliparity, smoking, excessive ingestion of alcohol or caffeine, high protein intake, high phosphate intake, hyperthyroidism, and chronic use of certain medications (e.g., corticosteroids, phenytoin). Postmenopausal women who do not take estrogen replacement therapy are at high risk because of estrogen deficiency, age-related bone loss, and a low peak bone mass. Osteoporosis occurs in men but less often than in women. Both men and women who take high doses of corticosteroids are at high risk because the drugs demineralize bone. In addition, renal transplant recipients can acquire osteoporosis from corticosteroid therapy, decreased renal function, increased parathyroid hormone secretion, and cyclosporine immunosuppressant therapy.

Osteopenia or early osteoporosis may be present and undetected unless radiography or a bone density measurement is done. If detected, treatment is needed to slow bone loss. If undetected or untreated, clinical manifestations of osteoporosis include shortened stature (a measurable loss of height), back pain, spinal deformity, or a fracture. Fractures often occur with common bending or lifting movements or falling.

Paget's Disease

Paget's disease is an inflammatory skeletal disease that affects older people. Its etiology is unknown. It is characterized by a high rate of bone turnover and results in bone deformity and pain. It is treated with non-narcotic analgesics and drugs that decrease bone resorption (e.g., bisphosphonates, calcitonin).

Bone is mineralized connective tissue that functions as structural support and a reservoir for calcium, phosphorus, magnesium, sodium, and carbonate. The role of bone in maintaining serum calcium levels takes precedence over its structural function (i.e., bone may be weakened or destroyed as calcium leaves bone and enters serum). Bone tissue is constantly being formed and broken down in a process called remodeling. During childhood, adolescence, and early adulthood, formation usually exceeds breakdown (resorption) as the person attains adult height and peak bone mass. After approximately 35 years of age, resorption is greater than formation. *Osteoporosis* results when bone strength (bone density and bone quality) is impaired, leading to increased porousness and vulnerability to fracture. Hormonal deficiencies, some diseases, and some medications (e.g., glucocorticoids) can also increase resorption, resulting in loss of bone mass and osteoporosis.

Individual Drugs

Calcium and Vitamin D Preparations

Calcium and vitamin D supplements are used to treat hypocalcemia and to prevent and treat osteoporosis. These drugs are described in the following sections, and names and dosages of individual drug preparations are listed in Table 25-1.

Calcium Preparations

An intravenous (IV) calcium salt (usually **calcium gluconate**) is given for acute, symptomatic hypocalcemia. An oral preparation (e.g., **calcium carbonate** or **citrate**) is given for asymptomatic, less severe, or chronic hypocalcemia. These preparations differ mainly in the amounts of calcium they contain and the routes by which they are given.

Even when serum calcium levels are normal, people who do not get enough calcium in their diets may need calcium supplements. Most diets in people of all ages, especially in young women and older adults, are thought to be deficient in calcium. Calcium supplements are also used in the prevention and treatment of osteoporosis.

Vitamin D Preparations

Vitamin D is used in chronic hypocalcemia if calcium supplements alone cannot maintain serum calcium levels within a normal range. It is also used to prevent deficiency states and treat hypoparathyroidism and osteoporosis. Although authorities agree that dietary intake is better than supplements, some suggest a vitamin D supplement for people who ingest less than the recommended amount. Supplementation recommendations include 400 international units daily for those 6 months to 24 years of age, 200 international units for those 25 to 50 years of age, 400 international units daily for those 51 to 70 years of age, and 600 international units for those 70 years of age and older. Supplementation of 800 international units daily is recommended for individuals at risk for vitamin D deficiency due to lack of sunlight exposure. If used, vitamin D supplements should be taken cautiously and not overused; excessive amounts can cause serious problems, including hypercalcemia.

Table 25-1	Drugs at a Glance: Calcium and Vitamin D Preparations

	ROUTES AND DOSAGE RANGES	
Generic/Trade Name	Adults	Children
Oral Calcium Products		
Calcium acetate (25% calcium) (PhosLo)	PO 2–4 tablets with each meal	Dosage not established
Calcium carbonate precipitated (40% calcium) (Os-Cal, Tums)	PO 1–1.5 g 3 times daily with meals (maximal dose, 8 g daily)	
Calcium citrate (21% calcium) (Citracal)	PO 1–2 tablets (200 mg calcium per tablet) 2–4 times daily	
Calcium gluconate (9% calcium)	PO 1–2 g 3 or 4 times daily	PO 500 mg/kg/d in divided doses
Parenteral Calcium Products		
Calcium chloride (10 mL of 10% solution contains 273 mg [13.6 mEq] of calcium)	IV 500 mg–1 g (5–10 mL of 10% solution) every 1–3 d, depending on clinical response or serum calcium measurements	2.7–5 mg/kg/dose every 4–6 h depending on clinical response or serum calcium measurements
Calcium gluconate (10 mL of 10% solution contains 93 mg [4.65 mEq] of calcium)	IV 5–20 mL of 10% solution	IV 500 mg/kg/d in divided doses
Vitamin D Preparations		
Calcitriol (Rocaltrol, Calcijex)	Dialysis patients, hypoparathyroidism, PO 0.25 mcg daily initially, then adjusted according to serum calcium levels (usual daily maintenance dose, 0.5–1 mcg)	Hypoparathyroidism, ≥6 y: PO 0.5–2 mcg daily 1–5 y: PO 0.25–0.75 mcg daily
Cholecalciferol (Delta-D)	PO 400–1000 IU daily	
Ergocalciferol (Calciferol, Drisdol)	Hypoparathyroidism, PO 50,000–200,000 units daily initially (average daily maintenance dose, 25,000–100,000 units)	
Paricalcitol (Zemplar)	Dialysis patients, 0.04–0.1 mcg/kg every other d initially; increased by 2–4 mcg at 2- to 4-week intervals, if necessary. Reduce dosage or stop therapy if hypercalcemia occurs.	

Drugs Used in Hypercalcemia and Selected Bone Disorders

Drugs used for hypercalcemia include bisphosphonates, calcitonin, corticosteroids, 0.9% sodium chloride IV infusion, and others. Drugs used for osteoporosis inhibit bone breakdown and demineralization and include *bisphosphonates*, calcitonin, estrogens, and antiestrogens. These drugs are described in the following sections, and most indications for use and dosages are listed in Table 25-2.

Bisphosphonates

Alendronate (Fosamax), **ibandronate** (Boniva), **pamidronate** (Aredia), **risedronate** (Actonel), and **zoledronate** (Zometa) are drugs that bind to bone and inhibit calcium resorption from bone. **Alendronate** (Fosamax PLUS D) is compounded to pro-

vide 2800 international units of vitamin D in a once-weekly dose. Although indications for use vary among the drugs, they are used mainly in the treatment of hypercalcemia and osteoporosis.

Bisphosphonates are poorly absorbed from the intestinal tract and must be taken on an empty stomach, with water at least 30 minutes before any other fluid, food, or medication. The drugs are not metabolized. The drug bound to bone is slowly released into the bloodstream. Most of the drug that is not bound to bone is excreted in the urine.

Calcitonin-salmon (Calcimar, Miacalcin) is used in the treatment of hypercalcemia, Paget's disease, and osteoporosis. In hypercalcemia, calcitonin lowers serum calcium levels by inhibiting bone resorption. Calcitonin is most likely to be effective in hypercalcemia caused by hyperparathyroidism,

Table 25-2	**Drugs at a Glance:** Drugs Used in Hypercalcemia and Selected Bone Disorders	

GENERIC/TRADE NAME	INDICATIONS FOR USE	ROUTES AND DOSAGE RANGES
Bisphosphonates		
Alendronate (Fosamax)	Osteoporosis: Prevention and treatment in postmenopausal women	Osteoporosis: *Postmenopausal women*: Prevention, PO 5 mg once daily or 35 mg once weekly; treatment, PO 10 mg once daily or 70 mg once weekly.
	Treatment in men and women with glucocorticoid-induced osteoporosis	*Men*: 10 mg once daily
		Glucocorticoid-induced, 5 mg once daily
	Paget's disease	Paget's disease, PO 40 mg daily for 6 mo; repeated if necessary
Ibandronate (Boniva)	Treatment and prevention of osteoporosis in postmenopausal women	PO 2.5 mg once daily or 150 mg every month
Pamidronate (Aredia)	Hypercalcemia of malignancy	Hypercalcemia, if IV 60 mg give over 4 h; if 90 mg give over 24 h
	Osteolytic lesions of breast cancer metastases or multiple myeloma	Osteolytic bone lesions; Breast cancer, IV 90 mg over 2 h every 3–4 wk; multiple myeloma, IV 90 mg over 4 h once monthly
	Paget's disease	Paget's disease, IV 30 mg over 4 h, daily for 3 doses
Risedronate (Actonel)	Osteoporosis, postmenopausal and glucocorticoid-induced, prevention and treatment	Prevention and treatment of osteoporosis, PO 5 mg once daily or 35 mg once weekly
	Paget's disease	Paget's disease, PO 30 mg once daily for 2 mo
Zoledronate (Zometa)	Hypercalcemia of malignancy	IV 4 mg over 15 min or longer
Selective Estrogen Receptor Modulator		
Raloxifene (Evista)	Osteoporosis: Prevention and treatment in postmenopausal women	PO 60 mg once daily
Calcitonin		
Calcitonin-salmon (Calcimar, Miacalcin)	Hypercalcemia	Hypercalcemia, Sub-Q, IM 4 IU/kg q12h; can be increased after 1 or 2 d to 8 IU/kg q12h; maximum dose, 8 IU/kg q6h
	Paget's disease	Paget's disease, Sub-Q, IM 50–100 IU/d
	Postmenopausal osteoporosis	Postmenopausal osteoporosis, Sub-Q, IM 100 IU/d; nasal spray (Miacalcin) 200 IU/d
Parathyroid Hormone		
Teriparatide (Forteo)	Osteoporosis	Sub-Q 20 mcg daily
Miscellaneous Agents		
Furosemide (Lasix)	Hypercalcemia	*Adults*: IV 80–100 mg q2h until a diuretic response is obtained or other treatment measures are initiated
		Children: IV 20–40 mg q4h until a diuretic response is obtained or other treatment measures are initiated
Phosphate salts (Neutra-Phos)	Hypercalcemia	PO 1–2 tablets 3 or 4 times daily, or contents of 1 capsule mixed with 75 mL of water 4 times daily
Prednisone or hydrocortisone	Hypercalcemia	Prednisone PO 20–50 mg twice daily (or equivalent dose of another glucocorticoid) for 5–10 d, then tapered to the minimum dose required to prevent hypercalcemia
		Hydrocortisone IM, IV 100–500 mg/d
		4–6 L/d
0.9% Sodium chloride injection	Acute hypercalcemia	

prolonged immobilization, or certain malignant neoplasms. In acute hypercalcemia, calcitonin may be used along with other measures to lower serum calcium levels rapidly. A single injection of calcitonin decreases serum calcium levels in approximately 2 hours, and its effects last approximately 6 to 8 hours.

In *Paget's disease*, calcitonin slows the rate of bone turnover, improves bone lesions on radiologic examination, and relieves bone pain. In osteoporosis, calcitonin prevents further bone loss in the presence of adequate calcium and vitamin D. In addition, calcitonin helps control pain in patients with osteoporosis or metastatic bone disease. Both subcutaneous injections and intranasal administration relieve pain within 1 to 12 weeks. The drug is given daily initially, then two to three times a week. The mechanism by which pain is reduced is unknown.

Estrogens and Antiestrogens

Estrogens are discussed here in relation to osteoporosis; see Chapter 27 for other uses and dosages. Estrogen replacement therapy (ERT) is beneficial for preventing postmenopausal osteoporosis. ERT is most beneficial immediately after menopause, when a period of accelerated bone loss occurs. Mechanisms by which ERT protects against bone loss and fractures are thought to include decreased bone breakdown, increased calcium absorption from the intestine, and increased calcitriol (active form of vitamin D that promotes absorption and use of calcium in bone building) concentration. Progestins have been used with estrogens in women with an intact uterus because of the increased risk of endometrial cancer with estrogen therapy alone. However, estrogen and estrogen–progestin combinations are no longer recommended because adverse effects are thought to outweigh benefits.

In postmenopausal osteoporosis, other drugs may be used instead of estrogen. Raloxifene (Evista) and tamoxifen (Nolvadex) act like estrogen in some body tissues and prevent the action of estrogen in other body tissues. Raloxifene is classified as a selective estrogen receptor modulator and is approved for prevention of postmenopausal osteoporosis. It has estrogenic effects in bone tissue, thereby decreasing bone breakdown and increasing bone mass density. It has antiestrogen effects in uterine and breast tissue. Tamoxifen, which is classified as an antiestrogen, is used to prevent and treat breast cancer. It also has estrogenic effects and can be used to prevent osteoporosis and cardiovascular disease, although it is not approved for these uses. Tamoxifen may help prevent osteoporosis in patients with breast cancer.

Parathyroid Hormone

Teriparatide (Forteo) is a recombinant DNA version of PTH. It is approved for the treatment of osteoporosis in women. Other drugs for osteoporosis slow bone loss, whereas teriparatide increases bone formation by increasing the number of bone-building cells (osteoblasts). Teriparatide also increases serum levels of calcium and calcitriol. In clinical trials, the drug increased vertebral bone mineral density and decreased vertebral fractures. It is recommended for use in patients with severe osteoporosis or those who have not responded adequately to other treatments, partly because osteosarcoma developed in some animals given high doses for long periods. No osteosarcoma developed in humans during clinical trials, but the longest of these trials was 2 years.

Teriparatide is rapidly and well absorbed after subcutaneous injection. Bioavailability is 95%, and peak serum levels occur in 30 minutes. The drug is metabolized and excreted through the liver, kidneys, and bone. It is not expected to accumulate in bone or other tissues, to interact significantly with other drugs, or to require dosage adjustment with renal or hepatic impairment. Adverse effects include nausea, headache, back pain, dizziness, syncope, and leg cramps.

Corticosteroids

Glucocorticoids (see Chap. 23) are used in the treatment of hypercalcemia due to malignancies or vitamin D intoxication. These drugs lower serum calcium levels by inhibiting cytokine release, by direct cytolytic effects on some tumor cells, by inhibiting calcium absorption from the intestine, and by increasing calcium excretion in the urine. Hydrocortisone or prednisone is often used. The serum calcium level decreases in approximately 5 to 10 days, and after it stabilizes, the dosage should be gradually reduced to the minimum needed to control symptoms of hypercalcemia. High dosage or prolonged administration leads to serious adverse effects.

Other Drugs for Hypercalcemia

Furosemide (Lasix) is a loop diuretic (see Chap. 53) that increases calcium excretion in urine by preventing its reabsorption in renal tubules. It can be given via IV route for rapid effects in acute hypercalcemia, but authorities do not agree about its use. Some recommend furosemide after extracellular fluid volume has been restored and saline diuresis occurs with IV infusion of several liters of 0.9% sodium chloride. Others recommend furosemide only if evidence of fluid overload is found or if heart failure occurs. Thiazide diuretics are contraindicated in patients with hypercalcemia because they decrease urinary excretion of calcium.

Phosphate salts (Neutra-Phos) inhibit intestinal absorption of calcium and increase deposition of calcium in bone. (Neutra-Phos is an oral combination of sodium phosphate and potassium phosphate.) Oral salts are effective in the treatment of hypercalcemia due to any cause. A potential adverse effect of phosphates is calcification of soft tissues due to deposition of calcium phosphate, which can lead to severe impairment of function in the kidneys and other organs. Phosphates should be given only when hypercalcemia is accompanied by hypophosphatemia (serum phosphorus < 3 mg/dL) and renal function is normal to minimize the risk of soft tissue calcification. Serum calcium, phosphorus, and creatinine levels should be monitored frequently, and the dose should be reduced if serum phosphorus exceeds 4.5 milligrams per deciliter or the product of serum calcium and phosphorus exceeds 60 milligrams per deciliter.

Sodium chloride (0.9%) injection (normal saline) is an IV solution that contains water, sodium, and chloride. It is included here because it is the treatment of choice for hypercalcemia and is usually effective. The sodium contained in the solution inhibits the reabsorption of calcium in renal tubules and thereby increases urinary excretion of calcium. The solution relieves the dehydration caused by vomiting and polyuria, and it dilutes the calcium concentration of serum and urine. Several liters are given daily. Patients should be monitored closely for signs of fluid overload, and serum calcium, magnesium, and potassium levels should be measured every 6 to 12 hours. Large amounts of magnesium and potassium are lost in the urine, and adequate replacement is essential.

Applying Your Knowledge 25-1

You are giving instructions to Ms. Taylor on the proper administration method for taking her alendronate. In addition to instructing Ms. Taylor to take this medication with water, what important instruction must you include for this patient?

Applying Your Knowledge 25-2

Patients like Ms. Taylor, who has osteoporosis, should take preventive measures in addition to taking their prescribed medication. One important measure is to increase the intake of foods that contain high levels of calcium. What dietary recommendations would you make to Ms. Taylor?

Nursing Process

Assessment

- Assess for risk factors and manifestations of hypocalcemia and calcium deficiency:
  - Assess dietary intake of dairy products, other calcium-containing foods, and vitamin D.
  - Check serum calcium reports for abnormal values. The normal total serum calcium level is approximately 8.5 to 10.5 mg/dL (SI units 2.2–2.6 mmol/L). Approximately half of the total serum calcium (e.g., 4–5 mg/dL) should be free ionized calcium, the physiologically active form. To interpret serum calcium levels accurately, serum albumin levels and acid–base status must be considered. Low serum albumin decreases the total serum level of calcium by decreasing the amount of calcium that is bound to protein; however, the ionized concentration is unaffected by serum albumin levels. Metabolic and respiratory alkalosis increase binding of calcium to serum proteins, thereby maintaining normal total serum calcium but decreasing the ionized values. Conversely, metabolic and respiratory acidosis decrease binding and therefore increase the concentration of ionized calcium.

- Check for *Chvostek's sign:* Tap the facial nerve just below the temple, in front of the ear. If facial muscles twitch, hyperirritability of the nerve is present, and tetany may occur.
- Check for *Trousseau's sign:* Constrict blood circulation in an arm (usually with a blood-pressure cuff) for 3 to 5 minutes. This produces ischemia and increased irritability of peripheral nerves, which causes spasms of the lower arm and hand muscles (carpopedal spasm) if tetany is present.
- Assess for conditions in which hypercalcemia is likely to occur (e.g., cancer, prolonged immobilization, vitamin D overdose).
- Observe for signs and symptoms of hypercalcemia in clients at risk. Electrocardiographic changes indicative of hypercalcemia include a shortened Q–T interval and an inverted T wave.
- Assess for risk factors and manifestations of osteoporosis, especially in postmenopausal women and men and women on chronic corticosteroid therapy.
  - If risk factors are identified, ask if preventive measures are being used (e.g., increasing calcium intake, exercise, medications).
  - If the patient is known to have osteoporosis, ask about duration and severity of symptoms, age at onset, location, whether fractures have occurred, what treatments have been performed, and response to treatments.
- If Paget's disease is suspected, assess for an elevated serum alkaline phosphatase level and abnormal bone scan reports.

Nursing Diagnoses

- Deficient Knowledge: Recommended daily amounts and dietary sources of calcium and vitamin D
- Deficient Knowledge: Disease process and drug therapy for osteoporosis
- Risk for Injury: Tetany, sedation, seizures from hypocalcemia
- Risk for Injury: Hypercalcemia related to overuse of supplements; hypocalcemia from aggressive treatment of hypercalcemia

Planning/Goals

The patient will

- Achieve and maintain normal serum levels of calcium
- Increase dietary intake of calcium-containing foods to prevent or treat osteoporosis
- Use calcium or vitamin D supplements in recommended amounts
- Comply with instructions for safe drug use
- Be monitored closely for therapeutic and adverse effects of drugs used to treat hypercalcemia

Nursing Process continues on page 402

■ Comply with procedures for follow-up treatment of hypocalcemia, hypercalcemia, or osteoporosis

■ Avoid preventable adverse effects of treatment for acute hypocalcemia or hypercalcemia

Interventions

Assist all patients in meeting the recommended daily requirements of calcium and vitamin D. With an adequate protein and calcium intake, enough phosphorus also is obtained.

■ The best dietary source is milk and other dairy products, including yogurt.

■ Unless contraindicated by the patient's condition, recommend that adults drink at least two 8-oz glasses of milk daily. This furnishes approximately half the daily calcium requirement; the remainder will probably be obtained from other foods.

■ Children need approximately four glasses of milk or an equivalent amount of calcium in milk and other foods to support normal growth and development.

■ Pregnant and lactating women also need approximately four glasses of milk or the equivalent to meet increased needs. Vitamin and mineral supplements are often prescribed during these periods.

■ Postmenopausal women who take estrogens need at least 1000 mg of calcium daily. Those who do not take estrogens need at least 1500 mg. Dosage adjusted to dietary calcium intake.

■ For patients who avoid or minimize their intake of dairy products because of the calories, identify low-calorie sources, such as skim milk and low-fat yogurt.

■ Milk that has been fortified with vitamin D is the best food source. Exposure of skin to sunlight is also needed to supply adequate amounts of vitamin D.

■ For people who are unable or unwilling to ingest sufficient calcium, a supplement may be needed to prevent osteoporosis.

Assist patients with hypercalcemia to decrease formation of renal calculi by forcing fluids to approximately 3000 to 4000 milliliters per day and preventing urinary tract infections.

Patient Guidelines for Drugs for Osteoporosis are presented in the accompanying display.

Evaluation

■ Check laboratory reports of serum calcium levels for normal values.

■ Interview and observe for relief of symptoms of hypocalcemia, hypercalcemia, or osteoporosis.

■ Interview and observe intake of calcium-containing foods.

■ Question about normal calcium requirements and how to meet them.

■ Interview and observe for accurate drug usage and compliance with follow-up procedures.

■ Interview and observe for therapeutic and adverse drug effects.

Principles of Therapy

Goal of Therapy

The goal of therapy is to restore normal calcium balance in the body. Drugs used for hypocalemia help correct calcium deficit, reduce the risk of *tetany* (prolonged and painful spasms of the voluntary muscles), and slow development of osteoporosis. Drugs used for hypercalcemia support treatment of the underlying condition and control serum calcium levels.

Drugs Used for Hypocalcemia

Drug Dosage and Administration

Calcium preparations and perhaps vitamin D are used to treat hypocalcemia. IV administration of calcium, usually 10 to 20 milliliters of 10% calcium gluconate (1–2 g of calcium), is necessary to treat acute, severe hypocalcemia, which is a medical emergency. Doses may be repeated, a continuous infusion may be given, or oral supplements may be used to avoid symptoms of hypocalcemia and maintain normal serum calcium levels (as measured every 4–6 hours). Once the hypocalcemia is stabilized, treatment is aimed at management of the underlying cause or prevention of recurrence. If hypocalcemia is caused by diarrhea or malabsorption, treatment of the underlying condition decreases loss of calcium from the body and increases absorption. Serum magnesium levels should also be measured, and, if hypomagnesemia is present, it must be treated before treatment of hypocalcemia can be effective.

Oral calcium supplements are preferred for less acute situations or for long-term treatment of chronic hypocalcemia. Vitamin D is given also if a calcium preparation alone cannot maintain serum calcium levels within a normal range. When vitamin D is given to treat hypocalcemia, dosage is determined by frequent measurement of serum calcium levels. Usually, higher doses are given initially, and lower doses are given for maintenance therapy. Calcium salts and vitamin D are combined in many over-the-counter preparations promoted as dietary supplements (Table 25-3). These preparations contain variable amounts of calcium and vitamin D. In general, intake of calcium should not exceed 2500 milligrams daily, from all sources, and intake of vitamin D should not exceed 400 international units daily. These mixtures are not indicated for maintenance therapy in chronic hypocalcemia.

Calcium supplements can decrease bone loss and fractures, especially in women. Calcium carbonate contains the most elemental calcium by weight (40%). It is inexpensive and available in a nonprescription form as the antacid Tums. Calcium citrate is reportedly better absorbed than calcium carbonate.

Effects of Calcium Preparations on Other Drugs

Calcium preparations and digoxin have similar effects on the myocardium. Therefore, if calcium is given to a patient taking digoxin, the risks of digitalis toxicity and cardiac dysrhythmias are increased. This combination must be used very cautiously. Oral calcium preparations decrease effects of oral tetracycline drugs by combining with the antibiotic and preventing its

Patient Teaching Guidelines | Drugs for Osteoporosis

General Considerations

■ Osteoporosis involves weak bones that fracture easily and may cause pain and disability.

■ Important factors in prevention and treatment include an adequate intake of calcium and vitamin D (from the diet, from supplements, or from a combination of both sources), regular weight-bearing exercise, and drugs that can slow bone loss.

■ It is better to obtain calcium and vitamin D from foods such as milk and other dairy products. Approximately 1000 to 1500 milligrams of calcium and a minimum of 400 IU of vitamin D are recommended daily.

■ If unable to get sufficient dietary calcium and vitamin D, consider supplements of these nutrients. Consult a health care provider about the types and amounts. For example, a daily multivitamin and mineral supplement may contain adequate amounts when added to dietary intake. If taking other supplements, avoid those containing bone meal because they may contain lead and other contaminants that are toxic to the human body. Do not take more than the recommended amounts of supplements; overuse can cause serious, life-threatening problems.

■ The main drugs approved for prevention and treatment of osteoporosis are the bisphosphonates (e.g., Fosamax, Actonel). These drugs help prevent the loss of calcium from bone, thereby strengthening bone and reducing the risks of fractures.

■ For people at high risk for development of osteoporosis (e.g., postmenopausal women, men and women who take an oral or inhaled corticosteroid such as prednisone or fluticasone [Flonase]), or those being treated for osteoporosis, a baseline measurement of bone mineral density and periodic follow-up measurements are needed. This is a noninvasive test that does not involve any injections or device insertions.

Self-Administration

■ If taking a calcium supplement, calcium carbonate 500 milligrams twice daily is often recommended. This can be obtained with the inexpensive over-the-counter antacid Tums, which contains 200 milligrams of calcium per tablet.

■ Do not take a calcium supplement with an iron preparation, tetracycline, ciprofloxacin, or phenytoin. Instead, take the drugs at least 2 hours apart to avoid calcium interference with absorption of the other drugs.

■ If taking both a calcium supplement and a bisphosphonate, take the calcium at least 2 hours after the bisphosphonate. Calcium, antacids, and other drugs interfere with absorption of bisphosphonate.

■ Take bisphosphonates with 6 to 8 ounces of water at least 30 minutes before any food, other fluid, or other medication. Beverages other than water and foods decrease absorption and effectiveness.

■ Take a bisphosphonate in an upright position and do not lie down for at least 30 minutes. This helps prevent esophageal irritation and stomach upset.

■ If taking a bisphosphonate, report new or worsening dysphagia, retrosternal pain, or heartburn to your health care provider. This may be an indication of esophageal irritation due to the bisphosphonate.

---

absorption. They should not be given at the same time or within 2 to 3 hours of each other.

Drugs Used for Hypercalcemia

Treatment of hypercalcemia depends largely on the cause and severity. When the cause is a tumor of parathyroid tissue, sur-gical excision is commonly used. When the cause is a malignant tumor, treatment of the tumor with surgery, radiation, or chemotherapy may reduce production of PTH. When the cause is excessive intake of vitamin D, the vitamin D preparation should be stopped immediately. Serum calcium levels should be measured periodically to monitor effects of therapy.

Drug Dosage and Administration

Acute hypercalcemia (e.g., severe symptoms or a serum calcium level > 12 mg/dL) is a medical emergency, and rehydration is a priority. An IV saline infusion (0.9% or 0.45% NaCl) of 4000 milligrams a day (or more if kidney function is adequate) is effective. After rehydration, furosemide may be given IV to increase renal excretion of calcium and prevent fluid overload. Because sodium, potassium, and water are also lost in the urine, these must be replaced in the IV fluids.

In mild hypercalcemia, further drug therapy is usually not necessary; most patients respond to the aforementioned treatment. In moderate to severe hypercalcemia, pamidronate or zoledronate may be the drug of choice. When pamidronate is given in a single IV infusion containing 60 or 90 milligrams, serum calcium levels decrease within 2 days, reach their lowest levels in approximately 7 days, and remain lower for 2 weeks or longer. Treatment can be repeated if hypercalcemia recurs. Zoledronate can be given over 15 minutes, and effects may last longer than those of pamidronate. Adverse effects of the two

Table 25-3	Selected Calcium/Vitamin D Combination Products	
GENERIC/ TRADE NAME	**CALCIUM (MG)*/ TABLET OR CAPSULE**	**VITAMIN D (IU)†/ TABLET**
Caltrate 600 + D and Caltrate Plus	600	200
Citracal caplets + D	315	200
Dical-D tablets	117	133
Dical-D wafers	233	200
Os-Cal 250 + D	250	125
Os-Cal 500 + D	500	125
Posture-D	600	125

*mg of elemental calcium; †IU, international units.

drugs are similar. Phosphates should not be used, unless hypophosphatemia is present. They are also contraindicated in patients with persistent urinary tract infections and an alkaline urine, because kidney stones composed of calcium phosphate are likely to form in such cases.

In chronic hypercalcemia, treatment of the underlying disease process and measures to control serum calcium levels (e.g., a high fluid intake and mobilization to help retain calcium in bone) are necessary. Oral phosphate administration may help if other measures are ineffective.

For patients receiving a calcium channel blocker (see Chap. 50), the drugs may be less effective in the presence of hypercalcemia. For calcium channel blocker overdose, replacement may require an hourly infusion after a bolus dose.

Drugs Used for Osteoporosis

To avoid or slow bone loss, preventive measures should be implemented in people of all ages, including a consistently adequate dietary intake of calcium to promote normal bone development and maintenance. In children, adolescents, and young adults, an adequate calcium intake promotes bone growth and peak bone mass. A well-stocked "reservoir" means that in later years, when bone loss exceeds formation, more bone can be lost before osteoporosis develops. Measures to prevent osteoporosis include the following:

■ Adequate calcium intake, which may slow the development of osteoporosis and fractures in postmenopausal women and men older than 40 years of age. Although dietary intake is much preferred, a supplement may be needed to ensure a daily intake of 1000 to 1500 milligrams, especially in adolescent girls, frail older adults, and those receiving corticosteroids.

■ Use of alendronate (Fosamax) and risedronate (Actonel), which are approved by the Food and Drug Administration for prevention of osteoporosis. (With alendronate, recommended dosage is smaller for prevention than for treatment.) Raloxifene (Evista) is approved for prevention and treatment of postmenopausal osteoporosis in women.

■ Adequate intake of vitamin D. However, supplementation is probably not indicated unless a deficiency can be demonstrated. Serum calcitriol can be measured in patients at risk for vitamin D deficiency, including older adults and those on chronic corticosteroid therapy.

■ Lifestyle changes, including regular exercise and smoking cessation. Numerous studies indicate that vigorous, weight-bearing exercise helps promote and maintain strong bone, and inactivity promotes bone weakening and loss. Smoking decreases the amount of active estrogen in the body and thus accelerates bone loss.

Preventive measures are necessary for patients on chronic corticosteroid therapy (e.g., prednisone 7.5 mg daily; equivalent amounts of other systemic drugs; high doses of inhaled drugs). For both men and women, most of the preceding guidelines apply (e.g., calcium supplements, regular exercise, a bisphosphonate drug). In addition, low doses and nonsystemic routes help prevent osteoporosis and other adverse effects. For men, corticosteroids decrease testosterone levels by approximately one half, and replacement therapy may be needed.

Preventive measures are also necessary for patients taking **phenytoin** (Dilantin) and phenobarbital, because these drugs may contribute to osteoporosis through their effects on calcium metabolism. These anticonvulsant medications increase hepatic metabolism of vitamin D, which leads to a decrease in calcium absorption in the intestine. Supplemental calcium and vitamin D as well as specific drugs for osteoporosis should be considered if bone density is low.

When bone loss is evident (from diagnostic tests of bone density or occurrence of fractures), several interventions may help slow further skeletal bone loss or prevent fractures. Most drugs used to treat osteoporosis decrease the rate of bone breakdown and thus slow the rate of bone loss. Alendronate (Fosamax) 10 milligrams daily or 70 milligrams weekly and risedronate (Actonel) 5 milligrams daily can increase bone mineral density, reduce risks of vertebral fractures, and slow progression of vertebral deformities and loss of height. One of these drugs is often used in combination with estrogen and calcium and vitamin D supplements. The drug teriparatide (Forteo) actually increases bone formation.

Patients diagnosed with osteoporosis require adequate calcium and vitamin D (at least the recommended dietary allowance), whether obtained from the diet or from supplements. Calcium 600 milligrams and vitamin D 200 international units once or twice daily are often recommended for postmenopausal women with osteoporosis, and pharmacologic doses of vitamin D are sometimes used to treat patients with serious osteoporosis. If such doses are used, caution should be exercised, because excessive amounts of vitamin D can cause hypercalcemia and hypercalciuria.

In addition, regular exercise and smoking cessation may be necessary. Treatment of men is similar to that of women, except that testosterone replacement may be required. In corticosteroid-induced osteoporosis, multiple treatment measures may be necessary, including increased dietary and supplemental calcium and possibly vitamin D supplementation, hormone replacement, corticosteroid dosage reduction, exercise, and a bisphosphonate or calcitonin to slow skeletal bone loss.

Use in Special Populations
Use in Children

Hypocalcemia is uncommon in children. However, inadequate calcium in the diet is thought to be common, especially in girls. Both inadequate calcium and exercise in children are risk factors for eventual osteoporosis. If hypocalcemia or dietary calcium deficiency develops, principles of using calcium or vitamin D supplements are the same as those in adults. Children should be monitored closely for signs and symptoms of adverse effects, including hypercalcemia. Hypercalcemia is probably most likely to occur in children with a malignant tumor. Guidelines for treating hypercalcemia in children are essentially the same as those for adults, with drug dosages adjusted. Safety, effectiveness, and dosage of pamidronate and zoledronate have not been established.

Use in Older Adults

Hypocalcemia is uncommon, because calcium moves from bone to blood to maintain normal serum levels. However, calcium deficiency commonly occurs because of long-term dietary deficiencies of calcium and vitamin D, impaired absorption of calcium from the intestine, lack of exposure to sunlight, and impaired liver or kidney metabolism of vitamin D to its active form. These and other factors lead to demineralization and weakening of bone (osteoporosis) and an increased risk of fractures. Postmenopausal women are at high risk for osteoporosis. Although osteoporosis also develops in older men, it occurs less often, at a later age, and to a lesser extent than in older women. Both men and women who take corticosteroids are at risk for osteoporosis. The risk is higher with systemic corticosteroids but may also occur with oral or inhaled drugs, especially at higher doses. In general, all older adults must continue their dietary intake of dairy products and other calcium-containing foods. Older adults with osteoporosis or risk factors for osteoporosis may need calcium supplements and a bisphosphonate or calcitonin to prevent or treat the disorder.

Hypercalcemia usually requires large amounts of IV 0.9% sodium chloride (e.g., 150–200 mL/hour). Older adults often have chronic cardiovascular disorders that may be aggravated by this treatment, and they should be monitored closely for signs of fluid overload, congestive heart failure, pulmonary edema, and hypertension.

Use in Patients With Renal Impairment

Patients with renal impairment or failure often have disturbances in calcium and bone metabolism. If hypercalcemia develops in patients with severely impaired renal function, hemodialysis or peritoneal dialysis with calcium-free solution is effective and safe. Calcium acetate may be used to prevent or treat hyperphosphatemia. The calcium reduces blood levels of phosphate by reducing its absorption from foods. That is, calcium binds with dietary phosphate to produce calcium phosphate, which is insoluble and excreted in feces. If vitamin D therapy is needed to treat osteomalacia associated with renal impairment, calcitriol (e.g., Rocaltrol) is preferred (see Table 25-1). Calcitriol is the active form of vitamin D and thus requires no metabolism.

None of the bisphosphonate drugs is recommended for use in severe renal impairment (e.g., serum creatinine > 5 mg/dL or creatinine clearance < 30 mL/minute). With alendronate, dosage does not need to be reduced in mild to moderate impairment (e.g., creatinine clearance 35–60 mL/minute). Pamidronate and zoledronate are nephrotoxic, and renal function should be closely monitored during their use.

Teriparatide (Forteo), a form of PTH, apparently does not require dosage adjustment in renal impairment.

Use in Patients With Hepatic Impairment

The bisphosphonates are not metabolized in the liver and are unlikely to affect liver function. Teriparatide (Forteo), a form of PTH, apparently does not require dosage adjustment in hepatic impairment.

Use in Home Care

Home care nurses have an excellent opportunity to promote health and prevent illness related to calcium and bone disorders. Nurses who assist in the care of any seriously ill patient should also be able to recognize and obtain immediate treatment for hypocalcemia or hypercalcemia. For example, hypercalcemia may occur in patients with cancer, especially cancers involving bone.

All members of a household should be assessed in relation to calcium and vitamin D intake because an adequate amount of these nutrients is needed throughout life. Intake of both calcium and vitamin D is often inadequate in children and adolescent girls, who may risk developing osteoporosis. It may be necessary to teach about dietary and supplemental sources of these nutrients as well as adverse effects of excessive amounts. Patients who are taking medications to prevent or treat osteoporosis may also require teaching or other assistance.

 Applying Your Knowledge 25-3

How Can You Avoid This Medication Error?

Ms. Taylor knows she cannot drink her morning coffee or eat her breakfast for 30 minutes after taking her alendronate. You tell her to get up and take her medication, then go back to bed for half an hour.

Nursing Actions   Drugs Used in Calcium and Bone Disorders

NURSING ACTIONS	RATIONALE/EXPLANATION
1. Administer accurately	
a. With calcium preparations:	
(1) Give oral preparations with or after meals.	To increase absorption
(2) Give intravenous (IV) preparations slowly (0.5–2 mL/min), check pulse and blood pressure closely, and monitor the electrocardiogram (ECG) if possible.	These solutions may cause dysrhythmias and hypotension if injected rapidly. They are also irritating to tissues.
(3) Do not mix IV preparations with any other drug in the same syringe.	Calcium reacts with some other drugs and forms a precipitate.
b. With bisphosphonates:	
(1) Give alendronate, ibandronate, and risedronate with 6–8 ounces of plain water, at least 30 minutes before the first food, beverage, or medication of the day.	To promote absorption and decrease esophageal and gastric irritation
(2) Give etidronate on an empty stomach, as a single dose or in divided doses. Avoid giving within 2 hours of ingesting dairy products, antacids, or vitamin or mineral preparations.	If gastrointestinal (GI) symptoms occur with the single dose, divided doses may relieve them. Substances containing calcium or other minerals decrease absorption of etidronate.
(3) Give IV pamidronate and zoledronate according to the manufacturers' instructions.	These drugs require reconstitution, diluting with IV fluids, and specific time intervals of administration.
c. Give calcitonin at bedtime.	To decrease nausea and discomfort from flushing
d. With phosphate salts, mix powder forms with water for oral administration. See package inserts for specific instructions.	
2. Observe for therapeutic effects	
a. With calcium preparations, observe for:	
(1) Relief of symptoms of neuromuscular irritability and tetany, such as decreased muscle spasms and decreased paresthesias	
(2) Serum calcium levels within the normal range (8.5–10.5 mg/dL)	
(3) Absence of Chvostek's and Trousseau's signs	
b. With alendronate or risedronate for osteoporosis, observe for improved bone mass density and absence of fractures.	Early osteopenia and osteoporosis are asymptomatic. Measurement of bone mass density is the only way to quantify bone loss.
c. With calcitonin, corticosteroids, pamidronate, or zoledronate for hypercalcemia, observe for:	
(1) Decreased serum calcium level	Calcitonin lowers serum calcium levels in about 2 hours after injection and effects last 6–8 hours. Corticosteroids require 10–14 days to lower serum calcium. Bisphosphonates lower serum calcium levels within 2 days, but may require a week or more to produce normal serum calcium levels.
(2) Decreased signs and symptoms of hypercalcemia	
3. Observe for adverse effects	
a. With calcium preparations, observe for hypercalcemia:	
(1) GI effects—anorexia, nausea, vomiting, abdominal pain, constipation	
(2) Central nervous system effects—apathy, poor memory, depression, drowsiness, disorientation	
(3) Other effects—weakness and decreased tone in skeletal and smooth muscles, dysphagia, polyuria, polydipsia, cardiac dysrhythmias	
(4) Serum calcium >10.5 mg/dL	
(5) ECG changes indicating hypercalcemia (a prolonged Q-T interval and an inverted T wave)	
b. With vitamin D preparations, observe for hypervitaminosis D and hypercalcemia (see above).	This is most likely to occur with chronic ingestion of high doses daily. In children, accidental ingestion may lead to acute toxicity.

NURSING ACTIONS	RATIONALE/EXPLANATION
c. With alendronate, ibandronate, and risedronate, observe for:	
(1) GI effects—abdominal distention, acid regurgitation, dysphagia, esophagitis, flatulence	Adverse effects are usually minor with the doses taken for prevention or treatment of osteoporosis, if the drugs are taken as directed. More severe effects may occur with the higher doses taken for Paget's disease.
(2) Other effects—headache, musculoskeletal pain, decreased serum calcium and phosphate	
d. With calcitonin, observe for nausea, vomiting, tissue irritation at administration sites, and allergic reactions.	Adverse effects are usually mild and transient. Nasal administration produces greater patient compliance than injections, with few adverse effects.
e. With drug therapy for hypercalcemia, observe for hypocalcemia.	Hypocalcemia may occur with vigorous treatment of hypercalcemia. This can be minimized by monitoring serum calcium levels frequently and adjusting drug dosages and other treatments.
f. With pamidronate and zoledronate, observe for:	
(1) GI effects—anorexia, nausea, vomiting, constipation	
(2) Cardiovascular effects—fluid overload, hypertension	
(3) Electrolyte imbalances—hypokalemia, hypomagnesemia, hypophosphatemia	
(4) Musculoskeletal effects—muscle and joint pain	
(5) Miscellaneous effects—fever, tissue irritation at IV insertion site, pain, anemia	
g. With etidronate, observe for anorexia, nausea, diarrhea, bone pain, fever, fluid overload, and increased serum creatinine.	Adverse effects are more frequent and more severe at higher doses. The drug is nephrotoxic and should not be used in patients with renal failure.
h. With phosphates, observe for nausea, vomiting, and diarrhea.	
4. Observe for drug interactions	
a. Drugs that *increase* effects of calcium:	
(1) Vitamin D	Increases intestinal absorption of calcium from both dietary and supplemental drug sources
(2) Thiazide diuretics	Reduce calcium losses in urine
b. Drugs that *decrease* effects of calcium:	
(1) Corticosteroids (prednisone, others), calcitonin, and phosphates	These drugs lower serum calcium levels by various mechanisms. They are used in the treatment of hypercalcemia.
c. Drugs that *increase* effects of vitamin D:	
(1) Thiazide diuretics	Thiazide diuretics administered to hypoparathyroid patients may cause hypercalcemia (potentiate vitamin D effects).
d. Drugs that *decrease* effects of vitamin D:	
(1) Phenytoin	Accelerates metabolism of vitamin D in the liver and may cause vitamin D deficiency, hypocalcemia, and rickets or osteomalacia. Increased intake of vitamin D may be needed.
(2) Cholestyramine resin (Questran)	May decrease intestinal absorption of vitamin D preparations
(3) Mineral oil	Mineral oil is a fat and therefore combines with fat-soluble vitamins, such as vitamin D, and prevents their absorption from the gastrointestinal tract.
e. Drugs that *decrease* effects of oral bisphosphonates:	
(1) Antacids and calcium supplements	These drugs interfere with absorption of bisphosphonates and should be taken at least 2 hours after a bisphosphonate.
f. Drug that *decreases* the effects of tiludronate:	
(1) Aspirin	Aspirin decreases the bioavailability of tiludronate by up to 50% when taken within 2 hours of tiludronate.
g. Drugs that alter effects of calcitonin:	
(1) Testosterone and other androgens *increase* effects.	Androgens and calcitonin have additive effects on calcium retention and inhibition of bone resorption (movement of calcium from bone to serum).
(2) Parathyroid hormone *decreases* effects.	Parathyroid hormone antagonizes or opposes calcitonin.
h. Drugs that *decrease* effects of phosphate salts:	
(1) Antacids containing aluminum and magnesium	Aluminum and magnesium may combine with phosphate and thereby prevent its absorption and therapeutic effect.

Key Concepts

- Hypoparathyroidism is most often caused by removal of or damage to the parathyroid glands during neck surgery.

- Hyperparathyroidism is most often caused by a tumor or hyperplasia of a parathyroid gland.

- Deficiency of vitamin D causes inadequate absorption of calcium and phosphorus.

- In general, intake of calcium should not exceed 2500 mg daily, from all sources, and intake of vitamin D should not exceed 400 international units daily.

- Calcium deficiency commonly occurs in the elderly because of long-term dietary deficiencies of calcium

and vitamin D, impaired absorption of calcium from the intestine, lack of exposure to sunlight, and impaired liver or kidney metabolism of vitamin D to its active form.

- Postmenopausal women are at high risk for osteoporosis.

- Both men and women who take corticosteroids are at risk for osteoporosis.

- For men, corticosteroids decrease testosterone levels by approximately one half, and replacement therapy may be needed.

Review and Application Exercises

Short Answer Exercises

1. What are the major physiologic functions of calcium?

2. What is the normal serum level of calcium?

3. What are some nursing interventions to prevent hypocalcemia?

4. What signs and symptoms may indicate hypocalcemia?

5. How is hypocalcemia treated?

6. What signs and symptoms may indicate hypercalcemia?

7. How is hypercalcemia treated?

8. Why is it important to have an adequate intake of calcium and vitamin D throughout life?

9. What are the main elements of prevention and treatment of osteoporosis?

NCLEX-Style Questions

10. To decrease nausea and discomfort from flushing with calcitonin, the nurse should instruct the patient to take the drug in which of the following ways?
    a. with a warm beverage
    b. with a glass of orange juice
    c. with breakfast
    d. at bedtime

11. Rapid administration of IV calcium may result in which of the following conditions?
    a. cardiac dysrhythmias
    b. nephrotoxicity
    c. ototoxicity
    d. pathologic fractures

12. Which of the following drugs is used to treat osteoporosis and can actually increase bone formation?
    a. teriparatide (Forteo)
    b. phosphate salts (Neutra-Phos)
    c. furosemide (Lasix)
    d. calcitriol (Rocaltrol)

13. If oral calcium preparations are given at the same time or within 2 to 3 hours of administration of antibiotics, they prevent absorption of which of the following antibiotics?
    a. penicillin
    b. cephalosporin
    c. tetracycline
    d. erythromycin

14. Alendronate is used in postmenopausal women for the prevention and treatment of osteoporosis. It acts to decrease plasma calcium levels by
    a. inhibiting calcium resorption from bone
    b. binding calcium in the blood
    c. promoting renal excretion of calcium
    d. limiting intestinal absorption of calcium

Selected References

Corwin, E. J. (2006). *Handbook of pathophysiology* (3rd ed.). Philadelphia: Lippincott Williams & Wilkins.

Djulbegovic, B., Wheatley, K., Ross, J., Clark, O., Bos, G., Goldschmidt, H., Cremer, F., Alsina, M., & Glasmacher, A. (2007). Bisphos-

phonates in multiple myeloma. *Cochrane Database of Systematic Reviews*, Issue 2. Art no.: CD003188.

Drug facts and comparisons. (Updated monthly). St. Louis, MO: Facts and Comparisons.

Gass, M., & Dawson-Hughes, B. (2006). Preventing osteoporosis-related fractures: An overview. *The American Journal of Medicine, 119,* 3S–11S.

Guyton, A. C., & Hall, J. E. (2006). *Textbook of medical physiology* (11th ed.). Philadelphia: W. B. Saunders.

Homik, J., Suarez-Almazor, M. E., Shea, B., Cranney, A., Wells, G., & Tugwell, P. (2007). Calcium and vitamin D for corticosteroid-induced osteoporosis. *Cochrane Database of Systematic Reviews,* Issue 2. Art no.: CD000952

Lacy, C. F., Armstrong, L. L., Goldman, M. P., & Lance, L. L. (2007). *Lexi-Comp's drug information handbook* (15th ed.). Hudson, OH: American Pharmaceutical Association.

Porth, C. M. (2004). *Pathophysiology: Concepts of altered health states* (7th ed.). Philadelphia: Lippincott Williams & Wilkins.

Antidiabetic Drugs

LEARNING OBJECTIVES

After studying this chapter, you will be able to:

1. Describe major effects of endogenous insulin on body tissues.
2. Discuss characteristics and uses of the various types of insulins and insulin analogs.
3. Discuss the relationships among diet, exercise, and drug therapy in controlling diabetes.
4. Differentiate types of oral agents used to manage diabetes mellitus in terms of mechanisms of action, indications for use, adverse effects, and nursing process implications.
5. Discuss the indications, characteristics, and benefits of amylin analogs, incretin mimetics, and dipeptidyl peptidase-4 (DPP-4) inhibitors.
6. Explain the benefits of maintaining glycemic control in preventing complications of diabetes mellitus.
7. State reasons for combinations of insulin and oral agents or different types of oral agents.
8. Assist patients or caregivers in learning how to manage diabetes care, including administration of medication agents used to manage diabetes mellitus.
9. Collaborate with nurse diabetes educators, dietitians, pharmacists, and others in teaching self-care activities to patients with diabetes.
10. Assess and monitor patients' conditions in relation to diabetes mellitus and their compliance with prescribed management strategies.
11. Discuss dietary and herbal supplements that affect blood sugar and diabetes control.
12. Review the National Cholesterol Education Program (NCEP) Adult Treatment Panel III (ATP III) guidelines for lipid management in high risk and/or diabetic states.

Applying Your Knowledge

Carwein Coulter is a 55 year-old African American with type 2 diabetes. He has been a diagnosed diabetic for at least 10 years and is overweight. Mr. Coulter's current daily medications include Novolin 70/30 insulin, glimepiride, and metformin. He has a sliding scale of insulin lispro for elevated blood glucose results.

Introduction

Insulin and oral hypoglycemic agents are two of the several types of medications used to lower blood *glucose* in diabetes mellitus. New drug therapies include amylin analogs, incretin mimetics, and dipeptidyl peptidase-4 (DPP-4) inhibitors. To assist readers in understanding the clinical use of these drugs, characteristics of endogenous insulin, diabetes mellitus, and the medications are described.

Endogenous Insulin

Insulin is a protein hormone secreted by beta cells in the pancreas. The average adult pancreas secretes 40 to 60 units of insulin daily. This includes a basal amount of 1 to 2 units per hour and additional amounts (4–6 units/hour) after meals or when the *blood glucose level* exceeds 100 milligrams per deciliter. In a fasting state, serum insulin levels are low and stored glucose and amino acids are used for energy needs of tissues that require glucose. After a meal, serum insulin levels increase and peak in a few minutes, then decrease to baseline levels in 2 to 3 hours.

Amylin, a pancreatic hormone secreted with insulin, delays gastric emptying, increases satiety, and suppresses *glucagon* secretion, thus complementing the effects of insulin on the blood sugar. A synthetic form of amylin, pramlintide (Symlin), has been developed to assist with glucose control in both type 1 and type 2 diabetic patients.

Insulin is secreted into the portal circulation and transported to the liver, where about half is used or degraded. The other half reaches the systemic circulation, where it circulates mainly in an unbound form and is transported to body cells.

At the cellular level (Fig. 26-1), insulin binds with and activates receptors on the cell membranes of about 80% of body cells. Liver, muscle, and fat cells have many insulin receptors and are primary tissues for insulin action. After insulin–receptor binding occurs, cell membranes become highly permeable to glucose and allow rapid entry of glucose into the cells. The cell membranes also become more permeable to amino acids, fatty acids, and electrolytes such as potassium, magnesium, and phosphate ions. Cellular metabolism is altered by the movement of these substances into the cells, by activation of some enzymes and inactivation of others, by movement of proteins between intracellular compartments, by changes in the amounts of proteins produced, and perhaps by other mechanisms. Overall, the changes in cellular metabolism stimulate anabolic effects (e.g., utilization and storage of glucose, amino acids, and fatty acids) and inhibit catabolic processes (e.g., breakdown of glycogen, fat, and protein). After binding to insulin and entering the cell, receptors may be degraded or recycled back to the cell surface.

Insulin is cleared from circulating blood in 10 to 15 minutes because of rapid binding to peripheral tissues or metabolic breakdown. The insulin that does not combine with receptors is metabolized in the liver, kidneys, plasma, and muscles. In the kidneys, insulin is filtered by the glomeruli and reabsorbed by the tubules, which also degrade it. Severe renal impairment slows the clearance of insulin from the blood.

Insulin plays a major role in metabolism of carbohydrate, fat, and protein (Box 26-1). These foodstuffs are broken down into molecules of glucose, lipids, and amino acids, respectively. The molecules enter the cells and are converted to energy for cellular activities. The energy can be used immediately or converted to storage forms for later use. When carrying out its metabolic functions, the overall effect of insulin is to lower blood glucose levels, primarily by the following mechanisms:

- In the liver, insulin acts to decrease breakdown of glycogen (glycogenolysis), form new glucose from fatty acids and amino acids (*gluconeogenesis*), and form ketone bodies (ketogenesis). At the same time, it acts to increase synthesis and storage of glycogen and fatty acids.

- In adipose tissue, insulin acts to decrease breakdown of fat (lipolysis) and to increase production of glycerol and fatty acids.

- In muscle tissue, insulin acts to decrease protein breakdown and amino acid output and to increase amino acid uptake, protein synthesis, and glycogen synthesis.

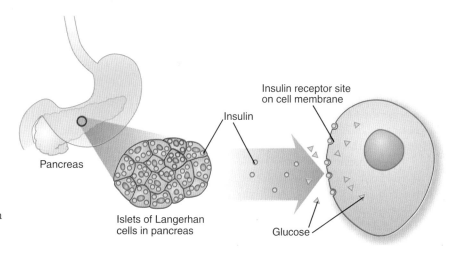

Figure 26-1 ▪ Normal glucose metabolism. After insulin binds with receptors on the cell membrane, glucose can move into the cell, promoting cellular metabolism and energy production.

Pancreas

Islets of Langerhan cells in pancreas

Insulin

Insulin receptor site on cell membrane

Glucose

Box 26-1	Effects of Insulin on Metabolism

Carbohydrate Metabolism

- Insulin increases glucose transport into the liver, skeletal muscle, adipose tissue, the heart, and some smooth muscle organs (such as the uterus); it must be present for muscle and fat tissues to use glucose for energy.
- Insulin regulates glucose metabolism to produce energy for cellular functions. If excess glucose is present after this need is met, it is converted to glycogen and stored for future energy needs or converted to fat and stored. The excess glucose transported to liver cells is converted to fat only after glycogen stores are saturated. When insulin is absent or blood glucose levels are low, these stored forms of glucose can be reconverted. The liver is especially important in restoring blood sugar levels by breaking down glycogen or by forming new glucose.

Fat Metabolism

- Insulin promotes transport of glucose into fat cells, where it is broken down. One of the breakdown products is alpha-glycerophosphate, which combines with fatty acids to form triglycerides. This is the mechanism by which insulin promotes fat storage.

- When insulin is lacking, fat is released into the bloodstream as free fatty acids. Blood concentrations of triglycerides, cholesterol, and phospholipids are also increased. The high blood lipid concentration probably accounts for the atherosclerosis that tends to develop early and progress more rapidly in people with diabetes mellitus. Also, when more fatty acids are released than the body can use as fuel, some fatty acids are converted into ketones. Excessive amounts of ketones produce acidosis and coma.

Protein Metabolism

- Insulin increases the total amount of body protein by increasing transport of amino acids into cells and synthesis of protein within the cells. The basic mechanism of these effects is unknown.
- Insulin potentiates the effects of growth hormone.
- Lack of insulin causes protein breakdown into amino acids, which are released into the bloodstream and transported to the liver for energy or gluconeogenesis. The lost proteins are not replaced by synthesis of new proteins; and protein wasting causes abnormal functioning of many body organs, severe weakness, and weight loss.

Regulation of Insulin Secretion

Insulin decreases blood sugar and regulates the amount of glucose available for cellular metabolism and energy needs, during both fasting and feeding. Insulin secretion involves coordination of various nutrients, hormones, the autonomic nervous system, and other factors.

Glucose is the major stimulus of insulin secretion; others include amino acids, fatty acids, ketone bodies (which are acidotic substances in themselves), and stimulation of $beta_2$-adrenergic receptors or vagal nerves. Oral glucose is more effective than intravenous (IV) glucose because glucose or food in the digestive tract stimulates vagal activity and induces the release of gastrointestinal (GI) hormones called incretins. Incretin hormones stimulate the release of insulin when glucose levels are normal or elevated. In addition, incretin hormones reduce glucagon production and delay gastric emptying. Two incretin hormones have been identified: glucose-dependent insulinotropic peptide (GIP) and glucagon-like peptide-1 (GLP-1). GLP-1 also appears to improve insulin sensitivity and may increase the formation of new beta cells in the pancreas. The therapeutic uses of incretin hormones have recently been investigated, and this has lead to the development of new drugs to treat diabetes mellitus.

Several hormones raise blood glucose levels and stimulate insulin secretion, including cortisol, glucagon, growth hormone, epinephrine, estrogen, and progesterone. Excessive, prolonged, endogenous secretion or administration of pharmacologic preparations of these hormones can exhaust the ability of pancreatic beta cells to produce insulin and thereby cause or aggravate diabetes mellitus.

Factors that inhibit insulin secretion include stimulation of pancreatic $alpha_2$-adrenergic receptors and stress conditions such as hypoxia, hypothermia, surgery, or severe burns.

Diabetes Mellitus

Diabetes mellitus is a chronic systemic disease characterized by metabolic and vascular abnormalities. Metabolic problems occur early in the disease process and are related to changes in the metabolism of carbohydrate, fat, and protein. A major clinical manifestation of disordered metabolism is hyperglycemia, or fasting blood glucose levels exceeding 126 milligrams per deciliter. An individual with a fasting blood glucose level between 100 and 125 milligrams per deciliter is said to have *impaired fasting glucose* (IFG) or *prediabetes*. The recommended blood glucose level for most people diagnosed with diabetes is from approximately 80 to 120 milligrams per deciliter before a meal, 180 milligrams per deciliter or less after a meal, and between 100 and 140 milligrams per deciliter at bedtime.

Vascular problems include atherosclerosis throughout the body. Macrovascular (moderate and large vessels) clinical manifestations include hypertension, myocardial infarction, stroke, and peripheral vascular disease. Changes in small blood vessels (microvasculature) especially affect the retina and kidney, resulting in retinopathy, blindness and nephropathy.

Classifications

The two major classifications are type 1 and type 2. Although both are characterized by hyperglycemia, they differ in onset, course, pathology, and treatment. Other types of diabetes may be induced by disease processes such as slowly progressing autoimmune disorders, certain drugs, and pregnancy.

Type 1

Type 1 diabetes, a common chronic disorder of childhood, results from an autoimmune disorder that destroys pancreatic beta cells. A certain subtype of type 1 diabetes mellitus, latent autoimmune diabetes of the adult (LADA), has been determined to occur with an onset during adulthood. Symptoms of traditional type 1 diabetes usually develop when 10% to 20% of functioning beta cells remain but may occur at any time if acute illness or stress increases the body's demand for insulin beyond the capacity of the remaining beta cells to secrete insulin. Eventually, all the beta cells are destroyed and no insulin is produced.

Type 1 may occur at any age but usually starts between 4 and 20 years of age. The peak incidence for girls is 10 to 12 years and for boys, 12 to 14 years. Type 1 usually has a sudden onset; produces severe symptoms; is difficult to control; produces a high incidence of complications, such as diabetic *ketoacidosis* (DKA) and renal failure; and requires administration of exogenous insulin. About 10% of people with diabetes have type 1.

Type 2

Type 2 is characterized by hyperglycemia and insulin resistance. The hyperglycemia results from increased production of glucose by the liver and decreased uptake of glucose in liver, muscle, and fat cells. Insulin resistance means that higher-than-usual concentrations of insulin are required. Thus, insulin is present but unable to work effectively (i.e., inhibits hepatic production of glucose and causes glucose to move from the bloodstream into liver, muscle, and fat cells). Most insulin resistance is attributed to impaired insulin action at the cellular level, possibly related to postreceptor, intracellular mechanisms.

Historically, the onset of type 2 diabetes occurred after 40 years of age. More recently, however, type 2 diabetes is increasing in prevalence among children and adolescents. Compared with type 1, it usually has a gradual onset, produces less severe symptoms initially, is easier to control, causes less DKA and renal failure but more myocardial infarctions and strokes, and does not necessarily require exogenous insulin because endogenous insulin is still produced. About 90% of people with diabetes have type 2; 20% to 30% of them require exogenous insulin at some point within their life time.

Type 2 is a heterogenous disease, and etiology probably involves multiple factors such as a genetic predisposition and environmental factors. Obesity is a major cause. With obesity and chronic ingestion of excess calories, along with a sedentary lifestyle, more insulin is required. The increased need leads to prolonged stimulation and eventual "fatigue" of pancreatic beta cells. As a result, the cells become less responsive to elevated blood glucose levels and less able to produce enough insulin to meet metabolic needs. Thus, insulin is secreted but is inadequate or ineffective, especially when insulin demand is increased by obesity, pregnancy, aging, or other factors.

A risk factor for the development of type 2 diabetes is the presence of the metabolic syndrome. *Metabolic syndrome* is characterized by a group of risk factors, including abdominal obesity (excessive fat tissue in and around the abdomen), hypertriglyceridemia, low HDL cholesterol, hypertension, and/ or impaired fasting glucose. People with the metabolic syndrome are at increased risk of coronary heart disease and other diseases related to plaque buildup in artery walls (e.g., stroke and peripheral vascular disease) and type 2 diabetes. The metabolic syndrome has become increasingly common in the United States. It is estimated that over 50 million Americans have it.

In the United States, African Americans, Hispanics, Native Americans, Native Alaskans, and some Asian Americans and Pacific Islanders are at high risk for development of type 2 diabetes. Prevalence rates are about 13.3% in African Americans and 13.9% in Hispanic Americans and 12.8% in American Indians and Alaska Natives compared with 8.7% in Caucasians. Undiagnosed diabetes is reportedly common in Mexican Americans.

Signs and Symptoms

Most signs and symptoms stem from a lack of effective insulin and the subsequent metabolic abnormalities. Their incidence and severity depend on the amount of effective insulin, and they may be precipitated by infection, rapid growth, pregnancy, or other factors that increase demand for insulin. Most early symptoms result from disordered carbohydrate metabolism, which causes excess glucose to accumulate in the blood (hyperglycemia). Hyperglycemia produces glucosuria, which, in turn, produces polydipsia, polyuria, dehydration, and polyphagia.

Glucosuria usually appears when the blood glucose level is approximately twice the normal value and the kidneys receive more glucose than can be reabsorbed. However, renal threshold varies, and the amount of glucose lost in the urine does not accurately reflect blood glucose. In children, glucose tends to appear in urine at much lower or even normal blood glucose levels. In older people, the kidneys may be less able to excrete excess glucose from the blood. As a result, blood glucose levels may be high with little or no glucose in the urine.

When large amounts of glucose are present, water is pulled into the renal tubule. This results in a greatly increased urine output (polyuria). The excessive loss of fluid in urine leads to increased thirst (polydipsia) and, if fluid intake is inadequate, to dehydration. Dehydration also occurs because high blood glucose levels increase osmotic pressure in the bloodstream and fluid is pulled out of the cells in the body's attempt to regain homeostasis.

Polyphagia (increased appetite) occurs because the body cannot use ingested foods. People with uncontrolled diabetes lose weight because of abnormal metabolism.

Complications

Complications of diabetes mellitus are common and potentially disabling or life threatening. Diabetes is a leading cause

Box 26-2	Acute Complications of Diabetes Mellitus

Diabetic Ketoacidosis (DKA)

This life-threatening complication occurs with severe insulin deficiency. In the absence of insulin, glucose cannot be used by body cells for energy and fat is mobilized from adipose tissue to furnish a fuel source. The mobilized fat circulates in the bloodstream, from which it is extracted by the liver and broken down into glycerol and fatty acids. The fatty acids are further changed in the liver to ketones (e.g., acetoacetic acid, acetone), which then enter the bloodstream and are circulated to body cells for metabolic conversion to energy, carbon dioxide, and water.

The ketones are produced more rapidly than body cells can use them, and their accumulation produces acidemia (a drop in blood pH and an increase in blood hydrogen ions). The body attempts to buffer the acidic hydrogen ions by exchanging them for intracellular potassium ions. Hydrogen ions enter body cells, and potassium ions leave the cells to be excreted in the urine. Another attempt to remove excess acid involves the lungs. Deep, labored respirations, called *Kussmaul's respirations*, eliminate more carbon dioxide and prevent formation of carbonic acid. A third attempt to regain homeostasis involves the kidneys, which excrete some of the ketones, thereby producing acetone in the urine.

DKA worsens as the compensatory mechanisms fail. Clinical signs and symptoms become progressively more severe. Early ones include blurred vision, anorexia, nausea and vomiting, thirst, and polyuria. Later ones include drowsiness, which progresses to stupor and coma, Kussmaul's respirations, dehydration and other signs of fluid and electrolyte imbalances, and decreased blood pressure, increased pulse, and other signs of shock.

Two major causes of DKA are omission of insulin and illnesses such as infection, trauma, myocardial infarction, or stroke.

Hyperosmolar Hyperglycemic Nonketotic Coma (HHNC)

HHNC is another type of diabetic coma that is potentially life threatening. It is relatively rare and carries a high mortality rate. The term *hyperosmolar* refers to an excessive amount of glucose, electrolytes, and other solutes in the blood in relation to the amount of water.

Like DKA, HHNC is characterized by hyperglycemia, which leads to osmotic diuresis and resultant thirst, polyuria, dehydration, and electrolyte losses, as well as neurologic signs ranging from drowsiness to stupor to coma. Additional clinical problems may include hypovolemic shock, thrombosis, renal problems, or stroke. In contrast with DKA, hyperosmolar coma occurs in people with previously unknown or mild diabetes, usually after an illness; occurs in hyperglycemic conditions other than diabetes (e.g., severe burns, corticosteroid drug therapy); and does not cause ketosis.

---

of myocardial infarction, stroke, blindness, leg amputation, and kidney failure. These complications result from hyperglycemia and other metabolic abnormalities that accompany a lack of effective insulin. The metabolic abnormalities associated with hyperglycemia can cause early, acute complications, such as DKA or hyperosmolar hyperglycemic nonketotic coma (HHNC; Box 26-2). Eventually, metabolic abnormalities lead to damage in blood vessels and other body tissues. For example, atherosclerosis develops earlier, progresses more rapidly, and becomes more severe in people with diabetes. Microvascular changes lead to nephropathy, retinopathy, and peripheral neuropathy. Other complications include musculoskeletal disorders, increased numbers and severity of infections, and complications of pregnancy.

Hypoglycemic Drugs

Insulin

Insulin is described in this section, and individual insulins are listed in Table 26-1.

Exogenous insulin used to replace endogenous insulin has the same effects as the pancreatic hormone. Insulin and its analogs (structurally similar chemicals) lower blood glucose levels by increasing glucose uptake by body cells, especially skeletal muscle and fat cells, and by decreasing glucose production in the liver.

The main clinical indication for insulin is treatment of diabetes mellitus. Insulin is the only effective drug treatment for type 1 diabetes because pancreatic beta cells are unable to secrete endogenous insulin and metabolism is severely impaired. Insulin is required for patients with type 2 diabetes who cannot control their disease with diet, weight control, and oral agents. It may be needed by anyone with diabetes during times of stress, such as illness, infection, or surgery. Insulin also is used to control diabetes induced by chronic pancreatitis, surgical excision of pancreatic tissue, hormones and other drugs, and pregnancy (gestational diabetes). In nondiabetic patients, insulin is used to prevent or treat hyperglycemia induced by IV parenteral nutrition and to treat hyperkalemia. In hyperkalemia, an IV infusion of insulin and dextrose solution causes potassium to move from the blood into the cells; it does not eliminate potassium from the body. The only clear-cut contraindication to the use of insulin is hypoglycemia, because of the risk of brain damage (Box 26-3).

All insulin in the United States is human insulin. Pork and bovine insulins, which were more antigenic, are no longer manufactured in the United States. The name human insulin means that the synthetic product is identical to endogenous insulin (i.e., has the same number and sequence of amino acids).

Table 26-1		Drugs at a Glance: Insulins

Generic/Trade Name	Characteristics	Routes and Dosage Ranges	Onset	Peak	Duration
			ACTION (H)		
Short-Acting Insulin					
Insulin injection (Humulin R, Novolin R)	■ A clear liquid solution with the appearance of water ■ The hypoglycemic drug of choice for diabetic patients experiencing acute or emergency situations, diabetic ketoacidosis, hyperosmolar nonketotic coma, severe infections or other illnesses, major surgery, and pregnancy ■ The only insulin preparation that can be given IV	Sub-Q, dosage individualized according to blood glucose levels. For sliding scale, 5–20 units before meals and bedtime, depending on blood glucose levels IV, dosage individualized. For ketoacidosis, regular insulin may be given by direct injection, intermittent infusion, or continuous infusion. One regimen involves an initial bolus injection of 10–20 units followed by a continuous low-dose infusion of 2–10 units/h, based on hourly blood and urine glucose levels.	$^1/_2$–1	2–3	5–7
Intermediate-Acting Insulins					
Isophane insulin suspension (NPH, Humulin N, Novolin N)	■ Commonly used for long-term administration ■ Modified by addition of protamine (a protein) and zinc ■ A suspension with a cloudy appearance when correctly mixed in the drug vial ■ Given *only* Sub-Q ■ Not recommended for use in acute situations ■ Hypoglycemic reactions are more likely to occur during mid to late afternoon	Sub-Q, dosage individualized. Initially, 7–26 units may be given once or twice daily.	1–1$^1/_2$	8–12	18–24
Insulin Mixtures					
NPH 70% **Regular 30%** (Humulin 70/30, Novolin 70/30)	■ Stable mixture ■ Onset, peak, and duration of action same as individual components	Sub-Q, dosage individualized			
NPH 50% **Regular 50%** (Humulin 50/50)	See Humulin 70/30, above	Sub-Q, dosage individualized			
Insulin Analogs					
Insulin lispro (Humalog)	■ A synthetic insulin of recombinant DNA origin, created by reversing two amino acids ■ Has a faster onset and a shorter duration of action than human regular insulin ■ Intended for use with a longer-acting insulin	Sub-Q, dosage individualized, 15 min before meals. May also be given in external insulin pumps	$^1/_4$	$^1/_2$–1$^1/_2$	6–8

(continued on page 416)

Table 26-1		Drugs at a Glance: Insulins (continued)			
				ACTION (H)	
Generic/Trade Name	**Characteristics**	**Routes and Dosage Ranges**	**Onset**	**Peak**	**Duration**
Insulin aspart (NovoLog)	Similar to lispro	Sub-Q, dosage individualized	$^1/_4$	1–3	3–5
Insulin glargine (Lantus)	▪ Long acting ▪ Provides basal amount of insulin ▪ Must *not* be diluted or mixed with any other insulin or solutions	Sub-Q, dosage individualized, once daily at bedtime	1.1	None	24
Insulin glulisine (Apidra)	▪ Clear, colorless solution ▪ More rapid onset of action and shorter duration of action than regular human insulin ▪ Should be used in regimens that include a longer-acting insulin or basal insulin analog ▪ May be mixed with NPH insulin for injection only. Draw up Apidra first, then NPH insulin. Do NOT mix Apidra with other insulins in Sub-Q infusion pumps.	Sub-Q by injection or continuous infusion pump, dosage individualized When used as a mealtime insulin, give up to 15 min before or within 20 min of beginning the meal.	$^1/_{12}$–$^1/_6$ (5–10 min)	1	4
Insulin levemir (Determir)	▪ Long acting ▪ Provides basal amount of insulin ▪ Must not be diluted or mixed with other insulins	Sub-Q once or twice daily, dosage individualized	1	None	6–23
Analog Mixture **Insulin lispro protamine 75%** **Insulin lispro 25%** (Humalog Mix 75/25)	▪ Same onset, peak, and duration as individual components	Sub-Q, dosage individualized			

NPH, isophane.

Insulin analogs are synthesized in the laboratory by altering the type or sequence of amino acids in insulin molecules. Insulin lispro (Humalog), insulin aspart (NovoLog), and insulin glulisine (Apidra) are short-acting products. Lispro, the first analog to be marketed, is identical to human insulin except for the reversal of two amino acids (lysine and proline). It is absorbed more rapidly and has a shorter half-life after subcutaneous (Sub-Q) injection than regular (short-acting) human insulin. As a result, it is similar to physiologic insulin secretion after a meal, more effective at decreasing postprandial hyperglycemia, and less likely to cause hypoglycemia before the next meal. Injection just before a meal produces hypoglycemic effects similar to those of an injection of conventional regular insulin given 30 minutes before a meal. Aspart has an even more rapid onset and shorter duration of action. The newest short-acting insulin analog, glulisine, has

the shortest onset time (5–10 minutes). In contrast, insulin glargine and insulin detemir are long-acting preparations used to provide a basal amount of insulin through 24 hours, similar to normal, endogenous insulin secretion.

Insulin cannot be given orally because it is a protein that is destroyed by proteolytic enzymes in the GI tract. Most insulins are given subcutaneously; regular insulin can also be administered intravenously.

Insulins differ in onset and duration of action. They are usually categorized as short, intermediate, or long acting. Short-acting insulins have a rapid onset and a short duration of action. Intermediate- and long-acting insulins (except for insulin glargine or detemir) are modified by adding protamine (a large, insoluble protein), zinc, or both to slow absorption and prolong drug action. Several mixtures of an intermediate- and a short-acting insulin are available and commonly used. U-100,

Box 26-3	Hypoglycemia: Characteristics and Management

Hypoglycemia may occur with insulin, meglitinides, oral sulfonylureas, amylin analogs (pramlintide [Symlin]), and incretin mimetics (exenatide [Byetta]). When hypoglycemia is suspected, the blood glucose level should be measured if possible, although signs and symptoms and the plasma glucose level at which they occur vary from person to person. Hypoglycemia is a blood glucose below 60 to 70 mg/dL and is especially dangerous at approximately 40 mg/dL or below. Central nervous system effects may lead to accidental injury or permanent brain damage; cardiovascular effects may lead to cardiac dysrhythmias or myocardial infarction. Causes of hypoglycemia include:

- Intensive insulin therapy (i.e., continuous subcutaneous [Sub-Q] infusion or three or more injections daily)
- Omitting or delaying meals
- An excessive or incorrect dose of insulin or an oral agent that causes hypoglycemia
- Altered sensitivity to insulin
- Decreased clearance of insulin or an oral agent (e.g., with renal insufficiency)
- Decreased glucose intake
- Decreased production of glucose in the liver
- Giving an insulin injection intramuscularly (IM) rather than Sub-Q
- Drug interactions that decrease blood glucose levels
- Increased physical exertion
- Ethanol ingestion

Hormones That Raise Blood Sugar

Normally, when hypoglycemia occurs, several hormones (glucagon, epinephrine, growth hormone, and cortisol) work to restore and maintain blood glucose levels. Glucagon and epinephrine, the dominant counter-regulatory hormones, act rapidly because they are activated as soon as blood glucose levels start declining. Growth hormone and cortisol act more slowly, about 2 hours after hypoglycemia occurs.

People with diabetes who develop hypoglycemia may have impaired secretion of these hormones, especially those patients with type 1 diabetes. Decreased secretion of glucagon is often evident in patients who have had diabetes for 5 years or longer. Decreased secretion of epinephrine also occurs in people who have been treated with insulin for several years. Decreased epinephrine decreases tachycardia, a common sign of hypoglycemia, and may delay recognition and treatment.

The Conscious Patient

Treatment of hypoglycemic reactions consists of immediate administration of a rapidly absorbed carbohydrate. For the conscious patient who is able to swallow, the carbohydrate is given orally. Foods and fluids that provide approximately 15 grams of carbohydrate include:

- Two sugar cubes or 1 to 2 teaspoons of sugar, syrup, honey, or jelly
- Two or three small pieces of candy or eight Lifesaver candies
- 4 oz of fruit juice, such as orange, apple, or grape

- 4 oz of ginger ale
- Coffee or tea with 2 teaspoons of sugar added
- Commercial glucose products (e.g., Glutose, B-D Glucose). These products must be swallowed to be effective.

Symptoms usually subside within 15 to 20 minutes. If they do not subside, the patient should take another 10 to 15 grams of oral carbohydrate. *If acarbose or miglitol has been taken with insulin or a sulfonylurea and a hypoglycemic reaction occurs, glucose (oral or intravenous [IV]) or glucagon must be given for treatment.* Sucrose (table sugar) and other oral carbohydrates do not relieve hypoglycemia because the presence of acarbose or miglitol prevents their digestion and absorption from the gastrointestinal tract.

The Unconscious Patient

For the unconscious patient, carbohydrate cannot be given orally because of the risks of aspiration. Therefore, the treatment choices are parenteral glucose or glucagon.

If the patient is in a health care facility where medical help is readily available, IV glucose in a 25% or 50% solution is the treatment of choice. It acts rapidly to raise blood glucose levels and arouse the patient. If the patient is at home or elsewhere, glucagon may be given if available and there is someone to inject it. A family member or roommate may be taught to give glucagon Sub-Q or IM. It can also be given IV. The usual adult dose is 0.5 to 1 milligram. Glucagon is a pancreatic hormone that increases blood sugar by converting liver glycogen to glucose. It is effective only when liver glycogen is present. Some clients cannot respond to glucagon because glycogen stores are depleted by conditions such as starvation, adrenal insufficiency, or chronic hypoglycemia. The hyperglycemic effect of glucagon occurs more slowly than that of IV glucose and is of relatively brief duration. If the patient does not respond to one or two doses of glucagon within 20 minutes, IV glucose is indicated.

Avoid Overtreatment

Caution is needed in the treatment of hypoglycemia. Although the main goal of treatment is to relieve hypoglycemia and restore the brain's supply of glucose, a secondary goal is to avoid overtreatment and excessive hyperglycemia. The patient having a hypoglycemic reaction should not use it as an excuse to eat high-caloric foods or large amounts of food. Health care personnel caring for the patient should avoid giving excessive amounts of glucose.

Posthypoglycemia Care

Once hypoglycemia is relieved, the person should have a snack or a meal. Slowly absorbed carbohydrate and protein foods, such as milk, cheese, and bread, are needed to replace glycogen stores in the liver and to prevent secondary hypoglycemia from rapid use of the carbohydrates given earlier. In addition, the episode needs to be evaluated for precipitating factors so that these can be minimized to prevent future episodes. Repeated episodes mean that the therapeutic regimen and patient compliance must be re-evaluated and adjusted if indicated.

the main insulin concentration in the United States, contains 100 units of insulin per milliliter of solution. It can be accurately measured only in an orange-tipped syringe designed for use with U-100 insulin.

With subcutaneous injection, insulin is absorbed most rapidly from the abdomen, followed by the upper arm, thigh, and buttocks. Absorption is delayed or decreased by injection into Sub-Q tissue with lipodystrophy or other lesions, by circulatory problems such as edema or hypotension, by insulin-binding antibodies (which develop after 2 or 3 months of insulin administration), and by injecting cold (i.e., refrigerated) insulin. Absorption may also be increased when administered in an extremity before the patient engages in a sport that requires use of the specific extremity (i.e., swimming, tennis, or jogging).

Temperature extremes can cause loss of potency. Insulin retains potency up to 36 months under refrigeration and 18 to 24 months at room temperature. At high temperatures (e.g., 100°F or 37.8°C), insulin loses potency in about 2 months. If frozen, insulin clumps or precipitates, cannot be measured accurately, and should be discarded.

Regular insulin and rapid-acting insulin analogs (Lispro, Aspart, Apidra) are appropriate insulins for continuous Sub-Q insulin infusion using external insulin pumps (Fig. 26-2). An insulin pump is a device that delivers a continuous supply of insulin. The pump is often programmed to deliver small steady doses of insulin throughout the day. This steady dosage is known as a basal rate. Additional doses, called boluses, are given to cover food or high blood glucose levels. The pump holds a reservoir of insulin that is delivered through a system of plastic tubing (infusion set). Most infusion sets are started with a guide needle, then the plastic cannula (a tiny, flexible tube) is left in place, taped with a dressing, and the needle is removed. Advantages of this method of insulin delivery include improved lifestyle flexibility and better control of blood glucose levels. Disadvantages include undetected interruptions in insulin delivery, resulting in the development of hyperglycemia and ketosis, and infection at the needle site. Hypoglycemia can also occur in pump users as with those administering insulin via Sub-Q injection. Insulin mixtures and intermediate-/long-acting insulins are not approved for use in continuous Sub-Q infusion pumps.

An inhaled insulin (Exubera) was approved by the Food and Drug Administration (FDA) in January 2006 for patients aged 18 or older with type 1 or type 2 diabetes and was used in combination with injections of intermediate- or long-acting insulin, with oral antidiabetic drugs, or alone with dietary changes. However, by October 2007, the drug manufacturer made a decision to cease production of Exubera, citing too few patients using inhaled insulin and the availability of other medications to lower blood sugar as reasons for discontinuing production. Patient concerns with Exubera included the large inhalation device (roughly the size of a flashlight), difficulty adjusting the dosage, cost, and the risk of lung disorders. Post marketing studies also identified concerns over increased risk of lung cancer, although the study results were confounded by previous use of tobacco. Currently, there are no FDA-approved inhaled insulins available; however, several drug manufacturers are working to develop new forms of insulin delivery, including mouth sprays, insulin patches, and inhalers.

Applying Your Knowledge 26-1

The main adverse effect of insulin 70/30 is hypoglycemia. At what time during a 24-hour period should you be especially alert to assess for the effects of hypoglycemia in Mr. Coulter?

Oral Hypoglycemic Medications

There are five types of oral antidiabetic agents, all of which may be used to treat type 2 diabetes when diet and exercise

Figure 26-2 ■ Continuous subcutaneous (Sub-Q) insulin infusion pump. The insulin dosage is programmed into the pump's computer and the appropriate amount of insulin is injected into the adipose tissue through a needle inserted into the Sub-Q area.

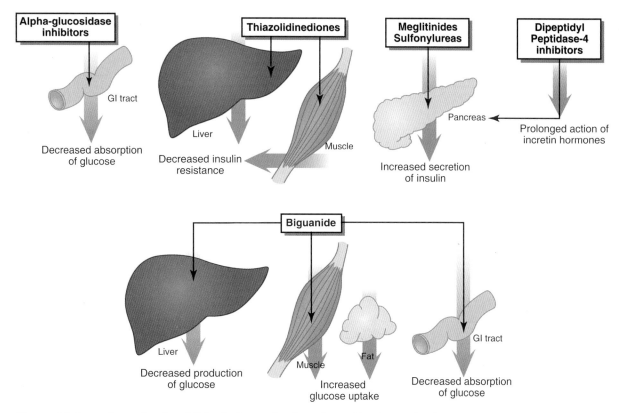

Figure 26-3 ■ Actions of oral antidiabetic drugs. The drugs lower blood sugar by decreasing absorption or production of glucose, by increasing secretion of insulin, or by increasing the effectiveness of available insulin (decreasing insulin resistance).

alone fail to control the disorder. The drugs lower blood sugar by different mechanisms (Fig. 26-3) and may be used in various combinations for additive effects. Some are also combined with insulin. These drugs are further described below and in Table 26-2.

Sulfonylureas

The sulfonylureas are the oldest and largest group of oral agents. They lower blood glucose mainly by increasing secretion of insulin. They may also increase peripheral use of glucose, decrease production of glucose in the liver, increase the number of insulin receptors, or alter postreceptor actions to increase tissue responsiveness to insulin. Because the drugs stimulate pancreatic beta cells to produce more insulin, they are effective only when functioning pancreatic beta cells are present.

First-generation drugs (e.g., acetohexamide, chlorpropamide, tolazamide, tolbutamide) have largely been replaced by the second generation and are not discussed further. The second-generation drugs, glipizide, glyburide, and glimepiride, are similar in therapeutic and adverse effects. The main adverse effect is hypoglycemia (see Box 26-3).

The sulfonylureas are chemically related to sulfonamide antibacterial drugs, well absorbed with oral administration, more than 90% bound to plasma proteins, and metabolized in the liver to inactive metabolites, which are excreted mainly by the kidneys (except for glyburide, which is excreted about equally in urine and bile). Therefore, this category of medications is contraindicated among patients with previous allergic sensitivities to sulfa-based medications.

A sulfonylurea may be given alone or with most other antidiabetic drugs in the treatment of type 2 diabetes, including insulin, acarbose, miglitol, metformin, pioglitazone, or rosiglitazone. Sulfonylureas are contraindicated in patients with hypersensitivity to them, with severe renal or hepatic impairment, and during pregnancy. They are unlikely to be effective during periods of stress, such as major surgery, severe illness, or infection. Insulin is usually required in these circumstances.

Alpha-Glucosidase Inhibitors

Acarbose and miglitol inhibit alpha-glucosidase enzymes (e.g., sucrase, maltase, amylase) in the GI tract and thereby delay digestion of complex carbohydrates into glucose and other simple sugars. As a result, glucose absorption is delayed and there is a smaller increase in blood glucose levels after a meal. The drugs are metabolized in the GI tract by digestive enzymes and intestinal bacteria. Some of the metabolites are absorbed systemically and excreted in urine; plasma concentrations are increased in the presence of renal impairment. An alpha-glucosidase inhibitor may be combined with insulin or an oral agent, usually a sulfonylurea. Alpha-glucosidase inhibitors are contraindicated in patients with hypersensitivity, DKA, hepatic cirrhosis, inflammatory or malabsorptive intestinal disorders, and severe renal impairment.

Table 26-2	Drugs at a Glance: Oral Drugs for Diabetes Mellitus	

GENERIC/TRADE NAME	CHARACTERISTICS	ROUTES AND DOSAGE RANGES
Sulfonylureas, Second Generation		
Glimepiride (Amaryl)	Onset of action, about 1 h; peak, 2–3 h	PO, initially 1–2 mg once daily, with breakfast or first main meal. Maximum starting dose, 2 mg or less. Maintenance dose, 1–4 mg once daily. After a dose of 2 mg is reached, increase dose in increments of 2 mg or less at 1- to 2-week intervals, based on blood glucose levels. Maximum recommended dose, 8 mg once daily In combination with insulin, PO 8 mg once daily with first main meal
Glipizide (Glucotrol, Glucotrol XL)	Onset of action, approximately 1–1.5 h; duration, 10–16 h	PO, initially 5 mg daily in a single dose, 30 min before breakfast Maximum dose, 40 mg daily In elderly, may start with 2.5 mg daily Extended-release: Give once daily with breakfast.
Glyburide (DiaBeta, Micronase, Glynase Pres Tab)	Onset of action, approximately 2–4 h; duration, 24 h. Glynase is better absorbed, acts faster (onset, about 1 h; duration, 24 h), and is given in smaller doses than other forms of glyburide.	PO, initially 2.5–5 mg daily in a single dose, with breakfast Maximum dose, 20 mg daily Glynase: PO, initially 1.5–3 mg daily with breakfast. Maximum dose, 12 mg daily
Alpha-Glucosidase Inhibitors		
Acarbose (Precose)	Delays digestion of carbohydrate foods when acarbose and food are present in GI tract at the same time	PO, initially 25 mg, 3 times daily with first bite of main meals; increase at 4- to 8-week intervals to a maximum dose of 50 mg 3 times daily (for patients weighing under 60 kg) if necessary, depending on 1-h postprandial blood glucose levels and tolerance. Patients weighing more than 60 kg may need doses up to 100 mg 3 times daily (the maximum dose).
Miglitol (Glyset)	Delays digestion of carbohydrates in the GI tract	PO, initially 25 mg 3 times daily with the first bite of each main meal, gradually increased if necessary Maximum dose, 100 mg 3 times daily
Biguanide		
Metformin (Glucophage, Glucophage XR))	Older adults are at higher risk for development of lactic acidosis, a rare but potentially fatal reaction. Thus, smaller doses and monitoring of renal function are recommended.	PO, initially 500 mg twice daily, with morning and evening meals; increase dose in increments of 500 mg/d every 2–3 wk if necessary, up to a maximum of 3000 mg daily, based on patient tolerance and blood glucose levels. In older patients, do not increase to maximum dose. Extended-release: PO once daily with the evening meal.
Glitazones		
Pioglitazone (Actos)	Increases effects of insulin; may be used alone or with insulin, metformin, or a sulfonylurea	PO 15–30 mg once daily

GENERIC/TRADE NAME	CHARACTERISTICS	ROUTES AND DOSAGE RANGES
Rosiglitazone (Avandia)	Increases effects of insulin; may be used alone or with metformin	PO 4–8 mg once daily, in 1 dose or 2 divided doses
Meglitinides		
Nateglinide (Starlix)	▪ Onset of action, within 20 min; peak, 1 h; duration, 3–4 h	PO 120 mg 3 times daily, 1–30 min before meals. Omit dose if skip a meal.
Repaglinide (Prandin)	▪ Onset of action, within 30 min; peak, 1 h; duration, approximately 3–4 h	PO 1–2 mg 15–30 min before each meal, increased to 4 mg before meals if necessary. Maximum dose, 16 mg daily. Omit a dose if skip a meal; add a dose if add a meal.
Combination Drugs*		
Glyburide/metformin (Glucovance)	▪ Available in preparations containing 1.25 mg glyburide and 250 mg metformin; 2.5 mg glyburide and 500 mg metformin; or 5 mg glyburide and 500 mg metformin	Initially, PO 1.25 mg/250 mg once or twice daily with meals. *Patients previously treated with glyburide or other sulfonylurea plus metformin:* Initially, PO 2.5 or 5 mg/500 mg twice daily with meals, not to exceed previous doses of separate drugs
Metformin/glipizide (Metaglip)	▪ Available as tablets containing metformin 250 or 500 mg and glipizide 2.5 or 5 mg	PO 2.5/250 mg once daily, increased if necessary
Rosiglitazone/metformin (Avandamet)	▪ Available in tablets containing 1, 2, or 4 mg rosiglitazone and 500 mg metformin and 2 or 4 mg rosiglitazone and 1000 mg metformin	PO, variable dose; maximum daily dose, 8 mg rosiglitazone and 2000 mg metformin
Pioglitazone/metformin (Acto Plus Met)	▪ Available as tablets containing pioglitazone 15 mg plus metformin 500 or 850 mg	PO, variable dose; maximum dose for pioglitazone is 45 mg daily and maximum dose for metformin is 2550 mg daily.
Pioglitazone/glimepiride (Duetact)	▪ Available as pioglitazone 30 mg plus glimepiride 2 mg or 4 mg.	PO, variable dose; maximum dose for pioglitazone is 45 mg daily and maximum dose for glimepiride is 8 mg daily.
Rosiglitazone/glimepiride (Avandaryl)	▪ Available as rosiglitazone 4 mg plus 1 mg, 2 mg or 4 mg glimepiride	PO, variable dose; maximum dose for rosiglitazone is 8 mg daily, maximum dose for glimepiride is 8 mg daily.
Sitagliptin/metformin (Janumet)	▪ Available as sitagliptin 100 mg plus metformin 1000 mg or 2000 mg	PO, variable dose; maximum dose for sitagliptin is 100 mg, maximum dose for metformin is 2000 mg.

*See Appendix A for additional combination drugs. GI, gastrointestinal

Biguanide

Metformin increases the use of glucose by muscle and fat cells, decreases hepatic glucose production, and decreases intestinal absorption of glucose. It is preferably called an antihyperglycemic rather than a hypoglycemic agent because it does not cause hypoglycemia, even in large doses, when used alone. Metformin is absorbed from the small intestine, circulates without binding to plasma proteins, and has a serum half-life of 1.3 to 4.5 hours. It is not metabolized in the liver and is excreted unchanged in the urine.

Metformin may be used alone or in combination with insulin or other oral agents. It is widely prescribed as the initial drug in obese patients with newly diagnosed type 2 diabetes, mainly because it does not cause weight gain as most other oral agents do. Metformin is considered to be weight neutral and ideal for overweight individuals with type 2 diabetes, who have been known to lose weight on this medication, further improving insulin sensitivity.

Metformin is contraindicated in patients with diabetes complicated by fever, severe infections, severe trauma, major surgery, acidosis, or pregnancy (insulin is indicated in these conditions). It is also contraindicated in patients with serious hepatic or renal impairment, cardiac or respiratory insufficiency, hypoxia, or a history of lactic acidosis because these conditions may increase production of lactate and the risk of potentially fatal lactic acidosis. A **BLACK BOX WARNING** alerts nurses to the dangers of lactic acidosis with metformin therapy in these individuals.

Thiazolidinediones (TZDs)

Thiazolidinediones include pioglitazone and rosiglitazone. They are sometimes called "glitazones" and are also referred to as insulin sensitizers. Thiazolidinediones decrease insulin resistance, a major factor in the pathophysiology of type 2 diabetes. The drugs stimulate receptors on muscle, fat, and liver cells. This stimulation increases or restores the effectiveness of circulating insulin and results in increased uptake of glucose by peripheral tissues and decreased production of glucose by the liver. Thiazolidinediones may be used as monotherapy with diet and exercise or in combination with insulin, metformin, a sulfonylurea, an amylin analog (pramlintide), or incretin mimetic (exenatide).

The drugs are contraindicated in patients with active liver disease or a serum alanine aminotransferase (ALT) level more than 2.5 times the upper limit of normal. They are also contraindicated in patients who are hypersensitive to them. The drugs should be used very cautiously, if at all, in patients at risk of developing congestive heart failure. Thiazolidinediones increase plasma volume and may cause fluid retention and heart failure. In one study, heart failure developed in 4.5% of glitazone users within 10 months and in 12.4% of users within 36 months. In people who did not take a thiazolidinedione, 2.6% developed heart failure within 10 months and 8.4% within 36 months. A **BLACK BOX WARNING** alerts health professionals to the risk of CHF in patients using pioglitazone and rosiglitazone. Furthermore, recent meta-analysis of several studies and clinical trials have raised concerns about increased risk of myocardial ischemic events including angina, myocardial infarction (heart attack), and heart-related deaths with rosiglitazone, prompting the FDA to issue an additional **BLACK BOX WARNING** regarding myocardial ischemia for this drug.

Meglitinides

Nateglinide and repaglinide are nonsulfonylureas that lower blood sugar by stimulating pancreatic secretion of insulin. They can be used as monotherapy with diet and exercise or in combination with metformin. These drugs should be taken just before or up to 30 minutes before a meal. If a meal is skipped, the drug dose should be skipped; if a meal is added, a drug dose should be added.

Meglitinides are well absorbed from the GI tract; peak plasma level occurs within 1 hour. They have a plasma half-life of 1 to 1.5 hours and are highly bound (>98%) to plasma proteins. They are metabolized in the liver; metabolites are excreted in urine and feces. Repaglinide is metabolized and removed from the bloodstream within 3 to 4 hours after a dose, nateglinide within about 6 hours. This decreases the workload of pancreatic beta cells (i.e., decreases duration of beta-cell stimulation), allows serum insulin levels to return to normal before the next meal, and decreases risks of hypoglycemic episodes.

New Types of Antidiabetic Drugs

There are several new classes of antidiabetic drugs that can be co-administered with traditional therapies to achieve better blood glucose control. Amylin analogs, incretin mimetics, and dipeptidyl peptidase-4 inhibitors are described below and in Table 26-3.

Table 26-3	Drugs at a Glance: New Antidiabetic Drugs	
GENERIC/TRADE NAME	**CHARACTERISTICS**	**ROUTES AND DOSAGE RANGES**
Amylin Analog **Pramlintide** (Symlin)	Given with insulin at mealtimes for type 1 and type 2 diabetes	Type 1: Sub-Q 15 mcg initially, titrate in 15-mcg increments to maintenance dose of 30–60 mcg. Preprandial short-acting insulins should be reduced by 50%. Type 2: Sub-Q 60 mcg initially, may increase to 120 mcg as tolerated. Preprandial short-acting insulins should be reduced by 50%.
Incretin Mimetic **Exenatide** (Byetta)	Given with metformin and/or a sulfonylurea for patients with type 2 diabetes to improve glucose control	Sub-Q 5 mcg twice daily before morning and evening meal. May be increased to 10 mcg twice daily if needed. No dosage adjustment required for concurrent metformin. Reduction of sulfonylurea dosage may be needed to prevent hypoglycemia.
Dipeptidyl peptidase-4 **(DPP-4) Inhibitor** **Sitagliptin** (Januvia)	Given alone or with metformin and/or thiazolidinediones for patients with type 2 diabetes to improve glucose control	PO 100 mg daily

Amylin Analog

Pramlintide (Symlin), a synthetic analog of amylin, is a peptide hormone secreted with insulin by the beta cells of the pancreas, important in the regulation of glucose control during the postprandial period. It is used as an adjunctive treatment with mealtime insulin for adult patients with type 1 or type 2 diabetes who have not achieved optimal glucose control with insulin therapy alone. Pramlintide slows gastric emptying, helping to regulate the postprandial rise in blood glucose. The drug also suppresses postprandial glucagon secretion, thus helping maintain better blood glucose control. Pramlintide increases the sense of satiety, possibly reducing food intake and promoting weight loss. Pramlintide and insulin therapy may be combined with metformin or sulfonylureas for patients with type 2 diabetes.

Pramlintide is given by subcutaneous injection before meals. Opened vials of pramlintide may be stored in a refrigerator or at room temperature for up to 28 days. It cannot be mixed in the same injection with mealtime insulin. Reduction in insulin dosages by 50% is required with initiation of pramlintide therapy to reduce the incidence of hypoglycemia. A **BLACK BOX WARNING** alerts nurses to the danger of severe insulin-induced hypoglycemia with pramlintide therapy, especially in type 1 diabetics. Nausea, another frequent adverse effect of pramlintide, tends to decrease with time and may be reduced with careful titration of the dosage to the therapeutic level. Pramlintide may delay the absorption of concurrently administered oral medications.

Incretin mimetic

Before starting a patient with type 2 diabetes on insulin, the provider should consider a new option for treatment of diabetes. Exenatide (Byetta), a synthetic GLP-1 analogue, is now used when oral medications, diet, and exercise together have not assisted in reaching the target A1C goal. Exenatide is administered subcutaneously twice a day and has been approved to be administered with oral medications such as sulfonylureas, metformin, and/or thiazolidinediones. Major advantages of exenatide over insulin are increased satiety and weight loss.

Exenatide acts as a natural helper hormone by stimulating the pancreas to secrete the right amount of insulin based on the food that was just eaten. This helps to reduce the problem of high blood glucose after meals. Exenatide also halts gluconeogenesis by the liver, keeping it from making too much glucose after a meal. Exenatide slows gastric emptying, which serves to reduce the sudden rise of blood glucose after a meal, and also quickly stimulates a feeling of satiety when eating. This fosters a sense of fullness which causes the patient to eat less and potentially lose weigh. Exenatide may reduce the absorption of concurrently administered oral medications.

Exenatide is available via a prefilled injection pen in two doses (5 or 10 mcg) and does not need to be adjusted base on blood glucose levels or the amount of food a patient was able to consume. The drug should be taken twice a day within 60 minutes of the morning and evening meal (at least 6 or more hours apart). Exenatide can be injected into the subcutaneous

Evidence-Based Practice

26-1 Use of Alternative Medicines in Diabetes Mellitus

It is well documented in the literature that a significant number of individuals with diabetes mellitus use complementary and alternative medicine (CAM). CAM includes acupuncture, relaxation techniques, massage, chiropractic, spiritual healing, herbal medicines, and vitamin supplements. Estimates of CAM use by patients with diabetes range as high as 57% in the literature and are comparable with CAM use by nondiabetic individuals. Studies reveal that generally diabetics use the same supplements and alternative remedies as nondiabetic individuals with the exception of increased use of chromium. The literature documents that some patients use CAM to lower blood glucose as well as to treat complications of diabetes; however, the majority of individuals report using CAM for a condition unrelated to diabetes. The use of CAM by diabetics raises several concerns. One obvious concern is the implications of using CAM in replacement of traditional therapies for diabetes such as insulin and oral hypoglycemic drugs; however, one study in the literature suggested that most diabetic patients use CAM in addition to traditional therapies rather than as a replacement for traditional medications. Another study documented that diabetic patients using CAM were more likely to also use preventive care practices such as obtaining a pneumococcal vaccination and visiting their health care provider on a regular basis. A second concern is the potential of CAM to do harm. With regard to herbal and vitamin supplements, harmful effects include potential interactions with traditional drugs as well as increased risk for hepatotoxicity, nephrotoxicity, and poor glycemic control. A third concern is the cost of CAM; one study reported that diabetics using CAM spend as much on the alternative therapies as they do on prescription drugs.

Because the use of CAM is widespread and has the potential for impacting blood glucose levels of diabetic patients, nurses should take careful drug histories, including questions about use of herbal and over-the-counter supplements. Nurses should also educate diabetic patients about the potential impact of complementary therapies on blood glucose levels when this information is available.

tissue of the upper arm or leg and the abdomen areas. It should be stored at all times in the original packaging in a refrigerator at 36 to 46°F, protected from light, kept dry, and discarded once opened after 30 days.

Major side effects of exenatide are GI distress and nauseas. Many patients experience nausea at first but should be encouraged to continue the medication if at all possible as nausea usually subsides and converts into a feeling of fullness. A rare but serious side effect is the development of acute pancreatitis. Patients should be taught to report unusual abdominal discomfort to their health care provider.

Dipeptidyl peptidase-4 (DPP-4) Inhibitors

Glucagon-like peptide-1 (GLP-1) has been known for some time to have an antidiabetic action via its ability to stimulate insulin secretion Recent advances have overcome the problems associated with short half-life and inactivation of the incretin hormone. A new medication, sitagliptin (Januvia), has been released that solves this problem. Januvia is a DPP-4 enzyme inhibitor, which results in a longer circulating half-life of GLP-1. Januvia has been found to not only balance the release of insulin and limit the release of additional glucose from the liver, it has also has been linked to increased beta cell neogenesis, inhibition of beta cell apoptosis, inhibition of glucagon secretion, delayed gastric emptying, and induction of satiety.

Sitagliptin is indicated solely for patients with type 2 diabetes mellitus in addition to exercise and proper diet. It is administered in the morning with or without food and comes in 25-, 50-, and 100-milligram doses. Common side effects of sitagliptin are upper respiratory tract infection, stuffy or runny nose, sore throat, and headache

Sitagliptin is contraindicated in patients with type 1 diabetes mellitus, patients receiving insulin, or patients who commonly produce ketones in their urine. Sitagliptin is *only* approved to be used alone or in combination with metformin and/or thiazolidinediones. It is to be strictly avoided with medications know to cause hypoglycemia (i.e., sulfonylureas or insulin). It is also contraindicated in ESRD, and dose adjustments are to be made in earlier stages of chronic kidney diseases.

Herbal and Dietary Supplements

Increasing numbers of people are choosing alternative medications to complement or, in some cases, to replace prescription medications. With most herbs and dietary supplements, even the commonly used ones (e.g., echinacea, St. John's wort), the effects on blood glucose levels are unknown; well-controlled, long-term studies of effects have not been done; and interactions with antidiabetic drugs are unknown. Thus, anyone with diabetes who wishes to take an herbal or dietary supplement should consult a health care provider, read product labels carefully, seek the most authoritative information available, and monitor blood glucose closely when starting the supplement. Described below are some products that reportedly affect blood sugar and that should be used cautiously, if at all, by patients with diabetes.

Supplements That May Increase Blood Glucose Levels

Bee pollen may cause hyperglycemia and decrease the effects of antidiabetic medications. It should not be used by people with diabetes.

Ginkgo biloba extract is thought to increase blood sugar in patients with diabetes by increasing hepatic metabolism of insulin and oral hypoglycemic drugs, thereby making the drugs less effective. It is not recommended for use.

Glucosamine, as indicated by animal studies, may cause impaired beta-cell function and insulin secretion similar to that observed in humans with type 2 diabetes. Long-term effects in humans are unknown, but the product is considered potentially harmful to people with diabetes or prediabetes. Adverse effects on blood sugar and drug interactions with

antidiabetic medications have not been reported. However, blood sugar should be monitored carefully. With chondroitin, which is often taken with glucosamine for osteoarthritis, there is no information about effects on blood sugar, use by diabetic patients, or interactions with antidiabetic drugs.

Supplements That May Decrease Blood Glucose Levels

Basil, which is commonly used in cooking, is also available as an herbal supplement. The amounts used in cooking are unlikely to affect blood sugar, but larger amounts may cause hypoglycemia or increase the hypoglycemic effects of insulin and oral antidiabetic drugs. The use of supplemental amounts should probably be avoided by people with diabetes. If used, blood glucose levels should be closely monitored.

Bay leaf is commonly used in cooking (it should be removed from the food before eating) and is also available as an extract made with ground leaves. It increases the effects of insulin and is sometimes recommended by nutritionists for diabetic diets. If used, blood glucose levels should be monitored closely

Cinnamon has been shown to improve glucose and lipid control in patients with type 2 diabetes, reducing fasting glucose, triglyceride, low-density lipoprotein, cholesterol, and total cholesterol levels. Patients with diabetes and prediabetes may benefit form the regular inclusion of cinnamon in their daily diet to prevent and control elevated glucose and blood lipid levels. Cinnamon may be a natural and inexpensive treatment for diabetes due to its molecular similarity to insulin.

Chromium is a trace mineral required for normal glucose metabolism. It may increase production of insulin receptors and insulin binding to the receptors, thereby increasing insulin effectiveness, lowering blood glucose levels, and decreasing insulin requirements in people with diabetes. It also may have beneficial effects on serum cholesterol levels. However, evidence for these effects is inconsistent, with some supporting and some negating the use of chromium supplements.

Chromium deficiency, considered rare in the United States, may play a role in the development of diabetes and atherosclerosis. If so, beneficial effects of a supplement may be more evident in a deficiency state. In one study of pregnant women and older adults with marginal levels of chromium, administration of a supplement improved glucose tolerance. At present, there is insufficient evidence to recommend routine chromium supplementation in diabetic patients. In nondiabetic patients, chromium supplements do not have hypoglycemic effects.

Echinacea has been studied in some clinical trials, but people with diabetes were excluded. It was concluded that diabetics should not take echinacea.

Garlic has been reported by some sources to have no known effects on blood glucose; others report a decrease in animals and humans. Some researchers also reported increased serum insulin and improvement in liver glycogen storage after garlic administration. There is a potential for additive hypoglycemic effects with antidiabetic drugs, although no apparent interactions have been reported.

Ginseng has been indicated in several studies (generally small and not well designed) to lower blood glucose levels in both diabetic and nondiabetic subjects. It may be useful in preventing diabetes or complications of diabetes. However, larger and longer studies are needed before general use can be recommended for diabetic or nondiabetic patients. For nondiabetic patients who use ginseng, the herb may need to be taken with a meal to prevent unintentional hypoglycemia. For diabetic patients, ginseng should be used very cautiously (if at all), with frequent monitoring of blood glucose and signs of hypoglycemia, because of possible additive effects with antidiabetic medications. Its use should also be accompanied by proper diet, physical activity, and antidiabetic medication.

Glucomannan, which is promoted as a diet aid and laxative, has hypoglycemic effects and should be avoided or used very cautiously by people with diabetes. If used, blood sugar levels should be monitored closely and lower doses of antidiabetic drugs may be needed.

Guar gum is a type of fiber that becomes gel-like upon contact with liquids (e.g., like Metamucil). It is used as a thickening agent in foods and drugs and is an ingredient in some over-the-counter weight-loss products. It should be used cautiously, if at all, by people with diabetes because it has hypoglycemic effects and slows GI motility. Several cases of esophageal and intestinal obstruction have been reported with weight-loss products.

Applying Your Knowledge 26-2

Mr. Coulter complains about feeling weak and confused. Your assessment reveals he is sweating and has tremors of his upper extremities. What action should you take?

Applying Your Knowledge 26-3

Mr. Coulter does not follow a prescribed diet. Even though he tells you that he gives himself his own insulin, he does not seem to be very knowledgeable about the use of the syringe and injection sites. He has not attended diabetic education classes because the time of the class interferes with his work schedule. What nursing diagnosis would be appropriate for Mr. Coulter?

Nursing Process

Assessment

Assess the patient's knowledge, attitude, and condition in relation to diabetes, the prescribed treatment plan, and complications. Assessment data should include past manifestations of the disease process and the patient's response to them; present status; and potential problem areas.

▪ *Historic data* include age at onset of diabetes, prescribed control measures and their effectiveness, the ease or difficulty of complying with the prescribed treatment, occurrence of complications such as ketoacidosis, and whether other disease processes have interfered with diabetes control.

▪ *Assess the patient's current status,* in relation to the following areas:
  ▪ **Diet.** Ask about the prescribed nutritional plan, who prepares the food, what factors help in following the diet, what factors interfere with following the diet, the current weight, and whether there has been a recent weight change. Also ask if herbal or other dietary supplements are used. If so, list each one by name and frequency of use. If a nutritionist is available, ask one to assess the patient's dietary practice and needs.
  ▪ **Activity.** Ask the patient to describe usual activities of daily living, including those related to work, home, and recreation, and whether he or she participates in a regular exercise program. If so, ask for more information about what, how often, how long, and so forth. If not, teaching is needed because exercise is extremely important in diabetes management.
  ▪ **Medication.** If the patient takes insulin, ask what kind; how much; who administers it; usual time of administration; sites used for injections; and if a hypoglycemic reaction to insulin has ever been experienced, how it was handled. This information helps to assess knowledge, usual practices, and teaching needs. If the patient takes an oral antidiabetic drug, ask the name, dosage, and time taken.
  ▪ **Monitoring methods.** Testing the blood for glucose and the urine for ketones (e.g., when blood sugar is elevated, when ill and unable to eat) are the two main methods of self-monitoring glycemic control. Ask about the method used, the frequency of testing, and the pattern of results. If possible, observe the patient performing and interpreting an actual test to assess accuracy.
  ▪ **Skin and mucous membranes.** Inspect for signs of infection and other lesions. Infections often occur in the axillary and groin areas because these areas have large numbers of microorganisms. Periodontal disease (pyorrhea) may be manifested by inflammation and bleeding of the gums. Women with diabetes are susceptible to monilial vaginitis and infections under the breasts. Check the sites of insulin injection for atrophy (dimpling or indentation), hypertrophy (nodules or lumps), and fibrosis (hardened areas). Check the lower leg for brown spots; these are caused by small hemorrhages into the skin and may indicate widespread changes in the blood vessels.

  Problems are especially likely to develop in the feet from infection, trauma, pressure, vascular insufficiency,

Nursing Process continues on page 426

and neuropathy. Therefore, inspect the feet for calluses, ulcers, and signs of infection. When such problems develop, sensory impairment from neuropathy may delay detection and impaired circulation may delay healing. Check pedal pulses, color, and temperature in both feet to evaluate arterial blood flow. Ankle edema may indicate venous insufficiency or impaired cardiac function.

■ **Eyes.** Ask about difficulties with vision and if eyes are examined regularly. Diabetic patients are prone to development of retinopathy, cataracts, and possibly glaucoma.

■ **Cardiovascular system.** Patients with diabetes have a high incidence of atherosclerosis, which makes them susceptible to hypertension, angina pectoris, myocardial infarction, peripheral vascular disease, and stroke. Therefore, check blood pressure and ask about chest pain and pain in the legs with exercise (intermittent claudication).

■ **Genitourinary system.** People with diabetes often have kidney and bladder problems. Assess for signs of urinary tract infection; albumin, white blood cells, or blood in urine; edema; increased urination at night; difficulty voiding; generalized itching; fatigue; and muscular weakness. Impotence may develop in men and is attributed to neuropathy.

■ Assess blood sugar reports for abnormal levels. Two or more fasting blood glucose levels greater than 126 mg/dL or two random levels greater than 200 mg/dL are diagnostic of diabetes. Decreased blood sugar levels are especially dangerous at 40 mg/dL or below.

■ Assess the glycosylated hemoglobin (also called *glycated hemoglobin* and *HbA*$_{1c}$) level when available. This test indicates glucose bound to hemoglobin in red blood cells (RBCs) when RBCs are exposed to hyperglycemia. The binding is irreversible and lasts for the lifespan of RBCs (approximately 120 days). The test reflects the average blood sugar during the previous 2 to 3 months. The goal is usually less than 7% (the range for people without diabetes is approximately 4%–6%). The test should be done every 3 to 6 months.

Test results are not affected by several factors that alter blood sugar levels, such as time of day, food intake, exercise, recently administered antidiabetic drugs, emotional stress, or patient cooperation. The test is especially useful with children; those whose diabetes is poorly controlled; those who do not test blood glucose regularly; and those who change their usual habits before a scheduled appointment with a health care provider so that their blood sugar control appears better than it actually is.

Nursing Diagnoses

■ Ineffective Tissue Perfusion, peripheral, related to atherosclerosis and vascular impairment

■ Disturbed Sensory Perception, visual and tactile, related to impaired vision or neuropathy

■ Ineffective Coping related to chronic illness and required treatment

■ Anxiety: Managing a chronic illness, finger sticks, insulin injections

■ Risk for Injury: Trauma, infection, hypoglycemia, hyperglycemia

■ Noncompliance related to inability or unwillingness to manage the disease process and required treatment

■ Deficient Knowledge: Disease process and management; administration and effects of antidiabetic drugs; interrelationships among diet, exercise, and antidiabetic drugs; and management of hypoglycemia, "sick days," and other complications

Planning/Goals

The patient will

■ Learn self-care activities

■ Manage drug therapy to prevent or minimize hypoglycemia and other adverse effects

■ Develop a consistent pattern of diet and exercise

■ Use available resources to learn about the disease process and how to manage it

■ Take antidiabetic drugs accurately

■ Self-monitor blood glucose and urine ketones appropriately

■ Keep appointments for follow-up and monitoring procedures by a health care provider

Interventions

Use nondrug measures to improve control of diabetes and to help prevent complications.

■ Assist the patient in maintaining the prescribed diet. Specific measures vary but may include teaching the patient and family about the importance of diet; referring the patient to a dietitian; and helping the patient identify and modify factors that decrease compliance with the diet. If the patient is obese, assist in developing a program to lose weight and then maintain weight at a more nearly normal level.

■ Assist the patient to develop and maintain a regular exercise program.

■ Perform and interpret blood tests for glucose accurately, and assist patient and family members to do so. Self-monitoring of blood glucose levels allows the patients to see the effects of diet, exercise, and hypoglycemic medications on blood glucose levels and may promote compliance.

Several products are available for home glucose monitoring. All involve obtaining a drop of capillary blood from a finger or forearm with a sterile lancet. The blood is placed on a semipermeable membrane that contains a reagent. The amount of blood glucose can be read with various machines (e.g., glucometers).

■ Test urine for ketones when the patient is sick, when blood glucose levels are above 200 mg/dL, and when episodes of nocturnal hypoglycemia are suspected. Also teach patients and family members to test urine when indicated.

■ Promote early recognition and treatment of problems by observing for signs and symptoms of urinary tract infection, peripheral vascular disease, vision changes, ketoacidosis, hypoglycemia, and others. Teach patients and families to observe for these conditions and report their occurrence.

■ Discuss the importance of regular visits to health care facilities for blood sugar measurements, weights, blood pressure measurements, and eye examinations.

■ Perform and teach correct foot care. Have the patient observe the following safeguards: avoid going barefoot, to prevent trauma to the feet; wear correctly fitted shoes; wash the feet daily with warm water, dry well, inspect for any lesions or pressure areas, and apply lanolin if the skin is dry; wear cotton or wool socks because they are more absorbent than synthetic materials; cut toenails straight across and only after the feet have been soaked in warm water and washed thoroughly. Teach the patient to avoid use of hot water bottles or electric heating pads; cutting toenails if vision is impaired; use of strong antiseptics on the feet; and cutting corns or calluses. Also teach the patient to report any lesions on the feet to the physician.

■ Help patients keep up with newer developments in diabetes care by providing information, sources of information, consultations with specialists, and other resources. However, do not overwhelm a newly diagnosed diabetic patient with excessive information or assume that a long-term diabetic patient does not need information.

Provide appropriate patient teaching for any drug therapy (see accompanying display).

Evaluation

■ Check blood sugar reports regularly for normal or abnormal values.

■ Check glycosylated hemoglobin reports when available.

■ Interview and observe for therapeutic and adverse responses to antidiabetic drugs.

■ Interview and observe for compliance with prescribed treatment.

■ Interview patients and family members about the frequency and length of hospitalizations for diabetes mellitus.

Principles of Therapy

Goals of Therapy

For most patients, the goals of treatment are to maintain blood glucose at normal or near-normal levels; promote normal metabolism of carbohydrate, fat, and protein; prevent acute and long-term complications; and prevent hypoglycemic episodes.

There is strong evidence that strict control of blood sugar delays the onset and slows progression of complications of diabetes. In addition to glycemic control, other measures can be used to help prevent complications of diabetes. Administration of angiotensin-converting enzyme (ACE) inhibitors (e.g., captopril) has protective effects on the kidneys in both type 1 and type 2 diabetes and in both normotensive and hypertensive people. Although ACE inhibitors are also used in the treatment of hypertension, their ability to delay nephropathy seems to be independent of antihypertensive effects. Additional measures to preserve renal function include effective treatment of hypertension, limited intake of dietary protein, prompt treatment of urinary tract infections, and avoidance of nephrotoxic drugs when possible.

Current research suggests a number of treatment strategies may be beneficial in reducing the cardiovascular disease risk associated with type 2 diabetes mellitus. Some clinicians are recommending the routine use of statins such as simvastatin to reduce the risk of occlusive arterial disease in all patients with diabetes regardless of cholesterol level. There is conflicting evidence regarding the effectiveness of thiazolidinediones in reducing the incidence of cardiovascular disease risk factors in patients with type 2 diabetes. Some clinical trials suggest that reducing insulin resistance through the use of thiazolidinediones has a cardioprotective benefit; however, recent safety data have shown a potentially significant increased risk of heart attack and heart-related deaths in patients taking rosiglitazone. The FDA has requested all approved oral antidiabetic drugs include labeling stating that no oral antidiabetic drug has been conclusively shown to reduce cardiovascular risk. Further studies are needed to resolve this question. Additional measures to reduce cardiovascular disease risk include reducing weight, controlling hypertension with an ACE inhibitor or angiotensin receptor blocker, use of aspirin therapy, and smoking cessation.

Treatment Regimens

When possible, it is desirable to have an interdisciplinary diabetes care team (e.g., physician, nurse diabetes educator, dietitian, perhaps others) work with the patient to design, monitor, and revise an individualized treatment plan. This is especially important for patients with newly diagnosed diabetes to assist them in learning to manage their disease and make appropriate lifestyle changes.

The best regimen for a particular patient depends on the type of diabetes, the patient's age and general condition, and the patient's ability and willingness to comply with the prescribed therapy. In type 1 diabetes, the only effective treatment measures are insulin, diet, and exercise. In type 2, the initial treatment of choice is diet, exercise, and weight control. If this regimen is ineffective, oral agents or insulin may be added.

Guidelines for Insulin Therapy

Choice of Insulin

When insulin therapy is indicated, the physician may choose from several preparations that vary in composition, onset,

Patient Teaching Guidelines | Antidiabetic Drugs

General Considerations

■ Wear or carry diabetic identification (e.g., a Medic-Alert necklace or bracelet) at all times, to aid treatment if needed.

■ Learn as much as you can about diabetes and its management. Few other diseases require as much adaptation in activities of daily living, and you must be well informed to control the disease, minimize complications, and achieve an optimal quality of life. Although much information is available from health care providers (physicians, nurses, nurse diabetes educators, nutritionists), an additional major resource is the

American Diabetes Association
1660 Duke St.
Alexandria, VA 22314
1-800-ADA-DISC
http://www.diabetes.org

■ In general, a consistent schedule of diet, exercise, and medication produces the best control of blood sugar levels and the least risk of complications.

■ Diet, weight control, and exercise are extremely important in managing diabetes. Maintaining normal weight and avoiding excessive caloric intake decrease the need for medication and decrease the workload of the pancreas. Exercise helps body tissues use insulin better, which means that glucose moves out of the bloodstream and into muscles and other body tissues. This promotes more normal blood glucose levels and decreases long-term complications of diabetes.

■ Take any antidiabetic medication as prescribed. If unable to take a medication, notify a health care provider. To control blood sugar most effectively, medications are balanced with diet and exercise. If you take insulin, you need to know what type(s) you are taking, how to obtain more, and how to store it. Unopened vials of insulin should be refrigerated. An opened vial may be stored at room temperature for 28 days. DO NOT freeze insulin. Regular and isophane (NPH) insulins and mixtures (e.g., Humulin) are available over-the-counter; Humalog, NovoLog, Lantus, Apidra, and Demetir require a prescription. Keep several days' supply of insulin and syringes on hand to allow for weather or other conditions that might prevent replacement of insulin or other supplies when needed.

If you take Byetta, you should store it in the original package in the refrigerator and discard unused portion after 30 days. Alert your health care provider if you experience acute abdominal discomfort while taking Byetta. If you take Symlin, opened vials can be kept in the refrigerator or at room temperature for up to 28 days.

■ You need to know the signs and symptoms of high blood sugar (hyperglycemia): increased blood glucose and excessive thirst, hunger, and urine output. Persistent hyperglycemia may indicate a need to change some aspect of the treatment program, such as diet or medication.

■ You need to know the symptoms of low blood sugar (hypoglycemia): sweating, nervousness, hunger, weakness, tremors, and mental confusion. Hypoglycemia may indicate too much medication or exercise or too little food. Treatment is a rapidly absorbed source of sugar, which

usually reverses symptoms within 10 to 20 minutes. If you are alert and able to swallow, take 4 ounces of fruit juice, 4 to 6 ounces of a sugar-containing soft drink, a piece of fruit or $1/3$ cup of raisins, two to three glucose tablets (5 grams each), a tube of glucose gel, 1 cup of skim milk, tea or coffee with 2 teaspoons of sugar, or eight Lifesaver candies. Avoid taking so much sugar that hyperglycemia occurs.

If you take acarbose (Precose) or miglitol (Glyset) along with insulin; glimepiride (Amaryl); glipizide (Glucotrol); or glyburide (DiaBeta, Glynase, Micronase) and a hypoglycemic reaction occurs, you must take some form of glucose (or glucagon) for treatment. Sucrose (table sugar) and other oral carbohydrates do not relieve hypoglycemia because the presence of acarbose or miglitol prevents their digestion and absorption from the gastrointestinal (GI) tract.

■ You need to have a family member or another person who is able to recognize and manage hypoglycemia in case you are unable to obtain or swallow a source of glucose. If you take insulin, glucagon should be available in the home and a caregiver should know how to give it.

■ The best way to prevent, delay, or decrease the severity of diabetes complications is to maintain blood sugar at a normal or near-normal level. Other measures include regular visits to health care providers, preferably a team of specialists in diabetes care; regular vision and glaucoma testing; and special foot care. In addition, if you have hypertension or elevated lipid levels, treatment can help prevent heart attacks and strokes.

■ Take only drugs prescribed by a physician who knows you have diabetes. Avoid other prescriptions and over-the-counter drugs unless these are discussed with the physician treating the diabetes because adverse reactions and interactions may occur. For example, nasal decongestants (alone or in cold remedies) and asthma medications may cause tachycardia and nervousness, which may be interpreted as hypoglycemia. In addition, liquid cold remedies and cough syrups may contain sugar and raise blood glucose levels.

■ If you wish to take any kind of herbal or dietary supplement, you should discuss this with the health care provider who is managing your diabetes. There has been little study of these preparations in relation to diabetes; many can increase or decrease blood sugar and alter diabetes control. If you start a supplement, you need to check your blood sugar frequently to see how it affects your blood glucose level.

■ Test blood regularly for glucose. A schedule individualized to your needs is best. Testing should be done more often when medication dosages are changed or when you are ill. Current blood glucose technology allows the selection of the fingertip or other location such as the forearm to obtain the blood sample. Glucose-concentrations measured at different sites may vary. The fingertips are the most accurate site and should be the preferred test site if hypoglycemia is suspected.

■ Reduce insulin dosage or eat extra food if you expect to exercise more than usual. Specific recommendations should be individualized and worked out with health care providers in relation to the type of exercise.

- Ask for written instructions about managing "sick days" and call your physician if unsure about what you need to do. Although each person needs individualized instructions, some general guidelines include the following:
  - Continue your antidiabetic medications unless instructed otherwise. Additional insulin also may be needed, especially if ketosis develops. Ketones (acetone) in the urine indicate insulin deficiency or insulin resistance.
  - Check blood glucose levels at least four times daily; test urine for ketones when the blood glucose level exceeds 250 mg/dL or with each urination. If unable to test urine, have someone else do it.
  - Rest, keep warm, do not exercise, and keep someone with you if possible.
  - If unable to eat solid food, take easily digested liquids or semiliquid foods. About 15 grams of carbohydrate every 1 to 2 hours is usually enough and can be provided by ½ cup of apple juice, applesauce, cola, cranberry juice, eggnog, Cream of Wheat cereal, custard, vanilla ice cream, regular gelatin, or frozen yogurt.
  - Drink 2 to 3 quarts of fluids daily, especially if you have a fever. Water, tea, broths, clear soups, diet soda, or carbohydrate-containing fluids are acceptable.
  - Record the amount of fluid intake as well as the number of times you urinate, vomit, or have loose stools.
  - Seek medical attention if a pre-meal blood glucose level is more than 250 mg/dL, if urine acetone is present, if you have fever above 100°F, if you have several episodes of vomiting or diarrhea, or if you have difficulty in breathing, chest pain, severe abdominal pain, or severe dehydration.

Self-Administration

- Use correct techniques for injecting insulin:
  - Follow instructions for times of administration as nearly as possible. Different types of insulin have different onsets, peaks, and durations of action. Accurate timing (e.g., in relation to meals), can increase beneficial effects and decrease risks of hypoglycemic reactions.
  - Wash hands; wash injection site, if needed.
  - Draw up insulin in a good light, being very careful to draw up the correct dose. If you have trouble seeing the syringe markers, get a magnifier or ask someone else to draw up the insulin. Prefilled syringes or cartridges for pen devices are also available.
  - Instructions may vary about cleaning the top of the insulin vial and the injection site with an alcohol swab and about pulling back on the plunger after injection to see if any blood enters the syringe. These techniques have been commonly used, but many diabetes experts do not believe they are necessary.
  - Inject straight into the fat layer under the skin, at a 90-degree angle. If very thin, pinch up a skinfold and inject at a 45-degree angle.
  - Rotate injection sites. Your health care provider may suggest a rotation plan. Many people rotate between the abdomen and the thighs. Insulin is absorbed fastest from the abdomen. Do not inject insulin within 2 inches of the "belly button" or into any skin lesions.
  - If it is necessary to mix two insulin preparations, ask for specific instructions about the technique and then follow it consistently. There is a risk of inaccurate dosage of both insulins unless measured very carefully. Commercial mixtures are also available for some combinations.
  - Change insulin dosage only if instructed to do so and the circumstances are specified.
  - Carry sugar, candy, or a commercial glucose preparation for immediate use if a hypoglycemic reaction occurs.
- Use correct technique for injecting amylin analogs and incretin mimetics:
  - Inject pramlintide (Symlin) subcutaneously into abdomen or thighs before meals. Do not mix in same syringe with insulin. Insulin dosages may be reduced by 50% when taking pramlintide.
  - Inject exenatide (Byetta) subcutaneously into abdomen, thigh, or upper arm within 60 minutes before morning and evening meal.
  - Rotate injection site of pramlintide and do not give in same site where insulin is administered.
- Take oral drugs as directed. Recommendations usually include the following:
  - Take glipizide or glyburide approximately 30 minutes before meals; take glimepiride with breakfast or the first main meal. Take Glucotrol XL with breakfast.
  - Take acarbose or miglitol with the first bite of each main meal. The drugs need to be in the GI tract with food because they act by decreasing absorption of sugar in the food. Starting with a small dose and increasing it gradually helps to prevent bloating, "gas pains," and diarrhea.
  - Take metformin (Glucophage) with meals to decrease stomach upset. Take Glucophage XR with the evening meal.
  - Take repaglinide (Prandin) or nateglinide (Starlix) about 15 to 30 minutes before meals (2, 3, or 4 times daily). Doses may vary from 0.5 to 4.0 milligrams, depending on fasting blood glucose levels. Dosage changes should be at least 1 week apart. If you skip a meal, you should skip that dose of repaglinide or nateglinide; if you eat an extra meal, you should take an extra dose.
  - Take pioglitazone (Actos), rosiglitazone (Avandia), and sitagliptin (Januvia) without regard to meals.
- If you take glimepiride, glipizide, glyburide, repaglinide or nateglinide, alone or in combination with other antidiabetic drugs, be prepared to handle hypoglycemic reactions (as with insulin, above). Acarbose, miglitol, metformin, pioglitazone, and rosiglitazone do not cause hypoglycemia when taken alone. Do not skip meals and snacks. This increases the risk of hypoglycemic reactions.
- If you exercise vigorously, you may need to decrease your dose of antidiabetic drug or eat more. Ask for specific instructions related to the type and frequency of the exercise.

duration of action, and other characteristics. Some factors to be considered include the following:

- Regular insulin (insulin injection) has a rapid onset of action and can be given IV. Therefore, it is the insulin of choice during acute situations, such as DKA, severe infection or other illness, and surgical procedures.

- Isophane insulin (NPH) is often used for long-term insulin therapy. For many patients, a combination of NPH and a short-acting insulin provides more consistent control of blood glucose levels. Although several regimens are used, a common one is a mixture of regular and NPH insulins administered before the morning and evening meals. A commercial mixture is more convenient and probably more accurate than a mixture prepared by a patient or caregiver, if the proportions of insulins are appropriate for the patient.

- Insulin lispro, aspart, or glulisine may be used instead of Sub-Q regular insulin in most situations, but safe usage requires both health care providers and patients to be aware of differences. Regular insulin, insulin aspart, and insulin glulisine are also approved for use in external insulin pumps that administer a Sub-Q continuous infusion.

- Insulin glargine or insulin detemir may be used to provide a basal amount of insulin over 24 hours, with a short-acting insulin or short-acting insulin analog at meal times.

Drug Dosage

Dosage of insulin must be individualized according to blood glucose levels. *Blood glucose meters* are devices that measure how much glucose is in the blood. A specially coated test strip containing a fresh sample of blood (obtained by pricking the skin, usually the finger or forearm, with a *lancet*) is inserted in the meter, which then measures the amount of glucose in the blood. The goal is to administer enough insulin to alleviate symptoms of hyperglycemia and to re-establish metabolic balance without causing hypoglycemia. An initial dose of 0.5 to 1 units per kilogram per day may be started and then adjusted to maintain blood glucose levels (tested before meals and at bedtime) of 90 to 130 milligrams per deciliter in adults (100–200 mg/dL in children younger than 5 years of age). However, many factors influence blood glucose response to exogenous insulin and therefore influence insulin requirements.

Factors that increase insulin requirements include weight gain, increased caloric intake, pregnancy, decreased activity, acute infections, hyperadrenocorticism (Cushing's disease), primary hyperparathyroidism, acromegaly, hypokalemia, and drugs such as corticosteroids, epinephrine, levothyroxine, and thiazide diuretics. Patients who are obese may require 2 units per kilogram per day because of resistance to insulin in peripheral tissues.

Factors that decrease insulin requirements include weight reduction; decreased caloric intake; increased physical activity; development of renal insufficiency; stopping administration of corticosteroids, epinephrine, levothyroxine, and diuretics; hypothyroidism; hypopituitarism; recovery from hyperthy-

roidism; recovery from acute infections; and the "honeymoon period" (see below), which may occur with type 1 diabetes.

People who need less than 0.5 units per kilogram per day may produce some endogenous insulin or their tissues may be more responsive to insulin because of exercise and good physical conditioning. Renal insufficiency decreases dosage requirements because less insulin is metabolized in the kidneys than with normal renal function. The "honeymoon period," characterized by temporary recovery of beta-cell function and production of insulin, may occur after diabetes is first diagnosed. Insulin requirements may decrease rapidly, and if the dosage is not decreased, severe hypoglycemic reactions may occur.

In acute situations, dosage of regular insulin needs frequent adjustments based on measurements of blood glucose. When insulin is given IV in a continuous infusion, 20% to 30% binds to the IV fluid container and the infusion tubing.

Dosage of insulin for long-term therapy is determined by blood glucose levels at various times of the day and is adjusted when indicated (e.g., because of illness or changes in physical activity). Titrating insulin dosage may be difficult and time consuming; it requires cooperation and collaboration between patients and health care providers.

Insulin pumps are being increasingly used, especially by adolescents and young adults who want flexibility in diet and exercise. These devices allow continuous Sub-Q administration of regular insulin, insulin aspart, or insulin glulisine. A basal amount of insulin is injected (e.g., 1 unit/hour or a calculated fraction of the dose used previously) continuously, with bolus injections before meals. This method of insulin administration maintains more normal blood glucose levels and avoids wide fluctuations. Candidates for insulin pumps include patients with diabetes that is poorly controlled with other methods and those who are able and willing to care for the devices properly. The MiniMed Paradigm* Real-Time System, the world's first integrated insulin pump and continuous glucose monitoring system, is now available in the United States and more than 20 other countries around the world (www.medtronic.com/Newsroom/NewsReleaseDetails.do? itemId=1164130391890&f…). The Guardian RT System displays glucose readings every 5 minutes and sounds an alarm when glucose levels reach high or low glucose limits preset by the clinical professional. The study completed on the RT System demonstrated that patients using Medtronic RT Continuous Glucose Monitoring technology had better control of their blood glucose than patients using fingersticks only.

Drug Administration
Timing of Insulin Administration

Many patients who take insulin need at least two injections daily to control hyperglycemia. A common regimen is one half to two thirds of the total daily dose in the morning before breakfast and the remaining one half or one third before the evening meal or at bedtime. With regular insulin before meals, it is very important that the medication be injected 30 to 45 minutes before meals so that the insulin is available when blood sugar increases after meals. With insulin lispro, aspart, or glulisine before meals, it is important to inject the medication about 15 minutes before eating. Insulin glargine or detemir is most commonly given at bedtime. However, it may be administered in the morning or in split doses as needed.

Selection of Subcutaneous Sites for Insulin Injections
Several factors affect insulin absorption from injection sites, including the site location, environmental temperature, and exercise or massage. Studies indicate that insulin is absorbed fastest from the abdomen, followed by the deltoid, thigh, and hip. Because of these differences, many clinicians recommend rotating injection sites within areas. This technique decreases rotations between areas and promotes more consistent blood glucose levels. With regard to temperature, insulin is absorbed more rapidly in warmer sites and environments. In relation to exercise, people who exercise should avoid injecting insulin into Sub-Q tissue near the muscles to be used. The increased blood flow that accompanies exercise promotes rapid absorption and may lead to hypoglycemia.

Timing of Food Intake

Patients receiving insulin need food at the peak action time of the insulin and at bedtime. The food is usually taken as a between-meal and a bedtime snack. These snacks help prevent hypoglycemic reactions between meals and at night. When hypoglycemia occurs during sleep, recognition and treatment may be delayed. This delay may allow the reaction to become more severe.

Use With Oral Antidiabetic Drugs

Insulin has been used successfully with all currently available types of oral agents (alpha-glucosidase inhibitors, biguanide, thiazolidinediones, meglitinides, and sulfonylureas).

Management of Diabetic Ketoacidosis

Insulin therapy is a major component of any treatment for DKA. Patients with DKA have a deficiency in the total amount of insulin in the body and a resistance to the action of the insulin that is available, probably due to acidosis, hyperosmolality, infection, and other factors. To be effective, insulin therapy must be individualized according to frequent measurements of blood glucose. Low doses, given by continuous IV infusion, are preferred in most circumstances.

Additional measures include identification and treatment of conditions that precipitate DKA, administration of IV fluids to correct hyperosmolality and dehydration, administration of potassium supplements to restore and maintain normal serum potassium levels, and administration of sodium bicarbonate to correct metabolic acidosis. Infection is one of the most common causes of DKA. If no obvious source of infection is identified, cultures of blood, urine, and throat swabs are recommended. When infection is identified, antimicrobial drug therapy may be indicated.

IV fluids, the first step in treating DKA, usually consist of 0.9% sodium chloride, an isotonic solution. Hypotonic solutions are usually avoided because they allow intracellular fluid shifts and may cause cerebral, pulmonary, and peripheral edema.

Although serum potassium levels may be normal at first, they fall rapidly after insulin and IV fluid therapy are begun. Decreased serum potassium levels are caused by expansion of extracellular fluid volume, movement of potassium into cells, and continued loss of potassium in the urine as long as hyperglycemia persists. For these reasons, potassium supplements are usually added to IV fluids. Because both hypokalemia and hyperkalemia can cause serious cardiovascular disturbances, dosage of potassium supplements must be based on frequent measurements of serum potassium levels. Also, continuous or frequent electrocardiogram monitoring is recommended.

Severe acidosis can cause serious cardiovascular disturbances, which usually stem from peripheral vasodilation and decreased cardiac output with hypotension and shock. Acidosis usually can be corrected by giving fluids and insulin; sodium bicarbonate may be given if the pH is less than 7.2. If used, sodium bicarbonate should be given slowly and cautiously. Rapid alkalinization can cause potassium to move into body cells faster than it can be replaced IV. The result may be severe hypokalemia and cardiac dysrhythmias. Also, giving excessive amounts of sodium bicarbonate can produce alkalosis.

Treatment of the Unconscious Patient

When a person with diabetes becomes unconscious and it is unknown whether the unconsciousness is caused by DKA or by hypoglycemia, the patient should be treated for hypoglycemia. If hypoglycemia is the cause, giving glucose may avert brain damage. If DKA is the cause, giving glucose does not harm the patient. Sudden unconsciousness in a patient who takes insulin is most likely to result from an insulin reaction producing hypoglycemia; DKA usually develops gradually over several days or weeks.

Hyperosmolar Hyperglycemic Nonketotic Coma (HHNC)

Treatment of HHNC is similar to that of DKA in that insulin, IV fluids, and potassium supplements are major components. Regular insulin is given by continuous IV infusion, and dosage is individualized according to frequent measurements of blood glucose levels. IV fluids are given to correct the profound dehydration and hyperosmolality, and potassium is given IV to replace the large amounts lost in urine during a hyperglycemic state.

Perioperative Insulin Therapy

Patients with diabetes who undergo major surgery have increased risks of both surgical and diabetic complications. Risks associated with surgery and anesthesia are greater if diabetes is not well controlled and complications of diabetes (e.g., hypertension, nephropathy, vascular damage) are already evident. Hyperglycemia and poor metabolic control are associated with increased susceptibility to infection, poor wound healing, and fluid and electrolyte imbalances. Risks of diabetic complications are increased because the stress of surgery increases insulin requirements and may precipitate DKA. Metabolic responses to stress include increased secretion of catecholamines, cortisol, glucagon, and growth hormone, all of which increase blood glucose levels. In addition to hyperglycemia, protein breakdown, lipolysis, ketogenesis, and insulin resistance occur. The risk of hypoglycemia is also increased.

The goals of treatment are to avoid hypoglycemia, severe hyperglycemia, ketoacidosis, and fluid and electrolyte imbalances. Maintenance of blood glucose levels between 120 and 180 milligrams per deciliter during the perioperative period is desirable. In general, mild hyperglycemia (e.g., blood glucose levels between 150 and 250 mg/dL) is considered safer for the patient than hypoglycemia, which may go unrecognized during anesthesia and surgery. Because surgery is a stressful event that increases blood glucose levels and the body's need for insulin, insulin therapy is usually required.

The goal of insulin therapy is to avoid ketosis from inadequate insulin and hypoglycemia from excessive insulin. Specific actions depend largely on the severity of diabetes and the type of surgical procedure. Diabetes should be well controlled before any type of surgery. Minor procedures usually require little change in the usual treatment program; major operations usually require a different medication regimen.

In general, regular, short-acting insulin is used with major surgery or surgery requiring general anesthesia. IV administration of insulin is preferred because it provides more predictable absorption than Sub-Q injections. For patients who use an intermediate-acting insulin, a different regimen using regular insulin in doses approximating the usual daily requirement is needed. For patients who usually manage their diabetes with diet alone or with diet and oral medications, insulin therapy may be started. Human insulin is preferred for temporary use to minimize formation of insulin antibodies. Small doses are usually required.

For elective major surgery, patients should be scheduled early in the day to avoid prolonged fasting. In addition, most authorities recommend omitting usual doses of insulin on the day of surgery and oral antidiabetic medications for 1 or 2 days before surgery. While the patient is NPO (nothing by mouth), before and during surgery, IV insulin is usually given. Along with the insulin, patients need adequate sources of carbohydrate. This is usually supplied by IV solutions of 5% or 10% dextrose at a rate of 5 grams of glucose per hour (D_5W at a rate of 100 mL/hour provides 5 g of glucose).

After surgery, IV insulin and dextrose may be continued until the patient is able to eat and drink. Several protocols exist for postoperative glucose control. Most involve continuous infusions of insulin with frequent blood glucose monitoring and subsequent titration of the insulin infusion to maintain a predetermined goal. Regular insulin can also be given Sub-Q every 4 to 6 hours, with frequent blood glucose measurements. Oral fluids and foods that contain carbohydrate should be resumed as soon as possible. When meals are fully tolerated, the preoperative insulin or oral medication regimen can be resumed. Additional regular insulin can be given for elevated blood glucose and ketone levels, if indicated.

Guidelines for Oral Antidiabetic Drug Therapy

Sulfonylureas

Sulfonylureas are not effective in all patients with type 2 diabetes, and many patients experience primary or secondary treatment failure. Primary failure involves a lack of initial response to the drugs. Secondary failure means that a therapeutic response occurs when the drugs are first given, but the drugs eventually become ineffective. Reasons for secondary failure may include decreased compliance with diet and exercise instructions, failure to take the drugs as prescribed, or decreased ability of the pancreatic beta cells to produce more insulin in response to the drugs.

Dosage of sulfonylureas is usually started low and increased gradually until the fasting blood glucose level is 110 milligrams per deciliter or less. The lowest dose that achieves normal fasting and postprandial blood sugar levels is recommended.

Sulfonylureas must be used cautiously in patients with impaired renal or hepatic function. They are usually not recommended for use during pregnancy because of risks of fetal hypoglycemia and death, congenital anomalies, and overt diabetes in women with gestational diabetes (because the drugs stimulate an already overstimulated pancreas).

Alpha-Glucosidase Inhibitors

Acarbose and miglitol should be taken at the beginning of a meal so they are present in the GI tract with food and able to delay digestion of carbohydrates. Low initial doses and gradual increases decrease GI upset (e.g., bloating, diarrhea) and promote patient compliance. Patients taking acarbose or miglitol should continue their diet, exercise, and blood glucose testing routines. Alpha-glucosidase inhibitors do not alter insulin secretion or cause hypoglycemia.

Biguanide

Renal function should be assessed before starting metformin and at least annually during long-term therapy. The drug should not be given initially if renal impairment is present; it should be stopped if renal impairment occurs during treatment. As with other antidiabetic drugs, patients taking metformin should continue their diet, exercise, and blood glucose testing regimens.

Parenteral radiographic contrast media containing iodine (e.g., Cholografin, Hypaque) may cause renal failure, and they have been associated with lactic acidosis in patients receiving metformin. Metformin should be discontinued at least 48 hours before diagnostic tests are performed with these materials and should not be resumed for at least 48 hours after the tests are done and tests indicate renal function is normal.

Thiazolidinediones

Liver function tests (e.g., serum aminotransferase enzymes) should be checked before starting therapy and periodically thereafter. In addition, patients should be monitored closely for edema and other signs of congestive heart failure.

Meglitinides

As with other antidiabetic drugs, patients taking one of these drugs should continue their diet, exercise, and blood glucose testing regimens. Dosage is flexible, depending on food intake, but patients should eat within a few minutes after taking a dose to avoid hypoglycemia.

Use With Insulin

All the currently available types of oral agents (alpha-glucosidase inhibitors, biguanide, thiazolidinediones, meglitinides, and sulfonylureas) have been used successfully with insulin.

 Applying Your Knowledge 26-4

How Can You Avoid This Medication Error?
Mr. Coulter is scheduled for a renal arteriogram. The nurse tells him to take his antidiabetic medication as usual.

Combination Drug Therapy for Type 2 Diabetes

Combination drug therapy is an increasing trend in type 2 diabetes that is not controlled by diet, exercise, and single-drug therapy. Useful combinations include drugs with different mechanisms of action, and several rational combinations are currently available. Most studies have involved combinations of two drugs; some three-drug combinations are also being used. All combination therapy should be monitored with periodic measurements of fasting plasma glucose and glycosylated hemoglobin levels. If adequate glycemic control is not achieved, oral drugs may need to be discontinued and insulin therapy started. Two-drug combinations include the following:

- **Insulin plus a sulfonylurea.** Advantages include lower fasting blood glucose levels, decreased glycosylated hemoglobin levels, increased secretion of endogenous insulin, smaller daily doses of insulin, and no significant change in body weight. The role of insulin analogs in combination therapy is not clear. One regimen, called BIDS, uses bedtime insulin, usually NPH, with a daytime sulfonylurea, usually glyburide.

- **Insulin plus a glitazone.** Thiazolidinediones increase the effectiveness of insulin, whether endogenous or exogenous.

- **Sulfonylurea plus acarbose or miglitol.** This combination is FDA approved for patients who do not achieve adequate glycemic control with one of the drugs alone.

- **Sulfonylurea plus metformin.** Glimepiride is FDA approved for this combination.

- **Sulfonylurea plus a glitazone.** The sulfonylurea increases insulin and the glitazone increases insulin effectiveness.

- **Metformin plus a meglitinide.** If one of the drugs alone does not produce adequate glycemic control, the other one may be added. Dosage of each drug should be titrated to the minimal dose required to achieve the desired effects.

- **Metformin plus a glitazone.** If metformin alone does not produce adequate glycemic control, a glitazone may be added. Pioglitazone is FDA approved for this combination.

- **Metformin or glitazone plus sitagliptin.** Sitagliptin may be added as adjunctive therapy with metformin or a glitazone to achieve desired glycemic control.

- **Metformin or sulfonylurea plus exenatide.** Exenatide may be added as adjunctive therapy with metformin or a sulfonylurea to achieve desired glycemic control.

- **Mealtime insulin plus metformin, glitazone, and/or sulfonylurea plus pramlintide.** Pramlintide may be given with mealtime insulin in type 2 diabetics to achieve better postprandial glucose control.

Use in Special Populations

Use in Diabetic Patients Who Are Ill

Illness may affect diabetes control in several ways. First, it causes a stress response. Part of the stress response is increased secretion of glucagon, epinephrine, growth hormone, and cortisol, hormones that raise blood glucose levels (by stimulating gluconeogenesis and inhibiting insulin action) and cause ketosis (by stimulating lipolysis and ketogenesis). Second, if the illness makes a person unable or unwilling to eat, hypoglycemia can occur. Third, if the illness affects GI function (e.g., causes vomiting or diarrhea), the person may be unable to drink enough fluids to prevent dehydration and electrolyte imbalance. In addition, hyperglycemia induces an osmotic diuresis that increases dehydration and electrolyte imbalances.

As a result of these potentially serious effects, an illness that would be minor in people without diabetes may become a major illness or medical emergency in people with diabetes. Everyone involved should be vigilant about recognizing and seeking prompt treatment for any illness. In addition, patients with diabetes (or their caregivers) should be taught how to adjust their usual regimens to maintain metabolic balance and prevent severe complications. The main goal during illness is to prevent complications such as severe hyperglycemia, dehydration, and DKA.

Use in Children

Diabetes, one of the most common chronic disorders of childhood, usually appears after 4 years of age and peaks in incidence at 10 to 12 years for girls and 12 to 14 years for boys. Approximately 75% of all newly diagnosed cases of type 1 diabetes occur in people under the age of 18. According to the Centers for Disease Control and Prevention, roughly 1 of every 400 to 600 children has type 1 diabetes. The incidence of type 2 diabetes in children and adolescents is increasing. The growing number of obese children is a major factor in this increase in type 2 diabetes among young people. Children of ethnic/minority groups such as Native Americans, Native Alaskans, African Americans, Mexican Americans, and Pacific Islanders are disproportionately affected.

Type 1 Diabetes

Insulin is the only drug indicated for use; it is required as replacement therapy because affected children cannot produce insulin. Effective management requires a consistent schedule of meals, snacks, blood glucose monitoring, insulin injections and dose adjustments, and exercise. Insulin injections must be given three or four times per day. Rotation of injection sites is important in infants and young children because of the relatively small areas for injection at each anatomic site and to prevent lipodystrophy. Young children usually adjust to injections and blood glucose monitoring better when the parents express less anxiety about these vital procedures.

A healthful, varied diet, rich in whole grains, fruits, and vegetables and limited in simple sugars, is recommended. According to the American Diabetes Association (2006), medical nutrition therapy should be tailored to a person's specific health issues and personal preferences to help maintain optimum health by controlling blood glucose levels, blood pressure, cholesterol, and other risk factors.

Food intake must be synchronized with insulin injections and usually involves three meals and three snacks, all at regularly scheduled times. Such a schedule is difficult to maintain in children, but it is extremely important in promoting normal growth and development. A major factor in optimal treatment is a supportive family in which at least one member is thoroughly educated about the disease and its management. Less-than-optimal treatment can lead to stunted growth, delayed puberty, and early development of complications such as retinopathy, nephropathy, or neuropathy.

Infections and other illnesses may cause wide fluctuations in blood glucose levels and interfere with metabolic control. For example, some infections cause hypoglycemia; others, especially chronic infections, may cause hyperglycemia and insulin resistance and may precipitate ketoacidosis. As a result, insulin requirements may vary widely during illness episodes and should be based on blood glucose and urine ketone levels. Hypoglycemia often develops in young children, partly because of anorexia and smaller glycogen reserves.

During illness, children are highly susceptible to dehydration, and an adequate fluid intake is very important. Many clinicians recommend sugar-containing liquids (e.g., regular sodas, clear juices, regular gelatin desserts) if blood glucose values are lower than 250 milligrams per deciliter. When blood glucose values are above 250 milligrams per deciliter, diet soda, unsweetened tea, and other fluids without sugar should be given.

Administration of insulin for infants and toddlers who weigh less than 10 kilograms or require less than 5 units of insulin per day can be difficult because small doses are hard to measure in a U-100 syringe. Use of diluted insulin allows more accurate administration. The most common dilution strength is U-10 (10 units/mL), and a diluent is available from insulin manufacturers for this purpose. Vials of diluted insulin should be clearly labeled and discarded after 1 month.

Avoiding hypoglycemia is a major goal in infants and young children because of potentially damaging effects on growth and development. For example, the brain and spinal cord do not develop normally without an adequate supply of glucose. Animal studies indicate that prolonged hypoglycemia results in decreased brain weight, numbers of neurons, and protein content. Myelinization of nerve cells is also decreased. Because complex motor and intellectual functions require an intact central nervous system, frequent, severe, or prolonged hypoglycemia can be a serious problem in infants, toddlers, and preschoolers. In addition, recognition of hypoglycemia may be delayed because signs and symptoms are vague and the children may be unable to communicate them to parents or caregivers. Because of these difficulties, most pediatric diabetologists recommend maintaining blood glucose levels between 100 and 200 milligrams per deciliter to prevent hypoglycemia. In addition, the bedtime snack and blood glucose measurement should never be skipped.

Signs and symptoms of hypoglycemia in older children are similar to those in adults (e.g., hunger, sweating, tachycardia). In young children, hypoglycemia may be manifested by changes in behavior, including severe hunger, irritability, and lethargy. In addition, mental functioning may be impaired in all age groups, even with mild hypoglycemia. Any time hypoglycemia is suspected, blood glucose should be tested.

Adolescents may resist adhering to their prescribed treatment regimens, and effective management may be especially difficult during this developmental period. Adolescents and young adults may delay, omit, or decrease dosage of insulin to fit in socially (e.g., by eating more, sleeping in, drinking alcohol) or to control their weight. Omitting or decreasing insulin dosage may lead to repeated episodes of ketoacidosis. Also, adolescent females may develop eating disorders.

A good resource is the Juvenile Diabetes Foundation (JDF), a not-for-profit health agency with support groups and other activities for families affected by diabetes: Juvenile Diabetes Foundation International, 120 Wall Street, New York, NY 10005-4001, 1-800-JDF-CURE, 1-800-223-1138, www.jdf.org.

Type 2 Diabetes

Type 2 diabetes is being increasingly identified in children. This trend is attributed mainly to obesity and inadequate exercise because most children with type 2 are seriously overweight and have poor eating habits. In addition, most are members of high-risk ethnic groups and have relatives with diabetes. These children are at high risk for development of serious complications during early adulthood, such as myocardial infarction during their fourth decade. Management involves exercise, weight loss, and a more healthful diet, and in some cases drug therapy including insulin may be indicated. Attention must also be given to treating comorbid conditions such as hypertension and hyperlipidemia.

Use in Older Adults

It is estimated that at least 20% of people over the age of 65 have diabetes. General precautions for safe and effective use of antidiabetic drugs apply to older adults, including close monitoring of blood glucose levels; however, control of cardiovascular risk factors may play a greater role in reducing morbidity and mortality in this population. In addition, older adults may have impaired vision, poor manual dexterity, or other problems that decrease their ability to perform needed tasks (e.g., self-administration of insulin, monitoring blood glucose levels, managing diet and exercise). They also may have other disorders and may take other drugs that complicate management of diabetes. For example, renal insufficiency may increase risks of adverse effects with antidiabetic drugs, and treatment with thiazide diuretics, corticosteroids, estrogens, and other drugs may cause hyperglycemia, thereby increasing dosage requirements for antidiabetic drugs.

With oral sulfonylureas, hypoglycemia is a concern for the older person. Drugs with a short duration of action and inactive metabolites are considered safer, especially with impaired liver or kidney function. Therapy usually should start with a low dose, which is then increased or decreased according to blood glucose levels and clinical response.

Few guidelines have been developed for the use of newer antidiabetic drugs in older adults. Insulin analogs appear to have some advantages over conventional insulin. Acarbose, miglitol, and metformin may not be as useful in older adults as in younger ones because of the high prevalence of impaired renal function. These drugs are relatively contraindicated in patients with renal insufficiency because they have a longer half-life and may accumulate. With metformin, dosage should be based on periodic tests of renal function, and the drug should be stopped if renal impairment occurs or if serum lactate increases. In addition, dosage should not be titrated to the maximum amount recommended for younger adults. Use of thiazolidinediones and metformin is often contraindicated in older adults who are more likely to have cardiovascular disorders that increase risks of fluid retention and congestive heart failure. With meglitinides, effects were similar in younger and older adults during clinical trials.

Use in Patients with Renal Impairment

Insulin. Frequent monitoring of blood glucose levels and dosage adjustments may be needed. It is difficult to predict dosage needs because, on the one hand, less insulin is degraded by the kidneys (normally about 25%) and this may lead to higher blood levels of insulin if dosage is not reduced. On the other hand, muscles and possibly other tissues are less sensitive to insulin, and this insulin resistance may result in an increased blood glucose level if dosage is not increased. Overall, vigilance is required to prevent dangerous hypoglycemia, especially in patients whose renal function is unstable or worsening.

Oral drugs. **Sulfonylureas** and their metabolites are excreted mainly by the kidneys; renal impairment may lead to accumulation and hypoglycemia. They should be used cautiously, with close monitoring of renal function, in patients with mild to moderate renal impairment, and are contraindicated in severe renal impairment. **Alpha-glucosidase inhibitors** are excreted by the kidneys and accu-

mulate in patients with renal impairment. However, dosage reduction is not helpful because the drugs act locally, within the GI tract. **Metformin** requires assessment of renal function before starting and at least annually during long-term therapy. It should not be given initially if renal impairment is present; it should be stopped if renal impairment occurs during treatment. **Meglitinides** do not require initial dosage adjustments, but increments should be made cautiously in patients with renal impairment or renal failure requiring hemodialysis. Renal function should be assessed before initiation of treatment with sitagliptin, and periodically during therapy. Dosage reductions must be made for patients with moderate to severe renal dysfunction.

Use in Patients With Hepatic Impairment

Insulin. There may be higher blood levels of insulin in patients with hepatic impairment because less insulin may be degraded. Careful monitoring of blood glucose levels and insulin dosage reductions may be needed to prevent hypoglycemia.

Oral drugs. **Sulfonylureas** should be used cautiously and liver function should be monitored. They are metabolized in the liver, and hepatic impairment may result in higher serum drug levels and inadequate release of hepatic glucose in response to hypoglycemia. With glipizide, initial dosage should be reduced in patients with liver failure. Glyburide may cause hypoglycemia in patients with liver disease. **Alpha-glucosidase inhibitors** require no precautions with hepatic impairment because acarbose is metabolized in the GI tract and miglitol is not metabolized. **Metformin** is not recommended for use in patients with clinical or laboratory evidence of hepatic impairment because risks of lactic acidosis may be increased. **Meglitinides** should be used cautiously and dosage increments should be made very slowly, because serum drug levels are higher, for a longer period of time, in patients with moderate to severe hepatic impairment. **Thiazolidinediones** have been associated with hepatotoxicity and require monitoring of liver enzymes. The drugs should not be given to patients with active liver disease or a serum ALT more than 2.5 times the upper limit of normal. After **glitazone** therapy is initiated, liver enzymes should be measured every 2 months for 1 year, then periodically.

Use in Patients With Critical Illness

Critically ill patients, with and without diabetes mellitus, often experience hyperglycemia associated with insulin resistance. Hyperglycemia may complicate the progress of the critically ill patient, resulting in increased complications such as postoperative infections, poor recovery, and increased mortality. Tight glycemic control is a key factor in preventing complications and improving mortality in the intensive care unit patient.

Insulin is more likely to be used in critical illness than any of the oral agents. Reasons include the greater ability to titrate dosage needs in patients who are often debilitated and unstable, with varying degrees of cardiovascular, liver, and kidney impairment. One important consideration with IV insulin therapy is that 30% or more of a dose may adsorb into containers of IV fluid or infusion sets. In addition, many critically ill patients are unable to take oral drugs.

Some critically ill patients are also at risk for serious hypoglycemia, especially if they are debilitated, sedated, or unable to recognize and communicate symptoms. Vigilant monitoring is essential for any patient who has diabetes and a critical illness.

Use in Home Care

Most diabetes care is delivered in ambulatory care settings or in the home, and any patient with diabetes may need home care. Hospitalization usually occurs only for complications, and patients are quickly discharged if possible. The home care nurse may need to assist patients of multiple age groups to learn self-care and assist caregivers to support patients' efforts or actively participate in diabetes management. Some aspects of the nursing role include mobilizing and coordinating health care providers and community resources, teaching and supporting patients and caregivers, monitoring the patient's health status and progress in disease management, assisting the patient to obtain diabetic supplies for monitoring and medication administration, and preventing or solving problems The person with diabetes has a tremendous amount of information to learn about living with this disease on a day-to-day basis. For most patients, the goal of diabetes education is self-care in terms of diet, exercise, medication administration, and blood glucose monitoring and prevention, recognition, and treatment of complications. For some patients, a parent or caregiver may assume most of the responsibility for diabetes management. Because of the amount and complexity of information, a multidisciplinary health care team that includes a nurse diabetes educator is preferred in home care as in other settings. The role of the home care nurse may include initial teaching or reinforcement and follow-up of teaching done by others.

Nursing Actions   Antidiabetic Drugs

NURSING ACTIONS	RATIONALE/EXPLANATION
1. Administer accurately a. With insulin: (1) Store the insulin vial in current use and administer insulin at room temperature. Refrigerate extra vials.	Cold insulin is more likely to cause lipodystrophy, local sensitivity reactions, discomfort, and delayed absorption. Insulin preparations are stable for months at room temperature if temperature extremes are avoided.
(2) Avoid freezing temperatures (32°F) or high temperatures (95°F or above).	Extremes of temperature decrease insulin potency and cause clumping of the suspended particles of modified insulins. This clumping phenomenon causes inaccurate dosage even if the volume is accurately measured.
(3) Discard insulin that has become discolored, turbid, or unusually viscous.	These changes suggest deterioration or contamination of the insulin.
(4) Use only an orange tipped insulin syringe calibrated to measure U-100 insulin.	For accurate measurement of the prescribed dose
(5) With isophane (NPH, Humulin N, Novolin N) intermediate insulins, be sure they are mixed to a uniform cloudy appearance before drawing up a dose.	These insulin preparations are suspensions, and the components separate on standing. Unless the particles are resuspended in the solution and distributed evenly, dosage will be inaccurate.

(6) When short-acting and isophane intermediate insulins must be mixed, prepare as follows:
    (a) Draw into the insulin syringe the amount of air equal to the total amount of both insulins.
    (b) Draw up the short-acting insulin first. Inject the equivalent portion of air, and aspirate the ordered dose.
    (c) With the intermediate vial, insert the remaining air (avoid injecting short-acting insulin into the intermediate vial), and aspirate the ordered dose.
    (d) Expel air bubbles, if present, and verify that the correct dosage is in the syringe.
	The insulins must be drawn up in the same sequence every time. Short-acting insulin should *always* be drawn up first, to avoid contamination of the short-acting insulin with the NPH. Because short-acting insulin combines with excess protamine in NPH, the concentration of short-acting insulin is changed when they are mixed. Following the same sequence also leaves the same type of insulin in the needle and syringe (dead space) every time. Although dead space is not usually a significant factor with available insulin syringes, it may be with small doses.

(e) Administer combined insulins *consistently* within 15 minutes of mixing or after a longer period; that is, do not give one dose within 15 minutes of mixing and another 2 hours or days after mixing.	Short-acting insulin combines with excess protamine when mixed with NPH insulin. This reaction occurs within 15 minutes of mixing and alters the amount of short-acting insulin present. After 15 minutes, the mixture is stable for approximately 1 month at room temperature and 3 months when refrigerated. Thus, to administer the same dose consistently, the mixture must be given at approximately the same time interval after mixing.

NURSING ACTIONS	RATIONALE/EXPLANATION
(7) Rotate injection sites systematically, within the same anatomic area (e.g., abdomen) until all sites are used. Avoid random rotation between the abdomen and thigh or arm, for example.	Frequent injection in the same site can cause tissue fibrosis, erratic absorption, and deposits of unabsorbed insulin. Also, if insulin is usually injected into fibrotic tissue where absorption is slow, injection into healthy tissue may result in hypoglycemia because of more rapid absorption. Further, deposits of unabsorbed insulin may initially lead to hyperglycemia. If dosage is increased to control the apparent hyperglycemia, hypoglycemia may occur. Rates of absorption differ among anatomic sites, and random rotation increases risks of hypoglycemic reactions.
(8) Inject insulin at a 90-degree angle into a subcutaneous pocket created by raising subcutaneous tissue away from muscle tissue. Avoid intramuscular injection.	Injection into a subcutaneous pocket is thought to produce less tissue irritation and better absorption than injection into subcutaneous tissue. Intramuscular injection should not be used because of rapid absorption.
(9) With insulin analogs, give aspart within 5 to 10 minutes of starting a meal; give lispro within 15 minutes before or immediately after a meal; give glulisine 15 minutes before meals or within 20 minutes of beginning the meal; give glargine once daily at bedtime; give levemir with evening meal or at bedtime for once a day dosing schedule.	Manufacturers' recommendations. Aspart, lispro and glulisine act rapidly; glargine is long acting.
b. With oral sulfonylureas: Give glipizide or glyburide 30 minutes before breakfast and the evening meal. Give glimepiride and Glucotrol XL with breakfast.	To promote absorption and effective plasma levels. Most of these drugs are given once or twice daily.
c. With acarbose and miglitol: Give at the beginning of each main meal, three times daily.	These drugs must be in the gastrointestinal (GI) tract when carbohydrate foods are ingested because they act by decreasing absorption of sugar in the foods.
d. With metformin: Give with meals. Give Glucophage XR with evening meal	To decrease GI upset
e. With pioglitazone, rosiglitazone, and sitagliptin: Give once daily, without regard to meals.	Manufacturers' recommendations
f. With repaglinide and nateglinide: Give 15 to 30 minutes before meals (2, 3, or 4 times daily). If the patient does not eat a meal, omit that dose; if the patient eats an extra meal, give an extra dose.	Dosage is individualized according to the levels of fasting blood glucose and glycosylated hemoglobin.
g. With pramlintide: Inject Sub-Q into abdomen or thigh before meals. Do not mix in same syringe with insulin. Insulin dosages will be reduced by 50%. Rotate injection sites and do not administer at same site where insulin is administered. Opened vials is can be kept in the refrigerator or at room temperature for up to 28 days.	Injection into arm results in variable absorption and is not recommended. Pramlintide and insulin are not compatible to mix in same syringe, and should not be given in same injection site.
h. With exenatide inject Sub-Q into abdomen, thigh or upper arm within 60 minutes of morning or evening meal. Store exenatide in the original package in the refrigerator for up to 30 days.	Manufacturers recommendations
2. Observe for therapeutic effects	
a. Improved blood glucose levels (fasting, preprandial, and postprandial) and glycosylated hemoglobin levels	The general goal is normal or near-normal blood glucose levels. However, specific targeted levels for individuals vary depending on intensity of treatment, risks of hypoglycemia, and other factors. Improved metabolic control can prevent or delay complications.
b. Absent or decreased ketones in urine (N = none)	In diabetes, ketonuria indicates insulin deficiency and impending diabetic ketoacidosis if preventive measures are not taken. Thus, always report the presence of ketones. In addition, when adequate insulin is given, ketonuria decreases. Ketonuria does not often occur with type 2 diabetes.
c. Absent or decreased pruritus, polyuria, polydipsia, polyphagia, and fatigue	These signs and symptoms occur in the presence of hyperglycemia. When blood sugar levels are lowered with antidiabetic drugs, they tend to subside.
d. Decreased complications of diabetes	

(continued on page 438)

Nursing Actions   Antidiabetic Drugs (continued)

NURSING ACTIONS	RATIONALE/EXPLANATION
3. Observe for adverse effects	
a. With insulin, sulfonylureas, meglitinides, exenatide and pramlintide:	
(1) Hypoglycemia	Hypoglycemia is more likely to occur with insulin than with oral agents and at peak action times of the insulin being used. Insulin plus pramlintide may produce severe hypoglycemia.
(a) Sympathetic nervous system (SNS) activation—tachycardia, palpitations, nervousness, weakness, hunger, perspiration	The SNS is activated as part of the stress response to low blood glucose levels. Epinephrine and other hormones act to raise blood glucose levels.
(b) Central nervous system impairment—mental confusion, incoherent speech, blurred or double vision, headache, convulsions, coma	There is an inadequate supply of glucose for normal brain function.
b. With insulin:	
(1) Local insulin allergy—erythema, induration, itching at injection sites	Uncommon with human insulin
(2) Systemic allergic reactions—skin rash, dyspnea, tachycardia, hypotension, angioedema, anaphylaxis	Uncommon; if a severe systemic reaction occurs, skin testing and desensitization are usually required.
(3) Lipodystrophy—atrophy and "dimpling" at injection site; hypertrophy at injection site	These changes in subcutaneous fat occur from too-frequent injections into the same site. They are uncommon with human insulin.
(4) Weight gain	This effect may decrease compliance with drug therapy, especially in adolescents and young-adult females.
c. With sulfonylureas:	
(1) Hypoglycemia and weight gain	Hypoglycemia occurs less often with oral agents than with insulin. It is more likely to occur in patients who are elderly, debilitated, or who have impaired renal and hepatic function. Weight gain may decrease drug compliance, especially in adolescents and young adult females.
(2) Allergic skin reactions—skin rash, urticaria, erythema, pruritus	These reactions may subside with continued use of the drug. If they do not subside, the drug should be discontinued.
(3) GI upset—nausea, heartburn	These are the most commonly reported adverse effects. If severe, reducing drug dosage usually relieves them.
(4) Miscellaneous—fluid retention and hyponatremia; facial flushing if alcohol is ingested; hematologic disorders (hemolytic or aplastic anemia, leukopenia, thrombocytopenia, others)	These are less common adverse effects.
d. With acarbose and miglitol: GI symptoms—bloating, flatulence, diarrhea, abdominal pain	These are commonly reported. They are caused by the presence of undigested carbohydrate in the lower GI tract. They can be decreased by low doses initially and gradual increases.
e. With metformin:	
(1) GI effects—anorexia, nausea, vomiting, diarrhea, abdominal discomfort, decreased intestinal absorption of folate and vitamin B_{12}	GI symptoms are common adverse effects. They may be minimized by taking the drug with meals and increasing dosage slowly.
(2) Allergic skin reactions—eczema, pruritus, erythema, urticaria	
(3) Lactic acidosis—drowsiness, malaise, respiratory distress, bradycardia and hypotension (if severe), blood lactate levels above 5 mmol/L, blood pH below 7.35	A rare but serious adverse effect (approximately 50% *fatal*). Most likely with renal or hepatic impairment, advanced age, or hypoxia. This is a medical emergency that requires hospitalization for treatment. Hemodialysis is effective in correcting acidosis and removing metformin. Lactic acidosis may be prevented by monitoring plasma lactate levels and stopping the drug if they exceed 3 mmol/L. Other reasons to stop the drug include decreased renal or hepatic function, a prolonged fast, or a very–low-calorie diet. The drug should be stopped immediately if a patient has a myocardial infarction or septicemia.

NURSING ACTIONS	RATIONALE/EXPLANATION
f. With pioglitazone and rosiglitazone:	
(1) Upper respiratory infections—pharyngitis, sinusitis	
(2) Liver damage or failure.	Few cases of liver failure have been reported, but the drugs are related to troglitazone (Rezulin), a drug that was taken off the market because of hepatotoxicity. Monitoring of liver enzymes is recommended during therapy.
(3) Fluid retention, edema, and congestive heart failure and with rosiglitazone risk of myocardial infarction and death.	Several reports indicate increased risks of developing or worsening heart failure and with rosiglitazone an increased risk of myocardial infarction and heart related death.
(4) Weight gain	
(5) Headache	
(6) Anemia	
g. With nateglinide and repaglinide:	
(1) Hypoglycemia	If occurs, usually of mild to moderate intensity
(2) Rhinitis, respiratory infection, influenza symptoms	These were the most commonly reported during clinical drug trials.
(3) Weight gain	This effect may decrease compliance with drug therapy, especially in adolescents and young-adult females.
h. With pramlintide and exenatide:	
(1) Nausea	Nausea is common. Nausea decreases with time in most patients. Pramlintide may require reduced dosage to control nausea.
i. With Byetta:	
(1) Acute abdominal discomfort	Acute pancreatitis is a rare but serious adverse effect.
4. Observe for drug interactions	
a. Drugs that *increase* effects of insulin:	
(1) Angiotensin-converting enzyme (ACE) inhibitors (e.g., captopril)	
(2) Alcohol	Increased hypoglycemia. Ethanol inhibits gluconeogenesis (in people with or without diabetes).
(3) Anabolic steroids	
(4) Antidiabetic drugs, oral	Oral agents are increasingly being used with insulin in the treatment of type 2 diabetes. The risks of hypoglycemia are greater with the combination but depend on the dosage of each drug and other factors that affect blood glucose levels.
(5) Antimicrobials (sulfonamides, tetracyclines)	
(6) Beta-adrenergic blocking agents (e.g., propranolol)	Increase hypoglycemia by inhibiting the effects of catecholamines on gluconeogenesis and glycogenolysis (effects that normally raise blood glucose levels in response to hypoglycemia). They also may mask signs and symptoms of hypoglycemia (e.g., tachycardia, tremors) that normally occur with a hypoglycemia-induced activation of the SNS.
b. Drugs that *decrease* effects of insulin:	These *diabetogenic* drugs may cause or aggravate diabetes because they raise blood sugar levels. Insulin dosage may need to be increased. Except with glucagon, hyperglycemia is an adverse effect of the drugs. Phenytoin and propranolol raise blood sugar by inhibiting insulin secretion; glucagon, a treatment for hypoglycemia, raises blood glucose by converting liver glycogen to glucose.
(1) Adrenergics (e.g., albuterol, epinephrine, others)	
(2) Corticosteroids (e.g., prednisone)	
(3) Estrogens and oral contraceptives	
(4) Glucagon	
(5) Levothyroxine (Synthroid)	
(6) Phenytoin (Dilantin)	
(7) Propranolol (Inderal)	
(8) Thiazide diuretics (e.g., hydrochlorothiazide)	
c. Drugs that *increase* effects of sulfonylureas:	
(1) Acarbose, miglitol, metformin, pioglitazone, rosiglitazone	One of these drugs may be used concomitantly with a sulfonylurea to improve glycemic control in patients with type 2 diabetes. There is an increased risk of hypoglycemia with the combinations.
(2) Alcohol (acute ingestion)	Additive hypoglycemia
(3) Cimetidine (Tagamet)	May inhibit metabolism of sulfonylureas, thereby increasing and prolonging hypoglycemic effects
(4) Insulin	Additive hypoglycemia

(continued on page 440)

Nursing Actions   Antidiabetic Drugs (continued)

NURSING ACTIONS	RATIONALE/EXPLANATION
d. Drugs that *decrease* effects of sulfonylureas:	
(1) Alcohol	Heavy, chronic intake of alcohol induces metabolizing enzymes in the liver. This accelerates metabolism of sulfonylureas, shortens their half-lives, and may produce hyperglycemia.
(2) Beta-blocking agents	Decrease hypoglycemic effects, possibly by decreasing release of insulin in the pancreas
(3) Corticosteroids, diuretics, epinephrine, estrogens, and oral contraceptives	These drugs have hyperglycemic effects.
(4) Glucagon	Raises blood glucose levels. It is used to treat severe hypoglycemia induced by insulin or oral antidiabetic agents.
(5) Nicotinic acid	Large doses have a hyperglycemic effect.
(6) Phenytoin (Dilantin)	Inhibits insulin secretion and has hyperglycemic effects
(7) Rifampin	Increases the rate of metabolism of sulfonylureas by inducing liver-metabolizing enzymes
(8) Thyroid preparations	Antagonize the hypoglycemic effects of oral antidiabetic drugs
e. Drugs that *decrease* effects of acarbose and miglitol:	
(1) Digestive enzymes	Decrease effects and should not be used concomitantly
(2) Intestinal adsorbents (e.g., charcoal)	Decrease effects and should not be used concomitantly
f. Drugs that *increase* effects of metformin:	
(1) Alcohol	Increases risk of hypoglycemia and lactic acidosis. Patients should avoid acute and chronic ingestion of excessive alcohol.
(2) Cimetidine	Increases risk of hypoglycemia. Cimetidine interferes with metabolism and increases blood levels of metformin.
(3) Furosemide	Increases blood levels of metformin
(4) Sulfonylurea hypoglycemic agents	The combination of these drugs is used to improve control of hyperglycemia in type 2 diabetes but it also increases risk of hypoglycemia.
g. Drugs that *increase* effects of pioglitazone:	
(1) Erythromycin, ketoconazole and related drugs	Inhibit cytochrome P450 3A4 enzymes that partially metabolize pioglitazone and may increase adverse effects. This interaction not reported with rosiglitazone, which is metabolized mainly by 2C8 and 2C9 enzymes.
h. Drugs that *increase* effects of nateglinide and repaglinide:	
(1) Nonsteroidal anti-inflammatory drugs and other agents that are highly bound to plasma proteins	May displace drugs from binding sites, therefore increasing their blood levels
(2) Beta blockers	
(3) Cimetidine, erythromycin, ketoconazole, miconazole	May inhibit hepatic metabolism of repaglinide and nateglinide and increase their blood levels
(4) Sulfonamides	
i. Drugs that *decrease* effects of nateglinide and repaglinide:	
(1) Adrenergics, corticosteroids, estrogens, niacin, oral contraceptives, thiazide diuretics	May cause hyperglycemia
(2) Carbamazepine, rifampin	Induce drug-metabolizing enzymes in the liver, which leads to faster inactivation
j. Drugs that may *increase* the effects of pramlintide and exenatide:	
(1) Anticholinergics	May further slow GI motility and intestinal absorption of drugs and/or nutrients.
(2) Alpha-glucosidase inhibitors	

Key Concepts

- The American Diabetes Association (ADA) suggests a target A1C of less than 7%.

- The ADA recommends re-evaluation of the management plan for anyone unable to achieve desired goals.

- A1C should be measured every 3 to 6 months.

- Exercise is perhaps the best therapy for the prevention of both type 2 diabetes and the metabolic syndrome. Exercise is an extremely strong hypoglycemic agent.

- Diabetes self-management education involves a continuum of services ranging from the teaching of survival skills to comprehensive self-management education programs to intensive management.

- Educational needs should be assessed at time of diagnosis and whenever there is poor clinical control or a major change in therapy.

- Licensed health care professionals with specific training in diabetes and training in education of people with diabetes should teach self-management education.

- Self-management education needs and plans should be documented in the medical record and acknowledged by all providers.

- Medical nutrition therapy is an integral component of diabetes management and of diabetes self-management education.

- A registered dietitian who is knowledgeable and skilled in implementing diabetes medical nutrition therapy should be the team member with primary responsibility for nutrition care and education.

- Self-monitoring of blood glucose(SMBG) is an important tool for achieving glycemic control.

- The frequency of SMBG should be individualized based on type of diabetes, glucose goals, and other factors.

- Weight loss is recommended to lower elevated blood glucose levels in overweight and obese persons with type 2 diabetes.

- Weight loss and weight maintenance therapy should use the combination of low-calorie diets, increased physical activity, and behavior therapy

- Annual influenza vaccine is recommended for all patients with diabetes.

- Pneumococcal vaccine is recommended for all patients with diabetes.

- Individuals who are at high risk for type 2 diabetes should be screened for disease.

- A fasting plasma glucose test (FPG) is the simplest and least expensive screening test.

- A FPG result of at least 126 milligrams per deciliter on two separate occasions is diagnostic of diabetes; values of 100 to 125 milligrams per deciliter are termed impaired fasting glucose, and values less than 100 milligrams per deciliter are considered normal.

- Individuals with impaired glucose tolerance can significantly reduce the risk of developing type 2 diabetes through intervention with diet and exercise.

- Medication therapy can involve oral hypoglycemic agents; insulin; newer agents such as amylin analogs, incretin mimetics, or dipeptidyl peptidase-4 inhibitors; or a combination of these therapies.

- Medication therapy is a therapeutic tool for use in lowering and maintaining blood glucose levels.

- Candidates for intensive insulin management must be motivated to improve glucose control and able to assume responsibility for their day-to-day care.

- Use of intensive insulin management should be initiated, monitored, and supported by a comprehensive diabetes team.

- Intensive insulin management is essential during pregnancy and recommended for all who wish to reduce their risk of diabetes complications.

Review and Application Exercises

Short Answer Exercises

1. What is the function of insulin in normal cellular metabolism?

2. What are the effects of insulin, cortisol, epinephrine, glucagon, and growth hormone on blood glucose levels?

3. What are the major differences between type 1 and type 2 diabetes?

4. What is the rationale for maintaining near-normal blood glucose levels? What is the major risk?

5. At what blood glucose range is brain damage most likely to occur?

6. Compare regular and NPH insulins in terms of onset, peak, and duration of action.

7. Describe major characteristics and uses of insulin analogs.

8. In a diabetic patient with typical signs and symptoms, distinguish between manifestations of hyperglycemia and hypoglycemia.

9. Contrast the five types of oral hypoglycemic agents in terms of mechanisms of action, indications for use, contraindications to use, and adverse effects.

10. For an adult patient newly diagnosed with type 2 diabetes, outline interventions to assist the patient in learning self-care.

11. Prepare a teaching plan for a patient starting insulin therapy and for a patient starting an oral hypoglycemic drug.

12. For a diabetic patient who reports using dietary and herbal supplements, analyze specific supplements in relation to their potential impact on blood sugar control.

NCLEX-Style Questions

13. Your patient is NPO for surgery at 10:00 A.M. He routinely receives 30 units of Humulin 70/30 every morning at 7:00 A.M. What is the appropriate nursing action in this situation?
    a. Administer 30 units of Humulin 70/30 Sub-Q.
    b. Hold the insulin because the patient is NPO.
    c. Give the patient a light breakfast and administer the insulin as ordered.
    d. Contact the physician for a pre-surgery insulin order.

14. The nurse knows that which of the following insulins cannot be administered in a continuous Sub-Q insulin infusion pump?
    a. regular insulin (Humulin R)
    b. insulin aspart (NovoLog)
    c. insulin glulisine (Apidra)
    d. insulin glargine (Lantus)

15. When teaching a newly diagnosed diabetic patient how to self-administer short- and intermediate-acting insulin Sub-Q, which of the following instructions is correct?
    a. The order of drawing up the two insulins into the syringe does not matter.
    b. Draw the short-acting insulin into the syringe first, followed by the intermediate-acting insulin.
    c. Draw the intermediate-acting insulin into the syringe first, followed by the short-acting insulin.
    d. You need to give yourself two injections because mixing these insulins together is unsafe.

16. An older person with type 2 diabetes who takes metformin presents to the emergency department with symptoms of drowsiness, malaise, respiratory distress, and bradycardia. As the nurse, you suspect
    a. hypoglycemia
    b. hyperglycemia
    c. lactic acidosis
    d. metabolic alkalosis

17. The nurse should be especially alert to the adverse effect of hypoglycemia in a type 2 diabetic patient taking which of the following oral hypoglycemics?
    a. sulfonylureas
    b. alpha-glucosidase inhibitors
    c. biguanide
    d. thiazolidinediones

Selected References

Ahren, B., & Schmitz, O. (2004). GLP-1 receptor agonists and DPP-4 inhibitors in the treatment of type 2 diabetes. *Hormone and Metabolic Research, 36*, 867–876.

American Diabetes Association. (2006). Position statement: Standards of medical in diabetes—2006. *Diabetes Care, 29*, S4–S42.

American Diabetes Association. (2007). *Prediabetes.* Retrieved May 22, 2007, from http://www.diabetes.org/pre-diabetes.jsp

American Heart Association. (2007). *Metabolic syndrome.* Retrieved May 22, 2007, from http://www.americanheart.org/presenter.jhtml?identifier=4756

Bond, A. (2006). Exenatide (Byetta) as a novel treatment option for type 2 diabetes mellitus. *Proceedings of the Baylor University Medical Center, 19*, 281–284. Retrieved May 6, 2007 from, http://www.byetta.com/index.jsp?reqNavId=0

Davies, M., Storms, F., Shutler, S., Bianchi-Biscay, M., & Gomis, R. (2005). Improvement of glycemic control in subjects with poorly controlled type 2 diabetes: Comparison of two treatment algorithms using insulin glargine. *Diabetes Care, 28*, 1282–1288.

Drug facts and comparisons. (Updated monthly). St. Louis, MO: Facts and Comparisons.

Fetrow, C. W., Avila, J. R., & Margolis, S. (2003). *Professional's handbook of complementary and alternative medicines.* Springhouse, PA: Springhouse.

Fink, M. P. (2004, May 6). The role of maintaining tight control of blood glucose in the ICU. *ACS Surgery: Principles and Practice.* Retrieved September 16, 2005, from http://www.medscape.com/viewarticle/474745.

Guven, S., Kuenzi, J. A., & Matfin, G. (2005). Diabetes mellitus and the metabolic syndrome. In C. M. Porth (Ed.), *Pathophysiology: Concepts of altered health states* (7th ed., pp. 987–1015). Philadelphia: Lippincott Williams & Wilkins.

Krantz, M. J. (2006). Implications of thiazolidinedione use and cardiovascular risk: Is it all about the sugar? *Pharmacotherapy, 26*, 1049; discussion, 1049–1050.

Nelson, S. E., & Palumbo, P. J. (2006). Addition of insulin to oral therapy in patients with type 2 diabetes. *American Journal of the Medical Sciences, 331*, 257–263.

Novo Nordisk Inc. (2005). *Levemir* [Package Insert]. Princeton, NJ.

Ovalle, F., & Bell, D. S. (2004). Effect of rosiglitazone versus insulin on the pancreatic beta-cell function of subjects with type 2 diabetes. *Diabetes Care, 27*, 2585–2589.

Zacker, R. J. (2004). Exercise: A key component of diabetes management. *Diabetes Spectrum, 17*, 142–144.

Estrogens, Progestins, and Hormonal Contraceptives

LEARNING OBJECTIVES

After studying this chapter, you will be able to:

1. Discuss the effects of endogenous estrogens and progestins.
2. Outline the benefits and risks of postmenopausal hormone replacement therapy.
3. Recognize adverse effects associated with estrogens, progestins, and hormonal contraceptives.
4. Apply nursing process with patients taking estrogens, progestins, and hormonal contraceptives.

Applying Your Knowledge

Vickie Dalquist is a 21-year-old student. She has chosen to use oral contraceptives to prevent unwanted pregnancy. Vickie takes Alesse. You are the nurse at the student health clinic.

Introduction

Estrogens and *progestins* are female sex hormones produced primarily by the ovaries and secondarily by the adrenal cortex in nonpregnant women. Small amounts of estrogens are also synthesized in the liver, kidney, brain, skeletal muscle, testes, and adipose tissue. In normal premenopausal women, estrogen synthesis in adipose tissue may be a significant source of the hormone. Some evidence indicates that a minimum body weight (about 105 lb) and fat content (16%–24%) are required for initiation and maintenance of the menstrual cycle. This view is supported by the observation that women with anorexia nervosa, chronic disease, or malnutrition and those who are long-distance runners usually have amenorrhea. With anorexia nervosa, regaining weight and body mass usually re-establishes normal menstrual patterns.

As with other steroid hormones, estrogens and progestins are synthesized from cholesterol. The ovaries and adrenal glands can manufacture cholesterol or extract it from the blood. Through a series of chemical reactions, cholesterol is converted to progesterone and then to androgens, testosterone, and androstenedione. The ovaries use these male sex hormones to produce estrogens. After formation, the hormones are secreted into the bloodstream in response to stimulation by the anterior pituitary gonadotropic hormones, follicle-stimulating hormone (FSH), and luteinizing hormone (LH). In the bloodstream, the hormones combine with serum proteins and are transported to target tissues where they enter body cells. They cross cell membranes easily because of their steroid structure and lipid solubility. Inside the cells, the hormones bind to estrogen or progestin receptors and regulate intracellular protein synthesis. Estrogen can enhance target-tissue responses to progesterone by increasing progesterone receptors. Progesterone seems to inhibit tissue responses to estrogen by decreasing estrogen receptors.

Estrogens

Three ovarian estrogens (estradiol, estrone, and estriol) are secreted in significant amounts. Estradiol is the major estrogen because it exerts more estrogenic activity than the other two estrogens combined. The main function of the estrogens is to promote growth in tissues related to reproduction and sexual characteristics in women. More specific effects of estrogens on body tissues are described in Box 27-1.

In nonpregnant women, between puberty and menopause, estrogens are secreted in a monthly cycle called the menstrual cycle. During the first half of the cycle, before ovulation, estrogens are secreted in progressively larger amounts. During the second half of the cycle, estrogens and progesterone are secreted in increasing amounts until 2 to 3 days before the onset of menstruation. At that time, secretion of both hormones decreases abruptly. When the endometrial lining of the uterus loses its hormonal stimulation, it is discharged vaginally as menstrual flow.

During pregnancy, the placenta in conjunction with the fetus produces large amounts of estrogen causing enlargement of the uterus and breasts, growth of glandular tissue in the breasts, and relaxation of ligaments and joints in the pelvis. All these changes are necessary for the growth and birth of the fetus.

Finally, estrogens are deactivated in the liver and readily excreted through the kidneys. Metabolites are also formed in the gastrointestinal tract, brain, skin, and other steroid target tissues. Most of the conjugates are excreted in urine, and some are excreted in bile and recirculated to the liver or excreted in feces.

Progesterone

In the nonpregnant woman, progesterone is secreted by the corpus luteum during the last half of the menstrual cycle, which occurs after ovulation. This hormone continues the changes in the endometrial lining of the uterus begun by estrogens during

---

Box 27-1	Effects of Endogenous Estrogens

Breasts

■ Stimulate growth at puberty by causing deposition of fat, formation of connective tissue, and construction of ducts. These ducts become part of the milk-producing apparatus after additional stimulation by progesterone.

Sexual Organs

■ Enlarge the fallopian tubes, uterus, vagina, and external genitalia at puberty, when estrogen secretion increases greatly
■ Cause the endometrial lining of the uterus to proliferate and develop glands that later nourish the implanted ovum when pregnancy occurs
■ Increase resistance of the epithelial lining of the vagina to trauma and infection

Skeleton

■ Stimulate skeletal growth so that, beginning at puberty, height increases rapidly for several years. Estrogen then causes the epiphyses to unite with the shafts of the long bones, and linear growth is halted. This effect of estrogen is stronger than the similar effect of testosterone in the male. Consequently, women stop growing in height several years earlier than men and on the average are shorter than men.
■ Conserve calcium and phosphorus for healthy bones and teeth. This action promotes bone formation and decreases bone loss.
■ Broaden the pelvis in preparation for childbirth

Skin and Subcutaneous Tissue

■ Increase vascularity in the skin. This leads to greater skin warmth and likelihood of bleeding in women.

■ Cause deposition of fat in subcutaneous tissue, especially in the breasts, thighs, and buttocks, which produces the characteristic female figure

Anterior Pituitary Gland

■ Decrease pituitary secretion of follicle-stimulating hormone and increase secretion of luteinizing hormone when blood levels are sufficiently high (negative feedback mechanism)

Metabolism

■ Affect metabolism of both reproductive and nonreproductive tissues. Estrogen receptors are found in female reproductive organs, breast tissue, bone, the brain, liver, heart, and blood vessels. They are also found in various tissues in men.
■ Increase protein anabolism, bone growth, and epiphyseal closure in young girls
■ Decrease bone resorption
■ Increase sodium and water retention, serum triglycerides, and high-density lipoproteins (HDL or "good" cholesterol)
■ Decrease low-density lipoproteins (LDL or "bad" cholesterol)
■ Increase the amount of cholesterol in bile and thereby increase gallstone formation

Blood Coagulation

■ Enhance coagulation by increasing blood levels of several clotting factors, including prothrombin and factors VII, IX, and X, and probably increase platelet aggregation the first half of the menstrual cycle. These changes provide for implantation and nourishment of a fertilized ovum. When fertilization does not take place, the estrogen and progesterone levels decrease and menstruation occurs.

If the ovum is fertilized, progesterone acts to maintain the pregnancy. The corpus luteum produces progesterone during the first few weeks of gestation. Then, the placenta produces the progesterone needed to maintain the endometrial lining of the uterus. In addition to its effects on the uterus, progesterone prepares the breasts for lactation by promoting development of milk-producing cells. Milk is not secreted, however, until the cells are further stimulated by prolactin from the anterior pituitary gland. Progesterone also may help maintain pregnancy by decreasing uterine contractility. This, in turn, decreases the risk of spontaneous abortion.

Progesterone, in general, has opposite effects on lipid metabolism compared with estrogen. That is, progestins decrease high-density lipoprotein cholesterol and increase low-density lipoprotein cholesterol, both of which increase risks of cardiovascular disease. Physiologic progesterone increases insulin levels but does not usually impair glucose tolerance. However, long-term administration of potent synthetic exogenous progestins, such as norgestrel, may decrease glucose tolerance and make diabetes mellitus more difficult to control. Like estrogen, progesterone is metabolized in the liver.

General Characteristics of Estrogens, Progestins, and Hormonal Contraceptives

Mechanisms of Action

Estrogens circulate in the bloodstream to target cells, where they enter cells and combine with receptor proteins in cell cytoplasm. The estrogen–receptor complex is then transported to the cell nucleus where it interacts with DNA to produce RNA and new DNA. These substances stimulate cell reproduction and production of various proteins. Progestins also diffuse freely into cells, where they bind to progesterone receptors.

Hormonal contraceptives act by several mechanisms. First, they inhibit hypothalamic secretion of gonadotropin-releasing hormone, which inhibits pituitary secretion of FSH and LH. When these gonadotropic hormones are absent, ovulation and therefore conception cannot occur. Second, the drugs produce cervical mucus that resists penetration of spermatozoa into the upper reproductive tract. Third, the drugs interfere with endometrial maturation and reception of ova that are released and fertilized. These overlapping mechanisms make the drugs highly effective in preventing pregnancy.

Indications for Use

Estrogens

Indications for use of exogenous estrogens include the following:

■ As a component in birth control pills and other contraceptive preparations. An estrogen, when combined with a progestin, is used widely in females ages 12 to 45 years to control fertility. If pregnancy does occur, estrogens are contraindicated because their use during pregnancy has been associated with the occurrence of vaginal cancer in female offspring and possible harmful effects on male offspring.

■ Menopause. Estrogens are prescribed to relieve symptoms of estrogen deficiency (e.g., atrophic vaginitis and vasomotor instability, which produces "hot flashes" or "hot flushes") and to prevent or treat osteoporosis. Such use is usually called estrogen replacement therapy (ERT). When estrogen is prescribed for women with an intact uterus, a progestin is also given to prevent unwanted thickening of the lining of the uterus and to decrease the risk of cancer of the uterus, a possible result of using estrogen alone. Both drug therapies are commonly referred to as hormone replacement therapy (HRT) or menopausal hormone therapy (MHT), terms used to describe the administration of one or more female hormones during menopause.

■ As replacement therapy in deficiency states. Deficiency states usually result from hypofunction of the pituitary gland or the ovaries and may occur anytime during the life cycle. For example, in the adolescent girl with delayed sexual development, estrogen can be given to produce the changes that normally occur at puberty. In the woman of reproductive age (approximately 12 to 45 years of age), estrogens are occasionally used in menstrual disorders, including amenorrhea and abnormal uterine bleeding due to estrogen deficiency.

Recent large-scale randomized controlled trials indicated that for estrogen-only and combined estrogen–progestin therapy risks are greater than benefits (Box 27-2).

Progestins

Progestins are most often used in combination with an estrogen in contraceptive products. They also are used to suppress ovarian function in dysmenorrhea, endometriosis, endometrial cancer, and uterine bleeding. These uses of progestins are extensions of the physiologic actions of progesterone on the neuroendocrine control of ovarian function and on the endometrium. For approximately 20 to 25 years, progestins were used in combination with estrogen for long-term HRT in postmenopausal women with an intact uterus. With HRT, the purpose of a progestin is to prevent endometrial cancer, which can occur with unopposed estrogenic stimulation. Currently, however, the combination is not recommended for long-term use because evidence indicated that the adverse effects outweigh the beneficial effects (see Box 27-2).

Hormonal Contraceptives

The primary clinical indication for the use of hormonal contraceptives is to control fertility and prevent pregnancy. Some products are used for contraception after unprotected sexual intercourse. These preparations also are used to treat menstrual disorders (e.g., amenorrhea, dysmenorrhea).

Box 27-2	Hormone Replacement Therapy in Postmenopausal Women

From the 1980s until mid-2002, long-term postmenopausal estrogen replacement therapy (ERT) was frequently recommended for women, with the expectation that it would manage menopausal symptoms, exert cardioprotective effects, prevent osteoporosis, and prolong life. Two large-scale randomized controlled trials, the Heart and Estrogen/Progestin Replacement Study (HERS) and the Women's Health Initiative (WHI), disputed this prevailing observational data and expert opinion.

The Heart and Estrogen–Progestin Replacement Studies, HERS and HERS II, involved postmenopausal women with an intact uterus who already had coronary heart disease (CHD). Results indicated that in women who had pre-existing heart disease, hormones provided no benefit in relation to preventing serious cardiovascular events; this increased interest in the NIH-funded WHI trials that were designed to evaluate primary prevention.

The WHI study was conducted in healthy women to determine if an estrogen–progestin combination (in women with an intact uterus) or estrogen alone (in postmenopausal women who have had a hysterectomy) would prevent the development of CHD.

Both arms of the WHI study were stopped in the interest of safety. The consensus was that with estrogen-only therapy in post-hysterectomy women the hormone increased the risk of stroke and offered no protection against heart disease. As with healthy women, the conclusion of the WHI was that the hormones should not be started or continued for preventive purposes in women with CHD because risks were greater than benefits.

In the arm of the study looking at postmenopausal women who have had a hysterectomy and thus do not need a progestin, estrogen-only therapy significantly increased the hazard of deep vein thrombosis and had no significant effect on the risk of colorectal or breast cancer. A reduced risk of hip and other fractures was reported. A related study also found that the hormone might also increase the risk of dementia and mild cognitive impairment in older women.

In summary, studies have demonstrated no evidence for HRT in secondary prevention of heart disease and showed increased rates of CHD, thromboembolic stroke, venous thromboembolism, dementia, and breast cancer, which outweigh the benefits of decreased risk of fracture and colon cancer. Thromboembolic disorders are most likely to occur during the first year of use; risks of developing breast cancer increase with the duration of drug use. The FDA recommended that HRT only be used for women with symptoms severe enough to warrant its use, at the lowest dose and for the shortest duration possible, to ease the menopausal transition.

Contraindications to Use

Because of their widespread effects on body tissues and reported adverse reactions, estrogens, progestins, and hormonal contraceptives are contraindicated in

- Known or suspected pregnancy, because *teratogenic* effects capable of interfering with the normal development of the fetus may result
- Thromboembolic disorders, such as thrombophlebitis, deep vein thrombosis, or pulmonary embolism
- Known or suspected cancers of breast or genital tissues, because the drugs may stimulate tumor growth. An exception is the use of estrogens for treatment of metastatic breast cancer in women at least 5 years postmenopause.
- Undiagnosed vaginal or uterine bleeding
- Fibroid tumors of the uterus
- Active liver disease or impaired liver function
- History of cerebrovascular disease, coronary artery disease, thrombophlebitis, hypertension, or conditions predisposing to these disease processes
- Women older than 35 years of age who smoke cigarettes. These women have a greater risk of thromboembolic disorders if they take hormonal contraceptives, possibly because of increased platelet aggregation with estrogen ingestion and cigarette smoking. In addition, estrogen increases hepatic production of blood clotting factors.
- Family history of breast or reproductive system cancer

Individual Drugs

When exogenous estrogens and progestins are administered for therapeutic purposes, they produce the same effects as endogenous hormones. Multiple preparations of estrogens and progestins are available for various purposes and routes of administration. Clinical indications, routes of administration, and dosages are discussed in the estrogens and progestins Drugs at a Glance tables.

Estrogens

Table 27-1 summarizes important drug information about estrogens. The most widely used synthetic steroidal estrogen is **ethinyl estradiol** (Estinyl), which is used in hormonal contraceptives. Ethinyl estradiol is well absorbed with oral administration and reaches peak plasma levels within 2 hours. It is 98% bound to plasma proteins, and its half-life varies from 6 to 20 hours. Ethinyl estradiol undergoes extensive first-pass hepatic metabolism and is further metabolized and conjugated in the liver; the conjugates are then excreted in bile and urine.

Transdermal estradiol patches (e.g., Climara, Estraderm, Vivelle) allow for absorption of estrogen through the skin to the bloodstream. The patches are applied weekly or biweekly depending on the preparation. Serum levels produced through transdermal application more closely mimic premenopausal estrogen levels compared with serum levels with oral estrogens.

Table 27-1	Drugs at a Glance: Estrogens

ROUTES AND DOSAGE RANGES FOR VARIOUS INDICATIONS

Generic/ Trade Name	Menopausal Symptoms	Female Hypogonadism	Prevention of Osteoporosis	Other
Conjugated estrogens (synthetic) (Cenestin)	PO 0.625–1.25 mg daily			
Conjugated estrogens (Premarin)	PO 0.3–1.25 mg daily for 21 d followed by 7 d without the drug	PO 2.5–7.5 mg daily in divided doses, cyclically, 20 d on, 10 d off the drug	PO 0.625 mg daily for 21 d, then 7 d without the drug	Dysfunctional uterine bleeding: IM or IV for emergency use, 25 mg, repeated in 6–12 h if necessary Atrophic vaginitis: Topically, 2.4 g of vaginal cream inserted daily
Estradiol (Estrace, Estring)	PO 1–2 mg daily for 3 wk, then 1 wk off or daily Monday through Friday, none on Saturday or Sunday as prescribed		PO 0.5 mg daily for 23 d and no drug for 5 d each month	Atrophic vaginitis: Cream, 2–4 g daily for 2 wk, then 1–2 g daily for 2 wk, then 1 g 1–3 times weekly; vaginal ring (Estring), 1 every 3 mo
Estradiol cypionate (Depo-Estradiol)	IM 1–5 mg every 3–4 wk	IM 1.5–2 mg at monthly intervals		
Estradiol hemihydrate (Vagifem)				Atrophic vaginitis: 1 tablet, inserted into vagina, daily for 2 wk, then twice weekly
Estradiol transdermal system (Estraderm, Climara, Vivelle)	Topically to skin, 1 patch 1 or 2 times per wk			
Estradiol valerate (Delestrogen)	IM 10–20 mg every 4 wk	IM 10–20 mg every 4 wk		
Estrone	IM 0.1–0.5 mg weekly in single or divided doses	IM 0.1–2 mg weekly		Dysfunctional uterine bleeding: IM 2–4 mg daily for several days until bleeding is controlled, followed by progestin for 1 wk
Estropipate (Ogen)	PO 0.625–5 mg daily, cyclically	PO 1.25–7.5 mg daily for 3 wk, followed by an 8- to 10-d rest period. Repeat as needed.	PO 0.625 mg daily for 25 d and no drug for 6 d each month	Ovarian failure: Same dosage as for female hypogonadism Atrophic vaginitis: Topically, 1–2 g vaginal cream daily

Rates of absorption vary, depending on the type of patch applied. The total amount of drug absorbed and the resulting plasma drug concentrations from transdermal estrogen can increase during exposure to heat, so patients should be advised to avoid prolonged sun exposure in the area of the patch.

Conjugated estrogens (Premarin) and some synthetic derivatives of natural estrogens (e.g., ethinyl estradiol) are chemically modified to be effective with oral administration. Conjugated estrogens are used to treat moderate to severe vasomotor and atrophic symptoms associated with menopause, to prevent postmenopausal osteoporosis, and as palliative treatment for metastatic breast carcinoma and advanced androgen-dependent prostatic cancer. Intravenous injection is used, in the absence of organic pathology, for the treatment of abnormal uterine bleeding caused by hormonal imbalance. Conjugated estrogens are well absorbed with oral administration and are released slowly over several hours. Degradation occurs very slowly in the liver, allowing for high intrinsic potency with these preparations.

Along with several cream formulations, a vaginal tablet (Vagifem) and a vaginal ring (Estring) of estrogen are available for topical application in treating atrophic vaginitis.

Nonsteroidal synthetic preparations are chemically altered to slow their metabolism in the liver. They are also less bound to serum proteins than naturally occurring hormones. As with conjugated estrogens, nonsteroidal synthetic preparations are well absorbed with oral administration and are released slowly over several hours. Degradation occurs very slowly in the liver, allowing for high intrinsic potency with these preparations.

The FDA has issued a **BLACK BOX WARNING** that estrogens increase the risk for developing cancer of the uterus. The warning instructs individuals who take estrogens with or without progestins that there is an increased risk of dementia, myocardial infarctions, strokes, breast cancer, and blood clots.

Progestins

Progestins (Table 27-2) are used as noncontraceptives and as oral contraceptives, both as estrogen–progestin combinations and as progestin-only preparations ("minipills"). The choice of a combination contraceptive product may be determined by the progestin component. Progestins with minimal androgenic activity are **desogestrel** and **norgestimate**, those with intermediate activity include **norethindrone** and **ethynodiol**, and those with high androgenic effects include **norgestrel**. Progestins are rapidly absorbed after oral administration and go through prompt hepatic degradation. The drug can reach maximum concentration in 1 to 2 hours. Drug half-life varies. During the first 6 hours, half-life is about 2 to 3 hours; thereafter, half-life extends to 8 to 9 hours. Metabolites are excreted primarily in the urine. Progestins administered intramuscularly are also rapidly absorbed, with a half-life of just a few minutes. Long-acting forms can maintain effective concentrations for 3 to 6 months; maximum concentrations can be achieved in 24 hours with a half-life of about 10 weeks. Gel preparations have sustained-release properties, and absorption is prolonged with half-lives of 1 to 2 days.

There is no evidence to suggest that use of progestins in the first trimester of pregnancy to prevent habitual abortion is safe. There is evidence that when the drug is given during the first 4 months of pregnancy fetal harm is possible.

Table 27-3 provides information about noncontraceptive estrogen–progestin combinations. Several noncontraceptive combination oral tablets are available for treatment of menopausal symptoms and osteoporosis. Two combination products (Combi-Patch and Ortho Evra) are available in transdermal patches for topical application.

Hormonal Contraceptives

Most hormonal contraceptives consist of a synthetic estrogen (e.g., ethinyl estradiol) and a synthetic progestin (e.g., norethindrone) (Table 27-4). Three different types of formulation for hormonal contraceptives are commonly prescribed: monophasic contraceptives containing fixed amounts of both

| Table 27-2 | **Drugs at a Glance:** Progestins |

Generic/ Trade Name	\multicolumn{4}{c}{ROUTES AND DOSAGE RANGES FOR VARIOUS INDICATIONS}
	Menstrual Disorders	**Endometriosis**	**Endometrial Cancer**	**Other**
Medroxyproges-terone acetate (Depo-Provera, Provera)	Dysfunctional uterine bleeding: PO 5–10 mg daily for 5–10 d, beginning on 16th or 21st d of cycle		IM 400–1000 mg weekly until improvement, then 400 mg monthly	
Megestrol acetate (Megace)	Amenorrhea: PO 5–10 mg daily for 5–10 d		PO 40–320 mg daily in 4 divided doses for at least 2 mo	Breast cancer: PO 160 mg daily in 4 divided doses for at least 2 mo
Norethindrone acetate (Aygestin)	Amenorrhea, dysfunctional uterine bleeding: PO 2.5–10 mg daily, starting on 5th d of menstrual cycle and ending on 25th d	PO 5 mg daily for 2 wk, increased by 2.5 mg daily every 2 wk to dose of 15 mg. Then give 10–15 mg daily for maintenance.		
Progesterone	Amenorrhea, dysfunctional uterine bleeding: IM 5–10 mg for 6–8 consecutive d			

Table 27-3			Drugs at a Glance: Noncontraceptive Estrogen–Progestin Combination	
TRADE NAME	**ESTROGEN**	**PROGESTIN**	**INDICATIONS FOR USE**	**ROUTES AND DOSAGE RANGES**
Activella	Estradiol 1 mg	Norethindrone 0.5 mg	Menopausal symptoms; prevention of osteoporosis	PO 1 tablet daily
Combi-Patch	Estradiol 0.05 mg	Norethindrone 0.14 or 0.25 mg	Estrogen deficiency states due to menopause, hypogonadism, castration, or primary ovarian failure	1 transdermal patch twice weekly
Femhrt	Ethinyl estradiol 5 mcg	Norethindrone 1 mg	Menopausal symptoms; prevention of osteoporosis	PO 1 tablet daily
Premphase	Conjugated estrogens 0.625 mg*	Medroxyprogesterone 5 mg	Menopausal symptoms; prevention of osteoporosis	PO 1 tablet of estrogen-only once daily on d 1–14, then 1 combination tablet once daily on d 15–28
Prempro	Conjugated estrogens 0.3, 0.45, 0.625 mg	Medroxyprogesterone 1.5. 2.5, or 5 mg	Menopausal symptoms; prevention of osteoporosis	PO 1 tablet once daily in dial packs 28s

*Also available with estrogen only.

estrogen and progestin components, and biphasics and triphasics containing either fixed amounts of estrogen and varied amounts of progestin or varied amounts of both estrogen and progestin. Biphasic and triphasic preparations mimic normal variations of hormone secretion, decrease the total dosage of hormones, and may decrease adverse effects. These contraceptives are dispensed in containers with color-coded tablets that must be taken in the correct sequence. Dispensers with 28 tablets contain 7 inactive or placebo tablets of a third color. A few contraceptives are progestin-only products. These are not widely used because they are less effective in preventing pregnancy and are more likely to cause vaginal bleeding, which makes them less acceptable to many women. Several combination products and alternative dosage forms are available to help individualize treatment and promote compliance. Table 27-4 outlines the trade names of hormonal contraceptives

Applying Your Knowledge 27-1

Vickie comes to the clinic for a routine visit. You review her medication history. Vickie asks about the different-colored pills in her contraceptive container. What is the best response?

Herbal and Dietary Supplement

Black cohosh is an herb used to self-treat symptoms of menopause, and reportedly is effective in relieving vasomotor instability. Most published information supports the benefit of the herb for the relief of menopause-related symptoms; however, clinical trials in this area have demonstrated methodologic limitations, and more definitive information regarding safety and efficacy are needed. The product apparently exerts a nonhormonal effect and does not affect the endometrium or estrogen-dependent cancers; however, its effects on bone and osteoporosis are unknown. Trade names include Remifemin, Estroven, Femtrol, and GNC Menopause Formula.

Adverse effects may include nausea, vomiting, dizziness, hypotension, and visual disturbances. Blood pressure should be monitored closely in hypertensive patients, because the herb may increase the hypotensive effects of antihypertensive drugs. Black cohosh is contraindicated in pregnancy and not recommended for use longer than 6 months for menopausal symptoms.

Overall, this herb may be considered in patients who refuse estrogen therapy recommended by a prescriber or have conditions in which estrogen is contraindicated. If Remifemin is taken, the recommended dosage is one tablet (standardized to contain 20 mg of herbal drug) twice daily. Other dosage forms are available, and dosage depends on the method of preparation.

Table 27-4	Hormonal Contraceptives	

Estrogen–Progestin Combination Products

Monophasics

Alesse	Low-Orgestrel	Ortho-Cept
Apri	Microgestin Fe 1/20	Ortho-Cyclen
Aviane	Microgestin Fe 1.5/30	Ortho-Novum 1/35
Brevicon	Modicon	Ortho-Novum 1/50
Demulen 1/35	Necon 0.5/35	Ovcon-35
Demulen 1/50	Necon 1/35	Ovcon-50
Desogen	Necon 1/50	Ovral-28
Levlen	Nordette	Yasmin
Levlite	Norinyl 1 + 35	Zovia 1/35E
Levora	Norinyl 1 + 50	Zovia 1/50E
Loestrin 21 1.5/30	Nortrel 0.5/35	
Loestrin Fe 1/20	Nortrel 1/35	
Loestrin Fe 1.5/30	Ogestrel	

Biphasics

Jenest-28	Necon 10/11
Mircette	Ortho-Novum 10/11

Triphasics

Estrostep 21	Tri-Levlen
Estrostep Fe	Tri-Norinyl
Ortho-Novum 7/7/7	Triphasil
Ortho Tri-Cyclen	Trivora-28

Progestin-Only Products

Depo-Provera	Ovrette
Micronor	Progestasert intrauterine
Norplant Subdermal System	Transdermal Preparation
Nor-QD	Ortho Evra

Emergency Contraceptive

Plan B

Applying Your Knowledge 27-2

Vickie comes back to the clinic and tells you that she has not had a menstrual period this past month. Further assessment reveals that Vickie may not have taken all of her pills in sequence and that she has been sexually active. She is about 3 weeks overdue for her period. What action would you take?

Applying Your Knowledge 27-3

Vickie is not pregnant and she decides to remain on oral contraceptives. She explains to you that she sometimes does not take her pill because they make her sick to her stomach. How do you respond?

Nursing Process

Assessment

Before drug therapy is started, patients need a thorough history and physical examination, including measurements of blood pressure, serum cholesterol, and triglycerides. These parameters must be monitored periodically as long as the drugs are taken.

- Assess for conditions in which estrogens and progestins are used (e.g., menstrual disorders, menopausal symptoms).
- Assess for conditions that increase risks of adverse effects or are contraindications for hormonal therapy (e.g., thromboembolic disorders, pregnancy).
- Record blood pressure with each outpatient contact or regularly with hospitalized patients. Increases are likely in premenopausal women, especially with oral contraceptives, but are unlikely in women who are postmenopausal who are receiving physiologic replacement doses.
- Check laboratory reports of cholesterol and triglyceride levels when available.
- Assess diet and presence of cigarette smoking. A high-fat diet increases the risks of gallbladder disease and perhaps other problems; cigarette smoking increases risks of thromboembolic disorders in women older than 35 years of age who take oral contraceptives.
- Assess the patient's willingness to comply with instructions about drug therapy and follow-up procedures.
- Assess for signs and symptoms of thromboembolic disorders regularly. These are most likely to occur in women older than 35 years of age who take oral contraceptives, women who are postmenopausal who receive combined estrogen–progestin HRT, and women or men who take large doses for cancer.

Nursing Diagnoses

- Disturbed Body Image in women, related to effects of hormone deficiency states
- Disturbed Body Image in men, related to feminizing effects and impotence from female hormones
- Excess Fluid Volume related to sodium and water retention
- Deficient Knowledge: Effects of hormonal therapy
- Risk for Injury related to increased risks of hypertension and gallbladder disease

Planning/Goals

The patient will

- Be assisted to cope with self-concept and body image changes
- Take the drugs accurately, for the length of time prescribed
- Experience relief of symptoms for which the drugs are given
- Avoid preventable adverse drug effects
- Keep appointments for monitoring of drug effects

Interventions

- Assist patients of childbearing age to choose an appropriate contraceptive method. If the choice is an estrogen–progestin combination, help the patient take it accurately.
- Help postmenopausal women plan for adequate calcium and vitamin D in the diet and adequate weight-bearing exercise to maintain bone strength and prevent osteoporosis.
- Assist patients in obtaining follow-up health care when indicated.
- Provide patient teaching for drug therapy (see accompanying displays).

Evaluation

- Interview and observe for compliance with instructions for taking the drugs.
- Interview and observe for therapeutic and adverse drug effects.

Principles of Therapy

Need for Continuous Supervision

Because estrogens, progestins, and hormonal contraceptives are often taken for years and may cause adverse reactions, patients taking these drugs need continued supervision by a health care provider. Before the drugs are prescribed, a complete medical history, a physical examination including breast and pelvic examinations and a Papanicolaou (Pap) test, uri-nalysis, and weight and blood pressure measurements are recommended. These examinations should be repeated at least annually as long as the patient is taking the drugs.

Drug Selection

Choice of preparation depends on the reason for use, desired route of administration, and duration of action. Conjugated estrogen (e.g., Premarin) is a commonly used oral estrogen, and medroxyprogesterone (e.g., Provera) is a commonly used oral progestin. Transdermal estradiol (e.g., Climara, Estraderm, Vivelle) allows for absorption of estrogen through the skin to the bloodstream. Two advantages have been recognized with this form of administration. Because the liver is bypassed, the total dose of estrogen is reduced. Additionally, the serum levels produced through transdermal application more closely mimic premenopausal estrogen levels compared with serum levels with oral estrogens.

The choice of a combination contraceptive product may be determined by the progestin component. Some progestins are more likely to cause weight gain, acne, and changes in blood lipids that increase risks of myocardial infarction or stroke. These adverse effects are attributed mainly to the androgenic activity of the progestin, and some progestins have more androgenic effects than others. Duration of action may also be a factor. Some crystalline suspensions of estrogens and oil solutions of both estrogens and progesterone prolong drug action by slowing absorption. Long-acting progestin contraceptive preparations such as the intramuscular depot medroxyprogesterone (Depo-Provera) last 3 months per injection, intrauterine progesterone lasts 1 year, and levonorgestrel subcutaneous implants (Norplant) last 5 years.

Drug Dosage

Although dosage needs vary with patients and the conditions for which the drugs are prescribed, a general rule is to use the smallest effective dose for the shortest effective time. Estrogens are often given cyclically. In one regimen, the drug is taken for 3 weeks and then omitted for 1 week; in another, it is omitted the first 5 days of each month. These regimens more closely resemble normal secretion of estrogen and avoid prolonged stimulation of body tissues. A progestin may be added for 10 days each month.

Drug Administration

Naturally occurring, nonconjugated estrogens (estradiol, estrone) and natural progesterone are given intramuscularly because they are rapidly metabolized if administered orally. Nonsteroidal synthetic preparations are usually administered orally or topically.

Drug Interactions

These drugs may interact with several drugs or drug groups to increase or decrease their effects. Most interactions have been reported with oral contraceptives.

Estrogens may decrease the effectiveness of sulfonylurea antidiabetic drugs (probably by increasing their metabolism);

Patient Teaching Guidelines | Hormone Replacement Therapy

General Considerations

- Hormone replacement therapy (HRT) relieves symptoms of menopause and helps to prevent or treat osteoporosis.
- Women receiving HRT should be under medical supervision and should have a physical examination at least annually to check blood pressure and breasts, pelvis, and other areas for possible adverse reactions when these drugs are taken for long periods.
- Women who have not had a hysterectomy should take both estrogen and progestin; the progestin component (e.g., Provera) prevents endometrial cancer, an adverse effect of estrogen-only therapy. Post-hysterectomy, women should take estrogen-only medications. However, the Women's Health Initiative study concluded that risks of adverse effects with estrogen-only therapy and estrogen–progestin combinations are greater than previously believed (see Box 27-2). Women who are considering HRT (e.g., for severe symptoms of menopause) should discuss their individual risks and potential benefits with their health care providers.
- Combined estrogen–progestin therapy may increase blood sugar levels in women with diabetes. This effect is attrib-

uted to progestin and is unlikely to occur with estrogen-only therapy.
- Women with diabetes should report increased blood glucose levels.

Self-Administration

- Take estrogens and progestins with food or at bedtime to decrease nausea, a common adverse reaction.
- Apply transdermal estrogen patches (Climara, Estraderm, Vivelle) to clean, dry skin, preferably the abdomen. Press the patch tightly for 10 seconds to get a good seal and rotate sites so that at least a week passes between applications to a site; avoid prolonged sun exposure to the area of the patch.
- Apply transdermal estrogen gel (Estrogel) to clean, dry skin, avoiding the breast; avoid fire, flame, or smoking until gel has dried because it is flammable.
- Weigh weekly and report sudden weight gain. Fluid retention and edema may occur and produce weight gain.
- Report any unusual vaginal bleeding.

Patient Teaching Guidelines | Oral Contraceptives

General Considerations

- Seek information about the use of oral contraceptives.
- Oral contraceptives are very effective at preventing pregnancy, but they *do not* prevent transmission of sexually transmitted diseases (e.g., acquired immunodeficiency syndrome, chlamydia, gonorrhea).
- See a health care provider every 6 to 12 months for blood-pressure measurement, breast and pelvic examinations, and other care as indicated. This is very important to monitor for adverse drug effects such as high blood pressure, gallbladder disease, and blood-clotting disorders.
- Do not smoke cigarettes. Cigarette smoking increases risks of blood clots in the legs, lungs, heart, or brain. The blood clots may cause heart attack, stroke, or other serious diseases.
- Several medications may reduce the effectiveness of oral contraceptives (i.e., increase the likelihood of pregnancy). These include several antibiotics (e.g., ampicillin, clarithromycin and similar drugs, rifampin, penicillin V, sulfonamides [e.g., Bactrim], tetracyclines, and antiseizure medications (e.g., carbamazepine, oxcarbazepine, phenytoin, topiramate). Inform all health care providers who prescribe medications for you that you are taking a birth control pill.
- Be prepared to use an additional or alternative method of birth control if a dose is missed, if you are unable to take the oral contraceptive because of illness, or if you have an infection for which an antibiotic is prescribed. For exam-

ple, add a different method of birth control while taking an antibiotic and for the remainder of that cycle.

Self-Administration

- Read, keep, and follow instructions in the package inserts that are dispensed with the drugs. These inserts provide information about safe and effective use of the drugs.
- Take oral contraceptives with meals or food or at bedtime to decrease nausea. (If using Ortho Evra, a contraceptive skin patch that lasts a week, follow package instructions for correct application.)
- Take at about the same time every day to maintain effective blood levels and establish a routine so that missed doses are less likely. Missing one dose may allow pregnancy to occur. If you forget to take one pill, take it as soon as you remember. If you do not remember until the next scheduled pill, you can take two pills at once. If you miss two pills in a row, you may take two pills for the next 2 days. If you miss more than two pills, notify your health care provider.
- Use sunscreen and protective clothing when outdoors. The drugs may cause photosensitivity, with increased likelihood of sunburn after short periods of exposure.
- Weigh weekly and report sudden weight gain. The drugs may cause fluid retention; decreasing salt intake may be helpful.
- Report any unusual vaginal bleeding; calf tenderness, redness, or swelling; chest pain; weakness or numbness in an arm or leg; or sudden difficulty with seeing or talking.

warfarin, an oral anticoagulant (by increasing hepatic production of several clotting factors); and phenytoin, an anticonvulsant (possibly by increasing fluid retention). Estrogens may increase the adverse effects and risks of toxicity with corticosteroids, ropinirole, and tacrine by inhibiting their metabolism. Ropinirole and tacrine should not be used concurrently with an estrogen.

Oral contraceptives decrease effects of some benzodiazepines (e.g., lorazepam, oxazepam, temazepam), insulin, sulfonylurea antidiabetic drugs, and warfarin. If one of these drugs is taken concurrently with an oral contraceptive, increased dosage may be needed for therapeutic effects. Contraceptives increase effects of several drugs by inhibiting their metabolism. These include alcohol, some benzodiazepines (e.g., alprazolam, triazolam), tricyclic antidepressants, beta blockers (e.g., metoprolol), caffeine, corticosteroids, and theophylline (a xanthine bronchodilator). If one of these drugs is taken concurrently with an oral contraceptive, the drug may accumulate to toxic levels. Dosage may need to be reduced.

Use for Specific Indications

Contraception

The most effective and widely used contraceptives are estrogen–progestin combinations (see Table 27-4). Estrogen–progestin contraceptive preparations are nearly 100% effective in preventing pregnancy when taken correctly.

Numerous preparations are available, with different components and different doses of components, so that a preparation can be chosen to meet individual needs. Most oral contraceptives contain an estrogen and a progestin. The estrogen dose is usually 30 to 35 micrograms. Smaller amounts (e.g., 20 mcg) may be adequate for small or underweight women; larger amounts (e.g., 50 mcg) may be needed for large or overweight women. Effects of estrogen components are similar when prescribed in equipotent doses, but progestins differ in progestogenic, estrogenic, antiestrogenic, and androgenic activity. Consequently, adverse effects may differ to some extent, and a patient may be able to tolerate one contraceptive better than another.

Current products contain small amounts of estrogen and cause fewer adverse effects than previous products. Despite the decreased estrogen dosage, oral contraceptives may still be safest when administered to nonsmoking women younger than 35 years of age who do not have a history of thromboembolic problems, diabetes mellitus, hypertension, or migraine. When estrogen is contraindicated, a progestin-only contraceptive may be used.

It is necessary to assess each patient's need and desire for contraception, as well as her willingness to comply with the prescribed regimen. Assessment includes determining a patient's knowledge about birth control, both pharmacologic and nonpharmacologic, and identifying patients in whom hormonal contraceptives are contraindicated or who are at increased risk for adverse drug effects. Compliance involves the willingness to take the drugs as prescribed and to have breast and pelvic examinations and blood pressure measurements every 6 to 12 months.

Emergency (Postcoital) Contraception

Plan B (levonorgestrel) is the only emergency contraceptive on the market used to avoid pregnancy after unprotected sexual intercourse. It should be used only as a backup method and is not used for routine birth control. The drug is marketed by prescription and over-the-counter (OTC), with the OTC only being sold to women 18 years and older.

Emergency contraception is most effective if started within 24 hours and no later than 72 hours after exposure. The drug is believed to act mainly by inhibiting ovulation; the drug may also have an effect on fertilization and implantation. Plan B does not appear to have an effect on pregnancy after implantation. Side effects include nausea, abdominal pain, fatigue, headache, menstrual changes, dizziness, breast tenderness, vomiting, and diarrhea. Menstrual bleeding flow and timing may be altered after taking Plan B, and a woman whose menstrual period is delayed for greater than a week from the expected time should get a pregnancy test and follow-up with a health care professional.

Menopause

Menopause usually occurs in women ages 48 to 55 years. A woman who has not menstruated for a full year is considered menopausal, although symptoms of estrogen deficiency and irregular periods start approximately 4 years before final cessation. Physiologic menopause results from the gradual cessation of ovarian function and the resultant decrease in estrogen levels. Surgical menopause results from excision of both ovaries and the sudden loss of ovarian estrogen. Although estrogens from the adrenal cortex and other sites are still produced, the amount is insufficient to prevent estrogen deficiency.

ERT prevents vasomotor instability ("hot flashes" or "hot flushes") and other menopausal symptoms. A commonly prescribed regimen is a conjugated estrogen (Premarin) 0.625 to 1.25 milligrams daily for 25 days of each month, with a progestin, such as Provera, 10 milligrams daily for 10 days of each month, on days 15 to 25 of the cycle. The main function of the progestin is to decrease the risk of endometrial cancer; thus, women who have had a hysterectomy do not need it. Another regimen uses estradiol as a transdermal patch (e.g., Climara, Estraderm, Vivelle), which releases the drug slowly, provides more consistent blood levels than oral formulations, and is applied weekly or biweekly, depending on the formulation. A newer synthetic conjugated estrogen (Cenestin) is also approved for short-term treatment of hot flashes and sweating; it is not approved for long-term use in preventing osteoporosis in postmenopausal women. In addition, selective serotonin reuptake inhibitors (see Chap. 10) have shown great potential in reducing vasomotor symptoms. In randomized clinical trials, venlafaxine (Effexor), paroxetine (Paxil), and fluoxetine (Prozac) have been shown to reduce hot flashes significantly.

Osteoporosis: Prevention and Treatment

Estrogen or estrogen–progestin therapy is effective and has been widely used to prevent or treat osteoporosis and prevent fractures in postmenopausal women (see Chap. 25). Estrogenic effects in preventing bone loss include decreased bone resorption (breakdown), increased intestinal absorption of calcium, and increased calcitriol concentration. Calcitriol is the active form of vitamin D, which is required for absorption of calcium.

Estrogen and progestin may be used less often for osteoporosis in future for two main reasons. First, recent evidence (see Box 27-2) indicates that the risks of estrogen–progestin and estrogen-only hormonal therapy outweigh the benefits. Second, there are other effective measures for prevention and treatment of osteoporosis, including calcium and vitamin D supplements, bisphosphonate drugs (e.g., alendronate, risedronate), and weight-bearing exercise. ERT is still considered for fracture prevention among women who are at high risk of fracture and who are unable to take other preventive medications.

Use in Special Populations

Use in Children

There is little information about the effects of estrogens in children, and the drugs are not indicated for use. Because estrogens cause epiphyseal closure, they should be used with caution before completion of bone growth and attainment of adult height. When hormonal contraceptives are given to adolescent girls, as in other populations, the smallest effective doses should be used.

Use in Older Adults

The short-term use (1–2 years) of estrogens or estrogens and progestins in postmenopausal women may be indicated for management of menopausal symptoms. Long-term use of estrogen-only therapy and estrogen–progestin combinations is no longer recommended for most women, because of potentially serious adverse effects.

Use in Patients With Hepatic Impairment

Estrogens are contraindicated in impaired liver function, liver disease, or liver cancer. Impaired liver function may lead to impaired estrogen metabolism, with resultant accumulation and adverse effects. In addition, women who have had jaundice during pregnancy have an increased risk of recurrence if they take estrogen-containing contraceptives. Any patient in whom jaundice develops when taking estrogen should stop taking the drug. Because jaundice may indicate liver damage, the cause should be investigated. Progestins are contraindicated in patients with impaired liver function or liver disease.

Use in Home Care

Estrogens, progestins, and hormonal contraceptives are usually self-administered. Home care nurses may encounter patients or family members taking one of the drugs when visiting the home for another purpose. It may be necessary to teach or assist patients to take the drugs as prescribed. In addition, patients may need encouragement to keep appointments for follow-up supervision and blood pressure monitoring. When visiting families that include adolescent girls or young women, home care nurses may need to teach about birth control measures or about preventing osteoporosis by improving diet and exercise patterns. In families that include postmenopausal women, home care nurses may need to teach about nonhormonal strategies for preventing or treating osteoporosis and cardiovascular disease.

 Applying Your Knowledge 27-4

How Can You Avoid This Medication Error?
Vickie returns to the clinic for a urinary tract infection. The physician prescribes an antibiotic. You send Vickie to the school pharmacy and then home.

Nursing Actions — Estrogens, Progestins, and Hormonal Contraceptives

NURSING ACTIONS	RATIONALE/EXPLANATION
1. Administer accurately	
a. Give oral estrogens, progestins, and contraceptive preparations after meals or at bedtime.	To decrease nausea, a common adverse reaction
b. With aqueous suspensions to be given intramuscularly, roll the vial between the hands several times.	To be sure that drug particles are evenly distributed through the liquid vehicle
c. Give oil preparations deeply into a large muscle mass, preferably gluteal muscles.	
d. With estradiol skin patches, apply to clean, dry skin of the abdomen, buttocks, upper inner thigh, or upper arm. Avoid breasts, waistline areas, and areas exposed to sunlight. Press with palm of hand for about 10 seconds. Rotate sites.	To facilitate effective absorption and adherence to the skin and avoid skin irritation
e. With Combi-Patch, apply to clean, dry skin of the lower abdomen; rotate sites.	Manufacturer's recommendation. Rotating sites decreases skin irritation.

NURSING ACTIONS	RATIONALE/EXPLANATION
f. With Ortho Evra patch, apply to abdomen, buttocks, upper torso (except breasts), or upper outer arm.	Manufacturer's recommendation
2. Observe for therapeutic effects	
a. With estrogens:	Therapeutic effects vary, depending on the reason for use.
(1) When given for menopausal symptoms, observe for decrease in hot flashes and vaginal problems.	
(2) When given for amenorrhea, observe for menstruation.	
(3) When given for female hypogonadism, observe for menstruation, breast enlargement, axillary and pubic hair, and other secondary sexual characteristics.	
(4) When given to prevent or treat osteoporosis, observe for improved bone density tests and absence of fractures.	
b. With progestins:	
(1) When given for menstrual disorders, such as abnormal uterine bleeding, amenorrhea, dysmenorrhea, premenstrual discomfort, and endometriosis, observe for relief of symptoms.	
3. Observe for adverse effects	
a. With estrogens:	
(1) Menstrual disorders—breakthrough bleeding, dysmenorrhea, amenorrhea	Estrogen drugs may alter hormonal balance.
(2) Gastrointestinal system—nausea, vomiting, abdominal cramps, bloating	Nausea commonly occurs but usually subsides within 1 to 2 weeks of continued therapy. When high doses of estrogens are used as postcoital contraceptives, nausea and vomiting may be severe enough to require administration of antiemetic drugs.
(3) Gallbladder disease	Postmenopausal women taking an estrogen are 2 to 4 times more likely than non-users to require surgery for gallbladder disease.
(4) Cardiovascular system—thromboembolic conditions such as thrombophlebitis, pulmonary embolism, cerebral thrombosis, and coronary thrombosis; edema and weight gain	Estrogens promote blood clotting by stimulating hepatic production of four clotting factors (II, VII, IX, X). Thromboembolic disorders are most likely to occur in women older than 35 years of age who take oral contraceptives and smoke cigarettes; postmenopausal women taking long-term estrogen and progestin therapy; and men or women who receive large doses of estrogens for cancer treatment. Edema and weight gain are caused by fluid retention.
(5) Central nervous system—headache, migraine headache, dizziness, mental depression	Estrogens may cause or aggravate migraine headache in some women; the mechanism is unknown.
(6) Cancer—endometrial and possibly breast cancer	When estrogens are used alone in postmenopausal women, they cause endometrial hyperplasia and may cause endometrial cancer. Women with an intact uterus should also be given a progestin, which opposes the effects of estrogen on the endometrium.
	Opinions differ regarding estrogens as a cause of breast cancer. Most studies indicate little risk; a few indicate some risk, especially with high doses for prolonged periods (i.e., 10 y or longer). However, estrogens do stimulate growth in breast cancers that have estrogen receptors.
b. With progestins:	
(1) Menstrual disorders—breakthrough bleeding	Irregular vaginal bleeding is a common adverse effect that decreases during the first year of use. This is a major reason that some women do not want to take progestin-only contraceptives.
(2) Cardiovascular system—decreased high-density lipoprotein and increased low-density lipoprotein cholesterol	These adverse effects on plasma lipids potentially increase the risks of cardiovascular disease.
(3) Gastrointestinal system—nausea, increased or decreased weight	Nausea may be decreased by taking with food.

(continued on page 456)

Nursing Actions | Estrogens, Progestins, and Hormonal Contraceptives (cont'd)

NURSING ACTIONS	RATIONALE/EXPLANATION
(4) Central nervous system—drowsiness, insomnia, mental depression	
(5) Miscellaneous effects—edema, weight gain	
c. Combined estrogen and progestin oral contraceptives:	
(1) Gastrointestinal effects—nausea, others	Nausea may be minimized by taking the drugs with food or at bedtime.
(2) Cardiovascular effects—thromboembolism, myocardial infarction, stroke, hypertension	These effects occurred with earlier oral contraceptives, which contained larger amounts of estrogen than those currently used, and are much less common in most people who take low-dose preparations. However, for women older than 35 years of age who smoke, there is an increased risk of myocardial infarction and other cardiovascular disorders, even with low-dose pills.
(3) Gallbladder disease—cholelithiasis and cholecystitis	Women who use oral contraceptives or estrogen–progestin hormone replacement therapy are several times more likely to develop gallbladder disease than non-users. This is attributed to increased concentration of cholesterol in bile acids, which leads to decreased solubility and increased precipitation of stones.
(4) Miscellaneous—edema, weight gain, headache	
4. Observe for drug interactions	
a. Drugs that *decrease* effects of estrogens, progestins, and oral contraceptives:	
(1) Anticonvulsants—carbamazepine, oxcarbazepine, phenytoin, topiramate	Decrease effects by inducing enzymes that accelerate metabolism of estrogens and progestins
(2) Antimicrobials	Most interactions with antimicrobials have been reported with oral contraceptives. Rifampin induces drug-metabolizing enzymes that accelerate drug inactivation. Other antimicrobials act mainly by disrupting the normal bacterial flora of the gastrointestinal tract and decreasing enterohepatic recirculation of estrogens. This action may decrease effectiveness of contraceptives or cause breakthrough bleeding. To prevent pregnancy from occurring during antimicrobial therapy, a larger dose of oral contraceptive or an additional or alternative form of birth control is probably advisable.
(a) Antibacterials—ampicillin, macrolides (erythromycin, clarithromycin, dirithromycin), metronidazole, penicillin V, rifampin, sulfonamides, tetracyclines, trimethoprim	
(b) Antifungals—fluconazole, itraconazole, ketoconazole	
(c) Antivirals—efavirenz, ritonavir, lopinavir/ritonavir combination	

Key Concepts

■ When exogenous estrogens and progestins are administered for therapeutic purposes, they produce the same effects as endogenous hormones.

■ Oral contraceptives are very effective at preventing pregnancy, but they do not prevent transmission of sexually transmitted diseases.

■ Cigarette smoking in individuals who use oral contraceptives increases risks of blood clots in the legs, lungs, heart, or brain.

■ Because estrogens cause epiphyseal closure, they should be used with caution in children before completion of bone growth and attainment of adult height.

■ When estrogens are used alone in postmenopausal women, they cause endometrial hyperplasia and may cause endometrial cancer. Women with an intact uterus should also be given a progestin, which opposes the effects of estrogen on the endometrium.

■ Most interactions with antimicrobials have been reported with oral contraceptives. To prevent pregnancy from occurring during antimicrobial therapy, a larger dose of oral contraceptive or an additional or alternative form of birth control is probably advisable.

■ Research has demonstrated no evidence for HRT in secondary prevention of heart disease and shown increased rates of CHD, thromboembolic stroke, venous thromboembolism, dementia, and breast cancer, which outweigh the benefits of decreased risk of fracture and colon cancer.

■ The FDA has issued a **BLACK BOX WARNING** that estrogens increase the risk for developing cancer of the uterus. The warning instructs individuals who take estrogens with or without progestins that there is an increased risk of dementia, myocardial infarctions, strokes, breast cancer, and blood clots.

Review and Application Exercises

Short Answer Exercises

1. What are the reproductive and nonreproductive functions of estrogens?

2. What are the functions of progestins?

3. What is considered the major mechanism of action of hormonal contraceptives?

4. What are the adverse effects of hormonal contraceptives, and how can they be prevented or minimized?

5. Outline the points you would make for and against HRT for a postmenopausal woman.

6. Prepare a teaching plan for a perimenopausal or postmenopausal woman about nonpharmacologic measures to manage menopausal symptoms and prevent osteoporosis.

NCLEX-Style Questions

7. Estrogen replacement therapy is prescribed to relieve severe menopausal symptoms of hot flashes or flushes, which are the result of
   a. insufficient gonadotropin secretion
   b. vasomotor instability
   c. high levels of estrogen
   d. decreased progesterone

8. Progesterone is a progestin concerned almost entirely with reproduction. In the nonpregnant women, progesterone is secreted by which of the following?
   a. corpus luteum
   b. hypothalamus
   c. anterior pituitary
   d. adrenal cortex

9. Black cohosh is an herbal preparation that has been used to self-treat symptoms of menopause. Due to the risk of adverse effects, patients should be monitored closely for which of the following conditions?
   a. dysrhythmias
   b. hypertension
   c. hypotension
   d. bradycardia

10. Patient teaching for a woman who will be using the transdermal estradiol patch Estraderm should include information about applying the patch to
   a. the skin daily
   b. clean and dry skin
   c. the same area for consistency
   d. the skin every 2 weeks

Selected References

Brett, K. M., & Keenan, N. L. (2007). Complementary and alternative medicine use among midlife women for reasons including menopause in the United States: 2002. *Menopause, 14*(2), 300–307.

Drug facts and comparisons. (Updated monthly). St. Louis, MO: Facts and Comparisons.

Guay, M. P., Dragomir, A., Pilon, D., Moride, Y., & Perreault, S. (2007). Changes in pattern of use, clinical characteristics and persistence rate of hormone replacement therapy among postmenopausal women after the WHI publication. *Pharmacoepidemiology & Drug Safety, 16*(1), 17–27.

Guyton, A. C., & Hall, J. E. (2006). *Textbook of medical physiology* (11th ed.). Philadelphia: W. B. Saunders.

Helenius, I. M., Korenstein, D., & Halm, E. A. (2007). Changing use of hormone therapy among minority women since the Women's Health Initiative. *Menopause, 14*(2), 216–222.

Lacy, C. F., Armstrong, L. L., Goldman, M. P., & Lance, L. L. (2007). *Lexi-Comp's drug information handbook* (15th ed.). Hudson, OH: American Pharmaceutical Association.

Low Dog, T. (2005). Menopause: a review of botanical dietary supplements. *American Journal of Medicine, 118*(Suppl. 12B), 98–108.

Mehring, P. M. (2005). The female reproductive system. In C. M. Porth (Ed.), *Pathophysiology: Concepts of altered health states* (7th ed., pp. 1051–1064). Philadelphia: Lippincott Williams & Wilkins.

Viscoli, C. M. (2005). Estrogen therapy and risk of cognitive decline: results from the Women's Estrogen for Stroke Trial (WEST). *American Journal of Obstetrics & Gynecology, 192*(2), 387–393.

Androgens and Anabolic Steroids

LEARNING OBJECTIVES

After studying this chapter, you will be able to:

1. Examine the effects of endogenous androgens.
2. Discuss uses and effects of exogenous androgens and anabolic steroids.
3. Identify potential consequences of abusing androgens and anabolic steroids.
4. Counsel patients about the physiologic effects of the dietary supplements androstenedione and dehydroepiandrosterone (DHEA).

Applying Your Knowledge

Barbara Watson is a 35-year-old woman. She has endometriosis. Ms. Watson is receiving danazol (Danocrine) 800 mg daily in two divided doses.

Introduction

Androgens are male sex hormones secreted by the testes in men, the ovaries in women, and the adrenal cortex of both sexes. Like the female sex hormones, the naturally occurring male sex hormones are steroids synthesized from cholesterol. The sex organs and adrenal glands can produce cholesterol or remove it from the blood. Cholesterol then undergoes a series of conversions to progesterone, androgenic prehormones, and testosterone. The androgens produced by the ovaries have little androgenic activity and are used mainly as precursor substances for the production of naturally occurring estrogens. The adrenal glands produce several androgens, including androstenedione and dehydroepiandrosterone (DHEA). Androstenedione and DHEA are weak androgens with little masculinizing effect that are mainly converted to estrogens.

Testosterone

Testosterone is normally the only important male sex hormone. It is secreted by the Leydig's cells in the testes in response to stimulation by luteinizing hormone from the anterior pituitary gland. The main functions of testosterone are related to the development of male sexual characteristics, reproduction, and metabolism (Box 28-1).

About 97% of the testosterone secreted by the testes binds to plasma albumin or to sex hormone–binding globulin and circulates in the blood for 30 minutes to several hours. The bound testosterone is either transferred to the tissues or broken down into inactive products that are excreted. Much of the testosterone that transfers to tissues undergoes intracellular conversion to dihydrotestosterone which combines with receptor proteins in the cytoplasm; a series of actions stimulate production of proteins. Almost all testosterone effects result from the increased formation of proteins throughout the body, especially in the cells of target organs and tissues responsible for development of male sexual characteristics.

Box 28-1	Effects of Testosterone on Body Tissues

Fetal Development

Large amounts of chorionic gonadotropin are produced by the placenta during pregnancy. Chorionic gonadotropin is similar to luteinizing hormone (LH) from the anterior pituitary gland. It promotes development of the interstitial or Leydig's cells in fetal testes, which then secrete testosterone. Testosterone production begins in the second month of fetal life. When present, testosterone promotes development of male sexual characteristics (e.g., penis, scrotum, prostate gland, seminal vesicles, and seminiferous tubules), and suppresses development of female sexual characteristics. In the absence of testosterone, the fetus develops female sexual characteristics.

Testosterone also provides the stimulus for the descent of the testes into the scrotum. This normally occurs after the seventh month of pregnancy, when the fetal testes are secreting relatively large amounts of testosterone. If the testes do not descend before birth, administration of testosterone or gonadotropic hormone, which stimulates testosterone secretion, produces descent in most cases.

Adult Development

Little testosterone is secreted in boys until 11 to 13 years of age. At the onset of puberty, testosterone secretion increases rapidly and remains at a relatively high level until about 50 years of age, after which it gradually declines.

▪ The testosterone secreted at puberty acts as a growth hormone to produce enlargement of the penis, testes, and scrotum until approximately 20 years of age. The prostate gland, seminal vesicles, seminiferous tubules, and vas deferens also increase in size and functional ability. Under the combined influence of testosterone and follicle-stimulating hormone (FSH) from the anterior pituitary gland, sperm production is initiated and maintained throughout the man's reproductive life.

▪ **Skin.** Testosterone increases skin thickness and activity of the sebaceous glands. Acne in the male adolescent is attributed to the increased production of testosterone.

▪ **Voice.** The larynx enlarges and deepens the voice of the adult man.

▪ **Hair.** Testosterone produces the distribution of hair growth on the face, limbs, and trunk typical of the adult man. In men with a genetic trait toward baldness, large amounts of testosterone cause alopecia (baldness) of the scalp.

▪ **Skeletal muscles.** Testosterone is largely responsible for the larger, more powerful muscles of men. This characteristic is caused by the effects of testosterone on protein metabolism. Testosterone helps the body retain nitrogen, form new amino acids, and build new muscle protein. At the same time, it slows the loss of nitrogen and amino acids formed by the constant breakdown of body tissues. Overall, testosterone increases protein anabolism (buildup) and decreases protein catabolism (breakdown).

▪ **Bone.** Testosterone makes bones thicker and longer. After puberty, more protein and calcium are deposited and retained in bone matrix. This causes a rapid rate of bone growth. The height of a male adolescent increases rapidly for a time, then stops as epiphyseal closure occurs. This happens when the cartilage at the end of the long bones in the arms and legs becomes bone. Further lengthening of the bones is then prevented.

Anterior Pituitary Function

High blood levels of testosterone decrease secretion of FSH and LH from the anterior pituitary gland. This, in turn, decreases testosterone production.

The portion of testosterone that does not become attached to tissues is converted into androsterone and DHEA by the liver. These are conjugated with glucuronic or sulfuric acid and excreted in the bile or urine.

Anabolic Steroids

Anabolic steroids are synthetic drugs with increased anabolic activity and decreased androgenic activity compared with testosterone. They were developed during attempts to modify testosterone so that its tissue-building and growth-stimulating effects could be retained while its masculinizing effects could be eliminated or reduced.

Abuse of Androgen and Anabolic Steroid Drugs

Drugs used to enhance athletic performance are termed *ergogenic* (causing an increase in muscular work capacity). Androgens and anabolic steroids are widely abused in attempts to enhance muscle development, muscle strength, and athletic performance. Because of their abuse potential, the drugs are Schedule III controlled substances. Although nonprescription sales of the drugs are illegal, they apparently are easily obtained.

Athletes are considered a high-risk group because some start taking the drugs as early as middle school and continue for years. The use of performance-enhancing drugs in nonathletes is also on the rise to improve performance outside of sports. The number of teens taking anabolic steroids is thought to be small in comparison with the number using marijuana, amphetamines, and other illegal drugs. However, the number is increasing, and long-term effects may be as serious as the effects that occur with use of other illegal drugs. Although steroids have a reputation for being dangerous to adult athletes, such as body builders and football players, they are considered even more dangerous for teens because teens are still growing. Anabolic steroids can stop bone growth and damage the heart, kidneys, and liver of adolescents. In addition to those who take steroids to enhance athletic performance, some males take the drugs to produce a more muscular appearance and impress females. Steroid abusers usually take massive doses and often take several drugs or combine injectable and oral drugs for maximum effects. The large doses produce potentially serious adverse effects in several body tissues:

- **Cardiovascular disorders** include hypertension, decreased high-density blood lipoproteins (HDL), and increased low-density lipoproteins (LDL), all of which promote heart attacks and strokes.

- **Liver disorders** include benign and malignant neoplasms, cholestatic hepatitis and jaundice, and peliosis hepatis, a disorder in which blood-filled cysts develop in the liver and may lead to hemorrhage or liver failure.

- **Central nervous system disorders** include aggression, hostility, combativeness, and dependence characterized by preoccupation with drug use, inability to stop taking the drugs, and withdrawal symptoms similar to those that occur with alcohol, cocaine, and narcotics. In some cases, psychosis may develop.

- **Reproductive system disorders** include decreased testicular function (e.g., decreased secretion of endogenous testosterone, decreased formation of sperm), testicular atrophy, and impotence in men. They include amenorrhea in women.

- **Metabolic disorders** include atherosclerosis-promoting changes in cholesterol metabolism and retention of fluids, with edema and other imbalances. Fluid and electrolyte retention contribute to the increased weight associated with drug use.

- **Dermatologic disorders** include moderate to severe acne in both sexes, depending on drug dosage.

Many of these adverse effects persist several months after the drugs are stopped and may be irreversible. Names of anabolic steroids include oxandrolone (Oxandrin), oxymetholone (Anadrol-50), and stanozolol (Winstrol).

General Characteristics of Androgens and Anabolic Steroids Used As Drugs

- When male sex hormones or androgens are given from exogenous sources for therapeutic purposes, they produce the same effects as the naturally occurring hormones. These effects include inhibition of endogenous sex hormones and sperm formation through negative feedback of pituitary luteinizing hormone (LH) and follicle-stimulating hormone (FSH).

- Male sex hormones given to women antagonize or reduce the effects of female sex hormones. Thus, administration of androgenic or anabolic steroids to women suppresses menstruation and causes atrophy of the endometrial lining of the uterus.

- Several dosage forms of androgens are available; they differ mainly in route of administration and pharmacokinetics.

- Naturally occurring androgens are given by injection because they are metabolized rapidly by the liver if given orally. Some esters of testosterone have been modified to slow the rate of metabolism and thus prolong action. For example, intramuscular (IM) testosterone cypionate and testosterone enanthate have slow onsets of action and last 2 to 4 weeks.

- Oral testosterone is extensively metabolized in its first pass through the liver, so that nearly half of a dose is lost before it reaches the systemic circulation. As a result, doses as high as 400 milligrams per day may be needed to produce adequate blood levels for full replacement therapy. Methyltestosterone is a synthetic formulation that is less extensively metabolized by the liver and more suitable for oral administration.

- Several transdermal formulations of testosterone are available. They have a rapid onset of action and last approximately 24 hours. A topical gel (a 10-g dose delivers 100 mg) produces normal serum testosterone levels within 4 hours after application, and absorption of testosterone into the blood continues for 24 hours. Steady-state serum concentrations occur by the second or third day of use. When the gel is discontinued, serum testosterone levels remain in the normal range for 24 to 48 hours but decrease to pretreatment levels within about 5 days.

- Androderm is applied to nonscrotal skin, and testosterone is continuously absorbed for 24 hours, with normal blood levels achieved during the first day of drug use. Applying the patch at night produces serum testosterone levels similar to those in healthy young men (i.e., higher concentrations in the morning and lower ones in the evening).

- Like endogenous testosterone, drug molecules are highly bound (98%) to plasma proteins and serum half-life varies (e.g., 8 days for IM testosterone cypionate, 9 hours for oral fluoxymesterone). The drugs are inactivated primarily in the liver. About 90% of a dose is excreted in urine as conjugates of testosterone and its metabolites. About 6% of a dose is excreted in feces.

- Danazol is a synthetic drug with weak androgenic activity. It is given orally, has a half-life of 4 to 5 hours, and is metabolized in the liver. Route of excretion is unknown.

- All synthetic anabolic steroids are weak androgens. Consequently, giving these drugs for anabolic effects also produces masculinizing effects. This characteristic limits the clinical usefulness of these drugs in women and children. Profound changes in growth and sexual development may occur if these drugs are given to young children.

Mechanism of Action

Like other steroid drugs, androgenic and anabolic drugs penetrate the cell membrane and bind to receptor proteins in the cell cytoplasm. The steroid–receptor complex is then transported to the nucleus, where it activates RNA and DNA production and stimulates cellular synthesis of protein.

Indications for Use

With male sex hormones, the most clear-cut indication for use is to treat androgen deficiency states (e.g., hypogonadism, cryptorchidism, impotence, oligospermia) in boys and men. Hypogonadism may result from hypothalamic–pituitary or testicular dysfunction. In prepubertal boys, administration of the drugs stimulates the development of masculine characteristics. In postpubertal men who become androgen deficient, the hormones re-establish and maintain masculine characteristics and functions.

In women, danazol (Danocrine) may be used to prevent or treat endometriosis or fibrocystic breast disease. Anabolic steroids are more often abused for body-building purposes than used for therapeutic effects.

Although some drug literature still lists metastatic breast cancer and some types of anemia as indications for use, androgens have largely been replaced by newer drugs for these purposes. In breast cancer, for example, androgens are second-line hormonal agents, after anti-estrogens (e.g., tamoxifen). In anemia associated with renal failure, synthetic erythropoietin is more effective and likely to be used.

Contraindications to Use

Androgens and anabolic steroids are contraindicated during pregnancy (because of possible masculinizing effects on a female fetus), in patients with pre-existing liver disease, and in men with prostate-gland disorders. Men with an enlarged prostate may have additional enlargement, and men with prostatic cancer may experience tumor growth. Although not contraindicated in children, these drugs must be used very cautiously and with x-ray studies performed approximately every 6 months to evaluate bone growth.

Individual Drugs

Clinical indications, routes, and dosage ranges are listed in Table 28-1.

Herbal and Dietary Supplements

Androstenedione and DHEA, androgens produced by the adrenal cortex, are also available as over-the-counter (OTC) dietary supplements. They are marketed as safe, natural, alternative androgens for building muscles. These products, which have weak androgenic activity, act mainly as precursors for the production of sex hormones. Androstenedione, for example, may be converted to testosterone by way of an enzyme found in most body tissues. However, it may also be converted to estrogens, and the testosterone that is produced may be further converted to estrogen (estradiol). In one study, young men with

Table 28-1	Drugs at a Glance: Androgens	
	ROUTES AND DOSAGE RANGES	
Generic/Trade Name	**Hypogonadism**	**Other**
Testosterone cypionate (Depo-Testosterone)	IM 50–200 mg every 2–4 wk	
Testosterone enanthate (Delatestryl)	IM 50–200 mg every 2–4 wk	
Testosterone gel (Androgel 1%)	5 g (50 mg of drug) once daily to skin of shoulders and upper arms or abdomen	
Testosterone pellets	Sub-Q 150–450 mg every 3–6 mo	*Delayed puberty:* Sub-Q lower dosage range, for a limited duration (e.g., every 3 mo for 2–3 doses)
Testosterone transdermal systems (Androderm)	Apply 2 Androderm systems (dose of 5 mg) nightly to back, abdomen, upper arm, or thigh	
Testolactone (Teslac)		*Breast cancer:* PO 250 mg 4 times daily
Fluoxymesterone (Halotestin)	PO 5–20 mg daily	
Methyltestosterone (Android, Testred)		*Cryptorchidism:* PO 30 mg daily; buccal tablets, 15 mg daily
Danazol		*Endometriosis:* PO 800 mg daily in 2 divided doses for 3–9 mo
		Fibrocystic breast disease: PO 100–400 mg daily in 2 divided doses for 3–6 mo

normal serum testosterone levels were given an androstenedione supplement for 8 weeks. The researchers found little effect on serum testosterone levels or muscle development with resistance training. They also found increased serum levels of estrone and estradiol, which indicate that a significant proportion of the androstenedione was converted to estrogens. Thus, taking a supplement for masculinizing effects may produce feminizing effects instead.

DHEA is available alone as oral capsules or tablets and in a topical cream with vitamins and herbs. Most DHEA products of plant origin are produced in Europe and China. They are marketed with numerous claims for health benefits, including inhibition of aging, atherosclerosis, cancer, diabetes mellitus, and osteoporosis. Most claims stem from laboratory and animal studies. A few small human studies have been done, most of which used a dose of 50 milligrams daily. Overall, there is no conclusive evidence that DHEA supplementation will prevent or treat such conditions. In addition, long-term effects in humans are unknown.

DHEA is contraindicated in men with prostate cancer or benign prostatic hypertrophy (BPH) and in women with estrogen-responsive breast or uterine cancer, because DHEA may stimulate growth of these tissues. Patients older than 40 years of age should be aggressively screened for hormonally sensitive cancers before taking DHEA.

Adverse effects of DHEA include aggressiveness, hirsutism, insomnia, and irritability. Whether large doses of the OTC products can produce some of the serious adverse effects associated with standard anabolic steroids is unknown.

Applying Your Knowledge 28-1

You are counseling Ms. Watson about her self-administration of danazol. What teaching points do you cover?

Nursing Process

Assessment

Before drug therapy is started, patients need a thorough history and physical examination. Periodic monitoring of the patient's condition is needed throughout drug therapy.

■ Assess for conditions in which androgens are used (e.g., deficiency states).

■ Assess for conditions that increase risks of adverse effects or are contraindications (e.g., pregnancy, liver disease, prostatic hypertrophy).

■ Check laboratory reports of liver function tests (the drugs may cause cholestatic jaundice and liver damage), serum electrolyte levels (the drugs may cause sodium and water retention), and serum lipid levels (the drugs may increase levels and aggravate atherosclerosis).

■ Assess weight and blood pressure regularly. These may be elevated by retention of sodium and water with resultant edema, especially in patients with congestive heart failure.

■ For children, check x-ray examination reports of bone growth status initially and approximately every 6 months while the drugs are being taken.

■ Assess the patient's attitude toward taking male sex hormones.

■ Assess the patient's willingness to comply with instructions for taking the drugs and follow-up procedures.

Nursing Diagnoses

■ Disturbed Body Image related to masculinizing effects and menstrual irregularities

■ Deficient Knowledge: Physiologic and psychological consequences of overuse and abuse of the drugs to enhance athletic performance

■ Noncompliance: Overuse of drugs or dietary supplements

■ Risk for Injury: Liver disease and other serious adverse drug effects

Planning/Goals

The patient will

■ Use the drugs for medical purposes only

■ Receive or take the drugs as prescribed

■ Avoid abuse of drugs or dietary supplements for body building

■ Be counseled regarding effects of overuse and abuse if identified as being at risk (e.g., athletes, especially weight lifters and football players)

■ Avoid preventable adverse drug effects

■ Comply with monitoring and follow-up procedures

Interventions

■ Assist patients to use the drug correctly (see accompanying patient teaching display).

■ Assist patient to reduce sodium intake if edema develops.

■ Record weight and blood pressure at regular intervals.

■ Participate in school or community programs to inform children, parents, coaches, athletic trainers, and others of the risks of inappropriate use of androgens, anabolic steroids, and related dietary supplements.

Evaluation

■ Interview and observe for compliance with instructions for taking prescribed drugs.

■ Interview and observe for therapeutic and adverse drug effects.

■ Question athletes about illegal use of the drugs.

■ Observe athletes for increased weight and behavioral changes that may indicate drug abuse.

Patient Teaching Guidelines | Androgens

General Considerations

- Take the drugs only if prescribed and as prescribed. Use by athletes for body building is inappropriate and, if not prescribed by a licensed prescriber, is illegal.
- Continue medical supervision as long as the drugs are being taken.
- Weigh once or twice weekly and record the amount. An increase may indicate fluid retention and edema.
- Practice frequent and thorough skin cleansing to decrease acne, which is most likely to occur in women and children.

Self-Administration

- Take oral preparations before or with meals, in divided doses.
- For buccal preparations:
  - Take in divided doses.

- Place the tablet between the cheek and gum and allow to dissolve (do not swallow).
- Avoid eating, drinking, or smoking while the tablet is in place.
- With transdermal systems:
  - Apply 2 Androderm systems nightly to clean, dry skin on back, abdomen, upper arm, or thigh. Do not apply to scrotum. Rotate sites, with 7 days between applications to a site. Press firmly into place for adherence.
  - Apply the prescribed amount of gel to clean, dry, intact skin of the shoulders and upper arms or the abdomen (do **not** apply to the genital area), once daily, preferably in the morning. Wash hands after application and allow sites to dry before dressing. After application, wait at least 1 hour and preferably 4 to 6 hours before showering or swimming.

Principles of Therapy

Duration of Therapy

Drug therapy with androgens may be short or long term, depending on the condition in question, the patient's response to treatment, and the incidence of adverse reactions. If feasible, intermittent rather than continuous therapy is recommended.

Effects of Androgens and Anabolic Steroids on Other Drugs

Androgens may increase effects of cyclosporine and warfarin, apparently by slowing their metabolism and increasing their concentrations in the blood. These combinations should be avoided if possible. However, if required, serum creatinine and cyclosporine levels should be monitored with cyclosporine and prothrombin time or international normalized ratio (INR) with warfarin.

Androgens also increase effects of sulfonylurea antidiabetic drugs. Concurrent use should be avoided if possible. If required, smaller doses of sulfonylureas may be needed, blood glucose levels should be monitored closely, and patients should be assessed for signs of hypoglycemia. Danazol inhibits metabolism of carbamazepine and increases risks of toxicity. Concurrent use should be avoided.

Applying Your Knowledge 28-2

You are assessing Ms. Watson for adverse effects of her danazol. What signs and symptoms do you assess?

Use in Special Populations

Use in Children

The main indication for use of androgens is for boys with established deficiency states. Because the drugs cause epiphyseal closure, hands and wrists should undergo x-ray examination every 6 months to detect bone maturation and prevent loss of adult height. Stimulation of skeletal growth continues for approximately 6 months after drug therapy is stopped. If premature puberty occurs (precocious sexual development, enlarged penis), the drug should be stopped. The drugs may cause or aggravate acne. Scrupulous skin care and other anti-acne treatment may be needed, especially in adolescent boys.

Use in Older Adults

The main indication for use of androgens is a deficiency state in men. In male adults, levels of total testosterone decrease by nearly 1% per year; bioavailable levels decrease by 2% per year, resulting in a reported prevalence of hypogonadism of 20% in men aged 60 to 69.

Older adults often have hypertension and other cardiovascular disorders that may be aggravated by the sodium and water retention associated with androgens and anabolic steroids. In men, the drugs may increase prostate size and interfere with urination, increase risk of prostatic cancer, and cause excessive sexual stimulation and priapism.

Use in Patients With Hepatic Impairment

Androgens and anabolic steroids are contraindicated in patients with pre-existing liver disease. Prolonged use of high doses may cause potentially life-threatening conditions such as peliosis hepatis, hepatic neoplasms, and hepatocellular carcinoma. In addition, androgen therapy should be discontinued if cholestatic hepatitis with jaundice occurs or if liver function tests become abnormal. Drug-induced jaundice is reversible when the medication is stopped.

Applying Your Knowledge 28-3

Ms. Watson's brother is visiting from out of town. Warren Watson is a 27-year-old body builder. He has an 11-year history of abusing a variety of anabolic steroids. Ms. Watson is worried about him and convinces him to come to the clinic for a checkup.

At the clinic, Mr. Watson states that he takes no medication. You measure his blood pressure to be 180/94 mm Hg. Mr. Watson says he has "white-coat syndrome" and that his blood pressure is never elevated except at the office. When approached about his high blood pressure, he refuses to be treated. What is your nursing responsibility?

Nursing Actions   Androgens and Anabolic Steroids

NURSING ACTIONS	RATIONALE/EXPLANATION
1. Administer accurately	
a. Give intramuscular preparations of testosterone, other androgens. and anabolic steroids deeply, preferably in the gluteal muscle.	
b. Give oral preparations before or with meals, in divided doses.	To decrease gastrointestinal disturbances
c. For buccal preparations:	
(1) Give in divided doses.	
(2) Place the tablet between the cheek and gum.	
(3) Instruct the patient not to swallow the tablet and not to drink, chew, or smoke until the tablet is completely absorbed.	Buccal preparations must be absorbed through the mucous membranes.
d. With transdermal systems:	
(1) Apply 2 Androderm systems nightly to clean, dry skin on back, abdomen, upper arm, or thigh. Do *not* apply to scrotum. Rotate sites, with 7 days between applications to a site. Press firmly into place for adherence.	Correct site selection and application are necessary for therapeutic effects. Scrotal skin is more permeable to testosterone than other skin areas.
(2) Apply Androgel 1% to shoulders and upper arms or abdomen, once daily, preferably in the morning.	Manufacturer's recommendation. Patients may prefer self-application. Skin should be clean, dry, and intact; hands should be washed after application; and showering and swimming should be avoided for at least 1 hour and preferably 4 to 6 hours after application.
e. Inject testosterone pellets (Testopel) subcutaneously.	Manufacturer's recommendation
2. Observe for therapeutic effects	
a. When the drug is given for hypogonadism, observe for masculinizing effects, such as growth of sexual organs, deepening of voice, growth of body hair, and acne.	
b. When the drug is given for anabolic effects, observe for increased appetite, euphoria, or statements of feeling better.	
3. Observe for adverse reactions	
a. Virilism or masculinizing effects:	
(1) In adult men with adequate secretion of testosterone—priapism, increased sexual desire, reduced sperm count, and prostate enlargement	
(2) In prepubertal boys—premature development of sex organs and secondary sexual characteristics, such as enlargement of the penis, priapism, pubic hair	
(3) In women—masculinizing effects include hirsutism, deepening of the voice, menstrual irregularities	
b. Jaundice—dark urine, yellow skin and sclera, itching	
c. Edema	More likely in patients who are elderly or who have heart or kidney disease
d. Hypercalcemia	More likely in women with advanced breast cancer
e. Difficulty voiding due to prostate enlargement	More likely in middle-aged or elderly men
f. Inadequate growth in height of children	
4. Observe for drug interactions	
a. Drugs that *decrease* effects of androgens:	
(1) Barbiturates	Increase enzyme induction and rate of metabolism
(2) Calcitonin	Decreases calcium retention and thus antagonizes calcium-retaining effects of androgens

Key Concepts

- The androgens produced by the ovaries have little androgenic activity and are used mainly as precursor substances for the production of naturally occurring estrogens.

- The main functions of testosterone are related to the development of male sexual characteristics, reproduction, and metabolism.

- Androgens and anabolic steroids are used to enhance athletic performance and are termed ergogenic (causing an increase in muscular work capacity); they are widely abused in attempts to enhance muscle development, muscle strength, and athletic performance.

- Because of their abuse potential, androgens and anabolic steroids are classified as Schedule III controlled substances.

- Androstenedione and DHEA, androgens produced by the adrenal cortex, are also available as over-the-counter (OTC) dietary supplements.

- Adverse effects of DHEA include aggressiveness, hirsutism, insomnia, and irritability.

- Because androgens cause premature epiphyseal closure, boys with established deficiency states receiving androgens should undergo x-ray examination every 6 months to detect bone maturation and prevent loss of adult height.

Review and Application Exercises

Short Answer Exercises

1. How does testosterone promote development of male sexual characteristics?

2. What is the major clinical indication for therapeutic use of testosterone and related androgens?

3. What is the difference between androgenic activity and anabolic activity?

4. What are the adverse effects of using large doses of anabolic steroids in body-building efforts?

5. If your 14-year-old brother said some friends were telling him to take drugs to increase muscle development and athletic ability, how would you reply? Justify your answer.

NYCLEX-Style Questions

6. The nurse knows that the most clear-cut therapeutic indication for use of male sex hormones is
   a. to treat androgen deficiency states in boys and men
   b. for body-building purposes
   c. to treat metastatic breast cancer
   d. to treat anemia associated with renal failure

7. Four patients in an endocrine clinic are ordered to begin androgen therapy. The nurse reviews each patient's current medications and identifies which patient as able to begin androgen therapy without the risk of a known drug interaction?
   a. patient 1, taking cyclosporine
   b. patient 2, taking warfarin
   c. patient 3, taking sulfonylureas
   d. patient 4, taking heparin

8. What percentage of testosterone secreted by the testes binds to plasma albumin or to sex hormone–binding globulin and circulates in the blood?
   a. 26%
   b. 49%
   c. 78%
   d. 97%

9. A 19-year-old female athlete presents for her first prenatal visit and tells the nurse she has been on androgen therapy to improve her distance running. She asks the nurse if she can continue taking the androgens to maintain her "competitive edge." The nurse should instruct the patient that
   a. She can continue taking androgens, because the drugs pose no risk to the fetus.
   b. She can continue taking androgens, but a higher dose will be required due to increased drug metabolism during pregnancy.
   c. She can continue taking androgens until the third trimester, when they must be discontinued because androgens cause an increased risk of premature rupture of membranes.
   d. She must stop taking androgens immediately, because they pose a risk to the fetus; she should discuss this with her health care provider at today's visit.

10. Which of the following statements by a male patient taking transdermal androgens indicates that further teaching is necessary?
    a. "I need to weigh myself once or twice weekly and record the amount."
    b. "I should wash my face and body thoroughly to decrease the risk of acne."
    c. "The patch systems should be applied nightly to skin on my back, abdomen, upper arm, or thigh."
    d. "I should apply the patch systems in the morning to the same site each and every day."

Selected References

Carpenter P.C. (2007). Performance-enhancing drugs in sport. *Endocrinology and Metabolism Clinics of North America, 36,* 481–495.

Choi B. G., & McLaughlin, M. A. (2007). Why men's hearts break: Cardiovascular effects of sex steroids. *Endocrinology and Metabolism Clinics, 36,* 365–377.

Cunningham G. R. (2006). Testosterone replacement therapy for late-onset hypogonadism. *Nature Clinical Practice Urology, 3,* 260–267.

Drug facts and comparisons. (Updated monthly). St. Louis, MO: Facts and Comparisons.

Goldstein, I. (2007). A clinical paradigm for the combined management of androgen insufficiency and erectile dysfunction. *Endocrinology and Metabolism Clinics, 36,* 435–452.

Guyton, A. C., & Hall, J. E. (2006). *Textbook of medical physiology* (11th ed.). Philadelphia: W. B. Saunders.

Lacy, C. F., Armstrong, L. L., Goldman, M. P., & Lance, L. L. (2007). *Lexi-Comp's drug information handbook* (15th ed.). Hudson, OH: Lexi-Comp.

Porth, C. M. (2005). *Pathophysiology: Concepts of altered health states* (7th ed.). Philadelphia: Lippincott Williams & Wilkins.

Chapter Outline

General Characteristics of Antimicrobial Drugs

KEY TERMS

- Antibacterial
- Antibiotic
- Antibiotic resistance
- Antibiotic-resistant
- Anti-infective
- Antimicrobial
- Bacteria
- Bactericidal
- Bacteriostatic
- Broad spectrum
- Colonization
- Community-acquired
- Detection of antigens
- Fungi
- Nosocomial
- Opportunistic
- Penicillin-binding proteins
- Postantibiotic effect
- Resistance
- Serology
- Susceptibility
- Viruses

LEARNING OBJECTIVES

After studying this chapter, you will be able to:

1. Identify populations who have an increased risk of infection.
2. Discuss common pathogens and methods of infection control.
3. Outline common and potentially serious adverse effects of antimicrobial drugs.
4. Identify patients at increased risk for adverse drug reactions.
5. Discuss ways to increase benefits and decrease hazards of antimicrobial drug therapy.
6. Discuss ways to minimize emergence of drug-resistant microorganisms.
7. State appropriate nursing implications for a patient receiving an antimicrobial drug.
8. Discuss important elements of using antimicrobial drugs in children, older adults, patients with renal or hepatic impairment, and patients with critical illness.

Applying Your Knowledge

Rosalie Kurth is a 72-year-old grandmother and retired factory worker. Her work in a dusty environment has led her to have chronic bronchitis. She has been treated multiple times over the years with antibiotic drugs for recurrent infections. Ms. Kurth cares for her two grandchildren, ages 3 and 5, while their mother works. Ms. Kurth's exposure to the multiple infective organisms of childhood has resulted in more frequent infections and the need for antibiotics.

Introduction

Antimicrobial drugs are used to prevent or treat infections caused by pathogenic (disease-producing) microorganisms. The human body and the environment contain many microorganisms, most of which do not cause disease and live in a state of balance with the human host. When the balance is upset and infection occurs, characteristics of the infecting microorganism(s) and the adequacy of host defense mechanisms are major factors in the severity of the infection and the person's ability to recover. Conditions that impair defense mechanisms increase the incidence and severity of infections and impede recovery. In addition, use of antimicrobial drugs may lead to serious infections caused by drug-resistant microorganisms. To help prevent infectious diseases and participate effectively in antimicrobial drug therapy, the nurse must be knowledgeable about microorganisms, host responses to microorganisms, and antimicrobial drugs.

Microorganisms and Infections

In an infection, microorganisms initially attach to host cell receptors (i.e., proteins, carbohydrates, lipids). For example, some bacteria have hairlike structures that attach them to skin and mucous membranes. Most microorganisms preferentially attach themselves to particular body tissues. The microorganisms may then invade tissues, multiply, and produce infection. A major characteristic of microorganisms is their ability to survive in various environments. Bacteria, for example, may form mutant strains, alter their structures and functions, or become embedded in a layer of mucus. These adaptations help protect them from normal body defense mechanisms and antimicrobial drugs. Drug-resistant bacterial strains can be produced in the presence of antimicrobial drugs. Classifications, normal microbial flora, and common pathogenic microorganisms are described in the following sections.

Classifications

Bacteria are subclassified according to whether they are aerobic (require oxygen) or anaerobic (cannot live in the presence of oxygen), their reaction to Gram's stain (gram positive or gram negative), and their shape (e.g., cocci, bacilli).

Viruses are intracellular parasites that survive only in living tissues. They are officially classified according to their structure but are more commonly described according to origin and the disorders or symptoms they produce. Human pathogens include adenoviruses, herpesviruses, and retroviruses (see Chap. 35).

Fungi are plant-like organisms that live as parasites on living tissue or as saprophytes on decaying organic matter. Approximately 50 species are pathogenic in humans (see Chap. 36).

Normal Microbial Flora

The human body normally has areas that are sterile and areas that are colonized with microorganisms. Sterile areas are body fluids and cavities, the lower respiratory tract (trachea, bronchi, lungs), much of the gastrointestinal (GI) and genitourinary tracts, and the musculoskeletal system. Colonized areas include the skin, upper respiratory tract, and colon.

Normal skin flora includes staphylococci, streptococci, diphtheroids, and transient environmental organisms. The upper respiratory tract contains staphylococci, streptococci, pneumococci, diphtheroids, and *Haemophilus influenzae*. The external genitalia contain skin organisms; the vagina contains lactobacilli, *Candida*, and *Bacteroides*. The colon contains *Escherichia coli*, *Klebsiella*, *Enterobacter*, *Proteus*, *Pseudomonas*, *Bacteroides*, clostridia, lactobacilli, streptococci, and staphylococci. Microorganisms that are part of the normal flora and nonpathogenic in one area of the body may be pathogenic in other parts of the body; for example, *E. coli* often cause urinary tract infections.

Normal flora protects the human host by occupying space and consuming nutrients. This interferes with the ability of potential pathogens to establish residence and proliferate. If the normal flora is suppressed by antimicrobial drug therapy, potential pathogens may thrive. For example, the yeast *Candida albicans* is a normal resident of the vagina and the intestinal tract. An antibacterial drug may destroy the normal bacterial flora without affecting the fungal organism. As a result, *C. albicans* can proliferate and cause infection. Much of the normal flora can cause disease under certain conditions, especially in elderly, debilitated, or immunosuppressed people. Normal bowel flora also synthesizes vitamin K and vitamin B complex.

Infectious Diseases

Colonization involves the presence of normal microbial flora or transient environmental organisms that do not harm the host. Infectious disease involves the presence of a pathogen plus clinical signs and symptoms indicative of an infection. These microorganisms are usually spread by direct contact with an infected person or contaminated hands, food, water, or objects. Box 29-1 describes common bacterial pathogens of humans. Accurate assessment and documentation of symptoms can aid diagnosis of infectious diseases.

Opportunistic Pathogens

Opportunistic microorganisms are usually normal endogenous or environmental flora and nonpathogenic. However, they become pathogens in hosts whose defense mechanisms are

---

| **Box 29-1** | **Common Bacterial Pathogens** |

Gram-Positive Bacteria

Staphylococci

Staphylococcus aureus organisms are part of the normal microbial flora of the skin and upper respiratory tract and also are common pathogens. Some people carry (are colonized with) the organism in the anterior nares. The organisms are spread mainly by direct contact with people who are infected or who are carriers. The hands of health care workers are considered a major source of indirect spread and nosocomial infections. The organisms also survive on inanimate surfaces for long periods of time.

S. aureus organisms cause boils, carbuncles, burn and surgical-wound infections, and internal abscesses. Burns or surgical wounds often become infected from patients' own nasal carriage or from health care personnel. The organisms cannot penetrate intact skin or mucous membranes. However, they can penetrate damaged tissues and produce endotoxins that destroy erythrocytes, leukocytes, platelets, fibroblasts, and other human cells. Also, many strains produce enterotoxins that cause food poisoning when ingested. The enterotoxins survive heating at temperatures high enough to kill the organisms, so reheating foods does not prevent food poisoning.

(continued on page 470)

| Box 29-1 | Common Bacterial Pathogens (continued) |

High-risk groups for staphylococcal infections include newborns, the elderly, and those who are malnourished, have diabetes, or are obese. In children, staphylococcal infections of the respiratory tract are most common in those younger than 2 years of age. In adults, staphylococcal pneumonia often occurs in people with chronic lung disease or as a secondary bacterial infection after influenza. The influenza virus destroys the ciliated epithelium of the respiratory tract and thereby aids bacterial invasion.

Staphylococcus species, non-*aureus* (SSNA) describes a group of organisms that are also part of the normal microbial flora of the skin and mucosal surfaces and are increasingly common pathogens. The most common member of this group involved in infections is *Staphylococcus epidermidis*. However, not all laboratories routinely further identify the specific organism when SSNA is identified, and microbiology laboratory reports may just report SSNA. For this discussion, we will use the term *SSNA* unless a specific reference needs to be made to *S. epidermidis*.

Infections due to SSNA are associated with the use of treatment devices such as intravascular catheters, prosthetic heart valves, cardiac pacemakers, orthopedic prostheses, cerebrospinal fluid shunts, and peritoneal catheters. SSNA infections include endocarditis, bacteremia, and other serious infections and are especially hazardous to neutropenic and immunocompromised patients. Treatment usually requires removal of any infected medical device as well as appropriate antibiotic therapy.

Streptococci

Certain streptococci are part of the normal microbial flora of the throat and nasopharynx in many healthy people. Infections are usually spread by inhalation of droplets from the upper respiratory tract of carriers or people with infections. However, these organisms do not cause disease unless the mucosal barrier is damaged by trauma, previous infection, or surgical manipulation. Such damage allows the organisms to enter the bloodstream and gain access to other parts of the body. For example, the organisms may cause endocarditis if they reach damaged heart valves.

Streptococcus pneumoniae organisms, often called *pneumococci*, are common bacterial pathogens. They cause pneumonia, sinusitis, otitis media, and meningitis. Pneumococcal pneumonia usually develops when the mechanisms that normally expel organisms inhaled into the lower airway (i.e., the mucociliary blanket and cough reflex) are impaired by viral infection, smoking, immobility, or other insults. When *S. pneumoniae* reach the alveoli, they proliferate, cause acute inflammation, and spread rapidly to involve one or more lobes. Alveoli fill with proteinaceous fluid, neutrophils, and bacteria. When the pneumonia resolves, there is usually no residual damage to the pulmonary parenchyma. Older adults have high rates of illness and death from pneumococcal pneumonia, which can often be prevented by pneumococcal vaccine. Pneumococcal vaccine (see Chap. 39) contains 23 strains of the pneumococci that cause most of the serious infections.

Pneumococcal sinusitis and otitis media usually follow a viral illness, such as the common cold. The viral infection injures the protective ciliated epithelium and fills the air spaces with nutrient-rich tissue fluid, in which the pneumococci thrive. *S. pneumoniae* is a common pathogen in bacterial sinusitis. In young children, upper respiratory tract infections may be complicated by acute sinusitis. With otitis media, most children have repeated episodes by 6 years of age and the pneumococcus causes approximately half of these cases. Recurrent otitis media during early childhood may result in reduced hearing acuity. Otitis media rarely occurs in adults.

Pneumococcal meningitis may develop from sinus or middle ear infections or an injury that allows organisms from the nasopharynx to enter the meninges. *S. pneumoniae* infection is a common cause of bacterial meningitis in adults. Other potential secondary complications include septicemia, endocarditis, pericarditis, and empyema.

Susceptible pneumococcal infections may be treated with penicillin G. For people who are allergic to penicillin, a cephalosporin or a macrolide may be effective. *S. pneumoniae* organisms are developing resistance such that empiric treatment must be based on the likelihood of multidrug-resistant *S. pneumoniae* (MDRSP). Rates of MDRSP vary by locale; if high, the organisms will be resistant to penicillin and also cross-resistant to other alternatives such as second- and third-generation cephalosporins and possibly macrolides. Alternatives include fluoroquinolones, vancomycin, telithromycin, or high doses of amoxicillin/clavulanate. Empiric treatment of meningitis where *S. pneumoniae* is known or suspected should include a third-generation cephalosporin (ceftriaxone or cefotaxime) plus vancomycin. Empiric treatment for pneumonia should include a fluoroquinolone or a macrolide in those areas with high penicillin and cephalosporin resistance rates.

Streptococcus pyogenes (beta-hemolytic streptococcus) organisms are often part of the normal flora of the skin and oropharynx. The organisms spread from person to person by direct contact with oral or respiratory secretions. They cause severe pharyngitis ("strep throat"), scarlet fever, rheumatic fever, and endocarditis. With streptococcal pharyngitis, people remain infected with the organism for weeks after symptoms resolve and thus serve as a reservoir for infection.

Enterococci

Enterococci are normal flora in the human intestine but are also found in soil, food, water, and animals. Although the genus *Enterococcus* contains approximately 12 species, the main pathogens are *Enterococcus faecalis* and *Enterococcus faecium*. Most enterococcal infections occur in hospitalized patients, especially those in critical care units. Risk factors for nosocomial infections include serious underlying disease, prior surgery, renal impairment, and the presence of urinary or vascular catheters. These organisms, especially *E. faecalis*, are usually secondary invaders in urinary tract or wound infections. Enterococci may also cause endocarditis. This serious infection occurs most often in people with underlying heart disease, such as an injured valve. When the organisms reach a heart valve, they multiply and release emboli of foreign particles into the bloodstream. Symptoms of endocarditis include fever, heart murmurs, enlarged spleen, and anemia. This infection is diagnosed by isolating enterococci from blood cultures. If not treated promptly and appropriately, often with ampicillin and gentamicin, enterococcal endocarditis may be fatal. Antimicrobial resistance is increasing among the enterococci, as it is among other gram-positive bacteria.

Gram-Negative Bacteria
Bacteroides

Bacteroides are anaerobic bacteria normally found in the digestive, respiratory, and genital tracts. They are the most common bacteria in the colon, where they greatly outnumber *Escherichia coli*. *Bacteroides fragilis*, the major human pathogen, causes intra-abdominal and pelvic abscesses (e.g., after surgery or trauma that allows fecal contamination of these tissues), brain abscesses (e.g., from bacteremia or spread from a middle-ear or sinus infection), and bacteremia, which may spread the organisms throughout the body.

Escherichia coli

E. coli inhabit the intestinal tract of humans. They are normally nonpathogenic in the intestinal tract but are common pathogens in other parts of the body. They may be beneficial by synthesizing vitamins and by competitively discouraging growth of potential pathogens.

E. coli cause most urinary tract infections. They also cause pneumonia and sepsis in immunocompromised hosts and meningitis and sepsis in newborns. *E. coli* pneumonia often occurs in debilitated patients after colonization of the oropharynx with organisms from their endogenous microbial flora. In healthy people, the normal gram-positive organisms of oral cavities attach to material that coats the surface of oral mucosa and prevents transient *E. coli* from establishing residence. Debilitated or severely ill people produce an enzyme that destroys the material that allows gram-positive flora to adhere to oral mucosa. This allows *E. coli* (and other gram-negative enteric bacteria) to compete successfully with the normal gram-positive flora and colonize the oropharynx. Then, droplets of the oral flora are aspirated into the respiratory tract, where impaired protective mechanisms allow survival of the aspirated organisms.

E. coli also cause enteric gram-negative sepsis, which is acquired from the normal enteric bacterial flora. When *E. coli* and other enteric organisms reach the bloodstream of healthy people, host defenses eliminate the organisms. When the organisms reach the bloodstream of people with severe illnesses and conditions such as neutropenia, the host is unable to mount adequate defenses and sepsis occurs. In newborns, *E. coli* are the most common gram-negative organisms causing nosocomial septic shock and meningitis.

In addition, *E. coli* often cause diarrhea and dysentery. One strain, called *O157:H7*, causes hemorrhagic colitis, a disease characterized by severe abdominal cramps, copious bloody diarrhea, and hemolytic-uremic syndrome (hemolytic anemia, thrombocytopenia, and acute renal failure). Hemolytic-uremic syndrome occurs most often in children. The main reservoir of this strain is the intestinal tract of animals, especially cattle, and several epidemics have been associated with ingestion of undercooked ground beef. Other sources include contaminated water and milk and person-to-person spread. Because it cannot survive in nature, the presence of *E. coli* in milk or water indicates fecal contamination.

Treatment of *E. coli* infections is complicated by increasing resistance to cephalosporins, commonly used agents. Resistance is mediated by production of extended-spectrum beta-lactamases, which inactivates the antibiotic. Effective treatments may include aminoglycosides, fluoroquinolones, or trimethoprim-sulfamethoxazole.

Klebsiella

Klebsiella organisms, which are normal bowel flora, may infect the respiratory tract, urinary tract, bloodstream, burn wounds, and meninges, most often as opportunistic infections in debilitated persons. *Klebsiella pneumoniae* are a common cause of pneumonia, especially in people with pulmonary disease, bacteremia, and sepsis.

Proteus

Proteus organisms are normally found in the intestinal tract and in decaying matter. They most often cause urinary tract and wound infections but may infect any tissue, especially in debilitated people. Infection usually occurs with antibiotic therapy, which decreases drug-sensitive bacteria and allows drug-resistant bacteria to proliferate.

Pseudomonas

Pseudomonas organisms are found in water, soil, skin, and intestines. They are found in the stools of some healthy people and possibly 50% of inpatients. *Pseudomonas aeruginosa*, the species most often associated with human disease, can cause infections of the respiratory tract, urinary tract, wounds, burns, meninges, eyes, and ears. Because of its resistance to many antibiotics, it can cause severe infections in people receiving antibiotic therapy for burns, wounds, and cystic fibrosis. *P. aeruginosa* colonizes the respiratory tract of most patients with cystic fibrosis and infects approximately 25% of burn patients. Infection is more likely to occur in hosts who are very young or very old or who have an impaired immune system. Sources of infection include catheterization of the urinary tract, trauma or procedures involving the brain or spinal cord, and contamination of respiratory ventilators.

Serratia

Serratia marcescens organisms are found in infected people, water, milk, feces, and soil. They cause serious nosocomial infections of the urinary tract, respiratory tract, skin, burn wounds, and bloodstream. They also may cause hospital epidemics and produce drug-resistant strains. High-risk patients include newborns, the debilitated, and the immunosuppressed.

(continued on page 472)

| Box 29-1 | Common Bacterial Pathogens (continued) |

Salmonella

Approximately 1400 *Salmonella* species have been identified; several are pathogenic to humans. The organisms cause gastroenteritis, typhoid fever, septicemia, and a severe, sometimes fatal type of food poisoning. The primary reservoir is the intestinal tract of many animals. Humans become infected through ingestion of contaminated water or food. Water becomes polluted by introduction of feces from any animal excreting salmonellae. Infection via food usually results from ingestion of contaminated meat or by hands transferring organisms from an infected source. In the United States, undercooked poultry and eggs are common sources.

Salmonella enterocolitis is a common cause of foodborne outbreaks of gastroenteritis. Diarrhea usually begins several hours after ingesting contaminated food and may continue for several days, along with nausea, vomiting, headache, and abdominal pain.

Shigella

Shigella species cause gastrointestinal problems ranging from mild diarrhea to severe bacillary dysentery. Humans, who seem to be the only natural hosts, become infected after ingestion of contaminated food or water. Effects of shigellosis are attributed to loss of fluids, electrolytes, and nutrients and to the ulceration that occurs in the colon wall.

---

impaired. Opportunistic infections are likely to occur in people with severe burns, cancer, human immunodeficiency virus (HIV) infection, indwelling intravenous (IV) or urinary catheters, and antibiotic or corticosteroid drug therapy. Opportunistic bacterial infections, often caused by drug-resistant microorganisms, are usually serious and may be life threatening. Fungi of the *Candida* genus, especially *C. albicans*, may cause life-threatening bloodstream or deep-tissue infections, such as abdominal abscesses. Viral infections may cause fatal pneumonia in people with renal or cardiac disorders, in those with HIV infection, and in those who have received bone marrow transplants.

Laboratory Identification of Pathogens

Laboratory tests of infected fluids or tissues can identify probable pathogens. Bacteria can be identified based on Gram's stain and culture. Gram's stain identifies microscopic appearance, including shape and color of the organisms. Culture involves growing a microorganism in the laboratory. Growth on selective culture media characterizes color, shape, and texture of the growing colonies. Identification of other microorganisms (e.g., intracellular pathogens such as chlamydiae and viruses) may require different techniques. *Serology* identifies infectious agents indirectly by measuring the antibody level (titer) in the serum of a diseased host. A tentative diagnosis can be made if the antibody level against a specific pathogen rises during the acute phase of the disease and falls during convalescence. *Detection of antigens* uses features of culture and serology but reduces the time required for diagnosis. Another technique to identify an organism involves polymerase chain reaction (PCR), which can detect whether DNA for a specific organism is present in a sample.

Community-Acquired Versus Nosocomial Infections

Infections are often categorized as community acquired or nosocomial. Because the microbial environments differ, the two types of infections often have different causes and require different antimicrobial treatment. As a general rule, *community-acquired* infections are less severe and easier to treat, although *antibiotic-resistant* strains are increasing (e.g., methicillin-resistant *Staphylococcus aureus* [MRSA]). *Nosocomial* infections may be more severe and difficult to manage because they often result from drug-resistant microorganisms and occur in people whose immunity is impaired. Drug-resistant strains of staphylococci, *Pseudomonas*, and *Proteus* are common causes of nosocomial infections.

Antibiotic-Resistant Microorganisms

The increasing prevalence of bacteria resistant to the effects of antibiotic drugs is a major public health concern (Box 29-2). *Antibiotic resistance* occurs in most human pathogens. Both gram-positive and gram-negative bacteria are producing more antibiotic-resistant strains. Examples of gram-positive organisms with increasing antibiotic resistance include staphylococci, streptococci, and enterococci. Gram-negative bacteria associated with high rates of antibiotic resistance include *Pseudomonas aeruginosa* and *Serratia*, *Enterobacter*, and *Acinetobacter* species. These organisms are inherently resistant to penetration of antibiotics and acquire resistance by multiple mechanisms. Infections caused by drug-resistant organisms often require more toxic and expensive drugs, lead to prolonged illness or hospitalization, and increase mortality rates.

Resistant microorganisms grow and multiply when susceptible organisms, including normal flora, are suppressed by antimicrobial drugs or when normal body defenses are impaired by immunosuppressive disorders or drugs. They may emerge during or after antimicrobial drug therapy.

Broad-spectrum antibiotics affect the bacteria for which they are prescribed, transient organisms, other pathogens, and normal flora. When the normal flora is suppressed, space and nutrients become available to support the growth of organisms resistant to the effects of that antibiotic. The resistant organisms soon become the predominant strain. After they are established, resistant bacteria can cause superinfection in the original host, spread to other hosts, and even spread their resistance properties for that antibiotic to other

Methicillin-Resistant and Vancomycin-Intermediate/Resistant *Staphylococcus* Species

Penicillin-resistant staphylococci developed in the early days of penicillin use because the organisms produced beta-lactamase enzymes (penicillinases) that destroyed penicillin. Methicillin was one of five drugs developed to resist the action of beta-lactamase enzymes and thus be effective in treating staphylococcal infections. Eventually, strains of *Staphylococcus aureus* became resistant to these drugs as well. The mechanism of resistance in methicillin-resistant *S. aureus* (MRSA) is alteration of penicillin-binding proteins (PBPs). PBPs, the target sites of penicillins and other beta-lactam antibiotics, are proteins required for maintaining integrity of bacterial cell walls. Susceptible *S. aureus* have five PBPs called 1, 2, 3, 3a or 3′, and 4. Beta-lactam antibiotics bind to these enzymes and produce defective bacterial cell walls, which kill the organisms. MRSA have an additional PBP called *2a* or *2′*. Methicillin cannot bind effectively to the PBPs and inhibit bacterial cell-wall synthesis except with very high drug concentrations. Consequently, minimum inhibitory concentrations (MICs) of methicillin increased to high levels that were difficult to achieve.

The term *MRSA* is commonly used but misleading because the organisms are widely resistant to penicillins (including all of the antistaphylococcal penicillins, not just methicillin) and cephalosporins. Many strains of MRSA are also resistant to erythromycin, clindamycin, tetracycline, and the aminoglycosides. MRSA frequently colonize nasal passages of health care workers and are increasing as a cause of nosocomial infections, especially in critical care units. In addition, the incidence of methicillin-resistant *Staphylococcus epidermidis* (MRSE, often reported as *methicillin-resistant SSNA*) isolates is increasing.

A major reason for concern about infections caused by MRSA and MRSE is that vancomycin is the drug of choice for treatment. However, vancomycin has been used extensively to treat or prevent infections caused by *S. aureus*, *S. epidermidis*, and enterococci, and vancomycin resistance is increasing in those species. In 1997, the first case of vancomycin-intermediate *S. aureus* (VISA) in the United States was detected. By 2002, the first cases of vancomycin-resistant *S. aureus* (VRSA) had been reported. Options to treat these infections are limited (linezolid, quinupristin-dalfopristin, daptomycin), and measures to reduce the incidence and prevent spread of the organisms are of paramount importance.

Penicillin-Resistant *Streptococcus pneumoniae* (Pneumococci)

Penicillin has long been the drug of choice for treating pneumococcal infections (e.g., community-acquired pneumonia; bacteremia; meningitis; and otitis media in children). However, penicillin-resistant strains and multidrug-resistant strains are being identified with increasing frequency. Risk factors for the development of resistant strains include frequent antibiotic use and prophylactic antibiotics. After they have developed, resistant strains spread to other people, especially in children's daycare centers and in hospital settings. Children in daycare centers are often colonized or infected with antibiotic-resistant *S. pneumoniae*. This is attributed to a high incidence of otitis media, which is often treated with a penicillin or cephalosporin. Resistant strains in adults and older clients are often associated with previous use of a penicillin or cephalosporin and hospitalization.

S. pneumoniae are thought to develop resistance to penicillin by decreasing the ability of their PBPs to bind with penicillin (and other beta-lactam antibiotics). Organisms displaying high-level penicillin resistance may be cross-resistant to second- and third-generation cephalosporins, amoxicillin/clavulanate, and the macrolides. In pneumococcal infections resistant to penicillins and cephalosporins, vancomycin, fluoroquinolones, macrolides, and telithromycin are drugs of choice. To decrease spread of resistant *S. pneumoniae*, the Centers for Disease Control and Prevention (CDC) have proposed:

- Improved surveillance to delineate prevalence by geographic area and assist clinicians in choosing appropriate antimicrobial therapy.
- Rational use of antimicrobials to reduce exposures to drug-resistant pneumococci. For example, prophylactic antibiotic therapy for otitis media may increase colonization and infection of young children with resistant organisms.
- Pneumococcal vaccination for people older than 2 years of age with increased risk of pneumococcal infection, and for all people older than 65 years of age.

Vancomycin-Resistant Enterococci (VRE)

Enterococci have intrinsic and acquired resistance to many antibacterial drugs. For example, penicillins and cephalosporins inhibit rather than kill the organisms at achievable concentrations, and aminoglycosides are ineffective if used alone. As a result, standard treatment of an enterococcal infection outside of the urinary tract has involved a combination of ampicillin and gentamicin. This combination is often successful because the ampicillin damages the bacterial cell wall and allows the aminoglycoside to penetrate the bacterial cell. For ampicillin-allergic clients, vancomycin is given with an aminoglycoside.

This treatment is becoming less effective because some strains of enterococci have developed resistance to ampicillin, gentamicin, and vancomycin. The incidence of multidrug-resistant enterococci and VRE has increased in recent years. Three major types (VanA, VanB, and VanC) of VRE have been described, with different patterns of antimicrobial susceptibility. Some strains remain susceptible to ampicillin, whereas others are only susceptible to linezolid, quinupristin-dalfopristin, chloramphenicol, or newer fluoroquinolones.

A major contributing factor to VRE is increased use of vancomycin to prevent or treat other infections such as staphylococcal (MRSA and MRSE) infections. Therefore, to decrease the spread of VRE, the CDC recommends limiting the use of vancomycin. Specific recommendations include avoiding or

(continued on page 474)

Box 29-2	Antibiotic-Resistant Staphylococci, Streptococci, and Enterococci (continued)

minimizing use in routine surgical prophylaxis; empiric therapy for febrile clients with neutropenia (unless the prevalence of MRSA or MRSE is high); systemic or local prophylaxis for intravascular catheter infection or colonization; selective decontamination of the gastrointestinal tract; eradication of MRSA colonization; primary treatment of antibiotic-associated colitis; and routine prophylaxis for very low birth weight infants or patients on continuous ambulatory peritoneal dialysis. Thorough hand hygiene and environmental cleaning are also important, because VRE can survive for long periods on hands, gloves, stethoscopes, and environmental surfaces. Personnel should remove or change gloves after contact with patients known to be colonized or infected with VRE. Stethoscopes should be used only with infected patients or cleaned thoroughly between patients if used for both VRE-infected and uninfected patients.

species of bacteria. In addition to resistance to the effects of one antibiotic, cross-resistance to similar antibiotics also occurs because most antibiotics are variations of a few basic types. Interruption or inadequate antimicrobial treatment of infections may also contribute to the emergence of antibiotic-resistant organisms. Patients often stop taking a prescribed antibiotic when symptoms subside or they feel better. In such circumstances, only the most susceptible bacteria are affected and resistant organisms can become established residents.

Infections often associated with high rates of resistance include lower respiratory tract infections and those infections associated with cystic fibrosis or osteomyelitis. These infections are often difficult to treat because they tend to recur, involve multiple or resistant organisms, and involve anatomic locations that antibiotics do not penetrate well. Patients who are malnourished, severely ill, immunosuppressed, or receiving mechanical ventilation are at high risk for infections, including those caused by antibiotic-resistant organisms.

Resistant organisms are especially likely to emerge in critical care units and large teaching hospitals, where seriously ill patients often require extensive antibiotic therapy. The constant presence of antibiotics provides an environment conducive to selection and replication of resistant organisms. Patients in critical care units are more at risk for infection with antibiotic-resistant organisms because of person-to-person transmission by health care workers or equipment.

Resistant organisms and the antibiotics to which they develop resistance vary in geographic areas, communities, and hospitals according to the use of particular antibiotics. Nationally, resistant bacterial strains of major concern include penicillin-resistant *Streptococcus pneumoniae*, methicillin-resistant *S. aureus* and *Staphylococcus epidermidis*, vancomycin-resistant enterococcus (VRE), extended-spectrum beta-lactamase (ESBL)–producing gram-negative bacilli, and multidrug-resistant tuberculosis (MDR-TB). All of these organisms are resistant to multiple antibiotics. The first four are described in Box 29-2; MDR-TB is discussed in Chapter 34. Viruses and fungi also develop resistance to antimicrobial drugs, as discussed in Chapters 35 and 36, respectively.

Mechanisms of Resistance

Bacteria have developed numerous ways to acquire resistance to antimicrobial drugs, including

- Production of enzymes that inactivate the drugs. For example, beta-lactamase enzymes change the chemical structure of penicillins and cephalosporins by opening the beta-lactam ring and preventing the antibiotic from binding with its target site (called *penicillin-binding proteins*) in the bacterial cell wall.

- Modification of target sites for the antibiotic. This is a mechanism of resistance used by bacteria against fluoroquinolones.

- Production of an alternative enzyme to bypass antibiotic activity (e.g., methicillin-resistant staphylococci)

- Changing their cell wall structure to reduce permeability. An example is alteration in porin channels among *P. aeruginosa* to produce imipenem resistance.

- Acquiring or increasing the ability to pump drug molecules out of the cell (efflux). Examples include some gram-positive cocci resistant to tetracyclines.

- Modification of a binding target for the antibiotic (e.g., macrolides)

Bacteria have efficient mechanisms for exchange of genetic material (DNA or plasmids) that allow them to spread antibiotic resistance from one bacterial strain to another, including different species or types of bacteria. Thus, when a new antibiotic is used, resistance may rapidly appear and be disseminated to multiple bacteria.

Host Defense Mechanisms

Although the numbers and virulence of microorganisms help determine whether a person acquires an infection, another major factor is the host's ability to defend itself against the would-be invaders.

Major defense mechanisms of the human body are intact skin and mucous membranes, various anti-infective secretions, mechanical movements, phagocytic cells, and the immune and inflammatory processes. The skin prevents penetration of foreign particles, and its secretions and normal bacterial flora inhibit growth of pathogenic microorganisms. Secretions of the GI, respiratory, and genitourinary tracts (e.g., gastric acid, mucus) kill, trap, or inhibit growth of microorganisms. Coughing, swallowing, and peristalsis help remove foreign particles and pathogens trapped in mucus, as does the movement of cilia. Phagocytic cells in various organs and tissues engulf and digest pathogens and cellular debris. The immune system produces lymphocytes and antibodies (see Chap. 38). The inflammatory process is the body's response to injury by microorganisms, foreign particles, chemical agents, or physical irritation of tissues. Inflammation localizes, destroys, dilutes, or removes the injurious agents so tissue healing can occur.

Many factors impair host defense mechanisms and predispose to infection by disease-producing microorganisms. These factors include the following:

▪ Breaks in the skin and mucous membranes related to trauma, inflammation, open lesions, or insertion of prosthetic devices, tubes, and catheters for diagnostic or therapeutic purposes
▪ Impaired blood supply
▪ Neutropenia and other blood disorders
▪ Malnutrition
▪ Poor personal hygiene
▪ Suppression of normal bacterial flora by antimicrobial drugs
▪ Suppression of the immune system and the inflammatory response by immunosuppressive drugs, cytotoxic antineoplastic drugs, and adrenal corticosteroids
▪ Diabetes mellitus and other chronic diseases
▪ Advanced age

Characteristics of Antimicrobial Drugs

Terms and Concepts

Several terms are used to describe these drugs. *Anti-infective* and *antimicrobial* include antibacterial, antiviral, and antifungal drugs; *antibacterial* and *antibiotic* refer to drugs used in bacterial infections and are often used interchangeably. Most of the drugs in this section are antibacterials. Antiviral and antifungal drugs are discussed in Chapters 35 and 36, respectively.

Additional terms for antibacterial drugs include *broad spectrum*, for those effective against several groups of microorganisms, and narrow spectrum, for those effective against a few groups. The action of an antibacterial drug is usually described as *bactericidal* (kills the microorganism) or *bacteriostatic* (inhibits growth of the microorganism). Whether a drug is bactericidal or bacteriostatic often depends on its concentration at the infection site and the susceptibility of the microorganism to the drug. Successful treatment with bacteriostatic antibiotics depends on the ability of the host's immune system to eliminate the inhibited bacteria and an adequate duration of drug therapy. Stopping an antibiotic prematurely can result in rapid resumption of bacterial growth. Bactericidal drugs are preferred in serious infections, especially in people with impaired immune function.

Mechanisms of Action

Most antimicrobial drugs act on a specific target in the infecting organism (Fig. 29-1). Almost any structure unique to infecting organism, such as proteins or nucleic acids, can be a target for antibiotics. Specific mechanisms of action of antimicrobial drugs include the following:

▪ Inhibition of bacterial cell wall synthesis or activation of enzymes that disrupt bacterial cell walls (e.g., penicillins, cephalosporins, vancomycin)
▪ Inhibition of protein synthesis by bacteria or production of abnormal bacterial proteins (e.g., aminoglycosides, clindamycin, macrolides, ketolides, tetracyclines). These drugs bind irreversibly to bacterial ribosomes, intracellular structures that synthesize proteins. When antimicrobial drugs are bound to the ribosomes, bacteria cannot synthesize the proteins necessary for cell walls and other structures.
▪ Disruption of microbial cell membranes (e.g., antifungals)
▪ Inhibition of organism reproduction by interfering with nucleic acid synthesis (e.g., fluoroquinolones, rifampin, anti–acquired immunodeficiency syndrome antivirals)
▪ Inhibition of cell metabolism and growth (e.g., sulfonamides, trimethoprim)

Indications for Use

Antimicrobial drugs are used to treat and prevent infections. Because laboratory tests (except Gram's stain and a rapid test for group A streptococci) to identify causative organisms usually take 24 hours or longer, empiric therapy against the most likely pathogens is often begun. After organisms are identified, more specific therapy is instituted. Prophylactic therapy is recommended to prevent the following:

▪ Group A streptococcal infections and possibly rheumatic fever, rheumatic heart disease, and glomerulonephritis. Penicillin is commonly used.

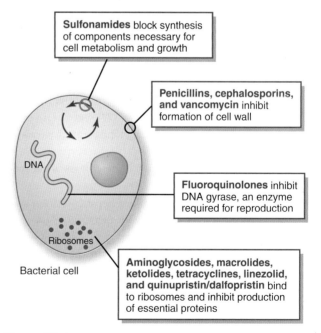

Figure 29-1 ▪ Actions of antibacterial drugs on bacterial cells.

■ Bacterial endocarditis in patients with cardiac valvular disease who are having dental, surgical, or other invasive procedures. Amoxicillin or ampicillin, with an aminoglycoside, is usually recommended for at-risk persons undergoing certain types of procedures.

■ Tuberculosis in patients with latent tuberculosis infection (see Chap. 34)

■ Perioperative infections in high-risk patients (e.g., those whose resistance to infection is lowered because of age, poor nutrition, disease, or drugs) and for high-risk surgical procedures (e.g., cardiac or GI surgery, certain orthopedic procedures, organ transplants)

■ Sexually transmitted diseases (e.g., gonorrhea, syphilis, chlamydial infections) after exposure has occurred

■ Recurrent urinary tract infections in premenopausal, sexually active women. A single dose of a fluoroquinolone or trimethoprim-sulfamethoxazole for two doses, taken after sexual intercourse, is often effective.

Nursing Process

Assessment

Assess for current or potential infection.

■ General signs and symptoms of infection are the same as those of inflammation, although the terms are not synonymous. *Inflammation* is the normal response to any injury; *infection* requires the presence of a microorganism. The two often occur together. Inflammation may weaken tissue, allowing microorganisms to invade and cause infection. Infection (tissue injury by microorganisms) arouses inflammation. Local signs include redness, heat, edema, and pain; systemic signs include fever and leukocytosis. Specific manifestations depend on the site of infection. Common sites are the respiratory tract, surgical or other wounds, and the genitourinary tract.

■ Assess each patient for the presence of factors that increase risks of infection (see "Host Defense Mechanisms," earlier).

■ Assess culture reports for causative organisms.

■ Assess susceptibility reports for appropriate antibacterial drug therapy.

■ Assess patients for drug allergies. If present, ask about specific signs and symptoms.

■ Assess baseline data about renal and hepatic function and other factors that aid monitoring for therapeutic and adverse drug effects.

■ Assess for characteristics that increase risks of adverse drug effects.

Nursing Diagnoses

■ Fatigue related to infection

■ Activity Intolerance related to fatigue

■ Diarrhea related to antimicrobial therapy

■ Imbalanced Nutrition: Less Than Body Requirements related to anorexia, nausea, and vomiting associated with antimicrobial therapy

■ Risk for Injury related to infection or adverse drug effects

■ Risk for Infection related to emergence of drug-resistant microorganisms

■ Deficient Knowledge: Methods of preventing infections

Planning/Goals

The patient will

■ Receive antimicrobial drugs accurately when given by health care providers or caregivers

■ Take drugs as prescribed and for the length of time prescribed when self-administered as an outpatient

■ Experience decreased fever, white blood cell (WBC) count, and other signs and symptoms of infection

■ Be monitored regularly for therapeutic and adverse drug effects

■ Receive prompt recognition and treatment of potentially serious adverse effects

■ Verbalize and practice measures to prevent future infections

■ Be safeguarded against nosocomial infections by health care providers

Interventions

■ Use measures to prevent and minimize the spread of infection.

■ Wash hands thoroughly and often. This is probably the most effective method of preventing infections.

■ Support natural defense mechanisms by promoting general health measures (e.g., nutrition, adequate fluid intake, rest, exercise).

■ Keep the patient's skin clean and dry, especially the hands, underarms, groin, and perineum, because these areas harbor large numbers of microorganisms. Also, take care to prevent trauma to the skin and mucous membranes. Damaged tissues are susceptible to infection.

■ Treat all body fluids (e.g., blood, aspirates from abdomen or chest) and body substances (e.g., sputum, feces, urine, wound drainage) as infectious. Major elements of standard precautions to prevent transmission of hepatitis B, HIV, and other pathogens include wearing gloves when likely to be exposed to any of these materials and thorough hand hygiene when the gloves are removed. Wear protective eyewear when a risk of spatter is present. Rigorous and consistent use of the recommended precautions helps to protect health care providers and patients.

■ Implement isolation procedures appropriately.

- To prevent spread of respiratory infections, have patients wash hands after coughing, sneezing, or contact with infected people; cover mouth and nose with tissues when sneezing or coughing and dispose of tissues by placing them in a paper bag and burning it; expectorate sputum (swallowing may cause reinfection); and avoid crowds when possible, especially during influenza season (approximately November through February). Recommend an annual influenza vaccine to high-risk populations (e.g., people with chronic diseases such as diabetes and heart, lung, or renal problems; older adults; health care personnel who are likely to be exposed). Pneumococcal vaccine (see Chap. 39) is recommended for the same populations.

- Assist or instruct patients at risk about pulmonary hygiene measures to prevent accumulation or promote removal of respiratory secretions. These measures include ambulating; turning; coughing and deep-breathing exercises; and incentive spirometry. Retained secretions are good culture media for bacterial growth.

- Use sterile technique when changing any dressing. If a wound is not infected, sterile technique helps prevent infection. If the wound is already infected, sterile technique avoids introducing new bacteria. For all but the smallest of dressings without drainage, remove the dressing with clean gloves, discard it in a moisture-proof bag, and wash hands before putting on sterile gloves to apply the new dressing.

- To minimize spread of infections, adhere to current established guidelines for isolatism precautions to prevent transmission of infections agents in health care settings published by the Centers for Disease Control and Prevention.

- For patients with infections, monitor temperature for increased or decreased fever, and monitor WBC count for decrease.

- For patients receiving antimicrobial therapy, maintain a total fluid intake of approximately 3000 mL/24 hours, if not contraindicated by the patient's condition. An adequate intake and avoidance of fluid volume deficit may help decrease drug toxicity, especially with aminoglycoside antibiotics. On the other hand, a patient receiving IV antibiotics, with 50 to 100 mL of fluid per dose, may be at risk for fluid volume overload.

- Assist patients with hand hygiene; maintaining nutrition and fluid balance; getting adequate rest; and handling secretions correctly. These measures help the body to fight the infection, prevent further infection, and enhance the effectiveness of anti-infective drugs.

- Assist patients in using antimicrobial drugs safely and effectively. Provide appropriate patient teaching (see accompanying display).

Evaluation

- Interview and observe for compliance with instructions for using antimicrobial drugs.
- Observe for adverse drug effects.
- Interview and observe for practices to prevent infection.

Applying Your Knowledge 29-1

Ms. Kurth tells you that she frequently takes her antibiotic for just long enough to feel better and then saves the rest of her medication for another illness. What teaching guidelines should you provide to her regarding safe and accurate self-administration of antibiotics?

Principles of Therapy

Goal of Therapy for Infections

The goal of treatment is to eradicate the causative microorganism and return the host to full physiologic functioning. This differs from the goal of most drug therapy, which is to relieve signs and symptoms rather than cure the underlying disorder.

Applying Your Knowledge 29-2

Ms. Kurth is hospitalized for acute infection and is receiving IV antibiotic medication. What are the nurse's responsibilities for accurate antibiotic administration?

Rational Use of Antimicrobial Drugs

Antimicrobials are among the most frequently used drugs worldwide. Their success in saving lives and decreasing severity and duration of infectious diseases has encouraged their extensive use. Authorities believe that much antibiotic use involves overuse, misuse, or abuse of the drugs. That is, an antibiotic is not indicated at all or the wrong drug, dose, route, or duration is prescribed. Inappropriate use of antibiotics increases adverse drug effects, infections with drug-resistant microorganisms, and health care costs. In addition, it decreases the number of effective drugs for serious or antibiotic-resistant infections.

Guidelines to promote more appropriate use of antimicrobial drugs include the following:

- Avoid the use of broad-spectrum antibacterial drugs to treat trivial or viral infections; use narrow-spectrum agents if they are likely to be effective. Give antibacterial drugs only when a significant bacterial infection is diagnosed or strongly suspected or when there is an established indication for prophylaxis. Antibacterial drugs are ineffective in viral infections and should not be used to treat them.

■ Collect specimens (e.g., sputum, urine) for culture and Gram's stain before giving the first dose of an antibiotic. For best results, specimens must be collected accurately and taken directly to the laboratory. If analysis is delayed, contaminants may overgrow pathogenic microorganisms.

■ Minimize antimicrobial drug therapy for fever unless other clinical manifestations or laboratory data indicate infection.

■ Use antimicrobial drugs in combination with other interventions to decrease microbial proliferation, such as universal precautions, medical isolation techniques, frequent and thorough hand hygiene, and preoperative skin and bowel cleansing.

■ Follow recommendations of the Centers for Disease Control and Prevention for prevention and treatment of infections, especially those caused by drug-resistant organisms (e.g., gonorrhea, penicillin-resistant streptococcal infections, MRSA, VRE, MDR-TB).

■ Consult infectious disease physicians, infection control nurses, and infectious disease pharmacists about local patterns of drug-resistant organisms and treatment of complicated infections.

Drug Selection

After an infection requiring treatment is diagnosed, numerous factors influence the choice of an antimicrobial drug or combination of drugs.

Empiric Therapy

Because most laboratory tests used to definitively identify causative organisms and to determine susceptibility to antibiotics require 48 to 72 hours, the physician usually prescribes for immediate administration a drug that is likely to be effective. This empiric therapy is based on an informed estimate of the most likely pathogen(s) given the patient's signs and symptoms and apparent site of infection. A single broad-spectrum antibiotic or a combination of drugs is often chosen.

Culture and Susceptibility Studies

Culture identifies the causative organism, and *susceptibility* tests determine which drugs are likely to be effective against the organism. One can then "match the drug to the bug." Culture and susceptibility studies are important in both suspected gram-positive and gram-negative infections because of the high incidence of drug-resistant microorganisms.

When a specific organism is identified by laboratory culture, tests can be performed to measure the organism's susceptibility to particular antibiotics. Laboratory reports indicate

Patient Teaching Guidelines | Antimicrobial Drugs

General Considerations

■ Wash hands often and thoroughly, especially before preparing food or eating and after exposure to any body secretions (e.g., urine, feces, sputum, nasal secretions). This is probably the most effective way to prevent infection and to avoid spreading an infection to others.

■ A balanced diet and adequate fluid intake, rest, and exercise also help the body to fight infection, prevent further infection, and increase the effectiveness of antimicrobial drugs.

■ Take all prescribed doses of an antimicrobial; do not stop when symptoms are relieved. If medication is stopped too soon, symptoms of the current infection may recur and new infections that are caused by antibiotic-resistant organisms and that are harder to treat may develop.

■ If problems occur with taking an antimicrobial drug, report them to a health care provider rather than stopping the drug.

■ Do not take antimicrobials left over from a previous illness or prescribed for someone else. Even if infection is present, the likelihood of having the appropriate drug on hand, and in adequate amounts, is extremely small. Thus, taking drugs not prescribed for the particular illness tends to maximize risks and minimize benefits. Also, if the infection is viral, antibacterial drugs are ineffective and should not be used.

■ Report any other drugs being taken to the prescribing physician. Drug interactions may occur, and changes in drug therapy may be indicated.

■ Report any drug allergies to all health care providers and wear a medical identification emblem that lists allergens.

■ Some antibiotics (e.g., ampicillin, nitrofurantoin, penicillin V, sulfonamides, tetracyclines) decrease the effectiveness of estrogens and oral contraceptives. Women taking these drugs should use another method of contraception. Inadequate blood levels of estrogen may be indicated by breakthrough bleeding.

Self-Administration

■ Unless instructed otherwise, take antimicrobial drugs at evenly spaced intervals around the clock. This helps maintain beneficial blood levels of most drugs.

■ Some oral antimicrobials should be taken on an empty stomach, approximately 1 hour before or 2 hours after meals. Food may decrease absorption and effectiveness. If the medication causes intolerable nausea or vomiting, a few bites of food may be taken.

■ Store most liquid preparations in the refrigerator, check expiration dates, and discard them when indicated. These preparations are stable and effective for a limited time.

■ Take the medications with a full glass of water. This helps tablets and capsules to dissolve better in the stomach and decreases stomach irritation.

■ Report nausea, vomiting, diarrhea, skin rash, recurrence of symptoms for which the antimicrobial drug was prescribed, or signs of new infection (e.g., fever, cough, sore mouth, drainage). These problems may indicate adverse effects of the drug, lack of therapeutic response to the drug, or another infection. Any of these requires evaluation and may indicate changes in drug therapy.

whether the organism is susceptible (S) or resistant (R) to the tested drugs. One indication of susceptibility is the minimum inhibitory concentration (MIC). The MIC is the lowest concentration of an antibiotic that prevents visible growth of microorganisms. Some laboratories report MIC instead of, or in addition to, S or R.

Susceptible organisms have low or moderate MICs that can be attained by giving usual doses of an antimicrobial agent. For the drug to be effective, its serum and tissue concentrations should usually exceed the MIC of an organism for a period of time. By how much and for how long drug concentrations need to exceed the MIC depend on the drug class and the bacterial species. With beta-lactam agents (e.g., penicillins, cephalosporins), the drug concentration usually needs to be maintained above the MIC of the infecting organism for a majority of the dosing interval. With the aminoglycosides (e.g., gentamicin, others), the drug concentration does not need to be maintained above the MIC of the organism for the entire dosing interval, because aminoglycosides have a *postantibiotic effect*. Postantibiotic effect is a persistent effect of an antimicrobial on bacterial growth after brief exposure of the organisms to a drug. Some studies demonstrate that large doses of aminoglycosides, given once daily, are as effective as more frequent dosing and may cause less nephrotoxicity.

Resistant organisms have high MICs and may require higher concentrations of drug than can be achieved in the body. In some cases the minimum bactericidal concentration (MBC) is reported, indicating no growth of the organism in the presence of a particular antibiotic. The MBC is especially desirable for infected hosts with impaired immune functions.

Patients' responses to antimicrobial therapy cannot always be correlated with the MIC of an infecting pathogen. Thus, reports of drug susceptibility testing must be applied in the context of the site of infection, the characteristics of the drug, and the clinical status of the patient.

Antibiotic Resistance Patterns

Because these patterns of resistance change in the community and agencies, continuing efforts must be made. *P. aeruginosa* is resistant to many antibiotics, and those strains resistant to gentamicin may be susceptible to amikacin, ceftazidime, imipenem, or aztreonam. Some gram-negative organisms have become increasingly resistant to aminoglycosides, third-generation cephalosporins, and aztreonam, but they may be susceptible to carbapenems or cefepime.

Organism Most Likely to Infect a Particular Site

For example, urinary tract infections are often caused by *E. coli*. Thus, a drug effective against this organism is indicated.

Ability to Penetrate Infected Tissues

Several antimicrobials are effective in urinary tract infections because they are excreted in the urine. However, the choice of an effective antimicrobial drug may be limited in infections of the brain, eyes, gallbladder, or prostate gland because many drugs are unable to reach therapeutic concentrations in these tissues.

Toxicity and Risk-to-Benefit Ratio

In general, the least toxic drug should always be used. However, for serious infections, more toxic drugs may be necessary.

Cost

If an older, less expensive drug meets the criteria for rational drug selection and is likely to be effective in a given infection, it should be used instead of a more expensive agent. For hospitals and nursing homes, personnel costs relating to preparation and administration should be considered as well as purchasing costs.

Combination Therapy

Antimicrobial drugs are often used in combination. Indications for combination therapy may include the following:

- Infections caused by multiple microorganisms (e.g., abdominal and pelvic infections)
- Nosocomial infections, which may be caused by many different organisms
- Serious infections in which a combination is synergistic (e.g., an aminoglycoside and an antipseudomonal penicillin for pseudomonal infections)
- Likely emergence of drug-resistant organisms if a single drug is used (e.g., in tuberculosis). Although drug combinations are widely used to prevent resistance, the only clearly effective use of combination therapy is for treatment of tuberculosis.
- Fever or other signs of infection in patients whose immune system is suppressed. Combinations of antibacterial plus antiviral and/or antifungal drugs may be needed.

Drug Dosage and Administration

Dosage (amount and frequency of administration) should be individualized according to characteristics of the causative organism, the chosen drug, and the patient's size and condition (e.g., type and severity of infection, ability to use and excrete the chosen drug). For example, dosage may need to be increased for more resistant organisms such as *P. aeruginosa* and for infections in which antibiotics have difficulty penetrating to the site of infection (e.g., meningitis). Dosage often must be reduced if the patient has renal impairment or other disorders that delay drug elimination.

Most antimicrobial drugs are given orally or IV for systemic infections. The route of administration depends on the patient's condition (e.g., location and severity of the infection, ability to take oral drugs) and the available drug dosage forms. In serious infections, the IV route is preferred for most drugs.

Duration of Therapy

Duration of therapy varies from a single dose to years, depending on the reason for use. For most acute infections, the average duration is approximately 7 to 10 days or until the recipient has been afebrile and asymptomatic for 48 to 72 hours.

Use in Special Populations

Perioperative Use

When used to prevent infections associated with surgery, a single dose of an antimicrobial medication is usually given within 1 hour of the first incision. This provides effective tissue concentrations during the procedure. If intraoperative contamination occurs, the patient should be treated for an infection. The choice of drug depends on the pathogens most likely to colonize the operative area. For most surgeries involving an incision through the skin, a first-generation cephalosporin such as cefazolin (Kefzol) with activity against *S. aureus* or *Streptococcus* species is commonly used. Repeated doses may be given during surgery for procedures of long duration, procedures involving insertion of prosthetic materials, and contaminated or infected operative sites. Postoperative antimicrobials are indicated with intraoperative contamination, traumatic wounds, or ruptured viscera.

Use in Children

Antimicrobial drugs are commonly used in hospitals and ambulatory settings for respiratory infections, otitis media, and other infections. General principles of pediatric (see Chap. 4) and antimicrobial drug therapy apply. Other guidelines include the following:

- Penicillins and cephalosporins are considered safe for most age groups. However, they are eliminated more slowly in neonates because of immature renal function and must be used cautiously and dosed appropriately for age. As with other classes of drugs, many penicillins and cephalosporins do not have Food and Drug Administration (FDA) approval for use in children (usually younger than 12 years of age). However, pediatric specialty references reflect the growing body of experience in using these drugs in younger children.

- Erythromycin, azithromycin (Zithromax), and clarithromycin (Biaxin) are considered safe.

- Aminoglycosides (e.g., gentamicin) may cause nephrotoxicity and ototoxicity in any patient population. Neonates are at high risk because of immature renal function.

- Tetracyclines are contraindicated in children younger than 8 years of age because of drug effects on teeth and bone (see Chap. 32).

- Clindamycin (Cleocin) warrants monitoring liver and kidney function when it is given to neonates and infants.

- Fluoroquinolones (e.g., ciprofloxacin [Cipro]) are contraindicated for use in children (<18 years of age) because weight-bearing joints have been impaired in young animals given the drugs. However, if fluoroquinolones are the only therapeutic option for a resistant pathogen, the prescriber may decide to use a fluoroquinolone in children.

- Trimethoprim-sulfamethoxazole (Bactrim) is used in children, although children younger than 2 months of age have not been evaluated.

- Linezolid (Zyvox) is considered safe for use in children.

Use in Older Adults

Antimicrobial drugs are commonly used in all health care settings for infections in older adults as in younger adults. General principles of geriatric (see Chap. 4) and antimicrobial drug therapy apply. Other guidelines include the following:

- Penicillins are usually safe. However, hyperkalemia may occur with large IV doses of penicillin G potassium (1.7 mEq potassium per 1 million units), and hypernatremia may occur with ticarcillin (Ticar), which contains 5.6 milliequivalents of sodium per gram. Hyperkalemia and hypernatremia are more likely to occur with impaired renal function.

- Cephalosporins (e.g., cefazolin) are considered safe but may cause or aggravate renal impairment, especially when other nephrotoxic drugs are used concurrently. Dosage of most cephalosporins should be reduced in the presence of renal impairment (see Chap. 30).

- Macrolides and ketolides (e.g., erythromycin, telithromycin) are usually safe. Dosage of clarithromycin should be reduced with severe renal impairment.

- Aminoglycosides (e.g., gentamicin) are contraindicated in the presence of impaired renal function if less toxic drugs are effective against causative microorganisms. Older adults are at increased risk of nephrotoxicity and ototoxicity from these drugs. Interventions to decrease adverse drug effects are described in Chapter 31.

- Tetracyclines (except doxycycline) and nitrofurantoin (Macrodantin) are contraindicated in the presence of impaired renal function if less toxic drugs are effective against causative organisms.

- Clindamycin may cause diarrhea and should be used with caution in the presence of GI disease, especially colitis.

- Trimethoprim-sulfamethoxazole (Bactrim, Septra) may be associated with an increased risk of severe adverse effects in older adults, especially those with impaired liver or kidney function. Severe skin reactions and bone marrow depression are the most frequently reported severe reactions.

- Daptomycin (Cubicin), quinupristin-dalfopristin (Synercid), tigecycline (Tygacil), and linezolid (Zyvox) are newer agents that may be used in older adults. Daptomycin dosage should be lowered in the presence of impaired renal function.

Use in Patients With Renal Impairment

Antimicrobial drug therapy requires close monitoring in patients with renal impairment. Many drugs are excreted primarily by the kidneys; some are nephrotoxic and may further damage the kidneys. In the presence of renal impairment, drugs may accumulate and produce toxic effects. Thus, dosage reductions are necessary for some drugs. Methods of calculating dosage are usually based on rates of creatinine clearance (CrCl). For some antibiotics, such as the aminoglycosides and vancomycin, serum drug concentrations should also be used to individualize dosage.

The following formula may be used to estimate CrCl:

Male: Weight in kilograms (IBW) × (140–age), divided by 72 × serum creatinine (in milligrams per 100 mL)

Female: 0.85 × above value

Dosage may be reduced by giving smaller individual doses, by increasing the time interval between doses, or both. Anti-infective drugs can be categorized as follows in relation to renal impairment:

■ Drugs that should be avoided in severe renal impairment (i.e., CrCl < 15–30 mL/minute) unless the infecting organism is sensitive only to a particular drug. These drugs include the tetracyclines (except doxycycline) and flucytosine.

■ Drugs that may exacerbate renal impairment and should not be used if safer alternatives are available. If used, dosage must be carefully adjusted, renal function must be closely monitored, and the patient must be closely observed for adverse effects. These drugs include aminoglycosides, amphotericin B, and the fluoroquinolones. Monitoring serum drug concentrations is recommended when using aminoglycoside antibiotics.

■ Drugs that require dosage reduction in severe renal impairment. These include penicillin G, ampicillin, most cephalosporins, fluoroquinolones, and trimethoprim-sulfamethoxazole.

■ Drugs that require little or no dosage adjustment. These include chloramphenicol, clindamycin, doxycycline, erythromycin, isoniazid, nafcillin, and rifampin.

An additional factor is important in patients with acute or chronic renal failure who are receiving hemodialysis or peritoneal dialysis: Some drugs are removed by dialysis, and an extra dose may be needed during or after dialysis. Patients with acute renal failure receiving continuous renal replacement therapy (CRRT) may also require adjustments in drug doses. Generally, CRRT is more effective at removing drugs than hemodialysis and peritoneal dialysis. Reference texts or scientific articles should be consulted to determine appropriate doses of antibiotics in these patients.

Use in Patients With Hepatic Impairment

Antimicrobial therapy in patients with liver impairment is not well defined. Some drugs are metabolized by the liver (e.g., cefoperazone, chloramphenicol, clindamycin, erythromycin), and dosage must be reduced in patients with severe liver impairment. Some are associated with elevations of liver enzymes and/or hepatotoxicity (e.g., certain fluoroquinolones, tetracyclines, isoniazid, rifampin). Laboratory monitoring may be helpful in high-risk populations.

Penicillins and other beta-lactam drugs rarely cause jaundice, hepatitis, or liver failure. However, acute liver injuries have been reported with the combination of amoxicillin-clavulanate (Augmentin), and some cases of cholestatic jaundice have been reported with ticarcillin-clavulanate (Timentin). Hepatotoxicity is attributed to the clavulanate component. These drugs are contraindicated in patients who have had cholestatic jaundice or hepatic dysfunction associated with their use and must be used with caution in patients with hepatic impairment.

Some fluoroquinolones have been associated with liver enzyme abnormalities and hepatotoxicity (e.g., hepatitis, liver impairment or failure). The drugs should be used cautiously in patients with or at risk for development of impaired liver function. The drug should be stopped if jaundice or any other symptoms of liver dysfunction develop.

Use in Patients With Critical Illness

Antimicrobials are frequently given in critical care units. Many patients have multiple organ impairments or chronic diseases with a superimposed acute illness or injury (e.g., surgery, trauma, burns). Thus, antimicrobial therapy is often more aggressive, complex, and expensive in critically ill patients than in other patients. In addition, measurement of plasma drug levels and dosage adjustment are often necessary to accommodate the changing physiology of a critically ill patient. Drug levels are usually measured after four or five doses are given so that steady-state concentrations have been reached.

Patients in critical care units are at high risk for acquiring nosocomial pneumonia because of the severity of their illness, duration of hospitalization, and antimicrobial drug therapy. The strongest predisposing factor is mechanical ventilation, which bypasses airway defenses against movement of microorganisms from the upper to the lower respiratory tract. Organisms often associated with nosocomial pneumonia are *S. aureus* and gram-negative bacilli. Bacterial pneumonia is usually treated with a broad-spectrum antibiotic until culture and susceptibility reports become available.

Selection of antibacterial drugs may be difficult because of frequent changes in antibiotic resistance patterns. Antibiotic rotation (i.e., switching preferred antibiotic or antibiotic classes used to treat infections, on a scheduled basis) has been successful in reducing rates of ventilator-associated pneumonia and mortality.

Use in Home Care

Infections are among the most common illnesses in all age groups, and they are often treated by antibiotic therapy at home, with medications administered by the patient or a family-member caregiver. If a home care nurse is involved, responsibilities may include teaching family members how to administer antibiotics (e.g., teaching a parent how to store and measure a liquid antibiotic), how to care for the person with an infection, and how to protect other people in the environment from the infection. General infection-control practices include frequent and thorough hand hygiene, use of gloves when indicated, and appropriate handling and disposal of body substances (e.g., blood, urine, feces, sputum, vomitus, wound drainage).

Increasingly, IV antibiotics are being given in the home. Any patient who needs more than a few days of IV antibiotic therapy may be a candidate for home care. Some infections that require relatively long-term IV antibiotic therapy include endocarditis, osteomyelitis, and some surgical-wound infections. Numerous people and agencies may be involved in providing this service. First, the patient and family need to be able and willing to manage some aspects of therapy and to provide space for necessary supplies. Second, arrangements must be made for procuring equipment, supplies, and medication. In some areas, nurses employed by equipment companies help families prepare and use IV infusion pumps. Medication is usually obtained from a local pharmacy in a unit-dose package ready for administration.

The role of the home care nurse includes teaching the patient and caregiver how to store and administer the medication, monitor the IV site, monitor the infection, manage problems, and report patient responses. Specific responsibilities may vary according to drug administration (intermittently or by continuous infusion), whether the patient has a peripheral or central IV line, and other factors. The family should be provided with detailed instructions and emergency telephone numbers of the home care nurse, the pharmacy, and the supply company.

Nursing Actions | Antimicrobial Drugs

NURSING ACTIONS	RATIONALE/EXPLANATION
1. Administer accurately	
a. Schedule at evenly spaced intervals around the clock.	To maintain therapeutic blood levels
b. Some oral antimicrobials should be given on an empty stomach, approximately 1 hour before or 2 hours after meals. Check specific recommendations.	To decrease binding to foods and inactivation by gastric acid
c. For oral and parenteral solutions from powder forms, follow label instructions for mixing and storing. Check expiration dates	Several antimicrobial drugs are marketed in powder forms because they are unstable in solution. When mixed, measured amounts of diluent must be added for drug dissolution and the appropriate concentration. Parenteral solutions are usually prepared in the pharmacy. Many solutions require refrigeration to prolong stability. None of the solutions should be used after the expiration date because drug decomposition is likely.
d. Give parenteral antimicrobial solutions alone; do not mix with any other drug in a syringe or intravenous (IV) solution.	To avoid chemical and physical incompatibilities that may cause drug precipitation or inactivation
e. Give intramuscular (IM) antimicrobials deeply into large muscle masses (preferably gluteal muscles), and rotate injection sites.	To decrease tissue irritation
f. For IV administration, use dilute solutions, giving direct injections slowly and intermittent infusions over 30–60 minutes. After infusions, flush the IV tubing with at least 10 milliliters of IV solution. For children, check instructions for individual drugs to avoid excessive concentrations and excessive fluids.	Most antimicrobials that are given IV can be given by intermittent infusion. Although instructions vary with specific drugs, most reconstituted drugs can be further diluted with 50–100 milliliters of IV fluid (D_5W, NS, D_5-1/4%, or D_5-1/2% NaCl). Dilution and slow administration minimize vascular irritation and phlebitis. Flushing ensures that the entire dose is given and prevents contact between drugs in the tubing.
2. Observe for therapeutic effects	
a. With local infections, observe for decreased redness, edema, heat, and pain.	Signs and symptoms of inflammation and infection usually subside within approximately 48 hours after antimicrobial therapy is begun.
b. With systemic infections, observe for decreased fever and white blood cell count, increased appetite, and reports of feeling better.	Although systemic manifestations of infection are similar regardless of the cause, local manifestations vary with the type or location of the infection.
c. With wound infections, observe for decreased signs of local inflammation and decreased drainage. Drainage also may change from purulent to serous.	
d. With respiratory infections, observe for decreased dyspnea, coughing, and secretions. Secretions may change from thick and colored to thin and white.	
e. With urinary tract infections, observe for decreased urgency, frequency, and dysuria. If urinalysis is done, check the laboratory report for decreased bacteria and white blood cells.	
f. Absence of signs and symptoms of infection when given prophylactically	

NURSING ACTIONS	RATIONALE/EXPLANATION
3. Observe for adverse effects	
a. Hypersensitivity	Reactions are more likely to occur in those with previous hypersensitivity reactions and those with a history of allergy, asthma, or hay fever.
(1) Anaphylaxis—hypotension, respiratory distress, urticaria, angioedema, vomiting, diarrhea	Hypersensitivity may occur with most antimicrobial drugs but is more common with penicillins. Anaphylaxis may occur with oral administration but is more likely with parenteral administration and may occur within 5–30 minutes of injection. Hypotension results from vasodilation and circulatory collapse. Respiratory distress results from bronchospasm or laryngeal edema.
(2) Serum sickness—chills, fever, vasculitis, generalized lymphadenopathy, joint edema and inflammation, bronchospasm, urticaria	This is a delayed allergic reaction, occurring 1 week or more after the drug is started. Signs and symptoms are caused by inflammation.
(3) Acute interstitial nephritis (AIN), hematuria, oliguria, proteinuria, pyuria	AIN is considered a hypersensitivity reaction that may occur with many antimicrobials, including penicillins, cephalosporins, aminoglycosides, sulfonamides, tetracyclines, and others. It is usually reversible if the causative agent is promptly stopped.
b. Superinfection	Superinfection is a new or secondary infection that occurs during antimicrobial therapy for a primary infection. Superinfections are common and potentially serious because responsible microorganisms are often drug-resistant staphylococci, gram-negative organisms (e.g., *Pseudomonas aeruginosa*), or fungi (e.g., *Candida*).
(1) Recurrence of systemic signs and symptoms (e.g., fever, malaise)	
(2) New localized signs and symptoms—redness, heat, edema, pain, drainage, cough	
(3) Stomatitis or "thrush"—sore mouth; white patches on oral mucosa; black, furry tongue	From overgrowth of fungi
(4) Pseudomembranous colitis—severe diarrhea characterized by blood, pus, and mucus in stools	May occur with most antibiotics. Antibiotics suppress normal bacterial flora and allow the overgrowth of *Clostridium difficile*. The organism produces a toxin that kills mucosal cells and produces superficial ulcerations that are visible with sigmoidoscopy. Discontinuing antibiotics and giving metronidazole or oral vancomycin are curative measures. However, relapses may occur.
(5) Monilial vaginitis—rash in perineal area, itching, vaginal discharge	From overgrowth of yeast organisms
c. Phlebitis at IV sites; pain at IM sites	Many antimicrobial parenteral solutions are irritating to body tissues.
d. Nausea and vomiting	These often occur with oral antimicrobials, probably from irritation of gastric mucosa.
e. Diarrhea	Commonly occurs; is caused by irritation of gastrointestinal mucosa and changes in intestinal bacterial flora; and may range from mild to severe. Pseudomembranous colitis is one type of severe diarrhea.
f. Nephrotoxicity	
(1) See AIN, earlier	More likely to occur in patients who are elderly or who have impaired renal function.
(2) Acute tubular necrosis (ATN)—increased blood urea nitrogen and serum creatinine, decreased creatinine clearance, fluid and electrolyte imbalances	Aminoglycosides are the antimicrobial agents most often associated with ATN.
g. Neurotoxicity—confusion, hallucinations, neuromuscular irritability, convulsive seizures	More likely with large IV doses of penicillins or cephalosporins, especially in patients with impaired renal function.
h. Bleeding—hypoprothrombinemia, platelet dysfunction	Most often associated with penicillins and cephalosporins.
4. Observe for drug interactions	See following chapters. The most significant interactions are those that alter effectiveness or increase drug toxicity.

Key Concepts

- Bacteria may form mutant strains, alter their structures and functions, or become embedded in a layer of mucus, allowing them to survive in various environments.

- Drug-resistant bacterial strains can be produced in the presence of antimicrobial drugs.

- Anti-infective and antimicrobial agents include antibacterial, antiviral, and antifungal drugs; antibacterial and antibiotic refer to drugs used in bacterial infections.

- The amount and frequency of anti-infective and antimicrobial agents should be individualized according to characteristics of the causative organism, the chosen drug, and the patient's size and condition (e.g., type and severity of infection, ability to use and excrete the chosen drug).

- For most surgeries involving an incision through the skin, a first-generation cephalosporin such as cefazolin (Kefzol) with activity against S. aureus or Streptococcus species is commonly used.

- Antimicrobial drug therapy requires close monitoring in patients with renal impairment as many drugs are excreted primarily by the kidneys and some are nephrotoxic and may further damage the kidneys.

- Schedule antibiotics at evenly spaced intervals around the clock, to maintain therapeutic blood levels.

- Check specific recommendations with regard to the administration of the antibiotic with food and other medication to decrease binding to food and drugs and prevent inactivation.

- Inappropriate use of antibiotics increases adverse drug effects, infections with drug-resistant microorganisms, and health care costs and reduces the number of available effective drugs for serious or antibiotic-resistant infections.

- Patient education related to antibiotic therapy should stress the importance of completing a full course of antibiotics as prescribed.

Review and Application Exercises

Short Answer Exercises

1. How does the body defend itself against infection?

2. When assessing a patient, what signs and symptoms may indicate an infectious process?

3. Do all infections require antimicrobial drug therapy? Why or why not?

4. With antimicrobial drug therapy, what is meant by the terms bacteriostatic, bactericidal, antimicrobial spectrum of activity, and minimum inhibitory concentration?

5. Why is it important to identify the organism causing an infection?

6. Why are infections of the brain, eye, and prostate gland more difficult to treat than infections of the GI, respiratory, and urinary tracts?

7. What factors promote the development of drug-resistant microorganisms, and how can they be prevented or minimized?

8. What are common adverse effects associated with antimicrobial drug therapy?

9. When teaching a patient about a prescribed antibiotic, a common instruction is to take all the medicine and not to stop prematurely. Why is this information important?

10. When a dose of an antibiotic is prescribed to prevent postoperative infection, should it be given before, during, or after surgery? Why?

11. What special precautions are needed for patients with renal or hepatic impairment or critical illness?

NCLEX-Style Questions

12. When teaching a mother about the antibiotic liquid preparation for her child's acute bronchitis, the nurse should do which of the following?
    a. Instruct the mother to administer the antibiotic until the child is afebrile.
    b. Tell the mother to expect the child's respiratory secretions to become thicker and darker as the infection responds to treatment.
    c. Instruct the mother to keep any remaining antibiotic liquid preparation for the next episode of bronchitis.
    d. Remind the mother that frequent hand hygiene after handling respiratory secretions is one way to reduce spread of infections.

13. The nurse should give which of the following instructions to patients taking oral antibiotics?
    a. Take oral antibiotics with a full glass of water.
    b. Always take an oral antibiotic after a full meal.
    c. If stomach upset occurs, take the oral antibiotic with a full, fatty meal.
    d. Do not refrigerate oral liquid antibiotic preparations.

14. Critically ill patients are at increased risk of infections due to resistant organisms for all the following reasons except
    a. They may have multiple medical conditions.
    b. Health care workers may spread resistant organisms on their hands in the closed environment.
    c. They have increased host defenses.
    d. Equipment used in critical care units may be a fomite for spread between people.

15. A patient is hospitalized with a large sacral wound and a urinary tract infection. The nurse should watch for which of the following signs that the patient is not responding appropriately to antibiotic treatment?
    a. decreased drainage from the wound
    b. increased bacteria and WBC counts on urinalysis
    c. decreased pain at the wound site
    d. increased activity tolerance

16. To decrease the spread of vancomycin-resistant enterococcus (VRE), the nurse caring for a patient with VRE should do all of the following except
    a. Use gloves when providing care involving direct patient contact.
    b. Thoroughly wash hands after contact with the patient.
    c. Clean equipment thoroughly after use by the patient.
    d. Ensure that the physician has prescribed vancomycin.

Selected References

Blumer, J. L., & Toltzis, P. (2005). Pediatric infectious disease. *Infectious Disease Clinics of North America, 19*(3), xiii–xv.

Corwin, E. J. (2006). *Handbook of pathophysiology* (3rd ed.). Philadelphia: Lippincott Williams & Wilkins.

Dunne, W.M., Jr. (2005). Mechanisms of Infectious disease. In C.M. Porth (Ed.), *Pathophysiology: Concepts of altered health states* (7th ed., pp. 341–361). Philadelphia: Lippincott Williams & Wilkins.

Guyton, A. C., & Hall, J. E. (2006). *Textbook of medical physiology* (11th ed.). Philadelphia: W. B. Saunders.

Lieberman, P. (Ed.), & the Joint Task Force on Practice Parameters. (2005). The diagnosis and management of anaphylaxis: An updated practice parameter. *Journal of Allergy and Clinical Immunology, 115*(3 Suppl. 2), S483–S523.

Siegel, J. D., Rhinehart, E., Jackson, M., & Chiarello, L. (2007). The Healthcare Infection Control Practices Advisory Committee. *Guideline for isolation precautions: Preventing transmission of infectious agents in health care settings.* Retrieved on September 14, 2007, from http://www.cdc.gov/ncidod/dhqp/pdf/guidelines/Isolation2007.pdf

Shoemaker, D. M., Jiang, P. P., Williamson, H., & Roland, W. E. (2007). Infectious diseases. In R. E. Rakel (Ed.), *Textbook of family medicine* (pp. 317–351). Philadelphia: Elsevier.

Solensky, R. (2006). Drug hypersensitivity. *Medical Clinics of North America, 90*(1), 233–60.

Beta-Lactam Antibacterials: Penicillins, Cephalosporins, and Other Drugs

LEARNING OBJECTIVES

After studying this chapter, you will be able to:

1. Describe general characteristics of beta-lactam antibiotics.
2. Discuss penicillins in relation to effectiveness, safety, spectrum of antibacterial activity, mechanism of action, indications for use, administration, observation of patient response, and teaching of patients.
3. Differentiate among extended-spectrum penicillins.
4. Question patients about allergies before the initial dose of a penicillin.
5. Describe characteristics of beta-lactamase inhibitor drugs.
6. State the rationale for combining a penicillin and a beta-lactamase inhibitor drug.
7. Discuss similarities and differences between cephalosporins and penicillins.
8. Differentiate cephalosporins in relation to antibacterial spectrum, indications for use, and adverse effects.
9. Describe major characteristics of carbapenem and monobactam drugs.
10. Apply principles of using beta-lactam antibacterials in selected patient situations.

Applying Your Knowledge

Verra Jang is a 32-year-old professional musician. She is being evaluated for chronic and frequent upper respiratory infections. She is scheduled for a bronchoscopy. The physician orders cefazolin 1 g IV immediately before the procedure.

Introduction

Beta-lactam antibacterials derive their name from the beta-lactam ring that is part of their chemical structure. An intact beta-lactam ring is essential for antibacterial activity. Several gram-positive and gram-negative bacteria produce beta-lactamase enzymes that disrupt the beta-lactam ring and inactivate the drugs. This is a major mechanism by which microorganisms acquire resistance to beta-lactam antibiotics. Penicillinase and cephalosporinase are beta-lactamase enzymes that act on penicillins and cephalosporins, respectively.

Despite the common element of a beta-lactam ring, characteristics of beta-lactam antibiotics differ widely because of variations in their chemical structures. The drugs may differ in antibacterial spectrum of activity, routes of administration, susceptibility to beta-lactamase enzymes, and adverse effects. Beta-lactam antibiotics include penicillins, cephalosporins, carbapenems, and monobactams, which are described in the following sections. Routes and usual dosage ranges are listed in the Drugs at a Glance tables.

Beta-lactam antibacterial drugs inhibit synthesis of bacterial cell walls by binding to proteins (penicillin-binding proteins) in bacterial cell membranes. This binding produces a defective cell wall that allows intracellular contents to leak out, destroying the microorganism. Beta-lactam antibiotics are most effective when bacterial cells are dividing.

Penicillins

The penicillins are effective, safe, and widely used antibacterial agents. The first antibiotic developed was penicillin, which was discovered from the *Penicillium* mold and serves as the prototype. When **P** penicillin was introduced, it was effective against many organisms, had to be given parenterally because it was destroyed by gastric acid, and injections were painful. With extensive use, strains of drug-resistant staphylococci appeared. Semisynthetic derivatives, formed by adding side chains to the penicillin nucleus, were developed to increase gastric acid stability, beta-lactamase stability, and antimicrobial spectrum of activity, especially against gram-negative microorganisms.

After absorption, penicillins are widely distributed and achieve therapeutic concentrations in most body fluids. Thera-peutic levels are not usually obtained in intraocular and cerebrospinal fluids (CSF) unless inflammation is present because normal cell membranes act as barriers to drug penetration. Penicillins are rapidly excreted by the kidneys and produce high drug concentrations in the urine (an exception is nafcillin, which is excreted by the liver).

Indications for Use

Clinical indications for use of penicillins include bacterial infections caused by susceptible microorganisms. As a class, penicillins usually are more effective in infections caused by gram-positive bacteria than those caused by gram-negative bacteria. However, their clinical uses vary significantly according to the subgroup or individual drug and microbial patterns of resistance. The drugs are often useful in skin/soft tissue, respiratory, gastrointestinal, and genitourinary infections. However, the incidence of resistance among streptococci, staphylococci, and other microorganisms continues to grow.

Contraindications to Use

Contraindications include hypersensitivity or allergic reactions to any penicillin preparation. An allergic reaction to one penicillin means the patient is allergic to all members of the penicillin class. The potential for *cross-allergenicity* (allergy to a drug of another class with similar chemical structure) with cephalosporins and carbapenems exists, although recent data suggest that the incidence is less than 1%, lower than previously thought. Administration of cephalosporins or carbapenems should be avoided in individuals with life-threatening allergic reactions to penicillin (anaphylaxis, laryngeal swelling angioedema, or hives).

Subgroups and Individual Penicillins

Table 30-1 provides pertinent information about individual penicillins.

| Table 30-1 | Drugs at a Glance: Penicillins |

	ROUTES AND USUAL DOSAGE RANGES	
Generic/Trade Name	**Adults**	**Children**
Penicillins G and V		
Penicillin G potassium and sodium (Pfizerpen)	IM 300,000–8 million units daily IV 6–20 million units daily by continuous or intermittent infusion every 2–4h. Up to 60 million units daily have been given in certain serious infections.	IM, IV 25,000–400,000 units/kg/d in divided doses q4–6h (maximum dose 24 million units/d)
Penicillin G benzathine (Bicillin LA)	IM 1.2–2.4 million units in a single dose Prophylaxis of recurrent rheumatic fever, IM 1.2 million units q 3–4 wk Treatment of syphilis, IM 2.4 million units (1.2 million units in each buttock) in a single dose.	IM 25,000–50,000 units/kg (maximum 2.4 million units) Prophylaxis of recurrent rheumatic fever, 25,000–50,000 units/kg times one dose q 3–4 wk (maximum 1.2 million units)

(continued on page 488)

Table 30-1	**Drugs at a Glance:** Penicillins (continued)

	ROUTES AND USUAL DOSAGE RANGES	
Generic/Trade Name	**Adults**	**Children**
Penicillin G procaine (Wycillin)	IM 600,000–4.8 million units daily in 1 or 2 doses	IM 25,000–50,000 units/kg/d in divided doses q12–24 h
Penicillin V (Veetids)	PO 125–500 mg q6–8h	*12 y and older:* same as adults *under 12 y:* PO 25–50 mg/kg/d every 6–8 h.
Penicillinase-Resistant (Antistaphylococcal) Penicillins Dicloxacillin	PO 125–1000 mg every 6 h	Not recommended in newborns *40 kg or less:* 12.5–100 mg/kg/d divided every 6 h *40 kg or more:* 125–500 mg every 6 h
Nafcillin	IM 500 mg every 4–6 h IV 500 mg–2 g every 4–6 h; maximum daily dose 18 g for serious infections.	IM 25 mg/kg every 12 h IV 50–200 mg/kg/d in divided doses every 4–6 h
Oxacillin	IM, IV, 250–2000 mg every 4–6 h	*40 kg or less:* IM, IV 100–200 mg/kg/d in divided doses every 6 h *more than 40 kg:* same as adults
Aminopenicillins Ampicillin (Principen)	PO, IM, IV 250–500 mg every 6 h. In severe infections, doses up to 2 g every 4 h may be given IV.	*Infants/children:* PO 50–100 mg/kg/d in divided doses every 6 h (maximum dose 2.4 g/d) IM, IV: 100–400 mg/kg/d in divided doses every 6 h (maximum dose 12 g/d)
Amoxicillin (Amoxil, Trimox)	PO 250–500 mg every 8 h or 500–875 mg every 12 h	*3 months or more:* PO 20–30 mg/kg/d in divided doses every 12 h *more than 3 months:* 20–50 mg/kg/d in divided doses every 8–12 h
Extended Spectrum (Antipseudomonal) Penicillins Carbenicillin indanyl sodium (Geocillin)	PO 1–2 tabs 4 times daily	PO 30–50 mg/kg/d in divided doses q6h
Ticarcillin (Ticar)	IM, IV 1–4 g q4–6h. IM injections should not exceed 2 g/injection.	*Infants/children:* IM 50–100 mg/kg/d in divided doses q6–8h. IV 50–300 mg/kg/d in divided doses q4–8h (maximum dose 24 g/d).
Piperacillin (Pipracil)	IM, IV 200–300 mg/kg/d in divided doses q4–6h. Usual adult dosage, 3–4 g q4–6h; maximum daily dose 24 g.	*less than 12 y:* Dosage not established
Penicillin–Beta-Lactamase Inhibitor Combinations Ampicillin-sulbactam (Unasyn)	IM, IV 1.5–3 g q6h	*1 y or older:* IV 100–400 mg/kg/d in divided doses q6h (maximum 8 g ampicillin/day; 12 g Unasyn) Doses up to 300 mg/kg/day may be given for severe infections in infants older than 1 month of age
Amoxicillin-clavulanate (Augmentin)	PO 250–500 mg q8h; or 875 mg q12h	*40 kg or more:* same as adults *less than 40 kg:* 20–90 mg/kg/d in divided doses q8–12h
Piperacillin-tazobactam (Zosyn)	IV 2.25–4.5 g q6–8h	IV 100 mg/kg/d q8h
Ticarcillin-clavulanate (Timentin)	IV 3.1 g q4–6h	*Weight less than 60 kg:* IV 200–300 mg/kg/d in divided doses q4–6h (maximum dose 18–24 g/d)

Penicillins G and V

Penicillin G (Pfizerpen, Bicillin, Wycillin) remains effective for a limited number of uses. Many strains of staphylococci and gonococci have acquired resistance to penicillin G, preventing its use for treatment of infections caused by these organisms. Some strains of streptococci have acquired resistance to penicillin G, although the drug is still effective in many streptococcal infections. It remains the drug of choice for the treatment of streptococcal pharyngitis, for prevention of recurrent attacks in patients who have had previous acute rheumatic fever due to group A streptococcus, and for treatment of neurosyphilis.

Penicillin G is not effective orally because it is inactivated by gastric acid. Several preparations of penicillin G are available for intravenous (IV) and intramuscular (IM) administration; however, it is important to note that the IV and IM forms of penicillin G can not be used interchangeably. Only aqueous preparations can be given IV. Preparations containing benzathine or procaine can be given only IM. A **BLACK BOX WARNING** alerts health care providers that inadvertent IV administration of penicillin G benzathine may result in cardiopulmonary arrest and death. Long-acting repository forms have additives that decrease their solubility in tissue fluids and delay their absorption.

Penicillin V (Veetids) is derived from penicillin G and has the same antibacterial spectrum. It is not destroyed by gastric acid and is given only by the oral route. It is well absorbed and produces therapeutic blood levels.

Penicillinase-Resistant (Antistaphylococcal) Penicillins

This group includes three drugs (**dicloxacillin, nafcillin**, and **oxacillin**) that are the drugs of choice for methicillin-susceptible *Staphylococcus aureus*. These drugs are formulated to resist the penicillinases that inactivate other penicillins. An older member of this group, methicillin, is no longer marketed for clinical use. However, susceptibility of bacteria to the antistaphylococcal penicillins is determined by exposing the bacteria to methicillin (methicillin susceptible or resistant) or oxacillin (oxacillin susceptible or resistant) in bacteriology laboratories. Although called "methicillin resistant," these staphylococcal microorganisms are also resistant to other antistaphylococcal penicillins.

Aminopenicillins

Ampicillin (Principen) is broad-spectrum, semisynthetic penicillin that is bactericidal for several types of gram-positive and gram-negative bacteria. It has been effective against enterococci, *Proteus mirabilis*, *Salmonella*, *Shigella*, and *Escherichia coli*, but resistant forms of these organisms are increasing. It is ineffective against penicillinase-producing staphylococci and gonococci.

Ampicillin is excreted mainly by the kidneys; thus, it is useful in some urinary tract infections (UTI). Because some is excreted in bile, it is useful in biliary tract infections not caused by biliary obstruction. It is used in the treatment of bronchitis, sinusitis, and otitis media.

P **Amoxicillin** (Amoxil, Trimox) is similar to ampicillin except it is only available orally. It is better absorbed and produces therapeutic blood levels more rapidly than oral ampicillin. It also causes less gastrointestinal distress.

The aminopenicillins are drugs of choice for prevention of bacterial endocarditis due to procedures that produce transient bacteremia.

Extended-Spectrum (Antipseudomonal) Penicillins

The drugs in this group (**carbenicillin** [Geocillin], **ticarcillin**, and **piperacillin**) have a broad spectrum of antimicrobial activity, especially against gram-negative organisms such as *Pseudomonas* and *Proteus* species and *E. coli*. For pseudomonal infections, one of these drugs is usually given concomitantly with an aminoglycoside or a fluoroquinolone (see Chap. 31). Carbenicillin is available as an oral formulation for UTI or prostatitis caused by susceptible pathogens. The other drugs are usually given by intermittent IV infusion, although most can be given IM.

Penicillin–Beta-Lactamase Inhibitor Combinations

Beta-lactamase inhibitors are drugs with a beta-lactam structure but little antibacterial activity. They bind with and inactivate the beta-lactamase enzymes produced by many bacteria (e.g., *E. coli*; *Klebsiella*, *Enterobacter*, and *Bacteroides* species; *S. aureus*). When combined with a penicillin, the beta-lactamase inhibitor protects the penicillin from destruction by the enzymes and extends the penicillin's spectrum of antimicrobial activity. Thus, the combination drug may be effective in infections caused by bacteria that are resistant to a beta-lactam antibiotic alone. Clavulanate, sulbactam, and tazobactam are the beta-lactamase inhibitors available in combinations with penicillins.

Unasyn is a combination of ampicillin and sulbactam available in vials with 1 gram of ampicillin and 0.5 grams of sulbactam, or 2 grams of ampicillin and 1 gram of sulbactam. **Augmentin** contains amoxicillin and clavulanate. It is available in 250-, 500-, and 875-milligram tablets, each of which contains 125 milligrams of clavulanate. Thus, two 250-milligram tablets are not equivalent to one 500-milligram tablet. It is also available as 1000-milligram extended-release tablets containing 62.5 milligrams of clavulanate. In addition, a chewable formulation is available as 400 milligrams of amoxicillin and 57 milligrams of clavulanate. Timentin is a combination of ticarcillin and clavulanate in an IV formulation containing 3 grams of ticarcillin and 100 milligrams of clavulanate. Zosyn is a combination of piperacillin and tazobactam in an IV formulation. Three dosage strengths are available, with 2 grams piperacillin and 0.25 grams tazobactam, 3 grams piperacillin and 0.375 grams tazobactam, or 4 grams piperacillin and 0.5 grams tazobactam.

Cephalosporins

Cephalosporins are a widely used group of drugs derived from a fungus. Although technically cefoxitin and cefotetan (cephamycins derived from a different fungus) are not cephalosporins, they are categorized with the cephalosporins because of their similarities to the group. Cephalosporins are broad-spectrum agents with activity against both gram-positive and gram-negative bacteria. Compared with penicillins, they are in general less active against gram-positive organisms but more active against gram-negative ones.

After they are absorbed, cephalosporins are widely distributed into most body fluids and tissues, with maximum concentrations in the liver and kidneys. Many cephalosporins do not reach therapeutic levels in CSF; exceptions are cefuroxime, a second-generation drug, and the third-generation agents. These drugs reach therapeutic levels when meninges are inflamed. Most cephalosporins are excreted through the kidneys. An exception includes ceftriaxone, which undergoes dual elimination via the biliary tract and kidneys. Cefotaxime is primarily metabolized in the liver to an active metabolite, desacetylcefotaxime, which is eliminated by the kidneys.

Indications for Use

Clinical indications for the use of cephalosporins include surgical prophylaxis and treatment of infections of the respiratory tract, skin and soft tissues, bones and joints, urinary tract, brain and spinal cord, and bloodstream (septicemia). In most infections with streptococci and staphylococci, penicillins are more effective and less expensive. In infections caused by MRSA, cephalosporins are not clinically effective even if in vitro testing indicates susceptibility. Infections caused by *Neisseria gonorrhoeae*, at one time susceptible to penicillin, are now treated with a third-generation cephalosporin such as ceftriaxone. Cefepime is indicated for use in sepsis; in severe infections of the lower respiratory and urinary tracts, skin and soft tissue, and female reproductive tract; and in febrile neutropenic patients. It may be used as monotherapy for all infections caused by susceptible organisms except *Pseudomonas aeruginosa*; a combination of drugs should be used for serious pseudomonal infections.

Contraindications to Use

A contraindication to the use of a cephalosporin is a previous severe anaphylactic reaction to a penicillin. Because cephalosporins are chemically similar to penicillins, there is a risk of cross-sensitivity. However, incidence of cross-sensitivity is low, especially in patients who have had delayed reactions (e.g., skin rash) to penicillins. Another contraindication is cephalosporin allergy. Immediate allergic reactions with anaphylaxis, bronchospasm, and urticaria occur less often than delayed reactions with skin rash, drug fever, and eosinophilia.

Classification

Tables 30-2 and 30-3 provide important information about oral and parenteral cephalosporins.

First-Generation Cephalosporins

The first cephalosporin, cephalothin, is no longer available for clinical use. However, it is used for determining susceptibility to first-generation cephalosporins, which have essentially the same spectrum of antimicrobial activity. These drugs are effective against streptococci; staphylococci (except MRSA); *Neisseria, Salmonella, Shigella, Escherichia, Klebsiella*, and *Bacillus* species; *Corynebacterium diphtheriae*; *P. mirabilis*; and *Bacteroides* species (except *Bacteroides fragilis*). They are not effective against *Enterobacter, Pseudomonas*, and *Serratia* species. Cefazolin is the drug of choice for surgical prophylaxis in most surgical procedures.

Second-Generation Cephalosporins

Second-generation cephalosporins are more active against some gram-negative organisms and against anaerobic organisms than the first-generation drugs. Thus, they may be effective in infections resistant to other antibiotics, including infections caused by *Haemophilus influenzae, Klebsiella* species, *E. coli*, and some strains of *Proteus*. Because each of these drugs has a different antimicrobial spectrum, susceptibility tests must be performed for each drug rather than for the entire group, as may be done with first-generation drugs. Cefoxitin (Mefoxin), for example, is active against *B. fragilis*, an anaerobic organism resistant to most drugs.

Third-Generation Cephalosporins

Third-generation cephalosporins further extend the spectrum of activity against gram-negative organisms. In addition to activity against the usual enteric pathogens (e.g., *E. coli, Proteus* and *Klebsiella* species), they are also active against several strains resistant to other antibiotics and to first- and second-generation cephalosporins. Thus, they may be useful in infections caused by unusual strains of enteric organisms such as *Citrobacter, Serratia*, and *Providencia* species. Another difference is that third-generation cephalosporins penetrate inflamed meninges to reach therapeutic concentrations in CSF. Thus, they may be useful in meningeal infections caused by common pathogens, including *H. influenzae, Neisseria meningitidis*, and *Streptococcus pneumoniae*. Although some of the drugs are active against *Pseudomonas* organisms, drug-resistant strains may emerge when a cephalosporin is used alone for treatment of pseudomonal infection.

Overall, cephalosporins gain gram-negative activity and lose gram-positive activity as they move from the first to the third generation. The second- and third-generation drugs are more active against gram-negative organisms because they are more resistant to the beta-lactamase enzymes (cephalosporinases) produced by some bacteria to inactivate cephalosporins.

Fourth-Generation Cephalosporins

Fourth-generation cephalosporins have a greater spectrum of antimicrobial activity and greater stability against breakdown by beta-lactamase enzymes compared with third-generation drugs. Cefepime is the first fourth-generation cephalosporin to be developed. It is active against both gram-positive and gram-negative organisms. With gram-positive organisms, it is active against streptococci and staphylococci (except for methicillin-resistant staphylococci). With gram-negative organisms, its activity against *P. aeruginosa* is similar to that of ceftazidime and its activity against Enterobacteriaceae is greater than that

Table 30-2   **Drugs at a Glance:** Oral Cephalosporins

Generic/ Trade Name	Characterstics/Indications	ROUTES AND USUAL DOSAGE RANGES Adults	Children
First Generation			
Cefadroxil (Duricef)	A derivative of cephalexin that has a longer half-life and can be given less often	PO 1–2 g twice daily	30 mg/kg/d in divided doses q12h
Cephalexin (Keflex)	First oral cephalosporin; still used extensively	PO 250–500 mg q6h, increased to 4 g q6h if necessary in severe infections	PO 25–50 mg/kg/d in divided doses q6h
Second Generation			
Cefaclor (Ceclor)	More active against *Hemophilus influenzae* and *Escherichia coli* than first-generation drugs	PO 250–500 mg q8h	PO 20–40 mg/kg/d in divided doses q8–12 h
Cefprozil (Cefzil)	Similar to cefaclor	PO 250–500 mg q12–24h	PO 7.5–15 mg/kg in divided doses q12 h
Cefuroxime (Ceftin)	1. Can also be given parenterally 2. The tablet may be crushed and added to a food (e.g., applesauce), but the crushed tablet leaves a strong, bitter, persistent aftertaste.	PO 250–500 mg q12h; IV, IM 750 mg–1.5 g every 6–8 h	*under 13 y:* PO 20–30 mg/kg/d in two divided doses. IM, IV 75–150 mg/kg/d in divided doses q8h (maximum dose 6 g/d) *13 y or older:* same as adults
Third Generation			
Cefdinir (Omnicef)	Indicated for bronchitis, pharyngitis, and otitis media caused by streptococci or *H. influenzae*	PO 300 mg q12h or 600 mg q24h for 10 d	*13 y or older,* PO same as adults *6 mo–12 y,* PO 7 mg/kg q12h or 14 mg/kg q24h for 10 d
Cefditoren pivoxil (Spectracef)	Indicated for pharyngitis, bacterial exacerbations of chronic bronchitis, and skin/skin structure infections	Bronchitis or pharyngitis, PO 400 mg twice daily (q12h) for 10 d Skin infections, PO 200 mg twice daily for 10 d	*12 y or older,* same as adults
Cefixime (Suprax)	First oral third-generation drug	PO 200 mg q12h or 400 mg q24h	Children ≥ 6mo: 8–20 mg/kg/d in divided doses every 12–24 h. (maximum dose 400 mg/d) PO give adult dose to children 50 kg of weight or 12 y or older
Cefpodoxime (Vantin)	Similar to cefixime except has some activity against staphylococci (except methicillin-resistant *Staphylococcus aureus*)	PO 200–400 mg q12h	PO 5 mg/kg q12h Give 10 mg/kg (400 mg or adult dose) to children 13 y or older with skin and soft-tissue infections
Ceftibuten .dax)	1. Indicated for bronchitis, otitis media, pharyngitis, or tonsillitis caused by streptococci or *H. influenzae* 2. Can be given once daily 3. Available in a capsule for oral use and an oral pediatric suspension that comes in two concentrations (90 mg/5 mL)	PO 400 mg daily for 10 d	9 mg/kg/d for 10 d (maximum dose 400 mg d.)

Table 30-3	**Drugs at a Glance:** Parenteral Cephalosporins

Generic/ Trade Name	Characteristics/ Indications	ROUTES AND USUAL DOSAGE RANGES	
		Adults	Children
First Generation **Cefazolin** (Kefzol, Ancef)	Active against streptococci, staphylococci, *Neisseria, Salmonella, Shigella, Escherichia, Klebsiella, Listeria, Bacillus, Hemophilus influenzae, Corynebacterium diphtheriae, Proteus mirabilis,* and *Bacteroides* (except *B. fragilis*)	IM, IV 250 mg–2 g q6–12h (maximum dose 12 g/d)	IM, IV 25–100 mg/kg/d in divided doses q6–8h (maximum dose 6 g/d)
Second Generation **Cefotetan** (Cefotan)	1. Effective against most organisms except *Pseudomonas* 2. Highly resistant to beta-lactamase enzymes	IV, IM 1–6 g/day in divided doses q12h Surgical prophylaxis, IV 1–2 g 30–60 min before surgery	Dosage not established
Cefoxitin (Mefoxin)	1. The first cephamycin (derived from a different fungus than cephalosporins) 2. A major clinical use may stem from increased activity against *B. fragilis,* an organism resistant to most other antimicrobial drugs.	IV 1–2 g q6–8h Surgical prophylaxis, IV 1 or 2 g 30–60 min before surgery	IV 80–160 mg/kg/d in divided doses q4–6h. Do not exceed 12 g/d.
Cefuroxime (Kefurox, Zinacef)	1. Similar to other second generation cephalosporins 2. Penetrates cerebrospinal fluid in presence of inflamed meninges	IV, IM, 750 mg–1.5 g q6–8h Surgical prophylaxis, IV 1.5 g 30–60 min before initial skin incision	*Neonates:* IM, IV 50–100 mg/kg/d in divided doses q 12h *<13 y:* PO 20–30 mg/kg/d in divided doses q12h. IM, IV 75–150 mg/kg/d in divided doses q8h (maximum dose 6 g/d).
Cefotaxime (Claforan)	1. Antibacterial activity against most gram-positive and gram-negative bacteria, including several strains resistant to other antibiotics 2. Recommended for serious infections caused by susceptible microorganisms	IV, IM 1–2 g q4–12h; maximum dose, 12 g/24 h	*Weight >50 kg:* same as adults *Weight <50 kg to 12y and age > 1 mo:* IV, IM 50–200 mg/kg/d, in divided doses q6–8h
Ceftazidime (Fortaz)	1. Active against gram-positive and gram-negative organisms 2. Especially effective against gram-negative organisms, including *Pseudomonas aeruginosa* and other bacterial strains resistant to aminoglycosides 3. Indicated for serious infections caused by susceptible organisms	IV, IM 500–2000mg q8–12h	*1 mo–12 y:* IV 30–50 mg/kg q8h, not to exceed 6 g/d
Ceftizoxime (Cefizox)	1. Broader gram-negative and anaerobic activity, especially against *B. fragilis* 2. More active against Enterobacteriaceae than cefoperazone 3. Dosage must be reduced with even mild renal insufficiency (CrCl < 80 mL/min).	IV, IM 1–4 g q8–12h	*more than 6 mo:* IV, IM 150–200 mg/kg/d in divided doses q6–8h(maximum dose 12 g/d)

Generic/ Trade Name	Characteristics/ Indications	ROUTES AND USUAL DOSAGE RANGES	
		Adults	Children
Ceftriaxone (Rocephin)	1. First third-generation cephalosporin approved for once-daily dosing 2. Antibacterial activity against most gram-positive and gram-negative bacteria, including several strains resistant to other antibiotics	IV, IM 1–2 g q12–24h	*Infants/children* IM, IV 50–100 mg/kg/d in 1–2 divided doses (maximun dose 4 g/d) Meningitis, IV, IM 100 mg/kg/d, not to exceed 4 g daily, in divided doses q12h
Fourth Generation Cefepime (Maxipime)	1. Indicated for urinary-tract infections caused by *Escherichia coli* or *Klebsiella pneumoniae*; skin and soft tissue infections caused by susceptible streptococci or staphylococci; pneumonia caused by *Streptococcus pneumoniae* or *P. aeruginosa*; complicated intra-abdominal infection and empiric therapy of febrile, neutropenic clients 2. Dosage must be reduced with renal impairment.	IV 1–2 g q6–12h IM 0.5–1 g q12h	IM, IV 50 mg/kg q8–12h, not to exceed recommended adult dose

of third-generation cephalosporins. Moreover, cefepime retains activity against strains of Enterobacteriaceae and *P. aeruginosa* that have acquired resistance to third-generation agents.

Applying Your Knowledge 30-1

Why is cefazolin the drug of choice for Ms. Jang's bronchoscopy?

....

Carbapenems

Carbapenems are broad-spectrum, bactericidal beta-lactam antimicrobials. Like other beta-lactam drugs, they inhibit synthesis of bacterial cell walls by binding with penicillin-binding proteins. The group consists of three drugs (Table 30-4).

Imipenem-cilastatin (Primaxin) is given parenterally and distributed in most body fluids. When given alone, the antibiotic imipenem is rapidly broken down by an enzyme (dehydropeptidase) in renal tubules and therefore reaches only low concentrations in the urine. Imipenem is formulated with cilastatin, which inhibits the destruction of imipenem by the enzyme. The addition of cilastatin increases the urinary concentration of imipenem, and reduces the potential renal toxicity of the antibacterial agent. Recommended doses indicate the amount of imipenem; the solution contains an equivalent amount of cilastatin.

The drug is effective in infections caused by a wide range of bacteria, including penicillinase-producing staphylococci, *E. coli*, *Proteus* species, *Enterobacter–Klebsiella–Serratia* species, *P. aeruginosa*, and *Enterococcus faecalis*. Its main use is treatment of infections caused by organisms resistant to other drugs. Adverse effects are similar to those of other beta-lactam antibiotics, including the risk of cross-sensitivity in patients with penicillin hypersensitivity. Central nervous system toxicity, including seizures, has been reported. Seizures are more likely in patients with a seizure disorder or when recommended doses are exceeded; however, they have occurred in other patients as well. To prepare the solution for IM injection, lidocaine, a local anesthetic, is added to decrease pain. This solution is contraindicated in people allergic to this type of local anesthetic or who have severe shock or heart block.

Meropenem (Merrem) has a broad spectrum of antibacterial activity and may be used as a single drug for empiric therapy before causative microorganisms are identified. It is effective against penicillin-susceptible staphylococci and *S. pneumoniae*, most gram-negative aerobes (e.g., *E. coli*, *H. influenzae*, *Klebsiella pneumoniae*, *P. aeruginosa*), and some anaerobes, including *B. fragilis*. It is indicated for use in intra-abdominal infections and bacterial meningitis caused by susceptible organisms. Adverse effects are similar to those of imipenem.

Ertapenem (Invanz) also has a broad spectrum of antibacterial activity, although it is more limited than imipenem and meropenem. It is approved for complicated intra-abdominal, skin and skin structure, acute pelvic, and urinary tract infections. It can be used to treat community-acquired pneu-

Table 30-4	**Drugs at a Glance:** Carbapenems and Monobactams	
	ROUTES AND USUAL DOSAGE RANGES	
Generic/Trade Name	**Adults**	**Children**
Carbapenems		
Ertapenem (Invanz)	IV 1 g once daily over 15–30 min	*3 mo–12 y*: IV, IM 15 mg/kg twice daily (maximum dose 1g/d)
Imipenem-cilastatin (Primaxin)	IV 250–1000 mg q6–8h (maximum dose 4g/d) IM 500–750 mg q12h	*>3 mo*: Non-CNS infections IV 15–25 mg/kg q6h
Meropenem (Merrem)	IV 1.5–6 g/d in divided doses q8h	*≥3 mo*: 60 mg/kg in divided doses q8h (maximum dose 6 g/d)
Monobactam aztreonam (Azactam)	For UTI: IM, IV 0.5–1.0 g q8–12h For moderate systemic infection: IM, IV 1 g q8–12h or IV 2 g q8–12h For meningitis: IV 2 g q6–8h	IM, IV 30 mg/kg q6–8h

UTI, urinary tract infection.

monia caused by penicillin-susceptible *S. pneumoniae.* Unlike imipenem and meropenem, ertapenem does not have in vitro activity against *P. aeruginosa* and Acinetobacter baumannii.

Ertapenem shares the adverse effect profile of the other carbapenems. Lidocaine is also used in preparation of the solution for IM injection to decrease pain with administration, and the same cautions should be used as with imipenem.

Monobactam

Aztreonam (Azactam) (see Table 30-4) is active against gram-negative bacteria, including Enterobacteriaceae and *P. aeruginosa,* and many strains that are resistant to multiple antibiotics. Activity against gram-negative bacteria is similar to that of the aminoglycosides, but the drug does not cause kidney damage or hearing loss. Aztreonam is stable in the presence of beta-lactamase enzymes. Because gram-positive and anaerobic bacteria are resistant to aztreonam, the drug's ability to preserve normal gram-positive and anaerobic flora may be an advantage over other antimicrobial agents.

Indications for use include infections of the urinary tract, skin and skin structures, and lower respiratory tract, as well as intra-abdominal and gynecologic infections and septicemia. Adverse effects are similar to those for penicillin, including possible hypersensitivity reactions.

Nursing Process

General aspects of the nursing process in antimicrobial drug therapy, as described in Chapter 29, apply to the patient receiving penicillins, cephalosporins, aztreonam, and car-

bapenems. In this chapter, only those aspects related specifically to these drugs are included.

Assessment

With penicillins, ask patients if they have ever taken a penicillin and, if so, whether they ever had a skin rash, hives, swelling, or difficulty breathing associated with the drug. With cephalosporins, ask patients if they have ever taken one of the drugs, as far as they know, and whether they ever had a severe reaction to penicillin. Naming a few cephalosporins (e.g., Ceclor, Keflex, Rocephin, Suprax) may help the patient identify previous usage.

Nursing Diagnoses

- Risk for Injury: Hypersensitivity reactions with penicillins or cephalosporins
- Risk for Injury: Renal impairment with cephalosporins
- Deficient Knowledge: Correct home care administration and usage of oral beta-lactams

Planning/Goals

The patient will

- Take oral beta-lactam antibacterials as directed
- Receive parenteral beta-lactam drugs by appropriate techniques to minimize tissue irritation
- Receive prompt and appropriate treatment if hypersensitivity reactions occur

Interventions

- After giving a penicillin parenterally in an outpatient setting, keep the patient in the area for at least 30 minutes.

Anaphylactic reactions are more likely to occur with parenteral than oral use and within a few minutes after injection.

- In any patient care setting, keep emergency equipment and supplies readily available.
- Monitor patient response to beta-lactam drugs.
- Monitor dosages of beta-lactam drugs for patients with impaired renal function.
- Provide patient teaching regarding drug therapy (see accompanying displays).

Evaluation

- Observe for improvement in signs of infection.
- Interview and observe for adverse drug effects.

Principles of Therapy

Goal of Therapy

The goal of antimicrobial therapy is to prevent or treat infections caused by pathogenic microorganisms.

Drug Selection

Choice of a beta-lactam antibacterial depends on the organism causing the infection, severity of the infection, and other factors.

Penicillins

Penicillin G or amoxicillin is the drug of choice in many infections. An antipseudomonal penicillin is indicated in *Pseudo-monas* infections. An antistaphylococcal penicillin is indicated in staphylococcal infections; antistaphylococcal drugs of choice are nafcillin for IV use and dicloxacillin for oral use.

Cephalosporins

First-generation drugs are often used for surgical prophylaxis, especially with prosthetic implants, because gram-positive organisms such as staphylococci cause most infections of surgical sites. They may also be used alone for treatment of infections caused by susceptible organisms in body sites where drug penetration and host defenses are adequate. Cefazolin (Kefzol) is a frequently used parenteral agent. It reaches a higher serum concentration, is more protein bound, and has a slower rate of elimination than other first-generation drugs. These factors prolong serum half-life, so cefazolin can be given less frequently. Cefazolin may also be administered IM.

Second-generation cephalosporins are also often used for surgical prophylaxis, especially for gynecologic and colorectal surgery. They are also used for treatment of intra-abdominal infections such as pelvic inflammatory disease, diverticulitis, penetrating wounds of the abdomen, and other infections caused by organisms inhabiting pelvic and colorectal areas.

Third-generation cephalosporins are recommended for serious infections caused by susceptible organisms that are resistant to first- and second-generation cephalosporins. They are often used in the treatment of infections caused by *E. coli*; *Proteus, Klebsiella*, and *Serratia* species; and other Enterobacteriaceae, especially when the infections occur in body sites not readily reached by other drugs (e.g., CSF, bone) and in patients with immunosuppression. Although effective against many *Pseudomonas* strains, these drugs should not be used alone in treating pseudomonal infections because *drug resistance* (inability to be eradicated by antibiotics) develops.

Patient Teaching Guidelines ▸ Oral Penicillins

General Considerations

- Do not take any penicillin if you have ever had an allergic reaction to penicillin in which you had difficulty breathing, swelling, or skin rash. However, some people call a minor stomach upset an allergic reaction which is incorrect, and are not given penicillin when that is the best antibiotic in a given situation.
- Complete the full course of drug treatment for greater effectiveness and prevention of secondary infection with drug-resistant bacteria.
- Follow instructions carefully about the dose and how often it is taken. Drug effectiveness depends on maintaining adequate blood levels.
- Penicillins often need more frequent administration than some other antibiotics, because they are rapidly excreted by the kidneys.

Self- or Caregiver Administration

- Take most penicillins on an empty stomach, 1 hour before or 2 hours after a meal. Penicillin V, amoxicillin, and Augmentin can be taken with food.

- Take each dose with a full glass of water; do not take with orange juice or with other acidic fluids (they may destroy the drug).
- Take at even intervals, preferably around the clock.
- Shake liquid penicillins well, to mix thoroughly and measure the dose accurately.
- Discard liquid penicillin after 1 week if stored at room temperature or after 2 weeks if refrigerated. Liquid forms deteriorate and should not be taken after their expiration dates.
- Report skin rash, hives, itching, severe diarrhea, shortness of breath, fever, sore throat, black tongue, or any unusual bleeding. These symptoms may indicate an allergy to penicillin.
- Augmentin: Take with meals to increase absorption and decrease gastrointestinal upset.

Patient Teaching Guidelines | Oral Cephalosporins

General Considerations

■ Inform your physician if you have ever had a severe allergic reaction to penicillin in which you had difficulty breathing, swelling, or skin rash. A small number of people are allergic to both penicillins and cephalosporins because the drugs are somewhat similar in their chemical structures.

■ Also inform your physician if you have had a previous allergic reaction to a cephalosporin (e.g., Ceclor, Keflex). If not sure whether a new prescription is a cephalosporin, ask the pharmacist before having the prescription filled.

■ Complete the full course of drug treatment for greater effectiveness and prevention of secondary infection with drug-resistant bacteria.

■ Follow instructions about dosing frequency; effectiveness depends on maintaining adequate blood levels.

Self- or Caregiver Administration

■ Take most oral drugs with food or milk to prevent stomach upset.

■ Take cefpodoxime (Vantin) and cefuroxime (Ceftin) with food to increase absorption.

■ Do not take cefaclor, cefdinir (Omnicef), or cefpodoxime (Vantin) with antacids containing aluminum or magnesium (e.g., Maalox, Mylanta) or with Pepcid, Tagamet, or Zantac. These drugs decrease absorption of these antibiotics and make them less effective. If necessary to take one of the drugs, take it 2 hours before or 2 hours after a dose of these antibiotics.

■ Shake liquid preparations well to mix thoroughly and measure the dose accurately.

■ Report the occurrence of diarrhea, especially if it is severe or contains blood, pus, or mucus. Cephalosporins can cause antibiotic-associated colitis and the drug may need to be stopped.

■ Inform the prescribing physician if you are breast-feeding. These drugs enter breast milk.

Fourth-generation drugs are most useful in serious gram-negative infections, especially infections caused by organisms resistant to third-generation drugs. Cefepime has the same indications for use as ceftazidime, a third-generation drug.

Drug Dosage and Administration

Choice of route and dosage depends mainly on the severity of the infection being treated. For serious infections, beta-lactam antibacterials are usually given IV in large doses. With penicillins, most must be given every 4 to 6 hours to maintain therapeutic blood levels, because the kidneys rapidly excrete them. The oral route is often used for less serious infections and for long-term prophylaxis of rheumatic fever. The IM route is rarely used in hospitalized patients but may be used in ambulatory settings. With cephalosporins, a few are sufficiently absorbed for oral administration; these are most often used in mild infections and UTI. Although some cephalosporins can be given IM, the injections may cause pain and irritation. Cefazolin is preferred for IM administration because it is less irritating to tissues.

Hypersensitivity to Penicillins

Before giving the initial dose of any penicillin preparation, ask the patient if he or she has ever taken penicillin and, if so, whether an allergic reaction occurred. Penicillin is the most common cause of drug-induced anaphylaxis, a life-threatening *hypersensitivity* (allergic) reaction, and a person known to be hypersensitive should be given another type of antibiotic.

In the rare instance in which penicillin is considered essential, a skin test may be helpful in assessing hypersensitivity. The reagents used in the skin test procedure are derivatives of the basic benzylpenicillin molecule. They are introduced into the epidermis by a skin prick or into the dermis by an intradermal injection. An immediate wheal-and-flare reaction confirms immediate hypersensitivity to penicillin. Allergic reactions, including fatal anaphylactic shock, have occurred with skin tests and after negative skin tests. If the scratch test is positive, desensitization may be accomplished by giving gradually increasing doses of penicillin.

Because anaphylactic shock may occur with administration of the penicillins, especially by parenteral routes, emergency drugs and equipment must be readily available. Treatment may require parenteral epinephrine, oxygen, and insertion of an endotracheal or tracheostomy tube if laryngeal edema occurs.

Applying Your Knowledge 30-2

The physician finds signs of infection during Ms. Jang's bronchoscopy and orders the patient to take amoxicillin 500 mg every 8 hours for 10 days, pending the results of the culture and susceptibility studies. Ms. Jang has the prescription filled and starts taking the medication. What should members of the health care team assess before Ms. Jang takes this medication?

Use of Penicillins in Specific Situations

Treatment of Streptococcal Infections

Clinicians should perform culture and susceptibility studies and be aware of local patterns of streptococcal susceptibility or resistance before prescribing penicillins for streptococcal infections. When used, penicillins should be given for the full prescribed course of treatment to prevent complications such as rheumatic fever, endocarditis, and glomerulonephritis.

Use in Combination With Probenecid

Probenecid (Benemid) can be given concurrently with penicillins to increase serum drug levels. Probenecid acts by blocking renal excretion of the penicillins. This action may be useful when high serum levels are needed with oral penicillins or when a single large dose is given IM for prevention or treatment of syphilis.

Use in Combination With Aminoglycosides

Aminoglycosides are often given concomitantly with penicillins for serious infections, such as those caused by *P. aeruginosa*. The drugs should not be admixed in a syringe or in an IV solution, because the penicillin inactivates the aminoglycoside.

Applying Your Knowledge 30-3

Ms. Jang has never before had a reaction to a medication and calls the office to report a skin rash and difficulty breathing. What action should you take?

Use in Special Populations

Perioperative Use of Cephalosporins

Some cephalosporins are used in surgical prophylaxis. The particular drug depends largely on the type of organism likely to be encountered in the operative area. First-generation drugs, mainly cefazolin, are used for procedures associated with gram-positive postoperative infections, such as prosthetic implant surgery. Second-generation cephalosporins (mainly cefotetan and cefoxitin) are often used for abdominal procedures, especially gynecologic and colorectal surgery, in which enteric gram-negative postoperative infections may occur. Third-generation drugs should not be used for surgical prophylaxis because they are less active against staphylococci than cefazolin, the gram-negative organisms they are most useful against are rarely encountered in elective surgery, widespread usage for prophylaxis promotes emergence of drug-resistant organisms, and they are very expensive.

When used perioperatively, cephalosporins should be given within 2 hours before the first skin incision is made so the drug has time to reach therapeutic serum and tissue concentrations. A single dose is usually sufficient, although repeat doses are necessary in patients undergoing a surgical procedure exceeding 4 hours or procedures involving major blood loss. Postoperative doses are rarely necessary but, if used, should generally not exceed 24 hours.

Use in Children

Penicillins and cephalosporins are widely used to treat infections in children and are generally safe. They should be used cautiously in neonates because immature kidney function slows their elimination. Dosages should be based on age, weight, severity of the infection being treated, and renal function. Specialized pediatric dosing references can provide guidance to dosing of most beta-lactams based on the child's age and weight.

Use in Older Adults

Beta-lactam antibacterials are relatively safe, although decreased renal function, other disease processes, and concurrent drug therapies increase the risks of adverse effects in older adults. With penicillins, hyperkalemia may occur with large IV doses of penicillin G potassium and hypernatremia may occur with ticarcillin. Hypernatremia is less likely with other antipseudomonal penicillins such as piperacillin. Cephalosporins may aggravate renal impairment, especially when other nephrotoxic drugs are used concurrently. Dosage of most cephalosporins must be reduced in the presence of renal impairment, depending on creatinine clearance (CrCl).

With aztreonam, imipenem-cilastatin, meropenem, and ertapenem, dose and frequency of administration are determined by renal status as indicated by CrCl.

Use in Patients With Renal Impairment

Beta-lactam antimicrobials are excreted mainly by the kidneys and may accumulate in the presence of renal impairment. Dosage of many beta-lactams must be decreased according to CrCl. In addition, some of the drugs are nephrotoxic. References should be consulted to determine dosages recommended for various levels of CrCl. Additional considerations are included in the following sections.

Penicillins

- Dosage of penicillin G, carbenicillin, piperacillin, piperacillin-tazobactam, and ticarcillin should be reduced.

- Patients on hemodialysis usually require an additional dose after treatment because hemodialysis removes substantial amounts and produces subtherapeutic serum drug levels.

- Carbenicillin, which is used to treat UTI, does not reach therapeutic levels in urine in patients with severe renal impairment (CrCl < 10 mL/minute).

- Nephropathy, such as interstitial nephritis, although infrequent, has occurred with all penicillins. It is most often associated with high doses of parenteral penicillins and is attributed to hypersensitivity reactions. Manifestations include fever, skin rash, eosinophilia, and possibly increased levels of blood urea nitrogen and serum creatinine.

- Electrolyte imbalances, mainly hypernatremia and hyperkalemia, may occur. Hypernatremia is most likely to occur when ticarcillin (5.6 mEq sodium/g) is given to patients with renal impairment or congestive heart failure. Hypokalemic metabolic acidosis may also occur with ticarcillin because potassium loss is enhanced by high sodium intake. Hyperkalemia may occur with large IV doses of penicillin G potassium (1.7 mEq/1 million units).

Cephalosporins

- Reduce dosage because usual doses may produce high and prolonged serum drug levels. In renal failure (CrCl < 20 to 30 mL/minute), dosage of all cephalosporins should be reduced.

- Cefotaxime is converted to active metabolites that are normally eliminated by the kidneys. These metabolites accumulate and may cause toxicity in patients with renal impairment.

Carbapenems

- Dosage of imipenem should be reduced in most patients with renal impairment and the drug is contraindicated in patients with severe renal impairment (CrCl of 5 mL/minute or less) unless hemodialysis is started within 48 hours. For patients already on hemodialysis, the drug may cause seizures and should be used very cautiously, if at all.
- Dosage of meropenem should be reduced with renal impairment (CrCl < 50 mL/minute).
- Dosage of ertapenem should be reduced to 500 milligram daily with renal impairment (CrCl < 30 mL/minute). For patients on hemodialysis, administer the daily dose after dialysis.

Monobactam

- After an initial loading dose, the dosage of aztreonam should be reduced by 50% or more in patients with CrCl of 30 milliliters per minute or less. Give at the usual intervals of 6, 8, or 12 hours.
- For serious or life-threatening infections in patients on hemodialysis, give 12.5% of the initial dose after each hemodialysis session, in addition to maintenance doses.

Use in Patients With Hepatic Impairment

- A few beta-lactam antibiotics may cause or aggravate hepatic impairment.
- Amoxicillin-clavulanate (Augmentin) should be used with caution in patients with hepatic impairment. It is contraindicated in patients who have had cholestatic jaundice and hepatic dysfunction with previous use of the drug. Cholestatic liver impairment usually subsides when the drug is stopped. Hepatotoxicity is attributed to the clavulanate component and has also occurred with ticarcillin-clavulanate (Timentin).
- Aztreonam, imipenem, meropenem, and ertapenem may cause abnormalities in liver function test results (i.e., elevated alanine and aspartate aminotransferases [ALT and AST] and alkaline phosphatase), but hepatitis and jaundice rarely occur.

Use in Patients With Critical Illness

Beta-lactam antimicrobials are commonly used in critical care units to treat pneumonia, bloodstream, wound, and other infections. The beta-lactam drugs are frequently given concomitantly with other antimicrobial drugs because critically ill patients often have multiorganism or nosocomial infections. Renal, hepatic, and other organ functions should be monitored in critically ill patients and drug dosages should be reduced when indicated.

With penicillins, the extended-spectrum drugs (e.g., piperacillin) and penicillin–beta-lactamase inhibitor combinations (e.g., Unasyn) are most likely to be used. With cephalosporins, third- and fourth-generation drugs are commonly used and are usually given by intermittent IV infusions every 8 or 12 hours. Continuous infusions of beta-lactam antibiotics also may be used. Blood levels of cephalosporins and penicillins need to be maintained above the minimum inhibitory concentration (MIC) of the microorganisms causing the infection being treated. Thus, continuous infusions may be of benefit with serious infections, especially those caused by relatively resistant organisms such as *Pseudomonas* or *Acinetobacter*.

Use in Home Care

Many beta-lactam antibiotics are given in the home setting. With oral agents, the role of the home care nurse is mainly to teach accurate administration and observation for therapeutic and adverse effects. With liquid suspensions for children, shaking to re-suspend medication and measuring with a measuring spoon or calibrated device are required for safe dosing. Household spoons should not be used because they vary widely in capacity. General guidelines for IV therapy are discussed in Chapter 29; specific guidelines depend on the drug being given.

 Applying Your Knowledge 30-4

How Can You Avoid This Medication Error?

Ms. Jang recovers from her allergic reaction to the penicillin. Her medical records now indicate that she is allergic to PCN. Her culture reports from the bronchoscopic examination have become available; her infection is caused by an organism sensitive to Zosyn. The on-call physician orders a dose of IV Zosyn. The nurse prepares the dose to be administered and starts the infusion. Ms. Jang experiences anaphylaxis and has to be resuscitated.

Nursing Actions   Beta-Lactam Antibacterials

NURSING ACTIONS	RATIONALE/EXPLANATION
1. Administer accurately 　a. With penicillins: 　　(1) Give most oral penicillins on an empty stomach, approximately 1 hour before or 2 hours after a meal. Penicillin V, amoxicillin, and amoxicillin/clavulanate may be given with food.	To decrease binding to foods and inactivation by gastric acid. The latter three drugs are not significantly affected by food.

NURSING ACTIONS	RATIONALE/EXPLANATION
(2) Give oral drugs with a full glass of water, preferably.	To promote absorption and decrease inactivation, which may occur in an acidic environment
(3) Give intramuscular (IM) penicillins deeply into a large muscle mass.	To decrease tissue irritation
(4) For intravenous (IV) administration, usually dilute reconstituted penicillins in 50–100 milliliters of 5% dextrose or 0.9% sodium chloride injection and infuse over 30–60 minutes.	To minimize vascular irritation and phlebitis
(5) Give reconstituted ampicillin IV or IM within 1 hour.	The drug is stable in solution for a limited time, after which effectiveness is lost.
b. With cephalosporins: (1) Give most oral drugs with food or milk. Cefpodoxime and cefuroxime should be taken with food. Chilling cefpodoxime improves flavor.	To decrease nausea and vomiting. Food delays absorption but does not affect the amount of drug absorbed. An exception is the pediatric suspension of ceftibuten, which must be given at least 1 hour before or 2 hours after a meal. Food increases the absorption of cefpodoxime and cefuroxime.
(2) Give IM drugs deeply into a large muscle mass.	The drugs are irritating to tissues and cause pain, induration, and possibly sterile abscess. The IM route is rarely used.
(3) For IV administration, usually dilute reconstituted drugs in 50–100 milliliters of 5% dextrose or 0.9% sodium chloride injection and infuse over 30 minutes.	These drugs are irritating to veins and cause thrombophlebitis. This can be minimized by using small IV catheters, large veins, adequate dilution, and slow infusion rates, and by changing venipuncture sites. Thrombophlebitis is more likely to occur with doses of more than 6 g/day for longer than 3 days.
c. With carbapenems: (1) For IV imipenem, mix reconstituted solution in 100 milliliters of 0.9% NaCl or 5% dextrose injection. Give 250- to 500-mg doses over 20–30 minutes; give 750-mg to 1-g doses over 40–60 minutes.	Manufacturer's recommendations
(2) For IM imipenem and ertapenem, mix with 1% lidocaine without epinephrine and inject deeply into a large muscle mass with a 21-gauge, 2-inch needle.	To decrease pain of injection
(3) For IV meropenem, give as an injection over 3–5 minutes or as an infusion over 15–30 minutes.	
(4) For IV ertapenem, mix in 50 milliliters of 0.9% sodium chloride and infuse over 30 minutes.	Manufacturer's recommendations
d. With aztreonam: (1) For IM administration, add 3 milliliters diluent per gram of drug, and inject into a large muscle mass.	
(2) For IV injection, add 6–10 milliliters sterile water, and inject into vein or IV tubing over 3–6 minutes.	
(3) For IV infusion, mix in at least 50 milliliters of 0.9% NaCl or 5% dextrose injection per gram of drug and give over 20–60 minutes.	
2. Observe for therapeutic effects a. Decreased signs of local and systemic infection b. Decreased signs and symptoms of the infection for which the drug is given c. Absence of signs and symptoms of infection when given prophylactically	See Chapter 29.
3. Observe for adverse effects a. Hypersensitivity—anaphylaxis, serum sickness, skin rash, urticaria	See Nursing Actions in Chapter 29 for signs and symptoms. Reactions are more likely to occur in those with previous hypersensitivity reactions and those with a history of allergy, asthma, or hay fever. Anaphylaxis is more likely with parenteral administration and may occur within 5–30 minutes of injection.
b. Phlebitis at IV sites and pain at IM sites	Parenteral solutions are irritating to body tissue.
c. Superinfection	See Chapter 29 for signs and symptoms.
d. Nausea and vomiting	May occur with all beta-lactam drugs, especially with high oral doses

(continued on page 500)

Nursing Actions   Beta-Lactam Antibacterials (continued)

NURSING ACTIONS	RATIONALE/EXPLANATION
e. Diarrhea, colitis, pseudomembranous colitis	Diarrhea commonly occurs with beta-lactam drugs and may range from mild to severe. The most severe form is pseudomembranous colitis, which is more often associated with ampicillin and the cephalosporins than other beta-lactams.
f. Nephrotoxicity (1) Acute interstitial nephritis (AIN)—hematuria, oliguria, proteinuria, pyuria	AIN may occur with any of the beta-lactams, especially with high parenteral doses of penicillins.
(2) Increased blood urea nitrogen and serum creatinine; casts in urine	More likely with cephalosporins, especially in patients who are older or who have impaired renal function, unless dosage is reduced
g. Neurotoxicity—confusion, hallucinations, neuromuscular irritability, convulsive seizures	More likely with large IV doses of penicillins, cephalosporins, or carbapenems, especially in patients with impaired renal function
h. Coagulation disorders and bleeding from hypoprothrombinemia or platelet dysfunction	Ticarcillin may cause decreased platelet aggregation. Cefoperazone and cefotetan may cause hypoprothrombinemia (by killing intestinal bacteria that normally produce vitamin K or a chemical structure that prevents activation of prothrombin) or platelet dysfunction. Bleeding can be treated by giving vitamin K. Vitamin K does not restore normal platelet function or normal bacterial flora in the intestines.
4. Observe for drug interactions a. Drugs that *increase* effects of penicillins: (1) Gentamicin and other aminoglycosides	Synergistic activity against *Pseudomonas* organisms when given concomitantly with extended-spectrum (antipseudomonal) penicillins Synergistic activity against enterococci that cause subacute bacterial endocarditis, brain abscess, meningitis, or urinary tract infection Synergistic activity against *Staphylococcus* aureus when used with nafcillin
(2) Probenecid (Benemid)	Decreases renal excretion of penicillins, thus elevating and prolonging penicillin blood levels
b. Drugs that *decrease* effects of penicillins: (1) Acidifying agents (ascorbic acid, cranberry juice, orange juice)	Most oral penicillins are destroyed by acids, including gastric acid. Amoxicillin and penicillin V are acid stable.
(2) Erythromycin	Erythromycin inhibits the bactericidal activity of penicillins against most organisms but potentiates activity against resistant strains of S. *aureus*.
(3) Tetracycline	These bacteriostatic antibiotics slow multiplication of bacteria and thereby inhibit the penicillins, which act against rapidly multiplying bacteria.
(4) Aminoglycosides, if admixed	The penicillin will inactivate the aminoglycoside.
c. Drugs that *increase* effects of cephalosporins: (1) Loop diuretics (furosemide, ethacrynic acid)	Increased renal toxicity
(2) Probenecid	Increases blood levels by decreasing renal excretion of the cephalosporins. This may be a desirable interaction to increase blood levels and therapeutic effectiveness or allow smaller doses.
d. Drugs that *decrease* effects of cephalosporins: (1) Antacids containing aluminum or magnesium (e.g., Mylanta) and histamine H$_2$ antagonists (e.g., cimetidine, ranitidine)	These drugs decrease absorption of cefaclor, cefdinir, and cefpodoxime. Give the drugs at least 2 hours apart.
e. Drugs that *increase* effects of carbapenems: (1) Probenecid	Probenecid minimally increases serum drug levels of carbapenems, but it is not recommended for concomitant use with any of the drugs.
(2) Cyclosporine	May increase central nervous system adverse effects of imipenem
f. Drugs that *alter* effects of aztreonam	Few documented, clinically significant interactions reported, but potential interactions are those that occur with other beta-lactam antibiotics.

Key Concepts

▪ Beta-lactam antibiotics include penicillins, cephalosporins, carbapenems, and monobactams.

▪ Choice of a beta-lactam antibacterial depends on the organism causing the infection, severity of the infection, and other factors.

▪ As a class, penicillins usually are more effective in infections caused by gram-positive bacteria than those caused by gram-negative bacteria.

▪ In the rare instance in which penicillin is considered essential, a skin test may be helpful in assessing hypersensitivity.

▪ Metabolic and electrolyte imbalances may occur in patients receiving penicillins who have renal impairment or congestive heart failure: hypernatremia and hypokalemic metabolic acidosis is most likely to occur when ticarcillin and hyperkalemia with large IV doses of penicillin G potassium.

▪ Probenecid (Benemid) blocks renal excretion of the penicillins and can be given concurrently with penicillins to increase serum drug levels.

Review and Application Exercises

Short Answer Exercises

1. How do beta-lactam drugs act against bacteria?

2. What adverse effects are associated with beta-lactam drugs, and how may they be prevented or minimized?

3. What are beta-lactamase enzymes, and what do they do to beta-lactam antibacterial drugs?

4. How are penicillins and other beta-lactam drugs excreted?

5. What are the main differences between penicillin G or V and antistaphylococcal and antipseudomonal penicillins?

6. What is the reason for combining clavulanate, sulbactam, or tazobactam with a penicillin?

7. When giving injections of penicillin in an outpatient setting, it is recommended to keep patients in the area and observe them for at least 30 minutes. Why?

8. When probenecid is given concurrently with a penicillin, what is its purpose?

9. What are the signs and symptoms of anaphylaxis?

10. For patients with renal impairment, which drugs in this chapter require reduced dosage?

11. Which drugs in this chapter may cause pseudomembranous (antibiotic-associated) colitis?

12. What are the signs, symptoms, and treatment of pseudomembranous colitis?

NCLEX-Style Questions

13. A nurse is preparing to administer the first dose of piperacillin-tazobactam (Zosyn) to a patient in an infusion clinic. The nurse should take which of the following precautions?
    a. Ask the patient about past allergic reactions to penicillins.
    b. Ask the patient about past allergic reactions to aminoglycosides.
    c. Mix the piperacillin-tazobactam with lidocaine to reduce pain of infusion.
    d. Instruct the patient to eat a snack to decrease stomach upset from piperacillin-tazobactam.

14. A woman is to receive Augmentin 500 mg PO q8h for bronchitis. The nurse retrieves two 250-mg tablets from the medication cart. This is incorrect for which of the following reasons?
    a. The amount of sulbactam in Augmentin 250 mg is 62.5 mg per tablet, twice the intended amount.
    b. This will provide twice the intended dose of clavulanate.
    c. The 250-mg tablets have less absorption than the 500-mg tablets.
    d. Augmentin can only be given IV, so giving tablets means that the wrong drug is being administered.

15. A nurse working in the neurointensive care unit is caring for a head-injury victim who has been experiencing seizures and now has *P. aeruginosa* pneumonia. The physician has prescribed imipenem 1 g IV q6h plus gentamicin for the pneumonia. Before administering the antibiotics, the nurse should do which of the following?

   a. Not admix the imipenem and gentamicin in the same IV bag to prevent inactivation of the gentamicin.

   b. Remind the physician of the patient's seizures and inquire whether a different antibiotic might be safer.

   c. Suggest to the physician that imipenem is used to treat gram-positive infections and will not be effective in this patient.

   d. Set the infusion pump to deliver the imipenem over 15 minutes.

16. In acute renal failure, doses of all of the following antibiotics must be reduced except

   a. nafcillin

   b. cefazolin

   c. meropenem

   d. aztreonam

17. Which of the following classes of cephalosporins has the best activity against gram-positive organisms?

   a. first-generation cephalosporins

   b. second-generation cephalosporins

   c. third-generation cephalosporins

   d. fourth-generation cephalosporins

Selected References

Antunez, C. (2006). Immediate allergic reactions to cephalosporins: Evaluation of cross-reactivity with a panel of penicillins and cephalosporins. *Journal of Allergy and Clinical Immunology, 117*(2), 404–410.

Corwin, E. J. (2006). *Handbook of pathophysiology* (3rd ed.). Philadelphia: Lippincott Williams & Wilkins.

Cunha, B. A. (2006). Antibiotic selection in the penicillin-resistant patient. *Medical Clinics of North America, 90*(6), 1257–1264.

Drug facts and comparisons. (Updated monthly). St. Louis, MO: Facts and Comparisons.

Elston, D. M. (2007). Methicillin-sensitive and methicillin-resistant *Staphylococcus aureus*: Management principles and selection of antibiotic therapy. *Dermatology Clinics, 25*(2), 157–164, vi.

Guyton, A. C., & Hall, J. E. (2006). *Textbook of medical physiology* (11th ed.). Philadelphia: W. B. Saunders.

Khardori, N. (2006). Antibiotics- past, present, and future. *Medical Clinics of North America, 90*(6), 1049–1076.

Lacy, C. F., Armstrong, L. L., Goldman, M. P., & Lance, L. L. (2007). *Lexi-Comp's drug information handbook* (15th ed.). Hudson, OH: American Pharmaceutical Association.

Pichichero, M. E. (2005). A review of evidence supporting the American Academy of Pediatrics recommendation for prescribing cephalosporin antibiotics for penicillin-allergic patients. *Pediatrics, 115,* 1048–1057.

Shoemaker, D. M., Jiang, P.P., Williamson, H., & Roland, W. E. (2007). Infectious diseases. In R. E. Rakel (Ed.), *Textbook of family medicine* (pp. 317–351), Philadelphia: Elsevier.

Aminoglycosides and Fluoroquinolones

LEARNING OBJECTIVES

After studying this chapter, you will be able to:

1. Identify characteristics of aminoglycosides and fluoroquinolones in relation to effectiveness, safety, spectrum of antimicrobial activity, indications for use, administration, and observation of patient responses.
2. Recognize factors influencing selection and dosage of aminoglycosides and fluoroquinolones.
3. State the rationale for the increasing use of single daily doses of aminoglycosides.
4. Discuss the importance of measuring serum drug levels during aminoglycoside therapy.
5. Describe measures to decrease nephrotoxicity and ototoxicity with aminoglycosides.
6. Describe characteristics, uses, adverse effects, and nursing process implications of fluoroquinolones.
7. Discuss principles of using aminoglycosides and fluoroquinolones in renal impairment and critical illness.

Applying Your Knowledge

Roger Dallas is an 84-year-old man who has been prescribed ciprofloxacin (Cipro) 500 mg PO every 12 hours to treat an infected leg wound. He has experienced arterial insufficiency to his lower extremities for many years, secondary to atherosclerosis. The medical plan is to clear the infection so that Mr. Dallas can have surgery to restore circulation to his lower extremities.

Introduction

The aminoglycosides have been widely used to treat serious gram-negative infections for many years. The quinolones are also older drugs originally used only for treatment of urinary tract infections (see Chap. 32). The fluoroquinolones are synthesized by adding a fluorine molecule to the quinolone structure. This addition increases drug activity against gram-negative microorganisms, broadens the antimicrobial spectrum to include several other microorganisms, and allows use of the drugs in treating systemic infections. General characteristics, mechanisms of action, indications for and contraindications to use, nursing process implications, and principles of therapy for these drugs are described in this chapter. Individual drugs, with routes of administration and dosage ranges, are listed in the Drugs at a Glance tables.

Aminoglycosides

Aminoglycosides (Table 31-1) are bactericidal agents with similar pharmacologic, antimicrobial, and toxicologic characteristics. They are used to treat infections caused by gram-negative microorganisms such as *Pseudomonas* and *Proteus* species, *Escherichia coli*, and *Klebsiella*, *Enterobacter*, and *Serratia* species.

These drugs are poorly absorbed from the gastrointestinal (GI) tract. Thus, when given orally, they exert local effects in the GI tract. They are well absorbed from intramuscular

Table 31-1	Drugs at a Glance: Aminoglycosides		

		ROUTES AND DOSAGE RANGES	
Generic/Trade Name	**Characteristics**	**Adults**	**Children**
Amikacin (Amikin)	Retains a broader spectrum of antibacterial activity than other aminoglycosides because it resists degradation by most enzymes that inactivate gentamicin and tobramycin Major clinical use is in infections caused by organisms resistant to other aminoglycosides (e.g., *Pseudomonas, Proteus, Escherichia coli, Klebsiella, Enterobacter, Serratia*), whether community or hospital acquired.	IM, IV 15–20 mg/kg q24h. Renal dosing: 5–7.5 mg/kg/d q8–24h	*Older children:* Same as adults *Neonates:* IM, IV 10 mg/kg initially, then 7.5 mg/kg q12h
Gentamicin (Garamycin)	Effective against several gram-negative organisms, although some strains have become resistant Acts synergistically with antipseudomonal penicillins against *Pseudomonas aeruginosa* and with ampicillin or vancomycin against enterococci	Conventional dosing IM, IV 1–2.5 mg/kg q8–24h depending on renal function. ODA dosing: 4–7 mg/kg/dose once daily	<5y: IM, IV 2.5 mg/kg q8h ≥5y: IM, IV 2–2.5 mg/kg q8h
Kanamycin (Kantrex)	Occasionally used to decrease bowel organisms before surgery, treat hepatic coma, or treat multidrug-resistant tuberculosis	IV, IM 15 mg/kg/d, in divided doses q8–12h	IV, IM same as adults
Neomycin	Given orally or topically to prepare GI tract for surgery Although poorly absorbed from GI tract, toxic levels may accumulate in presence of renal failure. Used topically, often in combination with other drugs, to treat infections of the eye, ear, and skin (burns, wounds, ulcers, dermatoses) When used for wound or bladder irrigations, systemic absorption may occur if the area is large or if drug concentration exceeds 0.1%.	PO, suppression of intestinal bacteria (with erythromycin 1 g) 1 g at 19, 18, and 9 h before surgery (3 doses); hepatic coma, 4–12 g daily in divided doses q4–6h for 5–6 d	
Streptomycin	May be used in a 4- to 6-drug regimen for treatment of multidrug-resistant tuberculosis	IM 15–30 mg/kg/d or 1–2g/d.	IM 20–40 mg/kg/d in 2 divided doses, q12h (maximum dose, 1 g/d)
Tobramycin	Similar to gentamicin in antibacterial spectrum, but may be more active against *Pseudomonas* organisms Often used with other antibiotics for septicemia and infections of burn wounds, other soft tissues, bone, the urinary tract, and the central nervous system	Conventional dosing: IM, IV 1–2.5 mg/kg q8–24h depending on renal function. ODA dosing: 4–7 mg/kg/dose once daily.	*under 5y:* IM, IV 2.5 mg/kg/dose q8h *5y or older:* 2–2.5 mg/kg/dose q8h

GI, gastrointestinal; ODA, once daily aminoglycoside.

injection sites and reach peak effects in 30 to 90 minutes if circulatory status is good. After intravenous (IV) administration, peak effects occur within 30 to 60 minutes. Plasma half-life is 2 to 4 hours with normal renal function.

After parenteral administration, aminoglycosides are widely distributed in extracellular fluid and reach therapeutic levels in blood, urine, bone, inflamed joints, and pleural and ascitic fluids. They accumulate in high concentrations in the proximal renal tubules of the kidney, leading to acute tubular necrosis. This damage to the kidney is termed *nephrotoxicity*. They also accumulate in high concentrations in the inner ear, damaging sensory cells in the cochlea (disrupting hearing) and the vestibular apparatus (disturbing balance). This damage to the inner ear is termed *ototoxicity*. They are poorly distributed to the central nervous system, intraocular fluids, and respiratory tract secretions.

Injected drugs are not metabolized; they are excreted unchanged in the urine, primarily by glomerular filtration. Oral drugs are excreted in feces.

Mechanism of Action

Aminoglycosides penetrate the cell walls of susceptible bacteria and bind irreversibly to 30S ribosomes, intracellular structures that synthesize proteins. As a result, the bacteria cannot synthesize the proteins necessary for their function and replication.

Indications for Use

The major clinical use of parenteral aminoglycosides is to treat serious systemic infections caused by susceptible aerobic gram-negative organisms. Many hospital-acquired infections are caused by gram-positive cocci and gram-negative organisms. These infections have become more common with control of other types of infections, widespread use of antimicrobial drugs, and diseases (e.g., acquired immunodeficiency syndrome [AIDS]) or treatments (e.g., radical surgery, therapy with antineoplastic or immunosuppressive drugs) that lower host resistance. Although they can occur anywhere, infections due to gram-negative organisms commonly involve the respiratory and genitourinary tracts, skin, wounds, bowel, and bloodstream. Any infection with gram-negative organisms may be serious and potentially life threatening. Management is difficult because the organisms are in general less susceptible to antibacterial drugs, and drug-resistant strains develop rapidly. In pseudomonal infections, an aminoglycoside is often given concurrently with an antipseudomonal penicillin (e.g., piperacillin) for synergistic therapeutic effects. The penicillin-induced breakdown of the bacterial cell wall makes it easier for the aminoglycoside to reach its site of action inside the bacterial cell. Decreased mortality has been demonstrated from combination antibiotic therapy in treatment of infections due to *Pseudomonas aeruginosa* and other multidrug-resistant gram-negative bacilli. However, routine use of combination antibiotic therapy containing an aminoglycoside has not been associated with decreased mortality in other gram-negative infections.

A second clinical use is for treatment of tuberculosis. Streptomycin may be used as part of a four- to six-drug regimen for treatment of multidrug-resistant tuberculosis (MDR-TR). However, it is considered a second-line agent because of increasing resistance and should only be used after susceptibility results confirm its usefulness. For patients who develop drug-induced hepatitis in response to first-line drugs, streptomycin or another second-line drug may be substituted until the hepatitis resolves or the causative antitubercular agent is identified.

A third clinical use is for synergistic action when combined with ampicillin, penicillin G, or vancomycin in the treatment of enterococcal and *Staphylococcus epidermidis* infections. Regimens for these infections, particularly meningitis or endocarditis, should include gentamicin in divided doses rather than once-daily dosing. Some strains are resistant to gentamicin, however, and microbiology results should be reviewed for each patient.

A final clinical use is oral administration to suppress intestinal bacteria. Neomycin and kanamycin may be given before bowel surgery and to treat hepatic coma. In hepatic coma, intestinal bacteria produce ammonia, which enters the bloodstream and causes encephalopathy. Drug therapy to suppress intestinal bacteria decreases ammonia production.

A few aminoglycosides are administered topically to the eye or to the skin. These are discussed in Chapters 63 and 64, respectively.

Contraindications to Use

Hypersensitivity to the aminoglycosides is a contraindication. Aminoglycosides are generally reserved for infections that have not responded to less toxic drugs. A **BLACK BOX WARNING** alerts health care professionals that these drugs are nephrotoxic and ototoxic and must be used very cautiously in the presence of renal impairment. Dosages are adjusted according to serum drug levels and creatinine clearance. The drugs must also be used cautiously in patients with myasthenia gravis and other neuromuscular disorders because muscle weakness may be increased.

Fluoroquinolones

Fluoroquinolones are synthetic bactericidal drugs with activity against gram-negative and gram-positive organisms. They may allow oral, ambulatory treatment of infections that previously required parenteral therapy and hospitalization. Most fluoroquinolones are given orally, after which they are well absorbed, achieve therapeutic concentrations in most body fluids, and are metabolized to some extent in the liver. The kidneys are the main route of elimination, with approximately 30% to 60% of an oral dose excreted unchanged in the urine. Dosage should be reduced in renal impairment.

Mechanism of Action

The drugs act by interfering with topoisomerase II (DNA gyrase) and topoisomerase IV, enzymes that are required for

Table 31-2	Drugs at a Glance: Fluoroquinolones	
GENERIC/TRADE NAME	**CHARACTERISTICS**	**ROUTES AND DOSAGE RANGES**
Ciprofloxacin (Cipro)	1. Effective in respiratory, urinary tract, gastrointestinal tract, and skin and soft-tissue infections as well as sexually transmitted diseases caused by chlamydiae and *Neisseria gonorrhoeae* organisms 2. Used as one of 4 to 6 drugs in treatment of multidrug-resistant tuberculosis 3. Used to treat anthrax infections	PO 250–750 mg q12h UTI/pyelonephritis; extended-release tablets 500 mg–1 g q24h IV 200–400 mg q12h
Gatifloxacin (Tequin)	Indicated for pneumonia, bronchitis, sinusitis, skin and soft tissue infections, urinary infections, pyelonephritis, and gonorrhea	PO, IV infusion 400 mg once daily. Give IV dose over 60 min; avoid rapid administration.
Gemifloxacin (Factive)	Indicated for acute bacterial exacerbation of chronic bronchitis and community-acquired pneumonia (mild to moderate severity)	PO 320 mg once daily for 5–7 d
Levofloxacin (Levaquin)	A broad-spectrum agent effective for treatment of bronchitis, cystitis, pneumonia, sinusitis, skin and skin-structure infections, and pyelonephritis	PO, IV 250–750 mg once daily. Infuse 250–500 mg IV dose slowly over 60 min. Infuse 750 mg IV dose over 90 min.
Moxifloxacin (Avelox)	Indicated for community-acquired pneumonia, sinusitis, bronchitis, skin and soft-tissue infections	PO, IV 400 mg once daily. Infuse IV dose slowly over 60 min.
Norfloxacin (Noroxin)	Used only for UTI	PO 400 mg twice daily
Ofloxacin (Floxin)	See ciprofloxacin, above	PO 200–400 mg q12h for 3–10 d Gonorrhea, PO 400 mg as a single dose

UTI, urinary tract infection.

synthesis of bacterial DNA and therefore are required for bacterial growth and replication.

Indications for Use

Fluoroquinolones are indicated for various infections caused by aerobic gram-negative and other microorganisms. Thus, they may be used to treat infections of the respiratory, genitourinary, and GI tracts as well as infections of bones, joints, skin, and soft tissues. Currently, the Centers for Disease Control and Prevention no longer recommends the use of fluoroquinolones for gonococcal disease, unless no other option exists and susceptibility can be confirmed. Because recommendations for treatment of gonorrhea change as resistance becomes more prevalent, consult www.cdc.gov/std for the most current recommendations.

Fluoroquinolones, specifically ciprofloxacin, are currently recommended as the first-line treatment for suspected *Bacillus anthracis* infections (anthrax) until culture and susceptibility results are available. Additional uses include treatment of MDR-TR (see Chap. 34), *Mycobacterium avium* complex

(MAC) infections in patients with acquired immune deficiency syndrome (AIDS; see Chap. 34), and fever in neutropenic cancer patients. Indications vary with individual drugs and are listed in Table 31-2.

Contraindications to Use

Fluoroquinolones are contraindicated in patients who have experienced a hypersensitivity reaction and in children younger than 18 years of age, if other alternatives are available. Limited data are available on the safety of fluoroquinolones in pregnant or lactating women; the drugs should not be used unless the benefits outweigh the potential risks.

Applying Your Knowledge 31-1

Mr. Dallas tells you that he is experiencing a moderate amount of indigestion and asks what he should use to treat it. What is the best response, taking into consideration Mr. Dallas's use of Cipro?

Nursing Process

General aspects of the nursing process as described in Chapter 29 apply to the patient receiving aminoglycosides and fluoroquinolones. In this chapter, only those aspects related specifically to these drugs are included.

Assessment

With aminoglycosides, assess for the presence of factors that predispose to nephrotoxicity or ototoxicity.

- Check laboratory reports of renal function (e.g., serum creatinine, creatinine clearance, blood urea nitrogen [BUN]) for abnormal values.
- Assess for impairment of balance or hearing, including audiometry reports if available.
- Analyze current medications for drugs that interact with aminoglycosides to increase risks of nephrotoxicity or ototoxicity.
- With fluoroquinolones, assess for the presence of factors that increase risks of adverse drug effects (e.g., impaired renal function, inadequate fluid intake, concomitant use of multivitamins or antacids, frequent or prolonged exposure to sunlight in usual activities of daily living).
- Assess laboratory tests (e.g., complete blood counts, tests of renal and hepatic function) for abnormal values.

Planning/Goals

The patient will

- Receive aminoglycoside dosages that are individualized by age, weight, renal function, and serum drug levels
- Have serum aminoglycoside levels monitored when indicated
- Have renal function tests performed regularly during aminoglycoside and fluoroquinolone therapy
- Be well hydrated during aminoglycoside and fluoroquinolone therapy
- Be observed regularly for adverse drug effects

Interventions

- With aminoglycosides, weigh patients accurately (dosage is based on ideal body weight) and monitor laboratory reports of BUN, serum creatinine levels, serum drug levels, and urinalysis for abnormal values.
- Force fluids to at least 2000 to 3000 mL daily if not contraindicated. Keeping the patient well hydrated reduces risks of nephrotoxicity with aminoglycosides and crystalluria with fluoroquinolones.
- Avoid concurrent use of other nephrotoxic drugs when possible.
- Provide appropriate teaching (see accompanying Patient Teaching Guidelines).

Evaluation

- Interview and observe for improvement in the infection being treated.
- Interview and observe for adverse drug effects.

Principles of Therapy

Drug Selection

The choice of aminoglycoside depends on local susceptibility patterns and specific organisms causing an infection. Gentamicin is often given for systemic infections if resistant microorganisms have not developed in the clinical setting. If gentamicin-resistant organisms have developed, amikacin or tobramycin may be given because they are usually less susceptible to drug-destroying enzymes. In terms of toxicity, the aminoglycosides cause similar effects.

The choice of fluoroquinolone is also determined by local susceptibility patterns and specific organisms because individual drugs differ somewhat in their antimicrobial spectra. The drugs cause similar adverse effects.

Drug Dosage: Aminoglycosides

Dosage of aminoglycosides must be carefully monitored based on serum concentrations. Two major dosing schedules are used: one involving multiple daily doses (conventional dosing) and one involving a single daily dose (once-daily aminoglycosides [ODA]). Single-dose regimen has gained favor over the traditional multiple-dose regimen, which takes advantage of the pharmacodynamic properties of aminoglycosides. These two regimens are described in the following sections. Multiple-dose regimens of aminoglycosides must be carefully monitored with evaluation of *peak serum drug levels* and *trough serum drug levels*. Once-daily regimens are monitored with random level (12-hour) serum evaluation.

Multiple Daily Dosing

An *initial loading dose*, based on patient weight and the desired peak serum concentration, is given to achieve therapeutic serum concentrations rapidly. If the patient is obese, lean or ideal body weight should be used because aminoglycosides are not significantly distributed in body fat. In patients with normal renal function, the recommended loading dose for gentamicin and tobramycin is 1 to 2.5 milligrams per kilogram of body weight; for amikacin the loading dose is 5 to 7.5 milligrams per kilogram.

Maintenance doses are based on serum drug concentrations. Peak serum concentrations should be assessed 30 to 60 minutes after drug administration (5–8 mcg/mL for gentamicin and tobramycin, 20–30 mcg/mL for amikacin). Measurement of both peak and trough levels helps to maintain therapeutic serum levels without excessive toxicity. For gentamicin and tobramycin, peak levels above 10 to 12 micrograms per milli-

Patient Teaching Guidelines | Oral Fluoroquinolones

General Considerations

- Avoid exposure to sunlight during and for several days after taking one of these drugs. Stop taking the drug and notify the prescribing physician if skin burning, redness, swelling, rash, or itching occurs. Sunscreen lotions do not prevent photosensitivity reactions.

- Be very careful if driving or doing other tasks requiring alertness or physical coordination. These drugs may cause dizziness or lightheadedness.

Self-Administration

- Take norfloxacin (Noroxin) levofloxacin solution and ofloxacin (Floxin) 1 hour before or 2 hours after meals on an

empty stomach. Ciprofloxacin (Cipro) may be taken with food to decrease GI upset. Gatifloxacin (Teguin), gemifloxacin (Factive), levofloxacin tabs, and moxifloxacin (Avelox) can be taken with or without regard to meals.

- Drink 2 to 3 quarts of fluid daily if able. This helps to prevent kidney problems.

- Do not take antacids containing magnesium or aluminum (e.g., Mylanta or Maalox); any products containing iron, magnesium, calcium (e.g., Tums), or zinc (e.g., multivitamins); sucralfate, or buffered didanosine preparations at the same time, or for several hours before or after a dose of the fluoroquinolone. (Consult product-specific information for individual drug recommendations.)

---

liter and trough levels above 2 micrograms per milliliter for prolonged periods have been associated with nephrotoxicity. For accuracy, blood samples must be drawn at the correct times and the timing of drug administration and blood sampling must be accurately documented and based on institutional recommendations.

With impaired renal function, dosage of aminoglycosides must be reduced. Methods of adjusting dosage include lengthening the time between doses or reducing doses. References should be consulted for specific recommendations on adjusting aminoglycoside doses for renal impairment. In urinary tract infections, smaller doses can be used than in systemic infections because the aminoglycosides reach high concentrations in the urine.

Single Daily Dosing

The use of once-daily aminoglycoside (ODA) dosing has replaced the common multiple daily dosing in many individuals unless contraindicated. This dosing method uses high doses (e.g., gentamicin, 4 to 7 mg/kg) to produce high initial drug concentrations, but a repeat dose is not administered until the serum concentration is quite low. The rationale for this dosing approach is a potential increase in efficacy with a reduced incidence of nephrotoxicity. Most patients can be successfully treated with one daily dose using this approach. However, certain populations are not appropriate due to age, renal function, and special situations. In general, the following circumstances contraindicate the use of a *single daily dosing* regimen: individuals aged 18 years of age or less, those pregnant or in the postpartum period, and those with endocarditis.

This practice evolved from increased knowledge about the concentration-dependent bactericidal effects and postantibiotic effects of aminoglycosides. *Concentration-dependent bactericidal effects* mean that the drugs kill more microorganisms with a large dose and high peak serum concentrations. *Postantibiotic effects* mean that aminoglycosides continue killing microorganisms even with low serum concentrations. These characteristics allow administration of high doses to achieve high peak serum concentrations and optimal killing of microorganisms. The

longer interval until the next dose allows the patient to eliminate the drug to very low serum concentrations for approximately 6 hours. During this low-drug period, the postantibiotic effect is active while there is minimal drug accumulation in body tissues. Monitoring of random level (12-hour) serum evaluation in a single dosing regimen replaces traditional peak and trough serum monitoring. Reported advantages of this regimen include increased bactericidal effects, less nephrotoxicity, reduced need for serum drug concentration data, and reduced nursing time for administration.

Guidelines for Reducing Toxicity of Aminoglycosides

In addition to the preceding recommendations, guidelines to decrease the incidence and severity of adverse effects include the following:

- Identify patients at high risk for adverse effects (e.g., neonates, older adults, patients with renal impairment, patients with disease processes or drug therapies that impair blood circulation and renal function).

- Keep patients well hydrated to decrease drug concentration in serum and body tissues. The drugs reach higher concentrations in the kidneys and inner ears than in other body tissues resulting in nephrotoxicity and ototoxicity. The goal of an adequate fluid intake is to decrease the incidence and severity of these adverse effects.

- Use caution with concurrent administration of diuretics. Diuretics may increase the risk of nephrotoxicity by decreasing fluid volume, thereby increasing drug concentration in serum and tissues. Dehydration is most likely to occur with loop diuretics such as furosemide.

- Give the drug for no longer than 10 days unless necessary for treatment of certain infections. Patients are most at risk when high doses are given for prolonged periods.

- Detect adverse effects early and reduce dosage or discontinue the drug. Changes in renal function tests that indicate nephrotoxicity may not occur until the patient has received an aminoglycoside for several days. If nephrotoxicity occurs, it is usually reversible if the drug is stopped. Early ototoxicity is detectable only with audiometry and is generally not reversible.

Mr. Dallas's wound is not responding to treatment. Due to his need for surgery, he is hospitalized for IV antibiotic therapy. His physician orders gentamicin IV once every 24 hours, to be dosed by the pharmacist. The medication is dosed and Mr. Dallas receives doses for 3 days. What assessments should you perform to observe for toxicity?

Drug Dosage: Fluoroquinolones

Recommended dosages of fluoroquinolones should not be exceeded in any patients, and dosages should be reduced in the presence of renal impairment.

Use in Special Populations

Use in Children

Aminoglycosides must be used cautiously in children as with adults. Dosage must be accurately calculated according to weight and renal function. Serum drug concentrations must be monitored and dosage adjusted as indicated to avoid toxicity. Neonates may have increased risk of nephrotoxicity and ototoxicity because of their immature renal function. Neomycin is not recommended for use in infants and children. Fluoroquinolones are not recommended for use in children if other alternatives are available because they have been associated with permanent damage in cartilage and joints in some animal studies.

Use in Older Adults

Because of impaired renal function, other disease processes (e.g., diabetes), and multiple-drug therapy, older adults are at high risk for development of aminoglycoside-induced nephrotoxicity and ototoxicity.

Aminoglycosides should not be given to older adults with impaired renal function if less toxic drugs are effective against causative organisms.

When the drugs are given, extreme caution is required. A **BLACK BOX WARNING** emphasizes the increased risk for ototoxicity with kanamycin in older adults. Interventions to decrease the incidence and severity of adverse drug effects, listed earlier in the section "Guidelines for Reducing Toxicity of Aminoglycosides," are especially important with older adults. In addition, prolonged therapy (>1 week) increases risk of toxicity and should be avoided when possible.

Fluoroquinolones are commonly used in older adults for the same indications as in younger adults. In older adults with normal renal function, the drugs should be accompanied by an adequate fluid intake and urine output to prevent drug crystals from forming in the urinary tract. In addition, urinary alkalinizing agents should be avoided because drug crystals form more readily in alkaline urine. In those with impaired renal function, a common condition in older adults, the drugs should be used cautiously and in reduced dosage. A **BLACK BOX WARNING** for fluoroquinolones has been issued by the FDA alerting health professionals to the increased risk of developing tendinitis and tendon rupture. The risk is greater for those over the age of 60, those with heart kidney and lung transplants, and those taking corticosteroidal medications; and necessitates discontinuation of the fluoroquinolone.

Use in Patients With Renal Impairment

Aminoglycosides are nephrotoxic and must be used very cautiously in patients with renal impairment. Both aminoglycosides and fluoroquinolones require dosage adjustments in renal impairment. Dosage guidelines have been established according to creatinine clearance and often involve lower dosages and prolonged intervals between doses (e.g., 36–72 hours). Guidelines for reducing nephrotoxicity of aminoglycosides are as listed previously.

With fluoroquinolones, reported renal effects include azotemia, crystalluria, hematuria, interstitial nephritis, nephropathy, and renal failure. Nephrotoxicity occurs less often than with aminoglycosides, and most cases of acute renal failure have occurred in older adults. It is unknown whether renal failure is caused by hypersensitivity or is a direct toxic effect of fluoroquinolones. Crystalluria rarely occurs in acidic urine but may occur in alkaline urine. Guidelines for reducing nephrotoxicity include using lower dosages, having longer intervals between doses, receiving adequate hydration, and avoiding substances that alkalinize the urine.

Use in Patients With Hepatic Impairment

With aminoglycosides, hepatic impairment is not a significant factor because the drugs are excreted through the kidneys. With fluoroquinolones, however, hepatotoxicity has been observed with some of the drugs. A **BLACK BOX WARNING** reports that trovafloxacin is associated with severe liver injury leading to liver transplantation or death and should be reserved for serious infections only. Clinical manifestations range from abnormalities in liver enzyme test results to hepatitis, liver necrosis, or hepatic failure.

Use in Patients With Critical Illness

Aminoglycosides and fluoroquinolones are often used in critically ill patients because this population has a high incidence of serious and difficult-to-treat infections. Aminoglycosides are usually given with other antimicrobials to provide broad-spectrum activity. Because critically ill patients are at high risk for development of nephrotoxicity and ototoxicity with aminoglycosides, guidelines for safe drug usage should be strictly followed. Renal function should be monitored to assess for needed dosage reductions in patients with renal dysfunction receiving aminoglycosides or fluoroquinolones. Because fluoroquinolones may be hepatotoxic, hepatic function should be monitored during therapy.

Fluoroquinolones are usually infused IV in critically ill patients. However, administration orally or by GI tube (e.g., nasogastric, gastrostomy, jejunostomy) may be feasible in some patients. Concomitant administration of antacids or enteral feedings decreases absorption.

Evidence-Based Practice

31-1 Home Antibiotic Therapy for Community-Acquired Pneumonia

An increasing number of individuals with community-acquired pneumonia (CAP) are being treated at home for a number of reasons, including increased availability and cost considerations of oral antibiotics. Oral drugs have demonstrated effectiveness and are the preferred route for individuals and family members, but management of individuals with oral drugs has widely varied. The American College of Chest Physicians position statement, cosponsored by the American Academy of Home Care Physicians, outlines recommendations for home care for patients with CAP. These include recommendations for evaluation and diagnosis in the home and the determination of the site of care and the plan of care and guidelines for monitoring and follow-up. Recommendations in the position statement take into consideration the best plan of care incorporating the best available evidence with clinician judgment and patient preferences.

Use in Patients With Diabetes Mellitus

Fluoroquinolones are associated with hyperglycemia and hypoglycemia. Older patients may be more at risk for these glucose disturbances. Severe hypoglycemia has occurred in patients receiving concomitant glyburide and fluoroquinolones. Although most cases have occurred in diabetic patients, severe cases of hyperglycemia have occurred in patients not previously diagnosed as diabetic. Gatifloxacin has been associated with hypoglycemic and hyperglycemic events more commonly than other fluoroquinolones. The explanation for an increased association with gatifloxacin is not currently known.

Use in Home Care

Parenteral aminoglycosides are usually given in a hospital setting. Oral fluoroquinolones are often self-administered at home. An increasing number of individuals with community-acquired pneumonia (CAP) are being treated at home. In a position statement by the American College of Chest Physicians, recommendations are outlined for the range of aspects of home care for patients with this condition (see Evidence-Based Practice Box 31-1).

Applying Your Knowledge 31-3

How Can You Avoid This Medication Error?

Taking into consideration Mr. Dallas's age and the concern about the possibility of heart disease, you restrict Mr. Dallas's fluid intake.

Nursing Actions Aminoglycosides and Fluoroquinolones

NURSING ACTIONS	RATIONALE/EXPLANATION
1. Administer accurately	
a. With aminoglycosides:	
(1) For intravenous (IV) administration, dilute the drug in 50–100 milliliters of 5% dextrose or 0.9% sodium chloride injection and infuse over 30–60 minutes. The concentration of gentamicin solution should not exceed 1 mg/mL.	To achieve therapeutic blood levels
(2) Give intramuscular aminoglycosides in a large muscle mass, and rotate sites.	To avoid local tissue irritation. This is less likely to occur with aminoglycosides than with most other antibiotics.
b. With fluoroquinolones:	
(1) Give IV infusions of levofloxacin over 60 to 90 minutes; with 250 or 500 mg infuse over 60 minutes. At 750 mg dose infuse over 90 minutes.	To decrease vein irritation and phlebitis
(2) When giving ciprofloxacin, gatifloxacin, or levofloxacin IV into a primary IV line (e.g., using piggyback apparatus or Y connector), stop the primary solution until ciprofloxacin is infused.	To avoid physical or chemical incompatibilities
2. Observe for therapeutic effects	
a. Decreased signs and symptoms of the infection for which the drug is being given	See Chapter 29.
3. Observe for adverse effects	
a. With aminoglycosides, observe for:	Adverse effects are more likely to occur with parenteral administration of large doses for prolonged periods. However, they may occur with oral administration in the presence of renal impairment and with usual therapeutic doses.

NURSING ACTIONS	RATIONALE/EXPLANATION
(1) Nephrotoxicity—casts, albumin, red or white blood cells in urine; decreased creatinine clearance; increased serum creatinine; increased blood urea nitrogen	Renal damage is most likely to occur in clients who are elderly; receive high doses or prolonged therapy; have prior renal damage; or receive other nephrotoxic drugs. This is the most serious adverse reaction. Risks of kidney damage can be minimized by using the drugs appropriately, detecting early signs of renal impairment, and keeping clients well hydrated.
(2) Ototoxicity—deafness or decreased hearing, tinnitus, dizziness, ataxia	This results from damage to the eighth cranial nerve. Incidence of ototoxicity is increased in older clients and in those with previous auditory damage; high doses or prolonged duration of therapy; and concurrent use of other ototoxic drugs. May be reversible with discontinuation of drug.
(3) Neurotoxicity—respiratory paralysis and apnea	This is caused by neuromuscular blockade and is more likely to occur after rapid IV injection, administration to a client with myasthenia gravis, or concomitant administration of general anesthetics or neuromuscular blocking agents (e.g., succinylcholine, tubocurarine). This effect also may occur if an aminoglycoside is administered shortly after surgery, due to the residual effects of anesthetics or neuromuscular blockers. Neostigmine or calcium may be given to counteract apnea.
(4) Hypersensitivity—skin rash, urticaria	This is an uncommon reaction except with topical neomycin, which may cause sensitization in as many as 10% of recipients.
(5) Nausea, vomiting, diarrhea, peripheral neuritis, paresthesias	Uncommon with parenteral aminoglycosides. Diarrhea often occurs with oral administration.
b. With fluoroquinolones, observe for:	The drugs are usually well tolerated.
(1) Hepatotoxicity (abnormal liver enzyme tests, hepatitis, hepatic failure)	Hepatotoxicity has been observed with most of the drugs.
(2) Allergic reactions (anaphylaxis, urticaria)	Uncommon, but some fatalities have been reported.
(3) Nausea, vomiting, diarrhea, pseudomembranous colitis	Nausea is the most common GI symptom.
(4) Headache, dizziness, confusion, tremors, hallucinations, depression, seizures	Uncommon, but may develop after first dose. Use caution in clients with known or suspected central nervous system disorders that lower seizure threshold.
(5) Crystalluria	Uncommon, but may occur with an inadequate fluid intake
(6) Photosensitivity (skin redness, rash, itching)	May occur with most fluoroquinolones with exposure to sunlight
(7) Glucose tolerance	Fluoroquinolones are associated with hyperglycemia and hypoglycemia. Older clients and those with diabetes are most at risk.
(8) QT prolongation	QT prolongation may result in life threatening dysrhythmias.
(9) Other	Adverse effects involving most body systems have been reported with one or more of the fluoroquinolones. Most have a low incidence (<1%) of occurrence.
4. Observe for drug interactions	
a. Drugs that *increase* effects of aminoglycosides:	The listed drugs increase toxicity.
(1) Amphotericin B, cephalosporins, cisplatin, cyclosporine, enflurane, vancomycin	These drugs are nephrotoxic alone and may increase nephrotoxicity of aminoglycosides.
(2) Loop diuretics (furosemide, bumetanide)	Increased ototoxicity
(3) Neuromuscular blocking agents (e.g., pancuronium, vecuronium)	Increased neuromuscular blockade with possible paralysis of respiratory muscles and apnea
b. Drugs that *decrease* effects of aminoglycosides:	
(1) Penicillins, when admixed directly in same syringe with aminoglycosides	Chemical inactivation of PCN
c. Drugs that *increase* effects of fluoroquinolones:	
(1) Cimetidine, probenecid	Cimetidine inhibits hepatic metabolism and probenecid inhibits renal excretion of fluoroquinolones. These actions may increase serum drug levels.
d. Drugs that *decrease* effects of fluoroquinolones:	
(1) Antacids, iron preparations, sucralfate, zinc preparations, buffered didanosine preparations, quinapril	These drugs interfere with absorption of fluoroquinolones from the GI tract.

Key Concepts

- The choice of aminoglycoside depends on local susceptibility patterns and specific organisms causing an infection.
- The major clinical use of parenteral aminoglycosides is to treat serious systemic infections caused by susceptible aerobic gram-negative organisms.
- Neomycin and kanamycin may be given to suppress intestinal bacteria before bowel surgery and to treat hepatic coma.
- Multiple-dose regimens (conventional dosing) of aminoglycosides must be carefully monitored with evaluation of peak and trough serum levels. Once-daily regimens are monitored with random level (12-hour) serum evaluation.
- Drugs reach higher concentrations in the kidneys and inner ears than in other body tissues; this is a major factor in nephrotoxicity and ototoxicity.
- Fluoroquinolones are associated with hyperglycemia and hypoglycemia and older patients may be more at risk for these glucose disturbances.

Review and Application Exercises

Short Answer Exercises

1. Why must aminoglycosides be given parenterally for systemic infections?
2. How are aminoglycosides excreted?
3. What are risk factors for aminoglycoside-induced nephrotoxicity and ototoxicity?
4. How would you assess a patient for nephrotoxicity or ototoxicity?
5. What is the reason for giving an aminoglycoside and an antipseudomonal penicillin in the treatment of serious infections caused by *P. aeruginosa*?
6. Why should an aminoglycoside and an antipseudomonal penicillin not be combined in a syringe or IV fluid for administration?
7. Which laboratory tests need to be monitored regularly for a patient receiving a systemic aminoglycoside?
8. What is the rationale for giving an oral aminoglycoside to treat hepatic coma?
9. What are the main clinical uses of fluoroquinolones?
10. What are adverse effects of fluoroquinolones, and how may they be prevented or minimized?
11. Why is it important to maintain an adequate fluid intake and urine output while taking a fluoroquinolone?
12. Why are fluoroquinolones not preferred drugs for children?

NCLEX-Style Questions

13. A hospitalized patient is scheduled to receive levofloxacin 500 mg PO at 9:00 A.M. The medication administration record also indicates that Maalox 30 mL PO and hydrochlorothiazide 25 mg PO are due at 9:00 A.M. The nurse should
    a. Administer all the medications as scheduled.
    b. Hold the Maalox until 11:00 A.M.
    c. Ask the physician to discontinue hydrochlorothiazide because of increased risk of ototoxicity.
    d. Administer the Maalox and levofloxacin, but hold the hydrochlorothiazide.

14. A critically ill patient is receiving tobramycin 1.5 mg/kg IV every 8 hours. The patient has recently stopped making urine, and the most recent laboratory results indicate that the creatinine level has risen from normal to 3.6 mg/dL. At the next scheduled administration time for tobramycin, the nurse should
    a. Administer half the prescribed dose.
    b. Hold the tobramycin and notify the physician.
    c. Administer tobramycin as prescribed.
    d. Draw a blood sample for testing the tobramycin level before the dose and then administer as prescribed.

15. An outpatient client has just been given a prescription for moxifloxacin 400 mg PO once daily for acute bronchitis. The nurse should teach the patient
    a. not to take moxifloxacin with a meal
    b. to restrict fluid intake to avoid fluid overload
    c. to take moxifloxacin with an antacid (e.g., Tums) to decrease the chance of stomach upset
    d. to avoid prolonged exposure to sunlight

16. A nursing home patient is brought to the emergency department with acute pyelonephritis. The emergency room physician prescribes ciprofloxacin 500 mg PO twice daily. The patient has a history of seizures and bradycardia. The nurse should
    a. Counsel the patient's caregiver to avoid administering the ciprofloxacin with the patient's anticonvulsant.
    b. Ask the physician to check blood levels of the patient's anticonvulsant(s) before giving the first dose of ciprofloxacin.
    c. Call the patient's seizure and dysrhythmia history to the physician's attention and inquire whether another type of antibiotic might be selected.
    d. Counsel the patient's caregiver to discontinue the ciprofloxacin after the patient's fever is gone.

17. A physician writes an order for gentamicin 7 mg/kg IV every 24 hours and ampicillin 500 mg IV every 6 hours. The patient has a diagnosis of endocarditis. This is not an ideal antibiotic regimen for endocarditis because
    a. Gentamicin should be dosed using the multiple daily dosing method for endocarditis.
    b. The addition of gentamicin to ampicillin increases the risk of treatment failure in endocarditis.
    c. The appropriate single daily dose of gentamicin is 15 mg/kg once daily.
    d. Streptomycin is the recommended aminoglycoside for use in endocarditis.

Selected References

Centers for Disease Control and Prevention. (2007). Update to CDC's sexually transmitted diseases treatment guidelines, 2006: Fluoroquinolones no longer recommended for treatment of gonococcal infections. *Morbidity and Mortality Weekly Report, 56*(14), 332–336.

Drug facts and comparisons. (Updated monthly). St. Louis, MO: Facts and Comparisons.

Lacy, C. F., Armstrong, L. L., Goldman, M. P., & Lance, L. L. (2007). *Lexi-Comp's drug information handbook* (15th ed.). Hudson, OH: American Pharmaceutical Association.

Ramsdell, J., Narsavage, G. L., & Fink, J. B. (2005). Management of community-acquired pneumonia in the home: an American College of Chest Physicians clinical position statement. *Chest, 127*(5), 1752–1763.

Schaad, U. B. (2005). Fluoroquinolone antibiotics in infants and children. *Infectious Disease Clinics of North America, 19*(3), 617–628.

Tetracyclines, Sulfonamides, and Urinary Agents

LEARNING OBJECTIVES

After studying this chapter, you will be able to:

1. Discuss major characteristics and clinical uses of tetracyclines.
2. Recognize doxycycline as the tetracycline of choice in renal failure.
3. Discuss characteristics, clinical uses, adverse effects, and nursing implications of selected sulfonamides.
4. Recognize trimethoprim-sulfamethoxazole as a combination drug that is commonly used for urinary tract and systemic infections.
5. Describe the use of urinary antiseptics in the treatment of urinary tract infections.
6. Teach patients strategies for preventing, recognizing, and treating urinary tract infections.

Applying Your Knowledge

Sharon Dee is an 18-year-old college student. She comes to the health clinic with complaints of urinary frequency and burning on urination. Her medication history includes ongoing, long-term treatment of acne with a tetracycline. She takes 250 mg of the drug PO daily. The physician diagnoses her with a urinary tract infection and prescribes trimethoprim-sulfamethoxazole (Bactrim) 160/800 mg PO every 12 hours for 10 days.

Introduction

Tetracyclines and sulfonamides are older, *broad-spectrum*, bacteriostatic drugs that are rarely used for systemic infections because of microbial resistance and the development of more effective or less toxic drugs. However, the drugs are useful in selected infections. Urinary antiseptics are used only in urinary tract infections (UTI). All of these drugs are described in this chapter and are listed in the Drugs at a Glance tables.

The *tetracyclines* are similar in pharmacologic properties and antimicrobial activity. They are effective against both gram-negative and gram-positive microorganisms, although they are usually not drugs of choice. Many gram-negative microorganisms have developed resistance to tetracyclines. Bacterial infections caused by *Brucella* and *Vibrio cholerae* are still treated by tetracyclines. The drugs also remain effective against rickettsiae, chlamydia, some protozoa, spirochetes, and others. Doxycycline (Vibramycin) is one of the drugs of choice for *Bacillus anthracis* (anthrax) and *Chlamydia trachomatis* and is used in respiratory tract infections due to *Mycoplasma pneumoniae*. Tetracyclines are widely distributed into most body tissues and fluids. The older tetracyclines are excreted mainly in urine, doxycycline is eliminated in urine and feces, and minocycline is eliminated mainly by the liver. Table 32-1 provides pertinent information about various tetracyclines.

Sulfonamides are bacteriostatic against a wide range of gram-positive and gram-negative bacteria, although increasing resistance is making them less useful. Susceptibility should be documented by culture and sensitivity testing, but sulfonamides may be active against *Streptococcus pyogenes*, some staphylococcal strains, *Haemophilus influenzae*, *Nocardia*, *C. trachomatis*, and toxoplasmosis. The combination of trimethoprim-sulfamethoxazole (Bactrim, Septra) is useful in bronchitis, UTIs due to Enterobacteriaceae, and *Pneumocystis jiroveci* infection (in high doses). Individual drugs vary in extent of systemic absorption and clinical indications. Some sulfonamides are well absorbed and can be used in systemic infections; others are poorly absorbed and exert more local effects. Table 32-2 summarizes key information about sulfonamides.

Urinary antiseptics may be bactericidal for sensitive organisms in the urinary tract because these drugs are concentrated in renal tubules and reach high levels in urine. They are not used in systemic infections because they do not attain therapeutic plasma levels. An additional drug, phenazopyridine

Table 32-1	Drugs at a Glance: Tetracyclines		

| | | ROUTES AND DOSAGE RANGES | |
Generic/Trade Name	Comments	Adults	Children
Tetracycline (Achromycin, others)	▪ Prototype drug ▪ Marketed under generic and numerous trade names	PO 250-500 mg q6h	*Older than 8 y:* PO 25–50 mg/kg/d in 4 divided doses
Demeclocycline (Declomycin)	▪ The tetracycline most likely to cause photosensitivity ▪ Primarily used to treat inappropriate secretion of antidiuretic hormone ▪ No longer recommended for treatment of gonorrhea	PO 150 mg q6h or 300 mg q12h	*Older than 8 y:* PO 8–12 mg/kg/d in 2–4 divided doses
Doxycycline (Vibramycin)	▪ Well absorbed from the gastrointestinal tract. Oral administration yields serum drug levels equivalent to those obtained by parenteral administration. ▪ Highly lipid soluble; therefore, reaches therapeutic levels in CSF, the eye, and the prostate gland ▪ Can be given in smaller doses and less frequently than other tetracyclines because of long serum half-life (approximately 18 h) ▪ Excreted by kidneys to a lesser extent than other tetracyclines and is considered safe for clients with impaired renal function	PO/IV 100 – 200 mg/day, in 1–2 divided doses.	*Older than 8 y:* PO, IV *Weight ≥45 kg:* same as adults *Weight <45 kg:* PO, IV 2–5 mg/kg/ day in 1–2 divided does (maximum dose 200 mg/day).
Minocycline (Minocin)	▪ Well absorbed after oral administration ▪ Like doxycycline, readily penetrates CSF, the eye, and the prostate gland ▪ Metabolized more than other tetracyclines, and smaller amounts are excreted in urine and feces	PO, 200 mg initially, then 100 mg q12h (maximum dose 400 mg/ day).	*Older than 8 y:* PO, 4 mg/kg initially, then 2 mg/kg q12h

CSF, cerebrospinal fluid

| Table 32-2 | Drugs at a Glance: Sulfonamides | | | |

Generic/Trade Name	Characteristics	Clinical indications	ROUTES AND DOSAGE RANGES	
			Adults	**Children**
Single Agents				
Sulfadiazine	■ A short-acting, rapidly absorbed, rapidly excreted agent for systemic infections ■ The addition of folinic acid may be recommended.	■ Nocardiosis ■ Toxoplasmosis	Toxoplasmosis, PO 2–6 g daily in divided doses q 6 h in conjunction with pyrimethamine Nocardiosis: 4–8 g/day for a minimum of 6 weeks	Toxoplasmosis, *older than 2 mo:* PO 75 mg/kg initially, then150 mg/kg/d in conjunction with pyrimethamine in 4–6 divided doses: maximal daily dose, 6 g
Sulfasalazine (Azulfidine)	■ Poorly absorbed ■ Does not alter normal bacterial flora in the intestine. Effectiveness in ulcerative colitis may be due to antibacterial (sulfapyridine) and anti-inflammatory (aminosalicylic acid) metabolites.	■ Ulcerative colitis/Crohn's disease ■ Rheumatoid arthritis	Ulcerative colitis, PO 3–4 g daily in 4 divided doses initially; 2 g daily in divided doses for maintenance; maximal daily dose, 4 g Rheumatoid arthritis, maintenance, PO 2 g daily in divided doses, q12h	PO 30–60 mg/kg/d in 2–6 divided doses initially, followed by 30 mg/kg/d in 4 divided doses; maximum daily dose, 2 g
Sulfisoxazole	■ Rapidly absorbed, rapidly excreted ■ Highly soluble and less likely to cause crystalluria than most other sulfonamides	■ UTI ■ Ocular infections	PO 2–4 g initially, then 4–8 g daily in 4–6 divided doses	*Older than 2 mo:* PO 75 mg/kg of body weight initially, then 120–150 mg/kg/d in 4–6 divided doses; maximal daily dose, 6 g
Combination Agent				
Trimethoprim-sulfamethox-azole (Bactrim,Septra, others) Dosage based on Trimethoprim Component	■ May exhibit synergistic effectiveness against many organisms (verify susceptibility first), including streptococci (*S. viridans*), staphylococci (*S. epidermidis, S. aureus*), *Escherichia coli, Salmonella, Shigella, Serratia, Klebsiella, Nocardia,* and others. Most strains of *Pseudomonas* are resistant.	■ Acute and chronic UTI ■ Acute exacerbations of chronic bronchitis ■ Acute otitis media caused by susceptible strains of *Hemophilus influenzae* and *Streptococcus pneumoniae* ■ Shigellosis ■ Infection by *Pneumocystis jiroveci* (prevention and treatment)	UTI, trimethoprim 160 mg and sulfamethoxazole 800 mg PO q12h for 10–14 d Shigellosis, same dose as abovefor 5 d Severe UTI, IV 8–10 mg (trimethoprim component)/kg/d in 2–4 divided doses, up to 14 d	UTI and otitis media, PO 8 mg/kg trimethoprim and 40 mg/kg sulfamethoxazole in 2 divided doses q12h for 10 d Shigellosis, same dose as above for 5 d Severe UTI, IV8–10 mg (trimethoprim component)/kg in 2–4 divided doses, q6–8h or q12h, up to 14 d

Generic/Trade Name	Characteristics	Clinical indications	ROUTES AND DOSAGE RANGES Adults	Children
	▪ The two drugs have additive antibacterial effects because they interfere with different steps in bacterial synthesis and activation of folic acid, an essential nutrient. ▪ The combination is less likely to produce resistant bacteria than either agent alone. ▪ Oral preparations contain different amounts of the two drugs, as follows: – "Regular" tablets contain trimethoprim 80 mg and sulfamethoxazole 400 mg. – Double-strength tablets (e.g., Bactrim D.S., Septra D.S.) contain trimethoprim 160 mg and sulfamethoxazole 800 mg. – Oral suspension contains trimethoprim 40 mg and sulfamethoxazole 200 mg in each 5 mL. ▪ IV preparation contains trimethoprim 80 mg and sulfamethoxazole 400 mg in 5 mL. ▪ Dosage must be reduced in renal insufficiency. ▪ The preparation is contraindicated if creatinine clearance is <15 mL/min.	▪ IV preparation indicated for *P. jiroveci* pneumonia, severe UTI, and shigellosis	*P. jiroveci* pneumonia, IV 15–20 mg (trimethoprim component)/kg/d in 3 or 4 divided doses, q6–8h up to 21 d; IV doses should be given over 60–90 min.	*P. jiroveci* pneumonia, IV 15–20 mg (trimethoprim component)/kg/d in 3 or 4 divided doses, q6–8h up to 21 d
Topical Sulfonamides **Mafenide** (Sulfamylon)	▪ Effective against most gram-negative and gram-positive organisms, especially *Pseudomonas aeruginosa* ▪ Application causes pain and burning. ▪ Mafenide is absorbed systemically and may produce metabolic acidosis.	Prevention of bacterial colonization and infection of severe burn wounds	Topical application to burned area, once or twice daily, in a thin layer	Same as adults

(continued on page 518)

| Table 32-2 | Drugs at a Glance: Sulfonamides (continued) |

Generic/Trade Name	Characteristics	Clinical indications	ROUTES AND DOSAGE RANGES	
			Adults	**Children**
Silver sulfadiazine (Silvadene)	■ Effective against most *Pseudomonas* species, the most common pathogen in severe burn sepsis; *E. coli*; *Klebsiella*; *Proteus*; staphylococci; and streptococci ■ Lower incidence of pain, burning, or itching than mafenide ■ Does not cause electrolyte or acid–base imbalances ■ Significant amounts may be absorbed systemically with large burned areas and prolonged use. Monitor for adverse effects common to sulfonamides.	Same as mafenide. Usually the preferred drug	1–2 times daily cover burned area with cream.	Same as mafenide

UTI, urinary tract infection.

(Pyridium), is given to relieve pain associated with UTI. It has no antibacterial activity.

Mechanisms of Action

Tetracyclines penetrate microbial cells by passive diffusion and an active transport system. Intracellularly, they bind to 30S ribosomes, like the aminoglycosides, and inhibit microbial protein synthesis. Sulfonamides act as antimetabolites of para-aminobenzoic acid (PABA), which microorganisms require to produce folic acid; folic acid, in turn, is required for the production of bacterial intracellular proteins. Sulfonamides enter into the reaction instead of PABA, compete for the enzyme involved, and cause formation of nonfunctional derivatives of folic acid. Thus, sulfonamides halt multiplication of new bacteria but do not kill mature, fully formed bacteria. With the exception of the topical sulfonamides used in burn therapy, the presence of pus, serum, or necrotic tissue interferes with sulfonamide action because these materials contain PABA. Some bacteria can change their metabolic pathways to use precursors or other forms of folic acid and thereby develop resistance to the antibacterial action of sulfonamides. After resistance to one sulfonamide develops, cross-resistance to others is common.

Indications for Use

A tetracycline is the drug of choice or an alternate (sometimes as part of combination therapy) in a few infections (e.g., brucellosis, chancroid, cholera, granuloma inguinale, psittacosis, Rocky Mountain spotted fever, syphilis, trachoma, typhus, gastroenteritis due to *V. cholerae* or *Helicobacter pylori*). Tetracyclines are also useful in treating some animal bites and Lyme disease. Other drugs (e.g., penicillins) are usually preferred in gram-positive infections, and many gram-negative organisms are resistant to tetracyclines. However, a tetracycline may be used if bacterial susceptibility is confirmed. Specific clinical indications for tetracyclines include

■ Treatment of uncomplicated urethral, endocervical, or rectal infections caused by *Chlamydia* organisms.

■ Adjunctive treatment, with other antimicrobials, in the treatment of pelvic inflammatory disease and sexually transmitted diseases.

■ Postexposure prophylaxis and treatment of anthrax. Doxycycline is the tetracycline of choice as part of a combination-drug regimen.

▪ Long-term treatment of acne. Tetracyclines interfere with the production of free fatty acids and decrease *Corynebacterium* in sebum. These actions decrease the inflammatory, pustular lesions associated with severe acne.

▪ As a substitute for penicillin in penicillin-allergic patients. Tetracyclines may be effective in treating syphilis. when penicillin cannot be given. They should not be substituted for penicillin in treating streptococcal pharyngitis because microbial resistance is common, and tetracyclines do not prevent rheumatic fever. In addition, they should not be substituted for penicillin in any serious staphylococcal infection because microbial resistance commonly occurs.

▪ Doxycycline may be used to prevent traveler's diarrhea due to enterotoxic strains of *Escherichia coli*.

▪ Demeclocycline (Declomycin) may be used to inhibit antidiuretic hormone in the treatment of chronic inappropriate antidiuretic hormone secretion.

Sulfonamides are commonly used to treat UTI (e.g., acute and chronic cystitis, asymptomatic bacteriuria) caused by *E. coli* and *Proteus* or *Klebsiella* organisms. In acute pyelonephritis, other agents are preferred. Trimethoprim-sulfamethoxazole is used in chronic bronchitis due to pneumococci, *H. influenzae*, and *Moraxella catarrhalis*. It is also the drug of choice for treatment and prophylaxis of *P. jiroveci* infection in patients with and without human immunodeficiency virus (HIV) infection. Additional uses of sulfonamides include ulcerative colitis and uncommon infections such as chancroid, lymphogranuloma venereum, nocardiosis, toxoplasmosis, and trachoma. Topical sulfonamides are used in prevention of burn wound infections and in treatment of ocular and other soft tissue infections. For specific clinical indications of individual drugs, see Table 32-2.

Urinary antiseptics are used only for UTI. Table 32-3 summarizes information about drugs used to treat UTI.

Contraindications to Use

Both tetracyclines (except doxycycline) and sulfonamides are contraindicated in patients with renal failure. Tetracyclines are also contraindicated in pregnant women and in children up to 8 years of age. In the fetus and young child, tetracyclines are deposited in bones and teeth along with calcium. If given during active mineralization of these tissues, tetracyclines can

Table 32-3	**Drugs at a Glance:** Miscellaneous Drugs for Urinary Tract Infections		

| | | ROUTES AND DOSAGE RANGES | |
Generic/Trade Name	**Characteristics**	**Adults**	**Children**
Nitrofurantoin (Furadantin, Macrodantin, Macrobid)	▪ Antibacterial activity against *E. coli* and most other organisms that cause UTI ▪ Used for short-term treatment of UTI or long-term suppression of bacteria in chronic, recurrent UTI ▪ Bacterial resistance develops slowly and to a limited degree. ▪ Contraindicated in severe renal disease	Macrodantin: PO 50–100 mg 4 times daily; Macrobid: 100 mg q12h for 7 d Prophylaxis of recurrent UTI in women, Macrodantin: PO 50–100 mg at bedtime	*Children older than 12 y:* Dual-release capsules: 100 mg q12h for 7 d *Children 1 mo and older:* PO macrocrystal capsules: 5–7 mg/kg/d in 4 divided doses for 7 d
Phenazopyridine (Pyridium)	▪ An azo dye that acts as a urinary tract analgesic and relieves symptoms of dysuria, burning, and frequency and urgency of urination, which occur with UTI ▪ It has no anti-infective action. ▪ It turns urine orange-red, which may be mistaken for blood. ▪ It is contraindicated in renal insufficiency and severe hepatitis.	PO 100–200 mg 3 times daily after meals	6–12 y: PO 12 mg/kg/d, in 3 divided doses after meals for 2 d

(continued on page 520)

Table 32-3   **Drugs at a Glance:** Miscellaneous Drugs for Urinary Tract Infections (continued)

Generic/Trade Name	Characteristics	ROUTES AND DOSAGE RANGES	
		Adults	Children
Trimethoprim (Proloprim)	■ A folate antagonist drug with antibacterial effects ■ Available as a single agent for treatment of UTI caused by susceptible strains of E. coli, and other gram-negative organisms ■ Most often used in a fixed-dose combination with sulfamethoxazole (Bactrim, Septra) ■ Contraindicated in clients with hypersensitivity to trimethoprim or megaloblastic anemia due to folate deficiency ■ Rash and pruritus are the most common adverse effects. Nausea, vomiting, thrombocytopenia, and leukopenia occasionally occur.	PO 100 mg q12h for 10 d or 200 mg q24h for 10 d	4 mg/kg/d in divided doses every 12 h

UTI, urinary tract infection.

interfere with tooth enamel formation, cause permanent discoloration (*mottling*) of tooth enamel, and depress bone growth. Increased photosensitivity is a common adverse effect, and patients should be warned to take precautions against sunburn while taking these drugs. Sulfonamides are also contraindicated in late pregnancy, lactation, children younger than 2 months of age (except for treatment of congenital toxoplasmosis), and people who have had hypersensitivity reactions to them or to chemically related drugs (e.g., thiazide diuretics, antidiabetic sulfonylureas). **Sulfasalazine** (Azulfidine) is contraindicated in people who are allergic to salicylates and in people with intestinal or urinary tract obstruction.

Nursing Process

General aspects of the nursing process in antimicrobial drug therapy, as described in Chapter 29, apply to the patient receiving tetracyclines, sulfonamides, and urinary antiseptics. In this chapter, only those aspects related specifically to these drugs are included.

Assessment

With tetracyclines, assess for conditions in which the drugs must be used cautiously or are contraindicated, such as impaired renal or hepatic function.

With sulfonamides, assess for signs and symptoms of disorders for which the drugs are used:

- For UTI, assess urinalysis reports for white blood cell and bacteria counts; urine culture reports for type of bacteria; and symptoms of dysuria, frequency, and urgency of urination.
- For burns, assess the size of the wound, amount and type of drainage, presence of edema, and amount of eschar.
- Ask patients specifically if they have ever taken a sulfonamide and, if so, whether they had an allergic reaction.

With urinary antiseptics, assess for signs and symptoms of UTI.

Nursing Diagnoses

- Risk for Injury: Hypersensitivity reaction, kidney, liver, or blood disorders with sulfonamides
- Deficient Knowledge: Correct administration and use of tetracyclines, sulfonamides, and urinary antiseptics

Planning/Goals

The patent will

- Receive or self-administer the drugs as directed

▪ Receive prompt and appropriate treatment if adverse effects occur

Interventions

▪ During tetracycline therapy for systemic infections, monitor laboratory tests of renal function for abnormal values.

▪ During sulfonamide therapy, encourage sufficient fluids to produce a urine output of at least 1200 to1500 mL daily. A high fluid intake decreases the risk of crystalluria (precipitation of drug crystals in the urine).

▪ Avoid urinary catheterization when possible. If catheterization is necessary, use sterile technique. The urinary tract is normally sterile except for the lower third of the urethra. Introduction of any bacteria into the bladder may cause infection.

▪ A single catheterization may cause infection. With indwelling catheters, bacteria colonize the bladder and produce infection within 2 to 3 weeks, even with meticulous care.

▪ When indwelling catheters must be used, measures to decrease UTI include using a closed drainage system; keeping the perineal area clean; forcing fluids, if not contraindicated, to maintain a dilute urine; and removing the catheter as soon as possible. Do not disconnect the system and irrigate the catheter unless obstruction is suspected. *Never* raise the urinary drainage bag above bladder level.

▪ Force fluids in anyone with a UTI unless contraindicated. Bacteria do not multiply as rapidly in dilute urine. In addition, emptying the bladder frequently allows it to refill with uninfected urine. This decreases the bacterial population of the bladder.

▪ Teach women to cleanse themselves from the urethral area toward the rectum after voiding or defecating to avoid contamination of the urethral area with bacteria from the vagina and rectum. Also, voiding after sexual intercourse helps cleanse the lower urethra and prevent UTI.

▪ Provide appropriate teaching related to any drug therapy (see accompanying displays).

Evaluation

▪ Interview and observe for improvement in the infection being treated.

▪ Interview and observe for adverse drug effects.

Applying Your Knowledge 32-1

Sharon needs to have adequate serum drug levels of Bactrim to treat her infection successfully. What instruction should you give Sharon in regard to fluid intake?

Principles of Therapy

Tetracyclines

Culture and susceptibility studies are needed before tetracycline therapy is started because many strains of organisms are either drug resistant or vary greatly in drug susceptibility. Cross-sensitivity and cross-resistance are common among tetracyclines. The oral route of administration is usually effective and preferred. Intravenous (IV) therapy is used when oral administration is contraindicated or for initial treatment of severe infections.

Tetracyclines decompose with age, exposure to light, and extreme heat and humidity. Because the breakdown products may be toxic, it is important to store these drugs correctly. Also, the manufacturer's expiration dates on containers should be noted, and outdated drugs should be discarded.

Sulfonamides and Urinary Antiseptics

Urine cultures and susceptibility tests are indicated in suspected UTI because of wide variability in possible pathogens and their susceptibility to antibacterial drugs. The best results

 Patient Teaching Guidelines **Oral Tetracyclines**

General Considerations
▪ Because tetracyclines inhibit rather than kill bacteria, they must be administered around the clock to achieve desired effects.
▪ These drugs increase sensitivity to sunlight and risks of sunburn. Avoid sunlamps, tanning beds, and intense or prolonged exposure to sunlight; if unable to avoid exposure, wear protective clothing and a sunblock preparation.
▪ Report severe nausea, vomiting, diarrhea, skin rash, or perineal itching. These symptoms may indicate a need for changing or stopping the tetracycline.

Self-Administration
▪ Take most tetracyclines on an empty stomach, at least 1 hour before or 2 hours after meals. Doxycycline and minocycline may be taken with food (except dairy products).
▪ Do not take with or within 2 hours of dairy products, antacids, or iron supplements. If an antacid must be taken, take at least 2 hours before or 4 hours after tetracycline.
▪ Take each dose with at least 8 ounces of water.

Patient Teaching Guidelines | Oral Sulfonamides

General Considerations

■ Sulfonamides inhibit rather than kill bacteria. Thus, it is especially important to take them as prescribed, for the length of time prescribed.

■ These drugs increase sensitivity to sunlight and risks of sunburn. Avoid sunlamps, tanning beds, and intense or prolonged exposure to sunlight; if unable to avoid exposure, wear protective clothing and a sunblock preparation.

■ Notify the prescribing physician if you have blood in urine, skin rash, difficulty in breathing, fever, or sore throat. These symptoms may indicate adverse drug effects and the need to change or stop the drug.

Self-Administration

■ Take oral sulfonamides with or without food with at least 8 ounces of water.

■ With oral suspensions, shake well, refrigerate after opening, and discard the unused portion after 14 days.

■ Drink 2 to 3 quarts of fluid daily, if able. A good fluid intake helps the drugs to be more effective, especially in urinary tract infections, and decreases the likelihood of damaging the kidneys.

are obtained with drug therapy indicated by the microorganisms isolated from each patient. With systemically absorbed sulfonamides, an initial loading dose may be given to produce therapeutic blood levels more rapidly. The amount is usually twice the maintenance dose.

Urine pH is important in drug therapy with sulfonamides and urinary antiseptics. With sulfonamide therapy, alkaline urine increases drug solubility and helps prevent *crystalluria*. It also increases the rate of sulfonamide excretion and the concentration of sulfonamide in the urine. The urine can be alkalinized by giving sodium bicarbonate. Alkalinization is not needed with sulfisoxazole (because the drug is highly soluble) or sulfonamides used to treat intestinal infections or burn wounds (because there is little systemic absorption).

Applying Your Knowledge 32-2

Sharon mentions that she is going to Florida for spring break. What precaution should you teach Sharon?

Use in Special Populations

Use in Children

Tetracyclines should not be used in children younger than 8 years of age because of their effects on teeth and bones. In teeth, the drugs interfere with enamel development and may cause a permanent yellow, gray, or brown discoloration. In bone, the drugs form a stable compound in bone-forming tissue and may interfere with bone growth.

Systemic sulfonamides are contraindicated during late pregnancy, lactation, and in children younger than 2 months of age. If a fetus or young infant receives a sulfonamide by placental transfer, in breast milk, or by direct administration, the drug displaces bilirubin from binding sites on albumin. As a result, bilirubin may accumulate in the bloodstream (hyperbilirubinemia) and central nervous system (kernicterus) and cause life-threatening toxicity.

Sulfonamides are often used to treat UTI in children older than 2 months of age. Few data are available regarding the effects of long-term or recurrent use of sulfamethoxazole in children younger than 6 years with chronic renal disease. Sulfamethoxazole is often given in combination with trimethoprim (Bactrim, Septra), although trimethoprim has not been established as safe and effective in children younger than 12 years of age.

Some clinicians recommend that asymptomatic bacteriuria be treated in children younger than 5 years of age to decrease risks of long-term renal damage. Treatment is the same as for symptomatic UTI.

Use in Older Adults

A major concern with the use of tetracyclines and sulfonamides in older adults is renal impairment, which commonly occurs in this population. Sulfonamides may cause additional renal impairment. As with younger adults, a fluid intake of 2 liters daily is needed to reduce formation of crystals and stones in the urinary tract.

With the combination of trimethoprim-sulfamethoxazole, older adults are at increased risk for severe adverse effects. Severe skin reactions and bone marrow depression are most often reported. Folic acid deficiency may also occur because both of the drugs interfere with folic acid metabolism.

Use in Patients With Renal Impairment

As discussed previously, most tetracyclines are contraindicated in patients with renal impairment. High concentrations of tetracyclines inhibit protein synthesis in human cells. This antianabolic effect increases tissue breakdown (catabolism) and the amount of waste products to be excreted by the kidneys. The increased workload can be handled by normally functioning kidneys, but waste products are retained when renal function is impaired. This leads to azotemia, increased blood urea nitrogen, hyperphosphatemia, hyperkalemia, and acidosis. If a tetracycline is necessary because of an organism's sensitivity or the host's inability to take other antimicrobial drugs, doxycycline or minocycline may be given.

Systemic sulfonamides should probably be avoided in patients with renal impairment, if other effective drugs are available. Acute renal failure (ARF) has occurred when the drugs or their metabolites precipitated in renal tubules and caused obstruction. ARF is rarely associated with newer sulfonamides, which are more soluble than older ones, but has increased with the use of sulfadiazine to treat toxoplasmosis in patients with acquired immunodeficiency syndrome (AIDS). Preventive measures include an intake of 2 to 3 liters of fluid daily.

Use in Patients With Hepatic Impairment

Tetracyclines are generally contraindicated in pregnant women because they may cause fatal hepatic necrosis in the mother (as well as interfere with bone and tooth development in the fetus). However, there are some situations where the benefit to the mother may outweigh the risk of liver dysfunction (e.g., rickettsial infections, ehrlichiosis, inhalational anthrax, and malaria). Tetracyclines must be used cautiously in the presence of liver or kidney impairment. Because tetracyclines are metabolized in the liver, hepatic impairment or biliary obstruction slows drug elimination. In patients with renal impairment, high IV doses (>2 g/day) have been associated with death from liver failure. If the drug is necessary to treat patients with known or suspected renal and hepatic impairment, renal and liver function test results should be monitored. In addition, hepatotoxic drugs should be avoided.

Sulfonamides cause cholestatic jaundice in a small percentage of patients and should be used with caution in patients with hepatic impairment.

Use in Patients With Critical Illness

Tetracyclines may be used to treat sepsis caused by rickettsial, chlamydial, or mycoplasma infection and pulmonary infection caused by M. pneumoniae or Legionella pneumophila. When necessary, doxycycline is the drug of choice because it can be given to patients with renal impairment, a common problem in critical care settings.

Sulfonamides are rarely used in critical care settings except topical silver sulfadiazine (Silvadene) used to treat burn wounds and trimethoprim-sulfamethoxazole used to treat P. jiroveci pneumonia. Although often given IV in critical care settings, oral or nasogastric tube administration of trimethoprim-sulfamethoxazole may be used in selected patients.

Applying Your Knowledge 32-3

While Sharon is in the clinic it would be prudent to review what she knows about her other medication. What dietary concerns should Sharon be aware of with regard to tetracycline's food–drug and drug–drug interactions?

Nursing Actions Tetracyclines, Sulfonamides, and Urinary Agents

NURSING ACTIONS	RATIONALE/EXPLANATION
1. Administer accurately	
a. With tetracyclines:	
(1) Give oral drugs with food that does not contain dairy products; do not give with or within 2 hours of dairy products, antacids, or iron supplements. Doxycycline and minocycline may be given with food.	To decrease nausea and other gastrointestinal (GI) symptoms. Tetracyclines combine with metallic ions (e.g., aluminum, calcium, iron, magnesium) and are not absorbed.
(2) For intravenous (IV) administration of Doxycycline, dilute with an appropriate type and amount of IV solution, and infuse over 1–4 hours. Avoid extravasation.	Rapid administration should be avoided. IV doses are usually mixed in hospital pharmacies. Doxycycline is very irritating to tissues.
b. With sulfonamides:	
(1) Give oral drugs before or after meals, with a full glass of water.	Absorption is better when taken on an empty stomach; however, taking with food decreases GI upset.
(2) Infuse IV trimethoprim-sulfamethoxazole (diluted in 125 mL of 5% dextrose in water) over 60–90 minutes. Do not mix with other drugs or solutions and flush IV lines to remove any residual drug.	Manufacturer's recommendations
(3) For topical sulfonamides to burn wounds, apply a thin layer with a sterile gloved hand after the surface has been cleansed of previously applied medication.	Burn wounds may be cleansed by whirlpool, shower, or spot cleansing with sterile saline, gauze pads, and gloves.
c. Give nitrofurantoin with meals.	Food decreases nausea, vomiting, and diarrhea.
2. Observe for therapeutic effects	Therapeutic effects depend on the reason for use.
a. With tetracyclines, observe for decreased signs and symptoms of the infection for which the drug is being given.	

(continued on page 524)

Nursing Actions — Tetracyclines, Sulfonamides, and Urinary Agents (continued)

NURSING ACTIONS	RATIONALE/EXPLANATION
b. With sulfonamides, observe for decreased symptoms of urinary tract infection (UTI); decreased diarrhea when given for ulcerative colitis or bacillary dysentery; lack of fever and wound drainage, and absence of infection and evidence of healing in burn wounds.	
c. With urinary antiseptics, observe for decreased symptoms of UTI.	
3. Observe for adverse effects	
a. Nausea, vomiting, diarrhea	Commonly occur with tetracyclines, sulfonamides, and urinary antiseptics, probably from local irritation of GI mucosa. After several days of an oral tetracycline, diarrhea may be caused by superinfection.
b. Hematologic disorders—anemia, neutropenia, thrombocytopenia	
c. Hypersensitivity—anaphylaxis, skin rash, urticaria, serum sickness	
d. Photosensitivity—sunburn reaction	This can be prevented or minimized by avoiding exposure to sunlight or other sources of ultraviolet light, wearing protective clothing, and using sunscreen lotions.
e. Thrombophlebitis at IV infusion sites	These drugs are irritating to tissues. Irritation can be decreased by diluting the drugs and infusing them at the recommended rates.
f. Nephrotoxicity—increased blood urea nitrogen and serum creatinine; hematuria; proteinuria; crystalluria	Nephrotoxicity is more likely to occur in people who already have impaired renal function. Keeping clients well hydrated may help prevent renal damage.
g. Hepatotoxicity—elevated aspartate aminotransferase and other enzymes	Hepatitis, cholestasis, and other serious liver disorders rarely occur with these drugs.
h. Superinfection—sore mouth; white patches on oral mucosa; black, furry tongue; diarrhea; skin rash; itching in the perineal area; pseudomembranous colitis	Superinfection may occur with tetracyclines because of their broad spectrum of antimicrobial activity. Signs and symptoms usually indicate monilial infection. Meticulous oral and perineal hygiene helps prevent these problems. The drug should be stopped if severe diarrhea occurs, with blood, mucus, or pus in stools.
i. Vertigo and dizziness	Occurs only with minocycline
j. Adverse effects of sulfonamides in human immunodeficiency virus (HIV)-infected patients—rash, fever, leukopenia, elevated transaminases, thrombocytopenia	Occurs in 20%–85% of HIV-infected patients
4. Observe for drug interactions	
a. Drugs that *decrease* effects of tetracyclines:	
(1) Aluminum, calcium, iron, or magnesium preparations(e.g., antacids, ferrous sulfate)	These metals combine with oral tetracyclines to produce insoluble, nonabsorbable compounds that are excreted in feces.
(2) Cathartics, didanosine	Decrease absorption
(3) Phenobarbital, carbamazepine, phenytoin, rifampin	These drugs induce drug-metabolizing enzymes in the liver and may speed up metabolism of doxycycline.
b. Drugs that *increase* effects of sulfonamides:	
(1) Alkalinizing agents (e.g., sodium bicarbonate)	Increase rate of urinary excretion, thereby raising levels of sulfonamides in the urinary tract and increasing effectiveness in UTIs
(2) Methenamine compounds, urinary acidifiers (e.g., ascorbic acid)	These drugs increase the risk of nephrotoxicity and should not be used with sulfonamides. They may cause precipitation of sulfonamide with resultant blockage of renal tubules.
(3) Salicylates (e.g., aspirin), nonsteroidal anti-inflammatory drugs (e.g., ibuprofen), oral anticoagulants, phenytoin, methotrexate	Increase toxicity by displacing sulfonamides from plasma proteinbinding sites, thereby increasing plasma levels of free drug
c. Drugs that *alter* effects of nitrofurantoin:	
(1) Antacids	May decrease absorption
(2) Acidifying agents	Increase antibacterial activity of nitrofurantoin by decreasing renal excretion. Nitrofurantoin is most active against organisms causing UTI when urine pH is 5.5 or less.

Key Concepts

■ The tetracyclines are effective against both gram-positive and gram-negative organisms, although they are usually not drugs of choice. Many gram-negative organisms have developed resistance to tetracyclines.

■ Sulfonamides are bacteriostatic against a wide range of gram-positive and gram-negative bacteria, although increasing resistance is making them less useful.

■ Sulfasalazine (Azulfidine) is contraindicated in people who are allergic to salicylates.

■ Urinary antiseptics may be bactericidal for sensitive organisms in the urinary tract because these drugs are concentrated in renal tubules and reach high levels in urine but are not used in systemic infections because they do not attain therapeutic plasma levels.

■ Both tetracyclines (except doxycycline) and sulfonamides are contraindicated in patients with renal failure.

Review and Application Exercises

Short Answer Exercises

1. What foods and drugs interfere with absorption of oral tetracyclines? How can interference be prevented or minimized?

2. What are potentially serious adverse effects of tetracyclines?

3. What is the rationale for long-term, low-dose administration of a tetracycline for acne?

4. Which tetracyclines may be given to patients with renal impairment?

5. Why are sulfonamides often effective in UTI?

6. What are major adverse effects of sulfonamides, and how may they be prevented or minimized?

7. What is the rationale for combining sulfamethoxazole and trimethoprim?

8. What are important characteristics of urinary antiseptics?

NCLEX-Style Questions

9. A 6-year-old child with bronchitis is being seen in the office by the pediatric nurse practitioner. The RN is asked to assess the child. During the nurse's assessment, the mother expresses concern about the expense of treatment. She asks if it is all right for her to use the leftover tetracycline that was prescribed for her 15-year-old son during his last bout of bronchitis. The appropriate response would *not* include:
   a. counseling the mother about the need to complete the full prescribed regimen of any antibiotic
   b. instructing the mother to use her son's old prescription, but at half the dose
   c. informing the mother of the adverse effects on tooth enamel for young children
   d. instructing the mother to discard her son's old tetracycline medication

10. An HIV-positive client is being seen for routine follow-up care in the physician's office. His chief complaints are fever and a severe rash. His medication regimen includes trimethoprim-sulfamethoxazole for prophylaxis of *P. jiroveci* (formerly called *carinii*) infection. The client asks if his symptoms could be due to his medication. The nurse's best response is
    a. The likelihood of the patient's fever and rash being drug-related is very low.
    b. A high percentage of patients with HIV receiving trimethoprim-sulfamethoxazole develop adverse reactions such as these.
    c. Adverse effects of trimethoprim-sulfamethoxazole in HIV-infected patients are rarely serious and usually self-limiting.
    d. The presence of fever and rash probably indicates that the trimethoprim-sulfamethoxazole regimen is ineffective.

11. Patient teaching about phenazopyridine should not include
    a. instruction that the drug is not an antibiotic and only relieves the symptoms of a UTI
    b. a warning that the drug causes a harmless orange-red discoloration of the urine
    c. counseling to take the drug after meals
    d. instruction that phenazopyridine will eradicate the UTI in 3 days

12. The nurse prepares to administer the 2:00 P.M. medications to a hospitalized patient. Scheduled for that time are doxycycline PO, Maalox PO, and ferrous sulfate PO. The nurse should
    a. change the doxycycline to IV to avoid drug interactions
    b. co-administer the doxycycline and ferrous sulfate but hold the Maalox until 4:00 P.M.
    c. reschedule the Maalox and ferrous sulfate to 4:00 P.M.
    d. give the medications with a glass of milk to decrease stomach irritation

13. Which of the following instructions should be given to clients prescribed either tetracycline or a sulfonamide medication?

a. Take with at least 8 ounces of water.

b. Direct exposure to the sun should be avoided, but use of tanning beds is acceptable during therapy.

c. Take the antibiotic until no longer febrile.

d. These medications are safe in late pregnancy.

Selected References

Bar-Or, D. (2005). Tetracycline: From antibiotic to antisepsis. *Critical Care Medicine, 33*, 1660–1601.

Chambers, H. F. (2001). Antimicrobial agents: Protein synthesis inhibitors and miscellaneous antibacterial agents. In J. G. Hardman & L. E. Limbird (Eds.), *Goodman & Gilman's the pharmacological basis of therapeutics* (10th ed., pp. 1239–1271). New York: McGraw-Hill.

Collins, J., Ali-Ibrahim, A., & Smoot, D. T. (2006). Antibiotic therapy for *Helicobacter pylori*. *Medical Clinics of North America, 90*, 1125–1140.

Drug facts and comparisons. (Updated monthly). St. Louis, MO: Facts and Comparisons.

Khardori, N. (2006). Antibiotics- past, present, and future. *Medical Clinics of North America, 90*, 1049–1076.

Lacy, C. F., Armstrong, L. L., Goldman, M. P., & Lance, L. L. (2007). *Lexi-Comp's drug information handbook* (15th ed.). Hudson, OH: American Pharmaceutical Association.

Shoemaker, D. M., Jiang, P. P, Williamson, H., & Roland, W. E. (2007). Infectious diseases. In R. E. Rakel (Ed.), *Textbook of family medicine* (pp. 317–351). Philadelphia: Elsevier.

Solensky, R. (2006). Drug hypersensitivity. *Medical Clinics of North America, 90*, 233–260.

Macrolides, Ketolides, and Miscellaneous Antibacterials

KEY TERMS

- Glycylcycline
- Gray syndrome
- Ketolides
- Lincosamide
- Lipopeptide
- MAC
- Macrolides
- MRSA
- MSSA
- Myelosuppression
- Oxazolidinone
- Red man syndrome
- SSNA
- Streptogramins
- VRE
- VREF

LEARNING OBJECTIVES

After studying this chapter, you will be able to:

1. Identify characteristics and specific uses of macrolide and ketolide antibacterials.
2. Compare and contrast macrolides and ketolides with other commonly used antibacterial drugs.
3. Apply principles of using macrolides and ketolides in selected patient situations.
4. Discuss characteristics and clinical indications for using chloramphenicol, clindamycin, daptomycin, linezolid, metronidazole, quinupristin-dalfopristin, rifaximin, spectinomycin, and vancomycin.
5. Discuss the roles of metronidazole and oral vancomycin in the treatment of pseudomembranous colitis.

Applying Your Knowledge

Juro Nikki is a 65-year-old man who has had chronic obstructive pulmonary disease for a number of years. He presents to the doctor's office with a respiratory tract infection. He is started on azithromycin 500 mg for one dose, then 250 mg PO daily for 4 days.

Introduction

The drugs described in this chapter are heterogeneous in their antimicrobial spectra, characteristics, and clinical uses. Some are used often; some are used only in specific circumstances. The macrolides, ketolides, and selected miscellaneous drugs are described in the following sections; names, routes, and dosage ranges of individual drugs are listed in the Drugs at a Glance tables.

Macrolides and Ketolides

Table 33-1 presents routes and dosage ranges for macrolides and ketolides.

The *macrolides*, which include erythromycin, **azithromycin** (Zithromax), and **clarithromycin** (Biaxin), have similar antibacterial spectra and mechanisms of action. Macrolides are widely distributed into body tissues and fluids and may be bacteriostatic or bactericidal, depending on drug concentration in infected tissues. They are effective against gram-positive cocci, including group A streptococci, pneumococci, and most staphylococci. They are also effective against species of

Table 33-1	Drugs at a Glance: Macrolides and Ketolides		

	USUAL ROUTES AND DOSAGE RANGES	
Generic/Trade Name	**Adults**	**Children**
Azithromycin (Zithromax)	Respiratory and skin infections: PO 500 mg as a single dose on day 1, then 250 mg once daily for 4 days (Zpak) Nongonococcal urethritis and cervicitis caused by *Chlamydia trachomatis*, 1 g as a single dose Prevention of MAC, PO 1200 mg once per week Treatment of MAC, PO 600 mg once daily Bacterial sinusitis: Tri-pak PO 500 mg daily for 3 days, or Zmax extended-release formula PO 2 g as a single dose CAP: IV 500 mg daily for at least 2 d followed by PO 500 mg daily for total of 7–10 d treatment	*6 mo to 2 y:* For otitis media, PO 10 mg/kg on day 1 (not to exceed 500 mg), then 5 mg/kg once daily for 4 days (not to exceed 250 mg/d) *2 y and older:* For pharyngitis/tonsillitis, PO 12 mg/kg (not to exceed 500 mg) once daily for 5 d
Clarithromycin (Biaxin, Biaxin XL)	PO 250–500 mg q12h for 7–14 d Prevention/treatment of MAC: PO 500 mg q12h or 1000 mg XL daily Extended-release: bronchitis and CAP PO 1000 mg daily for 7 d Acute maxillary sinusitis: PO 1000 mg daily for 14 d	PO 7.5 mg/kg, not to exceed 500 mg every 12 h Prevention/treatment of MAC: same as above
Erythromycin base (E-mycin)	PO 250–500 mg q6–12h Severe infections: up to 4 g daily in divided doses	PO 30–50 mg/kg/d in divided doses q6–12h
Erythromycin ethylsuccinate (E.E.S.)	PO 400–800 mg q6–12h Severe infections: up to 4 g daily in divided doses	PO 30–50 mg/kg/d in 2–4 divided doses
Erythromycin lactobionate	IV 15–20 mg/kg/d in divided doses q6h or 500 mg–1 g q6h or may be given as a continuous infusion over 24 h (maximum dose 4 g/d) Severe infections: up to 4 g daily in divided doses	15–50 mg/kg/d in divided doses q6h, not to exceed 4 g/d
Erythromycin stearate (Erythrocin stearate)	PO 250 mg q6h or 500 mg q12h Severe infections: up to 4 g daily in divided doses	PO 30–50 mg/kg/d in 2–4 divided doses
Telithromycin (Ketek)	CAP: PO 800 mg once daily for 7–10 d	

CAP, community-acquired pneumonia; MAC, Mycobacterium avium complex.

Corynebacterium, Treponema, Legionella, Chlamydia, Neisseria, and *Mycoplasma* and against some anaerobic species of organisms such as *Bacteroides* and *Clostridia.* Azithromycin and clarithromycin also are active against the atypical mycobacteria that cause *Mycobacterium avium* complex (MAC) disease. MAC disease (see Chap. 34) is an opportunistic infection that occurs mainly in people with advanced human immunodeficiency virus (HIV) infection. *Helicobacter pylori,* a pathogen implicated in peptic ulcer disease, is also treated by azithromycin or clarithromycin as part of a combination regimen (see Chap. 59).

P **Erythromycin,** the prototype, is now used less often because of microbial resistance, numerous drug interactions, and the development of newer macrolides. Erythromycin is metabolized in the liver and excreted mainly in bile; approximately 20% is excreted in urine. Depending on the specific salt formulation used, food can have a variable effect on the absorption of oral erythromycin. Compared with erythromycin, the newer drugs have enhanced antibacterial activity, require less frequent administration, and cause less nausea, vomiting, and diarrhea. Azithromycin is excreted mainly in bile, and clarithromycin is metabolized to an active metabolite in the liver, which is then excreted in urine.

Erythromycin is available in several preparations. Ophthalmic and topical preparations are discussed in Chapters 63 and 64, respectively.

A relative of the macrolides, **telithromycin** (Ketek) is the first member of the ketolide class. In addition to sharing the general spectrum of activity of the newer macrolides, it offers better activity against macrolide-resistant strains of *Streptococcus pneumoniae*, an increasingly common cause of infections in children and adults. Telithromycin is excreted by the liver and kidneys. Food does not affect the absorption of telithromycin.

Mechanism of Action

The macrolides and ketolides enter microbial cells and reversibly bind to the 50S subunits of ribosomes, thereby inhibiting microbial protein synthesis. *Ketolides* have a greater affinity for ribosomal RNA, expanding their antimicrobial spectrum compared with macrolides.

Indications for Use

The macrolides are widely used for treatment of respiratory tract and skin/soft tissue infections caused by streptococci and staphylococci. Erythromycin is also used as a penicillin substitute in patients who are allergic to penicillin; for prevention of rheumatic fever, gonorrhea, syphilis, pertussis, and chlamydial conjunctivitis in newborns (ophthalmic ointment); and to treat other infections (e.g., Legionnaire's disease, genitourinary infections caused by *Chlamydia trachomatis*, intestinal amebiasis caused by *Entamoeba histolytica*).

In addition, azithromycin is approved for treatment of urethritis and cervicitis caused by *C. trachomatis* organisms and is being used for the prevention and treatment of MAC disease. For acute bacterial sinusitis, azithromycin is approved for an abbreviated 3-day treatment duration.

Clarithromycin is approved for prevention and treatment of MAC disease. Clarithromycin is also approved to treat *H. pylori* infections associated with peptic ulcer disease.

The ketolide telithromycin is approved only for community-acquired pneumonia (including multidrug-resistant *S. pneumoniae*). The U.S. Food and Drug Administration (FDA) recently rescinded approval for two other indications, citing the risk of adverse effects (e.g., liver toxicity, loss of consciousness, and visual disturbances) outweighed the benefit of the medication.

Contraindications to Use

Macrolides and ketolides are contraindicated in people who have had hypersensitivity reactions. Telithromycin is contraindicated in people who have had hypersensitivity reactions to macrolides. All macrolides and telithromycin must be used with caution in patients with pre-existing liver disease. A **BLACK BOX WARNING** for erythromycin estolate and an FDA alert for telithromycin emphasizes the liver toxicity associated with these drugs. Use of erythromycin and telithromycin concurrently with drugs highly dependent on CYP3A4 liver enzymes for metabolism (e.g., pimozide) is contraindicated. The FDA has issued a **BLACK BOX WARNING** alerting health care professionals that telithromycin is contraindicated in patients with myasthenia gravis due to the potential for fatal and life-threatening respiratory failure.

Miscellaneous Antibacterial Drugs

Table 33-2 summarizes pertinent information about miscellaneous antibacterial drugs.

Table 33-2	**Drugs at a Glance: Miscellaneous Antibacterials**	
	ROUTES AND DOSAGE RANGES	
Generic/Trade Name	**Adults**	**Children**
Chloramphenicol (Chloromycetin)	IV 50–100 mg/kg/d in divided doses q6h (maximum dose 4 g/d)	Meningitis (infants older than 30 days and children): 50–100 mg/kg/d in divided doses q6h Other infections (infants older than 30 days and children): 50–75 mg/kg/d in divided doses q6h (maximum daily dose 4 g)
Clindamycin hydrochloride (Cleocin)	PO 150–450 mg q6–8h (maximum dose 1.8 g/d)	PO 8–16 mg/kg/d in divided doses q6–8h; up to 20 mg/kg/d in severe infections
Clindamycin phosphate (Cleocin phosphate)	IV, IM 1.2–1.8 g/d in 2–4 divided doses (maximum dose 4–8 g/d)	*Neonates:* 15–20 mg/kg/d in divided doses q6–8h

(continued on page 530)

Table 33-2	**Drugs at a Glance: Miscellaneous Antibacterials** (continued)	

	ROUTES AND DOSAGE RANGES	
Generic/Trade Name	**Adults**	**Children**
		1 mo and older: IM, IV 20–40 mg/kg/d in divided doses q6–8h; up to 40 mg/kg/d in severe infections
Clindamycin palmitate (Cleocin pediatric-75 mg/mL)		PO 8–25 mg/kg/d in divided doses q6–8h, the minimum dose is 37.5 mg q8h
Daptomycin (Cubicin)	Skin/soft tissue infections: IV 4 mg/kg q24h for 7–14 d MSSA, MRSA bacteremia or R-sided endo-carditis: 6 mg/kg/d for 2–6 wk	Dosage not established
Linezolid (Zyvox)	PO, IV 400–600 mg q12h for 10–28 d	*Neonates under 7 d:* PO, IV 10 mg/kg q12h *Children 7 d–11 y:* PO, IV 10 mg/kg q8h *12 y and older:* PO, IV 600 mg q12h
Metronidazole (Flagyl)	Anaerobic bacterial infection: PO, IV 500 mg q6–8h, not to exceed 4 g/d Surgical prophylaxis, colorectal surgery: IV 500 mg infused over 30–60 min within 0.5–1 h before surgery C. *difficile* colitis: PO 250–500 mg q6–8h for 10–14 d	Anaerobic infections in children *older than 7 d* and weighing 1200–2000 g: PO, IV 15 mg/kg/d in divided doses q12h Anaerobic infections in children *older than 7 d* and weighing *more than* 2000 g: 30 mg/kg/d in divided doses q12h *Children ≥ 1 mo:* PO 15–35 mg/kg/d in divided doses q8h; IV 30 mg/kg/d in divided doses q6h
Quinupristin-dalfopristin (Synercid)	IV 7.5 mg/kg over 60 min q12h for skin and skin-structure infections and q8h for VREF bacteremia	Same as adult Shunt infection due to VRE: 7.5 mg/kg/dose q8h
Rifaximin (Xifaxan)	PO 200 mg three times daily for 3 d	*12 y and older:* same as adult
Spectinomycin (Trobicin)	IM 2 g in a single dose (or 4 g in a single dose where antibiotic resistance is prevalent)	*45 kg and over:* Same as adult *under 45 kg:* IM 40 mg/kg single dose, maximum dose 2 g
Tigecycline (Tygacil)	IV 100 mg single dose initially; mainte-nance dose 50 mg q12h for 5–14 d	Dosage not established
Vancomycin (Vancocin)	Antibiotic-associated pseudomembranous colitis: PO 100–500 mg q6h (PO dose not for treating systemic infections) IV 20–45 mg/kg/d in divided doses (dose must be adjusted for renal impairment)	Antibiotic-associated pseudomembra-nous colitis: PO 40 mg/kg/d in divided doses q6–8h (PO dose not for treating systemic infections) *1 mo and older:* IV 10–15 mg/kg q6h

VREF, vancomycin-resistant Enterococcus faecium.

Chloramphenicol (Chloromycetin) is a broad-spectrum, bacteriostatic antibiotic that is active against most gram-positive and gram-negative bacteria, rickettsiae, chlamydiae, and treponemes. It acts by interfering with microbial protein synthesis. It is well absorbed and diffuses well into body tissues and fluids, including cerebrospinal fluid (CSF), but low drug levels are obtained in urine. It is metabolized in the liver and excreted in the urine.

Chloramphenicol is rarely used now to treat infections because of the effectiveness and low toxicity of alternative drugs. It is used in serious infections for which no adequate substitute drug is available. Specific infections include meningococcal, pneumococcal, or *Haemophilus meningitis* in penicillin-allergic patients; anaerobic brain abscess; *Bacteroides fragilis* infections; and rickettsial infections and brucellosis when tetracyclines are contraindicated. In infections due to vancomycin-resistant enterococci (*VRE*), chloramphenicol is effective against some strains. The FDA has issued a **BLACK BOX WARNING** reporting the development of serious and fatal blood dyscrasias with its use.

Clindamycin (Cleocin), a *lincosamide*, is similar to the macrolides in its mechanism of action and antimicrobial spectrum. Bacteriostatic in usual doses, it is effective against gram-positive cocci, including group A streptococci, pneumococci, most staphylococci, and some anaerobes such as *Bacteroides* and *Clostridia*. Clindamycin enters microbial cells and attaches to 50S subunits of ribosomes, thereby inhibiting microbial protein synthesis.

Clindamycin is often used to treat infections caused by *B. fragilis*. Because these bacteria are usually mixed with gram-negative organisms from the gynecologic or gastrointestinal (GI) tracts, clindamycin is usually given with another drug, such as an aminoglycoside or a fluoroquinolone, to treat mixed infections. The drug may be useful as a penicillin substitute in patients who are allergic to penicillin and who have serious streptococcal (including prevention of perinatal group B streptococcal disease), staphylococcal, or pneumococcal infections in which the causative organism is susceptible to clindamycin. A topical solution is used in the treatment of acne, and a vaginal cream is available. Clindamycin does not reach therapeutic concentrations in the central nervous system (CNS) and cannot be used for treating meningitis.

Clindamycin is well absorbed with oral administration and reaches peak plasma levels within 1 hour after a dose. It is widely distributed in body tissues and fluids, except CSF, and crosses the placenta. It is highly bound (90%) to plasma proteins. It is metabolized in the liver, and the metabolites are excreted in bile and urine. Dosage may need to be reduced in patients with severe hepatic failure to prevent accumulation and toxic effects. The FDA has issued a **BLACK BOX WARNING** for clindamycin reporting the development of severe colitis with its use that can be life-threatening.

Daptomycin (Cubicin) belongs to the *lipopeptide* class, a new class of antibiotics. It is a bactericidal agent effective only for gram-positive infections due to *Staphylococcus aureus* (including oxacillin-resistant strains), *Streptococcus pyogenes*, group B streptococci, and *Enterococcus faecalis* (vancomycin-susceptible strains only). In combination with gentamicin, daptomycin is synergistic in killing staphylococci and enterococci. Its mechanism of action is unique. The drug kills bacteria by inhibiting synthesis of bacterial proteins, DNA, and RNA. Indications are limited to the treatment of complicated skin and skin structure infections caused by the above organisms.

Available only for IV administration, the drug reaches target concentrations by the third daily dose. Daptomycin is excreted primarily by the kidneys. Information on use in children or during pregnancy and lactation is not known. Adverse musculoskeletal effects have been seen, primarily as increased serum creatine kinase (CK) levels. These effects are usually asymptomatic, but the drug should be discontinued in patients who develop muscle pain or weakness. The most common adverse effects are constipation, nausea, diarrhea, and vomiting.

Tigecycline (Tygacil) is a member of the *glycylcycline* class and is currently the only member in its class. Glycylcyclines are structurally related to tetracyclines and share many of their properties. Tigecycline binds to the 30S ribosomal subunit of susceptible bacteria, thus inhibiting protein synthesis. The drug is used for the treatment of complicated skin and skin structure infections caused by methicillin-resistant *Staphylococcus aureus* (MRSA) and vancomycin-sensitive *Enterococcus faecalis* as well as for treatment of complicated intra-abdominal infections. It is generally considered bacteriostatic and has demonstrated activity against a variety of gram-positive and gram-negative bacteria. Tigecycline is only administered intravenously. Because tigecycline is structurally similar to tetracycline, caution must be used in patients with prior hypersensitivity or severe adverse reactions associated with the use of tetracycline.

Tigecycline may be associated with antianabolic effects, pancreatitis, photosensitivity, pseudotumor cerebri, or superinfection. These potential adverse effects are due to structural similarities with tetracyclines. In addition, tigecycline may be associated with photosensitivity, and safety and efficacy has not been established in children younger than 18 years of age. The most common adverse effects appear to be gastrointestinal and include nausea, vomiting, and diarrhea. Others include hypertension, fever, headache, hypoproteinemia, abdominal pain, thrombocythemia, and increased liver enzymes. Use caution in patients with hepatic impairment. In severe impairment, a dosage adjustment may be necessary.

Linezolid (Zyvox) is a member of the *oxazolidinone* class, a newer class of antibiotics. It is active against aerobic gram-positive bacteria, in which it acts by inhibiting protein synthesis by a unique mechanism. Linezolid binds to the bacterial 23S ribosomal RNA of the 50S subunit, thus preventing an essential component of the bacterial translation process. The drug exhibits bactericidal activity against most staphylococci, enterococci, and streptococci. It is well absorbed orally, distributes widely, and undergoes hepatic elimination. Its effects in pregnancy and in children are largely unknown.

Linezolid is indicated for pneumonia (both community acquired and nosocomial), complicated and uncomplicated skin and skin structure infections, and vancomycin-resistant *Enterococcus faecium* (VREF) infections. The drug is bacteriostatic against enterococci (including *E. faecalis* and *E. faecium*) and staphylococci (including methicillin-resistant strains) and bactericidal for most streptococci.

Myelosuppression (e.g., anemia, leukopenia, pancytopenia, thrombocytopenia) is a serious adverse effect that may occur with prolonged therapy over 2 weeks. The patient's complete blood count should be monitored; if myelosuppression occurs, linezolid should be discontinued. Myelosuppression usually improves with drug discontinuation. Pseudomembranous colitis may also occur. Mild cases usually resolve with drug discontinuation; moderate or severe cases may require fluid and electrolyte replacement and an antibacterial drug that is effective against *Clostridium difficile* organisms. Hypertension may occur with the concomitant ingestion of linezolid and adrenergic drugs (e.g., dopamine, epinephrine). Patients receiving linezolid and selective serotonin reuptake inhibitors

(SSRIs) may be at risk for serotonin syndrome, characterized by fever and cognitive dysfunction. Because linezolid is a weak monoamine oxidase (MAO) inhibitor, patients should avoid food high in tyramine content (aged cheeses, fermented or air-dried meats, sauerkraut, soy sauce, tap beers, red wine) while taking the drug. An FDA alert (2007) noted an increased rate of deaths among individuals treated with linezolid for catheter-related bacteremia and catheter site infections and emphasized that linezolid is not approved for site infections or bacteremia due to catheters or for gram negative infections.

Metronidazole (Flagyl) is effective against anaerobic bacteria, including gram-negative bacilli such as *Bacteroides*, gram-positive bacilli such as *Clostridia*, and some gram-positive cocci. It is also effective against protozoa that cause amebiasis, giardiasis, and trichomoniasis (see Chap. 37). Metronidazole achieves therapeutic concentrations in body fluids and tissues and can be used to treat anaerobic brain abscesses. It is eliminated by the liver and kidneys.

Clinical indications for use include prevention or treatment of anaerobic bacterial infections (e.g., in colorectal surgery, intra-abdominal infections) and treatment of *C. difficile* infections associated with pseudomembranous colitis. As part of a combination regimen, it is also useful in treatment of infections due to *H. pylori*. It is contraindicated during the first trimester of pregnancy and must be used with caution in patients with CNS or blood disorders.

Quinupristin-dalfopristin (Synercid) belongs to a class of antimicrobials referred to as *streptogramins*. Both components are active antimicrobials that affect bacterial ribosomes to decrease protein synthesis. The combination is bacteriostatic against *E. faecium* (including vancomycin-resistant strains) and bactericidal against methicillin-susceptible strains of *S. aureus* (MSSA). It is not active against *E. faecalis*. The combination undergoes biliary excretion and fecal elimination.

Quinupristin-dalfopristin is indicated for skin and skin structure infections caused by *S. aureus* or group A streptococcus. It is also used for treatment of patients with serious or life-threatening infections associated with VREF bacteremia; however, a **BLACK BOX WARNING** reports that FDA approval for this use is based on the ability of the drug to clear bacteria from the bloodstream rather than its ability to cure the underlying infection. Further clinical studies are underway to verify the clinical benefits of quinupristin-dalfopristin for curing VREF infections.

Quinupristin-dalfopristin is a strong inhibitor of cytochrome P450 3A4 enzymes and therefore interferes with the metabolism of drugs such as cyclosporine, antiretrovirals, carbamazepine, and many others. Toxicity may occur with the inhibited drugs.

Rifaximin (Xifaxan) is a structural analog of rifampin. It is used in infectious (travelers') diarrhea due to *Escherichia coli* but is not effective in diarrhea due to *Campylobacter jejuni* (see Chap. 61). It is not known whether rifaximin is effective to treat diarrhea due to *Shigella* or *Salmonella* species. Because of its very limited systemic absorption (97% eliminated in feces),

rifaximin cannot be used to treat systemic infections, including infections due to invasive strains of *E. coli*. Therefore, diarrhea occurring with fever or bloody stools should be treated with alternative agents. After treatment with rifaximin is started, patients reporting worsening or persistent diarrhea for longer than 24 to 48 hours, fever, or blood in the stool should be treated with an alternative agent.

Spectinomycin (Trobicin) is used for treatment of gonococcal exposure or infection in people who are allergic to or unable to take the preferred regimen. It may be used during pregnancy when patients cannot tolerate cephalosporins. Spectinomycin has no activity against infections caused by *Chlamydia* organisms, which often accompany gonorrhea. Therefore, spectinomycin should be followed by adequate chlamydial treatment.

Vancomycin (Vancocin) is active only against gram-positive microorganisms. It acts by inhibiting cell wall synthesis. Parenteral vancomycin has been used extensively to treat infections caused by methicillin-resistant *S. aureus* (MRSA) and methicillin-resistant staphylococcal species non-aureus (SSNA, including *Staphylococcus epidermidis*) and endocarditis caused by *Streptococcus viridans* (in patients allergic to or with infections resistant to penicillins and cephalosporins) or *E. faecalis* (with an aminoglycoside).

S. pneumoniae remain susceptible to vancomycin, although vancomycin-tolerant strains have been identified. The drug has also been widely used for prophylaxis of gram-positive infections in patients who are at high risk of developing MRSA infections (e.g., those with diabetes, previous hospitalization, or MRSA in their nasal passages) and who require placement of long-term intravascular catheters and other invasive treatment or monitoring devices. Oral vancomycin is used only to treat staphylococcal enterocolitis and pseudomembranous colitis caused by *C. difficile*.

Partly because of this widespread use, VRE are being encountered more often, especially in critical care units, and treatment options for infections caused by these organisms are limited. To decrease the spread of VRE, the Centers for Disease Control and Prevention (CDC) recommend limiting the use of vancomycin. Specific recommendations include avoiding or minimizing use in empiric treatment of febrile patients with neutropenia (unless the prevalence of MRSA or SSNA is high), in initial treatment for *C. difficile* colitis (metronidazole is preferred), and as prophylaxis for surgery, low birth weight infants, intravascular catheter colonization or infection, and peritoneal dialysis.

For systemic infections, vancomycin is given IV and reaches therapeutic plasma levels within 1 hour after infusion. It is very important to give IV infusions slowly, over 1 to 2 hours, to avoid an adverse reaction characterized by hypotension, flushing, and skin rash. This reaction, sometimes called "*red man syndrome*," is attributed to histamine release. Vancomycin is excreted through the kidneys; dosage should be reduced in the presence of renal impairment. For bacterial colitis, vancomycin is given orally because it is not absorbed from the GI tract and acts within the bowel lumen. Large amounts of vancomycin are excreted in the feces after oral administration.

Nursing Process

Assessment

- Assess for infections that macrolides, ketolides, and the designated miscellaneous drugs are used to prevent or treat.
- Assess each patient for signs and symptoms of the specific current infection.
- Assess culture and susceptibility reports when available.
- Assess each patient for risk factors that increase risks of infection (e.g., immunosuppression) or risks of adverse drug reactions (e.g., impaired renal or hepatic function).

Nursing Diagnoses

- Deficient Knowledge related to type of infection and appropriate use of prescribed antimicrobial drugs
- Risk for Injury related to adverse drug effects
- Risk for Injury related to infection with antibiotic-resistant microorganisms

Planning/Goals

The patient will

- Take or receive macrolides, ketolides, and miscellaneous antimicrobials accurately, for the prescribed length of time
- Experience decreased signs and symptoms of the infection being treated
- Be monitored regularly for therapeutic and adverse drug effects
- Verbalize and practice measures to prevent recurrent infection

Interventions

- Use measures to prevent and minimize the spread of infection (see Chap. 29).
- Monitor for fever and other signs and symptoms of infection.
- Monitor laboratory reports for indications of the patient's response to drug therapy (e.g., white blood cell count [WBC], tests of renal function).
- Encourage fluid intake to decrease fever and maintain good urinary tract function.
- Provide foods and fluids with adequate nutrients to maintain or improve nutritional status, especially if febrile and hypermetabolic.
- Assist patients to prevent or minimize infections with streptococci, staphylococci, and other gram-positive organisms.
- Provide appropriate patient teaching for any drug therapy (see accompanying display).

Evaluation

- Interview and observe for improvement in the infection being treated.
- Interview and observe for adverse drug effects.

Applying Your Knowledge 33-1

What instructions should be given to Mr. Nikki with regard to drug–food or drug–drug interactions for him to accurately self-administer the azithromycin?

Principles of Therapy

Culture and Susceptibility Studies

Culture and susceptibility reports and local susceptibility patterns should be reviewed to determine if an antibiotic-resistant pathogen is present in the patient. This is particularly important before starting vancomycin, quinupristin-dalfopristin, daptomycin, or linezolid. These drugs have relatively narrow spectra of activity and appropriate indications for their use should be observed to decrease the likelihood of resistance.

Effects of Macrolides on Other Drugs

Erythromycin is metabolized by the cytochrome P450 3A4 isoenzymes in the liver. It interacts with other drugs metabolized by the same isoenzyme and interferes with the elimination of several drugs. As a result, the affected drugs are eliminated more slowly, their serum levels are increased, and they are more likely to cause adverse effects and toxicity unless dosage is reduced. Erythromycin in combination with potent inhibitors of CYP3A4 (e.g., fluconazole, diltiazem) increases the risk of sudden cardiac death. A partial list of other interacting drugs includes carbamazepine (Tegretol), cyclosporine (Sandimmune), digoxin (Lanoxin), disopyramide (Norpace), lopinavir-ritonavir (Kaletra), lovastatin (Mevacor), nevirapine (Viramune), pimozide (Orap), quinidine, rifampin (Rifadin), ritonavir (Norvir), simvastatin (Zocor), theophylline (Theo-Dur), triazolam (Halcion), and warfarin (Coumadin). These drugs represent a variety of drug classes.

Although they are less potent inhibitors of CYP3A than erythromycin, clarithromycin and telithromycin also interact with many of these drugs. Azithromycin is not a potent inhibitor of the CYP3A4 isoenzyme and is less prone to drug–drug interactions. However, caution should be used with all these agents.

Preventing Toxicity

Chloramphenicol

Blood dyscrasias (potentially serious and life-threatening) have occurred in patients taking chloramphenicol. The FDA has

Patient Teaching Guidelines | Macrolides and Ketolides

General Considerations

■ Complete the full course of drug therapy. The fastest and most complete relief of infections occurs with accurate usage of antibiotics. Moreover, inaccurate use may cause other, potentially more severe, infections.

■ These drugs are often given for infections of the respiratory tract or skin (e.g., bronchitis, pneumonia, cellulitis). Good hand hygiene can help prevent the development and spread of these infections.

■ Report symptoms of infection that recur or develop during antibiotic therapy. Such symptoms can indicate recurrence of the original infection (i.e., the antibiotic is not effective because it is the wrong drug or wrong dosage for the infection or it is not being taken accurately) or a new infection with antibiotic-resistant bacteria or fungi.

■ Report nausea, vomiting, diarrhea, abdominal cramping or pain, yellow discoloration of the skin or eyes (jaundice), dark urine, pale stools, or unusual tiredness. These symptoms may indicate liver damage, which sometimes occurs with these drugs.

■ Telithromycin (Ketek) may cause loss of consciousness and interfere with accommodation, resulting in visual disturbances such as blurred vision, difficulty focusing, and diplopia. This often occurs with the first or second dose. Caution should be used while driving, operating machinery, or engaging in other potentially hazardous activities. Report loss of consciousness or visual disturbances to your health care provider.

Self-Administration

■ Take each dose with 6 to 8 ounces of water, at evenly spaced time intervals, preferably around the clock.

■ With erythromycin, ask a health care provider if not instructed when to take the drug in relation to food. Erythromycin is available in several preparations. Some should be taken on an empty stomach (at least 1 hour before or 2 hours after meals) or may be taken with a small amount of food if gastrointestinal upset occurs. Some preparations may be taken without regard to meals.

■ Take azithromycin (Zithromax) tablets and oral suspension without regard to meals. Do not take with an antacid. Azithromycin ER should be taken on an empty stomach.

■ Take clarithromycin (Biaxin) regular tablets and the oral suspension without regard to meals. Take extended-release tablets (Biaxin XL) with food. With the oral suspension, do not refrigerate and shake well before measuring the dose.

■ Take telithromycin (Ketek) without regard to meals.

issued a **BLACK BOX WARNING** regarding this adverse effect. Irreversible bone marrow depression, which may lead to aplastic anemia, may appear weeks or months after therapy. A dose-related reversible bone marrow depression usually responds to discontinuation of the drug. Patients should be monitored with a complete blood count, platelet count, reticulocyte count, and serum iron test every 2 days. In addition, periodic measurements of serum drug levels are recommended when possible. Therapeutic levels are 5 to 20 micrograms per milliliter. Therapy should be discontinued as soon as possible, and the drug should not be used for trivial infections or for prophylaxis of infections. During therapy, it is recommended that the patient be hospitalized to facilitate close monitoring.

Clindamycin

If diarrhea develops in a patient receiving clindamycin, the drug should be stopped. The FDA has issued a **BLACK BOX WARNING** regarding the potential for severe and possible fatal colitis. If the diarrhea is severe and persistent, stools should be checked for WBCs, blood, mucus, and the presence of C. *difficile* toxin. Sigmoidoscopy can be done to more definitively determine whether the patient has pseudomembranous colitis, a potentially fatal adverse reaction. If lesions are seen on sigmoidoscopy, the drug should be stopped immediately. Although pseudomembranous colitis may occur with any antibiotic, it has often been associated with clindamycin therapy.

Applying Your Knowledge 33-2

Juro Nikki returns to the office with severe diarrhea and a fever. He is diagnosed with pseudomembranous colitis. His stool is positive for C. *difficile* secondary to antibiotic therapy. He is prescribed metronidazole 500 mg PO three times a day for 7 days. What adverse effects should you assess for in a patient receiving metronidazole?

Daptomycin

Unexplained increases in serum CK levels associated with symptoms of myopathy should prompt discontinuation of daptomycin. Concurrent use of daptomycin with other drugs that might produce rhabdomyolysis (e.g., statin cholesterol-lowering drug) may increase the risk of musculoskeletal toxicity. If possible, these drugs should not be used concomitantly.

Use in Special Populations

Use in Children

Erythromycin is usually considered safe for treatment of infections caused by susceptible organisms. Azithromycin and clarithromycin are used in young children for some infections (e.g., pharyngitis/tonsillitis, acute otitis media). Safety and effectiveness of telithromycin have not been established for children.

Dosage of chloramphenicol must be reduced in premature infants and in full-term infants less than 2 weeks of age because immature metabolism may lead to accumulation and adverse effects, including fatalities ("*gray syndrome*").

Clindamycin should be given to neonates and infants only if clearly indicated, and then liver and kidney function must be monitored. Diarrhea and pseudomembranous colitis may occur with topical clindamycin for treatment of acne. The safety and efficacy of metronidazole have been established in children only for the treatment of amebiasis, although the drug is used for other infections in pediatric patients without reported unusual adverse effects. Linezolid and vancomycin are used in children, including premature and full-term neonates, for the same indications as in adults. Monitoring serum drug levels is recommended with IV vancomycin.

With the newer drugs, such as daptomycin, quinupristin-dalfopristin, and rifaximin, there has been little or no experience with their use in children, and pediatric dosages have not been identified.

Use in Older Adults

Erythromycin is generally considered safe. Because it is metabolized in the liver and excreted in bile, it may be an alternative in patients with impaired renal function. Dosage reductions are not indicated with azithromycin and telithromycin but may be needed if clarithromycin is given to older adults with severe renal impairment. Dosage of vancomycin should be adjusted for impaired renal function in older adults as in other age groups.

Daptomycin, quinupristin-dalfopristin, and linezolid do not require dosage adjustment in older adults. The miscellaneous antibacterial drugs are used in older adults for the same indications as in younger adults.

Use in Patients With Renal Impairment

With the macrolides, dosage of erythromycin and azithromycin do not require reduction in renal impairment. However, clarithromycin dosage should be halved or the dosing interval doubled in patients with severe renal impairment (creatinine clearance [CrCl] < 30 mL/min). The dose of telithromycin for patients with severe renal impairment or those on dialysis has not been established.

Chloramphenicol concentrations may increase in patients with impaired renal function. Doses should be adjusted and serum levels monitored during therapy.

Dosage of clindamycin does not need reduction in renal impairment because it is excreted primarily by the liver. Daptomycin dosage should be reduced to every 48 hours in patients with CrCl of less than 30 milliliters per minute and in those undergoing dialysis. Dosage of vancomycin should be reduced because it is excreted mainly by the kidneys and accumulates in renal impairment. In addition, vancomycin may be nephrotoxic with IV administration, high serum concentrations, prolonged therapy, use in older adults or neonates, and concomitant use of other nephrotoxic drugs. Thus, in addition to reduced dosage, renal function and serum drug levels should

be monitored (therapeutic levels are 10–25 mcg/mL). Dosage of metronidazole, quinupristin-dalfopristin, and linezolid does not need to be reduced in patients with renal failure. The use of rifaximin in renal failure has not been studied.

Use in Patients With Hepatic Impairment

Erythromycin should be used cautiously, if at all, in patients with hepatic impairment. It is metabolized in the liver to an active metabolite that is excreted in the bile. Avoiding the drug or dosage reduction may be needed in liver failure. It has also been associated with cholestatic hepatitis. Symptoms, which may include nausea, vomiting, fever, and jaundice, usually occur after 1 to 2 weeks of drug administration and subside when the drug is stopped.

Other macrolides vary in their hepatic effects. Azithromycin is mainly eliminated unchanged in bile and could accumulate with impaired liver function, but dosage recommendations have not been established. It should be used with caution. Clarithromycin is metabolized in the liver to an active metabolite that is then excreted through the kidneys. Dosage reduction is not recommended for patients with hepatic impairment. The ketolide, telithromycin, does not need dosage adjustment in liver disease.

Clindamycin, chloramphenicol, and metronidazole should be used cautiously, if at all, in the presence of liver disease. Because these drugs are eliminated through the liver, they may accumulate and cause toxic effects. When feasible, other drugs should be substituted. If no effective substitutes are available, dosage should be reduced. Tigecycline should be adjusted in patients with severe hepatic impairment, and liver enzymes should be monitored closely. With daptomycin, quinupristin-dalfopristin, rifaximin, and linezolid, there are currently no recommendations to alter dosage in hepatic impairment.

Applying Your Knowledge 33-3

A common adverse reaction to many drugs is hepatotoxicity. This may occur with the administration of macrolides. What signs and symptoms should you teach the patient to monitor for and report to his primary care provider?

Use in Patients With Critical Illness

Erythromycin is seldom used in critical care settings, partly because broader spectrum bactericidal drugs are usually needed in critically ill patients and partly because it inhibits liver metabolism and slows elimination of several other drugs. For a critically ill patient who needs a macrolide antibiotic, one of the newer macrolides is preferred because they have broader spectra of antibacterial activity and fewer effects on the metabolism of other drugs.

Clindamycin should be used only when necessary (i.e., for serious infections caused by susceptible anaerobes) because critically ill patients may develop hepatic impairment and pseudomembranous colitis (also called antibiotic-associated colitis). These patients are at high risk for development of pseudomembranous colitis (the FDA has issued a **BLACK BOX WARNING**) because they often receive aggressive antibiotic therapy with multiple or broad-spectrum antibacterial drugs that destroy normal bowel microorganisms. Metronidazole is often used in critically ill patients with mixed infections. These patients are at risk for drug toxicity from accumulation of active metabolites. Vancomycin penetrates tissues well in critically ill patients and achieves therapeutic levels well above the minimum inhibitory concentration (MIC) for most staphylococci and enterococci. Plasma drug levels and renal function should be monitored. Although usually given by IV infusion, vancomycin is given orally to treat pseudomembranous colitis.

Quinupristin-dalfopristin, daptomycin, and linezolid are often used in critically ill patients because infections with resistant pathogens commonly occur in this population.

Use in Home Care

Most of the macrolides, telithromycin, and miscellaneous antibacterial drugs may be taken in the home setting. The role of the home care nurse is generally the same as with other antibiotic therapy; that is, the nurse may need to teach patients or caregivers about drug administration and expected effects. For patients taking oral metronidazole or vancomycin for pseudomembranous colitis, stool specimens may need to be collected and tested in the laboratory for the presence of C. *difficile* organisms or toxins.

Nursing Actions | Macrolides, Ketolides, and Miscellaneous Antibacterials

NURSING ACTIONS	RATIONALE/EXPLANATION
1. Administer accurately	
a. Give oral erythromycin preparations according to manufacturers' instructions, with 6–8 ounces of water, at evenly spaced intervals, around the clock.	Some should be taken on an empty stomach; some can be taken without regard to meals. Adequate water aids absorption; regular intervals help to maintain therapeutic blood levels.
b. With azithromycin, give the tablets or oral suspension without regard to meals. Give Azithromycin ER on an empty stomach. Do not give oral azithromycin with aluminum- or magnesium-containing antacids.	Antacids decrease absorption of tablets and the suspension.
c. With clarithromycin, give regular tablets and the oral suspension with or without food. Give the extended-release tablets (Biaxin XL) with food. Shake the suspension well before measuring the dose.	Manufacturer's recommendations All suspensions should be mixed well to measure accurately.
d. With telithromycin, give without regard to meals.	
e. For intravenous (IV) erythromycin, consult the manufacturer's instructions for dissolving, diluting, and administering the drug. Infuse continuously or intermittently (e.g., q6h over 30–60 min).	The IV formulation has limited stability in solution, and instructions must be followed carefully to achieve therapeutic effects. Also, instructions differ for intermittent and continuous infusions. IV erythromycin is the treatment of choice for Legionnaire's disease. Otherwise, it is rarely used.
f. With chloramphenicol:	
(1) Mix IV chloramphenicol in 50–100 milliliters of 5% dextrose in water and infuse over 15–30 minutes.	Do not administer intramuscularly (IM).
g. With clindamycin:	
(1) Give capsules with a full glass of water.	To avoid esophageal irritation
(2) Do not refrigerate reconstituted oral solution.	Refrigeration thickens the solution, making it difficult to measure and pour accurately.
(3) Give IM injections deeply, and rotate sites. Do not give more than 600 milligrams in a single injection.	To decrease pain, induration, and abscess formation
(4) For IV administration, dilute 300–600 milligrams in 50 milliliters of IV fluid and give over 10–20 minutes, or dilute 900 milligrams in 50–100 milliliters and give over 20 minutes. *Do not* give clindamycin undiluted or by direct injection.	Dilution decreases risks of phlebitis. Cardiac arrest has been reported with bolus injections of clindamycin.
h. With daptomycin:	
(1) Mix with normal saline or lactated Ringer's IV solution only.	The drug is incompatible with dextrose-containing IV solutions.
(2) Infuse over 30 minutes.	
i. With linezolid:	
(1) Give oral tablets and suspension without regard to meals.	Manufacturer's recommendations

NURSING ACTIONS	RATIONALE/EXPLANATION
(2) For IV administration, the drug is compatible with 5% dextrose, 0.9% sodium chloride, and lactated Ringer's solutions.	Note: Yellow color of infusion may intensify over time; however, this does not affect potency of medication.
(3) Infuse the drug over 30–120 minutes. If other drugs are being given through the same IV line, flush the line with one of the above solutions before and after linezolid administration.	
j. With IV metronidazole, check the manufacturer's instructions.	The drug requires specific techniques for preparation and administration.
k. With quinupristin-dalfopristin:	
(1) Give IV, mixed in a minimum of 250 milliliters of 5% dextrose solution and infused over 60 minutes.	Dilution in at least 250 milliliters of IV solution decreases venous irritation. A central venous catheter may also be used for drug administration to decrease irritation. Toxicity may increase with shorter infusion times.
(2) Do *not* mix the drug or flush the IV line with saline- or heparin-containing solutions.	The drug is incompatible with saline- and heparin-containing solutions.
l. Give rifaximin without regard to meals.	
m. With spectinomycin, administer by deep IM injection in upper outer quadrant of the gluteal muscle.	
n. With tigecycline infuse IV over 30–60 min. Flush line before and after administration with 0.9 NaCl injection or 5% dextrose injection.	Manufacturers recommendations
o. With vancomycin, dilute 500-milligram doses in 100 milliliters, and 1-gram doses in 200 milliliters of 0.9% NaCl or 5% dextrose injection and infuse over at least 60 minutes.	To decrease hypotension and flushing (i.e., "red man syndrome") that may occur with more rapid IV administration. This reaction is attributed to histamine release and may be prevented by prior administration of diphenhydramine, an antihistamine, or decreased rate of infusion. Dilution also decreases pain and phlebitis at the injection site.
2. Observe for therapeutic effects	See Chapter 29.
a. Decreased local and systemic signs of infection	
b. Decreased signs and symptoms of the specific infection for which the drug is being given	
3. Observe for adverse effects	
a. With macrolides and ketolides:	
(1) Nausea, vomiting, diarrhea	These are the most frequent adverse reactions, reportedly less common with azithromycin, clarithromycin, and telithromycin than with erythromycin.
(2) With IV erythromycin, phlebitis at the IV infusion site	The drug is very irritating to body tissues. Phlebitis can be minimized by diluting the drug well, infusing it slowly, and not using the same vein more than 48–72 hours, if possible.
(3) Hepatotoxicity—nausea, vomiting, abdominal cramps, fever, leukocytosis, abnormal liver function, cholestatic jaundice	More likely to occur with the estolate formulation of erythromycin; less likely to occur with the newer macrolides and ketolides than with erythromycin
(4) Allergic reactions—anaphylaxis, skin rash, urticaria	Potentially serious but infrequent
b. With chloramphenicol:	
(1) Bone marrow depression—anemia, leukopenia, thrombocytopenia	Blood dyscrasias are the most serious adverse reaction to chloramphenicol.
(2) Clinical signs of infection or bleeding	
c. With clindamycin:	
(1) Nausea, vomiting, diarrhea	These are the most frequent adverse effects and may be severe enough to require stopping the drug.
(2) Pseudomembranous colitis (also *called antibiotic- associated colitis*)—severe diarrhea, fever, stools containing neutrophils and shreds of mucous membrane	May occur with most antibiotics but is more common with oral clindamycin. It is caused by *Clostridium difficile*. The organism produces a toxin that kills mucosal cells and produces superficial ulcerations that are visible with sigmoidoscopy. Discontinuing the drug and giving oral metronidazole are curative measures. Do not give antidiarrheal medications.
d. With daptomycin:	
(1) Increases in serum creatine kinase, muscle pain or weakness	Daptomycin discontinuation may be warranted.

(continued on page 538)

Nursing Actions Macrolides, Ketolides, and Miscellaneous Antibacterials (continued)

NURSING ACTIONS	RATIONALE/EXPLANATION
e. With linezolid:	
(1) Nausea, vomiting, diarrhea	These are common effects.
(2) Bone marrow depression—anemia, leukopenia, thrombocytopenia (especially when used > 2wk)	Complete blood counts (CBCs) are recommended weekly to monitor for myelosuppression. If it occurs, the drug should be discontinued.
(3) Fever, cognitive dysfunction	Serotonin syndrome may occur if linezolid is taken in presence of SSRIs or tyramine containing foods.
f. With metronidazole:	
(1) Central nervous system effects—convulsive seizures, peripheral paresthesias, ataxia, confusion, dizziness, headache	Convulsions and peripheral neuropathy may be serious effects.
(2) GI effects—nausea, vomiting, diarrhea, unpleasant metallic taste. Disulfram (Antabuse) reaction with alcohol.	GI effects are most common. Disulfram reaction symptoms include flushing, headache, nausea, vomiting, chest/abdominal pain.
(3) Dermatologic effects—skin rash, pruritus, thrombophlebitis at infusion sites	
g. With quinupristin-dalfopristin:	
(1) IV infusion site reactions—pain, edema, inflammation	The most common adverse effects during clinical trials. Moderate to severe venous irritation can occur with administration through peripheral veins. This can be prevented by infusion through a central venous IV line.
(2) Nausea, vomiting, diarrhea	These effects occurred in 2.7%–4.6% of subjects in clinical trials. Most other adverse effects occurred in fewer than 1% of subjects.
h. With rifaximin:	
(1) Flatulence, headache, abdominal pain, nausea, constipation, vomiting	Occurred in ≥ 2% of subjects in clinical trials; however, with exeption of headache, symptom occurence was less than placebo group.
i. With vancomycin:	
(1) Nephrotoxicity—oliguria, increased blood urea nitrogen and serum creatinine	Most likely to occur with large doses, concomitant administration of an aminoglycoside antibiotic, or pre-existing renal impairment. Usually resolves when vancomycin is discontinued.
(2) Ototoxicity—hearing loss, tinnitus	Most likely to occur in people with renal impairment or a pre-existing hearing loss
(3) "Red man syndrome"—hypotension, skin flushing	Occurs with rapid infusion of IV vancomycin. Can be prevented by adequate dilution and infusing over 1–2 hours or premedicating with diphenhydramine (an antihistamine).
4. Observe for drug interactions	
a. Drugs that *increase* effects of erythromycin:	
(1) Chloramphenicol	The combination is effective against some strains of resistant *Staphylococcus aureus*.
(2) Streptomycin	The combination is effective against the enterococcus in bacteremia, brain abscess, endocarditis, meningitis, and urinary tract infection.
(3) Drugs that prolong the QT interval (e.g., cisapride, dofetilide, phenothiazines, pimozide, ranolazine)	May result in life-threatening dysrhythmias when taken with erythromycin.
b. Drugs that *increase* effects of clarithromycin:	
(1) Atazanavir, delavirdine, fluconazole, lopinavir, omeprazole, ritonavir, saquinavir	Inhibits metabolism of clarithromycin; dosage reductions of clarithromycin sometimes recommended.
c. Drugs that *decrease* effects of clarithromycin:	
(1) Efavirenz, nevirapine	Consider alternatives to clarithromycin.
d. Drugs that *decrease* effects of azithromycin:	
(1) Antacids	Antacids decrease peak serum levels.
e. Drugs that *decrease* effects of telithromycin:	
(1) Phenytoin, carbamazepine, phenobarbital, rifampin	Decrease in telithromycin levels may result, with loss of antibacterial effect.
f. Drugs that *decrease* effects of chloramphenicol:	
(1) Enzyme inducers (e.g., rifampin, phenobarbital)	Reduce serum levels, probably by accelerating liver metabolism of chloramphenicol

NURSING ACTIONS	RATIONALE/EXPLANATION
g. Drug that *decreases* effects of clindamycin: (1) Erythromycin	Delays absorptiom
h. Drugs that *increase* effects of daptomycin: (1) HMG-CoA reductase inhibitors (e.g., statin cholesterol-lowering drugs)	Potential to increase the musculoskeletal adverse effects of daptomycin
i. Drug that *increases* effects of metronidazole: (1) Cimetidine	Inhibits hepatic metabolism of metronidazole
j. Drugs that *decrease* effects of metronidazole: (1) Enzyme inducers (phenobarbital, phenytoin, prednisone, rifampin)	These drugs induce hepatic enzymes and decrease effects of metronidazole by accelerating its rate of hepatic metabolism.

Key Concepts

■ Macrolides, which include erythromycin, azithromycin and clarithromycin, inhibit microbial protein synthesis.

■ Erythromycin shares a similar antibacterial spectrum with penicillin, making it a good choice for patients with penicillin allergy.

■ The ketolide, telithromycin, is approved only for community-acquired pneumonia. Its mechanism of action is inhibition of microbial protein synthesis.

■ The ketolide, telithromycin, and a macrolide, erythromycin estolate, can cause severe liver injury.

■ Telithromycin is contraindicated in patients with myasthenia gravis due to the potential for fatal and life-threatening respiratory failure.

■ Chloramphenicol (Chloromycetin) is rarely used due to the possible development of serious and fatal blood dyscrasias with its use. It is effective against some strains of VRE.

■ Clindamycin belongs to the lincosamide class of antimicrobials, similar to macrolides in its mechanism of action and antimicrobial spectrum. A life-threatening adverse effect of clindamycin is the development of pseudomembranous colitis.

■ Daptomycin belongs to the lipopeptide class of antibiotics, which kills gram-positive bacteria by inhibiting synthesis of bacterial proteins, DNA, and RNA.

■ Tigecycline belongs to the glycylcycline class of antibiotics. It is similar to tetracycline in structure and properties and can be used to treat skin infections due to MRSA.

■ Linezolid belongs to the oxazolidinone class of antibiotics. It is effective against MRSA and VRE.

■ Quinupristin-dalfopristin belongs to the streptogramin class of antibiotics. It is indicated for VREF and MSSA.

■ Vancomycin is effective against gram-positive organisms only, including MRSA and SSNA.

■ Rifaximin is prescribed for travelers' diarrhea due to *Escherichia coli* infection.

■ Spectinomycin is an alternative treatment for gonococcal infection when patients are unable to take the preferred regime.

■ Metronidazole is effective against infections with anaerobic bacteria and some protozoa.

Review and Application Exercises

Short Answer Exercises

1. Why is erythromycin called a "penicillin substitute"?

2. What are adverse effects with erythromycin, and how may they be prevented or minimized?

3. How do the newer macrolides differ from erythromycin?

4. How does the ketolide differ from the macrolides?

5. How would you recognize pseudomembranous colitis in a patient? What would you do if you thought a patient might have it? Why?

6. Why is metronidazole preferred over vancomycin for initial treatment of pseudomembranous colitis?

7. Which antibacterial drug is considered the drug of choice for MRSA and SSNA?

8. What is "red man syndrome" and how can it be prevented or minimized?

9. What is the main clinical importance of the newer drugs, tigecycline, linezolid, daptomycin, rifaximin, and quinupristin-dalfopristin?

NCLEX-Style Questions

10. A 35-year-old man with HIV/AIDS is being seen for routine follow-up care. He is receiving highly active antiretroviral therapy (HAART). The patient was recently

hospitalized with an infection due to *Mycobacterium avium-intracellulare* (formerly known as *Mycobacterium avium* complex, or MAC) disease, and the physician now decides to place the patient on a preventive regimen. The best choice of drug would be

a. erythromycin

b. clarithromycin

c. azithromycin

d. telithromycin

11. A 19-year-old college student was seen in the student health center for severe diarrhea. The nurse practitioner diagnosed travelers' diarrhea based on the history given that the student had recently returned from Mexico. Rifaximin 200 mg orally three times daily for 3 days was prescribed. The student calls the office 4 days later and reports to the nurse that she has a fever and that the diarrhea has not resolved. The nurse should

a. Advise the student to return to the clinic for further tests and a different antibiotic.

b. Call the pharmacy and authorize one refill of rifaximin.

c. Advise the student that it takes up to 48 to 72 hours after the completion of treatment for the diarrhea to completely resolve.

d. Tell the student to continue to drink plenty of fluids and report back in 24 hours.

12. An 89-year-old man is admitted to the hospital from a nursing home with the diagnosis of pneumonia. The most likely pathogen is *Staphylococcus aureus*. He is also in acute renal failure with an estimated creatine clearance of 20 mL/min. Which of the following regimens would not require dosage adjustment because of the renal failure?

a. vancomycin + azithromycin

b. quinupristin-dalfopristin + azithromycin

c. daptomycin + telithromycin

d. linezolid + clarithromycin

13. A recent nurse graduate is preparing to administer vancomycin IV to a patient. She states the patient reported that he experienced flushing with his last dose of vancomycin. The nurse should

a. Infuse the vancomycin over 30 minutes to decrease the chance of a reaction.

b. Hold the vancomycin dose until the physician's rounds the following morning.

c. Dilute the vancomycin in 50 mL of normal saline solution and infuse over 60 minutes.

d. Contact the physician, report the reaction, and request an order for diphenhydramine pretreatment.

14. A patient is started on clarithromycin extended-release tablets (Biaxin XL) 500 mg every 24 hours for 7 days. The teaching plan for this patient should not include telling him to

a. Complete the full 7 days of treatment.

b. Perform thorough hand hygiene to decrease spread of infection.

c. Contact the physician if a rash, jaundice, or diarrhea develops.

d. Take on an empty stomach.

Selected References

Corwin, E. J. (2006). *Handbook of pathophysiology* (3rd ed.). Philadelphia: Lippincott Williams & Wilkins.

Cunha, B.A. (2006). New uses for older antibiotics: nitrofurantoin, amikacin, colistin, polymyxin B, doxycycline, and minocycline revisited. *Medical Clinics of North America, 90*, 1089–1107.

Doern, G. V. (2006). Macrolides and ketolides resistance with *Streptococcus pneumoniae. Medical Clinics of North America, 90,* 1109–1124.

Drug facts and comparisons. (Updated monthly). St. Louis, MO: Facts and Comparisons.

Guyton, A. C., & Hall, J. E. (2006). *Textbook of medical physiology* (11th ed.). Philadelphia: W. B. Saunders.

Lacy, C. F., Armstrong, L. L., Goldman, M. P., & Lance, L. L. (2007). *Lexi-Comp's drug information handbook* (15th ed.). Hudson, OH: American Pharmaceutical Association.

Drugs for Tuberculosis and *Mycobacterium avium* Complex (MAC) Disease

KEY TERMS

- Directly observed therapy (DOT)
- Extensively drug-resistant tuberculosis (XDR-TB)
- Hepatitis
- Jaundice
- Multidrug-resistant tuberculosis (MDR-TB)

LEARNING OBJECTIVES

After studying this chapter, you will be able to:

1. Describe characteristics of latent, active, and drug-resistant tuberculosis infections.
2. Identify populations at high risk for developing tuberculosis.
3. List characteristics, uses, effects, and nursing implications of using primary antitubercular drugs.
4. Describe the rationale for multiple-drug therapy in treatment of tuberculosis.
5. Discuss ways to increase adherence to antitubercular drug therapy regimens.
6. Discuss circumstances in which directly observed therapy (DOT) is needed.
7. Describe factors affecting drug therapy in multidrug-resistant (MDR-TB) and extensively drug-resistant tuberculosis (XDR-TB).
8. Describe *Mycobacterium avium* complex disease and the drugs used to prevent or treat it.

Applying Your Knowledge

Ramon Diaz is a 58-year-old homeless man. He is spending the night at a shelter where one of your coworkers volunteers one evening a month. Ramon has a productive cough. Your coworker notes that he has visibly lost weight since he was in the shelter 1 month ago. When she asks him how he feels, Ramon says he sweats a lot at night and thinks he has a fever. He is sent to the free clinic the next day, where his sputum test is positive for *Mycobacterium tuberculosis*. From the clinic, Ramon is sent to the county jail, where he will stay until his sputum test is negative. He is started on the following regimen:

> Isoniazid (INH) 300 mg PO daily for 6 months
>
> Rifampin 600 mg PO daily for 6 months
>
> Pyrazinamide 2000 mg daily for 2 months

The health department supplies his medication and is responsible for overseeing his course therapy. You are a nurse working for the health department.

Introduction

Tuberculosis (TB) is an infectious disease that usually affects the lungs but may affect lymph nodes, pleurae, bones, joints, kidneys, and the gastrointestinal tract. It is caused by *Mycobacterium tuberculosis*, the tubercle bacillus. In general, these bacilli multiply slowly, they may lie dormant in the body for many years, they resist phagocytosis and survive in phagocytic cells, and they develop resistance to antitubercular drugs.

Tuberculosis commonly occurs in many parts of the world. Authorities estimate that one-third of the world's population is infected with tuberculosis organisms and that tuberculosis is the cause of death in almost 2 million people every year. In the United States, active disease has decreased to a low level in American-born people; most new cases occur in foreign-born immigrants. There are also large numbers of people with inactive or latent TB infection. Contributing factors include increased exposure during a resurgence of active disease between 1985 and 1992, immigration from countries where the disease commonly occurs (e.g., Mexico, the Philippines, Vietnam, India, China), and increasing numbers of people with conditions or medications that depress the immune system.

Epidemiology of Tuberculosis

There are four phases in the initiation and progression of tuberculosis (Fig. 34-1):

1. **Transmission.** This occurs when an uninfected person inhales infected airborne particles that are exhaled by an infected person. Major factors affecting transmission are the number of bacteria expelled by the infected person and the closeness and duration of the contact between the infected and the uninfected person.

2. **Primary infection.** It is estimated that 30% of persons exposed to tuberculosis bacilli become infected and develop a mild, pneumonia-like illness that is often undiagnosed. About 6 to 8 weeks after exposure, those infected have positive reactions to tuberculin skin tests. Within approximately 6 months of exposure, spontaneous healing occurs as the bacilli are encapsulated in calcified tubercles.

3. **Latent tuberculosis infection (LTBI).** The immune system is able to stop bacterial growth in most people who become infected with TB bacteria. The bacteria become inactive, although they remain alive in the body and can become active later. People with inactive or latent TB infection have no symptoms, do not feel sick, do not spread TB to others, usually have a positive skin-test reaction, and can

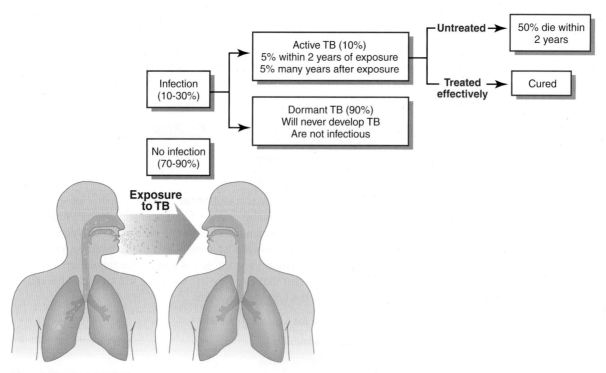

Figure 34-1 ■ Transmission of tuberculosis and progression from latent infection to reactivated disease. Among persons who are seronegative for the human immunodeficiency virus (HIV), approximately 30% of heavily exposed persons will become infected. In 5% of persons with latent infection, active disease will develop within 2 years, and in an additional 5%, progression to active disease will occur later. The rate of progression to active disease is dramatically increased among persons who are coinfected with HIV. (Adapted from Small, P. M., & Fujiwara, P. I. [2001]. Management of tuberculosis in the United States. *New England Journal of Medicine, 345,* 189–200.)

develop active TB disease years later if the latent infection is not effectively treated. In many people with LTBI, the infection remains inactive throughout their lives. In others, the TB bacteria become active and cause tuberculosis, usually when a person's immune system becomes weak as a result of disease, immunosuppressive drugs, or aging.

4. **Active tuberculosis.** This has long been thought to result almost exclusively from reactivation of latent infection, with only a few cases from new primary infections. However, more recent studies indicate that almost half of new TB cases may result from new infections or reinfections from exogenous sources.

Both reactivated and new infections are more likely to occur in people whose immune system is depressed by disease (e.g., human immunodeficiency virus [HIV] infection, diabetes mellitus, cancer) or from drug therapy (e.g., for cancer or organ transplantation). Among people with LTBI, signs and symptoms of active disease (e.g., cough that is persistent and often productive of sputum, chest pain, chills, fever, hemoptysis, night sweats, weight loss, weakness, lack of appetite, positive skin test, abnormal chest radiograph, positive sputum smear or culture) are estimated to develop in 5% within 2 years and in another 5% after 2 years. Among people with both HIV infection and latent or new primary TB infection, TB progresses more rapidly, often involves extrapulmonary sites, is more severe, and is often fatal.

Drug-Resistant Tuberculosis

In addition to LTBI, a major concern among public health and infectious-disease authorities is an increase in drug-resistant infections. Drug-resistant mutants of M. *tuberculosis* microorganisms are present in any infected person. When infected people receive antitubercular drugs, drug-resistant mutants are not killed or weakened by the drugs. Instead, they are able to reproduce in the presence of the drugs and to transmit the property of drug resistance to newly produced bacteria. Eventually, the majority of TB bacilli in the body are drug resistant. Once a drug-resistant strain of TB develops, it can be transmitted to other people just like a drug-susceptible strain.

The development of drug-resistant TB organisms has long been attributed mainly to poor patient adherence to prescribed antitubercular drug therapy, that is, when previously infected patients do not take the drugs and doses prescribed for the length of time prescribed. However, drug-resistant strains can be spread from one person to another, and there is increasing evidence that many drug-resistant infections are new infections, especially in people whose immune system is suppressed.

Multidrug-resistant tuberculosis (MDR-TB) indicates organisms that are resistant to isoniazid (INH) and rifampin, the most effective drugs available, with or without resistance to other antitubercular drugs. MDR-TB is associated with rapid progression, with 4 to 16 weeks from diagnosis to death, and a high death rate (50%–80%). It is also difficult and expensive to treat; most authorities recommend 24 months of drug therapy. Despite longer treatment with more drugs, the cure rate for MDR-TB is about 50% or less, compared with a cure rate of 90% or more for drug-susceptible strains of TB.

Some MDR-TB cases are now being described as *extensively drug-resistant TB (XDR-TB)*, an even more worrisome threat to public health. XDR-TB indicates resistance to the second-line drugs used to treat MDR-TB. Some cases are resistant to six or seven drugs, and there are essentially no effective drugs for their treatment.

Drug-resistant TB has been identified in many parts of the world, especially in Africa and Asia, and is a major concern in HIV-infected persons. Most cases in the United States occur among foreign-born persons. Factors contributing to the development of drug-resistant disease, whether acquired or new infection, include delayed diagnosis and delayed determination of drug susceptibility, which may take several weeks. In addition, some countries lack adequate laboratory facilities or do not test TB organisms for susceptibility to second-line antituberculosis drugs. These delays in effective treatment allow rapid disease progression and rapid transmission to others, especially to those with impaired immune systems.

Applying Your Knowledge 34-1

It is very important that the health department follow Mr. Diaz' treatment to ensure that he takes his prescribed medications. Why is it essential that Mr. Diaz take the full course of therapy?

Tuberculosis Control

An official joint statement from the Centers for Disease Control and Prevention (CDC), the American Thoracic Society (ATS), and the Infectious Diseases Society of America (IDSA) emphasizes continued treatment of active disease and expanded efforts to identify and treat latent infection (LTBI). For identification, tuberculin skin testing is recommended only for high-risk groups (Box 34-1). When LTBI is found in these groups, it should be treated to eradicate this reservoir of infection (Box 34-2). In addition, the statement recommends techniques for TB control among particular populations (e.g., children and adolescents, foreign-born persons, persons with HIV infection, homeless persons) and particular settings (e.g., health care facilities, prisons).

Cain et al. disagree with the CDC/ATS/IDSA recommendation that for foreign-born persons only those who have entered the United States during the previous 5 years be tested for LTBI. These authors say that over 50% of all reported TB cases in the United States occur in foreign-born persons and almost 25% of all reported cases occur in foreign-born persons who have lived in the country for longer than 5 years. Thus, they recommend testing for LTBI in the latter group as well.

Although local health departments are largely responsible for TB control programs, some authorities urge increased testing and treatment in primary-care settings and in settings where high-risk groups are found (e.g., homeless shelters).

Box 34-1	Targeted Tuberculin Testing for Latent Tuberculosis Infection (LTBI)

Purpose

To identify people with latent tuberculosis infection (LTBI) who are at high risk of developing active tuberculosis and who would benefit from treatment of LTBI, if detected.

Who Should Be Tested?

Numerous high-risk groups have been identified, including persons with the following circumstances or conditions:

- Having recent infection with *Mycobacterium tuberculosis* organisms
- Having close contact with someone diagnosed with infectious pulmonary TB
- Immigrating from areas of the world with high rates of TB.
- Belonging to younger age groups. Young children (e.g., under 5 years) with a positive skin test are at high risk for progression to active disease. The risk is also increased in adolescents and young adults.
- Belonging to older age groups, especially if also living or working in institutions with high-risk populations (e.g., hospitals, homeless shelters, correctional facilities, nursing homes, residential homes for patients with acquired immune deficiency syndrome [AIDS])
- Being homeless
- Being an injection drug user
- Having HIV infection or AIDS. HIV infection greatly increases the risk for progression of LTBI to active TB.
- Having chest radiographs that show fibrotic lesions in the lungs. Such lesions are likely to stem from prior, untreated, healed TB.
- Being underweight, especially if more than 10%–15% under ideal weight
- Having silicosis (a pulmonary disorder caused by inhalation of dust particles from mining or stonecutting). People with silicosis and a positive tuberculin test are about 30 times more likely to develop active disease than the general population.
- Having chronic renal failure and being on hemodialysis. These people are 10 to 25 times more likely to develop active disease than the general population.
- Having diabetes mellitus. These people are 2 to 4 times more likely to develop active TB than those without diabetes, and the risk is probably greater in those with insulin-dependent or poorly controlled diabetes.
- Having a history of gastrectomy (which is often accompanied by weight loss and malabsorption), jejunoileal bypass, renal or cardiac transplantation, carcinoma of the head or neck, lung cancer, lymphoma, or leukemia.
- Receiving high-dose corticosteroid therapy (e.g., prednisone >15 mg/d or equivalent amounts of other drugs for several weeks). These people may be at risk for reactivation of TB, but the exact risk is unknown. Lower doses and intermittent administration of corticosteroids are not associated with TB.

Where Should Testing Be Done?

Traditionally, local health departments have been responsible for testing, interpreting, and providing follow-up care; some

institutions have tested residents and employees, and some large businesses have tested employees. More recently, the Centers for Disease Control and Prevention (CDC) and other authorities have recommended that more testing be done in primary care settings and any other locations where high-risk individuals are. Such testing sites include neighborhood health centers, jails, homeless shelters, inner-city sites, methadone clinics, syringe and needle-exchange programs, and other community-based social service organizations. In the latter situations, local health departments are urged to assist local providers in developing, implementing, and evaluating TB screening programs appropriate for their communities.

Test Interpretation

Positive reactions differ according to the amount of induration (a nodule or area of hardened tissue, not to be confused with the area of redness, which may be larger than the area of induration) and characteristics of the group being tested, as follows:

- **Induration of 5 mm or more.** Persons at highest risk (e.g., close contacts of someone with active, infectious TB; those with HIV infection or risk factors for HIV infection; and those with chest radiographs that are consistent with previous TB)
- **Induration of 10 mm or more.** Persons at high risk (e.g., those with conditions or characteristics such as diabetes mellitus; silicosis; immunosuppressive drug therapy; leukemia; lymphoma; head or neck cancer; chronic renal failure; gastrectomy; jejunoileal bypass; low body weight; injecting drug users known to be seronegative for HIV infection; recent immigrants from countries that have high TB rates; residents and employees of prisons, long-term care institutions, and other congregate settings for high-risk populations; low-income groups; high-risk racial and ethnic groups; migrant farm workers; and infants, children, and adolescents exposed to adults in high-risk categories)
- **Induration of 15 mm or more.** Persons who are at low risk for developing TB and do not meet the criteria listed for the above groups. Routine testing is not recommended for low-risk groups.
- **False-positive reactions.** These may occur with infections caused by nontuberculous strains of mycobacteria or a previous intradermal injection of bacillus Calmette-Guérin (BCG), a live attenuated strain derived from *Mycobacterium bovis*. In many parts of the world, BCG is used as a vaccine against tuberculosis, especially in children. There is currently no reliable way to differentiate tuberculin reactions caused by vaccination with BCG from those caused by infection with *M. tuberculosis*. However, large areas of induration (>20 mm) are unlikely to result from BCG.
- **False-negative reactions.** These may occur with HIV infection or other conditions that suppress the immune system and inhibit the ability to react to the tuberculin antigen. Thus, a negative skin test may occur in the presence of tuberculosis infection.

Box 34-2	**Treatment of Latent Tuberculosis Infection (LTBI)**

Recommended Regimens for Adults

Isoniazid (INH) daily or twice weekly for 9 months is the preferred regimen, including persons with human immunodeficiency virus (HIV) infection or radiographic evidence of prior TB.

Isoniazid daily or twice weekly for 6 months. The main advantage of this regimen over the 9-month schedule is greater adherence because of the shorter length. It is also less costly. This regimen may be used for HIV-negative adults with normal chest radiographs; it is *not* recommended for HIV-positive persons, those less than 18 years of age, or those with fibrotic lesions as shown on chest radiographs.

Rifampin and pyrazinamide (RIF-PZA) daily or twice weekly for 2 months. This regimen may be used for contacts of patients with INH-resistant TB and for those who are unlikely to complete a longer course of treatment. Rifampin is contraindicated in HIV-positive patients who are receiving protease inhibitors or non-nucleoside reverse transcriptase inhibitors (NNRTIs), because rifampin greatly stimulates metabolism and decreases the effectiveness of the antiviral drugs. Rifabutin, which causes less enzyme induction than rifampin, may be substituted in some cases. Pyrazinamide is contraindicated during pregnancy.

This regimen was revised in 2001 because of several reports of liver failure and death. To reduce the risks of liver injury, the American Thoracic Society and the Centers for Disease Control and Prevention (CDC), with the endorsement of the Infectious Diseases Society of America, issued new recommendations for choosing patients and for more intensive clinical and laboratory monitoring, as follows:

1. The RIF-PZA regimen is not recommended for persons who have underlying liver disease or who have had INH-associated liver injury. It should be used with caution in patients who take other hepatotoxic medications or use alcohol, even if alcohol use is stopped during treatment. Persons being considered for treatment with this regimen should be informed about potential hepatotoxicity and asked whether they have had liver disease or adverse effects from INH.
2. The RIF-PZA regimen is recommended mainly for patients who are unlikely to complete longer courses of treatment and who can be monitored closely. (For other adults not infected with HIV, the 9-month daily regimen of INH is preferred, with 4 months of daily RIF as an acceptable alternative.)
3. The RIF-PZA regimen does increase risks of hepatotoxicity in patients with HIV infection. Still, INH daily for 9 months is the treatment of choice for HIV-infected persons with LTBI when completion of treatment can be assured.
4. Increase safety by limiting the pyrazinamide dose to less than 20 mg/kg/d and a maximum of 2 g/d; giving no more than a 2-week supply of rifampin and pyrazinamide at a time; and assessing patients at 2, 4, and 6 weeks of treatment for adherence, tolerance, and adverse effects, and at 8 weeks to document treatment completion. For non– English-speaking clients, health care providers who speak the patients'

language should instruct them to stop taking the drugs immediately and seek medical care if abdominal pain, emesis, jaundice, or other symptoms of hepatitis develop. Provider continuity is recommended for monitoring.

5. Perform liver function tests (e.g., serum aspartate and alanine aminotransferases [AST and ALT] and bilirubin) at baseline and at 2, 4, and 6 weeks. RIF-PZA treatment should be stopped and not resumed if enzyme levels are higher than five times the upper limit of normal in an asymptomatic person, are higher than normal range if symptoms of hepatitis are present, or if a serum bilirubin level is above normal range.

Rifampin daily for 4 months. This regimen is used mainly for patients who cannot tolerate INH or pyrazinamide.

Special Populations

1. Pregnant women. The preferred regimen for treatment of LTBI is INH, administered daily or twice weekly for 9 or 6 months. Pregnant women taking INH should also take pyridoxine supplementation. For HIV-positive women with higher risks of progression to active TB, treatment should not be delayed; for those with lower risks, some experts recommend waiting until after delivery to start treatment. In general, INH, rifampin, and ethambutol have good safety records in pregnancy. Pyrazinamide and streptomycin are contraindicated during pregnancy.
2. Children and adolescents. INH daily or twice weekly for 9 months is recommended. Infants and children under 5 years of age with LTBI are at high risk for progression to disease. They are also more likely than older children and adults to develop life-threatening forms of TB, including meningeal and disseminated disease. INH therapy appears to be more effective for children than adults, and the risk for INH-related hepatitis is minimal in infants, children, and adolescents, who generally tolerate the drug better than adults. Routine administration of pyridoxine is not recommended for children taking INH, but should be given to breast-feeding infants, children and adolescents with pyridoxine-deficient diets, and children who experience paresthesias when taking INH.

   Although few studies have been done in infants, children, and adolescents, rifampin alone, rifampin with INH, and rifampin with pyrazinamide have been used to treat LTBI with effectiveness. Although the optimal length of rifampin therapy in children with LTBI is unknown, the American Academy of Pediatrics (AAP) recommends 6 months.

   There have been no reported studies of any regimen for treatment for LTBI in HIV-infected children. The AAP recommends INH for 9 months; most experts recommend routine monitoring of serum liver enzyme concentrations and pyridoxine administration.
3. Contacts of patients with drug-susceptible TB and positive skin-test reactions (more than 5 mm) should be treated with one of the recommended regimens described above, regardless of age.

(continued on page 546)

| Box 34-2 | **Treatment of Latent Tuberculosis Infection (LTBI)** (continued) |

4. Contacts of patients with INH-resistant, rifampin-susceptible TB should generally be given rifampin and pyrazinamide for 2 months. For patients with intolerance to pyrazinamide, rifampin alone for 4 months is recommended. If rifampin cannot be used, rifabutin can be substituted.

5. Contacts of patients with multidrug-resistant (MDR)-TB who are at high risk for developing active TB are generally given pyrazinamide and ethambutol or pyrazinamide and a fluoroquinolone (levofloxacin or ofloxacin) for 6 to 12 months. Immunocompetent contacts may be observed without treatment or treated for 6 months; immunocompromised contacts (e.g., HIV-infected persons) should be treated for 12 months.

   For children exposed to MDR-TB, pyrazinamide and ethambutol are recommended for 9 to 12 months if the isolate is susceptible to both drugs. If these drugs cannot be used, two other drugs to which the infecting organism is likely susceptible should be given.

6. HIV-infected persons. With INH, the 9-month regimen is recommended. With rifampin, the drug is contraindicated or should be used with caution in persons who are taking protease inhibitors or NNRTIs. Rifabutin can be substituted for rifampin in some circumstances, but it should be used cautiously with saquinavir and nevirapine. Dosage of rifabutin needs to be reduced to one half the usual daily dose (i.e., from 300 mg/d to 150 mg/d) with indinavir or nelfinavir and to one fourth the usual dose (i.e., 150 mg every other day or 3 times a week) with ritonavir. Usual dosage (300 mg/d) can be given with nevirapine and 450 or 600 mg/d are needed with efavirenz. Rifapentine is not recommended as a substitute for rifampin because its safety, effectiveness, and interactions with anti-HIV medication have not been established.

7. Bacillus Calmette-Guérin (BCG)-vaccinated persons. A history of BCG vaccination should not influence the decision to treat LTBI.

Additional Recommendations

1. Before beginning treatment for LTBI, active TB should be ruled out by history, physical examination, chest radiography, and bacteriologic studies, if indicated.

2. Allow patients to participate in choosing a treatment regimen, when feasible, by discussing options and characteristics of each (e.g., the length and complexity, possible adverse effects, potential drug interactions).

3. Directly observed therapy (DOT) should be used consistently with intermittent regimens (e.g., twice weekly) and when possible with 2-month regimens and in certain settings (e.g., institutional settings, community outreach programs, and for persons living in households with patients who are receiving home-based DOT for active TB).

4. Try to ensure completion of treatment. This is determined by the total number of doses administered as well as the duration of therapy. For daily INH, the 9-month regimen should include at least 270 doses in 12 months and the 6-month regimen should include at least 180 doses in 9 months. For twice-weekly INH, the 9-month regimen should include at least 76 doses in 12 months and the 6-month regimen should include at least 52 doses in 9 months. For the 2-month regimen of daily rifampin (or rifabutin) and pyrazinamide, at least 60 doses should be given in 3 months. For the 4-month regimen of daily rifampin alone, at least 120 doses should be given in 6 months.

   These schedules allow minor interruptions in therapy although, ideally, patients should receive medication on a regular schedule until the course of therapy is completed. When doses are missed, the duration of therapy should be lengthened. When restarting therapy after interruptions, the original regimen may be continued as long as needed to complete the recommended duration of the particular regimen or a new regimen may be needed if interruptions were frequent or prolonged. If treatment is interrupted for longer than 2 months, the patient should be reassessed for active TB before restarting drug therapy.

In addition, authorities urge recognition and effective management of language, social, economic, transportation, and other barriers that limit access to health care and inhibit diagnosis and treatment.

Nurses have important roles to play in TB control. One role is to know and follow recommendations to prevent transmission (See "Guidelines for preventing the transmission of *Mycobacterium tuberculosis* in health-care settings," available at www.cdc.gov). Other roles include performing and reading tuberculin skin tests; managing TB clinics; tracking contacts of patients with active disease; assessing patients, homes, and other settings for risk factors; educating patients and families about TB infection and its treatment; administering antitubercular drugs (e.g., *directly observed therapy [DOT]*, in which a health care provider watches the patient take each dose of medication); and maintaining records (e.g., skin-test results,

patients starting or completing drug therapy, adherence or lack of adherence to prescribed treatment regimens).

In the United States, all citizens need to support efforts to maintain public health organizations and infrastructures to identify, treat, and monitor tuberculosis. The resurgence of active disease that occurred in the mid-1980s was due, at least in part, to decreased funding and a weakening of TB control measures at all levels of government. Strengthening those control measures has contributed to the present low level of active disease.

Worldwide, much work is needed to prevent further development and spread of drug-resistant TB. The development of XDR-TB indicates failure to adequately diagnose, prevent, and treat MDR-TB. One problem may be that effective drugs are not correctly prescribed, administered consistently, or even available. Another problem is that susceptibility testing for second-line drugs is not available or not widely used. In general, susceptibility testing of first-line drugs is performed, but testing of second-line drugs is usually limited to TB isolates from patients known or suspected to have drug-resistant TB. Drug-resistant TB is often not suspected until the patient has had 2 months or more of drug therapy (e.g., cultures remain positive for TB organisms after 2 or more months of treatment or susceptibility tests reveal drug resistance). The delay in identifying and treating drug-resistant TB allows additional spread of the disease. Additional problems include needs for better and internationally standardized tests for susceptibility testing of second-line drugs, new anti-TB drugs and drug therapy regimens, and better diagnostic tests for TB and MDR-TB. One newer diagnostic test, called microscopic-observation drug susceptibility (MODS), is reportedly faster and less expensive to perform.

Antitubercular Drugs

Antitubercular drugs are divided into primary (first-line) and second-line agents. The main primary drugs (isoniazid, rifampin, and pyrazinamide) are used to treat latent, active, and drug-resistant TB infection when possible. Ethambutol and streptomycin are also considered primary drugs. Because of their varied characteristics, these drugs are described individually below and their dosages are listed in Table 34-1.

Second-line drugs are used only for patients who are unable to tolerate first-line drugs or those who are infected with organisms that are resistant to first-line drugs. In general, second-line drugs are less effective, more toxic, or both.

Primary Drugs

P **Isoniazid** (also called INH), the most commonly used antitubercular drug and the prototype, is bactericidal, relatively inexpensive and nontoxic, and can be given orally or by injection. Although it can be used alone for treatment of LTBI, it must be used with other antitubercular drugs for treatment of active disease.

INH penetrates body cells and mycobacteria, kills actively growing intracellular and extracellular organisms, and inhibits

Table 34-1			Drugs at a Glance: Primary Antitubercular Drugs		
	DOSAGE RANGES (MAXIMUM DOSE)				
	ADULTS		**CHILDREN**		
Name/Route	**Daily**	**Twice/Wk**	**Daily**	**Twice/Wk**	**Comments**
Isoniazid (INH) PO or IM	5 mg/kg (300 mg)	15 mg/kg (900 mg)	10–20 mg/kg (300 mg)	20–40 mg/kg (900 mg)	*LTBI:* Given at least 6 mo; 9 mo preferred *Active TB:* Given at least 6 mo, with other drugs
Rifampin (Rifadin) PO or IV infusion	10 mg/kg (600 mg)	10 mg/kg (600 mg)	10–20 mg/kg (600 mg)	10–20 mg/kg (600 mg)	*LTBI:* Given 4 mo alone or 2 mo with pyrazinamide *Active TB:* Given for 6 mo, with other drugs
Pyrazinamide PO	15–30 mg/kg (2 g)	50–70 mg/kg (4 g)	15–30 mg/kg (2 g)	50–70 mg/kg (4 g)	*LTBI:* Given for 2 mo, with rifampin *Active TB:* Given for 2 mo, with INH and rifampin
Streptomycin IM	15 mg/kg (1 g)	25–30 mg/kg (1.5 g)	20–40 mg/kg (1 g)	25–30 mg/kg (1.5 g)	Used for active TB, with other drugs
Ethambutol (Myambutol) PO	15–25 mg/kg (2.5 g)	50 mg/kg (2.5 g)	15–25 mg/kg (2.5 g)	50 mg/kg (2.5 g)	Used for active TB, with other drugs, and MAC disease
Rifabutin (Mycobutin) PO	300 mg		Not established		Used to treat MAC disease and to substitute for rifampin in patients taking certain anti-HIV medications
Rifapentine (Priftin) PO		150 mg twice a wk for 2 mo, then once a wk for 4 mo	Not established		May be used instead of rifampin, with other drugs

HIV, human immunodeficiency virus; LTBI, latent tuberculosis infection; MAC, Mycobacterium avium complex; TB, tuberculosis.

the growth of dormant organisms in macrophages and tuberculous lesions. Its mechanism of action is to inhibit formation of cell walls in mycobacteria.

INH is well absorbed from the GI tract, with peak serum concentrations occurring 1 to 2 hours after a 300-milligram dose. It penetrates and reaches therapeutic concentrations in essentially all body fluids and cavities. Its half-life is 1 to 4 hours. It is acetylated in the liver to acetylisoniazid, which is excreted by the kidneys. Metabolism of INH is genetically determined; some people are "slow acetylators" and others are "rapid acetylators." A person's rate of acetylation affects response to INH. Slow acetylators have less N-acetyltransferase, the acetylating enzyme, in the liver. In these patients, INH is more likely to accumulate to toxic concentrations, and the development of peripheral neuropathy is more likely. However, there is no significant difference in the clinical effectiveness of INH. Rapid acetylators may require unusually high doses of INH. They also may be more susceptible to serious liver injury because of rapid formation of hepatotoxic metabolites. The drug is excreted in urine.

Potentially serious adverse effects include hepatotoxicity and peripheral neuropathy. Hepatotoxicity may be manifested by symptoms of *hepatitis* (e.g., anorexia, nausea, fatigue, malaise, *jaundice*) or elevated liver enzymes. The drug should be stopped if hepatitis develops or liver enzymes (e.g., alanine and aspartate aminotransferases [ALT and AST]) are more than five times the normal values. Hepatitis is more likely to occur during the first 8 weeks of INH therapy and in people who use alcohol. Patients receiving INH should be monitored monthly for signs and symptoms of hepatitis. Because of the risk of hepatotoxicity, INH should be used cautiously in patients with pre-existing liver disease. Peripheral neuropathy may be manifested by numbness and tingling in the hands and feet. It is most likely to occur in patients who are malnourished or older or who have alcoholism, diabetes mellitus, or uremia. Pyridoxine, 25 to 50 milligrams daily, is usually given with INH to minimize peripheral neuropathy.

Applying Your Knowledge 34-2

You will have multiple opportunities to assess Mr. Diaz when he receives his medication. For what adverse effects of INH do you plan to monitor Mr. Diaz?

Rifampin (Rifadin) is a rifamycin that is bactericidal for both intracellular and extracellular TB organisms. It kills mycobacteria by inhibiting synthesis of RNA and thereby causing defective, nonfunctional proteins to be produced. Its ability to penetrate intact cells contributes to its effectiveness in TB because mycobacteria are harbored in host cells. Rifampin and INH are synergistic in combination, eliminating tuberculosis bacilli from sputum and producing clinical improvement faster than any other drug regimen, unless organisms resistant to one or both drugs are causing the disease.

Rifampin is well absorbed with oral administration and diffuses well into body tissues and fluids, with highest concentrations occurring in the liver, lungs, gallbladder, and kidneys. Peak serum concentration occurs in 1 to 3 hours with oral administration and immediately with IV administration. The drug is metabolized in the liver and excreted primarily in bile; a small amount is excreted in urine. Its elimination half-life is approximately 3 hours with a 300-milligram dose and approximately 5 hours with a 600-milligram dose. Because it is a strong inducer of drug-metabolizing enzymes, its half-life becomes shorter with continued use.

Adverse effects include GI upset, skin rashes, hepatitis, and a harmless red-orange discoloration of urine, tears, sweat, and other body fluids. Soft contact lenses may be permanently stained.

Rifampin has many interactions with other drugs. It induces hepatic cytochrome P450 3A4 enzymes and accelerates the metabolism of numerous other drugs, thereby decreasing their serum concentrations, half-lives, and therapeutic effects. Affected drugs include anti–acquired immunodeficiency syndrome (AIDS) drugs (protease inhibitors [PIs] and non-nucleoside reverse transcriptase inhibitors [NNRTIs]; see Chap. 35), benzodiazepines, corticosteroids, cyclosporine, estrogens, fluconazole, methadone, metoprolol, phenytoin, propranolol, oral contraceptives, oral sulfonylureas, theophylline, verapamil, and warfarin. With warfarin, decreased anticoagulant effect occurs approximately 5 to 8 days after rifampin is started and lasts for 5 to 7 days after rifampin is stopped. With methadone, concurrent administration with rifampin may precipitate signs and symptoms of opiate withdrawal unless methadone dosage is increased.

Applying Your Knowledge 34-3

You are teaching Mr. Diaz about his medication. What adverse effect of rifampin should you include in your teaching so that Mr. Diaz does not become alarmed and stop taking his medication?

Rifabutin (Mycobutin) is another rifamycin that is active against mycobacteria. However, most rifampin-resistant strains are also resistant to rifabutin. The drug's two main uses are in patients with HIV infection, to treat *Mycobacterium avium* complex (MAC) disease; and to substitute for rifampin in patients who need both antitubercular and certain antiviral drugs. The major advantages of rifabutin over rifampin are a longer serum half-life (45 hours, on average) and reduced induction of hepatic drug-metabolizing enzymes. Rifabutin has no advantage over rifampin in treatment of TB but may be given concurrently with INH to patients who need prophylaxis against both *M. tuberculosis* and *M. avium*.

Rifabutin is well absorbed from the GI tract; a dose of 300 milligrams produces peak serum concentration in 23 hours. It is extensively metabolized in the liver (and to a lesser extent in the intestinal wall), and it is excreted in urine and bile.

Like rifampin, rifabutin causes a harmless red-orange discoloration of body fluids and permanent staining of soft contact lenses. Adverse effects include GI upset (nausea, vomiting, diarrhea), hepatitis, muscular aches, neutropenia, skin rash, and uveitis (an eye disorder with inflammation, pain, and impaired vision). Hepatotoxicity is rare. Adverse effects increase when rifabutin is administered with a drug that inhibits cytochrome P450 3A4 enzymes (e.g., clarithromycin) and inhibits rifabutin metabolism. Safety and effectiveness in children have not been established

Also similarly to rifampin, but to a lesser extent, rifabutin induces drug-metabolizing enzymes in the liver and accelerates the metabolism of numerous drugs. This action decreases concentration and clinical efficacy of beta blockers, corticosteroids, cyclosporine, digoxin, hormonal contraceptives, itraconazole, methadone, NNRTIs, oral hypoglycemic agents, phenytoin, PIs, theophylline, warfarin, and zidovudine. If these drugs are administered with rifabutin, their dosage may need to be increased.

Rifapentine (Priftin) is similar to rifampin in effectiveness, adverse effects, and enzyme induction activity. It may be used in the treatment of pulmonary TB and must be used with at least one other drug to which the causative organisms are susceptible. Its action has a slow onset and peaks in 5 to 6 hours. It is metabolized in the liver and excreted in urine and feces. It has a half-life of 14 hours. Rifapentine is infrequently used; its advantage over rifampin is that it can be given once weekly in the 4-month continuation phase of treatment for drug-susceptible tuberculosis.

Ethambutol (Myambutol) is a tuberculostatic drug that inhibits synthesis of RNA and thus interferes with mycobacterial protein metabolism. It may be a component in a four-drug regimen for initial treatment of active TB that may be caused by drug-resistant organisms. When culture and susceptibility reports become available (usually after several weeks), ethambutol may be stopped if the causative organisms are susceptible to INH and rifampin or continued if the organisms are resistant to INH or rifampin and susceptible to ethambutol. Ethambutol is not recommended for young children (e.g., under 5 years of age) whose visual acuity cannot be monitored but may be considered for children of any age when organisms are susceptible to ethambutol and resistant to other drugs. Mycobacterial resistance to ethambutol develops slowly.

Ethambutol is well absorbed from the GI tract, even when given with food. Dosage is based on body weight and should be changed during treatment if significant changes in weight occur. To obtain therapeutic serum levels, the total daily dose is given at one time. Drug action has a rapid onset, peaks in 2 to 4 hours, and lasts 20 to 24 hours. The drug has a half-life of 3 to 4 hours, is metabolized in the liver, and is excreted primarily by the kidneys. Dosage must be reduced with impaired renal function.

A major adverse effect is optic neuritis, an inflammatory, demyelinating disorder of the optic nerve that decreases visual acuity and ability to differentiate red from green. Tests of visual acuity and red–green discrimination are recommended before starting ethambutol and periodically during therapy. If optic neuritis develops, the drug should be promptly stopped. Recovery usually occurs when ethambutol is discontinued.

Pyrazinamide is used with INH and rifampin for the first 2 months of treating active TB. It is bactericidal against actively growing mycobacteria in macrophages, but its exact mechanism of action is unknown. It is well absorbed from the GI tract and penetrates most body fluids and tissues, including macrophages containing TB organisms. Its action has a rapid onset and it peaks in 2 hours. It is metabolized in the liver and excreted mainly through the kidneys. Its half-life is 9 to 10 hours.

The most common adverse effect is GI upset; the most severe adverse effect is hepatotoxicity, and the drug should not be given to a patient with pre-existing liver impairment unless it is considered essential. Patients without liver impairment should be assessed for symptoms of liver dysfunction every 2 weeks during the usual 8 weeks of therapy. If symptoms occur, liver enzymes (ALT and AST) should be measured. If significant liver damage is indicated, pyrazinamide should be stopped.

Pyrazinamide inhibits urate excretion. This characteristic causes hyperuricemia in most patients and may cause acute attacks of gout.

Streptomycin, an aminoglycoside antibiotic (see Chap. 31), acts only against extracellular organisms; it does not penetrate macrophages and tuberculous lesions. It may be used in a regimen of four drugs to treat active TB when the susceptibility of the causative organism is unknown or in a regimen of four to six drugs in the treatment of TB suspected or known to be resistant to INH, rifampin, or both. It may be discontinued when cultures become negative or after a few months of therapy.

Combination Primary Drugs

Rifamate and **Rifater** are combination products developed to increase convenience to patients and promote adherence to the prescribed drug therapy regimen (for drug-susceptible TB). Each Rifamate tablet contains INH 150 milligrams and rifampin 300 milligrams, and two tablets daily provide the recommended doses for a 6-month, short-course treatment regimen. Rifater contains INH 50 milligrams, rifampin 120 milligrams, and pyrazinamide 300 milligrams and is approved for the first 2 months of a 6-month, short-course treatment regimen. Dosage depends on weight, with four tablets daily for patients weighing 44 kilograms or less, five tablets daily for those weighing 45 to 54 kilograms, and six tablets daily for those weighing 55 kilograms or more. Rifater not only reduces the number of pills a patient has to take each day, it also prevents the patient from taking only one of the three medications, which can lead to MDR-TB.

Second-line Drugs

Para-aminosalicylic acid (PAS), **capreomycin** (Capastat), **cycloserine** (Seromycin), and **ethionamide** (Trecator SC) are diverse drugs that share tuberculostatic properties. They are indicated for use in disease caused by organisms resistant to primary drugs. They must be given concurrently with other drugs to inhibit emergence of resistant mycobacteria. These drugs are more costly, more toxic, and less effective than first-line drugs.

Other drugs used for the treatment of MDR-TB include aminoglycoside antibiotics (amikacin and kanamycin) and fluoroquinolones (ciprofloxacin, levofloxacin, moxifloxacin, ofloxacin). These drugs are not usually considered antitubercular drugs. However, they have activity against mycobacteria and may be a component of a four- to six-drug regimen to treat suspected or known MDR-TB.

Treatment of Active Tuberculosis

Adequate drug therapy of patients with active disease usually produces improvement within 2 to 3 weeks, with decreased fever and cough, weight gain, improved well-being, and improved chest radiographs. Treatment should generally be continued for at least 6 months or 3 months after cultures become negative. Most patients have negative sputum cultures within 3 to 6 months. If the patient is symptomatic or if the culture is positive after 3 months, noncompliance or drug resistance must be considered. Cultures that are positive after 6 months often include drug-resistant organisms, and an alternative drug therapy regimen is needed. With the increasing prevalence of MDR-TB, guidelines for treatment have changed and continue to evolve in the attempt to promote patient adherence to treatment and to manage MDR-TB, two of the major problems in drug therapy of tuberculosis.

The most commonly used regimen consists of INH, rifampin, and pyrazinamide daily for 2 months (the initial phase), followed by INH and rifampin (daily, two times weekly, or three times weekly) for 4 additional months (the continuation phase). If 4% or more of the tuberculosis isolates in the community are INH-resistant organisms, ethambutol or streptomycin should also be given until susceptibility reports become available. If the causative strain of M. *tuberculosis* is susceptible to INH, rifampin, and pyrazinamide, the regimen is continued as with the three-drug regimen described and the fourth drug (ethambutol or streptomycin) is discontinued. If rifampin is not used, an 18-month course of therapy is considered the minimum. In the absence of drug resistance, INH and rifampin in a 9-month regimen are effective; adding pyrazinamide for the initial 2 months of therapy allows the regimen to be shortened to 6 months.

For INH-resistant TB, the recommended regimen is rifampin, pyrazinamide, and ethambutol for 6 months. For rifampin-resistant TB, recommended regimens are INH and ethambutol for 18 months or INH, pyrazinamide, and streptomycin for 9 months. For MDR-TB, there is no standardized drug therapy regimen. Treatment of each patient must be individualized according to susceptibility reports. Such regimens usually include an aminoglycoside, a fluoroquinolone, and two to four additional drugs to which the causative organism is susceptible. The drugs should be given for 1 to 2 years after cultures become negative. Intermittent administration is not recommended for MDR-TB. For XDR-TB, it is difficult if not impossible to design a drug therapy program with a sufficient number of drugs known to be effective against the TB organism.

Directly observed therapy (DOT), in which a health care provider (or other responsible adult) observes the patient taking each dose of anti-TB drugs, is recommended for all drug regimens and considered mandatory in intermittent schedules, (e.g., two or three times weekly) and regimens for MDR-TB.

During pregnancy, a three-drug regimen of INH, rifampin, and ethambutol is usually used, with close monitoring of liver function tests. Pyrazinamide and streptomycin should not be used during pregnancy.

Mycobacterium avium Complex Disease

Mycobacterium *avium* and Mycobacterium *intracellulare* are different types of mycobacteria that resemble each other so closely that they are usually grouped together as *Mycobacterium avium* complex (MAC). These atypical mycobacteria are found in water (including natural water sources, indoor water systems, pools, and hot tubs) and soil throughout the United States as well as in animals. The organisms are thought to be transmitted by inhalation of droplets of contaminated water; there is no evidence of spread to humans from animals or other humans.

MAC rarely causes significant disease in immunocompetent people but causes an opportunistic pulmonary infection in approximately 50% of patients with advanced HIV infection. Symptoms include a productive cough, weight loss, hemoptysis, and fever. As the disease becomes disseminated through the body, chronic lung disease develops and the organism is found in the blood, bone marrow, liver, lymph nodes, and other body tissues.

The main drugs used in prevention of MAC disease are the macrolides azithromycin and clarithromycin (see Chap. 33) and rifabutin (described earlier in this chapter). Prophylactic drug therapy is recommended to be lifelong. For treatment, a three-drug regimen of azithromycin 250 milligrams daily or clarithromycin 1000 milligrams daily, rifampin or rifabutin (300 mg daily), and ethambutol (25 mg/kg/d for 2 months, then 15 mg/kg/d) is often used. The drugs may also be given two or three times weekly. Drug dosages are the same for intermittent regimens except that the larger dose of ethambutol is continued throughout. Streptomycin 500 to 1000 milligrams twice weekly is usually added for the initial 3 months of treatment when extensive MAC disease is present.

Nursing Process

Assessment

Assess for latent or active tuberculosis infection.

- For latent infection, identify high-risk patients (i.e., people who are close contacts of someone with active TB; are elderly or undernourished; have diabetes mellitus, silicosis, Hodgkin's disease, leukemia, or AIDS; are alcoholics; are receiving immunosuppressive drugs; or are immigrants from Southeast Asia and other parts of the world where the disease is endemic).

- For active disease, clinical manifestations include fatigue, weight loss, anorexia, malaise, fever, and a productive cough. In early phases, however, there may be no symptoms. If available, check diagnostic test reports for indications of TB (chest radiograph, tuberculin skin test, sputum smear and culture).

- In children, initial signs and symptoms may occur within a few weeks after exposure, before skin tests become positive, and resemble those of bacterial pneumonia. In addition, indications of disease in lymph nodes, GI and urinary tracts, bone marrow, and meninges may be present.

- In older adults, signs and symptoms of TB are often less prominent than in younger adults, or are similar to those in other respiratory disorders. Thus, an older adult is less likely to have fever, a positive skin test, significant sputum production, hemoptysis, or night sweats. However, mental status changes and mortality rates are higher in older than in younger adults.

- In patients with HIV infection, skin tests showing 5 mm of induration are considered positive. In addition, disease manifestations in patients with AIDS differ from those in people with undamaged immune systems. For example, malaise, weight loss, weakness, and fever are prominent. Other symptoms often resemble those of bacterial pneumonia, involve multiple lobes of the lungs, and involve extrapulmonary sites of infection.

- Assess candidates for antitubercular drug therapy for previous exposure and reaction to the primary drugs and for the current use of drugs that interact with the primary drugs.

- Assess for latent or active tuberculosis infection

- Assess for signs and symptoms of MAC disease, especially in patients with advanced HIV infection who have a CD4+ cell count of 100/mm^3 or less.

Nursing Diagnoses

- Anxiety or Fear related to chronic illness and long-term drug therapy

- Deficient Knowledge: Disease process and need for treatment

- Noncompliance related to adverse drug effects and need for long-term treatment

- Deficient Knowledge: Consequences of noncompliance with the drug therapy regimen

- Risk for Injury: Adverse drug effects

Planning/Goals

The patient will

- Take drugs as prescribed

- Keep appointments for follow-up care

- Report adverse drug effects

- Act to prevent spread of TB

Interventions

Assist patients to understand the disease process and the necessity for long-term treatment and follow-up. This is extremely important for the patient and the community, because lack of knowledge and failure to comply with the therapeutic regimen lead to disease progression and spread. The American Lung Association publishes many helpful pamphlets, written for the general public, that can be obtained from a local chapter and given to patients and their families. Do not use these as a substitute for personal contact, however.

Use measures to prevent the spread of tuberculosis:

- Isolate suspected or newly diagnosed hospitalized patients in a private room for 2 or 3 weeks, until drug therapy has rendered them noninfectious.

- Wear a mask with close contact, and perform thorough hand hygiene afterward.

- Have patients wear a mask when out of the room for diagnostic tests.

- Assist patients to take antitubercular drugs as prescribed, for the length of time prescribed.

Evaluation

- Observe for improvement in signs and symptoms of TB and MAC disease.

- Interview and observe for adverse drug effects; check laboratory reports of hepatic and renal function, when available.

- Question regarding compliance with instructions for taking antitubercular and anti-MAC drugs.

Principles of Therapy

Goals of Therapy

In general, the goals for treatment of TB are to cure patients with latent or active infection, to avoid the development of drug-resistant TB, and to minimize transmission of TB to other

Patient Teaching Guidelines ■ Isoniazid, Rifampin, and Pyrazinamide

■ Isoniazid (INH) is one of the most commonly used medications for tuberculosis infection. It is given to people with positive skin tests to prevent development of active disease. Vitamin B$_6$ (pyridoxine) is usually given along with the INH to prevent leg numbness and tingling. Take INH and pyridoxine in a single dose once daily. Take on an empty stomach if possible; if stomach upset occurs, the drugs may be taken with food.

■ For treatment of active disease, INH, rifampin, and pyrazinamide are usually given daily or twice weekly for 2 months; then the pyrazinamide is stopped and the others are continued for an additional 4 months.

■ For treatment of inactive or latent tuberculosis infection, various regimens of INH alone, rifampin and pyrazinamide, or rifampin alone may be used. Any one of these regimens can be effective in preventing active disease if the drugs are taken correctly and for the time prescribed.

■ INH, rifampin, and pyrazinamide can all cause liver damage. As a result, you should avoid alcoholic beverages and watch for signs and symptoms of hepatitis (e.g., nausea, yellowing of skin or eyes, dark urine, light-colored stools). If such symptoms occur, you should stop taking the drugs and report the symptoms to the health care provider managing the tuberculosis infection immediately. Blood tests of liver function will also be ordered. In some cases, liver failure has occurred, most often when patients continued to take the medications for a week or longer after symptoms of liver damage occurred.

■ Rifampin should be taken in a single dose, once daily or twice weekly, on an empty stomach, 1 hour before or 2 hours after a meal.

■ Rifampin causes a reddish discoloration of urine, tears, saliva, and other body secretions. This is harmless, except that soft contact lenses may be permanently stained.

■ Use all available resources to learn about tuberculosis and the medications used to prevent or treat the infection. This is extremely important because the information

can help you understand the reasons long-term treatment and follow-up care are needed. In addition to personal benefit, taking medications as prescribed can help your family and community by helping to prevent spread of tuberculosis. The American Lung Association publishes many helpful pamphlets that are available from local health departments and health care providers. Additional information is available on the Internet (e.g., the Centers for Disease Control and Prevention at http://www.cdc.gov).

■ Learn how to prevent spread of tuberculosis:
  ■ Cover mouth and nose when coughing or sneezing. This prevents expelling tuberculosis germs into the surrounding air, where they can be inhaled by and infect others.
  ■ Cough and expectorate sputum into at least two layers of tissue. Place the used tissues in a waterproof bag, and dispose of the bag, preferably by burning.
  ■ Wash hands after coughing or sneezing.

■ A nourishing diet and adequate rest help healing of infection.

■ Periodic visits to a health care provider are needed for follow-up care and to monitor medications.

■ The importance of taking medications as prescribed cannot be overemphasized. If not taken in the doses and for the length of time needed, there is a high likelihood for development of tuberculosis infection that is resistant to the most effective antituberculosis drugs. If this happens, treatment is much longer, very expensive, and requires strong drugs that cause more adverse effects. In addition, this very serious infection can be spread to family members and other close contacts. Thus, avoiding drug-resistant tuberculosis should be a strong incentive to complete the full course of treatment.

■ Rifampin decreases the effectiveness of oral contraceptive tablets; a different type of contraception should be used during rifampin therapy.

---

people. More specifically, the goal with latent TB infection is to prevent the development of active infection. The main goals with active infection are to decrease signs and symptoms, make the patient noninfectious, ensure adherence to the drug therapy regimen, and cure the patient (i.e., eliminate all TB organisms; at least 6 months of treatment are usually required). Secondary goals are to identify the person from whom the patient caught the infection (called the index case), identify other people infected by the index case or the new case of TB, and ensure that those persons are treated appropriately.

Drug-Susceptible Tuberculosis

Sputum culture and susceptibility reports require 6 to 8 weeks because the tubercle bacillus multiplies slowly. Consequently, initial drug therapy is based on other factors, such as the extent of disease, whether the patient has previously received antitubercular drugs, and whether multidrug-resistant strains are being found in the particular community.

Some general guidelines for pharmacologic treatment of TB are as follows:

■ Multiple drugs are required to effectively treat the infection and inhibit emergence of drug-resistant organisms.

■ Duration of drug therapy varies with the purpose, extent of disease, adherence to the drug therapy regimen, and clinical response. The trend in recent years, for treatment of both latent and active disease, is to give short courses of treatment (e.g., 6 months) when possible. Such regimens are more likely to be completed, and completion decreases the prevalence of drug-resistant disease in a community. In addition to the number of months of treatment, however, the total number of medication doses is also important. For example, the usual 6-month regimen for drug-susceptible TB consists of 182 doses of INH and rifampin and 56 doses of pyrazinamide. If treatment is interrupted for any reason, it is recommended that the drugs be continued so that the total number of doses is administered within a maximum time period of 9 months.

■ Fixed-dose combination tablets (e.g., Rifamate, Rifater) are recommended by some authorities, because they help to prevent the emergence of drug-resistant organisms. These formulations are more expensive than separate drugs.

Multidrug-Resistant Tuberculosis

Multidrug-resistant strains may occur anywhere. However, in the United States, they have been most evident in populations with AIDS, in closed environments (e.g., hospitals, prisons, long-term care facilities, homeless shelters), and in large urban areas.

Drug therapy regimens for people exposed to someone with MDR-TB or suspected of having MDR-TB should be designed in consultation with infectious-disease or tuberculosis specialists.

Treatment of MDR-TB requires concurrent administration of more drugs (e.g., four to six), for a longer period of time (e.g., 2 years or longer), than for drug-susceptible TB. The specific regimen is derived from cultures of infecting strains and susceptibility tests with primary and second-line drugs. It should include two or three drugs to which the isolate is sensitive and that the patient has not taken before.

All drug therapy for suspected or known MDR-TB should involve daily administration and DOT. Treatment is extremely expensive, even in the non-HIV population, and costs many thousand dollars more than the treatment of drug-susceptible TB.

XDR-TB may occur when treatment of MDR-TB is ineffective, for whatever reasons. Drug therapy for XDR-TB is extremely limited, because of the extensive resistance to both primary and second-line drugs.

Increasing Adherence to Antitubercular Drug Therapy

Failure to complete treatment regimens is a major problem in TB management because it increases the spread of the disease and the amount of drug-resistant disease in a community. There is more difficulty with getting patients to complete treatment for latent infection than for active disease. Identifying and treating LTBI requires several steps, including administering and reading skin tests; obtaining medical evaluations of infected persons; and initiating, monitoring, and completing treatment. Nonadherence is common in all of these aspects.

Strategies to Increase Adherence in TB Management

Supporting the use of short-course regimens, directly observed therapy (DOT), and intermittent drug administration. An additional strategy is to combine DOT with incentives and enablers (e.g., transportation, tokens or food coupons that are given to patients each time they appear at the health care facility for treatment).

Educating patients, family members, and contacts of patients. This may be especially important with treatment of LTBI. Most people are more motivated to take medications and schedule follow-up care when they have symptoms than when they feel well and have no symptoms. The importance of treatment for the future health of the individual, significant others, and the community must be emphasized. In addition, patients should be informed about common and potential adverse effects of drug therapy and what to do if they occur.

Providing support services and resources. These require substantial financial resources and may include more workers to provide DOT therapy at the patient's location; flexible clinic hours; reducing waiting times for patients; and assisting patients with child care, transportation, or other social service needs that encourage them to initiate and continue treatment. Lack of these services (e.g., clinics far from patients' homes, with inconvenient hours, long waiting times, unsupportive staff) may deter patients from being evaluated for a positive skin test, initiating treatment, or completing the prescribed treatment and follow-up care.

Individualizing treatment regimens. Treatment should be individualized whenever possible to increase patient convenience and minimize disruption of usual activities of daily living. Short-course regimens, intermittent dosing (e.g., two or three times weekly rather than daily), and fixed-dose combinations of drugs (e.g., Rifater, Rifamate) reduce the number of pills and the duration of therapy.

Promoting communication and continuity of care. With patients for whom English is not their primary language, it is desirable to have a health care worker who speaks their language or who belongs to their ethnic group. This worker may be able to more effectively teach patients and others, elicit cooperation with treatment, administer DOT, and be a consistent support person.

Monitoring Antitubercular Drug Therapy

There are two main methods of monitoring patient responses to treatment: clinical and laboratory.

Clinical monitoring is indicated for all patients. It includes teaching patients about signs and symptoms of adverse drug effects and which effects require stopping drug therapy and obtaining medical care (e.g., hepatotoxicity). It also includes regular assessment by a health care provider. Clinical monitoring should be repeated at each monthly visit. Patients should be assessed for signs of liver disease (e.g., loss of appetite, nausea, vomiting, dark urine, jaundice, fatigue, abdominal tenderness, easy bruising or bleeding) at least monthly if receiving INH alone or rifampin alone and at 2, 4, and 8 weeks if receiving rifampin and pyrazinamide. In addition to detecting adverse effects, these ongoing contacts are opportunities to reinforce teaching, assess adherence with therapy since the last visit, and observe for drug interactions. A standardized interview form may be helpful in eliciting appropriate information.

Laboratory monitoring mainly involves liver function tests (ALT, AST, bilirubin). Baseline measurements are indicated for patients with possible liver disorders, those infected with HIV, women who are pregnant or early postpartum (within 3 months of delivery), those with a history of liver disease (e.g., hepatitis or cirrhosis), those who use alcohol regularly, and those with risk factors for liver disease. Monitoring during therapy is indicated for patients who have abnormal baseline values or other risk factors for liver disease and those who develop symptoms of liver damage. Some clinicians recommend that INH be stopped for transaminase levels over three times the upper limit of normal if associated with symptoms and five times the upper limit of normal if the patient is asymptomatic.

Effects of Antitubercular Drugs on Other Drugs

Isoniazid (INH) increases risks of toxicity with several drugs by inhibiting their metabolism and increasing their blood levels. These include carbamazepine, fluconazole, haloperidol, phenytoin (effects of rifampin are opposite to those of INH and tend to predominate if both drugs are given with phenytoin), and vincristine. INH increases the risk of hepatotoxicity with most of these drugs; concurrent use should be avoided when possible or blood levels of the inhibited drug should be monitored. With vincristine, INH may increase peripheral neuropathy.

The rifamycins (rifampin, rifabutin, rifapentine) induce cytochrome P450 drug-metabolizing enzymes and therefore accelerate the metabolism and decrease the effectiveness of many drugs. Rifampin is the strongest inducer and may decrease the effects of angiotensin-converting enzyme (ACE) inhibitors, anticoagulants, antidysrhythmics, some antifungals (e.g., fluconazole), anti-HIV protease inhibitors (e.g., indinavir), anti-HIV NNRTIs (e.g., efavirenz, nevirapine), benzodiazepines, beta blockers, corticosteroids, cyclosporine, digoxin, diltiazem, estrogens and oral contraceptives, fexofenadine, fluoroquinolones, fluvastatin, haloperidol, lamotrigine, losartan, macrolide antibiotics, narcotic analgesics (e.g., methadone, morphine), nifedipine, ondansetron, phenytoin, propafenone, sertraline, sirolimus, sulfonylureas (e.g., glyburide), tacrolimus, tamoxifen, theophylline, thyroid hormones, toremifene, tricyclic antidepressants, verapamil, zaleplon, zidovudine, zolpidem, and other drugs. Rifapentine reportedly causes fewer drug interactions than rifampin but more than rifabutin. Rifabutin is a weaker enzyme inducer and may be substituted for rifampin in some cases, most often for patients who require anti-HIV medications.

Pyrazinamide may decrease effects of allopurinol and cyclosporine.

Use in Special Populations

Use in Patients With Human Immunodeficiency Virus (HIV) Infection

Tuberculosis is a common opportunistic infection in people with advanced HIV infection and may develop from an initial infection or reactivation of LTBI. For treatment of LTBI in patients with positive skin tests, INH daily or twice weekly for 9 months is effective.

Treatment of active disease is similar to that in persons who do not have HIV infection. Those with HIV infection who adhere to standard treatment regimens do not have an increased risk of treatment failure. Thus, these patients are usually treated with antitubercular drugs for 6 months like HIV-seronegative patients. The regimen may be longer if the bacteriologic (e.g., negative cultures) or clinical response (e.g., improvement in symptoms) is slow or inadequate.

A major difficulty with treatment of TB in patients with HIV infection is that rifampin interacts with many PIs and NNRTIs. If the drugs are given concurrently, rifampin decreases blood levels and therapeutic effects of the anti-HIV drugs. Rifabutin has fewer interactions and may be substituted for rifampin. The PIs indinavir and nelfinavir and most of the NNRTIs can be used with rifabutin. Ritonavir (PI) should not be used with rifabutin. Also, indinavir increases risks of rifabutin toxicity. Dosage of rifabutin should be decreased if given with indinavir.

Use in Children

Tuberculosis occurs in children of all ages. Infants and preschool children need early recognition and treatment because the disease can rapidly progress from primary infection to active pulmonary disease and perhaps to extrapulmonary involvement. TB is usually discovered during examination of a sick child or investigation of the contacts of someone with newly diagnosed active TB. Most children are infected in their home. Children in close contact with a patient with TB should receive skin testing, a physical examination, and a chest radiograph.

For treatment of LTBI, only one of the four regimens currently recommended for adults (INH for 9 months) is recommended for those under 18 years of age. For treatment of active disease, the prescribed regimens are similar to those used for adults. That is, the same primary drugs are used and may be given daily, twice weekly, or three times weekly with child-appropriate reductions in dosage. If the drug-susceptibility patterns of the M. *tuberculosis* strain causing the index case are known, the child is treated with those drugs; if this information is not available, the pattern of drug resistance in the community where the child likely became infected should be the guide for selecting the drug therapy regimen. As in adults, drug-susceptible TB is treated with INH, rifampin, and pyrazinamide for 2 months. Then, pyrazinamide is stopped and the INH and rifampin are continued for 4 more months. If drug-resistant organisms have been identified in the community, a fourth drug, ethambutol or streptomycin, should be given until the patient's culture and susceptibility reports become available. If pyrazinamide is not given, INH and rifampin are recommended for 9 months. When INH or rifampin cannot be used, therapy should continue for 12 to 24 months.

Drug-resistant TB in children is usually acquired from an adult family member or other close contact with active, drug-resistant disease. For children exposed to MDR-TB, there is no proven preventive therapy. Several regimens are used empirically, including ethambutol and pyrazinamide or ethionamide and cycloserine. When INH and rifampin cannot be given because of MDR-TB, drug therapy should continue for 24 months after sputum smears or cultures become negative. Fluoroquinolones (e.g., levofloxacin, others) are used for treatment of MDR-TB in adults but are not recommended for use in children. Patients with MDR-TB may require months of treatment before sputum smears become negative, and they are infectious during this period. To guide dosage and minimize adverse drug effects, serum drug levels should be measured periodically, especially in patients with GI, renal, or hepatic disease or in those with advanced HIV infection.

In children with HIV infection, the American Academy of Pediatrics recommends three drugs for at least 12 months. If drug-resistant or extrapulmonary disease is suspected, four drugs are indicated.

Overall, as with adults, drug therapy regimens vary with particular circumstances and continue to evolve. Health care providers must follow current recommendations of pediatric infectious-disease specialists.

Use in Older Adults

Although INH is the drug of choice for treatment of LTBI, its use is controversial in older adults. Because risks of drug-induced hepatotoxicity are higher in this population, some clinicians believe those patients with positive skin tests should have additional risk factors (e.g., recent skin-test conversion, immunosuppression, previous gastrectomy) before receiving INH. When INH is given, people who drink alcoholic beverages daily are most likely to sustain serious liver impairment.

For treatment of active disease caused by drug-susceptible organisms, INH, rifampin, and pyrazinamide are given, as in younger adults. Because all three drugs may cause hepatotoxicity, liver function tests should be monitored and the drugs discontinued if signs and symptoms of hepatotoxicity occur. For treatment of suspected or known MDR-TB, four to six drugs are used.

Use in Patients With Renal Impairment

Rifampin is mainly eliminated by the liver. However, up to 30% of a dose is excreted by the kidneys and dose reduction may be needed in patients with renal impairment. In addition, dosage of amikacin, capreomycin, cycloserine, ethambutol, fluoroquinolones, and streptomycin should be reduced in patients with impaired renal function. Cycloserine is contraindicated in severe renal impairment.

Use in Patients With Hepatic Impairment

Most antitubercular drugs are metabolized in the liver, and several (e.g., INH, rifampin, pyrazinamide) are hepatotoxic. Moreover, they are often used concomitantly, which increases risks of hepatotoxicity. To detect hepatotoxicity as early as possible, patients should be thoroughly instructed to report any signs of liver damage and health care providers who administer DOT or have any patient contact should observe for and ask about symptoms. For patients at risk of developing hepatotoxicity, serum ALT and AST should be measured before starting and periodically during drug therapy. If hepatitis occurs, these enzyme levels usually increase before other signs and symptoms develop.

With INH, mild increases in AST and ALT occur in approximately 10% to 20% of patients but are not considered significant and usually resolve without stopping the drug. Hepatitis and liver damage are more likely to occur during the first 8 weeks of INH therapy and in middle-aged and older adults. Patients should be assessed monthly for symptoms of hepatitis (anorexia, nausea, fatigue, malaise, jaundice). If symptoms occur or if AST and ALT increase significantly (more than five times the normal values), INH should be discontinued. INH should be used cautiously in patients with pre-existing liver disease.

With rifampin, liver damage is most likely to occur with pre-existing liver disease or concurrent use of other hepatotoxic drugs. Patients should be monitored at least monthly for symptoms of hepatotoxicity. AST and ALT may be measured before starting and periodically during rifampin therapy. If signs of liver damage occur, the drug should be stopped, serum AST and ALT should be measured, and medical evaluation should be done.

With pyrazinamide, the drug should not be given to a patient with pre-existing liver impairment unless it is considered absolutely essential. For patients without liver impairment, clinical monitoring for signs and symptoms of hepatotoxicity are recommended every 2 weeks. Serum ALT and AST may also be measured periodically. If significant symptoms or elevations of serum ALT and AST levels occur, the drug must be stopped.

Use in Home Care

The home care nurse has major roles to play in the health care of patients, families, and communities. With individual patients receiving antitubercular drugs for latent or active infection, the home care nurse needs to assist in taking the drugs as directed. Specific interventions vary widely and may include administering the drugs (DOT), teaching about the importance of taking the drugs and the possible consequences of not taking them (i.e., more severe disease, longer treatment regimens with more toxic drugs, spreading the disease to others), monitoring for adverse drug effects and assisting the patient to manage them or reporting them to the drug prescriber, assisting in obtaining the drugs and keeping follow-up appointments for blood tests and chest radiographs, and others. Family members may also need teaching related to preventing spread of the disease and assisting the patient to obtain adequate treatment. In relation to community needs, the nurse needs to be active in identifying cases, investigating contacts of newly diagnosed cases, and promoting efforts to manage tuberculosis effectively.

Nursing Actions   Antitubercular Drugs

NURSING ACTIONS	RATIONALE/EXPLANATION
1. Administer accurately	
a. Give isoniazid (INH), ethambutol, and rifampin in a single dose once daily, twice a week, or 3 times a week.	A single dose with the resulting higher blood levels is more effective. Also, less-frequent administration is more convenient for patients and more likely to be completed. Food delays absorption.
b. Give INH and rifampin on an empty stomach, 1 hour before or 2 hours after a meal, with a full glass of water. INH may be given with food if gastrointestinal (GI) upset occurs.	
c. Give parenteral INH by deep intramuscular (IM) injection into a large muscle mass, and rotate injection sites.	To decrease local pain and tissue irritation. Used only when patients are unable to take the medication orally.
d. Give IV rifampin by infusion, over 1–3 hours, depending on dose and volume of IV solution.	For a 600-mg dose, reconstitute with 10 mL of sterile water for injection; withdraw the entire amount and add it to 500 mL 5% dextrose or 0.9% sodium chloride solution; infuse over 3 hours.
e. Give rifabutin 300 mg once daily; if GI upset occurs, may give 150 mg twice daily.	Manufacturer's recommendation
f. Give rifapentine on an empty stomach when possible; may give with food if GI upset occurs.	Usually given twice weekly for 2 months, with 72 hours between doses, then once weekly for 4 months, along with other antitubercular drugs, for treatment of active TB.
g. Give secondary anti-TB drugs daily. See drug literature for specific instructions.	These drugs are used only to treat TB infection caused by organisms that are resistant to the primary anti-TB drugs.
2. Observe for therapeutic effects	Therapeutic effects are usually apparent within the first 2 or 3 weeks of drug therapy for active disease.
a. With latent infection, observe for the absence of signs and symptoms.	
b. With active disease, observe for clinical improvement (e.g., decreased cough, sputum, fever, night sweats, and fatigue; increased appetite, weight, and feeling of well-being; negative sputum smear and culture results; improvement in chest radiographs).	
3. Observe for adverse effects	
a. Nausea, vomiting, diarrhea	These symptoms are likely to occur with any of the oral antitubercular drugs.
b. Neurotoxicity:	
(1) Eighth cranial nerve damage—vertigo, tinnitus, hearing loss	A major adverse reaction to aminoglycoside antibiotics
(2) Optic nerve damage—decreased vision and color discrimination	The major adverse reaction to ethambutol
(3) Peripheral neuritis—tingling, numbness, paresthesias	Often occurs with INH but can be prevented by administering pyridoxine (vitamin B$_6$). Also may occur with ethambutol.
(4) Central nervous system changes—confusion, convulsions, depression	More often associated with INH, but similar changes may occur with ethambutol
c. Hepatotoxicity—increased serum alanine and aspartate aminotransferases (ALT and AST), and bilirubin; jaundice; other symptoms of hepatitis (e.g., anorexia, nausea, vomiting, abdominal pain)	May occur with INH, rifampin, and pyrazinamide, especially if the patient already has liver damage. Report these symptoms to the prescriber immediately, to prevent possible liver failure and death.
d. Nephrotoxicity—increased blood urea nitrogen and serum creatinine; cells in urine; oliguria	A major adverse reaction to aminoglycosides
e. Hypersensitivity—fever, tachycardia, anorexia, and malaise are early symptoms. If the drug is not discontinued, exfoliative dermatitis, hepatitis, renal abnormalities, and blood dyscrasias may occur.	Hypersensitivity reactions are more likely to occur between the third and eighth weeks of drug therapy. Early detection and drug discontinuation are necessary to prevent progressive worsening of the patient's condition. Severe reactions can be fatal.
f. Miscellaneous—rifampin, rifabutin, and rifapentine can cause:	
(1) a red-orange discoloration of body fluids, including urine and tears	The color change is harmless, but patients should avoid wearing soft contact lenses during therapy.
(2) permanent staining of soft contact lenses	
(3) increased sensitivity to sunlight	
(4) unplanned pregnancy, most often associated with rifampin, which makes hormonal birth control pills and implants less effective	Women who take rifampin should use a different form of birth control.

NURSING ACTIONS	RATIONALE/EXPLANATION
4. Observe for drug interactions	
a. Drugs that *increase* effects of antitubercular drugs:	
(1) Other antitubercular drugs	Potentiate antitubercular effects and risks of hepatotoxicity. These drugs are always used in combinations of two or more for treatment of active tuberculosis.
b. Drugs that *increase* effects of INH:	
(1) Alcohol	Increases risk of hepatotoxicity, even if use is stopped during INH therapy
(2) Carbamazepine	Accelerates metabolism of INH to hepatotoxic metabolites and increases risk of hepatotoxicity
c. Drug that *decreases* effects of INH:	
(1) Pyridoxine (vitamin B$_6$)	Decreases risk of peripheral neuritis
d. Drug that *decreases* effects of rifampin:	
(1) Ketoconazole	May decrease absorption

Key Concepts

- TB is a worldwide problem. Although not as extensive in the United States as in many other countries, the public health infrastructure for diagnosing and treating TB needs to be maintained.

- Multidrug resistant and extensively-drug resistant tuberculosis (MDR-TB and XDR-TB) are of increasing concern.

- Directly observed therapy (DOT) is recommended to prevent inadequate drug therapy and development of drug-resistant TB organisms.

- INH is the treatment of choice for LTBI.

- In drug-susceptible active TB, the treatment of choice is 2 months of INH, rifampin, and pyrazinamide, followed by 4 months of INH and rifampin.

- In drug-resistant TB, there is no standardized treatment regimen; treatment must be individualized for each patient according to drug susceptibility reports.

Review and Application Exercises

Short Answer Exercises

1. How do tuberculosis infections differ from other bacterial infections?

2. Why are patients with AIDS at high risk for developing tuberculosis?

3. What are the main risk factors for development of drug-resistant tuberculosis?

4. Who should receive INH to prevent tuberculosis? Who should not be given INH? Why?

5. When INH is given alone for treatment of LTBI, how long should it be taken?

6. If you worked in a health department with patients taking INH for treatment of LTBI, what are some interventions to promote patient adherence to the drug regimen?

7. Why is active, symptomatic tuberculosis always treated with multiple drugs?

8. In a patient with tuberculosis newly started on drug therapy, how could you explain the emergence of drug-resistant organisms and the importance of preventing this problem?

9. What are advantages and disadvantages of short-course (6–9 months) treatment programs?

10. What adverse effects are associated with INH, rifampin, pyrazinamide, and ethambutol, and how may they be prevented or minimized?

NCLEX-Style Questions

11. The nurse who is giving isoniazid (INH) anticipates an order for the following vitamin supplementation, which is usually given with isoniazid (INH).
    a. niacin
    b. pyridoxine
    c. vitamin D
    d. folate

12. The nurse knows to anticipate that the following adverse effect may be more likely to occur in patients receiving INH and rifampin.
    a. neurotoxicity
    b. hepatotoxicity
    c. nephrotoxicity
    d. ototoxicity

13. Patients taking INH should be taught by the nurse to avoid alcohol because of increased risks of
    a. severe central nervous system depression
    b. hepatitis
    c. drug-resistant M. *tuberculosis* organisms
    d. rapid drug metabolism

14. The family of a TB patient who is being treated asks the nurse when his symptoms will start to resolve with treatment. The nurse knows that the therapeutic effects of antitubercular drugs are usually evident in
    a. 3–5 days
    b. 7–10 days
    c. 2–3 weeks
    d. 6 weeks or longer

15. The nurse taking care of a patient with tuberculosis receives an order for a fluoroquinolone drug, ciprofloxacin. She knows that this drug may be used to treat
    a. inactive or latent tuberculosis
    b. active drug-susceptible tuberculosis
    c. MDR-TB
    d. nontuberculous mycobacterial infection

Selected References

American Thoracic Society, Centers for Disease Control and Prevention. (2000). Targeted tuberculin testing and treatment of latent tuberculosis infection. *American Journal of Respiratory and Critical Care Medicine, 161,* S221–S247.

American Thoracic Society, Centers for Disease Control and Prevention, Infectious Diseases Society of America. (2005). Controlling tuberculosis in the United States. *American Journal of Respiratory and Critical Care Medicine, 172,* 1169–1227.

Brooks, J. A. (2008). Management of patients with chest and lower respiratory tract disorders. In S. C. Smeltzer, B. G. Bare, J. L. Hinkle, & K. H. Cheever (Eds.), *Brunner & Suddarth's textbook of medical-surgical nursing* (11th ed., pp. 624–684). Philadelphia: Lippincott Williams & Wilkins.

Cain, K. P., Haley, C. A., Armstrong, L. R., Garman, K. N., Wells, C. D., Iademarco, M. F., et al. (2007). Tuberculosis among foreign-born persons in the United States: Achieving tuberculosis elimination. *American Journal of Respiratory and Critical Care Medicine, 175,* 75–79.

Chestnut, M. S., & Prendergast, T. J. (2007). Lung. In S. J. McPhee, M. A. Papadakis, & L. M. Tierney, Jr. (Eds.), *Current medical diagnosis and treatment 2007* (46th ed., pp. 222–315). New York: McGraw-Hill.

Drug facts and comparisons. (Updated monthly). St. Louis, MO: Facts and Comparisons.

Griffith, D. E., Aksamit, T., Brown-Elliott, B. A., Catanzareo, A., Daley, C., Gordin, F., et al. (2007). An official ATS/IDSA statement: Diagnosis, treatment, and prevention of nontuberculous mycobacterial diseases. *American Journal of Respiratory and Critical Care Medicine, 175,* 367–416.

Lacy, C. F., Armstrong, L. L., Goldman, M. P., & Lance, L. L. (2006). *Lexi-Comp's drug information handbook* (12th ed.). Hudson, OH: Lexi-Comp.

Marais, B. J., Gie, R. P., Schaaf, H. S., Beyers, N., Donald, R. R., & Starke, J. R. (2006). Childhood pulmonary tuberculosis: Old wisdom and new challenges. *American Journal of Respiratory and Critical Care Medicine, 173,* 1078–1090.

Munsiff, S. S., Kambili, C., & Ahuja, S. D. (2006). Rifapentine for the treatment of pulmonary tuberculosis. *Clinical Infectious Diseases, 43,* 1468–1475.

Pai, M. P., Momary, K. M., & Rodvold, K.A. (2006). Antibiotic drug interactions. *Medical Clinics of North America, 90,* 1223–1255.

Peloquin, C. A. (2005). Tuberculosis. In J. T. DiPiro, R. L. Talbert, G. C. Yee, G. R. Matzke, B. G. Wells, & L. M. Posey (Eds.), *Pharmacotherapy: A pathophysiologic approach* (6th ed., pp. 2015–2034). New York: McGraw-Hill.

Porth, C. M. (2005). Tuberculosis. In C. M. Porth (Ed.), *Pathophysiology: Concepts of altered health states* (7th ed., pp. 669–673). Philadelphia: Lippincott Williams & Wilkins.

Saukkonen, J. J., Cohn, D. L., Jasmer, R. M., Schenker, S., Jereb, J. A., Nolan, S. M., et al. (2006). An official ATS statement: Hepatotoxicity of antituberculosis therapy. *American Journal of Respiratory and Critical Care Medicine, 174,* 935–952.

Yew, W. W., & Leung, C. C. (2007). Update in tuberculosis 2006. *American Journal of Respiratory and Critical Care Medicine, 175,* 541–546.

CHAPTER 35

Antiviral Drugs

KEY TERMS

- Antiretroviral drugs
- Antiretroviral therapy (ART)
- Genital herpes
- HAART
- Herpesvirus
- Human immunodeficiency virus (HIV)
- Immunocompetent
- Immuno-compromised
- Retrovirus
- Viral hepatitis
- Viral load

LEARNING OBJECTIVES

After studying this chapter, you will be able to:

1. Describe characteristics of viruses and common viral infections.
2. Discuss difficulties in developing and using antiviral drugs.
3. Identify patients at risk for development of systemic viral infections.
4. Differentiate types of antiviral drugs used for various viral infections.
5. Describe selected antiviral drugs in terms of indications for use, adverse effects, and nursing process implications.
6. Discuss the rationale for using combinations of drugs in treating HIV infection.
7. Discuss guidelines for using antiviral drugs in special populations.
8. Teach patients strategies to prevent viral infections.

Applying Your Knowledge

Tony Bronowicz is a 32-year-old man who is HIV positive. He is following a drug regimen that consists of Combivir one capsule PO twice a day and ritonavir 600 mg PO twice a day. Mr. Bronowicz is currently hospitalized and you are his nurse.

Introduction

Viruses cause acquired immunodeficiency syndrome (AIDS), hepatitis, pneumonia, and other disorders that affect almost every body system. Many potentially pathogenic viral strains exist, including more than 150 that infect the human respiratory tract. Viruses can be spread by secretions from infected people, ingestion of contaminated food or water, breaks in skin or mucous membrane, sexual contact, pregnancy, breast-feeding, and organ transplantation. Viral infections vary from mild, localized disease with few symptoms to severe, systemic illness and death. Additional characteristics of viruses and viral infections are described in the following paragraphs; selected infections are described in Box 35-1.

- Viruses are intracellular parasites that gain entry to human host cells by binding to receptors on cell membranes. All human cells do not have receptors for all viruses; cells that lack receptors for a particular virus are resistant to infection by that virus. Thus, the locations and numbers of the receptors determine which host cells can be infected by a virus. For example, the mucous membranes lining the tracheobronchial tree have receptors for the influenza A virus; helper T lymphocytes and other white blood cells have CD4 molecules, which are the receptors for the *human immunodeficiency virus (HIV)*.
- Inside host cells, viruses use cellular metabolic activities for their own survival and replication. Viral replication involves dissolution of the protein coating and exposure of the genetic

559

Box 35-1 Selected Viral Infections

Avian Influenza A (H5N1)

In recent years, the highly pathogenic H5N1 subtype of influenza A has been found in numerous countries. It occurs mainly in birds and poultry, but a few hundred human cases have been confirmed. Most human cases occur after exposure to infected poultry or surfaces contaminated with poultry droppings. Because human infection may cause respiratory failure and has a high mortality rate, the possibility that these viral strains might mutate so that they infect humans more easily is a major public health concern. This virus is considered the most likely cause of a future worldwide influenza epidemic

Herpesvirus Infections

Cytomegalovirus Infection and Retinitis

Cytomegalovirus (CMV) infection is common, and most people become infected by adulthood. Infection is usually asymptomatic in healthy, *immunocompetent* adults. Like other herpesviruses, CMV can cause a primary infection, then remain latent in body tissues, probably for life. This means the virus can be shed in secretions of an asymptomatic host and spread to others by contact with infected saliva, blood, urine, semen, breast milk, and cervical secretions. It also means the virus may lead to an opportunistic infection when the host becomes immunosuppressed. During pregnancy, CMV is transmitted to the fetus across the placenta and may cause infection in the brain, inner ears, eyes, liver, and bone marrow. Learning disabilities and mental retardation can result from congenital CMV infection. Children spread the virus to each other in saliva or urine, whereas adolescents and adults transmit the virus mainly through sexual contact.

Major populations at risk for development of active CMV infection are patients with cancer who receive immunosuppressant drugs and organ transplant recipients, who must receive immunosuppressant drugs to prevent their body's rejection of the transplanted organ. Patients with advanced HIV infection are also at risk, but the incidence has decreased with highly active antiretroviral therapy (*HAART*). Systemic CMV infection occurs mainly from reactivation of endogenous virus, although it may occur from an exogenous source. Active CMV infection may cause cellular necrosis and inflammation in various body tissues. Common manifestations of disease include pneumonitis, hepatitis, encephalitis, adrenal insufficiency, gastrointestinal inflammation, and gastric ulcerations.

In the eye, CMV infection produces retinitis, usually characterized by blurred vision and decreased visual acuity. Visual impairment is progressive and irreversible and, if untreated, may result in blindness. CMV retinitis may also indicate systemic CMV infection or may be entirely asymptomatic.

Genital Herpes Infection

Genital herpes infection is caused by the herpes simplex virus (HSV) and produces recurrent, painful, blister-like lesions on skin and mucous membranes. HSV is usually transmitted from person to person by direct contact with open lesions or secretions, including genital secretions. Primary infection occurs at a site of viral entry, where the virus infects epithelial cells, produces progeny viruses, and eventually causes cell death. After primary infection, latent virus may become dormant within sensory nerve cells. In response to various stimuli (e.g., intense sunlight, emotional stress, febrile illness, menstruation), latent virus may become reactivated and lead to viral reproduction and shedding.

In the fetus, HSV may be transmitted from an infected birth canal, and neonatal herpes is a serious complication of maternal genital herpes. Neonatal herpes usually becomes evident within the first week of life and may be manifested by the typical clusters of blister-like lesions on skin or mucous membranes. Irritability, lethargy, jaundice, altered blood clotting, respiratory distress, seizures, or coma may also occur. The lesions may heal in 1 to 2 weeks, but neonatal herpes carries a high mortality rate. In immunosuppressed patients, HSV infection may result in severe, systemic disease.

Herpes Zoster

Herpes zoster is caused by the varicella-zoster virus, which is highly contagious and present worldwide. Most children in the United States are infected by early school age. The virus produces chickenpox on first exposure and is spread from person to person by the respiratory route or by contact with secretions from skin lesions. Recovery from the primary infection leaves latent infection in nerve cells. Reactivation of the latent infection (usually later in life) causes herpes zoster (more commonly known as "shingles"), a localized cluster of painful, blister-like skin lesions. The skin lesions have the same appearance as those of chickenpox and genital herpes. Over several days, the vesicles become pustules, then rupture and heal. Because the virus remains in sensory nerve cells, pain can persist for months after the skin lesions heal. Most cases of herpes zoster infection occur among the elderly and the immunocompromised.

Human Immunodeficiency Virus Infection

HIV infection is caused by a *retrovirus* that infects the immune system. Two types of HIV virus have been identified, HIV-1 and HIV-2. Most infections in the United States are caused by HIV-1; HIV-2 infections occur mainly in Africa. HIV binds to receptors on the surface of CD4+ cells (especially T lymphocytes or helper T cells). HIV entry and replication eventually results in cell death. Because CD4+ cells play major roles in regulating immune function, their destruction results in serious impairment of the immune system.

The initial phase of HIV infection is characterized by influenza-like symptoms (e.g., fever, chills, muscle aches) that may last several weeks. During this time, the virus undergoes rapid replication. The next phase is characterized by a dramatic decline in the rate of viral replication, attributed to a partially effective immune response. During this phase, no visible manifestations of HIV infection may be present. However, replication of HIV continues and antibodies may be detected in the serum. During this period, the person is seropositive (HIV+) and infectious but asymptomatic. Eventually, the immune system is substantially damaged and the rate of viral reproduction accelerates. When viral load and immunodeficiency reach significant levels, the illness is termed acquired human immunodeficiency syndrome (AIDS) and serious opportunistic infections occur. With effective drug therapy, viral load decreases and the CD4+ cell count increases, so that HIV-infected people may live for many years without progression to AIDS.

HIV infection occurs in all age groups and can spread to a new host during any phase of infection. The virus is commonly spread by sexual intercourse, injection of intravenous drugs with contaminated needles, mucous membrane contact with infected blood or body fluids, and perinatally from mother to fetus. Although the virus is found in most body fluids, infection has primarily been associated with exposure to blood, semen, or vaginal secretions. The virus is not spread through casual contact. Health care workers may be infected by needle-stick injuries. They should be aware that postexposure prophylaxis is available and may significantly reduce the risk of transmission.

Human Papilloma Virus (HPV) Infection

HPV infection, the most common sexually transmitted infection, is spread by contact with infected lesions. It affects both men and women and can cause genital warts and several types of cancer (e.g., cervical, vaginal, vulvar, anal, and penile). In women, 80% reportedly become infected within 5 years of becoming sexually active.

Respiratory Syncytial Virus Infection

RSV is a highly contagious virus that is present worldwide and infects most children by school age. Epidemics of RSV infection often occur in nurseries, daycare centers, and pediatric hospital units during winter months. RSV infects and destroys respiratory epithelium in the bronchi, bronchioles, and alveoli. It is spread by respiratory droplets and secretions, direct contact with an infected person, and contact with fomites, including the hands of caregivers.

RSV is the most common cause of bronchiolitis and pneumonia in infants and causes severe illness in those younger than 6 months of age. These infants usually have wheezing, cough, respiratory distress, and fever. The infection is usually self-limited and resolves in 1 to 2 weeks. Antiviral therapy with ribavirin is used in some cases. The mortality rate from RSV infection is low in children who are generally healthy but increases substantially in those with congenital heart disease or immunosuppression. Recurrent infection occurs but is usually less severe than primary infection. In older children, RSV infection produces much milder disease but may be associated with acute exacerbations of asthma.

In adults, RSV infection causes colds and bronchitis, with symptoms of fever, cough, and nasal congestion. Infection occurs most often in those with household or other close contact with children, including pediatric health care workers. In older adults, RSV infection may cause pneumonia requiring hospitalization. In immunocompromised patients, RSV infection may cause severe and potentially fatal pneumonia.

Viral Hepatitis

There are several types of *viral hepatitis*, and new hepatitis viruses are still being identified. Worldwide, viral hepatitis has increased in recent years. All hepatitis viruses have similar effects on the liver, although they differ in some other characteristics. Common types of viral hepatitis are described below. Vaccines are available to prevent hepatitis A and B (see Chap. 39).

Hepatitis A virus (HAV) is transmitted mainly by the fecal–oral route and close contact with an infected person; foodborne outbreaks also occur, usually from infected food handlers or contaminated produce in the United States. The virus survives for long periods in the environment (e.g., in water and soil) and on human hands and inanimate objects. It resists freezing, detergents, and acids but can be inactivated by chlorine and temperatures above 185°F.

The HAV reproduces only in liver and gastrointestinal cells, from which viral particles are released into blood and bile. The average incubation period is 25 to 30 days. The patient is infectious during the incubation period and for 7 to 10 days after symptoms develop. In infected adults, about 70% develop symptoms, including fever and jaundice, that may last as long as 2 months. Most recover without treatment and develop immunity against future HAV infections; 10% to 20% require hospitalization. In children, many are asymptomatic or develop flu-like or nonspecific symptoms without jaundice. However, even children with few or no symptoms may shed virus in their stools and be a source of community infection for as long as 6 months. The availability of hepatitis A vaccine has greatly decreased the number of reported cases. The vaccine is recommended for children and adults at increased risk of contracting the disease (e.g., travelers to certain countries, men who have sex with men, drug abusers, recipients of clotting factor replacement) and for persons with chronic liver disease.

Hepatitis B virus (HBV) can be transmitted by contact with contaminated blood and other body fluids (e.g., perinatally, during sexual contact with an infected person, by sharing needles during IV drug use, and undergoing acupuncture, hemodialysis, tattooing, or ear and body piercing). In addition, health care and public safety workers are at increased risk of developing HBV infection from injuries with contaminated equipment (e.g., contaminated needles) and from other exposures to infected body fluid. Any person exposed to infected body fluids should be evaluated for HBV infection; any person diagnosed with HBV infection should be evaluated for liver disease and for HIV infection. It is estimated that 70,000 Americans become infected with HBV every year and approximately 5,000 of them will die of the complications caused by the infection. Many Americans have chronic HBV infection; asymptomatic chronic carriers of HBV may transmit the infection to others. Hepatitis B can lead to cirrhosis, liver cancer, liver failure, and death.

(continued on page 562)

| **Box 35-1** | **Selected Viral Infections** (continued) |

The HBV can live up to 3 days on various surfaces that appear clean. The incubation period is 30 to 180 days. Increased hepatitis B surface antigens and liver enzymes (ALT, AST) occur before symptoms of HBV infection develop. After symptoms develop, antibodies to the viral antigens are produced and the presence of antigens and viral DNA in the patient's blood indicate that the patient is infectious.

Hepatitis C virus (HCV) can be transmitted by contact with contaminated blood or other body fluids. Persons at high risk of exposure include health care and public safety workers; IV drug users; those with multiple sex partners; those undergoing hemodialysis, tattoos, or body piercings; and those who received blood transfusions before 1990, when screening blood for HCV was started. In addition, pregnant women may trans-

mit the virus to their infants, and mothers with symptoms and high viral titers may transmit the virus to nursing infants.

The HCV incubation period is 14 to 80 days; infection is diagnosed by testing for viral DNA or antibodies. HCV infection affects people of all ages but is most often found among 20- to 39-year-olds. Infected persons can be asymptomatic for years, but most eventually develop chronic liver disease. In the United States, HCV infection is the leading cause of cirrhosis, liver cancer, and liver transplants. Effective drug therapy may cure HCV infection.

Other hepatitis viruses (e.g., D, G, and a "transfusion-transmissible" virus) have been identified; they, like HBV and HCV, are transmitted through contact with infected blood and body fluids.

material (deoxyribonucleic acid [DNA] or ribonucleic acid [RNA]). With DNA viruses, the viral DNA enters the host cell's nucleus, where it becomes incorporated into the host cell's chromosomal DNA. Then, host cell genes are coded to produce new viruses. In addition, the viral DNA incorporated with host DNA is transmitted to the host's daughter cells during host cell mitosis and becomes part of the inherited genetic information of the host cell and its progeny. With RNA viruses (e.g., HIV), viral RNA must be converted to DNA by an enzyme called reverse transcriptase before replication can occur.

After new viruses are formed, they are released from the infected cell either by budding out and breaking off from the cell membrane (leaving the host cell intact) or by causing lysis of the cell. When the cell is destroyed, the viruses are released into the blood and surrounding tissues, from which they can transmit the viral infection to other host cells.

▪ Viruses induce antibodies and immunity. Antibodies are proteins that defend against microbial or viral invasion. They are very specific (i.e., an antibody protects only against a specific virus or other antigen). For example, in a person who has had measles, antibody protection (immunity) develops against future infection by the measles virus, but immunity does not develop against other viral infections, such as chickenpox or hepatitis.

The protein coat of the virus allows the immune system of the host to recognize the virus as a "foreign invader" and to produce antibodies against it. This system works well for most viruses but does not work for the influenza A virus, which can alter its protein covering so much and so often that the immune system does not recognize it as foreign to the body. Thus, last year's antibody cannot recognize and neutralize this year's virus.

Antibodies against infecting viruses can prevent the viruses from reaching the bloodstream or, if they are already

in the bloodstream, prevent their invasion of host cells. After the virus has penetrated the cell, it is protected from antibody action, and the host depends on cell-mediated immunity (lymphocytes and macrophages) to eradicate the virus along with the cell harboring it.

▪ Viral infection may occur without signs and symptoms of illness. If illness does occur, the clinical course is usually short and self-limited. Recovery occurs as the virus is eliminated from the body. Some viruses (e.g., *herpesvirus*) can survive in host cells for many years and cause a chronic, latent infection that periodically becomes reactivated. Also, autoimmune diseases may be caused by viral alteration of host cells so that lymphocytes recognize the host's own tissues as being foreign.

▪ Symptoms usually associated with acute viral infections include fever, headache, cough, malaise, muscle pain, nausea and vomiting, diarrhea, insomnia, and photophobia. White blood cell counts usually remain normal. Other signs and symptoms vary with the type of virus and body organs involved.

Antiviral Drugs

Numerous vaccines have been developed (see Chap. 39) to prevent viral infections, and numerous drugs have been developed to treat HIV and other viral infections. Most antivirals inhibit viral reproduction but do not eliminate viruses from tissues. In general, available drugs are expensive, relatively toxic, and effective in a limited number of infections. Some may be useful in treating an established infection if given promptly and in chemoprophylaxis if given before or soon after exposure. Protection conferred by chemoprophylaxis is immediate but lasts only while the drug is being taken. Subgroups of antiviral drugs are described in the following sections; additional characteristics and dosage ranges are listed in Tables 35-1 and 35-2.

Table 35-1 **Drugs at a Glance:** Drugs for Prevention or Treatment of Selected Viral Infections

Generic/Trade Name	Indications for Use	ROUTES AND DOSAGE RANGES Adults	Children
Herpesvirus Infections			
Acyclovir (Zovirax)	Oral mucocutaneous lesions (e.g., cold sores, fever blisters) Genital herpes Herpes simplex encephalitis Varicella (chickenpox) in immunocompromised hosts Herpes zoster (shingles) in normal and immunocompromised hosts	Genital herpes, PO 200 mg q4h, 5 times daily for 10 d for initial infection; 400 mg 2 times daily to prevent recurrence of chronic infection; 200 mg q4h 5 times daily for 5 d to treat recurrence Herpes zoster, PO 800 mg q4h 5 times daily for 7–10 d Chickenpox, PO 20 mg/kg (maximum dose 800 mg) 4 times daily for 5 d Mucosal and cutaneous HSV infections in ICH, IV 5 mg/kg infused over 1 h, q8h for 7 d Varicella-zoster infections in ICH, IV 10 mg/kg, infused over 1 h, q8h for 7 d HSV encephalitis, IV 10 mg/kg, infused over 1 h, q8h for 10 d Topically to lesions q3h, 6 times daily for 7 d	*Under 12 y:* IV 10 or 20 mg/kg q8h for 7 or 10 d, depending on the condition being treated Chickenpox, weight above 40 kg, PO 800 mg 4 times daily for 5 d Chickenpox, 2 y and older and weight 40 kg or less, PO 20 mg/kg 4 times daily for 5 d *12 y and older:* topical, same as adults
Famciclovir (Famvir)	Acute herpes zoster Genital herpes	Herpes zoster, PO 500 mg q8h for 7 d Genital herpes, PO 125 mg twice daily for 5 d	
Foscarnet (Foscavir)	Treatment of CMV retinitis in persons with AIDS Treatment of acyclovir-resistant mucocutaneous HSV infections in ICH	CMV retinitis, IV 60 mg/kg q8h for 2–3 wk, depending on clinical response, then 90–120 mg/kg/d for maintenance HSV infections, IV 40 mg/kg q8–12h for 2–3 wk or until lesions are healed	Dosage not established
Ganciclovir (Cytovene)	CMV retinitis in ICH Prevention of CMV disease in patients with organ transplants or advanced HIV infection	CMV retinitis, IV 5 mg/kg q12h for 14–21 d, then 5 mg/kg once daily for 7 d/wk or 6 mg/kg once daily for 5 d/wk or PO 1000 mg 3 times daily for maintenance Prevention in transplant recipients, IV 5 mg/kg once daily 7 d/wk or 6 mg/kg once daily 5 d/wk Prevention in patients with HIV infection, PO 1000 mg 3 times daily	Dosage not established
Trifluridine (Viroptic)	Keratoconjunctivitis caused by herpes viruses	Topically to eye, 1% ophthalmic solution, 1 drop q2h while awake (maximum 9 drops/d) until re-epithelialization of corneal ulcer occurs; then 1 drop q4h (maximum 5 drops/d) for 7 d	*Older than 6 y,* same as adults

(continued on page 564)

Table 35-1   **Drugs at a Glance:** Drugs for Prevention or Treatment of Selected Viral Infections (continued)

Generic/Trade Name	Indications for Use	ROUTES AND DOSAGE RANGES	
		Adults	**Children**
Valacyclovir (Valtrex)	Herpes labialis, herpes zoster, and recurrent genital herpes in immunocompetent patients	Herpes labialis, PO 2 g twice daily for 1 d Herpes zoster, PO 1 g q8h for 7 d Recurrent genital herpes, PO 500 mg q12h daily for 5 d Reduce dosage with renal impairment	Herpes labialis, adolescents, PO, same as adults Dosage not established for children
Valganciclovir (Valcyte)	Prevention and treatment of CMV retinitis	PO 900 mg twice daily for 21 d	Dosage not established
Influenza Virus Infection **Amantadine** (Symmetrel)	Prevention or treatment of influenza A infection	PO 200 mg once daily or 100 mg twice daily Reduce dosage with renal impairment	*1–10 y and weight less than 40 kg:* PO 5 mg/kg/d; maximum dose 150 mg/d *10 y and older and weight 40 kg or over:* PO 100 mg twice daily
Oseltamivir (Tamiflu)	Prevention or treatment of influenza A infection	PO 75 mg once daily	*13 y and older or weight above 40 kg:* PO same as adults *1–12 y:* PO twice daily according to weight: 15 kg or less, 30 mg; above 15 kg to 23 kg or less, 45 mg; above 23 kg to 40 kg or less, 60 mg
Rimantadine (Flumadine)	Prevention or treatment of influenza A infection in adults Prophylaxis of influenza A in children	PO 100 mg twice daily	*10 y and older:* same as adults *Under 10 y:* 5 mg/kg once daily; maximum dose 150 mg
Zanamivir (Relenza)	Treatment of influenza A or B infection	Oral inhalation, 2 inhalations twice daily for 5 d	*7 y and older:* same as adults
Respiratory Syncytial Virus Infection **Ribavirin** (Virazole)	Treatment of hospitalized infants and young children with severe lower respiratory tract infections		Inhalation: diluted to a concentration of 20 mg/mL for 12–18 h/d for 3–7 d
Viral Hepatitis **Adefovir** (Hepsera)	Treatment of chronic hepatitis B	PO 10 mg once daily	Dosage not established
Entecavir (Baraclude)	Treatment of chronic hepatitis B	PO 0.5 mg once daily for patients beginning treatment; 1 mg daily for those who have developed resistance to lamivudine	Dosage not established
Lamivudine (Epivir HBV)	Treatment of chronic hepatitis B	PO 100 mg once daily	*2–17 y:* 3 mg/kg once daily; maximum dose, 100 mg
Ribavirin (Virazole)	Treatment of chronic hepatitis C (with peginterferon alfa 2a)	PO 800–1200 mg twice daily	PO 15 mg/kg twice daily
Telbivudine (Tyzeka)	Treatment of chronic hepatitis B	PO 600 mg once daily	*16 y and older:* same as adults

AIDS, acquired immunodeficiency syndrome; CMV, cytomegalovirus; HSV, herpes simplex virus; ICH, immunocompromised host.

Table 35-2 | **Drugs at a Glance:** Drugs for Human Immunodeficiency Virus Infection and Acquired Immunodeficiency Syndrome

Generic/Trade Name	Characteristics	ROUTES AND DOSAGE RANGES	
		Adults	Children
Nucleoside Reverse Transcriptase Inhibitors (NRTIs)			
Abacavir (Ziagen)	Well absorbed; 50% bound to plasma proteins; metabolized to inactive metabolites that are excreted in urine and feces **BBW:** Risks of serious hypersensitivity reactions, lactic acidosis, and hepatomegaly with steatosis	PO 300 mg twice daily	*Over 3 mo:* PO 8 mg/kg twice daily (maximum 300 mg twice daily)
Emtricitabine (Emtriva)	Well absorbed; metabolized in the liver and excreted mainly in urine **BBW:** Risks of lactic acidosis and hepatomegaly with steatosis	PO 200 mg (1 capsule) or 240 mg (24 mL of oral solution) once daily	*3 mo to 17 y:* Weight above 33 kg and can swallow capsule, PO 1 capsule once daily Oral solution, PO 6 mg/kg once daily (maximum dose, 240 mg or 24 mL daily)
Lamivudine (Epivir)	Used to treat HIV infection and chronic hepatitis B Well absorbed; mainly eliminated unchanged in urine Dosage should be reduced with renal impairment. **BBW:** Risks of lactic acidosis and hepatomegaly with steatosis	PO 150 mg twice daily Weight 60 kg (110 lbs) or less: PO 2 mg/kg twice daily	*12–16 y:* PO same as adults *3 mo to 12 y:* PO 4 mg/kg twice daily
P Zidovudine (AZT, ZVD, Retrovir)	Prototype NRTI Well absorbed, metabolized in the liver to an inactive metabolite, which is excreted in urine May cause peripheral neuropathy and pancreatitis **BBW:** Risks of severe anemia, neutropenia, lactic acidosis, and hepatomegaly with steatosis	PO 300 mg twice daily	*3 mo to 12 y:* 180 mg/m^2 q6h (not to exceed 200 mg q6h) Neonate born of HIV-infected mother who took the drug during pregnancy, labor, and delivery: PO 2 mg/kg q6h starting within 12 h of birth and continuing until 6 wk of age; IV 1.5 mg/kg q6h if unable to take oral drug
Nucleotide Reverse Transcriptase Inhibitor			
Tenofovir DF (Viread)	Used for salvage therapy after multiple drug failures Efficacious against hepatitis B **BBW:** Risks of lactic acidosis and hepatomegaly with steatosis	300 mg once daily	Dosage not established

(continued on page 566)

| Table 35-2 | | **Drugs at a Glance:** Drugs for Human Immunodeficiency Virus Infection and Acquired Immunodeficiency Syndrome (continued) |

Generic/Trade Name	Characteristics	ROUTES AND DOSAGE RANGES	
		Adults	Children
Non-Nucleoside Reverse Transcriptase Inhibitors (NNRTIs)			
Efavirenz (Sustiva)	Well absorbed; induces drug-metabolizing enzymes in the liver. May cause central nervous system side effects.	PO 600 mg at bedtime	*Weight over 40 kg:* PO same as adults *Age 3 y and over and weight 10–40 kg (22–88 lb):* PO 200–400 mg, depending on weight
Nevirapine (Viramune)	Well absorbed; induces drug-metabolizing enzymes in the liver **BBW:** Risks of hepatitis, hepatic necrosis, hepatic failure, and severe skin reactions	PO 200 mg once daily for 2 wk, then 200 mg twice daily	*2 mo to 8 y:* 4 mg/kg once daily for 14 d, then 7 mg/kg twice daily *8 y and older:* 4 mg/kg once daily for 14 d, then 4 mg/kg twice daily
Protease Inhibitors			
Atazanavir (Reyataz)	Well absorbed with few adverse effects May cause hyperbilirubinemia	PO 400 mg daily	Dosage not established
Darunavir (Prezista)	Must be taken with ritonavir and food to achieve therapeutic blood levels Highly bound to plasma proteins; metabolized in liver and excreted mainly in feces	PO 600 mg twice daily, with ritonavir 100 mg and food	Dosage not established
Fosamprenavir (Lexiva)	Prodrug formulation of amprenavir that allows for a reduced pill burden. A 700-mg tablet contains the equivalent of 600 mg of amprenavir.	Treatment-naïve: PO 1400 mg twice daily Treatment-experienced: PO 700 mg twice daily (with ritonavir 100 mg twice daily)	Dosage not established
Indinavir (Crixivan)	Well absorbed; metabolized in the liver; excreted mainly in feces May cause GI upset and kidney stones	PO 800 mg q8h	Dosage not established
Nelfinavir (Viracept)	Most common adverse effect is diarrhea, which can be controlled with over-the-counter drugs such as loperamide	PO 1250 mg twice daily	*1–13 y:* PO 20-30 mg/kg/dose, 3 times daily
Ritonavir (Norvir)	Metabolized in the liver; slows metabolism of many drugs **BBW:** Risk of serious adverse effects if given with certain other drugs, including antidysrhythmics (amiodarone, flecainide, propafenone, others), sedative-hypnotics (midazolam, triazolam), ergot derivatives, alfuzosin, voriconazole	PO 600 mg twice daily	PO 400 mg/m² daily

Generic/Trade Name	Characteristics	ROUTES AND DOSAGE RANGES	
		Adults	**Children**
Saquinavir (Invirase)	Not well absorbed; highly protein bound; metabolized in liver; excreted mainly in feces May produce fewer drug interactions than indinavir and ritonavir	PO 1200 mg 3 times daily	*16 y and older:* same as adults
Tipranavir (Aptivus)	Absorption increased with food; highly protein bound; metabolized in the liver mainly by CYP3A4 enzymes	PO 500 mg with ritonavir 200 mg twice daily	Dosage not established
Entry Inhibitors **Enfuvirtide** (Fuzeon)	Highly protein bound Adverse effects include injection site reactions, nausea, and diarrhea.	Sub-Q 90 mg (1 mL) twice daily into upper arm, anterior thigh, or abdomen	6-16 y: Sub-Q 2 mg/kg (maximum, 90 mg) twice daily, into upper arm, anterior thigh, or abdomen
Maraviroc (Selzentry)	Given with other antiretroviral drugs May cause hepatotoxicity	PO 150–600 mg twice daily, depending on other medications being taken	Dosage not established for children under 16 years of age
Combination Products **Atripla**	Tablets contain efavirenz 600 mg, emtricitabine 200 mg and tenofovir 300 mg	PO 1 tablet once daily	Not recommended
Combivir	Tablets contain zidovudine 300 mg and lamivudine 150 mg	PO 1 tablet twice daily	*12 y and older:* same as adults
Epzicom	Tablets contain abacavir 600 mg and lamivudine 300 mg	PO 1 tablet daily	Dosage not established
Kaletra	Tablets contain lopinavir 200 mg and ritonavir 50 mg Oral solution contains lopinavir 80 mg and ritonavir 20 mg/mL	PO 3 tablets twice daily	*Weight 7–15 kg:* 12/3 mg/kg twice daily *Weight 15-40 kg:* 10/2.5 mg/kg twice daily
Trizivir	Tablets contain zidovudine 300 mg, lamivudine 150 mg, and abacavir 300 mg	PO 1 tablet twice daily	Dosage not established
Truvada	Tablets contain emtricitabine 200 mg and tenofovir 300 mg	PO 1 tablet once daily	Dosage not established

BBW, black box warning; GI, gastrointestinal.

Drugs for Herpesvirus Infections

Acyclovir, famciclovir, and **valacyclovir** penetrate virus-infected cells, become activated by an enzyme, and inhibit viral DNA reproduction. They are used in the treatment of herpes simplex and herpes zoster infections. Acyclovir is used to treat genital herpes, in which it decreases viral shedding and the duration of skin lesions and pain. It does not eliminate inactive virus in the body and thus does not prevent recurrence of the disease unless oral drug therapy is continued. Acyclovir is also used for treatment of herpes simplex infections in *immunocompromised* patients. Prolonged or repeated courses of acyclovir therapy may result in the emergence of acyclovir-resistant viral strains, especially in immunocompromised patients. Acyclovir can be given orally, intravenously (IV), or applied topically to lesions. IV use is recommended for severe genital herpes in nonimmunocompromised patients and any herpes infections in immunocompromised patients. Oral and IV acyclovir are excreted mainly in urine, and dosage should be decreased in patients who are older or who have renal impairment.

Famciclovir and valacyclovir are oral drugs for herpes zoster and recurrent genital herpes. Famciclovir is metabolized to penciclovir, its active form, and excreted mainly in the urine. Valacyclovir is metabolized to acyclovir by enzymes in the liver and/or intestine and is eventually excreted in the urine. As with acyclovir, dosage of these drugs must be reduced in the presence of renal impairment.

Foscarnet, ganciclovir, and **valganciclovir** also inhibit viral reproduction after the drugs are activated by a viral enzyme found in virus-infected cells. The drugs are used to treat cytomegalovirus (CMV) retinitis. In addition, foscarnet is used to treat acyclovir-resistant mucocutaneous herpes simplex infections in people with impaired immune function. Valganciclovir and ganciclovir are used to prevent CMV disease, mainly in patients with organ transplants or HIV infection. Dosage of these drugs must be reduced with renal impairment. Ganciclovir causes granulocytopenia and thrombocytopenia in 20% to 40% of recipients, often during the first 2 weeks of therapy. If severe bone marrow depression occurs, ganciclovir should be discontinued; recovery usually occurs within a week of stopping the drug. Foscarnet should be used cautiously in patients with renal disease.

Trifluridine is applied topically to treat keratoconjunctivitis and corneal ulcers caused by the herpes simplex virus (herpetic keratitis). Trifluridine should not be used longer than 21 days because of possible ocular toxicity.

Drugs for HIV Infection (Antiretrovirals)

Antiretroviral therapy (ART) for treatment of HIV infection continues to evolve. In general, newer drugs and drug combinations are more effective in viral suppression, cause fewer serious adverse effects, and are more convenient for patients to take. Some of the older drugs are not recommended for initial treatment but may be used when drug-resistant infections develop with the newer drugs or are transmitted to other people. Testing for drug resistance is more often used; interactions among *antiretroviral drugs* and between antiretrovirals and other drugs continue to be complex.

Five classes of antiretroviral drugs currently exist: nucleoside reverse transcriptase inhibitors (NRTIs), nucleotide reverse transcriptase inhibitor, non-nucleoside reverse transcriptase inhibitors (NNRTIs), protease inhibitors, and entry inhibitors (see Table 35-2). The first four groups inhibit enzymes required for viral replication in human host cells; the entry inhibitors prevent the HIV from entering cells and causing infection (Fig. 35-1). To increase effectiveness and decrease viral mutations and emergence of drug-resistant viral strains, combinations of drugs are used. Recommendations for drug regimens change often; a good source for keeping up-to-date is www.aidsinfo.nih.gov.

Nucleoside Reverse Transcriptase Inhibitors (NRTIs)

The NRTIs are structurally similar to DNA components (adenosine, cytosine, guanosine, or thymidine) and thus easily enter human cells and viruses in human cells. For example, **P** **zidovudine**, the prototype, is able to substitute for thymidine. In infected cells, these drugs inhibit reverse transcriptase, an enzyme required by retroviruses to convert RNA to DNA and allow replication. The drugs are more active in slowing the

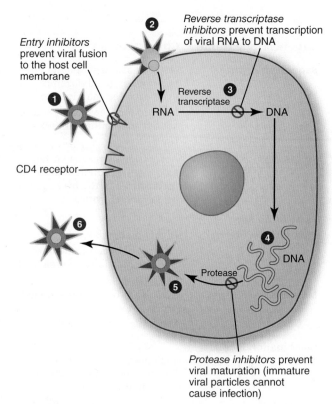

Figure 35-1 ■ Human immunodeficiency virus (HIV) entry into cells and replication; actions of anti-HIV drugs. (1) The virus attaches to receptors (e.g., CD4 molecules) and co-receptors (CCR5 molecules) on the host cell membrane. (2) The virus becomes uncoated and releases its RNA into the host cell. (3) The enzyme reverse transcriptase converts RNA to DNA, which is necessary for viral replication. (4) The DNA codes for protein synthesis, which produces immature viral particles. (5) The enzyme protease assembles the immature viral particles into mature viruses. (6) Mature viruses are released from the host cell.

progression of acute infection than in treating chronically infected cells. Thus, they do not cure HIV infection or prevent transmission of the virus through sexual contact or blood contamination. Didanosine (Videx) and stavudine (Zerit) are infrequently used and are not discussed further in this chapter.

Nucleotide Reverse Transcriptase Inhibitor

The one drug in this group, **tenofovir** (Viread), is similar to the NRTIs in that it inhibits the reverse transcriptase enzyme. However, it differs structurally, and this difference helps to prevent the development of drug-resistant viral strains.

Non-Nucleoside Reverse Transcriptase Inhibitors (NNRTIs)

The NNRTIs inhibit viral replication in infected cells by directly binding to reverse transcriptase and preventing its function. They are used in combination with NRTIs to treat HIV infection. Because the two types of drugs inhibit reverse transcriptase by different mechanisms, they may have synergistic antiviral effects. **Efavirenz** (Sustiva) is the most commonly used NNRTI, with **nevirapine** (Viramune) as an acceptable substitute in some circumstances. **Delavirdine** (Rescriptor) is the least effective of these drugs. It is not recommended for initial treatment but may be used to treat drug-resistant HIV strains. It is not discussed further in this chapter.

Protease Inhibitors (PIs)

The PIs exert their effects against HIV at a different phase of its life cycle than reverse transcriptase inhibitors. Protease is an HIV enzyme required to process viral protein precursors into mature particles that are capable of infecting other cells. The drugs inhibit the enzyme by binding to its protease-active site and cause the production of immature, noninfectious viral particles. These drugs are active in both acutely and chronically infected cells because they block viral maturation.

Two major concerns with PIs are viral resistance and drug interactions. Viral resistance develops fairly rapidly, with resistant strains developing in approximately half of the recipients within a year of drug therapy. Most PIs are metabolized in the liver by the cytochrome P450 enzyme system and should be used cautiously in patients with impaired liver function. In relation to drug interactions, PIs interfere with metabolism, increase plasma concentrations, and increase risks of toxicity of numerous other drugs metabolized by the cytochrome P450 enzymes in the liver.

Indinavir, ritonavir, and **saquinavir** are the oldest PIs. Ritonavir, the most potent cytochrome P450 inhibitor in the group, interacts with other PIs to increase their blood levels and therapeutic effectiveness. Thus, ritonavir is often given with other PIs (except nelfinavir) as a "booster." This usage allows fewer pills and less frequent administration but also increases risks of hyperlipidemia and drug interactions.

With other drugs, ritonavir may increase plasma concentrations of amiodarone, bupropion, clozapine, flecainide, meperidine, piroxicam, propafenone, propoxyphene, quinidine, rifabutin, and voriconazole. None of these drugs should be given concomitantly with ritonavir because high plasma concentrations may cause cardiac dysrhythmias, hematologic abnormalities, seizures, and other potentially serious adverse effects. In addition, ritonavir may increase sedation and respiratory depression when used concurrently with benzodiazepines (e.g., alprazolam, diazepam, triazolam) and zolpidem.

Indinavir increases plasma concentrations of several of the same drugs listed previously and should not be given concomitantly with them because of potential cardiac dysrhythmias or prolonged sedation. Saquinavir may produce fewer interactions because it inhibits the cytochrome P450 enzyme system to a lesser extent than indinavir and ritonavir. However, if saquinavir is given with clindamycin, quinidine, triazolam, or a calcium channel blocker, patients should be monitored closely for increased plasma levels and adverse drug effects.

Entry Inhibitors

HIV entry into human host cells requires two sequential steps, and a drug has been developed to block each step. First, the virus contains a glycoprotein on its surface that allows it to attach itself to CD4 receptors on human cells and fuse with the cell membrane. This initial binding and fusion is blocked by **enfuvirtide** (Fuzeon), which is also called a fusion inhibitor. Second, the HIV binds to another molecule on the surface of host cell membranes. This molecule, CCR5, is a co-receptor that enhances viral binding and fusion. **Maraviroc** (Selzentry) blocks the binding of the HIV to CCR5 and is also called a CCR5 antagonist.

Combination Drugs

Early antiretroviral drug regimens were very complex and involved the ingestion of many pills daily. Current regimens are simpler, partly because of newer drugs and partly because of more fixed-dose combinations of commonly used drugs. Combination products decrease the "pill burden" and promote adherence. A high degree of adherence is required to produce therapeutic effects and prevent the development of drug resistance.

 Applying Your Knowledge 35-1

How Can You Avoid This Medication Error?

Mr. Bronowicz complains of severe pain, so you notify the resident and receive an order for meperidine 50 mg IM for one dose. You prepare and administer the medication

Drugs for Influenza

Amantadine and **rimantadine** inhibit replication of the influenza A virus and are used to prevent or treat influenza A infections. Postexposure prophylaxis with these drugs may protect persons who have had direct contact with people infected with influenza A. Seasonal prophylaxis may be used in high-risk patients if the influenza vaccine cannot be given or may be ineffective. In epidemics, use of one of the drugs is recommended for patients at high risk who have not been vaccinated. The high-risk population includes older adults, those who have chronic lung disease, and those who have immunodeficiency disorders. During an epidemic, amantadine or rimantadine may be given for 2 weeks if the patient is vaccinated at the beginning of drug therapy or 4 to 8 weeks if the patient is un-vaccinated. Protection is lost within a few days after drug therapy is stopped. For treatment of influenza A infection, either drug may shorten the illness if started soon after onset and continued for 5 days. The drugs may also decrease viral shedding and spread.

Amantadine and rimantadine are well absorbed after oral administration. Amantadine is excreted in the urine unchanged. It accumulates in the body of older adults and others with impaired renal function, and dosage therefore should be reduced in these groups. Rimantadine is extensively metabolized, with small amounts excreted in the urine. The most common adverse effects of the drugs are gastrointestinal (anorexia, nausea) and central nervous system (CNS: nervousness, lightheadedness, difficulty concentrating) symptoms. CNS effects are more likely to occur with amantadine than rimantadine, and high plasma levels of amantadine have been associated with delirium, hallucinations, seizures, coma, and cardiac dysrhythmias. Amantadine has also been associated with exacerbations of pre-existing seizure disorders and psychiatric symptoms. Amantadine is teratogenic in animals, and neither drug has been established as safe for pregnant women.

Amantadine is also used in the treatment of Parkinson's disease and for extrapyramidal symptoms associated with the use of certain antipsychotic drugs (see Chap. 12).

Oseltamivir (Tamiflu) and **zanamivir** (Relenza) are approved for prevention or treatment of influenza A or B in patients with symptoms for 2 days or less. They may be more effective for prevention than treatment, with some reports indicating that they reduce symptoms by only 1 day and viral shedding by 2 days. When used, therapy should last for 5 days. Oseltamivir is an oral drug; zanamivir is a powder form for oral inhalation with a device called a Diskhaler. Zanamivir may cause bronchospasm in patients with asthma or chronic obstructive pulmonary disease. The drugs also have activity against avian influenza A (H5N1).

Drug for Respiratory Syncytial Virus Respiratory Tract Infections

Ribavirin is used mainly for the treatment of bronchiolitis or pneumonia caused by the respiratory syncytial virus (RSV). It is used in hospitalized infants and young children and given by inhalation with an aerosol device. The drug is not recommended for patients on ventilators because it precipitates and may block breathing tubes, including endotracheal tubes. Deterioration of pulmonary function is a common adverse effect. The drug is absorbed systemically after administration by aerosol. Most infants and children with RSV infections have mild, self-limited disease that does not involve the lower respiratory tract and therefore does not require hospitalization or ribavirin therapy.

Drugs for Viral Hepatitis Infections

Vaccines are available to prevent hepatitis A and hepatitis B, and the incidence of these infections has decreased with use of the vaccines. Still, viral hepatitis is an important cause of disability and death from liver disease as well as the major reason for liver transplantation. People at high risk of developing hepatitis include men who have sex with men, users of illicit drugs, and international travelers.

For treatment of hepatitis B, several drugs have been developed, including **adefovir, entecavir, interferon** (see Chap. 40), **lamivudine** (Epivir HBV), and **telbivudine**. Entecavir, lamivudine, and telbivudine are nucleoside analogs, all of which have **BLACK BOX WARNINGS** about increased risks of lactic acidosis and severe enlargement and accumulation of fat in the liver, including fatal cases. Because some patients experience exacerbation of hepatitis B symptoms when drug therapy is stopped, they should be monitored for several months. For treatment of chronic hepatitis C, a combination of ribavirin and peginterferon alfa-2a (see Chap. 40) is effective and may cure the infection.

Nursing Process

Assessment

- Assessment varies with the type of viral infection that is present or suspected.
- Assess renal function and adequacy of fluid intake.
- With HIV infection, assess baseline data to assist in monitoring response to drug therapy. Baseline data may include vital signs, weight and nutritional status, signs and symptoms of the disease, signs and symptoms of opportunistic infections associated with the disease and immunosuppression, and available reports of laboratory tests (e.g., complete blood count; CD4+ lymphocyte counts; plasma levels of viral RNA, blood urea nitrogen, and serum creatinine; liver function tests).
- With viral hepatitis, assess for risk factors, possible sources of exposure, and signs and symptoms of liver dysfunction.

Nursing Diagnoses

- Anxiety related to a medical diagnosis of serious viral infection (e.g., HIV infection, viral hepatitis)
- Altered Sexuality Patterns related to sexually transmitted viral infections (HIV infection, genital herpes)
- Disturbed Body Image related to sexually transmitted infection
- Social Isolation related to a medical diagnosis of HIV infection or genital herpes
- Deficient Knowledge: Disease process and methods of spread; availability of vaccines and other prophylactic interventions
- Risk for Injury: Recurrent infection; adverse drug effects; adverse drug interactions; infections and other problems associated with a compromised immune system in HIV infection; liver damage or failure with viral hepatitis

Planning/Goals

The patient will

- Receive or take antiviral drugs as prescribed
- Be safeguarded against new or recurrent infection
- Act to prevent spread of viral infection to others and recurrence in self
- Avoid preventable adverse drug effects and drug interactions
- Receive emotional support and counseling to assist in coping with HIV infection or genital herpes

Interventions

- Follow recommended policies and procedures for preventing spread of viral infections.

- Assist patients in learning ways to control spread and recurrence of viral infections.
- Assist patients to maintain immunizations against viral infections.
- For patients receiving systemic antiviral drugs, monitor serum creatinine and other tests of renal function, complete blood count, and fluid balance.
- For patients with HIV infection, assist to schedule their drug therapy regimen as conveniently as possible (to promote adherence), monitor for changes in baseline data during each contact, prevent opportunistic infections (e.g., herpes infections) when possible, and manage adverse effects of drug therapy to promote quality of life.

Evaluation

- Observe for improvement in signs and symptoms of the viral infection for which a drug is given.
- Interview outpatients regarding their compliance with instructions for taking antiviral drugs.
- Interview and observe for use of infection control measures.
- Interview and observe for adverse drug effects.
- Observe the extent and severity of any symptoms in patients with HIV infection or viral hepatitis.

Applying Your Knowledge 35-2

Mr. Bronowicz has been having a hard time with his drug regimen. He has difficulty with the proper timing of his medications. He also has complained about an upset stomach. What patient education should you provide to Mr. Bronowicz?

Principles of Therapy

Prevention of Viral Infections

General preventive measures include vaccination, hand hygiene, teaching patients with respiratory infections to cover their mouth and nose when coughing or sneezing, treatment of symptoms, and recognition and treatment of complications.

With sexually transmitted viral infections, spread of genital herpes can be prevented by avoiding sex when skin lesions are present and using condoms. HIV infection can be prevented by the consistent use of condoms and use of clean needles by IV drug users. In addition, anti-HIV medications can be given to prevent HIV infection after occupational (e.g., contaminated needle-stick injuries of health care personnel) or nonoccupational (e.g., sexual, drug use, accidental) exposure. For the latter group, those with high-risk exposure to an HIV-infected person should seek treatment within 72 hours. Drug therapy should be started as soon as possible and continued for 4 weeks. With human papilloma virus (HPV) infections, consistent use of condoms can prevent HPV infection. Although lesions may develop outside the area covered by a condom, such lesions are not considered a common or major source of infection spread. With hepatitis, prevention strategies include rigorous hand hygiene, avoiding contaminated water and food, avoiding contact with blood and body fluids, and avoiding injections, tattooing, or body piercing with contaminated needles.

Viral Vaccines

Viral vaccines are used to produce active immunity in patients before exposure or to control epidemics of viral disease in a community. Vaccines for prevention of cervical cancer, chickenpox, hepatitis A and B, herpes zoster, measles, mumps, poliomyelitis, rubella, smallpox, and yellow fever and for protection against influenza A, B, and avian influenza A (H5N1) and rabies are available (see Chap. 39). Live attenuated viral vaccines are generally safe and nontoxic. However, they should not be used in patients who are pregnant; immunodeficient; receiving high-dose, long-term corticosteroids; or receiving

---

Patient Teaching Guidelines ▸ Miscellaneous Antiviral Drugs

General Considerations

- Prevention is better than treatment, partly because medications used to treat viral infections may cause serious adverse effects. Thus, whenever possible, techniques to prevent viral infections should be employed.
  - Wash hands frequently and thoroughly; this helps prevent most infections.
  - Maintain immunizations against viral infections as indicated.
  - With genital herpes, avoid sexual intercourse when visible lesions are present and always wash hands after touching any lesion.
- Drugs may relieve symptoms but do not cure viral infections. For example, treatment of genital herpes does not

prevent transmission to others, and treatment of cytomegalovirus (CMV) retinitis may not prevent disease progression.

- Ask a health care provider for information about managing adverse drug effects.
- If taking foscarnet or ganciclovir for CMV retinitis, have eye examinations approximately every 6 weeks.

Self-Administration

- With acyclovir, famciclovir, and valacyclovir for genital herpes, start oral drugs for recurrent lesions as soon as signs and symptoms begin.
- Use gloves to apply acyclovir ointment to lesions.

Patient Teaching Guidelines | Antiretroviral Drugs

General Considerations

■ Prevention is better than treatment, partly because medications used to treat viral infections may cause serious adverse effects. Thus, whenever possible, techniques to prevent viral infections should be used.

- ■ Wash hands frequently and thoroughly; this helps prevent most infections.
- ■ Maintain immunizations against viral infections as indicated.
- ■ Always practice safer sex by using a condom.
- ■ In cases of intravenous drug use, use and promote the use of clean needles.

■ Drugs may relieve symptoms but do not cure human immunodeficiency virus (HIV) infection, prevent transmission of the virus, or prevent other illnesses associated with advanced HIV infection.

■ Effective treatment of HIV infection requires close adherence to drug therapy regimens involving several drugs and daily doses. Missing as few as one or two doses can decrease blood levels of antiretroviral drugs and result in increased HIV replication and development of drug-resistant viral strains.

■ It is generally recommended that herbal products not be used with antiretroviral medications. St. John's wort may decrease blood levels of some anti-HIV medications and make them less effective; echinacea should be avoided because it may stimulate viral replication.

■ Request information about adverse effects associated with the specific drugs you are taking and what you should do if they occur. Adverse effects vary among the drugs; some are potentially serious.

■ Have regular blood tests including viral load, CD4+ cell count, complete blood count, and others as indicated (e.g., tests of kidney and liver function).

■ Keep your health care providers informed about all medications being taken; do not take any other drugs (including drugs of abuse, herbal preparations, vitamin/mineral supplements, nonprescription drugs) without consulting a health care provider. These preparations may make anti-HIV medications less effective or more toxic.

Self-Administration

■ Take the medications exactly as prescribed. Do not change doses or stop the medications without consulting a health care provider. If a dose is missed, do not double the next dose. The drugs must be taken consistently to suppress HIV infection and minimize adverse drug effects.

■ These medications vary in their interactions with food and should be taken appropriately for optimal benefit. Unless otherwise instructed, take the drugs as follows:

- ■ Abacavir, Combivir, emtricitabine, famciclovir, fosamprenavir, Kaletra tablets, lamivudine, nevirapine, tenofovir, Trizivir, valacyclovir and zidovudine may be taken with or without food. However, do not take abacavir or efavirenz with a high-fat meal.
- ■ Take Atripla, efavirenz, entecavir, or indinavir on an empty stomach, 1 hour before or 2 hours after a meal.
- ■ Take atazanavir, darunavir, ganciclovir, Kaletra oral solution, nelfinavir, ritonavir, and tipranavir with food.
- ■ Take saquinavir within 2 hours after a meal.

■ To give nelfinavir to infants and young children, the oral powder can be mixed with a small amount of water, milk, or formula. After it is mixed, the entire amount must be taken to obtain the full dose. Acidic foods or juices (e.g., applesauce, orange juice, apple juice) should not be used because they produce a bitter taste.

---

antineoplastic or immunosuppressive drugs or radiation. Vaccines for influenza A and influenza B prevent infection in most patients. If infection does occur, less virus is shed in respiratory secretions. Thus, vaccination reduces transmission of influenza by decreasing the number of susceptible people and by decreasing transmission by immunized people who still become infected. The multiplicity of rhinoviruses (common cold), enteroviruses, and respiratory viruses hinders development of vaccines for these common diseases.

Use of Antibacterial Drugs in Viral Infections

Antibacterial drugs (e.g., antibiotics) should not be used to treat viral infections. They do have a role, however, in treating bacterial complications of viral infections. For example, bacterial pneumonia may develop as a complication of influenza.

Use of Antiretroviral Drugs in HIV Infection

■ The goals of drug therapy include reducing HIV-related morbidity and mortality, decreasing viral load to unde-

tectable levels (<400 copies/mL) as long as possible, halting disease progression, restoring immune function, and improving quality of life.

■ Treatment of HIV infection is complex, and recommendations change often as new drugs, new drug regimens, and research reports become available. Thus, when possible, clinicians with expertise in the care of HIV-infected patients should prescribe, supervise, and monitor drug therapy. Before starting drug therapy, clinicians should consult current treatment guidelines and individualize the regimen according to health status (e.g., impaired liver function, psychiatric illness, tuberculosis), dosing convenience (e.g., number of pills daily and frequency of administration), presence or absence of drug-resistant viral strains, potential adverse drug effects and drug interactions, the patient's likelihood of adhering to the drug therapy regimen, and other factors. Updated treatment guidelines are readily available via the Internet at www.aidsinfo.nih.gov and should be consulted regularly by health care personnel involved in treatment of patients with HIV infection.

- Benefits and risks of drug therapy must be clear to patients initiating drug therapy. A high degree of adherence to the prescribed regimen is required for viral suppression; nonadherence may lead to a lack of effectiveness and emergence of drug-resistant viral strains. Factors contributing to nonadherence include active substance abuse, depression, and lack of social support. The patient must also be able to tolerate or manage adverse drug effects.

- Evidence-based drug therapy for adults and adolescents is described in Evidence-Based Practice Box 35-1. Additional considerations include the following:

  - Combination antiretroviral therapy is the standard of care. A commonly used three-drug regimen includes two NRTIs and a protease inhibitor. Other options include two NRTIs and one NNRTI (most commonly efavirenz) or three NRTIs.

  - Potentially serious drug interactions, especially between protease inhibitors and other agents, are extensive and may require drug substitution or dose reduction to avoid toxicity.

  - Patients should be assessed for signs and symptoms of adverse drug effects approximately every 3 months during therapy.

  - Effective drug therapy usually produces significantly reduced plasma HIV RNA levels by 2 months and undetectable levels by 4 to 6 months. In addition, the CD4+ cell count usually increases faster during the first 3 months, then at an average of 100 to 150 cells/mm³ per year. Failure to obtain an undetectable viral load may result from nonadherence to the medication regimen, inadequate drugs or doses, drug-resistant viral strains, and other factors.

  - Laboratory tests are used to determine when to initiate drug therapy and to assess adherence and response to therapy. *Viral load* is a measure of the number of HIV RNA particles within the blood; it does not measure viral levels in tissues, where viral reproduction may be continuing. In untreated clients, measurement is recommended at the time of diagnosis, then every 3 to 4 months. In treated patients, HIV RNA levels should be assessed before and 2 to 8 weeks after starting drug therapy, then every 3 to 4 months.

    CD4+ cell counts are also assessed and used to monitor drug therapy. CD4+ cell counts should be measured at the time of diagnosis and every 3 to 6 months thereafter. Complete blood counts, electrolyte levels, fasting blood glucose and lipids, and tests of renal and hepatic function are also recommended.

  - Drug therapy should be continuous when at all possible. Studies indicate that interruptions in treatment allow viral growth and disease progression. In addition, patients receiving drug therapy for advanced HIV infection should continue medications during an opportunistic infection or malignancy, unless there are significant drug intolerances, toxicities, or interactions.

Evidence-Based Practice

35-1 Drug Therapy for HIV Infection in Adults and Adolescents

Treatment-Naïve Patients

- Initial antiretroviral drug therapy is recommended for all symptomatic patients and for asymptomatic patients with a CD4+ T-cell count below 350/mL, **before** the count falls to 200 cells/mL (Level of evidence A).
- A combination of three antiretroviral drugs is recommended for initial treatment of a previously untreated patient. Several combinations, often called highly active antiretroviral therapy (HAART), are possible. As of October 2006, the preferred regimen (Level of evidence A for all drugs) was
  - Efavirenz plus one of the following combinations:
  - Atazanavir + ritonavir
  - Fosamprenavir + ritonavir twice daily
  - Lopinavir/ritonavir twice daily
  - Tenofovir/emtricitabine
  - Zidovudine/lamivudine
- An alternative regimen (Level of evidence B for all drugs) consists of nevirapine rather than efavirenz, plus one of the following single drugs or combinations:
  - Atazanavir
  - Fosamprenavir
  - Fosamprenavir + ritonavir once daily
  - Lopinavir/ritonavir once daily
  - Abacavir/lamivudine
  - Didanosine + lamivudine
- Other options may be acceptable for individual patients, including nelfinavir, ritonavir-boosted saquinavir, and a combination of abacavir, zidovudine, and lamivudine.

Treatment-Experienced Patients

Treatment-experienced patients are those who have developed retroviral strains that are resistant to the drugs used earlier. Tests of drug susceptibility and design of a new drug therapy regimen with at least two active antiretroviral drugs is recommended (Level of evidence A). If two fully active drugs cannot be identified, clinicians may choose one of the following regimens (Level of evidence B):

- Add ritonavir to other protease inhibitors (except nelfinavir).
- Add a drug with activity against drug-resistant virus (e.g., a ritonavir-boosted protease inhibitor) and a drug with a new mechanism of action (e.g., HIV entry inhibitors such as enfuvirtide) to the current antiretroviral regimen. (Note: Tipranavir and darunavir are newer protease inhibitors approved for patients who are highly treatment-experienced or have HIV-1 strains resistant to multiple protease inhibitors.)

Sources: *www.aidsinfo.nih.gov;* Hammer, S. M., Saag, M. S., Schechter, M., Montaner, J. S. G., Schooley, R. T., Jacobson, D. M. et al. (2006). Treatment for adult HIV infection: 2006 Recommendations of the International AIDS Society—USA panel. *Journal of the American Medical Association, 296,* 827–843.

Applying Your Knowledge 35-3

During the course of therapy for Mr. Bronowicz, periodic laboratory tests will be done to monitor the effectiveness of drug therapy. What cell count is assessed and how often should it be monitored?

Use in Special Populations

Use in Children

The use of systemic antiviral drugs is more problematic in children because several of the available drugs have not been tested in this group, are not available in pediatric formulations, and/or do not have pediatric dosages.

Amantadine may be given to prevent or treat influenza A in children 1 year of age or older, and rimantadine is given only for prevention in children. Oseltamivir may be used in children 1 year and older. However, some serious adverse effects have been reported in children 16 years and younger who were taking oseltamivir. The adverse effects include neurologic and psychiatric problems (e.g., delirium, hallucinations, confusion, abnormal behavior, seizures, encephalitis) and a few severe skin reactions. Zanamivir may be used in children 7 years and older

Clinicians using anti-HIV drugs in children need to be experienced and up-to-date regarding recommendations. Some HIV infections in children result from perinatal transmission and HIV testing of pregnant women should be a part of routine perinatal care. HIV-seropositive females should receive zidovudine to prevent perinatal transmission. At 14 to 34 weeks of gestation, zidovudine should be administered at a dose of 100 milligrams PO five times a day until delivery. At delivery, a loading dose of 2 milligrams per kilogram of body weight should be given, followed by 1 milligram per kilogram every hour until birth. The infant is then given zidovudine 2 milligrams per kilogram every 6 hours for the first 6 weeks of life. If perinatal infection occurs, the infant usually develops symptoms (e.g., an opportunistic infection, failure to thrive) within the first 3 to 8 months of life. Zidovudine, which is approved for treatment of HIV infection in children, is usually the drug of choice. As in adults, anemia and neutropenia are common adverse effects of zidovudine.

In addition to zidovudine, several other drugs can be used in children, including abacavir, emtricitabine, enfuvirtide, efavirenz, lamivudine, nelfinavir, nevirapine, ritonavir, and the combination products Combivir, Kaletra, and Trizivir. Current drug literature should be consulted for age and weight ranges for individual drugs.

For older children and adolescents with HIV infection, additional factors need to be considered. A few are long-term survivors of perinatal HIV infection and their clinical course may differ from those infected later in life. However, many become infected during their teen years. The Centers for Disease Control and Prevention (CDC) estimate that half of the 40,000 new cases diagnosed each year occur in people 13 to 24 years of age.

In general, adult guidelines for anti-HIV drug therapy are appropriate for adolescents because those infected sexually or by injecting drugs follow a clinical course similar to that of adults. However, pediatric doses of antiretroviral drugs should be used for those in early puberty, and adult doses should usually be given for those in late puberty. Persuading adolescents to adhere to the drug therapy regimen may be especially difficult as they may not see the need for medications when they are asymptomatic, may experience adverse drug effects, want to fit in with their peer groups rather than being different, or have other barriers. Clinicians need to make the drug regimen as user friendly as possible and to use all available resources to promote adherence.

All adolescents with HIV infection, who are often sexually active, need information about prevention of HIV transmission. Female adolescents need additional information about contraception and drug interactions between anti-HIV medications and birth control pills.

Use in Older Adults

Antiviral drug selection and dosing should proceed cautiously with older adults, who often have impaired organ function, concomitant diseases, and other drug therapy. Most systemic antiviral drugs are excreted by the kidneys and renal impairment is common in older adults. Therefore, greater risks of toxicity exist. These risks may be minimized by dose reduction when indicated by decreased creatinine clearance. When amantadine is given to prevent or treat influenza A, dosage should be reduced with renal impairment, and older adults should be closely monitored for CNS (e.g., hallucinations, depression, confusion) and cardiovascular (e.g., congestive heart failure, orthostatic hypotension) effects.

HIV infection is increasing in those over 50 years of age, and there is little information about the effects of anti-HIV medications in older adults. As potent antiretroviral therapy extends the lifespan of HIV-infected patients, clinicians can expect to encounter greater numbers of older adults who take these medications. As a general rule, renal impairment may necessitate adjustment of NRTI and NNRTI doses, and hepatic impairment may affect dosing of protease inhibitors.

Use in Patients With Renal Impairment

Antiviral drugs should be used cautiously in patients with impaired renal function because some are nephrotoxic, most are eliminated by the kidneys, and many require dosage reductions because their elimination may be decreased. All patients with renal impairment should be monitored closely for abnormal renal function tests and drug-related toxicity. Renal effects and guidelines for usage of selected drugs are described in the following sections.

Nephrotoxic Drugs

■ Acyclovir may precipitate in renal tubules and cause renal impairment with high doses of oral drug or IV administration (e.g., to treat acute herpes zoster). This is most likely to occur in patients who are dehydrated and may be minimized by maintaining a high urine output. Although patients on hemodialysis usually need reduced doses, an additional dose is needed after dialysis because treatment removes up to 51% of serum acyclovir.

■ Foscarnet may cause or worsen renal impairment and should be used with caution in all patients. Manifestations of renal impairment are most likely to occur during the second week of induction therapy but may occur any time during treatment. Renal impairment may be minimized by monitoring renal function (e.g., at baseline; 2 or 3 times weekly during induction; at least every 1 or 2 weeks during maintenance therapy) and reducing dosage accordingly. The drug should be stopped if creatinine clearance drops below 0.4 milliliters per minute per kilogram. Adequate hydration should also be maintained throughout the course of drug therapy.

■ Indinavir may cause nephrolithiasis, flank pain, and hematuria. Symptoms usually subside with increased hydration and drug discontinuation. To avoid nephrolithiasis, patients on indinavir should consume 48 to 64 ounces of water or other fluid daily.

Drugs That Require Dosage Reduction

■ Amantadine, emtricitabine, entecavir, famciclovir, ganciclovir, lamivudine, telbivudine, and valacyclovir are eliminated mainly through the kidneys. In patients with renal impairment, they may accumulate, produce higher blood levels, have longer half-lives, and cause toxicity. For all of these drugs except famciclovir and emtricitabine, dosage should be reduced with creatinine clearance (CrCl) levels below 50 milliliters per minute. With famciclovir, dosage should be decreased with CrCl below 60 milliliters per minute. For patients receiving hemodialysis, dosages should be calculated according to CrCl, with daily doses given after dialysis. With emtricitabine, dosage is reduced by extending the dosage interval. Prescribers should consult manufacturers' recommendations.

■ Zidovudine dosage should be decreased in cases of severe renal impairment. Zidovudine is mainly metabolized in the liver to an inactive metabolite that is then eliminated renally (approximately 60%–75% of a dose); another 20% is excreted as unchanged drug in the urine. Thus, mild to moderate renal impairment does not lead to drug accumulation or a need for reduced dosage. With severe impairment, however, drug half-life is prolonged. Also, patients with renal impairment may be more likely to experience zidovudine-induced hematologic adverse effects because of decreased production of erythropoietin. Because of these

factors, it is recommended that the daily dosage be reduced by approximately 50% in patients with severe renal impairment (CrCl < 25 mL/minute) and patients on hemodialysis.

Use in Patients With Hepatic Impairment

The antiviral drugs of most concern in hepatic impairment are the anti-HIV agents, especially the protease inhibitors. Although most antiretroviral drugs have not been studied in patients with hepatic impairment, several are primarily metabolized in the liver and may produce high blood levels and cause adverse effects in the presence of liver dysfunction. In addition, patients with HIV infection may have concomitant liver disease that further impairs hepatic metabolism and elimination of the drugs. Although few guidelines are available, dosages should be individualized according to the severity of hepatic impairment and HIV infection, other drug therapies (for HIV infection, opportunistic infections, or other conditions), additional risk factors for drug toxicity, and the potential for drug interactions. In addition, all patients with hepatic impairment should be monitored closely for abnormal liver function tests (LFTs) and drug-related toxicity. Hepatic effects and considerations for usage of selected drugs are as follows:

■ Atazanavir, fosamprenavir, nelfinavir, nevirapine, ritonavir, saquinavir, and tenofovir may need dosage reductions in patients with impaired hepatic function.

■ Nevirapine may cause abnormal LFTs, and a few cases of fatal hepatitis have been reported. If moderate or severe LFT abnormalities occur, nevirapine administration should be discontinued until LFTs return to baseline. If liver dysfunction recurs when the drug is resumed, nevirapine should be discontinued permanently.

■ Zidovudine is eliminated slowly and has a longer half-life in patients with moderate to severe liver disease. Thus, daily doses should be reduced by 50% in patients with hepatic impairment.

Use in Home Care

Most antiviral drugs are self-administered or dosed by caregivers in the home. Precautions to prevent viral infections from occurring or spreading are important because of the close contact among members of a household. The home care nurse may need to teach infection-control precautions and to assess the immunization status of all household members. If immunizations are indicated, the nurse may need to teach about, encourage, provide, or facilitate their administration.

Home care of patients with HIV infection may include teaching patients and caregivers about the disease and its treatment, assisting with drug therapy for HIV or opportunistic infections, coordinating medical and social services, managing symptoms of infection or adverse drug effects, and preventing or minimizing opportunistic infections.

Nursing Actions Antiviral Drugs

NURSING ACTIONS	RATIONALE/EXPLANATION
1. Administer accurately	
a. Give oral drugs as recommended in relation to meals:	Manufacturers' recommendations to promote absorption and bioavailability
(1) Give abacavir, Combivir, emtricitabine, famciclovir, fosamprenavir, Kaletra tablets, lamivudine, nevirapine, tenofovir, Trizivir, valacyclovir, and zidovudine with or without food. However, do not give abacavir with a high-fat meal. Avoid antacids in combination with atazanavir.	
(2) Give Atripla, efavirenz, entecavir, or indinavir on an empty stomach, 1 hour before or 2 hours after a meal.	
(3) Give atazanavir, darunavir, ganciclovir, Kaletra oral solution, nelfinavir, ritonavir, and tipranavir with food.	
(4) Give saquinavir within 2 hours after a meal.	
b. To give nelfinavir to infants and young children, the oral powder can be mixed with a small amount of water, milk, or formula. After it is mixed, the entire amount must be taken to obtain the full dose.	Acidic foods or juices (e.g., orange juice, apple juice, applesauce) should not be used because they produce a bitter taste.
c. Give intravenous (IV) acyclovir, foscarnet, ganciclovir, and zidovudine over 1 hour.	To decrease tissue irritation and increased toxicity from high plasma levels
d. Give enfuvirtide Sub-Q in upper arm, anterior thigh or abdomen; apply ice or heat and massage the site after the injection.	See the manufacturer's instructions for reconstituting the drug powder.
e. When applying topical acyclovir, wear a glove.	To decrease local tissue irritation
2. Observe for therapeutic effects	
a. With acyclovir for genital herpes, observe for fewer recurrences when given for prophylaxis; observe for healing of lesions and decreased pain and itching when given for treatment.	
b. With amantadine, observe for absence of symptoms when given for prophylaxis of influenza A, and decreased fever, cough, muscle aches, and malaise when given for treatment.	
c. With ganciclovir or foscarnet for cytomegalovirus retinitis, observe for improved vision.	
d. With antiretroviral drugs, observe for improved clinical status and improved laboratory markers (e.g., decreased viral load, increased CD4+ cell count).	
3. Observe for adverse effects	
a. General effects—anorexia, nausea, vomiting, diarrhea, fever, headache	These effects occur with most systemic antiviral drugs and may range from mild to severe.
b. With IV acyclovir—phlebitis at injection site; skin rash; urticaria; increased blood urea nitrogen or serum creatinine; encephalopathy manifested by confusion, coma, lethargy, seizures, tremors	Encephalopathy is rare but potentially serious; other effects commonly occur.
c. With topical acyclovir—burning or stinging and pruritus	These effects are usually transient.
d. With amantadine and rimantadine—central nervous system (CNS) effects with anxiety, ataxia, dizziness, hyperexcitability, insomnia, mental confusion, hallucinations, slurred speech	CNS symptoms are more likely with amantadine and may be similar to those caused by atropine and CNS stimulants. Adverse reactions are more likely to occur in older adults and those with renal impairment.
e. With ganciclovir and foscarnet—bone marrow depression, renal impairment, neuropathy	
f. With protease inhibitor antiretroviral drugs—gastrointestinal distress, increased serum cholesterol and triglycerides	The most frequent adverse effects are the general ones listed above. Most are relatively mild. The dyslipidemia may increase risks of heart attack or stroke.
g. With NRTI antiretroviral drugs—hypersensitivity skin rash, peripheral neuropathy. Additional effects with zidovudine—severe anemia and neutropenia, pancreatitis	Anemia may occur within 2–4 weeks of starting zidovudine, neutropenia after 6–8 weeks. A complete blood count should be performed every 2 weeks. Filgrastim or sargramostim may be given to aid recovery of bone marrow function; blood transfusions may be given for anemia.

NURSING ACTIONS	RATIONALE/EXPLANATION
	Hematologic effects may occur in newborn infants when the mothers received zidovudine during pregnancy.
h. With enfuvirtide—injection site pain, hypersensitivity reactions	Injection site discomfort can be minimized by applying ice or heat and massaging the site after injection.
4. Observe for drug interactions	Antiviral drugs are given concurrently with many other drugs, especially in treatment of HIV infection, and significant interactions may occur.
a. Drugs that *increase* effects of amantadine and rimantadine:	
(1) Anticholinergics—atropine, first-generation antihistamines, antipsychotics, tricyclic antidepressants	These drugs add to the anticholinergic effects (e.g., blurred vision, mouth dryness, urine retention, constipation, tachycardia) of the antiviral agents.
(2) CNS stimulants	These drugs add to the CNS-stimulating effects (e.g., confusion, insomnia, nervousness, hyperexcitability) of the antiviral agents.
b. Drugs that *increase* effects of ganciclovir:	
(1) Imipenem-cilastatin	Increased risk of seizures; avoid the combination if possible.
(2) Nephrotoxic drugs (e.g., amphotericin B, cyclosporine)	Increased serum creatinine and potential nephrotoxicity
c. Drugs that *increase* effects of protease inhibitors:	In addition to the interactions listed here as occurring with PIs as a group, individual drugs may have additional interactions.
(1) Azole antifungals (fluconazole, itraconazole)	
(2) Clarithromycin	
(3) Other antiretrovirals	
d. Drugs that *decrease* effects of protease inhibitors:	
(1) Anticonvulsants (carbamazepine, phenytoin)	May decrease blood levels of PIs
(2) Rifamycins (rifampin, rifabutin)	Accelerate metabolism of PIs by inducing drug-metabolizing enzymes in the liver
(3) Other antiretrovirals	
e. Drug that *increases* the effects of lamivudine:	
(1) Trimethoprim-sulfamethoxazole	Decreases elimination of lamivudine
f. Drugs that *increase* effects of zidovudine:	
(1) Doxorubicin, vincristine, vinblastine	Increased bone marrow depression (anemia, neutropenia)
(2) Fluconazole	May increase blood levels
(3) Ganciclovir	Increased neutropenia
(4) Phenytoin, valproic acid	May increase blood levels
g. Drugs that *decrease* effects of zidovudine:	
(1) Acetaminophen	May decrease blood levels
(2) Rifampin, rifabutin	Accelerate metabolism of zidovudine and decrease blood levels
h. Drugs that *decrease* effects of nevirapine and efavirenz:	
(1) Rifamycins	Accelerate metabolism and decrease blood levels

Key Concepts

- Viral infections commonly occur in all age groups.

- Vaccinations, avoiding contact with people who have viral infections, and thorough hand hygiene are effective ways to prevent viral infections,

- Viral infections for which drug therapy is available include genital herpes, hepatitis B and C, HIV infection, and influenza.

- Because viruses are intracellular parasites, antiviral drugs are relatively toxic to human cells.

- Antiretroviral drugs are given in combination to increase effectiveness and decrease emergence of drug-resistant viruses.

Review and Application Exercises

Short Answer Exercises

1. What are the predominant effects of antiviral drugs on susceptible viruses?

2. Which viral infections may be prevented by administration of antiviral drugs?

3. What are the major adverse effects associated with commonly used antiviral drugs? How would you assess for each of these adverse effects?

4. Why is it important to monitor renal function in any patient receiving a systemic antiviral drug?

5. What is the advantage of combination drug therapy for HIV infection?

6. List nursing interventions to prevent or minimize adverse effects of anti-HIV drugs.

NCLEX-Style Questions

7. The nurse is admitting a patient transferred from a nursing home who has just been diagnosed with influenza type A. The nurse anticipates an immediate order for
   a. ganciclovir (Cytovene)
   b. amantadine (Symmetrel)
   c. nevirapine (Viramune)
   d. ritonavir (Norvir)

8. When counseling a patient with a first outbreak of genital herpes who has been prescribed 10 days of acyclovir (Zovirax), you tell her that this medication is being used to
   a. decrease fever
   b. decrease pain
   c. prevention of recurrence
   d. reduce number of lesions in recurrences

9. In caring for a pregnant woman who is HIV positive, which of the following drugs would you anticipate administering to prevent transmission of HIV to the fetus?
   a. zidovudine (AZT)
   b. adefovir (Hepsera)
   c. Fosamprenavir (Lexiva)
   d. ribavirin (Virazole)

10. A 21-year-old man is being started on a combination of antiretroviral drugs for treatment of AIDS. Which of the following statements indicates that he understands the nurse's accurate patient teaching?
    a. "The medicines inactivate the virus and prevent recurrence of the disease."
    b. "The medicines do not promote the development of drug-resistant viral strains."
    c. "The medicines slow the progression of the disease but do not cure it."
    d. "The medicines prevent the occurrence of opportunistic infections."

11. The nurse is preparing to administer enfuvirtide (Fuzeon) to a patient. He wants to know how it works. The nurse explains that it exerts its anti-HIV viral effects by
    a. inhibiting reverse transcriptase enzymes
    b. inhibiting protease enzymes
    c. having direct toxic effects on the virus in the bloodstream
    d. preventing the virus from attaching to human cells

Selected References

Brundage, S. C., & Fitzpatrick, A.N. (2006). Hepatitis A. *American Family Physician, 73,* 2162–2170.

Donegan, N. E. (2008). Management of patients with infectious diseases. In S. C. Smeltzer, B. G. Bare, J. L. Hinkle, & K. H. Cheever (Eds.), *Brunner & Suddarth's textbook of medical-surgical nursing* (11th ed., pp. 2474–2515). Philadelphia: Lippincott Williams & Wilkins.

Drug facts and comparisons. (Updated monthly). St. Louis, MO: Facts and Comparisons.

Durston, S. (2005). What you need to know about viral hepatitis. *Nursing 2005, 35,* 36–41.

Fletcher, C. V., & Kakuda, T. N. (2005). Human immunodeficiency virus infection. In J. T. DiPiro, R. L. Talbert, G. C. Yee, G. R. Matzke, B. G. Wells, & L. M. Posey (Eds.), *Pharmacotherapy: A pathophysiologic approach* (6th ed., pp. 2255–2277). New York: McGraw-Hill.

Goldrick, B. A., & Goetz, A. M. (2006). 'Tis the season for influenza. *Nurse Practitioner, 31,* 24–33.

Hammer, S. M., Saag, M. S., Schechter, M., Montaner, J. S. G., Schooley, R. T., Jacobson, D. M. et al. (2006). Treatment for adult HIV infection: 2006 Recommendations of the International AIDS Society—USA panel. *Journal of the American Medical Association, 296,* 827–843.

Lederman, M. M., Penn-Nicholson, A., Cho, M., & Mosier, D. (2006). Biology of CCR5 and its role in HIV infection and treatment. *Journal of the American Medical Association, 296,* 815–826.

Lee, L. S., Andrade, A. S. A., & Flexner, C. (2006). Interactions between natural health products and antiretroviral drugs: Pharmacokinetic and pharmacodynamic effects. *Clinical Infectious Diseases, 43,* 1052–1059.

Nokes, K. (2008). Management of patients with HIV infection and AIDS. In S. C. Smeltzer, B. G. Bare, J. L. Hinkle, & K. H. Cheever (Eds.), *Brunner & Suddarth's textbook of medical-surgical nursing* (11th ed., pp. 1814–1854). Philadelphia: Lippincott Williams & Wilkins.

Saag, M. S. (2006). Emtricitabine, a new antiretroviral agent with activity against HIV and hepatitis B virus. *Clinical Infectious Diseases, 42,* 126–131.

Shandera, W. X., & Koo, H. (2007). Infectious diseases: Viral and rickettsial. In S. J. McPhee, M. A. Papadakis, & L. M. Tierney, Jr. (Eds.), *Current medical diagnosis & treatment 2007* (46th ed., pp. 1378–1430). New York: McGraw-Hill.

Stark, S. W. (2006). HIV after age 55. *Nursing Clinics of North America, 41*, 469–479.

Stein, J. H. (2007). Cardiovascular risks of antiretroviral therapy. *New England Journal of Medicine, 356*, 1773–1775.

Sweeney, K. A. (2005). Acquired immunodeficiency syndrome. In C. M. Porth (Ed.), *Pathophysiology: Concepts of altered health states* (7th ed., pp. 427–445). Philadelphia: Lippincott Williams & Wilkins.

Wasley, A., Samandari, T., & Bell, B. P. (2005). Incidence of hepatitis A in the United States in the era of vaccination. *Journal of the American Medical Association, 294*, 194–201.

Working Group on Antiretroviral Therapy and Medical Management of HIV-Infected Children. (2006, Oct. 26). *Guidelines for the use of antiretroviral agents in pediatric HIV infection* (pp. 1–126). Retrieved June 2007, from http://aidsinfo.nih.gov/ContentFiles/PediatricGuidelines.pdf

Zolopa, A. R., & Katz, M. H. (2007). HIV infection. In S. J. McPhee, M. A. Papadakis, & L. M. Tierney, Jr. (Eds.), *Current medical diagnosis & treatment 2007* (46th ed., pp. 1346–1377). New York: McGraw-Hill.

36

Antifungal Drugs

LEARNING OBJECTIVES

After studying this chapter, you will be able to:

1. Describe characteristics of fungi and fungal infections.
2. Discuss antibacterial drug therapy and immunosuppression as risk factors for development of fungal infections.
3. Describe commonly used antifungal drugs in terms of indications for use, adverse effects, and nursing process implications.
4. Differentiate between adverse effects associated with systemic and topical antifungal drugs.
5. Teach patients about prevention and treatment of fungal infections.

Applying Your Knowledge

Charlotte Angelo, age 21, is on antibiotic therapy for a urinary tract infection. During the course of her therapy, she develops vaginal discharge and is diagnosed with a *Candida albicans* vaginal infection. The primary care provider prescribes fluconazole (Diflucan) 150 mg PO, one dose.

Introduction

Fungi

Fungi are *molds* and *yeasts* that are widely dispersed in the environment and are either saprophytic (i.e., obtain food from dead organic matter) or parasitic (i.e., obtain nourishment from living organisms). Molds are multicellular organisms composed of colonies of tangled strands. They form a fuzzy coating on various surfaces (e.g., the mold that forms on spoiled food, the mildew that forms in damp environments). Yeasts are unicellular organisms. Some fungi, called *dermatophytes*, can grow only at the cooler temperatures of body surfaces. Other fungi, called dimorphic, can grow as molds outside the body and as yeasts in the warm temperatures of the body. As molds, these fungi produce spores that can persist indefinitely in the environment and can be carried by the wind to distant locations. When these mold spores enter the body, most often by inhalation, they rapidly become yeasts that can invade body tissues. Dimorphic fungi include a number of human pathogens such as those that cause blastomycosis, histoplasmosis, and coccidioidomycosis.

Fungi that are pathogenic in humans exist in soil, decaying plants, and other environmental habitats or as part of the endogenous human flora. For example, *Candida albicans* organisms are part of the normal microbial flora of the skin, mouth, gastrointestinal (GI) tract, and vagina. Growth of *Candida* organisms is normally restrained by intact immune mechanisms and bacterial competition for nutrients. When these restraining forces are altered (e.g., by suppression of the immune system, antibacterial drug therapy), fungal overgrowth and opportunistic infection can occur. In addition, some fungi have characteristics that enhance their ability to cause disease. *Cryptococcus neoformans* organisms, for example, can become encapsulated, which allows them to evade the normal immune defense mechanism of phagocytosis. *Aspergillus* organisms produce protease, an enzyme that allows them to destroy structural proteins and penetrate body tissues.

Structurally, fungi are larger and more complex than bacteria. They have a thick, rigid cell wall, of which glucan is one of the components. Glucan is formed by the fungal enzyme, glucan synthetase. Fungi also have a cell membrane composed mainly of ergosterol, a lipid that is similar to cholesterol in human cell membranes. Within the cell membrane, structures are mostly the same as those in human cells (e.g., a nucleus, mitochondria, Golgi apparatus, ribosomes attached to endoplasmic reticulum, a cytoskeleton with microtubules and filaments).

Fungal Infections (Mycoses)

Fungal infections may be mild and superficial or life-threatening and systemic. Dermatophytes cause superficial infections of the skin, hair, and nails. They obtain nourishment from keratin, a protein in skin, hair, and nails. Dermatophytic infections include tinea pedis (athlete's foot) and tinea capitis (ringworm of the scalp) (see Chap. 64).

Systemic or invasive mycoses include the endemic mycoses that can cause disease (e.g., blastomycosis, coccidioidomycosis, histoplasmosis, sporotrichosis) in healthy hosts who are exposed to them in the environment and the opportunistic mycoses (e.g., aspergillosis, candidiasis, cryptococcosis) that cause serious infection mainly in immunosuppressed hosts. The fungi that cause endemic mycoses exist as molds in the environment; they grow in soil and decaying organic matter. Infection is acquired by inhalation of airborne spores from contaminated soil. Histoplasmosis, coccidioidomycosis, and blastomycosis usually occur as pulmonary disease but may be systemic. These infections often mimic common bacterial infections, and their severity is determined both by the extent of the exposure to the organism and by the immune status of the host. The fungi that cause opportunistic mycoses may be part of the normal body flora (e.g., *Candida* species) or exist in the environment (*Aspergillus*, *Cryptococcus*). Infection occurs after inhalation or inoculation of the fungus into body tissues.

Most fungal infections occur in healthy people but are more severe and invasive in *immunocompromised* hosts. Serious infections are increasing in incidence, largely because of human immunodeficiency virus (HIV) infections, the use of immunosuppressant drugs to treat patients with cancer or organ transplants, the use of indwelling intravenous catheters for prolonged drug therapy or parenteral nutrition, implantation of prosthetic devices, and widespread use of broad-spectrum antibacterial drugs. Characteristics of selected fungal infections are described in Box 36-1.

Box 36-1	Selected Fungal Infections

Aspergillosis occurs in debilitated and immunocompromised people, including those with leukemia, lymphoma, or acquired immunodeficiency syndrome (AIDS), and those with neutropenia. Invasive aspergillosis is a serious illness characterized by inflammatory granulomatous lesions, which may develop in the bronchi, lungs, ear canal, skin, or mucous membranes of the eye, nose, or urethra. It may extend into blood vessels, which leads to infection of the brain, heart, kidneys, and other organs. It is associated with thrombosis, ischemic infarction of involved tissues, and progressive disease. It is often fatal.

Allergic bronchopulmonary aspergillosis, an allergic reaction to inhaled aspergillus spores, may develop in people with asthma and cause bronchoconstriction, wheezing, dyspnea, cough, muscle aches, and fever. The condition is aggravated if the spores germinate and grow in the airways, thereby producing chronic exposure to the antigen and permanent fibrotic damage.

Aspergillus mold is widespread in the environment; spores are released into the air during soil excavations (e.g., for construction of buildings) or handling of decaying plant matter and are carried into most human environments. Spores have been found in water (e.g., hot water faucets, saunas, shower heads, swimming pools), public buildings and private homes (e.g., basements, bedding, humidifiers, ventilation ducts, potted plants, house dust), and foods (e.g., peppers and spices, pasta, peanuts, cashews, coffee beans). In hospitals, sources of infection include contaminated air from building renovations and new construction; hospital water, which may become aerosolized during activities such as patient showering; and cereals, powdered milk, tea, and soy sauce ingested by neutropenic patients. As *Aspergillus* molds grow, they produce toxins (e.g., aflatoxin, one of the strongest carcinogens known) that contaminate the food chain.

There are several species that cause invasive disease in humans, but *Aspergillus fumigatus* is the most common. *A. fumigatus* reproduces by releasing spores, which are small enough to reach the alveoli when inhaled. Most aspergillus organisms enter the body through the respiratory system, and pulmonary aspergillosis is acquired by inhalation of the spores. Other potential entry sites include damaged skin (e.g., burn wounds, intravenous catheter insertion sites), operative wounds, the cornea, and the ear.

Blastomycosis occurs with inhalation of spores from a fungus that grows in soil and decaying organic matter. The organism is widespread in the United States. Sporadic cases most often occur in adult males who have extensive exposure to woods and streams with vocational or recreational activities. The infection may be asymptomatic or produce pulmonary symptoms resembling pneumonia, tuberculosis, or lung cancer. It may also be systemic and involve other organs, especially the skin and bone. Skin lesions (e.g., pustules, ulcerations, abscesses) may progress over a period of years and eventually involve large areas of the body. Bone invasion, with arthritis and bone destruction, occurs in 25% to 50% of patients.

Blastomycosis can occur in healthy people with sufficient exposure but is more severe and more likely to involve multiple organs and central nervous system (CNS) disease in immunocompromised patients.

Candidiasis occurs in patients with malignant lymphomas, diabetes mellitus, or AIDS and in patients receiving antibiotic, antineoplastic, corticosteroid, and immunosuppressant drug therapy. *Candida* organisms are found in soil, on inanimate objects, in hospital environments, and in food. In the human body, they are found on skin and in the gastrointestinal (GI) and genitourinary tracts, including the urine of patients with indwelling bladder catheters. Historically, most infections arose from the normal endogenous organisms of the GI tract and were caused by *Candida albicans*. In recent years, however, the incidence of infections caused by other candidal strains has greatly increased. Oral, intestinal, vaginal, and systemic candidiasis can occur. Early recognition and treatment of local infections may prevent systemic candidiasis.

■ Oral candidiasis (thrush) produces painless white plaques on oral and pharyngeal mucosa. It often occurs in newborn infants who become infected during passage through an infected or colonized vagina. In older children and adults, thrush may occur as a complication of diabetes mellitus, as a result of poor oral hygiene, or after taking antibiotics or corticosteroids. It may also occur as an early manifestation of AIDS.

■ GI candidiasis often occurs after broad-spectrum antibacterial therapy, which destroys a large part of the normal flora of the intestine. The main symptom is diarrhea.

■ Vaginal candidiasis occurs in women who are pregnant, have diabetes mellitus, or take oral contraceptives or antibacterial drugs. The main symptom is a yellowish vaginal discharge. The infection may produce inflammation of the perineal area and spread to the buttocks and thighs.

■ Skin candidiasis occurs in people with continuously moist skinfolds or moist surgical dressings. The organism also may cause diaper rash and perineal rashes. Skin lesions are red and macerated.

■ Systemic or invasive candidiasis occurs when the organism gets into the bloodstream and is circulated throughout the body, with the brain, heart, kidneys, and eyes as the most common sites of infection. It occurs as a nosocomial infection in patients with serious illness or who are undergoing drug therapy that suppresses the immune system and may be fatal. Invasive infections may be present in any organ and may produce such disorders as urinary tract infection, endocarditis, and meningitis. It may be diagnosed by positive cultures of blood or tissue. Signs and symptoms depend on the severity of the infection and the organs affected and are indistinguishable from those occurring with bacterial infections.

The incidence of severe candidal infections has increased in recent years, in part because of increased numbers of neutropenic and immunodeficient patients. In addition, the frequent use of broad-spectrum antibiotics leads to extensive candidal colonization in debilitated patients, and the widespread use of medical devices (e.g., intravascular catheters, monitoring equipment, endotracheal tubes, urinary catheters) allows the organisms to reach sites that are normally sterile. People who use IV drugs also develop invasive candidiasis because the injections inoculate the fungi directly into the bloodstream.

Coccidioidomycosis is caused by an organism that grows as a mold in soil and decaying organic matter and is commonly found in the southwestern United States and northern Mexico. Infection results from inhalation of spores that convert to yeasts in the warm environment of the body and often cause asymptomatic or mild respiratory infection. However, the organism may cause acute pulmonary infection with fever, chest pain, cough, headache, and loss of appetite. Radiographs may show small nodules in the lung like those seen in tuberculosis. In some cases, chronic disease develops in which the organisms remain localized and cause large, organism-filled cavities in the lung. These cavities may become fibrotic and require surgical excision. In a few cases, severe, disseminated disease occurs, either soon after the primary infection or after years of chronic pulmonary disease. Disseminated coccidioidomycosis may produce acute or chronic meningitis or a generalized disease with lesions in many internal organs. Skin lesions appear as granulomas that may eventually heal or become ulcerations. Most patients with primary infection recover without treatment; patients with disseminated disease require long-term treatment.

Coccidioidomycosis may occur in healthy or immunocompromised people but is more severe and more likely to become systemic in immunocompromised patients. For example, patients with AIDS who live in endemic areas are highly susceptible to this infection. The severity of the disease also increases with intensity of exposure.

Cryptococcosis is caused by inhalation of spores of *Cryptococcus neoformans*, an organism found worldwide, especially in bird droppings. The spores have also been found in fruits, vegetables, and dairy products.

When cryptococcosis occurs in healthy people, the primary infection is localized in the lungs, is asymptomatic or produces mild symptoms, and heals without treatment. However, pneumonia may occur and lead to spread of the organisms by the bloodstream. When cryptococcosis occurs in immunocompromised people, it is likely to be more severe and to become disseminated to the CNS, skin, and other organs. People with AIDS are highly susceptible, and cryptococcosis is a frequent opportunistic infection in this population. Infection most often affects the lungs and CNS. Cryptococcal pneumonia in patients with AIDS has a high mortality rate. Cryptococcal meningitis, the most common manifestation of disseminated disease, often produces abscesses in the brain. Clinical manifestations include headache, dizziness, and neck stiffness, and the condition is often mistaken for brain tumor. Later symptoms include coma, respiratory failure, and death if the meningitis is not treated effectively.

Histoplasmosis is a common infection that occurs worldwide, especially in the central and mideastern United States. The causative fungus is found in soil and organic debris around chicken houses, bird roosts, and caves inhabited by bats. Exposure to spores may result from activities such as demolishing or

(continued on page 584)

Box 36-1	Selected Fungal Infections (continued)

remodeling old buildings or cleaning chicken coops. Spores can be picked up by the wind and spread over large areas. Histoplasmosis develops when the spores are inhaled into the lungs, where they rapidly develop into the tissue-invasive yeast cells that reach the bloodstream and become distributed throughout the body. In most cases, the organisms are destroyed or encapsulated by the host's immune system. The lung lesions heal by fibrosis and calcification and resemble the lesions of tuberculosis. Some people develop histoplasmosis years after the primary infection, probably from reactivation of a latent infection.

Clinical manifestations may vary widely. In people with a normal immune response, manifestations can be correlated with the extent of exposure. Most infections are asymptomatic or produce minimal symptoms for which treatment is not sought. When symptoms occur, they usually resemble an acute, influenza-like respiratory infection and improve within a few weeks. However, people exposed to large amounts of spores may have a high fever and severe pneumonia, which usually resolves with a low mortality rate. Some people, most often adult men with emphysema or other lung diseases, develop chronic pulmonary histoplasmosis with recurrent episodes of cough, fever, and weakness. In addition, histoplasmosis occasionally infects the liver, spleen, and other organs and is rapidly fatal if not treated effectively. The severe, disseminated form usually occurs in patients whose immune system is suppressed by diseases or drugs.

Pneumocystosis is caused by *Pneumocystis jirovecii*, an organism formerly considered a protozoan but now identified as a fungus. The organism is widespread in the environment, and most people are exposed at an early age. Infections are mild or asymptomatic in immunocompetent people. However, the organism can form cysts in the lungs, persist for long periods, and become activated in immunocompromised hosts. Activation produces an acute, life-threatening pneumonia (PCP) characterized by cough, fever, dyspnea, and presence of the organism in sputum. Groups at risk include human immunodeficiency virus (HIV) seropositive persons, those receiving corticosteroids or antineoplastics and other immunosuppressive drugs, and caregivers of infected people.

Sporotrichosis occurs when contaminated soil or plant material is inoculated into the skin through small wounds (e.g., thorn pricks) on the fingers, hands, or arms. It is most likely to occur among people who handle sphagnum moss, roses, or baled hay. Thus, infection is a hazard for gardeners and greenhouse workers. It can occur in both healthy and immunocompromised people but is more severe and disseminated in immunocompromised hosts.

Initial lesions, which are usually small, painless bumps resembling insect bites, occur 1 week to 6 months after inoculation. The subcutaneous nodule develops into a necrotic ulcer, which heals slowly as new ulcers appear in adjacent areas. Local lymphatic channels and lymph nodes also develop abscesses, nodules, and ulcers that may persist for years if the disease is not treated effectively. In immunocompromised people, sporotrichosis may spread to various tissues, including the meninges.

Antifungal Drugs

Development of drugs that are effective against fungal cells without being excessively toxic to human cells has been limited because fungal cells are similar to human cells. Most of the available drugs target the fungal cell membrane and produce potentially serious toxicities and drug interactions. In general, antifungal drugs disrupt the structure and function of fungal cell components (Fig. 36-1).

Polyenes (e.g., amphotericin B), azoles (e.g., fluconazole), and terbinafine act on ergosterol to disrupt fungal cell membranes. Amphotericin B (and nystatin) binds to ergosterol and forms holes in the membrane, causing leakage of fungal cell contents and lysis of the cell. The azole drugs bind to an enzyme that is required for synthesis of ergosterol. This action causes production of a defective cell membrane, which also allows leakage of intracellular contents and destruction of the cell. Both types of drugs also affect cholesterol in human cell membranes, a characteristic considered mainly responsible for the drugs' adverse effects.

Echinocandins (e.g., caspofungin) disrupt fungal cell walls rather than fungal cell membranes. They inhibit glucan synthetase, an enzyme required for synthesis of glucan. Glucan is a component of the fungal cell wall; its depletion leads to leakage of cellular contents and cell death. Because human cells do not contain cell walls, these drugs are less toxic than the polyene and azole antifungals.

Drugs for superficial fungal infections of skin and mucous membranes are often applied topically. Numerous preparations are available, many without a prescription. Drugs for systemic infections are given IV or orally. Patients with HIV infection or severe neutropenia due to treatment with cytotoxic cancer drugs require aggressive treatment of fungal infections, because they are at high risk for developing life-threatening systemic mycoses. Selected antifungal drugs are further described in the following sections. In addition, indications for use and dosage ranges are listed in Table 36-1.

Polyenes

Amphotericin B is active against most types of pathogenic fungi and is fungicidal or fungistatic, depending on the concentration in body fluids and the susceptibility of the causative fungus. Because of its toxicity, the drug is used only for serious fungal infections. It is usually given for 4 to 12 weeks.

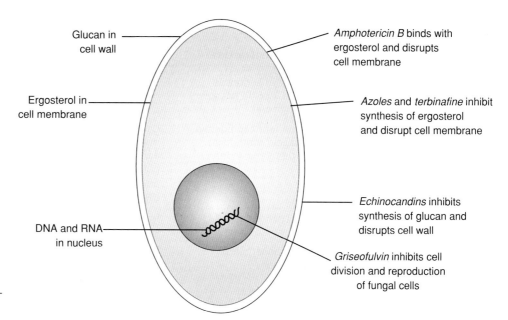

Fungal cell

Glucan in cell wall

Amphotericin B binds with ergosterol and disrupts cell membrane

Ergosterol in cell membrane

Azoles and *terbinafine* inhibit synthesis of ergosterol and disrupt cell membrane

Echinocandins inhibits synthesis of glucan and disrupts cell wall

DNA and RNA in nucleus

Griseofulvin inhibits cell division and reproduction of fungal cells

Figure 36-1 ■ Actions of antifungal drugs on fungal cells.

| Table 36-1 | **Drugs at a Glance:** Selected Antifungal Drugs |

Generic/Trade Name	Indications For Use	ROUTES AND DOSAGE RANGES	
		Adults	**Children**
Amphotericin B deoxycholate (Fungizone)	Serious, systemic fungal infections (e.g., candidiasis, histoplasmosis) Cutaneous candidiasis Oral candidiasis	IV, individualized according to disease severity and patient tolerance. Initial dose often 0.25 mg/kg/d, gradually increased to 0.5–1 mg/kg/d, infused over 2–6 h Topically to skin lesions, 2–4 times daily for 1–4 wk Oral suspension (100 mg/mL), 1 mL "swish and swallow" 4 times daily	Same as for adults for IV, skin preparations, and oral suspension
Amphotericin B lipid complex (Abelcet)	Systemic infections in patients who do not tolerate Fungizone	IV 5 mg/kg/d	Same as adults
Liposomal amphotericin B (AmBisome)	Systemic infections in patients who do not tolerate Fungizone Empiric treatment of presumed fungal infections in febrile, neutropenic patients	IV 3–5 mg/kg/d	Same as adults

(continued on page 586)

Table 36-1		**Drugs at a Glance:** Selected Antifungal Drugs (continued)	
		ROUTES AND DOSAGE RANGES	
Generic/Trade Name	**Indications For Use**	**Adults**	**Children**
Amphotericin B cholesteryl (Amphotec)	Systemic infections in patients who do not tolerate Fungizone	IV 3–4 mg/kg/d	Same as adults
Anidulafungin (Eraxis)	Treatment of candidemia, esophageal candidiasis, and other *Candida* infections	Candidemia IV infusion 200 mg initially, then 100 mg daily Esophageal candidiasis IV infusion 100 mg initially, then 50 mg daily	Dosage not established
Butoconazole (Femstat, Gynazole)	Vaginal candidiasis	Intravaginally, once daily for 3 d	
Caspofungin (Cancidas)	Invasive aspergillosis Candidiasis	IV infusion over 1 h, 70 mg initially, then 50 mg daily Hepatic impairment, 70 mg initially, then 35 mg daily	Safety and efficacy not established
Ciclopirox (Loprox, Penlac Nail Lacquer)	Tinea infections, cutaneous candidiasis, onychomycosis of fingernails and toenails	Tinea and candidal infections topically to skin lesions twice daily for 2–4 wk Onychomycosis topically once daily to affected nails	Safety not established for (1) cream or suspension under 10 years of age (2) Penlac for any age child (3) gel or shampoo under 16 years of age
Clotrimazole (Lotrimin, Mycelex, Gyne-Lotrimin)	Cutaneous dermatophytosis; oral, cutaneous, and vaginal candidiasis	Orally, 1 troche dissolved in mouth 5 times daily Topically to skin daily for 2–4 wk Intravaginally, once daily for 3–7 d	Same as adults
Econazole (Spectazole)	Tinea infections, cutaneous candidiasis	Topically to skin lesions, once or twice daily for 2–4 wk	Dosage not established
Fluconazole (Diflucan)	Oropharyngeal, esophageal, vaginal, and systemic candidiasis Prevention of candidiasis after bone marrow transplantation Cryptococcal meningitis	Oropharyngeal candidiasis, PO, IV 200 mg first day, then 100 mg daily for 2 wk Esophageal candidiasis, PO, IV, 200 mg first day, then 100 mg daily for at least 3 wk Vaginal candidiasis, PO 150 mg as a single dose Systemic candidiasis, PO, IV 400 mg first day, then 200 mg daily for at least 4 wk Prophylaxis, PO, IV 400 mg once daily Cryptococcal meningitis, PO, IV, 400 mg first day, then 200–400 mg/d for 10–12 wk	Oropharyngeal candidiasis, PO, IV 6 mg/kg first day, then 3 mg/kg/d for at least 2 wk Esophageal candidiasis, PO, IV, 6 mg/kg first day, then 3 mg/kg/d for at least 3 wk Systemic candidiasis, PO, IV 6–12 mg/kg/d Cryptococcal meningitis, PO, IV 12 mg/kg first day, then 6 mg/kg/d for 10–12 wk
Griseofulvin	Dermatophytosis (skin, hair, nails)	PO 250–500 mg daily	PO 5–10 mg/kg/d

		ROUTES AND DOSAGE RANGES	
Generic/Trade Name	**Indications For Use**	**Adults**	**Children**
Itraconazole (Sporanox)	Systemic fungal infections, including aspergillosis, in neutropenic and immuno-compromised hosts Onychomycosis Tinea infections	Systemic infection, PO 200 mg once or twice daily for 3 mo Blastomycosis, histoplasmosis, aspergillosis, IV 200 mg twice daily for 4 doses, then 200 mg/d Onychomycosis, Fingernail, PO 200 mg twice daily for 1 wk, no drug for 3 wk, then repeat dosage for 1 wk; toenail, PO 200 mg once daily for 12 consecutive wk Oral solution, 100–200 mg daily (10–20 mL), swish and swallow 3 times daily for 3–5 d Tinea infections, PO 100–200 mg daily for 1–4 wk	Safety and efficacy not established. 3–16-y-old patients have been treated with 100 mg daily for systemic infections and patients 6 mo–12 y have been treated with 5 mg/kg once daily for 2 wk without serious or unusual adverse effects.
Ketoconazole (Nizoral)	Candidiasis, histoplasmosis, coccidioidomycosis Cutaneous candidiasis Tinea infections	PO 200 mg once daily, increased to 400 mg once daily if necessary in severe infections Topically, once daily for 2–6 wk	*2 y and older:* PO 3.3–6.6 mg/kg/d as a single dose
Micafungin (Mycamine)	Treatment of esophageal candidiasis Prevention of *Candida* infections in patients undergoing hematopoietic stem cell transplantation (HSCT)	Treatment : IV infusion 150 mg daily Prevention: IV infusion 50 mg daily	Dosage not established
Miconazole (Monistat)	Dermatophytosis, cutaneous and vulvovaginal candidiasis	Topically, twice daily for 2–4 wk Intravaginally, vaginal cream, once daily at bedtime for 3–7 d; vaginal suppository, once daily at bedtime (1 d for 1200 mg; 3 d for 200 mg; 7 d for 100 mg)	
Naftifine (Naftin)	Tinea infections (athlete's foot, jock itch, ringworm)	Topically, once daily (cream) or twice daily (gel)	Safety and efficacy not established
Natamycin (Natacyn)	Fungal infections of the eye	Topically, 1 drop q1–2h for 3–4 d, then 1 drop 6–8 times daily for 14–24 d	Safety and efficacy not established
Nystatin (Mycostatin)	Candidiasis of skin, mucous membrane, and intestinal tract	Oral or intestinal infection, PO tablets 1–2 (500,000–1,000,000 units) 3 times daily; oral suspension, 4–6 mL (400,000–600,000 units) 4 times daily; oral troches 1–2 (200,000–400,000 units) 4–5 times daily Topically to skin lesions, 2–3 times daily Intravaginally, 1 vaginal tablet once daily for 14 d	*Older than 1 y:* PO oral suspension, same as adults; *infants,* 2 mL (200,000 units) 4 times daily Oral troches, same as adults for children old enough to suck on the lozenge until it dissolves

(continued on page 588)

| Table 36-1 | **Drugs at a Glance:** Selected Antifungal Drugs (continued) | | |

		ROUTES AND DOSAGE RANGES	
Generic/Trade Name	**Indications For Use**	**Adults**	**Children**
Oxiconazole (Oxistat)	Tinea infections	Topically to skin lesions, once or twice daily for 2–4 wk	Safety and efficacy not established
Posaconazole (Noxafil)	Treatment of oropharyngeal candidiasis Prevention of invaisve fungal infection	Prevention: PO 200 mg 3 times daily Oropharyngeal candidasis PO 100 mg twice daily initially, then 200 mg once daily for 13 days	Dosage not established
Sulconazole (Exelderm)	Tinea infections	Topically to skin lesions, once or twice daily for 3–4 wk	Safety and efficacy not established for children younger than 12 y
Terbinafine (Lamisil)	Tinea infections Onychomycosis of fingernails or toenails	Tinea infections, topically to skin, once or twice daily for at least 1 wk and no longer than 4 wk Fingernail infections, PO 250 mg daily for 6 wk Toenail infections, PO 250 mg daily for 12 wk	
Terconazole (Terazol)	Vaginal candidiasis	Intravaginally, 1 applicator once daily at bedtime for 7 doses (0.4% cream) or 3 doses (0.8% cream) Vaginal suppository, 1 daily at bedtime for 3 d	
Tioconazole (Vagistat)	Vaginal candidiasis	Intravaginally, 1 applicator at bedtime	
Tolnaftate (Tinactin)	Cutaneous mycoses (dermatophytosis)	Topically to skin lesions, twice daily for 2–6 wk	
Triacetin (Fungoid)	Dermatophytosis (e.g., athlete's foot), cutaneous candidiasis	Topically to skin lesions, 3 times daily	
Voriconazole (Vfend)	Esophageal candidiasis Invasive aspergillosis Other serious fungal infections	Esophageal candidiasis, PO 200 mg q12h for weight of ≥40 kg; 100 mg q12h for weight <40 kg. Give at least 14 d or 7 d after symptoms resolve. Aspergillosis and other serious infections, IV 6 mg/kg q12h for 2 doses (loading dose), then 4 mg/kg q12h (maintenance dose)	Safety and efficacy not established for children younger than 12 y
Zinc undecylenate (Desenex)	Dermatophytosis	Topically to skin twice daily for 2–4 wk	Same as for adults

Lipid formulations (Abelcet, AmBisome, Amphotec) reach higher concentrations in diseased tissues than in normal tissues, so that larger doses can be given to increase therapeutic effects. At the same time, they cause less damage to normal tissues and decrease adverse effects. These products are much more expensive than the deoxycholate formulation (Fungizone). They are most likely to be used for patients with pre-existing renal impairment or conditions in which other nephrotoxic drugs are routinely given (e.g., bone marrow transplant recipients) and when high doses are needed for difficult-to-treat infections. The lipid preparations differ in their characteristics and cannot be used interchangeably.

Amphotericin B must be given IV for systemic infections. After infusion, the drug is rapidly taken up by the liver and other organs. It is then slowly released back into the bloodstream. Despite its long-term use, little is known about its distribution and metabolic pathways. Drug concentrations in most body fluids are higher in the presence of inflammation; concentrations in cerebrospinal fluid (CSF) are low with or without inflammation. The drug has an initial serum half-life of 24 hours, which represents redistribution from the bloodstream to tissues. This is followed by a second elimination phase, with a half-life of 15 days, which represents elimination from tissue storage sites. Most of the drug is thought to be metabolized in the tissues; some is excreted in the urine and can be detected for several weeks.

Adverse effects include an infusion reaction (e.g., fever, chills, tachypnea). Nephrotoxicity is the most common and the most serious long-term adverse effect. The drug constricts afferent renal arterioles and reduces blood flow to the kidneys. Several strategies may decrease nephrotoxicity, such as keeping the patient well hydrated, giving 0.9% sodium chloride IV before drug administration, and avoiding the concomitant administration of other nephrotoxic drugs (e.g., aminoglycoside antibiotics). Hypokalemia and hypomagnesemia also occur and may require oral or IV mineral replacement. Additional adverse effects include anorexia, nausea, vomiting, anemia, and phlebitis at peripheral infusion sites. A central vein is preferred for administration.

Nystatin has the same mechanism of action as amphotericin B. However, it is used only for topical therapy of oral, intestinal, and vaginal candidiasis because it is too toxic for systemic use. Although given orally for oral or intestinal infections, the drug is not absorbed systemically and is excreted in the feces. With oral use, adverse effects include nausea, vomiting, and diarrhea; with vaginal application, adverse effects include local irritation and burning.

Azoles

The azoles are the largest group of commonly used antifungal agents. Many are used topically and some are available without a prescription for dermatologic (see Chap. 64) or vaginal use (e.g., butoconazole, clotrimazole, miconazole, terconazole, tioconazole). The main drugs discussed in this chapter are used systemically or both topically and systemically.

Systemic azoles include ketoconazole, fluconazole, itraconazole, posaconazole, and voriconazole. Compared with ketoconazole, the first azole, the other drugs have a broader spectrum of antifungal activity, better absorption with oral administration, better drug distribution in body tissues, fewer adverse effects, and fewer drug interactions. The most common adverse effects are nausea, diarrhea, and skin rash. In addition, all azoles may cause hepatotoxicity (e.g., hepatitis). Patients with impaired liver function or chronic use must be monitored closely. Azoles are contraindicated during pregnancy. The drugs also interact with cytochrome P450 enzymes to produce significant interactions with many other drugs (in which they usually decrease the metabolism and increase the risks of toxicity with affected drugs).

Applying Your Knowledge 36-1

What assessment should be made before Charlotte takes fluconazole (Diflucan)?

Ketoconazole (Nizoral) has largely been replaced by the newer drugs. It may still be used for long-term therapy, because it is less expensive than other azoles. It may also be used with cyclosporine and tacrolimus because it increases blood levels of these immunosuppressant drugs and allows smaller dosages in patients with organ transplants.

Fluconazole (Diflucan) is often the drug of choice for localized candidal infections (e.g., urinary tract infections, thrush) and is useful for systemic candidiasis. However, resistant strains of *Candida* organisms occur with extensive use of fluconazole. In vaginal candidiasis, a single oral dose of 150 milligrams is usually effective. Fluconazole is also used for long-term suppression of cryptococcal meningitis in patients with acquired immunodeficiency syndrome (AIDS), after initial use of amphotericin B.

Fluconazole can be given orally or IV. Oral drug is well absorbed, and the drug reaches therapeutic levels in most body fluids and tissues, including meninges. With a one-time loading dose of twice the usual daily dose, steady-state blood levels are reached in about 2 days; without a loading dose, 5 to 10 days are required. Once-daily dosing may be effective in some patients with normal renal function. Most of the drug is excreted as unchanged drug in urine; dosage may need to be reduced in patients with impaired renal function.

Fluconazole is usually well tolerated but may cause nausea, vomiting, diarrhea, abdominal pain, headache, and skin rash. In addition, elevation of liver enzymes and hepatic necrosis have been reported, and alopecia often occurs in patients receiving prolonged, high-dose treatment. Fluconazole increases the effects of several drugs, including cyclosporine, phenytoin, oral sulfonylureas, and warfarin, but has fewer interactions than ketoconazole and itraconazole.

Itraconazole (Sporanox) is a drug of choice for many fungal infections. It can be given orally or IV. Drug absorption may be decreased in patients with achlorhydria and in those receiving a concurrent antacid, histamine H$_2$ antagonist, or proton pump inhibitor. Serum levels should be measured to ensure adequate absorption. Drug concentrations are higher in visceral organs than in serum; little drug appears in urine or CSF.

Usual doses may cause GI upset and higher doses may cause hypokalemia, hypertension, edema, and heart failure. Itraconazole has many drug interactions. Drugs that increase the pH of gastric acid (e.g., antacids, histamine H$_2$ blockers, proton pump inhibitors) decrease absorption of itraconazole and should be given at least 2 hours after itraconazole. Drugs that induce drug-metabolizing enzymes (e.g., carbamazepine, phenytoin, rifampin) decrease serum levels of itraconazole. Itraconazole increases serum levels of cyclosporine, digoxin, oral sulfonylureas, and warfarin; it decreases serum levels of carbamazepine, phenytoin, and rifampin. There is a **BLACK BOX WARNING** about the risks of heart failure and drug interactions.

Posaconazole (Noxafil) is a second-generation azole with activity against *Candida* and *Aspergillus* species. It is available as an oral suspension; after administration, it reaches maximum concentration in the body in 3 to 5 hours and steady state in 7 to 10 days. It is highly protein bound and eliminated mainly in feces. Patients with severe vomiting and diarrhea or renal impairment should be monitored for breakthrough fungal infections. If given with drugs metabolized by the CYP3A4 enzymes in the liver, posaconazole increases blood levels and risks of adverse effects with the other drugs.

Voriconazole (Vfend) is a second-generation azole with activity against species of *Candida* and *Aspergillus*. It is well absorbed with oral administration and reaches peak serum levels in less than 2 hours. It is widely distributed in body tissues and metabolized in the liver by cytochrome P450 enzymes 2C9, 2C19, and 3A4. The metabolites are excreted renally. Transient visual disturbance is a common adverse effect, occurring in approximately 30% of recipients. Significant drug interactions include reduced voriconazole levels with enzyme inducers (e.g., rifampin, rifabutin, carbamazepine) and increased sirolimus levels with voriconazole administration, possibly to toxic levels. These drugs are contraindicated during voriconazole therapy and concomitant cyclosporine, tacrolimus, or warfarin administration requires vigilant monitoring. Dosage of voriconazole should be reduced with impaired liver function.

Applying Your Knowledge 36-2

The dose of Diflucan is not effective, and Charlotte returns to the office 2 weeks later with an active *C. albicans* infection. The primary care provider prescribes Diflucan 200 mg PO for one dose, then 100 mg PO daily for 14 days. What adverse effects should you monitor for in the patient taking Diflucan?

Echinocandins

The echinocandins have fungicidal activity against *Candida*, including azole-resistant organisms, and fungistatic activity against *Aspergillus*.

Anidulafungin (Eraxis) is used for *Candida* infections. It is moderately protein bound, has an elimination half-life of about 24 hours, and is excreted mainly in feces. It should be used cautiously with hepatic impairment. Adverse effects include a possible histamine-related reaction with dyspnea, flushing, hypotension, itching, and urticaria. This reaction is less likely to occur if the recommended infusion rate is not exceeded.

Caspofungin (Cancidas) is used for systemic *Candida* and *Aspergillus* infections. It is highly bound to plasma albumin, metabolized slowly, and excreted in feces and urine. It is usually well tolerated with doses of 50 milligrams per day. Adverse effects include fever, headache, nausea, skin rash, vomiting, and phlebitis at injection sites. Dosage must be reduced with moderate hepatic impairment; no dosage reduction is needed for renal impairment.

Cyclosporine increases the effects of caspofungin, including potential liver damage, and concomitant use is not recommended. Drugs that decrease effects include anti-HIV drugs (e.g., efavirenz, nelfinavir, nevirapine), anticonvulsants (e.g., carbamazepine, phenytoin), dexamethasone, and rifampin. Concurrent administration may significantly reduce caspofungin blood levels and therapeutic effectiveness unless dosage is increased (e.g., from the usual 50 mg to 70 mg daily).

Micafungin (Mycamine) is used to prevent or treat *Candida* infections. It is highly protein bound, metabolized in the liver, has an elimination half-life of 11 to 21 hours, and is excreted mainly in feces. It should be used cautiously with hepatic impairment. Adverse effects include liver and renal function changes and a possible histamine-related reaction with rash, itching, facial swelling, and vasodilation. Micafungin may increase blood levels and risks of toxicity of nifedipine and sirolimus.

Miscellaneous Antifungal Drugs

Griseofulvin is occasionally used for dermatophyte infections of the scalp and nails. Tinea infections of skin (e.g., ringworm) improve in 3 to 8 weeks; onychomycosis of toenails may require a year or more. Common adverse effects include GI upset (e.g., nausea, vomiting, diarrhea), fatigue, headache, insomnia, and skin rash. Hepatotoxicity may also occur.

Terbinafine (Lamisil) is a broad-spectrum antifungal that inhibits an enzyme needed for synthesis of ergosterol, a structural component of fungal cell membranes. It has fungicidal activity against dermatophytes and has been used mainly for topical treatment of ringworm infections and oral treatment of onychomycosis. Therapeutic effects may not be evident until months after drug therapy is stopped, because of the time required for growth of healthy nail. The drug is metabolized to inactive metabolites and excreted in the urine.

Common adverse effects with oral terbinafine include headache, diarrhea, and abdominal discomfort; skin reactions and liver failure may also occur with long-term use for onychomycosis. Hepatotoxicity is uncommon but has occurred in people with and without pre-existing liver disease and has led to liver transplant or death. The drug is not recommended for patients with chronic or active liver disease, and serum ALT and AST should be checked before starting the drug. There is a **BLACK BOX WARNING** regarding the risk of hepatotoxicity.

Nursing Process

Assessment

Assess for fungal infections. Specific signs and symptoms vary with location and type of infection as well as the immune state of the patient.

- Superficial lesions of skin, hair, and nails are usually characterized by pain, burning, and itching. Some lesions are moist; others are dry and scaling. They also may appear inflamed or discolored.

- Candidiasis occurs in warm, moist areas of the body. Skin lesions are likely to occur in perineal and intertriginous areas. They are usually moist, inflamed, pruritic areas with papules, vesicles, and pustules. Oral lesions are white patches that adhere to the buccal mucosa. Vaginal infection causes a cheesy vaginal discharge, burning, and itching. Intestinal infection causes diarrhea. Systemic infection causes chills and fever, myalgia, arthralgia, and prostration.

- Blastomycosis, coccidioidomycosis, and histoplasmosis may be asymptomatic or mimic influenza, pneumonia, or tuberculosis, with cough, fever, malaise, and other pulmonary manifestations. Severe histoplasmosis may also cause fever, anemia, enlarged spleen and liver, leukopenia, and GI tract ulcers.

- Cryptococcosis may involve the lungs, skin, and other body organs. In patients with AIDS or other immunosuppressant disorders, it often involves the central nervous system (CNS) and produces mental status changes, headache, dizziness, and neck stiffness.

- Sporotrichosis involves the skin and lymph nodes. It usually produces small nodules that look like insect bites initially and ulcerations later. Nodules and ulcers also may develop in local lymphatic channels and nodes. The infection can spread to other parts of the body in immunocompromised patients.

- Systemic mycoses produce severe symptoms and may be life-threatening. They are confirmed by recovery of organisms from specimens of body tissues or fluids.

Nursing Diagnoses

- Risk for Injury related to fungal infection
- Deficient Knowledge: Prevention of fungal infection; accurate drug usage

- Noncompliance related to the need for long-term therapy
- Risk for Injury: Adverse drug effects with systemic antifungal drugs

Planning/Goals

The patient will

- Take or receive systemic antifungal drugs as prescribed
- Apply topical drugs accurately
- Act to prevent recurrence of fungal infection
- Avoid preventable adverse effects from systemic drugs

Interventions

Use measures to prevent spread of fungal infections.

- Observe Standard Precautions while assessing or providing care to patients with skin lesions. Superficial infections (e.g., ringworm) are highly contagious and can be spread by sharing towels and hairbrushes. Systemic mycoses are not usually contagious.

- Decrease patient exposure to environmental fungi. For inpatients who are neutropenic or otherwise immunocompromised, do not allow soil-containing plants in the room and request regular cleaning and inspection of air-conditioning systems. Aspergillosis has occurred after inhalation of airborne mold spores from air-conditioning units and hospital water supplies. For outpatients, assist to identify and avoid areas of potential exposure (e.g., soil contaminated by chicken, bird, or bat droppings; areas where buildings are being razed, constructed, or renovated). If exposure is unavoidable, instruct to spray areas with water to minimize airborne spores and to wear disposable clothing and a face mask. For patients at risk of exposure to sporotrichosis (e.g., those who garden or work in plant nurseries), assist to identify risk factors and preventive measures (e.g., wearing gloves and long sleeves).

- For obese patients with skin candidiasis, apply dry padding to intertriginous areas to help prevent irritation and candidal growth.

- For patients with oropharyngeal ulcerations, provide soothing oral hygiene, nonacidic fluids, and soft, bland foods.

- For patients with systemic fungal infections, monitor respiratory, cardiovascular, and neurologic status at least every 8 hours. Provide comfort measures and medications (e.g., analgesics, antihistamines, antipyretics, antiemetics) for patients receiving IV amphotericin B.

Evaluation

- Observe for relief of symptoms for which an antifungal drug was prescribed.
- Interview outpatients regarding their compliance with instructions for using antifungal drugs.
- Interview and observe for adverse drug effects with systemic antifungal agents.

Patient Teaching Guidelines   Oral and Topical Antifungal Drugs

General Considerations

- If you have a condition or take a medicine that suppresses your immune system (e.g., bone marrow or organ transplant, leukemia, lymphoma, diabetes mellitus, human immunodeficiency virus [HIV] infection, cancer chemotherapy, corticosteroid therapy), avoid exposure to molds and fungi when possible, because serious, life-threatening infection may occur. To minimize exposure, avoid areas of building construction or renovation, avoid cleaning carpets or potentially moldy areas, and avoid potted plants and live flowers.
- With skin lesions, wash hands often and do not share towels, hairbrushes, or other personal items.
- With vaginal yeast infections, do not use over-the-counter medications repeatedly without consulting a health care provider. Recurrent infections may indicate inadequate treatment, reinfection, or a bacterial infection (for which an antifungal drug is not effective), and a different treatment may be needed.
- With histoplasmosis and other potentially serious fungal infections, avoid or minimize future exposure to chicken, pigeon, and bat droppings.
- If you work with plants (e.g., roses, sphagnum moss) or baled hay, prevent sporotrichosis by wearing gloves and long sleeves and avoiding injuries that cause breaks in the skin.

Self-Administration

- Use antifungal drugs as prescribed, to increase benefit and decrease adverse drug effects.

- With topical skin preparations, wash and dry the area before each application of medication.
- With vaginal antifungal preparations:
  - Read instructions.
  - Insert high into the vagina (except during pregnancy).
  - Continue use through menstruation (wear a minipad to avoid staining clothing; do not use a tampon).
  - Wash applicator with mild soap and rinse after each use.
  - Avoid sexual intercourse.
- With itraconazole (Sporanox) capsules, take after a full meal for best absorption. With the oral suspension, take on an empty stomach, usually by swishing in the mouth and then swallowing it.
- With oral posaconazole (Noxafil), take with a meal.
- With oral voriconazole (Vfend), take 1 hour before or after a meal.
- With nystatin suspension for mouth lesions (thrush), swish the medication around in the mouth (to increase drug contact with the lesions), then swallow the medication.
- With oral fluconazole (Diflucan), itraconazole (Sporanox), or terbinafine (Lamisil), notify a health care provider of unusual fatigue, loss of appetite, nausea, vomiting, jaundice, dark urine, pale stools, fever, abdominal pain, or diarrhea. These may be signs of liver damage or other adverse drug effects. Drug therapy may need to be discontinued.
- With griseofulvin, avoid prolonged exposure to sunlight or sunlamps; the drug may cause photosensitivity.
- With voriconazole, do not drive at night because vision may be blurred.

Principles of Therapy

Nonpharmacologic Treatment

Some fungal infections are asymptomatic or resolve spontaneously without treatment. In addition, some candidal infections respond to the removal of predisposing factors such as antibacterial drugs, corticosteroids or other immunosuppressant drugs, and indwelling IV or bladder catheters.

Drug Selection

Drug therapy for potentially serious fungal infections should be planned in consultation with an infectious-disease specialist when possible. Drug selection is determined mainly by the type of fungal infection. For serious infections, amphotericin B has long been the drug of choice, especially for invasive aspergillosis and systemic infections in immunocompromised hosts. However, azoles (e.g., fluconazole, itraconazole, voriconazole) and echinocandins (e.g., anidulafungin, caspofungin, micafungin) are increasingly being used for first-line treatment. The azoles are also used for initial therapy in less acutely ill patients and as long-term treatment after a brief initial course of amphotericin B. However, all azoles are contraindicated during pregnancy.

Drug Dosage and Administration

Dosages depend on illness severity, with large amounts required for systemic infections, especially in immunocompromised hosts. Routes are determined mainly by location and severity of infection. For example, local infections can often be treated by topical applications, whereas more serious or systemic infections require oral or IV routes.

Duration of Therapy

When antifungal drug therapy is required, it is usually long term, over weeks to months. In some cases, it may be continued for years or lifelong. If drug therapy is stopped too soon, relapse of the infection often occurs. However, in patients with AIDS, who often require long-term antifungal drug therapy, drug-resistant infections may develop. Fluconazole-resistant candidiasis is becoming increasingly recognized in this population. Patients with an impaired immune response often become reinfected after effective antifungal drug therapy and may require repeated courses.

Drug Treatment of Specific Infections

Aspergillosis. Itraconazole for approximately 1 year may be effective in mild to moderate infection. Amphotericin B is indicated for serious invasive disease, and large doses are required. Voriconazole or caspofungin may also be used.

Blastomycosis. Patients with skin, pulmonary, or other manifestations of systemic disease should receive systemic antifungal drug therapy to prevent further progression. Mild to moderate disease may be treated with itraconazole for 6 to 12 months. For severe disease and patients with CNS infection or immunosuppression, amphotericin B is the drug of first choice. After initial amphotericin B therapy and clinical improvement, itraconazole may be given for 6 to 12 months.

Candidiasis. Most mucocutaneous infections may be treated with local applications of drug. For oral candidiasis, clotrimazole troches are preferred; oral fluconazole, itraconazole, or nystatin suspension may also be used. Vaginal candidiasis may be treated with a single oral dose of fluconazole or multiple doses of vaginal tablets, creams, or suppositories containing butoconazole, clotrimazole, miconazole, terconazole, or tioconazole. Some of these preparations are available over-the-counter. One concern about self-treatment with nonprescription products is an incorrect diagnosis. Antifungal preparations do not help a bacterial vaginal infection. Pregnant patients should consult their obstetrician before using these drugs. Esophageal candidiasis should be treated with a systemically absorbed agent such as fluconazole or itraconazole. Systemic candidiasis may be treated with amphotericin B, an azole (e.g., fluconazole, itraconazole, voriconazole), or an echinocandin (e.g., anidulafungin, caspofungin). Fluconazole is usually preferred; amphotericin B may be preferred if the patient has previously received fluconazole or if the infection is caused by non-albicans *Candida*. Chronic systemic candidiasis usually requires months of drug therapy.

Coccidioidomycosis. Many coccidioidal infections are chronic in nature and require long-term drug therapy to control disease activity. Mild infections are usually treated with an oral azole (e.g., fluconazole, itraconazole) for 6 to 12 months. Amphotericin B is preferred for severe or disseminated disease and is usually given for 1 to 3 months. Patients with meningitis may require lifelong therapy with an azole drug to prevent recurrence.

Cryptococcosis. Amphotericin B followed by 6 to 12 months of oral fluconazole is used for treatment of meningitis. Patients with AIDS are usually given fluconazole long term to suppress recurrence.

Histoplasmosis. Itraconazole is the drug of choice for mild to moderate histoplasmosis, and amphotericin B is the drug of choice for severe disease. Patients who also have AIDS may be given itraconazole twice daily for 12 weeks, and then maintained on daily itraconazole to suppress recurrence.

Pneumocystis pneumonia (PCP). Trimethoprimsulfamethoxazole (TMP-SMZ, Bactrim) (see Chap. 32) is the drug of choice for prevention and treatment of PCP. Prophylaxis may be indicated for adults and adolescents with HIV and CD4+ cell counts of less than 200, organ transplant recipients, patients with leukemia or lymphoma who are receiving cytotoxic chemotherapy, and patients receiving high doses of corticosteroids (equivalent to 20 mg or more daily of prednisone) for longer than 2 weeks. Other drugs that may be used to prevent or treat PCP, usually in people who cannot tolerate TMP-SMZ, include atovaquone (Mepron), dapsone, pentamidine (Pentam 300, NebuPent), and trimetrexate (Neutrexin).

Sporotrichosis. Itraconazole, for 3 to 6 months, is the drug of choice for localized lymphocutaneous infection. Amphotericin B may be used to treat pulmonary, disseminated, and relapsing infections.

Characteristics and Usage of Amphotericin B

Amphotericin B has long been the gold standard of drug therapy for serious fungal infections. However, its use is problematic because of different preparations, special requirements for administration, and toxicity. These aspects are summarized below.

Preparations. The deoxycholate preparation (Fungizone), often called "conventional amphotericin B," is the oldest, most widely used form. Lipid preparations were developed to decrease the toxicity of the deoxycholate form, and three are currently available. These preparations have similar antifungal spectra, but they differ from the deoxycholate formulation and from each other in other respects.

Administration. These drugs should be reconstituted and prepared for IV administration in a pharmacy. Additional factors include the following:

- A test dose may be used to assess the patient's tolerance of the drug. Some authorities question the need for a test dose.

- Maintenance doses can be doubled and infused on alternate days. However, a single daily dose of Fungizone should not exceed 1.5 milligram per kilogram; overdoses can result in cardiorespiratory arrest.

- Small initial doses (e.g., 5–10 mg/day) are recommended for patients with impaired cardiovascular or renal function or a severe reaction to the test dose.

- Larger doses of lipid preparations are needed to achieve therapeutic effects similar to those of the deoxycholate preparation.

- Administer through a separate IV line when possible. If injecting into an existing IV line, the line should be flushed with 5% dextrose solution before and after drug administration (both deoxycholate and lipid formulations).

- An in-line filter may be used with Fungizone and AmBisome but should not be used with Abelcet or Amphotec.

- Prepared solutions should be infused within 8 hours of reconstitution.

Decreasing adverse effects. There are several recommendations for reducing toxicity of IV amphotericin B, but most have not been tested in controlled studies. Recommendations to decrease nephrotoxicity are listed below in "Use in Patients With Renal Impairment"; those to decrease fever and chills include premedication with acetaminophen, diphenhydramine, and a corticosteroid; and those to decrease phlebitis at injection sites include administering on alternate days, adding 500 to 2000 units of heparin to the infusion, rotating infusion sites, administering through a central vein, removing the needle after infusion, and using a pediatric scalp vein needle. Supplemental potassium may be used to treat hypokalemia, and recombinant erythropoietin may be used to treat anemia if the patient has a low plasma level of erythropoietin.

Applying Your Knowledge 36-3

A fungal infection that is severe or systemic may need to be treated with amphotericin B. Proper administration and assessment for adverse effects are part of the nurse's role. What adverse effects do you assess for in Charlotte while her amphotericin B is infusing?

Effects of Antifungals on Other Drugs

Amphotericin B increases effects of cyclosporine (nephrotoxicity), digoxin (risk of hypokalemia and cardiac dysrhythmias), nephrotoxic drugs (e.g., aminoglycoside antibiotics), skeletal muscle relaxants (amphotericin B–induced hypokalemia may enhance muscle relaxation), and thiazide and loop diuretics (risk of hypokalemia). Serum potassium levels should be monitored.

Azoles inhibit the metabolism of many drugs (by inhibiting cytochrome P450 drug-metabolizing enzymes in the liver and small intestine, especially 3A4 enzymes) and therefore increase their effects and risks of toxicity. These drugs include benzodiazepines (alprazolam, midazolam, triazolam), calcium channel blockers (felodipine, nifedipine), cyclosporine, phenytoin, statin cholesterol-lowering drugs (atorvastatin, simvastatin), sulfonylureas, tacrolimus, theophylline, warfarin, vincristine, and zidovudine.

Although the main concern about azole drug interactions is increased toxicity of inhibited drugs, ketoconazole may be given with cyclosporine and tacrolimus to decrease dosages and costs of the immunosuppressant drugs. There may also be a reduced risk of fungal infections, which commonly occur in people with an impaired immune system.

Fluconazole is apparently a less potent inhibitor of cytochrome P450 3A4 enzymes than ketoconazole and itraconazole. As a result, drug interactions with fluconazole are of lesser magnitude and usually occur only with dosages of 200 milligrams per day or more. However, fluconazole is a strong inhibitor of cytochrome P450 2C9 enzymes, and concurrent administration of losartan, phenytoin, or warfarin results in greater risks of toxicity with the inhibited drugs.

Caspofungin decreases serum levels of tacrolimus; serum levels of tacrolimus should be monitored. Micafungin increases blood levels and risks of toxicity with nifedipine and sirolimus. No significant interactions have been reported with anidulafungin.

Griseofulvin decreases the effects of cyclosporine, oral contraceptives, salicylates, and warfarin, probably by inducing hepatic drug-metabolizing enzymes and accelerating their metabolism.

Terbinafine is a strong inhibitor of cytochrome P450 2D6 enzymes and may increase the effects of propafenone, metoprolol, and desipramine and nortriptyline.

Use in Special Populations

Use in Children

Guidelines for the use of topical antifungal drugs in children are generally the same as those for adults. With most oral and intravenous agents for treatment of systemic fungal infections, safety, effectiveness, and guidelines for use have not been established. In addition, some agents have no established pediatric dosages and others have age restrictions. Despite these limitations, most antifungal drugs, including amphotericin B and the azoles, have been used successfully to treat children with serious fungal infections, without unusual or severe adverse effects. The safety and efficacy of echinocandins in children have not been established. Children receiving systemic antifungal drugs should be given the lowest effective dosage and be monitored closely for adverse effects.

Use in Older Adults

Specific guidelines for the use of antifungal drugs have not been established. The main concern is with oral or parenteral drugs because topical agents produce few adverse effects.

Virtually all adults receiving IV amphotericin B experience adverse effects. With the impaired renal and cardiovascular functions that usually accompany aging, older adults are especially vulnerable to serious adverse effects. They must be monitored closely to reduce the incidence and severity of nephrotoxicity, hypokalemia, and other adverse drug reactions. Lipid formulations of amphotericin B are less nephrotoxic than the conventional deoxycholate formulation and may be preferred for older adults. Azole drugs should probably be stopped if hypertension, edema, or hypokalemia occur. In addition, itraconazole has been associated with heart failure, a common condition in older adults. There is little information available about the effects of posaconazole, voriconazole, and the echinocandins (e.g., caspofungin) in older adults.

Use in Patients With Cancer

Patients with cancer are at high risk for development of serious, systemic fungal infections. In patients receiving cytotoxic anticancer drugs, antifungal therapy is often used to prevent or treat infections caused by *Candida* and *Aspergillus* organisms. For prophylaxis, topical, oral, or IV agents are given before and during periods of drug-induced neutropenia, often to prevent recurrence of infection that occurred during previous neutropenic episodes. For treatment, oral or IV drugs may be given at the onset of fever and neutropenia, when fever persists or recurs in a neutropenic patient despite appropriate antimicrobial therapy, or when maintenance therapy is needed after initial treatment of coccidioidomycosis, cryptococcosis, or histoplasmosis. These infections often relapse if antifungal drugs are discontinued. Patients must be closely monitored for adverse effects of antifungal drugs.

Use in Patients With Renal Impairment

Amphotericin B deoxycholate (Fungizone) is nephrotoxic. Renal impairment occurs in most patients (up to 80%) within the first 2 weeks of therapy but usually subsides with dosage reduction or drug discontinuation. Permanent impairment occurs in a few patients. Recommendations to decrease nephrotoxicity include hydrating patients with a liter of 0.9% sodium chloride solution IV and monitoring serum creatinine and blood urea nitrogen (BUN) at least weekly. If BUN exceeds 40 milligrams per deciliter or serum creatinine exceeds 3 milligrams per deciliter, the drug should be stopped or dosage should be reduced until renal function recovers. Another strategy is to give a lipid formulation (e.g., Abelcet, AmBisome, Amphotec), which is less nephrotoxic. For patients who already have renal impairment or other risk factors for development of renal impairment, a lipid formulation is indicated. Renal function should still be monitored frequently.

Caspofungin does not require dosage reduction for renal impairment and is not removed by hemodialysis. Fluconazole is mainly excreted in the urine as unchanged drug. For patients with a creatinine clearance (CrCl) above 50 milliliters per minute, full dosage may be given. For those with a CrCl of 50 milliliters per minute or less, dosage should be reduced by one half. However, for patients receiving hemodialysis, an extra dose may be needed because 3 hours of hemodialysis lowers plasma drug levels by approximately 50%. Itraconazole can be given to patients with mild to moderate renal impairment but is contraindicated in those with a CrCl of 30 milliliters per minute or less. It is not removed by hemodialysis. Voriconazole has been associated with acute renal failure; renal function should be closely monitored during use. Terbinafine clearance is reduced by 50% in patients with a CrCl of 50 milliliters per minute or less. Its use is not recommended.

Use in Patients With Hepatic Impairment

Although the main concern with amphotericin B is nephrotoxicity, it is recommended that liver function tests be monitored during use. Caspofungin dosage must be reduced with moderate hepatic impairment; the drug has not been studied in patients with severe hepatic impairment.

The azole antifungals may cause hepatotoxicity, ranging from mild elevations in ALT and AST to clinical hepatitis, cholestasis, hepatic failure, and death. Fatal hepatic damage has occurred mainly in patients with serious underlying conditions, such as AIDS or malignancy, and with multiple concomitant medications. The drugs are relatively contraindicated in patients with increased liver enzymes, active liver disease, or a history of liver damage with other drugs. They should be given only if expected benefits outweigh risks of liver injury. ALT, AST, and serum bilirubin should be checked before drug use, after several weeks of drug use, and every 1 to 2 months during long-term therapy. If ALT and AST increase to more than three times the normal range, the azole should be discontinued. Hepatotoxicity may be reversible if drug therapy is stopped.

Griseofulvin may cause hepatotoxicity, especially if given in large doses for prolonged periods. Terbinafine has been associated with liver failure, and its clearance is reduced by 50% in patients with hepatic cirrhosis. Its use is not recommended for patients with chronic or active liver disease, and liver function tests should be done in all patients before starting therapy. Hepatotoxicity has been reported in patients with and without pre-existing liver disease.

Use in Patients With Critical Illness

Amphotericin B, caspofungin, and the azoles are often used for serious fungal infections. Amphotericin B penetrates tissues well, except for CSF, and only small amounts are excreted in urine. With prolonged administration, the half-life increases from 1 to 15 days. Hemodialysis does not remove the drug. Lipid formulations may be preferred in critically ill patients because of less nephrotoxicity. Fluconazole penetrates tissues well, including CSF. Although IV administration may be necessary in many critically ill patients, the drug is well absorbed when administered orally or by nasogastric tube. Significantly impaired renal function may require reduced dosage, and impaired hepatic function may require discontinuation. When itraconazole is used in critically ill patients, a loading dose of 200 milligrams three times daily may be given for the first 3 days. Treatment should be continued for at least 3 months; inadequate treatment may lead to recurrent infection.

Use in Home Care

Antifungal drugs may be taken at home by various routes. For topical and oral routes, the role of the home care nurse may be teaching correct usage and encouraging patients to persist with the long-term treatment usually required. With IV antifungal drugs for serious infections, the home care nurse may need to assist in managing the environment, administering the drug, and monitoring for adverse effects. Because the immune function of these patients is often severely suppressed, protective interventions are needed. These may include teaching about frequent and thorough hand hygiene by patients, all members of the household, and visitors; safe food preparation and storage; removing potted plants and fresh flowers; and avoiding activities that generate dust in the patient's environment. In addition, air conditioning and air filtering systems should be kept meticulously clean and any plans for renovations should be postponed or canceled.

Nursing Actions   Antifungal Drugs

NURSING ACTIONS	RATIONALE/EXPLANATION
1. Administer accurately	
a. Give intravenous (IV) amphotericin B (Fungizone, Abelcet, AmBisome, and Amphotec) according to manufacturers' recommendations for each product:	This drug is given for serious, systemic fungal infections and unlikely to be commonly used in many health care settings.
(1) Follow recommendations for administration of test doses, if ordered.	Preparation, concentration, and infusion times vary among formulations. Solutions, including test doses, should be prepared in a pharmacy. Some clinicians may not use a test dose.
(2) Use an infusion pump.	To regulate flow accurately
(3) Use a separate IV line if possible; if using an existing line, flush with 5% dextrose in water before and after each infusion.	
(4) Fungizone IV—give in 5% dextrose in water, over 2–6 hours; use an in-line filter; do not mix with other IV medications.	
(5) Abelcet—give over 2 hours; do not use an in-line filter.	
(6) AmBisome—give over 2 hours or longer; may use an in-line filter.	
(7) Amphotec—give over at least 2 hours; do not use an in-line filter.	
(8) Apply cream or lotion liberally to skin lesions and rub in gently.	
b. Give azoles according to manufacturers' recommendations:	
(1) Give IV fluconazole as a continuous infusion at a maximum rate of 200 mg/h. Give IV voriconazole over 1 to 2 hours.	
(2) Shake oral suspensions of fluconazole, posaconazole, voriconazole before measuring the dose.	To resuspend medication in the liquid vehicle and ensure accurate dosage
(3) Give itraconazole capsules after a full meal; give the oral solution on an empty stomach and ask the patient to swish the medication in the mouth, then swallow it.	To decrease GI upset and increase absorption. The oral solution is used to treat oropharyngeal and esophageal candidiasis, and correct administration enhances contact with mucosal lesions.
(4) With posaconazole suspension, shake well and give with a full meal or liquid nutritional supplement.	To increase absorption
(5) Give oral voriconazole 1 h before or 2 h after a meal.	Manufacturer's recommendation
c. Review and follow manufacturers' instructions for IV administration of anidulafungin, caspofungin, and micafungin.	These drugs are given for serious, systemic fungal infections and unlikely to be commonly used in many health care settings.
2. Observe for therapeutic effects	
a. Decreased fever and malaise with systemic mycoses	Most antifungal drug therapy is long term, over weeks, months, or years. With skin infections, optimal therapeutic effects may occur 2–4 weeks after drug therapy is stopped. With nail infections, optimal effects may occur 6–9 months after drug therapy is stopped.
b. Healing of lesions on skin and mucous membranes	
c. Diminished diarrhea with intestinal candidiasis	
d. Decreased vaginal discharge and discomfort with vaginal candidiasis	
3. Observe for adverse effects	
a. With IV amphotericin B, observe for fever, chills, anorexia, nausea, vomiting, renal damage (elevated blood urea nitrogen and serum creatinine), hypokalemia, hypomagnesemia, headache, stupor, coma, convulsions, anemia from bone marrow depression, phlebitis at venipuncture sites, and anaphylaxis.	This is a highly toxic drug and most recipients develop adverse effects, including renal damage. Antipyretic and antiemetic drugs may decrease adverse reactions and promote patient comfort. Adequate hydration and lipid formulations may decrease renal damage. Anaphylaxis is uncommon; however, emergency medications and supplies should be available during infusions. If severe respiratory distress occurs, the drug should be stopped immediately.
b. With fluconazole, itraconazole, posaconazole, and voriconazole, observe for unusual fatigue, loss of appetite, nausea, vomiting, jaundice, dark urine, pale stools, fever, abdominal pain, or diarrhea.	These may be signs of liver damage or other adverse effects. Drug therapy may need to be discontinued.

NURSING ACTIONS	RATIONALE/EXPLANATION
c. With caspofungin 50 mg daily, observe for nausea, vomiting, and phlebitis at infusion sites. With larger doses (50–70 mg daily), observe for the above plus fever, headache, and abnormal laboratory reports (e.g., decreased white blood cells, hemoglobin, and hematocrit; increased serum potassium and liver aminotransferase enzymes).	The drug is usually well tolerated.
d. With griseofulvin, observe for GI symptoms, hypersensitivity (urticaria, photosensitivity, skin rashes, angioedema), headache, mental confusion, fatigue, dizziness, peripheral neuritis, and blood dyscrasias (leukopenia, neutropenia, granulocytopenia).	The incidence of serious reactions is low.
e. With oral terbinafine, observe for diarrhea, dyspepsia, headache, skin rash or itching, and liver enzyme abnormalities.	Elevated liver enzymes (alanine and aspartate aminotransferases [ALT and AST]) may indicate liver damage and may occur in patients with or without pre-existing liver disease. Adverse reactions are usually minimal with topical drugs, although hypersensitivity may occur.
f. With topical drugs, observe for skin rash and irritation.	
4. Observe for drug interactions	
a. Drugs that *increase* effects of amphotericin B:	
(1) Antineoplastic drugs	May increase risks of nephrotoxicity, hypotension, and bronchospasm
(2) Corticosteroids	May potentiate hypokalemia and precipitate cardiac dysfunction
(3) Zidovudine	Increases renal and hematologic adverse effects of the liposomal formulation. Renal and hematologic functions should be monitored closely.
(4) Nephrotoxic drugs (e.g., aminoglycoside antibiotics, cyclosporine)	Increase nephrotoxicity
b. Drug that *increases* effects of fluconazole:	
(1) Hydrochlorothiazide	Increases serum levels of fluconazole, attributed to decreased renal excretion
c. Drugs that *decrease* effects of fluconazole and posaconazole:	
(1) Cimetidine	Decreased absorption
(2) Rifampin	Accelerated metabolism from enzyme induction
d. Drugs that *decrease* effects of itraconazole:	
(1) Antacids, histamine H$_2$ antagonists, proton pump inhibitors	These drugs decrease gastric acid, which inhibits absorption. If required, they should be given at least 2 hours after the azole drug.
(2) Phenytoin, rifampin	Accelerate metabolism and decrease blood levels
e. Drugs that *increase* effects of voriconazole:	
(1) Cimetidine	
(2) Proton pump inhibitors	
(3) Protease inhibitors (anti-HIV drugs)	
f. Drugs that *decrease effects* of voriconazole	
(1) Phenytoin	Decrease serum levels, probably from accelerated metabolism
(2) Rifampin	
g. Drug that *increases* effects of caspofungin:	
(1) Cyclosporine	Increases serum levels
h. Drugs that *decrease* effects of caspofungin:	
(1) Enzyme inducers (efavirenz, nelfinavir, nevirapine, dexamethasone, carbamazepine, phenytoin, rifampin)	Decrease serum levels by accelerating caspofungin metabolism. The daily dose of caspofungin may need to be increased if given with one of these drugs.
i. Drugs that *decrease* effects of griseofulvin:	
(1) Enzyme inducers (e.g., rifampin)	Increase metabolism of griseofulvin
j. Drug that *increases* effects of terbinafine:	
(1) Cimetidine	Slows metabolism and elimination of terbinafine so that serum levels are increased
k. Drug that *decreases* effects of terbinafine:	
(1) Rifampin	Causes rapid metabolism and clearance of terbinafine

Key Concepts

- Serious fungal infections and infections with non-albicans *Candida* strains are increasing.

- Patients whose immune systems are suppressed are at high risk of serious fungal infections.

- Fungal infections often require long-term drug therapy.

- Systemic antifungal drugs may cause serious adverse effects. Nephrotoxicity is associated with amphotericin B; hepatotoxicity is associated with azole drugs.

- Liver function should be monitored with all systemic antifungal drugs; both hepatic and renal function should be monitored with amphotericin B.

Review and Application Exercises

Short Answer Exercises

1. What environmental factors predispose patients to development of fungal infections?

2. What signs and symptoms occur with candidiasis, and how would you assess for these?

3. Which fungal infections often mimic other respiratory infections?

4. What are the clinical indications for use of IV amphotericin B?

5. What are nursing interventions to decrease adverse effects of IV amphotericin B?

6. What are the differences between amphotericin B deoxycholate and the lipid formulations?

7. What are the clinical indications for use of oral antifungal drugs?

8. What are some early indications that a patient is developing nephrotoxicity or hepatotoxicity?

9. Which population groups are at high risk of developing serious fungal infections and what can be done to protect them?

NCLEX-Style Questions

10. The nurse caring for a patient with a serious fungal infection is aware that a major risk factor for these fungal infections is
    a. immunosuppression
    b. mild exposure to a causative organism
    c. poor hand hygiene technique
    d. taking an antibacterial drug for 5 days

11. The nurse knows that the following drug may be used to treat oral candidiasis (thrush)?
    a. terbinafine (Lamisil)
    b. flucytosine (Ancobon)
    c. fluconazole (Diflucan)
    d. butoconazole (Gynazole)

12. The nurse caring for a patient who has just been diagnosed with a serious fungal infection received an order to start IV amphotericin B. Which of the following is a major adverse effect of IV amphotericin B?
    a. bone marrow depression
    b. nephrotoxicity
    c. hepatotoxicity
    d. neurotoxicity

13. In administering an azole antifungal medication to a patient, as the nurse you are aware that a major adverse effect of the azole antifungal drugs is
    a. bone marrow depression
    b. nephrotoxicity
    c. hepatotoxicity
    d. neurotoxicity

14. Which of the following medications is often ordered to be given with IV amphotericin B to decrease infusion reactions?
    a. an antihistamine
    b. an antibacterial
    c. a diuretic
    d. a local anesthetic

Selected References

Brown, T. E. R., & Chin, T. W. F. (2005). Superficial fungal infections. In J. T. DiPiro, R. L. Talbert, G. C. Yee, G. R. Matzke, B. G. Wells, & L. M. Posey (Eds.), *Pharmacotherapy: A pathophysiologic approach* (6th ed., pp. 2145–2160). New York: McGraw-Hill.

Carver, P. L. (2005). Invasive fungal infections. In J. T. DiPiro, R. L. Talbert, G. C. Yee, G. R. Matzke, B. G. Wells, & L. M. Posey (Eds.), *Pharmacotherapy: A pathophysiologic approach* (6th ed., pp. 2161–2190). New York: McGraw-Hill.

Drug facts and comparisons. (Updated monthly) St. Louis, MO: Facts and Comparisons.

Morris, M. I., & Villman, M. (2006). Echinocandins in the management of invasive fungal infections, Part 1. *American Journal of Health-System Pharmacy, 63,* 1693–1703.

Morris, M. I., & Villman, M. (2006). Echinocandins in the management of invasive fungal infections, Part 2. *American Journal of Health-System Pharmacy, 63,* 1813–1820.

Shelburne, S. A., & Hamill, R. J. (2007). Infectious diseases: Mycotic. In S. J. McPhee, M. A. Papadakis, & L. M. Tierney, Jr. (Eds.), *Current medical diagnosis and treatment 2007* (46th ed., pp. 1567–1581). New York: McGraw-Hill.

Spanakis, E. K., Aperis, G., & Mylonakis, E. (2006). New agents for the treatment of fungal infections: Clinical efficacy and gaps in coverage. *Clinical Infectious Diseases, 43,* 1060–1068.

Spellberg, B. J., Filler, S. G., & Edwards, J. E., Jr. (2006). Current treatment strategies for disseminated candidiasis. *Clinical Infectious Diseases, 42,* 244–251.

Steinbach, W. J. (2005). Antifungal agents in children. *Pediatric Clinics of North America, 52,* 895–915.

Vazquez, J. A., & Sobel, J. D. (2006). Anidulafungin: A novel echinocandin. *Clinical Infectious Diseases, 43,* 215–222.

Antiparasitics

LEARNING OBJECTIVES

After studying this chapter, you will be able to:

1. Describe environmental and other major factors in prevention and recognition of selected parasitic diseases.
2. Discuss assessment and treatment of pinworm infestations and pediculosis in school-age children.
3. Teach preventive interventions to patients planning travel to a malarious area.

Applying Your Knowledge

Lacy Michelsen is a 35-year-old woman who is a missionary. She has just returned from a 2-year stay in a developing country. Ms. Michelsen comes to the clinic today with severe diarrhea, fever, chills, headache, and myalgia. She is diagnosed with giardiasis and malaria and is prescribed chloroquine 500 mg daily for 3 weeks and metronidazole 250 mg PO three times a day for 7 days.

Introduction

A *parasite* is a living organism that survives at the expense of another organism, called the host. Parasitic infestations are common human ailments worldwide. The effects of parasitic diseases on human hosts vary from minor to major and life threatening. Parasitic diseases discussed in this chapter are those caused by protozoa, helminths (worms), scabies, and pediculi (lice). Protozoa and helminths can infect the digestive tract and other body tissues; scabies and pediculi affect the skin.

Protozoal Infections

Amebiasis

Amebiasis is a common disease in Africa, Asia, and Latin America, but it can occur in any geographic region. In the United States, it is most likely to occur in residents of institutions for the mentally challenged, men who have sex with men, and residents or travelers in countries with poor sanitation.

Amebiasis is caused by the pathogenic protozoan *Entamoeba histolytica*, which exists in two forms, cysts and trophozoites. Cysts are inactive; resistant to drugs, heat, cold, and drying; and can survive outside the body for long periods. Amebiasis is transmitted by ingestion of food or water contaminated with human feces containing amebic cysts. After they are ingested, some cysts remain intact to be expelled in feces and continue the chain of infection, and some open in the ileum to release amebae, which produce trophozoites. Trophozoites are active amebae that feed, multiply, move about, and produce clinical manifestations of amebiasis. Trophozoites produce an enzyme that allows them to invade body tissues. They may form erosions and ulcerations in the intestinal wall with resultant diarrhea (this form of the disease is called intestinal amebiasis or amebic dysentery), or they may penetrate blood vessels and be carried to other organs, where they form abscesses. These abscesses are usually found in the liver (hepatic amebiasis) but also may occur in the lungs or brain.

Drugs used to treat amebiasis (*amebicides*) are classified according to their site of action. For example, chloroquine is a tissue or extraintestinal amebicide because it acts in the bowel wall, liver, and other tissues. Metronidazole (Flagyl) is effective in both intestinal and extraintestinal amebiasis. No amebicides are currently recommended for prophylaxis of amebiasis.

Giardiasis

Giardiasis is caused by *Giardia lamblia*, a common intestinal parasite. It is spread by food or water contaminated with human feces containing encysted forms of the organism or by contact with infected people or animals. Person-to-person spread often occurs among children in daycare centers, people in institutions, and men who have sex with men. The organism is also found in people who camp or hike in wilderness areas or who drink untreated well water in areas where sanitation is poor. Giardiasis may affect children more than adults and may cause community outbreaks of diarrhea.

Giardial infections occur 1 to 2 weeks after ingestion of the cysts and may be asymptomatic or produce diarrhea, abdominal cramping, and distention. If untreated, giardiasis may resolve spontaneously or progress to a chronic disease with anorexia, nausea, malaise, weight loss, and continued diarrhea with large, foul-smelling stools. Deficiencies of vitamin B_{12} and fat-soluble vitamins may occur. Adults and children older than 8 years of age with symptomatic giardiasis are usually treated with oral metronidazole.

Malaria

Malaria is a common cause of morbidity and mortality in many parts of the world, especially in tropical regions. In the United States, malaria is rare and affects travelers or immigrants from malarious areas.

Malaria is caused by four species of protozoa of the genus *Plasmodium*. The human being is the only natural reservoir of these parasites. All types of malaria are transmitted only by *Anopheles* mosquitoes. *Plasmodium vivax*, *Plasmodium malariae*, and *Plasmodium ovale* cause recurrent malaria by forming reservoirs in the human host. In these types of malaria, signs and symptoms may occur months or years after the initial attack. *Plasmodium falciparum* causes the most life-threatening type of malaria but does not form a reservoir. This type of malaria may be cured and prevented from recurring.

Plasmodia have a life cycle in which one stage of development occurs within the human body. When a mosquito bites a person with malaria, it ingests blood that contains gametocytes (male and female forms of the protozoan parasite). From these forms, sporozoites are produced and transported to the mosquito's salivary glands. When the mosquito bites the next person, the sporozoites are injected into that person's bloodstream.

From the bloodstream, the organisms lodge in the liver and other tissues, where they reproduce and form merozoites. The liver cells containing the parasite eventually rupture and release the merozoites into the bloodstream, where they invade red blood cells. After a period of growth and reproduction, merozoites rupture red blood cells, invade other erythrocytes, form gametocytes, and continue the cycle. After several cycles, clinical symptoms of malaria occur because of the large parasite burden. The characteristic cycles of chills and fever correspond to the release of merozoites from erythrocytes.

Antimalarial drugs act at different stages in the life cycle of plasmodial parasites. Some drugs (e.g., chloroquine) are effective against erythrocytic forms and are therefore useful in preventing or treating acute attacks of malaria. These drugs do not prevent infection with the parasite, but they do prevent clinical manifestations. Other drugs (e.g., primaquine) act against exoerythrocytic or tissue forms of the parasite to prevent initial infection and recurrent attacks or to cure some types of malaria. Combination drug therapy, administered concomitantly or consecutively, is common with antimalarial drugs.

Toxoplasmosis

Toxoplasmosis is caused by *Toxoplasma gondii*, a parasite spread by ingesting undercooked meat or other food containing encysted forms of the organism, by contact with feces from infected cats, and by congenital spread from mothers with acute infection. After infection, the organism may persist in tissue cysts for the life of the host. However, symptoms rarely occur unless the immune system is impaired or becomes impaired at a later time. Although symptomatic infection may occur in anyone with immunosuppression (e.g., people with cancer or organ transplantation), it is especially common and serious in people with AIDS, in whom it often causes encephalitis and death.

Trichomoniasis

The most common form of trichomoniasis is a vaginal infection caused by *Trichomonas vaginalis*. The disease is usually spread by sexual intercourse. Antitrichomonal drugs may be administered systemically (i.e., metronidazole) or applied locally as vaginal creams. Because trichomoniasis is transmitted by sexual intercourse, partners should be treated simultaneously to prevent reinfection.

Helminthiasis

Helminthiasis, or infestation with parasitic worms, often occurs in many parts of the world. Helminths are most often found in the gastrointestinal (GI) tract. However, several types penetrate body tissues or produce *larvae* that migrate to the blood, lymph channels, lungs, liver, and other body tissues. Helminthic infections are described in Box 37-1.

Drugs used for treatment of helminthiasis are called *anthelmintics*. Most anthelmintics act locally to kill or cause expulsion of parasitic worms from the intestines; some anthelmintics act systemically against parasites that have penetrated various body tissues. The goal of anthelmintic therapy

Box 37-1	**Helminthic Infections**

Hookworm infections are caused by *Necator americanus*, a species found in the United States, and *Ancylostoma duodenale*, a species found in Europe, the Middle East, and North Africa. Hookworm is spread by ova-containing feces from infected people. Ova develop into larvae when deposited on the soil. Larvae burrow through the skin (e.g., if the person walks on the soil with bare feet), enter blood vessels, and migrate through the lungs to the pharynx, where they are swallowed. Larvae develop into adult hookworms in the small intestine and attach themselves to the intestinal mucosa.

Pinworm infections (enterobiasis), caused by *Enterobius vermicularis*, are the most common parasitic worm infections in the United States. They are highly communicable and often involve schoolchildren and household contacts. Infection occurs from contact with ova in food or water or on bed linens. The female pinworm migrates from the bowel to the perianal area to deposit eggs, especially at night. Touching or scratching the perianal area deposits ova on hands and any objects touched by the contaminated hands.

Roundworm infections (ascariasis), caused by *Ascaris lumbricoides*, are the most common parasitic worm infections in the world. They occur most often in tropical regions but may occur wherever sanitation is poor. The infection is transmitted by ingesting food or water contaminated with feces from infected people. Ova are swallowed and hatch into larvae in the intestine. The larvae penetrate blood vessels and migrate through the lungs before returning to the intestines, where they develop into adult worms.

Tapeworms attach themselves to the intestinal wall and may grow as long as several yards. Segments called *proglottids*, which contain tapeworm eggs, are expelled in feces. Tapeworms are transmitted by ingestion of contaminated, raw, or improperly cooked beef, pork, or fish. Beef and fish tapeworm infections are not usually considered serious illnesses. Pork tapeworm, which is uncommon in the United States, is more serious because it produces larvae that enter the bloodstream and migrate to other body tissues (i.e., muscles, liver, lungs, and brain).

Threadworm infections (strongyloidiasis), caused by *Strongyloides stercoralis*, are potentially serious infections. This worm burrows into the mucosa of the small intestine, where the female lays eggs. The eggs hatch into larvae that can penetrate all body tissues.

Trichinosis, a parasitic worm infection caused by *Trichinella spiralis*, occurs worldwide. It is caused by ingestion of inadequately cooked meat, especially pork. Encysted larvae are ingested in infected pork. In the intestine, the larvae excyst, mature, and produce eggs that hatch into new larvae. The larvae enter blood and lymphatic vessels and are transported throughout the body. They penetrate various body tissues (e.g., muscles and brain) and evoke inflammatory reactions. Eventually, the larvae are re-encysted or walled off in the tissues and may remain for 10 years or longer.

Whipworm infections (trichuriasis) are caused by *Trichuris trichiura*. Whipworms attach themselves to the wall of the colon.

may be to eradicate the parasite completely or to decrease the magnitude of infestation ("worm burden").

Scabies and Pediculosis

Scabies and pediculosis are parasitic infestations of the skin. Scabies is caused by the "itch mite" (*Sarcoptes scabiei*), which burrows into the skin and lays eggs that hatch in 4 to 8 days. The burrows may produce visible skin lesions, most often between the fingers and on the wrists.

Pediculosis may be caused by one of three types of lice. *Pediculosis capitis* (head lice) is the most common type in the United States. It is diagnosed by finding louse eggs (nits) attached to hair shafts close to the scalp. *Pediculosis corporis* (body lice) is diagnosed by finding lice in clothing, especially in seams. *Pediculosis pubis* (pubic or crab lice) is diagnosed by the presence of nits in the pubic and genital areas. Although scabies and pediculosis are caused by different parasites, the conditions have several common characteristics:

■ They are more likely to occur in areas of poverty, overcrowding, and poor sanitation. However, they may occur in any geographic area and socioeconomic group.

■ They are highly communicable and transmitted by direct contact with an infected person or the person's personal effects (e.g., clothing, combs and hairbrushes, bed linens).

■ Pruritus is usually the major symptom. It results from an allergic reaction to parasite secretions. In addition to the intense discomfort associated with pruritus, scratching is likely to cause skin excoriation with secondary bacterial infection and formation of vesicles, pustules, and crusts.

■ They are treated with many of the same topical medications.

Antiparasitic Drugs

Antiparasitic drugs include amebicides, antimalarials, other antiprotozoal agents, anthelmintics, scabicides, and *pediculicides*. They are described below and in Table 37-1.

Antiprotozoal Agents

Amebicides

Chloroquine (Aralen) is used mainly for its antimalarial effects. When used as an amebicide, the drug is effective in extraintestinal amebiasis (i.e., hepatic amebiasis) but usually ineffective in intestinal amebiasis. Treatment is usually combined with an intestinal amebicide.

Iodoquinol (Yodoxin) is an iodine compound that acts against active amebae (trophozoites) in the intestinal lumen. It

Table 37-1	Drugs at a Glance: Antiparasitic Drugs

Generic/Trade Name	Indications for Use	ROUTES AND DOSAGE RANGES	
		Adults	**Children**
Amebicides			
Chloroquine (Aralen)	Extraintestinal amebiasis	PO 1 g/d for 2 d, then 500 mg/d for 2–3 wk	PO 20 mg/kg/d, in 2 divided doses, for 2 d, then 10 mg/kg/d for 2–3 wk
Iodoquinol (Yodoxin)	Intestinal amebiasis	Asymptomatic carriers, PO 650 mg/d Symptomatic intestinal amebiasis, PO 650 mg 3 times daily after meals for 20 d; repeat after 2–3 wk if necessary	PO 40 mg/kg/d in 3 divided doses for 20 d (maximum dose, 2 g/d); repeat after 2–3 wk if necessary
Metronidazole (Flagyl)	Intestinal and extraintestinal amebiasis Giardiasis Trichomoniasis	Amebiasis, PO 500–750 mg 3 times daily for 5–10 d Giardiasis, PO 250 mg 3 times daily for 7 d Trichomoniasis, PO 250 mg 3 times daily for 7 d, 1 g twice daily for 1 d, or 2 g in a single dose. Repeat after 4–6 wk, if necessary. *Gardnerella vaginalis* vaginitis, PO 500 mg twice daily for 7 d	Amebiasis, PO 35–50 mg/kg/d in 3 divided doses, for 10 d Giardiasis, PO 15 mg/kg/d in 3 divided doses, for 7 d
Tetracycline (Sumycin) and doxycycline (Vibramycin)	Intestinal amebiasis	PO 250–500 mg q6h, up to 14 d	PO 25–50 mg/kg/d in 4 divided doses, for 7 to 10 d
Tinidazole (Tindamax)	Amebiasis Giardiasis Trichomoniasis	Amebiasis, PO 2 g daily for 3–5 d Giardiasis and trichomoniasis, PO 2 g as a single dose	Amebiasis, 3 y and older, PO 50 mg/kg, up to 2 g, daily for 3–5 d Giardiasis and trichomoniasis, PO 50 mg/kg, up to 2 g, as a single dose
Antimalarial Agents			
Atovaquone/proguanil (Malarone)	Prevention and treatment of malaria	Prophylaxis, one adult tablet daily 1–2 d before and 7 d after travel Treatment, 4 adult tablets daily for 3 d	Prophylaxis, weight 11–40 kg, PO 1–3 pediatric tablets 1–2 d before and 7 d after travel Treatment, weight 40 kg or above, PO 1–4 adult tablets daily for 3 d; weight under 40 kg, PO 8 mg/kg according to the schedule for adults
Chloroquine phosphate (Aralen)	Prevention and treatment of malaria	Prophylaxis, PO 5 mg/kg weekly (maximum of 300 mg/wk), starting 2 wk before entering a malarious area and continuing for 8 wk after return Treatment, PO 1 g initially, then 500 mg after 6–8 h, then 500 mg daily for 2 d (total of 2.5 g in 4 doses)	Treatment, PO 10 mg/kg initially, then 5 mg/kg after 6 h, then 5 mg/kg/d for 2 d (total of 4 doses)

(continued on page 604)

Table 37-1	**Drugs at a Glance:** Antiparasitic Drugs (continued)		
		ROUTES AND DOSAGE RANGES	
Generic/Trade Name	Indications for Use	Adults	Children
Chloroquine with primaquine	Prophylaxis of malaria	PO 1 tablet weekly for 2 wk before entering and 8 wk after leaving malarious areas	PO same as adults for weight above 45 kg; 1/2 tablet for weight of 25–45 kg. For younger children, a suspension is prepared (e.g., 40 mg of chloroquine and 6 mg of primaquine in 5 mL). Dosages are then 2.5 mL for weight of 5–7 kg; 5 mL for 8–11 kg; 7.5 mL for 12–15 kg; 10 mL for 16–20 kg; and 12.5 mL for 21–24 kg. Dosages are given weekly for 2 wk before entering and 8 wk after leaving malarious areas.
Hydroxychloroquine (Plaquenil)	Erythrocytic malaria	Prophylaxis, PO 5 mg/kg, not to exceed 310 mg, once weekly for 2 wk before entering and 8 wk after leaving malarious areas Treatment of acute malaria, PO 620 mg initially, then 310 mg 6 h later, and 310 mg/d for 2 d (total of 4 doses)	Prophylaxis, PO 5 mg/kg once weekly for 2 wk before entering and 8 wk after leaving malarious areas Treatment of acute malaria, PO 10 mg/kg initially, then 5 mg/kg 6 h later, and 5 mg/kg/d for 2 doses (total of 4 doses)
Mefloquine (Lariam)	Prevention and treatment of malaria	Prophylaxis, PO 250 mg 1 wk before travel, then 250 mg weekly during travel and for 4 wk after leaving a malarious area Treatment, 1250 mg (5 tablets) as a single dose	Prophylaxis, PO 1/4 tablet for 15–19 kg weight; 1/2 tablet for 20–30 kg; 3/4 tablet for 31–45 kg; and 1 tablet for above 45 kg, according to the schedule for adults
Primaquine	Prevention of malaria	PO 26.3 mg (15 mg of primaquine base) daily for 14 d, beginning immediately after leaving a malarious area, or 79 mg (45 mg of base) once weekly for 8 wk. To prevent relapse, the same dose is given with chloroquine or a related drug daily for 14 d.	PO 0.3 mg of base/kg/d for 14 d, according to the schedule for adults, or 0.9 mg of base/kg/wk for 8 wk
Quinine	Treatment of malaria	PO 650 mg q8h for 10–14 d	PO 25 mg/kg/d in divided doses q8h for 10–14 d
Other Antiprotozoal Agent Nitazoxanide (Alinia)	Diarrhea caused by giardiasis or cryptosporidiosis	PO 500 mg q12h	12 y *and older,* PO 1 tab (500 mg) or 25 mL oral suspension q12h for 3d 4–11 y, PO 10 mL q12h for 3 d 12–47 mo, 5 mL q12h for 3 d
Anthelmintics Mebendazole (Vermox)	Treatment of hookworm, pinworm, roundworm, whipworm, and tapeworm infections	Most infections, PO 100 mg morning and evening for 3 consecutive d For pinworms, a single 100-mg dose may be sufficient. A second course may be given in 3 wk, if necessary	Same as adults

		ROUTES AND DOSAGE RANGES	
Generic/Trade Name	Indications for Use	Adults	Children
Pyrantel (Pin-Rid)	Treatment of round-worm, pinworm, and hookworm infections	Roundworms and pinworms, PO 11 mg/kg (maximum dose, 1 g) as a single dose; for hookworms, the same dose is given daily for 3 consecutive d. The course of therapy may be repeated in 1 mo, if necessary.	Same as adults
Ivermectin (Stromectol)	Treatment of strongyloidiasis	PO 200 mcg/kg as a single dose	*5 y and older,* PO 150 mcg/kg as a single dose
Scabicides and Pediculicides			
Lindane	Pediculosis Scabies	Scabies, apply to entire skin except the face, neck, and scalp; leave in place for 24 h; then remove by shower. Pediculosis, rub cream or lotion into affected area, leave in place for 12 h, then wash or shampoo (rub into the affected area for 4 min and rinse thoroughly).	Same as adults
Permethrin (Nix, Elimite)	Pediculosis Scabies	Scabies, massage Elimite into the skin over the entire body except the face, leave on for 8–14 h, wash off. Pediculosis, apply Nix after shampooing, rinsing, and towel-drying hair. Saturate hair and scalp, leave on for 10 min, rinse off with water.	Same as adults
Malathion (Ovide)	Pediculosis (head lice)	Apply to hair, rub in well to wet hair, then dry hair without cover-ing or using a hair dryer. After 8–12 h, shampoo, rinse, and comb hair with a fine-toothed comb to remove dead lice and eggs. If necessary, treatment can be repeated in 7–9 d.	*Above 2 y of age,* same as adults; *below 2 y,* safety and effective-ness not established

may be used alone in asymptomatic intestinal amebiasis to decrease the number of amebic cysts passed in the feces. When given for symptomatic intestinal amebiasis (e.g., amebic dysentery), it is usually given with other amebicides in concurrent or alternating courses. Iodoquinol is ineffective in amebic hepatitis and abscess formation. Its use is contraindicated with iodine allergy and liver disease.

Metronidazole (Flagyl) is effective against protozoa that cause amebiasis, giardiasis, and trichomoniasis and against anaerobic bacilli, such as *Bacteroides* and *Clostridia* (see Chap. 33). In amebiasis, metronidazole is amebicidal at intestinal and extraintestinal sites of infection. It is a drug of choice for all forms of amebiasis except asymptomatic intestinal amebiasis (in which amebic cysts are expelled in the feces). In trichomoniasis, metronidazole is more effective than any locally active agent.

Metronidazole is contraindicated during the first trimester of pregnancy and must be used with caution in patients with central nervous system (CNS) or blood disorders. Patients should also avoid all forms of ethanol while on this medication.

Tetracycline and **doxycycline** are antibacterial drugs (see Chap. 32) that act against amebae in the intestinal lumen by altering the bacterial flora required for amebic viability. One of these drugs may be used with other amebicides in the treatment of all forms of amebiasis except asymptomatic intestinal amebiasis.

Tinidazole (Tindamax), a chemical relative of metronidazole, is approved for the treatment of amebiasis, giardiasis, and trichomoniasis. It is metabolized in the liver by cytochrome P450 3A4 enzymes and should be used cautiously in people with impaired liver function. The most common adverse effects are a metallic/bitter taste and nausea.

What important information about contraindications to metronidazole should you teach to Ms. Michelsen?

Antimalarial Agents

Chloroquine is a widely used antimalarial agent. It acts against erythrocytic forms of plasmodial parasites to prevent or treat malarial attacks. When used for prophylaxis, it is given before, during, and after travel or residence in endemic areas. When used for treatment of malaria caused by *P. vivax*, *P. malariae*, or *P. ovale*, chloroquine relieves symptoms of the acute attack. However, the drug does not prevent recurrence of malarial attacks because it does not act against the tissue (exoerythrocytic) forms of the parasite. When used for treatment of malaria caused by *P. falciparum*, chloroquine relieves symptoms of the acute attack and eliminates the parasite from the body because *P. falciparum* does not form tissue reservoirs. Concern about chloroquine-resistant strains of *P. falciparum* has developed in many areas.

Chloroquine is also used in protozoal infections other than malaria, including extraintestinal amebiasis and giardiasis. It should be used with caution in patients with hepatic disease or severe neurologic, GI, ocular, or blood disorders.

Hydroxychloroquine (Plaquenil) is a derivative of chloroquine with essentially the same actions and uses with fewer adverse effects. It has also been used to treat rheumatoid arthritis and lupus erythematosus.

Chloroquine with **primaquine** is a mixture available in tablets containing chloroquine phosphate 500 milligrams (equivalent to 300 mg of chloroquine base) and primaquine phosphate 79 milligrams (equivalent to 45 mg of primaquine base). This combination is effective for prophylaxis of malaria and may be more acceptable to patients. It also may be more convenient for use in children because no pediatric formulation of primaquine is available.

Atovaquone and **proguanil** (Malarone) is a combination product with adult and pediatric formulations. The drugs inhibit different pathways in plasmodial reproduction. Malarone is used for prevention and treatment of malaria, including chloroquine-resistant strains.

Mefloquine (Lariam) is used to prevent *P. falciparum* malaria, including chloroquine-resistant strains, and to treat acute malaria caused by *P. falciparum* or *P. vivax*.

Primaquine is used to prevent the initial occurrence of malaria; to prevent recurrent attacks of malaria caused by *P. vivax*, *P. malariae*, and *P. ovale*; and to achieve "radical cure" (i.e., eradicating the tissue forms of the plasmodium and preventing survival of the blood forms) of these three types of malaria. It is especially effective in *P. vivax* malaria. When used to prevent initial occurrence of malaria (causal prophylaxis), primaquine is given concurrently with a suppressive agent (e.g., chloroquine, hydroxychloroquine) after the patient has returned from a malarious area.

Primaquine is not effective for treatment of acute attacks of malaria.

Quinine was the primary antimalarial drug for many years but has been largely replaced by synthetic agents that cause fewer adverse reactions. However, it may still be used in the treatment of chloroquine-resistant *P. falciparum* malaria. Quinine also relaxes skeletal muscles and has been used for prevention and treatment of nocturnal leg cramps.

Other Antiprotozoal Agent

Nitazoxanide (Alinia) is approved for treatment of diarrhea caused by giardiasis or cryptosporidiosis. It is the first drug approved for treatment of cryptosporidiosis, which may be life threatening in immunocompromised hosts.

Anthelmintics

Ivermectin (Stromectol) is used for numerous parasitic infections and is most active against strongyloidiasis. Ivermectin has also been used for the oral treatment of resistant lice infestations. The drug has relatively few adverse effects but may cause some nausea and vomiting.

Mebendazole (Vermox) is a broad-spectrum anthelmintic that is usually the drug of choice for treatment of hookworm, pinworm, roundworm, and whipworm infestations. It is also useful in tapeworm infection. The drug kills helminths by preventing uptake of the glucose necessary for parasitic metabolism. The helminths become immobilized and die slowly, so they may be expelled from the GI tract up to 3 days after drug therapy is completed. Mebendazole acts locally in the GI tract, and little drug is absorbed systemically. The drug is contraindicated during pregnancy because of teratogenic effects in rats; it is relatively contraindicated in children younger than 2 years of age.

Pyrantel (Pin-Rid) is effective in infestations of roundworms, pinworms, and hookworms. The drug acts locally to paralyze worms in the intestinal tract. Pyrantel is poorly absorbed from the GI tract, and most of an administered dose may be recovered in feces. Pyrantel is contraindicated in pregnancy and is not recommended for children younger than 1 year of age.

Scabicides and Pediculicides

Permethrin is the drug of choice for both pediculosis and scabies. Although a single application eliminates parasites and ova, two applications are generally recommended. For pediculosis, permethrin is available as a 1% over-the-counter liquid (Nix). For scabies, a 5% permethrin cream (Elimite) is available by prescription and a single application is curative. Permethrin is safer than other scabicides and pediculicides, especially for infants and children.

Permethrin is derived from a chrysanthemum plant, and people with a history of allergy to ragweed or chrysanthemum flowers should use it cautiously. The most frequent adverse effect is pruritus.

To avoid reinfection, close contacts should be treated simultaneously. With pediculosis, clothing and bedding should be sterilized by boiling or steaming, and seams of clothes should be examined to verify that all lice are eliminated.

Lindane is a second-line drug for scabies and pediculosis. It may be used for people who have hypersensitivity reactions or resistance to treatment with permethrin. It is applied topically, and substantial amounts are absorbed through intact skin. CNS toxicity has been reported with excessive use, especially in infants and children. The drug is available in a 1% concentration in a cream, lotion, and shampoo.

Malathion (Ovide) is a pediculicide used in the treatment of resistant head lice infestations, and **pyrethrin** preparations (e.g., RID) are available over-the-counter for treatment of pediculosis. These preparations require two applications approximately 10 days apart.

Nursing Process

Assessment

Assess for conditions in which antiparasitic drugs are used.

- Assess for exposure to parasites. Although exposure is influenced by many variables (e.g., geographic location, personal hygiene, environmental sanitation), some useful questions may include the following:
  - Does the person live in an institution, an area of poor sanitation, an underdeveloped country, a tropical region, or an area of overcrowded housing? These conditions predispose to parasitic infestations with lice, scabies, protozoa, and worms.
  - Are parasitic diseases present in the person's environment? For example, head lice, scabies, and pinworm infestations often affect school-age children and their families.
  - Has the person recently traveled (within the previous 1–3 weeks) in malarious regions? If so, were prophylactic measures used appropriately?
  - With vaginal trichomoniasis, assess in relation to sexual activity. The disease is spread by sexual intercourse, and sexual partners need simultaneous treatment to prevent reinfection.
  - With pubic (crab) lice, assess sexual activity. Lice may be transmitted by sexual and other close contact and by contact with infested bed linens.
- Assess for signs and symptoms. These vary greatly, depending on the type and extent of parasitic infestation.
  - **Amebiasis.** The person may be asymptomatic; have nausea, vomiting, diarrhea, abdominal cramping, and weakness; or experience symptoms from ulcerations of the colon or abscesses of the liver (amebic hepatitis) if the disease is severe, prolonged, and untreated. Amebiasis is diagnosed by identifying cysts or trophozoites of *E. histolytica* in stool specimens.

- **Malaria.** Initial symptoms may resemble those produced by influenza (e.g., headache, myalgia). Characteristic paroxysms of chills, fever, and copious perspiration may not be present in early malaria. During acute malarial attacks, the cycles occur every 36 to 72 hours. Additional manifestations include nausea and vomiting, splenomegaly, hepatomegaly, anemia, leukopenia, thrombocytopenia, and hyperbilirubinemia. Malaria is diagnosed by identifying the plasmodial parasite in peripheral blood smears (by microscopic examination).
- **Trichomoniasis.** Women usually have vaginal burning, itching, and yellowish discharge; men may be asymptomatic or have symptoms of urethritis. The condition is diagnosed by finding *T. vaginalis* organisms in a wet smear of vaginal exudate, semen, prostatic fluid, or urinary sediment (by microscopic examination). Cultures may be necessary.
- **Helminthiasis.** Light infestations may be asymptomatic. Heavy infestations produce symptoms according to the particular parasitic worm. Hookworm, roundworm, and threadworm larvae migrate through the lungs and may cause symptoms of pulmonary congestion. The hookworm may cause anemia by feeding on blood from the intestinal mucosa; the fish tapeworm may cause megaloblastic or pernicious anemia by absorbing folic acid and vitamin B_{12}. Large masses of roundworms or tapeworms may cause intestinal obstruction. The major symptom usually associated with pinworms is intense itching in the perianal area (pruritus ani). Helminthiasis is diagnosed by microscopic identification of parasites or ova in stool specimens. Pinworm infestation is diagnosed by identifying ova on anal swabs, obtained by touching the sticky side of cellophane tape to the anal area. (Early-morning swabs are best because the female pinworm deposits eggs during sleeping hours.)
- **Scabies and pediculosis.** Pruritus is the primary symptom. Secondary symptoms result from scratching and often include skin excoriation and infection (i.e., vesicles, pustules, and crusts). Pediculosis is diagnosed by visual identification of lice or ova (nits) on the patient's body or clothing.

Nursing Diagnoses

- Deficient Knowledge: Management of disease process and prevention of recurrence
- Deficient Knowledge: Accurate drug administration
- Imbalanced Nutrition: Less Than Body Requirements related to parasitic disease or drug therapy
- Self-Esteem Disturbance related to a medical diagnosis of parasitic infestation
- Noncompliance related to need for hygienic and other measures to prevent and treat parasitic infestations

Nursing Process continues on page 608

Planning/Goals

The patient will

- Experience relief of symptoms for which antiparasitic drugs were taken
- Self-administer drugs accurately
- Avoid preventable adverse effects
- Act to prevent recurrent infestation
- Keep appointments for follow-up care

Interventions

Use measures to avoid exposure to or prevent transmission of parasitic diseases.

- Environmental health measures include the following:
  - Sanitary sewers to prevent deposition of feces on surface soil and the resultant exposure to helminths
  - Monitoring of community water supplies, food-handling establishments, and food-handling personnel
  - Follow-up examination and possibly treatment of household and other close contacts of people with helminthiasis, amebiasis, trichomoniasis, scabies, and pediculosis
  - Mosquito control in malarious areas and prophylactic drug therapy for travelers to malarious areas. In addition, teach travelers to decrease exposure to mosquito bites (e.g., wear long-sleeved, dark clothing; use an effective insect repellent such as DEET; sleep in well-screened rooms or under mosquito netting). These measures are especially needed at dusk and dawn, the maximal feeding times for mosquitoes.
- Personal and other health measures include the following:
  - Maintain personal hygiene (i.e., regular bathing and shampooing, performing hand hygiene before eating or handling food and after defecation or urination).

- Avoid raw fish and undercooked meat. This is especially important for anyone with immunosuppression.
- Avoid contaminating streams or other water sources with feces.
- Control flies and avoid foods exposed to flies.
- With scabies and pediculosis infestations, drug therapy must be accompanied by measures to avoid reinfection or transmission to others. For example, close contacts should be examined carefully and treated if indicated. Clothes, bed linens, and towels should be washed and dried on hot cycles. Clothes that cannot be washed should be dry cleaned. With head lice, combs and brushes should be cleaned and disinfected; carpets and upholstered furniture should be vacuumed.
- With pinworms, clothing, bed linens, and towels should be washed daily on hot cycles. Toilet seats should be disinfected daily.
- Ensure follow-up measures, such as testing of stool specimens; vaginal examinations; anal swabs; smears; and cultures.
- With vaginal infections, avoid sexual intercourse, or have the male partner use a condom.

Evaluation

- Interview and observe for relief of symptoms.
- Interview outpatients regarding compliance with instructions for taking antiparasitic drugs and measures to prevent recurrence of infestation.
- Interview and observe for adverse drug effects.
- Interview and observe regarding food intake or changes in weight.

Patient Teaching Guidelines ▌ Antiparasitic Drugs

General Considerations

- Use measures to prevent parasitic infection or reinfection:
  - Support public health measures to maintain a clean environment (i.e., sanitary sewers, clean water, regulation of food-handling establishments and food-handling personnel).
  - When traveling to wilderness areas or to tropical or underdeveloped countries, check with the local health department about precautions needed to avoid parasitic infections.
  - Practice good hand hygiene and other personal hygienic practices.
  - When a family member or other close contact contracts a parasitic infection, be sure appropriate treatment and follow-up care are completed.
  - Avoid raw fish and undercooked meat.
  - With vaginal infections, avoid sexual intercourse or use a condom.

Self- or Caregiver Administration

- Use antiparasitic drugs as prescribed; their effectiveness depends on accurate use.
- Take atovaquone/proguanil, chloroquine and related drugs, iodoquinol, oral metronidazole, and tinidazole with or after meals. Food increases absorption of atovaquone and decreases gastrointestinal irritation with the other drugs.
- Avoid alcoholic beverages while taking metronidazole or tinidazole and for 3 days after the drugs are stopped. Flushing, headache, nausea, sweating, and vomiting, may occur if alcohol is ingested.
- Take or give most anthelmintics without regard to mealtimes or food ingestion. Mebendazole tablets should be chewed or crushed and mixed with food.
- Use pediculicides and scabicides as directed on the label or product insert. Instructions vary among preparations.

Ms. Michelsen should be taught measures to prevent parasitic infection or reinfection. What would you include in your teaching plan?

Principles of Therapy

Antiparasitic drugs should be used along with personal and public health control measures to prevent the spread of parasitic infestations. Specific measures vary according to the type of organism, the environment, and the host.

Many of the drugs described in this chapter are quite toxic; they should be used only when clearly indicated (i.e., laboratory documentation of parasitic infection).

Use in Special Populations

Use in Children

Children often receive an antiparasitic drug for head lice or worm infestations. These products should be used exactly as directed and with appropriate precautions to prevent reinfection. Malaria is usually more severe in children than in adults, and children should be protected from exposure when possible. When chemoprophylaxis or treatment for malaria is indicated, the same drugs are used for children as for adults, with appropriate dosage adjustments. The tetracyclines are an exception and should not be given to children younger than 8 years of age.

Use in Older Adults

Older adults are more likely to experience adverse effects of antiparasitic drugs because they often have impaired renal and hepatic function.

Use in Home Care

Most antiparasitic drugs are given in the home setting. The home care nurse may need to examine close contacts of the infected person and assess their need for treatment, assist parents and patients so that drugs are used appropriately, and teach personal and environmental hygiene measures to prevent reinfection. When children have parasitic infestations, the home care nurse may need to collaborate with daycare centers and schools to prevent or control outbreaks.

Nursing Actions Antiparasitics

NURSING ACTIONS	RATIONALE/EXPLANATION
1. Administer accurately	
a. Give atovaquone/proguanil, chloroquine and related drugs, iodoquinol, oral metronidazole, and tinidazole with or after meals.	Food improves absorption of atovaquone and decreases gastrointestinal (GI) irritation with the other drugs.
b. Give anthelmintics with or without food. Mebendazole tablets may be chewed, swallowed, or crushed and mixed with food.	Food does not decrease effectiveness of most anthelmintics.
c. For pediculicides and scabicides, follow the label or manufacturer's instructions.	Instructions vary among preparations.
2. Observe for therapeutic effects	
a. With chloroquine for acute malaria, observe for relief of symptoms and negative blood smears.	Fever and chills usually subside within 24–48 hours, and blood smears are negative for plasmodia within 24–72 hours.
b. With amebicides, observe for relief of symptoms and negative stool examinations.	Relief of symptoms does not indicate cure of amebiasis; laboratory evidence is required. Stool specimens should be examined for amebic cysts and trophozoites periodically for 6 months.
c. With anthelmintics, observe for relief of symptoms, absence of the parasite in blood or stool for three consecutive examinations, or a reduction in the number of parasitic ova in the feces.	The goal of anthelmintic drug therapy may be complete eradication of the parasite or reduction of the "worm burden."
d. With pediculicides, inspect affected areas for lice or nits.	For most patients, one treatment is effective; for some, a second treatment may be needed.
3. Observe for adverse effects	
a. With amebicides, observe for anorexia, nausea, vomiting, epigastric burning, diarrhea.	GI effects may occur with all amebicides.
b. With antimalarial agents, observe for nausea, vomiting, diarrhea, pruritus, skin rash, headache, central nervous system (CNS) stimulation.	These effects may occur with most antimalarial agents. However, adverse effects are usually mild because small doses are used for prophylaxis, and the larger doses required for treatment of acute attacks are given only for short periods.

(continued on page 610)

Nursing Actions   Antiparasitics (continued)

NURSING ACTIONS	RATIONALE/EXPLANATION
c. With metronidazole and tinidazole, observe for GI upset (e.g., nausea, diarrhea, unpleasant taste), dizziness, headache, peripheral neuropathy, seizures.	CNS effects are most serious; GI effects are most common.
d. With topical antitrichomonal agents, observe for hypersensitivity reactions (e.g., rash, inflammation), burning, and pruritus.	Hypersensitivity reactions are the major adverse effects.
e. With permethrin, observe for pruritus, burning, or tingling; with Lindane, observe for CNS stimulation (nervousness, tremors, insomnia, convulsions).	Antihistamines or topical corticosteroids may be used to decrease itching. CNS toxicity is more likely to occur with excessive use of Lindane (i.e., increased amounts, leaving in place longer than prescribed, or applying more frequently than prescribed).
4. Observe for drug interactions	Few clinically significant drug interactions occur because many antiparasitic agents are administered for local effects in the GI tract or on the skin. Most of the drugs also are given for short periods.
a. Drugs that *alter* effects of chloroquine: (1) Acidifying agents (e.g., ascorbic acid) (2) Alkalinizing agents (e.g,. sodium bicarbonate) (3) Monoamine oxidase (MAO) inhibitors	Accelerate urinary excretion Slow urinary excretion Increase risk of toxicity and retinal damage by inhibiting metabolism
b. Drugs that *alter* effects of metronidazole and tinidazole: (1) Enzyme inducers (e.g., phenytoin, rifampin) (2) Enzyme inhibitors (e.g., cimetidine)	Decrease effects by accelerating hepatic metabolism Increase effects by inhibiting hepatic metabolism
c. Drugs that *decrease* effects of atovaquone/proguanil: (1) Rifampin and other drugs that induce cytochrome P450 drug-metabolizing enzymes in the liver	Although few interactions have been reported, any enzyme-inducing drug can potentially decrease effects by accelerating hepatic metabolism.

Key Concepts

- Parasitic infestations injure host tissues.
- Travelers to malarious regions should generally receive chloroquine to prevent malaria and take precautions to avoid or minimize exposure to the causative mosquito.
- Personal and public health hygienic practices can prevent many parasitic infections and should be followed diligently.
- Antiparasitic drugs are usually given for local effects in the GI tract or on the skin.

Review and Application Exercises

Short Answer Exercises

1. What groups are at risk for development of parasitic infections (e.g., amebiasis, giardiasis, malaria, pediculosis, helminthiasis)?

2. What interventions are needed to prevent parasitic infections?

3. How would you assess for a parasitic infection in a patient who has been in an environment associated with a particular infestation?

4. How can you assess a patient's personal hygiene practices and environmental sanitation facilities?

5. How would you instruct a child's mother regarding treatment and prevention of reinfection with head lice or pinworms?

6. What are adverse effects of commonly used antiparasitic drugs, and how might they be prevented or minimized?

NCLEX-Style Questions

7. A patient being treated for amebiasis should be informed by the nurse that which of the following adverse drug effects may occur?
   a. dizziness and numbness of extremities
   b. weight gain and reduced urine output
   c. nausea, vomiting, and diarrhea
   d. low blood pressure and tachycardia, or a feeling of racing heartbeat

8. For a patient taking metronidazole (Flagyl) for trichomoniasis, which of the following statements indicates understanding of the nurse's instructions for safe drug usage?
   a. "I will limit my intake of caffeine."
   b. "I will eat a low-sodium diet for a week."
   c. "I will increase my daily intake of potassium."
   d. "I will not drink any alcoholic beverages."

9. The drug of choice for prevention or treatment of *Pneumocystis* pneumonia is
   a. trimethoprim-sulfamethoxazole (Bactrim)
   b. trimetrexate (Neutrexin)
   c. mebendazole (Vermox)
   d. permethrin (Nix, Elimite)

10. A usual drug of choice for prevention or treatment of malaria is
   a. chloroquine (Aralen)
   b. metronidazole (Flagyl)
   c. pentamidine (Pentam 300)
   d. pyrantel (Pin-Rid)

11. Patients taking antiparasitic drugs should be taught
   a. that adverse drug effects are often severe
   b. to have blood tests weekly
   c. ways to prevent reinfection
   d. that prior infection confers immunity to most parasitic infections

Selected References

Anandan, J. V. (2005). Parasitic diseases. In J. T. DiPiro, R. L. Talbert, G. C. Yee, G. R. Matzke, B. G. Wells, & L. M. Posey (Eds.), *Pharmacotherapy: A pathophysiologic approach* (6th ed., pp. 2067–2080). New York: McGraw-Hill.

Drug facts and comparisons. (Updated monthly). St. Louis, MO: Facts and Comparisons.

Dunne, W. M., Jr. (2005). Mechanisms of infectious disease. In C. M. Porth (Ed.), *Pathophysiology: Concepts of altered health states* (7th ed., pp. 341–364). Philadelphia: Lippincott Williams & Wilkins.

Goldsmith, R. S. (2007). Infectious diseases: Protozoal & helminthic. In S. J. McPhee, M. A. Papadakis, & L. M. Tierney, Jr. (Eds). *Current medical diagnosis and treatment 2007* (46th ed., pp. 1494–1566). New York: McGraw-Hill.

Griffith, K. S., Lewis, L. S., Mali, S., & Parise, M. E. (2007). Treatment of malaria in the United States: A systematic review. *Journal of the American Medical Association, 97,* 2264–2277.

Smeltzer, S. C., Bare, B. G., Hinkle, J. L., & Cheever, K. H. (Eds.). (2008). *Brunner & Suddarth's textbook of medical-surgical nursing* (11th ed.). Philadelphia: Lippincott Williams & Wilkins.

Drugs Affecting Hematopoiesis and the Immune System

Physiology of the Hematopoietic and Immune Systems

LEARNING OBJECTIVES

After studying this chapter, you will be able to:

1. Review hematopoiesis, body defense mechanisms, and immune mechanisms.
2. Differentiate between cellular and humoral types of immunity.
3. Describe the antigen–antibody reaction.
4. Discuss roles of various white blood cells in the immune response.
5. Describe the functions and roles of cytokines and hematopoietic growth factors.
6. Discuss selected factors that affect hematopoietic and immune system functions.
7. Discuss selected connections between the immune system and cancer.

Introduction

Hematopoietic and immune blood cells originate in bone marrow in stem cells, which are often called pluripotent stem cells because they are capable of becoming different types of cells. As these stem cells reproduce, some cells are exactly like the original cells and are retained in bone marrow to maintain a continuing supply. However, most reproduced stem cells differentiate to form other types of cells. The early offspring are committed to become a particular type of cell, and a committed stem cell that produces a cell type is called a colony-forming unit (CFU) (e.g., CFU-erythrocyte, CFU-granulocyte). Hematopoietic growth factors or cytokines control the reproduction, growth, and differentiation of stem cells and CFUs. They also initiate the processes required to produce fully mature cells. Overall, cytokines are involved in numerous physiologic responses, including *hematopoiesis*, cellular proliferation and differentiation, inflammation, wound healing, and cellular and humoral immunity.

Hematopoietic Cytokines

Cytokines are diverse substances produced mainly by bone marrow and white blood cells. They regulate many cellular activities by acting as chemical messengers among cells and as growth factors for blood cells.

Cytokines act by binding to receptors on target cells. After binding, the cytokine–receptor complexes trigger signal-transduction pathways that alter gene expression in the target cells. Cytokine actions and functions are affected by several factors. First, cytokines affect any cells they encounter that have cytokine receptors and are able to respond; they do not act in response to specific antigens. However, cytokine receptors are often expressed on a cell only after that cell has interacted with an *antigen*, so that cytokine activation is limited to antigen-activated lymphocytes. Second, the actions of most cytokines have been determined in laboratories by analysis of the effects of recombinant cytokines, often at nonphysiologic concentrations, and added individually to in vitro systems. Within the human body, however, cytokines rarely, if ever, act alone. Instead, a target cell is exposed to an environment containing a mixture of cytokines, which may have synergistic or antagonistic effects on each other. Third, cytokines often induce the synthesis of other cytokines. The resulting interactions among cytokines may profoundly alter physiologic responses. Fourth, proteins that act as cytokine antagonists are found in the bloodstream and other extracellular fluids. These proteins may bind directly to a cytokine and inhibit its activity or bind to a cytokine receptor but fail to activate the cell. The main groups of cytokines are colony-stimulating factors (CSFs), interferons, and interleukins. Especially important or clinically relevant cytokines are emphasized in this chapter.

Colony-Stimulating Factors (CSFs)

CSFs stimulate the production of red blood cells (erythropoietin), platelets (thrombopoietin), granulocytes (G-CSF), granulocyte–macrophages (GM-CSF), and monocyte–macrophages (M-CSF). In addition to granulocytes (neutrophils, basophils, and eosinophils), G-CSF also affects other blood cells (e.g., erythrocytes, platelet precursors, macrophages). Interleukin-3 (IL-3) is sometimes called multi-CSF because it stimulates the production of all types of blood cells.

Interferons

Interferons "interfere" with the ability of viruses in infected cells to replicate and spread to uninfected cells. They also inhibit reproduction and growth of other cells, including tumor cells, and activate natural killer (NK) cells. These antiproliferative and immunomodulatory activities play important roles in normal host defense mechanisms.

Interleukins (ILs)

ILs were initially named because they were thought to be produced by and to act only on leukocytes. However, they can be produced by body cells other than leukocytes and they can act on nonhematopoietic cells. Eighteen interleukins have been characterized and more have been identified. Especially important ILs include IL-3 (stimulates growth of stem-cell precursors of all blood cells), IL-2 (stimulates T and B lymphocytes), IL-12 (stimulates hematopoietic cells and lymphocytes), and IL-11 (stimulates platelets and other cells). Interleukin action may occur only when combined with another factor, may be suppressive rather than stimulatory (e.g., IL-10), or may involve a specific function (e.g., IL-8 mainly promotes movement of leukocytes into injured tissues as part of the inflammatory response).

Overview of Body Defense Mechanisms

The immune system is one of several mechanisms that protect the body from potentially harmful substances, including pathogenic microorganisms. The body's primary external defense mechanism is intact skin, which prevents entry of foreign substances and produces secretions that inhibit microbial growth. The mucous membranes lining the gastrointestinal (GI) and respiratory tracts are internal defense mechanisms that act as physical barriers and produce mucus that traps foreign substances so they may be expelled from the body. Mucous membranes also produce other secretions (e.g., gastric acid) that kill ingested microorganisms. Additional internal mechanisms include the normal microbial population, which is usually nonpathogenic and controls potential pathogens; and secretions (e.g., perspiration, tears, saliva) that contain lysozyme, an enzyme that destroys the cell walls of gram-positive bacteria.

If a foreign substance gets through defenses to penetrate body tissues and cause cellular injury, an inflammatory response begins immediately. Cellular injury may be caused by chemicals, hypoxia, ischemia, microorganisms, excessive heat or cold, radiation, and nutritional deficiencies or excesses. The cellular response to injury involves inflammation, a generalized reaction to any tissue damage, which attempts to remove the damaging agent and repair the damaged tissue. The hemodynamic aspect of inflammation includes vasodilation, which increases blood supply to the injured area, and increased capillary permeability, which allows fluid to leak into tissue spaces. The cellular aspect involves the movement of white blood cells (WBCs) into the area of injury. WBCs are attracted to the injured area by bacteria, tissue debris, plasma protein fractions (complement), and other substances, in a process called chemotaxis. After they reach the area, they phagocytize causative agents and tissue debris.

The final defense mechanism is the immune response, and an effective response involves lymphoid cells, inflammatory cells, and hematopoietic cells. The immune response stimulates production of antibodies and activated lymphocytes to destroy foreign invaders and mutant body cells (e.g., abnormal cells, cancer cells).

Inflammatory and immune responses interact in complex ways and share a number of processes, including phagocytosis. They produce their effects indirectly, through interactions among cytokines and other chemical mediators. Cytokines induce WBC replication, phagocytosis, antibody production, fever, inflammation, and tissue repair. Other chemical mediators (e.g., histamine, prostaglandins) are synthesized or released by mast cells and other cells. After they are activated, mediators may exert their effects on tissues locally or at distant target sites. They also may induce or enhance other mediators.

Immunity

Immunity indicates protection from a disease, and the main function of the immune system is host protection. To this end, the immune system detects and eliminates foreign substances that may cause tissue injury or disease. It also regulates tissue homeostasis and repair as cells of the immune system identify and remove injured, damaged, dead, or malignant cells.

To perform these functions, the immune system must be able to differentiate body tissues (self) from foreign substances (non-self). Self tissues are recognized by distinctive protein molecules on the surface membranes of body cells. These molecules or markers are encoded by a group of genes called the major histocompatibility complex (MHC). MHC markers are essential to immune system function because they regulate the antigens to which a person responds and allow immune cells (e.g., lymphocytes, *macrophages*) to recognize and communicate with each other. Non-self or foreign antigens are also recognized by distinctive molecules, called epitopes, on their surfaces. Epitopes vary widely in type, number, and ability to elicit an immune response.

A normally functioning immune system does not attack body tissues labeled as self but attacks non-self substances. An abnormally functioning immune system causes numerous diseases. When the system is hypoactive, immunodeficiency disorders develop because the person is highly susceptible to infectious and neoplastic diseases. When the system is hyperactive, it perceives ordinarily harmless environmental substances (e.g., foods, plant pollens) as harmful and induces allergic reactions. When the system is inappropriately activated (it loses its ability to distinguish between self and non-self, so an immune response is aroused against the host's own body tissues), the result is autoimmune disorders such as rheumatoid arthritis and systemic lupus erythematosus (SLE). Many other disorders, including diabetes mellitus, myasthenia gravis, and inflammatory bowel diseases, are thought to involve autoimmune mechanisms. To aid understanding of the immune response and drugs used to alter immune response, more specific characteristics, processes, and functions of the immune system are described.

Types of Immunity

Innate or natural immunity, which is not produced by the immune system, includes the general protective mechanisms described.

Adaptive or *acquired immunity* develops during gestation or after birth and may be active or passive. *Active immunity* is produced by the person's own immune system in response to a disease caused by a specific antigen or administration of an antigen (e.g., a vaccine) from a source outside the body, usually by injection. The immune response stimulated by the antigen produces activated lymphocytes and antibodies against the antigen. When an antigen is present for the first time, production of antibodies requires several days. As a result, the serum concentration of antibodies does not reach protective levels for

7 to 10 days, and the disease develops in the host. When the antigen is eliminated, the antibody concentration gradually decreases over several weeks.

The duration of active immunity may be brief (e.g., to influenza viruses), or it may last for years or a lifetime. Long-term active immunity has a unique characteristic called memory. When the host is re-exposed to the antigen, lymphocytes are activated and antibodies are produced rapidly, and the host does not contract the disease. This characteristic allows "booster" doses of antigen to increase antibody levels and maintain active immunity against some diseases.

Passive immunity occurs when antibodies are formed by the immune system of another person or animal and transferred to the host. For example, an infant is normally protected for several months by maternal antibodies received through the placenta during gestation. Also, antibodies previously formed by a donor can be transferred to the host by an injection of immune serum. These antibodies act against antigens immediately. Passive immunity is short-term, lasting only a few weeks or months.

Cellular and Humoral Immunity

Types of adaptive immunity are separated into cellular immunity (mainly involving activated T lymphocytes in body tissues) and humoral immunity (mainly involving B lymphocytes and antibodies in the blood). However, the two types are closely connected so that virtually all antigens elicit both cellular and humoral responses and most humoral (B cell) responses require cellular (T cell) stimulation.

Although most humoral responses occur when antibodies or B cells encounter antigens in blood, some occur when antibodies or B cells encounter antigens in other body fluids (e.g., tears, sweat, saliva, mucus, breast milk). The antibodies in body fluids other than blood are produced by a part of humoral immunity sometimes called the secretory or mucosal immune system. The B cells of the mucosal system migrate through lymphoid tissues of tear ducts, salivary glands, breasts, bronchi, intestines, and genitourinary structures. The antibodies (mostly immunoglobulin A [IgA]) secreted at these sites act locally rather than systemically. This local protection combats foreign substances, especially pathogenic microorganisms, that are inhaled, swallowed, or otherwise come in contact with external body surfaces. When the foreign substances bind to local antibodies, they are unable to attach to and invade mucosal tissue.

Antigens

Antigens are the foreign (non-self) substances (e.g., microorganisms, other proteins, polysaccharides) that initiate immune responses. Antigens have specific sites that interact with immune cells to induce the immune response. The number of antigenic sites on a molecule depends largely on its molecular weight. Large protein and polysaccharide molecules are complete antigens because of their complex chemical structure and multiple antigenic sites. Smaller molecules (e.g., animal danders, plant pollens, most drugs) are incomplete antigens (called haptens) and cannot act as antigens by themselves. However, they have antigenic sites and can combine with carrier substances to become antigenic. In discussions of hypersensitivity (allergic) conditions, antigens are often called allergens.

Immune Responses to Antigens

The immune response involves antigens that induce the formation of antibodies or activated T lymphocytes. The initial response occurs when an antigen is first introduced into the body. B lymphocytes recognize the antigen as foreign and develop antibodies against it. Antibodies are proteins called *immunoglobulins* (Ig) that interact with specific antigens.

Antigen–antibody interactions may result in formation of antigen–antibody complexes, agglutination (clumping) of cells, neutralization of bacterial toxins, destruction of pathogens or cells, attachment of antigen to immune cells, coating of the antigen so that it is more readily recognized by phagocytic cells (opsonization), or activation of *complement* (a group of plasma proteins activated by recognition of an antigen–antibody complex, bacteria, or viruses and essential to normal inflammatory and immunologic responses). Activated complement stimulates chemotaxis (movement of monocytes, neutrophils, basophils, and eosinophils toward the antigen) and the release of hydrolytic enzymes, actions that result in the destruction or inactivation of the invading antigen. With a later exposure to the antigen, *antibody* is rapidly produced. The number of exposures required to produce enough antibodies to bind a significant amount of antigen is unknown. Thus, an allergic reaction may occur with the second exposure or after several exposures, when sufficient antibodies have been produced.

Antigen–T lymphocyte interactions stimulate production and function of other T lymphocytes and help to regulate antibody production by B lymphocytes. T cells are involved in delayed hypersensitivity reactions, rejection of tissue or organ transplants, and responses to neoplasms and some infections.

Immune Cells

Immune cells (Fig. 38-1) are WBCs that circulate in the blood and lymphatic vessels or reside in lymphoid tissues. These cells are present in virtually all body tissues, and their ability to circulate throughout the body and to migrate between blood and lymphoid tissues are major components of host defenses. The cells are activated by exposure to an antigen. Although all WBCs play a role, neutrophils, monocytes, and lymphocytes are especially important in phagocytic and immune processes.

Neutrophils

Neutrophils are the major WBCs in the bloodstream and the body's main defense against pathogenic bacteria. They usually arrive at sites of tissue injury within 90 minutes. They localize the area of injury and phagocytize organisms or particles by releasing digestive enzymes and oxidative metabolites that kill engulfed pathogens or destroy other types of foreign particles. The number of neutrophils increases greatly during the inflammatory process. These cells circulate in the bloodstream for approximately 10 hours, then move into tissues, where they live for 1 to 3 days.

Eosinophils and Basophils

Eosinophils increase in number and activity during allergic reactions and parasitic infections. In parasitic infections, they bind to and kill the parasites. In hypersensitivity reactions, they produce enzymes that inactivate histamine and leukotrienes and may produce other enzymes that destroy antigen–antibody complexes. Despite these generally beneficial effects, eosinophils also may aggravate tissue damage by releasing cytotoxic substances. Basophils release histamine, a major chemical mediator in inflammatory and immediate hypersensitivity reactions. However, the function of basophils in normal immune responses is not well understood.

Monocytes

Monocytes arrive several hours after injury and usually replace neutrophils as the predominant WBC within 48 hours. They are the largest WBCs, and their lifespan is much longer than that of the neutrophils. Monocytes can phagocytize larger sizes and amounts of foreign material than neutrophils. In addition to their activity in the bloodstream, monocytes can leave blood vessels and enter tissue spaces, and are then called tissue macrophages. Tissue macrophages are widely distributed in connective tissue and in other areas (e.g., Kupffer's cells in the liver, alveolar macrophages in the lungs, others in the lymph nodes and spleen) and form the mononuclear phagocyte system. Both mobile and fixed monocyte–macrophages are important in inflammatory processes, and both can initiate the immune response by activating lymphocytes. They perform this function as part of *phagocytosis*, in which they engulf a circulating antigen (e.g., foreign material, cellular debris), break it into fragments, combine the fragments with MHC molecules, and return the antigenic fragments to the cell surface. The antigenic fragments are recognized as foreign material by circulating T and B lymphocytes, and an immune response is initiated. Because the monocytes prepare the antigen to interact with T and B lymphocytes, they are called antigen-presenting cells (APCs). In addition to phagocytosis, activated macrophages also secrete many products (e.g., enzymes, cytokines), remove antigen–antibody complexes, remove dying and dead host cells, and can destroy virus-infected cells and tumor cells.

Dendritic Cells

Dendritic cells are surface macrophages found in peripheral lymphoid and other tissues through which antigens enter the body (e.g., skin, mucosa, bronchial airways). They are star-shaped, with a large surface area through which they can recognize, capture, and ingest antigens. Their main function is the presentation of antigen to T lymphocytes, which activates the T cells and initiates the adaptive immune response. Dendritic

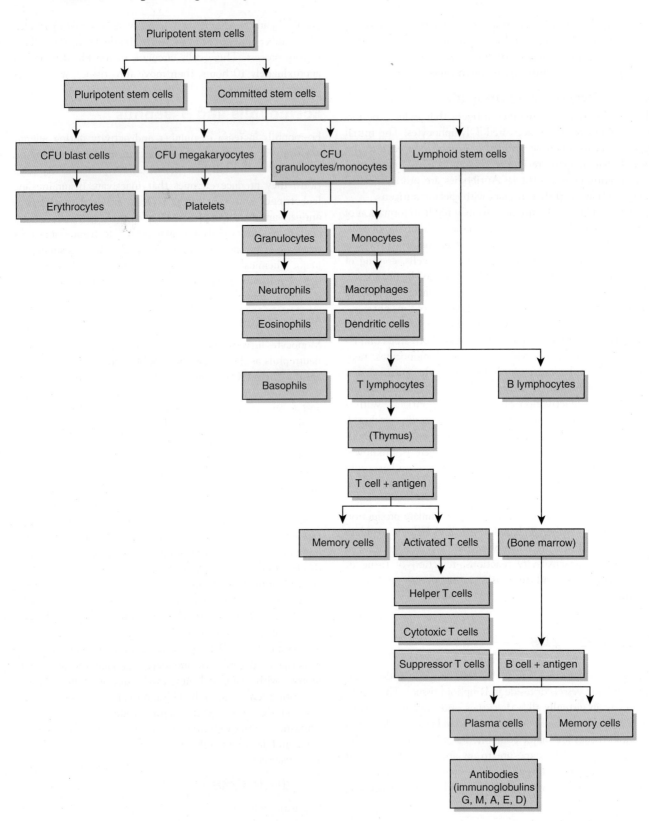

Figure 38-1 ▪ Hematopoiesis and formation of immune cells. CFU, colony-forming unit.

cells become active APCs when stimulated by injury or cytokines such as tumor necrosis factor–alpha (TNF-alpha) or interferon alfa. Activation also causes the antigen-containing cells to enter lymph vessels and migrate to regional lymph nodes, where T cells are located.

Lymphocytes

Lymphocytes are the main immune cells, and those in tissues are in dynamic equilibrium with those in circulating blood. These cells continuously travel through blood and lymph vessels from one lymphoid organ to another. The three types of lymphocytes are NK cells, T cells, and B cells.

Natural Killer Cells

Natural killer cells, so called because they do not need to interact with a specific antigen to become activated, destroy infectious microorganisms and malignant cells by releasing powerful chemicals. These cells are thought to provide the first line of defense against viral infections and other intracellular pathogens while adaptive immune responses are being generated. NK cells are sensitized by cytokines released from macrophages and dendritic cells. They function mainly by secreting interferon gamma, which activates macrophages and other cells. In addition to their ability to kill virus-infected cells, they are thought to kill certain tumor cells.

T Lymphocytes

T lymphocytes, the main regulators of the immune response, are involved in both cell-mediated and humoral immunity because they direct the activities of B cells and macrophages. T cells must be activated by antigens before they can fulfill their immune functions, and they have proteins on their cell-membrane surfaces that act as receptors for antigens.

Each T cell reacts only with a specific type of antigen and is capable of forming only one type of T cell. When a specific antigen attaches to cell-membrane receptors to form an antigen–antibody complex, the complex activates the T cell to form tremendous numbers of duplicate T cells (clones) that are exactly like the parent cell. T-cell clones are sensitized or activated T cells that are released into lymphatic ducts, carried to the blood, circulated through all tissue fluids, then returned to lymphatic ducts and recirculated. Additional participants in the activation process are phagocytic macrophages and helper T cells, which secrete cytokines that regulate the growth, reproduction, and function of lymphocytes.

T lymphocytes originate in stem cells in the bone marrow and differentiate into immune cells in the thymus gland. The thymus produces a substance called thymosin, which is necessary for T-cell maturation. When T cells bind with an antigen, specific genes are activated to produce substances that direct T-cell proliferation and differentiation. One such substance is IL-2, which stimulates T-cell DNA replication and mitosis. Cell division is necessary for production of large numbers of antigen-reactive cells and for cellular changes associated with the different subgroups of T cells. Specific types and functions of T cells include the following:

- Helper T cells (also called T_h or CD4+ cells), the largest subgroup, regulate virtually all immune functions by producing cytokines. The cytokines stimulate the growth of bone marrow and other cells of the immune system (e.g., cytotoxic T and B cells). They also activate macrophages and facilitate phagocytosis. Important cytokines include IL-2, -3, -4, -5, and -6; GM-CSF; and interferon gamma.

  Subsets of helper T cells have recently been identified as T_h1, T_h2, and suppressor T cells. Both T_h1 and T_h2 cells secrete IL-3 and GM-CSF but differ in the other cytokines they secrete. The T_h1 subset is responsible for many cell-mediated functions (e.g., delayed-type hypersensitivity reactions, activation of cytotoxic T cells) and for the production of IgG antibodies that promote recognition of antigens. These cells are also associated with excessive inflammation and tissue injury. The T_h2 subset stimulates the activation of eosinophils and stimulates B cells (e.g., to produce immunoglobulins such as IgM and IgE). These cells are also associated with hypersensitivity reactions. Suppressor T cells are thought to stop the immune response (i.e., decrease the activities of B cells and other T cells) when an antigen has been destroyed. This activity is important in preventing further tissue damage.

- Cytotoxic T cells (also called TC or CD8+ cells) are recruited and activated by helper T cells (i.e., helper T cells secrete IL-2, which is necessary for activation and proliferation of cytotoxic T cells). When activated by antigen and IL-2, cytotoxic T cells bind to antigens on the surfaces of target cells and damage or kill the target cells. After damaging the target cells, the cytotoxic cells can detach themselves and attack other target cells.

  Cytotoxic T cells persist in tissues for months and are especially lethal to virus-infected cells because virus particles become entrapped in the membranes of the cells and act as strong antigens that attract the T cells. These T cells can also destroy malignant cells, transplanted organs, and play a role in delayed hypersensitivity reactions.

B Lymphocytes

B cells are involved in humoral immunity; they secrete antibodies that can neutralize pathogens before their entry into host cells. B cells must be activated by antigens before they can fulfill their immune functions, and they have proteins on their cell-membrane surfaces that act as receptors for antigens. Each B lymphocyte reacts only with a specific type of antigen and is capable of forming only one type of antibody. When a specific antigen attaches to cell-membrane receptors to form an antigen–antibody complex, the complex activates the lymphocyte to form tremendous numbers of duplicate lymphocytes (clones) that are exactly like the parent cell. Clones of a B lymphocyte eventually secrete antibodies that circulate throughout the body.

B lymphocytes originate in stem cells in the bone marrow, differentiate into cells capable of forming antibodies (also in the bone marrow), and migrate to the spleen, lymph nodes, or other lymphoid tissue. In lymphoid tissue, the cells may be dormant until exposed to an antigen. In response to an antigen and IL-2 from helper T cells, B cells multiply rapidly, enlarge, and differentiate into plasma cells, which then produce antibodies (immunoglobulins [Ig]) to oppose the antigen. Immunoglobulins are secreted into lymph and transported to the bloodstream for circulation throughout the body. There are five main classes of immunoglobulins:

1. IgG is the most abundant immunoglobulin. It protects against bacteria, toxins, and viruses as it circulates in the bloodstream. Molecules of IgG combine with molecules of antigen, and the antigen–antibody complex activates complement. Activated complement causes an inflammatory reaction, promotes phagocytosis, and inactivates or destroys the antigen. IgG also crosses the placenta to provide maternally acquired antibodies (passive immunity) to the infant.

2. IgA is the main immunoglobulin in mucous membranes and body secretions. It is found in saliva, breast milk, and nasal, respiratory, prostatic, and vaginal secretions. It protects against antigens that gain access to these areas (e.g., it prevents attachment of viruses and bacteria to mucous membranes).

3. IgM protects against bacteria, toxins, and viruses that gain access to the bloodstream. It acts only in the bloodstream, because its large molecular size prevents its movement through capillary walls. It activates complement to destroy microorganisms.

4. IgE binds to mast cells and basophils. It is present in body fluids and readily enters body tissues. It is involved in parasitic infections and hypersensitivity reactions, including anaphylaxis. IgE sensitizes mast cells, which then release histamine and other chemical mediators that cause bronchoconstriction, edema, urticaria, and other manifestations of allergic reactions. IgE does not activate complement. The production of IgE is stimulated by T lymphocytes and IL-4, -5, and -6 and is inhibited by the interferons. Small amounts of IgE are present in the serum of nonallergic people; larger amounts are produced by people with allergies.

5. IgD is found on the cell membranes of B lymphocytes. It functions as an antigen receptor for initiating the differentiation and maturation of B lymphocytes.

Immune System Cytokines

Cytokines (Fig. 38-2) regulate the immune response by stimulating or inhibiting the activation, proliferation, and differentiation of various cells and by regulating the secretion of antibodies or other cytokines. They are secreted when immune cells are activated by antigens or other cytokines and are the primary means of communication between immune cells and other body tissues. Although the hematopoietic cytokines described include the immune system cytokines, the emphasis here is on those that affect immune cells. It is thought that

cytokines formed by activated macrophages enter the bone marrow, where they induce the synthesis and release of other cytokines that activate resting stem cells to produce more granulocytes and monocytes–macrophages. Newly formed granulocytes and monocytes leave the bone marrow and enter the circulating blood in approximately 3 days.

Cytokine binding to target cells elicits wide-ranging effects, including increased production of other cytokines. In general, the cytokines secreted by antigen-activated lymphocytes can affect the activity of most cells involved in the immune response. For example, cytokines produced by activated helper T cells influence the activity of B cells, cytotoxic T cells, NK cells, macrophages, granulocytes, and hematopoietic stem cells. As a result, a network of interacting cells is activated.

Some cytokines increase macrophage activity and phagocytosis. Some, especially IL-2, stimulate helper T cells and enhance the antiantigenic activity of the entire immune system. IL-4, -5, and -6 are especially important in B-cell activities.

Tumor necrosis factors (TNFs) are produced by activated macrophages and other cells and act on many immune and nonimmune target cells. They stimulate the inflammatory response and have cytotoxic effects on tumor cells. TNF-alpha stimulates production of cytokines; TNF-beta increases phagocytic activity of macrophages and neutrophils.

Patient-Related Factors That Influence Immune Function

Age

Fetuses and Neonates

During the first few months of gestation, the fetal immune system is deficient in antibody production and phagocytic activity. During the last trimester, the fetal immune system may be able to respond to infectious antigens, such as cytomegalovirus, rubella virus, and *Toxoplasma*. However, most fetal protection against infectious microorganisms is by maternal antibodies that reach the fetal circulation through the placenta.

At birth, the neonatal immune system is still immature, but IgG levels (from maternal blood) are near adult levels in umbilical cord blood. However, the source of maternal antibodies is severed at birth. Antibody titers in infants decrease over approximately 6 months as maternal antibodies are catabolized. Although the infant does start producing IgG, the rate of production is lower than the rate of breakdown of maternal antibodies. Cell-mediated immunity is functional at birth.

Older Adults

Both humoral and cell-mediated immune functions decline with aging, and this decline is probably a major factor in the older adult's increased susceptibility to infections and neoplasms. Lymphocytes are less able to proliferate in response

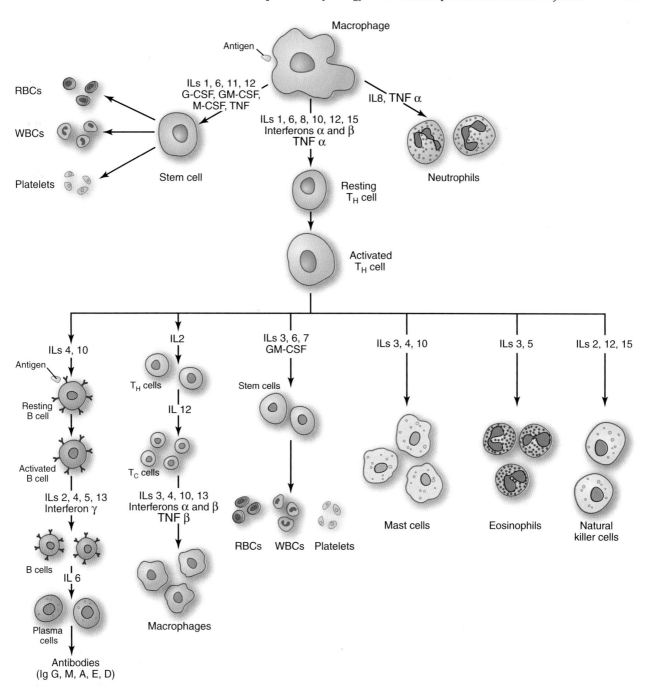

Figure 38-2 ▪ Macrophage and T-cell cytokines, their target cells, and the products of target cells. These elements overlap and interact to regulate the immune response. CSF, colony-stimulating factor; G-CSF, granulocyte–colony-stimulating factor; GM-CSF, granulocyte–macrophage colony-stimulating factor; Ig, immunoglobulin; IL, interleukin; M-CSF, monocyte–macrophage colony-stimulating factor; RBCs, red blood cells; Tc, cytotoxic T cell; Th, helper T cell; TNF, tumor necrosis factor; WBCs, white blood cells.

to antigenic stimulation, and a relative state of immunodeficiency prevails. With T lymphocytes, function is impaired, and the numbers in peripheral blood may be decreased. The functional impairment includes decreased activity of helper T cells. With B lymphocytes, the cells are less able to form antibodies in response to antigens. Abnormal antibody production results

from impaired function of B cells and helper T cells. Other aspects of immune system function also decline with age. For example, older adults have increased blood levels of antibodies against their own tissues (autoantibodies), which may account for the greater frequency of autoimmune diseases in this age group.

Impaired immune mechanisms have several implications for clinicians who care for older patients, including the following:

■ Older adults are more likely to develop infections (including reactivation of tuberculosis and herpes zoster) and less able to recover from them. Therefore, older adults need protective measures, such as rigorous personal hygiene; good nutrition; adequate exercise, rest, and sleep; minimal exposure to potential pathogens, when possible; and appropriate immunizations (e.g., influenza, pneumonia, tetanus). When an infection develops in older adults, signs and symptoms (e.g., fever, drainage) may be absent or less pronounced than in younger adults.

■ Older adults have impaired immune responses to antigens. Thus, achieving protective antibody titers may require higher doses of immunizing antigens in older adults than in younger adults.

■ Older adults often exhibit a less intense positive reaction in skin tests for tuberculosis (indicating a decreased delayed hypersensitivity response).

Nutritional Status

Nutritional status can have profound effects on immune function. Adequate nutrient intake contributes to immunocompetence (ability of the immune system to function effectively). Malnutrition contributes to immunodeficiency. A severe lack of calories or protein decreases numbers and functions of T cells, complement activity, neutrophil chemotaxis, and phagocytosis. An inadequate zinc intake can depress the functions of T and B cells. Zinc is a cofactor for many enzymes, some of which are found in lymphocytes and are required for lymphocyte function. Zinc deficiency also may result from inadequate absorption in the GI tract or excessive losses in urine, feces, or through the skin with such disorders as chronic renal disease, chronic diarrhea, burns, or severe psoriasis. Vitamin deficiencies may also depress T- and B-cell function because several (e.g., A, E, folic acid, pantothenic acid, pyridoxine) also are enzyme cofactors in lymphocytes.

Stress

There is evidence that stress depresses immune function and therefore increases risks for development of infection and cancer. The connection between the stress response and the immune response is thought to involve neuroendocrine mechanisms. The stress response is characterized by increased activity of catecholamine neurotransmitters in the central and autonomic nervous systems (e.g., norepinephrine, epinephrine) and increased secretion of cortisol from the adrenal cortex. Cortisol and other corticosteroids are well known to suppress immune function and are used therapeutically for that purpose. The immune response is affected by these neuroendocrine influences on lymphoid organs and lymphocyte functions because lymphocytes have receptors for many neurotransmitters and hormones.

Immune Disorders

Dysfunction of the immune system is related to many disease processes, including allergic, autoimmune, immunodeficiency, and neoplastic disorders. These disorders are described below to assist in understanding the use of drugs to alter immune functions.

Allergies

In allergic disorders, the body perceives normally harmless substances (e.g., foods, pollens) as antigens and mounts an immune response. More specifically, IgE binds to antigen on the surface of mast cells and causes the release of chemical mediators (e.g., histamine) that produce the allergic manifestations. These reactions may cause tissue damage ranging from mild skin rashes to life-threatening anaphylaxis.

Autoimmune Disorders

In autoimmune disorders, the body perceives its own tissues as antigens and elicits an immune response, usually chronic and inflammatory in nature. Hashimoto's thyroiditis, multiple sclerosis, myasthenia gravis, rheumatoid arthritis, systemic lupus erythematosus, and type 1 diabetes mellitus are considered autoimmune disorders. Autoimmune processes, which are similar to the processes elicited by pathogenic microorganisms and environmental antigens, may damage virtually every body tissue.

Immunodeficiency Disorders

Defects in any immune system components can compromise host protection and increase susceptibility to infections and malignant neoplasms. Immunodeficiency disorders can be inherited or acquired. Common causes of acquired disorders include infection with HIV, advanced age, cytotoxic anticancer chemotherapy, and immunosuppressive drugs used to treat transplant rejection or autoimmune disorders. The HIV paralyzes the immune system by targeting helper T cells, macrophages, and dendritic cells. More specifically, it decreases the numbers and almost all functions of T lymphocytes and several functions of B lymphocytes and monocytes. Advanced age is associated with reduced ability to produce T cells, and chemotherapy is often associated with permanent deficits in the numbers and functions of T cells.

Neoplastic Disorders

In neoplastic disease, immune cells lose their ability to recognize and destroy mutant cells or early malignant cells. This effect could result from immunodeficiency states or from cancer cells that are overwhelming in number or highly malignant. Mutant cells constantly occur during cell division, but few survive or lead to cancer. Most mutant cells simply die, some survive but retain the normal controls that prevent excessive growth, and some are destroyed by immune processes activated by the abnormal proteins found in most mutant cells.

Drugs That Alter Hematopoietic and Immune Responses

Drugs that modify the immune system (often called immuno-modulators) can enhance or restrict immune responses to various disease processes. Thus, they may be immunostimulants or immunosuppressants. Specific drug groups include hematopoietic growth factors, interferons, interleukins, and monoclonal antibodies. Interferons have antiviral and antiproliferative actions as well as immunomodulatory functions.

These drugs are heterogenous in their uses and characteristics. They are used to prevent or treat symptoms (e.g., anemia, neutropenia) caused by disease processes or their treatments, prevent or treat infections, prevent or treat rejection of transplanted tissues or organs, treat autoimmune disorders, and treat immunodeficiency disorders and cancer. In cancer, the drugs are used to modify host responses, to destroy tumor cells by suppressing their growth or killing the cells, or to modify tumor cell biology. Vaccines for melanoma and prostate cancer are being investigated.

Methods of modifying immune functions include administering exogenous antigens (e.g., immunizations, desensitization procedures), strengthening antigens (e.g., an antigen that is too weak to elicit an immune response), or suppressing the normal response to an antigen. In desensitization procedures, weak extracts of antigenic substances (e.g., foods, plant pollens, penicillin) are prepared as drugs and administered in small, increasing amounts so the patient develops a tolerance for the substances and avoids serious allergic reactions.

Overall, drugs can be given to stimulate immune responses (see Chap. 39), stimulate hematopoiesis and immune responses (see Chap. 40), suppress normal immune responses (see Chap. 41), and manage various aspects of oncologic disorders (see Chap. 42).

Key Concepts

- All hematopoietic and immune blood cells are derived from stem cells in the bone marrow.
- Hematopoietic growth factors include G-CSF, M-CSF, GM-CSF, erythropoietin, and thrombopoietin.
- Interferons alfa, beta, and gamma have antiviral and immunomodulating effects.
- Interleukins are important regulators of immune and inflammatory responses.
- T lymphocytes are major regulators of both humoral and cellular immunity.
- B cells produce antibodies in response to antigens. Immunoglobulins (Ig) A, D, G, E, and M are important in immune responses, including allergic disorders.
- Autoimmune disorders occur when the body erroneously perceives its own tissues as antigens and initiates an immune response.

Review and Application Exercises

Short Answer Exercises

1. What is the difference between innate and acquired immunity?
2. What are methods of producing active acquired immunity?
3. Which WBCs are phagocytes?
4. Describe phagocytosis.
5. Where are T lymphocytes formed, and what are their functions?
6. Where are B lymphocytes formed, and what are their functions?
7. What are antigens, and how do they elicit an immune response?
8. What are cytokines, and how do they function in the immune response?
9. What is complement, and how does it function in the immune response?
10. What are the main consequences of immunodeficiency states?

Selected References

Hall, P. D., & Hayney, M. S. (2005). Function and evaluation of the immune system. In J. T. DiPiro, R. L. Talbert, G. C. Yee, G. R. Matzke, B. G. Wells, & L. M. Posey (Eds.), *Pharmacotherapy: A pathophysiologic approach* (6th ed., pp. 1565–1579). New York: McGraw-Hill.

Sommer, C. (2005). The immune response. In C. M. Porth (Ed.), *Pathophysiology: Concepts of altered health states* (7th ed., pp. 365–385). Philadelphia: Lippincott Williams & Wilkins.

Immunizing Agents

LEARNING OBJECTIVES

After studying this chapter, you will be able to:

1. Discuss common characteristics of immunizations.
2. Discuss the importance of immunizations in promoting health and preventing disease.
3. Identify authoritative sources for immunization information.
4. Identify immunizations recommended for children.
5. Identify immunizations recommended for adults.
6. Discuss ways to promote immunization of all age groups.
7. Teach parents about recommended immunizations and record keeping.

Applying Your Knowledge

Deborah Stein is a 29-year-old woman who is planning a trip abroad this year. She is visiting her health care provider to plan for the necessary immunizations for her trip. She is unsure about her immunization history and she is new to this medical practice.

Introduction

Immune responses and types of immunity are described in Chapter 38. Many antigens that activate the immune response are microorganisms that cause infectious diseases. Early scientists observed that people who had certain diseases were thereafter protected despite repeated exposure to the disease. It was later discovered that protection stemmed from body substances called antibodies and that antibodies could also be induced by deliberate exposure to the antigen. *Immunization* involves administration of an antigen to induce antibody formation (for active immunity) or administration of serum from immune people (for passive immunity). Preparations used for immunization are biologic products prepared by pharmaceutical companies and regulated by the U.S. Food and Drug Administration (FDA). Widespread use of these products has dramatically decreased the incidence of many infectious diseases. See Box 39-1 for recent changes in recommendations for immunizations.

General Characteristics of Immunizing Agents

Some available agents are now infrequently used. These include the single vaccines for measles, mumps, and rubella, which have been largely replaced by the combination product containing all three vaccines (MMR). In addition, typhoid and yellow fever vaccines are used only in particular circumstances. These vaccines are not discussed further in this chapter.

Box 39-1	Recent Changes to Immunizations by Age Group

Newer immunization products and recent recommendations for various age groups include the following:

Children and Adolescents

- Rotavirus vaccine (Rotateq) to protect infants against rotavirus gastroenteritis, an infection that causes diarrhea, vomiting, and fever.
- A booster dose of tetanus and diphtheria toxoids and acellular pertussis vaccine (Tdap), recommended because protection against pertussis declines a few years after immunization with pertussis vaccine during infancy. Boostrix is used for persons aged 10 to 18 years, and Adacel is used for persons aged 11 to 64 years.
- Renewal of recommendations for four doses of pneumococcal vaccine (PCV7, Prevnar) for healthy young children. Two doses were recommended a few years ago because of a vaccine shortage.
- A second dose of chickenpox vaccine (e.g., Varivax) at 4 to 6 years old (first dose at 12–15 months). For adolescents, chickenpox vaccine for those who have never had chickenpox or been vaccinated previously; a second dose of chickenpox vaccine for adolescents who previously received a single dose
- A combined vaccine for measles, mumps, rubella, and chickenpox (Proquad) is available for use in children aged 12 months to 12 years. FDA approval has been requested for an additional combination vaccine (Pentacel) for diphtheria, tetanus, pertussis, polio, and *Haemophilus influenzae* type b (Hib). In clinical trials, Pentacel was administered at 2, 4, 6, and 15 to 18 months of age (4 doses) along with other recommended childhood vaccines.

- Hepatitis A vaccination for all children in the United States, with the first of two doses between 1 year and 2 years of age. It was formerly recommended for children in states with high rates of hepatitis A.
- Annual flu vaccination for children aged 6 months to 18 years and for household contacts, caregivers, and others who spend significant time with children from birth to 5 years.
- Human papilloma virus (HPV) vaccine (Gardasil) for all girls 11 or 12 years of age (can be given as early as 9 years) or up to 26 years of age if not received earlier, to help prevent HPV, a common sexually transmitted infection that can lead to genital warts and cervical cancer. Most effective if given before the person becomes sexually active.
- Meningococcal vaccine at 11 or 12 years of age. If not received earlier, recommended at entry to high school or college.

Adults

- Chickenpox vaccine for adults who never had the disease or vaccine; a second dose of vaccine for adults who previously received a single dose
- HPV vaccine if not previously received, up to age 26 years.
- Tdap booster vaccine (e.g., Adacel) is recommended for all adults under 65 years of age who have not already received Tdap, especially health professionals and those who have close contact with infants (under 1 year of age).
- Zoster vaccine (Zostavax) is available to prevent herpes zoster (shingles) in adults 60 years and older.

In general, immunizing agents are quite safe, and risks of the diseases they prevent are greater than the risks of the vaccines. However, risks and benefits for particular recipients should be considered because no vaccine is completely effective or completely safe. Some people may develop a disease after being immunized against it. However, if this happens, symptoms are usually less severe and complications are fewer than if the person had not been immunized. Adverse effects are usually mild and of short duration. Although the FDA evaluates vaccine safety before and after a vaccine is marketed, some adverse effects become apparent only after a vaccine is used in a large population.

Agents for Active Immunity

The biologic products used for *active immunity* are vaccines and toxoids. *Vaccines* are suspensions of microorganisms or their antigenic products that have been killed or attenuated (weakened or reduced in virulence) so they can induce antibody formation while preventing or causing very mild forms of the disease. Many vaccines produce long-lasting immunity. Attenuated live vaccines produce immunity, usually lifelong, that is

similar to that produced by natural infection. However, there is a small risk of producing disease with live vaccines, especially in people with impaired immune function. Vaccines developed with recombinant DNA technology have a low risk for causing active disease.

Toxoids are bacterial toxins or products that have been modified to destroy toxicity while retaining antigenic properties (i.e., ability to induce antibody formation). Immunization with toxoids is not permanent; scheduled repeat doses (boosters) are required to maintain immunity.

Additional components of vaccines and toxoids may include aluminum phosphate, aluminum hydroxide, or calcium phosphate. Products containing aluminum should be given intramuscularly only, because they cannot be given intravenously and greater tissue irritation occurs with subcutaneous injections. These additives are used to delay absorption and increase antigenicity.

For maximum effectiveness, vaccines and toxoids must be given before exposure to the pathogenic microorganism. They should also be given by the recommended route to ensure the desired immunologic response.

Indications for Use

Clinical uses of vaccines and toxoids include the following:

- Routine immunization of children against diphtheria, *H. influenzae* b infection, hepatitis A, hepatitis B, influenza A and B, measles (rubeola), mumps, pertussis, pneumococcal infection, poliomyelitis, rotavirus, rubella (German measles), tetanus, and varicella (chickenpox)
- Immunization of adolescents and adults against diphtheria, tetanus, and pertussis (Tdap rather than the previously used Td)
- Immunization of prepubertal girls or women of childbearing age against rubella. Rubella during the first trimester of pregnancy is associated with a high incidence of birth defects in the newborn.
- Immunization of people at high risk of serious morbidity or mortality from a particular disease. For example, pneumococcal vaccine is recommended for selected groups of people.
- Immunization of adults and children at high risk of exposure to a particular disease. For example, college freshmen who live in dormitories and military recruits may need immunization against meningococcal disease or mumps.

Contraindications to Use

Vaccines and toxoids are usually contraindicated during febrile illnesses; immunosuppressive drug therapy (see Chap. 41); immunodeficiency states; leukemia, lymphoma, or generalized malignancy; and pregnancy.

Applying Your Knowledge 39-1

What nursing assessments will the nurse perform to evaluate Ms. Stein for possible contraindications for immunization?

Agents for Passive Immunity

Immune serums are the biologic products used for *passive immunity*. They act rapidly to provide temporary (for 1–3 months) immunity in people exposed to or experiencing a particular disease. The goal of therapy is to prevent or modify the disease process (i.e., decrease the incidence and severity of symptoms).

Immune globulin products are made from the serum of individuals with high concentrations of the specific antibody or immunoglobulin (Ig) required. These products may consist of whole serum or of the immunoglobulin portion of serum in which the specific antibodies are concentrated. Immunoglobulin fractions are preferred over whole serum because they are more likely to be effective. Plasma used to prepare these products is negative for hepatitis B surface antigen (HBsAg). Hyperimmune serums are available for cytomegalovirus, hepatitis B, rabies, rubella, tetanus, varicella zoster (shingles), and respiratory syncytial virus infections.

Individual Immunizing Agents

Vaccines, toxoids, and immune serums are listed in Tables 39-1 and 39-2.

Nursing Process

Assessment

Assess the patient's immunization status by obtaining the following information:

- Determine the patient's previous history of diseases for which immunizing agents are available (e.g., measles, influenza).
- Ask if the patient has had previous immunizations.
  - For which diseases were immunizations received?
  - Which immunizing agent was received?
  - Were any adverse effects experienced? If so, what symptoms occurred, and how long did they last?
  - Was tetanus toxoid given for any cuts or wounds?
  - Did any foreign travel require immunizations?
- Determine whether the patient has any conditions that contraindicate administration of immunizing agents (e.g., malignancy, pregnancy, immunosuppressive drug therapy).
- For pregnant women not known to be immunized against rubella, serum antibody titer should be measured to determine resistance or susceptibility to the disease.
- For patients with wounds, assess the type of wound and determine how, when, and where it was sustained. Such information may reveal whether tetanus immunization is needed.
- For patients exposed to infectious diseases, try to determine the extent of exposure (e.g., household or brief, casual contact) and when it occurred.

Nursing Diagnoses

- Deficient Knowledge: Importance of maintaining immunizations for both children and adults
- Risk for Fluid Volume Deficit related to inadequate intake and febrile reactions to immunizing agent
- Noncompliance in obtaining recommended immunizations related to fear of adverse effects
- Risk for Injury related to hypersensitivity, fever, and other adverse effects

Planning/Goals

The patient will

- Avoid diseases for which immunizations are available and recommended
- Obtain recommended immunizations for children and self
- Keep appointments for immunizations

Nursing Process continues on page 628

Interventions

Use measures to prevent infectious diseases, and provide information about the availability of immunizing agents. General measures include those to promote health and resistance to disease (e.g., nutrition, rest, exercise). Additional measures include the following:

- Education of the public, especially parents of young children, regarding the importance of immunizations to personal and public health. Include information about the diseases that can be prevented and where immunizations can be obtained.

- Assisting patients in developing a system to maintain immunization records for themselves and their children. This is important because immunizations are often obtained at different places and over a period of years. Written, accurate, up-to-date records help to prevent diseases and unnecessary immunizations.

- Prevention of disease transmission. The following are helpful measures:
  - Hand hygiene (probably the most effective method)
  - Avoiding contact with people who have known or suspected infectious diseases, when possible
  - Using isolation techniques when appropriate
  - Using medical and surgical aseptic techniques
  - For someone exposed to rubeola, administration of measles vaccine within 48 hours to prevent the disease
  - For someone with a puncture wound or a dirty wound, administration of tetanus immune globulin to prevent tetanus, a life-threatening disease
  - For someone with an animal bite, washing the wound immediately with large amounts of soap and water. Health care should then be sought. Administration of rabies vaccine may be needed to prevent rabies, a life-threatening disease.
  - Explaining to the patient that contracting rubella or undergoing rubella immunization during pregnancy, especially during the first trimester, may cause severe birth defects in the infant. The goal of immunization is to prevent congenital rubella syndrome. Current recommendations are to immunize children against rubella at 12 to 15 months of age. It is recommended that previously unimmunized girls 11 to 13 years of age be immunized against rubella. Furthermore, nonpregnant women of childbearing age should have rubella antibody tests. If antibody concentrations are low, the woman should be immunized. Pregnancy should be avoided for 3 months after immunization.

Evaluation

- Interview and observe for symptoms.
- Interview and observe for adverse drug effects.
- Check immunization records when indicated.

Principles of Therapy

Keeping Up-to-Date With Immunization Recommendations

Recommendations regarding immunizations change periodically as additional information and new immunizing agents become available. Consequently, health care providers need to update their knowledge at least annually. The best source of information for current recommendations is the Centers for Disease Control and Prevention (CDC; www.cdc.gov). The main source of CDC recommendations is the Advisory Committee on Immunization Practices (ACIP; www.cdc.gov/nip/acip), which consists of experts appointed to advise the CDC on strategies to prevent vaccine-preventable diseases. Other sources of information include the American Academy of Pediatrics (AAP; www.aap.org) and the American Academy of Family Physicians (AAFP; www.aafp.org). Local health departments can also be consulted about routine immunizations and those required for foreign travel. These sources can also provide information on new vaccine releases, vaccine availability, and usage of specific vaccines.

Applying Your Knowledge 39-2

The nurse is unaccustomed to providing immunizations other than the usual childhood vaccines. How should you obtain current information for Ms. Stein and how often should the nurse update this information?

Storage of Vaccines

To maintain effectiveness of vaccines and other biologic preparations, the products must be stored properly. Most products require refrigeration at 2°C to 8°C (35.6°–46.4°F). Manufacturers' instructions for storage should be strictly followed.

 ### Applying Your Knowledge 39-3

How Can You Avoid This Medication Error?
The nurse looks in the supply area for vaccines to be administered to Ms. Stein at this visit. The MMR vaccine is on the shelf above the sink so the nurse prepares the injection and administers it to the patient.

Use in Special Populations

Use in Children

Routine immunization of children has reduced the prevalence of many common childhood diseases, and immunization rates have increased in recent years. By 4 to 6 years of age, children should have received vaccinations for chickenpox (varicella), diphtheria, hepatitis A and B, influenza, measles, mumps,

(text continues on page 637)

Table 39-1		Drugs at a Glance: Vaccines and Toxoids for Active Immunity	
		ROUTES AND DOSAGE RANGES	
Name/ Characteristics	**Indications for Use**	**Adults**	**Children**
Vaccines			
***Haemophilus influenzae b* (Hib)** (ActHIB, HibTITER, PedvaxHIB) Formed by conjugating a derivative of the organism with a protein. The protein increases antigenicity.	To prevent infection with Hib, a common cause of serious bacterial infections, including meningitis, in children younger than 5 y		ActHIB, HibTITER, IM, 2–6 mo, 0.5 mL every 2 mo for 3 doses;15 mo, 0.5-mL booster dose 7–11 mo, IM, 0.5 mL every 2 mo for 2 doses; 15 mo, 0.5-mL booster dose 12–14 mo, IM 0.5 mL as single dose; 15 mo, 0.5-mL booster dose, at least 2 mo after the first dose 15–71 mo, IM 0.5 mL as a single dose (no booster dose) Pedvax HIB, IM, 2–14 mo, 0.5 mL every 2 mo for 2 doses;12–15 mo, 0.5-mL booster dose; 15–71 mo, IM 0.5 mL as a single dose (no booster dose)
***Haemophilus influenzae b* (Hib) with hepatitis B** (Comvax) May be given at the same time as DTaP; measles, mumps, rubella (MMR); injected polio vaccine (IPV), but with separate syringes and in separate sites	Routine immunization of children 6 wk–15 mo of age born to HBsAg-negative mothers		IM, 0.5 mL at 2, 4, and 12–15 months of age
Hepatitis A (Havrix, Vaqta) More than 90% effective within 4 wk after first dose Contraindicated during febrile illness, immunosuppression Havrix adult form contains 1440 units in 1 mL; the pediatric form contains 360 or 720 units in 0.5 mL Vaqta adult form contains 50 units/mL; the pediatric form contains 25 units/0.5 mL The vaccines are interchangeable.	Workers in daycare centers, laboratories, food-handling establishments; men who have sex with men; IV drug users; military personnel; travelers to areas where hepatitis A is endemic; community residents during an outbreak; people with chronic liver disease (e.g., hepatitis B or C, cirrhosis)	Havrix, IM 1 mL initially and 6–12 mo later (total of 2 doses) Vaqta, IM in deltoid, 1 mL initially and 6–12 mo later (total of 2 doses)	Havrix, 1–18 y, IM, 360 units initially, 1 mo later, and 6–12 mo later (total of 3 doses) or 720 units initially and 6–12 mo later (total of 2 doses) Vaqta, IM, 25 units initially and 6–18 mo later (total of 2 doses)

(continued on page 630)

Table 39-1	**Drugs at a Glance:** Vaccines and Toxoids for Active Immunity (continued)		

| | | ROUTES AND DOSAGE RANGES | |
Name/ Characteristics	**Indications for Use**	**Adults**	**Children**
Hepatitis B (Engerix-B, Recombivax HB, Engerix-B) Approximately 96% effective in children and young adults and 88% in adults older than 40 y Duration of protection unknown; can measure serum antibody levels periodically	Pre-exposure immunization of high-risk groups, such as health care providers (nurses, physicians, dentists, laboratory workers); patients with cancer, organ transplants, hemodialysis, immunosuppressant drug therapy, or multiple infusions of blood or blood products; men who have sex with men; IV drug abusers; household contacts of hepatitis B virus carriers; residents and staff of institutions for mentally challenged people Persons requiring postexposure vaccine include infants born to carrier mothers, people with accidental exposure of skin or mucous membrane to infected blood (e.g., needlestick injuries), and household contacts or sexual partners of persons with acute hepatitis B infection	20 y and older: Engerix-B, IM, 1 mL initially and 1 mo and 6 mo later (3 doses) Predialysis and dialysis patients, IM, 2 mL initially and 1, 2, and 6 mo later (4 doses) Recombivax HB, IM, 1 mL initially and 1 mo and 6 mo later (3 doses) Predialysis and dialysis patients, IM, 1 mL initially and 1 mo and 6 mo later (3 doses)	*Neonates to 19 y:* Engerix-B IM 0.5 mL initially and 1 mo and 6 mo later (3 doses) *Neonates to 19 y:* Recombivax IM 0.5 mL initially and 1 mo and 6 mo later (3 doses)
Hepatitis A and hepatitis B (Twinrix) Contains hepatitis A and hepatitis B antigens	Adults exposed to hepatitis A or B (e.g., medical personnel, staff in institutional settings such as daycare centers, prisons) Adults at risk of exposure, including travelers to areas of high incidence; people with chronic liver disease; laboratory workers, police, emergency medical personnel, sanitation workers	IM 1 mL initially and 1 mo and 6 mo later (total of 3 doses)	
Human papillomavirus (HPV) (Gardasil) Because HPV is a common sexually transmitted infection, the vaccine is most effective when taken before becoming sexually active.	Prevention of diseases caused by HPV types 6, 11, 16, and 18 (cervical, vaginal and vulvar cancer; genital warts) in girls and women aged 9–26 y	IM 0.5 mL initially, 2 mo after first dose, and 6 mo after first dose (total of 3 doses)	9 y *and older;* same as adults
Influenza (Fluzone, Fluvirin, FluMist)	Annual immunization of most people, especially:	*All adults:* IM 0.5 mL in a single dose	Injectable form

Name/ Characteristics	Indications for Use	ROUTES AND DOSAGE RANGES	
		Adults	Children
Formulated annually to include current strains Provides protective antibody concentrations for about 6 mo Note: Fluvirin is indicated only in children 4 y and older. FluMist is indicated in healthy children and adolescents 5–17 y of age and in healthy adults 18–49 y of age (except during pregnancy).	Children between 6 months and 5 years old, Pregnant women, People older than 50 y, People who live in long-term health care facilities People with chronic medical conditions (e.g., diabetes, lung disease, HIV/AIDS) People living with or caring for young children, nursing-home residents, those with compromised immune systems, or those with chronic medical conditions	*Healthy adults 18–49 y:* Intranasal spray 0.5 mL per season	6–35 *mo:* IM, 0.25 mL, 1 dose if previously vaccinated; 2 doses at least 1 mo apart if first vaccination 3–8 *y:* IM, 0.5 mL, 1 dose if previously vaccinated; 2 doses at least 1 mo apart if first vaccination 9 *y and older:* IM, 0.5 mL in a single dose Intranasal spray 5–8 y (not previously vaccinated with FluMist): 0.5 mL per dose, 60 d apart for a total of 2 doses 5–8 y (previously vaccinated with FluMist): 0.5 mL in a single dose per season 9 *y and older:* 0.6 mL in a single dose per season
Measles, mumps, and rubella (MMR) Preferred and more commonly used than single immunizing agents Contains live, attenuated viruses that cause measles, mumps, and rubella Protects more than 95% of recipients for many years	Immunization at 12–15 mo and a second dose at 4–6 y	IM 0.5 mL	Same as adults
Measles, mumps, rubella, and varicella vaccine (Proquad)	Routine immunization of children 12 mo to 12 y of age		Sub-Q 0.5 mL as a single dose
Meningitis/meningococcal disease (Menactra; (menomune) Prevents invasive meningococcal infection caused by *Neisseria meningitidis* Provides protective levels of antibody within 7–10 d Note: A few cases of Guillain-Barré syndrome have been reported after Menactra administration.	Immunization of people at risk in epidemic or endemic areas Recommended for college students living in dormitories	Menomune, Sub-Q 0.5 mL Menactra, IM, 0.5 mL	Menomune, same as adults for children older than 2 y Menactra, same as adults for children 11 y and older

(continued on page 632)

Table 39-1 | **Drugs at a Glance:** Vaccines and Toxoids for Active Immunity (continued)

Name/ Characteristics	Indications for Use	ROUTES AND DOSAGE RANGES	
		Adults	Children
Pneumococcal polyvalent (Pneumovax 23, Pnu-Imune 23) Contains 23 strains of pneumococci, which cause most of the serious pneumococcal infections in the United States Protection begins about 3 wk after vaccination and lasts years. Not recommended for children under 2 y	Adults with disorders associated with risk of pneumococcal infection (e.g., cardiovascular or pulmonary disease, diabetes mellitus, Hodgkin's disease, multiple myeloma, cirrhosis, alcohol dependence, renal failure, immunosuppression) Adults 65 y and older who are otherwise healthy Children 2 y and older with chronic disease associated with risk of pneumococcal infection (e.g., asplenia, nephrotic syndrome, immunosuppression)	Sub-Q, IM 0.5 mL as a single dose; may be repeated after 5 y	Same as adults; may be repeated after 3 y
Pneumococcal 7-valent (Prevnar) Contains 7 *Streptococcus pneumoniae* antigens conjugated to a protein to increase antigenicity	To prevent life-threatening pneumococcal infections (e.g., bacteremia, meningitis, pneumonia) in young children		*Birth–6 mo*: IM 0.5 mL at 2, 4, and 6 mo and at 12–15 mo (4 doses) *7–11 mo*: IM 0.5 mL initially, at least 4 wk later, and after 1 y birthday (3 doses) *12–23 mo*: IM 0.5 ml initially and at least 2 mo later (2 doses) *24 mo–9 y*: IM 0.5 mL in a single dose
Poliomyelitis , inactivated (IPV) (IPOL)	Routine immunization of infants Immunization of adults not previously immunized and at risk of exposure (e.g., health care or laboratory workers)	Sub-Q, 0.5 mL monthly for 2 doses, than a third dose 6–12 mo later	Sub-Q, 0.5 mL at 2, 4, and 6–18 mo, and 4–6 y of age (4 doses) or at 2 and 4 mo (2 doses)
Rabies vaccine (Imovax, RabAvert) Immunity develops in 7–10 d and lasts 1 y or longer	Pre-exposure immunization in people at high risk of exposure (e.g., veterinarians, animal handlers) Postexposure prophylaxis in people who have been bitten by potentially rabid animals or who have skin scratches or abrasions exposed to animal saliva (e.g., animal licking of wound), urine, or blood	Pre-exposure, IM, 1.0 mL for 3 doses. The second dose is given 1 wk after the first; the third dose is given 3–4 wk after the first. Then, booster doses (1 mL) every 2–5 y based on antibody titers. Postexposure, IM, 1 mL for 5 doses. After the initial dose, other doses are given 3, 7, 14, and 28 d later.	Same as adults

Name/ Characteristics	Indications for Use	ROUTES AND DOSAGE RANGES	
		Adults	**Children**
Rotavirus (Rotateq) Can be given with most other childhood vaccines Adverse effects are usually mild diarrhea and vomiting. However, an earlier rotavirus vaccine was withdrawn because of an association with intussusception and a few cases have been reported after administration of Rotateq.	Prevention of rotavirus gastroenteritis in infants		PO 1 dose between 6 and 12 wk of age; a second and third dose at 4 to 10 wk intervals. The third dose should not be given after 32 wk of age.
Tuberculosis (bacillus Calmette-Guérin) (TICE BCG) Contains live, attenuated tuberculosis bacilli Converts negative tuberculin reactors to positive reactors; therefore, precludes use of the tuberculin skin test for screening or early diagnosis of tuberculosis Contraindicated in patients with impaired immune responses	People at high risk of exposure, including newborns of women with tuberculosis	Percutaneous, by multiple puncture disk, 0.2–0.3 mL	*Newborns:* percutaneous by multiple puncture disk, 0.1 mL *Older than 1 mo:* same as adults
Varicella (Varivax) Contains live, attenuated varicella virus Contraindicated in people with hematologic or lymphatic malignancy, immunosuppression, febrile illness, or pregnancy	Immunization of children 12 mo and older Immunization of adults	Sub-Q 0.5 mL, followed by a second dose of 0.5 mL 4–8 wk after the first dose	*12–15 mo:* Sub-Q 0.5 mL followed by a second dose at 4–6 y of age
Zoster vaccine (Zostavax) Redness, edema, tenderness at injection site were most common adverse reactions during clinical trials. Duration of protection unknown	Prevention of herpes zoster in adults 60 y and older	Sub-Q entire single-dose vial	
Toxoids			
Diphtheria and tetanus toxoids and acellular pertussis vaccine (DTaP, Tdap) (Adacel, Boostrix, Daptacel, Infanrix, Tripedia) The acellular pertussis vaccine decreases the adverse effects associated with the earlier pertussis vaccine.	Immunization of children aged 6 wk–7 y Booster dose for persons aged 10–18 y (Boostrix) or persons aged 11–64 y (Adacel)	IM 0.5 mL	IM 0.5 mL at approximately 2, 4, 6, and 18 mo of age and at 4–6 y Adacel or Boostrix IM 0.5 mL

(continued on page 634)

Table 39-1	Drugs at a Glance: Vaccines and Toxoids for Active Immunity (continued)		

		ROUTES AND DOSAGE RANGES	
Name/ Characteristics	**Indications for Use**	**Adults**	**Children**
DTaP and *Haemophilus influenzae* type B (DTaP-HIB) (TriHIBit)	Immunization of children 15–18 mo of age who have been previously immunized against diphtheria, tetanus, and pertussis		IM 0.5 mL
DTaP, hepatitis B, and polio (Pediarix)			IM 0.5 mL at 2, 4, and 6 mo of age (total of 3 doses)
Diphtheria and tetanus toxoids (pediatric type) (DT) Contains a larger amount of diphtheria antigen than "tetanus and diphtheria toxoids, adult type (Td)"	Routine immunization of infants and children 6 y and younger in whom pertussis vaccine is contraindicated (those who have adverse reactions to initial doses of DTaP vaccine		*Infants and children 6 y and younger*: IM 0.5 mL for 2 doses at least 4 wk apart, followed by a booster dose 1 y later and when the child starts school
Tetanus and diphtheria toxoids, (adult type) (Td) Contains a smaller amount of diphtheria antigen than "diphtheria and tetanus toxoids, pediatric type (DT)"	Primary immunization or booster doses in adults and children older than 6 y	IM 0.5 mL for 2 doses, at least 4 wk apart, followed by a booster dose 6–12 mo later and every 10 y thereafter	*Older than 6 y*: same as adults
Tetanus toxoid Protects about 100% of recipients for 10 y or more Usually given in combination (e.g., DTaP or DT) for primary immunization of infants and children 6 y of age or older Usually given alone or combined with diphtheria toxoid (e.g., Td adult type) for primary immunization of adults	Routine immunization of infants and young children Primary immunization of adults Prevention of tetanus in previously immunized people who sustain a potentially contaminated wound	Primary immunization in adults not previously immunized, IM 0.5 mL for 3 doses: initially, 4–8 wk later, then at 6–12 mo. Then, 0.5-mL booster dose every 10 y. Prophylaxis, IM 0.5 mL if wound contaminated and no booster dose was received for 5 y; 0.5 mL if wound is clean and no booster dose was received for 10 y	Same as adults

HBsAg, hepatitis B surface antigen.

Table 39-2	**Drugs at a Glance:** Immune Serums for Passive Immunity	
NAME/ CHARACTERISTICS	**INDICATIONS FOR USE**	**ROUTES AND DOSAGE RANGES**
Cytomegalovirus immune globulin, intravenous, human (CMV-IGIV) (CytoGam) Contains antibodies against CMV	Prevention of CMV infection in heart, kidney, liver, lung, and pancreas transplant recipients	Post-transplantation, IV infusion, 150 mg/kg within 72 h, then 100–150 mg/kg at 2, 4, 6, and 8 wk, then 50–100 mg/kg at 12 and 16 wk
Hepatitis B immune globulin, human (HBIG) (BayHep B, Nabi-HB) A solution of immunoglobulins that contains antibodies to HBsAg	To prevent hepatitis after exposure. Neonates born to HBsAg-positive or unknown-status mothers are given HBIG and the first dose of hepatitis B vaccine within 12 h of birth.	*Adults and children:* IM, 0.06 mL/kg (usual adult dose, 3–5 mL) as soon as possible after exposure, preferably within 7 d. Repeat dose in 1 mo.
Immune globulin (human) (IG; IGIM) (BayGam) Given IM only Commonly called "gamma globulin" Obtained from pooled plasma of normal donors Consists primarily of IgG, which contains concentrated antibodies Produces adequate serum levels of IgG in 2–5 d	To decrease the severity of hepatitis A, measles, and varicella after exposure To treat immunoglobulin deficiency	*Adults and children:* Exposure to hepatitis A, IM, 0.02 mL/kg Exposure to measles, IM, 0.25 mL/kg within 6 d of exposure Exposure to varicella, IM, 0.6–1.2 mL/kg Exposure to rubella (pregnant women only), IM, 0.55 mL/kg Immunoglobulin deficiency, IM, 1.3 mL/kg initially, then 0.6 mL/kg every 3–4 wk
Immune globulin intravenous (IGIV) (Polygam S/D, Panglobulin, Venoglobulin-S) Given IV only Provides immediate antibodies Half-life about 3 wk Mechanism of action in ITP unknown **BLACK BOX WARNING:** IGIV has been associated with renal dysfunction and failure and death. It should be used cautiously in patients with or at risk of developing renal impairment.	Immunodeficiency syndrome Idiopathic thrombocytopenic purpura (ITP)	See manufacturers' instructions
Rabies immune globulin (human) RIG (HyperRabS/D, Imogam) Gamma globulin obtained from plasma of people hyperim-munized with rabies vaccine Not useful in treatment of clinical rabies infection	Postexposure prevention of rabies, in conjunc-tion with rabies vaccine	*Adults and children:* IM, 20 units/kg (half the dose may be injected around the wound) as soon as possible after possible exposure (e.g., animal bite)

(continued on page 636)

Table 39-2   **Drugs at a Glance: Immune Serums for Passive Immunity** (continued)

NAME/ CHARACTERISTICS	INDICATIONS FOR USE	ROUTES AND DOSAGE RANGES
Respiratory syncytial virus immune globulin intravenous (human) (RSV-IGIV) (RespiGam) Reduces severity of RSV illness and the incidence and duration of hospitalization in high-risk infants May cause fluid overload Not established as safe and effective in children with congenital heart disease	Prevention of serious RSV infections in high-risk children less than 2 y of age (i.e., those with bronchopulmonary dysplasia or history of premature birth [gestation of 35 wk or less]) Treatment of RSV lower respiratory tract infections in hospitalized infants and young children	*Children*: IV infusion via infusion pump, 1.5 mL/kg/h for 15 min, then 3 mL/kg/h for 15 min, then 6 mL/kg/h until the infusion is completed, then once monthly, if tolerated. Maximum monthly dose, 750 mg/kg
Rh$_o$(D) immune globulin (human) (RhoGAM) Prepared from fractionated human plasma A sterile concentrated solution of specific immunoglobulin (IgG) containing anti-Rh$_o$(D)	To prevent sensitization in a subsequent pregnancy to the Rh$_o$(D) factor in an Rh-negative mother who has given birth to an Rh-positive infant by an Rh-positive father	*Obstetric use*: Inject contents of 1 vial IM for every 15 mL fetal packed red cell volume within 72 h after delivery, miscarriage, or abortion. Consult package instructions for blood typing and drug administration procedures.
Tetanus immune globulin (human) (BayTet) Solution of globulins from plasma of people hyperimmunized with tetanus toxoid Tetanus toxoid (Td) should also be given to initiate active immunization if minor wound and more than 10 y since Td, if major wound and more than 5 y since Td, or if Td primary immunization series was incomplete.	To prevent tetanus in patients with wounds possibly contaminated with *Clostridium tetani* and whose immunization history is uncertain or incomplete Treatment of tetanus infection	*Adults and children*: Prophylaxis, IM, 250 units as a single dose Treatment of clinical disease, IM 3000–6000 units in a single dose
Varicella-zoster immune globulin (human) (VZIG) The globulin fraction of human plasma Antibodies last 1 mo or longer.	Postexposure to chickenpox or shingles, to prevent or decrease severity of infections in children under 15 y of age who have not been immunized or who are immunodeficient because of illness or drug therapy Infants born to mothers who develop varicella 5 d before or 2 d after delivery and premature infants of less than 28 wk gestation	IM 125 units/10 kg up to a maximum of 625 units within 48 h after exposure if possible; may be given up to 96 h after exposure. Minimal dose, 125 units

CMV, cytomegalovirus; IgG, immunoglobulin G; RSV, respiratory syncytial virus; HBsAg, hepatitis B surface antigen.

Patient Teaching Guidelines Vaccinations

- Appropriate vaccinations should be maintained for adults as well as for children. Consult the Centers for Disease Control and Prevention (CDC) website (www.cdc.gov) or a health care provider periodically because recommendations for particular groups change fairly often.
- Maintain immunization records for yourself and all members of your family. This is important because immunizations are often obtained at different places and over a period of years. Written, accurate, up-to-date records help to prevent diseases and unnecessary immunizations.
- If a health care provider recommends an immunization and you do not know whether you have had the immunization or the disease, it is probably safer to take the immunization than to risk having the disease. Immunization after a previous immunization or after having the disease usually is not harmful.

- Most vaccines cause fever and soreness at the site of injection. Acetaminophen (e.g., Tylenol) can be taken two to three times daily for 24 to 48 hours (by adults and children) to decrease fever and discomfort.
- Women of childbearing age who receive a rubella (German measles) or a varicella (chickenpox) immunization must avoid becoming pregnant (i.e., must use effective contraceptive methods) for 3 months.
- After receiving varicella vaccine (to prevent chickenpox), avoid close contact with newborns, pregnant women, and anyone whose immune system is impaired. Vaccinated people may transmit the vaccine virus to susceptible close contacts.
- After receiving a vaccine, stay in the area for approximately 30 minutes. If an allergic reaction is going to occur, it will usually do so within that time.

pertussis (whooping cough), polio, pneumococcal diseases, rubella (German measles), tetanus, and *Haemophilus influenzae* and rotavirus infections. Because some vaccines are administered more than once, a child may receive more than 20 injections by 2 years of age. Two strategies to increase immunizations are the development of combination vaccines and the administration of multiple vaccines (in separate syringes and at different sites) at one visit to a health care provider when feasible. The combination vaccines decrease the number of injections, and giving multiple vaccines decreases the number of visits to a health care provider. Several combination vaccines are now available and continue to be developed. Studies indicate that these strategies are effective. In general, children's health care providers should follow the "Recommended Childhood Immunization Schedule" issued in January of each year by the CDC. In addition, current guidelines should be consulted about immunizations for children with chronic illnesses (e.g., asthma, heart disease, diabetes) or immunosuppression (e.g., from cancer, organ transplantation, or HIV infection). Dosages and schedules of administration for children whose immunizations begin in early infancy are listed in Table 39-1; different schedules are recommended for children 1 to 5 years of age and for those older than 6 years of age who are being immunized for the first time or who have missed doses.

Use in Healthy Adolescents, Young Adults, and Middle-Aged Adults

Adolescents who received all primary immunizations as infants and young children should have a second dose of varicella (chickenpox) vaccine, hepatitis A and hepatitis B vaccines (if not received earlier), a tetanus-diphtheria-pertussis booster (Tdap) between ages 11 and 18 years if 5 years since a tetanus-diphtheria (Td) booster, and meningococcal vaccine at 11 or 12 years of age. Adolescent girls should receive the human papilloma virus (HPV) vaccine if not received earlier. Young adults who are health care workers, are sexually active, or

belong to high-risk groups should receive varicella (chickenpox) vaccine or a second dose if they previously received a single dose; hepatitis A and hepatitis B vaccines if not previously received; a tetanus-diphtheria-pertussis booster (Tdap); MMR if not pregnant and rubella titer is inadequate or proof of immunization is unavailable; HPV vaccine (up to 26 years of age) if not previously received; and meningococcal vaccine if not previously received. In addition, young adults who are health care providers should have influenza vaccine annually. Middle-aged adults should maintain immunizations against tetanus-diphtheria-pertussis (Tdap); high-risk groups (e.g., those with chronic illness) and health care providers should receive hepatitis B vaccine once (if not previously taken) and influenza vaccine annually at 50 years of age and older. An additional vaccine to prevent zoster infections (shingles) is available for adults 60 years and older. Middle-aged adults (those born after 1956) should get at least one dose of measles-mumps-rubella (MMR) vaccine unless they have had either the vaccine or each of the three diseases.

Use in Older Adults

Older adults become more susceptible to some diseases, and influenza, pneumococcal infections, tetanus, and shingles can be especially serious in this population. The varicella-zoster virus, the same virus that causes chickenpox, causes shingles.

Recommended immunizations for older adults usually consist of a tetanus-diphtheria (Td) booster every 10 years, annual influenza vaccine, and a one-time administration of pneumococcal vaccine at 65 years of age. A second dose of pneumococcal vaccine may be given at 65 years if the first dose was given 5 years previously.

A newer tetanus-diphtheria-pertussis vaccine is recommended to replace the Td booster dose in adults up to 64 years of age, and a vaccine to prevent shingles is available for adults 60 years and older. As with younger adults, immunization for most other diseases is recommended for older adults at high risk of exposure.

Use in Patients With Immunosuppression

Compared with healthy, immunocompetent individuals, the antibody response to immunization is usually adequate but reduced in immunosuppressed people. Immunizations should be individualized. In general, those with diabetes mellitus or chronic pulmonary, renal, or hepatic disorders who are not receiving immunosuppressant drugs may be given both live attenuated and killed vaccines and toxoids to induce active immunity. However, they may need higher doses or more frequent administration to induce adequate immunity. With hepatitis B vaccine, for example, larger doses may be required initially and booster doses may be needed later if antibody concentrations fall.

Patients with active malignant disease may be given killed vaccines or toxoids but should not be given live vaccines (an exception is persons with leukemia who have not received chemotherapy for at least 3 months). When vaccines are used, they should be given at least 2 weeks before the start of chemotherapy or 3 months after chemotherapy is completed. Passive immunity with immunoglobulins may be used in place of active immunity.

Patients receiving a systemic corticosteroid in high doses (e.g., prednisone 20 mg or equivalent daily) or for longer than 2 weeks should wait at least 3 months before being given a live-virus vaccine. Immunizations are not contraindicated with short-term use (less than 2 weeks) or low to moderate doses (less than 20 mg of prednisone daily). In addition, long-term alternate-day therapy with short-acting agents; maintenance physiologic doses; and the use of topical, aerosol, or intra-articular injections are not contraindications to immunization.

Patients with HIV infection have less-than-optimal responses to immunizing agents because the disease produces major defects in cell-mediated and humoral immunity. Live bacterial (BCG, oral typhoid) or viral (MMR, varicella) vaccines should not be given because the bacteria or viruses may be able to reproduce and cause active infection. Persons with asymptomatic HIV infection should receive inactivated vaccines; those exposed to measles or varicella may be given immune globulin or varicella-zoster immune globulin for passive immunization.

For children with HIV infection, most routine immunizations (DTaP, IPV, MMR, Hib, influenza) are recommended. MMR is not recommended in children with severe immunosuppression, and varicella vaccine is recommended only for children with no evidence of immunosuppression. Pneumococcal vaccine is recommended for HIV-infected persons over 2 years of age.

Use in Patients With Cancer

For patients with active malignant disease, live vaccines should not be given. Although killed vaccines and toxoids may be given, antibody production may be inadequate to provide immunity. When possible, patients should receive needed immunizations 2 weeks before or 3 months after immunosuppressive radiation or chemotherapy treatments. For example, patients with Hodgkin's lymphoma who are more than 2 years old should be immunized with pneumococcal and Hib vaccines 10 to 14 days before therapy is started. In addition, patients who have not received chemotherapy for 3 to 4 weeks may have an adequate antibody response to influenza vaccine.

Nursing Actions | Immunizing Agents

NURSING ACTIONS	RATIONALE/EXPLANATION
1. Administer accurately	
a. Read the package insert and check the expiration date on all biologic products (e.g., vaccines, toxoids, human immune serums).	Concentration, dosage, and administration of biologic products often vary with the products. Avoid administration of expired products and use reconstituted products within designated time limits because they are usually stable for only a few hours.
b. Follow instructions for administering each vaccine.	Most vaccines are given by injection. In general, the vastus lateralis is the largest skeletal muscle mass in infants and is preferred for IM injections. The deltoid or vastus lateralis muscle may be used for older children and adults. Injection into the gluteal muscles is not recommended because the vaccine may be injected into fatty tissue and be less effective in arousing an immune response.
c. Check the patient's temperature before giving a vaccine.	Some immunizations are contraindicated during febrile illnesses.
d. Give IM human immune serum globulin with an 18- to 20-gauge needle, preferably in gluteal muscles. If the dose is 5 mL or more, divide it and inject it into two or more IM sites. Follow manufacturer's instructions for preparation and administration of intravenous (IV) formulations.	To promote absorption and minimize tissue irritation and other adverse reactions

NURSING ACTIONS	RATIONALE/EXPLANATION
e. Aspirate carefully before IM or Sub-Q injection of any immunizing agent.	To avoid inadvertent IV administration and greatly increased risks of severe adverse effects
f. Have aqueous epinephrine 1:1000 readily available before administering any vaccine.	For immediate treatment of allergic reactions
g. After administration of an immunizing agent in a clinic or office setting, have the patient stay in the area for at least 30 minutes. Provide patients with a Vaccine Information Statement (VIS).	To observe for allergic reactions, which usually occur within 30 minutes
2. Observe for therapeutic effects	
a. Absence of diseases for which immunized	
b. Decreased incidence and severity of symptoms when given to modify disease processes	
3. Observe for adverse effects	Most adverse effects are mild and transient. However, serious reactions occasionally occur. The risk of serious adverse effects from immunization is usually much smaller than the risk of the disease immunized against.
	Adverse effects may be caused by the immunizing agent or by foreign protein incorporated with the immunizing agent (e.g., egg protein in viral vaccines grown in chick embryos).
a. General reactions:	
(1) Pain, tenderness, redness at injection sites	Local tissue irritation may occur with injected immunizing agents.
(2) Fever, malaise, muscle aches	These adverse effects commonly occur with vaccines and toxoids.
(3) Anaphylaxis—cardiovascular collapse, shock, laryngeal edema, urticaria, angioneurotic edema, severe respiratory distress	Anaphylaxis occasionally occurs with immunizing agents. It is a medical emergency that requires immediate treatment with Sub-Q epinephrine (0.5 mL for adults; 0.01 mL/kg for children). Anaphylaxis is most likely to occur within 30 minutes after immunizing agents are injected.
(4) Serum sickness—urticaria, fever, arthralgia, enlarged lymph nodes	Serum sickness is a delayed hypersensitivity reaction that occurs several days or weeks after an injection of serum. Treatment is symptomatic. Symptoms are usually relieved by acetaminophen, antihistamines, and corticosteroids.
b. With DTaP:	
(1) Soreness, erythema, edema at injection sites	These effects are common.
(2) Anorexia, nausea	
(3) Severe fever, encephalopathy, seizures	These reactions are rare. If they occur, they are thought to be caused by the pertussis antigen, and further administration of pertussis vaccine or DTaP may be contraindicated.
c. With *Haemophilus influenzae* b vaccine—pain and erythema at injection sites	These effects occur in about 25% of recipients but are usually mild and resolve within 24 hours.
d. With hepatitis B vaccine:	
(1) Injection site soreness, erythema, induration	Soreness and fever commonly occur and can be relieved by acetaminophen or ibuprofen. Anaphylaxis and other severe reactions rarely occur.
(2) Fever	
(3) Anaphylaxis	
e. With influenza vaccine:	
(1) Via injection—pain, induration, and erythema at injection sites; flu-like symptoms such as chills, fever, malaise, muscle aches	Adverse effects can be minimized by giving acetaminophen at the time of immunization and at 4, 8, and 12 hours later. Injection site reactions and flu-like symptoms may start within 12 hours after vaccination.
(2) Via intranasal spray—runny nose, headache, cough, sore throat, irritability in children	
f. With MMR vaccine:	
(1) Mild symptoms of measles—cough, fever up to 39.4°C (102°F), headache, malaise, photophobia, skin rash, sore throat	These symptoms may occur 6–11 days after immunization.
(2) Febrile seizures	These are rare but are more likely to occur in children less than 2 years of age.
(3) Arthralgia (joint pain)	Joint pain has been reported in as many as 25% of adult females 2–6 weeks after receiving rubella vaccine.

(continued on page 640)

Nursing Actions | Immunizing Agents (continued)

NURSING ACTIONS	RATIONALE/EXPLANATION
(4) Anaphylaxis in recipients who are allergic to eggs	The measles and mumps viruses used in MMR vaccine are grown in chick-embryo cell cultures. Recipients who are allergic to eggs should be observed for 90 minutes after the vaccine is injected. MMR vaccine should be given only in a setting where personnel and equipment are available to treat anaphylaxis.
g. With pneumococcal vaccine: (1) Local effects—soreness, induration, and erythema at injection sites (2) Systemic effects—chills, fever, headache, muscle aches, nausea, photophobia, weakness	Local effects occur in 40%–90% of recipients; systemic effects occur less frequently.
h. With polio vaccine: (1) Soreness at injection sites (2) Fever (3) Anaphylaxis	Adverse effects are usually mild. Anaphylaxis rarely occurs. However, if it occurs within 24 hours after administration of polio vaccine, no additional doses of the vaccine should be given.
i. With varicella vaccine: (1) Early effects—transient soreness or erythema at injection sites (2) Late effect—a mild, maculopapular skin rash with a few lesions	Injection site reactions occur in 20%–35% of recipients; a skin rash develops in a few (about 8%) recipients within a month. Those who develop a rash from the vaccine have milder symptoms of shorter duration than those who develop varicella naturally.
j. With immune globulin intravenous (IGIV): (1) Chills; dizziness; dyspnea; fever; flushing; headache; nausea; urticaria; vomiting; tightness in chest; pain in chest, hip, or back (2) Renal dysfunction, acute renal failure, death	These effects are related to the rate of infusion. If they occur, the infusion should be stopped until the symptoms subside, then restarted at a slower rate. The symptoms can also be prevented or minimized by pre-infusion administration of acetaminophen and diphenhydramine or a corticosteroid. Acute renal failure is most likely to occur in patients older than 65 years of age; in those with pre-existing renal insufficiency, diabetes mellitus, volume depletion, or sepsis; or in those taking known nephrotoxic drugs.
4. Observe for drug interactions a. Drugs that *decrease* effects of vaccines in general: (1) Immunosuppressants (e.g., corticosteroids, antineoplastic drugs, phenytoin)	Vaccines may be contraindicated in patients receiving immunosuppressive drugs. These patients cannot produce sufficient amounts of antibodies for immunity and may develop the illness produced by the particular organism contained in the vaccine. The disease is most likely to occur with the live-virus vaccines (measles, mumps, rubella). Similar effects occur when the patient is receiving radiation and phenytoin, an anticonvulsant drug that suppresses immune responses.
b. Drugs that *decrease* effects of measles and MMR vaccines: (1) Immunosuppressants	May decrease effectiveness of immunization; patients may remain susceptible to measles despite immunization.
(2) Immune globulins (e.g., RIG, RSV-IGIV, VZIG, IGIV)	To avoid inactivation of the attenuated virus, give measles or MMR vaccine at least 14–30 days before or 6–8 weeks after the immune globulin. Alternatively, may check antibody titers or repeat the measles vaccine dose 3 months after immune globulin administration
(3) Interferon	May inhibit antibody response to the vaccine
c. Drug that *decreases* effects of meningococcal vaccine: (1) Measles vaccine	These vaccines should be given at least 1 month apart.
d. With varicella vaccine, salicylates may *increase* risk of Reye's syndrome.	Aspirin and other salicylates should be avoided for 6 weeks after vaccine administration because of potential for Reye's syndrome, which has been reported with salicylate use after natural varicella infection.

Key Concepts

■ Many infectious diseases can be prevented by immunizations.

■ Immunizations are needed for all age groups.

■ Children in the United States are much more likely to receive recommended immunizations than are adolescents and adults.

■ Health care providers who provide or participate in immunizations need to keep their knowledge base current with annual updates regarding recommendations from the CDC.

■ Health care providers need to assess and inform patients about recommended immunizations.

■ New immunizing products continue to be developed.

Review and Application Exercises

Short Answer Exercises

1. What is the difference between active immunity and passive immunity?

2. How do vaccines act to produce active immunity?

3. What are the sources and functions of immune serums?

4. List common childhood diseases for which immunizing agents are available.

5. Which immunizations are recommended for adults?

6. What are advantages of administering a combination of immunizing agents rather than single agents?

7. What are common adverse reactions to immunizing agents, and how may they be prevented or minimized?

8. Why should live vaccines not be given to people whose immune system is suppressed by drugs or diseases?

NCLEX-Style Questions

9. In explaining vaccines to a parent, the nurse knows that vaccines provide
   a. active immunity
   b. passive immunity
   c. innate immunity
   d. nonspecific immunity

10. The nurse caring for a patient with severe immunosuppression knows that this condition is a contraindication to

a. all injectable immunizations
b. the use of live bacterial or viral vaccines
c. the use of immune globulins for passive immunity
d. the use of most immunizing agents in children

11. To decrease fever and discomfort after an immunization, the nurse should advise that adults and children can take
   a. an opioid analgesic every 6 to 8 hours for 48 hours
   b. acetaminophen every 4 to 6 hours for at least 24 hours
   c. an antihistamine for 2 days before and 2 days after vaccine administration
   d. a sedative at bedtime to aid sleep

12. For a child receiving an immunization, the nurse should inform the parents that common after-effects may include
   a. skin rash and swelling
   b. redness and soreness at the injection site
   c. muscle weakness and difficulty in walking
   d. nausea, vomiting, and diarrhea

13. An adult patient has had an injury with skin penetration by a piece of dirty metal. He is seeking minor first aid care, but as the nurse you are concerned about prevention of tetanus. You know that adults should be given tetanus toxoid vaccine every
   a. year
   b. 2 years
   c. 5 years
   d. 10 years

Selected References

Brundage, S. C., & Fitzpatrick, A. N. (2006). Hepatitis A. *American Family Physician, 73,* 2162–2170.

Chaves, S. S., Gargiullo, P., Zhang, J. X., Civen, R., Guris, D., Mascola, L., & Seward, J. F. (2007). Loss of vaccine-induced immunity to varicella over time. *New England Journal of Medicine, 356,* 1121–1129.

Drug facts and comparisons. (Updated monthly). St. Louis, MO: Facts and Comparisons.

Goldrick, B. A., & Goetz, A. M. (2006). Tis the season for influenza. *Nurse Practitioner, 31,* 24–33.

Halperin, S. A. (2007). The control of pertussis—2007 and beyond. *New England Journal of Medicine, 356,* 110–113.

Hayney, M. S. (2005). Vaccines, toxoids, and other immunobiologics. In J. T. DiPiro, R. L. Talbert, G. C. Yee, G. R. Matzke, B. G. Wells, & L. M. Posey (Eds.), *Pharmacotherapy: A pathophysiologic approach* (6th ed., pp. 2231–2253). New York: McGraw-Hill.

Jacobs, R. A., & Cin-Hong, P. V. (2007). General problems in infectious diseases. In S. J. McPhee, M. A. Papadakis, & L. M. Tierney, Jr. (Eds.), *Current medical diagnosis and treatment 2007* (46th ed., pp. 1311–1345). New York: McGraw-Hill.

Morantz, C. (2006). ACIP updates recommendations for prevention of hepatitis B virus transmission. *American Family Physician, 73,* 1839–1845.

Morantz, C. A. (2006). Recommended childhood and adolescent immunization schedule, United States, 2006. *American Family Physician, 73,* 167.

Oxman, M. N., Levin, M. J., & Johnson, G. R. (2005). A vaccine to prevent herpes zoster and postherpetic neuralgia in older adults. *New England Journal of Medicine, 352,* 2271–2284.

Pichichero, M. E., Rennels, M. B., & Edwards, K. M. (2005). Combined tetanus, diphtheria, and 5-component pertussis vaccine for use in adolescents and adults. *Journal of the American Medical Association, 293,* 3003–3011.

Porth, C. M. (2005). *Pathophysiology: Concepts of altered health states* (7th ed.). Philadelphia: Lippincott Williams & Wilkins.

Smeltzer, S. C., Bare, B. G., Hinkle, J. L., & Cheever, K. H. (2008). *Brunner & Suddarth's textbook of medical-surgical nursing* (11th ed.). Philadelphia: Lippincott Williams & Wilkins.

Van Damme, P., & Van Herck, K. (2005). Effect of hepatitis A vaccination programs [Editorial]. *Journal of the American Medical Association, 294,* 246–248.

Wasley, A., Samandari, T., & Bell, B. P. (2005). Incidence of hepatitis A in the United States in the era of vaccination. *Journal of the American Medical Association, 294,* 194–201.

Hematopoietic and Immunostimulant Drugs

LEARNING OBJECTIVES

After studying this chapter, you will be able to:

1. Describe the goals and methods of enhancing hematopoietic and immune functions.
2. Discuss the use of hematopoietic agents in the treatment of anemia.
3. Discuss the use of filgrastim and sargramostim in neutropenia and bone marrow transplantation.
4. Describe the adverse effects and nursing process implications of administering filgrastim and sargramostim.
5. Discuss interferons in terms of clinical uses, adverse effects, and nursing process implications.

Applying Your Knowledge

Alice Paul is a 76-year-old woman who is being treated with chemotherapy for inoperable liver cancer. She receives a combination chemotherapy regimen every 6 weeks. She is in the oncologist's office for her routine laboratory work 10 days after chemotherapy and complains of severe fatigue. The results of her blood work are:

Hemoglobin 10.9 g
Hematocrit 32%
WBC 2000
ANC 800
Platelet count 120,000

Introduction

Adequate blood cell production and development (*hematopoiesis*) and immune system function (immunocompetence) are vital processes in the human body's ability to fight harmful invaders. Inadequate or impaired hematopoiesis or immune function (immunodeficiency) leads to high risks for infection and cancer. Efforts to enhance a person's own body systems to fight disease include the development of drugs to stimulate hematopoiesis and immune function. Drugs that stimulate immune function are called immunostimulants, biologic response modifiers, and immunomodulators. These drugs are given to restore normal function or to increase the ability of the immune system to eliminate potentially harmful invaders. Drugs available for therapeutic use include hematopoietic *colony-stimulating factors* (CSFs; e.g., darbepoetin alfa, epoetin alfa, filgrastim, sargramostim), several interferons, and two interleukins. These drugs, which are the primary focus of this chapter, are described in the following sections and in Table 40-1.

Table 40-1 **Drugs at a Glance:** Hematopoietic and Immunostimulant Agents

GENERIC/TRADE NAME	INDICATIONS FOR USE	ROUTES AND DOSAGE RANGES
Hematopoietic Agents		
Darbepoetin alfa (Aranesp)	Anemia associated with chronic renal failure (CRF)	Sub-Q, IV 0.45 mcg/kg once weekly, adjusted to achieve and maintain hemoglobin level no greater than 12 g/dL
Epoetin alfa (Epogen, Procrit)	Prevention and treatment of anemia associated with CRF or anticancer chemotherapy Reduction of blood transfusions in anemic patients undergoing elective noncardiac, nonvascular surgery	*CRF:* IV, Sub-Q 50–100 units/kg 3 times weekly to achieve or maintain a hematocrit of 30%–36% *Cancer chemotherapy:* Sub-Q 150–300 units/kg 3 times weekly *Surgery:* Sub-Q 300 units/kg/d for 10 d before surgery, on the day of surgery, and for 4 d after surgery
Colony-Stimulating Factors (CSFs)		
Filgrastim (G-CSF) (Neupogen)	To prevent infection in patients with neutropenia induced by cancer chemotherapy or bone marrow transplantation To mobilize stem cells from bone marrow to peripheral blood, where they can be collected and reinfused after chemotherapy that depresses bone marrow function To treat severe chronic neutropenia	*Myelosuppressive chemotherapy:* Sub-Q injection, IV infusion over 15–30 min, or continuous Sub-Q or IV infusion 5 mg/kg/d, up to 2 wk until ANC reaches 10,000/mm³ *Bone marrow transplantation:* IV or Sub-Q infusion, 10 mcg/kg/d initially, then titrated according to neutrophil count (5 mcg/kg/d if ANC over 1000/mm³ for 3 consecutive days; stop drug if over 1000/mm³ for 6 d. If ANC drops below 1000/mm³, restart filgrastim at 5 mcg/kg/d). *Collection of peripheral stem cells:* Sub-Q 10 mcg/kg/d for 6–7 d, with collection on the last 3 d of drug administration *Severe, chronic neutropenia:* Sub-Q 5 or 6 mcg/kg, once or twice daily, depending on clinical response and ANC
Pegfilgrastim (Neulasta)	To prevent infection in patients with neutropenia induced by cancer chemotherapy	Sub-Q 6 mg once per chemotherapy cycle. Do not give between 14 d before and 24 h after cytotoxic chemotherapy.
Sargramostim (GM-CSF) (Leukine)	After bone marrow transplantation to promote bone marrow function or to treat graft failure or delayed function Mobilization of stem cells in peripheral blood so they can be collected	*Bone marrow reconstitution:* IV infusion over 2 h, 250 mcg/m²/d, starting 2–4 h after bone marrow infusion, and continuing for 21 d *Graft failure or delay:* IV infusion over 2 h, 250 mcg/m²/d, for 14 d Course of treatment may be repeated after 7 d off therapy if engraftment has not occurred. *Mobilization of stem cells:* Sub-Q or IV over 24 h, 250 mcg/m²/d
Interferons		
Interferon alfa-2a (Roferon-A)	Chronic hepatitis C in adults* Hairy cell leukemia in adults* AIDS-related Kaposi's sarcoma in adults* Chronic myelogenous leukemia	*Hepatitis C:* Sub-Q, IM 3 million IU 3 times weekly for 12 mo *Hairy cell leukemia:* Sub-Q, IM Induction, 3 million IU daily for 16–24 wk Maintenance, 3 million IU 3 times weekly *Kaposi's sarcoma:* Sub-Q, IM

GENERIC/TRADE NAME	INDICATIONS FOR USE	ROUTES AND DOSAGE RANGES
		Induction, 36 million IU daily for 10–12 wk Maintenance, 36 million IU 3 times weekly *Chronic myelogenous leukemia (CML):* Sub-Q, IM 9 million IU daily
Peginterferon alfa-2a (Pegasys)	Chronic hepatitis B	Sub-Q, 180 mcg (1 mL) once weekly for 48 wk
	Chronic hepatitis C, with ribavirin	Sub-Q, 180 mcg once weekly for 24 wk for viral genotypes 2 and 3; for 48 wk for viral strains 1 and 4
Interferon alfa-2b (Intron A)	Hairy cell leukemia in adults* AIDS-related Kaposi's sarcoma in adults* Condylomata (genital warts) Chronic hepatitis B Chronic hepatitis C, alone or with ribavirin Malignant melanoma, after surgical excision, to delay recurrence and prolong survival Non-Hodgkin's lymphoma	*Hairy cell leukemia:* Sub-Q, IM Induction and maintenance, 2 million IU/m^2 3 times weekly up to 6 mo *Kaposi's sarcoma:* Sub-Q, IM Induction and maintenance, 30 million IU/m^2 3 times weekly *Hepatitis B:* Sub-Q, IM 5 million IU daily or 10 million IU 3 times weekly (total of 30–35 million IU per wk) for 16 wk *Hepatitis C:* Sub-Q, IM 3 million IU 3 times weekly for 16 wk–24 mo *Malignant melanoma:* induction IV, 20 million IU/m^2 on 5 consecutive d per week for 4 wk; maintenance, Sub-Q 10 million IU/m^2 3 times per week for 48 wk *Condylomata:* intralesionally 1 million IU/lesion (maximum of 5 lesions) 3 times weekly for 3 wk
Peginterferon alfa-2b (PEG-Intron)	Chronic hepatitis C, alone or with ribavirin	Sub-Q 1 mcg once weekly for 1 y
Interferon alfacon-1 (Infergen)	Chronic hepatitis C in adults*	Sub-Q 9 mcg 3 times weekly for 24 wk, with at least 48 h between doses
Interferon beta-1a (Avonex, Rebif)	Multiple sclerosis, to reduce frequency of exacerbations	*Avonex:* IM 30 mcg once per week *Rebif:* Sub-Q 8.8 mcg for 2 wk, then 22 mcg for 2 wk, then 44 mcg. Give all doses three times weekly, with at least 48 h between doses.
Interferon beta-1b (Betaseron)	Same as interferon beta-1a	Sub-Q 0.25 mg every other day
Interferon gamma-1b (Actimmune)	Reducing frequency and severity of serious infections associated with granulomatous disease	Sub-Q 50 mcg/m^2 if body surface area (BSA) is over 0.5 m^2; 1.5 mcg/kg if BSA is under 0.5 m^2, 3 times weekly
Vaccine Bacillus Calmette-Guérin (TICE BCG, TheraCys)	Bladder cancer	Intravesical instillation by urinary catheter, three vials, reconstituted according to manufacturer's instructions, then diluted further in 50 mL of sterile, preservative-free saline solution (total volume per dose, 53 mL). Repeat once weekly for 6 wk, then give one dose monthly for 6–12 mo (TICE BCG) or one dose at 3, 6, 12, 18, and 24 mo (TheraCys).

*18 y of age and older.

AIDS, acquired immunodeficiency syndrome; ANC, absolute neutrophil count; IV, international units.

Bacillus Calmette-Guérin (BCG) vaccine, used in the treatment of bladder cancer, is also discussed. Other drugs with immunostimulant properties are discussed in other chapters. These include traditional immunizing agents (see Chap. 39); levamisole (Ergamisol), which restores functions of macrophages and T cells and is used with fluorouracil in the treatment of intestinal cancer (see Chap. 42); and antiviral drugs used in the treatment of acquired immunodeficiency syndrome (AIDS) (see Chap. 35). Levamisole and antiviral drugs are more accurately called immunorestoratives because they help a compromised immune system regain normal function rather than stimulating "supranormal" function. In AIDS, the human immunodeficiency virus (HIV) causes severe immune system dysfunction, so the antiviral drugs indirectly improve immunologic function.

General Characteristics of Hematopoietic and Immunostimulant Drugs

■ Most hematopoietic and *immunostimulant* drugs are synthetic versions of endogenous cytokines (see Chap. 38). Techniques of molecular biology are used to delineate the type and sequence of amino acids and to identify the genes responsible for producing the substances. These genes are then inserted into bacteria (usually *Escherichia coli*) or yeasts capable of producing the substances exogenously.

■ Exogenous drug preparations have the same mechanisms of action as the endogenous products. Thus, CSFs bind to receptors on the cell surfaces of immature blood cells in the bone marrow and increase the number, maturity, and functional ability of the cells. Interferons, called alfa, beta, or gamma according to specific characteristics, also bind to specific cell-surface receptors and alter intracellular activities. In viral infections, they induce enzymes that inhibit protein synthesis and degrade viral ribonucleic acid. As a result, viruses are less able to enter uninfected cells, reproduce, and release new viruses.

In addition to their antiviral effects, interferons also have antiproliferative and immunoregulatory activities. They can increase expression of major histocompatibility complex (MHC) molecules, augment the activity of natural killer (NK) cells, increase the effectiveness of antigen-presenting cells in inducing the proliferation of cytotoxic T cells, aid the attachment of cytotoxic T cells to target cells, and inhibit angiogenesis (formation of blood vessels). Because of these characteristics, the interferons are used mainly to treat viral infections and cancers.

■ In cancer, the exact mechanisms by which interferons and interleukins exert antineoplastic effects are unknown. However, their immunostimulant effects are thought to enhance activities of immune cells (i.e., NK cells, T cells, B cells, and macrophages), induce tumor-cell antigens (which make tumor cells more easily recognized by immune cells), or alter the expression of oncogenes (genes that can cause a normal cell to change to a cancer cell). BCG vaccine is thought to act against cancer of the urinary bladder by stimulating the immune system and eliciting a local inflammatory response, but its exact mechanism of action is unknown.

■ Exogenous cytokines are given by subcutaneous (Sub-Q) or intravenous (IV) injection because they are proteins that would be destroyed by digestive enzymes if given orally. Darbepoetin alfa (Aranesp), epoetin alfa (Epogen, Procrit), filgrastim (Neupogen, Neulasta), and the interferons are often self- or caregiver-administered to ambulatory patients.

■ The drugs may produce adverse effects so that patients do not feel better when taking one of these drugs.

■ The combination of injections and adverse effects may lead to noncompliance in taking the drugs as prescribed.

■ All of the drugs are contraindicated for use in patients who have previously experienced hypersensitivity reactions to any component of the formulation.

Classifications and Individual Drugs

Hematopoietic Agents

Darbepoetin alfa (Aranesp) and **epoetin alfa** (Epogen, Procrit) are drug formulations of *erythropoietin*, a hormone from the kidney that stimulates bone marrow production of red blood cells. They are used to prevent or treat anemia associated with several conditions, including chronic renal failure and *myelosuppressive* anticancer chemotherapy (depresses bone marrow function). In chronic renal failure, epoetin has a serum half-life of 4 to 13 hours and produces detectable blood levels of erythropoietin within 24 hours with IV administration. With Sub-Q administration, peak serum levels occur within 5 to 24 hours and then decline slowly. Darbepoetin has a longer half-life (about 49 hours) in patients with chronic renal failure, and peak plasma levels occur in about 34 hours.

These erythropoiesis-stimulating drugs have been used to raise the hemoglobin and reduce the need for blood transfusions in many patients with anemia. However, studies indicated an increased risk of serious cardiovascular problems (e.g., hypertension, thromboembolic events) and death in patients with chronic renal failure and an increased risk of tumor progression and death in patients with cancer. These problems became evident when the drugs were used to achieve normal hemoglobin levels of 12 to 14 grams per deciliter. These results led the U.S. Food and Drug Administration (FDA) to issue a **BLACK BOX WARNING** advising prescribers to avoid using the drugs in patients with hemoglobin values of 12 grams per deciliter or above. In addition, when the drugs are used, they are prescribed at the lowest dose effective in raising hemoglobin levels just enough to avoid the need for blood transfusion, and hemoglobin levels are monitored regularly until they stabilize.

Colony-Stimulating Factors

Filgrastim (Neupogen) and **sargramostim** (Leukine) are drug formulations of granulocyte colony-stimulating factor (G-CSF) and granulocyte macrophage colony-stimulating factor (GM-CSF), respectively. They are used to stimulate blood cell production by the bone marrow in patients with bone marrow transplantation or chemotherapy-induced *neutropenia*. The drugs can reduce the incidence and severity of infections in neutropenic patients. G-CSF is also used to collect stem cells for transplantation, and GM-CSF is also used to promote growth of blood vessels (angiogenesis) in patients with ischemic heart disease. The drug apparently promotes growth of arterioles around blocked areas in coronary arteries. It may be more effective than drugs that stimulate capillary growth, because arterioles are larger and can carry more blood. Filgrastim is conjugated with polyethylene glycol, in a process called *pegylation*, to produce **pegfilgrastim** (Neulasta), a formulation that stays in the body longer and can be given less often than filgrastim. *When used to stimulate blood cell production, the drugs should be stopped when blood cell counts normalize.*

Interferons

Interferons alfa-2a and **alfa-2b**, structurally the same except for one amino acid, are used to treat hairy-cell leukemia (a type of B-cell leukemia in which the cells are covered with fine, hairlike structures), Kaposi's sarcoma associated with AIDS, and chronic hepatitis. Interferon alfa-2b is also approved for the treatment of genital warts (condylomata) associated with infection by human papillomavirus, non-Hodgkins lymphoma, and malignant melanoma. In chronic hepatitis, interferon alfa-2a or 2b may be combined with ribavirin, another antiviral drug, to increase effectiveness. In condylomata, interferon alfa-2b is injected directly into the lesions for several weeks.

The older preparations of interferon alfa have been largely replaced by peginterferon alfa for some clinical uses. These are interferons that have been conjugated with polyethylene glycol. Pegylation changes the pharmacokinetics of interferons so that they act longer and can be given less often. Peginterferons also provide constant blood levels, whereas unpegylated interferons provide fluctuating levels.

Interferon alfa-n1 and **alfacon-1** are approved for treatment of chronic hepatitis C, a condition that can lead to liver failure and liver cancer. **Interferon gamma** is used to treat chronic granulomatous disease, which involves impaired phagocytosis of ingested microbes and frequent infections. Drug therapy reduces the incidence and severity of infections. **Interferon beta** is used for multiple sclerosis, an autoimmune neurologic disorder in which the drug slows progression of neurologic dysfunction, prolongs remissions, and reduces the severity of relapses.

Systemic interferons are usually well absorbed, widely distributed, and eliminated primarily by the kidneys. Although the main adverse effects are flu-like symptoms, alfa interferons may also cause or aggravate serious, life-threatening neuropsychiatric (including depression and some reports of suicide), autoimmune, ischemic, and infectious disorders. Patients receiving the drugs should be closely monitored with clinical and laboratory examinations, and the drugs should be discontinued if persistently severe or worsening signs or symptoms of these disorders occur. In many cases, these disorders resolve after stopping interferon alfa.

Interleukins

Aldesleukin (Proleukin) is a recombinant DNA version of interleukin-2 (IL-2). It activates cellular immunity; produces tumor necrosis factor, interleukin-1 (IL-1), and interferon gamma; and inhibits tumor growth. It is used to treat metastatic kidney cancer and metastatic melanoma skin cancer. The drug is highly toxic and is contraindicated in patients with pre-existing serious cardiovascular or pulmonary impairment. It is given only to hospitalized patients and should be prescribed and administered by health professionals (e.g., oncology nurses) who are experienced in its use. Because the drug is likely to be given by few nurses, details about administration and patient monitoring are omitted in this chapter.

Oprelvekin (Neumega) is recombinant IL-11, which stimulates platelet production. It is used to prevent thrombocytopenia and reduce the need for platelet transfusions in patients with cancer who are receiving myelosuppressive chemotherapy. However, its usefulness is limited because it is ineffective in severe thrombocytopenia and is highly toxic. Because of infrequent use, details about administration and patient monitoring are omitted in this chapter.

Bacillus Calmette-Guérin

Bacillus Calmette-Guérin vaccine is a suspension of weakened *Mycobacterium bovis*, long used as an immunizing agent against tuberculosis. The drug's immunostimulant properties stem from its ability to stimulate cell-mediated immunity. It is used as a topical agent to treat superficial cancers of the urinary bladder, in which approximately 80% of patients achieve a therapeutic response. BCG is contraindicated in immunosuppressed patients because the live tubercular organisms may cause tuberculosis in this high-risk population.

Nursing Process

Assessment

- Assess the patient's status in relation to conditions for which hematopoietic and immunostimulant drugs are used (e.g., infection, neutropenia, cancer).
- Assess nutritional status, including appetite and weight.
- Assess functional abilities in relation to activities of daily living (ADLs).
- Assess adequacy of support systems for outpatients (e.g., transportation for clinic visits).
- Assess ability and attitude toward planned drug therapy and associated monitoring and follow-up.

Nursing Process continues on page 648

- Assess coping mechanisms of patient and significant others in stressful situations.
- Assess patient for factors predisposing to infection (e.g., skin lesions, invasive devices, cigarette smoking).
- Assess environment for factors predisposing to infection (e.g., family or health care providers with infections).
- Assess baseline values of laboratory and other diagnostic test reports to aid monitoring of responses to hematopoietic and immunostimulant drug therapy.

Nursing Diagnoses

- Risk for Injury: Infection related to drug-induced neutropenia, immunosuppression, malnutrition, chronic disease; bleeding related to anemia or thrombocytopenia
- Risk for Injury: Adverse drug effects
- Activity Intolerance related to weakness, fatigue from debilitating disease, or drug therapy
- Anxiety related to the diagnosis of cancer, hepatitis, multiple sclerosis, or HIV infection
- Deficient Knowledge: Disease process; hematopoietic and immunostimulant drug therapy

Planning/Goals

The patient will

- Participate in interventions to prevent or decrease infection
- Remain afebrile during immunostimulant therapy
- Experience increased immunocompetence as indicated by increased white blood cell (WBC) count (if initially leukopenic) or tumor regression
- Avoid preventable infections
- Experience relief or reduction of disease symptoms
- Maintain independence in ADLs when able; be assisted appropriately when unable
- Maintain adequate levels of nutrition and fluids, rest and sleep, and exercise
- Maintain or increase appetite and weight if initially anorexic and underweight
- Learn to self-administer medications accurately when indicated

Interventions

- Practice and promote good hand hygiene techniques by patients and all others in contact with the patient.
- Use sterile technique for all injections, IV site care, wound dressing changes, and any other invasive diagnostic or therapeutic measures.
- Screen staff and visitors for signs and symptoms of infection; if infection is noted, do not allow contact with the patient.

- Allow patients to participate in self-care and decision making when feasible.
- Use isolation procedures when indicated, usually when the neutrophil count is less than 500/mm³.
- Promote adequate nutrition, with nutritious fluids, supplements, and snacks when indicated.
- Promote adequate rest, sleep, and exercise (e.g., schedule frequent rest periods, avoid interrupting sleep when possible, individualize exercise or activity according to the patient's condition).
- Inform patients about diagnostic test results, planned changes in therapeutic regimens, and evidence of progress.
- Allow family members or significant others to visit patients when feasible.
- Monitor complete blood count (CBC) and other diagnostic test reports for normal or abnormal values. **Note that darbepoetin and epoetin should be stopped when the hemoglobin level approaches 12 grams and filgrastim and sargramostim should be stopped when white blood cell counts normalize.** Report test results to prescribers when indicated.
- Schedule drug administration, diagnostic tests, and other elements of care to conserve patients' energy.
- Consult other health care providers (e.g., physician, dietitian, social worker) on the patient's behalf when indicated.
- Assist patients to learn ways to prevent or reduce the incidence of infections (e.g., meticulous personal hygiene, avoiding contact with infected people).
- Assist patients to learn ways to enhance immune mechanisms and other body defenses by healthy lifestyle habits, such as a nutritious diet, adequate rest and sleep, and avoidance of tobacco and alcohol.
- Assist patients or caregivers in learning how to prepare and inject darbepoetin alfa, epoetin alfa, filgrastim, or an interferon, when indicated.

Evaluation

- Determine the number and type of infections that have occurred in neutropenic patients.
- Compare current CBC reports with baseline values for changes toward normal levels (e.g., WBC count 5000–10,000/mm³).
- Compare weight and nutritional status with baseline values for maintenance or improvement.
- Observe and interview for decreased numbers or severity of disease symptoms.
- Observe for increased energy and ability to participate in ADLs.
- Observe and interview outpatients regarding compliance with follow-up care.
- Observe and interview regarding the mental and emotional status of the patient and family members.

Patient Teaching Guidelines | Blood Cell and Immune System Stimulants

General Considerations

- Help your body maintain immune mechanisms and other defenses by healthy lifestyle habits, such as a nutritious diet, adequate rest and sleep, and avoidance of tobacco and alcohol.
- Practice meticulous personal hygiene and avoid people and circumstances in which you are exposed to infection.
- Keep appointments with health care providers for follow-up care, blood tests, and so forth.
- Inform any other physician, dentist, or health care provider about your condition and the medications you are taking.
- Several of these medications can be taken at home, even though they are taken by injection. If you are going to self-inject a medication at home, allow sufficient time to learn and practice the techniques under the supervision of a health care provider. Correct preparation and injection are necessary to increase beneficial effects and decrease adverse effects.
- With interferons, report the occurrence of depression or thoughts of suicide, dizziness, hives, itching, chest tightness, cough, difficulty breathing or wheezing, or visual problems. These symptoms may require that the drug be stopped or the dosage reduced. In addition, avoid pregnancy (use effective contraceptive methods), avoid prolonged exposure to sunlight, wear protective clothing, and use sunscreens.

Self- or Caregiver Administration

- Take the drugs as prescribed. Although this is important with all medications, it is especially important with these. Obtaining beneficial effects and decreasing adverse effects depend to a great extent on how the drugs are taken.
- Use correct techniques to prepare and inject the medications. Instructions for mixing the drugs should be followed exactly.
  - With interferons:
  - Store in the refrigerator.
  - Do not freeze or shake the drug vial.
  - Do not change brands (changes in dosage may result).
  - Take at bedtime to reduce some common adverse effects (e.g., flu-like symptoms such as fever, headache, fatigue, anorexia, nausea, and vomiting).
  - Take acetaminophen (e.g., Tylenol, others), if desired, to prevent or decrease fever and headache.
  - Maintain a fluid intake of 2 to 3 quarts daily.

Applying Your Knowledge 40-1

Mrs. Paul has a great risk for infection with her low WBC count and absolute neutrophil count. What should the nurse teach the patient about preventing infection?

Principles of Therapy

Drug Dosage

With darbepoetin and epoetin, dosage is adjusted to achieve and maintain a hemoglobin value of no more than 12 grams per deciliter (serious adverse effects may occur with values higher than 12 g/dL). Dosage should be reduced when the hemoglobin level approaches 12 grams per deciliter or increases by more than 1 gram per deciliter in any 2-week period. With interferons, optimal dosages have not been established. For patients who experience severe adverse reactions with interferon alfa, dosage should be reduced by 50% or administration stopped until the reaction subsides.

Laboratory Monitoring

With darbepoetin and epoetin, iron stores (transferrin saturation and serum ferritin) should be measured before and periodically during treatment. Hemoglobin should be measured twice weekly until stabilized and maintenance drug doses are established.

With most of the hematopoietic and immunostimulant drugs, a CBC with WBC differential and platelet count should be done before and during treatment to monitor response and prevent avoidable adverse reactions. With CSF, these tests are recommended twice weekly during drug administration. With interferons alfacon-1 and alfa-n1, tests of platelet and neutrophil counts, hemoglobin, serum creatinine, serum albumin, and thyroid-stimulating hormone are recommended for all patients before starting therapy, 2 weeks later, and periodically thereafter during the 24 weeks of therapy.

Use in Special Populations

Use in Patients With Cancer

Hematopoietic Agents

Darbepoetin and epoetin are often used to prevent or treat anemia in patients with cancer. Studies indicate that patients with cancer-related anemia and a hemoglobin of 10 grams per deciliter or less feel better and require fewer blood transfusions with use of the drugs. An adequate intake of iron is required for drug effectiveness and an iron supplement is usually necessary.

Despite the benefits, evidence indicates that these agents may stimulate tumor growth, mainly when the drugs are used to achieve normal hemoglobin levels of 12 to 14 grams per deciliter. As a result, prescribers are warned to avoid dosages that increase hemoglobin to above 12 grams per deciliter. In addition, because cancer-related anemia may have numerous causes, some authorities recommend a return to the original indication for use of these drugs in cancer, that is, for anemia induced by chemotherapy that depresses bone marrow function.

Colony-Stimulating Factors

Filgrastim, pegfilgrastim, and sargramostim are used to restore, promote, or accelerate bone marrow function in patients with cancer who are undergoing chemotherapy or bone marrow transplantation. With chemotherapy, many drugs cause bone marrow depression and result in anemia and neutropenia. Neutropenic patients are at high risk for bacterial, fungal and viral infections, which often stem from the normal microbial flora of the patient's body or environmental microorganisms. The patient is most vulnerable to infection when the neutrophil count falls below 500/mm^3. Filgrastim and pegfilgrastim help to prevent infection by reducing the incidence, severity, and duration of neutropenia associated with several chemotherapy regimens. Most patients taking these drugs have fewer days of fever, infection, and antimicrobial drug therapy. In addition, by promoting bone marrow recovery after a course of cytotoxic antineoplastic drugs, the drugs also may allow higher doses or more timely administration of subsequent antitumor drugs.

When filgrastim is given to prevent infection in neutropenic patients with cancer, the drug should be started at least 24 hours after the last dose of the antineoplastic agent and continued during the period of bone marrow suppression and recovery. CBC and platelet counts should be performed twice weekly during therapy, and the drug should be stopped if the neutrophil count exceeds 10,000/mm^3. Pegfilgrastim should not be given between 14 days before and 24 hours after cytotoxic chemotherapy.

When sargramostim is given to patients with cancer who have had bone marrow transplantation, the drug should be started 2 to 4 hours after the bone marrow infusion and at least 24 hours after the last dose of antineoplastic chemotherapy or 12 hours after the last radiotherapy treatment. CBC should be done twice weekly during therapy, and the neutrophil count should not exceed approximately 20,000/mm^3.

 Applying Your Knowledge 40-2

How Can You Avoid This Medication Error?
Mrs. Paul is having her blood work done 10 days before chemotherapy. The nurse administers pegfilgrastim for the low WBC according to the standing orders for a WBC below 5000. What should the nurse have taken into account before giving the injection?

Interferons

Interferon alfa has demonstrated antitumor effects in multiple myeloma, renal cell carcinoma, and others. In chronic myelogenous leukemia (CML), 70% response rates have been reported, and some patients undergo complete remission. Common solid tumors of the breast, lung, and colon are unresponsive.

In hairy-cell leukemia, interferons normalize WBC counts in 70% to 90% of patients. Drug therapy must be continued indefinitely to avoid relapse, which usually develops rapidly after the drug is discontinued. In AIDS-related Kaposi's sarcoma, larger doses are required than in other clinical uses, with resultant increases in toxicity. Interferon alfa is recommended for patients with CD4 cell counts higher than 200 per milliliter (CD4 cells are the helper T cells attacked by the AIDS virus), who have no systemic symptoms, and who have had no opportunistic infections. Approximately 40% of these patients achieve a therapeutic response that lasts 1 to 2 years. In addition to antineoplastic effects, data indicate that viral replication is suppressed in responding patients.

Bacillus Calmette-Guérin Vaccine

Bacillus Calmette-Guérin, when instilled into the urinary bladder of patients with superficial bladder cancer, causes remission in up to 82% of patients for an average of 4 years. Early, successful treatment of carcinoma in situ also prevents development of invasive bladder cancer. A specific protocol has been developed for administration of BCG solution, and it should be followed exactly.

Applying Your Knowledge 40-3

Epoetin alfa is prescribed for Mrs. Paul's anemia. What dietary consideration should the nurse be aware of?

Use in Patients Undergoing Bone Marrow and Stem Cell Transplantation

Filgrastim, pegfilgrastim, and sargramostim are used to treat patients who undergo bone marrow transplantation for Hodgkin's disease, non-Hodgkin's lymphoma, or acute lymphoblastic leukemia. Before receiving a bone marrow transplant, the patient's immune system is suppressed by anticancer drugs or irradiation. After transplantation, it takes 2 to 4 weeks for the engrafted bone marrow cells to mature and begin producing blood cells. During this time, the patient has virtually no functioning granulocytes and is at high risk for infection. Sargramostim promotes engraftment and function of the transplanted bone marrow, thereby decreasing risks of infection. If the graft is successful, the granulocyte count starts to rise in approximately 2 weeks. Sargramostim also is used to treat graft failure.

In stem cell transplantation, filgrastim or sargramostim is used to stimulate the movement of hematopoietic stem cells from the bone marrow to circulating blood, where they can be readily collected. Transplantation of large numbers of stem cells can lead to more rapid engraftment and recovery, with less risk of transplant failure and complications.

Use in Patients With Chronic Viral Hepatitis

Chronic hepatitis B and hepatitis C (see Chap. 35) may lead to liver failure (and a need for liver transplantation) or liver cancer. Hepatitis B becomes chronic in 5% to 10% of patients. Interferon alfa and lamivudine or other antiviral drugs may be used for treatment. Drug resistance may develop and active hepatitis may resume when the drugs are discontinued.

Hepatitis C most often affects young adults, 20 to 39 years old, although it may affect people of any age. It can remain asymptomatic for years, but 70% to 80% of infected people eventually develop chronic liver disease. Hepatitis C may be treated with a combination of an interferon (alfa-2b, pegylated alfa-2b, alfacon-1, or pegylated alfa-2a) and ribavirin; interferon monotherapy is used only when there are specific reasons not to use ribavirin. The current drug therapy of choice is peginterferon alfa-2a and ribavirin. Because peginterferon can be given once per week and maintains constant blood levels, it has largely replaced other interferons for both monotherapy and combination therapy for hepatitis C. The duration of drug therapy is determined by the particular strain of the causative virus. Genotypes 2 and 3 are more responsive and require 24 weeks of drug therapy, whereas genotypes 1 and 4 require 48 weeks.

Use in Children

There has been limited experience with hematopoietic and immunostimulant drugs in children (younger than 18 years of age), and the drugs' safety and effectiveness have not been established. Filgrastim and sargramostim have been used in children with therapeutic and adverse effects similar to those in adults. In clinical trials, filgrastim produced a greater incidence of subclinical spleen enlargement in children than in adults, but whether this affects growth and development or has other long-term consequences is unknown.

Little information is available about the use of interferons in children. Interferon alfa-2b may be used to treat chronic hepatitis B in children. It is given Sub-Q in doses of 3 million units per/m^2 three times per week for the first week, then 6 million units/m^2 three times per week for 16 to 24 weeks. Dosage should be reduced by 50% or the drug discontinued if serious adverse effects or laboratory abnormalities develop.

Use in Older Adults

In general, hematopoietic and immunostimulant agents have the same uses and responses in older adults as in younger adults. Older adults may be at greater risk of adverse effects, especially if large doses are used.

Use in Patients With Renal Impairment

Except for darbepoetin and epoetin, which are used to treat anemia in patients with chronic renal failure, little information is available about the use of hematopoietic and immunostimulant drugs in patients with renal impairment. In some patients with pre-existing renal impairment, sargramostim increased serum creatinine. Values declined to baseline levels when the drug was stopped or its dosage reduced. Renal function tests are recommended every 2 weeks in patients with pre-existing impairment.

Use in Patients With Hepatic Impairment

In some patients with pre-existing hepatic impairment, sargramostim increased serum bilirubin and liver enzymes. Values declined to baseline levels when the drug was stopped or its dosage reduced. Liver function tests are recommended every 2 weeks in patients with pre-existing impairment.

Interferons may aggravate hepatic impairment. Interferons alfa-2b, alfacon-1, and alfa-n1 are contraindicated in patients with signs and symptoms of liver disease (e.g., jaundice, ascites, bleeding disorders, or decreased serum albumin), autoimmune hepatitis, a history of autoimmune disease, or posttransplantation immunosuppression. Worsening of liver disease, with jaundice, hepatic encephalopathy, hepatic failure, and death, has occurred in these patients. The drugs should be discontinued in patients with signs and symptoms of liver failure.

Use in Home Care

Darbepoetin, epoetin, filgrastim, pegfilgrastim, and the interferons are often self-administered or given by a caregiver to chronically ill patients. The home care nurse may need to teach patients or caregivers accurate drug preparation and injection techniques as well as proper disposal of needles and syringes. Assistance may also be needed in obtaining appropriate laboratory tests (e.g., CBC, platelet count, tests of renal or hepatic function) to monitor patients' responses to the medications. Other interventions depend on the drug being taken. For example, epoetin is not effective unless sufficient iron is present, and most patients need an iron supplement. When an iron preparation is prescribed, the home care nurse may need to emphasize the importance of taking it. With filgrastim, the nurse may need to help the patient and family with techniques to reduce exposure to infection.

Nursing Actions — Hematopoietic and Immunostimulant Agents

NURSING ACTIONS	RATIONALE/EXPLANATION

1. Administer accurately
  a. Give darbepoetin intravenously (IV) or subcutaneously (Sub-Q) once weekly; omit the dose if the hemoglobin level is above 12 g/dL.
  b. Give epoetin IV or Sub-Q; do not shake the vial; and discard any remainder of multidose vials 21 days after opening. Omit the dose if the hemoglobin level is above 12g/dL.
	The drugs are preferably prepared in a pharmacy. When nurses or patients prepare the drugs, they should consult the manufacturer's instructions.
	
	Outpatients may be taught self-administration.

(continued on page 652)

Nursing Actions Hematopoietic and Immunostimulant Agents (continued)

NURSING ACTIONS	RATIONALE/EXPLANATION
	For patients with chronic renal failure on hemodialysis, epoetin can be given by bolus injection at the end of dialysis. For other patients with an IV line, the drug can be given IV. For patients without an IV line or who are ambulatory, the drug is injected Sub-Q.
	Shaking can inactivate the medication; the manufacturer does not ensure sterility or stability of multidose vials after 21 days.
c. Give filgrastim (Neupogen) according to indication for use: (1) With cancer chemotherapy, give by Sub-Q bolus injection, IV infusion over 15–30 minutes, or continuous Sub-Q or IV infusion. (2) For bone marrow transplantation, give by IV infusion over 4 hours or by continuous IV or Sub-Q infusion. (3) For collection of stem cells, give as a bolus or a continuous infusion. (4) For chronic neutropenia, give Sub-Q.	Manufacturer's recommendation
d. Give pegfilgrastim (Neulasta) Sub-Q only.	Manufacturer's recommendation
e. Give sargramostim by IV infusion over 2 hours, after reconstitution with 1 mL sterile water for injection and addition to 0.9% sodium chloride.	
f. With interferons: (1) Read drug labels carefully to ensure having the correct drug preparation. (2) Give most interferons Sub-Q, 3 times weekly, on a regular schedule (e.g., Mon., Wed., and Fri.), at about the same time of day, at least 48 hours apart. (3) Inject interferon for condylomata intralesionally into the base of each wart with a small-gauge needle. For large warts, inject at several points.	Available drugs have similar names but often differ in indications for use, dosages, and routes of administration. Manufacturer's recommendation Manufacturer's recommendation
g. With intravesical bacillus Calmette-Guérin (BCG): (1) Reconstitute solution (see Table 40-1). (2) Wear gown and gloves. (3) Insert a sterile urethral catheter and drain bladder. (4) Instill medication slowly by gravity. (5) Remove catheter. (6) Have the patient lie on abdomen, back, and alternate sides for 15 min in each position. Then, allow to ambulate but ask to retain solution for a total of 2 hours before urinating, if able. (7) Dispose of all equipment in contact with BCG solution appropriately. (8) Do not give if catheterization causes trauma (e.g., bleeding), and wait 1 week before a repeat attempt.	Reconstituted solution should be used immediately or refrigerated. Discard if not used within 2 hours. BCG contains live mycobacterial organisms and is infectious.
2. Observe for therapeutic effects a. With darbepoetin and epoetin, observe for increased red blood cells, hemoglobin, and hematocrit; increased energy and exercise capacity; improved quality of life. b. With parenteral interferons, observe for improvement in signs and symptoms.	Therapeutic effects depend on the dose and the patient's underlying condition. The goal is usually to achieve and maintain a hemoglobin of no more than 12 g/dL. With hairy-cell leukemia, hematologic tests may improve within 2 months, but optimal effects may require 6 months of drug therapy. With Kaposi's sarcoma, skin lesions may resolve or stabilize over several weeks. With chronic hepatitis, liver function tests may improve within a few weeks.
c. With intralesional interferon, observe for disappearance of genital warts.	Lesions usually disappear after several weeks of treatment.
3. Observe for adverse effects a. With darbepoetin and epoetin, observe for nausea, vomiting, diarrhea, arthralgias, hypertension, and other cardiovascular problems.	Hypertension commonly occurs. The drugs also increase risks of myocardial infarction and stroke, especially if they are used to achieve hemoglobin levels greater than 12 g/dL.

NURSING ACTIONS	RATIONALE/EXPLANATION
b. With filgrastim, observe for nausea, vomiting, diarrhea, mucositis, bone pain, and erythema at Sub-Q injection sites.	Bone pain occurs in approximately 25% of patients.
c. With pegfilgrastim, observe for bone pain, constipation, headache, muscle and joint pain, peripheral edema, and vomiting.	Bone pain occurs in approximately one-third to one-half of patients. Other effects occur in more than 10% of patients.
d. With sargramostim, observe for bone pain, fever, headache, muscle aches, generalized maculopapular skin rash, and fluid retention (peripheral edema, pleural effusion, pericardial effusion).	Pleural and pericardial effusions are more likely at doses greater than 20 mcg/kg/d. Adverse effects occur more often with sargramostim than filgrastim.
e. With interferons, observe for acute flu-like symptoms (e.g., fever, chills, fatigue, muscle aches, headache), nausea, vomiting, diarrhea, tissue damage at injection sites, chronic fatigue, depression, leukopenia, and increased liver enzymes. f. With intravesical BCG, assess for symptoms of bladder irritation (e.g., frequency, urgency, dysuria, hematuria) and systemic symptoms of fever, chills, and malaise.	Acute effects occur in most patients, increasing with higher doses and decreasing with continued drug administration. Injection site damage occurs with all the interferons but more commonly with interferon beta-1b and pegylated interferon alfa-2b. Fatigue and depression occur with long-term use. These effects occur in more than 50% of patients, usually starting a few hours after administration and lasting 2 to 3 days.
4. Observe for drug interactions a. Drugs that *increase* effects of sargramostim: (1) Corticosteroids, lithium	Note: No significant interactions have been reported with darbepoetin or epoetin. These drugs have myeloproliferative (bone-marrow stimulating) effects of their own, which may add to those of sargramostim.

Key Concepts

- A drug formulation of erythropoietin is given to increase red blood cells in patients with anemia associated with chronic renal failure or bone marrow–damaging anticancer drug therapy.
- Adverse effects of epoetin and darbepoetin include increased risks of hypertension, myocardial infarction, and stroke, especially when used to increase hemoglobin above 12 grams per deciliter.

- Filgrastim is used to increase white blood cells and decrease risks of infection in patients with or at high risk of severe neutropenia.
- Interferons are used mainly for viral hepatitis and certain types of cancer.
- Filgrastim and some interferons are conjugated with polyethylene glycol, in a process called pegylation, to prolong drug actions.

Review and Application Exercises

Short Answer Exercises

1. What are the hematopoietic, colony-stimulating cytokines, and how do they function in the body?

2. What are adverse effects of filgrastim and sargramostim, and how may they be prevented or minimized?

3. What are the clinical uses of pharmaceutical interferons?

4. What are the adverse effects of interferons, and how can they be prevented or minimized?

5. Describe the clinical uses of hematopoietic and immunostimulant drugs in the treatment of anemia, neutropenia, cancer, bone marrow transplantation, and chronic viral hepatitis.

NCLEX-Style Questions

6. The expected outcome of administering epoetin alfa (Epogen, Procrit) or darbepoetin alfa (Aranesp) to a patient with chronic renal failure is
   a. decreased bleeding
   b. increased WBC production
   c. increased RBC production
   d. improved renal function

7. The nurse who is administering epoetin alfa knows that most patients who take epoetin or darbepoetin also need to take
   a. iron
   b. potassium
   c. antacids
   d. analgesics

8. The nurse is caring for a patient who is undergoing chemotherapy for cancer. Filgrastim is ordered. The nurse explains to the patient that an expected outcome after the administration of filgrastim (Neupogen) is
   a. fewer infections
   b. decreased anemia
   c. longer life expectancy
   d. less nausea and vomiting

9. Interferon may be used to treat
   a. most types of cancer
   b. chronic hepatitis C
   c. flu-like symptoms
   d. mental depression

10. BCG for bladder cancer would be contraindicated for patients with a history of
    a. heart disease
    b. diabetes mellitus
    c. pulmonary fibrosis
    d. organ transplantation

Selected References

DiPiro, J. T., Talbert, R. L., Yee, G. C., Matzke, G. R., Wells, B. G., & Posey, L. M. (Eds.). (2005). *Pharmacotherapy: A pathophysiologic approach* (6th ed.). New York: McGraw-Hill.

Drug facts and comparisons. (Updated monthly). St. Louis, MO: Facts and Comparisons.

Kaushansky, K. (2006). Lineage-specific hematopoietic growth factors. *New England Journal of Medicine, 354,* 2034–2045.

Lacy, C. F., Armstrong, L. L., Goldman, M. P., & Lance, L. L. (2006). *Drug information handbook* (14th ed.). Hudson, OH: Lexi-Comp Inc.

McPhee, S. J., Papadakis, M. A., & Tierney, L. M., Jr. (2007). *Current medical diagnosis and treatment 2007.* New York: McGraw-Hill.

Porth, C. M. (2005). *Pathophysiology: Concepts of altered health states* (7th ed.). Philadelphia: Lippincott Williams & Wilkins.

Smeltzer, S. C., Bare, B. G., Hinkle, J. L., & Cheever, K. H. (Eds.). (2008). *Brunner & Suddarth's textbook of medical-surgical nursing* (11th ed.). Philadelphia: Lippincott Williams & Wilkins.

Susla, G. M., Suffredini, A. F., McAreavey, D., Solomon, M. A., Hoffman, W. D., & Nyquist, P. (2006). *The handbook of critical care drug therapy* (3rd ed.). Philadelphia: Lippincott Williams & Wilkins.

Immunosuppressants

LEARNING OBJECTIVES

After studying this chapter, you will be able to:

1. Describe characteristics and consequences of immunosuppression.
2. Discuss characteristics and uses of major immunosuppressant drugs in autoimmune disorders and organ transplantation.
3. Identify adverse effects of immunosuppressant drugs.
4. Discuss nursing interventions to decrease adverse effects of immunosuppressant drugs.
5. Teach patients, family members, and caregivers about safe and effective immunosuppressant drug therapy.
6. Assist patients and family members to identify potential sources of infection in the home care environment.

Applying Your Knowledge

Richard Kinney is a 58-year-old college administrator. He has had a long-standing history of hypertension that resulted in severe kidney damage. He required a kidney transplant 2 years ago. His current immunosuppressive drug regimen consists of prednisone, cyclosporine, sirolimus, and mycophenolate.

Introduction

Immunosuppressant drugs interfere with the production or function of immune cells and cytokines. The drugs are used to decrease an undesirable immune response.

The immune response is normally a protective mechanism (see Chap. 38) that helps the body defend itself against potentially harmful agents. However, disease processes develop when the immune system perceives normally harmless substances (e.g., allergens) or the person's own body tissues as harmful invaders and tries to eliminate them. This inappropriate activation of the immune response is a major factor in allergic and autoimmune disorders (e.g., rheumatoid arthritis [RA], Crohn's disease, psoriasis).

An appropriate but undesirable immune response occurs when foreign tissue is transplanted into the body. If the immune response is not suppressed, the body reacts as with other antigens and attempts to destroy the foreign tissue (*graft rejection reaction*). Although numerous advances have been made in *transplantation* technology, the immune response remains a major factor in determining the success or failure of transplantation.

Drugs used therapeutically as immunosuppressants comprise a diverse group, several of which also are used for other purposes. These include corticosteroids (see Chap. 23) and certain *cytotoxic* antineoplastic drugs (see Chap. 42). These drugs are discussed here in relation to their effects on the immune response. The drugs used to treat inflammatory autoimmune disorders or to prevent or treat transplant rejection reactions are the main focus of this chapter. These drugs are described in the following sections and in Table 41-1. To aid in the understanding of immunosuppressive drug therapy, selected inflammatory autoimmune disorders, tissue transplantation, and rejection reactions are described.

Autoimmune Disorders

Autoimmune disorders occur when a person's immune system loses its ability to differentiate between antigens on its own cells (called self-antigens or *autoantigens*) and antigens on foreign cells. As a result, an immune response is aroused against

host tissues. Autoantigens for some disorders have been identified as specific proteins and are found in affected tissues; in other disorders, the autoantigen is unknown. Even when the autoantigen is known, the mechanism by which it is altered to elicit an immune response is unclear. Potential mechanisms include genetic susceptibility and possible "triggering" events (e.g., tissue damage by microorganisms or trauma, similarities between autoantigens and foreign antigens). After an autoantigen is changed so that it is perceived as foreign or "nonself," the immune response may involve T lymphocytes in direct destruction of tissue, production of proinflammatory cytokines that

| **Table 41-1** | **Drugs at a Glance: Immunosuppressants** |

GENERIC/TRADE NAME	INDICATIONS FOR USE	ROUTES AND DOSAGE RANGES
Abatacept (Orencia)	Rheumatoid arthritis	IV, according to body weight, initially, at 2 and 4 wk after initial dose, then every 4 wk. Weight below 60 kg, 500 mg; 60–100 kg, 750 mg; above 100 kg, 1000 mg
Adalizumab (Humira)	Rheumatoid arthritis Crohn's disease	Sub-Q 40 mg every other week
Alefacept (Amevive)	Psoriasis	IM 15 mg once weekly for 12 wk; IV 7.5 mg once weekly for 12 wk
Anakinra (Kineret)	Rheumatoid arthritis	Sub-Q 100 mg once daily
Antithymocyte globulin (Atgam, equine; Thymoglobulin, rabbit) dasd	Atgam, prevent or treat renal transplant rejection; treat aplastic anemia Thymoglobulin, treat renal transplant rejection	Atgam, IV 15 mg/kg/d for 14 d, then every other day for 14 d (total of 21 doses) Thymoglobulin, IV 1.5 mg/kg/d for 7–14 d
Basiliximab (Simulect)	Prevent renal transplant rejection	*Adults:* IV 20 mg within 2 h before transplantation and 20 mg 4 d after transplantation (total of two doses) *Children (2–15 y):* IV 12 mg/m² up to a maximum of 20 mg for two doses as for adults
Cyclosporine (Sandimmune, Neoral)	Prevent rejection of solid organ (e.g., heart, kidney, liver) transplant Prevent and treat graft-versus-host disease in bone marrow/stem cell transplantation Psoriasis Rheumatoid arthritis	*Sandimmune:* PO 15 mg/kg 4–12 h before transplantation, then 15 mg/kg once daily for 1–2 wk, then decrease by 5% per week to a maintenance dose of 5–10 mg/kg/d; IV 5–6 mg/kg infused over 2–6 h *Neoral:* PO, the first dose in patients with new transplants is the same as the first oral dose of Sandimmune; later doses are titrated according to cyclosporine blood levels.
Daclizumab (Zenapax)	Prevent renal transplant rejection	IV 1 mg/kg over 15 min. First dose within 24 h before transplantation, then a dose every 14 d for four doses (total of five doses)
Efalizumab (Raptiva)	Psoriasis	Sub-Q 0.7 mg/kg initially, then 1 mg/kg once weekly
Etanercept (Enbrel)	Rheumatoid arthritis Psoriatic arthritis Ankylosing spondylitis Juvenile chronic arthritis	*Adults:* Sub-Q 25 mg twice weekly, 72–96 h apart *Children (4–17 y):* Sub-Q 0.4 mg/kg up to a maximum of 25 mg per dose, twice weekly, 72–96 h apart

GENERIC/TRADE NAME	INDICATIONS FOR USE	ROUTES AND DOSAGE RANGES
Infliximab (Remicade)	Crohn's disease Rheumatoid arthritis Psoriasis	IV infusion, 3–5 mg/kg initially, 2 and 6 wk later, then every 8 wk
Leflunomide (Arava)	Rheumatoid arthritis	PO 100 mg once daily for 3 d, then 20 mg once daily
Methotrexate (MTX) (Rheumatrex)	Severe rheumatoid arthritis unresponsive to other treatment Psoriasis	PO 7.5 mg/wk as single dose, or 2.5 mg q12h for 3 doses once weekly
Muromonab-CD3 (Orthoclone OKT3)	Treatment of renal, cardiac, and hepatic transplant rejection	IV 5 mg bolus injection once daily for 10–14 d
Mycophenolate mefetil (CellCept, Myfortic)	Prevent renal, cardiac, and hepatic transplant rejection	*Renal transplantation:* PO, IV 1 g twice daily *Cardiac and hepatic transplantation:* PO, IV 1.5 g twice daily *Extended-release tablets (Myfortic):* PO 720 mg twice daily
Omalizumab (Xolair)	Allergic asthma	Sub-Q variable, according to weight and serum IgE levels. See manufacturer's instructions.
Sirolimus (Rapamune)	Prevent renal transplant rejection	*Adults:* PO 6 mg as soon after transplantation as possible, then 2 mg daily *Children over 13 y:* PO 3 mg/m² as loading dose, then 1 mg/m² daily
Tacrolimus (Prograf)	Prevent heart, kidney, and liver transplant rejection	*Adults:* IV infusion, 25–50 mcg/kg/d, starting 6 h after transplantation or later, until the patient can tolerate oral drug PO 150–200 mcg/kg/d, in two divided doses q12h, with the first dose 8–12 h after stopping the IV infusion *Children:* IV 50–100 mcg/kg/d; PO 200–300 mcg/kg/d

IgE, immunoglobulin E.

attract and activate phagocytes, and stimulation of B lymphocytes to produce antibodies that lead to inflammation and tissue damage.

Knowledge about the roles of inflammatory cells and cytokines in the immunologic response to tissue injury has increased in recent years. One example involves tumor necrosis factor (TNF)-alpha, a cytokine that plays a major role in the response to infection. Functions of TNF include activation of monocytes, macrophages, and cytotoxic T cells; enhancement of natural killer (NK) cell functions; increased leukocyte movement into areas of tissue injury; increased phagocytosis by neutrophils; and stimulation of B and T lymphocytes. Despite beneficial effects of a "normal" amount of TNF, however, an excessive TNF response has been associated with the pathogenesis of *autoimmune disorders* such as RA and Crohn's disease.

In addition to the factors that activate an immune response, there are also factors that prevent the immune system from "turning off" the abnormal immune or inflammatory process. One of these factors may be an inadequate number of suppressor T cells, which are thought to be a subpopulation of helper or cytotoxic T cells. Another factor may be inadequate amounts of anti-inflammatory cytokines (e.g., interleukin [IL]-10).

In general, autoimmune disorders share inflammation as a major mechanism of tissue damage. Allergic asthma, Crohn's disease, psoriasis, psoriatic arthritis, and RA are inflammatory disorders that may be treated with immunosuppressant drugs.

Tissue and Organ Transplantation

Tissue and organ transplantation involves replacing diseased host tissue with healthy donor tissue. The goal of such treatment is to save or enhance the quality of the host's life. Skin and renal grafts are commonly performed; heart, liver, lung, pancreas, and bone marrow/stem cell transplantations are increasing. (Bone marrow cells from bone marrow aspiration can be used in transplants, but they have largely been replaced by hematopoietic stem cells mobilized from bone marrow into circulating blood, where they are easily retrieved.)

Although many factors affect graft survival, including the degree of matching between donor tissues and recipient tissues, drug-induced *immunosuppression* is a major part of transplantation protocols. The goal is to provide adequate immunosuppression. If immunosuppression is inadequate, graft rejection reactions occur with solid organ transplantation, and *graft-versus-host disease* (GVHD) occurs with bone marrow/stem cell transplantation. If immunosuppression is excessive, the patient develops serious infections and other adverse effects because the drug actions that slow the proliferation of activated lymphocytes also affect any rapidly dividing nonimmune cells. Serious complications can occur.

Rejection Reactions With Solid Organ Transplantation

A rejection reaction occurs when the host's immune system is stimulated to destroy the transplanted organ. The immune cells of the transplant recipient attach to the donor cells of the transplanted organ and react against the antigens of the donor organ. The rejection process involves T and B lymphocytes, antibodies, multiple cytokines, and inflammatory mediators. In general, T-cell activation and proliferation are more important in the rejection reaction than B-cell activation and formation of antibodies. Cytotoxic and helper T cells are activated; activated helper T cells stimulate B cells to produce antibodies and lead to a delayed hypersensitivity reaction. The antibodies injure the transplanted organ by activating complement, producing antigen–antibody complexes, or causing antibody-mediated tissue breakdown. This reaction can destroy the solid organ graft within 2 weeks if the recipient's immune system is inadequately suppressed by immunosuppressant drugs.

Rejection reactions are acute or chronic. Acute reactions may occur from 10 days to a few months after transplantation and mainly involve cellular immunity and proliferation of T lymphocytes. Characteristics include signs of organ failure and vasculitis lesions that often lead to arterial narrowing or obliteration. Treatment with immunosuppressant drugs is usually effective in ensuring short-term survival of the transplant but does not prevent chronic rejection. Chronic reactions occur after months or years of normal function, are caused by both cellular and humoral immunity, and do not respond to increased immunosuppressive drug therapy. Characteristics include fibrosis of blood vessels and progressive failure of the transplanted organ.

Rejection reactions produce general manifestations of inflammation and specific manifestations depending on the organ involved. With renal transplantation, for example, acute rejection reactions produce fever, flank tenderness over the graft organ site, and symptoms of renal failure (e.g., increased serum creatinine, decreased urine output, edema, weight gain, hypertension). Chronic rejection reactions are characterized by a gradual increase in serum creatinine levels over 4 to 6 months.

Bone Marrow/Stem Cell Transplantation and Graft-Versus-Host Disease

With bone marrow/stem cell transplantation, the donor cells mount an immune response (mainly by stimulating T lymphocytes) against antigens on the host's tissues, producing GVHD. Tissue damage is produced directly by the action of cytotoxic T cells or indirectly through the release of inflammatory mediators (e.g., complement) and cytokines (e.g., TNF-alpha and interleukins).

Acute GVHD occurs in 30% to 50% of patients, usually within 6 weeks. Signs and symptoms include delayed recovery of blood cell production in the bone marrow, skin rash, liver dysfunction (indicated by increased alkaline phosphatase, aminotransferases, and bilirubin), and diarrhea. The skin reaction is usually a pruritic maculopapular rash that begins on the palms and soles and may extend over the entire body. Liver involvement can lead to bleeding disorders and coma.

Chronic GVHD occurs when symptoms persist or occur 100 days or more after transplantation. It is characterized by abnormal humoral and cellular immunity, severe skin disorders, and liver disease. Chronic GVHD appears to be an autoimmune disorder in which activated T cells perceive self-antigens as foreign antigens.

Classifications and Individual Drugs

Drugs used as immunosuppressants are diverse agents with often overlapping mechanisms and sites of action (Fig. 41-1). Older drugs generally depress the immune system (i.e., are nonspecific and suppress the immune response to all antigens). This greatly increases risks of serious infections with bacteria, viruses, fungi, or protozoa during the immunosuppressed state. In addition, many immunosuppressant drugs slow the proliferation of activated lymphocytes and damage rapidly dividing nonimmune cells (e.g., mucosal cells, intestinal cells, bone marrow hematopoietic stem cells). As a result, serious, life-threatening complications can occur. For example, patients on long-term immunosuppressant drug therapy (e.g., with autoimmune disorders, organ transplantation) are at increased risk of serious infections, cancer (especially lymphoma), hypertension, and metabolic bone disease.

Extensive research has been done to develop drugs that modify the immune response (often called immunomodulators or biologic response modifiers). As a result, several drugs with more specific immunosuppressive actions are now available. Most are used in combination with older immunosuppressants for synergistic effects.

Immunosuppressants are discussed here as corticosteroids, cytotoxic antiproliferative agents, conventional antirejection agents, antibody preparations, cytokine inhibitors, and miscellaneous drugs. Indications for use and dosages of individual drugs are listed in Table 41-1; all of the drugs are contraindicated for people with hypersensitivity reactions to any component of the drug formulation.

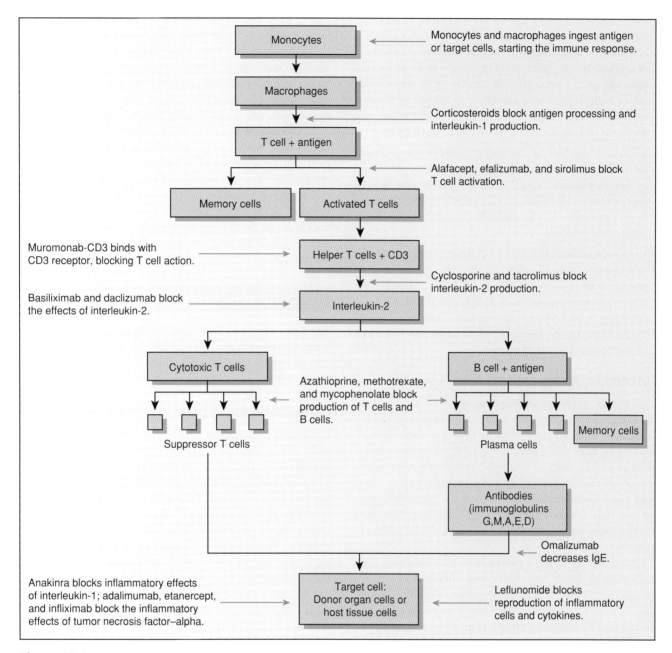

Figure 41-1 ■ Sites of action of immunosuppressant drugs. Available immunosuppressants inhibit the immune response by blocking that response at various sites.

Corticosteroids

Corticosteroids are potent anti-inflammatory drugs that suppress the immune response at multiple levels. In many disorders, they relieve signs and symptoms by decreasing the accumulation of lymphocytes and macrophages and the production of cell-damaging cytokines at sites of inflammatory reactions. Because inflammation is a common response to chemical mediators or antigens that cause tissue injury, the anti-inflammatory and immunosuppressive actions of corticosteroids often overlap and are indistinguishable. However, corticosteroid effects on the immune response are emphasized here. In general, the drugs suppress growth of all lymphoid tissue and therefore decrease formation and function of antibodies and T cells. For patients with autoimmune disorders, corticosteroids decrease inflammation but do not prevent tissue damage. For patients with transplanted tissues, a corticosteroid is usually given with other agents to prevent acute graft rejection. Specific effects include the following:

■ Increased numbers of circulating neutrophils (more are released from bone marrow and fewer leave the circulation to enter inflammatory exudates). In terms of neutrophil functions, corticosteroids increase chemotaxis and release of lysosomal enzymes.

- Decreased numbers of circulating basophils, eosinophils, and monocytes. The reduced availability of monocytes is considered a major factor in the anti-inflammatory activity of corticosteroids. Functions of monocyte–macrophages are also impaired. Corticosteroids suppress phagocytosis and initial antigen processing (necessary to initiate an immune response), impair migration to areas of tissue injury, and block the differentiation of monocytes to macrophages.

- Decreased numbers of circulating lymphocytes (immune cells), resulting from impaired production (i.e., inhibition of deoxyribonucleic acid [DNA], ribonucleic acid [RNA], and protein synthesis), sequestration in lymphoid tissues, or lysis of the cells. T cells are markedly reduced; B cells are moderately reduced.

- Impaired function of cellular (T-cell) and humoral (B-cell) immunity. Corticosteroids inhibit the production of immunostimulant cytokines (e.g., IL-1, IL-2) required for activation and expansion of lymphocytes and cytotoxic cytokines (e.g., TNF and interferons). When administered for 2 to 3 weeks, the drugs also reduce serum concentrations of immunoglobulins [Ig] G and A.

Cytotoxic, Antiproliferative Agents

Cytotoxic, antiproliferative drugs damage or kill cells that are able to reproduce, such as immunologically competent lymphocytes. These drugs are used primarily in cancer chemotherapy. However, in small doses, some also exhibit immunosuppressive activities and are used to treat autoimmune disorders and to prevent rejection reactions in organ transplantation. These drugs cause generalized suppression of the immune system and can kill lymphocytes and nonlymphoid proliferating cells (e.g., bone marrow blood cells, GI mucosal cells, germ cells in gonads).

Azathioprine is an antimetabolite that interferes with production of DNA and RNA and thus blocks cellular reproduction, growth, and development. Rapidly proliferating cells are most affected, including T and B lymphocytes, which normally reproduce rapidly in response to stimulation by an antigen. For many years, azathioprine was used to prevent rejection reactions to transplanted organs. However, it has largely been replaced by mycophenolate and is now rarely used for rheumatoid arthritis. Because of these declines in clinical uses, the drug is not discussed further in this chapter.

Methotrexate is a folate antagonist. It inhibits dihydrofolate reductase, the enzyme that converts dihydrofolate to the tetrahydrofolate required for biosynthesis of DNA and cell reproduction. The resultant DNA impairment inhibits production and function of immune cells, especially T cells. Methotrexate has long been used in the treatment of cancer. Other uses have evolved from its immunosuppressive effects, including treatment of autoimmune disorders (e.g., severe RA and psoriasis). It is also used (with cyclosporine) to prevent GVHD with bone marrow transplantation. Lower doses are given for these conditions than for cancers, and adverse drug

effects are fewer and less severe. CBC, platelet counts, and renal and liver function tests should be monitored.

Mycophenolate is used for prevention and treatment of rejection reactions with renal, cardiac, and hepatic transplantation. It inhibits proliferation and function of T and B lymphocytes. It has synergistic effects with corticosteroids and cyclosporine and is used in combination with these drugs.

After oral or intravenous administration, the drug is rapidly broken down to mycophenolic acid, the active component. Mycophenolic acid is further metabolized to inactive metabolites that are eliminated in bile and urine. Adverse effects include infection, neutropenia, and thrombocytopenia. For early detection of these effects, a CBC is recommended weekly during the first month, every 2 weeks during the second and third months, and monthly during the first year of drug administration.

Applying Your Knowledge 41-1

Mr. Kinney is prescribed mycophenolate. Related to the administration of mycophenolate, you should assess Mr. Kinney for what adverse effects?

Conventional Antirejection Agents

Cyclosporine, tacrolimus, and sirolimus are fungal metabolites with strong immunosuppressive effects. Cyclosporine and tacrolimus are chemically unrelated but have a similar action. They inhibit the synthesis of a cytokine, IL-2, which is required for activation of T cells and B cells. Sirolimus is structurally similar to tacrolimus. It inhibits T-cell activation and proliferation in response to several interleukins (e.g., IL-2, IL-4, IL-15). It also inhibits antibody production. Sirolimus and tacrolimus may have stronger immunosuppressant activity than cyclosporine.

By inhibiting helper–T-cell proliferation and cytokine expression, these three drugs reduce the activation of various cells involved in graft rejection, including cytotoxic T cells, NK cells, macrophages, and B cells. Consequently, they are widely used in heart, liver, kidney, and bone marrow transplantation.

Cyclosporine is used to prevent rejection reactions and prolong graft survival after solid organ transplantation (e.g., kidney, liver, heart, lung) or to treat chronic rejection in patients previously treated with other immunosuppressive agents. The drug inhibits both cellular and humoral immunity but affects T lymphocytes more than B lymphocytes. With T cells, cyclosporine reduces proliferation of helper and cytotoxic T cells and synthesis of several cytokines (e.g., IL-2, interferons). With B cells, cyclosporine reduces production and function to some extent, but considerable activity is retained.

Transplant rejection reactions mainly involve cellular immunity or T cells. With cyclosporine-induced deprivation of IL-2, T cells stimulated by the graft antigen do not undergo clonal expansion and differentiation, and graft destruction is inhibited. In addition to its use in solid organ transplantation, cyclosporine is used to prevent and treat GVHD, a complication of bone marrow transplantation. In GVHD, T lymphocytes from the transplanted marrow of the donor mount an immune response against the tissues of the recipient.

Cyclosporine is not well absorbed with oral administration. The drug is highly bound to plasma proteins, and approximately 50% is distributed in erythrocytes, so drug levels in whole blood are higher than those in plasma. Peak plasma levels occur 4 to 5 hours after a dose, and the elimination half-life is 10 to 27 hours. Cyclosporine is metabolized in the liver and excreted in bile; less than 10% is excreted unchanged in urine.

Because the drug is insoluble in water, other solvents are used in commercial formulations. Thus, it is prepared in alcohol and olive oil for oral administration and in alcohol and castor oil for IV administration. Anaphylactic reactions, attributed to the castor oil, have occurred with the IV formulation. Neoral is an oral formulation that is better absorbed than oral Sandimmune. The two formulations are not equivalent and cannot be used interchangeably.

Serum drug levels are used to regulate dosage and should be monitored closely. Subtherapeutic levels may lead to organ transplant rejection; high levels increase adverse effects. Nephrotoxicity is a major adverse effect. Acute nephrotoxicity may occur and progress to chronic nephrotoxicity and kidney failure. Renal function tests (serum creatinine, blood urea nitrogen) should be monitored throughout cyclosporine therapy. Liver function tests (bilirubin, aminotransferase enzymes) should also be done regularly to monitor for hepatotoxicity. In addition, many drugs interact with cyclosporine to increase or decrease its effects, both therapeutic and toxic.

Sirolimus is used to prevent renal transplant rejection. It inhibits T-cell activation and is given concomitantly with a corticosteroid and cyclosporine. It may have synergistic effects with cyclosporine because it has a different mechanism of action. However, the two drugs are metabolized by the same cytochrome P450 3A4 enzymes and cyclosporine increases blood levels of sirolimus, possibly to toxic levels. Consequently, the drugs should not be given at the same time; sirolimus should be taken 4 hours after a dose of cyclosporine.

Sirolimus is well absorbed with oral administration. Its action has a rapid onset and peaks within 1 hour. It has a long half-life of 62 hours. It is metabolized in the liver and excreted mainly in feces. Serum drug levels are monitored in patients who are likely to have altered drug metabolism (e.g., those 13 years and older who weigh less than 40 kg, those with impaired hepatic function, and those who also are receiving enzyme-inducing or inhibiting drugs).

Adverse effects include anemia, edema, hepatotoxicity, hypercholesterolemia, hypertension, infection, leukopenia, nephrotoxicity, and thrombocytopenia. Because of the high risk of infection, antimicrobial prophylaxis is recommended for cytomegalovirus (CMV) infection for 3 months and *Pneumocystis* pneumonia for 1 year after transplantation.

Tacrolimus is similar to cyclosporine in its mechanisms of action, pharmacokinetic characteristics, and adverse effects. It prevents rejection of transplanted organs by inhibiting proliferation of T lymphocytes. Many transplant centers now use tacrolimus rather than cyclosporine, mainly because cyclosporine is given with corticosteroids. Using tacrolimus may allow corticosteroids to be reduced or stopped, thereby decreasing the adverse effects of long-term corticosteroid therapy.

Tacrolimus is not well absorbed orally, so higher oral doses than IV doses must be given to obtain similar blood levels. With IV administration, action onset is rapid and peak action occurs in 1 to 2 hours; with oral administration, onset varies and peak action occurs in 1.5 to 3.5 hours. The drug is metabolized in the liver and intestine to several metabolites, which are excreted in bile and urine. It has a half-life of 6 hours. Impaired liver function may slow its metabolism and elimination.

Dosage varies according to clinical response, adverse effects, and blood concentrations. Serum drug levels are monitored, with therapeutic ranges of 10 to 20 nanograms per milliliter for 6 months after transplantation, then 5 to 15 nanograms per milliliter. Children metabolize tacrolimus more rapidly than adults and require higher doses (per kg of body weight) to maintain similar blood levels.

There are numerous potential drug interactions that increase or decrease blood levels and effects. Because tacrolimus is metabolized mainly by the cytochrome P450 enzymes that metabolize cyclosporine, drug interactions known to alter cyclosporine effects are likely to alter tacrolimus effects. For example, antacids and enzyme inducers (e.g., carbamazepine, phenytoin, rifampin) may reduce therapeutic effects, nephrotoxic drugs (e.g., amphotericin B, aminoglycoside antibiotics) may increase nephrotoxic effects, and enzyme inhibitors (e.g., erythromycin, fluconazole and related antifungals) may increase blood levels and toxic effects. Plasma drug levels and measurements of serum creatinine, potassium, and glucose are recommended to monitor for the adverse effects of nephrotoxicity, hyperkalemia, and hyperglycemia.

Antibody Preparations

Antibody (immunoglobulin) preparations are produced in the laboratory or derived from animals injected with human lymphoid tissue to stimulate an immune response. Such preparations are used in inflammatory autoimmune disorders, transplantation rejection reactions, and cancer.

The antibodies may be polyclonal or monoclonal. Polyclonal preparations are a mixture of antibodies (IgA, IgD, IgE,

IgG, IgM) produced by several clones of B lymphocytes. Each clone produces a structurally and functionally different antibody, even though the humoral immune response was induced by a single antigen. Monoclonal antibodies are produced in the laboratory by procedures that isolate and clone individual B lymphocytes, resulting in the production of identical antibody molecules. The antigen to which the desired antibody will respond is first injected into a mouse. The mouse mounts an immune response in which its B lymphocytes are stimulated to produce a specific antibody against that antigen. The B lymphocytes are then recovered from the spleen of the mouse and mixed with myeloma cells (a cell line that can live forever in culture) in polyethylene glycol. This treatment results in fusion of the cells and produces an antibody-secreting hybridoma, which can be cloned to produce large amounts of the desired antibody. The antibodies can be isolated from the culture and prepared for clinical use. Because the antibodies are proteins and would be destroyed if taken orally, they must be given by injection.

Older animal-derived antibodies (e.g., antithymocyte globulin, muromonab-CD3) are themselves antigenic; they usually elicit human antibodies against the animal cells within 2 weeks. Newer *murine* (mouse-derived) *antibodies* (e.g., basiliximab) have human antibodies added by recombinant DNA technology and are less likely to elicit an immune response. However, because the products are proteins, there is a risk of hypersensitivity reactions.

Because they are derived from one cell line or clone, monoclonal antibodies can be designed to suppress the specific components of the immune system that are causing tissue damage in particular disorders. They cause cell destruction by eliciting an antigen–antibody reaction, activating complement, targeting molecules on the cell surface that are necessary for growth or differentiation of that cell, or inhibiting proinflammatory cytokines.

Note that the generic names of monoclonal antibodies used as drugs end in "mab" and thus identify their origin.

Polyclonal Antibodies

Antithymocyte globulin (ATG) is a nonspecific immune globulin. ATG (equine: Atgam) obtained from horse serum is used to treat renal transplant rejection reactions and aplastic anemia in patients who are not considered candidates for bone marrow transplantation. ATG (rabbit: Thymoglobulin) is used to treat renal transplant rejection reactions. Both preparations have been issued **BLACK BOX WARNINGS** by the U.S. Food and Drug Administration (FDA) to restrict use to experienced prescribers.

ATG contains antibodies that destroy lymphoid tissues and decrease the number of circulating T cells, thereby suppressing cellular and humoral immune responses. In addition to its high concentration of antibodies against T lymphocytes, the preparation contains low concentrations of antibodies against other blood cells. With Atgam, a skin test is recommended before administration to determine whether the patient is allergic to horse serum. Because there is a high risk of anaphylactic reactions in recipients previously sensitized to horse serum, patients with positive skin tests should be desensitized before drug therapy is begun.

Monoclonal Antibodies

Alefacept (Amevive) and **efalizumab** (Raptiva) are monoclonal antibodies used to treat moderate to severe psoriasis. Psoriasis involves activated T lymphocytes that secrete inflammatory mediators. The drugs bind to receptors on the surface of T lymphocytes, inhibit the receptors from interacting with particular antigens, and thereby inhibit activation of T lymphocytes.

Alefacept is given IM or IV, usually once weekly for 12 weeks. Its half-life after IV administration is about 10 days. Common adverse effects include lymphopenia and injection-site reactions (e.g., edema, inflammation, pain). Efalizumab is given subcutaneously (Sub-Q) once weekly for 12 weeks. It reaches steady-state concentration in 4 weeks and is excreted over 3 weeks. Common adverse effects include headache, infection, lymphocytosis, and a first-dose reaction characterized by chills, fever, muscle aches, and nausea.

Basiliximab (Simulect) and **daclizumab** (Zenapax) are humanized IgE (i.e., a combination of human and mouse-derived antibodies). They are called IL-2 receptor antagonists because they bind to IL-2 receptors on the surface of activated lymphocytes. This action inhibits the ability of IL-2 to stimulate proliferation and cytokine production of lymphocytes, a critical component of the cellular immune response involved in rejection reactions. The drugs are used to prevent organ rejection in patients receiving renal transplants and are given in combination with cyclosporine and a corticosteroid.

Basiliximab is given IV and its effects last an average of 36 days. Its elimination half-life is about 7 days in adults, 9 days in children. Daclizumab is also given IV and its elimination half-life is about 20 days in adults, 13 days in children. Common adverse effects include constipation, diarrhea, edema, fever, headache, hypertension, infection, nausea, and vomiting.

Muromonab-CD3 (Orthoclone OKT3) is a *monoclonal antibody* that acts against an antigenic receptor called CD3, which is found on the surface membrane of most T cells in blood and body tissues. CD indicates clusters of differentiation or groups of cells with the same surface markers (antigenic receptors). The CD3 molecule is associated with the antigen recognition structure of T cells and is essential for T-cell activation. Muromonab-CD3 binds with its antigen (CD3) and therefore blocks all known functions of T cells containing the CD3 molecule. Because rejection reactions are mainly T-cell–mediated immune responses against antigenic (nonself) tissues, the drug's ability to suppress such reactions accounts for its therapeutic effects in treating renal, cardiac, and hepatic transplant rejection. It is usually given for 10 to 14 days. After treatment, CD3-positive T cells reappear rapidly and reach pretreatment levels within 1 week. The drug's name is derived from its source (murine or mouse cells) and its action (monoclonal antibody against the CD3 antigen). Because the drug is a protein and induces antibodies in most patients, decreased effectiveness and serious allergic reactions may occur if it is readministered later. Second courses of treatment must be undertaken cautiously.

Omalizumab (Xolair) is a humanized monoclonal antibody used to treat allergic asthma that is not relieved by inhaled corticosteroids. Allergic asthma is thought to be caused mainly by IgE. When stimulated by an allergen, IgE combines with a receptor on mast cells and basophils and causes the release of allergic and proinflammatory mediators. Omalizumab binds with the IgE and reduces the amount of IgE free to bind to the receptors on mast cells and basophils. This action inhibits IgE-induced tissue injury.

Omalizumab is given Sub-Q and slowly absorbed. Peak concentration is reached in about 1 week, and it has a half-life of 3 to 4 weeks. It is metabolized in the liver. Dosage and frequency of administration are determined by body weight and serum IgE level, which should be measured before the start of treatment and periodically during treatment. Common adverse effects include injection-site reactions and infections (e.g., viral, upper respiratory tract, pharyngitis, sinusitis). However, a **BLACK BOX WARNING** about the risk of anaphylaxis was added to drug literature in 2007. Reportedly, patients may develop anaphylaxis after any dose of the drug and as long as 24 hours after a dose is given. Health care providers should have medications and other supplies available for treatment of anaphylaxis, should observe patients for at least 2 hours after an injection, and should teach patients how to self-administer emergency treatment.

Cytokine Inhibitors

Two major cytokines in chronic, inflammatory autoimmune disorders are IL-1 and TNF-alpha. This knowledge led to the development of biologic agents directed against these cytokines. The cytokine inhibitors used as drugs (some of which are monoclonal antibodies, such as basiliximab and daclizumab) inhibit one of these cytokines to suppress inflammation and promote tissue repair in disorders such as RA, Crohn's disease, and psoriasis.

Cytokine inhibitors can greatly improve signs and symptoms of arthritis, Crohn's disease, and psoriasis. Despite their therapeutic effects, however, cytokine inhibitors also increase the risks of serious infections, especially the TNF-alpha inhibitors. A wide range of infections has occurred, including tuberculosis characterized by increased extrapulmonary and/or disseminated disease. Other serious infections include pneumococcal infections, necrotizing fasciitis, *Pneumocystis* pneumonia, and systemic fungal infections such as aspergillosis and cryptococcosis.

Interleukin Blocking Agent

Anakinra (Kineret) is a recombinant interleukin-receptor antagonist. It binds to the IL-1 receptor and thereby blocks the inflammatory effects of IL-1. It is used to treat moderate to severe RA in adults. It may be used alone or in combination with other disease-modifying antirheumatic drugs (except TNF blocking agents).

Anakinra is well absorbed with Sub-Q injection and reaches its peak concentration in 3 to 7 hours. Its elimination half-life is 4 to 6 hours. Common adverse effects include headache, injection-site reactions (redness, bruising, inflammation, pain), infection, nausea, diarrhea, decreased WBCs, sinusitis, and flulike symptoms.

Tumor Necrosis Factor–Alpha Blocking Agents

Adalimumab (Humira) is a recombinant monoclonal antibody that binds to TNF-alpha receptor sites and prevents endogenous TNF-alpha from binding to the sites and exerting its injurious effects. The drug is used to treat moderate to severe RA. In RA, the drug reduces the elevated levels of TNF-alpha in synovial fluid that are thought responsible for pain and joint destruction.

Adalimumab is given Sub-Q, peak serum concentration occurs within 2 to 5 days, and its elimination half-life is about 2 weeks. Excretion is decreased in patients over 40 years of age. Common adverse effects include injection-site reactions, upper respiratory tract infections, headache, nausea, and skin rash.

Etanercept (Enbrel) is a synthetic TNF receptor that binds with TNF and prevents it from binding with its "normal" receptors on cell surfaces. This action inhibits TNF activity in inflammatory and immune responses. The drug is used to treat moderate to severe RA in adults and children. In this condition, TNF is increased in joint synovial fluid and considered important in joint inflammation and destruction. Etanercept can be used in combination with methotrexate in patients who do not respond adequately to methotrexate alone.

Etanercept is given Sub-Q and reaches its peak concentration in about 3 days. Onset of action occurs within 2 to 3 weeks, and its elimination half-life is about 5 days. Common adverse effects include headache, injection-site reactions, and infections.

Infliximab (Remicade) is a humanized IgG monoclonal antibody used to treat RA and Crohn's disease. It inhibits TNF-alpha from binding to its receptors and thus neutralizes its actions. Infliximab's ability to neutralize TNF-alpha accounts for its anti-inflammatory effects.

Infliximab is given IV. Its half-life elimination is about 8 days, and its onset of action in Crohn's disease is about 2 weeks. Adverse effects include formation of autoimmune antibodies and hypersensitivity reactions. Dyspnea, hypotension, and urticaria have occurred. The drug should be administered in settings in which personnel and supplies (e.g., epinephrine, antihistamines, corticosteroids) are available for treatment of hypersensitivity reactions and should be discontinued if severe reactions occur. In addition, infections developed in approximately 21% of patients in clinical trials, and the drug may aggravate congestive heart failure.

Miscellaneous Immunosuppressants

Abatacept (Orencia) is used to treat RA. It inhibits activation of T lymphocytes in synovial membranes of joints affected by RA and thereby decreases inflammation and joint destruction. It may be used alone or with other anti-RA drugs except anakinra and TNF-alpha blocking agents. Common adverse effects include dizziness, headache, infections, and nausea.

Leflunomide (Arava) has antiproliferative and anti-inflammatory activities that are attributed to its effects on the immune system. The drug inhibits the synthesis of pyrimidines, which are components of DNA and RNA, and therefore blocks the expansion of T cells. Leflunomide is used to treat RA, in which it relieves signs and symptoms and slows the destruction of joint tissues.

After oral administration, leflunomide is metabolized to an active metabolite (called M1) that exerts most of the drug's effects. M1 has a half-life of about 2 weeks, and a loading dose of leflunomide is usually given for 3 days to achieve therapeutic blood levels more rapidly. The metabolite is highly bound to serum albumin and eliminated by further metabolism and renal or biliary excretion. Some of the M1 excreted in bile is reabsorbed, and this contributes to its long half-life. Most adverse effects in clinical trials were similar to those of placebos. With leflunomide, renal and liver function tests should be performed.

Nursing Process

Assessment

- Assess patients receiving or anticipating immunosuppressant drug therapy for signs and symptoms of current infection or factors predisposing them to potential infection (e.g., impaired skin integrity, invasive devices, cigarette smoking).

- Assess the environment for factors predisposing to infection (e.g., family or health care providers with infections, contact with young children, potential exposure to childhood infectious diseases).

- Assess nutritional status, including appetite and weight.

- Assess baseline values of laboratory and other diagnostic test results to aid monitoring of responses to immunosuppressant drug therapy. With pretransplantation patients, this includes assessing for impaired function of the diseased organ and for abnormalities that need treatment before surgery.

- Assess adequacy of support systems for transplant recipients.

- Assess posttransplantation patients for surgical wound healing, manifestations of organ rejection, and adverse effects of immunosuppressant drugs.

- Assess patients with autoimmune disorders (e.g., RA, Crohn's disease) for manifestations of the disease process and responses to drug therapy.

Nursing Diagnoses

- Risk for Injury: Adverse drug effects

- Risk for Injury: Infection and cancer related to immunosuppression and increased susceptibility

- Deficient Knowledge: Disease process and immunosuppressant drug therapy

- Anxiety related to the diagnosis of serious disease or need for organ transplantation

- Social Isolation related to activities to reduce exposure to infection

Planning/Goals

The patient will

- Participate in decision making about the treatment plan

- Receive or take immunosuppressant drugs correctly

- Verbalize or demonstrate essential drug information

- Participate in interventions to prevent infection (e.g., maintain good hygiene, avoid known sources of infection) while immunosuppressed

- Experience relief or reduction of disease symptoms

- Maintain adequate levels of nutrition and fluids, rest and sleep, and exercise

- Be assisted to cope with anxiety related to the disease process and drug therapy

- Keep appointments for follow-up care

- Have adverse drug effects prevented or recognized and treated promptly

- Maintain diagnostic test values within acceptable limits

- Maintain family and other emotional or social support systems

- Receive optimal instructions and information about the treatment plan, self-care in activities of daily living, reporting adverse drug effects, and other concerns

- Before and after tissue or organ transplantation, receive appropriate care, including prevention or early recognition and treatment of rejection reactions

Interventions

- Practice and emphasize good personal and hand hygiene techniques by patients and all others in contact with patients.

- Use sterile technique for all injections, IV site care, wound dressing changes, and any other invasive diagnostic or therapeutic measures.

- Screen staff and visitors for signs and symptoms of infection; if infection is noted, do not allow contact with the patient.

- Report fever and other manifestations of infection immediately.

- Allow patients to participate in decision making when possible and appropriate.

- Use isolation techniques according to institutional policies, usually after transplantation or when the neutrophil count is less than 500/mm^3.

- Assist patients to maintain adequate nutrition, rest and sleep, and exercise.

- Inform patients about diagnostic test results, planned changes in therapeutic regimens, and evidence of progress.

- Allow family members or significant others to visit patients when feasible.

- Monitor complete blood count (CBC) and other diagnostic test results related to blood, liver, and kidney function throughout drug therapy. Specific tests vary with the patient's health or illness status and the immunosuppressant drugs being taken.

- Schedule drug administration to maximize therapeutic effects and minimize adverse effects.

- Consult other health care providers (e.g., physician, dietitian, social worker) on the patient's behalf when indicated. Multidisciplinary consultation is essential for transplantation patients and desirable for patients with autoimmune disorders.

- Assist patients in learning strategies to manage day-to-day activities during long-term immunosuppression.

Evaluation

- Interview and observe for accurate drug administration.

- Interview and observe for personal hygiene practices and infection-avoiding maneuvers.

- Interview and observe for therapeutic and adverse drug effects with each patient contact.

- Interview regarding knowledge and attitude toward the drug therapy regimen, including follow-up care and symptoms to report to health care providers.

- Determine the number and types of infections that have occurred in the neutropenic patient.

- Compare current CBC and other reports with baseline values for acceptable levels, according to the patient's condition.

- Observe and interview outpatients regarding compliance with follow-up care.

- Interview and observe for organ function and absence of rejection reactions in posttransplantation patients.

Applying Your Knowledge 41-3

What are the specific teaching points to be covered with Mr. Kinney regarding proper self-administration of his medication?

Patient Teaching Guidelines | Immunosuppressant Drugs

General Considerations

- People taking medications that suppress the immune system are at high risk for development of infections. As a result, patients, caregivers, and others in the patient's environment need to wash their hands often and thoroughly, practice meticulous personal hygiene, avoid contact with infected people, and practice other methods of preventing infection.

- Report adverse drug effects (e.g., signs or symptoms of infection such as sore throat or fever, decreased urine output if taking cyclosporine, easy bruising or bleeding if taking methotrexate) to a health care provider.

- Try to maintain healthy lifestyle habits, such as a nutritious diet, adequate rest and sleep, and avoiding tobacco and alcohol. These measures enhance immune mechanisms and other body defenses.

- Carry identification that lists the drugs being taken; the dosage; the prescriber's name, address, and telephone number; and instructions for emergency treatment. This information is needed if an accident or emergency situation occurs.

- Inform all health care providers that you are taking these drugs.

- Maintain regular supervision by a health care provider. This is extremely important for evaluating health status, evaluating drug responses and indications for dosage change, detecting adverse drug reactions, and having blood tests or other monitoring tests when indicated.

- Take no other drugs, prescription or nonprescription, without notifying the prescriber who is managing immunosuppressant therapy. Immunosuppressant drugs may influence reactions to other drugs, and other drugs may influence reactions to the immunosuppressants. Thus, taking other drugs may decrease therapeutic effects or increase adverse effects. In addition, some vaccinations should be avoided while taking immunosuppressant drugs.

- People of reproductive capability who are sexually active should practice effective contraceptive techniques during immunosuppressive drug therapy. With methotrexate, use contraception during and for at least 3 months (men) or one ovulatory cycle (women) after stopping the drug. With mycophenolate, effective contraception should be continued for 6 weeks after the drug is stopped. With sirolimus, effective contraception must be used before, during, and for 12 weeks after drug therapy.

(continued on page 666)

■ Wear protective clothing and use sunscreens to decrease exposure of skin to sunlight and risks of skin cancers. Also, methotrexate and sirolimus increase sensitivity to sunlight and may increase sunburn.

Self-Administration

■ Follow instructions about taking the drugs. This is vital to achieving beneficial effects and decreasing adverse effects. If unable to take a medication, report to the prescriber or other health care provider; do not stop unless advised to do so. For transplant recipients, missed doses may lead to transplant rejection; for patients with autoimmune diseases, missed doses may lead to acute flare-ups of symptoms. In addition, take at approximately the same time each day to maintain consistent drug levels in the blood.

■ With cyclosporine oral solution, use the same solution consistently. The two available solutions (Neoral and Sandimmune) are not equivalent and cannot be used interchangeably. If a change in formulation is necessary, it should be made cautiously and only under supervision of the prescriber.

   Measure oral cyclosporine solution with the dosing syringe provided; add to orange or apple juice that is at room temperature (avoid grapefruit juice); stir well and drink at once (do not allow diluted solution to stand before drinking). Use a glass container, not plastic. Rinse the glass with more diluent to ensure the total dose is taken. Do not rinse the dosing syringe with water or other cleaning agents. Take on a consistent schedule with regard to time of day and meals.

   These are the manufacturer's recommendations. Mixing with orange or apple juice improves taste; grapefruit

juice should not be used because it affects metabolism of cyclosporine. The amount of fluid should be large enough to increase palatability, especially for children, but small enough to be consumed quickly. Rinsing ensures the entire dose is taken.

■ Take mycophenolate on an empty stomach; food decreases drug absorption by approximately 40%. Do not crush mycophenolate tablets and do not open or crush the capsules.

■ Take sirolimus consistently with or without food; do not mix or take the drug with grapefruit juice. Grapefruit juice inhibits metabolism and increases adverse effects. If also taking cyclosporine, take the sirolimus 4 hours after a dose of cyclosporine.

   If taking the oral solution, use the syringe that comes with the medication to measure and withdraw the dose from the bottle. Empty the dose into a glass or plastic container with at least 2 oz (1/4 cup or 60 mL) of water or orange juice. *Do not use any other liquid to dilute the drug.* Stir the mixture vigorously, and drink it immediately. Refill the container with at least 4 oz (1/2 cup or 120 mL) of water or orange juice, stir vigorously, and drink at once.

■ Take tacrolimus with food to decrease stomach upset.

■ If giving or taking an injected drug, be sure you understand how to mix and inject the medication correctly. With Enbrel, for example, rotate injection sites, give a new injection at least 1 inch from a previous injection site, and do not inject the medication into areas where the skin is tender, bruised, red, or hard. When possible, practice the required techniques and perform at least the first injection under supervision of a qualified health care professional.

Principles of Therapy

Risk–Benefit Factors

Immunosuppression is a serious, life-threatening condition that may result from disease or drug therapy. At the same time, immunosuppressant drugs are used to treat serious illnesses, and their use may be required. Rational use of the drugs requires thorough assessment of a patient's health status, clear-cut indications for use, a lack of more effective and safer alternative treatments, cautious administration, and vigilant monitoring of the patient's response. If a decision is then made that immunosuppressant drug therapy is indicated and benefits outweigh risks, the therapeutic plan must be discussed with the patient (i.e., reasons, expected benefits, consequences for the patient's health and lifestyle).

In addition to the specific risks of individual immunosuppressant drugs, general risks of immunosuppression include infection and cancer. Infection is a major cause of morbidity and mortality, especially in patients who are neutropenic (neutrophil count less than 1000/mm³) from cytotoxic immunosuppressant drugs, who take TNF inhibitors, or who have had bone marrow or solid organ transplantation. For those with solid organ transplantation, who must continue lifelong immuno-

suppression to avoid graft rejection, serious infection is a constant hazard. If efforts to prevent infections are unsuccessful, infections may be fatal unless recognized promptly and treated aggressively. Common infections are bacterial (gram-positive, such as *Staphylococcus aureus* or *S. epidermidis;* and gram-negative, such as *Escherichia coli, Klebsiella,* and *Pseudomonas* species), fungal (candidiasis, aspergillosis), or viral (CMV, herpes simplex, or herpes zoster). In addition, severe, disseminated tuberculosis is associated with the use of TNF inhibitors.

Cancer may result from immunosuppression. When T lymphocytes and NK cells are suppressed and unable to recognize and eliminate abnormal cells, the abnormal cells may undergo spontaneous malignant transformation and result in widespread and often aggressive malignancies. Most of the available information is related to posttransplant cancer development.

With early transplantations, major causes of death were graft rejection and infection. Now, improvements are leading to more transplants, older transplant recipients, and longer survival rates among recipients. One consequence of long-term survival and chronic immunosuppression is increased risk of developing a malignancy. The incidence is unknown but often estimated at 20% or more after 10 years of immunosuppression. As a result, cancer has become the second most common cause of mortality in transplant recipients.

The most common malignancies among transplant recipients are skin cancers and lymphomas. Other malignancies include solid organ tumors, some of which occur at similar rates in the general and posttransplant populations (e.g., brain, breast, lung, prostate) and some of which occur more often in the posttransplant population (e.g., renal cell cancer in renal transplant recipients; colon cancers; cervical, perineal/anal, and vulvar cancers in women). When breast cancer occurs posttransplantation, it often occurs at a younger age and grows more aggressively than in the general population. In addition, men with transplants are more likely to develop breast cancer than men in the general population.

When cancer develops, treatment includes reduced immunosuppressant drug therapy as well as treatment of the malignancy. Reducing dosages of immunosuppressant drugs increases risks of rejection reactions and the need for retransplantation.

Use in Autoimmune Disorders

Allergic Asthma

Allergic asthma is characterized by increased production of IgE in response to inhaled allergens. IgE molecules then interact with allergen molecules to form IgE–allergen complexes that damage tissues and produce signs and symptoms. Omalizumab (Xolair) combines with free IgE so that there is less IgE available to combine with allergens. It is second-line therapy for patients whose symptoms are not adequately controlled with inhaled corticosteroids.

Crohn's Disease

Crohn's disease is a chronic, recurrent, inflammatory bowel disorder that can affect any area of the GI tract. The inflammation is attributed to a mixture of inflammatory mediators (e.g., IL-1 and -6, TNF-alpha) produced by activated macrophages. The goal of treatment is to decrease inflammation and promote healing of bowel lesions. Several medications are effective, including corticosteroids, cyclosporine, metronidazole, and sulfasalazine. Because elevated concentrations of TNF-alpha are found in patients' stools and correlate with episodes of increased disease activity, infliximab (Remicade) is also used. Infliximab reduces infiltration of inflammatory cells, production of TNF-alpha in inflamed areas of the intestine, and the number of cells that can produce TNF-alpha. It is indicated for patients with moderate to severe disease who do not respond adequately to other treatment measures.

Psoriasis and Psoriatic Arthritis

Psoriasis is a skin disorder of unknown cause. It is thought that activated T lymphocytes produce cytokines that stimulate abnormal growth of affected skin cells and blood vessels. The accompanying inflammation results from infiltration of neutrophils and monocytes. Several medications (e.g., beta blockers, lithium) may precipitate or aggravate psoriasis. Corticosteroids and other immunosuppressants (e.g., cyclosporine, methotrexate) have long been used to treat psoriasis because they suppress inflammation and proliferation of T cells. Newer biologic immunosuppressants (e.g., alefacept, efalizumab) also reduce the activity of T lymphocytes and the inflammation of skin lesions.

Psoriatic arthritis is a type of arthritis associated with psoriasis that is similar to RA. It may be characterized by extensive and disabling joint damage, especially in hand and finger joints. Etanercept (Enbrel) is a TNF-alpha inhibitor approved for treatment.

Rheumatoid Arthritis

Rheumatoid arthritis is an abnormal immune response that leads to inflammation and damage of joint cartilage and bone. It is thought to involve the activation of T lymphocytes, release of inflammatory cytokines, and formation of antibodies. Research in recent years has delineated the roles of TNF-alpha and IL-1 in the pathophysiology of RA and led to the development of drugs directed against TNF-alpha (e.g., adalimumab, etanercept, infliximab) and IL-1 (e.g., anakinra).

These drugs are highly effective in relieving joint pain and inflammation and they also slow progression of RA, as measured by serial radiographs. Because of their ability to slow disease progression, they are called disease-modifying antirheumatic drugs (DMARDs). They act more rapidly than older DMARDs (e.g., methotrexate) and greatly improve the quality of life for patients with RA. However, their use is also associated with significant risks of serious infections, especially with the TNF-alpha blocking agents. To decrease the adverse effects of the TNF inhibitors, the following guidelines have been developed for patients receiving these drugs:

- Tuberculin testing before starting a TNF inhibitor and antitubercular prophylaxis for patients with positive skintest results
- Administration of pneumococcal and perhaps meningococcal vaccine
- Administration of trimethoprim-sulfamethoxazole (TMP-SMX) to prevent infection
- Consideration of fluconazole administration to patients at high risk of developing coccidioidomycosis and cryptococcosis
- Education of patients and caregivers to avoid potential exposures to infection in the community
- Provision of antibiotics for immediate initiation at home with the onset of fever or upper respiratory infection, followed by seeking emergency care

Use in Transplantation

Immunosuppressant drugs are used to prevent rejection of transplanted tissues, a reaction involving T and B lymphocytes and multiple inflammatory cytokines. Specific drug therapy protocols vary among transplantation centers and types of transplants; they continue to evolve in efforts to increase effectiveness and decrease complications of transplantation.

One strategy is to use combinations of immunosuppressant drugs. Combinations are rational because the drugs act on different components of the immune response and often have overlapping and synergistic effects. They may also allow lower doses of individual drugs, which usually cause fewer or less severe adverse effects.

A second strategy is to reduce the number of drugs and drug dosages after transplanted tissue is functioning and rejection has been successfully prevented or treated. Vigilant monitoring is required, to catch rejection reactions early, when restarting immunosuppressant drugs or increasing their dosage can still save the transplant.

A third strategy involves interventions to decrease adverse effects of immunosuppressant drug therapy such as worsening of pre-existing conditions (e.g., diabetes mellitus, hypertension) and development of new diseases (e.g., nephrotoxicity, osteoporosis, and malignancies). Regular screening tests for breast, colon, and prostate cancer are recommended, along with annual skin examination.

Drug Dosage

Immunosuppressant drugs are relatively toxic, and adverse effects occur more often and are more severe with higher doses. Thus, the general principle of using the smallest effective dose for the shortest period of time is especially important with immunosuppressant drug therapy. Dosage must be individualized according to the patient's serum drug levels and clinical response (i.e., improvement in signs and symptoms or occurrence of adverse effects). With corticosteroids, for example, high doses are usually given immediately after transplantation and during treatment of acute graft rejection reactions. Doses are usually tapered by 6 months after the transplantation, and long-term maintenance doses of prednisone are usually under 10 milligrams per day. For some patients, the drugs may be discontinued. With cyclosporine, higher doses are given for 3 months posttransplantation and may be given IV for a few days after surgery (at one third the oral dosage).

Drug Selection and Type of Transplant

Cardiac transplant recipients are usually given cyclosporine, prednisone, and mycophenolate. Tacrolimus may be used instead of cyclosporine. Renal transplant recipients are usually given high doses of IV methylprednisolone for a few days, then switched to prednisone. If cyclosporine is used, despite its unpredictable absorption and nephrotoxicity, it is given in low doses. After approximately 3 months, maintenance drug therapy may consist of mycophenolate, prednisone, and cyclosporine or tacrolimus. Liver transplant recipients are usually given methylprednisolone initially, with cyclosporine or tacrolimus. Treatment of rejection reactions may include high-dose corticosteroids and muromonab-CD3 or anti-thymocyte globulin for 7 to 14 days. Bone marrow/stem cell transplant recipients are usually given cyclosporine and a corticosteroid.

Use in Special Populations

Use in Children

Most immunosuppressants are used in children for the same disorders and with similar effects as in adults. Corticosteroids impair growth in children. As a result, some transplantation centers avoid prednisone therapy until a rejection episode occurs. When prednisone is used, administering it every other day may improve growth rates. Cyclosporine has been given to children as young as 6 months of age, and muromonab-CD3 has been used in children as young as 2 years of age. Mycophenolate has been used in a few children undergoing renal transplantation. In children with impaired renal function, recommended doses of mycophenolate cause a high incidence of adverse effects. Thus, dosage should be adjusted for the level of renal function. Tacrolimus has been used in children younger than 12 years of age who were undergoing liver transplantation. This usage indicates that children require relatively high doses because they metabolize the drug rapidly.

Little information is available about the use of newer immunosuppressants in children. Safety and effectiveness have not been established for basiliximab, daclizumab, infliximab, or leflunomide. Leflunomide is not recommended for children under 18 years of age. Etanercept is approved for children 4 to 17 years of age with juvenile RA. Most children in a 3-month study had an infection while receiving etanercept, but the infections were usually mild. Children reported abdominal pain, headache, nausea and vomiting with etanercept more often than adults. Other medications (e.g., a corticosteroid, methotrexate, a nonsteroidal anti-inflammatory drug, an analgesic) may be continued during treatment.

For children age 12 and older with allergic asthma, omalizumab is the only immunosuppressant drug approved for use. Dosages and frequency of administration are determined by body weight and serum levels of IgE. The drug is reportedly well tolerated in children.

Use in Older Adults

Immunosuppressants are used for the same purposes and produce similar therapeutic and adverse effects in older adults as in younger adults. Because older adults often have multiple disorders and organ impairments, it is especially important that drug choices, dosages, and monitoring tests are individualized. In addition, infections occur more commonly in older adults, and this tendency is increased with immunosuppressant therapy.

Use in Patients With Renal Impairment

Cyclosporine is nephrotoxic but commonly used in patients with renal and other transplants. Nephrotoxicity has been noted in 25% of renal, 38% of cardiac, and 37% of liver transplant recipients, especially with high doses. It usually subsides with decreased dosage or stopping the drug. In renal transplant recipients, when serum creatinine and blood urea nitrogen levels remain elevated, a complete evaluation of the patient must be done to differentiate cyclosporine-induced nephrotoxicity from a transplant rejection reaction. If renal function is deteriorating from cyclosporine, dosage reduction or a different immunosuppressant may be effective. If renal function is deteriorating from a rejection reaction, decreasing cyclosporine dosage would increase the severity of the reaction.

Methotrexate is mainly excreted in urine, so its half-life is prolonged in patients with renal impairment, with risks of accumulation to toxic levels and additional renal damage.

However, the risks are less with the small doses used for treatment of RA than for the high doses used in cancer chemotherapy. To decrease these risks, adequate renal function should be documented before the drug is given and patients should be well hydrated.

Mycophenolate produces higher plasma levels in renal transplant recipients with severe renal impairment than in patients with less severe renal impairment and healthy volunteers. Doses higher than 1 gram twice a day should be avoided in these patients.

Tacrolimus is associated with high rates of nephrotoxicity when given IV, so oral dosing is preferred.

Little information is available about the use of basiliximab, etanercept, infliximab, or leflunomide in patients with renal impairment. However, leflunomide metabolites are partly excreted renally and the drug should be used cautiously.

Use in Patients With Hepatic Impairment

Cyclosporine reportedly causes hepatotoxicity (e.g., elevated serum aminotransferases and bilirubin) in approximately 4% of renal and liver transplant recipients and 7% of cardiac transplant recipients. This is most likely to occur during the first month of therapy, when high doses of cyclosporine are usually given, and usually subsides with reduced dosage.

Methotrexate may cause hepatotoxicity, even in the low doses used in RA and psoriasis. Many clinicians recommend serial liver biopsies for patients on long-term, low-dose methotrexate. In addition, in patients with or without initial liver impairment, liver function tests should be performed to monitor patients for hepatotoxicity and to guide drug dosage. In general, methotrexate dosage should be decreased if bilirubin is between 3 and 5 milligrams per deciliter or aspartate aminotransferase (AST) is above 180 international units per liter, and the drug should be omitted if bilirubin is above 5 milligrams per deciliter.

Mycophenolate is metabolized in the liver to an active metabolite that is further metabolized to inactive metabolites. Liver impairment may interfere with these processes and affect both action and elimination.

Sirolimus is extensively metabolized in the liver and may accumulate in the presence of hepatic impairment. The maintenance dose should be reduced by 35%; it is not necessary to reduce the loading dose.

Tacrolimus is metabolized in the liver by the cytochrome P450 enzyme system. Impaired liver function may decrease presystemic (first-pass) metabolism of oral tacrolimus and produce higher blood levels. Also, the elimination half-life is significantly longer. As a result, dosage must be decreased in patients with impaired liver function.

There is little or no information about the use of basiliximab, daclizumab, etanercept, or infliximab in patients with liver impairment. Leflunomide may be hepatotoxic in patients with normal liver function and is not recommended for use in patients with liver impairment or positive serology tests for hepatitis B or C. The manufacturer's recommendations for use should be consulted.

Use in Home Care

With patients who are taking immunosuppressant drugs, a major role of the home care nurse is to assess the environment for potential sources of infection, assist patients and other members of the household to understand the patient's susceptibility to infection, and teach ways to decrease risks of infection. Although infections often develop from the patient's own body flora, other potential sources include people with infections, caregivers, water or soil around live plants, and raw fruits and vegetables. Meticulous environmental cleansing as well as personal and hand hygiene are required. In addition, the nurse may need to assist with clinic visits for monitoring and follow-up care.

Applying Your Knowledge 41-4

Mr. Kinney has a depressed immune system secondary to the medications necessary to prevent organ rejection. What is Mr. Kinney at risk to develop?

Nursing Actions Immunosuppressants

NURSING ACTIONS	RATIONALE/EXPLANATION
1. Administer accurately	
a. For prepared IV solutions, check for appropriate dilution, discoloration, particulate matter, and expiration time. If okay, give by infusion pump, for the recommended time.	IV drugs should be reconstituted and diluted in a pharmacy, and the manufacturers' instructions should be followed exactly. After they are mixed, most of these drugs are stable only for a few hours and some do not contain preservatives. Manufacturer's recommendations. Using a high-flow vein decreases phlebitis and thrombosis at the IV site. The filter is used to remove any insoluble particles.
b. Give antithymocyte globulin (diluted to a concentration of 1 mg/mL) IV, using an in-line filter and infusion pump, over at least 4 hours. After it is diluted, use within 24 hours.	
c. With basiliximab, infuse IV over 20–30 minutes. Use the reconstituted solution within 4 hours at room temperature or 24 hours if refrigerated.	The first dose is given within 2 hours before transplantation surgery and the second dose 4 days after transplantation.

(continued on page 670)

Nursing Actions Immunosuppressants (continued)

NURSING ACTIONS	RATIONALE/EXPLANATION
d. With IV cyclosporine, infuse over 2–6 hours.	IV drug is given to patients who are unable to take it orally; resume oral administration when feasible.
e. With oral cyclosporine solutions, measure doses with the provided syringe; add to room-temperature orange or apple juice (avoid grapefruit juice); stir well and have the patient drink at once (do not allow diluted solution to stand before drinking). Use a glass container, not plastic. Rinse the glass with more juice to ensure the total dose is taken. Do not rinse the dosing syringe with water or other cleaning agents. Give on a consistent schedule in relation to time of day and meals.	Manufacturers' recommendations. Mixing with orange or apple juice improves taste; grapefruit juice should not be used because it affects metabolism of cyclosporine. The amount of fluid should be large enough to increase palatability, especially for children, but small enough to be consumed quickly. Rinsing ensures the entire dose is taken.
f. Infuse reconstituted and diluted daclizumab IV over 15 minutes. After it is mixed, use within 4 hours or refrigerate up to 24 hours.	The first dose is given approximately 24 hours before transplantation, followed by a dose every 2 weeks for four doses (total of five doses).
g. With etanercept, inject 1 mL of the supplied Sterile Bacteriostatic Water for Injection into the vial, without shaking (to avoid excessive foaming). Give Sub-Q, rotating sites so that a new dose is injected at least 1 inch from an old site and never into areas where the skin is tender, bruised, red, or hard.	This drug may be administered at home, by a patient or a caregiver, with appropriate instructions and supervised practice in mixing and injecting the drug.
h. Infuse reconstituted and diluted infliximab over approximately 2 hours, starting within 3 hours of preparation (contains no antibacterial preservatives).	Infliximab should be prepared in a pharmacy because special equipment is required for administration.
i. Give muromonab-CD3 in an IV bolus injection once daily. Do not give by IV infusion or mix with other drug solutions.	Manufacturer's recommendations
j. Infuse IV mycophenolate over approximately 2 hours, within 4 hours of solution preparation (contains no antibacterial preservatives).	The IV drug must be reconstituted and diluted with 5% dextrose to a concentration of 6 mg/mL (1 g reconstituted drug in 140 mL or 1.5 g in 210 mL). Handle the drug cautiously to avoid contact with skin and mucous membranes. If such contact occurs, wash thoroughly with soap and water; rinse eyes with plain water.
k. Give oral mycophenolate on an empty stomach. Do not crush the tablets, do not open or crush the capsules, and ask patients to swallow the capsules whole, without biting or chewing.	Food decreases absorption. Avoid inhaling the powder from the capsules or getting on skin or mucous membranes. Such contacts produced teratogenic effects in animals.
l. With sirolimus, give 4 hours after a dose of cyclosporine, give consistently with or without food, and do not give with grapefruit juice. With oral sirolimus solution, use the oral-dose syringe to withdraw a dose from the bottle, empty the dose into a glass or plastic container with at least 60 mL of water or orange juice (do not use any other diluent), stir the mixture vigorously and ask the patient to drink it immediately, refill the container with at least 120 mL of water or orange juice, stir vigorously, and ask the patient to drink all of the fluid.	Serum drug levels of sirolimus are increased if the two drugs are taken at the same time; consistent timing in relation to food provides more consistent absorption and blood levels; grapefruit juice inhibits the enzymes that metabolize sirolimus, thereby increasing blood levels of drug and increasing risks of toxicity.
m. Give IV tacrolimus as a continuous infusion by infusion pump; give the first dose of oral tacrolimus 8–12 hours after stopping the IV infusion.	Oral tacrolimus can usually be substituted for IV drug 2–3 days after transplantation.

2. Observe for therapeutic effects

a. When a drug is given to suppress the immune response to organ transplants, therapeutic effect is the absence of signs and symptoms indicating rejection of the transplanted tissue.

b. When methotrexate is given for RA, observe for decreased pain.

Therapeutic effects usually occur within 3–6 weeks.

c. When adalimumab, etanercept, or infliximab is given for RA, observe for decreased symptoms and less joint destruction on x-ray examination reports.

NURSING ACTIONS	RATIONALE/EXPLANATION
d. When infliximab is given for Crohn's disease, observe for decreased symptoms.	
e. When alefacept or efalizumab is given for psoriasis, observe for improvement in skin lesions.	

3. Observe for adverse effects

NURSING ACTIONS	RATIONALE/EXPLANATION
a. Observe for infection (fever, sore throat, wound drainage, productive cough, dysuria, and so forth).	Risks are high in immunosuppressed patients, and frequency and severity increase with higher drug doses. Infections may be caused by almost any microorganism and may affect any part of the body, although respiratory and urinary tract infections may occur more often.
b. With antithymocyte globulin, observe for:	
(1) Anaphylaxis (chest pain, respiratory distress, hypotension, or shock)	An uncommon but serious allergic reaction that may occur anytime during therapy. If it occurs, stop the drug infusion, inject 0.3 mL epinephrine 1:1000 Sub-Q or IM, and provide other emergency care as indicated.
(2) Chills and fever	Fever occurs in approximately 50% of patients; it may be decreased by premedicating with acetaminophen, an antihistamine, or a corticosteroid.
c. With basiliximab and daclizumab, observe for nausea, vomiting, diarrhea, heartburn, abdominal distention.	GI symptoms were often reported in clinical trials. Other adverse effects were similar for basiliximab, daclizumab, and placebo groups. All patients were also receiving cyclosporine and a corticosteroid.
d. With cyclosporine, observe for:	
(1) Nephrotoxicity (increased serum creatinine and blood urea nitrogen [BUN], decreased urine output, edema, hyperkalemia)	This is a major adverse effect which often occurs 2–3 months after transplantation and results in a decreased level of renal function.
(2) Hepatotoxicity (increased serum enzymes and bilirubin)	The reported incidence is less than 8% after kidney, heart, or liver transplantation. It usually occurs during the first month, when high doses are used, and decreases with dosage reduction.
(3) Hypertension	This is especially likely to occur in patients with heart transplants and may require antihypertensive drug therapy. Do not give a potassium-sparing diuretic as part of the antihypertensive regimen because of increased risk of hyperkalemia.
(4) Anaphylaxis (with IV cyclosporine) (urticaria, hypotension or shock, respiratory distress)	This rarely occurs. If it does, the allergen is thought to be the castor oil component because people who had allergic reactions with the IV drug have later taken oral doses without allergic reactions. During IV administration, observe the patient continuously for the first 30 minutes and often thereafter. Stop the infusion if a reaction occurs, and give emergency care (e.g., epinephrine 1:1000).
(5) Central nervous system (CNS) toxicity (confusion, depression, hallucinations, seizures, tremor)	CNS effects are relatively uncommon and may be caused by factors other than cyclosporine (e.g., nephrotoxicity).
(6) Other (gingival hyperplasia, hirsutism)	Gingival hyperplasia can be minimized by thorough oral hygiene.
e. With infliximab, observe for:	
(1) Infusion reactions (fever, chills, pruritus, urticaria, chest pain)	
(2) GI upset (nausea, vomiting, abdominal pain)	
(3) Respiratory symptoms (bronchitis, chest pain, coughing, dyspnea)	
f. With leflunomide, observe for:	In clinical trials, adverse effects were similar to those occurring with placebo.
(1) GI upset (nausea, diarrhea)	
(2) Hepatotoxicity (elevation of transaminases)	
(3) Skin disorders (alopecia, rash)	
g. With methotrexate, observe for:	
(1) GI disorders (nausea, vomiting, diarrhea, ulcerations, bleeding)	
(2) Bone marrow depression (anemia, neutropenia, thrombocytopenia)	Monitor CBC regularly. Bone marrow depression is less likely to occur with the small doses used for inflammatory disorders than with doses used in cancer chemotherapy.
(3) Hepatotoxicity	Long-term, low-dose methotrexate may produce fatty changes, fibrosis, necrosis, and cirrhosis in the liver.

(continued on page 672)

Nursing Actions Immunosuppressants (continued)

NURSING ACTIONS	RATIONALE/EXPLANATION
h. With muromonab-CD3, observe for:	
(1) An acute reaction called the cytokine release syndrome (high fever, chills, chest pain, dyspnea, hypertension, nausea, vomiting, diarrhea)	This reaction is attributed to the release of cytokines by activated lymphocytes or monocytes. Symptoms may range from "flu-like" to serious cardiovascular and CNS disorders.
(2) Hypersensitivity (edema, difficulty in swallowing or breathing, skin rash, urticaria, rapid heart beat)	Symptoms usually occur within 30–60 minutes after a dose and may last several hours. The reaction is most likely to occur with the first dose, with dosage increases, and when restarting after a period without the drug.
(3) Nausea, vomiting, diarrhea	
i. With mycophenolate, observe for:	
(1) GI effects (nausea, vomiting, diarrhea)	GI effects are more likely when mycophenolate is started and may subside if dosage is reduced.
(2) Hematologic effects (anemia, neutropenia)	Monitor CBC reports regularly. Some renal and cardiac transplant recipients develop severe neutropenia, which may be related to mycophenolate, concomitant medications, viral infections, or a combination of these causes. If a patient has neutropenia, stop the drug or reduce the dose and start appropriate treatment as soon as possible.
(3) CNS effects (dizziness, headache, insomnia)	
j. With sirolimus, observe for:	Most adverse effects occurred in more than 10% of recipients.
(1) GI effects (abdominal pain, nausea, vomiting, constipation, diarrhea, hepatotoxicity)	However, patients were also receiving cyclosporine and a corticosteroid.
(2) Hematologic effects (anemia, leukopenia, thrombocytopenia, hypercholesterolemia)	
(3) Cardiovascular effects (edema, hypertension)	
(4) CNS effects (insomnia, headache, tremor)	
k. With tacrolimus, observe for:	
(1) Nephrotoxicity (increased serum creatinine, decreased urine output)	Nephrotoxicity has occurred in one third or more of liver transplant recipients who received tacrolimus. The risk is greater with higher doses.
(2) Neurotoxicity (minor effects include headaches, insomnia, nightmares, photophobia, tremors; major effects include expressive aphasia, confusion, coma, psychosis, encephalopathy, seizures)	Neurologic symptoms occur in approximately 10%–20% of patients receiving tacrolimus.
(3) Infection (cytomegalovirus (CMV) infection and others)	CMV infection commonly occurs.
(4) Hyperglycemia	Glucose intolerance may require insulin therapy.
4. Observe for drug interactions	Drug interactions have not been reported with the newer biologic immunosuppressants (adalimumab, alefacept, anakinra, basiliximab, daclizumab, etanercept, infliximab, omalizumab).
a. Drugs that *increase* effects of cyclosporine:	
(1) Aminoglycoside antibiotics (e.g., gentamicin), amphotericin B	Increased risk of nephrotoxicity
(2) Enzyme inhibitors, including azole antifungals (e.g., itraconazole), calcium channel blockers (e.g., nicardipine), macrolide antibiotics (e.g., erythromycin, clarithromycin), cimetidine	Decreased hepatic metabolism, increased serum drug levels, and increased risk of toxicity
b. Drugs that *decrease* effects of cyclosporine:	
(1) Enzyme inducers, including anticonvulsants (e.g., carbamazepine, phenytoin), rifampin	Drugs that induce CYP3A4 enzymes in the liver stimulate metabolism of cyclosporine and thereby reduce blood levels.
c. Drugs that *increase* effects of leflunomide:	
(1) Rifampin	Rifampin induces liver enzymes and accelerates metabolism of leflunomide to its active metabolite.
(2) Hepatotoxic drugs (e.g., methotrexate)	Additive hepatotoxicity
d. Drugs that *decrease* effects of leflunomide:	
(1) Charcoal	These drugs may be used to lower blood levels of leflunomide.
(2) Cholestyramine	

NURSING ACTIONS	RATIONALE/EXPLANATION
e. Drugs that *increase* effects of methotrexate: (1) Probenecid (2) Salicylates (3) Sulfonamides (4) Nonsteroidal anti-inflammatory drugs (NSAIDs) (5) Procarbazine (6) Alcohol and other hepatotoxic drugs	Probenecid, salicylates, and sulfonamides may increase both therapeutic and toxic effects. The mechanism is unknown but may involve slowing of methotrexate elimination through the kidneys or displacement of methotrexate from plasma protein-binding sites. NSAIDs are often used concomitantly with methotrexate by patients with rheumatoid arthritis. There may be an increased risk of GI ulceration and bleeding. Procarbazine may increase nephrotoxicity. Hepatotoxic drugs increase hepatotoxicity.
f. Drug that *decreases* effects of methotrexate: (1) Folic acid	Methotrexate acts by blocking folic acid. Its effectiveness is decreased by folic acid supplementation, alone or in multivitamin preparations.
g. Drugs that *increase* effects of mycophenolate: (1) Acyclovir, ganciclovir (2) Probenecid, salicylates	Increase blood levels of mycophenolate, probably by decreasing renal excretion Increase blood levels
h. Drug that *decreases* effects of mycophenolate: (1) Cholestyramine	Decreases absorption
i. Drugs that *increase* effects of sirolimus: (1) Cyclosporine (2) CYP3A4 enzyme inhibitors—azole antifungal drugs (e.g., itraconazole), calcium channel blockers (e.g., nicardipine, verapamil), macrolide antibiotics (e.g., erythromycin, clarithromycin), protease inhibitors (e.g., ritonavir, indinavir), cimetidine	Increases blood levels of sirolimus and should not be given at same time (give sirolimus 4 hours after a dose of cyclosporine) These drugs inhibit metabolism of sirolimus, which increases blood levels and risks of toxicity.
j. Drugs that *decrease* effects of sirolimus: (1) Enzyme inducers—anticonvulsants (e.g., carbamazepine, phenytoin), rifamycins (e.g., rifampin, rifabutin), St. John's wort	These drugs speed up the metabolism and elimination of sirolimus.
k. Drugs that *increase* effects of tacrolimus: (1) Nephrotoxic drugs (e.g., aminoglycoside antibiotics, amphotericin B, cisplatin, NSAIDs) (2) Antifungals (e.g., clotrimazole, itraconazole), erythromycin and other macrolides, calcium channel blockers (e.g., diltiazem, verapamil), cimetidine, danazol, methylprednisolone, metoclopramide (3) Angiotensin-converting enzyme inhibitors, potassium supplements	Increased nephrotoxicity These drugs may increase blood levels of tacrolimus, probably by inhibiting or competing for hepatic drug-metabolizing enzymes. Increased risk of hyperkalemia. Serum potassium levels should be monitored closely.
l. Drugs that *decrease* effects of tacrolimus: (1) Antacids (2) Enzyme inducers—carbamazepine, phenytoin, rifampin, rifabutin	With oral tacrolimus, antacids adsorb the drug or raise the pH of gastric fluids and increase its degradation. If ordered concomitantly, an antacid should be given at least 2 hours before or after tacrolimus. Induction of drug-metabolizing enzymes in the liver may accelerate metabolism of tacrolimus and decrease its blood levels.

Key Concepts

■ Immunosuppressants are used to decrease the immune response with allergic and autoimmune disorders and to avoid graft rejection after transplantation.

■ With current treatments, most transplant patients must maintain immunosuppressive drug therapy the rest of their lives.

■ Immunosuppressant drugs greatly increase risks of infection.

■ Cyclosporine and tacrolimus are similar drugs that are effective immunosuppressants, widely used in organ trans-

plantation, cause nephrotoxicity, and are subject to numerous drug interactions (enzyme-inhibiting drugs increase blood levels and enzyme-inducing drugs decrease blood levels).

■ Many transplant centers now prefer tacrolimus over cyclosporine.

■ Newer immunosuppressants have more specific effects on the immune system and may cause fewer or less severe adverse effects than older drugs.

Review and Application Exercises

Short Answer Exercises

1. List clinical indications for use of immunosuppressant drug therapy.

2. How do the different types of drugs exert their immunosuppressant effects?

3. What are major adverse effects of immunosuppressant drugs?

4. When assessing a patient receiving one or more immunosuppressant drugs, what specific signs and symptoms indicate adverse drug effects?

5. For a patient taking one or more immunosuppressant drugs, prepare a teaching plan related to safe and effective drug therapy.

NCLEX-Style Questions

6. In addition to organ transplantation, immunosuppressant drugs are used to treat
   a. serious infections
   b. Crohn's disease and rheumatoid arthritis
   c. gastroesophageal reflux disease (GERD)
   d. seizure disorders

7. After organ transplantation, immunosuppressants are given to prevent
   a. nephrotoxicity
   b. hepatotoxicity
   c. rejection reactions
   d. bleeding disorders

8. The family of a middle-aged patient who has received a kidney transplant has questions about the increased risk of cancer as a result of the need for long-term (lifelong) immunosuppressant drugs. The nurse is correct in informing the family that the most common malignancies that occur with immunosuppression include
   a. skin cancers and lymphomas
   b. cancers of the GI tract
   c. renal and liver cancers
   d. brain and spinal cord cancers

9. Patients taking immunosuppressant drugs should be taught
   a. ways to decrease infections
   b. to avoid weight gain
   c. to maintain a good fluid intake
   d. to increase rest and decrease exercise

Selected References

Bongartz, T., Sutton, A. J., Sweeting, M. J., Buchan, I., Matteson, E. L., & Montori, V. (2006). Anti-TNF antibody therapy in rheumatoid arthritis and the risk of serious infections and malignancies: Systematic review and meta-analysis of rare harmful effects in randomized controlled trials. *Journal of the American Medical Association, 295,* 2275–2285.

Johnson, H. J., & Schonder, K. S. (2005). Solid-organ transplantation. In J. T. DiPiro, R. L. Talbert, G. C. Yee, G. R. Matzke, B. G. Wells, & L. M. Posey (Eds.), *Pharmacotherapy: A pathophysiologic approach* (6th ed., pp. 1613–1643). New York: McGraw-Hill.

McPhee, S. J., Papadakis, M. A. & Tierney, L. M., Jr. (2007). *Current medical diagnosis and treatment 2007* (46th ed.). New York: McGraw-Hill.

Mutlu, G. M., Mutlu, E. A., Bellmeyer, A., & Rubinstein, I. (2006). Pulmonary adverse events of anti-tumor necrosis factor-alpha antibody therapy. *American Journal of Medicine, 119,* 639–646.

Perkins, J. B., & Yee, G. C. (2005). Hematopoietic stem cell transplantation. In J. T. DiPiro, R. L. Talbert, G. C. Yee, G. R. Matzke, B. G. Wells, & L. M. Posey (Eds.), *Pharmacotherapy: A pathophysiologic approach* (6th ed., pp. 2541–2558). New York: McGraw-Hill.

Porth, C. M. (2005). *Pathophysiology: Concepts of altered health states* (7th ed.). Philadelphia: Lippincott Williams & Wilkins.

Smeltzer, S. C., Bare, B. G., Hinkle, J. L., & Cheever, K. H. (2008). *Brunner & Suddarth's textbook of medical-surgical nursing* (11th ed.). Philadelphia: Lippincott Williams & Wilkins.

Drugs Used in Oncologic Disorders

KEY TERMS

- Alopecia
- Angiogenesis
- Anti-oncogenes
- Cancer
- Carcinomas
- Cell cycle
- Chemotherapy
- Cytotoxic
- Extravasation
- Leukemias
- Leukopenia
- Malignant
- Metastasis
- Mucositis
- Mutation
- Myelosuppression
- Nephropathy
- Neutropenia
- Oncogenes
- Proto-oncogenes
- Remission
- Sarcomas
- Stomatitis
- Thrombocytopenia

LEARNING OBJECTIVES

After studying this chapter, you will be able to:

1. Contrast normal and malignant cells.
2. Describe major types of antineoplastic drugs in terms of mechanism of action, indications for use, administration, and nursing process implications.
3. Discuss the rationales for using antineoplastic drugs in combination with each other, with surgical treatment, and with radiation therapy.
4. Discuss adverse drug effects and their prevention or management.
5. Assist patients/caregivers in preventing or managing symptoms associated with chemotherapy regimens.
6. Teach, promote, and practice reduction of risk factors for development of cancer; early recognition of cancer signs and symptoms; and early implementation of effective treatment measures.

Applying Your Knowledge

Julia Gardner is a 60-year-old retired teacher. She has been diagnosed with cancer in her right breast. Before her mastectomy, Ms. Gardner is receiving neoadjuvant chemotherapy. Ms. Gardner receives trastuzumab (Herceptin), doxorubicin, and paclitaxel (Taxol) IV every 3 weeks. She takes methotrexate PO 2 times a week.

Introduction

Oncology is the study of malignant neoplasms and their treatment. Drugs used in oncologic disorders include those used to kill, damage, or slow the growth of cancer cells and those used to prevent or treat adverse drug effects. Antineoplastic drug therapy is a major treatment modality for cancer, along with surgery and radiation therapy.

Major groups of anticancer drugs are the traditional cytotoxic agents (e.g., alkylating agents, antimetabolites, antitumor antibiotics, plant alkaloids), newer cytotoxic "biologic targeted therapies" (e.g., monoclonal antibodies, growth-factor inhibitors), and hormone inhibitors, which are not cytotoxic. In addition, several drugs are used to ameliorate the adverse effects of cytotoxic drugs (e.g., cytoprotectants, including some immunostimulants discussed in Chap. 40). To aid understanding of the drugs used in oncologic disorders, selected characteristics of cancer and the drugs are described below.

Cancer

The term *cancer* is used to describe many disease processes with the common characteristics of uncontrolled cell growth, invasiveness, and *metastasis*, as well as numerous etiologies, clinical manifestations, and treatments.

Normal Versus Malignant Cells

Normal cells reproduce in response to a need for tissue growth or repair and stop reproduction when the need has been met. The normal *cell cycle* is the interval between the "birth" of a cell and its division into two daughter cells (Fig. 42-1). The daughter cells may then enter the resting phase (G_0) or proceed through the reproductive cycle to form more new cells. Normal cells are also well differentiated in appearance and function and have a characteristic lifespan.

Malignant cells occupy space, take blood and nutrients away from normal tissues, and serve no useful purpose. They grow in an uncontrolled fashion and avoid the restraints (e.g., contact with other cells) that stop the growth of normal cells. They are undifferentiated, which means they have lost the structural and functional characteristics of the cells from which they originated. They are loosely connected, so that cells break off from the primary tumor and invade adjacent tissues. Loose cells also enter blood and lymph vessels, circulate through the body, and produce additional neoplasms at sites distant from the primary tumor.

A malignant cell develops from a transformed normal cell. The transformation may begin with a random *mutation* (abnormal structural change in the genetic material of a cell). A

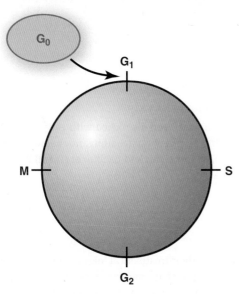

Figure 42-1 ■ Normal cell cycle. The normal cell cycle (the interval between the birth of a cell and its division into two daughter cells) involves several phases. During the resting phase (G_0), cells perform all usual functions except replication; that is, they are not dividing but are capable of doing so when stimulated. Different types of cells spend different lengths of time in this phase, after which they either reenter the cell cycle and differentiate or die. During the first active phase (G_1), ribonucleic acid (RNA) and enzymes required for production of deoxyribonucleic acid (DNA) are developed. During the next phase (S), DNA is synthesized for chromosomes. During G_2, RNA is synthesized, and the mitotic spindle is formed. Mitosis occurs in the final phase (M). The resulting two daughter cells may then enter the resting phase (G_0) or proceed through the reproductive cycle.

mutated cell may be destroyed by body defenses (e.g., an immune response) or it may replicate. When the mutated cell eludes destruction by the immune system and begins to reproduce, additional changes that occur during succeeding cell divisions may produce cells with progressively fewer normal and more malignant characteristics. It usually takes years for malignant cells to produce a clinically detectable neoplasm.

Development of Cancer

Cancer is a heterogeneous disease, and there are multiple causes, such as environmental factors (tobacco) and genetic factors. Genetic causes include mutation of genes, abnormal activation of genes that regulate cell growth and mitosis, or lack of tumor-suppressor genes. The abnormal genes, called *oncogenes*, are mutations of normal growth-regulating genes, called *proto-oncogenes*, which are present in all body cells. When proto-oncogenes are exposed to carcinogens and genetically altered to oncogenes, they may operate continuously and cause abnormal, disordered, and unregulated cell growth. Unregulated cell growth and proliferation increases the probability of neoplastic transformation of the cell. Tumors of the breast, colon, lung, and bone have been linked to activation of oncogenes.

Tumor-suppressor genes (*anti-oncogenes*) normally function to inhibit inappropriate cellular growth and proliferation. Abnormal tumor-suppressor genes (i.e., absent, damaged, mutated, or inactivated) may be inherited or result from exposure to carcinogens. When these genes are inactivated, a block to proliferation is removed and the cells begin unregulated growth. One tumor suppressor gene, p53, is present in virtually all normal tissues. When cellular deoxyribonucleic acid (DNA) is damaged, the p53 gene allows time for DNA repair and restricts proliferation of cells with abnormal DNA. Mutations of the p53 gene, a common genetic change in cancer, are associated with more than 90% of small cell lung cancers and more than 50% of breast and colon cancers. Mutant p53 proteins can also form complexes with normal p53 proteins and inactivate the function of the normal suppressor gene.

Thus, activation of oncogenes and inactivation of anti-oncogenes probably both play roles in cancer development. Multiple genetic abnormalities are characteristic of cancer cells and may occur concurrently or sequentially.

Overall, evidence indicates that neoplastic transformation is a progressive process involving several generations of cells, with each new generation becoming more like malignant cells. Thus, malignancy probably results from a combination of factors experienced over a person's lifetime, including random cell mutations, exposure to carcinogens, and host characteristics or lifestyle habits that increase susceptibility to cancer development. Some known carcinogens and risk factors are listed in Box 42-1.

After a cancer develops, factors influencing its growth include blood and nutrient supply, immune response, and hormonal stimulation (e.g., in tumors of the breast, uterus, ovary, and prostate). Malignant tumors are able to form new blood vessels (a process called *angiogenesis*) to support their growth.

Box 42-1	Carcinogens and Risk Factors

Environmental Carcinogens

Biologic carcinogens. Viruses linked to cancer include Epstein-Barr (Burkitt's lymphoma, Hodgkin's disease), hepatitis B and C (liver), herpes simplex II (cervix and vulva), human papilloma (cervix, penis, oral cavity, esophagus, larynx), human immunodeficiency (Kaposi's sarcoma), and human T-cell lymphotropic (T-cell leukemia or lymphoma). In addition, *Helicobacter pylori* bacteria are associated with gastric cancer and gastric lymphoma.

Radiation (e.g., from sunlight) can damage DNA and cause cell mutations.

Chemicals include many substances that can damage cellular structures and interfere with cell regulation. Industrial carcinogens include benzene (bladder cancer), hydrocarbons (lung and skin cancer), polyvinyl chloride (liver cancer), and other substances used in the production of various products. Workers who manufacture the products and people who live in the plant vicinity are most likely to be affected. Tobacco products, including cigarettes and smokeless products, contain numerous carcinogens and are associated with cancers of the lungs, mouth, pharynx, larynx, esophagus, and bladder.

Therapeutic drugs are associated with both hematologic and solid neoplasms. The alkylating antineoplastic drugs are associated with leukemia, lymphoma, and other cancers. The drugs damage DNA and interfere with growth or replication of tumor cells. At the same time, they may damage the DNA of normal cells and transform some of them into malignant cells. Immunosuppressants (e.g., azathioprine, cyclosporine, tacrolimus, corticosteroids) are associated with an increased risk of non-Hodgkin's lymphoma and skin cancer in renal transplant patients. Other patients taking immunosuppressant drugs (e.g., for rheumatoid arthritis) are at risk for lymphomas, squamous cell carcinoma of skin, and soft tissue sarcomas, but at lower rates than transplant recipients.

Sex hormones are growth factors for certain cells. In women, estrogens are associated with breast and endometrial cancer. The antiestrogen tamoxifen is associated with endometrial cancer. In men, androgens are associated with prostate cancer; and anabolic steroids, especially in high doses and with prolonged use, are associated with hepatic neoplasms.

Host Factors

Age. Except for a few early-childhood cancers, the risks of cancer increase with age.

Alcohol use is associated with cancers of the breast, head and neck, and liver.

Diet. A high-fat diet is associated with breast, colon, and prostate cancer; a low-fiber diet may increase risks of colon cancer.

Gender. Men are more likely to have leukemia and cancer of the urinary bladder, stomach, and pancreas; women are at risk of cancer of the breast, cervix, and endometrium. Lung and colon cancer occur equally in both sexes.

Geography and **ethnicity** are more environmental than hereditary or racial. Immigrants who adopt dietary and lifestyle habits of natives have similar risks and people who live in cities have greater risks because of greater exposure to air pollutants and other carcinogens. In the United States, African Americans have higher rates of multiple myeloma and cancers of the lung, prostate, esophagus, and pancreas than white people. In addition, African American women who develop breast cancer may have more aggressive, estrogen-receptor negative, high-grade tumors, and poorer survival rates than Hispanic and Caucasian women.

Heredity. In some families, there is a tendency toward development of cancer (e.g., close relatives of premenopausal women with breast cancer are at high risk for breast cancer).

Immunosuppression, whether caused by disease or drug therapy, is associated with an increased risk of lymphomas, skin cancers, and other malignancies.

Obesity is associated with increased risks of developing cancer of the breast, colon, endometrium, esophagus, liver, pancreas, and prostate gland.

Previous cancer is associated with a higher risk of other cancers in those who are treated with chemotherapy or radiation and survive. Secondary cancers are usually attributed to treatments that damage DNA and eventually transform normal cells into malignant cells.

Tobacco use is a major risk factor for cancers of the lung, esophagus, and head and neck. Chemicals in cigarette smoke cause most lung cancer, in smokers and other people exposed to cigarette smoke.

Classification of Malignant Neoplasms

Malignant neoplasms are classified according to the type of tissue involved and other characteristics. With the exception of the acute leukemias, they are considered chronic diseases.

Hematologic malignancies involve the bone marrow and lymphoid tissues; they include leukemias, lymphomas, and multiple myeloma. *Leukemias* are cancers of the bone marrow characterized by overproduction of abnormal white blood cells. The four main types are acute lymphocytic, acute myelogenous, chronic lymphocytic, and chronic myelogenous. Lymphomas are tumors of lymphoid tissue characterized by abnormal proliferation of the white blood cells normally found in lymphoid tissue. They usually develop within lymph nodes and may occur anywhere, because virtually all body tissues contain lymphoid structures. The two main types are Hodgkin's disease and non-Hodgkin's lymphoma. Multiple myeloma is a tumor of the bone marrow in which abnormal plasma cells proliferate. Because normal plasma cells produce antibodies and abnormal plasma cells cannot fulfill this function, the body's immune system is impaired. As the malignant cells expand, they crowd out normal cells, interfere with other bone marrow functions, infiltrate and destroy bone, and eventually metastasize to other tissues, such as the spleen, liver, and lymph nodes.

Solid neoplasms are composed of a mass of malignant cells (parenchyma) and a supporting structure of connective tissue, blood vessels, and lymphatics (stroma). The two major classifications are carcinomas and sarcomas. *Carcinomas* are derived from epithelial tissues (skin, mucous membrane, linings and coverings of viscera) and are the most common type of malignant tumors. They are further classified by cell type, such as adenocarcinoma or basal cell carcinoma. *Sarcomas* are derived from connective tissue (muscle, bone, cartilage, fibrous tissue, fat, blood vessels). They are subclassified by cell type (e.g., osteogenic sarcoma, angiosarcoma).

Grading and Staging of Malignant Neoplasms

When a malignant neoplasm is identified, it is further "graded" according to the degree of malignancy and "staged" according to tissue involvement. Grades 1 and 2 are similar to the normal tissue of origin and show cellular differentiation; grades 3 and 4 are unlike the normal tissue of origin, less differentiated, and more malignant. Staging indicates whether the neoplasm is localized or metastasized and which organs are involved. These characteristics assist in treatment (e.g., localized tumors are usually amenable to surgery, radiation, or chemotherapy combined with radiation [concurrent] therapy; metastatic disease requires systemic chemotherapy alone).

Effects of Cancer on the Host

Effects vary according to the location and extent of the disease process. There are few effects initially. As the neoplasm grows, effects occur when the tumor becomes large enough to cause pressure, distortion, or deficient blood supply in surrounding tissues; interfere with organ function; obstruct ducts and organs; and impair nutrition of normal tissues. More specific effects include anemia, malnutrition, pain, immunosuppression, infection, hemorrhagic tendencies, thromboembolism, hypercalcemia, cachexia, and various symptoms related to impaired function of affected organs and tissues.

Overview of Antineoplastic Drug Therapy

One definition of *chemotherapy* is the use of medications to treat cancer (rather than surgical or radiation therapy). However, the term is most often used to indicate the use of traditional cytotoxic antineoplastic drugs (as differentiated from biologic or hormonal therapy). Actually, except for hormone inhibitors that slow the growth of cancer cells stimulated by hormones, the purpose of all antineoplastic drugs is to damage or kill cancer cells (i.e., be cytotoxic). Most chemotherapy regimens involve a combination of drugs with different actions at the cellular level, which destroys a greater number of cancer cells and reduces the risk of the cancer developing drug resistance. Because drug resistance is a major problem, many newer drugs are recommended for use after initial drug therapy becomes ineffective (i.e., allows tumor progression).

Chemotherapy is usually administered in cycles, depending on the type of cancer and which drugs are used. Cycles involve taking the drugs daily, weekly, or monthly for a period of time, often with a recovery period following each treatment cycle. Recovery periods allow time for the patient's body to rest and produce new, healthy cells. Chemotherapy is often continued as long as it is effective and does not produce unacceptable toxicity.

Because the consequences of inappropriate or erroneous drug therapy may be fatal for patients (from the disease or the treatment), chemotherapy regimens should be managed by medical oncologists experienced in use of the drugs. Because of the drugs' toxicity, nurses who administer intravenous (IV) cytotoxic chemotherapy should be specially trained and certified in handling and administering the drugs safely and accurately.

Traditional Cytotoxic Antineoplastic Drugs

These drugs comprise the largest, oldest, and most diverse group of antineoplastic drugs. General characteristics and subgroups are described below; names, indications for use, dosages, and selected adverse effects of individual drugs are listed in Table 42-1.

General Characteristics

- Most drugs kill malignant cells by interfering with cell replication, with the supply and use of nutrients (e.g., amino acids, purines, pyrimidines), or with the genetic materials in the cell nucleus (DNA or RNA).

- The drugs act during the cell's reproductive cycle (Fig. 42-2). Some, called cell cycle–specific, act mainly during specific phases such as DNA synthesis or formation of the mitotic spindle. Others act during any phase of the cell cycle and are called cell cycle–nonspecific.

- *Cytotoxic* drugs are most active against rapidly dividing cells, both normal and malignant. Commonly damaged normal cells are those of the bone marrow, the lining of the gastrointestinal (GI) tract, and the hair follicles. Healthy cells usually recover fairly soon.

- Each drug dose kills a specific percentage of cells. To achieve a cure, all malignant cells must be killed or reduced to a small number that can be killed by the person's immune system.

- Antineoplastic drugs may induce drug-resistant malignant cells. Mechanisms may include inhibiting drug uptake or activation, increasing the rate of drug inactivation, pumping the drug out of the cell before it can act, increasing cellular repair of DNA damaged by the drugs, or altering metabolic pathways and target enzymes of the drugs. Mutant cells also may emerge.

- Most cytotoxic antineoplastic drugs are potential teratogens, and pregnancy should be avoided during and for several months after drug therapy is stopped.

Table 42-1 **Drugs at a Glance:** Cytotoxic Antineoplastic Drugs

GENERIC/ TRADE NAME	ROUTES AND DOSAGE RANGES*	CLINICAL USES	ADVERSE EFFECTS
Alkylating Drugs			
Nitrogen Mustard Derivatives			
Chlorambucil (Leukeran)	PO 0.1–0.2 mg/kg/d for 3–6 wk. Maintenance therapy, 0.03–0.1 mg/kg/d	Chronic lymphocytic leukemia, Hodgkin's and non-Hodgkin's lymphomas	Bone marrow depression, hepatotoxicity, secondary leukemia
Cyclophosphamide (Cytoxan)	Induction therapy, PO 1–5 mg/kg/d; IV 20–40 mg/kg in divided doses over 2–5 days. Maintenance therapy, PO 1–5 mg/kg daily	Hodgkin's disease; non-Hodgkin's lymphomas; leukemias; cancer of breast, lung, or ovary; multiple myeloma; neuroblastoma	Bone marrow depression, nausea, vomiting, alopecia, hemorrhagic cystitis, hypersensitivity reactions, secondary leukemia or bladder cancer
Ifosfamide (Ifex)	IV 1.2 g/m²/d for 5 consecutive d. Repeat every 3 wk or after white blood cell and platelet counts return to normal after a dose.	Germ cell testicular cancer	Bone marrow depression, hemorrhagic cystitis, nausea and vomiting, alopecia, CNS depression, seizures
Melphalan (Alkeran)	PO 6 mg/d for 2–3 wk, then 28 drug-free days, then 2 mg daily IV 16 mg/m² every 2 wk for 4 doses, then every 4 wk	Multiple myeloma, ovarian cancer	Bone marrow depression, nausea and vomiting, hypersensitivity reactions
Nitrosoureas			
Carmustine (BiCNU, Gliadel)	IV 150–200 mg/m² every 6 wk Wafer, implanted in brain after tumor resection	Hodgkin's disease, non-Hodgkin's lymphomas, multiple myeloma, brain tumors	Bone marrow depression, nausea, vomiting
Lomustine (CCNU)	PO 130 mg/m² every 6 wk	Hodgkin's disease, brain tumors	Nausea and vomiting, bone marrow depression
Platinum Compounds			
Carboplatin (Paraplatin)	IV infusion 360 mg/m² on day 1 every 4 wk	Palliation of ovarian cancer	Bone marrow depression, nausea and vomiting, nephrotoxicity
Cisplatin (Platinol)	IV 100 mg/m² once every 4 wk	Advanced carcinomas of testes, bladder, ovary	Nausea, vomiting, anaphylaxis, nephrotoxicity, bone marrow depression, ototoxicity
Oxaliplatin (Eloxatin)	IV infusion 85 mg/m² every 2 wk	Advanced colon cancer	Anaphylaxis, anemia, increased risk of bleeding or infection, cold-induced acute neurotoxicities
Antimetabolites			
Capecitabine (Xeloda)	PO 1250 mg/m² q12h for 2 wk, then a rest period of 1 wk, then repeat cycle	Metastatic breast cancer, colorectal cancer	Bone marrow depression, nausea, vomiting, diarrhea, mucositis, hand & foot syndrome
Cladribine (Leustatin)	IV infusion 0.09 mg/kg/d for 7 consecutive d	Hairy cell leukemia	Bone marrow depression, nausea, vomiting
Cytarabine (Cytosar-U)	IV infusion 100 mg/m²/d for 7 d	Leukemias of adults and children	Bone marrow depression, nausea, vomiting, anaphylaxis, mucositis, diarrhea

(continued on page 680)

Table 42-1 **Drugs at a Glance:** Cytotoxic Antineoplastic Drugs (continued)

GENERIC/ TRADE NAME	ROUTES AND DOSAGE RANGES*	CLINICAL USES	ADVERSE EFFECTS
Fludarabine (Fludara)	IV 25 mg/m²/d for 5 consecutive d; repeat every 28 d	Chronic lymphocytic leukemia	Bone marrow depression, nausea, vomiting, diarrhea
Fluorouracil (5-FU) (Adrucil, Efudex, Fluoroplex)	IV 12 mg/kg/d for 4 d, then 6 mg/kg every other day for 4 doses	Carcinomas of the breast, colon, stomach, and pancreas	Bone marrow depression, nausea, vomiting, mucositis
	Topical, apply to skin cancer lesion twice daily for several weeks	Solar keratoses, basal cell carcinoma	Pain, pruritus, burning at site of application
Gemcitabine (Gemzar)	IV 1000 mg/m² once weekly up to 7 wk or toxicity, withhold for 1 wk, then once weekly for 3 wk and withhold for 1 wk	Lung and pancreatic cancer	Bone marrow depression, nausea, vomiting, flu-like symptoms, skin rash
Mercaptopurine (Purinethol)	PO 2.5 mg/kg/d (100–200 mg for average adult)	Acute and chronic leukemias	Bone marrow depression, nausea, vomiting, mucositis
P **Methotrexate (MTX)** (Rheumatrex)	Acute leukemia in children, induction, PO, IV 3 mg/m²/d; maintenance, PO 30 mg/m² twice weekly	Leukemias; non-Hodgkin's lymphomas; osteosarcoma; choriocarcinoma of testes; cancers of breast, lung, head and neck	Bone marrow depression, nausea, vomiting, mucositis, diarrhea, fever, alopecia
	Choriocarcinoma, PO, IM 15 mg/m² daily for 5 d		
Pemetrexed (Alimta)	IV infusion 500 mg/m² over 10 min, every 21 d	Non–small cell lung cancer	Mucositis, skin rash
Antitumor Antibiotics **Bleomycin** (Blenoxane)	IV, IM, Sub-Q 0.25–0.5 units/kg once or twice weekly	Squamous cell carcinoma, Hodgkin's and non-Hodgkin's lymphomas, testicular carcinoma	Pulmonary toxicity, mucositis, alopecia, nausea, vomiting, hypersensitivity reactions
Dactinomycin (Actinomycin D, Cosmegen)	IV 15 mcg/kg/d for 5 d and repeated every 2–4 wk	Rhabdomyosarcoma, Wilms' tumor, choriocarcinoma, testicular carcinoma, Ewing's sarcoma	Bone marrow depression, nausea, vomiting. Extravasation may lead to tissue necrosis.
Daunorubicin conventional	IV 25–45 mg/m² daily for 3 d every 3–4 wk	Acute leukemias, lymphomas	Same as doxorubicin, below
Daunorubicin liposomal (DaunoXome)	IV infusion, 40 mg/m² every 2 wk	AIDS-related Kaposi's sarcoma	Bone marrow depression, nausea, vomiting
Doxorubicin conventional (Adriamycin)	Adults, IV 60–75 mg/m² every 21 d	Acute leukemias; lymphomas; carcinomas of breast, lung, and ovary	Bone marrow depression, alopecia, mucositis, GI upset, cardiomyopathy. Extravasation may lead to tissue necrosis.
	Children, IV 30 mg/m² daily for 3 d, repeated every 4 wk		
Doxorubicin liposomal (Doxil)	IV infusion, 20 mg/m², once every 3 wk	AIDS-related Kaposi's sarcoma	Bone marrow depression, nausea, vomiting, fever, alopecia
Epirubicin (Ellence)	IV infusion 120 mg/m² every 3–4 wk	Breast cancer	Cardiotoxicity
Idarubicin (Idamycin)	IV injection 12 mg/m²/d for 3 d, with cytarabine	Acute myeloid leukemia	Same as doxorubicin, above

GENERIC/ TRADE NAME	ROUTES AND DOSAGE RANGES*	CLINICAL USES	ADVERSE EFFECTS
Mitomycin (Mutamycin)	IV 20 mg/m^2 every 6–8 wk	Metastatic carcinomas of stomach and pancreas	Bone marrow depression, nausea, vomiting. Extravasation may lead to tissue necrosis.
Mitoxantrone (Novantrone)	IV infusion 12 mg/m^2 on days 1–3, for induction of remission in leukemia	Acute nonlymphocytic leukemia, prostate cancer	Bone marrow depression, congestive heart failure, nausea
Pentostatin (Nipent)	IV 4 mg/m^2 every other week	Hairy cell leukemia unresponsive to interferon alfa	Bone marrow depression, hepatotoxicity, nausea, vomiting
Valrubicin (Valstar)	Intravesically, 800 mg once weekly for 6 wk	Bladder cancer	Dysuria, urgency, frequency, bladder spasms, hematuria
Plant Alkaloids **Camptothecins** **Irinotecan** (Camptosar)	IV infusion, 125 mg/m^2 once weekly for 4 wk, then a 2-wk rest period; repeat regimen	Metastatic cancer of colon or rectum	Bone marrow depression, diarrhea
Topetecan (Hycamtin)	IV infusion 1.5 mg/m^2 daily for 5 consecutive days every 21 d	Advanced ovarian cancer, small-cell lung cancer	Bone marrow depression, nausea, vomiting, diarrhea
Podophyllotoxins **Etoposide** (VePesid)	IV 50–100 mg/m^2/d on days 1–5, or 100 mg/m^2/d on days 1, 3, and 5, every 3–4 wk PO 2 times the IV dose	Testicular cancer, small-cell lung cancer	Bone marrow depression, allergic reactions, nausea, vomiting, alopecia
Teniposide (Vumon)	IV infusion 165 mg/m^2 twice weekly for 8–9 doses	Acute lymphocytic leukemia in children	Same as etoposide, above
Taxanes **Docetaxel** (Taxotere)	IV infusion 60–100 mg/m^2, every 3 wk	Advanced breast cancer, non–small cell lung cancer	Bone marrow depression, nausea, vomiting, hypersensitivity reactions
Paclitaxel (Taxol)	IV infusion 135 mg/m^2 every 3 wk	Advanced ovarian cancer, advanced breast cancer, non–small cell lung cancer, AIDS-related Kaposi's sarcoma	Bone marrow depression, allergic reactions, hypotension, bradycardia, nausea, vomiting
Vinca Alkaloids **Vinblastine** (Velban)	Adults, IV 3.7–11.1 mg/m^2 (average 5.5–7.4 mg/m^2) weekly Children, IV 2.5–7.5 mg/m^2 weekly	Metastatic testicular carcinoma, Hodgkin's disease	Bone marrow depression, nausea, vomiting. Extravasation may lead to tissue necrosis.
Vincristine (Oncovin)	Adults, IV 1.4 mg/m^2 weekly Children, IV 2 mg/m^2 weekly	Hodgkin's and other lymphomas, acute leukemia, neuroblastoma, Wilms' tumor	Peripheral neuropathy. Extravasation may lead to tissue necrosis.
Vinorelbine (Navelbine)	IV injection 30 mg/m^2 once weekly	Non–small cell lung cancer	Bone marrow depression, peripheral neuropathy. Extravasation may lead to tissue necrosis.

(continued on page 682)

Table 42-1	Drugs at a Glance: Cytotoxic Antineoplastic Drugs (continued)

GENERIC/ TRADE NAME	ROUTES AND DOSAGE RANGES*	CLINICAL USES	ADVERSE EFFECTS
Miscellaneous Agents			
L-Asparaginase (Elspar)	IV 1000 IU/kg/d for 10 d	Acute lymphocytic leukemia	Hypersensitivity reactions, including anaphylaxis
Hydroxyurea (Hydrea)	PO 80 mg/kg as a single dose every third day or 20–30 mg/kg as a single dose daily	Chronic myelocytic leukemia, melanoma, ovarian cancer, head and neck cancer	Bone marrow depression, nausea, vomiting, peripheral neuritis
Ixabepilone (Ixempra)	IV infusion 40 mg/m² over 3h, every 3 wk	Advanced breast cancer	Bone marrow suppression, peripheral neuropathy nausea, vomiting, diarrhea, mucositis
Levamisole (Ergamisol)	PO 50 mg q8h for 3 d every 2 wk	Colon cancer, with fluorouracil	Nausea, vomiting, diarrhea
Procarbazine (Matulane)	PO 2–4 mg/kg/d for 1 wk, then 4–6 mg/kg/d	Hodgkin's disease	Bone marrow depression, mucositis, CNS depression

*Dosages may vary significantly or change often, according to use in different types of cancer and in different combinations.

AIDS, acquired immunodeficiency syndrome.

▪ Most antineoplastic drugs are given orally or IV; some are given topically, intrathecally, or by instillation into a body cavity.

▪ Doxorubicin and daunorubicin are available in conventional and liposomal preparations. The liposomal preparations increase drug concentration in malignant tissues and decrease concentration in normal tissues, thereby increasing effectiveness while decreasing toxicity (e.g., cardiotoxicity).

▪ Common adverse effects include *alopecia* (hair loss), anemia, bleeding, fatigue, *mucositis* (inflammation and erosion of oral mucous membrane), nausea and vomiting, *neutropenia* (low white blood cell count), and *thrombocytopenia* (low platelet count). Other problems may include damage to the heart, liver, lungs, kidneys, or nerves. In general, adverse effects depend on the specific drugs used and the patient's health status.

▪ With treatment of leukemias and lymphomas, a serious, life-threatening adverse effect called tumor lysis syndrome may occur. This syndrome occurs when large numbers of cancer cells are killed or damaged and release their contents into the bloodstream. As a result, hyperkalemia, hyperphosphatemia, hyperuricemia, hypomagnesemia, hypocalcemia, and acidosis develop. Signs and symptoms depend on the severity of the metabolic imbalances but may include GI upset, fatigue, altered mental status, hypertension, muscle cramps, paresthesias (numbness and tingling), tetany,

seizures, electrocardiographic changes (e.g., dysrhythmias), cardiac arrest, reduced urine output, and acute renal failure. The condition can be prevented or minimized by aggressive hydration with IV normal saline, alkalinization with IV sodium bicarbonate, and administration of allopurinol (e.g., 300 mg daily for adults and 10 mg/kg/d for children) to reduce uric acid levels. Maintaining a urine pH of 7 or more prevents renal failure from precipitation of uric acid crystals in the kidneys. Treatment of hyperkalemia may include IV dextrose and regular insulin (to drive potassium into cells) or Kayexalate to eliminate potassium in feces. Treatment of hyperphosphatemia may include administration of aluminum hydroxide or another phosphate-binding agent. Hemodialysis may be used if the other measures are ineffective.

▪ Many cytotoxic antineoplastic drugs have **BLACK BOX WARNINGS** about potentially serious adverse effects and special precautions for safe usage.

Indications for Use

Cytotoxic antineoplastic drugs are used to cure the disease, relieve symptoms, or induce or maintain *remission* (symptom-free period). In hematologic neoplasms, drug therapy is the treatment of choice because the disease is systemic rather than localized. In solid tumors, drug therapy may be used before or after surgery or radiation therapy and when metastasis occurs.

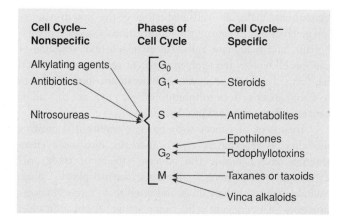

Figure 42-2 ■ Cell cycle effects of cytotoxic antineoplastic drugs.

Antineoplastic drugs are sometimes used in the treatment of nonmalignant conditions. For example, small doses of methotrexate (MTX) are used for rheumatoid arthritis and psoriasis.

Classifications and Mechanisms of Action

Cytotoxic antineoplastic drugs are usually classified in terms of their mechanisms of action (alkylating agents and antimetabolites) or their sources (plant alkaloids, antibiotics).

Alkylating Agents

Alkylating agents include nitrogen mustard derivatives, nitrosoureas, and platinum compounds. *Nitrogen mustard derivatives* (e.g., *cyclophosphamide*) interfere with cell division and the structure of DNA during all phases of the malignant cell cycle. As a result, they have a broad spectrum of activity. They are most effective in hematologic malignancies but also are used to treat breast, lung, and ovarian tumors. All of these drugs cause significant bone marrow depression (*myelosuppression*) and frequent complete blood counts (CBCs) are required.

Nitrosoureas also interfere with DNA replication and RNA synthesis and may inhibit essential enzymatic reactions of cancer cells. They are cell cycle–nonspecific and may be used in patients with GI, lung, and brain tumors. They are highly lipid soluble and therefore enter the brain and cerebrospinal fluid more readily than other antineoplastic drugs. They cause delayed bone marrow depression, with maximum *leukopenia* and thrombocytopenia occurring 5 to 6 weeks after drug administration. As a result, the drugs are given less often than other drugs, and CBCs are needed weekly for at least 6 weeks after a dose.

Platinum compounds are cell cycle–nonspecific agents that inhibit DNA, RNA, and protein synthesis. *Cisplatin* is used to treat advanced cancers of the bladder, ovary and testes. Adverse effects include severe nausea and vomiting and nephrotoxicity. Carboplatin is used to treat endometrial and ovarian carcinomas, and it produces bone marrow depression

as a major adverse effect. Oxaliplatin is used to treat colorectal cancer, with 5-fluorouracil and leucovorin. Adverse effects include anemia and peripheral neuropathy.

Antimetabolites

Antimetabolites are diverse drugs that are allowed to enter cancer cells because they are similar to metabolites or nutrients needed by the cells for reproduction. Inside the cell, the drugs replace normal metabolites or inhibit essential enzymes. These actions deprive the cell of substances needed for formation of DNA or cause formation of abnormal DNA. The drugs are cell cycle–specific because they exert their cytotoxic effects only during the S phase of the cell's reproductive cycle, when DNA is being synthesized.

This group includes folic acid antagonists (e.g., **P** methotrexate (prototype), pemetrexed), purine antagonists (e.g., *mercaptopurine*), and pyrimidine antagonists (e.g., *fluorouracil*). These drugs are most effective against rapidly growing tumors, and individual drugs vary in their effectiveness with different kinds of cancer. Toxic effects include bone marrow depression, mucositis and ulceration of the GI tract, and hair loss. Pemetrexed blocks folate and enzymes essential for cancer cell reproduction and may increase blood levels of homocysteine. Homocysteine is produced when proteins are broken down in the blood and elevated blood levels are considered a risk factor for coronary artery disease and stroke. Treatment with folic acid and vitamin B_{12} supplements, which can reduce homocysteine blood levels, is required for all patients taking the drug.

Applying Your Knowledge 42-1

Because Ms. Gardner is being treated as an outpatient, it is extremely important that an appropriate plan of care be made to allow her to care for the adverse effects of these medications at home. What are the most common adverse effects of the methotrexate and what nursing interventions should be anticipated?

Antitumor Antibiotics

These drugs (e.g., **doxorubicin**) bind to DNA so that DNA and RNA transcription is blocked. They are active in all phases of the cell cycle, and their cytotoxic effects are similar to those of the alkylating agents. Major toxicities are bone marrow depression and GI upset. Doxorubicin and related drugs also cause cardiotoxicity and tissue necrosis if *extravasation* (leaking of medication into soft tissues around the venipuncture site) occurs. Bleomycin may cause significant pulmonary toxicity.

Plant Alkaloids

Plant alkaloids include derivatives of camptothecin (e.g., *topotecan*), podophyllotoxin (e.g., *etoposide*), taxanes (e.g., paclitaxel), and plants of the *Vinca* genus (e.g., **vincristine**). These drugs vary in their characteristics and clinical uses.

Camptothecins (also called DNA topoisomerase inhibitors) inhibit an enzyme required for DNA replication and repair. They have activity in several types of cancers; dose-limiting toxicity is myelosuppression.

Podophyllotoxins act mainly in the G_2 phase of the cell cycle and prevent mitosis. Etoposide is used mainly to treat testicular and small cell lung cancer; teniposide is used mainly for childhood acute lymphocytic leukemia. Dose-limiting toxicity is myelosuppression.

Taxanes inhibit cell division (antimitotic effects). They are used mainly for advanced breast and ovarian cancers. Dose-limiting toxicity is neutropenia.

Vinca alkaloids are cell cycle–specific agents that stop mitosis. These drugs have similar structures but different antineoplastic activities and adverse effects. Vincristine is used to treat Hodgkin's disease, acute lymphoblastic leukemia, and non-Hodgkin's lymphomas. Vinblastine is used to treat Hodgkin's disease and choriocarcinoma; vinorelbine is used to treat non–small cell lung cancer. The drugs can cause severe tissue damage with extravasation. In addition, vinblastine and vinorelbine cause bone marrow depression, and vincristine causes peripheral nerve toxicity.

Miscellaneous Cytotoxic Agents

Miscellaneous agents vary in their sources, mechanisms of action, indications for use, and toxic effects. L-Asparaginase (Elspar) is an enzyme that inhibits protein synthesis and reproduction by depriving cells of required amino acids. It is used to treat acute lymphocytic leukemia and can cause allergic reactions, including anaphylaxis. **Pegaspargase** (Oncaspar) is a modified formulation for people who are hypersensitive to Elspar. **Hydroxyurea** acts in the S phase of the cell cycle to impair DNA synthesis. It is used to treat leukemia, melanoma, and advanced ovarian cancer. A major adverse effect is myelosuppression. **Ixabepilone** (Ixempra) is the first of a new class of antineoplastic drugs called epothilones. Epothilones, which are obtained from bacteria, stop growth of tumor cells by preventing cell division (antimitotic effects). Ixabepilone is a semisynthetic analog of epothilone approved for treatment of advanced breast cancer, alone or with capecitabine. Adverse effects include bone marrow suppression, hypersensitivity reactions, and peripheral neuropathy. **Procarbazine** inhibits DNA, RNA, and protein synthesis. It is used to treat Hodgkin's disease. It is a monoamine oxidase inhibitor and may cause hypertension if given with adrenergic drugs, tricyclic antidepressants, or foods with high tyramine content (see Chap. 10). Common adverse effects include leukopenia and thrombocytopenia.

Biologic Targeted Antineoplastic Drugs

Two major mechanisms in cancer development are thought to be failure of the immune system to eliminate mutant, prema-

lignant, and malignant cells and failure of the growth-regulating mechanisms to control the proliferation of mutant, premalignant, and malignant cells. As increased understanding of cancer-cell biology has evolved in recent years, much research has focused on biologic agents to stimulate the immune system to fight cancer cells or to inhibit biologic processes that allow cancer cells to grow and proliferate.

Treatment of cancer with biologic agents is a growing modality as researchers try to increase anticancer effectiveness and decrease the adverse effects of traditional cytotoxic chemotherapy. Biologic antineoplastic drugs include immunotherapy drugs and drugs that "target" biologic processes of malignant cells. Some immunologic anticancer drugs are discussed in Chapter 40 (e.g., bacillus Calmette-Guérin vaccine for bladder cancer; interferon alfa for AIDS-related Kaposi's sarcoma, selected leukemias, malignant melanoma, and non-Hodgkin's lymphoma; and interleukin-2 for renal cell carcinoma). Other available drugs are monoclonal antibodies, tyrosine kinase inhibitors, and a proteasome inhibitor. These drugs are described below and in Table 42-2.

Monoclonal Antibodies

Monoclonal antibodies (see Chap. 41) are produced from one cell line. Early murine (mouse-derived) antibodies produced problems as hosts' immune systems reacted against the foreign protein. Most newer drugs are humanized and target specific cellular components. In cancer, these drugs act by one of three main mechanisms: blocking a receptor and preventing the over-expressed growth factor receptors from signaling for cell division, attaching to a cell receptor so that the body's own immune system can kill the cell, or carrying chemotherapy or radioisotopes to the cancer cells and causing cell death.

Alemtuzumab (Campath) and **rituximab** (Rituxan) bind to an antigen on normal T and B lymphocytes and malignant lymphoid cells to activate antibody- and complement-mediated cytotoxicity. **Bevacizumab** (Avastin), **cetuximab** (Erbitux), **panitumumab** (Vectibix), and **trastuzumab** (Herceptin) bind to growth factors or growth factor receptors found on blood vessels, colorectal cancer cells, and breast cancer cells, respectively, to prevent the growth factors from becoming activated and stimulating cell growth. For example, bevacizumab was developed to bind with vascular endothelial growth factor (VEGF) and inhibit the formation of the new blood vessels required for tumor growth (antiangiogenesis). In addition, trastuzumab was developed to bind with human epidermal growth factor receptor 2 (HER2), of which 25% to 30% of women with breast cancer have an excessive number.

Gemtuzumab ozogamicin (Mylotarg), **ibritumomab tiuxetan** (Zevalin), and **tositumomab and iodine I-131 tositumomab** (Bexxar) are conjugated with a radioisotope or toxin to increase anticancer effectiveness.

Table 42-2	Drugs at a Glance: Biologic Antineoplastic Drugs

GENERIC/TRADE NAMES	ROUTES AND DOSAGE RANGES	CLINICAL USES	ADVERSE EFFECTS
Monoclonal Antibodies			
Alemtuzumab (Campath IH)	IV infusion, initially, 3 mg/d as a 2-h infusion; increase to 10 mg/d, then to 30 mg/d as tolerated. Maintenance, 30 mg/d 3 times weekly on alternate days for up to 12 wk	Chronic lymphocytic leukemia in patients previously treated with alkylating agents and fludarabine	Allergic infusion reactions (dyspnea, fever, chills, skin rash), immunosuppression, hypotension, hypertension, peripheral edema, nausea, vomiting, diarrhea, mucositis
Bevacizumab (Avastin)	IV infusion, 5 mg/kg once every 14 d until disease progression is detected	Colorectal cancer	Heart failure, hemorrhage, hypertension, diarrhea, leukopenia, pain, dyspnea, dermatitis, stomatitis, vomiting
Cetuximab (Erbitux)	IV infusion, initially, 400 mg/m^2 over 2 h; maintenance, 250 mg/m^2 over 1 h once weekly	Metastatic colorectal cancer	Anemia, leukopenia, infusion reaction, nausea, diarrhea, stomatitis, vomiting, dyspnea, fever
Gemtuzumab ozogamicin (Mylotarg)	IV infusion, 9 mg/m^2, for 2 doses, 14 d apart	Acute myeloid leukemia	Chills, fever, nausea, vomiting, diarrhea
Ibritumomab tiuxetan (Zevalin)	See literature	Non-Hodgkin's lymphoma, with rituximab	Severe or fatal infusion reaction, severe bone marrow depression
Panitumumab (Vectibix)	IV infusion, 6 mg/kg over 60 min every 14 days. Doses over 1000 mg should be given over 90 min.	Metastatic colorectal cancer	Infusion reactions, skin rash, pulmonary fibrosis, nausea, vomiting, diarrhea
Rituximab (Rituxan)	IV infusion, 375 mg/m^2 once weekly for 4 doses	Non-Hodgkin's lymphoma	Hypersensitivity reactions, cardiac dysrhythmias
Tositumomab and Iodine 131-Itositumomab (Bexxar)	See literature	Non-Hodgkin's lymphoma	Fever, chills, nausea, vomiting, skin rash, headache, cough, infection, pain
Trastuzumab (Herceptin)	IV infusion, 4 mg/kg initially, then 2 mg/kg once weekly	Metastatic breast cancer	Cardiotoxicity (dyspnea, edema, heart failure)
Growth Factor and Tyrosine Kinase Inhibitors			
Dasatinib (Sprycel)	PO 70 mg twice daily	Chronic myelogenous leukemia Acute lymphoblastic leukemia	Anemia, diarrhea, dyspnea, edema, fever, infection, nausea, pain, skin rash
Erlotinib (Tarceva)	PO 150 mg daily	Non–small cell lung cancer, brain glioma	Nausea, vomiting, diarrhea, skin rash
Imatinib (Gleevec)	Adults, PO 400–800 mg/d Children, 3 y and older, PO 260–340 mg/m^2/d	Chronic myeloid leukemia, gastrointestinal stromal tumors (GIST)	Dyspnea, edema, heart failure, hemorrhage, nausea, vomiting, diarrhea, neutropenia, thrombocytopenia
Lapatanib (Tykerb)	PO 1250 mg (5 tablets) once daily on days 1 to 21, with capecitabine PO 2000 mg/m^2/d (in 2 doses, 12 h apart) on days 1 to 14 in a repeating 21-d cycle	Advanced breast cancer	Diarrhea, dyspnea, insomnia, nausea, vomiting, stomatitis

(continued on page 686)

Table 42-2	Drugs at a Glance: Biologic Antineoplastic Drugs (continued)		
GENERIC/TRADE NAMES	**ROUTES AND DOSAGE RANGES**	**CLINICAL USES**	**ADVERSE EFFECTS**
Sorafenib (Nexavar)	PO 400 mg twice daily	Advanced renal cell cancer, advanced liver cell cancer	Hypertension, skin rash, alopecia, anemia, nausea, vomiting, diarrhea
Sunitinib (Sutent)	PO 50 mg daily for 4 wk, followed by 2 wk off drug	Advanced renal cell cancer, gastrointestinal stromal tumors (GIST)	Hypertension, skin rash, diarrhea, anemia, neutropenia, nausea and vomiting
Temsirolimus (Torisel)	IV infusion, 25 mg over 30–60 min once per week	Advanced renal cell cancer	Anorexia, diarrhea, edema, mucositis, nausea, skin rash
Proteasome Inhibitor **Bortezomib (Velcade)**	IV injection, 1.3 mg/m^2, twice weekly for 2 wk, followed by a 10-d rest period	Multiple myeloma	Edema, nausea, vomiting, diarrhea, anemia, neutropenia, thrombocytopenia

Serious adverse effects of these drugs include a potentially fatal hypersensitivity-type infusion reaction (e.g., chills, fever, bronchospasm, dyspnea, skin rash or urticaria) and bone marrow depression (e.g., anemia, leukopenia, thrombocytopenia). To prevent or decrease infusion reactions, premedication with diphenhydramine (Benadryl) and acetaminophen is recommended. With alemtuzumab, a very high risk of infection results because the drug depletes normal B and T lymphocytes. As a result, prophylactic antimicrobial drugs are recommended during and for 3 months after alemtuzumab administration. Severe cardiotoxicity, including heart failure, has also been reported, more often with bevacizumab and trastuzumab. With trastuzumab, patients at higher risk of cardiotoxicity include those 60 years and older and those who have received doxorubicin (or a related drug) or cyclophosphamide. Left ventricular function should be evaluated in all patients before and during treatment and trastuzumab should be discontinued in those who develop significant decreases.

Monoclonal antibodies, which may be used alone or in combination with traditional cytotoxic antineoplastic drugs and other treatment modalities, have become an integral part of treatment plans for a variety of cancers. They and other biologic targeted therapies continue to be developed and tested for clinical use.

Applying Your Knowledge 42-2

Ms. Gardner asks why she must take the Herceptin because there are such serious concerns about an allergic reaction to the monoclonal antibodies. How would you respond?

Growth Factor and Tyrosine Kinase Inhibitors

Growth factors such as epidermal growth factor (EGF, which stimulates the growth of epithelial cells in the skin and other organs) and platelet-derived growth factor (PDGF, which stimulates the proliferation of vascular smooth muscle and endothelial cells) bind to receptors on cell membrane surfaces or within cells and initiate intracellular events that result in cell growth. EGF is normally produced in the kidneys and salivary glands and is found in almost all body fluids. When EGF binds to the external portion of the EGF receptor, it stimulates gene expression, cell proliferation, programmed cell death (apoptosis), and angiogenesis.

The EGF receptor (EGFR; also called the tyrosine kinase receptor), which is found in normal body cells and some malignant cells, has three distinctive areas (Fig. 42-3). One area is on the cell membrane surface and available to combine with EGF. A second area crosses the cell membrane. A third, an intracellular area, contains tyrosine kinase enzymes. Tyrosine kinase enzymes play an important role in the proliferation and differentiation of cells.

Erlotinib (Tarceva) inhibits the tyrosine kinase enzyme portion of the EGFR. This action inhibits cell proliferation and induces cell death. The drug is used to treat advanced non–small cell lung cancer, the most common type of lung cancer, which is known to over-express the EGFR. It is also used to treat malignant glioma, a type of brain tumor. Adverse effects include skin rash, diarrhea, nausea, and vomiting. In addition, interstitial lung disease has been reported in some patients, with a few deaths. Patients should be monitored for acute onset or worsening of dyspnea and pneumonitis. If interstitial lung disease is confirmed, erlotinib should be discontinued.

Imatinib (Gleevec) inhibits several tyrosine kinase enzymes that are essential to the growth of some cancer cells,

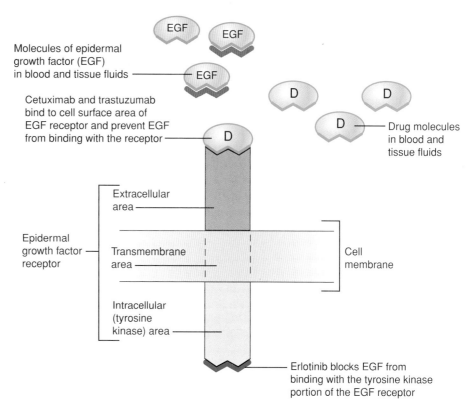

Figure 42-3 ▪ Actions of selected biologic targeted drugs. These drugs prevent epidermal growth factor (EGF) from combining with its receptors and thereby prevent or decrease cell growth. Cetuximab and trastuzumab bind with the extracellular portion of the EGF receptor; erlotinib blocks the intracellular (tyrosine kinase) portion of the EGF receptor.

including an abnormal type of tyrosine kinase thought to be the main cause of chronic myelogenous leukemia (CML) and the tyrosine kinases activated by PDGF and stem cell factor (SCF). This action inhibits cell proliferation and induces cell death. The drug is used to treat CML and a rare type of cancer called gastrointestinal stromal tumor (GIST). It is well absorbed with oral administration, and peak serum levels are reached in 2 to 4 hours. It is highly protein bound, its elimination half-life is 18 hours, it is metabolized in the liver, and it is excreted mainly in feces. Adverse effects include anemia, cardiotoxicity, edema, musculoskeletal pain, and nausea

Dasatinib (Sprycel), **lapatinib** (Tykerb), **sorafenib** (Nexavar), **sunitinib** (Sutent), and **temsirolimus** (Torisel) are newer tyrosine kinase inhibitors with varying indications for use and adverse effects (see Table 42-2). Most are recommended for use after disease progression with imatinib or other treatment.

Most of these drugs are metabolized mainly by cytochrome P450 3A4 enzymes and interact with drugs that induce (e.g., rifampin, phenytoin) or inhibit (e.g., clarithromycin, itraconazole) these enzymes. Dosage may need to be increased with concurrent administration of inducers or decreased with concurrent use of inhibitors.

Proteasome Inhibitor

Proteasomes are enzyme complexes in the cytoplasm and nucleus of all body cells, both normal and malignant. These enzymes regulate intracellular proteins. **Bortezomib** (Velcade) inhibits proteasomes, affects multiple proteins within cells, and is thought to have multiple mechanisms of cytotoxicity (e.g., preventing formation of new blood vessels in tumors and accelerating death of malignant cells). In general, the drug leads to cell cycle arrest, delayed tumor growth, and cell death. It is indicated for treatment of multiple myeloma in patients whose disease progressed during previous treatment.

Bortezomib is moderately protein bound (83%) and metabolized by several cytochrome P450 enzymes in the liver. The drug should be used with caution in patients with impaired hepatic or renal function. Adverse effects include peripheral neuropathy, which may be increased with previous use of neurotoxic agents or pre-existing peripheral neuropathy. Dosage adjustment may be needed.

Antineoplastic Hormone Inhibitor Drugs

The main hormonal agents used in the treatment of cancer are the corticosteroids (see Chap. 23) and drugs that block the production or activity of estrogens and androgens. Corticosteroids suppress or kill malignant lymphocytes and are most useful in the treatment of leukemias, lymphomas, and multiple myeloma. They are also used to treat complications of cancer (e.g., brain metastases, hypercalcemia). Prednisone and dexamethasone are commonly used. Sex-hormone blocking drugs are used mainly to control tumor growth and relieve symptoms. They are not cytotoxic and adverse effects are usually mild.

Sex hormones are growth factors in some malignancies (e.g., estrogens in breast and uterine cancer, androgens in prostate cancer). The hormones may be normally produced within the body or administered as drugs. For example, oral contraceptives and long-term estrogen replacement therapy are associated with breast cancer.

Surgery or antihormonal drugs may be used to decrease hormonal stimulation of cancer growth. Estrogens and androgens are normally produced from cholesterol through a series of chemical conversions involving the hypothalamus, anterior pituitary, adrenal glands, and ovaries in females and testes in males. Preventing production anywhere along this path or blocking estrogens and androgens from combining with their receptors in target tissues can decrease the growth of cells stimulated by the hormones. Excision of the ovaries or testes (surgical castration) and antihormonal drugs (medical or chemical castration) are commonly used. The ovaries are most likely to be removed in premenopausal women with breast cancer and the testes may be removed in men with prostate cancer. In general, currently used drugs interfere with hormone production or hormone action at the cellular level (Fig. 42-4).

The main hormone inhibitor drugs are the antiestrogens, aromatase inhibitors, antiandrogens, and luteinizing hormone–releasing hormone (LHRH; also known as gonadotropin-releasing hormone [GnRH]) analogs. These are described as follows and in Table 42-3.

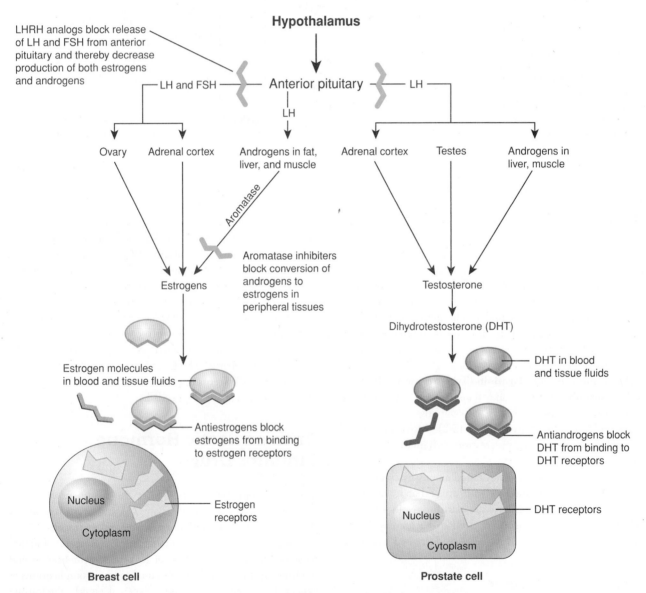

Figure 42-4 ■ Actions of hormone inhibitor drugs. Drugs used to treat breast cancer block the production of estrogens (e.g., LHRH analogs, aromatase inhibitors) or prevent estrogens from binding to receptors in breast cancer cells (antiestrogens). Drugs used to treat prostate cancer block the production of androgens (e.g., LHRH analogs) or prevent DHT, the active form of testosterone, from binding to receptors in prostate cancer cells (antiandrogens).

Table 42-3	Drugs at a Glance: Antineoplastic Hormone Inhibitors		

GENERIC/TRADE NAMES	ROUTES AND DOSAGE RANGES	CLINICAL USES	ADVERSE EFFECTS
Antiestrogens			
Fulvestrant (Faslodex)	IM 250 mg once monthly (one 5-mL or two 2.5-mL injections)	Advanced breast cancer in postmenopausal women	GI upset, hot flashes, injection site reactions
Tamoxifen	PO 20 mg once or twice daily	Breast cancer, after surgery or radiation; prophylaxis in high-risk women; and treatment of metastatic disease	Hot flashes, nausea, vomiting, vaginal discharge, risk of endometrial cancer in nonhysterectomized women
Toremifene (Fareston)	PO 60 mg once daily	Metastatic breast cancer in postmenopausal women	Hot flashes, nausea, hypercalcemia, tumor flare
Aromatase Inhibitors			
Anastrazole (Arimidex)	PO 1 mg once daily	Breast cancer in postmenopausal women	Nausea, hot flashes, edema
Exemestane (Aromasin)	PO 25 mg once daily	Breast cancer in postmenopausal women	Hot flashes, nausea, depression, insomnia, anxiety, dyspnea, pain
Letrozole (Femara)	PO 2.5 mg once daily	Breast cancer in postmenopausal women	Nausea, hot flashes
Antiandrogens			
Bicalutamide (Casodex)	PO 500 mg once daily (with goserelin or leuprolide)	Advanced prostatic cancer	Nausea, vomiting, diarrhea, hot flashes, pain, breast enlargement
Flutamide (Eulexin)	PO 250 mg every 8 h	Advanced prostatic cancer	Nausea, vomiting, diarrhea, hot flashes, hepatotoxicity
LHRH Analogs			
Nilutamide (Nilandron)	PO 300 mg daily for 30 d, then 150 mg daily	Advanced breast cancer in postmenopausal women	Diarrhea, GI bleeding, heart failure, hyperglycemia
Goserelin (Zoladex)	Sub-Q implant, 3.6 mg every 28 d or 10.8 mg every 12 wk	Advanced prostatic or breast cancer, endometriosis	Hot flashes, transient increase in bone pain
Leuprolide (Eligard, Lupron, Viadur)	Sub-Q 7.5 mg/mo IM 7.5 mg/mo, 22.5 mg/3 mo, or 30 mg/4 mo	Advanced prostatic cancer	Same as for goserelin, above
Triptorelin (Trelstar LA, Trelstar Depot)	IM implant 65 mg/12 mo IM 3.75 mg/28 d or 11.25 mg/3 mo	Advanced prostatic cancer	Same as for goserelin and leuprolide, above

GI, gastrointestinal.

Antiestrogens

Antiestrogens (also called estrogen receptor modulators) used in the treatment of cancer include **fulvestrant** (Faslodex), **tamoxifen** (Nolvadex), and **toremifene** (Fareston). These drugs bind to estrogen receptors in normal and malignant cells. In breast cancer, the drugs compete with estrogen for receptor binding sites and thereby decrease the estrogen growth-stimulating action on malignant cells. Tamoxifen has been widely used to prevent recurrence of breast cancer after surgical excision and to treat metastatic breast cancer in postmenopausal women with receptor-positive disease. For prevention, the drug is usually taken for 2 to 5 years.

Tamoxifen becomes ineffective after about 5 years, and several studies indicate greater effectiveness when an aromatase inhibitor is given instead of tamoxifen after 2 to 5 years. Although antiestrogens and aromatase inhibitors both block the growth of breast tumors that respond to estrogen, their mechanisms of action are different. For example, tamoxifen inhibits the ability of breast cancer cells to use estrogen for growth, whereas an aromatase inhibitor inhibits the production of estrogen in fat, muscle, and other tissues. Adverse effects of antiestrogens include increased risk of blood clots or stroke, vaginal bleeding, and muscle cramps.

Sexually active premenopausal women who take tamoxifen should use effective nonhormonal contraception during and for 2 months after tamoxifen is discontinued. (Premenopausal women may also be treated with an LHRH analog, which may be as effective as antiestrogen therapy.)

Aromatase Inhibitors

Anastrazole (Arimidex), **exemestane** (Aromasin), and **letrozole** (Femara) are aromatase inhibitors used to prevent or treat recurrence of estrogen-responsive breast cancer in postmenopausal women. Aromatase is an enzyme that catalyzes the production of estrogen in the ovaries of premenopausal women and in fat, liver, and muscle cells of postmenopausal or castrated women. Thus, inhibiting aromatase reduces estrogen levels in the blood and target tissues, including the breast.

Earlier, an aromatase inhibitor was used after 5 years of tamoxifen therapy. Later studies with letrozole or exemestane indicate that changing to an aromatase inhibitor after 2 or 3 years of tamoxifen therapy is more effective in decreasing recurrent breast cancer. Letrozole following tamoxifen is the current standard of care, and exemestane is being considered as first-line therapy (instead of tamoxifen) for metastatic breast cancer in postmenopausal women.

Adverse effects include nausea, diarrhea, headache, hot flashes, joint pain, bone loss and fractures, and vision disturbances. Because aromatase inhibitors promote bone loss, these drugs may not be appropriate for women at high risk of bone fractures.

Antiandrogens

Bicalutamide (Casodex), **flutamide** (Eulexin), and **nilutamide** (Nilandron) are used to treat prostate cancer, usually with an LHRH analog (see below). The drugs bind to androgen receptors in cells of the prostate gland and thereby block dihydrotestosterone (DHT) stimulation of malignant cell growth.

In the prostate gland, normal cell growth and differentiation depends on the presence of androgens, specifically DHT, the active form of testosterone. These androgens are produced mainly by the testes and the adrenal glands through a series of chemical conversions also involving the hypothalamus and anterior pituitary. In prostate cancer, androgenic stimulation of tumor growth can be reduced by surgical excision of the organs involved in androgen production (usually the testes) or administering drugs that inhibit the production or action of androgens (e.g., antiandrogens, LHRH analogs). Adverse drug effects include hot flashes, breast enlargement and tenderness, nausea, vomiting, constipation, diarrhea, and pain.

Luteinizing Hormone–Releasing Hormone (LHRH) Analogs

Goserelin (Zoladex), **leuprolide** (Eligard, Lupron, Viadur), and **triptorelin** (Trelstar) are synthetic versions of the hypothalamic LHRH that initiates production of both estrogens and androgens. Therapeutic doses of LHRH analogs initially increase the release of luteinizing hormone (LH) and follicle-stimulating hormone (FSH) from the anterior pituitary, then decrease their release by down-regulating receptors. Inhibiting the release of LH and FSH reduces the production of ovarian estrogen in women to postmenopausal levels and testicular testosterone in men to castration levels. These effects occur within 2 to 4 weeks after drug therapy is begun. In premenopausal women with estrogen receptor–positive breast cancer, medical castration with these drugs is increasingly being used instead of surgical excision of the ovaries. One of these drugs is usually combined with an antiestrogen. In men with prostate cancer, these drugs reduce androgens to the levels seen with surgical excision of the testes. In metastatic prostate cancer, an LHRH analog is often given with an antiandrogen to increase effectiveness. Goserelin is approved for treatment of both breast and prostate cancer; leuprolide and triptorelin are approved only for prostate cancer.

Adverse effects are basically those of estrogen or testosterone deficiency and may include nausea and hot flashes. The drugs may also cause or aggravate depression. Impotence occurs in men but may be reversible when the drug is discontinued. When given for prostate cancer, the drugs may cause increased bone pain and increased difficulty in urinating during the first few weeks of use.

Cytoprotectant Drugs

Cytoprotectants reduce the adverse effects of cytotoxic drugs, which may be severe, debilitating, and life threatening (Box 42-2). Severe adverse effects may also limit drug dosage or frequency of administration, thereby limiting the effectiveness of chemotherapy. Several cytoprotectants are available to protect certain body tissues from one or more adverse effects and allow a more optimal dose and schedule of cytotoxic agents. To be effective, administration and scheduling must be precise in relation to administration of the cytotoxic agent. A cytoprotective agent does not prevent or treat all adverse effects of a particular cytotoxic agent and it may have adverse effects of its own.

Amifostine produces a metabolite that combines with cisplatin and decreases cisplatin-induced renal damage. **Dexrazoxane** decreases cardiac toxicity of doxorubicin. **Erythropoietin, filgrastim, oprelvekin,** and **sargramostim** (see Chap. 40) stimulate the bone marrow to produce blood cells. Erythropoietin stimulates production of red blood cells and is used for anemia; oprelvekin stimulates production of platelets and may be used to prevent thrombocytopenia; filgrastim and sargramostim stimulate production of white blood cells and are

Box 42-2	Management of Chemotherapy Complications

Complications of anticancer drug therapy range from minor to life threatening. Vigilant efforts toward prevention or early detection and treatment are needed.

- **Nausea** and **vomiting** commonly occur and are treated with antiemetics (see Chap. 62). With traditional cytotoxic chemotherapy, the drugs are most effective when started before drug administration and continued on a regular schedule for 24 to 48 hours afterward. An effective regimen is a serotonin receptor antagonist (e.g., ondansetron) and a corticosteroid (e.g., dexamethasone), given orally or IV. Other measures include a benzodiazepine (e.g., lorazepam) for anticipatory nausea and vomiting and limiting oral intake for a few hours. Guidelines have not been developed for managing nausea and vomiting with the biologic antineoplastic drugs.
- **Anorexia** interferes with nutrition. Well-balanced meals, with foods the patient is able and willing to eat, and nutritional supplements, to increase intake of protein and calories, are helpful.
- **Fatigue** is often caused or aggravated by anemia and can be treated with administration of erythropoietin. Alternating periods of activity and rest and an adequate diet may also be helpful.
- **Alopecia** occurs with cyclophosphamide, doxorubicin, MTX, and vincristine. Counsel patients taking these drugs that hair loss is temporary and that hair may grow back a different color and texture; suggest the purchase of wigs, hats, and scarves before hair loss is expected to occur; and instruct women to use a mild shampoo and avoid rollers, permanent waves, hair coloring, and other treatments that damage the hair.
- *Mucositis* (also called *stomatitis*) often occurs with the antimetabolites, antibiotics, plant alkaloids, and growth factor/tyrosine kinase inhibitors. It usually lasts 7 to 10 days and may interfere with nutrition; lead to oral ulcerations, infections, and bleeding; and cause pain. Nurse or patient interventions to minimize or treat mucositis include the following:
  - Brush the teeth after meals and at bedtime with a soft toothbrush and floss once daily. Stop brushing and flossing if the platelet count drops below 20,000/mm³ because gingival bleeding is likely. Teeth may then be cleaned with soft, sponge-tipped or cotton-tipped applicators.
  - Rinse the mouth several times daily, especially before meals (to decrease unpleasant taste and increase appetite) and after meals (to remove food particles that promote growth of microorganisms). One suggested solution is 1 teaspoon of table salt and 1 teaspoon of baking soda in 1 quart of water. Commercial mouthwashes are not recommended, because their alcohol content causes drying of oral mucous membranes.
  - Encourage the patient to drink fluids. Systemic dehydration and local dryness of the oral mucosa contribute to the development and progression of mucositis. Pain and soreness contribute to dehydration. Fluids usually tolerated include tea, carbonated beverages, ices (e.g.,

popsicles), and plain gelatin desserts. Fruit juices may be diluted with water, ginger ale, Sprite, or 7-Up to decrease pain, burning, and further tissue irritation. Drinking fluids through a straw may be more comfortable, because this decreases contact of fluids with painful ulcerations.
  - Encourage the patient to eat soft, bland, cold, nonacidic foods. Although individual tolerances vary, it is usually better to avoid highly spiced or rough foods.
  - Remove dentures entirely or for at least 8 hours daily because they may irritate oral mucosa.
  - Inspect the mouth daily for signs of inflammation and lesions.
  - Give medications for pain. Local anesthetic solutions, such as viscous lidocaine, can be taken a few minutes before meals. Because the mouth and throat are anesthetized, swallowing and detecting the temperature of hot foods may be difficult, and aspiration or burns may occur. Doses should not exceed 15 mL every 3 hours or 120 mL in 24 hours. If systemic analgesics are used, they should be taken 30 to 60 minutes before eating.
  - For oral infections resulting from mucositis, local or systemic antimicrobial drugs are used. Fungal infections with *Candida albicans* can be treated with antifungal tablets, suspensions, or lozenges. Severe infections may require systemic antibiotics, depending on the causative organism as identified by cultures of mouth lesions.
- **Infection** is common because the disease and its treatment lower host resistance to infection.
  - If fever occurs, especially in a neutropenic patient, possible sources of infection are usually cultured and antibiotics are started immediately.
  - Severe neutropenia can be prevented or its extent and duration minimized by administering filgrastim or sargramostim to stimulate the bone marrow to produce leukocytes. A protective environment may be needed to decrease exposure to pathogens.
  - Instruct the patient to avoid exposure to infection by avoiding crowds, anyone with a known infection, and contact with fresh flowers, soil, animals, or animal excrement.
  - Frequent and thorough hand hygiene by the patient and everyone involved in his or her care is necessary to reduce exposure to pathogenic microorganisms.
  - The patient should take a bath daily and put on clean clothes. In addition, the perineal area should be washed with soap and water after each urination or defecation.
  - When venous access devices are used, take care to prevent them from becoming sources of infection. For implanted catheters, inspect and cleanse around exit sites according to agency policies and procedures. Use strict sterile technique when changing dressings or flushing the catheters. For peripheral intravenous lines, the same principles of care apply, except that sites should be changed every 3 days or if signs of phlebitis occur.
  - Avoid indwelling urinary catheters when possible. When they are necessary, cleanse the perineal area

(continued on page 692)

Box 42-2	Management of Chemotherapy Complications (continued)

with soap and water at least once daily and provide sufficient fluids to ensure an adequate urine output.

■ Help the patient maintain a well-balanced diet. Oral hygiene and analgesics before meals may increase food intake. High-protein, high-calorie foods and fluids can be given between meals. Nutritional supplements can be taken with or between meals. Provide fluids with high nutritional value (e.g., milkshakes or nutritional supplements) if the patient can tolerate them and has an adequate intake of water and other fluids.

■ **Bleeding** may be caused by thrombocytopenia and may occur spontaneously or with minor trauma. Precautions should be instituted if the platelet count drops to 50,000/mm³ or below. Measures to avoid bleeding include giving oprelvekin to stimulate platelet production and prevent thrombocytopenia; avoiding trauma, including venipuncture and injections, when possible; using an electric razor for shaving; checking skin, urine, and stool for blood; and for platelet counts less than 20,000/mm³, stop brushing and flossing the teeth.

■ **Extravasation.** Several drugs (called vesicants) cause severe inflammation, pain, ulceration, and tissue necrosis if they leak into soft tissues around veins. Thus, efforts are needed to prevent extravasation or to minimize tissue damage if it occurs.

■ Identify patients at risk for extravasation, including those who are unable to communicate (e.g., sedated patients, infants), have vascular impairment (e.g., from multiple attempts at venipuncture), or have obstructed venous drainage after axillary node surgery.

■ Be especially cautious with the anthracyclines (e.g., doxorubicin) and the vinca alkaloids (e.g., vincristine). Choose peripheral IV sites carefully, avoiding veins that are small or located in an edematous extremity or near a joint. Inject the drugs slowly (1–2 mL at a time) into the tubing of a rapidly flowing IV infusion, for rapid dilution and detection of extravasation. Observe

the venipuncture site for swelling and ask the patient about pain or burning. After a drug has been injected, continue the rapid flow rate of the IV fluid for 2 to 5 minutes to flush the vein.

■ If using a central IV line, do not give the drug unless patency is indicated by a blood return. Using a central line does not eliminate the risk of extravasation.

■ When extravasation occurs, the drug should be stopped immediately. Techniques to decrease tissue damage include aspirating the drug (about 5 mL of blood, if able) through the IV catheter before it is removed, elevating the involved extremity, and applying warm (with dacarbazine, etoposide, vinblastine, and vincristine) or cold (with daunorubicin and doxorubicin) compresses. Nurses involved in cytotoxic chemotherapy must know the procedure to be followed if extravasation occurs so that it can be instituted immediately.

■ **Hyperuricemia** from rapid breakdown of malignant cells can lead to kidney damage. Risks of *nephropathy* can be decreased by high fluid intake, high urine output, alkalinizing the urine with sodium bicarbonate, and giving allopurinol to inhibit uric acid formation.

■ **Hand-foot syndrome** (also called palmar-plantar erythrodysesthesia or erythema) is a sunburn type of skin reaction with redness, tenderness, and possibly peeling, numbness, and tingling of palms and soles. It is associated with some traditional cytotoxic drugs (e.g., capecitabine, doxorubicin, fluorouracil) and some growth factor/tyrosine kinase inhibitors (e.g., lapatinib, sorafenib, sunitinib). It is attributed to leakage of drug from capillaries into the palms and soles; heat and friction increase leakage. Management efforts involve decreasing heat and friction (e.g., minimizing exposure of hands and feet to hot water), avoiding increased pressure (e.g., from long walks, squeezing small implements in cooking, gardening, etc.), or applying ice packs for 15 or 20 minutes at a time. Acetaminophen may be taken for discomfort.

used to reduce neutropenia and infection. **Leucovorin** is used with high-dose MTX. **Mesna** is used with ifosfamide, which produces a metabolite that causes hemorrhagic cystitis. Mesna combines with and inactivates the metabolite and thereby decreases cystitis. Dosages and routes of administration for these medications are listed in Table 42-4.

Nursing Process

Assessment

■ Assess all patients for risk factors, screening behaviors, and/or manifestations of cancer, in order to prevent cancer, if possible, or recognize and seek treatment for cancer as early as possible. Risk factors include use of tobacco

products (including inhalation of secondhand cigarette smoke in home or work environments), drinking more than one drink a day (for women) or two drinks a day (for men), being overweight, damage to skin unprotected by sunscreen, and unsafe sexual behaviors. Screening behaviors include the use of breast self-examinations, regular mammograms, colonoscopy when indicated, measurement of prostate-specific antigen (PSA), and so forth.

■ Assess the patient's condition before chemotherapy is started and often during treatment. Useful information includes the type, grade, and stage of the tumor as well as the signs and symptoms of cancer. General manifestations include anemia, malnutrition, weight loss, pain, and infection; specific manifestations depend on the organs affected.

Table 42-4	**Drugs at a Glance:** Cytoprotective Agents	
GENERIC/TRADE NAME	**CLINICAL USE**	**ROUTES AND DOSAGE RANGES**
Amifostine (Ethyol)	Reduction of cisplatin-induced renal toxicity	IV infusion 910 mg/m² once daily within 30 min of starting chemotherapy
Dexrazoxane (Zinecard)	Reduction of doxorubicin-induced cardiomyopathy in women with metastatic breast cancer who have received a cumulative dose of 300 mg/m² and need additional doxorubicin	IV 10 times the amount of doxorubicin (e.g., dexrazoxane 500 mg/m² per doxorubicin 50 mg/m²), then give doxorubicin within 30 min of completing dexrazoxane dose
Erythropoietin (Epogen, Procrit)	Treatment of chemotherapy-induced anemia	Sub-Q 150–300 units/kg 3 times weekly, adjusted to maintain desired hematocrit
Filgrastim (Neupogen)	Treatment of chemotherapy-induced neutropenia	Sub-Q, IV 5 mcg/kg/d, at least 24 h after cytotoxic chemotherapy, up to 2 wk or an absolute neutrophil count of 10,000/mm³
Leucovorin (Wellcovorin)	"Rescue" after high-dose methotrexate for osteosarcoma Advanced colorectal cancer, with 5-fluorouracil	"Rescue," PO, IV, IM 15 mg q6h for 10 doses, starting 24 h after methotrexate begun Colorectal cancer, IV 20 mg/m² or 200 mg/m², followed by 5-fluorouracil, daily for 5 d, repeated every 28 d
Mesna (Mesnex)	Prevention of ifosfamide-induced hemorrhagic cystitis	IV, 20% of ifosfamide dose for 3 doses (at time of ifosfamide dose, then 4 h and 8 h after ifosfamide dose)
Oprelvekin (Neumega)	Prevention of thrombocytopenia	Sub-Q 50 mcg/kg once daily, usually for 10–21 d
Sargramostim (Leukine)	Myeloid reconstitution after bone marrow transplant; to decrease chemotherapy-induced neutropenia	IV infusion 250 mcg/m²/d until absolute neutrophil count is above 1500/mm³ for 3 d, up to 42 d

■ Assess for other diseases and organ dysfunctions (e.g., cardiac, renal, hepatic) that influence response to chemotherapy.

■ Assess emotional status, coping mechanisms, family relationships, financial resources, and social support mechanisms. Anxiety and depression are common features during cancer diagnosis and treatment.

■ Assess laboratory test results before chemotherapy to establish baseline data and during chemotherapy to monitor drug effects.

■ **Blood tests for tumor markers** (tumor-specific antigens on cell surfaces). Alpha-fetoprotein is a fetal antigen normally present during intrauterine and early postnatal life but absent in adulthood. Increased amounts may indicate hepatic or testicular cancer. Carcinoembryonic antigen (CEA) is secreted by several types of malignant cells (e.g., colorectal cancer). A rising level may indicate tumor progression and levels that are elevated before surgery and disappear after surgery indicate adequate tumor excision. If CEA levels rise later, it probably indicates tumor recurrence. With chemotherapy, falling CEA levels indicate effective-ness. Other tumor markers are immunoglobulins (elevated levels may indicate multiple myeloma) and PSA (elevated levels may indicate prostatic cancer).

■ **CBC** to check for anemia, leukopenia, and thrombocytopenia because most cytotoxic antineoplastic drugs cause bone marrow depression. A CBC and white blood cell differential are done before each cycle of chemotherapy to determine dosage and frequency of drug administration, to monitor bone marrow function so fatal bone marrow depression does not occur, and to assist the nurse in planning care. For example, the patient is very susceptible to infection when the leukocyte count is low, and bleeding is likely when the platelet count is low.

■ **Other tests.** These include tests of kidney and liver function, serum calcium, uric acid, and others, depending on the organs affected by the cancer or its treatment.

Nursing Diagnoses

■ Pain, nausea and vomiting, weakness, and activity intolerance related to disease process or chemotherapy

■ Imbalanced Nutrition: Less Than Body Requirements related to disease process or chemotherapy

Nursing Process continues on page 694

- Anxiety related to the disease, its possible progression, and its treatment
- Ineffective Family Coping related to illness and treatment of a family member
- Deficient Fluid Volume related to chemotherapy-induced nausea, vomiting, and diarrhea
- Risk for Injury: Infection related to drug-induced neutropenia; bleeding related to drug-induced thrombocytopenia; stomatitis related to damage of GI mucosal cells
- Deficient Knowledge about cancer chemotherapy and managing adverse drug effects

Planning/Goals

The patient will

- Receive assistance in coping with the diagnosis of cancer
- Experience reduced anxiety and fear
- Receive chemotherapy accurately and safely
- Experience reduction of tumor size, change of laboratory values toward normal, or other therapeutic effects of chemotherapy
- Experience minimal bleeding, infection, nausea and vomiting, and other consequences of chemotherapy
- Maintain adequate food and fluid intake and body weight
- Receive assistance in activities of daily living when needed
- Be informed about community resources for cancer care (e.g., Hospice, Reach to Recovery, other support groups)

Interventions

- Participate in and promote efforts to prevent cancer.
  - Follow and promote the diet recommended by the American Cancer Society (i.e., decrease fat, eat at least five servings of fruits and vegetables daily, increase intake of dietary fiber, minimize intake of salt-cured or smoked foods).
  - Promote weight control. Obesity may contribute to the development of several cancers, including breast and endometrial cancer in women.
  - Identify cancer-causing agents in homes and workplaces and strategies to reduce exposure to them when possible.
  - Strengthen host defenses by promoting a healthful lifestyle (e.g., good nutrition, adequate rest and exercise, stress management techniques, avoiding or minimizing alcohol and tobacco use).
  - Avoid smoking cigarettes and being around smokers. Passive smoking increases risk of lung cancer in spouses of smokers and risks of brain cancer, lymphomas, and acute lymphogenous leukemia in children of smokers.
  - Minimize exposure to sunlight, use sunscreens liberally, and wear protective clothing to prevent skin cancer.

- Participate in and promote cancer screening tests in non-symptomatic people, especially those at high risk, to detect cancer before signs and symptoms occur. These tests include regular examination of breasts, cervix (Pap test), testicles, and skin and tests for colon cancer such as hemoccult tests on stool and colonoscopy. Early recognition of risk factors, premalignant tissue changes (dysplasia), biochemical tumor markers, and beginning malignancies may be life saving; early treatment can greatly reduce the suffering and problems associated with advanced cancer.
- For patients receiving cytotoxic anticancer drugs, try to prevent or minimize the incidence and severity of adverse reactions (see Box 42-2).
- Provide supportive care to patients and families. Physiologic care includes pain management, comfort measures, and assistance with nutrition, hygiene, ambulation, and other activities of daily living as needed. Psychological care includes allowing family members or significant others to be with the patient and participate in care when desired, and keeping patients and families informed.

Evaluation

- Monitor drug administration for accuracy.
- Observe and interview for therapeutic effects of chemotherapy.
- Compare current laboratory reports with baseline values for changes toward normal values.
- Compare weight and nutritional status with baseline values for maintenance or improvement.
- Observe and interview for adverse drug effects and interventions to prevent or manage them.
- Observe and interview for effective pain management and other symptom control.

Principles of Therapy

Overview of Cancer Treatment

For many patients, cancer treatment involves surgery, radiation, and chemotherapy during the course of their disease. Surgery is used to excise localized tumors, which may be curative, and to treat complications of cancer, such as bowel obstruction. Radiation therapy is used to treat most types of cancer. It may be used alone for some malignancies, such as Hodgkin's disease or cervical cancer. It may be used with surgery to reduce the need for radical surgery, to eliminate malignant cells (e.g., positive lymph nodes) that remain after surgery, with chemotherapy to control growth of tumors, and to relieve symptoms in patients with metastatic bone or brain involvement.

Chemotherapy may be used to eliminate or control the growth of malignant cells or to relieve symptoms and improve the patient's quality of life. It is most effective when started

Patient Teaching Guidelines | Managing Chemotherapy

- There are many different chemotherapy drugs, and the ones used for a particular patient depend on the type of malignancy, its location, and other factors. Some are taken orally at home; many are given intravenously, in outpatient clinics, by nurses who are specially trained to administer the medications and monitor your condition. The medications are usually given in cycles such as every few weeks.

- The goal of chemotherapy is to be as effective as possible with tolerable side effects. Particular side effects vary with the medications used; some increase risks of infection, and some cause anemia, nausea, or hair loss. All of these can be managed effectively, and several medications can help prevent or minimize side effects. In addition, some helpful activities are listed below.

  - Keep all appointments for chemotherapy, blood tests, and check-ups. This is extremely important. Chemotherapy effectiveness depends on its being given on time; blood tests help to determine when the drugs should be given and how the drugs affect your body tissues.

  - Do everything you can to avoid infection, such as avoiding other people who have infections and washing your hands frequently and thoroughly. If you have a fever, chills, sore throat, or cough, notify your oncologist.

  - Try to maintain or improve your intake of nutritious food and fluids; this will help you feel better and maintain your weight at a more optimal level to promote healing. A dietitian can be helpful in designing a diet to meet your needs and preferences.

  - If your chemotherapy may cause bleeding, you can decrease the likelihood by shaving with an electric razor, avoiding aspirin and other nonsteroidal anti-inflammatory drugs (including over-the-counter Advil, Aleve, and others), and avoiding injections, cuts, and other injuries when possible. If you notice excessive bruising, bleeding gums when you brush your teeth, or blood in your urine or bowel movement, notify your oncologist immediately.

  - If hair loss is expected with the medications you take, you can use wigs, scarves, and hats. These should be purchased before starting chemotherapy, if possible. Hair loss is temporary; your hair will grow back!

- Inform any other physician, dentist, or health care provider that you are taking chemotherapy before any diagnostic test or treatment is begun. Some procedures may be contraindicated or require special precautions.

- If you are of childbearing age, effective contraceptive measures should be carried out during and a few months after chemotherapy.

- For medications taken at home, instructions for taking the drugs should be followed exactly for the most beneficial effects.

- Although specific instructions vary with the drugs you are taking, the following are a few precautions with some commonly used drugs:

- With **cyclophosphamide**, take the tablets on an empty stomach. If severe stomach upset occurs, take with food. Also, drink 2 or 3 quarts of fluid daily, if possible, and urinate often, especially at bedtime. If blood is seen in the urine or signs of cystitis occur (e.g., burning with urination), report to a health care provider. The drug is irritating to the bladder lining and may cause cystitis. High fluid intake and frequent emptying of the bladder help to decrease bladder damage.

- With **doxorubicin**, the urine may turn red for 1 to 2 days after drug administration. This discoloration is harmless; it does not indicate bleeding. Also, report to a health care provider if you have edema, shortness of breath, and excessive fatigue. Doxorubicin may need to be stopped if these symptoms occur.

- With **fluorouracil**, drink plenty of liquids while taking.

- With **methotrexate**, avoid alcohol, aspirin, and prolonged exposure to sunlight.

- With **oxaliplatin**, avoid exposure to cold during, and for 3 to 5 days after, drug administration. This helps prevent or minimize nerve damage that may cause numbness, tingling, and pain in the throat or hands. Swallowing and daily activities that require hand grasping may be impaired.

- With **vincristine**, eat high-fiber foods, such as whole cereal grains, if you are able, to prevent constipation. Also try to maintain a high fluid intake. A stool softener or bulk laxative may be prescribed for daily use.

---

before extensive tumor growth or when the tumor burden has been reduced by surgical excision or radiation therapy. When solid tumors metastasize, they become systemic diseases and are not accessible to surgical excision or radiation therapy. Neoadjuvant chemotherapy is used before surgery or radiation, to reduce the size of tumors; adjuvant chemotherapy is used after surgery or radiation to destroy or reduce microscopic metastases (e.g., in the treatment of patients with carcinomas of the breast, colon, lung, ovaries, or testes). Palliative chemotherapy is used in advanced cancer to relieve symptoms and treat or prevent complications.

Drug Selection

Drug therapy for a particular patient depends on the type and stage of cancer, the effectiveness of particular drugs in that type

and stage of cancer, and the patient's age and health status, including liver and kidney function. Most regimens use combinations of drugs because they are more effective, less toxic, and less likely to cause drug resistance than single agents. Numerous combinations have been developed for use in specific types of cancer. Effective combinations include drugs that act by different mechanisms, act at different times in the reproductive cycle of malignant cells, and differ in their adverse effects. Bleomycin is often combined with myelosuppressive drugs because it rarely causes myelosuppression. However, it can cause severe allergic reactions with hypotension and pulmonary toxicity (e.g., interstitial pneumonitis, pulmonary fibrosis). Increasingly, biologic drugs such as monoclonal antibodies and tyrosine kinase inhibitors are being added to traditional cytotoxic drug regimens.

Drug Dosage

Dosage must be calculated and regulated carefully to minimize toxicity. The patient's age, functional status, nutritional status, blood count, kidney and liver function, and previous chemotherapy or radiation therapy must be considered. Additional guidelines include the following:

■ High doses, to the limits of tolerance of normal tissues (e.g., bone marrow), are usually most effective.

■ Doses are usually calculated according to body surface area, which includes both weight and height, and are expressed as milligrams of drug per square meter of body surface area (mg/m^2). Doses also can be expressed as milligrams per kilogram of body weight (mg/kg). Because doses based on body surface area consider the patient's size, they are especially important for children. If the patient's weight changes more than a few pounds during treatment, doses should be recalculated.

■ Dosage may be reduced for neutropenia, thrombocytopenia, stomatitis, diarrhea, and renal or hepatic impairment that reduces the patient's ability to eliminate the drugs.

■ Total dose limits for doxorubicin (550 mg/m^2) and bleomycin (450 units) should not be exceeded.

Drug Administration

■ Dosage schedules are largely determined by clinical trials and should be followed as exactly as possible.

■ Many antineoplastic drugs are given on an intermittent or cyclic schedule, according to pharmacokinetic principles of cancer chemotherapy. However, certain chemotherapeutic agents (e.g., 5-fluorouracil) are ideally administered continuously.

■ Each antineoplastic drug should be used in the schedule, route, and dosage judged to be most effective for a particular type of cancer. With combinations of drugs, the recommended schedule should be followed precisely because safety and effectiveness may be schedule dependent. When chemotherapy is used as an adjuvant to surgery, it usually should be started as soon as possible after surgery, given in maximal tolerated doses just as if advanced disease were present, and continued for several months.

■ IV drugs should be given by experienced personnel who ensure free flow of fluid to the vein and verify adequate blood return. Infusion should be through a large, upper-extremity vein. When possible, veins of the antecubital fossa, wrist, dorsum of the hand, and the arm where an axillary lymph node dissection has been done should be avoided. An indwelling central venous catheter is often inserted for patients who have poor peripheral venous access, who require many doses of chemotherapy, or who require continuous infusions.

■ With bleomycin, a test dose of 1 to 2 milligrams should be given subcutaneously before starting full doses. Severe allergic reactions with hypotension may occur.

■ With paclitaxel and docetaxel, premedication is needed to decrease severe hypersensitivity reactions with dyspnea, hypotension, angioedema, and urticaria. A few deaths have occurred despite premedication. With paclitaxel, one regimen is oral dexamethasone 20 milligrams at 12 and 6 hours before, with IV diphenhydramine (Benadryl) 50 milligrams and cimetidine 300 milligrams, famotidine 20 milligrams, or ranitidine 50 milligrams at 30 to 60 minutes before. Additional paclitaxel is contraindicated for patients who experience severe hypersensitivity reactions. With docetaxel, an oral corticosteroid (e.g., dexamethasone 8 mg twice daily) is recommended for 3 days, starting 1 day before docetaxel administration. This reduces risk and severity of hypersensitivity reactions and fluid retention.

■ Premedication with diphenhydramine and acetaminophen is recommended before administration of several antineoplastic monoclonal antibodies to decrease potentially serious allergic reactions to drug infusions.

Hormone Inhibitor Therapy

Sex hormone inhibitors (e.g., antiestrogens, aromatase inhibitors, antiandrogens, LHRH analogs) are often used to treat breast or prostate cancer. Decreasing the hormones that stimulate tumor growth in these tissues can decrease symptoms and prolong survival.

In some patients with breast cancer, the presence of receptors for estrogen indicates a likely response to drugs that decrease estrogen availability. After initial surgery and/or radiation therapy, tamoxifen or a related drug is often used to treat breast cancers in patients with estrogen receptors because it inhibits estrogen binding to estrogen receptors. However, tumors may become resistant to tamoxifen because of mutations in receptors that alter receptor functions. An aromatase inhibitor drug (e.g., letrozole, exemestane) is increasingly being used after 2 to 5 years of tamoxifen therapy and is being investigated for use as first-line therapy instead of tamoxifen. In patients with prostate cancer, antiandrogens (e.g., bicalutamide) and LHRH analogs decrease androgen availability.

When both hormone inhibitor and cytotoxic drug therapies are needed, they are not given concurrently because hormone antagonists decrease malignant cell growth and cytotoxic agents are most effective when the cells are actively dividing. In patients with breast cancer, a hormone-inhibiting drug is usually given before cytotoxic chemotherapy in metastatic disease and after chemotherapy when used for adjuvant treatment.

Planning With Patient and Family

Patients with cancer and their families should be provided with information about their disease, their treatment options, and the preferred treatment. When cytotoxic chemotherapy is recommended, discussions should include expected benefits, adverse drug effects and their prevention or management, specific information about when and how the drugs will be administered, and the importance of regular blood tests to monitor drug effects. For those with Internet access, helpful information can be obtained at

CancerNet: http://www.cancer.gov/cancer_information

Cancer News on the Net: http://www.cancernews.com/default2.asp

OncoLink: http://cancer.med.upenn.edu

Applying Your Knowledge 42-3

Ms. Gardner still appears concerned about a possible adverse reaction to the Herceptin. What should you tell her about the precautions taken when administering this drug?

Safety Precautions With Cytotoxic Antineoplastic Drugs

Most cytotoxic antineoplastic drugs are carcinogenic, mutagenic, and teratogenic. Exposure during pregnancy increases risks of fetal abnormalities, ectopic pregnancy, and spontaneous abortion. In addition, parenteral solutions are irritating to the skin and mucous membranes and may cause contact dermatitis, cough, nausea, vomiting, and diarrhea. As a result, guidelines have been established for nurses who administer these drugs, to increase the safety of both patients and nurses. These guidelines include the following:

- Ensure appropriate orders (e.g., be sure the prescriber is qualified to write chemotherapy orders; do not accept verbal or telephone orders).

- Do not give injectable drugs unless certified to administer chemotherapy.

- Check all IV drug preparations for appropriate dilution, dosage that corresponds to the prescriber's order, absence of precipitates, expiration dates, and so forth.

- Avoid direct contact with solutions for injection by wearing gloves, face shields, and protective clothing (e.g., disposable, liquid-impermeable gowns).

- If handling a powder form of a drug, avoid inhaling the powder.

- Do not prepare the drugs in eating areas (to decrease risks of oral ingestion).

- Dispose of contaminated materials (e.g., needles, syringes, ampules, vials, IV tubing and bags) in puncture-proof containers labeled "Warning: Hazardous Material."

- Wear gloves when handling patients' clothing, bed linens, or excreta. Blood and body fluids are contaminated with drugs or metabolites for about 48 hours after a dose.

- Wash hands thoroughly after exposure or potential exposure.

- Wear a respiratory mask and follow recommended procedures for cleaning up spills.

Use in Special Populations

Use in Children

Children are at risk for a wide range of malignancies, including acute leukemias, lymphomas, brain tumors, Wilms' tumor, and sarcomas of muscle and bone. In recent years, however, there have been rapid advances in cancer care for children and high cure rates for many pediatric malignancies. Many of the advances have resulted from the systematic enrollment of children in well-designed clinical trials.

Chemotherapy should be designed, ordered, and supervised by pediatric oncologists. Dosage of cytotoxic drugs should be based on body surface area because this takes size into account. Special efforts are needed to maintain nutrition, organ function, psychological support, growth and development, and other aspects of health status during and after therapy. Long-term follow-up care is needed for survivors because of increased risk of health problems associated with the cancer or its treatment. For example, children who receive an anthracycline drug (e.g., doxorubicin) are at increased risk of developing cardiotoxic effects (e.g., heart failure) during treatment or after receiving the drug. Efforts to reduce cardiotoxicity include using alternative drugs when effective, giving smaller cumulative doses of anthracycline drug, and observing patients closely so that early manifestations can be recognized and treated before heart failure occurs. In addition, after successful chemotherapy, children are at increased risk for development of cancers in adulthood (e.g., leukemia). After radiation therapy, they are at increased risk of developing breast, thyroid, or brain cancer. Children treated for Hodgkin's disease seem to have the highest risk of developing a new cancer later.

Most of the newer anticancer drugs (e.g., targeted therapies such as monoclonal antibodies and tyrosine kinase inhibitors) are used to treat malignancies that do not commonly occur in children and little is known about their effects in children.

Use in Older Adults

Aging is a risk factor for developing cancer, and the number of new cancer cases is about 10 times greater in people 65 years and older. Currently, 60% of all malignant tumors occur in persons aged 65 years and older. Although they are likely to have chronic cardiovascular, renal, and other disorders (comorbidities) that increase their risks of serious adverse effects, they should not be denied the potential benefits of traditional cytotoxic chemotherapy on the basis of age alone. In addition to comorbidities, issues that impact treatment include access to care, financial and transportation issues, functional status, need for independence, and social support. Physiologic changes of decreased renal function, impaired hepatic blood flow, and decreased cardiac reserve also add to the challenge of managing cancer in older adults. Vigilance is needed to maximize benefits and minimize hazards of antineoplastic drug administration. For example, older adults are more sensitive to the neurotoxic effects of vincristine and need reduced dosages of some drugs (e.g., cyclophosphamide, MTX) if renal function is impaired. Creatinine clearance (CrCl) should be monitored; serum creatinine level is not a reliable indicator of renal function in older adults because of their decreased muscle mass. Many antineoplastic drugs are metabolized by the liver; decreased liver blood flow and decreased liver size can lead to accumulation of drug due to decreased clearance, resulting in increased toxicity.

Estrogen- and androgen-inhibiting drugs are often used in older adults to treat breast or prostate cancer. The drugs may be used with or instead of other treatment modalities and are usually well tolerated. Newer biologic agents (targeted therapies) are commonly used to treat lung, colorectal, breast, and hematologic malignancies in older adults.

Use in Patients With Renal Impairment

Some antineoplastic drugs are nephrotoxic (e.g., cisplatin, MTX), and many are excreted through the kidneys. In the presence of impaired renal function, risks of further impairment or accumulation of toxic drug levels are increased. Thus, renal function should be monitored carefully during therapy and drug dosages are often reduced according to CrCl levels. Renal effects of selected cytotoxic chemotherapy drugs and precautions to reduce nephrotoxicity are described in the following paragraphs.

Carmustine and *lomustine* are associated with azotemia and renal failure, usually with long-term IV administration and large cumulative doses. *Cisplatin* is nephrotoxic, and acute overdosage can cause renal failure. Because nephrotoxicity is increased with repeated doses, cisplatin is given at 3- or 4-week intervals and blood tests of renal function (e.g., creatinine, urea nitrogen, electrolytes) are measured before each course of therapy. Renal function is usually allowed to return to normal before another dose is given. Nephrotoxicity may be reduced by the use of amifostine or IV hydration and mannitol. *Cyclophosphamide* may cause hemorrhagic ureteritis and renal tubular necrosis with IV doses above 50 milligrams per kilogram. These effects usually subside when the drug is stopped. *Ifosfamide* may cause hemorrhagic cystitis, manifested by hematuria. Cystitis can be reduced by the use of mesna, vigorous hydration, and delaying drug administration if a predose urinalysis shows hematuria.

Irinotecan dosage should be reduced in patients with moderate renal impairment (CrCl 20–39 mL/minute). *Melphalan* should be reduced in dosage when given IV. *Mercaptopurine* should be reduced in dosage. MTX use in patients with impaired renal function may lead to accumulation of toxic amounts or additional renal damage. The patient's renal status should be evaluated before and during MTX therapy. If significant renal impairment occurs, the drug should be discontinued or reduced in dosage until renal function improves. In patients who receive high doses for treatment of osteosarcoma, MTX may cause renal damage leading to acute renal failure. Nephrotoxicity is attributed to precipitation of MTX and a metabolite in renal tubules. Renal

impairment may be reduced by monitoring renal function closely, ensuring adequate hydration, alkalinizing the urine, and measuring serum drug levels. *Procarbazine* may cause more severe adverse effects if given to patients with impaired renal function. Hospitalization is recommended for the first course of treatment.

Many other drugs should be used with caution in patients with renal impairment. *L-Asparaginase* often increases blood urea nitrogen; acute renal failure and fatal renal insufficiency have been reported. *Bleomycin* is rarely associated with nephrotoxicity, but its elimination half-life is prolonged in patients with a CrCl of less than 35 milliliters per minute. *Cytarabine* is detoxified mainly by the liver. However, patients with renal impairment may have more central nervous system (CNS)-related adverse effects, and dosage reduction may be needed. *Gemcitabine* was associated with mild proteinuria and hematuria during clinical trials, and hemolytic-uremic syndrome (HUS) was reported in a few patients. HUS may be manifested by anemia, elevated bilirubin and reticulocyte counts, and renal failure. The drug should be stopped immediately if HUS occurs; hemodialysis may be required.

Bortezomib should be used with caution; most other biologic drugs have not been studied in relation to renal impairment.

Use in Patients With Hepatic Impairment

Some antineoplastic drugs are hepatotoxic and many are metabolized in the liver. With impaired hepatic function, risks of further impairment or accumulation of toxic drug levels are increased. Hepatic function should be monitored with most drugs and dosage reduction is needed with some. However, abnormal values for the usual liver function tests (e.g., serum aspartate aminotransferase [AST] and alanine aminotransferase [ALT], bilirubin, alkaline phosphatase) may indicate liver injury but do not indicate decreased ability to metabolize drugs. Patients with metastatic cancer often have impaired liver function.

Hepatotoxic drugs include the anthracyclines (e.g., doxorubicin), MTX, paclitaxel, and vincristine. Hepatic effects of selected drugs are described below.

L-Asparaginase is hepatotoxic in most patients; it may increase pre-existing hepatic impairment and hepatotoxicity of other medications. Signs of liver impairment, which usually subside when the drug is discontinued, include increased AST, ALT, alkaline phosphatase, and bilirubin and decreased serum albumin, cholesterol, and plasma fibrinogen. *Capecitabine* blood levels are significantly increased with hepatic impairment, and patients with liver metastases should be monitored closely. *Carmustine* may increase AST, ALT, alkaline phosphatase, and bilirubin when given IV. *Cisplatin* may cause a transient increase in liver enzymes and bilirubin. *Cytarabine* may cause CNS-related adverse effects in patients with impaired liver function. The drug should be used with caution and dosage may need to be reduced. *Dacarbazine* is hepatotoxic, and a few cases of hepatic-vein thrombosis and fatal liver necrosis have been reported. *Daunorubicin*, liposomal formulation, should be reduced in dosage according to serum bilirubin (e.g., bilirubin 1.2–3 mg/dL, give three fourths the normal dose; bilirubin above 3 mg/dL, give one half the normal dose). Doxorubicin toxicity is increased with impaired hepatic function. Liver function tests should be done before drug administration, and dosage of both regular and liposomal formulations should be reduced according to the serum bilirubin (e.g., bilirubin 1.2 to 3 mg/dL, give one half the normal dose; bilirubin above 3 mg/dL, give one fourth the normal dose).

Gemcitabine increased serum aminotransferases in most patients during clinical trials. *Idarubicin* should not be given to patients with a serum bilirubin above 5 milligrams per deciliter. *Irinotecan* may cause abnormal liver function tests in patients with liver metastases. *Mercaptopurine* causes hepatotoxicity, especially with higher doses (above 2.5 mg/kg/day) and in combination with doxorubicin. Encephalopathy and fatal liver necrosis have occurred. The drug should be stopped if signs of hepatotoxicity (e.g., jaundice, hepatomegaly) occur. Serum aminotransferases, alkaline phosphatase, and bilirubin should be monitored weekly initially, then monthly. MTX may cause acute (increased serum aminotransferases, hepatitis) and chronic (fibrosis and cirrhosis) hepatotoxicity. Chronic toxicity is potentially fatal. It is more likely to occur after prolonged use (e.g., 2 years or longer) and after a total dose of at least 1.5 grams. Liver function tests should be closely monitored in patients with pre-existing liver damage or impaired hepatic function.

Paclitaxel may cause more toxicity in patients with impaired hepatic function. *Procarbazine* causes more toxic effects in patients with hepatic impairment. Hospitalization is recommended for the first course of therapy. *Topotecan* is cleared from plasma more slowly in patients with hepatic impairment. *Vinblastine* and *vincristine* may cause more toxicity with hepatic impairment, and dosage should be reduced 50% for patients with a direct serum bilirubin value above 3 milligrams per deciliter. *Bortezomib* should be used with caution in patients with impaired hepatic function. With *imatinib*, liver function tests should be monitored at baseline and at least monthly. The drug should be stopped for elevated bilirubin (3 times the upper limit of normal) or elevated transaminases (5 times the upper limit of normal) until values return to normal. The drug may then be resumed at a reduced dose, with continuous monitoring during treatment.

Other drugs that should be used with caution include the antineoplastic hormone inhibitors. The antiandrogens include bicalutamide, flutamide, and nilutamide. *Bicalutamide* is excreted slowly in patients with severe hepatic impairment and should be used with caution in patients with moderate to severe hepatic impairment, with periodic liver function tests during long-term therapy. *Flutamide* is associated with serum aminotransferase abnormalities, cholestatic jaundice,

hepatic encephalopathy, hepatic necrosis, and a few deaths. Liver function tests should be performed periodically and at the first sign or symptom of liver dysfunction (e.g., pruritus, dark urine, jaundice). Flutamide should be discontinued if jaundice develops in patients who do not have liver metastases or if serum aminotransferase levels increase more than two to three times the upper limit of normal. Liver damage usually subsides if flutamide is discontinued or if dosage is reduced. Nilutamide may cause hepatitis or increases in liver enzymes. Liver enzymes should be checked at baseline and every 3 months. If symptoms of liver injury occur or if aminotransferases increase over two to three times the upper limits of normal, nilutamide should be discontinued.

Medroxyprogesterone should be stopped if manifestations of impaired liver function develop. *Tamoxifen* is associated with changes in liver enzyme levels and occasionally more severe liver damage, including fatty liver, cholestasis, hepatitis, and hepatic necrosis. *Toremifene's* elimination half-life is prolonged in patients with hepatic cirrhosis or fibrosis.

Bortezomib should be used with caution in patients with impaired hepatic function; most other biologic agents have not been studied in relation to impaired hepatic function.

Use in Home Care

Patients may receive parenteral cytotoxic drugs as outpatients and return home, or these and other antineoplastic drugs may be administered at home by the patient or a caregiver. The home care nurse may be involved in a wide range of activities associated with antineoplastic drug therapy, including administering the drugs, administering other drugs to prevent or manage adverse effects, and assessing patient and family responses to therapy. In addition, a major role involves teaching about the disease process, management of pain and other symptoms, the anticancer drugs, prevention or management of adverse drug effects, preventing infection, maintaining food and fluid intake, and other aspects of care. If a patient is receiving erythropoietin or oprelvekin subcutaneously, the patient or a caregiver may need to be taught injection technique.

The home care nurse also needs to teach patients and caregivers about safe handling of the traditional cytotoxic agents, including items contaminated with the drugs and patient body fluids or excreta. Precautions need to be similar to those used in health care agencies.

Applying Your Knowledge 42-4

Ms. Gardner has a long drive to the clinic to receive her chemotherapy and has to arrange with a friend or relative to bring her. Ms. Gardner arrives at the clinic and you look for her orders. You are unable to locate any written orders so you call the physician, who gives you the orders over the telephone.

Nursing Actions   Antineoplastic Drugs

NURSING ACTIONS	RATIONALE/EXPLANATION
1. Administer accurately a. With oral drugs, follow specific instructions for individual drugs. b. With **intravenous (IV) cytotoxic drugs**, general instructions include the following: (1) Compare labels on prepared solutions to medication orders in terms of the drug, concentration, expiration date, and instructions for administration. (2) Follow instructions for administering each drug. Common methods include injecting the drug into the tubing of a rapidly flowing IV or infusing the drug over a specified period of minutes to hours. (3) For patients with a long-term venous access device (e.g., Hickman or Groshong catheter), follow agency protocols for drug administration and catheter care. (4) Follow agency protocols for skin exposure or spills of cytotoxic drug solutions. c. With **monoclonal antibodies**, general instructions include the following: (1) Compare labels on prepared solutions to medication orders in terms of the drug, concentration, expiration date, and instructions for administration. (2) Administer by IV infusion; do *not* give as an IV push or bolus injection; do *not* mix with any other drugs. (3) Follow instructions *exactly* re: rates of infusion. (4) Pre-medicate with diphenhydramine and acetaminophen when ordered. d. With **growth factor/tyrosine kinase inhibitors**: (1) Ask patients to swallow dasatinib tablets whole, without crushing or chewing. (2) Give imatinib with a meal and large glass of water. Tablets may be dissolved in water or apple juice (50 mL for 100-mg tablet) for patients unable to swallow the tablets. Stir and have the patient drink the suspension immediately. (3) Give lapatinib once daily, 1 h before or 1 h after a meal e. With **bortezomib**, give the reconstituted solution as a bolus IV injection. f. With **hormonal drugs**: (1) Give goserelin and leuprolide according to the manufacturers' instructions. (2) Give letrozole, tamoxifen, and toremifene without regard to meals; give exemestane after a meal. (3). Give fulvestrant intramuscularly, into buttock, as a single 5-mL injection or as two 2.5-mL injections.	These drugs are usually taken at home by patients or administered by a caregiver. These drugs should be given only by nurses who are certified to do so, who administer the drugs regularly, and who maintain their knowledge base about antineoplastic drug therapy. Drug solutions should be prepared in a pharmacy. Because the drugs are highly toxic, every precaution must be taken to ensure safe and accurate administration. Long-term devices decrease the number of venipunctures a patient must undergo but require special care to maintain patency and prevent infection. These solutions are hazardous materials that require special handling. These drugs should be prepared in a pharmacy. They may be given in an outpatient setting but recipients must be closely monitored. To ensure accurate administration of these diverse products. Manufacturer's recommendations Recommended rates vary according to the individual drugs and whether the first or later doses are being given. To prevent allergic-type infusion reactions, which are associated with alemtuzumab, cetuximab, gemtuzumab, panitumumab, and rituximab. Manufacturer's recommendations Manufacturer's recommendations Manufacturer's recommendations The drug is reconstituted with 3.5 mL of 0.9% sodium chloride injection, preferably in a pharmacy. These drugs require specific techniques. Manufacturer's recommendations
2. Observe for therapeutic effects a. Increased appetite b. Increased feelings of well-being c. Improved mobility d. Decreased pain e. Laboratory and diagnostic tests that indicate improvement	Therapeutic effects depend to a large extent on the type of malignancy being treated. They may not become evident for several weeks after drug therapy is begun. With traditional cytotoxic drugs, some patients experience anorexia, nausea, and vomiting for 2 to 3 weeks after each cycle of drug therapy.

NURSING ACTIONS	RATIONALE/EXPLANATION
3. Observe for adverse effects	
a. With traditional cytotoxic drugs:	Cytotoxic drugs may have adverse effects on any body tissue. These effects range from common to rare, from relatively mild to life threatening, and occur with usual dosage ranges. Myelosuppressive effects are used to guide drug therapy.
(1) Hematologic effects: bone marrow depression with anemia, leukopenia, and thrombocytopenia; decreased antibodies and lymphocytes	For most drugs, white blood cell (WBC) and platelet counts reach their lowest points (nadirs) 7 to 14 days after drug administration and return toward normal after 21 days. Normal leukocyte and platelet counts indicate recovery of bone marrow function. Anemia may occur later because the red blood cell lives longer than WBCs and platelets. Most of these drugs have immunosuppressant effects, which impair body defenses against infection.
(2) Gastrointestinal (GI) effects—anorexia, nausea, vomiting, diarrhea, constipation, oral and intestinal mucositis and mucosal ulcerations, oral candidiasis	Nausea and vomiting are common, usually occur within a few hours of drug administration, and often subside within 12 to 24 hours. Constipation is most likely to occur with vincristine. Mucositis may occur anywhere in the GI tract; may interfere with nutrition and cause significant discomfort; may lead to infection, hemorrhage, or perforation; and may require that drug therapy be stopped.
(3) Dermatologic effects—alopecia, dermatitis, hand-foot syndrome (redness, tenderness of palms and soles), phlebitis at injection sites	Hair loss may occur over several weeks. Hand-foot syndrome is associated with capecitabine, doxorubicin, and fluorouracil. Some drugs cause tissue necrosis if they leak into tissues around the injection site.
(4) Renal effects:	
(a) Hyperuricemia and uric acid nephropathy	When malignant cells are destroyed, they release uric acid into the bloodstream. Uric acid crystals may precipitate in the kidneys and cause impaired function or failure.
(b) With cisplatin, nephrotoxicity (increased blood urea nitrogen [BUN] and serum creatinine; decreased creatinine clearance)	Decreasing the dose or frequency of administration, vigorous hydration, and amifostine administration can reduce the incidence of nephrotoxicity.
(c) With cyclophosphamide or ifosfamide, hemorrhagic cystitis (blood in urine, dysuria, burning on urination)	Drug metabolites are thought to irritate bladder mucosa; the drug is stopped if this occurs. Cystitis can be decreased by an ample fluid intake. In addition, mesna is given with ifosfamide.
(5) Pulmonary effects—cough, dyspnea, chest x-ray examination changes	Adverse effects on the lungs are associated mainly with bleomycin and methotrexate. With bleomycin, pulmonary toxicity may be severe and progress to pulmonary fibrosis.
(6) Cardiovascular effects—heart failure (dyspnea, edema, fatigue), dysrhythmias, electrocardiographic changes	Cardiomyopathy is associated mainly with doxorubicin and related drugs. This is a life-threatening adverse reaction.
(7) Central nervous system effects—peripheral neuropathy with vincristine, manifested by muscle weakness, numbness and tingling of extremities, foot drop, and decreased ability to walk	This common effect of vincristine may worsen for several weeks after drug administration. There is usually some recovery of function eventually.
(8) Endocrine effects—menstrual irregularities, sterility in men and women	
b. With monoclonal antibodies:	Although these drugs act more specifically than traditional cytotoxic drugs, they may still affect normal cells and produce serious adverse effects.
(1) Hypersensitivity-type infusion reactions—chills, fever, bronchospasm, dyspnea, skin rash or urticaria	These products are proteins and may contain other components capable of arousing an allergic reaction. Premedication with diphenhydramine (Benadryl) and acetaminophen is recommended with most of the drugs (e.g., alemtuzumab, cetuximab, panitumumab, gemtuzumab, rituximab).
(2) Hematologic effects—bone marrow depression (anemia, leukopenia, thrombocytopenia); high risk of infection, with chills, fever, respiratory, and other symptoms	These effects occur with most of the drugs and leukopenia may be especially severe with alemtuzumab, for which prophylactic antimicrobial drugs are recommended during and for 2 to 3 months after drug administration.
(3) GI effects—anorexia, nausea, vomiting, stomatitis, diarrhea	These effects commonly occur.

(continued on page 702)

Nursing Actions   Antineoplastic Drugs (continued)

NURSING ACTIONS	RATIONALE/EXPLANATION
(4) Cardiovascular effects—hypertension, hypotension, peripheral edema, heart failure, especially with alemtuzumab, bevacizumab, gemtuzumab, and trastuzumab	Severe cardiotoxicity leading to heart failure may be more likely to occur with bevacizumab and trastuzumab. With trastuzumab, cardiotoxicity is most likely to develop in patients who are 60 years or older and those who have received doxorubicin or cyclophosphamide. Left ventricular function should be monitored and trastuzumab should be discontinued in those who develop significantly decreased ejection fractions.
(5) Miscellaneous effects with most of the drugs—joint and muscle pain, weakness, dyspnea, headache, dizziness	
c. With growth factor and tyrosine kinase inhibitors	
(1) GI effects—anorexia, nausea, vomiting, diarrhea, mucositis	These are common effects, especially diarrhea.
(2) Dermatologic effects—skin rash, pruritus, hand-foot syndrome (redness, tenderness, tingling of palms and soles)	A variety of skin disorders may occur with all currently available drugs; hand-foot syndrome is associated with sorafenib, sunitinib, and temsirolimus.
(3) Cardiovascular effects—bleeding, fluid retention, edema, heart failure, hypertension	Bleeding is associated with erlotinib and imatinib; fluid retention and edema with dasatinib, imatinib, and temsirolimus; heart failure with imatinib; hypertension with sorafenib.
(4) Miscellaneous effects—dyspnea, fatigue, fever, joint and muscle pain, neutropenia	Fatigue is associated with all of the drugs; dyspnea with dasatinib, erlotinib and temsirolimus; neutropenia with dasatinib and imatinib.
d. With bortezomib—dehydration, edema, fever, hypotension, nausea, vomiting, skin rash, peripheral neuropathy	The risk of neuropathy may be increased with previous use of neurotoxic agents or pre-existing peripheral neuropathy.
e. With hormone inhibitors:	
(1) Aromatase inhibitors—hot flashes, fatigue, headache, nausea, musculoskeletal pain	Hot flashes and nausea are the most common adverse effect of drugs that decrease estrogen.
(2) Antiestrogens—hot flashes, nausea, fluid retention, weight loss, musculoskeletal pain, vaginal discharge and menstrual irregularities in premenopausal women	
(3) LHRH analogs—headache, depression, hot flashes, sexual dysfunction in males and females, infections in females	Hot flashes were the most commonly reported effect in both males and females; headache and depression were reported more often in females than in males.
(4) Antiandrogens—hot flashes, breast tenderness and enlargement, chest pain, heart failure, weight gain, muscle pain, neuropathy	
4. Observe for drug interactions	
a. Drugs that *increase* effects of cytotoxic antineoplastic drugs:	
(1) Anticoagulants, oral	Increased risk of bleeding
(2) Bone marrow depressants	Increased bone marrow depression
(3) Other antineoplastic drugs	Additive cytotoxic effects, both therapeutic and adverse
b. Drugs that *increase* effects of cyclophosphamide:	
(1) Anesthetics, inhalation	Lethal combination. Cyclophosphamide should be stopped at least 12 hours before general inhalation anesthesia is to be given.
(2) Carbamazepine, phenytoin, rifampin	These drugs induce liver enzymes, which accelerate transformation of the drug into its active metabolites
(3) Other myelosuppressive antineoplastic drugs	Increased bone marrow depression
c. Drug that *increases* the effect of mercaptopurine: Allopurinol	Allopurinol increases formation of the active mercaptopurine metabolite; doses of mercaptopurine must be reduced to one third to one fourth the usual dose.
d. Drugs that *increase* effects of methotrexate (MTX):	
(1) Alcohol	Additive liver toxicity. Avoid concomitant use.
(2) Aspirin, nonsteroidal anti-inflammatory drugs (NSAIDs), phenytoin, procarbazine, sulfonamides	Potentiate MTX by displacing it from protein-binding sites in plasma. Salicylates also block renal excretion of methotrexate. This may cause pancytopenia and liver toxicity.
(3) Other hepatotoxic drugs	Additive liver toxicity

NURSING ACTIONS	RATIONALE/EXPLANATION
(4) Other antineoplastic drugs	Additive cytotoxic effects, both therapeutic and adverse. Cisplatin may induce renal damage that impairs MTX excretion, increases blood levels, and increases toxicity.
(5) Trimethoprim-sulfamethoxazole (TMP-SMX, Bactrim)	Increased MTX toxicity; avoid concurrent administration if possible.
e. Drug that *decreases* effects of methotrexate (MTX): Leucovorin (folinic acid)	Leucovorin antagonizes the toxic effects of MTX and is used as an antidote for high-dose MTX regimens or for overdose. It must be given exactly at the specified time, before affected cells become too damaged to respond.
f. Drugs that *increase* effects of vinca alkaloids: (1) Erythromycin increases vinblastine toxicity; itraconazole increases vincristine toxicity.	These drugs probably inhibit metabolism of vinblastine and vincristine.
g. Drugs that *alter* effects of monoclonal antibodies: (1) Paclitaxel may increase blood levels and effects of trastuzumab.	Limited information is available about interactions with these drugs.
h. Drugs that *alter* effects of growth factor and tyrosine kinase inhibitor drugs: (1) Enzyme inhibitors (e.g., cimetidine, clarithromycin, itraconazole, others) *increase* effects; enzyme inducers (e.g., carbamazepine, phenytoin, rifampin, others) *decrease* effects. (2) With imatinib, chronic use of acetaminophen may increase risks of hepatotoxicity. i. Drugs that *alter* effects of hormone inhibitors: (1) With tamoxifen and toremifene, enzyme inhibitors increase effects and enzyme inducers decrease effects (see h. (1), above). (2) With flutamide, amiodarone, fluoroquinolones, and fluvoxamine may increase effects; carbamazepine and rifampin may decrease effects. (3) With nilutamide, fluconazole, fluvoxamine, gemfibrozil, isoniazid, and omeprazole may increase effects; carbamazepine and rifampin may decrease effects.	Most interactions are thought to occur with drugs metabolized by CYP3A4 enzymes. If the biologic drugs are given concurrently with an enzyme inhibitor, dosage may be decreased; if given with an enzyme inducer, dosage may be increased.

Key Concepts

■ Traditional cytotoxic antineoplastic drugs are nonselective in their effect on proliferating cells; therefore bone marrow toxicity is a common adverse effect of many cytotoxic drugs. These drugs kill the same fraction of cells with each cycle of chemotherapy treatment; repeated cycles of cytotoxic drugs potentially lower the number of cancer cells to a level where a person's immune responses are able to take over and destroy the remaining cancer cells.

■ Biologic targeted antineoplastic agents are designed to specifically attack a target that is expressed exclusively, or disproportionally, in the cancer cell.

■ Hormonal therapies that block the effects of estrogen (in an estrogen-responsive tumor) and androgen (in an androgen-responsive tumor), respectively, are essential in the treatment of breast and prostate cancers.

■ Cancer in older adults presents a unique challenge, due in part to the presence of comorbidities and the physical, biologic, and physiologic changes that occur with normal aging. Until recently, older adults were excluded from participating in clinical trials.

Review and Application Exercises

Short Answer Exercises

1. List major characteristics of malignant cells.

2. Which common cancers are attributed mainly to environmental factors? Which are attributed to genetic factors?

3. Which cytotoxic antineoplastic drugs are associated with serious adverse effects (e.g., bone marrow suppression, cardiotoxicity, hepatotoxicity, nephrotoxicity, neurotoxicity)?

4. Which drugs are associated with second malignancies?

5. How do the newer biologic agents differ from traditional cytotoxic drugs?

6. What is the basis for the anticancer effects of hormone inhibiting drugs?

7. For which cytotoxic drugs are cytoprotective drugs available?

8. List at least one intervention to prevent or minimize each of the following adverse effects of traditional cytotoxic chemotherapy: anemia, bleeding, infection, nausea and vomiting, neutropenia, stomatitis.

9. What measures are used to prevent or decrease the allergic infusion reactions associated with several antineoplastic monoclonal antibodies?

NCLEX-Style Questions

10. A priority nursing diagnosis to include in your care plan for a patient receiving cytotoxic chemotherapy is
    a. Risk for Impaired Skin Integrity
    b. Risk for Injury: Infection
    c. Body Image Disturbance related to alopecia
    d. Ineffective Family Coping

11. For a patient receiving a drug that causes bone marrow depression, which of the following should be especially emphasized with the patient and family members or caregivers?
    a. Wash hands often and avoid people with colds, flu, or other infections.
    b. Fatigue and weakness are uncommon.
    c. More nausea and vomiting may occur when the blood cell counts are low.
    d. Take acetaminophen for fever.

12. In explaining cytotoxic therapy to a family member of a patient who is to receive this treatment, the nurse explains that it
    a. damages both malignant and nonmalignant cells
    b. causes few adverse effects
    c. stimulates growth of cancer cells
    d. must be given daily

13. Antineoplastic hormone inhibitor drugs used in the treatment of cancer
    a. are highly cytotoxic to both cancer cells and normal cells
    b. target specific antigens or vital processes of cancer cells
    c. slow the growth of some cancer cells
    d. protect normal cells from cytotoxic drugs

14. The nurse who is giving a vesicant antineoplastic drug knows that the drug can
    a. cause minor skin irritation
    b. cause extensive tissue damage
    c. only be given through a central IV line
    d. be given by deep intramuscular injection if diluted with normal saline

Selected References

Bonosky, K., & Miller, R. (2005). Hypersensitivity reactions to oxaliplatin: What nurses need to know. *Clinical Journal of Oncology Nursing, 9,* 325–330.

Bouchardy, C., Rapiti, E., Blagojevic, S., Vlastos, A., & Vlastos, G. (2007). Older female cancer patients: Importance, causes, and consequences of undertreatment. *Journal of Clinical Oncology, 25,* 1858–1869.

Breslin, S. (2007). Cytokine-release syndrome: Overview and nursing implications. *Clinical Journal of Oncology Nursing, 11* (Suppl. 1), 37–42.

Demosthenes, M., Scherpereel, A., Copin, M. C., Colin, G., Brun, L., Lafitte, J. J., & Marquette, C. H. (2007). Fatal interstitial lung disease associated with oral erlotinib therapy for lung cancer. *BMC Cancer, 7.* Retrieved August 21, 2007, from http://www.biomedcentral.com/1471-2407/7/150

Drug facts and comparisons. (Updated monthly). St. Louis, MO: Facts and Comparisons.

Gobel, B. H. (2007). Nursing considerations of bevacizumab use in multiple tumor types. *Oncology Nursing Forum, 34,* 693–701.

Izzedine, H., Billemont, B., Thibault, F., & Rixe, O. (2007). New challenges in kidney cancer therapy: Sunitinib. *Annals of Oncology, 18* (Suppl. 9), 83–86.

Lacouture, M. E. (2007). Insights into the pathophysiology and management of dermatologic toxicities to EGFR-targeted therapies in colorectal cancer. *Cancer Nursing, 30* (Suppl. 4), 17–29.

Lacy, C. F., Armstrong, L. L., Goldman, M. P., et al. (2006). *Lexi-Drug information handbook* (14th ed.). Hudson, OH: Lexi-Comp.

Lynch, T. J., Kim, E. S., Eaby, B., Garey, J., West, D. P., & Lacouture, M. E. (2007). Epidermal growth factor receptor inhibitor-associated cutaneous toxicities: An evolving paradigm in clinical management. *Oncologist 2007, 12,* 610–621.

McGregor, L. M., Metzger, M. L., Sanders, R., & Santana, V. M. (2007). Pediatric cancers in the new millennium: Dramatic progress, new challenges. *Oncology, 21,* 809–820.

Morse, L., & Calarese, P. (2006). EGFR-targeted therapy and related skin toxicity. *Seminars in Oncology Nursing, 22,* 152–162.

O'Dea, D., Handy, C. M., & Wexler, A. (2006). Ocular changes with oxaliplatin. *Clinical Journal of Oncology Nursing, 10,* 227–229.

Oncology Nursing Society and Geriatric Oncology Consortium. (2007). Joint position on cancer care for older adults. *Oncology Nursing Forum, 34,* 623–624.

Polovich, M., White, J. M., & Kelleher, L. O. (2005). *Chemotherapy and biotherapy guidelines and recommendations for practice* (2nd ed.). Pittsburg, PA: Oncology Nursing Society.

Porth, C. M. (2005). *Pathophysiology: Concepts of altered health states* (7th ed.). Philadelphia: Lippincott Williams & Wilkins.

Reb, A. M. (2006). Physiology of aging. In D. G. Cope & A. M. Reb (Eds.), *An evidence-based approach to the treatment and care of the older adult with cancer* (pp. 41–55). Pittsburg, PA: Oncology Nursing Society.

Rokita, S. A. (2008). Oncology: Nursing management in cancer care. In S. C. Smeltzer & B. G. Bare (Eds.), *Brunner & Suddarth's textbook of medical-surgical nursing* (11th ed., pp. 380–446). Philadelphia: Lippincott Williams & Wilkins.

Seiwert, T. Y., Salama, J. K., & Vokes, E. E. (2007). The concurrent chemoradiation paradigm: General principles. *Nature Clinical Practice Oncology, 4,* 86–100.

Wilkes, G. M., & Barton-Burke, M. (2007). *2007 Oncology Nursing Drug Handbook.* Sudbury, MA: Jones and Bartlett.

Drugs Affecting the Respiratory System

Physiology of the Respiratory System

KEY TERMS

- Alveolar–capillary membrane
- Alveoli
- Apneustic center
- Cilia
- Diffusion
- Perfusion
- Pneumotaxic center
- Surfactant
- Ventilation

LEARNING OBJECTIVES

After studying this chapter, you will be able to:

1. Review roles and functions of the main respiratory tract structures in oxygenation of body tissues.
2. Describe the role of carbon dioxide in respiration.
3. List common signs and symptoms affecting respiratory function.
4. Identify general categories of drugs used to treat respiratory disorders.

Overview of the Respiratory System

The respiratory system helps meet the basic human need for oxygen (O_2). Oxygen is necessary for energy for cellular metabolism. When the oxygen supply is inadequate, cell function is impaired; when oxygen is absent, cells die. Permanent brain damage occurs within 4 to 6 minutes of anoxia. In addition to providing oxygen to all body cells, the respiratory system also removes carbon dioxide (CO_2), a major waste product of cell metabolism. Excessive accumulation of CO_2 damages or kills body cells and produces respiratory acidosis.

The efficiency of the respiratory system depends on the quality and quantity of air inhaled, the patency of air passages, the ability of the lungs to expand and contract, and the ability of O_2 and CO_2 to cross the alveolar–capillary membrane. In addition to the respiratory system, the circulatory, nervous, and musculoskeletal systems have important functions in respiration. Additional characteristics of the respiratory system and the process of respiration are described in the following sections.

Respiration

Respiration is the process of gas exchange by which O_2 is obtained and CO_2 is eliminated. This gas exchange occurs between the lung and the blood across the *alveolar–capillary membrane* and between the blood and body cells. More specifically, the four parts of respiration are:

- *Ventilation*—the movement of air between the atmosphere and the alveoli of the lungs
- *Perfusion*—blood flow through the lungs
- *Diffusion*—the process by which O_2 and CO_2 are transferred between alveoli and blood and between blood and body cells
- Regulation of breathing by the respiratory muscles and nervous system

Respiratory Tract

The respiratory tract is a series of branching tubes with progressively smaller diameters. These tubes (nose, pharynx, larynx, trachea, bronchi, and bronchioles) function as air passageways and air "conditioners" that filter, warm, and humidify incoming air. Most of the conditioning is done by the ciliated mucous membrane that lines the entire respiratory tract, except the pharynx and alveoli. *Cilia* are tiny, hair-like projections that sweep mucus toward the pharynx to be expectorated or swallowed. The mucous membrane secretes mucus, which forms a protective blanket and traps foreign particles, such as bacteria and dust.

When air is inhaled through the nose, it is conditioned by the nasal mucosa. When the nasal passages are blocked, the mouth serves as an alternate airway. The oral mucosa may warm and humidify air but cannot filter it.

Pharynx, Larynx, and Trachea

Air passes from the nasal cavities to the pharynx (throat). Pharyngeal walls are composed of skeletal muscle, and their lining is composed of mucous membrane. The pharynx contains the palatine tonsils, which are large masses of lymphatic tissue. The pharynx is a passageway for food, fluids, and air. Food and fluids go from the pharynx to the esophagus, and air passes from the pharynx into the trachea.

The larynx is composed of nine cartilages joined by ligaments and controlled by skeletal muscles. It contains the vocal cords and forms the upper end of the trachea. It closes on swallowing to prevent aspiration of food and fluids into the lungs.

The trachea is the passageway between the larynx and the main stem bronchi. It is a cartilaginous tube lined with ciliated epithelium and mucus-secreting cells. Cilia and mucus help to protect and defend the lungs.

Lungs

The lungs begin where the trachea divides into the right and left mainstem bronchi and contain the remaining respiratory structures. They are divided into five lobes, each with a secondary bronchus. The lobes are further subdivided into bronchopulmonary segments supplied by smaller bronchi. The bronchopulmonary segments contain lobules, which are the functional units of the lung (the site where gas exchange takes place). Each lobule is supplied by a bronchiole, an arteriole, a venule, and a lymphatic vessel. Blood enters the lobules through a pulmonary artery and exits through a pulmonary vein. Lymphatic structures surround the lobule and aid in the removal of plasma proteins and other particles from interstitial spaces.

The mainstem bronchi branch into smaller bronchi, then into bronchioles. Bronchioles are approximately the size of a pencil lead and do not contain cartilage or mucus-secreting glands. The walls of the bronchioles contain smooth muscle, which is controlled by the autonomic nervous system. Stimulation of parasympathetic nerves causes constriction; stimulation of sympathetic nerves causes relaxation or dilation.

The epithelial lining of the bronchioles becomes thinner with progressive branchings until only one cell layer is apparent. The bronchioles give rise to the *alveoli*, which are grape-like clusters of air sacs surrounded by capillaries.

The alveoli are composed of two types of cells. Type I cells are flat, thin epithelial cells that fuse with capillaries to form the alveolar–capillary membrane across which gas exchange occurs. Oxygen enters the bloodstream to be transported to body cells; CO_2 enters the alveoli to be exhaled from the lungs. Type II cells produce *surfactant*, a lipoprotein substance that

decreases the surface tension in the alveoli and aids lung inflation. The alveoli also contain macrophages that help to protect and defend the lungs.

The lungs are encased in a membrane called the pleura, which is composed of two layers. The inner layer, which adheres to the surface of the lung, is called the visceral pleura. The outer layer, which lines the thoracic cavity, is called the parietal pleura. The potential space between the layers is called the pleural cavity. It contains fluid that allows the layers to glide over each other and minimizes friction.

The lungs expand and relax in response to changes in pressure relationships (intrapulmonic and intrapleural pressures). Elastic tissue in the bronchioles and alveoli allows the lungs to stretch or expand to accommodate incoming air. This ability is called compliance. The lungs also recoil (like a stretched rubber band) to expel air. Some air remains in the lungs after expiration, which allows gas exchange to continue between respirations.

In addition to exchanging O_2 and CO_2, the lungs synthesize, store, release, remove, metabolize, or inactivate a variety of biologically active substances. These substances, which may be locally released or carried in blood or tissue fluids, participate in both physiologic and pathologic processes. Specific substances that may be released from the lungs include biogenic amines (e.g., catecholamines, histamine, serotonin), arachidonic acid metabolites (e.g., prostaglandins, leukotrienes), angiotensin-converting enzyme, and heparin. The amines are important in regulating smooth muscle tone (i.e., constriction or dilation) in the airways and blood vessels. Prostaglandins and leukotrienes are important in inflammatory processes. Angiotensin-converting enzyme converts angiotensin I to angiotensin II, which is important in regulating blood pressure. Heparin helps to dissolve blood clots, especially in the capillaries, where small clots are trapped. The lungs also process peptides, lipids, hormones, and drugs and inactivate bradykinin.

Lung Circulation

The pulmonary circulatory system transports O_2 and CO_2. After oxygen enters the bloodstream across the alveolar–capillary membrane, it combines with hemoglobin in red blood cells for transport to body cells, where it is released. Carbon dioxide combines with hemoglobin in the cells for return to the lungs and elimination from the body.

The lungs receive the total cardiac output of blood and are supplied with blood from two sources, the pulmonary and bronchial circulations. The pulmonary circulation provides for gas exchange because the pulmonary arteries carry deoxygenated blood to the lungs and the pulmonary veins return oxygenated blood to the heart. The bronchial arteries arise from the thoracic aorta and supply the air passages and supporting structures. The bronchial circulation also warms and humidifies incoming air and can form new vessels and develop collateral circulation when normal vessels are blocked (e.g., in pulmonary embolism). The latter ability helps to keep lung tissue alive until circulation can be restored.

Capillaries in the lungs are lined by a single layer of epithelial cells called endothelium. Once thought to be a passive conduit for blood, it is now known that the endothelium performs several important functions. First, it forms a barrier that prevents leakage of water and other substances into lung tissue. Second, it participates in the transport of respiratory gases, water, and solutes. Third, it secretes vasodilating substances such as nitric oxide and prostacyclin. Nitric oxide also regulates smooth muscle tone in the bronchi, and prostacyclin also inhibits platelet aggregation. When pulmonary endothelium is injured (e.g., by endotoxins or drugs such as bleomycin, an anticancer drug), these functions are impaired.

Nervous System's Role in Respiration

The nervous system regulates the rate and depth of respiration by the respiratory center in the medulla oblongata, the *pneumotaxic center* in the pons, and the *apneustic center* in the reticular formation. The respiratory center is stimulated primarily by increased CO_2 in the fluids of the center. (However, excessive CO_2 depresses the respiratory center.) When the center is stimulated, the rate and depth of breathing are increased, and excessive CO_2 is exhaled. A lesser stimulus to the respiratory center is decreased oxygen in arterial blood.

The nervous system also operates several reflexes important to respiration. The cough reflex is especially important because it helps protect the lungs from foreign particles, air pollutants, bacteria, and other potentially harmful substances. A cough occurs when nerve endings in the respiratory tract mucosa are stimulated by dryness, pressure, cold, irritant fumes, or excessive secretions.

Musculoskeletal System's Role in Respiration

The musculoskeletal system participates in chest expansion and contraction. Normally, the diaphragm and external intercostal muscles expand the chest cavity and are called muscles of inspiration. The abdominal and internal intercostal muscles are the muscles of expiration.

Summary of Respiratory Function

Overall, normal respiration requires

1. Atmospheric air containing at least 21% O_2.
2. Adequate ventilation. Ventilation, in turn, requires patent airways, expansion and contraction of the chest, expansion and contraction of the lungs, and maintenance of a normal range of intrapulmonic and intrapleural pressures.
3. Adequate diffusion of O_2 and CO_2 through the alveolar–capillary membrane. Factors influencing diffusion include the thickness and surface area of the membrane and pressure differences between gases on each side of the membrane.
4. Adequate perfusion or circulation of blood and sufficient hemoglobin to carry needed O_2.

In addition, normal breathing occurs 16 to 20 times per minute and is quiet, rhythmic, and effortless. Approximately 500 milliliters of air is inspired and expired with a normal breath (tidal volume); deep breaths or "sighs" occur 6 to 10 times per hour to ventilate more alveoli. Fever, exercise, pain, and emotions such as anger increase respirations. Sleep or rest and various medications, such as antianxiety drugs, sedatives, and opioid analgesics, slow respiration.

Disorders of the Respiratory System

The respiratory system is subject to many disorders that interfere with respiration and other lung functions. These disorders may be caused by agents that reach the system through inhaled air or through the bloodstream and include respiratory tract infections, allergic disorders, inflammatory disorders, and conditions that obstruct airflow (e.g., excessive respiratory tract secretions, asthma, other chronic obstructive pulmonary diseases). Injury to the lungs by various disorders (e.g., anaphylaxis, asthma, mechanical stimulation such as hyperventilation, pulmonary thromboembolism, pulmonary edema, acute respiratory distress syndrome) is associated with the release of histamine and other biologically active chemical mediators from the lungs. These mediators often cause inflammation and constriction of the airways.

The ciliated epithelial cells of the larger airways, the type I epithelial cells of the alveoli, and the capillary endothelial cells of the alveolar area are especially susceptible to injury. When they are injured, cellular functions are impaired (e.g., decreased mucociliary clearance). Common signs and symptoms of respiratory disorders include cough, increased secretions, mucosal congestion, and bronchospasm. Severe disorders or inadequate treatment may lead to cell necrosis or respiratory failure.

Drug Therapy

In general, drug therapy is more effective in relieving respiratory symptoms than in curing the underlying disorders that cause the symptoms. Major drug groups used to treat respiratory symptoms are bronchodilating and anti-inflammatory agents (see Chap. 44), antihistamines (see Chap. 45), and nasal decongestants, antitussives, and cold remedies (see Chap. 46).

Key Concepts

- When the oxygen supply is inadequate, cell function is impaired; when oxygen is absent, cells die.

- The efficiency of the respiratory system depends on the quality and quantity of air inhaled, the patency of air passages, the ability of the lungs to expand and contract, and the ability of O_2 and CO_2 to cross the alveolar–capillary membrane.

- The nervous system regulates the rate and depth of respiration by the respiratory center in the medulla oblongata, the pneumotaxic center in the pons, and the apneustic center in the reticular formation.

- The respiratory system is subject to many disorders that interfere with respiration and other lung functions, including respiratory tract infections, allergic disorders, inflammatory disorders, and conditions that obstruct airflow.

- Major drug groups used to treat respiratory symptoms are bronchodilating and anti-inflammatory agents, antihistamines, and nasal decongestants, antitussives, and cold remedies.

Review and Application Exercises

Short Answer Exercises

1. What is the main function of the respiratory system?

2. Where does the exchange of oxygen and carbon dioxide occur?

3. List factors that stimulate rate and depth of respiration.

4. List factors that depress rate and depth of respiration.

5. What are common signs and symptoms of respiratory disorders for which drug therapy is often used?

Selected References

Corwin, E. J. (2006). *Handbook of pathophysiology* (3rd ed.). Philadelphia: Lippincott Williams & Wilkins.

Guyton, A. C., & Hall, J. E. (2006). *Textbook of medical physiology* (11th ed.). Philadelphia: W. B. Saunders.

Porth, C. M. (2005). *Pathophysiology: Concepts of altered health states* (7th ed.). Philadelphia: Lippincott Williams & Wilkins.

Drugs for Asthma and Other Bronchoconstrictive Disorders

KEY TERMS

- Adrenergic drugs
- Anticholinergics
- Asthma
- Beta$_2$-adrenergic agonists
- Bronchitis
- Bronchospasm
- Corticosteroids
- Emphysema
- Hyperreactivity
- Leukotrienes
- Mast cells
- Occupational asthma

LEARNING OBJECTIVES

After studying this chapter, you will be able to:

1. Describe the main pathophysiologic characteristics of asthma and other bronchoconstrictive disorders.
2. Discuss the uses and effects of bronchodilating drugs, including adrenergics, anticholinergics, and xanthines.
3. Differentiate between short-acting and long-acting inhaled beta$_2$-adrenergic agonists in terms of uses and nursing process implications.
4. Discuss the uses of anti-inflammatory drugs, including corticosteroids, leukotriene modifiers, and mast cell stabilizers.
5. Discuss reasons for using inhaled drugs when possible.
6. Differentiate between "quick relief" and long-term control of asthma symptoms.
7. Discuss the use of antiasthmatic drugs in special populations.
8. Teach patients self-care and long-term control measures.

Applying Your Knowledge

Lynne Albright is a 48-year-old woman who has adult-onset asthma. Her medications include zafirlukast and salmeterol/fluticasone (Advair) daily. She uses an albuterol inhaler as needed. Ms. Albright is a professor in women's studies for a large university. You are the on-site nurse for the campus.

Introduction

The drugs described in this chapter are used to treat respiratory disorders characterized by bronchoconstriction, inflammation, mucosal edema, and excessive mucus production (asthma, bronchitis, and emphysema). Asthma is emphasized because of its widespread prevalence, especially in urban populations. Compared with Caucasians, African Americans and Hispanics have a higher prevalence and African Americans have a higher death rate from asthma. However, the differences are usually attributed to urban living and lesser access to health care rather than race or ethnic group. *Occupational asthma* (i.e., asthma resulting from repeated and prolonged exposure to industrial inhalants) is also a major health problem. Persons with occupational asthma often have symptoms while in the work environment, with improvement on days off and during vacations. Symptoms sometime persist after termination of exposure. Asthma may occur at any age but is especially common in children and older adults. Children who are exposed to allergens and airway irritants such as tobacco smoke during infancy are at high risk for development of asthma.

Asthma

Symptoms

Asthma is an airway disorder characterized by bronchoconstriction, inflammation, and *hyperreactivity* to various stimuli. Resultant symptoms include dyspnea, wheezing, chest tightness, cough, and sputum production. Wheezing is a high-pitched, whistling sound caused by turbulent airflow through an obstructed airway. Thus, any condition that produces significant airway occlusion can cause wheezing. However, a chronic cough may be the only symptom for some people with asthma. Symptoms vary in incidence and severity from occasional episodes of mild respiratory distress, with normal functioning between "attacks," to persistent, daily, or continual respiratory distress if not adequately controlled. Inflammation and damaged airway mucosa are chronically present, even when patients appear symptom free.

Acute symptoms of asthma may be precipitated by numerous stimuli, and hyperreactivity to such stimuli may initiate both inflammation and bronchoconstriction. Viral infections of the respiratory tract are often the causative agents, especially in infants and young children whose airways are small and easily obstructed. Asthma symptoms may persist for days or weeks after the viral infection resolves. In about 25% of patients with asthma, aspirin and other nonsteroidal anti-inflammatory drugs (NSAIDs) can precipitate an attack. Some patients are allergic to sulfites and may experience life-threatening asthma attacks if they ingest foods processed with these preservatives (e.g., beer, wine, dried fruit). The U.S. Food and Drug Administration (FDA) has banned the use of sulfites on foods meant to be served raw, such as open salad bars. Patients with severe asthma should be cautioned against ingesting food and drug products containing sulfites or metabisulfites.

Gastroesophageal reflux disease (GERD), a common disorder characterized by heartburn and esophagitis, is also associated with asthma. Asthma that worsens at night may be associated with nighttime acid reflux. Although the precise mechanism of pulmonary symptoms of GERD in asthma is not known, there are suggestions that microaspirations or a vagally mediated, reflex type of bronchoconstriction may be involved. Asthma may also aggravate GERD, because antiasthma medications that dilate the airways also relax muscle tone in the gastroesophageal sphincter and may increase acid reflux. It has been suggested that in individuals with inadequate control of their asthma symptoms, a trial of an H_2-blocker or proton-pump inhibitor therapy may be of benefit.

Additional precipitants may include allergens (e.g., pollens, molds), airway irritants and pollutants (e.g., chemical fumes, cigarette smoke, automobile exhaust), cold air, and exercise. Acute episodes of asthma may last minutes to hours.

Pathophysiology

Bronchoconstriction (also called *bronchospasm*) involves strong muscle contractions that narrow the airways. Airway smooth muscle extends from the trachea through the bronchioles. It is wrapped around the airways in a spiral pattern, and contraction causes a sphincter type of action that can completely occlude the airway lumen. Bronchoconstriction is aggravated by inflammation, mucosal edema, and excessive mucus and may be precipitated by the numerous stimuli described above.

When lung tissues are exposed to causative stimuli, *mast cells* release substances that cause bronchoconstriction and inflammation. Mast cells are found throughout the body in connective tissues and are abundant in tissues surrounding capillaries in the lungs. When sensitized mast cells in the lungs or eosinophils in the blood are exposed to allergens or irritants, multiple cytokines and other chemical mediators (e.g., acetylcholine, cyclic guanosine monophosphate [GMP], histamine, interleukins, leukotrienes, prostaglandins, serotonin) are synthesized and released. These chemicals act directly on target tissues of the airways, causing smooth muscle constriction, increased capillary permeability and fluid leakage, and changes in the mucus-secreting properties of the airway epithelium.

Bronchoconstrictive substances are antagonized by cyclic adenosine monophosphate (cyclic AMP). Cyclic AMP is an intracellular substance that initiates various intracellular activities, depending on the type of cell. In lung cells, cyclic AMP inhibits release of bronchoconstrictive substances and thus indirectly promotes bronchodilation. In mild to moderate asthma, bronchoconstriction is usually recurrent and reversible, either spontaneously or with drug therapy. In advanced or severe asthma, airway obstruction becomes less reversible and worsens because chronically inflamed airways undergo structural changes (e.g., fibrosis, enlarged smooth muscle cells, enlarged mucous glands), called "airway remodeling," that inhibit their function.

National Asthma Education and Prevention Program (NAEPP)

Because of asthma's significance as a public health problem, the National Heart, Lung, and Blood Institute (NHLBI) of the National Institutes of Health (NIH) established the NAEPP. The NAEPP assembled a group of experts who established "Guidelines for the Diagnosis and Management of Asthma." After nearly a decade, these guidelines (Box 44-1) were updated in 2007, including an expanded portion on childhood asthma. Further distinction is placed on the importance of classifying asthma severity and assessing asthma control. The guidelines are the current "standard of care" for adults and children with asthma and center around four essential components of asthma care: assessment and monitoring, patient education, control of factors contributing to asthma severity, and pharmacologic treatment. Additional information can be obtained from http://www.nhlbi.nih.gov.

Chronic Bronchitis and Emphysema

Chronic *bronchitis* and *emphysema*, commonly called chronic obstructive pulmonary disease (COPD), usually develop after long-standing exposure to airway irritants such as cigarette smoke. In these conditions, bronchoconstriction and

| Box 44-1 | National Asthma Education and Prevention Program (NAEPP) Expert Panel Guidelines* |

Definition

Asthma is "a chronic inflammatory disorder of the airways in which many cells and cellular elements play a role: in particular, mast cells, eosinophils, T lymphocytes, macrophages, neutrophils, and epithelial cells. In susceptible individuals, this inflammation causes recurrent episodes of wheezing, breathlessness, chest tightness, and coughing, particularly at night or in the early morning."

Goals of Therapy

1. Minimal or no chronic symptoms day or night
2. Minimal or no exacerbations
3. No limitations on activities; for children, no school/parent's work missed
4. Minimal use of short-acting inhaled beta$_2$ agonist (<1 time per day, <1 canister/month)
5. Minimal or no adverse effects from medications

General Recommendations

- Establish and teach patients/parents/caregivers about quick relief measures and long-term control measures. Assist to identify and control environmental factors that aggravate asthma.
- For acute attacks, gain control as quickly as possible (a short course of systemic corticosteroids may be needed); then step down to the least medication necessary to maintain control.
- Review the treatment regimen every 1 to 6 months. If control is adequate and goals are being met, a gradual stepwise reduction in medication may be possible. If control is inadequate, the treatment regimen may need to be changed. For example, frequent or increasing use of a short-acting beta$_2$ agonist (>2 times a week with intermittent asthma; daily or increasing use with persistent asthma) may indicate the need to initiate or increase long-term control therapy. However, first reassess patients' medication techniques (e.g., correct use of inhalers), adherence, and environmental control measures.

Quick Relief for Acute Exacerbations

- **Adults and children > 5 years:** Short-acting, inhaled, beta$_2$ agonist, 2–4 puffs as needed. If symptoms are severe, patients may need up to 3 treatments at 20-minute intervals or a nebulizer treatment. A short course of a systemic corticosteroid may also be needed.
- **Children 5 years and younger:** Short-acting beta$_2$ agonist by nebulizer or face mask and spacer or holding chamber. Alternative: oral beta$_2$ agonist. With viral respiratory infections, the beta$_2$ agonist may be needed q4–6h up to 24 hours or longer and a systemic corticosteroid may be needed.

Long-Term Control

- **Step 1 Mild Intermittent** (symptoms 2 days/week or less or 2 nights/month or less): No daily medication needed; treat acute exacerbations with an inhaled beta$_2$ agonist and possibly a short course of a systemic corticosteroid.
- **Step 2 Mild Persistent** (symptoms >2/week but <1×/day or >2 nights/month):

- **Adults and children > 5 years:** Low-dose inhaled corticosteroid. Alternatives: cromolyn or nedocromil, a leukotriene modifier, or sustained-release theophylline to maintain a serum theophylline drug level of 5–15 mcg/mL.
- **Children 5 years and younger:** Administer the inhaled corticosteroid by a nebulizer or metered-dose inhaler (MDI) with a holding chamber. Alternatives: cromolyn (via nebulizer or MDI with holding chamber) or a leukotriene modifier.
- **Step 3 Moderate Persistent** (symptoms daily and >1 night/week):
  - **Adults and children > 5 years:** Low- to medium-dose inhaled corticosteroid and a long-acting beta$_2$ agonist. Alternatives: increase corticosteroid dose or continue low to medium dose of corticosteroid and add a leukotriene modifier or theophylline.
  - **Children < 5 years:** Low-dose inhaled corticosteroid and a long-acting beta$_2$ agonist or medium-dose inhaled corticosteroid.
- **Step 4 Severe Persistent** (symptoms continual during daytime hours and frequent at night):
  - **Adults and children > 5 years:** High-dose inhaled corticosteroid and long-acting beta$_2$ agonist and, if necessary, a systemic corticosteroid (2 mg/kg/d, not to exceed 60 mg/d). Reduce systemic corticosteroid when possible.
  - **Children < 5 years:** Same as for adults and older children.

Low (L), Medium (M), and High (H) Doses of Inhaled Corticosteroids:

	Adults (mcg)	Children (12 y and younger) (mcg)
Beclomethasone (42 or 84 mcg/puff)	L: 168–504 M: 504–840 H: >840	L: 84–336 M: 336–672 H: >672
Beclomethasone (40–80 mcg/puff)	L: 80–240 M: 240–480 H: >480	L: 80–160 M: 160–320 H: >320
Budesonide (200 mcg/inhalation)	L: 200–600 M: 600–1200 H: >1200	L: 200–400 M: 400–800 H: >800
Budesonide inhalation suspension for nebulization (child dose only)		L: 0.5 mg M: 1.0 mg H: 2.0 mg
Flunisolide (250 mcg/puff)	L: 500–1000 M: 1000–2000 H: >2000	L: 500–750 M: 1000–1250 H: >1250
Fluticasone aerosol (44, 110, or 220 mcg/puff)	L: 88–264 M: 264–660 H: >660	L: 88–176 M: 176–440 H: >440
Fluticasone powder (50, 100, or 250 mcg/puff)	L: 100–300 M: 300–600 H: >600	L: 100–200 M: 200–400 H: >400
Triamcinolone acetonide (100 mcg/puff)	L: 400–1000 M: 1000–2000 H: >2000	L: 400–800 M: 800–1200 H: >1200

*Adapted from NAEPP Expert Panel Report 3 (NIH Publication No. 08-4051, 2007).

inflammation are more constant and less reversible than with asthma. Anatomic and physiologic changes occur over several years and lead to increasing dyspnea, activity intolerance, and reduced quality of life. These conditions usually affect middle-aged or older adults.

Drug Therapy

Two general classifications of drugs are used for asthma management: long-term (prophylactic) control medications to achieve and maintain control of persistent asthma and quick relief (rescue) medications used during periods of acute symptoms and exacerbations. Specifically, two major groups of drugs used to treat asthma, acute and chronic bronchitis, and emphysema are bronchodilators and anti-inflammatory drugs. Bronchodilators are used to prevent and treat bronchoconstriction; anti-inflammatory drugs are used to prevent and treat inflammation of the airways. Reducing inflammation also reduces bronchoconstriction by decreasing mucosal edema and mucous secretions that narrow airways and by decreasing airway hyperreactivity to various stimuli. The drugs are described in the following sections; pharmacokinetic characteristics of inhaled drugs are listed in Table 44-1.

Bronchodilators

Table 44-2 lists routes and dosage ranges of the bronchodilators.

Adrenergics

Adrenergic drugs (see Chap. 17) stimulate beta$_2$-adrenergic receptors in the smooth muscle of bronchi and bronchioles. The receptors, in turn, stimulate the enzyme adenyl cyclase to increase production of cyclic AMP. The increased cyclic AMP produces bronchodilation. Some beta-adrenergic drugs (e.g., epinephrine) also stimulate beta$_1$-adrenergic receptors in the heart to increase the rate and force of contraction. Cardiac stimulation is an adverse effect when the drugs are given for bronchodilation. These drugs are contraindicated in patients with cardiac tachydysrhythmias and severe coronary artery disease; they should be used cautiously in patients with hypertension, hyperthyroidism, diabetes mellitus, and seizure disorders.

Epinephrine may be injected subcutaneously in an acute attack of bronchoconstriction, with therapeutic rescue effects in approximately 5 minutes and lasting for approximately 4 hours. However, an inhaled selective beta$_2$ agonist is the drug of choice in this situation. Epinephrine is also available without prescription in a pressurized aerosol form (e.g., Primatene). Almost all over-the-counter aerosol products promoted for use in asthma contain epinephrine. These products are often abused and may delay the patient from seeking medical attention. Patients should be cautioned that excessive use may produce hazardous cardiac stimulation and other adverse effects.

Albuterol and **levalbuterol** are short-acting *beta$_2$-adrenergic agonists* used for prevention and treatment of bronchoconstriction. These drugs act more selectively on beta$_2$ receptors and cause less cardiac stimulation than epinephrine. Most often taken by inhalation, they are also the most effective bronchodilators and the treatment of first choice to relieve acute asthma. Because the drugs can be effectively delivered by aerosol or nebulization, even to young children and to patients on mechanical ventilation, there is seldom a need to give epinephrine or other nonselective adrenergic drugs by injection.

The beta$_2$ agonists are usually self-administered by metered-dose inhalers (MDIs). Although most drug references still list a regular dosing schedule (e.g., every 4 to 6 hours),

Table 44-1	Pharmacokinetics of Selected Inhaled Antiasthma Medications				
	ACTION				
Generic Name	Onset (min)	Peak (hours)	Duration (hours)	Metabolism/Excretion	Half-Life (Hours)
Adrenergics					
Albuterol	5	0.5–2	4–6	Liver/urine	2–4
Levalbuterol	5–10	1	3–6	Liver/urine	3–4
Salmeterol	30–48 COPD 120	2–4	12	Liver/feces	5.5
Anticholinergic					
Ipratropium	1–3	1.5–2	≤ 4		1.6
Corticosteroids					
Beclomethasone	Rapid	1–2 wk		Liver/feces	2.3–6
Budesonide	Immediate	Rapid	8–12	Liver/urine (60%) & feces	2.8
Flunisolide	Slow	10–30	4–6	Liver/renal (50%), feces (40%)	1–2
Fluticasone	Slow		24	Liver/feces & urine	3.1

Table 44-2	Drugs at a Glance: Bronchodilating Drugs

ROUTES AND DOSAGE RANGES

Generic/Trade Name	Adults	Children
Bronchodilators **Adrenergics** **Albuterol** (Proventil, Ventolin, AccuNeb)	Inhalation* aerosol (90 mcg/actuation): 1–2 oral inhalations q4–6h; prevention of exercise-induced bronchospasm, 2 inhalations 1 min before exercise Inhalation solution via nebulizer, 2.5 mg 3–4 times daily (in 2.5 mL sterile saline, over 5–15 min) Regular tablets: PO 2–4 mg 3–4 times daily Extended-release tablets: Proventil Repetabs PO 4–8 mg q12h, initially. Increase if necessary to a maximum of 32 mg/d, in divided doses, q12h.	*Inhalation aerosol:* 4 y and older (12 y and older for Proventil), same as adults Nebulizer solution, 12 y and older, same as adults; 2–12 y (AccuNeb), 1.25 mg 3–4 times daily, as needed, over 5–15 min *Regular tablets:* 12 y and older, same as adults; 6–12 y, 2 mg 3–4 times daily *Extended-release tablets:* 12 y and older, same as adults: 6–12 y: PO 4 mg q12h initially; increase if necessary to a maximum of 24 mg/d, in divided doses, q12h.
Epinephrine (Adrenalin, Bronkaid)	Aqueous solution (epinephrine 1:1000), Sub-Q 0.3–0.5 mg; dose may be repeated after 20 min if necessary for 3 doses Inhalation by inhaler, one or two inhalations 4–6 times per day Inhalation by nebulizer, 1–3 inhalations of 2.25% racemic epinephrine in 2.5 mL normal saline up to q3h	Aqueous solution (epinephrine 1:1000), Sub-Q 0.01 mL/kg q4h as needed. A single dose should not exceed 0.5 mL. Inhalation, same as adults for both inhaler and nebulizer
Formoterol (Foradil)	Oral inhalation by special inhaler (Aerolizer), 12 mcg (contents of 1 capsule) twice daily, q12h	5 y and older, same as adults
Levalbuterol (Xopenex, MDI: Xopenex HFA)	Nebulizer, 0.63–1.25 mg 3 times daily, q6–8h MDI: 1–2 puffs q4–6h	12 y and older, same as adults 6–11 y: Nebulizer, 0.31 mg 3 times daily, q6–8h MDI ≥4 y same as adults
Metaproterenol (Alupent)	Inhalation,* 2–3 puffs (0.65 mg/dose), q3–4h; maximum dose, 12 inhalations/d	Inhalation, not recommended for use in children <12 y
Salmeterol (Serevent)	Inhalation powder: 1 inhalation (50 mcg) q12h	<12 y, dosage not established Inhalation powder: 4 y and older, same as adults
Terbutaline	PO 2.5–5 mg q6–8h; maximum dose, 15 mg/d Sub-Q 0.25 mg, repeated in 15–30 min if necessary, q4–6h	PO 2.5 mg 3 times per day for children 12 y and older; maximum dose, 7.5 mg/d Sub-Q dosage not established
Anticholinergics **Ipratropium** bromide (Atrovent)	Two inhalations (36 mcg) from the metered-dose inhaler 4 times per day	Dosage not established
Tiotropium (Spiriva)	One tablet (18 mcg) in HandiHaler once daily	Dosage not established
Xanthines **Short-acting theophylline** (Aminophylline)	PO, 500 mg initially, then 200–300 mg q6–8h; IV infusion, 6 mg/kg over 30 min, then 0.1–1.2 mg/kg/h	PO, 7.5 mg/kg initially, then 5–6 mg/kg q6–8h; IV infusion, 6 mg/kg over 30 min, then 0.6–0.9 mg/kg/h

Generic/Trade Name	ROUTES AND DOSAGE RANGES	
	Adults	**Children**
Anticholinergics **Xanthines** **Long-acting theophylline** (Theochron, others)	PO, 150–300 mg q8–12h; maximal dose 13 mg/kg or 900 mg daily, whichever is less	PO, 100–200 mg q8–12h; maximal dose, 24 mg/kg/d
Combination Drugs **Fluticasone/Salmeterol** (Advair)	Oral inhalation, one inhalation, twice daily	12 y *and older:* same as adults
Ipratropium/Albuterol (Combivent, DuoNeb)	Aerosol: two inhalations 4 times daily Nebulizing solution: 1 vial 4 times daily, increased to 6 times daily if necessary	Dosage not established

Short-acting adrenergic bronchodilators are used mainly by inhalation, as needed, rather than on a regular schedule.

MDI, multidose inhaler.

asthma experts recommend that the drugs be used when needed (e.g., to treat acute dyspnea or prevent dyspnea during exercise). If these drugs are overused, they lose their bronchodilating effects because the beta$_2$-adrenergic receptors become unresponsive to stimulation. This tolerance does not occur with the long-acting beta$_2$ agonists.

Formoterol and **salmeterol** are long-acting beta$_2$-adrenergic agonists used only for prophylaxis of acute bronchoconstriction. They are not effective in acute attacks because they have a slower onset of action than the short-acting drugs (up to 20 minutes for salmeterol). Effects last 12 hours and the drugs should *not* be taken more frequently. If additional bronchodilating medication is needed, a short-acting agent (e.g., albuterol) should be used. The FDA has issued a **BLACK BOX WARNING** that initiating salmeterol in individuals with significantly worsening or acutely deteriorating asthma may be life-threatening.

Metaproterenol is a relatively selective, intermediate-acting beta$_2$-adrenergic agonist that may be given orally or by MDI. It is used to treat acute bronchospasm and to prevent exercise-induced asthma. In high doses, metaproterenol loses some of its selectivity and may cause cardiac and central nervous system (CNS) stimulation.

Terbutaline is a relatively selective beta$_2$-adrenergic agonist that is a long-acting bronchodilator. When given subcutaneously, terbutaline loses its selectivity and has little advantage over epinephrine. Muscle tremor is the most frequent side effect with this agent.

Anticholinergics

Anticholinergics (see Chap. 20) block the action of acetylcholine in bronchial smooth muscle when given by inhalation. This action reduces intracellular GMP, a bronchoconstrictive substance.

Ipratropium was formulated to be taken by inhalation for maintenance therapy of bronchoconstriction associated with chronic bronchitis and emphysema. Improved pulmonary function usually occurs in a few minutes. Ipratropium acts synergistically with adrenergic bronchodilators and may be used concomitantly. It improves lung function about 10% to 15% over an inhaled beta$_2$ agonist alone. Ipratropium may also be used to treat rhinorrhea associated with allergic rhinitis and the common cold. It is available as a nasal spray for such usage. Ipratropium is poorly absorbed and produces few systemic effects. However, cautious use is recommended in patients with narrow-angle glaucoma and prostatic hypertrophy. The most common adverse effects are cough, nervousness, nausea, gastrointestinal upset, headache, and dizziness.

Tiotropium (Spiriva) was approved to be taken once daily by inhalation for maintenance therapy of bronchoconstriction associated with chronic bronchitis and emphysema. Tiotropium has differences in its pharmacokinetic and pharmacologic properties that may make it superior to ipratropium as an anticholinergic agent. The primary adverse effect of tiotropium is dry mouth, though other effects include headache, dizziness, abdominal pain, constipation, diarrhea, flulike symptoms, and chest pain. Cautious use is recommended in patients with narrow-angle glaucoma.

Xanthines

The main xanthine used clinically is **theophylline.** Despite many years of use, the drug's mechanism of action is unknown. Various mechanisms have been proposed, such as inhibiting phosphodiesterase enzymes that metabolize cyclic AMP, increasing endogenous catecholamines, inhibiting calcium ion movement into smooth muscle, inhibiting prostaglandin synthesis and release, or inhibiting the release of bronchoconstrictive substances from mast cells and leukocytes. In addition to bronchodilation, other effects that may be beneficial in asthma and COPD include inhibiting pulmonary edema by decreasing vascular permeability, increasing the ability of cilia to clear mucus from the airways, strengthening contractions of the diaphragm, and decreasing inflammation. Theophylline also increases cardiac output, causes peripheral vasodilation, exerts a mild diuretic effect, and stimulates the CNS. The cardiovascular and CNS effects are adverse effects. Serum drug levels should be monitored to help regulate dosage and avoid adverse effects. Theophylline preparations are contraindicated in patients with acute gastritis and peptic ulcer disease; they should be used cautiously in those with cardiovascular disorders that could be aggravated by drug-induced cardiac stimulation.

Theophylline was formerly used extensively in the prevention and treatment of bronchoconstriction associated with asthma, bronchitis, and emphysema. Now it is considered a second-line agent that may be added in severe disease inadequately controlled by first-line drugs. Numerous dosage forms of theophylline are available. Theophylline ethylenediamine (aminophylline) contains approximately 85% theophylline and is the only formulation that can be given intravenously (IV). However, IV aminophylline is not recommended for emergency treatment of acute asthma because studies indicate little, if any, added benefit in adults or children. Oral theophylline preparations may be used for long-term treatment. Most formulations contain anhydrous theophylline (100% theophylline) as the active ingredient, and sustained-action tablets (e.g., Theochron) are more commonly used than other formulations. Theophylline is metabolized in the liver; metabolites and some unchanged drug are excreted through the kidneys.

 Applying Your Knowledge 44-1

How Can You Avoid This Medication Error?
Ms. Albright is having difficulty breathing and visits the on-site clinic. You assist her in the administration of her inhaled bronchodilator, the Advair.

Anti-Inflammatory Agents

Table 44-3 provides routes and dosage ranges of anti-inflammatory antiasthmatic drugs.

Corticosteroids

Corticosteroids (see Chap. 23) are used in the treatment of acute and chronic asthma and other bronchoconstrictive disorders. They suppress the release of inflammatory mediators, block the generations of cytokines, and decrease the recruitment of airway eosinophils. Beneficial effects of suppressing airway inflammation include decreased mucus secretion, decreased edema of airway mucosa, and repair of damaged epithelium, with subsequent reduction of airway reactivity. Corticosteroids increase the number and sensitivity of beta$_2$-adrenergic receptors, which restores or increases the effectiveness of beta$_2$-adrenergic bronchodilators. The number of beta$_2$ receptors increases within approximately 4 hours, and improved responsiveness to beta$_2$ agonists occurs within approximately 2 hours.

In acute, severe asthma, a systemic corticosteroid in relatively high doses is indicated in patients whose respiratory distress is not relieved by multiple doses of an inhaled beta$_2$ agonist (e.g., every 20 minutes for 3 to 4 doses). The corticosteroid may be given IV or orally, and IV administration offers no therapeutic advantage over oral administration. After the drug is started, pulmonary function usually improves in 6 to 8 hours. Most patients achieve substantial benefit within 48 to 72 hours and the drug is usually continued for 7 to 10 days. Multiple doses are usually given because studies indicate that maintaining the drug concentration at steroid receptor sites in the lung is more effective than high single doses. High single or pulse doses do not increase therapeutic effects; they may increase risks of developing myopathy and other adverse effects, however. In some infants and young children with acute, severe asthma, oral prednisone for 3 to 10 days has relieved symptoms and prevented hospitalization.

Corticosteroids are the most consistently effective long-term control medications for asthma. In chronic asthma, a corticosteroid is usually taken by inhalation, on a daily schedule. It is often given concomitantly with one or more bronchodilators and may be given with another anti-inflammatory drug such as a leukotriene modifier or a mast cell stabilizer. In some instances, the other drugs allow smaller doses of the corticosteroid. For acute flare-ups of symptoms during treatment of chronic asthma, a systemic corticosteroid may be needed temporarily to regain control.

In early stages of the progressive disease, patients with COPD are unlikely to need corticosteroid therapy. In later stages, however, they usually need periodic short-course therapy for episodes of respiratory distress. When needed, the corticosteroid is given orally or parenterally because effectiveness of inhaled corticosteroids has not been established in COPD (see Evidence-Based Practice Box 23-1: Efficacy of Corticosteroids on the Outcome in Patients With Acute Exacerbations of COPD).

In end-stage COPD, patients often become "steroid-dependent" and require daily doses because any attempt to reduce dosage or stop the drug results in respiratory distress. Such patients experience numerous serious adverse effects of prolonged systemic corticosteroid therapy.

Corticosteroids should be used with caution in patients with peptic ulcer disease, inflammatory bowel disease, hypertension, congestive heart failure, and thromboembolic disorders. However, they cause fewer and less severe adverse effects when taken in short courses or by inhalation than when taken systemically for long periods of time.

Beclomethasone, budesonide, flunisolide, fluticasone, mometasone, and **triamcinolone** are topical corticosteroids for inhalation. Most inhaled drugs are being reformulated (indicated with "HFA" secondary to the propellant being used). Topical administration minimizes systemic absorption and adverse effects. These preparations may substitute for or allow reduced dosage of systemic corticosteroids. In people with

Table 44-3 **Drugs at a Glance:** Anti-Inflammatory Antiasthmatic Drugs

Generic/Trade Name	ROUTES AND DOSAGE RANGES	
	Adults	**Children**
Corticosteroids		
Beclomethasone (QVAR)	Oral inhalation, two inhalations (0.84 mg/dose) three or four times daily; maximum, 20 inhalations/24 h	6–12 y: Oral inhalation, one or two inhalations three or four times per day; maximum dose, 10 inhalations/24 h
Beclomethasone (Beconase AQ)	1 spray in each nostril 2–4 times/day or 2 sprays in each nostril twice daily (total dose 168–336 mcg/day)	
Budesonide (Pulmocort Turbuhaler)	Oral inhalation, 200–400 mcg twice daily	6 y: Oral inhalation 200 mcg twice daily
Flunisolide (AeroBid, Aerospan-not inter changeable)	Aerobid: Oral inhalation, two inhalations (0.50 mg/dose) twice daily, morning and evening; maximum dose, four inhalations twice daily (2 mg) Aerospan: two inhalations twice daily; maximum eight inhalations daily	Aerobid: 6–15 y: Oral inhalation, two inhalations twice daily; maximum eight inhalation daily Aerospan: 6–11y: Oral inhalation: one inhalation twice daily; maximum four times daily
Fluticasone (Flonase)	4 sprays in each nostril once daily (265 mcg/day)	12 y and older: Same as adults 4–11 y: 1 spray in each nostril once daily; may increase to 2 sprays in each nostril for desired effect
Fluticasone aerosol (Flovent)	Aerosol, 88–440 mcg twice daily	Dosage not established
Fluticasone powder (Flovent Rotadisk)	Powder, 100–500 mcg twice daily	12 y and older: Same as adults 4–11 y: Powder, 50–100 mcg twice daily
Hydrocortisone sodium phosphate and sodium succinate	IV 100–200 mg q4–6h initially, then decreased or switched to an oral dosage form	IV 1–5 mg/kg q4–6h
Methylprednisolone sodium succinate	IV 10–40 mg q4–6h for 48–72 h	IV 0.5 mg/kg q4–6h
Mometasone (Asmanex Twisthaler, Nasonex)	Nasal inhalation two sprays (50 mcg/spray) in each nostril once daily	12 y and older: Same as adults 2–11 y: 1 spray (50 mcg) in each nostril once daily
Prednisone	PO 20–60 mg/d	PO 2 mg/kg/d initially
Triamcinolone (Azmacort)	Oral inhalation, two (100 mcg/puff) inhalations 3 or 4 times per day or four inhalations twice daily; maximum dose, 16 inhalations (1600 mcg)/24 h	6–12 y: one or two (100 mcg/puff) inhalations 3 or 4 times per day or two to four inhalations twice daily; maximum dose, 12 inhalations/24 h
Leukotriene Modifiers		
Montelukast (Singulair)	PO 10 mg once daily in the evening or at bedtime	15 y and older: Same as adults 6–14 y: PO 5 mg once daily in the evening 2–5 y: 4 mg once daily
Zafirlukast (Accolate)	PO 20 mg twice daily, 1 h before or 2 h after a meal	12 y and older: Same as adults 5–11 y: PO 10 mg twice daily
Mast Cell Stabilizers		
Cromolyn (Intal)	Nebulizer solution, oral inhalation, 20 mg 4 times daily Aerosol spray, oral inhalation, two sprays 4 times daily	2 y and older: Same as adults 5 y and older: Same as adults

asthma who are taking an oral corticosteroid, the oral dosage is reduced slowly (over weeks to months) when an inhaled corticosteroid is added. The goal is to give the lowest oral dose necessary to control symptoms. Beclomethasone, flunisolide, and fluticasone also are available in nasal solutions for treatment of allergic rhinitis, which may play a role in bronchoconstriction. Because systemic absorption occurs in patients using inhaled corticosteroids (about 20% of a dose), high doses should be reserved for those otherwise requiring oral corticosteroids.

Hydrocortisone, prednisone, and **methylprednisolone** are given to patients who require systemic corticosteroids. Prednisone is given orally; hydrocortisone and methylprednisolone may be given IV to patients who are unable to take an oral medication.

Applying Your Knowledge 44-2

Ms. Albright has a friend who takes prednisone for his breathing problems. She asks why she isn't taking the same medication. How should you respond?

Leukotriene Modifiers

Leukotrienes are strong chemical mediators of bronchoconstriction and inflammation, the major pathologic features of asthma. They can cause sustained constriction of bronchioles and immediate hypersensitivity reactions. They also increase mucus secretion and mucosal edema in the respiratory tract. Leukotrienes are formed by the lipoxygenase pathway of arachidonic acid metabolism (Fig. 44-1) in response to cellular injury. They are designated by LT; the letter B, C, D, or E; and the number of chemical bonds in their structure (e.g., LTB4, LTC4, and LTE4, also called slow releasing substances of anaphylaxis, or SRS-A, because they are released more slowly than histamine).

Leukotriene modifier drugs were developed to counteract the effects of leukotrienes and are indicated for long-term treatment of asthma in adults and children. The drugs help to prevent acute asthma attacks induced by allergens, exercise, cold air, hyperventilation, irritants, and aspirin or NSAIDs. They are not effective in relieving acute attacks. However, they may be continued concurrently with other drugs during acute episodes.

The leukotriene modifiers include two agents, **montelukast** and **zafirlukast,** classed as leukotriene receptor antagonists. Zafirlukast and montelukast improve symptoms and pulmonary function tests (PFTs), decrease nighttime symptoms, and decrease the use of beta$_2$ agonist drugs. They are effective with oral administration, can be taken once or twice a day, can be used with bronchodilators and corticosteroids, and elicit a high degree of patient adherence and satisfaction.

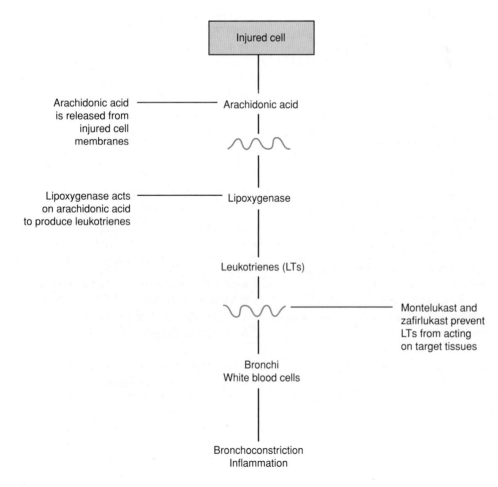

Figure 44-1 ■ Formation of leukotrienes and actions of leukotriene-modifying drugs.

However, they are less effective than low doses of inhaled corticosteroids.

Montelukast and zafirlukast are well absorbed with oral administration. They are metabolized in the liver by the cytochrome P450 enzyme system and may interact with other drugs metabolized by this system. Most metabolites are excreted in the feces. Zafirlukast is excreted in breast milk and should not be taken during lactation. The most common adverse effects reported in clinical trials were headache, nausea, diarrhea, and infection.

Mast Cell Stabilizers

Cromolyn and **nedocromil** stabilize mast cells and prevent the release of bronchoconstrictive and inflammatory substances when mast cells are confronted with allergens and other stimuli. The drugs are utilized as an alternative, but not preferred, medication for prophylaxis of acute asthma attacks in patients with of mild persistent asthma; they are not effective in acute bronchospasm or status asthmaticus and should not be used in these conditions. Use of one of these drugs may allow reduced dosage of bronchodilators and corticosteroids and can be used prior to exercise or exposure to known allergens.

The drugs are taken by inhalation. Cromolyn is available in a metered-dose aerosol and a solution for use with a power-operated nebulizer. A nasal solution is also available for prevention and treatment of allergic rhinitis.

Mast cell stabilizers are contraindicated in patients who are hypersensitive to the drugs. They should be used with caution in patients with impaired renal or hepatic function. Also, the propellants in the aerosols may aggravate coronary artery disease or dysrhythmias.

Immunosuppressant Monoclonal Antibody

Omalizumab (Xolair) works by binding to immunoglobulin E (IgE), blocking receptors on the surfaces of mast cells and basophils. This prevents IgE from attaching to the cells, thus preventing the release of substances in the body that can trigger an allergic reaction and preventing the development of inflammation. As an immunomodifier, omalizumab is indicated as adjunctive therapy in patients with allergic asthma whose symptoms do not respond adequately to inhaled steroids. Due to the risk of anaphylaxis the FDA has issued a **BLACK BOX WARNING** for omalizumab. The drug should only be administered to patients in a health care setting under direct medical supervision by provider who can initiate treatment of life-threatening anaphylaxis. Further discussion of this drug is found in Chapter 41.

Herbal and Dietary Supplements

Numerous preparations are promoted to relieve symptoms of asthma, and patients with asthma are increasingly using alternative and complementary therapies. Many herbal preparations are used traditionally, and tradition varies by culture. As with most herbal treatments, few clinical studies support their use though some herbs used are similar to asthma preparations in their chemical properties. For example, caffeine is a xanthine and therefore has bronchodilating effects similar to, but weaker than, those of theophylline. In addition to herbal preparations for the long-term treatment of asthma, vitamins and minerals are used frequently (i.e., vitamins C, B_6, E, and magnesium, selenium).

In general, herbal and dietary therapies in asthma, as in other disorders, have not been studied in controlled clinical trials and should be avoided. Because asthma can result in death in a matter of minutes, patients should be counseled *not* to use dietary or herbal supplements in place of prescribed bronchodilating and anti-inflammatory medications. Delays in appropriate treatment can have serious, even fatal, consequences.

Applying Your Knowledge 44-3

Ms. Albright comes into the clinic and you suspect she is experiencing respiratory distress. You focus your assessment on what signs/symptoms?

Nursing Process

Assessment

Assess the patient's pulmonary function.

■ General assessment factors include rate and character of respiration, skin color, arterial blood gas analysis, and pulmonary function tests. Abnormal breathing patterns (e.g., rate below 12 or above 24 per minute, dyspnea, cough, orthopnea, wheezing, "noisy" respirations) may indicate respiratory distress. Severe respiratory distress is characterized by tachypnea, dyspnea, use of accessory muscles of respiration, and hypoxia. Early signs of hypoxia include mental confusion, restlessness, anxiety, and increased blood pressure and pulse rate. Late signs include cyanosis and decreased blood pressure and pulse. Hypoxemia is confirmed if arterial blood gas analysis shows decreased partial pressure of oxygen (PO_2).

■ In acute bronchospasm, a medical emergency, the patient is in obvious and severe respiratory distress. A characteristic feature of bronchospasm is forceful expiration or wheezing.

■ If the patient has chronic asthma, try to determine the frequency and severity of acute attacks; factors that precipitate or relieve acute attacks; antiasthmatic medications taken occasionally or regularly; allergies; and condition between acute attacks, such as restrictions in activities of daily living due to asthma.

Nursing Process continues on page 722

- If the patient has chronic bronchitis or emphysema, assess for signs of respiratory distress, hypoxia, cough, amount and character of sputum, exercise tolerance (e.g., dyspnea on exertion, dyspnea at rest), medications, and nondrug treatment measures (e.g., breathing exercises, chest physiotherapy).

Nursing Diagnoses

- Impaired Gas Exchange related to bronchoconstriction and excessive mucus production
- Activity Intolerance related to impaired gas exchange and fatigue
- Risk for Injury: Severe bronchospasm with asthma and adverse effects with antiasthmatic drugs
- Noncompliance: Overuse of adrenergic bronchodilators
- Deficient Knowledge: Factors precipitating bronchoconstriction and strategies to avoid precipitating factors
- Deficient Knowledge: Accurate self-administration of drugs, including use of inhalers

Planning/Goals

The patient will

- Self-administer bronchodilating and other drugs accurately
- Experience relief of symptoms
- Avoid preventable adverse drug effects
- Avoid overusing bronchodilating drugs
- Avoid exposure to stimuli that cause bronchospasm when possible
- Avoid respiratory infections when possible

Interventions

Use measures to prevent or relieve bronchoconstriction when possible. General measures include those to prevent respiratory disease or promote an adequate airway. A specific monitoring plan should be in place, whether peak-flow or symptom monitoring. Some measures include the following:

- Use mechanical measures for removing excessive respiratory tract secretions and preventing their retention. Effective measures include coughing, deep breathing, percussion, and postural drainage.
- Help the patient identify and avoid exposure to conditions that precipitate bronchoconstriction. For example, allergens may be removed from the home, school, or work environment; cigarette smoke should be avoided when possible. When bronchospasm is precipitated by exercise, prophylaxis by prior inhalation of bronchodilating agents is better than avoiding exercise, especially in children.
- Assist patients with asthma to identify early signs of difficulty, including increased need for beta-adrenergic agonists, activity limitations, and waking at night with asthma symptoms.

- Monitor peak expiratory flow rate (PEFR) when indicated. Portable meters are available for use in clinics, physicians' offices, and patients' homes. This is an objective measure of airflow/airway obstruction and helps to evaluate the patient's treatment regimen.
- Assist patients with moderate to severe asthma in obtaining meters and learning to measure PEFR. Patients with a decreased PEFR may need treatment to prevent acute, severe respiratory distress.
- Assist patients and at least one family member in managing acute attacks of bronchoconstriction, including when to seek emergency care.
- Try to prevent or reduce anxiety, which may aggravate bronchospasm. Stay with the patient during an acute asthma attack if feasible. Patients experiencing severe and prolonged bronchospasm (status asthmaticus) should be admitted or transferred to a hospital intensive care unit.
- With any patients who smoke cigarettes, encourage cessation of smoking and provide information, resources, and assistance in doing so. Emphasize the health benefits of improved respiratory function.
- In addition, provide appropriate patient teaching related to drug therapy (see accompanying display).

Evaluation

- Observe for relief of symptoms and improved arterial blood gas values.
- Interview and observe for correct drug administration, including use of inhalers.
- Interview and observe for tachydysrhythmias, nervousness, insomnia, and other adverse drug effects.
- Interview about and observe behaviors to avoid stimuli that cause bronchoconstriction and respiratory infections.

Principles of Therapy

Drug Selection and Administration

Choice of drug and route of administration are determined largely by the severity of the disease process and the patient's response to therapy. Some guidelines include the following:

- A selective, short-acting, inhaled beta$_2$-adrenergic agonist (e.g., albuterol) is the initial drug of choice for acute bronchospasm.
- Because aerosol products act directly on the airways, drugs given by inhalation can usually be given in smaller doses and produce fewer adverse effects than oral or parenteral drugs.
- Ipratropium and tiotropium, the anticholinergic bronchodilators, are most useful in the long-term management of COPD. They are ineffective in relieving acute

Patient Teaching Guidelines | Antiasthmatic Drugs

General Considerations

▪ Asthma and other chronic lung diseases are characterized by constant inflammation of the airways and periodic or persistent labored breathing from constriction or narrowing of the airways. Antiasthmatic drugs are often given in combination to combat these problems. Thus, it is extremely important to know the type and purpose of each drug.

▪ Except for the short-acting, inhaled bronchodilators (e.g., albuterol), antiasthmatic medications are used long term to control symptoms and prevent acute asthma attacks. This means they must be taken on a regular schedule and continued when symptom free.

▪ When an asthma attack (i.e., acute bronchospasm with shortness of breath, wheezing respirations, cough) occurs, the only fast-acting, commonly used medication to relieve these symptoms is an inhaled, short-acting bronchodilator (e.g., albuterol). Other inhaled and oral drugs are not effective and should not be used.

▪ Try to prevent symptoms. For example, respiratory infections can precipitate difficulty in breathing. Avoiding infections (e.g., by good hand hygiene, avoiding people with infections, annual influenza vaccinations, and other measures) can prevent acute asthma attacks. If you are allergic to tobacco smoke, perfume, or flowers, try to avoid or minimize exposure.

▪ A common cause of acute asthma attacks is not taking medications correctly. Some studies indicate that one third to two thirds of patients with asthma do not comply with instructions for using their medications. Factors that contribute to noncompliance with drug therapy include long-term use, expense, and adverse effects. If you have difficulty taking medications as prescribed, discuss the situation with a health care provider. Cheaper medications or lower doses may be effective alternatives. Just stopping the medications may precipitate acute breathing problems.

▪ If unable to prevent symptoms, early recognition and treatment may help prevent severe distress and hospitalizations. Signs of impending difficulty include increased needs for bronchodilator inhalers, activity limitations, waking at night because of asthma symptoms, and variability in the peak expiratory flow rate (PEFR), if you use a PEFR meter at home. The first treatment is to use a short-acting, inhaled bronchodilator. If this does not improve breathing, seek emergency care.

▪ Keep adequate supplies of medications on hand. Missing a few doses of long-term control or "preventive" medications may precipitate an acute asthma attack; not using an inhaled bronchodilator for early breathing difficulty may lead to more severe problems and the need for emergency treatment or hospitalization.

▪ Be sure you can use your metered-dose inhalers correctly. According to several research studies, many patients do not.

▪ Drinking 2 to 3 quarts of fluids daily helps thin secretions in the throat and lungs and makes them easier to remove.

▪ Avoid tobacco smoke and other substances that irritate breathing passages (e.g., aerosol hair spray, antiperspirants, cleaning products, and automobile exhaust) when possible.

▪ Avoid excessive intake of caffeine-containing fluids such as coffee, tea, and cola drinks. These beverages may increase bronchodilation but also may increase heart rate and cause palpitations, nervousness, and insomnia with bronchodilating drugs.

▪ Take influenza vaccine annually and pneumococcal vaccine at least once if you have chronic lung disease.

▪ Inform all health care providers about the medications you are taking and do not take over-the-counter drugs or herbal supplements without consulting a health care provider. Some drugs can decrease beneficial effects or increase adverse effects of antiasthmatic medications. For example, over-the-counter nasal decongestants, asthma remedies, cold remedies, and antisleep medications can increase the rapid heartbeat, palpitations, and nervousness often associated with bronchodilators. With herbal remedies, none are as effective as standard antiasthmatic medication, and they may cause serious or life-threatening adverse effects.

Self-Administration

▪ Follow instructions carefully. Better breathing with minimal adverse effects depends on accurate use of prescribed medications. If help is needed with metered-dose inhalers, consult a health care provider.

▪ Use short-acting bronchodilator inhalers as needed, not on a regular schedule. If desired effects are not achieved or if symptoms worsen, inform the prescribing physician. Do not increase dosage or frequency of taking medication. Overuse increases adverse drug effects and decreases drug effectiveness.

▪ If taking formoterol or salmeterol, which are long-acting, inhaled bronchodilators, do not use more often than every 12 hours. If constricted breathing occurs, use a short-acting bronchodilator inhaler between doses of a long-acting drug. Salmeterol does not relieve acute shortness of breath because it takes approximately 20 minutes to start acting and 1 to 4 hours to achieve maximal bronchodilating effects.

▪ If taking an oral or inhaled corticosteroid, take on a regular schedule, at approximately the same time each day. The purpose of these drugs is to relieve inflammation in the airways and prevent acute respiratory distress. They are not effective unless taken regularly.

▪ If taking oral theophylline, take fast-acting preparations before meals with a full glass of water, at regular intervals around the clock. If gastrointestinal upset occurs, take with food. Take long-acting preparations every 8 to 12 hours; do not chew or crush.

▪ Take zafirlukast 1 hour before or 2 hours after a meal; montelukast and zileuton may be taken with or without food. Take montelukast in the evening or at bedtime. This schedule provides maximum beneficial effects during the night and early morning, when asthma symptoms often occur or worsen.

▪ Use inhalers correctly:
  1. Shake well immediately before each use.
  2. Remove the cap from the mouthpiece.
  3. Exhale to the end of a normal breath.
  4. With the inhaler in the upright position, place the mouthpiece just inside the mouth, and use the lips to

(continued on page 724)

form a tight seal or hold the mouthpiece approximately two finger-widths from the open mouth.

5. While pressing down on the inhaler, take a slow, deep breath for 3 to 5 seconds, hold the breath for approximately 10 seconds, and exhale slowly.

6. Wait 3 to 5 minutes before taking a second inhalation of the drug.

7. Rinse the mouth with water after each use.

8. Rinse the mouthpiece and store the inhaler away from heat.

9. If you have difficulty using an inhaler, ask your provider about a spacer device (a tube attached to the inhaler that makes it easier to use).

---

bronchospasm by themselves, but they add to the bronchodilating effects of adrenergic drugs.

- Theophylline is used less often than formerly and is now considered a second-line drug. When used, it is usually given orally in an extended-release formulation for chronic disorders, such as COPD. IV aminophylline is no longer used to treat acute asthma attacks.

- Cromolyn is used prophylactically; it is ineffective in acute bronchospasm.

- Because inflammation has been established as a major component of asthma, an inhaled corticosteroid is being used early in the disease process, often with a bronchodilator or mast cell stabilizer. In acute episodes of bronchoconstriction, a corticosteroid is often given orally or IV for several days.

- In chronic disorders, inhaled corticosteroids should be taken on a regular schedule. These drugs may be effective when used alone or with relatively small doses of an oral corticosteroid. Optimal schedules of administration are not clearly established, but more frequent dosing (e.g., every 6 hours) may be more effective than less frequent dosing (e.g., every 12 hours), even if the total amount is the same. As with systemic glucocorticoid therapy, the recommended inhaled corticosteroid dose is the lowest amount required to control symptoms. High doses suppress adrenocortical function but much less so than systemic drugs. Small doses may impair bone metabolism and predispose adults to osteoporosis by decreasing calcium deposition and increasing calcium resorption from bone. In children, chronic administration of corticosteroids may retard growth. Local adverse effects (oropharyngeal candidiasis, hoarseness) can be decreased by reducing the dose, administering less often, rinsing the mouth after use, or using a spacer device. These measures decrease the amount of drug deposited in the oral cavity. The inhaled drugs are well tolerated with chronic use.

- A common regimen for treatment of moderate asthma is an inhaled corticosteroid on a regular schedule, two to four times daily, and a short-acting, inhaled beta$_2$-adrenergic agonist as needed for prevention or treatment of bronchoconstriction. For more severe asthma, an inhaled corticosteroid is continued, and both a short-acting and a long-acting beta$_2$ agonist may be given. A leukotriene modifier may also be added to the regimen to further control symptoms and reduce the need for corticosteroids and inhaled bronchodilators.

- Multidrug regimens are commonly used, and one advantage is that smaller doses of each agent can usually be given. This may decrease adverse effects and allow dosages to be increased when exacerbation of symptoms occurs. Available combination inhalation products include Combivent (albuterol and ipratropium) and Advair (salmeterol and fluticasone). Advair, which was developed to treat both inflammation and bronchoconstriction, was more effective than the individual components at the same doses and as effective as concurrent use of the same drugs at the same doses. In addition, the combination reduced the corticosteroid dose by 50% and was more effective than higher doses of fluticasone alone in reducing asthma exacerbations. The combination improved symptoms within 1 week. Additional combination products are likely to be marketed and may improve patient compliance with prescribed drug therapy.

Drug Dosage

Dosage of antiasthmatic drugs must be individualized to attain the most therapeutic effects and the fewest adverse effects. Larger doses of bronchodilators and corticosteroids (inhaled, systemic, or both) are usually required to relieve the symptoms of acute, severe bronchoconstriction or status asthmaticus. Then, doses should be reduced to the smallest effective amounts for long-term control.

Dosage of theophylline preparations should be based mainly on serum theophylline levels (therapeutic range is 5–15 mcg/mL; toxic levels are 20 mcg/mL or above). Blood for serum levels should be drawn 1 to 2 hours after immediate-release dosage forms and about 4 hours after sustained-release forms are taken. In addition, children and cigarette smokers usually need higher doses to maintain therapeutic blood levels because they metabolize theophylline rapidly, and patients with liver disease, congestive heart failure, chronic pulmonary disease, or acute viral infections usually need smaller doses because these conditions impair theophylline metabolism. For obese patients, theophylline dosage should be calculated on the basis of lean or ideal body weight because theophylline is not highly distributed in fatty tissue.

Toxicity: Recognition and Management

With antiasthmatic drugs, signs and symptoms of overdose and toxicity are probably most likely to occur when patients with acute or chronic bronchoconstrictive disorders overuse bronchodilators in their efforts to relieve dyspnea. General management of acute poisoning includes early recognition of signs and symptoms, stopping the causative drug, and instituting other treatment measures as indicated. Specific measures include the following:

▪ **Bronchodilator overdose.** With inhaled or systemic adrenergic bronchodilators, major adverse effects are excessive cardiac and CNS stimulation. Symptoms of cardiac stimulation include angina, tachycardia, and palpitations; serious dysrhythmias and cardiac arrest have also been reported. Symptoms of CNS stimulation include agitation, anxiety, insomnia, seizures, and tremors. Severe overdoses may cause delirium, collapse, and coma. In addition, hypokalemia, hyperglycemia, and hypotension or hypertension may occur. Management includes discontinuing the causative medications and using general supportive measures. Emesis, gastric lavage, or activated charcoal may be useful with oral drugs if benefit exceeds risk. For cardiac symptoms, monitor blood pressure, pulse, and electrocardiogram. Cautious use of a beta-adrenergic blocking drug (e.g., propranolol) may be indicated. However, a nonselective beta blocker may induce bronchoconstriction.

▪ **Theophylline overdose.** Signs and symptoms include anorexia, nausea, vomiting, agitation, nervousness, insomnia, tachycardia and other dysrhythmias, and tonic-clonic convulsions. Ventricular dysrhythmias or convulsions may be the first sign of toxicity. Serious adverse effects rarely occur at serum drug levels below 20 micrograms per milliliter. Overdoses with sustained-release preparations may cause a dramatic increase in serum drug concentrations much later (12 hours or longer) than the immediate-release preparations. Early treatment helps but does not prevent these delayed increases in serum drug levels.

In patients without seizures, induce vomiting unless the level of consciousness is impaired. In these patients, precautions to prevent aspiration are needed, especially in children. If overdose is identified within an hour of drug ingestion, gastric lavage may be helpful if unable to induce vomiting or vomiting is contraindicated. Administration of activated charcoal and a cathartic is also recommended, especially for overdoses of sustained-release formulations if benefit exceeds risk.

In patients with seizures, treatment includes securing the airway, giving oxygen, injecting IV diazepam (0.1–0.3 mg/kg, up to 10 mg), monitoring vital signs, maintaining blood pressure, providing adequate hydration, and monitoring serum theophylline levels until below 20 micrograms per milliliter. Also, symptomatic treatment of dysrhythmias may be needed.

▪ **Leukotriene modifiers and mast cell stabilizers.** These drugs seem relatively devoid of serious toxicity. There have been few reports of toxicity in humans and little clinical experience in managing it. If toxicity occurs, general supportive and symptomatic treatment is indicated.

Use in Special Populations

Use in Children

The American Academy of Pediatrics endorses the clinical practice guidelines established by the NAEPP (see Box 44-1). In general, antiasthmatic medications are used in children and adolescents for the same indications as for adults. With adrenergic bronchodilators, recommendations for use vary according to route of administration, age of the child, and specific drug formulations. However, even infants and young children can be treated effectively with aerosolized or nebulized drugs. In addition, some oral drugs can be given to children as young as 2 years and most can be given to children 6 to 12 years of age.

With theophylline, use in children should be closely monitored because dosage needs and rates of metabolism vary widely. In children younger than 6 months, especially premature infants and neonates, drug elimination may be prolonged because of immature liver function. Except for preterm infants with apnea, theophylline preparations are not recommended for use in this age group. Children 6 months to 16 years of age, approximately, metabolize theophylline more rapidly than younger or older patients. Thus, they may need higher doses than adults in proportion to size and weight. If the child is obese, the dosage should be calculated on the basis of lean or ideal body weight because the drug is not highly distributed in fatty tissue. Long-acting dosage forms are not recommended for children younger than 6 years of age. Children may become hyperactive and disruptive from the CNS-stimulating effects of theophylline. Tolerance to these effects usually develops with continued use of the drug.

Corticosteroids are being used earlier in children as in adults and inhaled corticosteroids are first-line drugs for treatment of persistent bronchoconstrictive disorders. The effectiveness and safety of inhaled corticosteroids in children older than 3 years of age is well established; few data are available on the use of inhaled drugs in those younger than 3 years. Major concerns about long-term use in children include decreased adrenal function, growth, and bone mass. Most corticosteroids are given by inhalation, and dosage, type of inhaler device, and characteristics of individual drugs influence the extent and severity of these systemic effects.

Adrenal insufficiency is most likely to occur with systemic or high doses of inhaled corticosteroids. Dose-related inhibition of growth has been reported in short and intermediate studies, but long-term studies have found few, if any, decreases in expected adult height. Inhaled corticosteroids have not been associated with significant decreases in bone mass, but more studies of high doses and of drug therapy in adolescents are needed. Bone growth should be monitored closely in children taking corticosteroids. Although inhaled corticosteroids are the most effective anti-inflammatory medications available for asthma, high doses in children are still of concern. The risk of high doses is especially great in children with other allergic conditions that require topical corticosteroid drugs. The risk can be decreased by using the lowest effective dose, administration techniques that minimize swallowed drug, and other antiasthmatic drugs to reduce corticosteroid dose.

Leukotriene modifiers have not been extensively studied in children and adolescents. With montelukast, the 10-milligram film-coated tablet is recommended for adolescents 15 years of age and older and a 4-milligram chewable tablet is recommended for children 2 to 5 years of age. Safety and effectiveness of zafirlukast in children younger than 12 years have not been established.

Cromolyn aerosol solution may be used in children 5 years of age and older, and nebulizer solution is used with children 2 years and older.

Use in Older Adults

Older adults often have chronic pulmonary disorders for which bronchodilators and antiasthmatic medications are used. As with other populations, administering the medications by inhalation and giving the lowest effective dose decrease adverse effects. The main risks with adrenergic bronchodilators are excessive cardiac and CNS stimulation.

Theophylline use must be carefully monitored because drug effects are unpredictable. On the one hand, cigarette smoking and drugs that stimulate drug-metabolizing enzymes in the liver (e.g., phenobarbital, phenytoin) increase the rate of metabolism and therefore dosage requirements. On the other hand, impaired liver function, decreased blood flow to the liver, and some drugs (e.g., cimetidine, erythromycin) impair metabolism and therefore decrease dosage requirements. Adverse effects include cardiac and CNS stimulation. Safety can be increased by measuring serum drug levels and adjusting dosage to maintain therapeutic levels of 5 to 15 micrograms per milliliter. If the patient is obese, dosage should be based on lean or ideal body weight because theophylline is not highly distributed in fatty tissue.

Corticosteroids increase the risks of osteoporosis and cataracts in older adults. Leukotriene modifiers usually are well tolerated by older adults, with pharmacokinetics and effects similar to those in younger adults. With zafirlukast, however, blood levels are higher and elimination is slower than in younger adults.

Use in Patients With Renal Impairment

Bronchodilating and anti-inflammatory drugs can usually be given without dosage adjustments in patients with impaired renal function. Beta agonists may be given by inhalation or parenteral routes. Theophylline can be given in usual doses, but serum drug levels should be monitored. Most corticosteroids are eliminated by hepatic metabolism, and dosage reductions are not needed in patients with renal impairment. No data are available about the use of montelukast, and no dosage adjustments are recommended for zafirlukast.

Cromolyn is eliminated by renal and biliary excretion; the drug should be given in reduced doses, if at all, in patients with renal impairment.

Use in Patients With Hepatic Impairment

Montelukast and zafirlukast produce higher blood levels and are eliminated more slowly in patients with hepatic impairment. However, no dosage adjustment is recommended for patients with mild to moderate hepatic impairment.

Cromolyn is eliminated by renal and biliary excretion; the drug should be given in reduced doses, if at all, in patients with hepatic impairment.

Use in Patients With Critical Illness

Acute, severe asthma (status asthmaticus) is characterized by severe respiratory distress and requires emergency treatment. Beta$_2$ agonists should be given in high doses and as often as every 20 minutes for 1 to 2 hours (by MDIs with spacer devices or by compressed-air nebulization). However, high doses of nebulized albuterol have been associated with tachycardia, hypokalemia, and hyperglycemia. After symptoms are controlled, dosage can usually be reduced and dosing intervals extended. High doses of systemic corticosteroids are also given for several days, IV or orally. If the patient is able to take an oral drug, there is no therapeutic advantage to IV administration.

When respiratory function improves, efforts to prevent future episodes are needed. These efforts may include identifying and avoiding suspected triggers, evaluation and possible adjustment of the patient's treatment regimen, and assessment of the patient's adherence to the prescribed regimen.

Use in Home Care

Most of the drugs discussed in this chapter are used in the home setting; omalizumab should be administered only in the health care setting due to the risk of life-threatening anaphylaxis with administration. A major role of the home care nurse is to assist patients in using the drugs safely and effectively. Several studies have indicated that many people do not use MDIs and other inhalation devices correctly. The home care nurse needs to observe a patient using an inhalation device when possible. If errors in technique are assessed, further education may be needed. With inhaled medications, a spacer device may be useful, especially for children and older adults, because less muscle coordination is required to administer a dose. Adverse effects may be minimized as well.

For patients with asthma, especially children, assess the environment for potential triggers of acute bronchospasm, such as cigarette smoking. In addition, assist patients to recognize and treat (or get help for) exacerbations before respiratory distress becomes severe.

With theophylline, the home care nurse needs to assess the patient and the environment for substances that may affect metabolism of theophylline and decrease therapeutic effects or increase adverse effects. In addition, the nurse needs to reinforce the importance of not exceeding the prescribed dose, not crushing long-acting formulations, reporting adverse effects, and keeping appointments for follow-up care.

Nursing Actions — Drugs for Asthma and Other Bronchoconstrictive Disorders

NURSING ACTIONS	RATIONALE/EXPLANATION
1. Administer accurately	
a. Be sure patients have adequate supplies of inhaled bronchodilators and corticosteroids available for self-administration. Observe technique of self-administration for accuracy and assist if needed.	
b. Give immediate-release oral theophylline before meals with a full glass of water, at regular intervals around the clock. If gastrointestinal upset occurs, give with food.	To promote dissolution and absorption. Taking with food may decrease nausea and vomiting.
c. Give sustained-release theophylline q8–12h, with instructions not to chew or crush.	Sustained-release drug formulations should never be chewed or crushed because doing so causes immediate release of potentially toxic doses.
d. Give zafirlukast 1 hour before or 2 hours after a meal; montelukast may be given with or without food.	The bioavailability of zafirlukast is reduced approximately 40% if taken with food. Food does not significantly affect the bioavailability of montelukast.
e. Give montelukast in the evening or at bedtime.	This schedule provides high drug concentrations during the night and early morning, when asthma symptoms tend to occur or worsen.
2. Observe for therapeutic effects	
a. Decreased dyspnea, wheezing, and respiratory secretions	Relief of bronchospasm and wheezing should be evident within a few minutes after giving subcutaneous epinephrine, or aerosolized adrenergic bronchodilators.
b. Reduced rate and improved quality of respirations	
c. Reduced anxiety and restlessness	
d. Therapeutic serum levels of theophylline (5–15 mcg/mL)	
e. Improved arterial blood gas levels (normal values: PO_2, 80 to 100 mm Hg; PCO_2, 35 to 45 mm Hg; pH, 7.35 to 7.45)	
f. Improved exercise tolerance	
g. Decreased incidence and severity of acute attacks of bronchospasm with chronic administration of drugs	
3. Observe for adverse effects	
a. With adrenergic bronchodilators, observe for tachycardia, dysrhythmias, palpitations, restlessness, agitation, insomnia.	These signs and symptoms result from cardiac and central nervous system (CNS) stimulation.
b. With ipratropium and tiotropium, observe for cough or exacerbation of symptoms.	Ipratropium and tiotropium produce few adverse effects because they are not absorbed systemically.
c. With xanthine bronchodilators, observe for tachycardia, dysrhythmias, palpitations, restlessness, agitation, insomnia, nausea, vomiting, convulsions.	Theophylline causes cardiac and CNS stimulation. Convulsions occur at toxic serum concentrations (>20 mcg/mL). They may occur without preceding symptoms of toxicity and may result in death. IV diazepam (Valium) may be used to control seizures. Theophylline also stimulates the chemoreceptor trigger zone in the medulla oblongata to cause nausea and vomiting.
d. With inhaled corticosteroids, observe for hoarseness, cough, throat irritation, and fungal infection of mouth and throat.	Inhaled corticosteroids are unlikely to produce the serious adverse effects of long-term systemic therapy (see Chap. 23).
e. With cromolyn, observe for dysrhythmias, hypotension, chest pain, restlessness, dizziness, convulsions, CNS depression, anorexia, nausea and vomiting. Sedation and coma may occur with overdosage.	Some of the cardiovascular effects are thought to be caused by the propellants used in the aerosol preparation.
4. Observe for drug interactions	
a. Drugs that *increase* effects of bronchodilators:	
(1) Monoamine oxidase inhibitors	These drugs inhibit the metabolism of catecholamines. The subsequent administration of bronchodilators may increase blood pressure.
(2) Erythromycin, clindamycin, cimetidine	These drugs may decrease theophylline clearance and thereby increase plasma levels.

(continued on page 728)

Nursing Actions — Drugs for Asthma and Other Bronchoconstrictive Disorders (continued)

NURSING ACTIONS	RATIONALE/EXPLANATION
b. Drugs that *decrease* effects of bronchodilators:	
(1) Lithium	Lithium may increase excretion of theophylline and therefore decrease therapeutic effectiveness.
(2) Phenobarbital	This drug may increase the metabolism of theophylline by way of enzyme induction.
(3) Propranolol, other nonselective beta blockers	These drugs may cause bronchoconstriction and oppose effects of bronchodilators.
c. Drugs that alter effects of zafirlukast:	
(1) Aspirin	Increases blood levels
(2) Erythromycin, theophylline	Decrease blood levels

Key Concepts

■ A specific monitoring plan for patients with asthma should be in place, whether through peak-flow or symptom monitoring.

■ Two general classifications of drugs are used for asthma management: long-term control medications to achieve and maintain control of persistent asthma and quick relief medications used during periods of acute symptoms and exacerbations.

■ Two major groups of drugs used to treat asthma, acute and chronic bronchitis, and emphysema are bronchodilators and anti-inflammatory drugs.

■ A selective, short-acting, inhaled beta$_2$-adrenergic agonist (e.g., albuterol) is the initial rescue drug of choice for acute bronchospasm; subcutaneous epinephrine may also be considered.

■ Because aerosol products act directly on the airways, drugs given by inhalation can usually be given in smaller doses and produce fewer adverse effects than oral or parenteral drugs.

■ Asthma may aggravate GERD, because antiasthma medications that dilate the airways also relax muscle tone in the gastroesophageal sphincter and may increase acid reflux.

■ Almost all over-the-counter aerosol products promoted for use in asthma contain epinephrine, which may produce hazardous cardiac stimulation and other adverse effects.

■ Cigarette smoking and drugs that stimulate drug-metabolizing enzymes in the liver (e.g., phenobarbital, phenytoin) increase the rate of metabolism and therefore dosage requirements of aminophylline.

■ Due to the risk of anaphylaxis the FDA has issued a **BLACK BOX WARNING** for omalizumab.

■ The FDA has issued a **BLACK BOX WARNING** that initiating salmeterol in individuals with significantly worsening or acutely deteriorating asthma may be life-threatening.

Review and Application Exercises

Short Answer Exercises

1. What are some causes of bronchoconstriction, and how can they be prevented or minimized?

2. How do beta-adrenergic agonists act as bronchodilators?

3. What adverse effects are associated with bronchodilators, and how can they be prevented or minimized?

4. For what effects are corticosteroids used in the treatment of bronchoconstrictive respiratory disorders?

5. How does cromolyn act to prevent acute asthma attacks?

6. What are the main elements of treating respiratory distress from acute bronchospasm?

NCLEX-Style Questions

7. The nurse notes that a patient's serum theophylline level is 25 mcg/mL and that a scheduled dose of the medication is due. The nurse should
   a. Hold the scheduled dose, contact the health care provider, and assess the patient for signs of theophylline toxicity.
   b. Administer the dose as scheduled.
   c. Administer only half of the dose and repeat the theophylline level in 4 hours.
   d. Hold the dose until the next meal and administer at that time.

8. A patient, taking a short-acting inhaled bronchodilator and a steroid inhaler at the same scheduled time, asks the nurse if the order of administration of the inhalers matters. The best response by the nurse is
   a. "You should not take both inhalers at the same time."
   b. "The short-acting inhaled bronchodilator should be used first, followed by the steroid inhaler."
   c. "Either medication can effectively be used first."
   d. "The steroid inhaler should be used first, followed by the short-acting inhaled bronchodilator."

9. A patient on a steroid inhaler complains of anorexia and discomfort when he eats. The nurse reports this to the care provider, and the patient is diagnosed with oropharyngeal candidiasis. This is an adverse affect that can be decreased by all of the following except
   a. reducing the dose
   b. administering the drug more frequently
   c. rinsing the mouth after use
   d. using a spacer device

10. Montelukast is effective in relieving the inflammation and bronchoconstriction associated with acute asthmatic attacks through which principal action?
   a. stabilizing mast cells
   b. blocking leukotriene receptors
   c. binding to immunoglobulin E (IgE)
   d. decreasing prostaglandin synthesis

Selected References

Drug facts and comparisons. (Updated monthly). St. Louis, MO: Facts and Comparisons.

Guyton, A. C., & Hall, J. E. (2006). *Textbook of medical physiology* (11th ed.). Philadelphia: W. B. Saunders.

Hanania, N. A. (2007). Update on the pharmacologic therapy for chronic obstructive pulmonary disease. *Clinics in Chest Medicine, 28,* 589–607.

Lacy, C. F., Armstrong, L. L., Goldman, M. P., & Lance, L. L. (2007). *Lexi-Comp's drug information handbook* (15th ed.). Hudson, OH: American Pharmaceutical Association.

Mark, J. D. (2007). Asthma. In D. Rakel (Ed.), *Integrative medicine* (2nd ed., pp. 347–358). Philadelphia: Saunders Elsevier.

Mathur, S. K., & Busse, W. W. (2006). Asthma: Diagnosis and management. *Medical Clinics of North America, 90,* 39–60.

National Asthma Education and Prevention Program. (2007, August). *Expert panel report 3: Guidelines for the diagnosis and management of asthma* (NIH Publication No. 08-4051). Bethesda, MD: National Institutes of Health, National Heart, Lung, and Blood Institute. Retrieved August 30, 2007, from http://www.nhlbi.nih.gov/guidelines/asthma/asthgdln.pdf

Ogawa, Y. (2006). The role of leukotrienes in airway inflammation. *Journal of Allergy and Clinical Immunology, 118,* 789–798.

Sin, D. D., Man, J., Sharpe, H., Gan, Q. W., & Man, S. F. M. (2004). Pharmacological management to reduce exacerbations in adults with asthma: A systematic review and meta-analysis. *Journal of the American Medical Association, 292,* 367–376.

Weiler, J. M. (2007). American Academy of Allergy, Asthma & Immunology Work Group report: Exercise-induced asthma. *Journal of Allergy and Clinical Immunology, 119,* 1349–1358.

Wood-Baker, R. R., Gibson, P., Hannay, M., Walters, E. H., & Walters, J. A. E. (2007). Systemic corticosteroids for acute exacerbations of chronic obstructive pulmonary disease. *The Cochrane Database of Systematic Reviews, Issue 2.*

LEARNING OBJECTIVES

After studying this chapter, you will be able to:

1. Delineate effects of histamine on selected body tissues.
2. Describe the types of hypersensitivity or allergic reactions.
3. Discuss allergic rhinitis, allergic contact dermatitis, and drug allergies as conditions for which antihistamines are commonly used.
4. Identify the effects of histamine that are blocked by histamine$_1$ (H$_1$) receptor antagonist drugs.
5. Differentiate first- and second-generation antihistamines.
6. Describe antihistamines in terms of indications for use, adverse effects, and nursing process implications.
7. Discuss the use of antihistamines in special populations.

Applying Your Knowledge

Lakisha Whitehead, age 32, suffers from seasonal allergies. You work at a community health clinic. Ms. Whitehead comes to the clinic seeking your advice about what medication might provide relief of her symptoms of runny nose and eyes, nasal congestion, and productive cough.

Introduction

Antihistamines are drugs that antagonize the action of histamine. Thus, to understand the use of these drugs, it is necessary to understand histamine and its effects on body tissues, characteristics of allergic reactions, and selected conditions for which antihistamines are used.

Histamine and Its Receptors

Histamine is the first chemical mediator to be released in immune and inflammatory responses. It is synthesized and stored in most body tissues, with high concentrations in tissues exposed to environmental substances (e.g., the skin and mucosal surfaces of the eye, nose, lungs, and gastrointestinal [GI] tract). It is also found in the central nervous system (CNS). In these tissues, histamine is located mainly in secretory granules of mast cells (tissue cells surrounding capillaries) and basophils (circulating blood cells).

Histamine is discharged from mast cells and basophils in response to certain stimuli (e.g., allergic reactions, cellular injury, extreme cold). After it is released, it diffuses rapidly into other tissues, where it interacts with histamine receptors on target organs, called H$_1$ and H$_2$. H$_1$ receptors are located mainly on smooth muscle cells in blood vessels and the respiratory and GI tracts. When histamine binds with these receptors and stimulates them, effects include

- Contraction of smooth muscle in the bronchi and bronchioles (producing bronchoconstriction and respiratory distress)

- Stimulation of vagus nerve endings to produce reflex bronchoconstriction and cough

- Increased permeability of veins and capillaries, which allows fluid to flow into subcutaneous tissues and form edema

- Increased secretion of mucous glands. Mucosal edema and increased nasal mucus produce the nasal congestion characteristic of allergic rhinitis and the common cold.

- Stimulation of sensory peripheral nerve endings to cause pain and pruritus. Pruritus is especially prominent with allergic skin disorders.

- Dilation of capillaries in the skin, to cause flushing

When H_2 receptors are stimulated, the main effects are increased secretion of gastric acid and pepsin, increased rate and force of myocardial contraction, and decreased immunologic and proinflammatory reactions (e.g., decreased release of histamine from basophils, decreased movement of neutrophils and basophils into areas of injury, inhibited T- and B-lymphocyte function). Stimulation of both H_1 and H_2 receptors causes peripheral vasodilation (with hypotension, headache, and skin flushing) and increases bronchial, intestinal, and salivary secretion of mucus.

Hypersensitivity (Allergic) Reactions

In predisposed individuals, harmless environmental antigens that do not cause a reaction in most people may trigger an adaptive immune response, immunologic memory, and, on subsequent exposure to the environmental antigen, inflammation responses (see Chap. 38). *Hypersensitivity*, or allergic, reactions are exaggerated responses by the immune system that produce tissue injury and may cause serious disease. The mechanisms that eliminate pathogens in adaptive immune responses are essentially identical to those of natural immunity. Allergic reactions may result from specific antibodies, sensitized T lymphocytes, or both, formed during exposure to an antigen. Treatments and interventions are covered in other chapters.

Types of Responses to Cell-Mediated Invasion

Hypersensitivity reactions are grouped into four types according to the mechanisms by which they are produced. The substances that produce the effect for types I, II, and III hypersensitivity reactions are antibody molecules. The substances responsible for type IV reactions are antigen-specific T cells.

Type I (also called immediate hypersensitivity because it occurs within minutes of exposure to the antigen) is an immunoglobulin E (IgE)-induced response triggered by the interaction of antigen with antigen-specific IgE bound on mast cells, causing mast cell activation. Histamine and other mediators are released immediately, and cytokines, chemokines, and leukotrienes are synthesized after activation. Anaphylaxis is a type I response that may be mild (characterized mainly by urticaria, other dermatologic manifestations, or rhinitis) or severe and life threatening (characterized by respiratory distress and cardiovascular collapse). It is uncommon and does not occur on first exposure to an antigen; it occurs with a second or later exposure, after antibody formation was induced by an earlier exposure. Severe anaphylaxis (sometimes called anaphylactic shock; see Chap. 51) is characterized by cardiovascular collapse from profound vasodilation and pooling of blood in the splanchnic system so that the patient has severe hypotension and functional hypovolemia. Respiratory distress often occurs from laryngeal edema and bronchoconstriction. Urticaria often occurs because the skin has many mast cells that release histamine. Anaphylaxis is a systemic reaction that usually involves the respiratory, cardiovascular, and dermatologic systems. Severe anaphylaxis may be fatal if not treated promptly and effectively.

Type II responses are mediated by IgG or IgM generating direct damage to the cell surface. These cytotoxic reactions include blood transfusion reactions, hemolytic disease of newborns, autoimmune hemolytic anemia, and some drug reactions. Hemolytic anemia (caused by destruction of erythrocytes) and thrombocytopenia (caused by destruction of platelets), both type II hypersensitivity responses, are adverse effects of certain drugs (e.g., penicillin, methyldopa, heparin).

Type III is an IgG- or IgM-mediated reaction characterized by formation of antigen–antibody complexes that induce an acute inflammatory reaction in the tissues. *Serum sickness*, the prototype of these reactions, occurs when excess antigen combines with antibodies to form immune complexes. The complexes then diffuse into affected tissues, where they cause tissue damage by activating the complement system and initiating the immune response. If small amounts of immune complexes are deposited locally, the antigenic material can be phagocytized and digested by white blood cells and macrophages without tissue destruction. If large amounts are deposited locally or reach the bloodstream and become deposited in blood vessel walls, the lysosomal enzymes released during phagocytosis may cause permanent tissue destruction.

Type IV hypersensitivity (also called delayed hypersensitivity because of the lag time from exposure to antigen until the response is evident) is a cell-mediated response in which sensitized T lymphocytes react with an antigen to cause inflammation mediated by release of lymphokines, direct cytotoxicity, or both. The classic type IV hypersensitivity reaction is the tuberculin test, but similar reactions occur with contact dermatitis and some graft rejection.

Allergic Rhinitis

Allergic rhinitis is inflammation of nasal mucosa caused by a type I hypersensitivity reaction to inhaled allergens. It is a very common disorder characterized by nasal congestion, itching, sneezing, and watery drainage. Itching of the throat, eyes, and ears often occurs as well.

There are two types of allergic rhinitis. Seasonal disease (often called hay fever) produces acute symptoms in response to the protein components of airborne pollens from trees, grasses, and weeds, mainly in spring or fall. Perennial disease produces chronic symptoms in response to nonseasonal allergens such as dust mites, animal dander, and molds. Actually, mold spores can cause both seasonal and perennial allergies because they are present year round, with seasonal increases. Some people have both types, with chronic symptoms plus acute seasonal symptoms.

People with a personal or family history of other allergic disorders are likely to have allergic rhinitis. When nasal mucosa is inflamed, symptoms can be worsened by nonallergenic irritants such as tobacco smoke, strong odors, air pollution, and climatic changes.

Allergic rhinitis is an immune response in which normal nasal breathing and filtering of air brings inhaled antigens into contact with mast cells and basophils in nasal mucosa, blood vessels, and submucosal tissues. With initial exposure, the inhaled antigens are processed by lymphocytes that produce IgE, an antigen-specific antibody that binds to mast cells. With later exposures, the IgE interacts with inhaled antigens and triggers the breakdown of the mast cell. This breakdown causes the release of histamine and other inflammatory mediators such as prostaglandins and leukotrienes (Fig. 45-1). These mediators, of which histamine may be the most important, dilate and engorge blood vessels to produce nasal congestion, stimulate secretion of mucus, and attract inflammatory cells (e.g., eosinophils, lymphocytes, monocytes, macrophages). In people with allergies, mast cells and basophils are increased in both number and reactivity. Thus, these cells may be capable of releasing large amounts of histamine and other mediators.

Allergic rhinitis that is not effectively treated may lead to chronic fatigue, impaired ability to perform usual activities of daily living, difficulty sleeping, sinus infections, postnasal drip, cough, and headache. In addition, this condition is a strong risk factor for asthma.

Allergic Contact Dermatitis

Allergic contact dermatitis is a type IV hypersensitivity reaction resulting from direct contact with antigens to which a person has previously become sensitized (e.g., poison ivy or poison oak, cosmetics, hair dyes, metals, drugs applied topically to the skin). This reaction, which may be acute or chronic, usually occurs more than 24 hours after re-exposure to an antigen and may last from days to weeks.

Figure 45-1 ▪ Type I hypersensitivity reaction: allergic rhinitis. **(A)** The first exposure of mast cells in nasal mucosa to inhaled antigens (e.g., pollens from weeds, grasses, trees) leads to the formation of immunoglobulin E (IgE) antibody molecules. These molecules then bind to the surface membranes of mast cells. This process sensitizes mast cells to the effects of inhaled antigens (allergens). **(B)** When sensitized mast cells are re-exposed to inhaled pollens or other antigens, they release histamine and other chemical mediators, which then act on nasal mucosa to produce characteristic symptoms of allergic rhinitis.

Affected areas of the skin are usually inflamed, warm, edematous, intensely pruritic, and tender to touch. Skin lesions are usually erythematous macules, papules, and vesicles (blisters) that may drain, develop crusts, and become infected. Lesion location may indicate the causative antigen.

Allergic Food Reactions

Typically, food allergies are an immune response to the ingestion of a protein. Some food allergens such as shellfish, fish, corn, seeds, bananas, egg, milk, soy, peanut, and tree nuts have a higher inherent risk for triggering anaphylaxis than others. However, many other foods have been identified as allergens, including certain fruits and vegetables. Commonly, children allergic to milk, eggs, wheat, or soy outgrow their allergy. Exclusive breast-feeding has been found to be protective against the development of food allergies in early life but to increase the risk of food allergies as the individual ages. There is no known preventive strategy to prevent food allergies except to delay introducing allergy-prone foods to infants until the gastrointestinal tract has had time to mature. The timing for this varies from food to food and from infant to infant. The most common food allergy among adults is shellfish, often first presenting later in life.

Allergic Drug Reactions

Virtually any drug may induce an immunologic response in susceptible people, and any body tissues may be affected. Allergic drug reactions are complex and diverse and may include any of the types of hypersensitivity described previously. A single drug may induce one or more of these states and multiple symptoms. There are no specific characteristics that identify drug-related reactions, although some reactions commonly attributed to drugs (e.g., skin rashes, drug fever, hematologic reactions, hepatic reactions) rarely occur with plant pollens and other naturally occurring antigens. Usually, however, the body responds to a drug as it does to other foreign materials (antigens). In addition, some reactions may be caused by coloring agents, preservatives, and other additives rather than the drug itself. It may be difficult to recognize in an individual with atypical, resolving, or partially treated symptoms, as when skin signs such as urticaria are absent or masked by medications.

Allergic drug reactions should be considered when new signs and symptoms develop or when they differ from the usual manifestations of the illness being treated, especially if a reaction

■ Follows ingestion of a drug, especially one known to produce allergic reactions

■ Is unpredictable and occurs in only a few patients when many patients receive the suspected drug

■ Occurs approximately 7 to 10 days after initial exposure to the suspected drug (to allow antibody production)

■ Follows a previous exposure to the same or similar drug (sensitizing exposure)

■ Occurs minutes or hours after a second or subsequent exposure

■ Occurs after small doses (reduces the likelihood that the reaction is due to dose-related drug toxicity)

■ Occurs with other drugs that are chemically or immunologically similar to the suspected drug

■ Produces signs and symptoms that differ from the usual pharmacologic actions of the suspected drug

■ Produces signs and symptoms usually considered allergic in nature (e.g., anaphylaxis, urticaria, serum sickness)

■ Produces similar signs and symptoms to previous allergic reactions to the same or a similar drug

■ Increases eosinophils in blood or tissue

■ Resolves within a few days of discontinuing the suspected drug

Virtually all drugs have been implicated in *anaphylactic reactions*. Penicillins and other antimicrobials, radiocontrast media, aspirin and other nonsteroidal anti-inflammatory drugs, and antineoplastics such as L-asparaginase and cisplatin are more common offenders. Less common causes include anesthetics (local and general), opioid analgesics, skeletal muscle relaxants used with general anesthetics, and vaccines. Approximately 10% of severe anaphylactic reactions are fatal. In many cases, it is unknown whether clinical manifestations are immunologic or nonimmunologic in origin.

Serum sickness is a delayed hypersensitivity reaction most often caused by drugs, such as antimicrobials. In addition, many drugs that produce anaphylaxis also produce serum sickness. With initial exposure to the antigen, symptoms usually develop within 7 to 10 days and include urticaria, lymphadenopathy, myalgia, arthralgia, and fever. The reaction usually resolves within a few days but may be severe or even fatal. With repeated exposure to the antigen, after prior sensitization of the host, accelerated serum sickness may develop within 2 to 4 days, with similar but often more severe signs and symptoms.

Systemic lupus erythematosus (SLE) is an autoimmune disorder that may be idiopathic from nondrug causes or induced by hydralazine, procainamide, isoniazid, and other drugs. Clinical manifestations vary greatly, depending on the location and severity of the inflammatory and immune processes, and may include skin lesions, fever, pneumonia, anemia, arthralgia, arthritis, nephritis, and others. Drug-induced lupus produces less renal and CNS involvement than idiopathic SLE.

Fever often occurs with allergic drug reactions. It may occur alone, with a skin rash and eosinophilia, or with other drug-induced allergic reactions such as serum sickness, SLE, vasculitis, and hepatitis. Dermatologic conditions (e.g., skin rash, urticaria, inflammation) commonly occur with allergic drug reactions and may be the first and most visible manifestations.

Pseudoallergic Drug Reactions

Pseudoallergic drug reactions resemble immune responses (because histamine and other chemical mediators are released), but they do not produce antibodies or sensitized T lymphocytes. *Anaphylactoid reactions* are like anaphylaxis in terms of immediate occurrence, symptoms, and life-threatening severity. The main difference is that they are not antigen–antibody reactions and therefore may occur on first exposure to the causative agent. The drugs bind directly to mast cells, activate the cells, and cause the release of histamine and other vasoactive chemical mediators. Contrast media for radiologic diagnostic tests are often implicated.

General Characteristics of Antihistamines

There are several classes of antihistamines: alkylamines (brompheniramine, chlorpheniramine, etc.), ethanolamines (carbinoxamine, clemastine, etc.), ethylenediamines (tripelennamine, pyrilamine), phenothiazines (methdilazine, promethazine, etc.), piperazines (cyclizine, hydroxyzine, etc.), piperidines (azatadine, cyproheptadine), and the miscellaneous

group. The term *antihistamine* generally indicates classic or traditional drugs. With increased knowledge about histamine receptors, these drugs are often called H_1 receptor antagonists. These drugs prevent or reduce most of the physiologic effects that histamine normally induces at H_1 receptor sites. Thus, they

■ Inhibit smooth muscle constriction in blood vessels and the respiratory and GI tracts

■ Decrease capillary permeability

■ Decrease salivation and tear formation

The drugs are similar in effectiveness as histamine antagonists but differ in adverse effects. These are the antihistamines discussed in this chapter. Cimetidine (Tagamet), ranitidine (Zantac), famotidine (Pepcid), and nizatidine (Axid) are H_2 receptor antagonists or blocking agents used to prevent or treat peptic ulcer disease. These are discussed in Chapter 59. Selected H_1 antagonists are described in the following sections and in Table 45-1.

Table 45-1	**Drugs at a Glance: Commonly Used Antihistamines**		
		ROUTES AND DOSAGE RANGES	
GeneriC/Trade Name	**Indications for use**	**Adults**	**Children**
First Generation			
Brompheniramine (LoHist)	Allergic rhinitis	1–2 tablets (6–12 mg) q12h	*12 y and older:* Same as adults. 6–12 1 tablet (6 mg) q12h
Chlorpheniramine (Chlor-Trimeton)	Allergic rhinitis	PO 4 mg q4–6h; maximal dose, 24 mg in 24 h. Timed-release forms, PO 8 mg q8–12h or 12 mg q12h; maximal dose, 24 mg in 24 h	*12 y and older:* Same as adults 6–12 y: PO 2 mg q4–6h; maximal dose, 12 mg in 24 h 2–6 y: PO 1 mg q4–6h Timed-release forms, ≥12 y: PO 8 mg q8–12h or 12 mg q12h; maximal dose, 24 mg in 24 h
Clemastine (Tavist)	Allergic rhinitis Urticaria/angioedema	Allergic rhinitis, PO 1.34 mg twice daily, increased up to a maximum of 8.04 mg daily, if necessary. Urticaria/angioedema, PO 2.68 mg one to three times daily	Allergic rhinitis, 6–12 y (syrup only): PO 0.67 mg twice daily, increased up to a maximum of 4.02 mg daily, if necessary Urticaria/angioedema, 6–12 y (syrup only): PO 1.34 mg twice daily
Cyproheptadine	Hypersensitivity reactions (allergic rhinitis, conjunctivitis, dermatitis)	PO 4 mg q8h initially, increase if necessary. Maximal dose 0.5 mg/kg/d	(Calculate total daily dosage as 0.25 mg/kg or 8 mg/m²) 7–14 y: PO 4 mg q8–12h; maximal dose, 16 mg/d 2–6 y: 2 mg q8–12h; maximal dose, 12 mg/d
Dexchlorpheniramine	Hypersensitivity reactions (allergic rhinitis, conjunctivitis, dermatitis)	Regular tablets and syrup, PO 2 mg q4–6h Timed-release tablets, PO 4–6 mg at bedtime or q8–12h	*12 y and older:* Same as adults 6–11 y: PO 1 mg q4–6h 2–5 y: PO 0.5 mg q4–6h Timed-release tablets, *12 y and older:* Same as adults; 6–12 y: 4 mg once daily, at bedtime

(continued on page 736)

Table 45-1		**Drugs at a Glance:** Commonly Used Antihistamines (continued)	
		ROUTES AND DOSAGE RANGES	
Generic/Trade Name	**Indications for use**	**Adults**	**Children**
P Diphenhydramine (Benadryl)	Hypersensitivity reactions (allergic rhinitis, conjunctivitis, dermatitis) Motion sickness Parkinsonism Insomnia Antitussive (syrup only)	Hypersensitivity reaction, motion sickness, parkinsonism, PO 25–50 mg q4–8h; IV or deep IM 10–50 mg, increased if necessary to a maximal daily dose of 400 mg Insomnia, PO 50 mg at bedtime Syrup for cough, PO 25 mg (10 mL) q4h, not to exceed 100 mg (40 mL) in 24 h	*Weight greater than 10 kg (22 lbs):* PO 12.5–25 mg q6–8h, 5 mg/kg/d, or 150 mg/m2/d; IV 5 mg/kg/d, or 150 mg/m²/d. Maximum oral or parenteral dosage, 300 mg daily Insomnia, ≥12 y: Same as adults Syrup for cough, 6–12 y: PO 12.5 mg (5 mL) q4h, not to exceed 50 mg (20 mL) in 24 h; 2–6 y: PO 6.25 mg (2.5 mL) q4h, not to exceed 25 mg (10 mL) in 24 h
Hydroxyzine (Vistaril)	Pruritus Sedation Antiemetic	PO 25 mg q6–8h; IM 25–100 mg as needed	*older than 6 y:* PO 50–100 mg daily in divided doses *under 6 y:* PO 50 mg daily in divided doses
Phenindamine (Nolahist)	Allergic rhinitis	PO 25 mg q4–6h; maximal dose 150 mg in 24 h	*12 y or older:* Same as adults *6–11 y:* PO 12.5 mg q4–6h; maximal dose 75 mg in 24 h
Promethazine (Phenergan)	Hypersensitivity reactions (allergic rhinitis, conjunctivitis, dermatitis) Sedation Antiemetic Motion sickness	PO, IM, rectally, 25 mg q4–6h as needed	*2 y or older:* 12.5 mg q4–6h as needed
Triprolidine (Zymine)	Allergic rhinitis	PO 10 mL (1.2 mg/5 mL) q4–6h, not to exceed 40 mL/ 24 h	*12 y or older:* Same as adults *6–12 y:* 5 mL q4–6h, not to exceed 20 mL/24h *4–6 y:* 3.75 mL q4–6h, not to exceed 15 mL/24h *2–4 y:* 2.5 mL q4–6h, not to exceed 10 mL/24h *4 m–2 y:* 1.25 mL q4–6h, not to exceed 5 mL/24h
Second Generation **Azelastine** (Astelin)	Allergic rhinitis	Nasal inhalation, two sprays per nostrils q12h	*12 y or older:* Same as adults
Cetirizine (Zyrtec)	Allergic rhinitis Chronic idiopathic urticaria	PO 5–10 mg once daily Renal or hepatic impairment, PO 5 mg once daily	*6 y or older:* Same as adults *6 mo–5y:* PO 2.5 mg (one-half tsp) once daily
Desloratadine (Clarinex)	Allergic rhinitis Chronic idiopathic urticaria	5 mg once daily	*12 y or older:* Same as adults *12 y or younger:* Dosage not established
Fexofenadine (Allegra)	Allergic rhinitis	PO 60 mg twice daily Renal impairment, PO 60 mg once daily	*12 y or older:* Same as adults *6–11 y:* PO 30 mg twice daily
Loratadine (Claritin)	Allergic rhinitis Chronic idiopathic urticaria	PO 10 mg once daily Renal or hepatic impairment, PO 10 mg every other day	*6 y or older:* Same as adults *2–5 y:* PO 5 mg daily

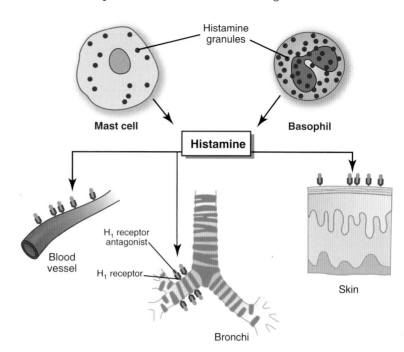

Figure 45-2 ▪ Action of antihistamine drugs. Histamine$_1$ (H$_1$) receptor antagonists bind to H$_1$ receptors. This prevents histamine from binding to its receptors and acting on target tissues.

Mechanism of Action

Antihistamines are structurally related to histamine and occupy the same receptor sites as histamine, which prevents histamine from acting on target tissues (Fig. 45-2). Thus, the drugs are effective in inhibiting vascular permeability, edema formation, bronchoconstriction, and pruritus associated with histamine release. They do not prevent histamine release or reduce the amount released.

Indications for Use

Antihistamines are used for a variety of allergic and nonallergic disorders to prevent or reverse target organ inflammation and its effects on organ function. The drugs can relieve symptoms but do not relieve the hypersensitivity.

- Allergic rhinitis. Of people with seasonal allergic rhinitis, 75% to 95% experience some relief of sneezing, rhinorrhea, nasal congestion, and conjunctivitis with the use of antihistamines. People with perennial allergic rhinitis usually experience decreased nasal congestion and drying of nasal mucosa. However, many people require an additional drug to relieve symptoms. Cromolyn, ipratropium, and several corticosteroids are available in intranasal preparations for this purpose. These drugs, with dosage ranges for adults and children, are listed in Table 45-2.

- Anaphylaxis. Antihistamines are helpful in treating urticaria and pruritus but are not effective in treating bronchoconstriction and hypotension. Epinephrine, rather than an antihistamine, is the drug of choice for treating severe anaphylaxis.

- Allergic conjunctivitis. This condition, which is characterized by redness, itching, and tearing of the eyes, is often associated with allergic rhinitis. Antihistamine eye medications may be given (see Chap. 63).

- Drug allergies and pseudoallergies. Antihistamines may be given to prevent or treat reactions to drugs. When used for prevention, they should be given before exposure (e.g., before a diagnostic test that uses an iodine preparation as a contrast medium, before an intravenous infusion of amphotericin B). When antihistamines are used for treatment, giving the antihistamine and stopping the causative drug usually relieve signs and symptoms within a few days.

- Transfusions of blood and blood products. Premedication with an antihistamine is often used to prevent allergic reactions.

- Dermatologic conditions. Antihistamines are the drugs of choice for treatment of allergic contact dermatitis and acute urticaria (a vascular reaction of the skin characterized by papules or wheals and severe itching, often called hives). Urticaria often occurs because the skin has many mast cells to release histamine. Other indications for use include drug-induced skin reactions, pruritus ani, and pruritus vulvae. Systemic drugs are used; topical preparations are not recommended because they often induce skin rashes themselves. With pruritus, oral cyproheptadine and hydroxyzine (Vistaril) are especially effective.

- Miscellaneous. Some antihistamines are commonly used for nonallergic disorders, such as motion sickness, nausea and vomiting (e.g., promethazine, hydroxyzine; see Chap. 62), and sleep (e.g., diphenhydramine). The active ingredient in over-the-counter (OTC) sleep aids (e.g., Compoz, Sominex) is a sedating antihistamine. Antihistamines are also common ingredients in OTC cold remedies (see Chap. 46).

Contraindications to Use

Antihistamines are contraindicated or must be used with caution in pregnant women and patients with hypersensitivity to

Table 45-2	Drugs at a Glance: Intranasal Drugs for Allergic Rhinitis	
	ROUTES AND DOSAGE RANGES	
GeneriC/Trade Name	**Adults**	**Children**
Anticholinergic **Ipratropium** (Atrovent nasal spray)	2 sprays (42 mcg or 84 mcg) per nostril 2–4 times daily	12 y *and older:* Same as adults
Corticosteroids **Beclomethasone** (Beconase)	1 inhalation (42 mcg) in each nostril 2–4 times daily	12 y *and older:* Same as adults 6–12 y: 1 inhalation in each nostril 3 times daily
Budesonide (Rhinocort)	256 mcg daily as 2 sprays per nostril twice daily or 4 sprays per nostril once daily	6 y *and older:* Same as adults
Flunisolide (Nasalide, Nasarel)	2 sprays (50 mcg) in each nostril 2 times daily, increase to 3 times daily if necessary	6–14 y: 1 spray (25 mcg) in each nostril 3 times daily or 2 sprays per nostril (50 mcg) 2 times daily
Fluticasone (Flonase)	2 sprays (50 mcg each) per nostril once daily (200 mcg daily)	4 y *and older:* 1 spray per nostril per day (100 mcg daily)
Mometasone (Nasonex)	2 sprays (50 mcg each) per nostril once daily (200 mcg daily)	12 y *and older:* Same as adults 3–11 y: 1 spray per nostril once daily (100 mcg daily)
Triamcinolone (Nasacort, Nasacort AQ)	2 sprays (55 mcg/spray) in each nostril once daily	6 y *and older:* Same as adults initially, then reduce to 1 spray per nostril per day
Mast Cell Stabilizer **Cromolyn** (Nasalcrom)	1 spray in each nostril 3–6 times daily, q4–6h	6 y *and older:* Same as adults

the drugs, narrow-angle glaucoma, prostatic hypertrophy, stenosing peptic ulcer, and bladder neck obstruction.

Classifications and Individual Drugs

First-Generation H₁ Receptor Antagonists

These chemically diverse antihistamines (also called nonselective or sedating agents) bind to both central and peripheral H₁ receptors and can cause CNS depression or stimulation. They usually cause CNS depression (drowsiness, sedation) with therapeutic doses and may cause CNS stimulation (anxiety, agitation) with excessive doses, especially in children. They also have substantial *anticholinergic effects* (e.g., cause dry mouth, urinary retention, constipation, blurred vision).

Brompheniramine, **chlorpheniramine** (Chlor-Trimeton), and **dexchlorpheniramine** cause minimal drowsiness. P **Diphenhydramine** (Benadryl), the prototype of first-generation antihistamines, causes a high incidence of drowsiness and anticholinergic effects. **Hydroxyzine** (Vistaril) and **promethazine** (Phenergan) are strong CNS depressants and cause extensive drowsiness.

First-generation antihistamines are usually well absorbed after oral administration. Immediate-release oral forms act within 15 to 60 minutes and last 4 to 6 hours. Enteric-coated or sustained-release preparations last 8 to 12 hours. Most drugs are given orally; a few may be given parenterally. These drugs are primarily metabolized by the liver, with metabolites and small amounts of unchanged drug excreted in urine within 24 hours. Several of these drugs are available without prescription. Brompheniramine, chlorpheniramine, and diphenhydramine are available alone and in combination with adrenergic nasal decongestants, analgesics, and allergy, cold, and sinus remedies.

Second-Generation H₁ Receptor Antagonists

Second-generation H₁ antagonists (also called selective or nonsedating agents) were developed mainly to produce less sedation than the first-generation drugs. They cause less CNS depression because they are selective for peripheral H₁ receptors and do not cross the blood–brain barrier. Loratadine (Claritin) and cetirizine (Zyrtec) are available for OTC sales. Proponents of OTC availability usually argue that the drugs are safer than the first-generation drugs that have been available OTC for many years.

Azelastine (Astelin) is the only antihistamine formulated as a nasal spray for topical use. When applied to nasal mucosa, it produces peak levels in 2 to 3 hours and lasts 12 to 24 hours. It is metabolized in the liver to an active metabolite and is excreted mainly in feces. The other drugs are well absorbed with oral administration and have a rapid onset of action. **Cetirizine** (Zyrtec) is an active metabolite of hydroxyzine that causes less drowsiness than hydroxyzine. It reaches maximal serum concentration in 1 hour and is about 93% protein bound. About half of a dose is metabolized in the liver; the other half is excreted unchanged in the urine. **Fexofenadine** (Allegra) reaches peak serum concentrations in about 2.5 hours, is 60% to 70% protein bound, and 95% is excreted unchanged in bile and urine. **Loratadine** (Claritin) effects occur within 1 to 3 hours, reach a maximum in 8 to 12 hours, and last 24 hours or longer. Loratadine is metabolized in the liver and its long duration of action is due, in part, to an active metabolite. The patent for loratadine expired in December 2002, clearing the way for generic formulations. **Desloratadine** (Clarinex), an active metabolite of loratadine and marketed by the manufacturer of Claritin, seems to offer no advantage over loratadine or other second-generation drugs.

Nursing Process

Assessment

- Assess the patient's condition in relation to disorders for which antihistamines are used. For the patient with known allergies, try to determine the factors that precipitate or relieve allergic reactions and specific signs and symptoms experienced during a reaction.

- Assess every patient for a potential hypersensitivity reaction. For example, it is standard practice on first contact to ask a patient if he or she has any food, drug, or other allergies. The health care provider is likely to get more complete information by asking patients about allergic reactions to specific drugs (e.g., antibiotics such as penicillin, local anesthetics) rather than asking if they are allergic to or cannot take any drugs.

    If a drug allergy is identified, ask about specific signs and symptoms as well as any drugs currently being taken. With previous exposure and sensitization to the same or a similar drug, immediate allergic reactions may occur. With a new drug, antibody formation and allergic reactions usually require a week or longer. Most reactions appear within a month of starting a drug.

    When a suspected allergic reaction occurs (e.g., skin rash, fever, edema, dyspnea), interview the patient or consult medical records about the drug, dose, route, and time of administration. In addition, evaluate all the drugs a patient is taking as a potential cause of the reaction. This assessment may involve searching drug literature to see if the suspected drug is associated with allergic reactions, and discussion with physicians and pharmacists.

Nursing Diagnoses

- Risk for Injury related to drowsiness with first-generation antihistamines
- Deficient Knowledge: Safe and accurate drug use
- Deficient Knowledge: Strategies for minimizing exposure to allergens and irritants

Planning/Goals

The patient will

- Experience relief of symptoms
- Take antihistamines accurately
- Avoid hazardous activities if sedated from antihistamines
- Avoid preventable adverse drug effects
- Avoid taking sedative-type antihistamines with alcohol or other sedative drugs

Interventions

- For patient's with known allergies, assist in identifying and avoiding precipitating factors when possible. If it is a drug allergy, encourage the patient to carry a medical alert device that identifies the drug.

- Monitor the patient closely for excessive drowsiness during the first few days of therapy with antihistamines known to cause sedation.

- Encourage a fluid intake of 2000 to 3000 mL daily, if not contraindicated.

- Because antihistamines are most effective before exposure to the stimulus that causes histamine release, assist patient's in learning when to take the drugs (e.g., during seasons of high pollen and mold counts).

- When indicated, obtain an order and administer an antihistamine before situations known to elicit allergic reactions (e.g., blood transfusions, diagnostic tests that involve contrast media).

- For patients who have experienced an allergic or pseudoallergic drug reaction, assist them in learning about the drug thought responsible (including the generic and commonly used trade names), suitable alternatives for future drug therapy, and potential sources of the drug.

- For children with allergies, provide all family members, daycare, and school with an emergency plan.

- Provide appropriate patient teaching regarding any drug therapy (see accompanying display).

Evaluation

- Observe for relief of symptoms.
- Interview and observe for correct drug usage.
- Interview and observe for excessive drowsiness.

Ms. Whitehead starts taking OTC loratadine. What patient teaching points are appropriate?

Principles of Therapy

Prevention of Histamine-Releasing Reactions

When possible, avoiding exposure to known allergens can prevent allergic reactions. If antihistamine therapy is required, it is more effective if started before exposure to allergens because the drugs can then occupy receptor sites before histamine is released.

Drug Selection

▪ Choosing an antihistamine is based on the desired effect, duration of action, adverse effects, and other characteristics of available drugs. For most people, a second-generation drug is the first drug of choice. However, they are quite expensive. If costs are prohibitive for a patient, a first-generation drug may be used with minimal daytime sedation if taken at bedtime or in low initial doses, with gradual increases over a week or two. Azelastine nasal spray also causes little sedation, but it leaves an unpleasant taste. Overall, safety should be the determining factor. Some studies have shown cognitive and performance impairment with the first-generation drugs even when the person does not feel drowsy or impaired.

▪ For treatment of acute allergic reactions, a rapid-acting agent of short duration is preferred.

▪ For chronic allergic symptoms (e.g., allergic rhinitis), long-acting preparations provide more consistent relief. A patient may respond better to one antihistamine than to another. Thus, if one does not relieve symptoms or produces excessive sedation, another may be effective.

▪ For treatment of the common cold, studies have demonstrated that antihistamines do not relieve symptoms and are

Patient Teaching Guidelines | Antihistamines

General Considerations

▪ Some antihistamines should not be taken by people with glaucoma, peptic ulcer, urinary retention, or pregnancy. Inform your physician if you have any of these conditions or, for over-the-counter (OTC) antihistamines, read the label to see if you should avoid a particular drug.

▪ Antihistamines may dry and thicken respiratory tract secretions and make them more difficult to remove. Thus, do not take diphenhydramine (Benadryl), which is available OTC, if you have active asthma, bronchitis, or pneumonia.

▪ Some antihistamines cause drowsiness or dizziness and impair mental alertness, judgment, and physical coordination, especially during the first few days. Do not smoke, drive a car, operate machinery, or perform other tasks requiring alertness and physical dexterity until drowsiness has worn off, to avoid injury.

▪ Avoid using sedating antihistamines with other sedative-type drugs (e.g., alcohol, medications to relieve nervousness or produce sleep), to avoid adverse effects and dangerous drug interactions. Alcohol and other drugs that depress brain function may cause excessive sedation, respiratory depression, and death.

▪ Do not take more than one antihistamine at a time (e.g., two prescription drugs, two OTC drugs, or a combination of prescription and OTC drugs) because adverse effects are likely. If you do not know whether a particular medication is an antihistamine, consult a health care provider. For example, many OTC cold remedies and "nighttime" or "PM" allergy or sinus preparations contain an antihistamine. In addition, the active ingredient in OTC sleep aids is a sedating antihistamine, usually diphenhydramine (Benadryl).

▪ Avoid prolonged exposure to sunlight and use sunscreens and protective clothing; some antihistamines may increase sensitivity to sunlight and risks of skin damage from sunburn.

▪ Report adverse effects, such as excessive drowsiness. The physician may be able to change drugs or dosages to decrease adverse effects.

▪ Store antihistamines out of reach of children to avoid accidental ingestion.

▪ If you experience an allergic reaction to a medication, obtain information about the drug thought responsible (including its various names), acceptable alternatives for future drug therapy, and potential sources of the drug. In addition, read the list of ingredients on labels of OTC drug preparations, inform all health care providers about the drug reaction before taking any newly prescribed drug, and wear a medical alert device that lists drugs to be avoided. Note that people may be allergic to additives (e.g., dyes, binders, others) rather than the active drug.

Self-Administration

▪ Take antihistamines only as prescribed or as instructed on packages of OTC preparations to increase beneficial effects and decrease adverse effects. If you miss a dose, do not take a double dose.

▪ Take most antihistamines with meals to decrease stomach upset. Take loratadine (Claritin) on an empty stomach for better absorption; cetirizine (Zyrtec) and desloratadine (Clarinex) may be taken with or without food.

▪ Do not chew or crush sustained-release tablets and do not open sustained-release capsules. Such actions can cause rapid drug absorption, high blood levels, and serious adverse effects, rather than the slow absorption and prolonged action intended with these products.

not recommended. However, an antihistamine is often included in prescription and OTC combination products for the common cold.

Applying Your Knowledge 45-2

Ms. Whitehead returns to the clinic. She states, "The medication makes me feel better, but it is so expensive. I have a hard time affording it." What advice can you offer?

Use in Special Populations

Use in Children

First-generation antihistamines (e.g., diphenhydramine) may cause drowsiness and decreased mental alertness in children as in adults. Young children may experience paradoxical excitement. These reactions may occur with therapeutic dosages. In overdosage, hallucinations, convulsions, and death may occur. Close supervision and appropriate dosages are required for safe drug usage in children.

Diphenhydramine is not recommended for use in newborn infants (premature or full-term) or children with chickenpox or a flu-like infection. When used in young children, doses should be small because of drug effects on the brain and nervous system. Promethazine should not be used in children with hepatic disease, Reye's syndrome, a history of sleep apnea, or a family history of sudden infant death syndrome.

The second-generation drugs vary in recommendations for use according to age groups. Cetirizine and loratadine may be used in children 2 years and older. Syrup formulations are available for use in younger children. Azelastine may be used in children 5 years and older, fexofenadine may be used in children 6 years of age and older, and desloratadine may be used in children 12 years and older.

 Applying Your Knowledge 45-3

How Can You Avoid This Medication Error?
During her visit, Ms. Whitehead tells you that her 18-month-old daughter has a cold. Last night, she gave her daughter a dose of the loratadine to relieve her symptoms and help the child get some rest.

Use in Older Adults

First-generation antihistamines (e.g., diphenhydramine) may cause confusion (with impaired thinking, judgment, and memory), dizziness, hypotension, sedation, syncope, unsteady gait, and paradoxical CNS stimulation in older adults. These effects, especially sedation, may be misinterpreted as senility or mental depression. Older men with prostatic hypertrophy may have difficulty voiding while taking these drugs. Some of these adverse reactions derive from anticholinergic effects of the drugs and are likely to be more severe if the patient is also tak-

ing other drugs with anticholinergic effects (e.g., tricyclic antidepressants, older antipsychotic drugs, some antiparkinson drugs). Despite the increased risk of adverse effects, however, diphenhydramine is sometimes prescribed as a sleep aid for occasional use in older adults. As with many other drugs, smaller-than-usual dosages are indicated.

In general, second-generation antihistamines should be used for older adults. They are much safer because they do not impair consciousness, thinking, or ability to perform activities of daily living (e.g., driving a car or operating various machines).

Use in Patients With Renal Impairment

Little information is available about using antihistamines in patients with impaired renal function. With diphenhydramine, the dosing interval should be extended to 12 to 18 hours in patients with severe kidney failure. With cetirizine (5 mg once daily), desloratadine (5 mg every other day), fexofenadine (60 mg once daily), and loratadine (10 mg every other day), recommended doses for initial use are approximately one half of those used for young and middle-aged adults. No data are available regarding use of azelastine. However, because the drug is metabolized in the liver and excreted mainly in feces, it is unlikely that a dosage reduction is needed in patients with renal impairment.

Use in Patients With Hepatic Impairment

Little information is available about using antihistamines in patients with impaired hepatic function. With diphenhydramine, single doses are probably safe, but the effects of multiple doses have not been studied in this population. With promethazine, cholestatic jaundice has been reported, and the drug should be used with caution. With cetirizine (5 mg once daily) and loratadine (10 mg every other day), smaller-than-usual doses are recommended. No data are available regarding use of azelastine. However, because the drug is metabolized in the liver and excreted mainly in feces, cautious use and a possible dosage reduction may be needed in patients with hepatic impairment.

Use in Patients With Critical Illness

Antihistamines are not often used in the treatment of patients with critical illness. Most are given orally, and many critically ill patients are unable to take oral drugs. Diphenhydramine may be given by injection, usually as a single dose, to a patient who is having a blood transfusion or a diagnostic test to prevent allergic reactions. Hydroxyzine or promethazine may be given by injection for nausea and vomiting or to provide sedation but are not usually the first drugs of choice for these indications.

Use in Home Care

Antihistamines are often taken in the home setting, especially for allergic rhinitis and other allergic disorders. Most people are familiar with the uses and side effects of antihistamines. The home care nurse is unlikely to be involved in antihistamine drug therapy unless visiting a patient for other care and purposes. If a first-generation drug is being used, the home care nurse needs to assess for drowsiness and safety hazards in the environment (e.g., operating a car or other potentially hazardous machinery). In most people, tolerance develops to the sedative effects within a few days if they are not taking other sedative-type drugs or alcoholic beverages.

If a patient has an allergic disorder, the home care nurse may need to assist in identifying and alleviating environmental allergens (e.g., cigarette smoke, animal dander, dust mites).

Nursing Actions Antihistamines

NURSING ACTIONS	RATIONALE/EXPLANATION
1. Administer accurately	
a. Give most oral antihistamines with food; give loratadine on an empty stomach; give cetirizine or desloratadine with or without food.	To decrease gastrointestinal (GI) effects of the drugs
b. Give intramuscular antihistamines deeply into a large muscle mass.	To decrease tissue irritation
c. Inject intravenous (IV) antihistamines slowly, over a few minutes.	Severe hypotension may result from rapid IV injection.
d. When a drug is used to prevent motion sickness, give it 30–60 minutes before travel.	
2. Observe for therapeutic effects	Therapeutic effects depend on the reason for use.
a. A verbal statement of therapeutic effect (relief of symptoms)	
b. Decreased nausea and vomiting when given for antiemetic effects	
c. Decreased dizziness and nausea when taken for motion sickness	
d. Drowsiness or sleep when given for sedation	
3. Observe for adverse effects	
a. First-generation drugs	
(1) Sedation	Drowsiness due to central nervous system (CNS) depression is the most common adverse effect.
(2) Paradoxical excitation—restlessness, insomnia, tremors, nervousness, palpitations	This reaction is more likely to occur in children. It may result from the anticholinergic effects of antihistamines.
(3) Convulsive seizures	Antihistamines, particularly the phenothiazines, may lower the seizure threshold.
(4) Dryness of mouth, nose, and throat; blurred vision; urinary retention; constipation	Due to anticholinergic effects
(5) GI distress—anorexia, nausea, vomiting	
b. Second-generation drugs	Adverse effects are few and mild.
(1) Drowsiness	Drowsiness and dry mouth are more likely to occur with cetirizine; headache is more likely to occur with loratadine; desloratadine and fexofenadine reportedly produce minimal adverse effects.
(2) Dry mouth	
(3) Fatigue	
(4) Headache	
(5) GI upset	
4. Observe for drug interactions	Note: No documented drug interactions have been reported with intranasal azelastine or oral cetirizine or desloratadine.
a. Drugs that *increase* effects of first-generation antihistamines:	
(1) Alcohol and other CNS depressants (e.g., antianxiety and antipsychotic agents, opioid analgesics, sedative-hypnotics)	Additive CNS depression. Concomitant use may lead to drowsiness, lethargy, stupor, respiratory depression, coma, and death.
(2) Monoamine oxidase inhibitors	Inhibit metabolism of antihistamines, leading to an increased duration of action; increased incidence and severity of sedative and anticholinergic adverse effects.
(3) Tricyclic antidepressants	Additive anticholinergic side effects
b. Drugs that *increase* effects of loratadine:	All of these drugs increase plasma levels of loratadine by decreasing its metabolism.
(1) Macrolide antibacterials (azithromycin, clarithromycin, erythromycin)	
(2) Azole antifungals (fluconazole, itraconazole, ketoconazole, miconazole)	
(3) Cimetidine	
c. Drugs that may *decrease* effects of fexofenadine:	
(1) Rifampin	Rifampin may induce enzymes that accelerate metabolism of fexofenadine.

Key Concepts

- Virtually any drug may induce an immunologic response in susceptible people, and any body tissues may be affected

- Allergic rhinitis is inflammation of nasal mucosa caused by a type I hypersensitivity reaction to inhaled allergens.

- Some food allergens such as shellfish, egg, milk, peanuts, and tree nuts have a higher inherent risk for triggering anaphylaxis than others.

- First-generation antihistamines (e.g., diphenhydramine) may cause drowsiness and decreased mental alertness in children as in adults.

- First-generation antihistamines have substantial anticholinergic effects (e.g., cause dry mouth, urinary retention, constipation, blurred vision).

- Second-generation H_1 antagonists cause less CNS depression because they are selective for peripheral H_1 receptors and do not cross the blood–brain barrier.

- Azelastine (Astelin) is the only antihistamine formulated as a nasal spray for topical use.

- Patients with drug allergies should wear a medical alert bracelet identifying the drug.

- For children with allergies, provide all family members, daycare, and school with an emergency plan.

Review and Application Exercises

Short Answer Exercises

1. Describe several factors that cause histamine release from cells.

2. What signs and symptoms are produced by the release of histamine?

3. How do antihistamines act to block the effects of histamine?

4. Differentiate between H_1 and H_2 receptor antagonists in terms of pharmacologic effects and clinical indications for use.

5. In general, when should an antihistamine be taken to prevent or treat allergic disorders?

6. Compare and contrast the first- and second-generation antihistamines.

NCLEX-Style Questions

7. In explaining options for antihistamine medications to a patient, the nurse knows that second-generation H_1 antagonists differ from first-generation antagonists in that they
   a. cause greater CNS sedation
   b. are available only by prescription
   c. are less expensive
   d. do not cross the blood–brain barrier

8. Your patient has asked for an antihistamine to relieve his symptoms of an upper respiratory infection. You explain to him that studies have demonstrated that for treatment of the common cold, antihistamines
   a. are effective in relieving cold symptoms
   b. do not relieve symptoms and are not recommended
   c. should be compounded with other products to be effective
   d. relieve nonallergenic symptoms only

9. The nurse in the emergency room anticipates an order of a severe allergic reaction with anaphylaxis, knowing that the drug of choice for severe allergic reactions with anaphylaxis is
   a. atropine
   b. cimetidine (Tagamet)
   c. epinephrine
   d. loratadine (Claritin)

10. The nurse who receives an order to administer diphenhydramine (Benadryl) knows that this medication is recommended for use in
    a. premature or full-term infants
    b. adults to prevent allergic reactions
    c. children with chickenpox
    d. children with a flu-like infection

11. Due to the action of antihistamines on target tissues, these drugs are effective in producing all of the following actions except
    a. inhibiting vascular permeability
    b. reducing pruritus
    c. minimizing edema formation
    d. preventing histamine release

Selected References

Corwin, E. J. (2006). *Handbook of pathophysiology* (3rd ed.). Philadelphia: Lippincott Williams & Wilkins.

Drug facts and comparisons. (Updated monthly). St. Louis, MO: Facts and Comparisons.

Guyton, A. C., & Hall, J. E. (2006). *Textbook of medical physiology* (11th ed.). Philadelphia: W. B. Saunders.

Joint Task Force on Practice Parameters, American Academy of Allergy, Asthma and Immunology, American College of Allergy, Asthma and Immunology, Joint Council of Allergy, Asthma and Immunology. (2005). The diagnosis and management of anaphylaxis: An updated practice parameter. *Journal of Allergy and Clinical Immunology, 115*(3 Suppl 2), S483–S523.

Karch, A. M. (2007). *2008 Lippincott's nursing drug guide*. Philadelphia: Lippincott Williams & Wilkins.

Kobrynski, L. J. (2007). Anaphylaxis. *Clinical Pediatric Emergency Medicine, 8*, 110–116.

Lacy, C. F., Armstrong, L. L., Goldman, M. P., & Lance, L. L. (2007). *Lexi-Comp's drug information handbook* (15th ed.). Hudson, OH: American Pharmaceutical Association.

Matheson, M. C., Erbas, B., Balasuriya, A., Jenkins, M. A., Wharton, C. L., Tang, M. L., Abramson, M. J., Walters, E. H., Hopper, J. L., & Dharmage, S. C. (2007). Breast-feeding and atopic disease: a cohort study from childhood to middle age. *Journal of Allergy and Clinical Immunology, 120*, 1051–1057.

Porth, C. M. (2005). *Pathophysiology: Concepts of altered health states* (7th ed.). Philadelphia: Lippincott Williams & Wilkins.

Simons, F. E. (2007). Risk assessment in anaphylaxis: Current and future approaches. *Journal of Allergy and Clinical Immunology, 120*(1 Suppl), S2–S24.

Nasal Decongestants, Antitussives, and Cold Remedies

LEARNING OBJECTIVES

After studying this chapter, you will be able to:

1. Describe characteristics of selected upper respiratory disorders and symptoms.
2. Review decongestant and adverse effects of adrenergic drugs.
3. Describe general characteristics and effects of antitussive agents.
4. Discuss the advantages and disadvantages of using combination products to treat the common cold.
5. Evaluate over-the-counter allergy, cold, cough, and sinus remedies for personal or patients' use.
6. Use the nursing process in the care of individuals with the common cold.

Applying Your Knowledge

Archie Hobbs is a 45-year-old welder at an industrial plant. As the occupational nurse for the facility, you observe a high rate of people with colds. Archie comes to the health office complaining about his nasal congestion and cough.

Introduction

The drugs discussed in this chapter are used to treat upper respiratory disorders and symptoms such as the common cold, sinusitis, nasal congestion, cough, and excessive secretions. Some of these diverse drugs are discussed more extensively in other chapters; they are discussed here in relation to their use in upper respiratory conditions.

Common Respiratory Disorders

The Common Cold

The common cold, a viral infection of the upper respiratory tract, is the most common respiratory tract infection. Adults usually have two to four colds per year; schoolchildren may have as many as 10 annually. Colds can be caused by many types of virus, most often the rhinovirus. Shedding of these viruses by infected people, mainly from nasal mucosa, can result in rapid spread to other people.

The viruses can enter the body through mucous membranes. Cold viruses can survive for several hours on the skin and hard surfaces, such as wood and plastic. There may also be airborne spread from sneezing and coughing, but this source is considered secondary. After the viruses gain entry, the incubation period is generally 5 days, the most contagious period is about 3 days after symptoms begin, and the cold usually lasts near 7 days. Because of the way cold viruses are spread, frequent and thorough hand hygiene (by both infected and uninfected people) is the most important protective and preventive measure. The tendency for overmedication and inappropriate use of antibiotics with the common cold are widespread and pose significant risk for complications and drug resistance.

Sinusitis

Sinusitis is inflammation of the paranasal sinuses, air cells that connect with the nasal cavity and are lined by similar mucosa. As in other parts of the respiratory tract, ciliated mucous membranes help move fluid and microorganisms out of the sinuses and into the nasal cavity. This movement becomes impaired when sinus openings are blocked by nasal swelling, and the impairment is considered a major cause of sinus infections. Another contributing factor is a lower oxygen content in the sinuses, which aids the growth of microorganisms and impairs local defense mechanisms. *Rhinitis* (inflammation and congestion of nasal mucosa) and upper respiratory tract infections are the most common causes of sinusitis. Symptoms may include moderate to severe headache, tenderness or pain in the affected sinus area, and fever.

Applying Your Knowledge 46-1

Mr. Hobbs works in an area with many other people. What should you emphasize to help prevent the further spread of infection throughout the plant?

Common Signs and Symptoms of Respiratory Disorders

Nasal Congestion

Nasal congestion is manifested by obstructed nasal passages ("stuffy nose") and nasal drainage ("runny nose"). It is a prominent symptom of the common cold and rhinitis (including allergic rhinitis; see Chap. 45). Nasal congestion results from dilation of the blood vessels in the nasal mucosa and engorgement of the mucous membranes with blood. At the same time, nasal membranes are stimulated to increase mucus secretion. Related symptomatic terms are *rhinorrhea* (secretions discharged from the nose) and rhinitis (inflammation of nasal mucosa, usually accompanied by nasal congestion, rhinorrhea, and sneezing).

Cough

Cough is a forceful expulsion of air from the lungs. It is normally a protective reflex for removing foreign bodies, environmental irritants, or accumulated secretions from the respiratory tract. The cough reflex involves central and peripheral mechanisms. Centrally, the cough center in the medulla oblongata receives stimuli and initiates the reflex response (deep inspiration, closed glottis, buildup of pressure within the lungs, and forceful exhalation). Peripherally, cough receptors in the pharynx, larynx, trachea, or lungs may be stimulated by air, dryness of mucous membranes, or excessive secretions. A cough is productive when secretions are expectorated; it is nonproductive when it is dry and no sputum is expectorated.

Cough is a prominent symptom of respiratory tract infections (e.g., the common cold, influenza, bronchitis, pharyngitis) and chronic obstructive pulmonary diseases (e.g., emphysema, chronic bronchitis).

Increased Secretions

Increased secretions may result from excessive production or decreased ability to cough or otherwise remove secretions from the respiratory tract. Secretions may seriously impair respiration by obstructing airways and preventing air flow to and from alveoli, where gas exchange occurs. Secretions also may cause atelectasis (a condition in which part of the lung is airless and collapses) by blocking airflow, and they may cause or aggravate infections by supporting bacterial growth.

Respiratory disorders characterized by retention of secretions include influenza, pneumonia, upper respiratory infections, acute and chronic bronchitis, emphysema, and acute attacks of asthma. Nonrespiratory conditions that predispose to secretion retention include immobility, debilitation, cigarette smoking, and postoperative status. Surgical procedures involving the chest or abdomen are most likely to be associated with retention of secretions because pain may decrease the patient's ability to cough, breathe deeply, and ambulate.

General Characteristics Of Drugs Used In/For Respiratory Disorders

Numerous drugs are available and widely used to treat the symptoms of respiratory disorders. Many are nonprescription drugs and can be obtained alone or in combination products. Available products include nasal decongestants, antitussives, and expectorants.

Nasal Decongestants

Nasal *decongestants* are used to relieve nasal obstruction and discharge. Adrenergic (sympathomimetic) drugs are most often used for this purpose (see Chap. 17). These agents relieve nasal congestion and swelling by constricting arterioles and reducing blood flow to nasal mucosa. Oxymetazoline (Afrin) is a commonly used nasal spray; pseudoephedrine (Sudafed) is taken orally. Rebound nasal swelling can occur with excessive or extended use of nasal sprays.

Nasal decongestants are most often used to relieve rhinitis associated with respiratory infections or allergies. They also may be used to reduce local blood flow before nasal surgery and to aid visualization of the nasal mucosa during diagnostic examinations.

These drugs are contraindicated in patients with severe hypertension or coronary artery disease because of their cardiac stimulating and vasoconstricting effects. They also are contraindicated for patients with narrow-angle glaucoma and those taking tricyclic or monoamine oxidase inhibitor antidepressants. They must be used with caution in the presence of cardiac dysrhythmias, hyperthyroidism, diabetes mellitus, glaucoma, and prostatic hypertrophy.

 Applying Your Knowledge 46-2

How Can You Avoid This Medication Error?

Mr. Hobbs has been sick for more than 7 days. He feels that he is getting worse. When you ask him what medication he is taking, he reports that he is using a nasal spray that you had recommended the last time he was congested.

Antitussives

Antitussive agents suppress cough by depressing the cough center in the medulla oblongata or the cough receptors in the throat, trachea, or lungs. Centrally acting antitussives include narcotics (e.g., codeine, hydrocodone) and non-narcotics (e.g., dextromethorphan). Locally acting agents (e.g., throat lozenges, cough drops) may suppress cough by increasing the flow of saliva and by containing demulcents or local anesthetics to decrease irritation of pharyngeal mucosa. Flavored syrups are often used as vehicles for other drugs.

The major clinical indication for use of antitussives is a dry, hacking, nonproductive cough that interferes with rest and sleep. It is not desirable to suppress a productive cough because the secretions need to be removed. Although antitussives continue to be used and adults report beneficial effects in reducing cough, antitussives, particularly dextromethorphan, has not been demonstrated to be effective in children and adolescents. The American Academy of Pediatrics and several other groups advise against the use of antitussives in children and adolescents.

Expectorants

Expectorants are agents given orally to liquefy respiratory secretions and allow for their easier removal. Guaifenesin is the most commonly used expectorant, because the drug reduces the viscosity of tenacious secretions by increasing respiratory tract fluid. It is available alone and as an ingredient in many combination cough and cold remedies, although research studies do not support its effectiveness and many authorities do not recommend its use.

Mucolytics

Mucolytics are administered by inhalation to liquefy mucus in the respiratory tract. Solutions of mucolytic drugs may be nebulized into a face mask or mouthpiece or instilled directly into the respiratory tract through a tracheostomy. Sodium chloride solution and acetylcysteine (Mucomyst) are the only agents recommended for use as mucolytics. Acetylcysteine is effective within 1 minute after inhalation, and maximal effects occur within 5 to 10 minutes. It is effective immediately after direct instillation. Oral acetylcysteine is widely used in the treatment of acetaminophen overdosage (see Chap. 7).

Cold Remedies

Many combination products are available for treating symptoms of the common cold. Many of the products contain an antihistamine, a nasal decongestant, and an analgesic. Some contain antitussives, expectorants, and other agents as well. Many cold remedies are over-the-counter (OTC) formulations. Commonly used ingredients include chlorpheniramine (antihistamine), pseudoephedrine (adrenergic nasal decongestant), acetaminophen (analgesic and antipyretic), dextromethorphan (antitussive), and guaifenesin (expectorant). Although antihistamines are popular OTC drugs because they dry nasal secretions, they are not recommended because they can also dry lower respiratory secretions and worsen secretion retention and cough. The use of OTC products containing pseudoephedrine to manufacture methamphetamine has increased at an alarming rate. Most states have passed laws placing these products behind pharmacy counters to restrict and control sales.

Many products come in several formulations, with different ingredients, and are advertised for different purposes (e.g., allergy, sinus disorders, multisymptom cold and flu remedies). For example, allergy remedies contain an antihistamine; "nondrowsy" or "daytime" formulas contain a nasal decongestant, but do not contain an antihistamine; "PM" or "night" formulas contain a sedating antihistamine to promote sleep; pain, fever, and multisymptom formulas usually contain acetaminophen; and "maximum strength" preparations usually refer only to the amount of acetaminophen per dose, usually 1000 milligrams for adults. In addition, labels on OTC combination products list ingredients by generic name, without identifying the type of drug. As a result of these bewildering products, consumers, including nurses and other health care providers, may not know what medications they are taking or whether some drugs increase or block the effects of other drugs.

The use of antivirals for cold treatment has also increased in popularity. **Oseltamivir** (Tamiflu) limits spread of virus within the respiratory tract and may also prevent virus penetration of respiratory secretions to initiate replication. Oseltamivir has activity against influenza A and B. Although the drug was effective in community-acquired colds caused by rhinoviruses in two placebo-controlled trials, there is not sufficient evidence to support its use in viral upper respiratory tract infections.

Applying Your Knowledge 46-3

Mr. Hobbs also complains of a productive cough. He has been taking chlorpheniramine to treat it. What advice should you give to Mr. Hobbs with regard to the appropriate treatment of a productive cough?

Individual Drugs

Individual decongestants, antitussives, expectorants, and mucolytics are listed in Table 46-1; selected combination products are listed in Table 46-2.

Herbal and Dietary Supplements

Several supplements are commonly used to prevent or treat symptoms of the common cold. While labeled as "natural," these supplements have effects with or on prescription medications. In general, there is limited or no support for such use.

Echinacea preparations differ in chemical composition depending on which of the nine species or parts of the plant (e.g., leaves, roots, whole plant) are used as well as the season of harvesting. Also, which constituents of the plants are phar-

macologically active is unclear. A Cochrane review concluded that there is no conclusive evidence that echinacea products effectively treat or prevent the common cold.

Vitamin C is used to reduce the incidence and severity of colds and influenza. No unequivocal evidence suggests that vitamin C shortens the duration of colds and alleviates its symptoms in adults, although clinical trials with adults have been partially positive. The therapeutic benefit of vitamin C in reducing cold incidence and severity in children has not been demonstrated.

Zinc gluconate lozenges are marketed as a cold remedy. However, some studies indicate beneficial effects and others do not. Most of the studies suggesting benefit are considered flawed in methodology. For example, although some studies were supposed to be blind, the lozenges' distinctive taste likely allowed the drug to be distinguished from a placebo. More recently, nasal zinc preparations (Cold-Eeze, Zycam) have been developed, and the possible risk of loss of smell posed by nasal zinc likely outweighs any benefit.

Table 46-1 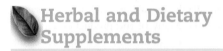	**Drugs at a Glance:** Nasal Decongestants, Antitussives, Expectorants and Mucolytics	
	ROUTES AND DOSAGE RANGES	
Generic/Trade Name	**Adults**	**Children**
Nasal Decongestants		
Naphazoline (Privine) 0.05% spray or drops	Topically, 1–2 sprays or drops no more often than q6h. Maximum, 4 doses/24 h; not to exceed 3 continuous d	12 y *and older:* Same as adults *under 12 y:* Not recommended
Oxymetazoline (Afrin) 0.05% spray	Topically, 2–3 sprays in each nostril, q10–12h. Maximum, 2 doses/24 h	6 y *and older:* Same as adults *under 6 y:* Not recommended
Phenylephrine (Neo-Synephrine)	PO 10–20 mg q4h. Maximum, 120 mg/24 h Topically, 1–2 sprays or drops of 0.25%, 0.5%, or 1% solution in each nostril no more often than q4h. Maximum, 6 doses/24 h. not to exceed 3 continuous d	12 y *and older:* Same as adults 6–11 y: PO 10 mg q4h. Maximum, 60 mg/24 h Topically, 1–2 sprays or drops of 0.25% solution in each nostril no more often than q4h. Maximum, 6 doses/24 h. Not to exceed 3 continuous d 2–5 y: Topically, 1–2 sprays or drops of 0.125% solution no more often than q4h. Maximum 6 doses/24 h. Not to exceed 3 continuous d
Pseudoephedrine (Sudafed, Dimetapp)	Regular tablets, PO 30 mg q4–6 h Extended-release tablets, PO 120 mg q12h or 240 mg q24h. Maximum, 240 mg in 24 h	12 y *and older:* Same as adults for regular and extended-release tablets 6–12 y: 30 mg q4–6h. Maximum, 120 mg/24 h 2–5 y: PO 15 mg q4–6h. Maximum, 60 mg/24 h *under 2 y:* PO: 4 mg/kg /day in divided doses q6 h
Narcotic Antitussive		
Codeine	PO 10–20 mg q4–6h. Maximum, 120 mg/24 h	6–12 y: PO 5–10 mg q4–6h. Maximum, 60 mg/24 h 2–6 y: PO 2.5–5 mg q4–6h. Maximum, 30 mg/24 h

ROUTES AND DOSAGE RANGES

Generic/Trade Name	Adults	Children
Hydrocodone bitrartate (Hycodan)	PO 1 (5 mg) tablet q4–6h up to 6 daily	Not recommended
Non-Narcotic Antitussive		
Dextromethorphan (Benylin DM, others)	Liquid, lozenges, and syrup, 10–30 mg q4–8h. Maximum, 120 mg/24 h Sustained-action liquid (Delsym), PO 60 mg q12h	*12 y and older:* Same as adults *6–12 y:* 5–10 mg q4h or 15 mg q6–8h; Maximum, 60 mg/24 h *2–6 y:* 2.5–7.5 mg q4–8h. Maximum, 30 mg/24 h Sustained-action liquid, *6–12 y:* 30 mg q12h *2–5 y:* 15 mg q12h
Expectorant		
Guaifenesin (glyceryl guaiacolate) (Robitussin, others)	PO 100–400 mg q4h. Maximum, 2400 mg/24 h	*12 y and older:* Same as adults *6–12 y:* PO 100–200 mg q4h. Maximum, 1200 mg/24 h *2–6 y:* PO 50–100 mg q4h. Maximum, 600 mg/24 h
Mucolytic		
Acetylcysteine (Mucomyst)	Nebulization, 1–10 mL of a 20% solution or 2–20 mL of a 10% solution q2–6h Instillation, 1–2 mL of a 10% or 20% solution q1–4h Acetaminophen overdosage, PO 140 mg/kg initially, then 70 mg/kg q4h for 17 doses; dilute a 10% or 20% solution to a 5% solution with cola, fruit juice, or water	Acetaminophen overdosage, see literature

Table 46-2		**Drugs at a Glance:** Representative Multi-Ingredient Nonprescription Cold, Cough, and Sinus Remedies			

	INGREDIENTS				
Trade Name	**Antihistamine**	**Nasal Decongestant**	**Analgesic**	**Antitussive**	**Expoectorant**
Actifed Cold & Allergy	Triprolidine 2.5 mg/tablet	Pseudoephedrine 60 mg/tablet			
Advil Cold and Sinus Tablets		Pseudoephedrine 30 mg/tablet	Ibuprofen 200 mg/tablet		
Cheracol D Cough Liquid				Dextromethorphan 10 mg/5 mL	Guaifenesin 100 mg/5 mL
Comtrex Cold & Sinus Tablets	Brompheniramine 2 mg/tablet	Pseudoephedrine 30 mg/tablet	Acetaminophen 500 mg/tablet		
Contac Day & Night Cold & Flu Tablets	(Night) Diphen-hydramine 50 mg/tablet	Pseudoephedrine 60 mg/tablet	Acetaminophen 650 mg/tablet	(Day) Dex-tromethorphan 30 mg/tablet	
Coricidin D Cold, Flu & Sinus Tablets	Chlorpheniramine 2 mg/tablet	Pseudoephedrine 30 mg/tablet	Acetaminophen 325 mg/tablet		

(continued on page 750)

| Table 46-2 | **Drugs at a Glance:** Representative Multi-Ingredient Nonprescription Cold, Cough, and Sinus Remedies (continued) | | | | |

	INGREDIENTS				
Trade Name	**Antihistamine**	**Nasal Decongestant**	**Analgesic**	**Antitussive**	**Expoectorant**
Dimetapp Cold and Allergy Elixir	Brompheniramine 1 mg/5 mL	Pseudoephedrine 15 mg/5 mL			
Dristan Cold Formula	Chlorpheniramine 2 mg/tablet	Phenylephrine 5 mg/tablet	Acetaminophen 325 mg/tablet		
Motrin Sinus Tablets		Pseudoephedrine 30 mg/tablet	Ibuprofen 200 mg/tablet		
Robitussin Cold and Flu Tablets		Pseudoephedrine 10 mg/tablet	Acetaminophen 325 mg/tablet	Dextromethorphan 30 mg/tablet	Guaifenesin 200 mg/tablet
Sinutab Sinus Allergy Maximum Strength Tablets	Chlorpheniramine 2 mg/tablet	Pseudoephedrine 30 mg/tablet	Acetaminophen 500 mg/tablet	Dextromethorphan 10 mg/tablet	
TheraFlu Flu, Cold, and Cough Powder	Chlorpheniramine 4 mg/pack	Pseudoephedrine 60 mg/pack	Acetaminophen 650 mg/pack	Dextromethorphan 20 mg/pack	
Vicks NyQuil Cold & Flu Capsules	Doxylamine 6.25 mg/capsule	Pseudoephedrine 30 mg/capsule	Acetaminophen 250 mg/capsule	Dextromethorphan 10 mg/capsule	

Nursing Process

Assessment

Assess the patient's condition in relation to disorders for which the drugs are used.

- With nasal congestion, observe for decreased ability to breathe through the nose. If nasal discharge is present, note the amount, color, and thickness. Question the patient about the duration and extent of nasal congestion and factors that precipitate or relieve the symptom.

- With coughing, a major assessment factor is whether the cough is productive of sputum or dry and hacking. If the cough is productive, note the color, odor, viscosity, and amount of sputum. In addition, assess factors that stimulate or relieve cough and the patient's ability and willingness to cough effectively.

- Assess fluid intake and hydration status.

Nursing Diagnoses

- Risk for Injury related to cardiac dysrhythmias, hypertension, and other adverse effects of nasal decongestants
- Noncompliance: Overuse of nasal decongestants
- Deficient Knowledge: Appropriate use of single- and multi-ingredient drug formulations

Planning/Goals

The patient will

- Experience relief of symptoms
- Take drugs accurately and safely
- Avoid overuse of decongestants
- Avoid preventable adverse drug effects
- Act to avoid recurrence of symptoms

Interventions

Encourage patients to use measures to prevent or minimize the incidence and severity of symptoms:

- Avoid smoking cigarettes or breathing secondhand smoke, when possible. Cigarette smoke irritates respiratory tract mucosa, and this irritation causes cough, increased secretions, and decreased effectiveness of cilia in cleaning the respiratory tract.

- Avoid or limit exposure to crowds, especially during winter when the incidence of colds and influenza is high.

- Avoid contact with people who have colds or other respiratory infections. This is especially important for patients with chronic lung disease, because upper respiratory infections may precipitate acute attacks of asthma or bronchitis.

- Maintain a fluid intake of 2000 to 3000 mL daily unless contraindicated by cardiovascular or renal disease.

- Maintain nutrition, rest, activity, and other general health measures.
- Practice good hand hygiene techniques.
- Annual vaccination for influenza is recommended for patients who are elderly or have chronic respiratory, cardiovascular, or renal disorders.
- Provide appropriate teaching related to drug therapy (see accompanying display).

Evaluation

- Interview and observe for relief of symptoms.
- Interview and observe for tachycardia, hypertension, drowsiness, and other adverse drug effects.
- Interview and observe for compliance with instructions about drug use.

Principles Of Therapy

Drug Selection and Administration

Choice of drugs and routes of administration are influenced by several patient- and drug-related variables. Some guidelines include the following:

- Single-drug formulations allow flexibility and individualization of dosage, whereas combination products may contain unneeded ingredients and are more expensive. However, many people find combination products more convenient to use.
- With nasal decongestants, topical preparations (i.e., nasal solutions or sprays) are often preferred for short-term use. They are rapidly effective because they come into direct contact with nasal mucosa. If used longer than the recommended 3 days or in excessive amounts, however, these products may produce rebound nasal congestion. Oral drugs

Patient Teaching Guidelines — Nasal Decongestants, Anticough Medications, and Multi-Ingredient Cold Remedies

General Considerations

- These drugs may relieve symptoms but do not cure the disorder causing the symptoms.
- An adequate fluid intake, humidification of the environment, and sucking on hard candy or throat lozenges can help relieve mouth dryness and cough.
- Over-the-counter (OTC) cold remedies should not be used longer than 1 week. Do not use nose drops or sprays more often or longer than recommended. Excessive or prolonged use may damage nasal mucosa and produce chronic nasal congestion.
- Do not increase dosage if symptoms are not relieved by recommended amounts.
- See a health care provider if symptoms persist longer than 1 week.
- Inform health care providers about any herbal supplements that are being taken.
- Read the labels of OTC allergy, cold, and sinus remedies for information about ingredients, dosages, conditions or other medications with which the drugs should not be taken, and adverse effects.
- Do not combine two drug preparations containing the same or similar active ingredients. For example, pseudoephedrine is the nasal decongestant component of most prescription and OTC sinus and multi-ingredient cold remedies. The recommended dose for immediate-release preparations is usually 30 to 60 mg of pseudoephedrine; doses in extended-release preparations are usually 120 mg. Taking more than one preparation containing pseudoephedrine (or phenylephrine, a similar drug) may increase dosage to toxic levels and cause irregular heartbeats and extreme nervousness.
- Note that many combination products contain acetaminophen or ibuprofen as pain relievers. If you are taking

another form of one of these drugs (e.g., Tylenol or Advil), there is a risk of overdosage and adverse effects. Acetaminophen can cause liver damage; ibuprofen is a relative of aspirin that can cause gastrointestinal upset and bleeding. Thus, you need to be sure your total daily dosage is not excessive (with Tylenol, above four doses of 1000 mg each; with ibuprofen, above 2400 mg).

- Individuals with diabetes mellitus should read OTC labels for sugar content because many decongestants and cough medicines may contain sucrose, glucose, or corn syrup as a base.

Self-Administration

- Take medications as prescribed or as directed on the labels of OTC preparations. Taking excessive amounts or taking recommended amounts too often can lead to serious adverse effects.
- Do not chew or crush long-acting tablets or capsules (e.g., those taken once or twice daily). Such actions can cause rapid drug absorption, high blood levels, and serious adverse effects, rather than the slow absorption and prolonged action intended with these products.
- For OTC drugs available in different dosage strengths, start with lower recommended doses rather than "maximum strength" formulations or the highest recommended doses. It is safer to see how the drugs affect you, then increase doses if necessary and not contraindicated.
- With topical nasal decongestants:
  1. Use only preparations labeled for intranasal use. For example, phenylephrine (Neo-Synephrine) is available in both nasal and eye formulations. The two types of solutions cannot be used interchangeably. In addition, phenylephrine preparations may contain 0.125%, 0.25%, 0.5%, or 1% of drug. Be sure the

(continued on page 752)

are preferred for long-term use (>7 days). For patients with cardiovascular disease, topical nasal decongestants are usually preferred. Oral agents are usually contraindicated because of cardiovascular effects (e.g., increased force of myocardial contraction, increased heart rate, increased blood pressure).

■ Antihistamines are clearly useful in allergic conditions (e.g., allergic rhinitis; see Chap. 45), but their use to relieve cold symptoms is controversial. First-generation antihistamines (e.g., chlorpheniramine, diphenhydramine) have anticholinergic effects that may reduce sneezing, rhinorrhea, and cough. Also, their sedative effects may aid sleep. Many multi-ingredient cold remedies contain an antihistamine.

■ Cough associated with the common cold usually stems from postnasal drainage and throat irritation. Most antitussives are given orally as tablets or cough syrups. Syrups serve as vehicles for antitussive drugs and may exert antitussive effects of their own by soothing irritated pharyngeal mucosa. Dextromethorphan is the antitussive drug of choice in most circumstances and is the antitussive ingredient in almost all OTC cough remedies (often designated by "DM" on the product label). However, as discussed previously, some authorities question the effectiveness of antitussives and do not recommend them for use in children or adults.

■ Ipratropium (Atrovent), an anticholinergic drug, in a 0.06% nasal spray, is U.S. Food and Drug Administration (FDA) approved for treatment of rhinorrhea associated with the common cold.

■ Cromolyn, a mast cell stabilizer, used by oral or intranasal inhalation, seems effective in reducing the symptoms and duration of the common cold but it is not FDA approved for this purpose. In one study, it was used every 2 hours for the first 2 days, then 4 times daily. The nasal solution (Nasalcrom) is available OTC.

■ For treatment of excessive respiratory tract secretions, mechanical measures (e.g., coughing, deep breathing, ambu-

lation, chest physiotherapy, forcing fluids) are more likely to be effective than expectorant drug therapy.

Use in Special Populations

Use in Children

Upper respiratory infections with nasal congestion, sore throat, cough, and increased secretions are common in children, and the drugs described in this chapter are often used. Several OTC cough and cold medicines for use in infants have been recalled voluntarily by U.S. manufacturers due to concerns about possible misuse that could result in overdoses. Recommendations from consumer groups advising against the use of OTC cough and cold medicines in children less than 2 years of age have been submitted to the FDA. More research is needed regarding dosage, safety, and effectiveness of cough and cold mixtures in children. Some considerations include the following:

Evidence-Based Practice

46-1 Cough and the Common Cold

The American College of Chest Physicians (ACCP) published evidence-based clinical practice guidelines regarding cough and the common cold. Pharmacologic recommendations include the following:

■ Treatment of individuals with the common cold experiencing acute cough, postnasal drip, and throat clearing with a first-generation antihistamine/decongestant preparation (sustained-release pseudoephedrine and brompheniramine) is recommended. Naproxen can also be taken to help decrease cough in this group.

■ Newer generation, nonsedating antihistamines are ineffective for reducing cough and should not be used in individuals with the common cold (ACCP, 2006).

- Most–upper respiratory infections are viral in origin, and antibiotics are not generally recommended. For sore throat, a throat culture for streptococcus organisms should be performed and the results obtained before an antibiotic is prescribed. For bronchitis, which is almost always viral, antibiotics are not usually indicated unless pneumonia is suspected or the cough lasts 10 to 14 days without improvement.
- Cough medicines are not considered effective by some authorities.
- With nasal decongestants, pseudoephedrine is considered effective in children older than 5 years of age, but research studies are inconclusive about its effectiveness in younger children. One consideration is that the low doses found in children's preparations may be insufficient to produce therapeutic effects. As a result, some pediatricians do not recommend usage, whereas others say the drug may be useful in some children.
- Nasal congestion may interfere with an infant's ability to nurse. Phenylephrine nasal solution, applied just before feeding time, is usually effective. However, excessive amounts or too-frequent administration of topical agents may result in rebound nasal congestion and systemic effects of cardiac and central nervous system stimulation. Therefore, the drug should be given to infants only when recommended by a pediatric specialist.
- Parents often administer a medication (e.g., acetaminophen, ibuprofen) for pain and fever when a child has cold symptoms, whether the child has pain and fever or not.

Some pediatricians suggest treating fevers above 101 degrees if the child seems uncomfortable but not to treat them otherwise. Parents may need to be counseled that fever is part of the body's defense mechanism and may help the child recover from an infection.

Use in Older Adults

A major consideration is that older adults are at high risk of adverse effects from oral nasal decongestants (e.g., hypertension, cardiac dysrhythmias, nervousness, insomnia). Adverse effects from topical agents are less likely, but rebound nasal congestion and systemic effects may occur with overuse. Older adults with significant cardiovascular disease should avoid the drugs. Also, as in other populations, antitussives and expectorants have questionable effectiveness.

Use in Home Care

These drugs are used primarily in home settings, and household members may ask the home care nurse for advice about OTC remedies for conditions such as allergies, colds, coughs, and sinus headaches. Before recommending a particular product, the nurse needs to assess the intended recipient for conditions or other medications that contraindicate the product's use. For example, the nasal decongestant component may cause or aggravate cardiovascular disorders (e.g., hypertension). In addition, other medications the patient is taking need to be evaluated in terms of potential drug interactions with the remedy. The home care nurse also must emphasize the need to read the label of any OTC medication for ingredients, precautions, contraindications, drug interactions, administration instructions, and so forth.

Nursing Actions Nasal Decongestants, Antitussives, and Cold Remedies

NURSING ACTIONS	RATIONALE/EXPLANATION
1. Administer accurately	
a. With topical nasal decongestants:	
(1) Use only preparations labeled for intranasal use.	Intranasal preparations are usually dilute, aqueous solutions prepared specifically for intranasal use. Some agents (e.g., phenylephrine) are available in ophthalmic solutions as well. The two types of solutions cannot be used inter-changeably.
(2) Use the drug concentration ordered.	Some drug preparations are available in several concentrations. For example, phenylephrine preparations may contain 0.125%, 0.25%, 0.5%, or 1% of drug.
(3) For instillation of nose drops, have the patient lie down or sit with the neck hyperextended. Instill medication without touching the dropper to the nares. Rinse the medication dropper after each use.	To avoid contamination of the dropper and medication
(4) For nasal sprays, have the patient sit, squeeze the container once to instill medication, avoid touching the spray tip to the nares, and rinse the spray tip after each use.	Most nasal sprays are designed to deliver one dose when used correctly. If necessary, secretions may be cleared and a second spray used. Correct usage and cleansing prevents contamination and infection.
(5) Give nasal decongestants to infants 20–30 minutes before feeding.	Nasal congestion interferes with an infant's ability to suck.
b. Administer cough syrups undiluted and instruct the patient to avoid eating and drinking for approximately 30 minutes.	Part of the therapeutic benefit of cough syrups stems from soothing effects on pharyngeal mucosa. Food or fluid removes the medication from the pharynx.

(continued on page 754)

Nursing Actions — Nasal Decongestants, Antitussives, and Cold Remedies (continued)

NURSING ACTIONS	RATIONALE/EXPLANATION
2. Observe for therapeutic effects	Therapeutic effects depend on the reason for use.
a. When nasal decongestants are given, observe for decreased nasal obstruction and drainage.	
b. With antitussives, observe for decreased coughing.	The goal of antitussive therapy is to suppress nonpurposeful coughing, not productive coughing.
c. With cold and allergy remedies, observe for decreased nasal congestion, rhinitis, muscle aches, and other symptoms.	
3. Observe for adverse effects	
a. With nasal decongestants, observe for:	
(1) Tachycardia, cardiac dysrhythmias, hypertension	These effects may occur with any of the adrenergic drugs (see Chap. 17). When adrenergic drugs are used as nasal decongestants, cardiovascular effects are more likely to occur with oral agents. However, topically applied drugs also may be systemically absorbed through the nasal mucosa or by being swallowed and absorbed through the gastrointestinal tract. Adverse effects on nasal mucosa are more likely to occur with excessive or long-term (>10 d) use.
(2) Rebound nasal congestion, chronic rhinitis, and possible ulceration of nasal mucosa	
b. With antitussives, observe for:	
(1) Excessive suppression of the cough reflex (inability to cough effectively when secretions are present)	This is a potentially serious adverse effect because retained secretions may lead to atelectasis, pneumonia, hypoxia, hypercarbia, and respiratory failure.
(2) Nausea, vomiting, constipation, dizziness, drowsiness, pruritus, and drug dependence	These are adverse effects associated with narcotic agents (see Chap. 6). When narcotics are given for antitussive effects, however, they are given in relatively small doses and are unlikely to cause adverse reactions.
(3) Nausea, drowsiness, and dizziness with non-narcotic antitussives	Adverse effects are infrequent and mild with these agents.
c. With combination products (e.g., cold remedies), observe for adverse effects of individual ingredients (i.e., antihistamines, adrenergics, analgesics, and others).	Adverse effects are rarely significant when the products are used as prescribed. There may be subtherapeutic doses of one or more component drugs, especially in over-the-counter formulations. Also, the drowsiness associated with antihistamines may be offset by stimulating effects of adrenergics. Ephedrine, for example, has central nervous system (CNS)–stimulating effects.
4. Observe for drug interactions	
a. Drugs that *increase* effects of nasal decongestants:	These interactions are more likely to occur with oral decongestants than topically applied drugs.
(1) Cocaine, digoxin, general anesthetics, monoamine oxidase (MAO) inhibitors, other adrenergic drugs, thyroid preparations, and xanthines	Increased risks of cardiac dysrhythmias
(2) Antihistamines, epinephrine, ergot alkaloids, MAO inhibitors, methylphenidate	Increased risks of hypertension due to vasoconstriction
b. Drugs that *increase* antitussive effects of codeine:	
(1) CNS depressants (alcohol, antianxiety agents, barbiturates, and other sedative-hypnotics)	Additive CNS depression. Codeine is given in small doses for antitussive effects, and risks of significant interactions are minimal.
c. Drugs that *alter* effects of dextromethorphan:	
(1) MAO inhibitors	This combination is contraindicated. Apnea, muscular rigidity, hyperpyrexia, laryngospasm, and death may occur.
d. Drugs that may *alter* effects of combination products for coughs, colds, and allergies:	Interactions depend on the individual drug components of each formulation. Risks of clinically significant drug interactions are increased with use of combination products.
(1) Adrenergic (sympathomimetic) agents (see Chap. 17)	
(2) Antihistamines (see Chap. 45)	
(3) CNS depressants (see Chaps. 6, 8, and 13)	
(4) CNS stimulants (see Chap. 15)	

Key Concepts

- Most upper respiratory infections are viral in origin, and antibiotics are not generally recommended.

- Retention of secretions commonly occurs with influenza, pneumonia, upper respiratory infections, acute and chronic bronchitis, emphysema, and acute attacks of asthma.

- Nonrespiratory conditions that predispose to secretion retention include immobility, debilitation, cigarette smoking, and postoperative status.

- An adequate fluid intake, humidification of the environment, and sucking on hard candy or throat lozenges can help relieve mouth dryness and cough.

- Rebound nasal swelling can occur with excessive or extended use of nasal sprays.

- First-generation antihistamines (e.g., chlorpheniramine, diphenhydramine) have anticholinergic effects that may reduce sneezing, rhinorrhea, and cough.

- There is limited or no support for the use of dietary or herbal supplements to prevent or treat symptoms of the common cold.

- Several OTC cough and cold medicines for use in infants have been recalled voluntarily due to concerns about possible misuse that could result in overdoses.

Review and Application Exercises

Short Answer Exercises

1. How do adrenergic drugs relieve nasal congestion?

2. Who should usually avoid OTC nasal decongestants and cold remedies?

3. What are advantages and disadvantages of multi-ingredient cold remedies?

4. In a patient with a productive cough, what are nondrug interventions to promote removal of secretions?

5. A patient who uses echinacea, vitamin C, or zinc lozenges asks you what you think about the products as cold remedies. How would you reply?

NCLEX-Style Questions

6. A common mucolytic used to liquefy mucus in the respiratory tract is
   a. acetylcysteine (Mucomyst)
   b. ipratropium (Atrovent)
   c. dextromethorphan
   d. pseudoephedrine (Sudafed)

7. In caring for a patient with nasal congestion, the nurse knows that adrenergic drugs are used as nasal decongestants to relieve symptoms by

   a. constricting arterioles and reducing blood flow to nasal mucosa
   b. stimulating air movement in the lungs
   c. stabilizing mast cells
   d. initiating the cough reflex

8. As the nurse caring for a patient with nasal congestion who is using the over-the-counter decongestant oxymetazoline (Afrin), you counsel the patient that this medication should only be used for the time recommended on the package and not for longer use because excessive use may produce
   a. copious lower respiratory tract secretions
   b. ringing in the ears
   c. rebound nasal congestion
   d. a suppressed cough reflex

9. Cold remedies listed as "nondrowsy" or labeled as being "daytime" formulas do not contain
   a. a nasal decongestant
   b. a first-generation antihistamine
   c. a pain reliever
   d. any of the above

Selected References

Bolser, D. C. (2006). Cough suppressant and pharmacologic protussive therapy: ACCP evidence-based clinical practice guidelines. *Chest, 129*(1 Suppl), 238S–249S.

Corwin, E. J. (2006). *Handbook of pathophysiology* (3rd ed.). Philadelphia: Lippincott Williams & Wilkins.

Drug facts and comparisons. (Updated monthly). St. Louis, MO: Facts and Comparisons.

Guyton, A. C., & Hall, J. E. (2006). *Textbook of medical physiology* (11th ed.). Philadelphia: W. B. Saunders.

Karch, A. M. (2007). *2008 Lippincott's nursing drug guide*. Philadelphia: Lippincott Williams & Wilkins.

Lacy, C. F., Armstrong, L. L., Goldman, M. P., & Lance, L. L. (2007). *Lexi-Comp's drug information handbook* (15th ed.). Hudson, OH: American Pharmaceutical Association.

Porth, C. M. (2005). *Pathophysiology: Concepts of altered health states* (7th ed.). Philadelphia: Lippincott Williams & Wilkins.

Pratter, M. R. (2006). Cough and the common cold: ACCP evidence-based clinical practice guidelines. *Chest, 129*(1 Suppl), 72S–74S.

Simasek, M., & Blandino, D. A. (2007). Treatment of the common cold. *American Family Physician, 75*, 515–520.

Chapter Outline

Physiology of the Cardiovascular System

LEARNING OBJECTIVES

After studying this chapter, you will be able to:

1. Recognize the functions of the heart, blood vessels, and blood in supplying oxygen and nutrients to body tissues.
2. Describe the role of vascular endothelium in maintaining homeostasis.
3. Discuss atherosclerosis as the basic disorder causing many cardiovascular disorders for which drug therapy is required.
4. Manage the care of individuals with cardiovascular disorders for which drug therapy is a major treatment modality.

Introduction

The cardiovascular or circulatory system is composed of the heart, blood vessels, and blood. The general functions of the system are to carry oxygen, nutrients, hormones, antibodies, and other substances to all body cells and to remove waste products of cell metabolism (carbon dioxide and others). The efficiency of the system depends on the heart's ability to pump blood, the patency and functions of blood vessels, and the quality and quantity of blood.

Heart

The heart is a hollow, muscular organ that functions as a two-sided pump to circulate 5 to 6 liters of blood through the body every minute. Major components and characteristics are identified in Figure 47-1 and described in the following sections.

Chambers of the Heart

The heart has four chambers: two atria and two ventricles. The *atria* are receiving chambers. The right atrium receives deoxygenated blood from the upper part of the body by way of the superior vena cava, from the lower part of the body by way of the inferior vena cava, and from veins and sinuses within the heart itself. The left atrium receives oxygenated blood from the lungs through the pulmonary veins. The *ventricles* are distributing chambers. The right ventricle sends deoxygenated blood through the pulmonary circulation. It is small and thin walled because it contracts against minimal pressure. The left ventricle pumps oxygenated blood through the systemic circuit. It is much more muscular and thick walled because it contracts against relatively high pressure. The right atrium and right ventricle form one pump, and the left atrium and left ventricle form another. A muscular wall called the *septum* separates the right and left sides of the heart.

Layers of the Heart

The layers of the heart are the endocardium, myocardium, and epicardium. The *endocardium* is the membrane lining the heart chambers. It is continuous with the endothelial lining of blood vessels

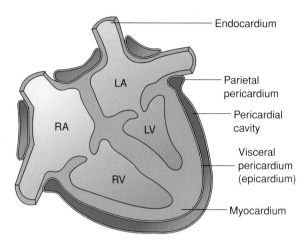

Figure 47-1 ▪ Layers of the heart, showing the visceral pericardium, the pericardial cavity, and the parietal pericardium. RA, right atrium; LA, left atrium; RV, right ventricle; LV, left ventricle.

entering and leaving the heart, and it covers the heart valves. The *myocardium* is the strong muscular layer of the heart that provides the pumping power for circulation of blood. The *epicardium* is the outer, serous layer of the heart. The heart is enclosed in a fibroserous sac called the *pericardium*.

Heart Valves

Heart valves function to maintain the one-way flow of blood and prevent backflow. The mitral valve separates the left atrium and left ventricle. The tricuspid valve separates the right atrium and right ventricle. The pulmonic valve separates the right ventricle and pulmonary artery. The aortic valve separates the left ventricle and aorta.

Conduction System

The heart contains special cells that can carry electrical impulses much more rapidly than ordinary muscle fibers. This special conduction system consists of the sinoatrial (SA) node, the atrioventricular node, bundle of His, right and left bundle branches, and Purkinje fibers. The SA node, the normal pacemaker of the heart, generates a burst of electrical energy approximately 60 to 100 times each minute under normal circumstances. The electrical current flows over the heart in an orderly way to produce contraction of both atria, then both ventricles. An expanded discussion of cardiac conduction is found in Chapter 49.

A unique characteristic of the heart is that any cell in any chamber can generate its own electrical impulse to contract. For example, the ventricles can beat independently, but at a rate of less than 40 beats per minute. This provides a backup mechanism should the SA node fail to fire, with an inherent rate that does not compete with SA node firing. In addition, the heart does not require nervous stimulation to contract. However, the autonomic nervous system does influence heart rate. Sympathetic nerves increase heart rate (through the release of epinephrine and norepinephrine); parasympathetic nerves (by way of the vagus nerve) decrease heart rate.

Blood Supply

The heart receives its blood supply from the coronary arteries. Coronary arteries originate at the base of the aorta in the aortic cusps and fill during *diastole*, the resting or filling phase of the cardiac cycle. Coronary arteries branch into smaller arteries that supply specific parts of the myocardium, without an overlapping supply from other arterial branches. However, artery-to-artery anastomoses occur between many adjacent vessels. These anastomotic arteries may not supply sufficient blood to the heart if a major artery is suddenly occluded, but they may dilate to considerable size when disease (usually coronary atherosclerosis) develops slowly. The resultant *collateral circulation* may provide a sufficient blood supply for myocardial function, at least during rest.

Blood Vessels

There are three types of blood vessels: arteries, veins, and capillaries. Arteries and veins are similar in that they have three layers. The intima, the inner lining, is composed of a layer of endothelial cells next to the blood (to provide a smooth surface for blood circulation) and an elastic layer that joins the media. The media is the middle layer of muscle and elastic tissue. The adventitia is the outer layer of connective tissue.

Blood vessel walls are composed of two types of cells, smooth muscle cells and endothelial cells. Vascular smooth muscle functions to maintain blood pressure and blood flow. It contracts and relaxes in response to numerous stimuli, including local and circulating mediators. Contractile properties also vary among blood vessels, with some being more responsive to stimuli than others. Overall, regulation of tone in vascular smooth muscle depends on the intracellular concentration of calcium ions. Increased intracellular calcium leads to increased vascular tone. There are several mechanisms by which calcium ions can enter the cell.

Endothelial cells, once thought to be passive conduits for blood flow, are now known to perform two extremely important functions in maintaining homeostatic processes. One function is structural, in which the cells act as a permeability barrier and regulate passage of molecules and cells across the blood vessel wall. The second function is metabolic, in which the cells secrete opposing mediators that maintain a balance between bleeding and clotting of blood (including activation and inhibition of platelet functions and fibrinolysis), constriction and dilation of blood vessels, and promotion and inhibition of vascular cell growth and inflammation. Selected mediators are listed in Table 47-1; some are discussed in more detail in later chapters.

Arteries

Arteries and arterioles contain a well-developed layer of smooth muscle (the media) and are sometimes called resistance vessels. Their efficiency depends on their patency and

Table 47-1	Endothelial Mediators That Regulate Cardiovascular Function	

PROMOTING FACTORS	INHIBITING FACTORS
Vasomotor Tone	
Vasodilators	**Vasoconstrictors**
Endothelial-derived hyperpolarizing factor (EDHF)	Angiotensin II
Nitric oxide (also called endothelial-derived relaxing factor, or EDRF)	Endothelin
	Endothelium-derived constricting factor
Prostacyclin (prostaglandin I_2)	Platelet-derived growth factor
	Thromboxane A_2
Blood Coagulation	
Procoagulants	**Anticoagulants**
Tissue factor	Heparin sulfate
Von Willebrand factor	Thrombomodulin
Platelet activators	**Platelet inhibitors**
Platelet-activating factor	Nitric oxide
Von Willebrand factor	Prostacyclin
Profibrinolytic factors	**Antifibrinolytic factor**
Tissue plasminogen activator (t-PA)	Plasminogen activator inhibitor-1
Urokinase-type plasminogen activator	
Cell Growth	
Angiotensin II	Heparin
Endothelin	Nitric oxide
Platelet-derived growth factor	Prostacyclin
Inflammation	
Proinflammatory factors	**Anti-inflammatory factors**
Cellular and intercellular adhesion molecules	Nitric oxide
Monocyte chemotactic protein-1	
Interleukin-8	

ability to constrict or dilate in response to various stimuli. The degree of constriction or dilation (vasomotor tone) determines peripheral vascular resistance, which is a major determinant of blood pressure.

Veins

Veins and venules have a thin media and valves that assist blood flow against gravity. They are sometimes called capacitance vessels, because blood may accumulate in various parts of the venous system. Their efficiency depends on patency, competency of valves, and the contraction and relaxation action of muscles around veins.

Capillaries

Capillaries, the smallest blood vessels, connect the arterial and venous segments of the circulation. They consist of a single layer of connected endothelial cells and a few smooth muscle cells. Gases, nutrients, cells, and waste products are exchanged between blood and extracellular fluid across capillary walls. The endothelial lining acts as a semipermeable membrane to regulate the exchange of plasma solutes with extracellular fluid. Lipid-soluble materials diffuse directly through the capillary cell membrane; water and water-soluble materials enter and leave the capillary through the junctions or gaps between endothelial cells.

Lymphatics

Lymphatic vessels, which are composed mainly of endothelium, parallel the veins and empty into the venous system. They drain tissue fluid that has filtered through the endothelium of capillaries and venules from the plasma. They then carry lymphocytes, large molecules of protein and fat, microorganisms, and other materials to regional lymph nodes.

Blood

Blood functions to nourish and oxygenate body cells, protect the body from invading microorganisms, and initiate hemostasis when a blood vessel is injured. Specific functions and components are listed in the following sections.

Functions

- Transports oxygen to cells and carbon dioxide from cells to lungs for removal from the body
- Transports absorbed food products from the gastrointestinal tract to tissues; at the same time, carries metabolic wastes from tissues to the kidneys, skin, and lungs for excretion
- Transports hormones from endocrine glands to other parts of the body
- Transports leukocytes and antibodies to sites of injury, infection, and inflammation
- Assists in regulation of body temperature by transferring heat produced by cell metabolism to the skin, where it can be released
- Transports platelets to injured areas for hemostasis

Components

- Plasma comprises approximately 55% of the total blood volume, and it is more than 90% water. Other components are
  - Serum albumin, which helps maintain blood volume by exerting colloid osmotic pressure
  - Fibrinogen, which is necessary for hemostasis
  - Gamma globulin, which is necessary for defense against microorganisms
  - Less than 1% antibodies, nutrients, metabolic wastes, respiratory gases, enzymes, and inorganic salts
- Solid particles or cells comprise approximately 45% of total blood volume. Cells include erythrocytes (red blood cells or RBCs), leukocytes (white blood cells or WBCs), and thrombocytes (platelets). The bone marrow produces all RBCs, 60% to 70% of WBCs, and all platelets. Lymphatic tissues (spleen and lymph nodes) produce 20% to 30% of WBCs, and reticuloendothelial tissues (spleen, liver, lymph nodes) produce 4% to 8% of WBCs. Cell characteristics include the following:
  - Erythrocytes function primarily to transport oxygen. Almost all oxygen (95%–97%) is transported in combination with hemoglobin; very little is dissolved in blood. The lifespan of a normal RBC is approximately 120 days.
  - Leukocytes function primarily as a defense mechanism against microorganisms. They leave the bloodstream to enter injured tissues and phagocytize the injurious agent. They also produce antibodies. The lifespan of a normal WBC is a few hours.
  - Platelets are fragments of large cells, called megakaryocytes, found in the bone marrow. Platelets are essential for blood coagulation. For example, when a blood vessel is injured, platelets adhere to each other and the edges of the injury to form a cluster of activated platelets (i.e., a platelet thrombus or "plug") that adheres to the vessel wall and prevents leakage of blood. In addition, the clus-

tered platelets release substances (e.g., adenosine diphosphate, thromboxane A_2, von Willebrand factor) that promote recruitment and aggregation of new platelets.

Platelets have no nucleus and cannot replicate. If not used, they circulate for approximately a week before being removed by phagocytic cells of the spleen.

Cardiovascular Disorders

Cardiovascular disorders, which are common causes of morbidity and mortality, often stem from blood vessel abnormalities. In turn, most vascular diseases result from the malfunction of endothelial cells or smooth muscle cells. Dysfunctional endothelium is considered a major factor in atherosclerosis, acute coronary syndromes (symptomatic myocardial ischemia, asymptomatic myocardial infarction [MI], and MI with or without ST-segment elevation), hypertension, and thromboembolic disorders. The main cause of endothelial dysfunction is injury to the blood vessel wall from trauma or disease processes. The injury alters the normal regulatory forces and leads to vasospasm, thrombosis, growth of the intimal layer of the blood vessel, rupture of atherosclerotic plaque, tissue ischemia and infarction, and dysrhythmias. Pathologic changes in the structure of the capillary and venular endothelium also result in the accumulation of excess fluid in interstitial space (edema), a common symptom of cardiovascular and other disorders.

Overall, cardiovascular disorders may involve any structure or function of the cardiovascular system. Because the circulatory system is a closed system, a disorder in one part of the system eventually disturbs the function of all other parts.

Drug Therapy Used for Cardiovascular Disorders

Cardiovascular disorders usually managed with drug therapy include atherosclerosis, heart failure, cardiac dysrhythmias, ischemia, myocardial infarction, hypertension, hypotension, and shock. Peripheral vascular disease and valvular disease are usually managed surgically. Blood disorders that respond to drug therapy include certain types of anemia and coagulation disorders.

The goal of drug therapy in cardiovascular disorders is to restore homeostasis or physiologic balance between opposing factors (e.g., coagulant vs. anticoagulant, vasoconstriction vs. vasodilation). Cardiovascular drugs may be given to increase or decrease cardiac output, blood pressure, and heart rate; to alter heart rhythm; to increase or decrease blood clotting; to alter the quality of blood; and to decrease chest pain of cardiac origin. In addition, these drugs may be given for palliation of symptoms without alteration of the underlying disease process.

Key Concepts

- The efficiency of the cardiovascular system depends on the heart's ability to pump blood, the patency and functions of blood vessels, and the quality and quantity of blood.

- Heart valves function to maintain the one-way flow of blood and prevent backflow.

- A unique characteristic of the heart is that any cell in any chamber can generate its own electrical impulse to contract at an inherent rate that does not compete with SA node firing; this provides a backup mechanism should the SA node fail to fire.

- Coronary arteries originate at the base of the aorta in the aortic cusps and fill during diastole, the resting or filling phase of the cardiac cycle.

- Blood functions to nourish and oxygenate body cells, protect the body from invading microorganisms, and initiate hemostasis when a blood vessel is injured.

- Dysfunctional endothelium is considered a major factor in atherosclerosis, acute coronary syndromes, hypertension, and thromboembolic disorders.

- The goal of drug therapy in cardiovascular disorders is to restore homeostasis or physiologic balance between opposing factors (e.g., coagulant vs. anticoagulant, vasoconstriction vs. vasodilation).

- Cardiovascular drugs may be given to increase or decrease cardiac output, blood pressure, and heart rate; to alter heart rhythm; to increase or decrease blood clotting; to alter the quality of blood; and to decrease chest pain of cardiac origin.

Review and Application Exercises

Short Answer Exercises

1. How does the heart muscle differ from skeletal muscle?

2. What is the normal pacemaker of the heart?

3. In what circumstances do other parts of the heart take over as pacemaker?

4. What is the effect of parasympathetic (vagal) stimulation on the heart?

5. What is the effect of sympathetic stimulation on the heart and blood vessels?

6. List five chemical mediators produced by endothelial cells and their roles in maintaining cardiovascular function.

7. How does endothelial cell dysfunction contribute to cardiovascular disorders?

Selected References

Corwin, E. J. (2006). *Handbook of pathophysiology* (3rd ed.). Philadelphia: Lippincott Williams & Wilkins.

Elesber, A. A. (2007). Coronary endothelial dysfunction and hyperlipidemia are independently associated with diastolic dysfunction in humans. *American Heart Journal, 153,* 1081–1087.

Guyton, A. C., & Hall, J. E. (2006). *Textbook of medical physiology* (11th ed.). Philadelphia: W. B. Saunders.

Kusmirek, S. L., & Gold, M. R. (2007). Sudden cardiac death: The role of risk stratification. *American Heart Journal, 153*(4 Suppl), 25–33.

Porth, C. M. (2005). *Pathophysiology: Concepts of altered health states* (7th ed.). Philadelphia: Lippincott Williams & Wilkins.

CHAPTER 48

Drug Therapy for Heart Failure

KEY TERMS

- Catecholamines
- Decompensation
- Diastolic dysfunction
- Digitalis toxicity
- Digitalization
- Endothelin
- Inotropic
- Loading dose
- Maintenance dose
- Renin
- Systolic dysfunction
- Therapeutic index
- Ventricular remodeling

LEARNING OBJECTIVES

After studying this chapter, you will be able to:

1. Recognize major manifestations of heart failure (HF).
2. Discuss the role of endothelial dysfunction in HF.
3. Differentiate the types of drugs used to treat HF.
4. Identify the role of digoxin in the management of HF and atrial fibrillation.
5. List characteristics of digoxin in terms of effects on myocardial contractility and cardiac conduction, indications for use, principles of therapy, and nursing process implications.
6. Differentiate digitalizing and maintenance doses of digoxin.
7. Explain the roles of potassium chloride, lidocaine, atropine, and digoxin immune fab in the management of digoxin toxicity.

Applying Your Knowledge

Clara Motsinger is a 70-year-old woman who has HF. She has been treated with an ACE inhibitor and a diuretic for several years, but this drug regimen has now failed to control her HF. Her cardiologist has added digoxin 0.125 mg daily (tablets) to her treatment regimen.

Introduction

Heart failure (HF) is a complex clinical condition that occurs when the heart cannot pump enough blood to meet tissue needs for oxygen and nutrients. It may result from impaired myocardial contraction during systole (*systolic dysfunction*), impaired relaxation and filling of ventricles during diastole (*diastolic dysfunction*), or a combination of systolic and diastolic dysfunction. HF has also been referred to as congestive heart failure (CHF) because frequently there is congestion (fluid accumulation) in the lungs and peripheral tissues. Many patients, however, do not have congestive symptoms; therefore, *heart failure* is the preferred term.

Causes of Heart Failure

At the cellular level, HF stems from dysfunction of contractile myocardial cells and the endothelial cells that line the heart and blood vessels (see Chap. 47). Vital functions of the endothelium include maintaining equilibrium between vasodilation and vasoconstriction, coagulation and anticoagulation, and cellular growth promotion and inhibition. Endothelial dysfunction allows processes that narrow the blood vessel lumen (e.g., buildup of atherosclerotic plaque, growth of cells, inflammation, activation of platelets) and lead to blood-clot formation and vasoconstriction that further narrow the blood vessel lumen. These are major factors in coronary artery disease and hypertension, the most common conditions leading to HF.

Other causative factors include hyperthyroidism, excessive intravenous (IV) fluids or blood transfusions, and drugs that decrease the force of myocardial contraction (e.g., antidysrhythmic drugs) or cause retention of sodium and water (e.g., corticosteroids, estrogens, nonsteroidal anti-inflammatory agents). These factors impair the pumping ability or increase the workload of the heart so an adequate cardiac output cannot be maintained.

Compensatory Mechanisms of Heart Failure

As the heart fails, the low cardiac output and inadequately filled arteries activate the neurohormonal system by several feedback mechanisms. One mechanism is increased sympathetic activity and circulating *catecholamines* (neurohormones), which increases the force of myocardial contraction, increases heart rate, and causes vasoconstriction. The effects of the baroreceptors in the aortic arch and carotid sinus that normally inhibit undue sympathetic stimulation are blunted in patients with HF, and the effects of the high levels of circulating catecholamines are intensified. Endothelin, a neurohormone secreted primarily by endothelial cells, is the most potent endogenous vasoconstrictor and may exert direct toxic effects on the heart and result in myocardial cell proliferation.

Another mechanism is activation of the renin–angiotensin–aldosterone system. *Renin* is an enzyme produced in the kidneys in response to impaired blood flow and tissue perfusion. When released into the bloodstream, renin stimulates the production of angiotensin II, a powerful vasoconstrictor. Arterial vasoconstriction impairs cardiac function by increasing the resistance (afterload) against which the ventricle ejects blood. This raises filling pressures inside the heart, increases stretch and stress on the myocardial wall, and predisposes to subendocardial ischemia. In addition, patients with severe HF have constricted arterioles in cerebral, myocardial, renal, hepatic, and mesenteric vascular beds. This results in increased organ hypoperfusion and dysfunction. Venous vaso-

constriction limits venous capacitance, resulting in venous congestion and increased diastolic ventricular filling pressures (preload). Angiotensin II also promotes sodium and water retention by stimulating aldosterone release from the adrenal cortex and the release of vasopressin (antidiuretic hormone) from the posterior pituitary gland.

All of these mechanisms combine to increase blood volume and pressure in the heart chambers, stretch muscle fibers, and produce dilation, hypertrophy, and changes in the shape of the heart (a process called *cardiac or ventricular remodeling*) that make it contract less efficiently. Overall, the compensatory mechanisms increase preload (amount of venous blood returning to the heart), workload of the heart, afterload (amount of resistance in the aorta and peripheral blood vessels that the heart must overcome to pump effectively), and blood pressure. These compensatory mechanisms that initially preserve cardiac function result in progressive deterioration of myocardial function over time.

Signs and Symptoms of Heart Failure

Cardinal manifestations of HF are dyspnea and fatigue, which can lead to exercise intolerance and fluid retention, resulting in pulmonary congestion and peripheral edema. Patients with compensated (asymptomatic) HF usually have no symptoms at rest and no edema; dyspnea and fatigue occur only with activities involving moderate or higher levels of exertion. Symptoms that occur with minimal exertion or at rest and are accompanied by ankle edema and distention of the jugular vein (from congestion of veins and leakage of fluid into tissues) reflect *decompensation* (symptomatic HF). Acute, severe cardiac decompensation is manifested by pulmonary edema, a medical emergency that requires immediate treatment. Two models currently exist for classification of HF. The New York Heart Association (NYHA) classifies HF based on functional limitations. A newer system of staging HF, proposed by the American College of Cardiology (ACC) and the American Heart Association (AHA), is based on the progression of HF. These classifications complement each other and are often used together to determine and evaluate therapy (Table 48-1).

Table 48-1	Classifying Signs and Symptoms of Heart Failure to Determine Treatment	
NEW YORK HEART ASSOCIATION (NYHA) CLASSIFICATION	**AMERICAN COLLEGE OF CARDIOLOGY (ACC)/AMERICAN HEART ASSOCIATION (AHA) GUIDELINES**	**RECOMMENDATIONS**
	Stage A. Patient at high risk for developing heart failure (HF) but without structural heart disease or signs and symptoms of HF.	■ Treat hypertension, lipid disorders, diabetes. ■ Encourage patient to stop smoking and to exercise regularly. ■ Discourage use of alcohol, illicit drugs.

NEW YORK HEART ASSOCIATION (NYHA) CLASSIFICATION	AMERICAN COLLEGE OF CARDIOLOGY (ACC)/AMERICAN HEART ASSOCIATION (AHA) GUIDELINES	RECOMMENDATIONS
		■ ACE inhibitor or angiotensin receptor blocker if indicated
Class I. Ordinary physical activity does not cause undue fatigue, palpitations, dyspnea, or angina.	*Stage B.* Structural heart disease, but without signs and symptoms of HF.	■ All stage A therapies ■ Beta-blocker unless contraindicated ■ Implantable defibrillator, if indicated
Class II. Slight limitation of physical activity but asymptomatic at rest. Ordinary physical activity causes fatigue, palpitations, dyspnea, or anginal pain.	*Stage C.* Structural heart disease with prior or current signs and symptoms of HF.	■ All stage A and B therapies ■ Sodium-restricted diet ■ Diuretics for fluid retention ■ Digoxin
Class III. Marked limitation of physical activity, but typically asymptomatic at rest. Less-than-ordinary physical activity causes fatigue, palpitations, dyspnea, or angina.		■ Avoid or withdraw antiarrhythmic agents, most calcium channel blockers, and nonsteroidal anti-inflammatory drugs. ■ Consider aldosterone antagonists, angiotensin receptor blockers, hydralazine, and nitrates. ■ Biventricular pacing
Class IV. Unable to perform any physical activity without discomfort; symptoms may be present at rest. Discomfort increases with physical activity.	*Stage D.* End-stage disease requiring specialized treatment strategies, such as mechanical circulatory support, continuous inotropic infusion, or heart transplant.	■ All therapies for stages A, B, and C ■ Permanent mechanical support ■ Continuous inotropic therapy ■ Heart transplant ■ Hospice care

Hunt, S. A., Abraham, W. T., Chin, M. H., Feldman, F. A., Francis, G. S., Ganiats, T. G., Jessup, M., et al. (2005). ACC/AHA 2005 guideline update for the diagnosis and management of chronic heart failure in the adult- summary article: A report of the American College of Cardiology/American Heart Association Task Force on Practice Guidelines (writing committee to revise the 2001 Guidelines for the Evaluation and Management of Heart Failure). Retrieved September 30, 2007, from http://www. acc. org/quality and science/clinical/ guidelines/failure/date/–wkt. pdf

Drug Therapy for Heart Failure

Several drugs are used to treat acute HF. A diuretic, in combination with an angiotensin-converting enzyme (ACE) inhibitor or angiotensin II receptor blocker (ARB), is first-line therapy for chronic failure. Digoxin, a beta-adrenergic blocking agent, or an aldosterone inhibitor may be added to the ACE inhibitor or ARB and diuretic regimen.

Drug therapy for HF continues to evolve as the pathophysiologic mechanisms are better understood and research studies indicate more effective regimens. Combinations of drugs are commonly used in efforts to improve circulation, alter the compensatory mechanisms, and reverse heart damage. Most of the drugs used to treat HF are also used in other disorders and are discussed in other chapters; their effects in HF are described in Box 48-1. The primary focus of this chapter is inotropic agents, which include digoxin (a cardiac glycoside) and the phosphodiesterase inhibitor milrinone. An additional classification of drugs, human B-type natriuretic peptides, is also presented. These drugs are discussed in the following sections and in Table 48-2.

Inotropes

Cardiac Glycosides (Digoxin)

Digoxin (Lanoxin) is the only commonly used digitalis glycoside. In the following discussion, the terms *digitalization* and *digitalis toxicity* refer to digoxin.

General Characteristics

When digoxin is given orally, absorption varies among available preparations. Lanoxicaps, which are liquid-filled capsules, and the elixir used for children are better absorbed than tablets. With tablets, the most frequently used formulation, differences in bioavailability are important because a person who is stabilized on one formulation may be underdosed or overdosed if another formulation is taken. Differences are attributed to the rate and extent of tablet dissolution rather than amounts of digoxin. In addition to drug dosage forms, other factors that may decrease digoxin absorption include the presence of food in the GI tract, delayed gastric emptying, malabsorption syndromes, and concurrent administration of some drugs (e.g., antacids, cholestyramine).

Box 48-1	Additional Drugs Used to Treat Heart Failure

Adrenergics

Dopamine or dobutamine (see Chaps. 17 and 51) may be used in acute, severe heart failure (HF) when circulatory support is required, usually in a critical care unit. Given by intravenous (IV) infusion, these drugs strengthen myocardial contraction (inotropic or cardiotonic effects) and increase cardiac output. Dosage or flow rate is titrated to hemodynamic effects; minimal effective doses are recommended because of vasoconstrictive effects. The drugs also cause tachycardia and hypertension and increase cardiac workload and oxygen consumption.

Angiotensin-Converting Enzyme (ACE) Inhibitors

Captopril and other ACE inhibitors (see Chap. 52) are drugs of first choice in treating patients with chronic HF. ACE inhibitors are usually given in combination with a diuretic. All of the drugs have similar effects, but captopril, enalapril, lisinopril, quinapril, and ramipril are Food and Drug Administration (FDA)-approved for treatment of HF. Some clinicians use captopril initially because it has a short half-life and is rapidly eliminated when stopped, then switch to a long-acting drug if captopril is tolerated by the patient. Digoxin, a beta-adrenergic blocking agent, or an aldosterone inhibitor may be added to the ACE-inhibitor/diuretic regimen.

These drugs improve cardiac function and decrease mortality. They also relieve symptoms, increase exercise tolerance, and delay further impairment of myocardial function and progression of HF (i.e., ventricular dilatation and enlargement [ventricular remodeling]). They act mainly to decrease activation of the renin–angiotensin–aldosterone system, a major pathophysiologic mechanism in HF. More specifically, the drugs prevent inactive angiotensin I from being converted to angiotensin II. Angiotensin II produces vasoconstriction and retention of sodium and water; inhibition of angiotensin II decreases vasoconstriction and retention of sodium and water. Thus, major effects of the drugs are dilation of both veins and arteries, decreased preload and afterload, decreased workload of the heart, and increased perfusion of body organs and tissues.

During ACE-inhibitor therapy, patients usually need to see a health care provider frequently for dosage titration and monitoring of serum creatinine and potassium levels for increases. Elevated creatinine levels may indicate impaired renal function, in which case dosage needs to be reduced; elevated potassium levels indicate hyperkalemia, an adverse effect of the drugs.

Angiotensin II Receptor Blockers (ARBs)

Losartan and other angiotensin receptor blockers (see Chap. 52) are similar to ACE inhibitors in their effects on cardiac function, although the mechanism of action is at the angiotensin II receptor site rather than inhibiting the conversion of angiotensin I to angiotensin II. All ARBs are approved for treatment of hypertension; however, only valsartan has received FDA approval for treatment of patients with moderate to severe HF and those unable to tolerate an ACE

inhibitor due to adverse effects such as cough. Studies indicate that the addition of an ARB to a regimen that includes ACE inhibitors may result in a decrease in hospitalizations, but does not reduce the mortality rate.

Beta-Adrenergic Blocking Agents

Although beta blockers (see Chaps. 18, 49, and 52) were formerly considered contraindicated, numerous research studies indicate they decrease morbidity (i.e., symptoms and hospitalizations) and mortality in patients with chronic HF. The change evolved from a better understanding of the mechanisms causing chronic HF.

Beta blockers suppress activation of the sympathetic nervous system and the resulting catecholamine excess that eventually damages myocardial cells, reduces myocardial beta receptors, and reduces cardiac output. As a result, over time, ventricular remodeling regresses, the heart returns toward a more normal shape and function, and cardiac output increases.

Beta blockers are not recommended for patients in acute HF because of the potential for an initial decrease in myocardial contractility. A beta blocking agent is started after normal blood volume is restored and edema and other symptoms are relieved. The goal of beta blocker therapy is to shrink the ventricle back to its normal size (reverse remodeling). The beta blocker is added to the ACE-inhibitor/diuretic regimen, usually near the end of a hospital stay or as outpatient therapy. Most studies have been done with bisoprolol, carvedilol, or metoprolol; it is not yet known whether some beta blockers are more effective than others. When used in patients with chronic HF, recommendations include starting with a low dose (because symptoms may initially worsen in some patients), titrating the dose upward at approximately 2-week intervals, and monitoring closely. Significant hemodynamic improvement usually requires 2 to 3 months of therapy, but effects are long lasting. Beneficial effects can be measured by increases in the left ventricular ejection fraction (i.e., cardiac output).

The FDA has issued a **BLACK BOX WARNING** for patients with coronary artery disease withdrawing from oral forms of atenolol, metoprolol, nadolol, propranolol, and timolol; abrupt withdrawal has resulted in exacerbation of angina, the incidence of ventricular dysrhythmias, and the occurrence of myocardial infarctions.

Diuretics

Diuretics (see Chap. 53) are used in treating both acute and chronic HF. Thiazides (e.g., hydrochlorothiazide) can be used for mild diuresis in patients with normal renal function; loop diuretics (e.g., furosemide) should be used in patients who have impaired renal function or who need strong diuresis.

For patients in acute HF, which is characterized by fluid accumulation, a diuretic is the initial treatment. It acts to decrease plasma volume (extracellular fluid volume) and increase excretion of sodium and water, thereby decreasing preload. With early or mild HF, starting or increasing the dose of an oral thiazide may be effective. With moderate to severe HF (pulmonary edema), an IV loop diuretic is indicated.

IV furosemide also has a vasodilatory effect that helps relieve vasoconstriction (afterload). Although diuretic therapy relieves symptoms, it does not improve left ventricular function and decrease mortality rates. Some patients may also need drugs to increase myocardial contractility and vasodilators to decrease preload, afterload, or both.

In patients with chronic HF, an oral diuretic is a common component of treatment regimens. Depending on the severity of symptoms or degree of HF, the regimen may also include an ACE inhibitor or ARB, a beta blocker, and digoxin.

Potassium-sparing diuretics (e.g., amiloride, triamterene) are often given concurrently with potassium-losing diuretics (e.g., thiazides or loop diuretics) to help maintain normal serum potassium levels. Concomitant use of ACE inhibitors and nonsteroidal anti-inflammatory drugs and the presence of diabetes mellitus increase risks of hyperkalemia.

With all diuretic therapy, serum potassium levels must be measured periodically to monitor for hypokalemia and hyperkalemia. Both hypokalemia and hyperkalemia are cardiotoxic and impair heart function.

Aldosterone Antagonist

Increasingly, spironolactone has being added to the drug regimen for patients with moderate to severe HF since the publication of the randomized Aldactone evaluation study (RALES). The study demonstrated that the addition of spironolactone to ACE inhibition decreases mortality in HF. Increased aldosterone, a major factor in the pathophysiology of HF, results in increased interstitial fibrosis that may decrease systolic function and increase the risk of ventricular dysrhythmias. Spironolactone is an aldosterone antagonist that reduces the aldosterone-induced retention of sodium and water and

impaired vascular function. Although ACE inhibitors also decrease aldosterone initially, this effect is transient. Spironolactone is given in a daily dose of 12.5 to 25 mg, along with standard doses of an ACE inhibitor, a loop diuretic, and usually digoxin. In patients with adequate renal function (i.e., serum creatinine 2.5 mg/dL or less), the addition of spironolactone usually allows smaller doses of loop diuretics and potassium supplements. Overall, studies indicate that the addition of spironolactone improves cardiac function and reduces symptoms, hospitalizations, and mortality. A second drug, eplerenone, is approved for use in the management of HF after a myocardial infarction to improve survival.

Vasodilators

Vasodilators are essential components of treatment regimens for HF, and the beneficial effects of ACE inhibitors and angiotensin II receptor antagonists stem significantly from their vasodilating effects (i.e., preventing or decreasing angiotensin-induced vasoconstriction). Other vasodilators may also be used. Venous dilators (e.g., nitrates) decrease preload; arterial dilators (e.g., hydralazine) decrease afterload. Isosorbide dinitrate and hydralazine may be combined to decrease both preload and afterload. The combination has similar effects to those of an ACE inhibitor or an ARB, but may not be as well tolerated by patients. Nitrates are discussed in Chapter 50; hydralazine and other vasodilators are discussed in Chapter 52.

Oral vasodilators usually are used in patients with chronic HF and parenteral agents are reserved for those who have severe HF or are unable to take oral medications. Vasodilators should be started at low doses, titrated to desired hemodynamic effects, and discontinued slowly to avoid rebound vasoconstriction.

Table 48-2	**Drugs at a Glance:** Drugs for Heart Failure

	ROUTES AND DOSAGE RANGES	
Generic/Trade Name	**Adults**	**Children**
Inotropic Agents		
Cardiac Glycoside		
Digoxin (Lanoxin)	Digitalizing dose, PO 0.75–1 mg in 3 or 4 divided doses over 24 h; IV 0.5–0.75 mg in divided doses over 24 h. Maintenance dose, PO, IV 0.125–0.5 mg/d (average, 0.25 mg)	> 10 y: Same as adult. 2–10 y: Digitalizing dose, PO 0.02–0.04 mg/kg in 4 divided doses over 24 h. Maintenance dose, PO, IV approximately 20%–35% of the digitalizing dose or a maximum dose of 100–150 mcg/d 1 mo–2 y: Digitalizing dose, PO 0.035–0.06 mg/kg in 4 divided doses over 24 h; IV, 0.035–0.05 mg/kg in 4 divided doses over 24 h. Maintenance dose, PO, IV, approximately 20%–35% of the digitalizing dose *Newborns:* Digitalizing dose, PO 0.025–0.035 mg/kg in 4 divided doses over 24 h. Maintenance dose, PO, IV, approximately 20%–35% of the digitalizing dose.

(continued on page 768)

Table 48-2	**Drugs at a Glance:** Drugs for Heart Failure (continued)	

	ROUTES AND DOSAGE RANGES	
Generic/Trade Name	Adults	Children
Phosphodiesterase Inhibitor **Milrinone** (Primacor)	IV bolus infusion (loading dose), 50 mcg/kg over 10 min IV continuous infusion (maintenance dose), 0.375–0.75 mcg/kg/min, diluted in 0.9% or 0.45% NaCl or 5% dextrose solution	Not established
Human B-Type Natriuretic Peptide **Nesiritide** (Natrecor)	IV bolus infusion (loading dose), 2 mcg/kg followed by continuous infusion of 0.01 mcg/kg/min. Use for >48 hours not studied.	Safety not established

Therapeutic serum levels of digoxin are 0.5 to 2 nanograms per milliliter; toxic serum levels are above 2. In the elderly and in the presence of renal failure, therapeutic serum levels are 0.5 to 1.3 nanograms per milliliter. Research in the past decade has suggested that serum levels of 1.0 nanograms per milliliter or less are more appropriate in those with HF. However, toxicity may occur at virtually any serum level. Dosage must be reduced in the presence of renal failure because most of the digoxin (60%–70%) is excreted unchanged by the kidneys to prevent drug accumulation and toxicity. The remainder is metabolized or excreted by nonrenal routes.

Mechanisms of Action

In HF, digoxin exerts a cardiotonic or positive *inotropic* effect that improves the contractility and pumping ability of the heart. The mechanism by which digoxin increases the force of myocardial contraction is thought to be inhibition of Na,K-adenosine triphosphatase (Na,K-ATPase), an enzyme in cardiac cell membranes that decreases the movement of sodium out of myocardial cells after contraction. As a result, calcium enters the cell in exchange for sodium, causing additional calcium to be released from intracellular binding sites increasing myocardial contractility. Overall, digoxin helps to relieve symptoms and decrease hospitalizations but does not prolong survival. In HF, it is given concomitantly with a diuretic and an ACE inhibitor or ARB.

In patients with atrial dysrhythmias (see Chap. 49), digoxin slows the rate of ventricular contraction (negative chronotropic effect). Negative chronotropic effects are probably caused by several factors. First, digoxin has a direct depressant effect on cardiac conduction tissues, especially the atrioventricular node. This action decreases the number of electrical impulses allowed to reach the ventricles from supraventricular sources. Second, digoxin indirectly stimulates the vagus nerve. Third, increased efficiency of myocardial contraction and vagal stimulation decrease compensatory tachycardia that results from the sympathetic nervous system response to inadequate circulation.

Indications for Use

The clinical uses of digoxin include management of HF, atrial fibrillation, and atrial flutter. Digoxin may be used in patients with acute or chronic conditions, for digitalization, or for maintenance therapy. Although the use of digoxin in patients with normal sinus rhythm has been questioned, studies indicate improved ejection fraction and exercise tolerance in patients who receive digoxin. In addition, in patients with HF who are stabilized on digoxin, a diuretic, and an ACE inhibitor or ARB, symptoms worsen if digoxin is discontinued.

Contraindications to Use

Digoxin is contraindicated in patients with severe myocarditis, ventricular tachycardia, or ventricular fibrillation and must be used cautiously in those with acute myocardial infarction, heart block, Adams-Stokes syndrome, Wolff-Parkinson-White syndrome (risk of fatal dysrhythmias), electrolyte imbalances (hypokalemia, hypomagnesemia, hypercalcemia), and renal impairment.

Administration and Digitalization

Digoxin is given orally or IV. Although it can be given intramuscularly, this route is not recommended because pain and muscle necrosis may occur at injection sites. When given orally, onset of action occurs in 30 minutes to 2 hours, and peak effects occur in approximately 6 hours. When given IV, the onset of action occurs within 10 to 30 minutes, and peak effects occur in 1 to 5 hours.

In the heart, maximum drug effect occurs when a steady-state tissue concentration has been achieved. This occurs in approximately 1 week (five half-lives) unless loading doses are given for more rapid effects. Traditionally, a *loading dose* is called a digitalizing dose. Digitalization (administration of an amount sufficient to produce therapeutic effects) may be accomplished rapidly by giving a total dose of 0.75 to 1.5 milligrams of digoxin in divided doses, 6 to 8 hours apart, over a 24-hour period. Because rapid digitalization engenders higher risks of toxicity, it is usually done for atrial tachydysrhythmias, with continuous cardiac monitoring, rather than for HF. Slow digitalization may be accomplished by initiating therapy with a *maintenance dose* of digoxin. When digoxin is discontinued, elimination of the drug requires approximately 1 week.

Applying Your Knowledge 48-1

Ms. Motsinger is due for her first dose of digoxin. Her physician has decided to digitalize the patient. What does digitalization involve and why would this be desirable in Ms. Motsinger's case?

Digoxin Toxicity

Digoxin has a narrow *therapeutic index* so a dose adequate for therapeutic effects may produce signs of toxicity. Individuals with hypokalemia can develop digoxin toxicity even when digoxin levels are not considered elevated. Signs of toxicity include potentially life-threatening heart rhythm disturbances, ranging from very slow to rapid ventricular rhythms. Other side effects include nausea, vomiting, loss of appetite, abdominal discomfort, blurred vision, and mental changes. Digoxin toxicity may result from many contributing factors:

■ Accumulation of larger-than-necessary maintenance doses

■ Rapid loading or digitalization, whether by one or more large doses or frequent administration of small doses

■ Impaired renal function, which delays excretion of digoxin

■ Age extremes (young or old)

■ Electrolyte imbalance (e.g., hypokalemia, hypomagnesemia, hypercalcemia)

■ Hypoxia due to heart or lung disease, which increases myocardial sensitivity to digoxin

■ Hypothyroidism, which slows digoxin metabolism and may cause accumulation

■ Concurrent treatment with other drugs affecting the heart, such as quinidine, verapamil, or nifedipine

Applying Your Knowledge 48-2

Ms. Motsinger has been taking digoxin for 2 days. You must assess her drug level before administration of digoxin; blood for the test was drawn this morning. What should her drug level be to be in the therapeutic range?

Phosphodiesterase Inhibitors

Milrinone IV (Primacor) is the most commonly used cardiotonic–inotropic agent for short-term management of acute, severe HF that is not controlled by digoxin, diuretics, and vasodilators. The drug increases levels of cyclic adenosine monophosphate (cAMP) in myocardial cells by inhibiting phosphodiesterase, the enzyme that normally metabolizes cAMP. Milrinone also relax vascular smooth muscle to produce vasodilation and decrease preload and afterload. In HF, inotropic and vasodilator effects increase cardiac output. The effects of this drug are additive to those of digoxin and may be synergistic with those of adrenergic drugs (e.g., dobutamine). There is a time delay before the drug reaches therapeutic serum levels as well as inter-individual variability in therapeutic doses.

Milrinone is a potent inotropic agent that is given IV by bolus injection followed by continuous infusion. Flow rate is titrated to maintain adequate circulation. Milrinone can be used alone or with other drugs such as dobutamine and nitroprusside. Its dosage should be reduced in the presence of renal impairment. Dose-limiting adverse effects of the drugs include tachycardia, atrial or ventricular dysrhythmias, and hypotension. Hypotension is more likely to occur in patients who are hypovolemic. Milrinone has a long half-life of approximately 80 hours and may accumulate with prolonged infusions.

Human B-Type Natriuretic Peptide (Nesiritide)

Nesiritide (Natrecor) is the first in this class of drugs to be used in the management of acute HF. Produced by recombinant DNA technology, nesiritide is identical to endogenous human B-type natriuretic peptide (BNP), which is secreted primarily by the ventricles in response to fluid and pressure overload. This drug acts to compensate for deteriorating cardiac function by reducing preload and afterload, increasing diuresis and secretion of sodium, suppressing the renin–angiotensin–aldosterone system, and decreasing secretion of the neurohormones *endothelin* and norepinephrine. Onset of action is immediate with peak effects attained in 15 minutes with a bolus dose followed by continuous IV infusion. Administration should be by a separate IV line because nesiritide is incompatible with many other drugs. Hemodynamic monitoring of pulmonary artery pressure is indicated to determine drug effectiveness. Clearance of the drug is proportional to body weight and partially by the kidneys; however, no adjustment in dosing is required for age, gender, race/ethnicity, or renal function impairment.

Nursing Process

Assessment

Assess patients for current or potential HF.

■ Identify risk factors for HF.

■ **Cardiovascular disorders:** atherosclerosis, hypertension, coronary artery disease, myocardial infarction, cardiac dysrhythmias, and cardiac valvular disease

Nursing Process continues on page 770

- **Noncardiovascular disorders:** severe infections, hyperthyroidism, pulmonary disease (e.g., cor pulmonale—right-sided HF resulting from lung disease)
- **Other factors:** excessive amounts of IV fluids, rapid infusion of IV fluids or blood transfusions, advanced age

◼ Interview and observe for signs and symptoms of **chronic HF.** Within the clinical syndrome of HF, clinical manifestations vary from few and mild to many and severe, including the following:

- **Mild HF:** Common signs and symptoms of mild HF are ankle edema, dyspnea on exertion, and fatigue with ordinary physical activity. Edema results from increased venous pressure, which allows fluids to leak into tissues; dyspnea and fatigue result from tissue hypoxia.

- **Moderate or severe HF:** More extensive edema, dyspnea, and fatigue at rest are likely to occur. Additional signs and symptoms include orthopnea, postnocturnal dyspnea, and cough (from congestion of the respiratory tract with venous blood); mental confusion (from cerebral hypoxia); oliguria and decreased renal function (from decreased blood flow to the kidneys); and anxiety.

◼ Observe for signs and symptoms of **acute** HF. Acute pulmonary edema indicates acute HF and is a medical emergency. Pulmonary edema occurs when left ventricular failure results in accumulation of blood and fluid in pulmonary veins and tissues. Causes include acute myocardial infarction, cardiac dysrhythmias, severe hypertension, acute fluid or salt overload, and certain drugs (e.g., quinidine and other cardiac depressants; propranolol and other antiadrenergics; phenylephrine, norepinephrine, and other alpha-adrenergic stimulants). As a result, the person experiences severe dyspnea, hypoxia, hypertension, tachycardia, hemoptysis, frothy respiratory tract secretions, and anxiety.

Assess patients for signs and symptoms of atrial tachydysrhythmias.

◼ Record the rate and rhythm of apical and radial pulses. Atrial fibrillation, the most common atrial dysrhythmia, is characterized by tachycardia, pulse deficit (faster apical rate than radial rate), and a very irregular rhythm. Fatigue, dizziness, and fainting may occur.

◼ Check the electrocardiogram (ECG) for abnormal P waves, rapid rate of ventricular contraction, and QRS complexes of normal configuration but irregular intervals.

Assess baseline vital signs; weight; edema; laboratory results for potassium, magnesium, and calcium levels; and other tests of cardiovascular function when available.

Assess a baseline ECG before digoxin therapy when possible. If a patient is in normal sinus rhythm, later ECGs may aid recognition of digitalis toxicity (i.e., drug-induced dysrhythmias). If a patient has an atrial tachydysrhythmia and is

receiving digoxin to slow the ventricular rate, later ECGs may aid recognition of therapeutic and adverse effects. For patients who are already receiving digoxin at the initial contact, a baseline ECG can still be valuable because changes in later ECGs may promote earlier recognition and management of drug-induced dysrhythmias.

Nursing Diagnoses

◼ Ineffective Tissue Perfusion related to decreased cardiac output
◼ Anxiety related to chronic illness and lifestyle changes
◼ Impaired Gas Exchange related to venous congestion and fluid accumulation in lungs
◼ Activity intolerance related to impaired gas exchange and fatigue
◼ Imbalanced Nutrition: Less Than Body Requirements related to digoxin-induced anorexia, nausea, and vomiting
◼ Noncompliance related to the need for long-term drug therapy and regular medical supervision
◼ Deficient Knowledge: Managing drug therapy regimen safely and effectively

Planning/Goals

The patient will

◼ Take digoxin and other medications safely and accurately
◼ Experience improved breathing and less fatigue and edema
◼ Maintain serum digoxin levels within therapeutic ranges
◼ Be closely monitored for therapeutic and adverse effects, especially during digitalization; when dosage is being changed; and when other drugs are added to or removed from the management regimen
◼ Keep appointments for follow-up monitoring of vital signs, serum potassium levels, serum digoxin levels, and renal function

Interventions

◼ Use measures to prevent or minimize HF and atrial dysrhythmias. In the broadest sense, preventive measures include sensible eating habits (a balanced diet; avoiding excess saturated fat and salt; weight control), avoiding cigarette smoking, and regular exercise. In the patient at risk for development of HF and dysrhythmias, preventive measures include the following:

- Treatment of hypertension
- Avoidance of hypoxia
- Weight control
- Avoidance of excess sodium in the diet
- Avoidance of fluid overload, especially in elderly patients

- Maintenance of management programs for HF, atrial dysrhythmias, and other cardiovascular or noncardiovascular disorders
- Monitor vital signs, weight, urine output, and serum potassium level regularly, and compare with baseline values.
- Monitor ECGs when available, and compare with baseline or previous tracings.
- Provide appropriate teaching related to drug therapy (see accompanying display).

Evaluation

- Interview and observe for relief of symptoms (weight loss, increased urine output, less extremity edema, easier breathing, improved activity tolerance and self-care ability, slower heart rate).
- Observe serum drug levels for normal or abnormal values, when available.
- Interview regarding compliance with instructions for taking the drug.
- Interview and observe for adverse drug effects, especially cardiac dysrhythmias.

 Applying Your Knowledge 48-3

How Can You Avoid This Medication Error?
You are giving Ms. Motsinger her morning medication. The pharmacy has sent Lanoxicaps for today's dose of digoxin. You administer the 0.125-mg capsule.

Principles of Therapy

Goals of Therapy

The goals for patients with compensated HF are to maintain function as nearly normal as possible and to prevent symptomatic (acute, congestive, or decompensated) HF, hospitalizations, and death. When symptoms (decompensation) occur, the goals are to relieve symptoms, restore function, and prevent progressive cardiac deterioration.

Nonpharmacologic Management Measures

- Prevent or treat conditions that precipitate cardiac decompensation and failure (e.g., fluid and sodium retention, factors that impair myocardial contractility or increase cardiac workload).
- Restrict dietary sodium intake to reduce edema and other symptoms and allow a decrease in diuretic dosage. For most patients, sodium restriction need not be severe. A common order, "no added salt," may be accomplished by avoiding

obviously salty foods (e.g., ham, potato chips, snack foods) and by not adding salt during cooking or eating. For patients with more severe HF, dietary intake may be more restricted (e.g., no more than 2 g daily). A major source of sodium intake is table salt: A level teaspoonful contains 2300 milligrams of sodium.

- If hyponatremia (serum sodium < 130 mEq/L) develops from sodium restrictions and diuretic therapy, fluids may need to be restricted (e.g., 1.5 L/day or less) until the serum sodium level increases. Severe hyponatremia (<125 mEq/L) may lead to dysrhythmias.
- For patients who are obese, weight loss is desirable to decrease systemic vascular resistance and myocardial oxygen demand.
- Reduce physical activity in patients with symptomatic HF. This decreases the workload and oxygen consumption of the myocardium. If bed rest is instituted, antithrombotic measures such as compression stockings/devices or heparin therapy should be prescribed to prevent deep vein thrombosis.
- Administer oxygen, if needed, to relieve dyspnea, improve oxygen delivery, reduce the work of breathing, and decrease constriction of pulmonary blood vessels (which is a compensatory measure in patients with hypoxemia).
- Prepare patient and family for heart transplant, if indicated.

Pharmacologic Management

Drug Selection

A combination of drugs is the standard of care for both acute and chronic HF. Specific drug components depend on the patient's symptoms and hemodynamic status.

Acute Heart Failure

For acute HF, the first drugs of choice may include an IV loop diuretic, a cardiotonic–inotropic agent (e.g., digoxin, dobutamine, milrinone), and vasodilators (e.g., nitroglycerin and hydralazine or nitroprusside). For patients with decompensated acute HF, nesiritide may be used for initial treatment (<48 hours) or may be given in combination with diuretics, inotropes, or vasodilators. These combinations reduce preload and afterload and increase myocardial contractility.

In acute HF, there is a high risk of hypokalemia because large doses of potassium-losing diuretics are often given. Serum potassium levels should be monitored regularly and supplemental potassium may be needed.

Chronic Heart Failure

For chronic HF, an ACE inhibitor or ARB and a diuretic are the basic standard of care. Digoxin, a beta-adrenergic blocking agent, and spironolactone may also be added. Although the use of digoxin in patients with normal sinus rhythm has been questioned, studies indicate improved ejection fraction and exercise tolerance in patients who receive digoxin. In addition, in patients stabilized on digoxin, a diuretic, and an ACE inhibitor or ARB, symptoms worsen if digoxin is discontinued.

Patient Teaching Guidelines　Digoxin

General Considerations

- This drug is prescribed for two types of heart disease. One type is heart failure, in which digoxin strengthens your heartbeat and helps to relieve such symptoms as ankle swelling, shortness of breath, and fatigue. The other type is a fast heartbeat called *atrial fibrillation*, in which digoxin slows the heartbeat and decreases symptoms such as fatigue. Because these are chronic conditions, digoxin therapy is usually long term. Ask your health care provider why you are being given digoxin and what effects you can expect, both beneficial and adverse.

- It is extremely important to take digoxin (and other cardiovascular medications) as prescribed, usually once daily. The drug must be taken regularly to maintain therapeutic blood levels, but overuse can cause serious adverse effects.

- Precautions to increase the drug's safety and effectiveness include the following:

  - As a general rule, *do not* miss a dose. It is helpful to develop a routine of taking the medication at approximately the same time each day and maintaining a written record, such as a dated checklist. If you forget a dose at the usual time and remember it within a few hours (approximately 6), go ahead and take the daily dose.

  - *Do not* take an extra dose. For example, do not take a double dose to make up for a missed dose.

  - *Do not* take other prescription or nonprescription (e.g., antacids, cold remedies, diet pills) drugs without consulting the health care provider who prescribed digoxin. Many drugs interact with digoxin to increase or decrease its effects.

  - You will need periodic physical examinations, electrocardiograms, and blood tests to check digoxin and electrolyte (sodium, potassium, magnesium) levels to monitor your response to digoxin and see whether changes in dosage are needed.

- Digoxin is often one drug in a management regimen of several drugs for heart disease. The drugs are all needed to help the heart and blood vessels work better. Together, the drugs help maintain a balance in the cardiovascular system. As a result, changing any aspect of one of the drugs can upset the balance and lead to symptoms. For example, stopping one drug because of adverse effects can lead to problems. If you think a drug needs to be stopped or its dosage reduced, talk with a health care provider. Do not

make changes on your own; serious illness or even death could result.

- Small doses (e.g., 0.125 milligrams [125 micrograms] daily or every other day) are usually given to older adults, and other people with impaired kidney function. Digoxin is eliminated through the kidneys; it can accumulate and cause adverse effects if dosage is not reduced in patients with kidney impairment.

- You may need to limit your salt (sodium chloride) intake and get an adequate supply of potassium. Follow your health care provider's recommendations about any diet changes. People taking digoxin are often taking a diuretic, a drug that increases urine production and loss of sodium and potassium from the body. If potassium levels get too low, adverse effects of digoxin are more likely to occur. However, too much potassium can also be harmful. Do not use salt substitutes (potassium chloride) without consulting a health care provider.

- Report adverse drug effects (e.g., undesirable changes in heart rate or rhythm, nausea and vomiting, or visual problems) to a health care provider. These symptoms may indicate that digoxin dosage needs to be reduced.

- Use the same brand and type of digoxin all the time. For example, whether using generic digoxin or trade-name Lanoxin tablets, get the same one each time a prescription is refilled. In addition, there is a capsule form and a liquid form. These forms and concentrations are different and cannot be used interchangeably. Underdoses and overdoses may occur. Lanoxin tablets are the most commonly used formulation.

Self- or Caregiver Administration

- If instructed to do so by your health care provider, count your pulse before each dose. In some circumstances, you may be advised to skip that scheduled dose. *Do not* skip doses unless specifically instructed to do so.

- Take or give digoxin tablets approximately the same time each day to maintain more even blood levels and help in remembering to take the drug. The tablets may be crushed and can be taken with or after food, if desired, although milk and dairy products may delay absorption.

- Digoxin capsules should be swallowed whole.

- If taking or giving a liquid form of digoxin, it is extremely important to measure it accurately. A few drops more could produce overdosage, with serious adverse effects; a few drops less could produce underdosage, with a loss or decrease of therapeutic effects.

In chronic HF, hypokalemia may be less likely to occur because lower doses of potassium-losing diuretics are usually being given. In addition, there may be more extensive use of potassium-sparing diuretics (e.g., amiloride, triamterene) and the aldosterone antagonist, spironolactone. Note, however, that hyperkalemia must also be prevented because it is cardiotoxic. Overall, these drugs improve patients' quality of life by decreasing their symptoms and increasing their ability to function in activities of daily living. They also decrease hospitalizations and deaths from HF.

Digoxin Dosage and Administration

Digoxin dosages must be interpreted with consideration of specific patient characteristics including age, weight, gender, renal function, general health state, and concurrent drug therapy. Loading or digitalizing doses are necessary for initiating therapy as digoxin's long half-life make therapeutic serum levels difficult to obtain without loading. Loading doses should be used cautiously in patients who have taken digoxin within the previous 2 or 3 weeks. Maintenance doses, which are much smaller than loading doses, are always used for long-term therapy. They may be safely used to initiate digoxin therapy, but therapeutic serum levels may not be achieved for weeks. In general, larger doses of digoxin are needed to slow the heart rate in atrial tachydysrhythmias than to increase myocardial contractility in HF. A small group of individuals (about 10%) have digoxin-metabolizing bacteria in their colons require larger doses of digoxin to reach therapeutic serum levels. Members of this group are at risk for development of digoxin toxicity if they are concomitantly given antibacterial drugs that destroy colonic bacteria.

When converting from the oral to IV route, the dosage of digoxin should be reduced by 20% to 30%. When a maintenance dose is given IV, the onset and peak occur earlier, although the duration of action remains the same. Cardiac monitoring should be used in patients receiving IV loading regimens.

Smaller doses (loading and maintenance) should be given to patients who are elderly or have hypothyroidism. Because metabolism and excretion of digoxin are delayed in such people, the drug may accumulate and cause toxicity if dosage is not reduced. Dosage also should be reduced in patients with hypokalemia, extensive myocardial damage, or cardiac conduction disorders. These conditions increase risks of digoxin-induced dysrhythmias.

Dosage can be titrated according to patient response. In HF, severity of symptoms, ECGs, and serum drug concentrations are useful. In atrial fibrillation, dosage can be altered to produce the desired decrease in the ventricular rate of contraction. Optimal dosage is the lowest amount that relieves signs and symptoms of HF or alters heart rate and rhythm toward normal without producing toxicity.

Digoxin dosage must be reduced by approximately half in patients with renal failure to avoid drug accumulation and toxicity. Dosage should be based on signs and symptoms of toxicity, creatinine clearance, and serum drug levels.

Dosage of digoxin must be reduced by approximately half when certain drugs are given concurrently to avoid drug accumulation and toxicity. For example, amiodarone, quinidine, nifedipine, and verapamil slow digoxin excretion and increase serum digoxin levels.

When a hospitalized patient is unable to take a daily maintenance dose of digoxin at the scheduled time because of diagnostic tests, treatment measures, or other reasons, the dose should usually be given later rather than omitted. If the patient is having surgery, the nurse often must ask the surgeon whether the drug should be given on the day of surgery (i.e., orally with a small amount of water or parenterally) and if the drug should be reordered after surgery. Many patients require continued digoxin therapy. However, if a dose is missed, probably no ill effects will occur because the pharmacologic actions of digoxin persist longer than 24 hours.

Electrolyte balance must be monitored and maintained during digoxin therapy, particularly normal serum levels of potassium (3.5–5 mEq/L), magnesium (1.5–2.5 mg/100 mL), and calcium (8.5–10 mg/100 mL). Hypokalemia and hypomagnesemia increase cardiac excitability and ectopic pacemaker activity, leading to dysrhythmias; hypercalcemia enhances the effects of digoxin. These electrolyte abnormalities increase the risk of digoxin toxicity. Hypocalcemia increases excitability of nerve and muscle cell membranes and causes myocardial contraction to be weak (leading to a decrease in digoxin effect).

Digoxin Toxicity: Recognition and Management

Digitalis toxicity is one of the most commonly encountered drug-related reasons for hospitalization. Digoxin has a narrow therapeutic index (a small difference between toxic and therapeutic doses), and the endpoint of effective therapy is often difficult to define and measure. Recognition of digoxin toxicity may be difficult because of nonspecific early manifestations (e.g., anorexia, nausea, confusion) and the similarity between the signs and symptoms of heart disease for which digoxin is given and the signs and symptoms of digoxin intoxication. Continued atrial fibrillation with a rapid ventricular response may indicate inadequate dosage. However, other dysrhythmias may indicate toxicity. Premature ventricular contractions commonly occur. Serum drug levels and ECGs may be helpful in verifying suspected toxicity. Blood for serum digoxin testing should be drawn just before a dose. Drug distribution to tissues requires about 6 hours after a dose is given; if the blood is drawn before 6 hours, the level may be high.

When digoxin toxicity occurs, management may include any or all of the following interventions, depending on the patient's condition:

- Digoxin should be discontinued, not just reduced in dosage. Most patients with mild or early toxicity recover completely within a few days after the drug is stopped.

- If serious cardiac dysrhythmias are present, several drugs may be used, including

  - **Potassium chloride**, if serum potassium level is low. It is a myocardial depressant that acts to decrease myocardial excitability. The dose depends on the severity of toxicity, serum potassium level, and patient response. Potassium is contraindicated in renal failure and should be used with caution in the presence of cardiac conduction defects.

  - **Lidocaine**, an antidysrhythmic local anesthetic agent used to decrease myocardial irritability

  - **Atropine** or **isoproterenol**, used in the management of bradycardia or conduction defects

  - Other antidysrhythmic drugs may be used but are in general less effective in digoxin-induced dysrhythmias than in dysrhythmias due to other causes.

  - **Digoxin immune fab** (Digibind) is a digoxin-binding antidote derived from antidigoxin antibodies produced in sheep. It is recommended only for serious toxicity. It combines with digoxin and pulls digoxin out of tissues and into the bloodstream. This causes serum digoxin levels to be high, but the drug is bound to the antibody and therefore inactive. Digoxin immune fab is given IV, as a bolus injection if the patient is in danger of immediate cardiac arrest, but preferably over 15 to 30 minutes. Dosage varies and is calculated according to the amount of digoxin ingested or serum digoxin levels (see manufacturer's instructions).

Use in Special Populations

Use in Children

Digoxin is commonly used in children for the same indications as for adults and should be prescribed or supervised by a pediatric cardiologist when possible. The response to a given dose varies with age, size, and renal and hepatic function. There may be little difference between a therapeutic dose and a toxic dose. Very small amounts are often given to children. These factors increase the risks of dosage errors in children. In a hospital setting, institutional policies may require that each dose be verified with another nurse before it is administered. Liquid digoxin must be precisely measured in a syringe and the dose should not be rounded. ECG monitoring is desirable when digoxin therapy is started.

As in adults, dosage of digoxin should be individualized and carefully titrated. Digoxin is primarily excreted by the kidneys, and dosage must be reduced with impaired renal function. In general, divided daily doses should be given to infants and children younger than 10 years, and adult dosages adjusted to their weight should be given to children older than 10 years of age. Larger doses are usually needed to slow a too-rapid ventricular rate in children with atrial fibrillation or flutter. Differences in bioavailability of different preparations (parenterals, capsules, elixirs, and tablets) must be considered when switching from one preparation to another.

Neonates vary in tolerance of digoxin depending on their degree of maturity. Premature infants are especially sensitive to drug effects. Dosage must be reduced, and digitalization should be even more individualized and cautiously approached than in more mature infants and children. Early signs of toxicity in newborns are undue slowing of sinus rate, sinoatrial arrest, and prolongation of the P–R interval.

Use in Older Adults

Digoxin is widely used and a frequent cause of adverse effects in older adults. Reduced dosages are usually required because of decreased liver or kidney function, decreased lean body weight, and advanced cardiovascular disease. All of these characteristics are common in older adults. Impaired renal function leads to slower drug excretion and increased risk of accumulation. Dosage must be reduced by approximately 50% with renal failure or concurrent administration of amiodarone, quinidine, nifedipine, or verapamil. These drugs increase serum digoxin levels and increase risks of toxicity if dosage is not reduced. The most commonly recommended dose is 0.125 milligrams daily. Antacids decrease absorption of oral digoxin and should not be given at the same time.

Use in Patients With Renal Impairment

Digoxin should be used cautiously, in reduced dosages, because renal impairment delays its excretion. Both loading and maintenance doses should be reduced. Patients with advanced renal impairment can achieve therapeutic serum concentrations with a dosage of 0.125 milligrams three to five times per week.

In addition, in patients with reduced blood flow to the kidneys (e.g., fluid volume depletion, acute HF), digoxin may be reabsorbed in renal tubules. As a result, less digoxin is excreted through the kidneys and maintenance doses may need even greater decreases than those calculated according to creatinine clearance. Thus, digoxin toxicity develops more often and lasts longer in renal impairment. Patients with renal impairment who are receiving digoxin, even in small doses, should be monitored closely for adverse effects, and serum digoxin levels should be monitored periodically.

With milrinone, which is also excreted primarily by the kidneys, renal impairment significantly increases elimination half-life, drug accumulation, and adverse effects. Dosage should be reduced according to creatinine clearance (see manufacturer's instructions).

Use in Patients With Hepatic Impairment

Hepatic impairment has little effect on digoxin clearance, and no dosage adjustments are needed.

Use in Patients With Critical Illness

Critically ill patients often have multiple cardiovascular and other disorders that require drug therapy. Acute HF may be the primary critical illness. It may also be precipitated by other illnesses or treatments that alter fluid balance, impair myocardial contractility, or increase the workload of the heart beyond its capacity to accommodate. Management is often symptomatic, with choice of drug and dosage requiring careful titration and frequent monitoring of the patient's response. Cardiotonic, diuretic, and vasodilator drugs are often required. All of the drugs should be used with caution in critically ill patients.

Use in Home Care

Most digoxin is taken at home, and the home care nurse shares responsibility for teaching patients how to use the drug effectively and circumstances to be reported to a health care provider. Accurate dosing is vitally important because underuse may cause recurrence of symptoms and overuse may cause toxicity. Either condition may be life threatening and require emergency care. The home care nurse also needs to monitor patients' responses to the drug and changes in conditions or drug therapy that increases risks of toxicity.

When patients are receiving a combination of drugs for management of HF, the nurse needs to assist them in understanding that the different types of drugs have different actions and produce different responses. As a result, they work together to be more effective and maintain a more balanced state of cardiovascular function. Changing drugs or dosages can upset the balance and lead to acute and severe symptoms that require hospitalization and may even cause death from HF. Thus, it is extremely important that they take all the medications as prescribed. If unable to take the medications for any reason, patients or caregivers should notify the prescribing health care provider. They should be instructed not to wait until symptoms become severe before seeking care.

Use in Patients Taking Herbal and Dietary Supplements

Use of nonprescription herbal and dietary supplements is frequently not reported by the patient even though one third of the adults in the United States use these agents. Significant interactions can occur between supplements and prescribed drugs. Natural licorice blocks the effects of spironolactone and causes sodium retention and potassium loss, effects that may worsen HF and potentiate the effects of digoxin. Hawthorn should be used cautiously as it may increase the effects of ACE inhibitors and digoxin. Use of ginseng can result in digoxin toxicity. Patients may utilize herbs such as dandelion root and juniper berries for their diuretic effect. Herbal and dietary supplements should not be taken instead of prescribed drug therapies.

Nursing Actions — Cardiotonic-Inotropic Drugs

NURSING ACTIONS	RATIONALE/EXPLANATION
1. Administer accurately	
a. With digoxin:	
(1) Read the drug label and the health care provider's order carefully when preparing a dose.	For accurate administration
(2) Give only the ordered dosage form (e.g., tablet, Lanoxicap, or elixir).	Digoxin formulations vary in concentration and bioavailability and *cannot* be used interchangeably.
(3) Check the apical pulse before each dose. If the rate is less than 60 in adults, 70 in older children, or 100 in younger children and infants, omit the dose, and notify the health care provider.	Bradycardia is an adverse effect.
(4) Have the same nurse give digoxin to the same patients when possible because it is important to detect changes in rate and rhythm (*see Observe for therapeutic effects* and *Observe for adverse effects,* later).	
(5) Give oral digoxin with food or after meals.	This may minimize gastric irritation and symptoms of anorexia, nausea, and vomiting. However, these symptoms probably arise from drug stimulation of chemoreceptors in the medulla rather than as a direct irritant effect of the drug on the gastrointestinal (GI) tract.
(6) Inject intravenous (IV) digoxin slowly (over at least 5 min).	Digoxin should be given slowly because the diluent, propylene glycol, has toxic effects on the cardiac conduction system if given too rapidly. Digoxin may be given undiluted or diluted with a fourfold or greater volume of sterile water for injection, 0.9% sodium chloride injection, or 5% dextrose injection. If diluted, use the solution immediately.
b. With milrinone:	
(1) Dilute with 0.9% or 0.45% sodium chloride or 5% dextrose solution; use the diluted solution within 24 hours.	Manufacturer's recommendations
(2) Give the loading dose by bolus infusion over 10 minutes.	
(3) Give maintenance infusions at a standard rate of 0.5 mcg/kg/min; this rate may be increased or decreased according to response.	Manufacturer's recommendations
c. With nesiritide:	
(1) Dilute with 5 mL of 0.9% or 0.45% sodium chloride or 5% dextrose solution from a 250 mL IV container; add mixed drug to the container and use diluted solution within 24 hours.	Manufacturer's recommendations
(2) Prime infusion tubing with 25 mL prior to connecting to the patient; withdraw a bolus loading dose from infusion solution.	Manufacturer's recommendations
(3) Give a bolus injection of 2 mcg/kg over 1 minute.	
(4) Give the maintenance infusion at a rate of 0.01 mcg/kg/min.	
(5) Do not mix with any other drug solution; administer through a separate line.	Incompatible with most drugs

(continued on page 776)

Nursing Actions Cardiotonic-Inotropic Drugs (continued)

NURSING ACTIONS	RATIONALE/EXPLANATION
2. Observe for therapeutic effects a. When the drugs are given in heart failure (HF), observe for: (1) Fewer signs and symptoms of pulmonary congestion (dyspnea, orthopnea, cyanosis, cough, hemoptysis, crackles, anxiety, restlessness)	The pulmonary symptoms that develop with HF are a direct result of events initiated by inadequate cardiac output. The left side of the heart is unable to accommodate incoming blood flow from the lungs. The resulting back pressure in pulmonary veins and capillaries causes leakage of fluid from blood vessels into tissue spaces and alveoli. Fluid accumulation may result in severe respiratory difficulty and pulmonary edema, a life-threatening development. The improved strength of myocardial contraction resulting from cardiotonic-inotropic drugs reverses this potentially fatal chain of events. Diuresis and decreased edema result from improved circulation and increased renal blood flow.
(2) Decreased edema—absence of pitting, decreased size of ankles or abdominal girth, decreased weight (3) Increased tolerance of activity	Indicates a more adequate supply of blood to tissues
b. When digoxin is given in atrial dysrhythmias, observe for: (1) Gradual slowing of the heart rate to 70 to 80 beats/min	In patients with atrial fibrillation, slowing of the heart rate and elimination of the pulse deficit are clinical indicators that digitalization has been achieved.
(2) Elimination of the pulse deficit (3) Change in rhythm from irregular to regular	
3. Observe for adverse effects a. With digoxin observe for:	There is a high incidence of adverse effects with digoxin therapy. Therefore, every patient receiving digoxin requires close observation. Severity of adverse effects can be minimized with early detection and treatment.
(1) Cardiac dysrhythmias:	Digoxin toxicity may cause any type of cardiac dysrhythmia. These are the most serious adverse effects associated with digoxin therapy. They are detected as abnormalities in electrocardiograms and in pulse rate or rhythm.
(a) Premature ventricular contractions (PVCs)	PVCs are among the most common digoxin-induced dysrhythmias. They are not specific for digoxin toxicity because there are many possible causes. They are usually perceived as "skipped" heartbeats by patients.
(b) Bradycardia	Excessive slowing of the heart rate is an extension of the drug's therapeutic action of slowing conduction through the atrioventricular (AV) node and probably depressing the sinoatrial node as well.
(c) Paroxysmal atrial tachycardia with heart block	Electrocardiogram study is necessary for identification of nodal rhythms and heart block.

(d) AV nodal tachycardia
    (e) AV block (second- or third-degree heart block)
  (2) Anorexia, nausea, vomiting
	These GI effects commonly occur with digoxin therapy. Because they are caused at least in part by stimulation of the vomiting center in the brain, they occur with parenteral and oral administration. The presence of these symptoms raises suspicion of digitalis toxicity, but they are not specific because many other conditions may cause anorexia, nausea, and vomiting. Also, patients receiving digoxin are often taking other medications that cause these side effects, such as diuretics and potassium supplements.

(3) Headache, drowsiness, confusion	These central nervous system effects are most common in older adults.
(4) Visual disturbances (e.g., blurred vision, photophobia, altered perception of colors, flickering dots)	These are due mainly to drug effects on the retina and may indicate acute toxicity.
b. With milrinone, observe for ventricular dysrhythmias, hypotension, and headache.	Ventricular dysrhythmias reportedly occur in 12% of patients, hypotension and headache in approximately 3% of patients.

NURSING ACTIONS	RATIONALE/EXPLANATION
c. With nesiritide, observe for hypotension, headache, nausea, back pain, ventricular tachycardia, dizziness, anxiety, insomnia, bradycardia, and vomiting.	Hypotension occurs in approximately 11% of patients; headache in 8%; nausea and back pain in 4%; and other adverse effects in 1%–3%.
4. Observe for drug interactions	Most significant drug interactions increase risks of toxicity. Some alter absorption or metabolism to produce under-digitalization and decreased therapeutic effect.
a. Drugs that *increase* effects of digoxin: (1) Adrenergic drugs (e.g., ephedrine, epinephrine, isoproterenol)	Increase risks of cardiac dysrhythmias
(2) Antidysrhythmics (e.g., amiodarone, propafenone, quinidine)	Decrease clearance of digoxin, thereby increasing serum digoxin levels and risks of toxicity. Dosage of digoxin should be reduced if one of these drugs is given concurrently (25% with propafenone and 50% with amiodarone and quinidine).
(3) Anticholinergics	Increase absorption of oral digoxin by slowing transit time through the GI tract
(4) Calcium preparations	Increase risks of cardiac dysrhythmias. IV calcium salts are contraindicated in digitalized patients.
(5) Calcium channel blockers (e.g., diltiazem, felodipine, nifedipine, verapamil)	Decrease clearance of digoxin, thereby increasing serum digoxin levels and risks of toxicity. Dosage of digoxin should be reduced 25% if verapamil is given concurrently.
b. Drugs that *decrease* effects of digoxin: (1) Antacids, cholestyramine, colestipol, laxatives, oral aminoglycosides (e.g., neomycin)	Decrease absorption of oral digoxin

Key Concepts

- Heart failure may result from impaired myocardial contraction during systole (systolic dysfunction), impaired relaxation and filling of ventricles during diastole (diastolic dysfunction), or a combination of systolic and diastolic dysfunction.
- The most common conditions leading to HF are coronary artery disease and hypertension.
- Cardinal manifestations of HF are dyspnea and fatigue, which can lead to exercise intolerance and fluid retention, resulting in pulmonary congestion and peripheral edema.
- Beta blockers are not recommended for patients in acute HF because of the potential for an initial decrease in myocardial contractility.

- For acute HF, the first drugs of choice may include an IV loop diuretic, a cardiotonic–inotropic agent (e.g., digoxin, dobutamine, milrinone), and vasodilators (e.g., nitroglycerin and hydralazine or nitroprusside).
- Digitalis toxicity is one of the most commonly encountered drug-related reasons for hospitalization because the drug has a narrow therapeutic index and the endpoint of effective therapy is often difficult to define and measure.
- The normal digoxin level is 0.5 to 2.0 ng/mL. Toxic serum levels are greater than 2 ng/mL; however, toxicity may occur at any serum level.

Review and Application Exercises

Short Answer Exercises

1. What signs and symptoms usually occur with HF? How would you assess for these?
2. What are the physiologic effects of digoxin on the heart?
3. How does digoxin produce or assist diuresis?
4. Differentiate between a loading dose of digoxin and a daily maintenance dose.
5. Why do nurses need to check heart rate and rhythm before giving digoxin?
6. When is it appropriate to withhold a dose of digoxin?
7. What are adverse effects associated with digoxin, and how may they be prevented or minimized?
8. Why is it important to maintain a therapeutic serum potassium level during digoxin therapy?
9. What is the specific antidote for severe digoxin toxicity?

NCLEX-Style Questions

10. A 65-year-old patient that you are caring for develops digoxin toxicity 1 month after beginning 0.25 mg of digoxin PO daily. Which factor will affect the duration of such an adverse reaction?
    a. daily drug dosage
    b. half-life of the drug
    c. form of the drug prescribed
    d. duration of therapy

11. A 5-year-old child that you are caring for has an order to be placed on digoxin. You know that the electrolyte imbalance that will place her at the greatest risk for digoxin toxicity is
    a. hyponatremia
    b. hyperkalemia
    c. hypocalcemia
    d. hypokalemia

12. When administering the daily dose of digoxin 0.125 mg PO to a patient with a history of type 1 diabetes mellitus who is now in heart failure, it is most important for the nurse to
    a. give it with orange juice
    b. monitor for dysrhythmias
    c. administer it 1 hour before the morning insulin
    d. withhold it if the apical pulse rate is less than 80 beats per minute

13. A 44-year-old patient develops blurring of the vision with yellow spots in his visual fields while taking digoxin. The nurse recognizes that the visual changes may indicate
    a. a need for a vision exam
    b. adjustment of the retina to the drug
    c. acute toxicity
    d. therapeutic effects

14. As the nurse prepares to administer a scheduled dose of digoxin to an adult patient, she reviews lab results from earlier in the day and notes that the plasma level of digoxin is 1.5 ng/mL. Based on this report, the nurse should
    a. Withhold the drug and notify the health care provider during rounds.
    b. Withhold the drug and notify the health care provider immediately.
    c. Administer Digibind to counteract the toxicity.
    d. Check the patient's pulse and if it is greater than 60 beats per minute, administer the dose of digoxin.

Selected References

Drug facts and comparisons. (Updated monthly). St. Louis, MO: Facts and Comparisons.

Ferri, F. F. (2007). *Practical guide to the care of the medical patient* (7th ed.). Philadelphia: Elsevier Mosby.

Gabardi, S. (2005). Drug dosing in chronic kidney disease. *Medical Clinics of North America, 89,* 649–687.

Hunt, S. A., Abraham, W. T., Chin, M. H., Feldman, F. A., Francis, G. S., Ganiats, T. G., Jessup, M., et al. (2005). ACC/AHA 2005 guideline update for the diagnosis and management of chronic heart failure in the adult—summary article: A report of the American College of Cardiology/American Heart Association Task Force on Practice Guidelines (writing committee to revise the 2001 Guidelines for the Evaluation and Management of Heart Failure). Retrieved September 30, 2007, from http://www.acc.org/qualityandscience/clinical/guidelines/failure/indexupdate101705_pkt.pdf

Karch, A. M. (2007). *2008 Lippincott's nursing drug guide.* Philadelphia: Lippincott Williams & Wilkins.

Kurien, S. (2006). Effects of standard heart failure therapy and concomitant treatment with intravenous furosemide or inotropes (dobutamine, dopamine, and/or milrinone) on renal function and mortality in patients treated with nesiritide. *American Journal of Cardiology, 98,* 1627–1630.

Kutzleb, J., & Reiner, D. (2006). The impact of nurse-directed patient education on quality of life and functional capacity in people with heart failure. *Journal of the American Academy of Nurse Practitioners, 18,* 116–123.

Lacy, C. F., Armstrong, L. L., Goldman, M. P., & Lance, L. L. (2007). *Lexi-Comp's drug information handbook* (15th ed.). Hudson, OH: American Pharmaceutical Association.

Morris, S. A. (2006). Digoxin therapy for heart failure: an update. *American Family Physician, 74,* 613–618.

Rich, M. W. (2006). Heart failure in older adults. *Medical Clinics of North America, 90,* 863–885, xi.

Smith, L. (2007). Diagnosis and management of chronic heart failure in adults (2007). *American Family Physician, 75,* 742–755.

Strunk, A. (2006). Impact of the history of congestive heart failure on the utility of B-type natriuretic peptide in the emergency diagnosis of heart failure: results from the Breathing Not Properly Multinational Study. *American Journal of Medicine, 119,* 69.e1-11.

Trupp, R. J. (2007). Building the foundation of excellence in heart failure nursing. *Progress in Cardiovascular Nursing, 22,* 180–182.

Antidysrhythmic Drugs

KEY TERMS

- Absolute refractory period
- Antidysrhythmic
- Arrhythmias
- Automaticity
- Dysrhythmias
- Ectopic
- Excitability
- Relative refractory period

LEARNING OBJECTIVES

After studying this chapter, you will be able to:

1. Provide an overview of the cardiac electrophysiology and specific cardiac dysrhythmias effecting rhythm.
2. Discuss the roles of sodium channel, beta-adrenergic, potassium channel, and calcium channel blockers along with two unclassified drugs in the management of dysrhythmias.
3. Describe the nursing process implications and actions related to caring for patients using selected antidysrhythmic drugs.
4. Describe principles of therapy to include nonpharmacologic and pharmacologic measures to manage tachydysrhythmias.
5. Differentiate between supraventricular and ventricular dysrhythmias in terms of etiology and hemodynamic effect on the patient.
6. Discuss the effects of dysrhythmias in special populations.

Applying Your Knowledge

Tyrone Brown is a 74-year old man with cardiovascular disease. He has just undergone cardiac bypass surgery for three coronary artery bypasses. During the postoperative period, Mr. Brown develops premature ventricular complexes (PVCs) and atrial fibrillation (AF).

Introduction

Antidysrhythmic agents are medications used for prevention and treatment of cardiac dysrhythmias. *Dysrhythmias*, sometimes called *arrhythmias*, are abnormalities in heart rate or rhythm. They become significant when they interfere with cardiac function and the ability to perfuse body tissues. To aid in understanding of antidysrhythmic drug therapy, the physiology of the cardiac conduction system is reviewed.

Cardiac Electrophysiology

The heart is an electrical pump. The "electrical" activity resides primarily in the specialized tissues that can generate and conduct an electrical impulse. Although impulses are conducted through muscle cells, the rate is much slower. The mechanical or "pump" activity resides in contractile tissue. Normally, these activities result in effective cardiac contraction and distribution of blood throughout the body. Each heartbeat occurs at regular intervals and consists of four events: *stimulation* from an electrical impulse, *transmission* of the electrical impulse to adjacent conductive or contractile tissue, *contraction* of atria and then ventricles, and *relaxation* of atria and then ventricles.

Automaticity

Automaticity is the heart's ability to generate an electrical impulse. Any part of the conduction system can spontaneously start an impulse, but the sinoatrial (SA) node normally has the fastest rate of automaticity and therefore the faster rate of spontaneous impulse formation. With this faster rate of electrical discharge or depolarization than other parts of the conduction system, the SA node serves as the pacemaker site.

Initiation of an electrical impulse depends predominately on the movement of sodium and calcium ions into a myocardial cell and movement of potassium ions out of the cell. Normally, the cell membrane becomes more permeable to sodium and opens channels to allow rapid movement into the cell. Calcium ions follow sodium ions into the cell at a slower rate and through different channels. As sodium and calcium ions move into cells, potassium ions move out of cells. The movement of the ions changes the membrane from its resting state of electrical neutrality to an activated state of electrical energy buildup. After the electrical energy is discharged (depolarization), muscle contraction occurs.

The ability of a cardiac muscle cell to respond to an electrical stimulus is called *excitability*. The stimulus must reach a certain threshold to cause contraction. After contraction, sodium and calcium ions return to the extracellular space, potassium ions return to the intracellular space, muscle relaxation occurs, and the cell prepares for the next electrical stimulus followed by contraction.

Following contraction there is also a period of decreased excitability (called the *absolute refractory period*) during which the cell cannot respond to a new stimulus. Before the resting membrane potential is reached, a stimulus greater than normal can evoke a response in the cell. This period is called the *relative refractory period*.

Conductivity

Conductivity is the ability of cardiac tissue to transmit electrical impulses. The orderly, rhythmic transmission of impulses to all cells is needed for effective myocardial contraction. The cardiac conduction system is shown in Figure 49-1. Normally, electrical impulses originate in the SA node and are transmitted through internodal pathways to the atrioventricular (AV) node, where the impulse is delayed for a period of time. Then the impulse travels through the bundle of His, bundle branches, Purkinje fibers, and throughout the ventricular muscle.

Cardiac Dysrhythmias

Cardiac dysrhythmias can originate in any part of the conduction system or from atrial or ventricular muscle. They result from disturbances in electrical impulse formation (automaticity), conduction (conductivity), or both. The characteristic of automaticity allows myocardial cells other than the SA node to depolarize and initiate the electrical impulse that culminates in contraction. This may occur when the SA node fails to initiate an impulse or does so too slowly. When the electrical impulse arises anywhere other than the SA node, it is an abnormal or *ectopic* focus. If the ectopic focus depolarizes at a rate faster than the SA node, the ectopic focus becomes the dominant pacemaker. Ectopic pacemakers may be activated by hypoxia, ischemia, or hypokalemia. Ectopic foci indicate myocardial irritability (increased responsiveness to stimuli) and potentially serious impairment of cardiac function.

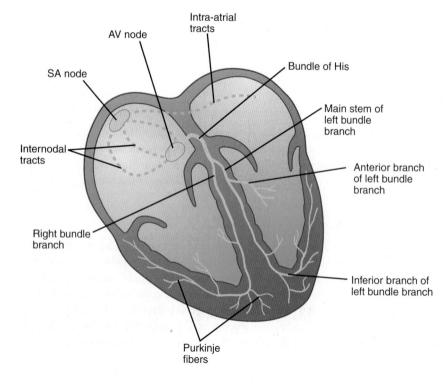

Intra-atrial tracts

AV node

SA node

Bundle of His

Main stem of left bundle branch

Internodal tracts

Anterior branch of left bundle branch

Right bundle branch

Inferior branch of left bundle branch

Purkinje fibers

Figure 49.1 ■ The conducting system of the heart. Impulses originating in the SA node are transmitted through the atria, into the AV node to the bundle of His, and by way of Purkinje fibers through the ventricles.

Dysrhythmias may be clinically significant if they interfere with cardiac function (i.e., the heart's ability to pump sufficient blood to body tissues). The normal heart can maintain an adequate cardiac output with ventricular rates ranging from 40 to 150 beats per minute. The diseased heart, however, may not be able to maintain an adequate cardiac output with heart rates below 60 or above 120 beats per minute. Dysrhythmias are usually categorized by rate, location, or patterns of conduction. Various types of dysrhythmias are described in Box 49-1.

General Characteristics of Antidysrhythmic Drugs

Antidysrhythmic drugs alter the heart's electrical conduction system. Atropine for bradydysrhythmias is discussed in Chapter 20; digoxin and its use in treating atrial fibrillation (A-Fib) are discussed in Chapter 48. The focus of this chapter is the drugs used for *tachydysrhythmias*. These drugs are described in the following sections and listed in Table 49-1.

Clinical use of antidysrhythmic drugs for tachydysrhythmias has undergone changes. One change is that the goal of drug therapy is to prevent or relieve symptoms or prolong survival, not just suppress dysrhythmias. This change resulted from study outcomes in which patients treated for some dysrhythmias had a higher mortality rate than patients who did not receive antidysrhythmic drug therapy. The higher mortality rate was attributed to prodysrhythmic effects (i.e., worsening existing dysrhythmias or causing new dysrhythmias).

Another change is the greater use of nonpharmacologic management of dysrhythmias. These treatments include destroying dysrhythmogenic areas within the heart with radio waves through radiofrequency catheter ablation or surgical procedures, thereby implanting devices for sensing, cardioverting, defibrillating, and/or pacing the patient (e.g., the implantable cardioverter–defibrillator [ICD]).

Indications for Use

Antidysrhythmic drug therapy is commonly indicated in the following conditions:

- Conversion of atrial fibrillation (A-Fib) or atrial flutter to normal sinus rhythm (NSR)
- Maintaining NSR after conversion from A-Fib or atrial flutter
- Suppression of a fast or irregular ventricular rate which alters the cardiac output. Altered cardiac output leads to symptoms of decreased coronary, cerebral, and/or systemic circulation.
- Presence of dangerous dysrhythmias that may be fatal if not quickly terminated. For example, ventricular tachycardia may cause cardiac arrest.

Mechanisms of Action

Drugs used for the treatment of rapid dysrhythmias mainly reduce automaticity (spontaneous depolarization of myocardial cells, including ectopic pacemakers), slow conduction of electrical impulses through the heart, and prolong the refractory period of myocardial cells (so they are less likely to be prematurely activated by adjacent cells). Several different groups of drugs perform one or more of these actions. They are classified according to their mechanisms of action and effects on the conduction system, even though they differ in other respects. Additionally, some drugs have characteristics of more than one classification.

Classifications and Individual Drugs

Class I Sodium Channel Blockers

Class I drugs block cardiac sodium channels and slow conduction velocity, prolonging refractoriness and decreasing automaticity of sodium-dependent tissue. This results in a membrane-stabilizing effect and decreases formation and conduction of electrical impulses.

Class IA

Class IA drugs have a broad spectrum of *antidysrhythmic* effects that block sodium and potassium channels. They are used for maintenance of normal sinus rhythm (NSR) after conversion of atrial fibrillation (A-Fib) or atrial flutter; treatment of symptomatic premature ventricular contractions (PVCs), supraventricular tachycardia (SVT), and ventricular tachycardia (VT); and prevention of ventricular fibrillation (V-Fib).

P **Quinidine**, the prototype, reduces automaticity, slows conduction, and prolongs the refractory period. Quinidine is well absorbed after oral administration. Therapeutic serum levels (2–5 mcg/mL) are attained within 1 hour and persist for 6 to 8 hours. Quinidine is highly bound to serum albumin and has a half-life of about 6 hours. It is metabolized by the liver (about 80%) and excreted in the urine (about 20%). In alkaline urine (i.e., pH > 7), renal excretion of quinidine decreases, and serum levels may rise. Serum levels greater than 5 micrograms per milliliter are toxic. Quinidine is usually contraindicated in patients with severe, uncompensated heart failure or with heart block because it depresses myocardial contractility and conduction through the AV node.

Procainamide is related to the local anesthetic procaine and is similar to quinidine in actions and uses. Quinidine may be preferred for long-term use because procainamide produces a high incidence of adverse effects, including a syndrome resembling lupus erythematosus. Procainamide has a short duration of action (3–4 hours); sustained-release tablets (Procanbid) prolong action to about 6 hours. Therapeutic serum levels are 4 to 8 micrograms per milliliter.

Disopyramide is similar to quinidine in pharmacologic actions and may be given orally to adults with ventricular tachydysrhythmias. It is well absorbed after oral administration and reaches peak serum levels (2–8 mcg/mL) within 30 to 60 minutes. Toxic serum level is greater than 8 micrograms per milliliter. Drug half-life is 4 to 10 hours. Disopyramide is

Box 49-1	Types of Dysrhythmias

Sinus bradycardia

Premature ventricular contractions (the third beat)

Sinus tachycardia

Ventricular tachycardia

Atrial flutter

Ventricular fibrillation

Atrial fibrillation (Lead II view)

Table 49-1 **Drugs at a Glance:** Antidysrhythmic Drugs

	ROUTES AND DOSAGE RANGES	
Drugs for Tachydysrhythmias	**Adults**	**Children**

Class I Sodium Channel Blockers

Class 1A

Maintenance of normal sinus rhythm (NSR) after conversion of atrial fibrillation (A-Fib) or atrial flutter; treatment of symptomatic premature ventricular contractions (PVCs), supraventricular tachycardia (SVT), and ventricular tachycardia (VT); prevention of ventricular fibrillation (V-fib).

Quinidine	PO 100–600 mg q4–6h; maximum dose, 3–4 g/d; maintenance dose, PO 200–600 mg q4-6h, or extended-action tablets, 324–972 mg q8–12h	Safety and efficacy not established PO 30 mg/kg/d in doses every q4–6h
Procainamide (Pronestyl, Procanbid)	PO loading dose 1 g initially, then 250–500 mg q3–6h (500–1000 mg q6h for sustained-release tablets) IM loading dose, 500–1000 mg followed by oral maintenance doses IV loading dose 50–100 mg; may repeat q5–10 min or 15–18 mg/kg (max 1–1.5 g); then maintenance infusion 3–4 mg/min	PO 15–50 mg/kg/d in divided doses q3–6h IV loading dose 3–6 mg/kg over 5 min (max 100 mg); may repeat q5–10 min to max total dose of 15 mg/kg; then maintenance dose of 20–80 mcg/kg/min; max 2 g/d
Disopyramide (Norpace)	PO (weighing 50 kg and more) 150 mg q6h (300 mg q12h extended release); (weighing less than 50 kg) 100 mg q6h (200 mg q12h with extended release)	12–18 y: 6–15 mg/kg/d in 4 divided doses 5–11 y: 10–15 mg/kg/d in 4 divided doses 1–4 y: 10–20 mg/kg/d in 4 divided doses <1 y: 10–30 mg/kg/d in 4 divided doses

Class 1B

Treatment of symptomatic premature ventricular contractions (PVCs) and ventricular tachycardia (VT); prevention of ventricular fibrillation (V-fib).

Lidocaine (Xylocaine)	IV 1 mg/kg bolus, not to exceed 50–100 mg, as a single bolus injection at 25–50 mg/min, may be repeated in 5 min; give no more than 200–300 mg in 1 h followed by a continuous infusion of 1–4 mg/min; maximum dose IM 4.3 mg/kg as a single dose; may repeat in 60–90 min	IV injection 0.5–1 mg/kg bolus, may repeat but total dose not to exceed 3–5 mg/kg; followed by IV infusion of 10–50 mcg/kg/min
Mexiletine (Mexitil)	PO 200 mg q8h initially, increased by 50–100 mg every 2–3 d if necessary to a maximum of 1200 mg/d	1.4–5 mg/kg per dose, given every 8 h
Tocainide (Tonocard)	PO 400 mg q8h initial dose; 1.2–1.8 g/d in divided doses q8h maintenance dose	Safety and efficacy not established
Phenytoin (Dilantin)	PO, loading dose 250 mg 4 times a day for 1 day; 250 mg 2 times a day for 2 days; maintenance dose 300–400 mg/d 1–4 times per day IV loading dose 1.25 mg/kg q5min; may repeat up to total dose of 15 mg/kg	PO 5–10 mg/kg/d in 2–3 divided doses IV loading dose 1.25 mg/kg q5 min; may repeat up to total dose of 15 mg/kg; maintenance dose 5–10 mg/kg/d in 2–3 divided doses

Class IC

Treatment of life-threatening ventricular tachycardia (VT) or ventricular fibrillation (V-fib) and supraventricular tachycardia (SVT) unresponsive to other drugs

(continued on page 784)

Table 49-1	**Drugs at a Glance:** Antidysrhythmic Drugs (continued)	

	ROUTES AND DOSAGE RANGES	
Drugs for Tachydysrhythmias	**Adults**	**Children**
Flecainide (Tambocor)	PO 100 mg q12h initially, increased by 50 mg q12h every 4 d until effective; maximum dose, 400 mg/d	Initial 1–3 mg/kg/d in 3 divided doses; usual 3–6 mg/kg/d in 3 divided doses up to 8 mg/kg/d
Propafenone (Rythmol)	PO 150 mg q8h initially, increase at 3–4 day intervals to 225 mg q8h, then to 300 mg q8h; maximum dose of 900 mg/d PO (extended release) 225 mg q12h initially, may increase at 5 day intervals; maximum 425 mg q12h	Safety and efficacy not established
Moricizine (Ethmozine)	PO 200–300 mg q8h; maximum dose 900 mg/d	Safety and efficacy not established
Class II Beta-Adrenergic Blockers		
Treatment of supraventricular tachycardia		
Acebutolol (Sectral) Beta$_1$	PO 200 mg q12h, increased gradually to 600–1200 mg/d in 2 divided doses	Safety and efficacy not established
Atenolol (Tenormin) Beta$_1$	IV push 5 mg over 5 min; may repeat in 10 min. Give IV infusion over 15 min PO 50–100 mg/d	No dosing for this indication
Bisoprolol (Zebeta) Beta$_1$	PO 2.5–5 mg/d. May increase up to 20 mg/d.	Safety and efficacy not established
Carteolol (Cartrol) Beta$_1$ Beta$_2$	PO 2.5–10 mg/d	No dosing for this indication
Esmolol (Brevibloc) Beta$_1$	IV 500 mcg/kg/min initially as a loading dose for 1 min, followed by a maintenance dose of 50 mcg/kg/min over 4 min. If no response in 5 min, repeat the same loading dose, and increase maintenance doses to 100 mcg/kg/min for 4 min, continue to increase by 50 mcg/kg/min up to 200 mcg/kg/min for 4 min. Once desired response is attained, stop leading dose and increase infusion by no more than 25 mcg/kg/min. Average maintenance dose 100 mcg/kg/min. Infusion administered over 24–48 h.	IV infusion 500 mcg/kg/min initially as a loading dose over 1 min, with a maximum dose of 50–250 mcg/kg/min
Metoprolol (Lopressor) Beta$_1$	IV injection 1–5 mg over 1 min every 2 min for 3 doses, followed by 50 mg PO q6h for 48 h. Begin oral dose 15 min after last IV dose. PO 50–450 mg/d	Safety and efficacy not established
Nadolol (Corgard) Beta$_1$	PO 40 mg/d, may increase by 40–80 mg at 3–7 day intervals. Maximum 240–360 mg/d	Safety and efficacy not established
Propranolol (Inderal) Beta$_1$ Beta$_2$	PO 10–20 mg q6-8h; may gradually increase dose to 40–320 mg/d IV 0.5–3 mg repeat once in 2 min, additional doses at intervals of at least 4 h; maximum 5 mg total	PO 0.5–1 mg/kg/d in divided doses q6–8 h; may increase every 3–5 days; usual dose 2–4 mg/kg/d; maximum 16 mg/kg/d

	ROUTES AND DOSAGE RANGES	
Drugs for Tachydysrhythmias	**Adults**	**Children**
		IV injection 0.01–0.1 mg/kg slow IVP over 10 min, with a maximum dose of 3 mg; infant maximum dose of 1 mg
Sotalol (Betapace) *Beta$_1$ Beta$_2$*	PO 80 mg q12h initially, titrated to response; average dose, 160–320 mg daily. See manufacturer's recommendations for dosing in renal failure.	Safety and efficacy not established
Timolol (Blocadren) *Beta$_1$ Beta$_2$*	PO 10 mg twice a day beginning 1–4 wk after infarction	Safety and efficacy not established
Class III Potassium Channel Blockers Treatment of ventricular tachycardia (VT) and ventricular fibrillation (V-fib); conversion of atrial flutter or atrial fibrillation to sinus rhythm; maintenance of sinus rhythm (amiodarone)		
Amiodarone (Cordarone)	Loading dose, IV 150 mg over 10 min (15 mg/min), then 360 mg over the next 6 h (1 mg/min), then 540 mg over the next 18 h (0.5 mg/min); maintenance dose, IV 720 mg/24 h (0.5 mg/min) Loading dose, PO 800–1600 mg/d for 1–3 wk, with a gradual decrease to 600–800 mg/d for 1 month; maintenance dose, PO 400 mg/d	IV safety and efficacy not established Loading dose, PO 10–15 mg/kg/d in 1–2 divided doses for up to 14 d or until dysrhythmia controlled. Dose should then be reduced to 5 mg/kg/d once daily for several weeks. Minimal maintenance dose, PO 2.5 mg/kg/d for 5–7 d/wk
Dofetilide (Tikosyn)	IV 500 mcg twice daily with creatinine clearance > 60 mL/min, adjusted to manage adverse effects	Safety and efficacy not established
Ibutilide (Corvert)	Weight > 60 kg: IV infusion over 10 min, 1 mg Weight < 60 kg: IV infusion over 10 min, 0.01 mg/kg The dose can be repeated once, after 10 min, if necessary.	Safety and efficacy not established
Sotalol (Betapace) *Class II and class III effects*	PO 80 mg q12h initially, titrated to response; average dose, 160–320 mg daily. See manufacturer's recommendations for dosing in renal failure.	Safety and efficacy not established
Class IV Calcium Channel Blockers Treatment of supraventricular tachycardia		
Diltiazem (Cardizem)	IV injection 0.25 mg/kg (average dose 20 mg) over 2 min. A second dose of 0.35 mg/kg (average, 25 mg) may be given in 15 min, and an IV infusion of 5–15 mg/h may be given up to 24 h, if necessary.	Safety and efficacy not established
Verapamil (Calan, Isoptin)	PO 40–120 mg q6–8h IV 5–10 mg initially, then 10 mg 30 min later, if necessary	1–15 y: IV injection 0.1–0.3 mg/kg (usual range 2–5 mg for a single dose) over 2 min with continuous ECG monitoring; repeat in 30 min if necessary <1 y: IV injection 0.1–0.2 mg/kg (usual range, 0.75–2.0 mg for a single dose) over 2 min with continuous ECG monitoring
Unclassified Adenosine is used to treat supraventricular tachycardia; magnesium sulfate is used to treat torsades de pointes		
Adenosine (Adenocard)	IV 6 mg given rapidly over 1–2 sec. If first dose does not slow the	*Neonates:* Initial IV dose 0.05 mg/kg. If first dose does not slow the

(continued on page 786)

Table 49-1	Drugs at a Glance: Antidysrhythmic Drugs (continued)	

	ROUTES AND DOSAGE RANGES	
Drugs for Tachydysrhythmias	**Adults**	**Children**
	supraventricular tachycardia within 1–2 min, give 12 mg rapidly, and repeat one time, if necessary.	supraventricular tachycardia within 1–2 min, increase dose by 0.25 mg/kg. *Infants and children:* 0.1 mg/kg. If first dose does not slow the supraventricular tachycardia, give 0.2 mg/kg.
Magnesium sulfate	IV 1–2 g (2–4 mL of 50% solution), diluted in 10 mL of 5% dextrose solution	Safety and efficacy not established for treatment of torsades de pointes

ECG, electrocardiogram; IVP, intravenous push.

excreted by the kidneys and the liver in almost equal proportions. Dosage must be reduced in renal insufficiency based on creatinine clearance. The U.S. Food and Drug Administration (FDA) has issued a **BLACK BOX WARNING** for disopyramide due to its known prodysrhythmic properties; the drug should be reserved for patients with life-threatening ventricular dysrhythmias.

Class IB

Class IB drugs shorten the repolarization phase.

P **Lidocaine** as an antidysrhythmic is the prototype of class IB drugs. It is the drug of choice for treating serious ventricular dysrhythmias associated with acute myocardial infarction, cardiac catheterization, cardiac surgery, and digitalis-induced ventricular dysrhythmias. Lidocaine decreases myocardial irritability (automaticity) in the ventricles. It has little effect on atrial tissue and thus is not useful in treating atrial dysrhythmias. It differs from quinidine in that it

- Must be given by injection
- Does not decrease AV conduction with usual therapeutic doses
- Has a rapid onset and short duration of action. After intravenous (IV) administration of a bolus dose, therapeutic effects occur within 1 to 2 minutes and last approximately 10 to 20 minutes. This characteristic is advantageous in emergency management but limits lidocaine use to intensive care settings.
- Is metabolized in the liver; thus dosage must be reduced in patients with hepatic insufficiency or right-sided heart failure to avoid drug accumulation and toxicity.
- Uncommonly does not have serious adverse reactions

Therapeutic serum levels of lidocaine are 1.5 to 6 micrograms per milliliter. Toxic serum levels are greater than 6 micrograms per milliliter. Lidocaine is contraindicated in patients allergic to related local anesthetics (e.g., procaine). Anaphylactic reactions may occur in sensitized individuals.

Mexiletine is an oral analog of lidocaine with similar pharmacologic actions. The drug is used to suppress ventricu-

lar tachycardia or ventricular fibrillation. It is well absorbed from the GI tract, and peak serum levels are obtained within 3 hours. Taking the drug with food delays but does not decrease absorption.

Tocainide is used for the suppression and prevention of ventricular dysrhythmias, including frequent unifocal and multifocal PVCs. It is rapidly and completely absorbed following oral administration and is metabolized in the liver and excreted in the urine. Therapeutic serum levels are 4 to 10 micrograms per milliliter, and toxic serum levels have not been established.

Phenytoin may be used to treat dysrhythmias produced by digoxin intoxication. Phenytoin decreases automaticity and improves conduction through the AV node. Decreased automaticity helps control dysrhythmias, whereas enhanced conduction may improve cardiac function. Further, because heart block may result from digoxin, quinidine, or procainamide, phenytoin may relieve dysrhythmias without intensifying heart block. Phenytoin is not a cardiac depressant. Its only quinidine-like action is to suppress automaticity; otherwise, it counteracts the effects of quinidine and procainamide largely by increasing the rate of conduction. Phenytoin also has a longer half-life (22–36 hours) than other antidysrhythmic drugs. Given IV, a therapeutic plasma level (10–20 mcg/mL) can be obtained rapidly. Given orally, however, the drug may not reach a steady-state concentration for approximately 1 week unless loading doses are given initially.

Applying Your Knowledge 49-1

You are assigned to care for Mr. Brown. He is prescribed lidocaine and started on IV lidocaine to control his PVCs. What therapeutic level should you monitor for?

Class IC

Class 1C drugs have no effect on the repolarization phase but slow conduction velocity and the refractory period. **Flecainide** and **propafenone** are oral agents that greatly decrease conduction in the ventricles. Along with **moricizine,** these drugs may cause new dysrhythmias or aggravate pre-existing dysrhythmias, sometimes causing sustained VT or V-Feb; thus therapy should be initiated in hospitalized patients with continuous electrocardiographic (ECG) monitoring. These effects are more likely to occur with high doses and rapid dose increases. The drugs are recommended for use in life-threatening ventricular dysrhythmias.

Class II Beta-Adrenergic Blockers

These agents (see Chap. 18) exert antidysrhythmic effects by slowing the sympathetic nervous system stimulation of beta receptors in the heart, slowing the SA and AV nodal conduction. Blockage of receptors in the SA node and ectopic pacemakers decreases automaticity and blockage of receptors in the AV node increases the refractory period. The drugs are effective for management of dysrhythmias resulting from excessive sympathetic activity. They are most often used to slow the ventricular rate of contraction in atrial flutter and A-Fib.

As a class II, beta-adrenergic blockers are being used more extensively because of their effectiveness in reducing mortality in post–myocardial infarction and heart failure patients. Reduced mortality may result from the drugs' ability to prevent ventricular fibrillation.

Propranolol may be given orally for chronic therapy to prevent ventricular dysrhythmias, especially those precipitated by exercise. It may be given IV for life-threatening dysrhythmias or for those occurring during anesthesia. **Esmolol** has a rapid onset and short duration of action. It is given IV for SVT and A-Fib or atrial flutter, especially during anesthesia, surgery, or other emergency situations when the ventricular rate must be reduced rapidly. It is not used for chronic therapy.

Dizziness is usually the first sign of impending hypotension. If pulse is 60 or less or systolic BP is 90 mmHg or less, withhold the beta-adrenergic blocker and contact a physician. **Acebutolol** may be given orally for chronic therapy to prevent ventricular dysrhythmias, especially those precipitated by exercise. A variety of beta-adrenergic blockers are listed in Table 49-1 that may be used for the treatment of dysrhythmias.

Class III Potassium Channel Blockers

These drugs act to prolong duration of the action potential, slow repolarization, and prolong the refractory period in both atria and ventricles. This is accomplished by blocking the cardiac potassium channels. Although the drugs share a common mechanism of action, they are very different drugs.

Although classified as a potassium channel blocker, **amiodarone** also has electrophysiologic characteristics of sodium channel blockers, beta blockers, and calcium channel blockers. Thus, it has vasodilating effects and decreases systemic vascular resistance, it prolongs conduction in all cardiac tissues and decreases heart rate, and it decreases contractility of the left ventricle.

Intravenous and oral amiodarone differ in their electrophysiologic effects. When given IV, the major effect is slowing conduction through the AV node and prolonging the effective refractory period. Thus, it is given IV mainly for acute suppression of refractory, hemodynamically destabilizing ventricular tachycardia and ventricular fibrillation. The drug has assumed an increasing role as a preferred agent in the American Heart Association Advanced Cardiac Life Support (ACLS) algorithm for this purpose. It is given orally to treat recurrent ventricular tachycardia or ventricular fibrillation and to maintain an NSR after conversion of A-Fib and atrial flutter. Low doses (100–200 mg/day) may prevent recurrence of A-Fib with less toxicity than higher doses of amiodarone or usual doses of other agents.

Amiodarone is extensively metabolized in the liver and produces active metabolites. The drug and its metabolites accumulate in the liver, lungs, fat, skin, and other tissues. With IV administration, the onset of action usually occurs within several hours. With oral administration, the action may be delayed from 3 days up to 3 weeks. Because of its long serum half-life, loading doses are usually given. These loading doses reduce the time required for therapeutic effects. However, effects may persist for several weeks after the drug is discontinued.

Amiodarone is an iodine-rich drug that has been associated with thyroid dysfunction, with hypothyroidism occurring more frequently than hyperthyroidism. Other adverse effects include serious, potentially fatal pulmonary toxicity (pulmonary fibrosis, pneumonitis, acute respiratory distress syndrome [ARDS]) which may begin with progressive dyspnea and cough with crackles, decreased breath sounds, pleurisy, heart failure, or hepatotoxicity. The FDA has issued a **BLACK BOX WARNING** for amiodarone recommending use only in patients with life-threatening dysrhythmias due to this substantial toxicity potential.

Corneal microdeposits are noted in almost all patients treated for more than 2 months and can lead to blurry vision. Most adverse effects are considered dose dependent and reversible. However, maintenance dose selection is difficult because absorption and elimination are variable.

When oral amiodarone is used long term, it also increases the effects of numerous drugs, worsening existing dysrhythmias or producing new dysrhythmias. Other drug interactions include beta blockers, oral anticoagulants, digoxin, and phenytoin.

Dofetilide is indicated for the maintenance of NSR in symptomatic patients who are in A-Fib of more than 1 week's duration. Adverse effects increase with decreasing creatinine clearance levels so renal function must be assessed and initial dosage is dependent on creatinine clearance levels. High dosages in patients with renal dysfunction result in drug accumulation and prodysrhythmia (torsades de pointes). The drug has an elimination half-life of approximately 8 hours with the kidneys being the major route of elimination. The drug should initially be administered in a setting with personnel and equipment available for emergency use.

Ibutilide is indicated for management of recent onset of A-Fib or atrial flutter, in which the goal is conversion to NSR. The drug enhances the efficacy of cardioversion. Ibutilide is structurally similar to sotalol but lacks clinically significant beta-blocking activity. Ibutilide is widely distributed and has an elimination half-life of about 6 hours. Most of a dose is metabolized, and the metabolites are excreted in urine and feces. Adverse effects include supraventricular and ventricular dysrhythmias (particularly torsades de pointes) and hypotension. Ibutilide should be administered in a setting with personnel and equipment available for emergency use.

Sotalol has both beta-adrenergic–blocking and potassium channel–blocking activity. Beta-blocking effects predominate at lower doses and class III effects predominate at higher doses. The drug is well absorbed after oral administration, and peak serum level is reached in 2 to 4 hours. It has an elimination half-life of approximately 12 hours, and 80% to 90% is excreted unchanged by the kidneys. Sotalol is approved for prevention or management of ventricular tachycardia and fibrillation. It has also been used, usually in smaller doses, to prevent or treat A-Fib. However, it is less effective than amiodarone in the prophylaxis of A-Fib. It is contraindicated in patients with asthma, sinus bradycardia, heart block, cardiogenic shock, heart failure, and previous hypersensitivity to sotalol. Dosage should be individualized, reduced with renal impairment, and increased slowly (e.g., every 2 to 3 days with normal renal function, at longer intervals with impaired renal function). Dysrhythmogenic effects are most likely to occur when therapy is started or when dosage is increased. Heart failure may occur in patients with markedly depressed left ventricular systolic function. Most adverse effects are attributed to beta-blocking activity.

Like amiodarone, sotalol may be preferred over a class I agent because it is more effective in reducing recurrent ventricular tachycardia, ventricular fibrillation, and death.

Applying Your Knowledge 49-2

Mr. Brown's AF is converted to NSR pharmacologically. The physician prescribes amiodarone at 200 mg PO daily. Why is Mr. Brown given this drug and what adverse effects should you monitor?

· ·

Class IV Calcium Channel Blockers

Calcium channel blockers (see Chap. 50) block the movement of calcium into conductile and contractile myocardial cells by inhibiting the influx of calcium through its channels, causing a slower conduction through the sinus and AV nodes. As antidysrhythmic agents, they act primarily against tachycardias at SA and AV nodes because the cardiac cells and slow channels that depend on calcium influx are found mainly at these sites. Thus, they reduce automaticity of the SA and AV nodes, slow conduction, and prolong the refractory period in the AV node. They are effective only in supraventricular tachycardias.

Diltiazem and **verapamil** are the only calcium channel blockers approved for management of dysrhythmias. Both drugs may be given IV to terminate acute paroxysmal

supraventricular tachycardia (PSVT), usually within 2 minutes, and in A-Fib and atrial flutter. They are also effective in exercise-related tachycardias. When given IV, the drugs act within 15 minutes and last up to 6 hours. Oral verapamil may be used in the chronic management of the aforementioned dysrhythmias. Diltiazem and verapamil are metabolized by the liver, and metabolites are primarily excreted by the kidneys. The drugs are contraindicated in digoxin toxicity because they may worsen heart block. If used with propranolol or digoxin, caution must be exercised to avoid further impairment of myocardial contractility. Do not use IV verapamil with IV propranolol; potentially fatal bradycardia and hypotension may occur.

Unclassified Drugs

Adenosine, a naturally occurring component of all body cells, differs chemically from other antidysrhythmic drugs but acts like the calcium channel blockers. It depresses conduction at the AV node and is used to restore NSR in patients with PSVT; it is ineffective in other dysrhythmias. The drug has a very short duration of action (serum half-life is less than 10 seconds) and a high degree of effectiveness. It must be given by a rapid bolus injection, preferably through a central venous line. If given slowly, it is eliminated before it can reach cardiac tissues and exert its action.

Magnesium sulfate is given IV in the management of several dysrhythmias, including prevention of recurrent episodes of torsades de pointes and management of digitalis-induced dysrhythmias. Its antidysrhythmic effects may derive from imbalances of magnesium, potassium, and calcium.

Hypomagnesemia increases myocardial irritability and is a risk factor for both atrial and ventricular dysrhythmias. Thus, serum magnesium levels should be monitored in patients at risk and replacement therapy instituted when indicated. However, in some instances, the drug seems to have antidysrhythmic effects even when serum magnesium levels are normal.

Nursing Process

Assessment

- Assess the patient's condition in relation to cardiac dysrhythmias.

- Identify conditions or risk factors that may precipitate dysrhythmias. These include the following:

  - Hypoxia

  - Electrolyte imbalances (e.g., hypokalemia, hypomagnesemia, hypocalcemia)

  - Acid–base imbalances

  - Acute coronary syndrome (angina pectoris, myocardial infarction)

- ▫ Cardiac valvular disease
- ▫ Febrile illness
- ▫ Respiratory disorders (e.g., chronic lung disease)
- ▫ Exercise
- ▫ Emotional upset
- ▫ Excessive ingestion of caffeine-containing beverages (e.g., coffee, tea, colas)
- ▫ Cigarette smoking
- ▫ Drug therapy use of digoxin, antidysrhythmic drugs, CNS stimulants, anorexiants, and tricyclic antidepressants
- ▫ Hyperthyroidism

- ■ Observe for clinical signs and symptoms of dysrhythmias. Mild or infrequent dysrhythmias may be perceived by the patient as palpitations or skipped heartbeats. More severe dysrhythmias may produce manifestations that reflect decreased cardiac output and other hemodynamic changes, as follows:

  - ▫ Hypotension, bradycardia or tachycardia, and irregular rhythm
  - ▫ Shortness of breath, dyspnea, and cough from impaired respiration
  - ▫ Syncope or mental confusion from reduced cerebral blood flow
  - ▫ Chest pain from decreased coronary artery blood flow. Angina pectoris or myocardial infarction may occur.
  - ▫ Oliguria from decreased renal blood flow

- ■ When ECG monitoring is available (e.g., 12-lead ECG or continuous ECG monitoring), assess for indications of dysrhythmias.

Nursing Diagnoses

- ■ Decreased Cardiac Output related to ineffective rhythm of the heart
- ■ Decreased Tissue Perfusion, cerebral and peripheral, related to compromised cardiac output or medication-induced hypotension
- ■ Activity Intolerance related to weakness and fatigue
- ■ Impaired Gas Exchange related to decreased tissue perfusion
- ■ Anxiety related to potentially serious illness
- ■ Deficient Knowledge: Pharmacologic and nonpharmacologic management of dysrhythmias
- ■ Excess Fluid Volume: Peripheral edema and pulmonary congestion related to alteration in cardiac output

Planning/Goals

The patient will

- ■ Receive or take antidysrhythmic drugs accurately
- ■ Avoid conditions that precipitate dysrhythmias, when feasible
- ■ Experience improved heart rate, circulation, and activity tolerance
- ■ Be monitored for therapeutic and adverse drug effects
- ■ Avoid preventable adverse drug effects
- ■ Have adverse drug effects promptly recognized and treated if they occur
- ■ Keep follow-up appointments for monitoring responses to treatment measures

Interventions

- ■ Use measures to detect, prevent, and/or minimize dysrhythmias.
- ■ Treat underlying disease processes that contribute to dysrhythmia development. These include cardiovascular (e.g., acute myocardial infarction) and noncardiovascular (e.g., chronic lung disease) disorders.
- ■ Prevent or treat other conditions that predispose to dysrhythmias (e.g., hypoxia, electrolyte imbalance, pain, acid-base imbalance, fluid alterations).
- ■ Help the patient understand the negative effects of cigarette smoking, overeating, excessive coffee drinking, and other habits that may cause or aggravate dysrhythmias. Encourage patient to avoid such behaviors. Long-term supervision and counseling may be needed.
- ■ For the patient receiving antidysrhythmic drugs, implement measures to minimize the incidence and severity of acute dysrhythmias and help the patient comply with drug therapy.
- ■ Monitor heart rate and rhythm and blood pressure every 4 to 6 hours (or as often as is the standard for the care environment where seeing the patient).
- ■ Check laboratory reports of serum electrolytes and serum drug levels when available. Report and treat abnormal values using established protocols and/or physician orders.
- ■ Provide appropriate patient teaching related to drug therapy (see accompanying display).

Evaluation

- ■ Check vital signs for improved heart rate and rhythm.
- ■ Interview and observe for relief of symptoms and improved functioning in activities of daily living.
- ■ Interview and observe for irregular rhythms, hypotension, and other adverse drug effects.
- ■ Interview and observe for compliance with instructions for taking antidysrhythmic drugs and other aspects of care.

Patient Teaching Guidelines | Antidysrhythmic Drugs

General Considerations

■ A fast heartbeat normally occurs in response to exercise, fever, and other conditions so that more blood can be pumped and carried to body tissues. An irregular heartbeat occurs occasionally in most individuals. However, when you are prescribed a long-term medication to slow or regularize your heartbeat, this means that you have a potentially serious condition. In addition, the medications can cause potentially serious adverse effects. So, it is extremely important that you take the medications exactly as prescribed. Taking extra doses is dangerous; skipping doses or waiting longer between doses may lead to loss of control of the heart problem.

■ You may be given a drug classified as an antidysrhythmic or a drug from another group that has antidysrhythmic effects (e.g., a beta blocker such as propranolol, a calcium channel blocker such as verapamil or diltiazem, or digoxin). Instructions should be provided for the specific drug ordered.

■ Be sure you know the names (generic and brand) of the medication, why you are receiving it, and what effects you can expect (therapeutic and adverse).

■ You will need continued medical supervision, along with periodic measurements of heart rate and blood pressure, blood tests, and electrocardiograms.

■ Try to learn the triggers for your irregular heartbeats and avoid them when possible (e.g., excessive caffeinated beverages, strenuous or excessive exercise).

■ Avoid over-the-counter cold and asthma remedies, appetite suppressants, and antisleep preparations. These drugs are stimulants that can cause or aggravate irregular heartbeats.

Self- or Caregiver Administration

■ Take or give medications at evenly spaced intervals to maintain adequate blood levels. Take your medications at the same time each day.

■ Take or give amiodarone, mexiletine, and quinidine with food to decrease gastrointestinal symptoms.

■ Do not crush or chew sustained-release tablets or capsules.

■ Report dizziness or fainting spells. This may mean the medication is decreasing your blood pressure too much, which is more likely to occur when starting or increasing the dose of an antidysrhythmic drug. Drug dosages may need to be adjusted.

 Applying Your Knowledge 49-3

How Can You Avoid This Medication Error?

While Mr. Brown is receiving his IV lidocaine, his heart rate decreases to 52 beats per minute with continued PVCs. You continue to monitor the IV and the ECG.

Principles of Therapy

Nonpharmacologic Management of Dysrhythmias

Nonpharmacologic management is preferred, at least initially, for several dysrhythmias. For example, sinus tachycardia usually results from such disorders as dehydration, fever, infection, or hypotension and intervention and management should attempt to relieve the underlying cause. For PSVT with mild or moderate symptoms, Valsalva's maneuver, carotid sinus massage, or other measures to increase vagal tone are preferred. For ventricular fibrillation, immediate defibrillation is the initial management of choice.

In addition to these strategies, others are being increasingly used. The impetus for nonpharmacologic management developed mainly from studies demonstrating that antidysrhythmic drugs could worsen existing dysrhythmias, cause new dysrhythmias, and cause higher mortality rates in patients receiving the drugs than patients not receiving the drugs. Current technology allows clinicians to insert pacemakers and defibrillators (e.g., ICD) to control bradydysrhythmias or

tachydysrhythmias and to use radio waves (radiofrequency catheter ablation) or surgery to deactivate ectopic foci.

Patients with stable coronary heart disease can benefit from practicing transcendental meditation, which appears to help control certain physiologic factors associated with the metabolic syndrome. Metabolic syndrome is characterized by insulin resistance, elevated blood pressure, visceral obesity, and dyslipidemia. These signs are considered an indicator of risk for coronary heart disease. The study suggests that the transcendental meditation practice modulates the physiologic response to stress by affecting neurohumoral pathways that play a role in the syndrome.

Nonpharmacologic management for atrial fibrillation specifically is determined based on the following criteria. Some patients with persistent atrial fibrillation will satisfy criteria for either an initial rate-control or a rhythm-control strategy (e.g., age > 65 years but also symptomatic):

■ Indications are regarded weighing the potential advantages and disadvantages of each strategy of which the patient concurs

■ Account for comorbidities

■ Appropriate antithrombotic treatment is used.

A rate-control strategy is the preferred initial option in patients with the following conditions with persistent atrial fibrillation:

■ Age greater than 65 years

■ Coronary artery disease

■ Contraindications to antiarrhythmic drugs

▪ Unsuitable for cardioversion

▪ No history of heart failure

A rhythm-control strategy is the preferred initial option in patients with the following conditions with persistent atrial fibrillation:

▪ Those who are symptomatic

▪ Younger patients

▪ First time presenters with lone atrial fibrillation

▪ Those with atrial fibrillation due to a precipitated event that is being treated or corrected

▪ Those with heart failure

Patients unsuitable for cardioversion include those with

▪ Contraindications to anticoagulation

▪ Structural heart disease (e.g., large left atrium, mitral stenosis) that precludes long-term maintenance of sinus rhythm

▪ Long duration of atrial fibrillation > 12 months

▪ Multiple failed attempts at cardioversion and/or relapses, even with use of antiarrhythmic drugs or nonpharmacologic approaches

▪ Ongoing but reversible cause of atrial fibrillation (e.g., thyrotoxicosis)

Pharmacologic Management of Dysrhythmias

Rational drug therapy for cardiac dysrhythmias requires accurate identification of the dysrhythmia, understanding of the basic mechanisms causing the dysrhythmia, observation of the hemodynamic and ECG effects of the dysrhythmia, knowledge of the pharmacologic actions of specific antidysrhythmic drugs, and the expectation that therapeutic effects will outweigh potential adverse effects. Even when these criteria are met, antidysrhythmic drug therapy is somewhat empiric. Although some dysrhythmias usually respond to particular drugs, different drugs or combinations of drugs are often required. General trends and guidelines for drug therapy of supraventricular and ventricular dysrhythmias (which may result from prolonged QT intervals) are described in the following sections. General trends include the following:

▪ Cardiotoxic effects occur most commonly with IV administration, particularly at high concentrations, and are observed as conduction changes (widening of the QRS complex, prolonging of the QT interval, flattened T waves, and disappearance of the P wave) ventricular tachycardia, or frequent PVCs.

▪ Patients with the highest priority for QT interval monitoring are those started on a drug that has been shown to cause the malignant ventricular dysrhythmia, torsades de pointes.

▪ Patients treated in hospital units are at higher risk than outpatients, who are started on the same prodysrhythmic drugs, for a number of reasons.

▪ Older adults are hospitalized patients who may receive intravenous administration of a QT-prolonging drug or multiple QT-prolonging drugs.

▪ Females and the elderly are both risk factors for torsades de pointes.

▪ Hospitalized patients have additional risk factors for torsades de pointes.

• Impaired elimination due to renal or hepatic dysfunction

• Electrolyte abnormalities (especially hypokalemia or hypomagnesemia)

• Heart disease (left-ventricular hypertrophy or heart failure)

• Dysrhythmias with slow rates

• Recent conversion of atrial fibrillation

• Catheter ablation of rapid tachycardias

• Neurologic disorders (especially subarachnoid hemorrhage).

▪ Class II and class III drugs are being used increasingly, because of demonstrated benefits in relieving symptoms and decreasing mortality rates in patients with heart disease.

Treatment of Supraventricular Tachydysrhythmias

▪ **Propranolol** and other beta blockers are being increasingly used for tachydysrhythmias, especially in patients with myocardial infarction, heart failure, or exercise-induced dysrhythmias. In addition to controlling dysrhythmias, the drugs decrease the mortality rate in these patients. Also, a beta blocker is the management of choice if a rapid heart rate is causing angina or other symptoms in a patient with known coronary artery disease.

▪ Atrial fibrillation is the most common dysrhythmia. Management priorities include rate and rhythm control.

  ▪ In patients with permanent atrial fibrillation, who need treatment for rate control

  • Beta blockers or rate-limiting calcium antagonists are preferred for initial treatment

  • Digoxin is only considered as monotherapy in sedentary patients

  ▪ In patients with permanent atrial fibrillation, where monotherapy is inadequate

  • Control of the heart rate only during normal activities

    - Beta blockers or rate-limiting calcium antagonists are given with digoxin

  • Control of the heart rate during both normal activities and exercise

    - Calcium antagonists that are rate-limiting are administered with digoxin

■ Management may involve conversion to NSR by electrical or pharmacologic means or long-term drug therapy to slow and control the rate of ventricular response. Advantages of conversion to NSR include improvement of symptoms and decreased risks of heart failure or thromboembolic problems. If pharmacologic conversion is chosen, IV **adenosine, dofetilide, ibutilide, verapamil,** or **diltiazem** may be used. After being converted to NSR, patients usually require long-term drug therapy.

■ Low-dose **amiodarone** is a pharmacologic choice for preventing recurrent A-Fib after electrical or pharmacologic conversion. The low doses cause fewer adverse effects than the higher ones used for life-threatening ventricular dysrhythmias.

In addition to amiodarone, other drugs used to slow the heart rate include a **beta blocker, digoxin, verapamil,** or **diltiazem.** In most patients, a beta blocker, verapamil, or diltiazem may be preferred. In patients with heart failure, digoxin may be preferred. In addition, the class IC agents **flecainide** or **propafenone** may be used to suppress paroxysmal atrial flutter and fibrillation in patients with minimal or no heart disease.

IV **adenosine, ibutilide, verapamil,** or **diltiazem** may be used to convert PSVT to an NSR. These drugs block conduction across the AV node.

Treatment of Ventricular Dysrhythmias

Treatment of asymptomatic PVCs and nonsustained ventricular tachycardia is not recommended. Treatment of symptomatic ventricular tachycardia is treated with **amiodarone, lidocaine,** and then **procainamide.** However, concurrent electrotherapy offers better outcomes in this unstable population. **Moricizine** is infrequently used in the United States because of its potential for causing undesirable cardiac events. It may be used to treat life-threatening ventricular dysrhythmias (e.g., sustained ventricular tachycardia) that have not responded to safer drugs.

Use in Special Populations

Use in Children

Antidysrhythmic drugs are less often needed in children than in adults, and their use has decreased with increased use of catheter ablative techniques. Catheter ablation uses radio waves to destroy dysrhythmia-producing foci in cardiac tissue and reportedly causes fewer adverse effects and complications than long-term antidysrhythmic drug therapy.

Antidysrhythmic drug therapy is also less clear-cut in children. However, pediatric cardiologists have used various drugs and developed guidelines for their use, especially dosages. As with adults, the drugs should be used only when clearly indicated, and children should be monitored closely because all of the drugs can cause adverse effects, including hypotension and new or worsened dysrhythmias.

Supraventricular tachydysrhythmias are the most common sustained dysrhythmias in children. IV adenosine, digoxin, procainamide, or propranolol can be used acutely to terminate supraventricular tachydysrhythmias. Adenosine is administered like the adult dosing for children over 50 kilograms. For children weighing less than 50 kilograms, initially 0.1 milligram per kilogram IV push is given, with a maximum dose administration of 6 milligrams. If this initial dose if ineffective, a repeat dose of 0.2 milligrams per kilogram, up to the maximum of 12 milligrams, may be administered IV push.

Considerations for IV digoxin include that premature infants are more susceptible to toxicity. Digoxin or a beta blocker may be used for long-term management of supraventricular tachydysrhythmias. In addition, IV procainamide and verapamil do not have age-related precautions noted for use in children.

Propranolol is the beta blocker most commonly used in children. It is one of the few antidysrhythmic drugs available in a liquid solution. When given IV, antidysrhythmic effects are rapid, and patients require careful monitoring for bradycardia and hypotension.

Lidocaine may be used to treat ventricular dysrhythmias precipitated by cardiac surgery or digitalis toxicity. Class I or III drugs are usually started in a hospital setting, at lower dosage ranges, because of prodysrhythmic effects. Prodysrhythmia is more common in children with structural heart disease or significant dysrhythmias. In general, serum levels should be monitored medications. Serious adverse reactions to lidocaine are uncommon.

As in adults, most antidysrhythmic drugs and their metabolites are excreted through the kidneys and may accumulate in children with impaired renal function.

Use in Older Adults

Cardiac dysrhythmias are common in older adults, but in general only those causing symptoms of circulatory impairment should be treated with antidysrhythmic drugs. Compared with younger adults, older adults are more likely to experience serious adverse drug effects, including aggravation of existing dysrhythmias, production of new dysrhythmias, hypotension, and heart failure. Cautious use is required, and dosage usually needs to be reduced to compensate for heart disease or impaired drug-elimination processes. Many elderly have an increased sensitivity to medications, this is true for antidysrhythmics.

Use in Patients With Renal Impairment

Antidysrhythmic drug therapy in patients with renal impairment should be very cautious, with close monitoring of drug effects (e.g., plasma drug levels, ECG changes, symptoms that may indicate drug toxicity). The kidneys excrete most antidysrhythmic drugs and their metabolites. As a result, decreased renal perfusion or other renal impairment can reduce drug elimination and lead to accumulation and adverse effects if dosage is not reduced. As a general rule, dosage of digoxin, disopyramide, lidocaine, procainamide, propafenone, quinidine, and sotalol should be reduced in patients with significant impairment of renal function. Dosage of adenosine, amiodarone, ibutilide, and mexiletine does not require reduction.

Use in Patients With Hepatic Impairment

As with renal impairment, antidysrhythmic drug therapy in patients with hepatic impairment should be very cautious, with close monitoring of drug effects (e.g., plasma drug levels, ECG changes, symptoms that may indicate drug toxicity).

Amiodarone may be hepatotoxic and cause serious, sometimes fatal, liver disease. Hepatic enzyme levels are often elevated without accompanying symptoms of liver impairment. However, liver enzymes should be monitored regularly, especially in patients receiving relatively high maintenance doses. If enzyme levels are above three times the normal range or double in a patient whose baseline levels were elevated, dosage reduction or drug discontinuation should be considered.

Hepatic impairment increases plasma half-life of several antidysrhythmic drugs, and dosage usually should be reduced. Dosages of digoxin, disopyramide, propafenone, and quinidine should be reduced in patients with impairment of hepatic function. Dosages of adenosine and ibutilide are unlikely to need reductions in patients with hepatic impairment.

Use in Patients With Critical Illness

Critically ill patients often have multiple cardiovascular and other disorders that increase their risks for development of acute, serious, and potentially life-threatening dysrhythmias. They may also have refractory dysrhythmias that require strong, potentially toxic antidysrhythmic drugs. Thus, antidysrhythmic drugs are often given IV in critical care settings for rapid reversal of a fast rhythm. After reversal, IV or oral drugs may be given to prevent recurrence of the dysrhythmia.

Because serious problems may stem from either dysrhythmias or their treatment, health care providers should be adept in preventing, recognizing, and treating conditions that predispose to the development of serious dysrhythmias (e.g., electrolyte imbalances, hypoxia). If dysrhythmias cannot be prevented, early recognition and treatment are needed.

Overall, any antidysrhythmic drug therapy in critically ill patients is preferably performed or at least initiated in critical care units or other facilities with appropriate equipment and personnel. For example, nurses who work in emergency departments or critical care units must be certified in cardiopulmonary resuscitation and ACLS. With ACLS, the American Heart Association and others have developed algorithms to guide drug therapy of dysrhythmias.

Use in Home Care

Patients receiving chronic antidysrhythmic drug therapy are likely to have significant cardiovascular disease. With each visit, the home care nurse needs to assess the patient's physical, mental, and functional status and evaluate pulse and blood pressure. In addition, patients and caregivers should be taught to report symptoms (e.g., dizziness or fainting, chest pain) and avoid over-the-counter agents unless discussed with a health care provider.

Nursing Actions Antidysrhythmic Drugs

NURSING ACTIONS	RATIONALE/EXPLANATION
1. Administer accurately	
a. Check apical and radial pulses before each dose. Hold the dose and check with the physician if marked changes are noted in rate, rhythm, or quality of pulses.	Bradycardia may indicate impending heart block or cardiovascular collapse.
b. Check blood pressure at least once every shift, usually every 4 hours is the standard for hospitalized patients.	To detect hypotension, which is most likely to occur when antidysrhythmic drug therapy is being initiated or altered
c. During intravenous (IV) administration of antidysrhythmic drugs, maintain continuous cardiac monitoring and check blood pressure about every 1–5 minutes, depending on the onset of action.	For early detection of hypotension and impending cardiac collapse. These drug side effects are more likely to occur with IV use.
d. Give oral drugs at evenly spaced intervals.	To maintain adequate blood levels
e. With oral amiodarone, give once daily or in two divided doses if stomach upset occurs.	
f. With IV amiodarone, mix and give loading and maintenance infusions according to the manufacturer's instructions.	Specific instructions are required for accurate mixing and administration, partly because concentrations and infusion rates vary. The drug should be given in a critical care setting, by experienced personnel, preferably through a central venous catheter.
g. Give mexiletine and quinidine with food.	To decrease gastrointestinal (GI) symptoms
h. Give lidocaine parenterally only, as a bolus injection or a continuous drip. Use only solutions labeled "For cardiac dysrhythmias," and do not use solutions containing epinephrine. Give an IV bolus over 2 minutes.	Lidocaine solutions that contain epinephrine are used for local anesthesia only. They should never be given IV to patients with cardiac dysrhythmias because the epinephrine can cause or aggravate dysrhythmias. Rapid injection (within approximately 30 sec) produces transient blood levels several times greater than therapeutic range limits. Therefore, there is increased risk of toxicity without a concomitant increase in therapeutic effectiveness.

(continued on page 794)

Nursing Actions | Antidysrhythmic Drugs (continued)

NURSING ACTIONS	RATIONALE/EXPLANATION
2. Observe for therapeutic effects a. Conversion to normal sinus rhythm	After a single oral dose, peak plasma levels are reached in approximately 1–4 hours with quinidine, procainamide, and propranolol and in 6–12 hours with phenytoin. Equilibrium between plasma and tissue levels is reached in 1 or 2 days with quinidine, procainamide, and propranolol; in approximately 1 week with phenytoin; in 1–3 weeks with amiodarone; and in just a few minutes with IV lidocaine.
b. Improvement in rate, rhythm, and quality of apical and radial pulses and the electrocardiogram (ECG) c. Signs of increased cardiac output—blood pressure near normal range, urine output more adequate, no complaints of dizziness	
d. Serum drug levels (mcg/mL) within therapeutic ranges (Table 49-2)	Serum drug levels must be interpreted in light of the patient's clinical status.
3. Observe for adverse effects a. Heart block—may be indicated on the ECG by a prolonged PR interval or presence of more P waves than QRS complexes; or presence of bundle branch block noted in a prolonged QRS complex	Due to depressant effects on the cardiac conduction system
b. Dysrhythmias—aggravation of existing dysrhythmia, tachycardia, bradycardia, premature ventricular contractions, ventricular tachycardia, or fibrillation	Because they affect the cardiac conduction system, antidysrhythmic drugs may worsen existing dysrhythmias or cause new dysrhythmias.
c. Hypotension	Due to decreased cardiac output
d. Additional adverse effects with specific drugs: (1) Disopyramide—mouth dryness, blurred vision, urinary retention, heart failure, prodysrhythmic effects other anticholinergic effects	These effects commonly occur.
(2) Lidocaine—drowsiness, agitation, muscle twitching, seizures, paraesthesias and prodysrhythmic effects	Most adverse reactions result from drug effects on the central nervous system (CNS). Convulsions are most likely to occur with high doses. Hypersensitivity reactions may occur in individuals who are allergic to related local anesthetic agents. CNS changes are caused by depressant effects.
(3) Phenytoin—nystagmus, ataxia, slurring of speech, tremors, drowsiness, confusion, gingival hyperplasia	
(4) Propranolol—bradycardia, hypotension, depression, nightmares, fatigue, sexual dysfunction	The beta-adrenergic blocking action of propranolol blocks the normal sympathetic nervous system response to activity and exercise. Patients may have symptoms caused by deficient blood supply to body tissues.
(5) Quinidine—diarrhea, hypotension, nausea, vomiting, cinchonism, fever, thrombocytopenia, prodysrhythmic effects	These are the most frequent adverse effects.
(6) Tocainide—drowsiness, agitation, muscle twitching, seizures, paresthesias, prodysrhythmic effects, nausea, vomiting, diarrhea, agranulocytosis	
4. Observe for drug interactions a. Drugs that *increase* effects of antidysrhythmics:	These drugs may potentiate therapeutic effects or increase risk of toxicity.
(1) Antidysrhythmic agents	When antidysrhythmic drugs are combined, there are additive cardiac depressant effects.
(2) Antihypertensives, diuretics, phenothiazine antipsychotic agents	Additive hypotension
(3) Cimetidine	Decreases metabolism and increases blood concentrations of calcium channel blockers, lidocaine, metoprolol, phenytoin, propranolol
b. Drugs that *decrease* effects of antidysrhythmic agents: (1) Atropine sulfate	Atropine is used to reverse propranolol-induced bradycardia.
(2) Phenytoin, rifampin	Decreases effects by inducing drug-metabolizing enzymes in the liver and accelerating the metabolism of quinidine, disopyramide, and mexiletine

Table 49-2	Therapeutic Serum Drug Level Ranges of Common Antidysrhythmics	
DRUG	**THERAPEUTIC RANGE (mcg/mL)**	
Class IA		
Quinidine	2–5	
Procainamide	4–8	
Disopyramide	2–8	
Class IB		
Lidocaine	1.5–6	
Mexiletine	0.5–2	
Tocainide	4–10	
Phenytoin	10–20	
Class IC		
Flecainide	0.2–1	
Propafenone	0.06–1	
Class II		
Propranolol	0.05–0.1	
Class III		
Amiodarone	0.5–2.5	
Class IV		
Verapamil	0.08–0.3	

Key Concepts

■ Atrial fibrillation is the most common dysrhythmia.

■ Initiation of an electrical impulse depends predominately on the movement of sodium and calcium ions into a myocardial cell and movement of potassium ions out of the cell.

■ Quinidine, the prototype of class IA antidysrhythmics, reduces automaticity, slows conduction, and prolongs the refractory period. Phenytoin may be used to treat dysrhythmias produced by digoxin intoxication.

■ Lidocaine is the prototype of class IB antidysrhythmics used for treating serious ventricular dysrhythmias associated with acute myocardial infarction, cardiac catheterization, cardiac surgery, and digitalis-induced ventricular dysrhythmias.

■ Flecainide, propafenone, and moricizine are class 1C drugs and have no effect on the repolarization phase but greatly decrease conduction in the ventricles.

■ As a class II drug, beta-adrenergic blockers are being used more extensively because of their effectiveness in reducing mortality in post–myocardial infarction and heart failure patients.

■ As class IV drugs, diltiazem and verapamil are the only calcium channel blockers approved for management of dysrhythmias.

■ The FDA has issued a **BLACK BOX WARNING** for disopyramide due to its known prodysrhythmic properties; the drug should be reserved for patients with life-threatening ventricular dysrhythmias.

■ Amiodarone is a potassium channel blocker that prolongs conduction in all cardiac tissues and decreases heart rate, and it decreases contractility of the left ventricle.

■ The FDA has issued a **BLACK BOX WARNING** for amiodarone recommending use only in patients with life-threatening dysrhythmias due to the risk of developing potentially fatal pulmonary toxicity with its use.

Review and Application Exercises

Short Answer Exercises

1. Which tissues in the heart are able to generate an electrical impulse and therefore serve as a pacemaker?

2. What risk factors predispose a patient to development of dysrhythmias?

3. Name interventions that patients or health care providers can perform to decrease risks of dysrhythmias.

4. Differentiate the hemodynamic effects of common dysrhythmias.

5. What are the classes of antidysrhythmic drugs?

6. How do beta-adrenergic blocking agents act on the conduction system to slow heart rate?

7. What are common and potentially serious adverse effects of antidysrhythmic drugs?

NCLEX-Style Questions

8. The clinical use of class III agents is increasing over the use of class I agents for patients with heart disease, because they are associated with
   a. less ventricular fibrillation
   b. increased mortality
   c. more sustained effects
   d. mild adverse effects

9. A patient being monitored in the critical care unit has been receiving quinidine. The nurse notes that the patient's serum quinidine level is 8 mcg/mL, and the patient has developed diarrhea. The most appropriate action by the nurse is to
   a. Hold the medication and report the findings to the health care prescriber immediately.
   b. Administer the medication as ordered.
   c. Anticipate that the dosage of the medication will be increased.
   d. Anticipate that the dosage of the medication will be decreased.

10. Mr. Conley, age 53, is about to be discharged from the hospital after treatment for recurrent ventricular fibrillation unresponsive to other agents. To prevent further ventricular ectopy, the health care provider prescribes amiodarone (Cordarone), 1000 mg PO daily as a loading dose for 2 weeks. Why is such a large loading dose required?
    a. Most of the drug is destroyed in the GI tract.
    b. Males require larger dosages because of their faster metabolisms.
    c. A history of ventricular dysrhythmia necessitates a higher dose.
    d. The drug has a long serum half-life.

11. Phenytoin, an anticonvulsant, may be used to treat dysrhythmias produced by
    a. digoxin toxicity
    b. quinidine intoxication
    c. lidocaine overdose
    d. procainamide toxicity

12. Ms. Ferguson, age 58, is admitted to the coronary care unit for treatment of an acute anterior myocardial infarction. That evening, she experiences frequent runs of ventricular tachycardia. The health care provider tells the nurse to prepare an IV bolus dose of lidocaine. Why is lidocaine administered IV instead of orally?
    a. Lidocaine absorption is too erratic when administered orally.
    b. Lidocaine is inactivated by hydrochloric acid.
    c. Most of an absorbed oral dose undergoes first-pass metabolism in the liver.
    d. Onset of action for oral lidocaine is over 8 hours.

Selected References

Camm, A. J., Savelieva, I., & Lip, G. Y. H. on behalf of the Guideline Development Group for the NICE clinical guideline for the management of atrial fibrillation. (2007). Rate control in the medical management of atrial fibrillation. *Heart, 93,* 35–38.

Day, J. J., Doshi, N. D., Belott, P., Birgersdotter-Green, U., Behboodikhah, M., Ott, P., et al. (2007). Inductionless or limited shock testing is possible in most patients with implantable cardioverter-defibrillators/cardiac resynchronization therapy defibrillators. *Circulation, 115,* 2382–2389.

DeVoe,, J. & Judkins, D. Z. What is the best approach to the evaluation of resting tachycardia for an adult? *Journal of Family Physicians, 56,* 59–61.

Dobrzynski, H., Boyett, M. R., & Anderson, R. H. (2007). New insights into pacemaker activity: Promoting understanding of sick sinus syndrome. *Circulation, 115,* 1921–1932.

Drew, B. (2007). Pulling it all together: Case studies on ECG monitoring. *AACN Advanced Critical Care, 18,* 305–317.

Heist, E. K., & Ruskin, J. N. (2005). Drug-induced proarrhythmia and use of QTc-prolonging agents: Clues for clinicians. *Heart Rhythm, 2*(2suppl), S1–S8.

Kayyali, A., & Lindsey, H. (2007). Informing Practice. *American Journal of Nursing, 107,* 72A–72B.

Paul-Labrador, M., Polk, D., Dwyer, J. H., et al. (2006). Effects of a randomized controlled trial of transcendental meditation on components of metabolic syndrome in subjects, with coronary heart disease. *Archives of Internal Medicine, 166,* 1218–1224.

Smellie, W. S. A., & Coleman, J. J. (2007). Cases in primary care laboratory medicine: Pitfalls of testing and summary of guidance on safety monitoring with amiodarone and digoxin. *BMJ, 334,* 312–315.

KEY TERMS

- Atherosclerosis
- Angina pectoris
- Coronary artery disease
- Metabolic syndrome
- Myocardial infarction

LEARNING OBJECTIVES

After studying this chapter, you will be able to:

1. Describe the types, causes, and effects of angina pectoris.
2. Describe general characteristics and types of antianginal drugs.
3. Discuss nitrate antianginals in terms of indications for use, routes of administration, adverse effects, nursing process implications, and drug tolerance.
4. Differentiate between short-acting and long-acting dosage forms of nitrate antianginal drugs.
5. Teach patients ways to prevent, minimize, or manage acute anginal attacks.
6. Use the nursing process in the care of individuals on antianginal and adjunctive therapy for treatment of myocardial ischemia.

Applying Your Knowledge

Richard Gerald is a 72-year-old man with a history of hypertension, coronary artery disease (CAD), and a myocardial infarction (MI). He stopped smoking and began a regular exercise program after his MI.

Introduction

Angina pectoris is a clinical syndrome characterized by episodes of chest pain. It occurs when there is a deficit in myocardial oxygen supply (myocardial ischemia) in relation to myocardial oxygen demand. It is most often caused by atherosclerotic plaque in the coronary arteries but may also be caused by coronary vasospasm. The development and progression of atherosclerotic plaque is called *coronary artery disease* (CAD). Atherosclerotic plaque narrows the lumen, decreases elasticity, and impairs dilation of coronary arteries. The result is impaired blood flow to the myocardium, especially with exercise or other factors that increase the cardiac workload and need for oxygen.

The continuum of CAD progresses from angina to *myocardial infarction* (MI). There are three main types of angina: classic angina, variant angina, and unstable angina (Box 50-1). The Canadian Cardiovascular Society classifies patients with angina according to the amount of physical activity they can tolerate before anginal pain occurs (Box 50-2). These categories can assist in clinical assessment and evaluation of therapy.

Classic anginal pain is usually described as substernal chest pain of a constricting, squeezing, or suffocating nature. It may radiate to the jaw, neck, or shoulder; down the left or both arms; or to the back. The discomfort is sometimes mistaken for arthritis or for indigestion, because the pain may be associated with nausea, vomiting, dizziness, diaphoresis, shortness of breath, or fear of

797

Box 50-1	Types of Angina Pectoris

Classic

Classic angina (also called *stable*, *typical*, or *exertional angina*) occurs when atherosclerotic plaque obstructs coronary arteries and the heart requires more oxygenated blood than the blocked arteries can deliver. Chest pain is usually precipitated by situations that increase the workload of the heart, such as physical exertion, exposure to cold, and emotional upset. Recurrent episodes of classic angina usually have the same pattern of onset, duration, and intensity of symptoms. Pain is usually relieved by rest, a fast-acting preparation of nitroglycerin, or both.

Variant

Variant angina (also called *atypical*, *Prinzmetal's*, or *vasospastic angina*) is caused by spasms of the coronary artery that decrease blood flow to the myocardium. The spasms occur most often in coronary arteries that are already partly blocked by atherosclerotic plaque. Variant angina usually occurs during rest or with minimal exercise and often occurs at night. It often occurs at the same time each day. Pain is usually relieved by nitroglycerin. Long-term management includes avoidance of conditions that precipitate vasospasm, when possible (e.g., exposure to cold, smoking, and emotional stress), as well as antianginal drugs.

Unstable

Unstable angina (also called *rest*, *preinfarction*, and *crescendo angina*) is a type of myocardial ischemia that falls between classic angina and myocardial infarction. It usually occurs in patients with advanced coronary atherosclerosis and produces increased frequency, intensity, and duration of symptoms. It often leads to myocardial infarction.

Unstable angina usually develops when a minor injury ruptures atherosclerotic plaque. The resulting injury to the endothelium causes platelets to aggregate at the site of injury, form a thrombus, and release chemical mediators that cause vasoconstriction (e.g., thromboxane, serotonin, platelet-derived growth factor). The disrupted plaque, thrombus, and vasoconstriction combine to obstruct blood flow further in the affected coronary artery. When the plaque injury is mild, blockage of the coronary artery may be intermittent and cause silent myocardial ischemia or episodes of anginal pain at rest. Thrombus formation and vasoconstriction may progress until the coronary artery is completely occluded, producing myocardial infarction. Endothelial injury, with subsequent thrombus formation and vasoconstriction, may also result from therapeutic procedures (e.g., angioplasty, atherectomy).

The Agency for Healthcare Research and Quality, in its clinical practice guidelines for the management of angina, defines unstable angina as meeting one or more of the following criteria:

- Anginal pain at rest that usually lasts longer than 20 minutes
- Recent onset (<2 months) of exertional angina of at least Canadian Cardiovascular Society Classification (CCSC) class III severity
- Recent (<2 months) increase in severity as indicated by progression to at least CCSC class III

However, myocardial ischemia may also be painless or silent in a substantial number of patients. Overall, the diagnosis is usually based on chest pain history, electrocardiographic evidence of ischemia, and other signs of impaired cardiac function (e.g., heart failure).

Because unstable angina often occurs hours or days before acute myocardial infarction, early recognition and effective management are extremely important in preventing progression to infarction, heart failure, or sudden cardiac death.

Box 50-2	Canadian Cardiovascular Society Classification of Patients with Angina Pectoris

Class I: Ordinary physical activity (e.g., walking, climbing stairs) does not cause angina. Angina occurs with strenuous, rapid, or prolonged exertion at work or recreation.

Class II: Slight limitation of ordinary activity. Angina occurs on walking or climbing stairs rapidly, walking uphill, walking or stair climbing after meals, or in cold, in wind, or under emotional stress. Walking more than two blocks on the level and climbing more than one flight of ordinary stairs at a normal pace and in normal conditions can elicit angina.

Class III: Marked limitations of ordinary physical activity. Angina occurs on walking one or two blocks on the level and climbing one flight of stairs in normal conditions and at a normal pace.

Class IV: Inability to carry on any physical activity without discomfort—anginal symptoms may be present at rest.

impending doom. The discomfort is usually brief, typically lasting 5 minutes or less until the balance of oxygen supply and demand is restored.

Current research indicates that gender differences exist in the type and quality of cardiac symptoms, with women reporting epigastric or back discomfort. Additionally, older adults may have atypical symptoms of CAD and may experience "silent" ischemia that may delay them from seeking professional help. Individuals with diabetes mellitus may present without classic angina, although they may experience related symptoms. The American Heart Association has released guidelines for the management of angina.

Numerous overlapping factors contribute to the development and progression of CAD. To aid understanding of drug therapy for angina, these factors are described in the following sections.

Coronary Atherosclerosis

Atherosclerosis begins with accumulation of lipid-filled macrophages (i.e., foam cells) on the inner lining of coronary arteries. Foam cells, which promote growth of atherosclerotic plaque, develop in response to elevated blood cholesterol levels. These early lesions progress to fibrous plaques containing foam cells covered by smooth muscle cells and connective tissue. Advanced lesions also contain hemorrhages, ulcerations, and scar tissue. Factors contributing to plaque development and growth include endothelial injury, lipid infiltration (i.e., cholesterol), recruitment of inflammatory cells (mainly monocytes and T lymphocytes), and smooth muscle cell proliferation. Endothelial injury may be the initiating factor in plaque formation because it allows monocytes, platelets, cholesterol, and other blood components to come in contact with and stimulate abnormal growth of smooth muscle cells and connective tissue in the arterial wall.

Atherosclerosis commonly develops in the coronary arteries. As the plaque lesions develop over time, they become larger and extend farther into the lumen of the artery. The lesions may develop for decades before they produce symptoms of reduced blood flow. Eventually, a partially or completely occluded artery precipitates myocardial ischemia. Thus, serious impairment of blood flow may occur with a large atherosclerotic plaque or a relatively small plaque with superimposed vasospasm and thrombosis. If stenosis blocks approximately 80% of the artery, blood flow cannot increase in response to increased need; if stenosis blocks 90% or more of the artery, blood flow is impaired when the patient is at rest.

When coronary atherosclerosis develops slowly, collateral circulation develops to increase blood supply to the heart. Collateral circulation develops from anastomotic channels that connect the coronary arteries and allow perfusion of an area by more than one artery. Endothelium-derived relaxing factors such as nitric oxide (NO) can dilate collateral vessels and facilitate regional myocardial blood flow. Although collateral circulation may prevent myocardial ischemia in the patient at rest, it has limited ability to increase myocardial perfusion with increased cardiac workload.

Myocardial ischemia impairs blood flow to the myocardium, especially with exercise, mental stress, exposure to cold, or other factors that increase the cardiac workload. Most individuals with myocardial ischemia have advanced coronary atherosclerosis. Hypertension is also a major risk factor for myocardial ischemia.

Myocardial Ischemia

Myocardial ischemia occurs when the coronary arteries are unable to provide sufficient blood and oxygen for normal cardiac functions. Also known as ischemic heart disease, CAD, and coronary heart disease, myocardial ischemia may present as an acute coronary syndrome with three main consequences. One consequence is unstable angina, with the occurrence of pain (symptomatic myocardial ischemia). A second is MI that is silent or asymptomatic and diagnosed by biochemical markers only. A third is MI, with or without ST-segment elevation, which occurs when the ischemia is persistent or severe.

Resultant Cardiovascular Impairments

With normal cardiac function, coronary blood flow can increase to meet needs for an increased oxygen supply with exercise or other conditions that increase cardiac workload. When coronary arteries are partly blocked by atherosclerotic plaque, vasospasm, or thrombi, blood flow may not be able to increase sufficiently.

The endothelium of normal coronary arteries synthesizes numerous substances (see Chap. 47) that protect against vasoconstriction and vasospasm, bleeding and clotting, inflammation, and excessive cell growth. Impaired endothelium (e.g., by rupture of atherosclerotic plaque or the shear force of hypertension) leads to vasoconstriction, vasospasm, clot formation, formation of atherosclerotic plaque, and growth of smooth muscle cells in blood vessel walls.

One important substance produced by the endothelium of coronary arteries is NO (also called endothelium-derived relaxing factor). NO, which is synthesized from the amino acid arginine, is released by shear stress on the endothelium, sympathetic stimulation of exercise, and interactions with acetylcholine, histamine, prostacyclin, serotonin, thrombin, and other chemical mediators. NO relaxes vascular smooth muscle and inhibits adhesion and aggregation of platelets. When the endothelium is damaged, these vasodilating and antithrombotic effects are lost. At the same time, production of strong vasoconstrictors (e.g., angiotensin II, endothelin-1, thromboxane A_2) is increased. In addition, inflammatory cells enter the injured area and growth factors stimulate growth of smooth muscle cells. All of these factors participate in blocking coronary arteries.

Sympathetic nervous system stimulation normally produces dilation of coronary arteries, tachycardia, and increased myocardial contractility to handle an increased need for oxygenated blood. Atherosclerosis of coronary arteries, especially if severe, may cause vasoconstriction as well as decrease blood flow by obstruction.

In a healthy heart, about two thirds of the energy (adenosine triphosphate [ATP] production), for cellular function is obtained from the free fatty acid pathway; additional energy is obtained from glucose oxidation and lactate. In hypoxic conditions myocardial cells speed up glucose uptake to produce adequate ATP. Severe ischemia rapidly induces an imbalance between the cardiac supply and demand causing alterations in contraction and electrical conduction, resulting in failure and dysrhythmias. At the cellular level, hypoxia increases anaerobic metabolism with resultant cellular acidosis. The free fatty acid pathway is slowed down, resulting in less ATP production. These metabolic changes lead to disruption of cell homeostasis and ultimately, cell death.

Nonpharmacologic Management of CAD

Nonpharmacologic management of angina and MI include risk factor modification, patient education, and revascularization procedures. For patients at any stage of CAD development, irrespective of symptoms of myocardial ischemia, optimal management involves lifestyle changes and medications, if necessary, to control or reverse risk factors for disease progression. *The Third Report of the National Cholesterol Education Program Expert Panel on Detection, Evaluation, and Treatment of High Blood Cholesterol in Adults* (NCEP III) defines *metabolic syndrome* as a cluster of several cardiovascular risk factors linked with obesity: elevated waist circumference, elevated triglycerides, reduced high-density lipoprotein cholesterol, elevated blood pressure, and elevated fasting glucose. These risk factors frequently produce an additive effect on CAD and result in significant morbidity and mortality. Thus, efforts are needed to assist patients in reducing blood pressure, weight, and serum cholesterol levels, when indicated, and developing an exercise program. For patients with diabetes mellitus, glucose and blood pressure control can reduce the microvascular changes associated with the condition.

In addition, patients should avoid circumstances known to precipitate acute attacks, and those who smoke should stop. Smoking is harmful to patients because

- Nicotine increases catecholamines which, in turn, increase heart rate and blood pressure.

- Carboxyhemoglobin, formed from the inhalation of carbon monoxide in smoke, decreases delivery of blood and oxygen to the heart, decreases myocardial contractility, and increases the risks of life-threatening cardiac dysrhythmias (e.g., ventricular fibrillation) during ischemic episodes.

- Both nicotine and carbon monoxide increase platelet adhesiveness and aggregation, thereby promoting thrombosis.

- Smoking increases the risks for MI, sudden cardiac death, cerebrovascular disease (e.g., stroke), peripheral vascular disease (e.g., arterial insufficiency), and hypertension. It also reduces high-density lipoprotein, the "good" cholesterol.

Additional nonpharmacologic management strategies include surgical revascularization (e.g., coronary artery bypass graft) and interventional procedures that reduce blockages (e.g., percutaneous transluminal coronary angioplasty [PTCA], intracoronary stents, laser therapy, rotational atherectomy). Additionally, the use of supersaturated oxygen (SSO_2) has shown significant improvement in limiting myocardial damage in patients with anterior MIs. In the AMIHOT II trial, infusing SSO_2 into the previously blocked artery after performing an angioplasty procedure reduced infarct zone size by 6.5%.

Nonpharmacologic management improves patient outcomes. However, most patients still require antianginal and other cardiovascular medications to manage their disease.

Drug Management

Drugs used for myocardial ischemia are the organic nitrates, the beta-adrenergic blocking agents, and the calcium channel blocking agents. These drugs relieve anginal pain by reducing myocardial oxygen demand or increasing blood supply to the myocardium. A new classification of drug, metabolic modulators, appears to increase the heart's effectiveness in energy production to preserve cardiac function without decreasing heart rate or blood pressure. The drug class is approved as second-line therapy in patients who continue to experience angina despite treatment with another class of antianginal medications. Nitrates, beta blockers, and metabolic modulators are described in the following sections; dosage ranges for these drugs are listed in Table 50-1. Calcium channel blockers are described in a following section; indications for use and dosage ranges are listed in Table 50-2.

Antianginal Drugs: Classifications and Individual Drugs

Organic Nitrates

General Characteristics

Organic nitrates relax smooth muscle in blood vessel walls. This action produces vasodilation, which relieves anginal pain by several mechanisms. First, dilation of veins reduces venous pressure and venous return to the heart. This decreases blood volume and pressure within the heart (preload), which in turn decreases cardiac workload and oxygen demand. Second, nitrates dilate coronary arteries at higher doses and can increase blood flow to ischemic areas of the myocardium. Third, nitrates dilate arterioles, which lowers peripheral vascular resistance (afterload). This results in lower systolic blood pressure and, consequently, reduced cardiac workload. The prototype and most widely used nitrate is **nitroglycerin.**

Nitrates are converted to NO in vascular smooth muscle. NO activates guanylate cyclase, an enzyme that catalyzes formation of cyclic guanine monophosphate, which decreases calcium levels in vascular smooth muscle cells. Because intracellular calcium is required for contraction of vascular smooth muscle, the result of decreased calcium is vasodilation.

Table 50-1	Drugs at a Glance: Nitrate, Beta-Blocker, and Metabolic Modulator Antianginal Drugs	

GENERIC/TRADE NAME	INDICATIONS FOR USE	ROUTES AND DOSAGE RANGES
Nitrates		
P Nitroglycerin (Nitro-Bid, others)	Relieve acute angina Prevent exercise-induced angina Long-term prophylaxis to decrease the frequency and severity of acute anginal episodes	PO immediate-release tablets, 2.5–9 mg 2 or 3 times per day PO sustained-release tablets or capsules, 2.5 mg 3 or 4 times per day SL 0.15–0.6 mg PRN for chest pain Translingual spray, one or two metered doses (0.4 mg/dose) sprayed onto oral mucosa at onset of anginal pain, to a maximum of 3 doses in 15 min Transmucosal tablet, 1 mg q3–5h while awake, placed between upper lip and gum or cheek and gum Topical ointment, 1/2–2 inches q4–8h; do not rub in Topical transdermal disc, applied once daily IV 5–10 mcg/min initially, increased in 10- to 20-mcg/min increments up to 100 mcg/min or more if necessary to relieve pain
Isosorbide dinitrate (Isordil)	Treatment and prevention of angina	SL 2.5–10 mg PRN or q2–4h PO regular tablets, 5–40 mg 4 times/d PO chewable tablets, 5–10 mg q2–3h PO sustained-release capsules, 40 mg q6–12h
Isosorbide mononitrate (Ismo, Imdur)	Treatment and prevention of angina	PO 5–20 mg twice daily, with first dose on arising and the second dose 7 h later PO extended-release tablets (Imdur), 30–60 mg once daily in the morning, increased after several days; maximum dose 240 mg once daily
Beta Blockers		
P Propranolol (Inderal)	Long-term management of angina, to reduce frequency and severity of anginal episodes	PO 10–80 mg 2 to 4 times per day IV 0.5–3 mg q4h until desired response is obtained
Atenolol (Tenormin)	Long-term management of angina, to reduce frequency and severity of anginal episodes	PO 50 mg once daily, initially, increased to 100 mg/d after 1 wk if necessary
Metoprolol (Lopressor)	Long-term management of angina, to reduce frequency and severity of anginal episodes	PO 100–450 mg/d in 2–3 divided doses
Nadolol (Corgard)	Long-term management of angina, to reduce frequency and severity of anginal episodes	PO 40–240 mg/d in a single dose
Metabolic Modulator		
Ranolazine (Ranexa)	Long-term management of angina, not responsive to other antianginal medications	PO 500 mg twice daily, if needed; maximum recommended dose is 1000 mg twice daily

SL, sublingual.

Table 50-2		**Drugs at a Glance:** Calcium Channel Blockers

GENERIC/TRADE NAME	INDICATIONS FOR USE	ROUTES AND DOSAGE RANGES
Amlodipine (Norvasc)	Angina Hypertension	PO 5–10 mg once daily
Diltiazem (Cardizem)	Angina Hypertension Atrial fibrillation and flutter PSVT	Angina or hypertension, immediate-release, PO 60–90 mg 4 times daily before meals and at bedtime Hypertension, sustained-release only, PO 120–180 mg twice daily Dysrhythmias (Cardizem IV only), IV injection 0.25 mg/kg (average dose 20 mg) over 2 min with a second dose of 0.35 mg/kg (average dose 25 mg) in 15 min if necessary, followed by IV infusion of 5–15 mg/h up to 24 h
Felodipine (Plendil)	Hypertension	PO 5–10 mg once daily
Isradipine (DynaCirc)	Hypertension	PO 2.5–5 mg twice daily
Nicardipine (Cardene)	Angina Hypertension	Angina, immediate-release only, PO 20–40 mg 3 times daily Hypertension, immediate-release, same as for angina, above; sustained-release, PO 30–60 mg twice daily
Nifedipine (Adalat, Procardia)	Angina Hypertension	Angina, immediate-release, PO 10–30 mg 3 times daily; sustained-release, PO 30–60 mg once daily Hypertension, sustained-release only, 30–60 mg once daily
Nimodipine (Nimotop)	Subarachnoid hemorrhage	PO 60 mg q4h for 21 consecutive days. If patient unable to swallow, aspirate contents of capsule into a syringe with an 18-gauge needle, administer by nasogastric tube, and follow with 30 mL normal saline.
Nisoldipine (Sular)	Hypertension	PO, initially 20 mg once daily, increased by 10 mg/wk or longer intervals to a maximum of 60 mg daily. Average maintenance dose, 20–40 mg daily. Adults with liver impairment or >65 y, PO, initially 10 mg once daily
Verapamil (Calan, Isoptin)	Angina Atrial fibrillation or flutter PSVT Hypertension	Angina, PO 80–120 mg 3 times daily Dysrhythmias, PO 80–120 mg 3 to 4 times daily; IV injection, 5–10 mg over 2 min or longer, with continuous monitoring of electrocardiogram and blood pressure Hypertension, PO 80 mg 3 times daily or 240 mg (sustained-release) once daily

PSVT, paroxysmal supraventricular tachycardia.

The NO derived from nitrate medications can be considered a replacement or substitute for the NO that a damaged endothelium can no longer produce.

Clinical indications for nitroglycerin and other nitrates are management and prevention of acute chest pain caused by myocardial ischemia. For acute angina and prophylaxis before a situation deemed likely to precipitate acute angina, fast-acting preparations (sublingual or chewable tablets,

transmucosal spray or tablet) are used. For management of recurrent angina, long-acting preparations (oral and sustained-release tablets or transdermal ointment and discs) are used. However, they may not be effective long term because tolerance develops to their hemodynamic effects. Intravenous (IV) nitroglycerin is used to manage angina that is unresponsive to organic nitrates via other routes or beta-adrenergic blocking agents. It also may be used to control blood pressure in perioperative or emergency situations and to reduce preload and afterload in severe heart failure.

Contraindications include hypersensitivity reactions, severe anemia, hypotension, and hypovolemia. The drugs should be used cautiously in the presence of head injury or cerebral hemorrhage because they may increase intracranial pressure. Additionally, males taking nitroglycerin or any other nitrate should not take phosphodiesterase enzyme type 5 inhibitors such as sildenafil (Viagra) and vardenafil (Levitra) for erectile dysfunction. Nitrates and phosphodiesterase enzyme type 5 inhibitors decrease blood pressure and the combined effect can produce profound, life-threatening hypotension.

Individual Nitrates

P Nitroglycerin (Nitro-Bid, others), the prototype drug, is used to relieve acute angina pectoris, prevent exercise-induced angina, and decrease the frequency and severity of acute anginal episodes. Oral dosage forms are rapidly metabolized in the liver, and relatively small proportions of doses reach the systemic circulation. In addition, oral doses act slowly and do not help relieve acute chest pain.

For these reasons, several alternative dosage forms have been developed, including transmucosal tablets and sprays administered sublingually or buccally, transdermal ointments and adhesive discs applied to the skin, and an IV preparation. When given sublingually, nitroglycerin is absorbed directly into the systemic circulation. It acts within 1 to 3 minutes and lasts 30 to 60 minutes. When applied topically to the skin, nitroglycerin is also absorbed directly into the systemic circulation. However, absorption occurs at a slower rate, and topical nitroglycerin has a longer duration of action than other forms. It is available in an ointment, which is effective for 4 to 8 hours, and in a transdermal disc, which is effective for about 12 hours. An IV form of nitroglycerin is used to relieve acute anginal pain that does not respond to other agents. Regardless of the route, nitroglycerin has a half-life of 1 to 5 minutes, supporting the beneficial use of transdermal patches and sustained-release tablets.

Isosorbide dinitrate (Isordil) is used to reduce the frequency and severity of acute anginal episodes. When given sublingually or in chewable tablets, it acts in about 2 minutes, and its effects last 2 to 3 hours. When higher doses are given orally, more drug escapes metabolism in the liver and produces systemic effects in approximately 30 minutes. Therapeutic effects last about 4 hours after oral administration. The effective oral dose is usually determined by increasing the dose until headache occurs, indicating the maximum tolerable dose. Sustained-release capsules also are available.

Isosorbide mononitrate (Ismo, Imdur) is the metabolite and active component of isosorbide dinitrate. It is well absorbed after oral administration and almost 100% bioavailable. Unlike other oral nitrates, this drug is not subject to first-pass hepatic metabolism. Onset of action occurs within 1 hour, peak effects occur between 1 and 4 hours, and the elimination half-life is approximately 5 hours. It is used only for prophylaxis of angina; it does not act rapidly enough to relieve acute attacks.

⊘ **Applying Your Knowledge 50-1**

How Can You Avoid This Medication Error?

Mr. Gerald is prescribed nitroglycerin in both sublingual form and as a transdermal patch. While reviewing his medication instructions with Mr. Gerald, the nurse learns he has had a history of erectile dysfunction and has sildenafil medication in the medicine cabinet that was prescribed for him before his MI. The nurse leaves the patient information instructions for the nitroglycerin with Mr. Gerald and leaves the room.

Beta-Adrenergic Blocking Agents
General Characteristics

Beta-adrenergic blocking agents are often prescribed in a variety of clinical conditions. Their actions, uses, and adverse effects are discussed in Chapter 18. In this chapter, the drugs are discussed only in relation to their use in angina pectoris.

Sympathetic stimulation of beta$_1$ receptors in the heart increases heart rate and force of myocardial contraction, both of which increase myocardial oxygen demand and may precipitate acute anginal attacks. Beta-blocking drugs prevent or inhibit sympathetic stimulation. Thus, the drugs reduce heart rate and myocardial contractility, particularly when sympathetic output is increased during exercise. A slower heart rate may improve coronary blood flow to the ischemic area. Beta blockers also reduce blood pressure, which in turn decreases myocardial workload and oxygen demand. Studies indicate that beta blockers are more effective than nitrates or calcium channel blockers in decreasing the likelihood of silent ischemia and improving the mortality rate after transmural MI. In angina pectoris, beta-adrenergic blocking agents are used in long-term management to decrease the frequency and severity of anginal attacks, decrease the need for sublingual nitroglycerin, and increase exercise tolerance. When a beta blocker is being discontinued after prolonged use, it should be tapered in dosage and gradually discontinued or rebound angina can occur.

These drugs should not be given to patients with known or suspected coronary artery spasms because they may intensify the frequency and severity of vasospasm. This probably results from unopposed stimulation of alpha-adrenergic receptors, which causes vasoconstriction, when beta-adrenergic receptors are blocked by the drugs. Patients who continue to smoke may have reduced efficacy with the use of beta blockers. Patients with asthma should be observed for bronchospasm from blockage of beta$_2$ receptors in the lung. Beta blockers should be used with caution in patients with diabetes mellitus because they can conceal signs of hypoglycemia (except for sweating).

Individual Drugs

P Propranolol, the prototype beta blocker, is used to reduce the frequency and severity of acute attacks of angina. It is usually added to the antianginal drug regimen when nitrates do not prevent anginal episodes. It is especially useful in preventing exercise-induced tachycardia, which can precipitate anginal attacks.

Propranolol is well absorbed after oral administration. It is then metabolized extensively in the liver; a relatively small proportion of an oral dose (approximately 30%) reaches the systemic circulation. For this reason, oral doses of propranolol are much higher than IV doses. Onset of action is 30 minutes after oral administration and 1 to 2 minutes after IV injection. Because of variations in the degree of hepatic metabolism, patients vary widely in the dosages required to maintain a therapeutic response.

Atenolol, metoprolol, and **nadolol** have the same actions, uses, and adverse effects as propranolol, but they have long half-lives and can be given once daily. They are excreted by the kidneys, and dosage must be reduced in patients with renal impairment.

Applying Your Knowledge 50-2

In addition to nitroglycerin, the physician prescribes metoprolol. Mr. Gerald understands why nitroglycerin is beneficial to his condition. He asks about the metoprolol and why he needs to take this medication. How should you respond?

Calcium Channel Blocking Agents

Calcium channel blockers act on contractile and conductive tissues of the heart and on vascular smooth muscle. For these cells to function normally, the concentration of intracellular calcium must be increased. This is usually accomplished by movement of extracellular calcium ions into the cell (through calcium channels in the cell membrane) and release of bound calcium from the sarcoplasmic reticulum in the cell. Thus, calcium plays an important role in maintaining vasomotor tone, myocardial contractility, and conduction. Calcium channel blocking agents prevent the movement of extracellular calcium into the cell. As a result, coronary and peripheral arteries are dilated, myocardial contractility is decreased, and the conduction system is depressed in relation to impulse formation (automaticity) and conduction velocity (Fig. 50-1).

In angina pectoris, the drugs improve the blood supply to the myocardium by dilating coronary arteries and decrease the workload of the heart by dilating peripheral arteries. In variant angina, calcium channel blockers reduce coronary artery vasospasm. In atrial fibrillation or flutter and other supraventricular tachydysrhythmias, **diltiazem** and **verapamil** slow the rate of ventricular response. In hypertension, the drugs lower blood pressure primarily by dilating peripheral arteries.

Calcium channel blockers are well absorbed after oral administration but undergo extensive first-pass metabolism in the liver. Most of the drugs are more than 90% protein bound and reach peak plasma levels within 1 to 2 hours (6 hours or longer for sustained-release forms). Most also have short elimination half-lives (<5 hours), so doses must be given three or

Figure 50-1 ■ Calcium channel blockers: mechanism of action. **(A)** During muscle relaxation, potassium ions are inside the muscle cell and calcium and sodium ions are outside the muscle cell. **(B)** For muscle contraction to occur, potassium ions leave the cell and sodium and calcium ions enter the cell through open channels in the cell membrane. **(C)** When calcium channels are blocked by drug molecules, muscle contraction is decreased because calcium ions cannot move through the cell membrane into the muscle cell.

four times daily unless sustained-release formulations are used. **Amlodipine** (30–50 hours) and **felodipine** (11–16 hours) have long elimination half-lives and therefore can be given once daily. The drugs are metabolized in the liver, and dosage should be reduced in patients with severe liver disease. Dosage reductions are not required with renal disease.

The calcium channel blockers approved for use in the United States vary in their chemical structures and effects on body tissues. Seven of these are chemically dihydropyridines, of which **P** nifedipine is the prototype. Diltiazem and verapamil differ chemically from the dihydropyridines and each other. Nifedipine and related drugs act mainly on vascular smooth muscle to produce vasodilation, whereas verapamil and diltiazem have greater effects on the cardiac conduction system.

The drugs also vary in clinical indications for use; most are used for angina or hypertension, and only diltiazem and verapamil are used to manage supraventricular tachydysrhythmias.

In patients with CAD, the drugs are effective as monotherapy but are commonly prescribed in combination with beta blockers. In addition, **nimodipine** is approved for use only in subarachnoid hemorrhage, in which it decreases spasm in cerebral blood vessels and limits the extent of brain damage. In animal studies, nimodipine exerted greater effects on cerebral arteries than on other arteries, probably because it is highly lipid soluble and penetrates the blood–brain barrier.

Contraindications to use include second- or third-degree heart block, cardiogenic shock, and severe bradycardia, heart failure, or hypotension. The drugs should be used cautiously with milder bradycardia, heart failure, or hypotension and with renal or hepatic impairment.

Applying Your Knowledge 50-3

Mr. Gerald has had anginal pain at rest and his physician prescribes diltiazem. He asks what this new medication will do for him. How do you respond?

Metabolic Modulator

General Characteristics

A metabolic modulator is a miscellaneous second-line cardiovascular agent used in chronic angina in combination with amlodipine, beta blockers, or nitrates. The drug does not relieve acute anginal attacks but is given to patients with chronic angina who have not had adequate antianginal responses with other agents. Although the mechanism of action is not clearly understood, **ranolazine,** the only drug currently in the drug class is thought to be a partial fatty acid oxidation (PFox) inhibitor, increasing the efficiency of ATP production in the presence of hypoxia. The drug decreases ischemia but does not possess negative inotropic (contractility) or chronotropic (rate) effects; minimal effects on heart rate and blood pressure were reported during clinical trials. Ranolazine is also a late sodium channel inhibitor.

Individual Drugs

Ranolazine (Ranexa) represents the new classification of a metabolic modulator used in individuals with chronic angina. The drug is labeled for use in combination with amlodipine, beta blockers, or nitrates. After oral administration, peak plasma concentrations are reached within 2 to 5 hours. The drug is rapidly and extensively metabolized in the liver. Due to a risk of dose-dependent QT prolongation on electrocardiogram, ranolazine is reserved for the treatment of patients with chronic angina who have not achieved a satisfactory antianginal response with traditional drugs. Baseline and follow-up electrocardiography should be performed to evaluate the QT interval. Ranolazine is contraindicated in patients with pre-existing QT prolongation. The drug can be taken with or without meals and, because it is an extended-release tablet, should be swallowed whole and not crushed, chewed, or broken. Avoid giving with grapefruit juice. If a dose is missed, it should be taken at the next scheduled time; no dose should be doubled.

Adjunctive Antianginal Drugs

In addition to antianginal drugs, several other drugs may be used to control risk factors and prevent progression of myocardial ischemia to MI and sudden cardiac death:

- **Aspirin.** This drug has become the standard of care because of its antiplatelet (i.e., antithrombotic) effects. Recommended doses vary from 81 mg daily to 325 mg daily or every other day; apparently all doses are beneficial in reducing the possibility of myocardial reinfarction, stroke, and death. **Clopidogrel** (see Chap. 54), 75 mg/day, is an acceptable alternative for individuals with aspirin allergy.

- **Antilipemics.** These drugs (see Chap. 55) may be needed by patients who are unable to lower serum cholesterol levels sufficiently with a low-fat diet. **Lovastatin** or a related "statin" is often used. The goal is usually to reduce the serum cholesterol level below 200 mg/dL and low-density lipoprotein cholesterol to below 130 mg/dL.

- **Antihypertensives.** These drugs (see Chap. 52) may be needed for patients with hypertension. Because beta blockers and calcium channel blockers are used to manage hypertension as well as angina, one of these drugs may be effective for both disorders.

Nursing Process

Assessment

Assess the patient's condition in relation to angina pectoris. Specific assessment data vary with each patient but usually should include the following:

- During the initial nursing history interview, try to answer the following questions:

  - How long has the patient been taking antianginal drugs? For what purpose are they being taken (prophylaxis, treatment of acute attacks, or both)?

  - What is the frequency and duration of acute anginal attacks? Has either increased recently? (An increase could indicate worsening coronary atherosclerosis and increased risk of MI.)

  - Do symptoms other than chest pain occur during acute attacks (e.g., sweating, nausea)?

  - Are there particular activities or circumstances that provoke acute attacks? Do attacks ever occur when the patient is at rest? Where does the patient fit in the Canadian Cardiovascular Society classification system?

  - What measures relieve symptoms of acute angina?

Nursing Process continues on page 806

- If the patient takes nitroglycerin, ask how often it is required, how many tablets are needed for relief of pain, how often the supply is replaced, and where the patient stores or carries the drug.

- Assess blood pressure and pulse, electrocardiogram (ECG) reports, serum cholesterol, and cardiac enzyme reports. Elevated cholesterol is a significant risk factor for coronary atherosclerosis and angina, and the risk is directly related to the degree of elevation. Cardiac enzyme levels, such as troponin, creatine kinase (CK), lactate dehydrogenase (LDH), and aspartate aminotransferase (AST), should all be normal in patients with angina.

- During an acute attack, assess the following:

  - Location and quality of the pain. Chest pain is nonspecific. It may be a symptom of numerous disorders, such as pulmonary embolism, esophageal spasm or inflammation (heartburn), costochondritis, or anxiety. Chest pain of cardiac origin is caused by myocardial ischemia and may indicate angina pectoris or MI.

  - Precipitating factors. For example, what was the patient doing, thinking, or feeling just before the onset of chest pain?

  - Has the patient had invasive procedures to diagnose or treat his or her CAD (e.g., cardiac catheterization, angioplasty, revascularization surgery)?

Nursing Diagnoses

- Decreased Cardiac Output related to altered stroke volume or drug therapy

- Acute pain in chest related to inadequate perfusion of the myocardium

- Activity Intolerance related to chest pain

- Deficient Knowledge related to management of disease process and drug therapy

- Ineffective Individual Coping related to chronic disease process

- Sexual Dysfunction related to fear of precipitating chest pain

Planning/Goals

The patient will

- Receive or take antianginal drugs accurately

- Experience relief of acute chest pain

- Have fewer episodes of acute chest pain

- Have increased activity tolerance

- Identify and manage situations that precipitate anginal attacks

- Be closely monitored for therapeutic and adverse effects, especially when drug therapy is started

- Avoid preventable adverse effects

- Verbalize essential information about the disease process, needed dietary and lifestyle changes to improve health status, and drug therapy

- Recognize signs and symptoms that necessitate professional intervention

- Keep appointments for follow-up care and monitoring

Interventions

Use the following measures to prevent acute anginal attacks.

- Assist in preventing, recognizing, and managing contributory disorders, such as atherosclerosis, hypertension, hyperthyroidism, hypoxia, and anemia. For example, hypertension is a common risk factor for CAD and morbidity and mortality increase progressively with the degree of either systolic or diastolic elevation. Management of hypertension reduces morbidity and mortality rates. However, most studies indicate that the reductions stem more from fewer strokes, less renal failure, and less heart failure, than from less CAD.

- Help the patient recognize and avoid precipitating factors (e.g., heavy meals, strenuous exercise) when possible. If anxiety is a factor, relaxation techniques or psychological counseling may be helpful.

- Help the patient develop a more healthful lifestyle in terms of diet and weight control, adequate rest and sleep, regular exercise, and not smoking. Ideally, these self-help interventions are practiced before illness occurs; they can help prevent or delay illness. However, most individuals are unmotivated until illness develops, and perhaps after it develops as well. These interventions are beneficial at any stage of CAD. For example, for a patient who already has angina, a supervised exercise program helps develop collateral circulation. Smoking has numerous ill effects on the patient with angina and decreases effectiveness of antianginal drugs.

During an acute anginal attack in a patient known to have angina or CAD, take the following actions.

- Assume that any chest pain may be of cardiac origin.

- Have the patient lie down or sit down to reduce cardiac workload and provide rest.

- Check vital signs and compare them with baseline values.

- Record the characteristics of chest pain and the presence of other signs and symptoms.

- Have the patient take a fast-acting nitroglycerin preparation (previously prescribed), up to three sublingual tablets or three oral sprays, each 5 minutes apart, as necessary.

- If chest pain is not relieved with rest and nitroglycerin, assume that an MI has occurred until proven otherwise. In a health care setting, keep the patient at rest and notify the client's physician immediately. Outside of a health care setting, call 911 for immediate assistance.

■ Leave sublingual nitroglycerin at the bedside of hospitalized patients (per hospital policy). The tablets or spray should be within reach so that they can be used immediately. Record the number of tablets used daily, and ensure that an adequate supply is available.

Provide appropriate patient teaching related to drug therapy (see accompanying display).

Evaluation

■ Observe and interview for relief of acute chest pain.

■ Observe and interview regarding the number of episodes of acute chest pain.

■ Identify CAD lifestyle factors that are being successfully modified or require modification (e.g., diet, weight, activity, smoking cessation).

■ Interview regarding success and compliance with drug therapy.

Principles of Therapy

Goals of Therapy

The goals of drug therapy are to relieve acute anginal pain, reduce the number and severity of acute anginal attacks, improve exercise tolerance and quality of life, delay progression of CAD, prevent MI, and prevent sudden cardiac death.

Drug Selection and Dosage

For relief of acute angina and prophylaxis before events that cause acute angina, nitroglycerin (sublingual tablets or translingual spray) is usually the primary drug of choice. Sublingual or chewable tablets of isosorbide dinitrate also may be used. For long-term prevention or management of recurrent angina, oral or topical nitrates, beta-adrenergic blocking agents, or calcium channel blocking agents are used. Combination drug therapy with a nitrate and one of the other drugs is common and effective. Patients taking one or more long-acting antianginal drugs should carry a short-acting drug as well to be used for acute attacks.

Dosage of all antianginal drugs should be individualized to achieve optimal benefit and minimal adverse effects. This is usually accomplished by starting with relatively small doses and increasing them at appropriate intervals as necessary. Doses may vary widely among individuals.

Tolerance to Long-Acting Nitrates

Patients who take long-acting dosage forms of nitrates on a regular schedule develop tolerance to the vasodilating (antianginal) effects of the drug. The patients more likely to develop tolerance are those on high-dose, uninterrupted therapy. Although tolerance decreases the adverse effects of hypotension, dizziness, and headache, therapeutic effects also may be

decreased. As a result, episodes of chest pain may occur more often or be more severe than expected. In addition, short-acting nitrates may be less effective in relieving acute pain.

Opinions seem divided about the best way to prevent or manage nitrate tolerance. Some authorities recommend using short-acting nitrates when needed and avoiding the long-acting forms. Others recommend using the long-acting forms for 12 to 16 hours daily during active periods and omitting them during inactive periods or sleep. Thus, a dose of an oral nitrate or topical ointment would be given every 6 hours for three doses daily, allowing a rest period of 6 hours without a dose. Transdermal discs should be removed at bedtime. If anginal symptoms occur during sleeping hours, short-acting nitrates may be beneficial in relieving the symptoms. All nitrates should be administered at the lowest effective dosage.

Use in Special Populations

Use in Children

The safety and effectiveness of antianginal drugs have not been established for children. Nitroglycerin has been given IV for heart failure and intraoperative control of blood pressure, with the initial dose adjusted for weight and later doses titrated to response.

Use in Older Adults

The prevalence of CAD increases with age and is the major cause of disability, morbidity, and mortality in older adults. The elderly have a higher incidence of multivessel coronary disease, decreased left ventricular function, and comorbid conditions. Antianginal drugs are often used because cardiovascular disease and myocardial ischemia are common problems in older adults. Traditional antianginal drugs that act via hemodynamic mechanisms (e.g., beta blockers, calcium antagonists, nitrates) can pose a problem in older adults because of the associated higher risk of drug interaction and greater incidence of adverse drug effects. Adverse effects, such as hypotension and syncope, are likely to occur, and they may be more severe than in younger adults. Blood pressure and ability to ambulate safely should be closely monitored, especially when drug therapy is started or dosages are increased. Ambulatory patients also should be monitored for their ability to take the drugs correctly.

With calcium channel blockers, older adults may have higher plasma concentrations of verapamil, diltiazem, nifedipine, and amlodipine. This is attributed to decreased hepatic metabolism of the drugs, probably because of decreased hepatic blood flow. In addition, older adults may experience more hypotension with verapamil, nifedipine, and felodipine than younger patients. Blood pressure should be monitored with these drugs.

Use in Patients With Renal Impairment

Little information is available about the use of antianginal drugs in patients with impaired renal function. A few studies indicate that advanced renal failure may alter the pharmacokinetics of calcium channel blockers. Although the pharmacokinetics of diltiazem and verapamil are quite similar in patients

Patient Teaching Guidelines | Antianginal Drugs

General Considerations

■ Angina is chest pain that occurs because your heart is not getting enough blood and oxygen. The most common causes are hypertension and atherosclerosis of the coronary arteries. The chest pain usually lasts less than 5 minutes and episodes can be managed for years without causing permanent heart damage. However, if the pain is severe or prolonged, a heart attack and heart damage may develop. You need to seek information about your heart condition to prevent or decrease episodes of angina and prevent a heart attack.

■ Several types of drugs are used in angina, and you may need a combination of drugs for the best effects. Most patients take one or more long-acting drugs to prevent anginal attacks and a fast, short-acting drug (usually nitroglycerin tablets that you dissolve under your tongue, or a nitroglycerin solution that you spray into your mouth) to relieve acute attacks. You should seek emergency care immediately if rest and three sublingual tablets or oral sprays 5 minutes apart do not relieve your chest pain. The long-acting medications are not effective in relieving sudden anginal pain.

■ As with any medications for serious or potentially serious conditions, it is extremely important to take antianginal medications as prescribed. Do not increase dosage or discontinue the drugs without specific instructions from your health care provider.

■ With sublingual nitroglycerin tablets, keep them in the original container; carry them so that they are always within reach but not where they are exposed to body heat; and replace them approximately every 6 months because they become ineffective.

■ It may be helpful to record the number and severity of anginal episodes, the number of nitroglycerin tablets required to relieve the attack, and the total number of tablets taken daily. Such a record can help your health care provider know when to change your medications or your dosages.

■ Headache and dizziness may occur with nitrate antianginal drugs, especially sublingual nitroglycerin. These effects are usually temporary and dissipate with continued therapy. If dizziness occurs, avoid strenuous activity and stand up slowly for approximately an hour after taking the drugs. If headache is severe, you may take aspirin or acetaminophen with the nitrate drug. Do not reduce drug dosage or take the drug less often to avoid headache; loss of effectiveness may occur.

■ Keep family members or support individuals informed about the location and use of antianginal medications in case help is needed.

■ Avoid over-the-counter decongestants, cold remedies, and diet pills, which stimulate the heart and constrict blood vessels and thus may cause angina.

■ With nitrate antianginal drugs, avoid alcohol. Both the drugs and alcohol dilate blood vessels and an excessive reduction in blood pressure (with dizziness and fainting) may occur with the combination.

■ With a metabolic modulator, avoid concurrent intake of grapefruit juice: Grapefruit juice increases serum drug levels.

■ Several calcium channel blockers are available in both immediate-acting and long-acting (sustained-release) forms. The brand names often differ very little (e.g., Procardia is a brand name of immediate-release nifedipine; Procardia XL is a long-acting formulation). It is extremely important that the correct formulation is used consistently.

Self- or Caregiver Administration

■ Take or give as instructed; specific instructions differ with the type of antianginal drug being taken.

■ Take or give antianginal drugs on a regular schedule, at evenly spaced intervals. This increases drug effectiveness in preventing acute attacks of angina.

■ With nitroglycerin and other nitrate preparations:

■ Use according to instructions for the particular dosage form. The dosage forms were developed for specific routes of administration and are not interchangeable.

■ For sublingual nitroglycerin tablets, place them under the tongue until they dissolve. Take at the first sign of an anginal attack, before severe pain develops. If chest pain is not relieved in 5 minutes, dissolve a second tablet under the tongue. If pain is not relieved within another 5 minutes, dissolve a third tablet. If pain continues or becomes more severe, notify your health care provider immediately or report to the nearest hospital emergency room. Sit down when you take the medications. This may help to relieve your pain and prevent dizziness from the drug.

■ For the translingual solution of nitroglycerin, spray onto or under the tongue; do not inhale the spray.

■ For transmucosal tablets of nitroglycerin, place them under the upper lip or between the cheek and gum and allow them to dissolve slowly over 3 to 5 hours. Do not chew or swallow the tablets.

■ Take oral nitrates on an empty stomach with a glass of water. Oral isosorbide dinitrate is available in regular and chewable tablets; be sure each type is taken appropriately. Do not crush or chew sustained-release nitrate tablets.

■ For sublingual isosorbide dinitrate tablets, place them under the tongue until they dissolve.

■ If an oral nitrate and topical nitroglycerin are being used concurrently, stagger the times of administration. This minimizes dizziness from low blood pressure and headache, which are common adverse effects of nitrate drugs.

■ For nitroglycerin ointment, use the special paper to measure the dose. Place the ointment on a nonhairy part of the upper body and apply with the applicator paper. Cover the area with plastic wrap or tape. Rotate application sites (because the ointment can irritate the skin) and wipe off the previous dose before applying a new dose. Wash hands after applying the ointment.

■ The measured paper must be used for accurate dosage. The paper is used to apply the ointment because the drug is readily absorbed through the skin. Skin contact should be avoided except on the designated area of the body. Plastic wrap or tape aids absorption and prevents removal of the drug. It also prevents soiling of clothes and linens.

- For nitroglycerin patches, apply at the same time each day to clean, dry, hairless areas on the upper body or arms. Rotate sites. Avoid applying below the knee or elbow or in areas of skin irritation or scar tissue. Correct application is necessary to promote effective and consistent drug absorption. The drug is not as well absorbed from distal portions of the extremities because of decreased blood flow. Rotation of sites decreases skin irritation. Also, used patches must be disposed of properly because there is enough residual nitroglycerin to be harmful, especially to children and pets.
- With sustained-release forms of calcium channel blockers, which are usually taken once daily, do not take more often than prescribed and do not crush or chew.

with normal and impaired renal function, caution is still advised. With verapamil, about 70% of a dose is excreted as metabolites in urine.

Dosage reductions are considered unnecessary with verapamil and diltiazem but may be needed with nifedipine and several other dihydropyridine derivatives. With nifedipine, protein binding is decreased and the elimination half-life is prolonged with renal impairment. In a few patients, reversible elevations in blood urea nitrogen and serum creatinine have occurred. With nicardipine, plasma concentrations are higher in patients with renal impairment, and dosage should be reduced.

Use in Patients With Hepatic Impairment

Nitrates, beta blockers (see Chap. 18), and calcium channel blockers are metabolized in the liver, and all should be used with caution in patients with significant impairment of hepatic function from reduced blood flow or disease processes.

With oral nitrates, it is difficult to predict effects. On the one hand, first-pass metabolism is reduced, which increases the bioavailability (amount of active drug) of a given dose. On the other hand, the nitrate reductase enzymes that normally deactivate the drug may increase if large doses are given. In this case, more enzymes are available and the drug is metabolized more rapidly, possibly reducing therapeutic effects of a given dose. Relatively large doses of oral nitrates are sometimes given to counteract the drug tolerance (reduced hemodynamic effects) associated with chronic use. In addition, metabolism of nitroglycerin and isosorbide dinitrate normally produces active metabolites. Thus, if metabolism is reduced by liver impairment, drug effects may be decreased and shorter in duration.

A metabolic modulator is contraindicated in patients with hepatic impairment. Prolongation of QT interval may be more significant in patients with liver dysfunction.

With calcium channel blockers, impairment of liver function has profound effects on the pharmacokinetics and pharmacodynamics of most of these drugs. Thus, the drugs should be used with caution, dosages should be substantially reduced, and patients should be closely monitored for drug effects (including periodic measurements of liver enzymes). These recommendations stem from the following effects:

- An impaired liver produces fewer drug-binding plasma proteins such as albumin. This means that a greater proportion of a given dose is unbound and therefore active.
- In patients with cirrhosis, bioavailability of oral drugs is greatly increased and metabolism (of both oral and parenteral drugs) is greatly decreased. Both of these effects increase plasma levels of drug from a given dose (essentially an overdose). The effects result from shunting of blood around the liver so that drug molecules circulating in the bloodstream do not come in contact with drug-metabolizing enzymes and therefore are not metabolized. For example, the bioavailability of verapamil, nifedipine, felodipine, and nisoldipine is approximately double and their clearance is approximately one third that of patients without cirrhosis.
- Although hepatotoxicity is uncommon, clinical symptoms of hepatitis, cholestasis, or jaundice and elevated liver enzymes (e.g., alkaline phosphatase, creatine kinase [CK], lactate dehydrogenase [LDH], aspartate aminotransferase [AST], alanine aminotransferase [ALT]) have occurred, mainly with diltiazem, nifedipine, and verapamil. These changes resolve if the causative drug is stopped.

Use in Patients With Critical Illness

Antianginal drugs have multiple cardiovascular effects and may be used alone or in combination with other cardiovascular drugs in patients with critical illness. They are probably used most often to manage severe angina, severe hypertension, or serious cardiac dysrhythmias. For example, IV nitroglycerin may be used for angina and hypertension; an IV beta blocker or calcium channel blocker may be used to improve cardiovascular function with angina, hypertension, or supraventricular tachydysrhythmias. With any of these drugs, dosage must be carefully titrated and patients must be closely monitored for hypotension and other drug effects.

In addition, absorption of oral drugs or topical forms of nitroglycerin may be impaired in patients with extensive edema, heart failure, hypotension, or other conditions that impair blood flow to the gastrointestinal tract or skin.

Use in Home Care

The role of the home care nurse may vary, depending largely on the severity of the patient's illness. Initially, the nurse should assess the frequency and severity of anginal attacks and how the attacks are managed. In addition, the nurse can assess the home setting for lifestyle and environmental factors that may precipitate myocardial ischemia. When causative factors are identified, plans can be developed to avoid or minimize them. Other aspects of home care may include monitoring the patient's response to antianginal medications; teaching patients and caregivers how to use, store, and replace medications to ensure a constant supply; and discussing circumstances for which the patient should seek emergency care.

Nursing Actions   Antianginal Drugs

NURSING ACTIONS	RATIONALE/EXPLANATION
1. Administer accurately	
a. Check blood pressure and heart rate before each dose of an antianginal drug. Withhold the drug if systolic blood pressure is below 90 mm Hg. If the dose is omitted, record and report to the health care provider.	Hypotension is an adverse effect of antianginal drugs. Bradycardia is an adverse effect of propranolol and nadolol. Dosage adjustments may be necessary if these effects occur.
b. Give antianginal drugs on a regular schedule, at evenly spaced intervals.	To increase effectiveness in preventing acute attacks of angina
c. If oral nitrates and topical nitroglycerin are being used concurrently, stagger times of administration.	To minimize risks of additive hypotension and headache
d. For sublingual nitroglycerin and isosorbide dinitrate, instruct the patient to place the tablets under the tongue until they dissolve.	
e. For oral isosorbide dinitrate, regular and chewable tablets are available. Be sure each type of tablet is taken appropriately.	
f. For sublingual nitroglycerin, check the expiration date on the container.	Sublingual tablets of nitroglycerin are volatile. After the bottle has been opened, they become ineffective after approximately 6 months and should be replaced.
g. To apply nitroglycerin ointment, use the special paper to measure the dose. Place the ointment on a nonhairy part of the body, and apply with the applicator paper. Cover the area with plastic wrap or tape. Rotate application sites and wipe off previous ointment before applying a new dose.	The measured paper must be used for accurate dosage. The paper is used to apply the ointment because the drug is readily absorbed through the skin. Skin contact should be avoided except on the designated area of the body. Plastic wrap or tape aids absorption and prevents removal of the drug. It also prevents soiling of clothes and linens. Application sites should be rotated because the ointment can irritate the skin.
h. For nitroglycerin patches, apply at the same time each day to clean, dry, hairless areas on the upper body or arms. Rotate sites. Avoid applying below the knee or elbow or in areas of skin irritation or scar tissue.	To promote effective and consistent drug absorption. The drug is not as well absorbed from distal portions of the extremities because of decreased blood flow. Rotation of sites decreases skin irritation.
i. For intravenous (IV) nitroglycerin, dilute the drug and give by continuous infusion, with frequent monitoring of blood pressure and heart rate. Use only with the special administration set supplied by the manufacturer to avoid drug adsorption onto tubing.	The drug should not be given by direct IV injection. The drug is potent and may cause hypotension. Dosage (flow rate) is adjusted according to response (pain relief or drop in systolic blood pressure of 20 mm Hg).
j. With IV verapamil, inject slowly, over 2–3 minutes.	To decrease hypotension and other adverse effects
2. Observe for therapeutic effects	
a. Relief of chest pain with acute attacks	Sublingual nitroglycerin usually relieves pain within 5 minutes. If pain is not relieved, two additional tablets may be given, 5 minutes apart. If pain is not relieved after three tablets, report to the health care provider or seek emergency care.
b. Reduced incidence and severity of acute attacks with prophylactic antianginal drugs	
c. Increased exercise tolerance	
3. Observe for adverse effects	
a. With nitrates, observe for hypotension, dizziness, lightheadedness, tachycardia, palpitations, and headache.	Adverse effects are extensions of pharmacologic action. Vasodilation causes hypotension, which in turn causes dizziness from cerebral hypoxia and tachycardia from compensatory sympathetic nervous system stimulation. Hypotension can decrease blood flow to coronary arteries and precipitate angina pectoris or myocardial infarction. Hypotension is most likely to occur within an hour after drug administration. Vasodilation also causes headache, the most common adverse effect of nitrates.
b. With beta-adrenergic blocking agents, observe for hypotension, bradycardia, bronchospasm, and heart failure.	Beta blockers lower blood pressure by decreasing myocardial contractility and cardiac output. Excessive bradycardia may contribute to hypotension and cardiac dysrhythmias. Bronchospasm is more likely to occur in patients with asthma or other chronic respiratory problems.

NURSING ACTIONS	RATIONALE/EXPLANATION
c. With calcium channel blockers, observe for hypotension, dizziness, lightheadedness, weakness, peripheral edema, headache, heart failure, pulmonary edema, nausea, and constipation. Bradycardia may occur with verapamil and diltiazem; tachycardia may occur with nifedipine and nicardipine.	Adverse effects result primarily from reduced smooth muscle contractility. These effects, except constipation, are much more likely to occur with nifedipine and other dihydropyridines. Nifedipine may cause profound hypotension, which activates the compensatory mechanisms of the sympathetic nervous system and the renin–angiotensin–aldosterone system. Peripheral edema may require the administration of a diuretic. Constipation is more likely to occur with verapamil. Diltiazem reportedly causes few adverse effects.
4. Observe for drug interactions	
a. Drugs that *increase* effects of antianginal drugs:	
(1) Antidysrhythmics, antihypertensive drugs, diuretics, phenothiazine antipsychotic agents	Additive hypotension
(2) Cimetidine	May increase beta-blocking effects of propranolol by slowing its hepatic clearance and elimination. Increases effects of all calcium channel blockers by inhibiting hepatic metabolism and increasing serum drug levels.
(3) Digoxin	Additive bradycardia when given with beta-blocking agents
(4) With nitrates, PDE type 5 inhibitors like Viagra (contraindicated)	Potentially life-threatening hypotension may occur.
b. Drugs that *decrease* effects of antianginal drugs:	
(1) Adrenergic drugs (e.g., epinephrine, isoproterenol)	Adrenergic drugs, which stimulate beta receptors, can reverse bradycardia induced by beta blockers.
(2) Anticholinergic drugs	Drugs with anticholinergic effects can increase heart rate, offsetting slower heart rates produced by beta blockers.
(3) Calcium salts	May decrease therapeutic effectiveness of calcium channel blockers
(4) Carbamazepine, phenytoin, rifampin	May decrease effects of calcium channel blockers by inducing hepatic enzymes and thereby increasing their rate of metabolism

Key Concepts

◼ Angina pectoris results from deficit in myocardial oxygen supply (myocardial ischemia) in relation to myocardial oxygen demand, most often caused by atherosclerotic plaque in the coronary arteries.

◼ The goals of antianginal drug therapy are to relieve acute anginal pain, reduce the number and severity of acute anginal attacks, improve exercise tolerance and quality of life, delay progression of CAD, prevent MI, and prevent sudden cardiac death.

◼ Because oral nitroglycerin is rapidly metabolized in the liver, relatively small proportions reach systemic circulation; transmucosal, transdermal, and IV preparations are more effective.

◼ Common drugs used for myocardial ischemia are the organic nitrates, the beta-adrenergic blocking agents, and the calcium channel blocking agents.

◼ Beta blockers are more effective than nitrates or calcium channel blockers in decreasing the likelihood of silent ischemia and improving the mortality rate after transmural MI.

◼ Traditional antianginal drugs that act via hemodynamic mechanisms (e.g., beta blockers, calcium antagonists, nitrates) can pose a problem in older adults because of the associated higher risk of drug interaction and greater incidence of adverse drug effects.

◼ Patients who take long-acting dosage forms of nitrates on a regular schedule develop tolerance to the vasodilating (antianginal) effects of the drug.

◼ In angina pectoris, calcium channel blockers improve blood supply to the myocardium by dilating coronary arteries and decrease the workload of the heart by dilating peripheral arteries; in variant angina, the drugs reduce coronary artery vasospasm.

◼ Aspirin, antilipemics, and antihypertensives are used in conjunctional with antianginal drugs to prevent progression of myocardial ischemia to MI.

◼ Starting with relatively small doses of antianginal drugs and increasing them at appropriate intervals as necessary should achieve optimal benefit and minimal adverse effects.

Review and Application Exercises

Short Answer Exercises

1. What is angina pectoris?

2. What is the role of endothelial dysfunction in the development of coronary artery atherosclerosis and myocardial ischemia?

3. How do nitrates relieve angina?

4. Develop a teaching plan for a patient who is beginning nitrate therapy.

5. How do beta blockers relieve angina?

6. Why should beta blockers be tapered and discontinued slowly in patients with angina?

7. How do calcium channel blockers relieve angina?

8. Develop a teaching plan for a patient taking a calcium channel blocker.

NCLEX-Style Questions

9. The nurse removes a patient's transdermal nitroglycerin disc at bedtime as ordered to minimize nitrate tolerance. The patient awakens during the night and complains of anginal symptoms. The nurse's first action is to
   a. Notify the health care provider.
   b. Apply a new transdermal disc.
   c. Obtain further history of complaints.
   d. Administer a short-acting nitrate as ordered.

10. The health care provider prescribes nitroglycerin 2% ointment, 1.5-inch dose every 4 hours. To accurately apply the ointment, the patient should be instructed to
    a. Rub the ointment into the skin to enhance absorption.
    b. Leave previous ointment on for 4 hours after applying a new dose.
    c. Rotate application sites to decrease skin irritation.
    d. Place the ointment on a distal part of the lower body to increase absorption.

11. Concurrent use of nitrates in any form or route of administration with phosphodiesterase enzyme inhibitors produces
    a. enhanced erectile potential
    b. significant tachycardia
    c. severe hypotensive effects
    d. mild bronchodilation

12. A patient who is taking metoprolol (Lopressor) is seen in the cardiac clinic following an MI and reports that he continues to smoke. The nurse recognizes that smoking may contribute to what effect on beta-blocking activity?
    a. reduce the efficacy
    b. potentiate an increase in intracranial pressure
    c. precipitate ventricular fibrillation
    d. increase the incidence of side effects

13. A patient with angina pectoris, being discontinued from his beta blockers, asks the nurse, "Why can't I just stop taking the drug today if it's not working anyway?" The nurse instructs the patient that failure to taper the drug slowly may lead to
    a. worsening of his angina symptoms
    b. significant bronchoconstriction
    c. development of congestive heart failure
    d. drug fever

14. In caring for a patient with chronic angina who has been prescribed the new drug, ranolazine (Ranexa), the nurse is correct in counseling that
    a. This drug may be crushed if necessary.
    b. This drug must not be taken with beta blockers.
    c. This drug must not be taken with meals.
    d. This drug should not be taken with grapefruit juice.

Selected References

Anderson, J. L., Adams, C. D., Antman, E. M., Bridges, C. R., Califf, R. M., Casey, D. E. Jr., et al. (2007). ACC/AHA 2007 guidelines for the management of patients with unstable angina/non–ST-elevation myocardial infarction: a report of the American College of Cardiology/American Heart Association Task Force on Practice Guidelines (writing committee to revise the 2002 Guidelines for the Management of Patients With Unstable Angina/Non–ST-Elevation Myocardial Infarction). *Circulation, 116,* e148–e304.

Corwin, E. J. (2006). *Handbook of pathophysiology* (3rd ed.). Philadelphia: Lippincott Williams & Wilkins.

Drug facts and comparisons. (Updated monthly). St. Louis, MO: Facts and Comparisons.

Gabardi, S. (2005). Drug dosing in chronic kidney disease. *Medical Clinics of North America, 89,* 649–687.

Gibler, W. B. (2005). Practical implementation of the guidelines for unstable angina/non-st-segment elevation myocardial infarction in the emergency department. *Annals of Emergency Medicine, 46,* 185–197.

Guyton, A. C., & Hall, J. E. (2006). *Textbook of medical physiology* (11th ed.). Philadelphia: W. B. Saunders.

Hilas, O. (2007). Ranolazine (Ranexa) for chronic angina. *American Family Physician, 75,* 544–546.

Junnila, J. L. (2006). Coronary artery disease screening, treatment, and follow-up. *Primary Care, 33,* 863–885, vi.

Karch, A. M. (2007). *2008 Lippincott's nursing drug guide.* Philadelphia: Lippincott Williams & Wilkins.

Kitakaze, N., et al. (2007). Patients given ANP post heart-attack have lower infarct size, fewer reperfusion injuries. *Lancet, 370,* 1483–1493.

Lacy, C. F., Armstrong, L. L., Goldman, M. P., et al. (2007). *Lexi-Comp's drug information handbook* (15th ed.). Hudson, OH: Lexi-Comp.

Marzilli, M., Affinito, S., & Focardi, M. (2006). Changing scenario in chronic ischemic heart disease: Therapeutic implications. *American Journal of Cardiology, 98,* 3J–7J.

National Institutes of Health Expert Panel. (2001). *Third report of the National Cholesterol Education Program (NCEP) Expert Panel on Detection, Evaluation, and Treatment of High Blood Cholesterol in Adults (Adult Treatment Panel III)* (NIH Publication No. 01-3670). Bethesda, MD: National Institutes of Health.

Waters, D. D. (2008). Acute coronary syndrome: Unstable angina and non-ST segment elevation myocardial infarction. In Goldman (Ed.), *Cecil medicine* (23rd ed.). Retrieved November 1, 2007, from http://www.mdconsult.com/das/book/body/80877982-10/0/1492/301. html?tocnode=53600597&fromURL=301.html

Drugs Used in Hypotension and Shock

KEY TERMS

- Anaphylactic shock
- Cardiogenic shock
- Distributive shock
- Hypovolemic shock
- Neurogenic shock
- Septic shock
- Vasogenic shock

LEARNING OBJECTIVES

After studying this chapter, you will be able to:

1. Identify patients at risk for development of hypovolemia and shock.
2. Identify common causes of hypotension and shock.
3. Discuss an assessment of a patient in shock.
4. Describe therapeutic and adverse effects of vasopressor drugs used in the management of hypotension and shock.

Applying Your Knowledge

Karim Alrashed is a 65 year-old man who has been admitted to ICU suffering from hypovolemic shock. He has had aggressive fluid resuscitation; however, his BP remains low. The physician orders IV dopamine to keep his systolic BP above 90 mm Hg.

Introduction

Shock is a clinical condition of insufficient perfusion of cells and vital organs, causing tissue hypoxia. Clinical symptoms depend on the degree of impaired perfusion of vital organs (e.g., brain, heart, kidneys). Common signs and symptoms include oliguria, heart failure, mental confusion, cool extremities, and coma. Most, but not all, people in shock are hypotensive. An additional consequence of inadequate blood flow to tissues is that cells change from aerobic (oxygen-based) to anaerobic metabolism. Lactic acid produced by anaerobic metabolism leads to generalized metabolic acidosis and eventually to organ failure and death if blood flow is not promptly restored.

Types of Shock

There are three general categories of shock that are based on the circulatory mechanisms involved. These mechanisms are intravascular volume, the ability of the heart to pump, and vascular tone.

Hypovolemic shock involves a loss of intravascular fluid volume that may be due to actual blood loss or relative loss from fluid shifts within the body.

Cardiogenic shock occurs when the myocardium has lost its ability to contract efficiently and maintain an adequate cardiac output.

Distributive or *vasogenic* shock is characterized by massive vasodilation, which results in a relative hypovolemia. Distributive shock is further divided into anaphylactic, neurogenic, and septic shock.

- *Anaphylactic* shock is due to massive vasodilation caused by release of histamine in response to a severe allergic reaction.
- *Neurogenic* shock is due to massive vasodilation caused by a suppression of the sympathetic nervous system.

■ *Septic* shock is due to massive vasodilation caused by release of mediators of the inflammatory process in response to overwhelming infection. Almost any organism that gains access to the bloodstream can cause septic shock, but the most often is associated with gram-negative and gram-positive bacterial infections and fungi.

It is important to know the etiology of shock because management varies among the types. The types of shock, with their causes and symptoms, are summarized in Table 51-1.

General Characteristics of Antishock Drugs

Drugs used in the management of shock are primarily the adrenergic drugs, which are discussed more extensively in Chapter 17. In this chapter, the drugs are discussed only in relation to their use in hypotension and shock. In these conditions, drugs with alpha-adrenergic activity (e.g., norepinephrine, phenylephrine) are used to increase peripheral vascular resistance and raise blood pressure. Drugs with beta-adrenergic activity (e.g., dobutamine) are used to increase myocardial contractility and heart rate, which in turn raises blood pressure. Some drugs have both alpha- and beta-adrenergic activity (e.g., dopamine, epinephrine). In many cases, a combination of drugs is used, depending on the type of shock and the patient's response to treatment. In an emergency, the drugs may be used to maintain adequate perfusion of vital organs until sufficient fluid volume is replaced and circulation is restored.

Adrenergic drugs with beta activity may be relatively contraindicated in shock states precipitated or complicated by cardiac dysrhythmias. Beta-stimulating drugs are used cautiously

Table 51-1	Types of Shock	
TYPE OF SHOCK	**POSSIBLE CAUSES**	**CLINICAL MANIFESTATION**
Hypovolemic	Trauma Gastrointestinal bleed Genital-urinary bleed Ruptured aneurysms Third spacing Dehydration	Hypotension Tachycardia Cool, clammy skin Diaphoresis Pallor Oliguria
Cardiogenic	Acute myocardial infarction Cardiac surgery Dysrhythmias Cardiomyopathy Heart failure Ventricular aneurysm Ventricular hypertrophy Ventricular dysfunction	Signs and symptoms of heart failure Signs and symptoms of decreased cardiac output
Distributive		
Anaphylactic	Chemicals Contrast dyes Drugs Insect bites Foods	Hypotension Hives Bronchospasm, dyspnea, cough, stridor, wheezing Nausea, abdominal cramping, abdominal pain Flushing, warm to hot skin Restlessness, change in level of consciousness
Neurogenic	Spinal cord damage Spinal anesthesia Insulin shock Severe pain Drugs	Hypotension Bradycardia Hypothermia Neurologic deficit Warm, dry skin
Septic	Infection (e.g., urinary tract, upper respiratory infections) Immunosuppression Invasive procedures	Hypotension Cool or warm, dry skin Hypothermia or hyperthermia

in cardiogenic shock after myocardial infarction because increased contractility and heart rate will increase myocardial oxygen consumption and extend the area of infarction. Individual drugs are described in the following section; indications for use and dosage ranges are listed in Table 51-2.

Individual Drugs

Dobutamine is a synthetic catecholamine developed to provide less vascular activity than dopamine. It acts mainly on beta$_1$ receptors in the heart to increase the force of myocardial contraction with a minimal increase in heart rate. Dobutamine also may increase blood pressure with large doses. It is less

likely to cause tachycardia, dysrhythmias, and increase myocardial oxygen consumption than dopamine. It is most useful in cases of shock that require increased cardiac output without the need for blood pressure support. It is recommended for short-term use only. It may be used with dopamine to augment the beta$_1$ activity that is sometimes overridden by alpha effects when dopamine is used alone at doses greater than 20 micrograms per kilogram per minute.

Dobutamine has a short plasma half-life and therefore must be administered by continuous intravenous (IV) infusion. A loading dose is not required because the drug has a rapid onset of action and reaches steady state within approximately 10 minutes after the infusion is begun. It is rapidly metabolized to inactive metabolites.

Dopamine is a naturally occurring catecholamine that functions as a neurotransmitter. Dopamine exerts its actions by stimulating alpha, beta, or dopaminergic receptors, depending on the dose being used. In addition, dopamine acts indirectly by releasing norepinephrine from sympathetic nerve endings and the adrenal glands. Peripheral dopamine receptors are located in splanchnic and renal vascular beds. At doses

| Table 51-2 | Drugs at a Glance: Drugs Used for Hypotension and Shock |

Generic/Trade Name	Indications for Use/Action	ROUTES AND DOSAGE RANGES	
		Adults	**Children**
Dobutamine (Dobutrex)	Management of cardiac decompensation Increase cardiac output	IV 2.5–20 mcg/kg/min, increased to 40 mcg/kg/min if necessary Reconstitute the 250-mg vial with 10 mL of sterile water or 5% dextrose injection. The resulting solution should be diluted to 250–500 mL with IV solution before administering (5000 mcg/mL). Add 250 mg of drug to 500 mL of diluent for a concentration of 500 mcg/mL.	2–15 mcg/kg/min
Dopamine (Intropin)	Acute hypotension and shock Increase cardiac output	IV 1 mcg/kg/min initially, gradually increasing to 50 mcg/kg/min Prepare by adding 200 mg of dopamine to 250 mL of IV fluid for a final concentration of 800 mcg/mL or to 500 mL IV fluid for a final concentration of 400 mcg/mL	1–20 mcg/kg/min
Epinephrine (Adrenalin)	Treat anaphylactic shock Reverse bronchoconstriction Increase cardiac output Treat cardiac arrest	IV 1–10 mcg/min. Prepare the solution by adding 2 mg (2 mL) of epinephrine injection 1:1000 to 250 or 500 mL of IV fluid. The final concentration is 8 or 4 mcg/mL, respectively.	IV infusion, 0.01 mcg/kg/min.

Generic/Trade Name	Indications for Use/Action	ROUTES AND DOSAGE RANGES	
		Adults	**Children**
Metaraminol	Treat hypotension due to spinal anesthesia	IM 2–10 mg IV injection, 0.5–5 mg IV infusion, add 15–500 mg of metaraminol to 250 or 500 mL of IV fluid. Adjust flow rate (dosage) to maintain the desired blood pressure.	IM 0.1 mg/kg IV injection, 0.01 mg/kg IV infusion, 1 mg/25 mL of diluent. Adjust flow rate to maintain the desired blood pressure.
Milrinone (Primacor)	Inotropic agent Increase cardiac output in cardiogenic shock	IV injection (loading dose), 50 mcg/kg over 10 min IV infusion (maintenance dose), 0.375–0.75 mcg/kg/min diluted in 0.9% or 0.45% sodium chloride or 5% dextrose solution. Maximum dose, 0.59–1.13 mg/kg/d	Safety and efficacy not established
Norepinephrine (Levophed)	Stimulate beta and alpha receptors Treat hypotension Increase cardiac output	IV infusion, 0.5–1 mcg/min initially, titrate to a maximum of 30 mcg/min. Prepare solution by adding 4 mg to 250 mL of IV fluid. Final concentration not > 128 mcg/mL.	IV infusion, 0.05–0.1 mcg/kg/min; maximum 1-2 mcg/kg/min Range 0.5–3 mcg/min
Phenylephrine (Neo-Synephrine)	Stimulate alpha receptors Treat hypotension	IM, Sub-Q: 2–5 mg/dose q1–2h IV injection: 0.1–0.5 mg every 10–15 min. IV infusion: 100–180 mcg/min initially, then 40–60 mcg/min Prepare solution by adding 10 mg of phenylephrine to 250 or 500 mL of IV fluid. Final concentration is 20 or 40 mcg/mL, respectively.	IM, Sub-Q: 0.1 mg/kg q1–2h IV injection: 5–20 mcg/kg/dose q10–15 min IV infusion : 0.1-0.5 mcg/kg/min Titrate to effect

greater than 10 micrograms per kilogram per minute, beta receptors are stimulated, and there is an increase in heart rate, myocardial contractility, and blood pressure. At the highest doses (20–50 mcg/kg/min), beta activity remains, but increasing alpha stimulation (vasoconstriction) may overcome its actions.

Dopamine is useful in hypovolemic and cardiogenic shock. Adequate fluid therapy is necessary for the maximal pressor effect of dopamine. Acidosis decreases the effectiveness of dopamine.

Epinephrine is a naturally occurring catecholamine produced by the adrenal glands. At low doses, epinephrine stimulates beta receptors, which increases cardiac output by increasing the rate and force of myocardial contractility. It also causes bronchodilation. Larger doses act on alpha receptors to increase blood pressure.

Epinephrine is the drug of choice for management of anaphylactic shock because of its rapid onset of action and antiallergic effects. It prevents the release of histamine and other mediators that cause symptoms of anaphylaxis, thereby reversing vasodilation and bronchoconstriction. In early management of anaphylaxis, it may be given subcutaneously to produce therapeutic effects within 5 to 10 minutes, with peak activity in approximately 20 minutes.

Epinephrine is also used to manage other kinds of shock and is usually given by continuous IV infusion. However, bolus doses may be given in emergencies, such as cardiac arrest. Epinephrine may produce excessive cardiac stimulation, ventricular dysrhythmias, and reduced renal blood flow. Epinephrine has an elimination half-life of about 2 minutes and is rapidly inactivated to metabolites, which are then excreted by the kidneys.

Metaraminol is used mainly for hypotension associated with spinal anesthesia. It acts indirectly by releasing norepinephrine from sympathetic nerve endings. Thus, its vasoconstrictive actions are similar to those of norepinephrine, except that metaraminol is less potent and has a longer duration of action.

Milrinone is discussed in Chapter 48 as a treatment for heart failure. It is also used to manage cardiogenic shock in combination with other inotropic agents or vasopressors. It increases cardiac output and decreases systemic vascular resistance without significantly increasing heart rate or myocardial oxygen consumption. The increased cardiac output improves renal blood flow, which then leads to increased urine output, decreased circulating blood volume, and decreased cardiac workload.

Norepinephrine (Levophed) is a pharmaceutical preparation of the naturally occurring catecholamine norepinephrine. It stimulates alpha-adrenergic receptors and thus increases blood pressure primarily by vasoconstriction. It also stimulates beta$_1$ receptors and therefore increases heart rate, force of myocardial contraction, and coronary artery blood flow. It is useful in cardiogenic and septic shock, but reduced renal blood flow limits its prolonged use. As with all drugs used to manage shock, blood pressure should be monitored frequently during infusion.

Phenylephrine (Neo-Synephrine) is an adrenergic drug that stimulates alpha-adrenergic receptors. As a result, it constricts arterioles and raises systolic and diastolic blood pressures. Phenylephrine resembles epinephrine but has fewer cardiac effects and a longer duration of action. Reduction of renal and mesenteric blood flow limits prolonged use.

Applying Your Knowledge 51-2

The IV infusion of dopamine infiltrates and the physician orders phentolamine to be administered. What is the purpose of this drug?

Nursing Process

Assessment

- Assess the patient's condition in relation to hypotension and shock.
- Check blood pressure; heart rate; urine output; skin temperature and color of extremities; level of consciousness; orientation to person, place, and time; and adequacy of respiration. Abnormal values are not specific indicators of hypotension and shock, but they may indicate a need for further evaluation. In general, report blood pressure less than 90 mm Hg systolic, mean blood pressure greater than 65 mmHg, heart rate greater than 100 beats/minute, and urine output less than 30 mL/hour.
- Assess electrocardiogram and cardiac status for alterations in rhythm or rate.
- Monitor and optimize hemodynamic status noting and acting on indications of impaired cardiac function. Trend mixed venous oxygen saturation (SVO$_2$), stroke index

(SI), cardiac index (CI), pulmonary artery occlusive pressure (PAOP), and central venous pressure (CVP) values for effectiveness of treatments and indications for progress of patient toward goals.

- Monitor available laboratory reports for abnormal values (e.g., decreased oxygen saturation levels indicate decreased oxygenation of tissues; abnormal arterial blood gases may indicate metabolic acidosis; an increased hematocrit may indicate hypovolemia; an increased eosinophil count may indicate anaphylaxis; the presence of bacteria in blood cultures may indicate sepsis; increased serum creatinine and blood urea nitrogen may indicate impending renal failure).

Nursing Diagnoses

- Decreased Cardiac Output related to altered stroke volume
- Ineffective Tissue Perfusion: Decreased related to compromised cardiac output
- Deficient Fluid Volume related to fluid loss or vasodilation
- Anxiety related to potentially life-threatening illness
- Risk for Injury: Myocardial infarction, stroke, or renal damage related to decreased blood flow to vital organs

Planning/Goals

- Improve tissue perfusion and relief of symptoms
- Improve hemodynamic status signs
- Guard against recurrence of hypotension and shock if possible
- Assess for therapeutic and adverse effects of adrenergic drugs
- Avoid preventable adverse effects of adrenergic drugs

Interventions

- Use measures to prevent or minimize hypotension and shock.
- General measures include those to maintain the airway, maintain fluid balance, control hemorrhage, manage infections, prevent hypoxia, and control other causative factors.
- Recognize impending shock so management can be initiated early. Do not wait until symptoms are severe. The earlier the management, the greater the likelihood of reversing shock and preventing end-stage organ damage.
- Recognize and manage the underlying cause of shock in a particular patient (e.g., replacing fluids; preventing further loss of blood or other body fluids).
- Monitor patients during shock and vasopressor drug therapy.
- Titrate adrenergic drug infusions to maintain blood pressure and tissue perfusion without causing hypertension.
- Check hemodynamic indices, including SVO$_2$, SI, CI, PAOP, and CVP, every hour and blood pressure and pulse

constantly or at least every 5 to 15 minutes during acute shock and titration of vasopressor drug therapy. Intra-arterial monitoring is more reliable than cuff blood-pressure measurements in shock conditions.

- Monitor mental status, distal pulses, urine output, and skin temperature and color closely to assess tissue perfusion.

- Administer all vasoactive medications via a central access line. Assess venipuncture sites frequently for signs of infiltration or extravasation. If peripheral sites are present, have phentolamine (Regitine), an alpha-adrenergic blocking agent that reverses vasoconstriction, readily available in any setting where IV adrenergic drugs are used. If infiltration occurs, instill phentolamine through the IV catheter prior to removal. If catheter has been removed, phentolamine may be administered subcutaneously, around the area of extravasation.

- Keep family members informed about patient status and management measures, including drug therapy, monitoring equipment, and the need for close observation of vital signs, IV infusion site, and urine output.

- Provide patient teaching regarding drug therapy.

Evaluation

- Observe for improved hemodynamic status, vital signs, color and temperature of skin, urine output, and mental responsiveness.

Principles of Therapy

Goal of Therapy

The goal of adrenergic drug therapy in hypotension and shock is to restore and maintain adequate tissue perfusion, especially to vital organs.

Drug Selection

The choice of drug depends primarily on the pathophysiology involved. For cardiogenic shock and decreased cardiac output, dobutamine is given. With severe heart failure characterized by decreased cardiac output and high peripheral vascular resistance, vasodilator drugs (e.g., nitroprusside, nitroglycerin) may be given along with the cardiotonic drug. The combination increases cardiac output and decreases cardiac workload by decreasing preload and afterload. However, vasodilators should not be used alone because of the risk of severe hypotension and further compromising tissue perfusion. Milrinone may be given when other drugs fail.

For distributive shock characterized by severe vasodilation and decreased peripheral vascular resistance, a vasopressor drug, such as norepinephrine, is the first drug of choice. Drug dosage must be carefully titrated to avoid excessive vasocon-striction and hypertension, which causes impairment rather than improvement in tissue perfusion.

Guidelines for Management of Hypotension and Shock

The overall goal in the treatment of hypotension and shock is to maximize oxygen delivery to the tissues by maintaining vascular volume and optimal hemoglobin levels. Volume replacement is administered to optimize the SVO_2 (saturation of venous oxygen, thus mixed venous oxygen consumption) yet avoid hypothermia. Depending on the rationale for the volume loss, fluid is administered to reach specific end-points. Crystalloid fluids may consist of normal saline or lactated Ringer's. Colloids consist of albumin, plasma protein fraction, dextran, or hetastarch. Blood and blood products are also colloids but usually have specific indications for administration of these products.

The overall type of shock determines the type of volume replacement. In hypovolemic shock, blood products are administered if hemorrhage is present. If the hypovolemia is pure volume loss, a combination of crystalloids and colloids may be administered. In addition, neurogenic shock is initially treated with crystalloids and colloids. Burn victims are usually treated with crystalloids; sepsis and anaphylaxis patients are usually treated with crystalloids, at least initially. Following the initial fluid resuscitation, medications are administered to produce the desired effect.

Vasopressor drugs are less effective in the presence of inadequate blood volume, electrolyte abnormalities, and acidosis. These conditions also must be treated if present. In addition, normalizing the blood pH and body temperature facilitates the release of oxygen and unloads it from hemoglobin to the cells with a shift of the oxyhemoglobin dissociation curve to the right.

Minimal effective doses of adrenergic drugs are recommended because of the extreme vasoconstrictive effects that can produce lactic acidosis at the cell level and create metabolic acidosis. Because catecholamine drugs have short half-lives, varying the flow rate of IV infusions can easily control dosage. Dosage and flow rates usually are titrated to maintain SVO_2 values. Such titration depends on frequent and accurate measurement of evidence-based parameters.

Cardiogenic shock may be complicated by pulmonary congestion, for which diuretic drugs are indicated and IV fluids are contraindicated (except to maintain a patent IV line). Use of the intra-aortic balloon pump (IABP) may be indicated if the patient is unable to respond with the use of medications. Other support may be ordered (e.g., left ventricular assist device).

Anaphylactic shock is often managed by nonadrenergic drugs as well as epinephrine. For example, the histamine-induced cardiovascular symptoms (e.g., vasodilation and increased capillary permeability) are thought to be mediated through both types of histamine receptors.

Septic shock due to bacterial infection requires appropriate antibiotic therapy in addition to other management measures (see Section 5). If an abscess is the source of infection, it must be surgically drained.

Use in Special Populations

Use in Children

Little information is available about adrenergic drugs for the management of hypotension and shock in children. Children who lose up to one fourth of their circulating blood volume may produce minimal changes in arterial blood pressure and a relatively low heart rate. In general, management is the same as for adults, with drug dosages adjusted for weight.

Use in Older Adults

Older adults often have disorders such as atherosclerosis, peripheral vascular disease, and diabetes mellitus and may not demonstrate common symptoms of volume depletion (e.g., thirst, skin turgor changes). Also, when adrenergic drugs are given, the vasoconstricting effects may decrease blood flow and increase risks of tissue ischemia and thrombosis. Careful monitoring of vital signs, skin color and temperature, urine output, and mental status is essential. In addition, in older adults the contractility of the myocardial protein fibers is altered; thus this age-related phenomenon is considered.

Use in Patients With Renal Impairment

Although adrenergic drugs may be life saving, they can reduce renal blood flow and cause renal failure because of their vasoconstrictive effects. Renal impairment may occur in patients with previously normal renal function and may be worsened in patients whose renal function is already impaired.

Most adrenergic drugs are metabolized in the liver, and the metabolites are excreted in the urine. However, little accumulation of the drugs or metabolites is likely because the drugs have short half-lives.

Use in Patients With Hepatic Impairment

Catecholamine drugs are metabolized by monoamine oxidase (MAO) and catechol-O-methyl transferase (COMT). MAO is widely distributed in most body tissues, whereas COMT is located mainly in the liver. Thus, the drugs are eliminated mainly by liver metabolism and must be used cautiously in patients with impaired liver function. Patients should be monitored closely, and drug dosage should be adjusted as symptoms warrant. However, the half-life of most adrenergic drugs is very brief, and this decreases the chances of drug accumulation in hepatically impaired patients.

Use in Patients With Critical Illness

The adrenergic catecholamines (e.g., dobutamine, dopamine, epinephrine, norepinephrine) are widely used in patients with a low cardiac output that persists despite adequate fluid replacement and correction of electrolyte imbalance.

By improving circulation, the drugs also help to prevent tissue injury from ischemia (e.g., renal failure).

Although the drugs may be used initially in almost any setting, most patients with hypotension and shock are managed in critical care units. Dobutamine is usually the cardiotonic agent of choice in critically ill patients. Dopamine varies in clearance rate in adult and pediatric patients. However, this variance may result from the use of non–steady-state plasma concentrations in calculating the clearance rate. When a dopamine IV infusion is started, it may take 1 to 2 hours to achieve a steady-state plasma level. Relatively large doses of dopamine are given for cardiotonic and vasoconstrictive effects.

Epinephrine and norepinephrine are also widely used in critically ill patients. Recommended infusion rates in critically ill patients vary from 1 to 10 micrograms per minute for epinephrine and from 0.05 to 0.30 micrograms per minute for norepinephrine. All patients receiving drugs for management of hypotension and shock should be closely monitored regarding hemodynamic status, vital signs, drug dosage, relevant laboratory test results, as well as other indicators of clinical status.

Continuous invasive hemodynamic monitoring using a mixed venous oxygen pulmonary artery catheter and an arterial catheter is indicated to titrate drug dosage and monitor response to drug therapy. Close monitoring of the critically ill is essential as these patients often have multiple organ impairments and are clinically unstable.

 Applying Your Knowledge 51-3

How Can You Avoid This Medication Error?
Mr. Alrashed's BP remains below 90 mm Hg and his physician orders norepinephrine to be administered. The nurse retrieves the solution from the medication storage machine and hangs the brownish colored solution.

Evidence-Based Practice

51-1 Polyclonal Intravenous Immunoglobulin Therapy with Sepsis

A meta-analysis was done to evaluate the effect of polyclonal intravenous immunoglobulin therapy on death in critically ill adult patients with sepsis. The main rationale for this treatment for individuals with primary or secondary antibody deficiency (as with sepsis) is antibody substitution. Polyclonal intravenous immunoglobulin therapy was associated with an overall survival benefit (risk ratio, 0.74 [95% CI, 0.62 to 0.89]) compared with placebo or no intervention. A survival benefit was observed for patients with sepsis who received polyclonal intravenous immunoglobulin therapy compared with those who received placebo or no intervention. Substituting polyclonal antibodies could assist the immunocompromised individuals resist the attacks of pathogenic microbes.

Nursing Actions — Drugs Used in Hypotension and Shock

NURSING ACTIONS	RATIONALE/EXPLANATION
1. Administer accurately	
a. Use a large vein for the venipuncture site.	To decrease risk of extravasation
b. Dilute drugs for continuous infusion in 250 or 500 mL of intravenous (IV) fluid. For use of other IV fluids, consult drug manufacturers' literature. Dilute drugs for bolus injections to at least 10 mL with sodium chloride or water for injection.	To avoid adverse effects, which are more likely to occur with concentrated drug solutions
c. Use a dedicated IV line setup.	This allows the adrenergic drug solution to be regulated or discontinued without disruption of other IV lines.
d. Use an infusion pump.	To administer the drug at a consistent rate and prevent alterations in hemodynamic function
e. Discard any solution with a brownish color or precipitate.	Most of the solutions are stable for 24–48 hours. Epinephrine and isoproterenol decompose on exposure to light, producing a brownish discoloration.
f. Start the adrenergic drug slowly, and increase as necessary to obtain desired outcome in hemodynamic function.	Flow rate (dosage) is titrated according to patient response.
g. Stop the drug gradually.	Abrupt discontinuance of pressor drugs may cause rebound hypotension.
h. Manage the patient, not the monitor.	Monitor values and trend parameters before adjusting medication dosage.
2. Observe for therapeutic effects	
a. SVO$_2$ normal is 60–75. SI is 25–45 mL/beat/m^2. CI is 2.5–4.0 L/min/m^2. PAOP is 8–12 mm Hg, CVP is 2–6 mm Hg.	These levels are adequate for tissue perfusion.
b. Mean blood pressure of >65 mm Hg	However, higher levels may be necessary to maintain cerebral blood flow in older adults.
c. Heart rate of 60–100 beats/minute, improved quality of peripheral pulses	These indicate improved tissue perfusion and cardiovascular function.
d. Improved urine output	Increased urine output indicates improved blood flow to the kidneys.
e. Improved skin color and temperature	These indicate improved peripheral tissue perfusion.
f. Pulmonary capillary wedge pressure between 15 and 20 mm Hg in cardiogenic shock	Higher levels are required to maintain cardiac output in cardiogenic shock.
3. Observe for adverse effects	
a. Bradycardia	Reflex bradycardia may occur with norepinephrine, metaraminol, and phenylephrine.
b. Tachycardia	This is more likely to occur with dopamine, but may occur with epinephrine.
c. Dysrhythmias	Serious dysrhythmias may occur with any of the agents used in hypotension and shock. Causes may include high doses that result in excessive adrenergic stimulation of the heart, low doses that result in inadequate perfusion of the myocardium, or the production of lactic acid by ischemic tissue.
d. Hypertension	This is most likely to occur with high doses of norepinephrine, metaraminol, and phenylephrine.
e. Hypotension	This is most likely to occur with lower doses of dopamine due to vasodilation.
f. Angina pectoris—chest pain, dyspnea, palpitations	All pressor agents may increase myocardial oxygen consumption and induce myocardial ischemia.
g. Tissue necrosis if extravasation occurs	This may occur with solutions containing dopamine, norepinephrine, metaraminol, and phenylephrine due to local vasoconstriction and impaired blood supply. Tissue necrosis may be prevented by injecting 5–10 mg of phentolamine (Regitine) through the catheter preferably or subcutaneously around the area of extravasation. Phentolamine is most effective if injected within 12 hours after extravasation.

(continued on page 822)

Nursing Actions   Drugs Used in Hypotension and Shock (continued)

NURSING ACTIONS	RATIONALE/EXPLANATION
4. Observe for drug interactions	
a. Drugs that *increase* effects of pressor agents:	
(1) General anesthetics (e.g., halothane)	Halothane and other halogenated anesthetics increase cardiac sensitivity to sympathomimetic drugs and increase the risks of cardiac dysrhythmias.
(2) Anticholinergic drugs (e.g., atropine)	Atropine and other drugs with anticholinergic activity may potentiate the tachycardia that often occurs with pressor agents.
(3) Monoamine oxidase (MAO) inhibitors (e.g., tranylcypromine)	All effects of exogenously administered adrenergic drugs are magnified in patients taking MAO inhibitors because MAO is the circulating enzyme responsible for metabolism of adrenergic agents.
(4) Oxytocics (e.g., oxytocin)	The risk of severe hypertension is increased.
b. Drugs that *decrease* effects of pressor agents:	
(1) Beta-blocking agents (e.g., propranolol)	Beta-blocking agents antagonize the cardiac stimulation of some pressor agents (e.g., dobutamine). Decreased heart rate, myocardial contractility, and blood pressure may result.

Key Concepts

- Shock is a clinical condition of insufficient perfusion of cells and vital organs, causing tissue hypoxia.

- The overall goal in the treatment of hypotension and shock is to maximize oxygen delivery to the tissues by maintaining vascular volume and optimal hemoglobin levels.

- For all drugs used to manage shock, blood pressure should be monitored frequently during infusion.

- In hypotension and shock, drugs with alpha-adrenergic activity (e.g., norepinephrine, phenylephrine) are used to increase peripheral vascular resistance and raise blood pressure.

- The adrenergic catecholamines (e.g., dobutamine, dopamine, epinephrine, norepinephrine) are widely used in patients with a low cardiac output that persists despite adequate fluid replacement and correction of electrolyte imbalance. Dobutamine is usually the cardiotonic agent of choice in critically ill patients.

Review and Application Exercises

Short Answer Exercises

1. How do adrenergic drugs improve circulation in hypotension and shock?

2. Which adrenergic drug should be readily available for management of anaphylactic shock?

3. What are major adverse effects of adrenergic drugs?

4. How would you assess the patient for therapeutic or adverse effects of an adrenergic drug being given by continuous IV infusion?

5. Why is it important to prevent extravasation of adrenergic drug infusions into tissues surrounding the vein?

6. In hypovolemic shock, should fluid volume be replaced before or after an adrenergic drug is given? Why?

NCLEX-Style Questions

7. During administration of dopamine, a patient complains of pain at the infusion site. The nurse should recognize that the

   a. Patient is hypersensitive to the drug, and infusion should be stopped.

   b. Infusion rate is too fast and should be slowed.

   c. Medication should be stopped, phentolamine should be infused, and the infusion site should be changed.

   d. Medication is probably not effective and therefore patient response should be assessed once all the medication is infused.

8. A patient in cardiogenic shock is started on dobutamine (Dobutrex). The health care provider's order reads dobutamine 10 mcg/kg/min IV. What effect should the nurse expect after beginning drug therapy?
   a. enhanced cardiac contraction and contractility via stimulation of $alpha_1$, $beta_1$, and $beta_2$ receptors
   b. dilated blood vessels via stimulation of dopamine receptors
   c. increased cardiac output through stimulation of $beta_1$ receptors
   d. constricted blood vessels and increased cardiac output through stimulation of $alpha_1$ receptors

9. A patient receiving norepinephrine (Levophed) for shock has an arterial line in place. The patient's blood pressure has been near 90/42 mm Hg for most of the morning. The blood pressure reading on the continuous monitor suddenly shows a blood pressure of 130/80. The nurse should
   a. Decrease the rate of the norepinephrine.
   b. Call the health care provider.
   c. Stop the norepinephrine infusion.
   d. Confirm the blood pressure with a manual reading.

10. A patient who is in anaphylactic shock presents to the emergency department. The nurse should anticipate that the drug of choice for this type of shock would be
   a. dobutamine
   b. dopamine
   c. isoproterenol
   d. epinephrine

Selected References

Deitch, E. A., Livingston, D. H., Lavery, R. F., Monaghan, S. R., Bongu, A., & Machiedo, G. W. (2007). Hormonally active women tolerate shock-trauma better than do men: A prospective study of over 4000 trauma patients. *Annals of Surgery, 246,* 447–455.

Jones, A. E., Focht, A., Horton, J. H., & Kline, J. A. (2007). Prospective external validation of the clinical effectiveness of an emergency department-based early goal-directed therapy protocol for severe sepsis and septic shock. *Chest, 132,* 425–432.

Remick, D. G. (2007). Pathophysiology of sepsis. *American Journal of Pathology, 170,* 1435–1444.

Sahjian, M., & Frakes, M. (2007). Crush injuries: Pathophysiology and current treatment. *The Nurse Practitioner, 32,* 13–18.

Turgeon, A. F., Hutton, B., Fergusson, D. A., McIntyre, L. M., Tinmouth, A. A., Cameron, D. W., & Hébert, P. C. (2007). Meta-analysis: Intravenous immunoglobulin in critically ill adult patients with sepsis. *Annals of Internal Medicine, 146,* 193–203.

LEARNING OBJECTIVES

After studying this chapter, you will be able to:

1. Describe factors that control blood pressure.
2. Define/describe hypertension.
3. Identify patients at risk for development of hypertension and its sequelae.
4. Discuss nonpharmacologic measures to control hypertension.
5. Review the effects of alpha-adrenergic blockers, beta-adrenergic blockers, calcium channel blockers, and diuretics in hypertension.
6. Discuss angiotensin-converting enzyme inhibitors and angiotensin II receptor blockers in terms of mechanisms of action, indications for use, adverse effects, and nursing process implications.
7. Describe the rationale for using combination drugs in the management of hypertension.
8. Discuss interventions to increase therapeutic effects and minimize adverse effects of antihypertensive drugs.
9. Discuss the use of antihypertensive drugs in special populations.

Applying Your Knowledge

Harold Olms is a 55-year-old, African-American man. He is married, has four children, and works as an automobile salesman. Mr. Olms has experienced hypertension for the past 15 years. His current drug regimen to keep his blood pressure at less than 140/90 mm Hg consists of

Valsartan 80 mg PO daily
Amlodipine 10 mg PO daily
Hydrochlorothiazide 12.5 mg PO daily

Introduction

Antihypertensive drugs are used to treat hypertension, a common, chronic disorder affecting an estimated 50 to 60 million adults and an unknown number of children and adolescents in the United States. Hypertension increases risks of myocardial infarction, heart failure, cerebral infarction and hemorrhage, and renal disease. To understand hypertension and antihypertensive drug therapy, it is necessary first to understand the physiologic mechanisms that normally control blood pressure, characteristics of hypertension, and characteristics of antihypertensive drugs.

Regulation of Blood Pressure

Arterial blood pressure reflects the force exerted on arterial walls by blood flow. Blood pressure normally remains constant because of homeostatic mechanisms that adjust blood flow to meet tissue needs. The two major determinants of arterial blood pressure are cardiac output (systolic pressure) and peripheral vascular resistance (diastolic pressure).

Cardiac output equals the product of the heart rate and stroke volume (CO = HR (SV). Stroke volume is the amount of blood ejected with each heartbeat (approximately 60–90 mL). Thus, cardiac output depends on the force of myocardial contraction, blood volume, and other factors. Peripheral vascular resistance is determined by local blood flow and the degree of constriction or dilation in arterioles and arteries (vascular tone).

Autoregulation of Blood Flow

Autoregulation is the ability of body tissues to regulate their own blood flow. Local blood flow is regulated primarily by nutritional needs of the tissue, such as lack of oxygen or accumulation of products of cellular metabolism (e.g., carbon dioxide, lactic acid). Local tissues produce vasodilating and vasoconstricting substances to regulate local blood flow. Important tissue factors include histamine, bradykinin, serotonin, and prostaglandins.

Histamine is found mainly in mast cells surrounding blood vessels and is released when these tissues are injured. In some tissues, such as skeletal muscle, mast cell activity is mediated by the sympathetic nervous system (SNS), and histamine is released when SNS stimulation is blocked or withdrawn. In this case, vasodilation results from increased histamine release and the withdrawal of SNS vasoconstrictor activity. *Bradykinin*

is released from a protein in body fluids. Kinins dilate arterioles, increase capillary permeability, and constrict venules. *Serotonin* is released from aggregating platelets during the blood clotting process. It causes vasoconstriction and plays a major role in control of bleeding. *Prostaglandins* are formed in response to tissue injury and include vasodilators (e.g., prostacyclin) and vasoconstrictors (e.g., thromboxane A_2).

An important component of regulating local blood flow is the production of several vasoactive substances by the endothelial cells that line blood vessels. Vasoconstricting substances, which increase vascular tone and blood pressure, include angiotensin II, endothelin-1, and thromboxane A_2. Vasodilating substances, which decrease vascular tone and blood pressure, include nitric oxide and prostacyclin. Excessive vasoconstrictors or deficient vasodilators may contribute to the development of atherosclerosis, hypertension, and other diseases. Injury to the endothelial lining of blood vessels (e.g., by the shear force of blood flow with hypertension, by rupture of atherosclerotic plaque) leads to vasoconstriction, vasospasm, thrombus formation, and thickening of the blood vessel wall. All of these factors narrow the blood vessel lumen and increase peripheral vascular resistance.

Overall, regulation of blood pressure involves a complex, interacting, overlapping network of hormonal, neural, and vascular mechanisms, and any condition that affects heart rate, stroke volume, or peripheral vascular resistance affects arterial blood pressure. Many of these mechanisms are compensatory effects that attempt to restore balance when hypotension or hypertension occurs. The mechanisms are further described in Box 52-1 and are referred to in the following discussion of antihypertensive drugs and their actions in lowering high blood pressure.

Box 52-1	Mechanisms That Regulate Blood Pressure

Neural

Neural regulation of blood pressure mainly involves the sympathetic nervous system (SNS). In the heart, SNS neurons control heart rate and force of contraction. In blood vessels, SNS neurons control muscle tone by maintaining a state of partial contraction, with additional constriction or dilation accomplished by altering this basal state. When hypotension and inadequate tissue perfusion occur, the SNS is activated and produces secretion of epinephrine and norepinephrine by the adrenal medulla; constriction of blood vessels in the skin, gastrointestinal tract, and kidneys; and stimulation of beta-adrenergic receptors in the heart, which increases heart rate and force of myocardial contraction. All of these mechanisms act to increase blood pressure and tissue perfusion, especially of the brain and heart.

The SNS is activated by the vasomotor center in the brain, which constantly receives messages from baroreceptors and chemoreceptors located in the circulatory system. Adequate function of these receptors is essential for rapid and short-term

regulation of blood pressure. The vasomotor center interprets the messages from these receptors and modifies cardiovascular functions to maintain adequate blood flow.

More specifically, baroreceptors detect changes in pressure or stretch. For example, when a person moves from a lying to a standing position, blood pressure falls and decreases stretch in the aorta and arteries. This elicits increased heart rate and vasoconstriction to restore adequate circulation. The increased heart rate occurs rapidly and blood pressure is adjusted within 1 to 2 minutes. This quick response prevents orthostatic hypotension with dizziness and possible syncope. (Antihypertensive medications may blunt this response and cause orthostatic hypotension.)

Chemoreceptors, which are located in the aorta and carotid arteries, are in close contact with arterial blood and respond to changes in the oxygen, carbon dioxide, and hydrogen ion content of blood. Although their main function is to regulate ventilation, they also communicate with the vasomotor center and can induce vasoconstriction. Chemoreceptors are

(continued on page 826)

| Box 52-1 | Mechanisms That Regulate Blood Pressure (continued) |

stimulated when blood pressure drops to a certain point because oxygen is decreased and carbon dioxide and hydrogen ions are increased in arterial blood.

The central nervous system (CNS) also regulates vasomotor tone and blood pressure. Inadequate blood flow to the brain results in ischemia of the vasomotor center. When this occurs, neurons in the vasomotor center stimulate widespread vasoconstriction in an attempt to raise blood pressure and restore blood flow. This reaction, the CNS ischemic response, is an emergency measure to preserve blood flow to vital brain centers. If blood flow is not restored within 3 to 10 minutes, the neurons of the vasomotor center are unable to function, the impulses that maintain vascular muscle tone stop, and blood pressure drops to a fatal level.

Hormonal

The renin–angiotensin–aldosterone (RAA) system and vasopressin are important hormonal mechanisms in blood pressure regulation.

The *RAA system* is activated in response to hypotension and acts as a compensatory mechanism to restore adequate blood flow to body tissues. Renin is an enzyme that is synthesized, stored, and released from the kidneys in response to decreased blood pressure, SNS stimulation, or decreased sodium concentration in extracellular fluid. When released into the bloodstream, where its action lasts 30 to 60 minutes, renin converts angiotensinogen (a plasma protein) to angiotensin I. Angiotensin-converting enzyme (ACE) in the endothelium of pulmonary blood vessels then acts on angiotensin I to produce angiotensin II. Angiotensin II strongly constricts arterioles (and weakly constricts veins), increases peripheral resistance, and increases blood pressure by direct vasoconstriction, stimulation of the SNS, and stimulation of catecholamine release from the adrenal medulla. It also stimulates secretion of aldosterone from the adrenal cortex, which then causes the kidneys to retain sodium and water. Retention of sodium and water increases blood volume, cardiac output, and blood pressure.

Vasopressin, also called antidiuretic hormone or ADH, is a hormone secreted by the posterior pituitary gland that regulates reabsorption of water by the kidneys. It is released in response to decreased blood volume and decreased blood pressure. It causes retention of body fluids and vasoconstriction, both of which act to raise blood pressure.

Vascular

The endothelial cells that line blood vessels synthesize and secrete several substances that play important roles in regulating cardiovascular functions, including blood pressure. These substances normally maintain a balance between vasoconstriction and vasodilation. When the endothelium is damaged (e.g., by trauma, hypertension, hypercholesterolemia, or atherosclerosis), the resulting imbalance promotes production of vasoconstricting substances and also causes blood vessels to lose their ability to relax in response to dilator substances. In addition, changes in structure of endothelial and vascular smooth muscle cells (vascular remodeling) further impair vascular functions.

Vasoconstrictors increase vascular tone (i.e., constrict or narrow blood vessels so that higher blood pressure is required to pump blood to body tissues). Vasoconstricting substances produced by the endothelium include angiotensin II, endothelin-1, platelet-derived growth factor (PDGF), and thromboxane A_2. Endothelin-1 is the strongest endogenous vasoconstrictor known. Angiotensin II and thromboxane A_2 can also be produced by other types of cells, but endothelial cells can produce both. Thromboxane A_2, a product of arachidonic acid metabolism, also promotes platelet aggregation and thrombosis.

Vasodilators decrease vascular tone and blood pressure. Major vasodilating substances produced by the endothelium include nitric oxide and prostacyclin (prostaglandin I2)

Nitric oxide (NO) is a gas that can diffuse through cell membranes, trigger biochemical reactions, and then dissipate rapidly. It is formed by the action of the enzyme NO synthase on the amino acid l-arginine and continually released by normal endothelium. Its production is tightly regulated and depends on the amount of ionized calcium in the fluid portion of endothelial cells. Several substances (e.g., acetylcholine, bradykinin, catecholamines, substance P, and products of aggregating platelets such as adenosine diphosphate and serotonin) act on receptors in endothelial cell membranes to increase the cytosolic concentration of ionized calcium, activate NO synthase, and increase NO production. In addition, increased blood flow or blood pressure increases shear stress at the endothelial surface and stimulates production of NO.

Once produced, endothelium-derived NO produces vasodilation primarily by activating guanylyl cyclase in vascular smooth muscle cells and increasing intracellular cyclic 3,5′-guanosine monophosphate as a second messenger. NO also inhibits platelet aggregation and production of platelet-derived vasoconstricting substances. Because NO is released into the vessel wall (to relax smooth muscle) and into the vessel lumen (to inactivate platelets), it is thought to have protective effects against vasoconstriction and thrombosis.

NO is also produced in leukocytes, fibroblasts, and vascular smooth muscle cells and may have pathologic effects when large amounts are produced. In these tissues, NO seems to have other functions, such as modifying nerve activity in the nervous system.

Prostacyclin is synthesized and released from endothelium in response to stimulation by several factors (e.g., bradykinin, interleukin-1, serotonin, thrombin, PDGF). It produces vasodilation by activating adenylyl cyclase and increasing levels of cyclic adenosine monophosphate in smooth muscle cells. In addition, like NO, prostacyclin also inhibits platelet aggregation and production of platelet-derived vasoconstricting substances. The vasodilating effects of prostacyclin may occur independently or in conjunction with NO.

Overall, excessive vasoconstrictors or deficient vasodilators may contribute to the development of atherosclerosis, hypertension, and other diseases. Injury to the endothelial lining of blood vessels (e.g., by the shear force of blood flow with hypertension or by rupture of atherosclerotic plaque) decreases vasodilators and leads to vasoconstriction, vasospasm, thrombus formation, and thickening of the blood vessel wall. All of these factors require the blood to flow through a narrowed lumen and increase blood pressure.

Vascular Remodeling

Vascular remodeling is similar to the left ventricular remodeling that occurs in heart failure (see Chap. 48). It results from endothelial dysfunction and produces a thickening of the blood vessel wall and a narrowing of the blood vessel lumen. Thickening of the wall makes blood vessels less flexible and less able to respond to vasodilating substances. There are also changes in endothelial cell structure (i.e., the connections between endothelial cells become looser) that lead to increased permeability. The mechanisms of these vascular changes, which promote and aggravate hypertension, are described below.

As discussed in previous chapters, normal endothelium helps maintain a balance between vasoconstriction and vasodilation, procoagulation and anticoagulation, proinflammation and antiinflammation, and progrowth and antigrowth. In the inflammatory process, normal endothelium acts as a physical barrier against the movement of leukocytes into the subendothelial space. Endothelial products such as nitric oxide may also inhibit leukocyte activity. However, inflammatory cytokines such as tumor necrosis factor–alpha and interleukin-1 activate endothelial cells to produce adhesion molecules (which allow leukocytes to adhere to the endothelium), interleukin-8 (which attracts leukocytes to the endothelium and allows them to accumulate in subendothelial cells), and foam cells (lipid-filled monocyte/macrophages that form fatty streaks, the beginning lesions of atherosclerotic plaque). Although activation of endothelial cells may be a helpful component of the normal immune response, the resulting inflammation may contribute to disease development.

In terms of cell growth, normal endothelium limits the growth of vascular smooth muscle that underlies the endothelium and forms the vessel wall. Growth-inhibiting products of the endothelium include nitric oxide, which also inhibits platelet activation and production of growth-promoting substances. When the endothelium is damaged, endothelial cells become activated and also produce growth-promoting products. Other endothelial products (e.g., angiotensin II and endothelin-1) may also stimulate growth of vascular smooth muscle cells. Thus, damage or loss of endothelial cells stimulates growth of smooth muscle cells in the intimal layer of the blood vessel wall.

Response to Hypotension

When hypotension (and decreased tissue perfusion) occurs, the SNS is stimulated, the hormones epinephrine and norepinephrine are secreted by the adrenal medulla, angiotensin II and aldosterone are formed, and the kidneys retain fluid. These compensatory mechanisms raise the blood pressure. Specific effects include the following:

- Constriction of arterioles, which increases peripheral vascular resistance

- Constriction of veins and increased venous tone

- Stimulation of cardiac beta-adrenergic receptors, which increases heart rate and force of myocardial contraction

- Activation of the renin–angiotensin–aldosterone mechanism

Response to Hypertension

When arterial blood pressure is elevated, the following sequence of events occurs:

- Kidneys excrete more fluid (increase urine output).

- Fluid loss reduces both extracellular fluid volume and blood volume.

- Decreased blood volume reduces venous blood flow to the heart and therefore decreases cardiac output.

- Decreased cardiac output reduces arterial blood pressure.

- The vascular endothelium produces vasodilating substances (e.g., nitric oxide, prostacyclin), which reduce blood pressure.

Hypertension

Hypertension is persistently high blood pressure that results from abnormalities in regulatory mechanisms. It is usually defined as a systolic pressure above 140 mm Hg or a diastolic pressure above 90 mm Hg on multiple blood pressure measurements.

Primary or essential hypertension (that for which no cause can be found) makes up 90% to 95% of known cases. Secondary hypertension may result from renal, endocrine, or central nervous system disorders and from drugs that stimulate the SNS or cause retention of sodium and water. Primary hypertension can be controlled with appropriate therapy; secondary hypertension can sometimes be cured by surgical therapy.

The Seventh Report of the Joint National Committee on Prevention, Detection, Evaluation, and Treatment of High Blood Pressure (JNC 7), guidelines published in 2003, classified blood pressures in adults (in mm Hg) as follows:

- Normal = systolic < 120 <u>and</u> diastolic < 80

- Prehypertension = systolic 120–139 <u>or</u> diastolic 80–89

- Stage 1 hypertension = systolic 140–159 <u>or</u> diastolic 90–99

- Stage 2 hypertension = systolic >160 <u>or</u> diastolic 100 or more

This classification is markedly different from the four stages previously defined. The addition of a prehypertension stage targets individuals who are twice as likely to progress to hypertension as those with lower pressure values. Stages 3 and 4 have been eliminated. These newer guidelines also recommend a goal blood pressure for those with diabetes or renal disease of less than 130/80 mm Hg. A systolic pressure of 140 or above, with a diastolic pressure below 90, is called isolated systolic hypertension and is more common in the elderly. New JNC8 guidelines are expected to be released in 2009.

Hypertension profoundly alters cardiovascular function by increasing the workload of the heart and causing thickening and sclerosis of arterial walls. As a result of increased cardiac workload, the myocardium hypertrophies as a compensatory mechanism and heart failure eventually occurs. As a result of endothelial dysfunction and arterial changes (vascular remodeling), the arterial lumen is narrowed, blood supply to tissues is decreased, and risks of thrombosis are increased. In addition, necrotic areas may develop in arteries, and these may rupture with sustained high blood pressure. The areas of most serious damage are the heart, brain, kidneys, and eyes. These are often called target organs.

Initially and perhaps for years, primary hypertension may produce no symptoms. If symptoms occur, they are usually vague and nonspecific. Hypertension may go undetected, or it may be incidentally discovered when blood pressure measurements are taken as part of a routine physical examination, screening test, or assessment of other disorders. Eventually, symptoms reflect target organ damage. Hypertension is often discovered after a person experiences angina pectoris, myocardial infarction, heart failure, stroke, or renal disease.

Hypertensive emergencies are episodes of severely elevated blood pressure that may be an extension of malignant (rapidly progressive) hypertension or caused by cerebral hemorrhage, dissecting aortic aneurysm, renal disease, pheochromocytoma, or eclampsia. These require immediate management, usually with intravenous (IV) antihypertensive drugs, to lower blood pressure. Symptoms include severe headache, nausea, vomiting, visual disturbances, neurologic disturbances, disorientation, and decreased level of consciousness (drowsiness, stupor, coma). Hypertensive emergencies require immediate blood pressure reduction with parenteral antihypertensive drugs to limit damage to target organs. Hypertensive urgencies are episodes of marked elevation in blood pressure without target organ damage and are often managed with oral drugs. The goal of management is to lower blood pressure within 24 hours. In most instances, it is better to lower blood pressure gradually and to avoid wide fluctuations in blood pressure.

Antihypertensives: Classifications and Individual Drugs

Drugs used in the management of primary hypertension belong to several different groups, including *angiotensin-converting enzyme* (ACE) *inhibitors*; *angiotensin II receptor blockers* (ARBs), also called angiotensin II receptor antagonists (AIIRAs); *antiadrenergics*; calcium channel blockers; *diuretics*; and direct *vasodilators*. In general, these drugs act to decrease blood pressure by decreasing cardiac output or peripheral vascular resistance.

Antihypertensive agents are shown in Table 52-1; antihypertensive–diuretic combination products are listed in Table 52-2. Adult dosages are based on product labeling and JNC 7 recommendations. Pediatric dosages are based on product labeling and recommendations from the National High Blood Pressure Education Program Working Group on High Blood Pressure in Children and Adolescents (2004).

Angiotensin-Converting Enzyme Inhibitors

Angiotensin-converting enzyme (also called kininase) is mainly located in the endothelial lining of blood vessels, which is the site of production of most angiotensin II. This same enzyme also metabolizes bradykinin, an endogenous substance with strong vasodilating properties.

ACE inhibitors block the enzyme that normally converts angiotensin I to the potent vasoconstrictor angiotensin II. By blocking production of angiotensin II, the drugs decrease vasoconstriction (having a vasodilating effect) and decrease aldosterone production (reducing retention of sodium and water). In addition to inhibiting formation of angiotensin II, the drugs also inhibit the breakdown of bradykinin, prolonging its vasodilating effects. These effects and possibly others help to prevent or reverse the remodeling of heart muscle and blood vessel walls that impairs cardiovascular function and exacerbates cardiovascular disease processes. Because of their effectiveness in hypertension and beneficial effects on the heart, blood vessels, and kidneys, these drugs are increasing in importance and use. Widely used to treat heart failure and hypertension, the drugs may also decrease morbidity and mortality in other cardiovascular disorders. They improve post–myocardial infarction survival when added to the standard therapy of aspirin, a beta blocker, and a thrombolytic.

ACE inhibitors may be used alone or in combination with other antihypertensive agents, such as thiazide diuretics. Although the drugs can cause or aggravate proteinuria and renal damage in nondiabetic people, they decrease proteinuria and slow the development of nephropathy in diabetic patients.

Most ACE inhibitors (captopril, enalapril, fosinopril, lisinopril, ramipril, and quinapril) also are used in the management of heart failure because they decrease peripheral vascular resistance, cardiac workload, and ventricular remodeling. **P Captopril** and other ACE inhibitors are recommended as first-line agents for treating hypertension in diabetic patients, particularly those with type 1 diabetes and/or diabetic nephropathy, because they reduce proteinuria and slow progression of renal impairment.

ACE inhibitors are well absorbed with oral administration, produce effects within 1 hour that last approximately 24 hours, have prolonged serum half-lives with impaired renal function, and most are metabolized to active metabolites that are excreted in urine and feces. These drugs are well tolerated, with a low incidence of serious adverse effects (e.g., neutropenia, agranulocytosis, proteinuria, glomerulonephritis, angioedema).

Table 52-1	Drugs at a Glance: Antihypertensive Drugs	

	ROUTES AND DOSAGE RANGES	
Generic/Trade Name	**Adults**	**Children 1–17 Years of Age (Unless Otherwise Stated)**
Angiotensin-Converting Enzyme (ACE) Inhibitors		
Benazepril (Lotensin)	PO 10 mg once daily initially, increased to 40 mg daily if necessary, in 1 or 2 doses	
P **Captopril** (Capoten)	PO 25 mg, 2 to 3 times daily initially, gradually increased to 50, 100, or 150 mg 2 to 3 times daily, if necessary; maximum dose, 450 mg/d	PO 1.5 mg/kg/d in divided doses, q8h; maximum dose, 6 mg/kg/d Neonates: PO 0.03–0.15 mg/kg/d, q8–24h; maximum dose, 2 mg/kg/d
Enalapril (Vasotec)	PO 5 mg once daily, increased to 10–40 mg daily, in 1 or 2 doses, if necessary	PO 0.15 mg q12–24h
Fosinopril (Monopril)	PO 10 mg once daily initially, increased to 40 mg daily if necessary in 1 or 2 doses	
Lisinopril (Prinivil, Zestril)	PO 10 mg once daily, increased to 40 mg if necessary	
Moexipril (Univasc)	PO initial dose 7.5 mg (3.75 mg for those who have renal impairment or are taking a diuretic). Maintenance dose, 7.5–30 mg daily, in 1 or 2 doses, adjusted according to blood-pressure control	
Perindopril (Aceon)	PO 4–16 mg daily, in 1 or 2 doses	
Quinapril (Accupril)	PO 10 mg once daily initially, increased to 20, 40, or 80 mg daily if necessary, in 1 or 2 doses. Wait at least 2 wk between dose increments.	
Ramipril (Altace)	PO 2.5 mg once daily, increased to 20 mg daily if necessary, in 1 or 2 doses	
Trandolapril (Mavik)	PO initial dose 1 mg once daily (0.5 mg for those who have hepatic or renal impairment or are taking a diuretic; 2 mg for African Americans). Maintenance dose, 2–4 mg daily, in a single dose, adjusted according to blood-pressure control	
Angiotensin II Receptor Blockers		
Candesartan (Atacand)	PO 16 mg once daily initially, increased if necessary to a maximum of 32 mg daily, in 1 or 2 doses	
Irbesartan (Avapro)	PO 150 mg once daily initially, increased up to 300 mg once daily, if necessary	
Losartan (Cozaar)	PO 50 mg once daily initially (25 mg for those who have hepatic impairment or are taking a diuretic). Maintenance dose, 35–100 mg daily, in 1 or 2 doses, adjusted according to blood-pressure control	
Olmesartan (Benicar)	PO 20 mg once daily initially, increased to 40 mg after 2 wk	
Telmisartan (Micardis)	PO 40 mg once daily initially, increased to a maximum of 80 mg daily if necessary	

(continued on page 830)

Table 52-1	Drugs at a Glance: Antihypertensive Drugs (continued)	

	ROUTES AND DOSAGE RANGES	
Generic/Trade Name	**Adults**	**Children 1–17 Years of Age (Unless Otherwise Stated)**
Valsartan (Diovan)	PO 80 mg once daily initially, when used as monotherapy in clients who are not volume depleted. Maintenance dose may be increased. However, adding a diuretic is more effective than increasing dose beyond 80 mg.	
Antiadrenergic Agents **Alpha₁-adrenergic Blocking Agents**		
Doxazosin (Cardura)	PO 1 mg once daily initially, increased to 2 mg, then to 4, 8, and 16 mg daily if necessary	
Prazosin (Minipress)	PO 1 mg 2 to 3 times daily initially, increased if necessary to 20 mg in divided doses. Average maintenance dose, 6–15 mg daily	
Terazosin (Hytrin)	PO 1 mg at bedtime initially, may be increased gradually. Usual maintenance dose, 1–5 mg once daily	
Alpha₂ Agonists		
Clonidine (Catapres)	PO 0.1 mg 2 times daily initially, gradually increased up to 2.4 mg daily, if necessary. Average maintenance dose, 0.2–0.8 mg daily	PO 5–25 mcg/kg/d, in divided doses, q6h; increase at 5- to 7-day intervals, if needed
Guanfacine (Tenex)	PO 1 mg daily at bedtime, increased to 2 mg after 3–4 wk, then to 3 mg if necessary	
Methyldopa	PO 250 mg 2 or 3 times daily initially, increased gradually until blood pressure is controlled or a daily dose of 3 g is reached	PO 10 mg/kg/d in 2 to 4 divided doses initially, increased or decreased according to response. Maximum dose, 65 mg/kg/d or 3 g daily, whichever is less
Beta-Adrenergic Blocking Agents		
Acebutolol (Sectral)	PO 400 mg once daily initially, increased to 800 mg daily if necessary	
Atenolol (Tenormin)	PO 50 mg once daily initially, increased in 1–2 wk to 100 mg once daily, if necessary	
Bisoprolol (Zebeta)	PO 5 mg once daily, increased to a maximum of 20 mg daily if necessary	
Metoprolol (Lopressor)	PO 50 mg twice daily, gradually increased in weekly or longer intervals if necessary. Maximum dose, 450 mg daily	
Nadolol (Corgard)	PO 40 mg once daily initially, gradually increased if necessary. Average dose, 80–320 mg daily	
Pindolol (Visken)	PO 5 mg 2 or 3 times daily initially, increased by 10 mg/d at 3- to 4-wk intervals to a maximum of 60 mg daily	
Propranolol (Inderal)	PO 40 mg twice daily initially, gradually increased to 160–640 mg daily	PO 1 mg/kg/d initially, gradually increased to a maximum of 10 mg/kg/d
Timolol (Blocadren)	PO 10 mg twice daily initially, increased gradually if necessary. Average daily dose, 20–40 mg; maximal daily dose, 60 mg	

ROUTES AND DOSAGE RANGES

Generic/Trade Name	Adults	Children 1–17 Years of Age (Unless Otherwise Stated)
Alpha–Beta-Adrenergic Blocking Agents		
Carvedilol (Coreg)	PO 6.25 mg twice daily for 7–14 days, then increase to 12.5 mg twice daily for 7–14 days, then increase to a maximal dose of 25 mg twice daily if tolerated and needed	
Labetalol (Trandate, Normodyne)	PO 100 mg twice daily, increased by 100 mg twice daily every 2–3 days if necessary. Usual maintenance dose, 200–400 mg twice daily. Severe hypertension may require 1200–2400 mg daily.	
	IV injection, 20 mg slowly over 2 min, followed by 40–80 mg every 10 min until the desired blood pressure is achieved or 300 mg has been given	
	IV infusion, add 200 mg to 250 mL of 5% dextrose or 0.9% sodium chloride solution and infuse at a rate of 2 mg/min. Adjust flow rate according to blood pressure, and substitute oral labetalol when blood pressure is controlled.	
Calcium Channel Blocking Agents		
Amlodipine (Norvasc)	PO 5–10 mg once daily	
Diltiazem (sustained release) (Cardizem SR)	PO 60–120 mg twice daily. Extended-release tablets; swallow whole, do not crush or chew.	
Felodipine (Plendil)	PO 5–10 mg once daily. Extended-release tablets; swallow whole, do not crush or chew.	
Isradipine (DynaCirc)	PO 2.5–5 mg twice daily	
Nicardipine (Cardene, Cardene SR, Cardene IV)	PO 20–40 mg three times daily	
	Sustained-release, PO 30–60 mg twice daily; IV infusion 5–15 mg/h	
Nifedipine (Adalat, Procardia, Procardia XL)	Sustained-release only, PO 30–60 mg once daily, increased over 1–2 wk if necessary	
Nisoldipine (Sular)	PO, 20 mg once daily initially, increased by 10 mg/wk or longer intervals to a maximum of 60 mg daily. Average maintenance dose, 20–40 mg daily	
	Adults with liver impairment or >65 y, PO, 10 mg once daily initially	
Verapamil (Calan, Calan SR, Isoptin SR)	Immediate-release, PO 80 mg 3 times daily	IV, see manufacturer's instructions
	Sustained-release, PO 240 mg once daily	
	IV, see manufacturer's instructions	
Other Vasodilators		
Fenoldopam (Corlopam)	IV infusion, initial dose based on body weight, then flow rate titrated to achieve desired response. Mix with 0.9% sodium chloride or 5% dextrose to a concentration of 40 mcg/mL (e.g., 40 mg of drug [4 mL of concentrate] in 1000 mL of IV fluid).	

(continued on page 832)

Table 52-1	Drugs at a Glance: Antihypertensive Drugs (continued)	

	ROUTES AND DOSAGE RANGES	
Generic/Trade Name	**Adults**	**Children 1–17 Years of Age (Unless Otherwise Stated)**
Hydralazine (Apresoline)	Chronic hypertension, PO 10 mg 4 times daily for 2–4 d, gradually increased up to 300 mg/d, if necessary	Chronic hypertension, 0.75 mg/kg/d initially in 4 divided doses. Gradually increase over 3–4 wk to a maximal dose of 7.5 mg/kg/d if necessary.
	Hypertensive crisis, IM, IV 10–20 mg, increased to 40 mg if necessary. Repeat dose as needed.	Hypertensive crisis, IM, IV 0.1–0.2 mg/kg every 4–6 h as needed
Minoxidil (Loniten)	PO 5 mg once daily initially, increased gradually until blood pressure is controlled. Average daily dose, 10–40 mg; maximal daily dose, 100 mg in single or divided doses	<12 y, PO 0.2 mg/kg/d initially as a single dose, increased gradually until blood pressure is controlled. Average daily dose, 0.25–1.0 mg/kg; maximal dose, 50 mg/d
Sodium nitroprusside (Nipress)	IV infusion 0.5–10 mcg/kg/min; average dose, 3 mcg/kg/min. Prepare solution by adding 50 mg of sodium nitroprusside to 250–1000 mL of 5% dextrose in water, and cover promptly to protect from light.	Same as for adults

However, a persistent cough develops in approximately 10% to 20% of patients and may lead to stopping the drug. Also, acute hypotension may occur when an ACE inhibitor is started, especially in patients with fluid volume deficit. This reaction may be prevented by starting with a low dose taken at bedtime or by stopping diuretics and reducing dosage of other antihypertensive drugs temporarily. Hyperkalemia may develop in patients who have diabetes mellitus or renal impairment or who are taking nonsteroidal anti-inflammatory drugs, potassium supplements, or potassium-sparing diuretics.

These drugs are contraindicated during pregnancy and should be discontinued when pregnancy is recognized. The U.S. Food and Drug Administration (FDA) has issued a **BLACK BOX WARNING** during pregnancy for drugs that directly affect the renin-angiotensin system as their use can cause injury and even death to a developing fetus.

Angiotensin II Receptor Blockers

Angiotensin II receptor blockers (ARBs) were developed to block the strong blood pressure–raising effects of angiotensin II. Instead of decreasing production of angiotensin II, as the ACE inhibitors do, these drugs compete with angiotensin II for tissue binding sites and prevent angiotensin II from combining with its receptors in body tissues. Although multiple types of receptors have been identified, the AT1 receptors located in brain, renal, myocardial, vascular, and adrenal tissue determine most of the effects of angiotensin II on cardiovascular and renal functions. ARBs block the angiotensin II AT1 receptors and decrease arterial blood pressure by decreasing systemic vascular resistance (Fig. 52-1).

These drugs are similar to ACE inhibitors in their effects on blood pressure and hemodynamics and are as effective as ACE inhibitors in the management of hypertension and probably heart failure. They are less likely to cause hyperkalemia than ACE inhibitors, and the occurrence of a persistent cough is rare. Overall, the drugs are well tolerated, and the incidence of most adverse effects is similar to that of placebo. However, the FDA has issued a **BLACK BOX WARNING** during pregnancy for drugs that directly affect the renin-angiotensin system as their use can cause injury and even death to a developing fetus.

P Losartan, the first ARB, is readily absorbed and rapidly metabolized by the cytochrome P450 liver enzymes to an active metabolite. Both losartan and the metabolite are highly bound to plasma albumin, and losartan has a shorter duration of action than its metabolite. When losartan therapy is started, maximal effects on blood pressure usually occur within 3 to 6 weeks. If losartan alone does not control blood pressure, a low dose of a diuretic may be added. A combination product of losartan and hydrochlorothiazide is available.

Antiadrenergics

Antiadrenergic (sympatholytic) drugs inhibit activity of the SNS. When the SNS is stimulated (see Chap. 16), the nerve impulse travels from the brain and spinal cord to the ganglia. From the ganglia, the impulse travels along postganglionic fibers to effector organs (e.g., heart, blood vessels). Although SNS stimulation produces widespread effects in the body, the effects relevant to this discussion are the increases in heart rate, force of myocardial contraction, cardiac output, and blood pressure that occur. When the nerve impulse is inhibited or blocked at any location along its pathway, the result is decreased blood pressure (see Chap. 18).

Alpha$_1$-adrenergic receptor blocking agents (e.g., *prazosin*) dilate blood vessels and decrease peripheral vascular

Table 52-2 — Drugs at a Glance: Oral Antihypertensive Combination Products*

			COMPONENTS			
Trade Name	Angiotensin II Receptor Blocker	Angiotensin-Converting Enzyme Inhibitor	Beta Blocker	Calcium channel Blocker	Diuretic	Non–Beta-Blocker Antiadrenergic	Dosage Ranges
Avalide	Irbesartan 150 or 300 mg				HCTZ 12.5 mg		1 tablet once daily
Capozide		Captopril 25 or 50 mg			HCTZ 15 or 25 mg		1 tablet 2 to 3 times daily
Corzide			Nadolol 40 or 80 mg		Bendroflume-thiazide 5 mg		1 tablet daily
Diovan HCT	Valsartan 80 or 160 mg				HCTZ 12.5 mg		1 tablet daily
Hyzaar	Losartan 50 mg				HCTZ 12.5 mg		1 tablet once daily
Inderide			Propranolol 40 or 80 mg		HCTZ 25 mg		1–2 tablets twice daily
Lexxel		Enalapril 5 mg		Felodipine 5 mg			1–2 tablets once daily
Lopressor HCT			Metoprolol 50 or 100 mg		HCTZ 25 or 50 mg		1–2 tablets daily
Lotensin HCT		Benazepril 5, 10, or 20 mg			HCTZ 12.5 or 25 mg		1 tablet daily
Lotrel		Benazepril 10 or 20 mg		Amlodipine 2.5 or 5 mg			1 capsule daily
Minizide					Polythiazide 0.5 mg	Prazosin 1, 2, or 5 mg	1 capsule 2 to 3 times daily
Prinzide		Lisinopril 20 mg			HCTZ 12.5 or 25 mg		1 tablet daily
Tarka		Trandolapril 1, 2, or 4 mg		Verapamil 180 or 240 mg			1 tablet daily
Tenoretic			100 mg		Chlorthalidone 25 mg		1 tablet daily
Vaseretic		Enalapril 5 mg			HCTZ 12.5 mg		1–2 tablets daily
Zestoretic		Lisinopril 10 or 20 mg	Timolol 10 mg		HCTZ 12.5 or 25 mg		1 tablet daily
Ziac		Bisoprolol 2.5, 5, or 10 mg			HCTZ 6.25 mg		1 tablet daily

*Note that one trade-name product may be available in multiple formulations, with variable amounts of antihypertensive, diuretic, or both components.
HCTZ, hydrochlorothiazide.

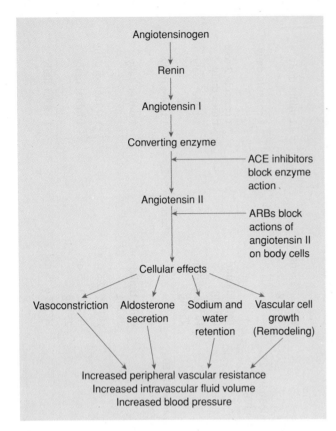

Figure 52-1 ■ Angiotensin-converting enzyme (ACE) inhibitors inhibit angiotensin-converting enzyme and thereby prevent formation of angiotensin II. Angiotensin II receptor blockers (ARBs) prevent angiotensin II from connecting with its receptors and thereby prevent it from acting on body tissues containing those receptors (e.g., blood vessels, adrenal cortex).

resistance. These drugs can be used alone or in multidrug regimens. One adverse effect, called the *first-dose phenomenon*, results in orthostatic hypotension with palpitations, dizziness, and perhaps syncope 1 to 3 hours after the first dose or an increased dose. To prevent this effect, first doses and first increased doses are taken at bedtime. Another effect, associated with long-term use or higher doses, leads to sodium and fluid retention and a need for concurrent diuretic therapy. Centrally acting sympatholytics (e.g., *clonidine*) stimulate presynaptic alpha$_2$ receptors in the brain and are classified as alpha$_2$ receptor agonists. When these drugs are taken, less norepinephrine is released and sympathetic outflow from the vasomotor center is reduced. Stimulation of presynaptic alpha$_2$ receptors peripherally may also contribute to the decreased sympathetic activity. Reduced sympathetic activity leads to decreased cardiac output, heart rate, peripheral vascular resistance, and blood pressure. Chronic use of clonidine and related drugs may result in sodium and fluid retention, especially with higher doses.

Beta-adrenergic blocking agents (e.g., *propranolol*) decrease heart rate, force of myocardial contraction, cardiac output, and renin release from the kidneys. The FDA has

issued a **BLACK BOX WARNING** for in patients with CAD withdrawing from oral forms of atenolol, metoprolol, nadolol, propranolol, and timolol; abrupt withdrawal has resulted in exacerbation of angina, the incidence of ventricular dysrhythmias and the occurrence of MIs.

Other antiadrenergics include alpha blockers (*phentolamine* and *phenoxybenzamine*), which occasionally are used in hypertension resulting from catecholamine excess. Individual antiadrenergic drugs are discussed in Chapter 18 and listed in Tables 18-1 and 18-2.

Calcium Channel Blocking Agents

Calcium channel blockers (e.g., *verapamil*) are used for several cardiovascular disorders. The mechanism of action and use in the management of tachydysrhythmias and angina pectoris are discussed in Chapters 49 and 50, respectively. In hypertension, the drugs mainly dilate peripheral arteries and decrease peripheral vascular resistance by relaxing vascular smooth muscle.

Most of the available drugs are approved for use in hypertension. **Nifedipine**, a short-acting calcium channel blocker, has been used to treat hypertensive emergencies or urgencies, often by puncturing the capsule and squeezing the contents under the tongue or having the patient bite and swallow the capsule. Such use is no longer recommended, because this practice is associated with an increased risk of adverse cardiovascular events precipitated by a rapid and severe decrease in blood pressure.

As a group, the calcium channel blockers are well absorbed from the gastrointestinal tract following oral administration and are highly bound to protein. The drugs are metabolized in the liver and excreted in urine.

Diuretics

Antihypertensive effects of diuretics are usually attributed to sodium and water depletion. In fact, diuretics usually produce the same effects as severe dietary sodium restriction. In many cases of hypertension, diuretic therapy alone may lower blood pressure. When diuretic therapy is begun, blood volume and cardiac output decrease. With long-term administration of a diuretic, cardiac output returns to normal, but there is a persistent decrease in peripheral vascular resistance. This has been attributed to a persistent small reduction in extracellular water and plasma volume, decreased receptor sensitivity to vasopressor substances such as angiotensin, direct arteriolar vasodilation, and arteriolar vasodilation secondary to electrolyte depletion in the vessel wall. In moderate or severe hypertension that does not respond to a diuretic alone, the diuretic may be continued and another antihypertensive drug added, or monotherapy with a different type of antihypertensive drug may be tried.

Thiazide diuretics (e.g., *hydrochlorothiazide*) are most commonly used in the management of hypertension. Loop diuretics (e.g., *furosemide*) or potassium-sparing diuretics (e.g., *spironolactone*) may be useful in some circumstances. Diuretics are discussed in Chapter 53 and listed in Table 53-1.

Vasodilators (Direct Acting)

Vasodilator antihypertensive drugs directly relax smooth muscle in blood vessels, resulting in dilation and decreased peripheral vascular resistance. They also reduce afterload and may be used in management of heart failure. *Hydralazine* and *minoxidil* act mainly on arterioles; *nitroprusside* acts on arterioles and venules. These drugs have a limited effect on hypertension when used alone because the vasodilating action that lowers blood pressure also stimulates the SNS and triggers reflexive compensatory mechanisms (vasoconstriction, tachycardia, and increased cardiac output), which raise blood pressure. This effect can be prevented during long-term therapy by also giving a drug that prevents excessive sympathetic stimulation (e.g., propranolol, an adrenergic blocker). These drugs also cause sodium and water retention, which may be minimized by concomitant diuretic therapy. The FDA has issued a **BLACK BOX WARNING** for minoxidil as the drug can exacerbate angina and precipitate pericardial effusion (which can progress to cardiac tamponade).

Applying Your Knowledge 52-1

Mr. Olms is noncompliant with his drug regimen. How should you react?

Nursing Process

Assessment

Assess the patient's condition in relation to hypertension.

- Identify conditions and risk factors that may lead to hypertension. These include
  - Obesity
  - Elevated serum cholesterol (total and low-density lipoprotein) and triglycerides
  - Cigarette smoking
  - Sedentary lifestyle
  - Family history of hypertension or other cardiovascular disease
  - African-American race
  - Renal disease (e.g., renal artery stenosis)
  - Adrenal disease (e.g., hypersecretion of aldosterone, pheochromocytoma)
  - Other cardiovascular disorders (e.g., atherosclerosis, left ventricular hypertrophy)
  - Diabetes mellitus
  - Use of oral contraceptives, corticosteroids, appetite suppressants, nasal decongestants, nonsteroidal anti-inflammatory agents
  - Neurologic disorders (e.g., brain damage)

- Observe for signs and symptoms of hypertension.
  - Check blood pressure accurately and repeatedly. As a rule, multiple measurements in which systolic pressure is greater than 140 mm Hg, and/or diastolic pressure is greater than 90 mm Hg, are necessary to establish a diagnosis of hypertension.

    The importance of accurate blood pressure measurements cannot be overemphasized because there are many possibilities for errors. Some ways to improve accuracy and validity include using correct equipment (e.g., proper cuff size), having the patient rested and in the same position each time blood pressure is measured (e.g., sitting or supine with arm at heart level), and using the same arm for repeated measurements.

- In most cases of early hypertension, elevated blood pressure is the only clinical manifestation. If symptoms do occur, they are usually nonspecific (e.g., headache, weakness, fatigue, tachycardia, dizziness, palpitations, epistaxis).

- Eventually, signs and symptoms occur as target organs are damaged. Heart damage is often evidenced as angina pectoris, myocardial infarction, or heart failure. Chest pain, tachycardia, dyspnea, fatigue, and edema may occur. Brain damage may be indicated by transient ischemic attacks or strokes of varying severity with symptoms ranging from syncope to hemiparesis. Renal damage may be reflected by proteinuria, increased blood urea nitrogen (BUN), and increased serum creatinine. Ophthalmoscopic examination may reveal hemorrhages, sclerosis of arterioles, and inflammation of the optic nerve (papilledema). Because arterioles can be visualized in the retina of the eye, damage to retinal vessels may indicate damage to arterioles in the heart, brain, and kidneys.

Nursing Diagnoses

- Decreased Cardiac Output related to disease process or drug therapy
- Ineffective Coping related to long-term lifestyle changes and drug therapy
- Noncompliance related to lack of knowledge about hypertension and its management, costs and adverse effects of drug therapy, and psychosocial factors
- Disturbed Body Image related to the need for long-term management and medical supervision
- Fatigue related to antihypertensive drug therapy
- Deficient Knowledge related to hypertension, antihypertensive drug therapy, and nondrug lifestyle changes
- Sexual Dysfunction related to adverse drug effects

Nursing Process continues on page 836

Planning/Goals

The patient will

- Receive or take antihypertensive drugs correctly

- Be monitored closely for therapeutic and adverse drug effects, especially when drug therapy is started, when changes are made in choice of drugs, and when dosages are increased or decreased

- Use nondrug measures to assist in blood pressure control

- Avoid, manage, or report adverse drug reactions

- Verbalize or demonstrate knowledge of prescribed drugs and recommended lifestyle changes

- Keep follow-up appointments

Interventions

Implement measures to prevent or minimize hypertension. Preventive measures are mainly lifestyle changes to reduce risk factors. These measures should be started in childhood and continued throughout life. After hypertension is diagnosed, lifetime adherence to a therapeutic regimen may be necessary to control the disease and prevent complications. The nurse's role is important in the prevention, early detection, and management of hypertension. Some guidelines for intervention at community, family, and personal levels include the following:

- Participate in programs to promote healthful lifestyles (e.g., improving eating habits, increasing exercise, managing stress more effectively, avoiding cigarette smoking).

- Participate in community screening programs, and make appropriate referrals when abnormal blood pressures are detected. If hypertension develops in women taking oral contraceptives, the drug should be discontinued for 3 to 6 months to see whether blood pressure decreases without antihypertensive drugs.

- Help the hypertensive patient comply with prescribed therapy (see accompanying patient teaching display). Noncompliance is high among patients with hypertension. Reasons given for noncompliance include lack of symptoms; lack of motivation and self-discipline to make needed lifestyle changes (e.g., lose weight, stop smoking, restrict salt intake); perhaps experiencing more symptoms from medications than from hypertension; the cost of therapy; and the patient's failure to realize the importance of effective management, especially as related to prevention of major cardiovascular diseases (myocardial infarction, stroke, and death). In addition, several studies have shown that compliance decreases as the number of drugs and number of doses increase.

The nurse can help increase compliance by teaching the patient about hypertension, helping the patient make necessary lifestyle changes, and maintaining supportive interpersonal relationships. Losing weight, stopping

smoking, and other changes are most likely to be effective if attempted one at a time.

- Use recommended techniques for measuring blood pressure. Poor techniques are too often used (e.g., the patient's arm up or down rather than at heart level; cuff applied over clothing, too loosely, deflated too rapidly, or reinflated before completely deflated; a regular-sized cuff used on large arms that need a large cuff; using the stethoscope diaphragm rather than the bell). It is disturbing to think that antihypertensive drugs may be prescribed and dosages changed on the basis of inaccurate blood pressures.

Evaluation

- Observe for blood pressure measurements within goal or more nearly normal ranges.

- Observe and interview regarding compliance with instructions about drug therapy and lifestyle changes.

Observe and interview regarding adverse drug effects.

Principles of Therapy

Therapeutic Regimens

After the diagnosis of hypertension is established, a therapeutic regimen must be designed and implemented. The goal of management for most patients is to achieve and maintain blood pressure below 140/90 mm Hg. The target blood pressure for diabetic patients is 130/80 mm Hg. If the goal cannot be achieved, lowering blood pressure to any extent is still considered beneficial in decreasing the incidence of coronary artery disease and stroke.

The Joint National Committee on Prevention, Detection, Evaluation, and Treatment of High Blood Pressure (JNC 7) recommends management guidelines in which initial interventions are lifestyle modifications (i.e., reduction of weight and sodium intake, regular physical activity, moderate alcohol intake, and no smoking) to maintain normal blood pressure or for those in the prehypertension group. If these modifications do not produce goal blood pressure or substantial progress toward goal blood pressure, antihypertensive drug therapy should be initiated and the lifestyle modifications should be continued. The JNC 7 guidelines suggest thiazide diuretics be used as first-line therapy, either alone (monotherapy) or with a beta blocker, ACE inhibitor, ARB, or calcium channel blocker. If the initial drug (and dose) does not produce the desired blood pressure, options for further management include increasing the drug dose, substituting another drug, or adding a second drug from a different group. If the response is still inadequate, a second or third drug may be added, including a diuretic if not previously prescribed. When current management is ineffective, reassess the patient's compliance with lifestyle modifications and drug therapy. In addition, review other factors that may decrease the therapeutic response, such as the use of

Patient Teaching Guidelines | Antihypertensive Drugs

General Considerations

■ Hypertension is a major risk factor for heart attack, stroke (sometimes called brain attack), and kidney failure. Although it rarely causes symptoms unless complications occur, it can be controlled by appropriate management. Consequently, you need to learn all you can about the disease process, the factors that cause or aggravate it, and its management. In few other conditions is your knowledge and understanding about your condition as important as with hypertension.

■ For many people, lifestyle changes (i.e., a diet to avoid excessive salt and control weight and fat intake; regular exercise; and avoiding smoking) may be sufficient to control blood pressure. If drug therapy is prescribed, these measures should be continued.

■ When drug therapy is needed, your prescriber will try to choose a drug and develop a regimen that works for you. There are numerous antihypertensive drugs and many can be taken once a day, which makes their use more convenient and less disruptive of your usual activities of daily living. You may need several office visits to find the right drug or combination of drugs and the right dosage. Changes in drugs or dosages may also be needed later, especially if you develop other conditions or take other drugs that alter your response to the antihypertensive drugs.

■ Antihypertensive drug therapy is usually long term, may require more than one drug, and may produce side effects. You need to know the brand and generic names of any prescribed drugs and how to take each drug for optimal benefit and minimal adverse effects.

■ Antihypertensive drugs must be taken as prescribed for optimal benefits, even if you do not feel well when a medication is started or when dosage is increased. *No antihypertensive drug should be stopped abruptly. If problems develop, they should be discussed with the health care provider who is treating the hypertension.* If treatment is stopped, blood pressure usually increases gradually as the medications are eliminated from the body. However, sometimes blood pressure rapidly increases to pretreatment levels or even higher. With any of these situations, you are at risk of a heart attack or stroke. In addition, stopping one drug of a multidrug regimen may lead to increased adverse effects as well as decreased antihypertensive effectiveness. To avoid these problems, antihypertensive drugs should be tapered in dosage and discontinued gradually, as directed by your health care provider.

■ Blood pressure measurements are the only way you can tell if your medication is working. Thus, you may want to monitor your blood pressure at home, especially when starting drug therapy, changing medications, or changing dosages. If so, a blood pressure machine may be purchased at a medical supply store. Follow instructions regarding use, take your blood pressure approximately the same time(s) each day (e.g., before morning and evening meals), and keep a record to show to your health care provider.

■ People sometimes feel dizzy or faint while taking antihypertensive medications. This usually means your blood pressure drops momentarily and is most likely to occur when you start a medication, increase dosage, or stand up suddenly from a sitting or lying position. This can be prevented or decreased by moving to a standing position slowly, sleeping with the head of the bed elevated, wearing elastic stockings, exercising legs, avoiding prolonged standing, and avoiding hot baths. If episodes still occur, you should sit or lie down to avoid a fall and possible injury.

■ It is very important to keep appointments for follow-up care.

Self-or Caregiver Administration

■ Take or give antihypertensive drugs at prescribed time intervals, about the same time each day. For example, take once-daily drugs as close to every 24 hours as you can manage; twice-a-day drugs should be taken every 12 hours. If ordered four times daily, take approximately every 6 hours. Taking doses too close together can increase dizziness, weakness, and other adverse effects. Taking doses too far apart may not control blood pressure adequately and may increase risks of heart attack or stroke.

■ Take oral captopril on an empty stomach. Food decreases drug absorption.

■ Take most oral antihypertensive agents with or after food intake to decrease gastric irritation. Candesartan (Atacand), irbesartan (Avapro), losartan (Cozaar), telmisartan (Micardis), and valsartan (Diovan) may be taken with or without food.

■ With prazosin, doxazosin, or terazosin, take the first dose and the first increased dose at bedtime to prevent dizziness and possible fainting.

■ With the clonidine skin patch, apply to a hairless area on the upper arm or torso once every 7 days. Rotate sites.

over-the-counter appetite suppressants, dietary or herbal supplements, or nasal decongestants, which raise blood pressure.

The World Health Organization and the International Society of Hypertension guidelines for management of hypertension include considering age, ethnicity, and concomitant cardiovascular disorders when choosing an antihypertensive drug; starting with a single drug, in the lowest available dose; changing to a drug from a different group, rather than increasing dosage of the first drug or adding a second drug, if the initial drug is ineffective or not well tolerated; and using long-acting drugs (i.e., a single dose effective for 24 hours). The guidelines also note that many patients require two or more drugs to achieve adequate blood pressure control. When this is the case, fixed-dose combinations or long-acting agents may be preferred, as they decrease the number of drugs and doses that are required and may increase compliance.

Applying Your Knowledge 52-2

The JNC 7 has identified specific management guidelines for the patient with hypertension. What should you teach a patient with hypertension relative to the guidelines?

Drug Selection

Because many effective antihypertensive drugs are available, choices depend primarily on patient characteristics and responses. Some general guidelines are as follows.

ACE inhibitors may be effective alone in Caucasian hypertensive patients or in combination with a diuretic in African-American hypertensive patients. They are also recommended for hypertensive adults with diabetes mellitus and kidney damage because they slow the progression of albuminuria. Based on research studies that indicate reduced morbidity and mortality from cardiovascular diseases, these drugs are increasingly being prescribed as a component of a multidrug regimen.

ARBs have therapeutic effects similar to those of ACE inhibitors, with fewer adverse effects. They may be used in most patients with hypertension.

Antiadrenergics may be effective in any hypertensive population. Alpha agonists and antagonists are most often used in multidrug regimens in stage 2 hypertension, because they may cause postural hypotension and syncope. Clonidine is available in a skin patch that is applied once a week and reportedly reduces adverse effects and increases compliance. An additional advantage of transdermal clonidine is that patients who cannot take oral medications can use it. A disadvantage of this system is a delayed onset of effect (2–3 days), so other antihypertensive medications must also be given during the first 2 to 3 days of clonidine transdermal therapy. Other disadvantages include cost, a 20% incidence of local skin rash or irritation, and a 2- to 3-day delay in "offset" of action when transdermal therapy is discontinued.

Beta adrenergic blockers are the drugs of first choice for patients younger than 50 years of age with high-renin hypertension, tachycardia, angina pectoris, myocardial infarction, or left ventricular hypertrophy. Most beta blockers are approved for use in hypertension and are probably equally effective. However, the cardioselective drugs (see Chap. 18) are preferred for hypertensive patients who also have asthma, peripheral vascular disease, or diabetes mellitus. Research studies demonstrate reduced morbidity and mortality with diuretics and beta blockers used in combination, especially after a myocardial infarction.

Calcium channel blockers may be used for monotherapy or in combination with other drugs. They may be especially useful for hypertensive patients who also have angina pectoris or other cardiovascular disorders. The JNC 7 recommends that calcium channel blockers be considered the drug of first choice in African Americans with stage 2 hypertension. Note that sustained-release forms of nifedipine, diltiazem, verapamil and other long-acting drugs (e.g., amlodipine, felodipine) are recommended rather than the short-acting forms because they do not cause precipitous lowering of pressure.

Diuretics are preferred for initial therapy in all patients, but specifically in older and African-American hypertensive patients. They should be included in any multidrug regimen for these and other populations. Thiazide and related diuretics are equally effective. Hydrochlorothiazide is most commonly used.

Evidence-Based Practice

52-1 Enhanced Compliance With Fixed-Dose Combinations of Antihypertensive Medications.

A meta-analysis of nine studies (11,925 patients) was performed exploring compliance with medication administration using fixed-dose combinations compared with a regimen of drugs given individually (e.g., 1 pill of lisinopril plus hydrochlorothiazide versus lisinopril and hydrochlorothiazide given as 2 separate pills). A subgroup analysis of four retrospective studies on hypertension from this group showed individuals who were prescribed fixed-dose combinations of antihypertensive medications reduced the likelihood of noncompliance by 24% over those who took the same medications as individual pills. Since evidence now suggests that the majority of individuals with hypertension will require combinations of antihypertensive medications to achieve optimal blood pressure control, simplifying the drug regimen with fixed-combination drugs can improve compliance and produce better health outcomes (Bangalore, Kamalakkannan, Parkar, & Messerli, 2007).

Diazoxide, usually in parenteral form, is indicated for short-term treatment of malignant hypertension. Loop diuretics are indicated in those with renal insufficiency. Potassium-sparing diuretics may precipitate hyperkalemia. Recently, the selective aldosterone blocker, eplerenone, has demonstrated efficacy in African Americans.

Vasodilators are used in combination with a beta blocker and a diuretic to prevent hypotension-induced compensatory mechanisms (stimulation of the SNS and fluid retention) that raise blood pressure.

Combination products usually combine two drugs with different mechanisms of action (e.g., a thiazide or related diuretic plus a beta blocker or other antiadrenergic, an ACE inhibitor, an ARB, or a calcium channel blocker). Most are available in various formulations (see Table 52-2). Potential advantages of fixed-dose combination products include comparable or improved effectiveness, smaller doses of individual components, fewer adverse effects, improved compliance, and possibly decreased costs (see Evidence-Based Practice Box 52-1:Enhanced Compliance with Fixed-Dose Combinations of Antihypertensive Medications.

Drug Dosage

Dosage of antihypertensive drugs must be titrated according to individual response. Dosage should be started at minimal levels and increased if necessary. Lower doses decrease the incidence and severity of adverse effects.

For many patients, it may be more beneficial to change drugs or add another drug rather than increase dosage. Two or three drugs in small doses may be more effective and cause fewer adverse effects than a single drug in large doses. When two or more drugs are given, the dose of each drug may need to be reduced.

Patients who maintain control of their blood pressure for 1 year or so may be candidates for reduced dosages or reduced numbers of drugs. Any such adjustments must be gradual and carefully supervised by a health care provider. Expected benefits include fewer adverse effects and greater compliance.

Dietary Management of Blood Pressure

Key behavioral determinants of blood pressure are related to dietary consumption of calories and salt; the prevalence of hypertension rises proportionally to average body mass index. The Dietary Approaches to Stop Hypertension (DASH) study demonstrated that patients with prehypertension or stage 1 hypertension can reduce their blood pressures by adhering to a diet abundant in fresh fruits and vegetables and low-fat dairy products even without restricting calorie or sodium intake. The effects of the DASH diet demonstrate blood pressure–lowering effects that parallel the degree of benefit from drug monotherapy, can be augmented by dietary sodium restriction, and are observed in all ethnic groups, particularly African Americans. Information regarding the DASH diet can be obtained at www.nhlbi.nih.gov/health/public/heart/hbp/dash/.

Therapeutic regimens for hypertension may include sodium restriction. Severe restrictions usually are not acceptable to patients; however, moderate restrictions (4–6 g of salt a day) are beneficial and more easily implemented. Avoiding heavily salted foods (e.g., cured meats, sandwich meats, pretzels, potato chips) and not adding salt to food at the table can achieve this. Research and clinical observations indicate the following:

■ Sodium restriction alone reduces blood pressure.

■ Sodium restriction potentiates the antihypertensive actions of diuretics and other antihypertensive drugs. Conversely, excessive sodium intake decreases the antihypertensive actions of all antihypertensive drugs. Patients with unrestricted salt intake who are taking thiazides may lose excessive potassium and become hypokalemic.

■ Sodium restriction may decrease dosage requirements of antihypertensive drugs, thereby decreasing the incidence and severity of adverse effects.

Use in Special Populations

Use in Various Ethnic Groups

Nearly 70% of the familial considerations related to blood pressure are credited to shared genes rather than to shared environment. For most antihypertensive drugs, there have been few research studies comparing their effects in different genetic or ethnic groups. However, several studies indicate that beta blockers have greater effects in people of Asian heritage compared with their effects in Caucasians. For hypertension, Asians in general need much smaller doses because they metabolize and excrete beta blockers slowly. Other populations known to metabolize beta blockers slowly include Arab and Egyptian Americans and possibly German Americans. In

African Americans, diuretics are effective and recommended as initial drug therapy; calcium channel blockers, alpha$_1$ receptor blockers, and the alpha–beta blocker labetalol are reportedly equally effective in African Americans and Caucasians. ACE inhibitors, some ARBs (e.g., losartan, telmisartan), and beta blockers are less effective as monotherapy in African Americans. When beta blockers are used, they are usually one component of a multidrug regimen, and higher doses may be required. Overall, African Americans are more likely to have severe hypertension and require multiple drugs as a result of having low circulating renin, increased salt sensitivity, and a higher incidence of obesity.

Use in Children

Most principles of managing adult hypertension apply to managing childhood and adolescent hypertension; some additional management elements should be considered.

Routine blood pressure measurement is especially important for children who are overweight or who have a hypertensive parent. Increased blood pressure in children often correlates with hypertension in young adults.

In recent years, increased blood pressure measurements during routine pediatric examinations have led to the discovery of significant asymptomatic hypertension and the realization that mild elevations in blood pressure are more common during childhood, especially in adolescents, than previously thought. Hypertension in children and adolescents may indicate underlying disease processes (e.g., cardiac, endocrine, renovascular, renal parenchymal disorders) or the early onset of primary hypertension.

The National High Blood Pressure Education Program Working Group on High Blood Pressure in Children and Adolescents produced the fourth report on the diagnosis, evaluation, and treatment of high blood pressure in children and adolescents in 2004. These guidelines established parameters for blood pressure in children and adolescents of comparable age, body size (height and weight), and sex. Normal blood pressure is defined as systolic and diastolic values less than the 90th percentile; prehypertension is defined as an average of systolic or diastolic pressures within the 90th to 95th percentiles; hypertension is defined as pressures beyond the 95th percentile. Blood pressure values obtained with a child or adolescent should be compared with norms and recorded in permanent health care records. Measurements are recorded on three or more occasions. Multiple accurate measurements are especially important in diagnosing hypertension because blood pressure may be more labile in children and adolescents.

Children have a greater incidence of secondary hypertension than adults. In general, the higher the blood pressure and the younger the child, the greater the likelihood of secondary hypertension. Diagnostic tests may be needed to rule out renovascular disease or coarctation of the aorta in those younger than 18 years of age with blood pressure above 140/90 mm Hg and young children with blood pressures above the 95th percentile for their age group. Oral contraceptives may cause secondary hypertension in adolescents.

The goals of management are to reduce blood pressure to below the 95th percentile and prevent the long-term effects of persistent hypertension. As in adults, prevention of obesity, avoiding excessive sodium intake, and exercise are important nonpharmacologic measures. Obese adolescents who lose weight may lower their blood pressure, especially when they also increase physical activity.

Most children with secondary hypertension require drug therapy, which should be directed at the cause of hypertension if known. Drug therapy should be cautious and conservative because few studies have been done in children and long-term effects are unknown. The fewest drugs and the lowest doses should be used. Thus, if an initial drug is ineffective, it may be better to give a different single drug than to add a second drug to the regimen.

Based on the current recommendations of the National High Blood Pressure Education Program Working Group on High Blood Pressure in Children and Adolescents released in 2004, guidelines for choosing drugs include the following:

- Beta blockers are used in children of all ages and are the preferential drug for children with hypertension and migraine headache; they should probably be avoided in children with resting pulse rates under 60.

- Thiazide diuretics may be used, and they do not commonly produce hyperglycemia, hyperuricemia, or hypercalcemia in children as they do in adults.

- ACE inhibitors have been used to treat hypertension in children 6 years of age and over. The safety and efficacy of these drugs is continually being documented with studies and clinical practice. ACE inhibitors are preferred for managing hypertension in children who also have coexisting diabetes, microalbuminuria, or proteinuric renal diseases. Also, because of teratogenic effects, these drugs should be used very cautiously, if at all, in adolescent girls who may be sexually active.

- ARBs may be used in children 6 years of age or older who do not tolerate ACE inhibitors in the same way the JNC 7 recommends for adults. Further research and documentation regarding safety and efficacy are continuing.

- Calcium channel blockers are used in treating acute and chronic childhood hypertension. With chronic hypertension, immediate-release forms have a short duration of action and require frequent administration. Amlodipine may be given once daily and has specific pediatric labeling information.

- Hydralazine seems to be less effective in childhood and adolescent hypertension than in adult disease.

- Fixed-dose combination preparations, with the exception of bisoprolol and hydrochlorothiazide, have not had extensive study and are not recommended for routine use.

Although all patients with primary hypertension need regular supervision and assessment of blood pressure, this is especially important with young children and adolescents because of growth and developmental changes.

Use in Older Adults

Most principles of managing hypertension in other populations apply to older adults (>65 years). In addition, the following factors require consideration.

There are basically two types of hypertension in older adults. One is systolic hypertension, in which systolic blood pressure is above 140 mm Hg but diastolic pressure is below 90 mm Hg. The other type, systolic–diastolic hypertension, involves elevations of both systolic and diastolic pressures. Both types increase cardiovascular morbidity and mortality, especially heart failure and stroke, and should be treated.

Nonpharmacologic management should be tried alone or with drug therapy. For example, weight reduction, limited alcohol intake, moderate sodium restriction, and smoking cessation may be the initial treatment of choice if the patient is hypertensive and overweight.

If antihypertensive drug therapy is required, drugs used for younger adults may be used alone or in combination. A diuretic is usually the drug of first choice in older adults and may be effective alone. ACE inhibitors and calcium channel blocking agents may also be effective as monotherapy; beta blockers are usually less effective as monotherapy. Some ACE inhibitors (e.g., lisinopril, ramipril, quinapril, moexipril) or their active metabolites produce higher plasma concentrations in older adults than in younger ones. This is attributed to decreased renal function rather than age itself. Additional guidelines include the following:

- The goal of drug therapy for systolic–diastolic hypertension is usually a systolic pressure below 140 mm Hg and a diastolic below 90 mm Hg in patients with no other complications. For those with diabetes or renal failure, the goal is a systolic pressure below 130 mm Hg and a diastolic below 80 mm Hg. However, the latter goal may be difficult for most patients to meet because it requires rather stringent lifestyle restrictions and may require the use of two or more antihypertensive drugs.

- Older adults may be especially susceptible to the adverse effects of antihypertensive drugs because their homeostatic mechanisms are less efficient. For example, if hypotension occurs, the mechanisms that raise blood pressure are less efficient and syncope may occur. In addition, renal and liver function may be reduced, making accumulation of drugs more likely.

- Initial drug doses should be approximately half of the recommended doses for younger adults, and increases should be smaller and spaced at longer intervals. Lower drug dosages (e.g., hydrochlorothiazide 12.5 mg daily) are often effective and reduce risks of adverse effects.

- Blood pressure should be reduced slowly to facilitate adequate blood flow through arteriosclerotic vessels. Rapid lowering of blood pressure may produce cerebral insufficiency (syncope, transient ischemic attacks, stroke).

■ A further incentive for successful management of hypertension in older patients is the benefit of reducing the incidence of dementia with antihypertensives.

■ If blood pressure control is achieved and maintained for approximately 6 to 12 months, drug dosage should be gradually reduced, if possible.

Use in Patients With Renal Impairment

Antihypertensive drugs are frequently required by patients with renal impairment ranging from mild insufficiency to end-stage failure. A temporary decrease in renal function may occur in these patients when blood pressure is initially lowered. Guidelines include the following considerations:

■ In hypertensive patients with primary renal disease or diabetic nephropathy, drug therapy may slow progression of renal impairment.

■ Diuretics are usually required because sodium retention is an important element of hypertension in these patients. Loop diuretics, such as furosemide, are more often used, and relatively large doses may be required. Thiazides are usually contraindicated because they are ineffective if serum creatinine is above 2 mg/dL. However, metolazone, a thiazide-related drug, may be used and relatively large doses may be required.

■ ACE inhibitors are usually effective in patients with renal impairment, but responses may vary and the following factors should be considered Careful monitoring is required, especially during the first few weeks of therapy, to prevent irreversible renal failure. For some patients, it may not be possible to normalize blood pressure and maintain adequate renal perfusion.

■ In patients with severe atherosclerosis, especially those with stenosis of renal arteries, ACE inhibitors can impair renal blood flow and worsen renal impairment (i.e., increase BUN and serum creatinine). This may require discontinuing the drug or a reduction in dosage.

■ Approximately 25% of patients taking an ACE inhibitor for heart failure experience an increase in BUN and serum creatinine levels. These patients usually do not require drug discontinuation unless they have severe, pre-existing renal impairment. In patients with severe heart failure, whose renal function may depend on the activity of the renin–angiotensin–aldosterone system, management with an ACE inhibitor may worsen renal impairment. However, acute renal failure rarely occurs.

■ The mechanisms are unclear, but ACE inhibitors also have renal protective effects in hypertensive patients with some renal impairment and patients with diabetic nephropathy. A possible mechanism is less damage to the endothelium and less vascular remodeling (i.e., less narrowing of the lumen and less thickening of the vessel wall).

■ The elimination half-life of most ACE inhibitors and their active metabolites is prolonged in patients with renal impairment. Dosage may need to be reduced with benazepril, lisinopril, quinapril, and ramipril. Fosinopril requires no dosage adjustment as it is excreted by the hepatobiliary pathway.

■ All ARBs are metabolized by the liver and do not need dose reduction with renal impairment.

■ Most beta blockers are eliminated primarily by the kidneys and serum half-life is prolonged in patients with renal impairment. Most of the drugs should be used with caution and in reduced dosages. Dosage of metoprolol does not need to be reduced. An additional consideration is that cardiac output and blood pressure should not be lowered enough to impair renal blood flow and aggravate renal impairment.

■ None of the commonly used calcium channel blockers is significantly cleared by the kidney and does not require a dosage adjustment as half-life is not altered significantly in renal impairment. Verapamil or diltiazem may be preferred to other calcium channels blockers due to their ability to limit proteinuria. Calcium channel blockers are effective and well tolerated in renal impairment, and they maintain renal blood flow even during blood pressure reduction in most patients. However, cautious use is still recommended because several agents produce active metabolites that are excreted by the kidneys (see "Use in Patients With Renal Impairment," Chap. 53).

Use in Patients With Hepatic Impairment

Little information is available about the use of antihypertensive drugs in patients with impaired hepatic function. However, many of the drugs are metabolized in the liver and hepatic impairment can increase and prolong plasma concentrations.

Patients who have jaundice or marked elevations of hepatic enzymes while taking an ACE inhibitor should have the drug discontinued as the drugs have been associated with cholestatic jaundice and can progress to hepatic necrosis and possible death. In addition, therapeutic effects can be decreased with several of the drugs (e.g., fosinopril, quinapril, ramipril) because less of a given dose is converted to an active metabolite. Fosinopril may require a dosage adjustment with hepatic impairment as it is excreted by the hepatobiliary pathway. Clearance of fosinopril, quinapril, and probably other ACE inhibitors that are metabolized is reduced in patients with alcoholic or biliary cirrhosis.

ARBs should be used cautiously in patients with biliary tract obstruction or hepatic impairment. For some of these drugs (e.g., candesartan, irbesartan, valsartan), dosage reduction is unnecessary. However, a lower starting dose is recommended for losartan because plasma concentrations of the drug and its active metabolite are increased and clearance is decreased approximately 50%. With telmisartan, plasma concentrations are increased and bioavailability approaches 100%. In addition, the drug is eliminated mainly by biliary excretion, and patients with biliary tract obstruction or hepatic impairment have reduced clearance. The drug should be used with caution, but dosage forms that allow dosage reduction below 40 milligrams are not available. Thus, an alternative drug should probably be considered for patients with hepatic impairment.

Beta blockers that normally undergo extensive first-pass hepatic metabolism (e.g., acebutolol, metoprolol, propranolol, timolol) may produce excessive blood levels in patients with cirrhosis because the blood containing the drug is shunted around the liver into the systemic circulation. Dosage should be started at a low dose and titrated carefully in these patients. Dosage of bisoprolol and pindolol should also be reduced in patients with cirrhosis or other hepatic impairment.

Calcium channel blockers should be used with caution, dosages should be substantially reduced, liver enzymes should be monitored periodically, and patients should be closely monitored for drug effects (see "Use in Patients With Hepatic Impairment," Chap. 50).

Use in Patients Undergoing Surgery

Drug therapy should be continued until surgery and restarted as soon as possible after surgery. If patients cannot take drugs orally, parenteral diuretics, antiadrenergic agents, ACE inhibitors, calcium channel blockers, or vasodilators may be given to avoid the rebound hypertension associated with abrupt discontinuance of some antiadrenergic antihypertensive agents. Transdermal clonidine also may be used. The anesthesiologist and surgeon must be informed about the patient's hypertension and medication status.

Use in Patients With Critical Illness

Antihypertensive drugs are frequently prescribed for patients with critical illness and must be used cautiously, usually with reduced dosages and careful monitoring of responses. In many cases, the drugs are continued during critical illnesses caused by both cardiovascular and noncardiovascular disorders. If the patient cannot take oral drugs, drug choices are narrowed because many commonly used drugs are not available in a dosage form that can be given parenterally, by gastrointestinal tube, or topically (e.g., like a clonidine skin patch). Thus, patients' drug therapy must usually be re-titrated. In one way, this may be more difficult, because critically ill patients are often unstable in their conditions and responses to drug therapy. In another way, it may be easier in a critical care unit, where hemodynamic monitoring is commonly used. The goal of management is usually to maintain adequate tissue perfusion while avoiding both hypotension and hypertension.

Antihypertensive drugs are also used to treat hypertensive urgencies and emergencies, which involve dangerously high blood pressures and actual or potential damage to target organs. Although there are risks with severe hypertension, there are also risks associated with lowering blood pressure excessively or too rapidly, including stroke, myocardial infarction, and acute renal failure. Thus, the goal of management is usually to lower blood pressure over several minutes to several hours, with careful titration of drug dosage to avoid precipitous drops.

Urgencies can be treated with oral antihypertensive agents such as captopril 25 to 50 milligrams every 1 to 2 hours or clonidine 0.2 milligrams initially, then 0.1 milligrams hourly until diastolic blood pressure falls below 110 mm Hg or 0.7 milligrams has been given.

A hypertensive emergency, defined as a diastolic pressure of 120 mm Hg or higher and target organ damage, requires an IV drug. The goal of management is usually to lower diastolic pressure to 100 to 110 mm Hg and maintain it there for several days to allow adjustment of the physiologic mechanisms that normally regulate blood pressure. Then, the blood pressure can be lowered to normotensive levels.

Several drugs can be given to treat a hypertensive emergency. Fenoldopam is a fast-acting drug indicated only for short-term use (<48 hours) in hospitalized patients. Dosage is calculated according to body weight and desired effects on blood pressure. Administration is by an infusion pump, with frequent monitoring of blood pressure. Nitroglycerin is especially beneficial in patients with both severe hypertension and myocardial ischemia. The dose is titrated according to blood pressure response and may range from 5 to 100 micrograms per minute. Tolerance develops to IV nitroglycerin over 24 to 48 hours. Nitroprusside, which has a rapid onset and short duration of action, is given as a continuous infusion at a rate of 0.5 to 8 micrograms per kilogram of body weight per minute. Intra-arterial blood pressure should be monitored during the infusion. Nitroprusside is metabolized to thiocyanate, and serum thiocyanate levels should be measured if the drug is given longer than 72 hours. The infusion should be stopped after 72 hours if the serum thiocyanate level is more than 12 milligrams per deciliter; it should be stopped at 48 hours in patients with renal impairment. Symptoms of thiocyanate toxicity (e.g., nausea, vomiting, muscle twitching or spasm, seizures) can be reversed with hemodialysis. Other drugs that may be used include IV hydralazine, labetalol, and nicardipine; see Table 52-1.

Use in Home Care

Antihypertensive drugs are commonly self-administered in the home setting. The home care nurse is most likely to be involved when making home visits for other reasons. Whether the patient or another member of the household is taking antihypertensive medications, the home care nurse may be helpful in teaching about the drugs, monitoring for drug effects, and promoting compliance with the prescribed regimen (pharmacologic and lifestyle modifications).

Noncompliance with prescribed antihypertensive drug therapy is a major problem, and consequences may be catastrophic. The home care nurse is well situated to assess for actual or potential barriers to compliance. For example, several antihypertensive medications are quite expensive and patients may not take the drugs at all or they may take fewer than the prescribed number of doses. If the nurse's assessment reveals this sort of situation, he or she may contact the prescribing health care provider and discuss the possibility of using less expensive drugs. If the provider is unwilling to try alternative drugs, the nurse may be able to identify resources for obtaining the needed medications.

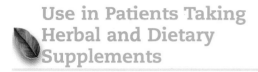

Use in Patients Taking Herbal and Dietary Supplements

Use of nonprescription herbal and dietary supplements is frequently not reported by the patient even though one third of adults in the United States use these agents. Significant interactions can occur between herbs or dietary supplements and prescribed drugs. Many nonprescription medications such as antihistamines, cold/cough preparations, and weight loss products can decrease the effectiveness of antihypertensive drugs or worsen hypertension. Caffeine, by its stimulating effects, may increase blood pressure. Yohimbe, used to treat erectile dysfunction, is a central nervous system stimulant and can affect blood pressure.

Applying Your Knowledge 52-3

Mr. Olms asks you why amlodipine was chosen to control his hypertension. What is the most appropriate response?

Nursing Actions Antihypertensive Drugs

NURSING ACTIONS	RATIONALE/EXPLANATION
1. Administer accurately a. Give oral captopril and moexipril on an empty stomach, 1 hour before meals.	Food decreases drug absorption.
b. Give most other oral antihypertensives with or after food intake.	To decrease gastric irritation
c. Give angiotensin II receptor blockers with or without food.	Food does not impair drug absorption.
d. For intravenous injection of propranolol or labetalol, the patient should be attached to a cardiac monitor. In addition, parenteral atropine and isoproterenol (Isuprel) must be readily available.	For early detection and management of excessive myocardial depression and dysrhythmias. Atropine may be used to treat excessive bradycardia. Isoproterenol may be used to stimulate myocardial contractility and increase cardiac output.
e. Give the first dose and the first increased dose of prazosin, doxazosin, and terazosin at bedtime.	To prevent orthostatic hypotension and syncope
f. For administration of fenoldopam and nitroprusside, use the manufacturers' instructions to develop a unit protocol for preparation of infusion solutions, dosages, flow rates, durations of use, and monitoring of blood pressure during infusion.	These drugs are used to lower blood pressure rapidly in hypertensive emergencies, usually in an emergency department or critical care unit. They also have specific requirements for preparation and administration. A protocol established beforehand can save valuable time in an emergency situation.
2. Observe for therapeutic effects a. Decreased blood pressure. The usual goal is a normal blood pressure (i.e., less than 140/90 mm Hg).	The choice of drugs and drug dosages often requires adjustment to maximize beneficial effects and minimize adverse effects. Thus, optimal therapeutic effects may not occur immediately after drug therapy is begun.
3. Observe for adverse effects	Adverse effects are most likely to occur in patients who are elderly, have impaired renal function, and are receiving multiple antihypertensive drugs or large doses of antihypertensive drugs.
a. Orthostatic hypotension, dizziness, weakness	This is an extension of the expected pharmacologic action. Orthostatic hypotension results from drug blockage of compensatory reflexes (vasoconstriction, decreased venous pooling in extremities and increased venous return to the heart) that normally maintain blood pressure in the upright position. This adverse reaction may be aggravated by other conditions that cause vasodilation (e.g., exercise, heat or hot weather, and alcohol consumption).
b. Sodium and water retention; increased plasma volume; perhaps edema and weight gain	These effects result from decreased renal perfusion. This reaction can be prevented or minimized by concurrent administration of a diuretic.
c. Prolonged atrioventricular conduction, bradycardia	Due to increased vagal tone and stimulation
d. Gastrointestinal disturbances, including nausea, vomiting, and diarrhea	These effects are more likely to occur with hydralazine, methyldopa, propranolol, and captopril.
e. Mental depression (with reserpine)	Apparently caused by decreased levels of catecholamines and serotonin in the brain

(continued on page 844)

Nursing Actions · Antihypertensive Drugs (continued)

NURSING ACTIONS	RATIONALE/EXPLANATION
f. Bronchospasm (with nonselective beta blockers)	The drugs may cause bronchoconstriction and are contraindicated in patients with asthma and other bronchoconstrictive lung disorders.
g. Hypertensive crisis (with abrupt withdrawal of clonidine or guanabenz)	This may be prevented by tapering dosage over several days before stopping the drug.
h. Cough and hyperkalemia with angiotensin-converting enzyme (ACE) inhibitors	A chronic, nonproductive cough is a relatively common adverse effect; hyperkalemia occurs in 1%–4% of patients.
4. Observe for drug interactions	
a. Drugs that *increase* effects of antihypertensives:	
(1) Other antihypertensive agents	Combinations of two or three drugs with different mechanisms of action are often given for their additive effects and efficacy in controlling blood pressure when a single drug is ineffective.
(2) Alcohol, other central nervous system depressants (e.g., opioid analgesics, phenothiazine antipsychotics)	These drugs have hypotensive effects when used alone and increased hypotension occurs when they are combined with antihypertensive drugs.
(3) Digoxin	Additive bradycardia with beta blockers
b. Drugs that *decrease* effects of antihypertensives:	
(1) Adrenergics	These drugs stimulate the sympathetic nervous system and raise blood pressure. They include over-the-counter nasal decongestants, cold remedies, bronchodilators, and appetite suppressants.
(2) Antacids	May decrease bioavailability of ACE inhibitors, especially captopril. Give antacids 2 hours before or after ACE inhibitors.
(3) Nonsteroidal anti-inflammatory drugs, oral contraceptives	These drugs tend to increase blood pressure by causing retention of sodium and water.

Key Concepts

- Hypertension is defined in adults as a systolic pressure above 140 mm Hg or a diastolic pressure above 90 mm Hg on multiple blood pressure measurements.

- Key behavioral determinants of blood pressure are related to dietary consumption of calories and salt; the prevalence of hypertension rises proportionally to average body mass index.

- Alpha$_1$-adrenergic receptor blocking agents should be administered at bedtime to minimize the first-dose phenomenon.

- ACE inhibitors and ARBs are equally effective at controlling blood pressure.

- Beta-adrenergic blockers are the drugs of first choice for patients younger than 50 years of age with high-renin hypertension, tachycardia, angina pectoris, myocardial infarction, or left ventricular hypertrophy.

- In general, individuals with hypertension of Asian descent require much smaller doses of beta blockers because they metabolize and excrete the drugs slowly.

- African Americans are more likely to have severe hypertension and require multiple drugs as a result of having low circulating renin, increased salt sensitivity, and a higher incidence of obesity.

- The FDA has issued a **BLACK BOX WARNING** for patients with CAD withdrawing from oral forms of atenolol, metoprolol, nadolol, propranolol, and timolol; abrupt withdrawal has resulted in exacerbation of angina, the incidence of ventricular dysrhythmias, and the occurrence of MIs.

- The FDA has issued a **BLACK BOX WARNING** for ACE inhibitors and ARBs during pregnancy as their use can cause injury and even death to a developing fetus.

- The FDA has issued a **BLACK BOX WARNING** for minoxidil as the drug can exacerbate angina and precipitate effusion (which can progress to cardiac tamponade).

Review and Application Exercises

Short Answer Exercises

1. Describe the physiologic mechanisms that control blood pressure.

2. What are common factors that raise blood pressure?

3. Why is it important to measure blood pressure accurately and repeatedly?

4. How do ACE inhibitors, ARBs, alpha- and beta-adrenergic blockers, calcium channel blockers, and direct vasodilators lower blood pressure?

5. What are adverse effects of each group of antihypertensive drugs, and how may they be prevented or minimized?

6. List at least two major considerations in using antihypertensive drugs in children, older adults, and patients who have renal or hepatic impairment.

7. How would you assess a patient being treated for hypertension for compliance with the prescribed lifestyle and drug therapy regimen?

NCLEX-Style Questions

8. In administering a newly initiated order for an ACE inhibitor to a patient, discharge instructions will include letting her know that which of the following is a common adverse reaction to therapy with an ACE inhibitor?
a. tinnitus
b. dry, nonproductive, persistent cough
c. muscle weakness
d. constipation

9. A patient with a history of hypertension comes to the emergency department with double vision and a blood pressure of 240/120 mm Hg. The physician prescribes sodium nitroprusside (Nipress) by continuous infusion and continual blood pressure monitoring. The nurse understands that this drug's immediate action is to lower blood pressure by
a. increasing peripheral vascular resistance
b. increasing cardiac output
c. dilating venous and arterial vessels
d. decreasing heart rate

10. Which of the following is indicated for initial drug therapy in a patient newly diagnosed with uncomplicated hypertension (stage 1)?
a. calcium channel blocker
b. potassium-sparing diuretic
c. direct-acting vasodilator
d. thiazide diuretic

11. Orthostatic or postural hypotension is a potential outcome that places the elderly at risk for injury from falls. Instructions given to the patient to decrease this effect of antihypertensive therapy include
a. Take the dose in the early afternoon.
b. Change position slowly when rising from bed or chair.
c. Increase fluid intake by 500 mL/day.
d. Decrease the dose until symptoms disappear.

12. Single-drug therapy with an ACE inhibitor would be least effective in
a. children
b. the elderly
c. Hispanics
d. African Americans

Selected References

American Heart Association. (2007). Treatment of hypertension in the prevention and management of ischemic heart disease: A scientific statement from the American Heart Association. *Circulation, 115,* 2761–2788.

Bangalore, S., Kamalakkannan, G., Parkar, S., & Messerli, F. H. (2007). Fixed-dose combinations improve medication compliance: a meta-analysis. *American Journal of Medicine, 120,* 713–719.

Drug facts and comparisons. (Updated monthly). St. Louis, MO: Facts and Comparisons.

Gabardi, S. (2005). Drug dosing in chronic kidney disease. *Medical Clinics of North America, 89,* 649–687.

Joint National Committee on Prevention, Detection, Evaluation, and Treatment of High Blood Pressure. (2003). *The seventh report of the Joint National Committee on Prevention, Detection, Evaluation, and Treatment of High Blood Pressure: The JNC 7 report.* Retrieved October 30, 2007, from http://www.nhlbi.nih.gov/guidelines/hypertension

Karch, A. M. (2007). *2008 Lippincott's nursing drug guide.* Philadelphia: Lippincott Williams & Wilkins.

National High Blood Pressure Education Program Working Group on High Blood Pressure in Children and Adolescents (2004). *The Fourth Report on the Diagnosis, Evaluation, and Treatment of High Blood Pressure in Children and Adolescents.* Retrieved September 28, 2005, from http://www.pediatrics.org/cgi/content/full/114/2/S2/555

Porth, C. M. (2005). *Pathophysiology: Concepts of altered health states* (7th ed., pp. 505–533). Philadelphia: Lippincott Williams & Wilkins.

Skidmore-Roth, L. (2004). *Mosby's handbook of herbs & natural supplements* (2nd ed.). St. Louis, MO: Mosby.

Victor, R. G. (2008). Arterial hypertension. In L. Goldman (Ed.), *Cecil medicine* (23rd ed). Retrieved November 1, 2007, from http://www.mdconsult.com/das/book/body/80877982-10/0/1492/286.html?tocnode=53600337&fromURL=286.html

White, W. B. (2005). Update on the drug treatment of hypertension in patients with cardiovascular disease. *American Journal of Medicine, 118,* 695–705.

World Health Organization, International Society of Hypertension (ISH) Writing Group. (2003). ISH Statement on management of hypertension. *Journal of Hypertension, 21,* 1983–1992.

LEARNING OBJECTIVES

After studying this chapter, you will be able to:

1. List characteristics of diuretics in terms of mechanism of action, indications for use, principles of therapy, and nursing process implications.
2. Discuss major adverse effects of thiazide, loop, and potassium-sparing diuretics.
3. Identify patients at risk for developing adverse reactions to diuretic administration.
4. Recognize commonly used potassium-losing and potassium-sparing diuretics.
5. Discuss the rationale for using combination products containing a potassium-losing and a potassium-sparing diuretic.
6. Discuss the rationale for concomitant use of a loop diuretic and a thiazide or related diuretic.
7. Teach patients to manage diuretic therapy effectively.
8. Discuss important elements of diuretic therapy in special populations.

Applying Your Knowledge

Agnes Bass is a 68-year-old woman who has lower-leg edema. She is being treated with furosemide 40 mg PO daily.

Introduction

Diuretics are drugs that increase renal excretion of water, sodium, and other electrolytes, thereby increasing urine formation and output. They are important therapeutic agents widely used in the management of both edematous (e.g., heart failure, renal and hepatic disease) and nonedematous (e.g., hypertension, ophthalmic surgery) conditions. Diuretics are also useful in preventing renal failure by their ability to sustain urine flow. To aid understanding of diuretic drug therapy, renal physiology related to drug action and characteristics of edema are reviewed.

Renal Physiology

The primary function of the kidneys is to regulate the volume, composition, and pH of body fluids. The kidneys receive approximately 25% of the cardiac output. From this large amount of blood flow, the normally functioning kidney is efficient in retaining substances needed by the body and eliminating those not needed.

The Nephron

The *nephron* is the functional unit of the kidney; each kidney contains approximately 1 million nephrons. Each nephron is composed of a glomerulus and a tubule (Fig. 53-1). The glomerulus is a network of capillaries that receives blood from the renal artery. Bowman's capsule is a thin-walled structure that surrounds the glomerulus, then narrows and continues as the tubule. The tubule is a thin-walled structure of epithelial cells surrounded by peritubular capillaries. The tubule is divided into three main segments, the proximal tubule, loop of Henle, and distal tubule, which differ in structure and function. The tubules are often called *convoluted tubules* because of their many twists and turns. The convolutions provide a large surface area that brings the blood flowing through the peritubular capillaries and the glomerular filtrate flowing through the tubular lumen into close proximity. Consequently, substances can be readily exchanged through the walls of the tubules.

The nephron functions by three processes: glomerular filtration, tubular reabsorption, and tubular secretion. These processes normally maintain the fluid volume, electrolyte concentration, and pH of body fluids within a relatively narrow range. They also remove waste products of cellular metabolism. A minimum daily urine output of approximately 400 milliliters is required to remove normal amounts of metabolic end products.

Glomerular Filtration

Arterial blood enters the glomerulus by the afferent arteriole at the relatively high pressure of approximately 70 mm Hg. This pressure pushes water, electrolytes, and other solutes out of the capillaries into Bowman's capsule and then to the proximal tubule. This fluid, called *glomerular filtrate*, contains the same components as blood except for blood cells, fats, and proteins that are too large to be filtered.

The glomerular filtration rate (GFR) is about 180 liters per day, or 125 milliliters per minute. Most of this fluid is reabsorbed as the glomerular filtrate travels through the tubules. The end product is about 2 liters of urine daily. Because filtration is a nonselective process, the reabsorption and secretion processes determine the composition of the urine. After it is formed, urine flows into collecting tubules, which carry it to the renal pelvis, then through the ureters, bladder, and urethra for elimination from the body.

Blood that does not become part of the glomerular filtrate leaves the glomerulus through the efferent arteriole. The efferent arteriole branches into the peritubular capillaries that eventually empty into veins, which return the blood to systemic circulation.

Tubular Reabsorption

The term *reabsorption,* in relation to renal function, indicates movement of substances from the tubule (glomerular filtrate) to the blood in the peritubular capillaries. Most reabsorption occurs in the proximal tubule. Almost all glucose and amino acids are reabsorbed; about 80% of water, sodium, potassium, chloride, and most other substances is reabsorbed. As a result, about 20% of the glomerular filtrate enters the loop of Henle. In the descending limb of the loop of Henle, water is reabsorbed; in the ascending limb, sodium is reabsorbed. A large fraction of the total amount of sodium (up to 30%) filtered by the glomeruli is reabsorbed in the loop of Henle. Additional sodium is reabsorbed in the distal tubule, primarily by the exchange of sodium ions for potassium ions secreted by epithelial cells of tubular walls. Final reabsorption of water occurs in the distal tubule and small collecting tubules. The remaining water and solutes are now appropriately called urine.

Antidiuretic hormone from the posterior pituitary gland promotes reabsorption of water from the distal tubules and the

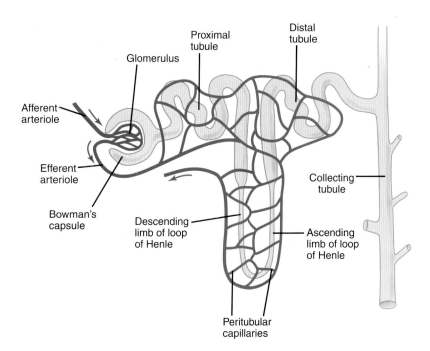

Figure 53-1 ■ The nephron is the functional unit of the kidney.

Glomerulus

Proximal tubule

Distal tubule

Afferent arteriole

Efferent arteriole

Bowman's capsule

Descending limb of loop of Henle

Peritubular capillaries

Collecting tubule

Ascending limb of loop of Henle

collecting ducts of the kidneys. This conserves water needed by the body and produces more concentrated urine. Aldosterone, a hormone from the adrenal cortex, promotes sodium–potassium exchange mainly in the distal tubule and collecting ducts. Thus, aldosterone promotes sodium reabsorption and potassium loss.

Tubular Secretion

The term *secretion*, in relation to renal function, indicates movement of substances from blood in the peritubular capillaries to glomerular filtrate flowing through the renal tubules. Secretion occurs in the proximal and distal tubules, across the epithelial cells that line the tubules. In the proximal tubule, uric acid, creatinine, hydrogen ions, and ammonia are secreted; in the distal tubule, potassium ions, hydrogen ions, and ammonia are secreted. Secretion of hydrogen ions is important in maintaining acid–base balance in body fluids.

Alterations in Renal Function

Many clinical conditions alter renal function. In some conditions, excessive amounts of substances (e.g., sodium, water) are retained; in others, needed substances (e.g., potassium, proteins) are eliminated. These conditions include cardiovascular, renal, hepatic, and other disorders that may be managed with diuretic drugs.

Edema

Edema is the excessive accumulation of fluid in body tissues. It is a symptom of many disease processes and may occur in any part of the body. Additional characteristics include the following:

- Edema formation results from one or more of the following mechanisms that allow fluid to leave the bloodstream (intravascular compartment) and enter interstitial (third) spaces:
  - Increased capillary permeability occurs as part of the response to tissue injury. Thus, edema may occur with burns and trauma or allergic and inflammatory reactions.
  - Increased capillary hydrostatic pressure results from a sequence of events in which increased blood volume (from fluid overload or sodium and water retention) or obstruction of venous blood flow causes a high venous pressure and a high capillary pressure. This is the primary mechanism for edema formation in heart failure, pulmonary edema, and renal failure.
  - Decreased plasma oncotic pressure may occur with decreased synthesis of plasma proteins (caused by liver disease or malnutrition) or increased loss of plasma proteins (caused by burn injuries or the nephrotic syndrome). Plasma proteins are important in keeping fluids within the bloodstream. When plasma proteins are lacking, fluid seeps through the capillaries and accumulates in tissues.
- Edema interferes with blood flow to tissues. Thus, it interferes with delivery of oxygen and nutrients and removal of

metabolic waste products. If severe, edema may distort body features, impair movement, and interfere with activities of daily living.

- Specific manifestations of edema are determined by its location and extent. A common type of localized edema occurs in the feet and ankles (dependent edema), especially with prolonged sitting or standing. A less common but more severe type of localized edema is pulmonary edema, a life-threatening condition that occurs with circulatory overload (e.g., of intravenous [IV] fluids, blood transfusions) or acute heart failure. Generalized massive edema (anasarca) interferes with the functions of many body organs and tissues.

General Characteristics of Diuretic Drugs

Diuretic drugs act on the kidneys to decrease reabsorption of sodium, chloride, water, and other substances. Major subclasses are the thiazides and related diuretics, loop diuretics, and potassium-sparing diuretics, which act at different sites in the nephron (Fig. 53-2).

Major clinical indications for diuretics are edema, heart failure, and hypertension. In edematous states, diuretics mobilize tissue fluids by decreasing plasma volume. In hypertension, the exact mechanism by which diuretics lower blood pressure is unknown, but antihypertensive action is usually attributed to sodium depletion. Initially, diuretics decrease blood volume and cardiac output. With chronic use, cardiac output returns to normal, but there is a persistent decrease in plasma volume and peripheral vascular resistance. Sodium depletion may have a vasodilating effect on arterioles.

The use of diuretic agents in the management of heart failure and hypertension is discussed further in Chapters 48 and 52, respectively. Types of diuretics are described in the following section, and individual drugs are listed in Table 53-1.

Types of Diuretics and Individual Drugs

Thiazide and Related Diuretics

Thiazide diuretics are synthetic drugs that are chemically related to the sulfonamides and differ mainly in their duration of action. **Hydrochlorothiazide** is the most commonly used; chlorothiazide is the only one that can be given IV. Related diuretics are nonthiazides whose pharmacologic actions are essentially the same as those of the thiazides; they include chlorthalidone, and metolazone.

Thiazides and related diuretics are frequently prescribed in the long-term management of heart failure and hypertension. They act to decrease reabsorption of sodium, water, chloride, and bicarbonate in the distal convoluted tubule. Most sodium

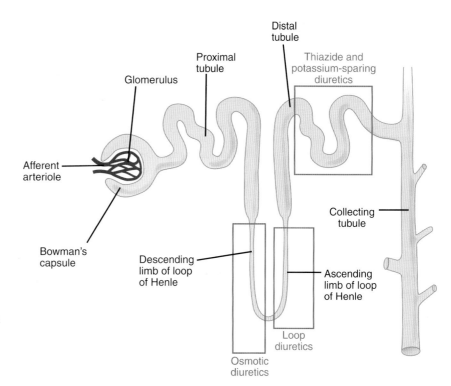

Figure 53-2 ■ Diuretic sties of action in the nephron. Diuretics act at different sites in the nephron to decrease reabsorption of sodium and water and to increase urine output.

is reabsorbed before it reaches the distal convoluted tubule and only a small amount is reabsorbed at this site. Thus, these drugs are not strong diuretics. In addition, they are ineffective when immediate diuresis is required (because of their slow onset of action) and relatively ineffective with decreased renal function. They work efficiently only when urine flow is adequate.

A dose of diuretic that yields a near-maximum diuretic response is called the *ceiling dose* or threshold. The ceiling dose is dependent on the type of diuretic and the extent of an individual's disease. Thiazide diuretics have a ceiling threshold. As the maximum effect is reached, a subsequent increase in dose does not enhance efficacy. In addition, there is a direct correlation between the dosage increase and the possible onset of adverse effects. When the diuretic dose is less than at ceiling, postdiuresis fluid retention results.

These drugs are well absorbed, widely distributed in body fluids, and highly bound to plasma proteins. They accumulate only in the kidneys. Diuretic effects usually occur within 2 hours, peak at 4 to 6 hours, and last 6 to 24 hours. Antihypertensive effects usually last long enough to allow use of a single daily dose. Most of the drugs are excreted unchanged by the kidneys within 3 to 6 hours; some (e.g., chlorthalidone) have longer durations of action (48–72 hours), attributed to slower excretion.

Thiazides and related drugs must be used cautiously in patients allergic to sulfonamide drugs as there is a known cross-sensitivity of some sulfonamide-allergic patients to a sulfonamide nonantibiotic. They must be used cautiously during pregnancy because they cross the placenta and may have adverse effects on the fetus by compromising placental perfusion.

Loop Diuretics

Loop diuretics inhibit sodium and chloride reabsorption in the ascending limb of the loop of Henle, where reabsorption of most filtered sodium occurs. Thus, these potent drugs produce significant diuresis, their sodium-losing effect being up to 10 times greater than that of thiazide diuretics. Dosage can be titrated upward as needed to produce greater diuretic effects. Overall, loop diuretics are the most effective and versatile diuretics available for clinical use.

Loop diuretics may be given orally or IV. After oral administration, diuretic effects occur within 30 to 60 minutes, peak in 1 to 2 hours, and last 6 to 8 hours. After IV administration, diuretic effects occur within 5 minutes, peak within 30 minutes, and last about 2 hours. Thus, the drugs produce extensive diuresis for short periods, after which the kidney tubules regain their ability to reabsorb sodium. Actually, the kidneys reabsorb more sodium than usual during this postdiuretic phase, so a high dietary intake of sodium can cause sodium retention and reduce or cancel the diuretic-induced sodium loss. Thus, dietary sodium restriction is required to achieve optimum therapeutic benefits. The drugs are metabolized and excreted by the kidneys, and drug accumulation does not occur even with repeated doses.

Loop diuretics are the diuretics of choice when rapid effects are required (e.g., in pulmonary edema) and when renal function is impaired (creatinine clearance < 30 mL/min). The drugs are contraindicated during pregnancy unless absolutely necessary. The pharmacologic characteristics of all loop diuretics are similar; use of another loop diuretic after a lack of response to one loop diuretic at adequate doses is not

Table 53-1	Drugs at a Glance: Diuretic Agents

	ROUTES AND DOSAGE RANGES	
Generic (trade) Name	**Adults**	**Children**
Thiazide and Related Diuretics		
Chlorothiazide (Diuril)	PO 500–2000 mg/d divided in 1 to 2 times doses Elderly, PO 500 mg once daily or 1 g 3 times/wk IV 250–1000 mg once or twice daily; maximum dose 1000 mg	PO 22 mg/kg/d in 2 divided doses Infants <6 mo, 20–40 mg/kg/d in 2 divided doses; maximum dose 375 mg/d IV dosing not well established
Chlorthalidone (Hygroton, Thalitone)	PO 25–100 mg/d Elderly, PO 12.5–25 mg/d or every other day	Not approved in children
Hydrochlorothiazide (Esidrix, Oretic)	Edema: PO 25–100 mg/d; maximum dose 200 mg/d Hypertension: PO 12.5–50 mg 1 or 2 times daily Elderly, PO 12.5–25 mg/d	PO 2 mg/kg/d in two divided doses Infants <6 mo, 2–3 mg/kg/d in 2 divided doses
Indapamide (Lozol)	Edema: PO 2.5–5 mg/d Hypertension: PO 1.25 mg in morning may increase to 5 mg/d	Dosage not established
Metolazone (Zaroxolyn)	Edema: PO 2.5–20 mg/d, depending on severity of condition and response Hypertension: 2.5 mg/d Elderly: 2.5 mg/d or every other day	Dosage not established
Loop Diuretics		
Bumetanide (Bumex)	PO 0.5–2 mg daily as a single dose. May be repeated q4–6h to a maximal dose of 10 mg, if necessary. Giving on alternate days or for 3–4 d with rest periods of 1–2 d is recommended for long-term control of edema. IV, IM 0.5–1 mg, repeated in 2–3 h if necessary, to a maximal daily dose of 10 mg. Give IV injections over 1–2 min.	Not recommended for children <18 y
Ethacrynic acid (Edecrin)	Edema, PO 50–100 mg daily, increased or decreased according to severity of condition and response. Maximal daily dose, 400 mg Rapid mobilization of edema, IV 50 mg or 0.5–1 mg/kg injected slowly to a maximum of 100 mg/dose	PO 25 mg daily No recommended parenteral dose in children
P **Furosemide** (Lasix)	Edema, PO 20–80 mg as a single dose initially. If an adequate diuretic response is not obtained, dosage may be gradually increased by 20- to 40-mg increments at intervals of 6–8 h. For maintenance, dosage range and frequency of administration vary widely and must be individualized. Maximal daily dose, 600 mg Hypertension, PO 40 mg twice daily, gradually increased if necessary Rapid mobilization of edema, IV 20–40 mg initially, injected slowly. This dose may be repeated in 2 h. With acute pulmonary edema, initial dose is usually 40 mg, which may be repeated in 60–90 min.	PO 2 mg/kg 1 or 2 times daily initially, gradually increased by increments of 1–2 mg/kg per dose if necessary at intervals of 6–8 h. Maximal daily dose, 6 mg/kg IV 1 mg/kg initially. If diuretic response is not adequate, increase dosage by 1 mg/kg no sooner than 2 h after previous dose. Maximal dose, 6 mg/kg

	ROUTES AND DOSAGE RANGES	
Generic (trade) Name	**Adults**	**Children**
	Acute renal failure, IV 40 mg initially, increased if necessary. Maximum dose, 1–2 g/24 h	
	Hypertensive crisis, IV 40–80 mg injected over 1–2 min. With renal failure, much larger doses may be needed.	
Torsemide (Demadex)	PO, IV 5–20 mg once daily	
Potassium-Sparing Diuretics		
Amiloride (Midamor)	PO 5–20 mg daily	Dosage not established
Spironolactone (Aldactone)	PO 25–200 mg daily	PO 3.3 mg/kg/d in divided doses
Triamterene (Dyrenium)	PO 100–300 mg daily in divided doses	PO 2–4 mg/kg/d in divided doses
Osmotic Agents		
Glycerin (Osmoglyn)	PO 1–1.5 g/kg of body weight, usually given as a 50% or 75% solution, 1–2 h before ocular surgery	Same as adults
Mannitol (Osmitrol)	Diuresis, IV infusion 50–200 g over 24 h, flow rate adjusted to maintain a urine output of 30–50 mL/h	Same as adults
	Oliguria and prevention of renal failure, IV 50–100 g	
	Reduction of intracranial or intraocular pressure, IV 1.5–2 g/kg, given as a 20% solution, over 30–60 min	

indicated. Instead, combining diuretics with different sites of action should be considered if aggressive diuresis is required.

P **Furosemide** is the most commonly used loop diuretic and serves as the prototype for the group. **Bumetanide** may be used to produce diuresis in some patients who are allergic to or no longer respond to furosemide. It is more potent than furosemide on a drug weight basis, and large doses can be given in small volumes. These drugs differ mainly in potency and produce similar effects at equivalent doses (e.g., furosemide 40 mg = bumetanide 1 mg).

Potassium-Sparing Diuretics

Sodium is normally reabsorbed in the distal tubule in exchange for potassium and hydrogen ions. *Potassium-sparing diuretics* act at the distal tubule to decrease sodium reabsorption and potassium excretion. This group includes three drugs. One is **spironolactone,** an aldosterone antagonist. Aldosterone is a hormone secreted by the adrenal cortex. It promotes retention of sodium and water and excretion of potassium by stimulating the sodium–potassium exchange mechanism in the distal tubule. Spironolactone blocks the sodium-retaining effects of aldosterone, and aldosterone must be present for spironolactone to be effective. The other two drugs, **amiloride** and **triamterene,** act directly on the distal tubule to decrease the exchange of sodium for potassium, and have similar diuretic activity.

Potassium-sparing diuretics are weak diuretics when used alone. Thus, they are usually given in combination with potassium-losing diuretics to increase diuretic activity and decrease potassium loss. They are contraindicated in the presence of renal insufficiency because their use may cause hyperkalemia through the inhibition of aldosterone and subsequent retention of potassium. Hyperkalemia is the major adverse effect of these drugs; patients receiving potassium-sparing diuretics should *not* be given potassium supplements and *should not be* encouraged to eat foods high in potassium or allowed to use salt substitutes. Salt substitutes contain potassium chloride rather than sodium chloride.

Osmotic Diuretics

Osmotic diuretics produce rapid diuresis by increasing the solute load (osmotic pressure) of the glomerular filtrate. The increased osmotic pressure causes water to be pulled from extravascular sites into the bloodstream, thereby increasing blood volume and decreasing reabsorption of water and electrolytes in the renal tubules. **Mannitol** is useful in managing oliguria or anuria, and it may prevent acute renal failure during prolonged surgery, trauma, or infusion of cisplatin, an antineoplastic agent. Mannitol is effective even when renal circulation and GFR are reduced (e.g., in hypovolemic shock, trauma, dehydration). Other important clinical uses of hyperosmolar agents include reduction of intracranial pressure before or after neurosurgery, reduction of intraocular pressure before certain types of ophthalmic surgery, and urinary excretion of toxic substances. Further information is found in Table 53-1.

Table 53-2	Drugs at a Glance: Combination Diuretic Products		
TRADE NAME	**THIAZIDE (POTASSIUM-LOSING) DIURETIC**	**POTASSIUM-SPARING DIURETIC**	**ADULT DOSAGE**
Aldactazide 25/25	HCTZ 25 mg	Spironolactone 25 mg	PO 1–8 tablets daily
Aldactazide 50/50	HCTZ 50 mg	Spironolactone 50 mg	PO 1–4 tablets daily
Dyazide, Maxzide 25 mg	HCTZ 25 mg	Triamterene 37.5 mg	Hypertension, PO 1 capsule bid initially, then adjusted according to response Edema, PO 1–2 capsules bid
Maxzide	HCTZ 50 mg	Triamterene 75 mg	PO 1 tablet daily
Moduretic	HCTZ 50 mg	Amiloride 5 mg	PO 1–2 tablets daily with meals

bid, twice a day; HCTZ, hydrochlorothiazide.

Combination Products

Thiazide and related diuretics are available in numerous fixed-dose combinations with nondiuretic antihypertensive agents (see Chap. 52) and with potassium-sparing diuretics (see Table 53-2 for combination diuretic products). A major purpose of the antihypertensive combinations is to increase patient convenience and compliance with drug therapy regimens. A major purpose of the diuretic combinations is to prevent potassium imbalances.

Applying Your Knowledge 53-1

While caring for Ms. Bass, she tells you that she enjoys snacks like potato chips and pretzels. What response would you have?

Applying Your Knowledge 53-2

Ms. Bass has spironolactone added to her treatment regimen to increase diuresis. Why was this added to her regimen instead of increasing her dose of furosemide?

Nursing Process

Assessment

Assess the patient's status in relation to baseline data and conditions in which diuretic drugs are used.

- Useful baseline data include serum electrolytes, creatinine, glucose, blood urea nitrogen (BUN), and uric acid, because diuretics may alter these values. Other data are

blood pressure readings, weight, amount and appearance of urine output, and measurement of edematous areas such as ankles or abdomen.

- Observe for edema. Visible edema often occurs in the feet and legs of ambulatory patients. Rapid weight gain may indicate fluid retention.

  - With heart failure, numerous signs and symptoms result from edema of various organs and tissues. For example, congestion in the gastrointestinal (GI) tract may cause nausea and vomiting; liver congestion may cause abdominal pain and tenderness; and congestion in the lungs (pulmonary edema) causes rapid, labored breathing; hypoxemia; frothy sputum; and other manifestations of severe respiratory distress.

  - Cerebral edema may be manifested by confusion, headache, dizziness, convulsions, unconsciousness, bradycardia, or failure of the pupils to react to light.

  - Ascites, which occurs with hepatic cirrhosis, is an accumulation of fluid in the abdominal cavity. The abdomen appears much enlarged.

- With heart failure, fatigue and dyspnea, in addition to edema, are common symptoms.

- Hypertension (blood pressure greater than 140/90 mm Hg on several measurements) may be the only clinical manifestation present.

Nursing Diagnoses

- Excess Fluid Volume in edematous patients, related to retention of sodium and water

- Deficient Fluid Volume related to increased diuresis during diuretic drug therapy

- Imbalanced Nutrition: Less Than Body Requirements related to excessive loss of potassium with thiazide and loop diuretics
- Risk for Injury: Hypotension and dizziness as adverse drug effects
- Deficient Knowledge related to the need for and correct use of diuretics
- Sexual Dysfunction related to adverse drug effects

Planning/Goals

The patient will

- Take or receive diuretic drugs as prescribed
- Experience reduced edema and improved control of blood pressure
- Reduce dietary intake of sodium and increase dietary intake of potassium
- Avoid preventable adverse drug effects
- Keep appointments for follow-up monitoring of blood pressure, edema, and serum electrolytes

Interventions

Promote measures to prevent or minimize conditions for which diuretic drugs are used.

- With edema, helpful measures include the following:
  - Decreasing dietary sodium intake
  - Losing weight, if obese
  - Elevating legs when sitting
  - Avoiding prolonged standing or sitting
  - Wearing support hose or elastic stockings
  - Treating the condition causing edema
- With heart failure and in older adults, administer IV fluids or blood transfusions carefully to avoid fluid overload and pulmonary edema. Fluid overload may occur with rapid administration or excessive amounts of IV fluids.
- With hypertension, helpful measures include decreasing dietary sodium intake, exercising regularly, and losing weight, if obese.
- With edematous patients, interventions to monitor fluid losses include weighing under standardized conditions, measuring urine output, and measuring edematous sites such as the ankles or the abdomen. After the patient reaches "dry weight," these measurements stabilize and can be done less often.
- With patients who are taking digoxin, a potassium-losing diuretic, and a potassium supplement, help them understand that the drugs act together to increase therapeutic effectiveness and avoid adverse effects (e.g., hypokalemia, digoxin toxicity). Thus, stopping or changing dosage of one of these drugs can lead to serious illness.

Provide patient teaching regarding drug therapy (see accompanying display).

Evaluation

- Observe for reduced edema and body weight.
- Observe for reduced blood pressure.
- Observe for increased urine output.
- Monitor serum electrolytes for normal values.
- Interview regarding compliance with instructions for diet and drug therapy.
- Monitor compliance with follow-up appointments in outpatients.

Principles of Therapy

Drug Selection

The choice of diuretic drug depends primarily on the patient's condition.

- **Thiazides and related diuretics** are the drugs of choice for most patients who require diuretic therapy, especially for long-term management of heart failure and hypertension. All the drugs in this group have similar effects. For most patients, hydrochlorothiazide is effective.
- A **loop diuretic** (e.g., furosemide) is preferred when rapid diuretic effects are required or when renal impairment is present.
- A **potassium-sparing diuretic** may be given concurrently with a potassium-losing diuretic to prevent or manage hypokalemia and to augment the diuretic effect. The two drugs can be given separately or in a fixed-dose combination product (see Table 53-2).
- Two **potassium-losing diuretics** are sometimes given concurrently when an inadequate diuretic response occurs with one of the drugs. The combination of a loop and a thiazide diuretic has synergistic effects because the drugs act in different segments of the renal tubule. The synergistic effects probably result from the increased delivery of sodium to the distal tubule (where thiazides act) because a loop diuretic blocks sodium reabsorption in the loop of Henle. A commonly used combination is furosemide and hydrochlorothiazide (chlorothiazide can be given IV in patients who are unable to take an oral drug). Furosemide and metolazone have also been used. Because a thiazide–loop diuretic combination can induce profound diuresis, with severe sodium, potassium, and volume depletion, its use should be reserved for hospitalized patients who can be closely monitored. If used for ambulatory patients, the thiazide diuretic should be given in very low doses or only occasionally to avoid serious adverse events.

Drug Dosage and Administration

Dosage of diuretics depends largely on the patient's condition and response and should be individualized to administer the minimal effective amount.

Patient Teaching Guidelines Diuretics

General Considerations

■ Diuretics increase urine output and are commonly used to manage hypertension, heart failure, and edema (swelling) from heart, kidney, liver, and other disorders.

■ While taking a diuretic drug, you need to maintain regular medical supervision so drug effects can be monitored and dosages adjusted when indicated.

■ Reducing sodium intake in your diet helps diuretic drugs be more effective and allows smaller doses to be taken. Smaller doses are less likely to cause adverse effects. Thus, you need to avoid excessive table salt and obviously salty foods (e.g., ham, packaged sandwich meats, potato chips, dill pickles, most canned soups). These foods may aggravate edema or hypertension by causing sodium and water retention.

■ Diuretics may cause blood potassium imbalances, and either too little or too much damages heart function. Periodic measurements of blood potassium and other substances is one of the major reasons for regular visits to a health care provider.

Too little potassium (hypokalemia) may result from the use of potassium-losing diuretics such as hydrochlorothiazide, furosemide (Lasix), and several others. To prevent or treat hypokalemia, your doctor may prescribe a potassium chloride supplement or a combination of a potassium-losing and a potassium-saving diuretic (either separately or as a combined product such as Dyazide, Maxzide, or Aldactazide). He or she may also recommend increased dietary intake of potassium-containing foods (e.g., bananas, orange juice).

Too much potassium (hyperkalemia) can result from the use of potassium-saving diuretics, the overuse of potassium supplements, or from the use of salt substitutes. Potassium-saving diuretics are not a major cause of hyperkalemia because they are usually given along with a potassium-losing diuretic. If potassium supplements are prescribed, they should be taken as directed. You should **not** use salt substitutes without consulting your primary health care provider because they contain potassium chloride instead of sodium chloride. Hyperkalemia is most likely to occur in people with decreased kidney function, which often occurs in older adults and people with diabetes.

■ With diuretic therapy, you will have increased urination, which usually lasts only a few days or weeks if you do not have edema. If you do have edema (e.g., in your ankles), you can expect weight loss and decreased swelling as well as increased urination. It is a good idea to check and record your weight 2 to 3 times per week (at same time of day with similar amount of clothing). Rapid changes in weight often indicate gain or loss of fluid.

■ Some commonly used diuretics may increase blood sugar levels and cause or aggravate diabetes. If you have diabetes, you may need larger doses of your antidiabetic medications.

■ Diuretics may cause sensitivity to sunlight. Thus, you need to avoid prolonged exposure to sunlight, use sunscreens, and wear protective clothing.

■ Do not drink alcoholic beverages or take other medications without the approval of your health care provider.

■ If you are taking a diuretic to lower your blood pressure, especially with other antihypertensive drugs, you may feel dizzy or faint when you stand up suddenly. This can be prevented or decreased by changing positions slowly. If dizziness is severe, notify your health care provider.

Self- or Caregiver Administration

■ Take or give a diuretic early in the day, if ordered daily, to decrease nighttime trips to the bathroom. Fewer bathroom trips means less interference with sleep and less risk of falls. Ask someone to help you to the bathroom if you are elderly, weak, dizzy, or unsteady in walking (or use a bedside commode).

■ Take or give most diuretics with or after food to decrease stomach upset. Torsemide (Demadex) may be taken without regard to meals.

■ If you are taking digoxin, a potassium-losing diuretic, and a potassium supplement, it is very important that you take these drugs as prescribed. This is a common combination of drugs for patients with heart failure and the drugs work together to increase beneficial effects and avoid adverse effects. Stopping or changing the dose of one of these medications while continuing the others can lead to serious illness.

■ With hydrochlorothiazide, smaller doses (e.g., 12.5–25 mg daily) are effective for most people and produce fewer adverse effects (e.g., hypokalemia) than larger doses. Some of the fixed-dose combinations of hydrochlorothiazide and a potassium-sparing diuretic contain 50 mg of hydrochlorothiazide. As a result, despite the convenience of a combination product, it may be better to give the drugs separately so that dosage can be titrated to the patient's needs.

■ Patients who do not achieve an adequate diuretic response with usual doses of an oral drug may need larger doses or an IV drug.

■ With torsemide, which is highly bioavailable after oral administration, oral and IV doses are equivalent and patients may be switched from one route to the other without changing dosage.

■ In liver disease, small doses of all diuretics are usually indicated because diuretic-induced electrolyte imbalances may precipitate or aggravate hepatic coma.

■ In renal disease, furosemide is often given in large doses to achieve a diuretic response. Bumetanide may be a useful alternative, because it can be given in smaller dose volumes.

■ When metolazone is given concurrently with furosemide, the initial dose is usually metolazone 2.5 to 10 mg. The dose is then doubled every 24 hours until the desired response is achieved. If an adequate diuretic effect occurs with the first dose of metolazone, the dose of furosemide can be decreased. Hydrochlorothiazide 50 mg may also be used with furosemide and may be safer than metolazone because of its shorter duration of action.

Use in Edema

When diuretics are used to manage patients with edema, the underlying cause of the edema should be addressed, not just the edema itself. When treating such patients, it is preferable to aim for a weight loss of approximately 2 pounds (1 kg) per day. Rapid and excessive diuresis may cause dehydration and decreased blood volume with circulatory collapse. In some patients, giving a diuretic every other day or 3 to 5 days per week may be effective and is less likely to cause electrolyte imbalances.

Use With Digoxin

When digoxin and diuretics are given concomitantly, as is common for patients with heart failure, the risk of digoxin toxicity is increased. Digoxin toxicity is related to diuretic-induced hypokalemia. Potassium is a myocardial depressant and antidysrhythmic; it has essentially opposite cardiac effects to those of digoxin. In other words, extracellular potassium decreases the excitability of myocardial tissue, but digoxin increases excitability. The higher the serum potassium, the less effective a given dose of digoxin will be. Conversely, decreased serum potassium increases the likelihood of digoxin-induced cardiac dysrhythmias, even with small doses and therapeutic serum levels of digoxin.

Supplemental potassium chloride, a potassium-sparing diuretic, and other measures to prevent hypokalemia are often used to maintain normal serum potassium levels (3.5–5.0 mEq/L).

Prevention and Management of Potassium Imbalances

Potassium imbalances (see Chap. 57) may occur with diuretic therapy. Hypokalemia and hyperkalemia are cardiotoxic and should be prevented when possible.

- *Hypokalemia* (serum potassium level < 3.5 mEq/L) may occur with potassium-losing diuretics (e.g., hydrochlorothiazide, furosemide). Measures to prevent or manage hypokalemia include the following:

  - Giving low doses of the diuretic (e.g., 12.5–25 mg daily of hydrochlorothiazide)

  - Giving supplemental potassium, usually potassium chloride, in an average dosage range of 20 to 60 mEq daily. Sustained-release tablets are usually better tolerated than liquid preparations.

  - Giving a potassium-sparing diuretic along with the potassium-losing drug

  - Increasing food intake of potassium. Many texts advocate this approach as preferable to supplemental potassium or combination diuretic therapy, but its effectiveness is not clearly established. Although the minimal daily requirement of potassium is unknown, usual recommendations are 40 to 50 mEq daily for the healthy adult. Potassium loss with diuretic drugs may be several times this amount.

Some foods (e.g., bananas) have undeserved reputations for having high potassium content; actually, large amounts must be ingested. To provide 50 mEq of potassium daily, estimated amounts of certain foods include 1000 milliliters of orange juice, 1600 milliliters of apple or grape juice, 1200 milliliters of pineapple juice, four to six bananas, or 30 to 40 prunes. Some of these foods are high in calories and may be contraindicated, at least in large amounts, for obese patients. Also, the amount of carbohydrate in these foods may be a concern for patients with diabetes mellitus.

- Restricting dietary sodium intake. This reduces potassium loss by decreasing the amount of sodium available for exchange with potassium in renal tubules.

- *Hyperkalemia* (serum potassium level > 5 mEq/L) may occur with potassium-sparing diuretics. The following measures help prevent hyperkalemia:

  - Avoiding use of potassium-sparing diuretics and potassium supplements in patients with renal impairment

  - Avoiding excessive amounts of potassium chloride supplements

  - Avoiding salt substitutes

  - Maintaining urine output, the major route for eliminating potassium from the body

Use in Special Populations

Use in Children

Although they have not been extensively studied in children, diuretics are commonly used to manage heart failure, which often results from congenital heart disease; hypertension, which is usually related to cardiac or renal dysfunction; bronchopulmonary dysplasia and respiratory distress syndrome, which are often associated with pulmonary edema; and edema, which may occur with cardiac or renal disorders such as the nephrotic syndrome.

With most thiazides, safety and effectiveness have not been established for use in children. Hydrochlorothiazide is used in doses of approximately 2.2 milligrams per kilogram of body weight per day. IV chlorothiazide usually is not recommended. Thiazides do not commonly cause hyperglycemia, hyperuricemia, or hypercalcemia in children, as they do in adults.

Although metolazone, a thiazide-related drug, is not usually recommended, it is sometimes used. Metolazone has some advantages over a thiazide because it is a stronger diuretic, causes less hypokalemia, and can produce diuresis in renal failure. In children, it is most often used with furosemide, in which case it is most effective when given 30 to 60 minutes before the furosemide.

Furosemide is the loop diuretic used most often in children. Oral therapy is preferred when feasible, and doses above 6 milligrams per kilogram of body weight per day are not recommended. In preterm infants, furosemide stimulates production of prostaglandin E_2 in the kidneys and may increase the incidence of patent ductus arteriosus and neonatal respiratory distress syndrome. In neonates, furosemide may be given with indomethacin to prevent nonsteroidal anti-inflammatory drug–induced nephrotoxicity during therapeutic closure of a patent ductus arteriosus. In both preterm and full-term infants, furosemide half-life is prolonged but becomes shorter as renal and hepatic functions develop.

Adverse effects of furosemide include fluid and electrolyte imbalances (e.g., hyponatremia, hypokalemia, fluid volume deficit) and ototoxicity. Serum electrolytes should be closely monitored in children because of frequent changes in kidney function and fluid distribution associated with growth and development. Ototoxicity, which is associated with high plasma drug levels (>50 mcg/mL), can usually be avoided by dividing oral doses and by slow injection or continuous infusion of IV doses.

Safety and effectiveness of bumetanide and torsemide have not been established. However, bumetanide may cause less ototoxicity and thus may be preferred for children who are taking other *ototoxic* drugs (e.g., premature and ill neonates are often given gentamicin, an aminoglycoside antibiotic). Bumetanide may also cause less hypokalemia. The half-life of bumetanide is about 2 hours in critically ill infants and 1 hour in children.

Spironolactone is the most widely used potassium-sparing diuretic in children. It is used with other diuretics to decrease potassium loss and hypokalemia. Spironolactone accumulates in renal failure, and dosage should be reduced. It usually should not be used in severe renal failure.

Use in Older Adults

Thiazide diuretics are often prescribed for the management of hypertension and heart failure, which are common in older adults. Older adults are especially sensitive to adverse drug effects, such as hypotension and electrolyte imbalance. Thiazides may aggravate renal or hepatic impairment. With rapid or excessive diuresis, myocardial infarction, renal impairment, or cerebral thrombosis may occur from fluid volume depletion and hypotension. The smallest effective dose is recommended, usually a daily dose of 12.5 to 25 milligrams of hydrochlorothiazide or equivalent doses of other thiazides and related drugs. Risks of adverse effects may exceed benefits at doses of hydrochlorothiazide greater than 25 milligrams.

With loop diuretics, older adults are at greater risk of excessive diuresis, hypotension, fluid volume deficit, and possibly thrombosis or embolism. Rapid diuresis may cause urinary incontinence. With potassium-sparing diuretics, hyperkalemia is more likely to occur in older adults because of the renal impairment that occurs with aging.

Use in Patients With Renal Impairment

Most patients with renal impairment require diuretics as part of their drug therapy regimens. In these patients, the diuretic response may be reduced and edema of the GI tract may limit absorption of oral medications.

Thiazides may be useful in managing edema due to renal disorders such as nephrotic syndrome and acute glomerulonephritis. However, their effectiveness decreases as the GFR decreases, and the drugs become ineffective when the GFR is less than 30 milliliters per minute. The drugs may accumulate and increase adverse effects in patients with impaired renal function. Thus, renal function tests should be performed periodically. If progressive renal impairment becomes evident (e.g., a rising serum creatinine or BUN), a thiazide usually should be discontinued and metolazone, indapamide, or a loop diuretic may be given. Metolazone and indapamide are thiazide-related diuretics that may be effective in patients with significantly impaired renal function.

Loop diuretics are effective in patients with renal impairment. However, in chronic renal failure, they have lower peak concentrations at their site of action, which decreases diuresis. Renal elimination of the drugs is also prolonged. If renal dysfunction becomes more severe during treatment (e.g., oliguria, increases in BUN or creatinine), the diuretic may need to be discontinued. If high doses of furosemide are used, a volume-controlled IV infusion at a rate of 4 milligrams or less per minute may be used. For continuous infusion, furosemide should be mixed with normal saline or lactated Ringer's solution because D5W may accelerate degradation of furosemide. If IV bumetanide is given to patients with chronic renal impairment, a continuous infusion (e.g., 12 mg over 12 hours) produces more diuresis than equivalent-dose intermittent injections. Continuous infusion also produces lower serum drug levels and therefore may decrease adverse effects.

Potassium-sparing diuretics are contraindicated in patients with renal impairment because of the high risk of hyperkalemia. If they are used at all, frequent monitoring of serum electrolytes, creatinine, and BUN is needed.

Use in Patients With Hepatic Impairment

Diuretics are often used to manage edema and ascites in patients with hepatic impairment. These drugs must be used with caution because diuretic-induced fluid and electrolyte imbalances may precipitate or worsen hepatic encephalopathy and coma. In patients with cirrhosis, diuretic therapy should be initiated in a hospital setting, with small doses and careful monitoring. To prevent hypokalemia and metabolic alkalosis, supplemental potassium or spironolactone may be needed.

Use in Patients With Critical Illness

Fast-acting, potent diuretics such as furosemide and bumetanide are the most likely diuretics to be used in critically ill patients (e.g., those with pulmonary edema). In patients with severe renal impairment, high doses are required to produce diuresis. Large doses may produce fluid volume depletion and worsen renal function. Although IV bolus doses of the drugs are often given, continuous IV infusions may be more effective and less likely to produce adverse effects in critically ill patients.

Use in Home Care

Diuretics are often taken in the home setting. The home care nurse may need to assist patients and caregivers in using the drugs safely and effectively, monitor patient responses (e.g., with each home visit, assess nutritional status, blood pressure, weight, use of over-the-counter medications that may aggravate edema or hypertension), and provide information as indicated. In some cases, the home care nurse may need to assist the patient in obtaining medications or blood for blood tests (e.g., serum potassium levels).

Nursing Actions Diuretics

NURSING ACTIONS	RATIONALE/EXPLANATION
1. Administer accurately	
a. Give in the early morning if ordered daily.	So that peak action will occur during waking hours and not interfere with sleep
b. Take safety precautions. Keep a bedpan or urinal within reach. Keep the call light within reach, and be sure the patient knows how to use it. Assist to the bathroom anyone who is elderly, weak, dizzy, or unsteady in walking.	Mainly to avoid falls
c. Give amiloride and triamterene with or after food.	To decrease gastrointestinal (GI) upset
d. Give intravenous (IV) injections of furosemide and bumetanide over 1–2 minutes; give torsemide over 2 minutes.	To decrease or avoid high peak serum levels, which increase risks of adverse effects, including ototoxicity
e. Give high-dose furosemide continuous IV infusions at a rate of 4 mg/min or less.	To decrease or avoid high peak serum levels, which increase risks of adverse effects, including ototoxicity
2. Observe for therapeutic effects	
a. Decrease or absence of edema, increased urine output, decreased blood pressure	Most oral diuretics act within 2 hours; IV diuretics act within minutes. Optimal antihypertensive effects occur in approximately 2–4 weeks.
(1) Weigh the patient daily while edema is present and two to three times weekly thereafter. Weigh under standard conditions: early morning before eating or drinking, after urination, with the same amount of clothing, and using the same scales.	Body weight is a very good indicator of fluid gain or loss. A weight change of 2.2 lb (1 kg) may indicate a gain or loss of 1000 mL of fluid. Also, weighing assists in dosage regulation to maintain therapeutic benefit without excessive or too rapid fluid loss.
(2) Record fluid intake and output every shift for hospitalized patients.	Normally, oral fluid intake approximates urinary output (1500 mL/24 h). With diuretic therapy, urinary output may exceed intake, depending on the amount of edema or fluid retention, renal function, and diuretic dosage. All sources of fluid gain, including IV fluids, must be included; all sources of fluid loss (perspiration, fever, wound drainage, GI tract drainage) are important. Patients with abnormal fluid losses have less urine output with diuretic therapy. Oliguria (decreased excretion of urine) may require stopping the drug. Output greater than 100 mL/h may indicate that side effects are more likely to occur.
(3) Observe and record characteristics of urine.	Dilute urine may indicate excessive fluid intake or greater likelihood of fluid and electrolyte imbalance due to rapid diuresis. Concentrated urine may mean oliguria or decreased fluid intake.
(4) Assess for edema daily or with each patient contact: ankles for the ambulatory patient, sacral area and posterior thighs for patients at bed rest. Also, it is often helpful to measure abdominal girth, ankles, and calves to monitor gain or loss of fluid.	Expect a decrease in visible edema and size of measured areas. If edema reappears or worsens, a thorough reassessment of the patient is in order. Questions to be answered include: (1) Is the prescribed diuretic being taken correctly? (2) What type of diuretic and what dosage is ordered? (3) Is there worsening of the underlying condition(s) that led to edema formation? (4) Has other disease developed?
(5) In patients with heart failure or acute pulmonary edema, observe for decreased dyspnea, crackles, cyanosis, and cough.	Decreased fluid in the lungs leads to improved respirations as more carbon dioxide and oxygen gas exchange takes place and greater tissue oxygenation occur.

(continued on page 857)

Nursing Actions **Diuretics** (continued)

NURSING ACTIONS	RATIONALE/EXPLANATION
(6) Record blood pressure 2 to 4 times daily when diuretic therapy is initiated.	Although thiazide diuretics do not lower normal blood pressure, other diuretics may, especially with excessive or rapid diuresis.
3. Observe for adverse effects	Major adverse effects are fluid and electrolyte imbalances.
a. With potassium-losing diuretics (thiazides, bumetanide, furosemide), observe for:	
(1) Hypokalemia (a) Serum potassium levels below 3.5 mEq/L (b) Electrocardiographic (ECG) changes (e.g., low voltage, flattened T wave, depressed ST segment) (c) Cardiac dysrhythmias; weak, irregular pulse (d) Hypotension (e) Weak, shallow respirations (f) Anorexia, nausea, vomiting (g) Decreased peristalsis or paralytic ileus (h) Skeletal muscle weakness (i) Confusion, disorientation	Potassium is required for normal muscle function. Thus, potassium depletion causes weakness of cardiovascular, respiratory, digestive, and skeletal muscles. Patients most likely to have hypokalemia are those who are taking large doses of diuretics, potent diuretics (e.g., furosemide), or adrenal corticosteroids; those who have decreased food and fluid intake; or those who have increased potassium losses through vomiting, diarrhea, chronic laxative or enema use, or GI suction. Clinically significant symptoms are most likely to occur with a serum potassium level below 3 mEq/L.
(2) Hyponatremia, hypomagnesemia, hypochloremic alkalosis, changes in serum and urinary calcium levels	In addition to potassium, sodium chloride, magnesium, and bicarbonate also are lost with diuresis. Thiazides and related diuretics cause hypercalcemia and hypocalciuria. They have been used to prevent calcium nephrolithiasis (kidney stones). Furosemide and other loop diuretics tend to cause hypocalcemia and hypercalciuria.
(3) Dehydration (a) Poor skin turgor, dry mucous membranes (b) Oliguria, urine of high specific gravity (c) Thirst (d) Tachycardia; hypotension (e) Decreased level of consciousness (f) Elevated hematocrit (above 45%)	Fluid volume depletion occurs with excessive or rapid diuresis. If it is prolonged or severe, hypovolemic shock may occur.

(4) Hyperglycemia—blood glucose above 120 mg/100 mL, polyuria, polydipsia, polyphagia, glycosuria	Hyperglycemia is more likely to occur in patients with known or latent diabetes mellitus. Larger doses of hypoglycemic agents may be required. The hyperglycemic effect may be reversible when diuretic therapy is discontinued.
	   Long-term use of a thiazide or loop diuretic may alter glucose metabolism. One mechanism is thought to involve diuretic-induced hypokalemia and hypomagnesemia, which then leads to decreased postprandial insulin release. Another mechanism may be development or worsening of insulin resistance.
	   Because glucose intolerance is an important risk factor for coronary artery disease, diuretics should be used with caution in prediabetic or diabetic hypertensive patients.

(5) Hyperuricemia—serum uric acid above 7.0 mg/100 mL	Hyperuricemia is usually asymptomatic except for patients with gout, a predisposition toward gout, or chronic renal failure. Apparently, decreased renal excretion of uric acid allows its accumulation in the blood.
(6) Pulmonary edema (with osmotic diuretics)	Pulmonary edema is most likely to occur in patients with heart failure who cannot tolerate the increased blood volume produced by the drugs.
(7) Ototoxicity (with furosemide and ethacrynic acid)	Reversible or transient hearing impairment, tinnitus, and dizziness are more common, although irreversible deafness may occur. Ototoxicity is more likely to occur with high serum drug levels (e.g., high doses or use in patients with severe renal impairment) or when other ototoxic drugs (e.g., aminoglycoside antibiotics) are being taken concurrently.
b. With potassium-sparing diuretics (spironolactone, triamterene, amiloride), observe for: (1) Hyperkalemia (a) Serum potassium levels above 5 mEq/L	Hyperkalemia is most likely to occur in patients with impaired renal function or those who are ingesting additional potassium (e.g., salt substitutes).

NURSING ACTIONS	RATIONALE/EXPLANATION
(b) ECG changes (i.e., prolonged P-R interval; wide QRS complex; tall, peaked T wave; depressed ST segment) (c) Cardiac dysrhythmias, which may progress to ventricular fibrillation and asystole	

4. Observe for drug interactions
  a. Drugs that *increase* effects of diuretics:
    (1) Aminoglycoside antibiotics
    (2) Antihypertensive agents
	Additive ototoxicity with ethacrynic acid
	
	Additive hypotensive effects. In addition, angiotensin-converting enzyme inhibitor therapy significantly increases risks of hyperkalemia with spironolactone.

(3) Corticosteroids
  b. Drugs that *decrease* effects of diuretics:
    (1) Nonsteroidal anti-inflammatory drugs (e.g., aspirin, ibuprofen, others)
    (2) Oral contraceptives
    (3) Vasopressors (e.g., epinephrine, norepinephrine)
	Additive hypokalemia
	
	These drugs cause retention of sodium and water.
	
	Retention of sodium and water
	These drugs may antagonize hypotensive effects of diuretics by decreasing responsiveness of arterioles.

Key Concepts

- Diuretic drugs act on the kidneys to decrease reabsorption of sodium, chloride, water, and other substances.

- A body weight change of 2.2 pounds (1 kg) may indicate a gain or loss of 1000 mL of fluid.

- Excessive table salt and salty foods (e.g., ham, packaged sandwich meats, potato chips, dill pickles, most canned soups) may aggravate edema or hypertension.

- Loop diuretics have a sodium-losing effect up to 10 times greater than that of thiazide diuretics.

- Potassium-sparing diuretics are contraindicated in patients with renal impairment because of the high risk of hyperkalemia.

- There is a known cross-sensitivity of some sulfonamide-allergic patients to a sulfonamide nonantibiotic, such as thiazides.

- Thiazides and related diuretics are the drugs of choice for most patients who require diuretic therapy, especially for long-term management of heart failure and hypertension.

- High-dose furosemide continuous IV infusions should be given at a rate of 4 mg/min or less to decrease or avoid risks of adverse effects, including ototoxicity.

- When digoxin and diuretics are given concomitantly, the risk of digoxin toxicity is increased due to diuretic-induced hypokalemia.

Review and Application Exercises

Short Answer Exercises

1. What are clinical indications for the use of diuretics?

2. What is the general mechanism by which diuretics act?

3. How can you assess a patient for therapeutic effects of a diuretic?

4. Compare and contrast the main groups of diuretics in terms of adverse effects.

5. Why should serum potassium levels be monitored during diuretic therapy?

6. Which prescription and over-the-counter drugs may decrease the effects of a diuretic?

7. For a patient who is starting diuretic therapy, what are important points to teach the patient about safe and effective drug usage?

8. For a patient who is taking a potassium-losing diuretic and a potassium chloride supplement, explain the possible consequences of discontinuing one drug while continuing the other.

NCLEX-Style Questions

9. A patient receives furosemide 80 mg IV for symptoms of severe heart failure. The nurse recognizes that administering the drug slowly IV push will reduce the likelihood of which of the following adverse effects of drug therapy?
   a. hyponatremia
   b. hypokalemia
   c. fluid volume deficit
   d. ototoxicity

10. A patient who is taking an oral hypoglycemic for management of his type 2 diabetes mellitus is started on hydrochlorothiazide. The nurse should monitor for which of the following serum laboratory changes?
    a. hypocalcemia
    b. hypercalciuria
    c. hyperglycemia
    d. hypernatremia

11. A nurse is instructing a patient on dietary considerations while taking spironolactone (Aldactone). Which of the following statements made by the patient indicates that further teaching is necessary?
    a. "I should not eat foods high in potassium while taking this medication."
    b. "I should use a salt substitute instead of regular salt."
    c. "I should call my nurse practitioner if I have any significant adverse effects from my medications."
    d. "I should not take large amounts of potassium chloride supplements."

12. What assessment finding in a patient with heart failure receiving furosemide (Lasix) would indicate an improvement in her fluid volume status?
    a. absence of crackles on auscultation of lungs
    b. complaints of proximal nocturnal dyspnea
    c. bounding radial pulse
    d. decrease in hematocrit

13. Mrs. Conley, age 53, has had hypertension for 10 years and admits that she does not comply with her prescribed antihypertensive therapy. Recently, she has begun to experience shortness of breath and ankle swelling. The nurse practitioner diagnoses renal insufficiency. What classification of diuretic is the drug of choice for the nurse practitioner to first prescribe for Mrs. Conley?
    a. thiazide
    b. loop
    c. osmotic
    d. potassium-sparing

Selected References

Drug facts and comparisons. (Updated monthly). St. Louis, MO: Facts and Comparisons.

Ferri, F. F. (2007). *Practical guide to the care of the medical patient* (7th ed.). Philadelphia: Elsevier Mosby.

Gabardi, S. (2005). Drug dosing in chronic kidney disease. *Medical Clinics of North America, 89*, 649–687.

Karch, A. M. (2007). 2008 *Lippincott's nursing drug guide*. Philadelphia: Lippincott Williams & Wilkins.

Lacy, C. F., Armstrong, L. L., Goldman, M. P., & Lance, L. L. (2007). *Lexi-Comp's drug information handbook* (15th ed.). Hudson, OH: American Pharmaceutical Association.

Porth, C. M. (2005). *Pathophysiology: Concepts of altered health states* (7th ed.). Philadelphia: Lippincott Williams & Wilkins.

Sica, D. A. (2007). Use of diuretics in the treatment of heart failure in the elderly. *Clinics in Geriatric Medicine, 23*, 107–121.

Drugs That Affect Blood Coagulation

KEY TERMS

- Anticoagulant
- Antiplatelet
- Embolus
- Fibrinolysin
- Hemostasis
- Plasmin
- Plasminogen
- Thrombogenesis
- Thrombolysis
- Thrombolytic
- Thrombus

LEARNING OBJECTIVES

After studying this chapter, you will be able to:

1. Describe important elements in the physiology of hemostasis and thrombosis.
2. Discuss potential consequences of blood clotting disorders.
3. Compare and contrast heparin and warfarin in terms of indications for use, onset and duration of action, route of administration, blood tests used to monitor effects, and nursing process implications.
4. Discuss antiplatelet agents in terms of indications for use and effects on blood coagulation.
5. Describe thrombolytic agents in terms of indications and contraindications for use, routes of administration, and major adverse effects.
6. Describe systemic hemostatic agents for treating overdoses of anticoagulant and thrombolytic drugs.
7. Use the nursing process in the care of patients on anticoagulant, antiplatelet, and thrombolytic agents.

Applying Your Knowledge

Andrew Dusseau is a 45-year-old man who has suffered an acute myocardial infarction with the complication of atrial fibrillation. He is started on a heparin IV. You are the nurse providing his care.

Introduction

Anticoagulant, antiplatelet, and thrombolytic drugs are used in the prevention and management of thrombotic and thromboembolic disorders. Thrombosis involves the formation (*thrombogenesis*) or presence of a blood clot (*thrombus*) in the vascular system. Blood clotting is a normal body defense mechanism to prevent blood loss. Thus, thrombogenesis may be life saving when it occurs as a response to hemorrhage; however, it may be life threatening when it occurs at other times, because the thrombus can obstruct a blood vessel and block blood flow to tissues beyond the clot. When part of a thrombus breaks off and travels to another part of the body, it is called an *embolus*.

Atherosclerosis is the basic disease process that often leads to pathologic thrombosis. Atherosclerosis begins with accumulation of lipid-filled macrophages (i.e., foam cells) on the inner lining of arteries. Foam cells develop in response to elevated blood lipid levels and eventually become fibrous plaques (i.e., foam cells covered by smooth muscle cells and connective tissue). Advanced atherosclerotic lesions also contain hemorrhages, ulcerations, and scar tissue.

Atherosclerosis can affect any organ or tissue but often involves the arteries supplying the heart, brain, and legs. Over time, plaque lesions become larger and extend farther into the lumen of the artery. Eventually, a thrombus may develop at plaque sites and partially or completely occlude an artery. In coronary arteries, a thrombus may precipitate myocardial ischemia (angina or infarction) (see Chap. 50); in carotid or cerebral arteries, a thrombus may precipitate a stroke; in peripheral arteries, a thrombus in peripheral circulation may cause intermittent claudication (pain in the legs with exercise) or acute occlusion. Thus, serious impairment of blood flow may occur with a large atherosclerotic plaque or a relatively small plaque with superimposed vasospasm and thrombosis. Consequences and clinical manifestations of thrombi and emboli depend primarily on their location and size.

Normally, thrombi are constantly being formed and dissolved (*thrombolysis*), but the blood remains fluid and flow is not significantly obstructed. If the balance between thrombogenesis and thrombolysis is upset, thrombotic or bleeding disorders result. Thrombotic disorders occur much more often than bleeding disorders and are emphasized in this chapter; bleeding disorders may result from excessive amounts of drugs that inhibit clotting. To aid understanding of drug therapy for thrombotic disorders, normal hemostasis, endothelial functions in relation to blood clotting, platelet functions, blood coagulation, and characteristics of arterial and venous thrombosis are described.

Hemostasis

Hemostasis is prevention or stoppage of blood loss from an injured blood vessel and is the process that maintains the integrity of the vascular compartment. It involves activation of several mechanisms, including vasoconstriction, formation of a platelet plug (a cluster of aggregated platelets), sequential activation of clotting factors in the blood (Fig. 54-1), and growth of fibrous tissue (fibrin) into the blood clot to make it more stable and to repair the tear (opening) in the damaged blood vessel. Overall, normal hemostasis is a complex process involving numerous interacting activators and inhibitors, including endothelial factors, platelets, and blood coagulation factors (Box 54-1).

Clot Lysis

When a blood clot is being formed, *plasminogen* (an inactive protein found in many body tissues and fluids) is bound to fibrin and becomes a component of the clot. After the outward blood flow is stopped and the tear in the blood vessel is repaired, plasminogen is activated by plasminogen activator (produced by endothelial cells or the coagulation cascade) to produce plasmin. *Plasmin* is an enzyme that breaks down the fibrin meshwork that stabilizes the clot; this fibrinolytic or thrombolytic action dissolves the clot.

Thrombotic and Thromboembolic Disorders

Thrombosis may occur in both arteries and veins. Arterial thrombosis is usually associated with atherosclerotic plaque, hypertension, and turbulent blood flow. These conditions damage arterial endothelium and activate platelets to initiate the coagulation process. Arterial thrombi cause disease by obstructing blood flow. If the obstruction is incomplete or temporary, local tissue ischemia (deficient blood supply) occurs. If the obstruction is complete or prolonged, local tissue death (infarction) occurs.

Venous thrombosis is usually associated with venous stasis. When blood flows slowly, thrombin and other procoagulant substances present in the blood become concentrated in local areas and initiate the clotting process. With a normal rate of blood flow, these substances are rapidly removed from the blood, primarily by Kupffer's cells in the liver. A venous thrombus is less cohesive than an arterial thrombus, and an embolus can easily become detached and travel to other parts of the body.

Venous thrombi cause disease by two mechanisms. First, thrombosis causes local congestion, edema, and perhaps inflammation by impairing normal outflow of venous blood (e.g., thrombophlebitis, deep vein thrombosis [DVT]). Second, embolization obstructs the blood supply when the embolus becomes lodged. The pulmonary arteries are common sites of embolization.

Drugs Used in Thrombotic and Thromboembolic Disorders: Classifications and Individual Drugs

Drugs given to prevent or treat thrombosis alter some aspect of the blood coagulation process (see Fig. 54-1). Anticoagulants are widely used in thrombotic disorders. They are more effective in preventing venous thrombosis than arterial thrombosis. Antiplatelet drugs are used to prevent arterial thrombosis. Thrombolytic agents are used to dissolve thrombi and limit tissue damage in selected thromboembolic disorders. These drugs are described in the following sections and in Table 54-1.

Anticoagulants

Anticoagulant drugs are given to prevent formation of new clots and extension of clots already present. They do not dissolve formed clots, improve blood flow in tissues around the clot, or prevent ischemic damage to tissues beyond the clot. Heparins and warfarin are commonly used anticoagulants; argatroban and lepirudin are additional agents. Clinical indications include prevention or management of thromboembolic disorders, such as thrombophlebitis, DVT, and pulmonary embolism. The main adverse effect is bleeding.

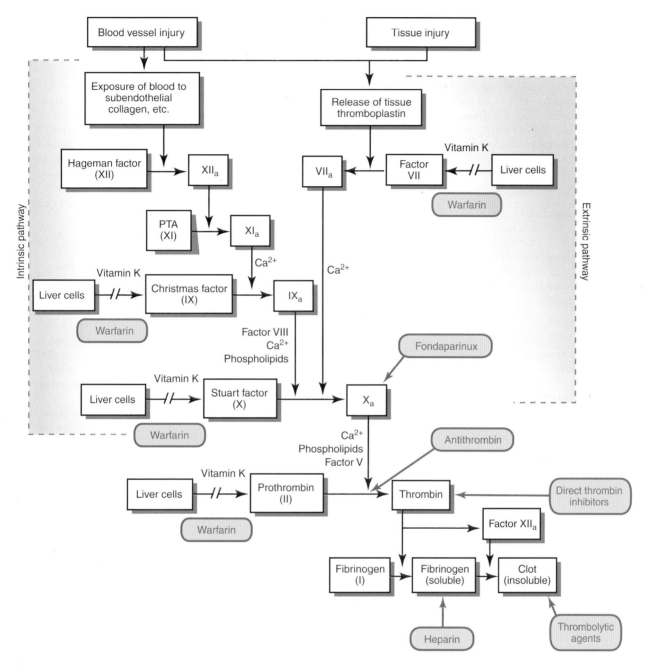

Figure 54-1 ■ Details of the intrinsic and extrinsic clotting pathways. The sites of action of some of the drugs that can influence these processes are shown in red.

Heparin

Heparin is a pharmaceutical preparation of the natural anticoagulant produced primarily by mast cells in pericapillary connective tissue. Endogenous heparin is found in various body tissues, most abundantly in the liver and lungs. Exogenous heparin is obtained from bovine lung or porcine intestinal mucosa and standardized in units of biologic activity.

Heparin combines with antithrombin III (a natural anticoagulant in the blood) to inactivate clotting factors IX, X, XI, and XII; inhibit the conversion of prothrombin to thrombin; and prevent thrombus formation (see Fig. 54-1). After thrombosis has developed, heparin can inhibit additional coagulation by inactivating thrombin, preventing the conversion of

fibrinogen to fibrin, and inhibiting factor XIII (the fibrin-stabilizing factor). Other effects include inhibiting factors V and VIII and platelet aggregation.

Heparin acts immediately after intravenous (IV) injection and within 20 to 30 minutes after subcutaneous (Sub-Q) injection. It is metabolized in the liver and excreted in the urine, primarily as inactive metabolites. Heparin does not cross the placental barrier and is not secreted in breast milk, making it the anticoagulant of choice for use during pregnancy and lactation.

Prophylactically, low doses of heparin are given to prevent DVT and pulmonary embolism in patients at risk for development of these disorders, such as the following:

Box 54-1	Hemostasis and Thrombosis

The blood vessels and blood normally maintain a balance between procoagulant and anticoagulant factors that favor anticoagulation and keeps the blood fluid. Injury to blood vessels and tissues causes complex reactions and interactions among vascular endothelial cells, platelets, and blood coagulation factors that shift the balance toward procoagulation and thrombosis.

Endothelial Cells

Normal endothelium helps to prevent thrombosis by producing anticoagulant factors, inhibiting platelet reactivity, and inhibiting activation of the coagulation cascade. However, endothelium promotes thrombosis if the blood vessel wall is damaged, function is altered, or when blood flow is altered or becomes static. After a blood clot is formed, the endothelium also induces its dissolution and restoration of blood flow.

Platelets

The only known function of platelets is hemostasis. Platelets (also called thrombocytes) are produced in the bone marrow and released into the bloodstream, where they circulate for approximately 7 to 10 days before they are removed by the spleen. They contain no nuclei and therefore cannot repair or replicate themselves.

The cell membrane of a platelet contains a coat of glycoproteins that prevents the platelet from adhering to normal endothelium but allows it to adhere to damaged areas of endothelium and collagen in the blood vessel wall. Breakdown of the cell membrane releases arachidonic acid (which can be metabolized to produce thromboxane A_2) and allows leakage of platelet contents (e.g., thromboplastin and other clotting factors), which function to stop bleeding.

When platelets come in contact with a damaged vascular surface, they become activated and aggregate at a site of injury to help plug a hole in a torn blood vessel. Aggregated platelets release substances that recruit new platelets and stimulate additional aggregation. This activity helps the platelet plug become large enough to block blood flow out of a damaged blood vessel. If the opening is small, the platelet plug can stop blood loss. If the opening is large, a platelet plug and a blood clot are both required to stop the bleeding. Platelets usually disappear from a blood clot within 24 hours and are replaced by fibrin.

Blood Coagulation

The blood coagulation process represented in Figure 54-1 causes hemostasis within 1 to 2 minutes. It involves sequential activation of clotting factors that are normally present in blood and tissues as inactive precursors and formation of a meshwork of fibrin strands that cements blood components together to form a stable, dense clot. Major phases include release of thromboplastin by disintegrating platelets and damaged tissue; conversion of prothrombin to thrombin, which requires thromboplastin and calcium ions; and conversion of fibrinogen to fibrin by thrombin.

Blood coagulation results from activation of the intrinsic or extrinsic coagulation pathway. Both pathways, which are activated when blood passes out of a blood vessel, are needed for normal hemostasis. The intrinsic pathway occurs in the vascular system; the extrinsic pathway occurs in the tissues. Although the pathways are initially separate, the terminal steps (i.e., activation of factor X and thrombin-induced formation of fibrin) are the same leading to the formation of thrombin, which then activates fibrinogen to form fibrin, and the clot is complete.

- Patients with major illnesses (e.g., acute myocardial infarction, heart failure, serious pulmonary infections, stroke)
- Patients having major abdominal or thoracic surgery
- Patients with a history of thrombophlebitis or pulmonary embolism, including pregnant women
- Patients having gynecologic surgery, especially if they have been taking estrogens or oral contraceptives or have other risk factors for DVT
- Patients expected to be on bed rest or to have limited activity for longer than 5 days

Therapeutically, heparin is used for management of acute thromboembolic disorders (e.g., DVT, thrombophlebitis, pulmonary embolism). In these conditions, the aim of therapy is to prevent further thrombus formation and embolization. Heparin is also used in disseminated intravascular coagulation (DIC), a life-threatening condition characterized by widespread clotting, which depletes the blood of coagulation factors. The depletion of coagulation factors then produces widespread bleeding. The goal of heparin therapy in DIC is to prevent blood coagulation long enough

for clotting factors to be replenished and thus be able to control hemorrhage. Heparin is also used to prevent clotting during cardiac and vascular surgery, extracorporeal circulation, hemodialysis, and blood transfusions, and in blood samples to be used in laboratory tests.

Contraindications include GI ulcerations (e.g., peptic ulcer disease, ulcerative colitis), intracranial bleeding, dissecting aortic aneurysm, blood dyscrasias, severe kidney or liver disease, severe hypertension, polycythemia vera, and recent surgery of the eye, spinal cord, or brain. Heparin should be used with caution in patients with hypertension, renal or hepatic disease, alcoholism, history of GI ulcerations, drainage tubes (e.g., nasogastric tubes, indwelling urinary catheters), threatened abortion, endocarditis, and any occupation with high risks of traumatic injury.

Disadvantages of heparin are its short duration of action and the subsequent need for frequent administration, the necessity for parenteral injection (because it is not absorbed from the gastrointestinal [GI] tract), and local tissue reactions at injection sites.

Table 54-1	**Drugs at a Glance:** Anticoagulant, Antiplatelet, and Thrombolytic Agents	

GENERIC/TRADE NAME	INDICATIONS FOR USE	ROUTES AND DOSAGE RANGES (ADULTS, UNLESS SPECIFIED)
Anticoagulants		
Heparin	Prevention and management of thromboembolic disorders (e.g., DVT, pulmonary embolism, atrial fibrillation with embolization)	*Adults:* IV injection, 5000 units initially, followed by 5000–10,000 units q4–6h, to a maximum dose of 25,000 units/d; IV infusion, 5000 units (loading dose), then 15–25 units/kg/h DIC, IV injection, 50–100 units/kg q4h; IV infusion, 20,000–40,000 units/d at initial rate of 0.25 units/kg/min, then adjusted according to aPTT; Sub-Q 10,000–12,000 units q8h, or 14,000–20,000 units q12h Low-dose prophylaxis, Sub-Q 5000 units 2 h before surgery, then q12h until discharged from hospital or fully ambulatory *Children:* DIC, IV injection, 25–50 units/kg q4h; IV infusion, 50 units/kg initially, followed by 100 units/kg q4h or 20,000 units/m^2 over 24 h
Argatroban (Argatroban)	Thrombosis prophylaxis or management in heparin-induced thrombocytopenia; adjunct to PTCA	IV continuous infusion 2 mcg/kg/min
Bivalirudin (Angiomax)	Patients with unstable angina undergoing PTCA; acute coronary syndrome	IV bolus dose of 0.75 mg/kg followed by 4-h infusion at rate of 1.75 mg/kg/min
Dalteparin (Fragmin)	Prophylaxis of DVT in patients having hip replacement surgery; also patients at high risk of thromboembolic disorders who are having abdominal surgery	Abdominal surgery, Sub-Q 2500 IU 1–2 h before surgery and then once daily for 5–10 days after surgery Hip replacement surgery, Sub-Q 2500 IU 1–2 h before surgery and the evening of surgery (at least 6 h after first dose) and then 5000 IU once daily for 5 days
Enoxaparin (Lovenox)	Prevention and management of DVT and pulmonary embolism Management of unstable angina, to prevent myocardial infarction	DVT prophylaxis in patients having hip or knee replacement surgery, Sub-Q 30 mg twice daily, with first dose within 12–24 h after surgery and continued until risk of DVT diminished or until adequately anticoagulated on warfarin Abdominal surgery, Sub-Q 40 mg once daily with first dose given 2 h before surgery, for 7–10 days DVT/pulmonary embolism management, outpatients, Sub-Q 1 mg/kg q12h; inpatients, 1 mg/kg q12h or 1.5 mg/kg q24h Unstable angina 1 mg/kg q12h in conjunction with oral aspirin (100–325 mg once daily)
Fondaparinux (Arixtra)	Prevention of DVT following hip fracture surgery or knee or hip replacement	Sub-Q 2.5 mg daily, with first dose 6–8 h after surgery and continuing for a maximum of 11 days

(continued on page 866)

Table 54-1 **Drugs at a Glance:** Anticoagulant, Antiplatelet, and Thrombolytic Agents (continued)

GENERIC/TRADE NAME	INDICATIONS FOR USE	ROUTES AND DOSAGE RANGES (ADULTS, UNLESS SPECIFIED)
Lepirudin (Refludan)	Heparin alternative for anticoagulation in patients with heparin-induced thrombocytopenia and associated thromboembolic disorders	IV injection, 0.4 mg/kg over 15–20 sec, followed by continuous IV infusion of 0.15 mg/kg for 2–10 days or longer if needed
Warfarin (Coumadin)	Long-term prevention or management of venous thromboembolic disorders, including DVT, PE, and embolization associated with atrial fibrillation and prosthetic heart valves. May also be used after myocardial infarction to decrease reinfarction, stroke, venous thromboembolism, and death	PO 2–5 mg/d for 2–3 days, then adjusted according to the international normalized ratio (INR); average maintenance daily dose, 2–5 mg
Antiplatelet Agents		
Aspirin	Prevention of myocardial infarction Prevention of thromboembolic disorders in patients with prosthetic heart valves or TIAs	PO 81–325 mg daily
Abciximab (ReoPro)	Used with PTCA to prevent rethrombosis of treated arteries Intended for use with aspirin and heparin	IV bolus injection, 0.25 mg/kg 10–60 min before starting PTCA, then a continuous IV infusion of 10 mcg/min for 12 h
Anagrelide (Agrylin)	Essential thrombocythemia, to reduce the elevated platelet count, the risk of thrombosis, and associated symptoms	PO 0.5 mg 4 times daily or 1 mg twice daily initially, then titrate to lowest dose effective in maintaining platelet count <600,000/mm^3
Cilostazol (Pletal)	Intermittent claudication, to increase walking distance (before leg pain occurs)	PO 100 mg twice daily, 30 min before or 2 h after breakfast and dinner; reduce to 50 mg twice daily with concurrent use of fluconazole, itraconazole, erythromycin, or diltiazem
Clopidogrel (Plavix)	Reduction of atherosclerotic events (myocardial infarction, stroke, vascular death) in patients with atherosclerosis documented by recent stroke, recent myocardial infarction, or established peripheral artery disease	PO 75 mg once daily with or without food
Dipyridamole (Persantine)	Prevention of thromboembolism after cardiac valve replacement, given with warfarin	PO 25–75 mg 3 times per day, 1 h before meals
Dipyridamole and aspirin (Aggrenox)	Reduction of stroke risk in patients with previous TIA or thrombotic event	PO 1 capsule (200 mg extended-release dipyridamole/25 mg aspirin) twice daily
Eptifibatide (Integrilin)	Acute coronary syndromes, including patients who are to be managed medically and those undergoing PTCA	IV bolus injection, 180 mcg/kg, followed by continuous infusion of 2 mcg/kg/min. See manufacturer's instructions for preparation and administration.
Ticlopidine (Ticlid)	Prevention of thrombosis in patients with coronary artery or cerebral vascular disease (e.g., patients who have had stroke precursors or a completed thrombotic stroke)	PO 250 mg twice daily with food
Tirofiban (Aggrastat)	Acute coronary syndromes, with heparin, for patients who are to be managed medically or those undergoing PTCA Acute myocardial infarction Pulmonary embolism	IV infusion, 0.4 mcg/kg/min for 30 min, then 0.1 mcg/kg/min. Patients with severe renal impairment (creatinine clearance <30 mL/min) should receive half the usual rate of infusion. See manufacturer's instructions for preparation and administration.

GENERIC/TRADE NAME	INDICATIONS FOR USE	ROUTES AND DOSAGE RANGES (ADULTS, UNLESS SPECIFIED)
Thrombolytic Agents		
Alteplase (Activase)	Acute ischemic stroke Acute myocardial infarction Pulmonary emboli	IV infusion, 100 mg over 3 h (first hour, 60 mg with a bolus of 6–10 mg over 1–2 min initially; second hour, 20 mg; third hour, 20 mg)
Drotrecogin alfa, activated (Xigris)	Reduction of mortality in severe sepsis	IV infusion of 24 mcg/kg/h for 96 h
Reteplase, recombinant (Retavase)	Acute myocardial infarction	IV injection, 10 units over 2 min, repeated in 30 min. Inject into a flowing IV infusion line that contains no other medications.
Streptokinase (Streptase)	Management of acute, severe pulmonary emboli or iliofemoral thrombophlebitis Used to dissolve clots in arterial or venous cannulas or catheters May be injected into a coronary artery to dissolve a thrombus if done within 6 h of onset of symptoms	IV 250,000 units over 30 min, then 100,000 units/h for 24–72 h
Tenecteplase (TNKase)	Acute myocardial infarction	IV bolus dose based on weight, 30 mg (for <60 kg) not to exceed 50 mg (>90 kg)
Urokinase (Abbokinase)	Coronary artery thrombi Pulmonary emboli Clearance of clogged IV catheters	IV 4400 units/kg over 10 min, followed by continuous infusion of 4400 units/kg/h for 12 h For clearing IV catheters, see manufacturer's instructions.

aPTT, activated partial thromboplastin time; DIC, disseminated intravascular coagulation; DVT, deep vein thrombosis; PE, pulmonary embolism; PTCA, percutaneous transluminal coronary angioplasty or atherectomy; TIA, transient ischemic attack.

Heparin-induced thrombocytopenia (HIT) may occur in 1% to 3% of those receiving heparin and is a very serious adverse effect of heparin. HIT is an immune-mediated process that results in development of antibodies that activate platelets. The activated platelets are rapidly consumed by the reticuloendothelial system, thereby triggering a subsequent release of procoagulant microparticles that cause platelet aggregation and a hyperthrombotic state. All patients exposed to any heparin at therapeutic or prophylactic doses or minute amounts in heparin flushes or on heparin-coated catheters, as well as those receiving low–molecular-weight heparin, are at risk. All heparin administration must be discontinued and anticoagulation managed with a direct thrombin inhibitor such as argatroban.

Low–Molecular-Weight Heparins

Standard heparin is a mixture of high– and low–molecular-weight fractions, but most anticoagulant activity is attributed to the low–molecular-weight portion. **Low–molecular-weight heparins** (LMWHs) contain the low–molecular-weight fraction and are as effective as IV heparin in treating thrombotic disorders. Indications for use include prevention or management of thromboembolic complications associated with surgery

or ischemic complications of unstable angina and myocardial infarction. Currently available LMWHs (dalteparin, enoxaparin) differ from standard heparin and each other and are not interchangeable.

LMWHs are given Sub-Q and do not require close monitoring of blood coagulation tests. These characteristics allow outpatient anticoagulant therapy, an increasing trend. The drugs are also associated with less thrombocytopenia than standard heparin. However, platelet counts should be monitored during therapy.

Applying Your Knowledge 54-1

Before providing care for Mr. Dusseau, you review his chart (medical diagnosis and medication orders). What is the main reason for patients to receive an anticoagulant and for what adverse effect should you monitor Mr. Dusseau?

Warfarin

Warfarin is the most commonly used oral anticoagulant. It acts in the liver to prevent synthesis of vitamin K–dependent clotting factors (i.e., factors II, VII, IX, and X). Warfarin is similar to vitamin K in structure and therefore acts as a competitive antagonist to hepatic use of vitamin K. Anticoagulant effects do not occur for 3 to 5 days after warfarin is started because clotting factors already in the blood follow their normal pathway of elimination. Warfarin has no effect on circulating clotting factors or on platelet function.

Warfarin is well absorbed after oral administration. It is highly bound to plasma proteins (98%), mainly albumin. It is metabolized in the liver and primarily excreted as inactive metabolites by the kidneys.

Warfarin is most useful in long-term prevention or management of venous thromboembolic disorders, including DVT, pulmonary embolism, and embolization associated with atrial fibrillation and prosthetic heart valves. In addition, warfarin therapy after myocardial infarction may decrease reinfarction, stroke, venous thromboembolism, and death. Smaller doses are being used now than formerly, with similar antithrombotic effects and decreased risks of bleeding.

Like heparin, warfarin is contraindicated in patients with GI ulcerations, blood disorders associated with bleeding, severe kidney or liver disease, severe hypertension, and recent surgery of the eye, spinal cord, or brain. It should be used cautiously in patients with mild hypertension, renal or hepatic disease, alcoholism, history of GI ulcerations, drainage tubes (e.g., nasogastric tubes, indwelling urinary catheters), and occupations with high risks of traumatic injury. In addition, warfarin is contraindicated during pregnancy. The U.S. Food and Drug Administration (FDA) has issued a **BLACK BOX WARNING** with warfarin due to its risk of causing major or fatal bleeding.

Direct Thrombin Inhibitors

Direct thrombin inhibitors (DTIs) have benefits over agents like heparin and warfarin, including the inhibition of both circulating and clot-bound thrombin. Heparin and warfarin are indirect inhibitors of thrombin. The DTIs exert their effect by interacting directly with the thrombin molecule without the need of a cofactor, such as heparin cofactor II or antithrombin. As such, they inhibit thrombin's ability to convert soluble fibrinogen to fibrin and to activate the fibrin-generating factors V, VIII, and IX. Because thrombin also stimulates platelets, DTIs also have antiplatelet activity.

Currently, the parenteral agents **lepirudin, bivalirudin,** and **argatroban** are available for clinical use; others, including oral forms, are undergoing clinical trials. These drugs provide advantages over heparin, including inhibition of both circulating and clot-bound thrombin, a more predictable dose-response anticoagulant effect, inhibition of thrombin-induced platelet aggregation, and the lack of production of immune-mediated thrombocytopenia. The drugs are available for heparin-induced thrombocytopenia, acute coronary syndrome, prophylaxis and treatment of venous thromboembolism, and management of atrial fibrillation. The DTIs are less suitable for long-term treatment since they are administered by injection, lack widely available option for therapeutic drug monitoring, and have no pharmacologic antidote available to reverse their effects.

Other Anticoagulant Drugs

Fondaparinux is the first of a new class of pentasaccharide antithrombotic agents that produces anticoagulant effects by directly binding to circulating and clot-bound factor Xa, accelerating the activity of antithrombin and inhibiting thrombin production. It is appreciated for its simple dosing regimen, no need for coagulation monitoring, and potentially a lower risk of heparin-induced thrombocytopenia compared with LMWH. It is used in the prevention of DVT in patients having surgery for hip fracture or joint replacement surgery of the knee or hip.

Antiplatelet Drugs

Antiplatelet drugs prevent one or more steps in the prothrombotic activity of platelets. As described previously, platelet activity is very important in both physiologic hemostasis and pathologic thrombosis. Arterial thrombi, which are composed primarily of platelets, may form on top of atherosclerotic plaque and block blood flow in the artery. They may also form on heart walls and valves and embolize to other parts of the body.

Drugs used clinically for antiplatelet effects act by a variety of mechanisms to inhibit platelet activation, adhesion, aggregation, or procoagulant activity. These include drugs that block platelet receptors for thromboxane A_2, adenosine diphosphate (ADP), glycoprotein (GP) IIb/IIIa, and phosphodiesterase.

Thromboxane A_2 Inhibitors

Aspirin is a commonly used analgesic–antipyretic–anti-inflammatory drug (see Chap. 7) with potent antiplatelet effects. Aspirin exerts pharmacologic actions by inhibiting synthesis of prostaglandins. In this instance, aspirin acetylates cyclooxygenase, the enzyme in platelets that normally synthesizes thromboxane A_2, a prostaglandin product that causes platelet aggregation. Thus, aspirin prevents formation of thromboxane A_2 and thromboxane A_2–induced platelet aggregation and thrombus formation. A single dose of 300 to 600 milligrams or multiple doses of 30 milligrams (e.g., daily for several days) inhibit the cyclooxygenase in circulating platelets almost completely. These antithrombotic effects persist for the life of the platelet (7–10 days). Aspirin may be used long term for prevention of myocardial infarction or stroke and in patients with prosthetic heart valves. It is also used for the immediate treatment of suspected or actual acute myocardial infarction, for transient ischemic attacks (TIAs), and for evolving thrombotic strokes. Adverse effects are uncommon with the small doses used for antiplatelet effects. However, there is an increased risk of bleeding, including hemorrhagic stroke. Because approximately 85% of strokes are thrombotic, the benefits of aspirin or other antiplatelet agents are thought to outweigh the risks of hemorrhagic strokes (approximately 15%). No antidote exists for the effects of aspirin because it produces irreversible platelet effects; platelet transfusion may be required.

Nonsteroidal anti-inflammatory drugs (NSAIDs), including **ibuprofen** and many other aspirin-related drugs, inhibit cyclooxygenase reversibly. Their antiplatelet effects subside when the drugs are eliminated from the circulation and the drugs usually are not used for antiplatelet effects. However, patients who take an NSAID daily (e.g., for arthritis pain) may not need to take additional aspirin for antiplatelet effects. **Acetaminophen** does not affect platelets in usual doses (see Chap. 7).

Adenosine Diphosphate Receptor Antagonists

The adenosine diphosphate receptor antagonists, **clopidogrel** (Plavix) and **ticlopidine** (Ticlid), irreversibly block the adenosine diphosphate (ADP) receptor on platelet cell membranes. This effectively prevents platelet aggregation for the lifespan of the platelet. The drug class is indicated for reduction of myocardial infarction, stroke, and vascular death in patients with atherosclerosis; clopidogrel reportedly causes fewer or less severe adverse effects than ticlopidine.

With clopidogrel, platelet inhibition can be demonstrated 2 hours after a single dose, but the onset of action is slow, so that a loading-dose is usually administered. The FDA has recently approved a 300-milligram tablet of clopidogrel for a loading dose for appropriate patients. Clopidogrel is rapidly absorbed after oral administration with a half-life of about 8 hours, but its effect can be seen as soon as 2 hours after a 300-milligram loading dose. The most common adverse effects associated with the use of clopidogrel are pruritus, rash, purpura, and diarrhea; thrombotic thrombocytopenic purpura, hemorrhage, and severe neutropenia have also been reported.

Ticlopidine is indicated for prevention of thrombotic stroke in people who have had stroke precursor events (e.g., TIAs) or a completed thrombotic stroke. Ticlopidine is considered a second-line drug for patients who cannot take aspirin. The adverse effects (e.g., neutropenia, diarrhea, skin rashes) and greater cost make it prohibitive for use by many patients. Contraindications include active bleeding disorders (e.g., GI bleeding from peptic ulcer, intracranial bleeding), neutropenia, thrombocytopenia, severe liver disease, and hypersensitivity to the drug. No antidote exists for the effects of the adenosine diphosphate receptor antagonists as they produce irreversible platelet effects. Platelet transfusion should be considered in patients who take these drugs and have hemorrhagic complications.

Glycoprotein IIb/IIIa Receptor Antagonists

Abciximab is a monoclonal antibody that prevents the binding of fibrinogen, von Willebrand factor, and other molecules to GP IIb/IIIa receptors on activated platelets. This action inhibits platelet aggregation.

Abciximab is used with percutaneous transluminal coronary angioplasty or removal of atherosclerotic plaque to prevent rethrombosis of treated arteries. It is used with aspirin and heparin and is contraindicated in patients who have recently received an oral anticoagulant or IV dextran. Other contraindications include active bleeding, thrombocytopenia, history of a serious stroke, surgery or major trauma within the previous 6 weeks, uncontrolled hypertension, or hypersensitivity to drug components.

Eptifibatide and **tirofiban** inhibit platelet aggregation by preventing activation of GP IIb/IIIa receptors on the platelet surface and the subsequent binding of fibrinogen and von Willebrand factor to platelets. Antiplatelet effects occur during drug infusion and stop when the drug is stopped. The drugs are indicated for acute coronary syndrome (e.g., unstable angina, myocardial infarction) in patients who are to be treated medically or by angioplasty or atherectomy.

Drug half-life is approximately 2.5 hours for eptifibatide and 2 hours for tirofiban; the drugs are cleared mainly by renal excretion. With tirofiban, plasma clearance is approximately 25% lower in older adults and approximately 50% lower in patients with severe renal impairment (creatinine clearance < 30 mL/minute).

The drugs are contraindicated in patients with hypersensitivity to any component of the products; current or previous bleeding (within previous 30 days); a history of thrombocytopenia after previous exposure to tirofiban; a history of stroke within 30 days or any history of hemorrhagic stroke; major surgery or severe physical trauma within the previous month; severe hypertension (systolic blood pressure > 180 mm Hg with tirofiban or >200 mm Hg with eptifibatide, or diastolic blood pressure > 110 mm Hg with either drug); a history of intra-cranial hemorrhage, neoplasm, arteriovenous malformation, or aneurysm; a platelet count less than 100,000 cubic millimeter; serum creatinine 2 milligrams per deciliter or above (for the 180 mcg/kg bolus and the 2 mcg/kg/min infusion) or 4 milligrams per deciliter or above (for the 135 mcg/kg bolus and the 0.5 mcg/kg/min infusion); or dependency on dialysis (eptifibatide).

Bleeding is the most common adverse effect, with most major bleeding occurring at the arterial access site for cardiac catheterization. If bleeding occurs and cannot be controlled with pressure, the drug infusion and heparin should be discontinued.

These drugs should be used cautiously if given with other drugs that affect hemostasis (e.g., warfarin, thrombolytics, other antiplatelet drugs).

Phosphodiesterase Inhibitor

Cilostazol inhibits phosphodiesterase, an enzyme that metabolizes cyclic adenosine monophosphate (cAMP). This inhibition increases intracellular cAMP, which then inhibits platelet aggregation and produces vasodilation. The drug reversibly inhibits platelet aggregation induced by various stimuli (e.g., thrombin, ADP, collagen, arachidonic acid, epinephrine, shear stress). It is indicated for management of intermittent claudication. Symptoms usually improve within 2 to 4 weeks but may take as long as 12 weeks. The drug is contraindicated in patients with heart failure.

Cilostazol is highly protein bound (95%–98%), mainly to albumin; extensively metabolized by hepatic cytochrome P450 enzymes; and excreted in urine (74%) and feces. The drug and two active metabolites accumulate with chronic administration and reach steady state within a few days. The most common adverse effects are diarrhea and headache.

Other Agents

Anagrelide inhibits platelet aggregation induced by cAMP phosphodiesterase, ADP, and collagen. However, it is indicated only to reduce platelet counts for patients with essential thrombocythemia (a disorder characterized by excessive numbers of platelets). Doses to reduce platelet production are smaller than those required to inhibit platelet aggregation.

Dipyridamole inhibits platelet adhesion, but its mechanism of action is unclear. It is used for prevention of thromboembolism after cardiac valve replacement and is given with warfarin. The combination of dipyridamole and aspirin is indicated for prevention of stroke in those who have had stroke precursors (TIAs) or a previously completed thrombotic stroke.

Thrombolytic Agents

Thrombolytic agents are given to dissolve thrombi. They stimulate conversion of plasminogen to plasmin (also called *fibrinolysin*), a proteolytic enzyme that breaks down fibrin, the framework of a thrombus. The main use of thrombolytic agents is for management of acute, severe thromboembolic disease, such as myocardial infarction, pulmonary embolism, and iliofemoral thrombosis.

The goal of thrombolytic therapy is to re-establish blood flow as quickly as possible and prevent or limit tissue damage. Drugs with shorter half lives increase the risk of rethrombosis or infarction. Anticoagulant drugs, such as heparin and warfarin, and antiplatelet agents are given following thrombolytic therapy to decrease reformation of a thrombus. Thrombolytic drugs are also used to dissolve clots in arterial or venous cannulas or catheters.

Streptokinase and **urokinase** are enzymes that break down fibrin. They are used mainly to lyse coronary artery clots in acute myocardial infarction. Streptokinase may also be used to dissolve clots in vascular catheters and to treat acute, severe pulmonary emboli or iliofemoral thrombophlebitis. Urokinase is recommended for use in patients allergic to streptokinase. As with other anticoagulants and thrombolytic agents, bleeding is the main adverse effect.

Alteplase, reteplase, and **tenecteplase** are tissue plasminogen activators used mainly in acute myocardial infarction to dissolve clots obstructing coronary arteries and re-establish perfusion of tissues beyond the thrombotic area. The drugs bind to fibrin in a clot and act locally to dissolve the clot. The most common adverse effect is bleeding, which may be internal (e.g., intracranial, GI, genitourinary) or external (e.g., venous or arterial puncture sites, surgical incisions). The drugs are contraindicated in the presence of bleeding, a history of stroke, central nervous system surgery or trauma within the previous 2 months, and severe hypertension.

Drotrecogin alfa is a recombinant version of human activated protein C that is approved for use in severe sepsis or septic shock. Severe sepsis is characterized by an excessive inflammatory reaction to infection, inappropriate blood clot formation, and impaired breakdown of clots. Drotrecogin alfa is given for its thrombolytic effects, along with other therapies for inflammation and infection. The major adverse effect is bleeding.

Drugs Used to Control Bleeding

Anticoagulant, antiplatelet, and thrombolytic drugs profoundly affect hemostasis, and their major adverse effect is bleeding. As a result, systemic hemostatic agents (antidotes) may be needed to prevent or treat bleeding episodes. Antidotes should be used cautiously because overuse can increase risks of recurrent thrombotic disorders. These drugs are described in this section and in Table 54-2.

Table 54-2	Drugs at a Glance: Systemic Hemostatic Drugs	
GENERIC/TRADE NAME	**INDICATIONS FOR USE**	**DOSAGE (ADULTS, UNLESS SPECIFIED)**
Aminocaproic acid (Amicar)	Control bleeding caused by overdoses of thrombolytic agents or bleeding disorders caused by hyperfibrinolysis (e.g., cardiac surgery, blood disorders, hepatic cirrhosis, prostatectomy, neoplastic disorders)	PO, IV infusion, 5 g initially, followed by 1.0 to 1.25 g/h for 8 h or until bleeding is controlled; maximum dose, 30 g/24 h
Protamine sulfate	Treatment of heparin overdosage	Depends on the amount of heparin given within the previous 4 h
Tranexamic acid (Cyklokapron)	Control bleeding caused by overdoses of thrombolytic agents Prevent or decrease bleeding from tooth extraction in patients with hemophilia	PO 25 mg/kg 3 to 4 times daily, starting 1 d before surgery, or IV 10 mg/kg immediately before surgery, followed by 25 mg/kg PO 3 to 4 times daily for 2–8 d
Vitamin K (Mephyton)	Antidote for warfarin overdosage	PO 10–20 mg in a single dose

Aminocaproic acid and tranexamic acid are used to stop bleeding caused by overdoses of thrombolytic agents. Aminocaproic acid also may be used in other bleeding disorders caused by hyperfibrinolysis (e.g., in cardiac surgery, blood disorders, hepatic cirrhosis, prostatectomy, neoplastic disorders). Tranexamic acid also is used for short periods (2–8 days) in patients with hemophilia to prevent or decrease bleeding from tooth extraction. Dosage of tranexamic acid should be reduced in the presence of moderate or severe renal impairment.

Protamine sulfate is an antidote for standard heparin and LMWHs. Because heparin is an acid and protamine sulfate is a base, protamine neutralizes heparin activity. Protamine dosage depends on the amount of heparin administered during the previous 4 hours. Each milligram of protamine neutralizes approximately 100 units of heparin or dalteparin and 1 milligram of enoxaparin. A single dose should not exceed 50 milligrams. The FDA has issued a **BLACK BOX WARNING** with the use of protamine sulfate due to the risk of severe hypotension, cardiovascular collapse, noncardiogenic pulmonary edema, catastrophic pulmonary vasoconstriction, and pulmonary hypertension with its use.

The drug is given by slow IV infusion over at least 10 minutes (to prevent or minimize adverse effects of hypotension, bradycardia, and dyspnea). Protamine effects occur immediately and last for approximately 2 hours. A second dose may be required because heparin activity lasts approximately 4 hours.

Protamine sulfate can cause severe hypotensive and anaphylactoid reactions. Thus, it should be given in settings with equipment and personnel for resuscitation and management of anaphylactic shock.

Vitamin K is the antidote for warfarin overdosage. An oral dose of 10 to 20 milligrams usually stops minor bleeding and returns the international normalized ratio (INR; see "Drug Dosage and Administration: Regulation of Heparin and Warfarin Dosage," below) to a normal range within 24 hours.

Nursing Process

Assessment

Assess the patient's status in relation to thrombotic and thromboembolic disorders.

- Risk factors for thromboembolism include
  - Immobility (e.g., limited activity or bed rest for more than 5 days)
  - Obesity
  - Cigarette smoking
  - History of thrombophlebitis, DVT, or pulmonary emboli
  - Congestive heart failure
  - Pedal edema
  - Lower limb trauma

  - Myocardial infarction
  - Atrial fibrillation
  - Mitral or aortic stenosis
  - Prosthetic heart valves
  - Abdominal, thoracic, pelvic, or major orthopedic surgery
  - Atherosclerotic heart disease or peripheral vascular disease
  - Use of oral contraceptives
- Signs and symptoms of thrombotic and thromboembolic disorders depend on the location and size of the thrombus.
  - DVT and thrombophlebitis usually occur in the legs. The conditions may be manifested by edema (the affected leg is often measurably larger than the other) and pain, especially in the calf when the foot is dorsiflexed (Homans' sign). If thrombophlebitis is superficial, it may be visible as a red, warm, tender area following the path of a vein.
  - Pulmonary embolism, if severe enough to produce symptoms, is manifested by chest pain, cough, hemoptysis, tachypnea, and tachycardia. Massive emboli cause hypotension, shock, cyanosis, and death.
  - DIC is usually manifested by bleeding, which may range from petechiae or oozing from a venipuncture site to massive internal bleeding or bleeding from all body orifices.

Nursing Diagnoses

- Ineffective Tissue Perfusion related to thrombus or embolus or drug-induced bleeding
- Acute Pain related to tissue ischemia
- Impaired Physical Mobility related to bed rest and pain
- Ineffective Coping related to the need for long-term prophylaxis of thromboembolic disorders or fear of excessive bleeding
- Anxiety related to fear of myocardial infarction or stroke
- Deficient Knowledge related to anticoagulant or antiplatelet drug therapy
- Risk for Injury related to drug-induced impairment of blood coagulation

Planning/Goals

The patient will

- Receive or take anticoagulant and antiplatelet drugs correctly
- Be monitored closely for therapeutic and adverse drug effects, especially when drug therapy is started and when changes are made in drugs or dosages
- Use nondrug measures to decrease venous stasis and prevent thromboembolic disorders

Nursing Process continues on page 872

- Act to prevent trauma from falls and other injuries
- Inform any health care provider when taking an anticoagulant or antiplatelet drug
- Avoid or report adverse drug reactions
- Verbalize or demonstrate knowledge of safe management of anticoagulant drug therapy
- Keep follow-up appointments for tests of blood coagulation and drug dosage regulation
- Avoid preventable bleeding episodes

Interventions

Use measures to prevent thrombotic and thromboembolic disorders.

- Have the patient ambulate and exercise legs regularly, especially after surgery.
- For patients who cannot ambulate or do leg exercises, do passive range-of-motion and other leg exercises several times daily when changing the patient's position or performing other care.
- Have the patient wear elastic stockings. Elastic stockings should be removed every 8 hours and replaced after inspecting the skin. Improperly applied elastic stockings can impair circulation rather than aid it. For patients on bed rest, intermittent pneumatic compression devices can also be used.
- Avoid trauma to lower extremities.
- Maintain adequate fluid intake (1500–3000 mL/day) to avoid dehydration and hemoconcentration.
- Assist patients to promote good blood circulation (e.g., exercise) and avoid situations that impair circulation (e.g., wearing tight clothing, crossing the legs at the knees, prolonged sitting or standing, bed rest, placing pillows under the knees when in bed).

For the patient receiving anticoagulant therapy, implement safety measures to prevent trauma and bleeding.

- For patients who cannot ambulate safely because of weakness, sedation, or other conditions, keep the call light within reach, keep bed rails elevated, and assist in ambulation.
- Provide an electric razor for shaving.
- Avoid intramuscular injections, venipunctures, and arterial punctures when possible.
- Avoid intubations when possible (e.g., nasogastric tubes, indwelling urinary catheters).

For the patient receiving tirofiban or eptifibatide:

- Monitor the femoral artery access site closely. This is the most common site of bleeding.
- Avoid invasive procedures as much as possible (e.g., arterial and venous punctures, intramuscular injections,

urinary catheters, nasotracheal suction, nasogastric tubes). If venipuncture must be done, avoid sites where pressure cannot be applied (e.g., subclavian or jugular veins).

- While the vascular sheath is in place, keep patients on complete bed rest with the head of the bed elevated 30 degrees and the affected limb restrained in a straight position.
- Discontinue heparin for 3 to 4 hours and be sure the activated clotting time is less than 180 seconds or the activated partial thromboplastin time (aPTT) is less than 45 seconds before removing the vascular sheath.
- After the vascular sheath is removed, apply pressure to the site and observe closely. For outpatients, be sure there is no bleeding for at least 4 hours before hospital discharge.

For the patient receiving a thrombolytic drug or a revascularization procedure for acute myocardial infarction:

- Monitor closely for bleeding.
- Assist the patient and family to understand the importance of diligent efforts to reverse risk factors contributing to coronary artery disease (e.g., diet and perhaps medication to lower serum cholesterol to less than 200 mg/dL and low-density lipoprotein cholesterol to less than 130 mg/dL; weight reduction if overweight; control of blood pressure if hypertensive; avoidance of smoking; stress-reduction techniques; exercise program designed and supervised by a health care provider).
- Assist the patient and family to understand the importance of complying with medication orders to prevent reinfarction and other complications, and continued medical supervision (see accompanying Patient Teaching Guidelines).

Evaluation

- Observe for signs and symptoms of thromboembolic disorders or bleeding.
- Check blood coagulation tests for therapeutic ranges.
- Observe and interview regarding compliance with instructions about drug therapy.
- Observe and interview regarding adverse drug effects.

Principles of Therapy

Drug Selection

Choices of anticoagulant and antiplatelet drugs depend on the reason for use and other drug and patient characteristics.

- Heparin is the anticoagulant of choice in acute venous thromboembolic disorders because the anticoagulant effect begins immediately with IV administration.

- Warfarin is the anticoagulant of choice for long-term maintenance therapy (i.e., several weeks or months) because it can be given orally.

- Aspirin has long been the most widely used antiplatelet drug for prevention of myocardial reinfarction and arterial thrombosis in patients with TIAs and prosthetic heart valves. However, clopidogrel may be more effective than aspirin.

- When anticoagulation is required during pregnancy, heparin is used because it does not cross the placenta. Warfarin is contraindicated during pregnancy as it crosses the placenta and may produce fatal fetal hemorrhage.

- Various combinations of antithrombotic drugs are used concomitantly or sequentially (e.g., abciximab is used with aspirin and heparin; thrombolytic drugs are usually followed with heparin and warfarin).

Drug Dosage and Administration: Regulation of Heparin and Warfarin Dosage

Heparin dosage is regulated by the activated partial thromboplastin time (aPTT), which is sensitive to changes in blood clotting factors, except factor VII. Thus, normal or control values indicate normal blood coagulation; therapeutic values

Patient Teaching Guidelines ■ Drugs to Prevent or Treat Blood Clots

General Considerations

- Antiplatelet and anticoagulant drugs are given to people who have had, or who are at risk of having, a heart attack, stroke, or other problems from blood clots. For prevention of a heart attack or stroke, you are most likely to be given an antiplatelet drug (e.g., aspirin, clopidogrel) or warfarin (Coumadin). For home management of deep vein thrombosis, which usually occurs in the legs, you are likely to be given heparin injections for a few days, followed by warfarin for long-term therapy. These medications help to prevent the blood clot from getting larger, traveling to your lungs, or recurring later.

- All of these drugs can increase your risk of bleeding, so you need to take safety precautions to prevent injury.

- To help prevent blood clots from forming and decreasing blood flow through your arteries, you need to reduce risk factors that contribute to cardiovascular disease. This can be done by a low-fat, low-cholesterol diet (and medication if needed) to lower total cholesterol to below 200 mg/dL and low-density lipoprotein cholesterol to below 130 mg/dL; weight reduction if overweight; control of blood pressure if hypertensive; avoidance of smoking; stress-reduction techniques; and regular exercise.

- To help prevent blood clots from forming in your leg veins, avoid or minimize situations that slow blood circulation, such as wearing tight clothing; crossing the legs at the knees; prolonged sitting or standing; and bed rest. For example, on automobile trips, stop and walk around every 1 to 2 hours; on long plane trips, exercise your feet and legs at your seat and walk around when you can.

- Following instructions regarding these medications is extremely important. Too little medication increases your risk of problems from blood clot formation; too much medication can cause bleeding.

- While taking any of these medications, you need regular medical supervision and periodic blood tests. The blood tests can help your health care provider regulate drug dosage and maintain your safety.

- You need to take the drugs as directed; avoid taking other drugs without the health care provider's knowledge and consent; inform any health care provider (including dentists) that you are taking an antiplatelet or anticoagulant drug before any invasive diagnostic tests or treatments are begun; and keep all appointments for continuing care.

- With warfarin therapy, you need to avoid walking barefoot; avoid contact sports; use an electric razor; avoid injections when possible; and carry an identification card, necklace, or bracelet (e.g., MedicAlert) stating the name of the drug and the health care provider's name and telephone number. Also, avoid large amounts of certain vegetables (e.g., broccoli, brussels sprouts, cabbage, cauliflower, chives, collard greens, kale, lettuce, mustard greens, peppers, spinach, turnips, and watercress), tomatoes, bananas, or fish; these foods contain vitamin K and may decrease anticoagulant effects.

- For home management of deep vein thrombosis, both warfarin and enoxaparin (Lovenox) are given for 3 months or longer. With Lovenox, you need an injection, usually every 12 hours. You or someone close to you may be instructed in injecting the medication, or a visiting nurse may do the injections, if necessary.

  Even if a nurse is not needed to give the injections, one will usually visit your home each day to perform a finger stick blood test. The results of this test determine your daily dose of warfarin. After the blood test and the warfarin dose stabilize, the blood tests are done less often (e.g., every 2 weeks).

- Report any sign of bleeding (e.g., excessive bruising of the skin; blood in urine or stool). If superficial bleeding occurs, apply direct pressure to the site for 3 to 5 minutes or longer if necessary.

Self-Administration

- Take aspirin with food or after meals, with 8 oz of water, to decrease stomach irritation. However, stomach upset is uncommon with the small doses used for antiplatelet effects. Do not crush or chew coated tablets (long-acting preparations).

- Take cilostazol (Pletal) 30 minutes before or 2 hours after morning and evening meals for better absorption and effectiveness.

- Take ticlopidine (Ticlid) with food or after meals to decrease GI upset. Clopidogrel (Plavix) may be taken with or without food.

- With Lovenox, wash hands and cleanse skin to prevent infection; inject deep under the skin, around the navel, upper thigh, or buttocks; and change the injection site daily. If excessive bruising occurs at the injection site, rubbing an ice cube over an area before the injection may be helpful.

indicate low levels of clotting factors and delayed blood coagulation. During heparin therapy, the aPTT should be maintained at approximately 1.5 to 2.5 times the control or baseline value. The normal control value is 25 to 35 seconds; therefore, therapeutic values are 45 to 70 seconds, approximately. With continuous IV infusion, blood for the aPTT may be drawn at any time; with intermittent administration, blood for the aPTT should be drawn approximately 1 hour before a dose of heparin is scheduled. Monitoring of aPTT is not necessary with low-dose standard heparin given Sub-Q for prophylaxis of thromboembolism or with the LMWHs (e.g., enoxaparin).

Applying Your Knowledge 54-2

Mr. Dusseau's aPTT is measured to regulate the amount of heparin he receives. What is the aPTT goal for a therapeutic value?

Warfarin dosage is regulated according to the INR, for which therapeutic values are 2.0 to 3.0 in most conditions. An average daily dose of 4 to 5 milligrams maintains a therapeutic INR; stopping warfarin returns an elevated INR to normal in approximately 4 days in most patients.

The INR is based on prothrombin time (PT). PT is sensitive to changes in three of the four vitamin K–dependent coagulation factors. Thus, normal or control values indicate normal levels of these factors; therapeutic values indicate low levels of the factors and delayed blood coagulation. A normal baseline or control PT is approximately 12 seconds; a therapeutic value is approximately 1.5 times the control, or 18 seconds.

When warfarin is started, PT and INR should be assessed daily until a stable daily dose is reached (the dose that maintains PT and INR within therapeutic ranges and does not cause bleeding). Thereafter, PT and INR are determined every 2 to 4 weeks for the duration of oral anticoagulant drug therapy. If the warfarin dose is changed, PT and INR measurements are needed more often until a stable daily dose is again established.

For many years, PT was used to regulate warfarin dosage. PT is determined by adding a mixture of thromboplastin and calcium to citrated plasma and measuring the time (in seconds) it takes for the blood to clot. However, values vary among laboratories according to the type of thromboplastin and the instrument used to measure PT. The INR system standardizes PT by comparing a particular thromboplastin with a standard thromboplastin designated by the World Health Organization. Advantages of the INR include consistent values among laboratories, more consistent warfarin dosage with less risk of bleeding or thrombosis, and more consistent reports of clinical trials and other research studies. Some laboratories report both PT and INR.

Warfarin dosage may need to be reduced in patients with biliary tract disorders (e.g., obstructive jaundice), liver disease (e.g., hepatitis, cirrhosis), malabsorption syndromes (e.g., steatorrhea), hyperthyroidism, or fever. These conditions increase

anticoagulant drug effects by reducing absorption of vitamin K, decreasing hepatic synthesis of blood clotting factors, or increasing the breakdown of clotting factors. Despite these influencing factors, however, the primary determinant of dosage is the PT and INR.

Warfarin interacts with many other drugs to cause increased, decreased, or unpredictable anticoagulant effects (see Nursing Actions). Thus, warfarin dosage may need to be increased or decreased when other drugs are given concomitantly. Most drugs can be given if warfarin dosage is titrated according to the PT or INR and altered appropriately when an interacting drug is added or stopped. INR or PT measurements and vigilant observation are needed whenever a drug is added to or removed from a drug therapy regimen containing warfarin.

⊘ Applying Your Knowledge 54-3

How Can You Avoid This Medication Error?
In anticipation of Mr. Dusseau's discharge from the hospital, the physician changes his medication from heparin to warfarin. The order is for warfarin 5 mg PO daily and for evaluation of baseline PT and INR. You administer the warfarin and order the blood work for the next morning.

Thrombolytic Therapy

▪ Thrombolytic therapy should be performed only by experienced personnel in an intensive care or diagnostic/interventional setting with cardiac and other monitoring devices in place.

▪ All of the available agents are effective with recommended uses. Thus, the choice of a thrombolytic agent depends mainly on risks of adverse effects and costs. All of the drugs may cause bleeding. Alteplase may act more specifically on the fibrin in a clot and cause less systemic depletion of fibrinogen, but this agent is very expensive. Streptokinase, the least expensive agent, may cause allergic reactions because it is a foreign protein. Combination therapy (e.g., with alteplase and streptokinase) may also be used.

▪ Before a thrombolytic agent is begun, INR, aPTT, platelet count, and fibrinogen should be checked to establish baseline values and to determine if a blood coagulation disorder is present. Two or 3 hours after thrombolytic therapy is started, the fibrinogen level can be measured to determine that fibrinolysis is occurring. Alternatively, INR or aPTT can be checked for increased values because the breakdown products of fibrin exert anticoagulant effects.

▪ Major factors in decreasing risks of bleeding are selecting recipients carefully, avoiding invasive procedures when possible, and omitting anticoagulant or antiplatelet drugs while thrombolytics are being given. If bleeding does occur, it is most likely from a venipuncture or invasive procedure site, and local pressure may control it. If bleeding cannot be controlled or involves a vital organ, the thrombolytic drug should be stopped and fibrinogen replaced with whole blood plasma or cryoprecipitate. Aminocaproic acid or tranexamic acid may also be given.

- When the drugs are used in acute myocardial infarction, cardiac dysrhythmias may occur when blood flow is re-established. Therefore, antidysrhythmic drugs should be readily available.

Use in Special Populations

Use in Children

Little information is available about the use of anticoagulants in children. Heparin solutions containing benzyl alcohol as a preservative should not be given to premature infants because fatal reactions have been reported. When given for systemic anticoagulation, heparin dosage should be based on the child's weight (approximately 50 units/kg). Extreme caution should be used to ensure that the vial concentration of heparin is correct. Fatalities in infants have been reported with over-dosing of heparin. Safety and effectiveness of LMWHs (e.g., enoxaparin) have not been established in children.

Warfarin is given to children after cardiac surgery to prevent thromboembolism, but doses and guidelines for safe, effective use have not been developed. Accurate drug administration, close monitoring of blood coagulation tests, safety measures to prevent trauma and bleeding, avoiding interacting drugs, and informing others in the child's environment (e.g., teachers, baby-sitters, health care providers) are necessary.

Antiplatelet and thrombolytic drugs have no established indications for use in children.

Use in Older Adults

Older adults often have atherosclerosis and thrombotic disorders, including myocardial infarction, thrombotic stroke, and peripheral arterial insufficiency, for which they receive an anticoagulant or an antiplatelet drug. They are more likely than younger adults to experience bleeding and other complications of anticoagulant and antiplatelet drugs. For example, aspirin or clopidogrel is commonly used to prevent thrombotic stroke, but both drugs increase risks of hemorrhagic stroke.

With standard heparin, general principles for safe and effective use apply. With LMWHs, elimination may be delayed in older adults with renal impairment and the drugs should be used cautiously. They should also be used with caution in patients taking a platelet inhibitor (e.g., aspirin, clopidogrel) to prevent myocardial infarction or thrombotic stroke or an NSAID for arthritis pain. NSAIDs, which are commonly used by older adults, also have antiplatelet effects. Patients who take an NSAID daily may not need low-dose aspirin for antithrombotic effects.

With warfarin, dosage should be reduced because impaired liver function and decreased plasma proteins increase the risks of bleeding. Also, many drugs interact with warfarin to increase or decrease its effect, and older adults often take multiple drugs. Starting or stopping any drug may require that warfarin dosage be adjusted.

Use in Patients With Renal Impairment

Most anticoagulant, antiplatelet, and thrombolytic drugs may be used in patients with impaired renal function. For example, heparin and warfarin can be used in usual dosages, and thrombolytic agents (e.g., streptokinase, urokinase) may be used to dissolve clots in IV catheters or vascular access sites for hemodialysis. Dosage of LMWHs should be reduced in patients with severe renal impairment (creatinine clearance < 30 mL/minute) because they are excreted by the kidneys and elimination is slowed. In addition, home management of DVT with LMWHs and warfarin is contraindicated in patients with severe renal impairment. Guidelines for the use of other drugs include the following:

- Anagrelide may be given to patients with renal impairment (e.g., serum creatinine < 2 mg/dL) if potential benefits outweigh risks. Patients receiving this medication should be monitored closely for signs of renal toxicity.

- Cilostazol is probably safe to use in patients with mild or moderate renal impairment. However, severe renal impairment alters drug protein binding and increases blood levels of metabolites.

- Clopidogrel does not need dosage reduction in patients with renal impairment.

- Eptifibatide does not need dosage reduction in patients with mild to moderate renal impairment. No data are available for patients with severe impairment or those on hemodialysis.

- Lepirudin is excreted by the kidneys and may accumulate in patients with impaired renal function. Dosage should be reduced.

- Ticlopidine may be more likely to cause bleeding in patients with renal impairment because the plasma drug concentration is increased and elimination is slower.

- Tirofiban clearance from plasma is decreased approximately 50% in patients with severe renal impairment (e.g., creatinine clearance < 30 mL/minute), including those receiving hemodialysis. Dosage must be reduced by approximately 50%.

Use in Patients With Hepatic Impairment

Little information is available about the use of most anticoagulant, antiplatelet, and thrombolytic drugs in patients with impaired liver function. However, such drugs should be used very cautiously because these patients may already be predisposed to bleeding due to decreased hepatic synthesis of clotting factors. Additional considerations include the following:

- Warfarin is more likely to cause bleeding in patients with liver disease, because of decreased synthesis of vitamin K. In addition, warfarin is eliminated only by hepatic metabolism and may accumulate with liver impairment.

- LMWHs are contraindicated for home management of DVT in patients with severe liver disease because of high risks of excessive bleeding.

■ Anagrelide is metabolized in the liver and may accumulate with hepatic impairment. Patients with evidence of impairment (e.g., bilirubin or aspartate aminotransferase more than 1.5 times the upper limit of normal) should receive anagrelide only if potential benefits outweigh potential risks. When anagrelide is given, patients should be closely monitored for signs of hepatotoxicity.

■ Clopidogrel is metabolized in the liver and may accumulate with hepatic impairment. It should be used cautiously.

■ Dipyridamole is metabolized in the liver and excreted in bile.

Use in Home Care

Antiplatelet agents and warfarin are used for long-term prevention or management of thromboembolism and are often taken at home. For prevention, antiplatelet agents and warfarin are usually self-administered at home, with periodic office or clinic visits for blood tests and other follow-up care.

For home management of DVT, warfarin may be self-administered, but a nurse usually visits, performs a fingerstick INR, and notifies the prescriber, who then prescribes the appropriate dose of warfarin. Precautions are needed to decrease risks of bleeding. The risk of bleeding has lessened in recent years because of the lower doses of warfarin being used. In addition, bleeding during warfarin therapy may be caused by medical conditions other than anticoagulation.

Heparin may also be taken at home. Standard heparin may be taken Sub-Q, but use of LMWHs for home management of venous thrombosis has become standard practice. Enoxaparin is approved by the Food and Drug Administration for outpatient use. Daily visits by a home care nurse may be needed if the patient or a family member is unable or unwilling to inject the medication. Platelet counts should be done before and every 2 to 3 days during heparin therapy. Heparin should be discontinued if the platelet count falls below 100,000 or to less than half the baseline value.

Most home management regimens involve a structured protocol. Patients and family members should be educated about the disorder (usually DVT), including the potential consequences of either overcoagulation or undercoagulation and the need for blood tests.

The home care nurse needs to assess patients in relation to knowledge about prescribed drugs and ability and willingness to comply with instructions for taking the drugs, obtaining blood tests when indicated, and taking safety precautions. In addition, assess the environment for risk factors for injury. Interventions vary with patients, environments, and assessment data but may include reinforcing instructions for safe use of the drugs, assisting patients to obtain laboratory tests, and teaching how to observe for signs and symptoms of bleeding.

Use of Herbal and Dietary Supplements

Many commonly used herbs and supplements have a profound effect on drugs used for anticoagulation. Multivitamin supplements may contain 25 to 28 micrograms of vitamin K and should be taken consistently to avoid fluctuating vitamin K levels. Doses of vitamin C in excess of 500 milligrams per day may lower INR, and vitamin E in excess of 400 international units per day may increase warfarin effects. Herbs commonly used that may increase the effects of warfarin include alfalfa, celery, clove, feverfew, garlic, ginger, ginkgo, ginseng, and licorice. Patients taking warfarin should be questioned carefully about their use of herbs as well as vitamin or mineral supplements.

Applying Your Knowledge 54-4

After 6 months of treatment with warfarin, the physician orders Mr. Dusseau to change to aspirin therapy. What is the purpose of aspirin therapy?

Nursing Actions — Drugs That Affect Blood Coagulation

NURSING ACTIONS	RATIONALE/EXPLANATION

1. Administer accurately
  a. With standard heparin:
    (1) When handwriting a heparin dose, write out "units" rather than using the abbreviation "U."
    (2) Check dosage and vial label carefully.
	This is a safety precaution to avoid erroneous dosage. For example, 1000 U (1000 units) may be misread as 10,000 units. Underdosage may cause thromboembolism, and overdosage may cause bleeding. In addition, heparin is available in several concentrations (1000, 2500, 5000, 10,000, 15,000, 20,000, and 40,000 units/mL).

(3) For subcutaneous (Sub-Q) heparin:
      (a) Use a 26-gauge, ½-inch needle.
      (b) Leave a small air bubble in the syringe to follow dose.
	To minimize trauma and risk of bleeding
	Locks drug into subcutaneous space and minimizes trauma

NURSING ACTIONS	RATIONALE/EXPLANATION
(c) Grasp a skinfold and inject the heparin into it, at a 90-degree angle, without aspirating.	To give the drug in a deep subcutaneous or fat layer, with minimal trauma
(d) Do not massage site after injection.	
(4) For intermittent intravenous (IV) administration:	
(a) Give by direct injection into a heparin lock or tubing injection site.	These methods prevent repeated venipunctures.
(b) Dilute the dose in 50–100 mL of any IV fluid (usually 5% dextrose in water).	
(5) For continuous IV administration:	This is usually the preferred method because it maintains consistent serum drug levels and decreases risks of bleeding.
(a) Use a volume-control device and an infusion-control device.	To regulate dosage and flow rate accurately
(b) Add only enough heparin for a few hours. One effective method is to fill the volume-control set (e.g., Volutrol) with 100 mL of 5% dextrose in water and add 5000 units of heparin to yield a concentration of 50 units/mL. Dosage is regulated by varying the flow rate. For example, administration of 1000 units/h requires a flow rate of 20 mL/h. Another method is to add 25,000 units of heparin to 500 mL of IV solution.	To avoid inadvertent administration of large amounts. Whatever method is used, it is desirable to standardize concentration of heparin solutions within an institution. Standardization is safer, because it reduces risks of errors in dosage.
b. With low–molecular-weight heparins:	
(1) Give by deep Sub-Q injection, into an abdominal skin fold, with the patient lying down, using the same technique as standard heparin. Do not rub the injection site.	To decrease bruising
(2) Rotate sites.	
c. After the initial dose of warfarin, check the international normalized ratio (INR) before giving a subsequent dose. Do not give the dose if the INR is above 3.0. Notify the health care provider.	The INR is measured daily until a maintenance dose is established, then periodically throughout warfarin therapy. An elevated INR indicates a high risk of bleeding.
d. Give ticlopidine with food or after meals; give cilostazol 30 minutes before or 2 hours after morning and evening meals; give clopidogrel with or without food.	
e. With eptifibatide, tirofiban, and thrombolytic agents, follow manufacturers' instructions for reconstitution and administration.	These drugs require special preparation and administration techniques.
2. Observe for therapeutic effects	
a. With prophylactic heparins and warfarin, observe for the absence of signs and symptoms of thrombotic disorders.	
b. With therapeutic heparins and warfarin, observe for decrease or improvement in signs and symptoms (e.g., less edema and pain with deep vein thrombosis, less chest pain and respiratory difficulty with pulmonary embolism).	
c. With prophylactic or therapeutic warfarin, observe for an INR between 2.0 and 3.0.	Frequency of INR determinations varies, but the test should be done periodically in all patients taking warfarin.
d. With therapeutic heparin, observe for an activated partial thromboplastin time of 1.5 to 2 times the control value.	
e. With anagrelide, observe for a decrease in platelet count.	Platelet counts should be done every 2 days during the first week of management and weekly until a maintenance dose is reached. Counts usually begin to decrease within the first 2 weeks of therapy.
f. With aspirin, clopidogrel, and other antiplatelet drugs, observe for the absence of thrombotic disorders (e.g., myocardial infarction, stroke).	
g. With cilostazol, observe for ability to walk farther without leg pain (intermittent claudication).	Improvement may occur within 2–4 weeks or take as long as 12 weeks.
3. Observe for adverse effects	
a. Bleeding:	Bleeding is the major adverse effect of anticoagulant drugs. It may occur anywhere in the body, spontaneously or in response to minor trauma.
	With eptifibatide and tirofiban, most major bleeding occurs at the arterial access site for cardiac catheterization.
(1) Record vital signs regularly.	Hypotension and tachycardia may indicate internal bleeding.

(continued on page 878)

NURSING ACTIONS	RATIONALE/EXPLANATION
(2) Check stools for blood (melena).	Gastrointestinal (GI) bleeding is fairly common; risks are increased with intubation. Blood in stools may be bright red, tarry (blood that has been digested by GI secretions), or occult (hidden to the naked eye but present with a guaiac test). Hematemesis also may occur.
(3) Check urine for blood (hematuria).	Genitourinary bleeding also is fairly common; risks are increased with catheterization or instrumentation. Urine may be red (indicating fresh bleeding) or brownish or smoky gray (indicating old blood). Or bleeding may be microscopic (red blood cells are visible only on microscopic examination during urinalysis).
(4) Inspect the skin and mucous membranes daily.	Bleeding may occur in the skin as petechiae, purpura, or ecchymoses. Surgical wounds, skin lesions, parenteral injection sites, the nose, and gums may be bleeding sites.
(5) Assess for excessive menstrual flow. b. Other adverse effects:	
(1) With heparin, tissue irritation at injection sites, transient alopecia, reversible thrombocytopenia, paresthesias, and hypersensitivity	These effects are uncommon. They are more likely to occur with large doses or prolonged administration.
(2) With warfarin, dermatitis, diarrhea, and alopecia	These effects occur only occasionally. Warfarin has been given for prolonged periods without toxicity.
(3) With anagrelide, adverse cardiovascular effects (e.g., tachycardia, vasodilation, heart failure)	These effects are most likely to occur in patients with known heart disease.
(4) With clopidogrel and ticlopidine, GI upset, skin rash, neutropenia, and thrombocytopenia	Neutropenia and thrombocytopenia are more likely to occur with ticlopidine than clopidogrel.
c. With thrombolytic drugs, observe for bleeding with all uses and reperfusion dysrhythmias when used for acute myocardial infarction.	Bleeding is most likely to occur at sites of venipuncture or other invasive procedures. Reperfusion dysrhythmias may occur when blood supply is restored to previously ischemic myocardium.
4. Observe for drug interactions	
a. Drugs that *increase* risks of bleeding with anticoagulant, antiplatelet, and thrombolytic agents:	These drugs are often used concurrently or sequentially to decrease risks of myocardial infarction or stroke.
(1) Any one of these drugs in combination with any other drug that affects hemostasis	
(2) A combination of these drugs	
b. Drugs that *increase* effects of heparins:	
(1) Antiplatelet drugs (e.g., aspirin, clopidogrel, others)	
(2) Warfarin	Additive anticoagulant effects and increased risks of bleeding
(3) Parenteral penicillins and cephalosporins	Some may affect blood coagulation and increase risks of bleeding.
c. Drugs that *decrease* effects of heparins:	
(1) Antihistamines, digoxin, tetracyclines	These drugs antagonize the anticoagulant effects of heparin. Mechanisms are not clear.
(2) Protamine sulfate	The antidote for heparin overdose
d. Drugs that *increase* effects of warfarin:	
(1) Analgesics (e.g., acetaminophen, aspirin and other nonsteroidal anti-inflammatory drugs)	Mechanisms by which drugs may increase effects of warfarin include inhibiting warfarin metabolism, displacing warfarin from binding sites on serum albumin, causing antiplatelet effects, inhibiting bacterial synthesis of vitamin K in the intestinal tract, and others.
(2) Androgens and anabolic steroids	
(3) Antibacterial drugs (e.g., aminoglycosides, erythromycin, fluoroquinolones, isoniazid, metronidazole, penicillins, cephalosporins, rimethoprim-sulfamethoxazole, tetracyclines)	
(4) Antifungal drugs (e.g., fluconazole, ketoconazole, miconazole), including intravaginal use	
(5) Antiseizure drugs (e.g., phenytoin)	
(6) Cardiovascular drugs (e.g., amiodarone, beta blockers, loop diuretics, gemfibrozil, lovastatin, propafenone, quinidine)	
(7) Gastrointestinal drugs (e.g., cimetidine, omeprazole)	
(8) Thyroid preparations (e.g., levothyroxine)	

NURSING ACTIONS	RATIONALE/EXPLANATION
e. Drugs that *decrease* effects of warfarin:	
(1) Antacids and griseofulvin	May decrease GI absorption
(2) Carbamazepine, disulfiram, rifampin	These drugs activate liver metabolizing enzymes, which accelerate the rate of metabolism of warfarin.
(3) Cholestyramine	Decreases absorption
(4) Diuretics	Increase synthesis and concentration of blood clotting factors
(5) Estrogens, including oral contraceptives	Increase synthesis of clotting factors and have thromboembolic effect
(6) Vitamin K	Restores prothrombin and other vitamin K–dependent clotting factors in the blood. Antidote for overdose of warfarin.
f. Drug that may *increase* or *decrease* effects of warfarin:	
(1) Alcohol	Alcohol may induce liver enzymes, which decrease effects by accelerating the rate of metabolism of the anticoagulant drug. However, with alcohol-induced liver disease (i.e., cirrhosis), effects may be increased owing to impaired metabolism of warfarin.
g. Drugs that *increase* effects of cilostazol:	
(1) Diltiazem	These drugs inhibit the main cytochrome P450 enzyme (CYP3A4) that metabolizes cilostazol. Grapefruit juice also inhibits drug metabolism and should be avoided.
(2) Erythromycin	
(3) Itraconazole, ketoconazole	

Key Concepts

- Anticoagulant drugs are given to prevent formation of new clots and extension of clots already present.
- Antiplatelet drugs are used to prevent arterial thrombosis.
- Thrombolytic agents are used to dissolve thrombi and limit tissue damage in selected thromboembolic disorders.
- No antidote exists for the effects of aspirin or the adenosine diphosphate receptor antagonists because both produce irreversible platelet effects; platelet transfusion may be required.
- Warfarin dosage is regulated according to the INR (derived from prothrombin time [PT]), for which a therapeutic value is between 2.0 to 3.0 in most conditions; a therapeutic PT value is approximately 1.5 times the control, or 18 seconds.
- Herbs commonly used that may increase the effects of warfarin include alfalfa, celery, clove, feverfew, garlic, ginger, ginkgo, ginseng, and licorice.
- Vitamin K (Mephyton) is the antidote for warfarin.
- The FDA has issued a **BLACK BOX WARNING** with warfarin due to its risk of causing major or fatal bleeding.

- Currently available LMWHs (dalteparin, enoxaparin) differ from standard heparin and each other and are not interchangeable.
- During heparin therapy, the aPTT should be maintained at approximately 1.5 to 2.5 times the control or baseline value.
- Monitoring of aPTT is not necessary with low-dose standard heparin given Sub-Q for prophylaxis of thromboembolism or with the LMWHs.
- Protamine sulfate is the antidote for standard heparin and LMWHs.
- The FDA has issued a **BLACK BOX WARNING** with the use of protamine sulfate due to the risk of severe hypotension, cardiovascular collapse, noncardiogenic pulmonary edema, catastrophic pulmonary vasoconstriction, and pulmonary hypertension with its use.
- When the thrombolytic agents are used in acute myocardial infarction, cardiac dysrhythmias may occur when blood flow is re-established; antidysrhythmic drugs should be readily available.

Review and Application Exercises

Short Answer Exercises

1. What are the major functions of the endothelium, platelets, and coagulation factors in hemostasis and thrombosis?

2. What are the indications for use of heparin and warfarin?

3. How do heparin and warfarin differ in mechanism of action, onset and duration of action, and method of administration?

4. List interventions to protect patients from anticoagulant-induced bleeding.

5. When is it appropriate to use protamine sulfate as an antidote for heparin?

6. When is it appropriate to use vitamin K as an antidote for warfarin?

7. How do antiplatelet drugs differ from heparin and warfarin?

8. For what conditions are antiplatelet drugs indicated?

9. When is it appropriate to use a thrombolytic drug?

10. How do aminocaproic acid and tranexamic acid stop bleeding induced by thrombolytics?

11. Compare and contrast nursing care needs of patients receiving anticoagulant therapy in hospital and home settings.

NCLEX-Style Questions

12. In explaining the use of warfarin to a patient, the nurse is correct in telling her all of the following, except
    a. Warfarin is a vitamin K antagonist.
    b. Warfarin does not cross the placenta.
    c. Warfarin is used for long-term anticoagulation therapy.
    d. Warfarin is metabolized by the liver.

13. The nurse is reviewing the laboratory results of a hospitalized patient receiving IV heparin therapy for pulmonary embolism. The aPTT is 38 seconds. The nurse should
    a. not give the next dose because the level is too high
    b. continue the present order because the level is appropriate
    c. notify the provider that the aPTT is low and the dose should be increased
    d. request an order for warfarin now that the patient is heparinized

14. The nurse explains to a patient that aspirin suppresses blood clotting by
    a. inactivating thrombin
    b. promoting fibrin degradation
    c. decreasing synthesis of clotting factors
    d. decreasing platelet aggregation

15. A patient's Port-a-Cath has become occluded with thrombus. The nurse expects which agent will likely be used to lyse the clot?
    a. protamine sulfate
    b. tirofiban
    c. streptokinase
    d. enoxaparin

16. Clopidogrel is indicated for
    a. reduction of myocardial infarction, stroke, and vascular death in patients with atherosclerosis
    b. adjunctive therapy to warfarin for DVT
    c. heparin-induced thrombocytopenia
    d. patients in whom bleeding is a consideration

Selected References

Barman, N. (2006). Antithrombotic therapy for percutaneous coronary intervention. *Cardiology Clinics, 24,* 175–199, v–vi.

Di Niso, M., Middeldorp, S., & Büller, H. R. (2005). Direct thrombin inhibitors. *New England Journal of Medicine, 8,* 1028–1040.

Drug facts and comparisons. (Updated monthly). St. Louis, MO: Facts and Comparisons.

Gaspard, K. J. (2005). Disorders of hemostasis. In C. M. Porth (Ed.), *Pathophysiology: Concepts of altered health states* (7th ed., pp. 287–298). Philadelphia: Lippincott Williams & Wilkins.

Karch, A. M. (2007). *2008 Lippincott's nursing drug guide.* Philadelphia: Lippincott Williams & Wilkins.

Kiernan, T.J. (2007). Thrombolysis in acute myocardial infarction: Current status. *Medical Clinics of North America, 91,* 617–637.

Lacy, C. F., Armstrong, L. L., Goldman, M. P., & Lance, L. L. (2007). *Lexi-Comp's drug information handbook* (15th ed.). Hudson, OH: American Pharmaceutical Association.

Nguyen, T. A., Diodati, J. G., & Pharand, C. (2005). Resistance to clopidogrel: A review of the evidence. *Journal of the American College of Cardiology, 45,* 1157–1164.

Nutescu, E. A., Shapiro, N. L., & Chevalier, A.(2006). New anticoagulant agents: Direct thrombin inhibitors. *Clinics in Geriatric Medicine,22,* 33–56, viii.

Shorr, A. F. (2007). The pharmacoeconomics of deep vein thrombosis treatment. *American Journal of Medicine, 120* (10 Suppl 2), S35–S41.

Shorr, A. F., Jackson, W. L., Moores, L. K., & Warkentin, T. E. (2007). Minimizing costs for treating deep vein thrombosis: The role for fondaparinux. *Journal of Thrombosis and Thrombolysis, 23,* 229–236.

Drugs for Dyslipidemia

KEY TERMS

- Central adiposity
- Cholesterol
- Dyslipidemia
- Hyperlipo proteinemias
- Lipoproteins
- Metabolic syndrome

LEARNING OBJECTIVES

After studying this chapter, you will be able to:

1. Recognize the role of dyslipidemia in the metabolic syndrome.
2. Identify sources and functions of cholesterol and triglycerides.
3. Describe dyslipidemic drugs in terms of mechanism of action, indications for use, major adverse effects, and nursing process implications.
4. Educate patients about pharmacologic and nonpharmacologic measures to prevent or reduce dyslipidemia.
5. Use the nursing process in the care of patients with dyslipidemia.

Applying Your Knowledge

Lewis Watkins is a 62-year-old man who has had elevated cholesterol and triglyceride levels during his two previous visits to the physician. He has tried diet modification and increasing exercise; however, his lipid levels remain elevated. His physician decides to prescribe atorvastatin 10 mg PO daily and gemfibrozil 600 mg PO bid. You are the home care nurse assigned to his care.

Introduction

Dyslipidemic drugs are used in the management of patients with elevated blood lipids, a major risk factor for atherosclerosis and vascular disorders such as coronary artery disease, strokes, and peripheral arterial insufficiency. These drugs have proven efficacy and are being used increasingly to reduce morbidity and mortality from coronary heart disease and other atherosclerosis-related cardiovascular disorders. To understand clinical use of these drugs, it is necessary to understand characteristics of blood lipids, metabolic syndrome, and types of blood lipid disorders.

Blood Lipids

Blood lipids, which include cholesterol, phospholipids, and triglycerides, are derived from the diet or synthesized by the liver and intestine. Most *cholesterol* is found in body cells, where it is a component of cell membranes and performs other essential functions. In cells of the adrenal glands, ovaries, and testes, cholesterol is required for the synthesis of steroid hormones (e.g., cortisol, estrogen, progesterone, testosterone). In liver cells, cholesterol is used to form cholic acid which is conjugated with other substances to form bile salts; bile salts promote absorption and digestion of fats. In addition, a small amount of cholesterol is found in blood serum. Serum cholesterol is the portion of total body cholesterol involved in formation of atherosclerotic plaques. Unless a person has a genetic disorder of lipid metabolism, the amount of cholesterol in the blood is strongly related to dietary intake of saturated fat. Phospholipids are essential components of cell membranes, and triglycerides provide energy for cellular metabolism.

Blood lipids are transported in plasma by specific proteins called *lipoproteins*. Each lipoprotein contains cholesterol, phospholipid, and triglyceride bound to protein. The lipoproteins vary in density and amounts of lipid and protein. Density is determined mainly by the amount of protein, which is more dense than fat. Thus, density increases as the proportion of protein increases. The lipoproteins are differentiated according to these properties, which can be measured in the laboratory. For example, high-density lipoprotein (HDL) cholesterol contains larger amounts of protein and smaller amounts of lipid; low-density lipoprotein (LDL) cholesterol contains less protein and larger amounts of lipid. Other plasma lipoproteins are chylomicrons and very–low-density lipoproteins (VLDL).

Additional characteristics of lipoproteins are described in Box 55-1.

Metabolic Syndrome

Metabolic syndrome is a group of cardiovascular risk factors linked with obesity. *The Third Report of the National Cholesterol Education Program Expert Panel on Detection, Evaluation, and Treatment of High Blood Cholesterol in Adults* (NCEP III) clustered several elements of metabolic syndrome: elevated waist circumference (*central adiposity*), elevated triglycerides, reduced high-density lipoprotein cholesterol, elevated blood pressure, and elevated fasting glucose. These risk factors frequently produce an additive effect on cardiovascular,

---

Box 55-1	Types of Lipoproteins

Chylomicrons, the largest lipoprotein molecules, are synthesized in the wall of the small intestine. They carry recently ingested dietary cholesterol and triglycerides that have been absorbed from the gastrointestinal tract. Hyperchylomicronemia normally occurs after a fatty meal, reaches peak levels in 3 to 4 hours, and subsides within 12 to 14 hours. Chylomicrons carry triglycerides to fat and muscle cells, where the enzyme lipoprotein lipase breaks down the molecule and releases fatty acids to be used for energy or stored as fat. This process leaves a remnant containing cholesterol, which is then transported to the liver. Thus, chylomicrons transport triglycerides to peripheral tissues and cholesterol to the liver.

Low-density lipoprotein (LDL) cholesterol, sometimes called "bad cholesterol," transports approximately 75% of serum cholesterol and carries it to peripheral tissues and the liver. LDL cholesterol is removed from the circulation by receptor and nonreceptor mechanisms. The receptor mechanism involves the binding of LDL cholesterol to receptors on cell surface membranes. The bound LDL molecule is then engulfed into the cell, where it is broken down by enzymes and releases free cholesterol into the cytoplasm.

Most LDL cholesterol receptors are located in the liver. However, nonhepatic tissues (e.g., adrenal glands, smooth muscle cells, endothelial cells, and lymphoid cells) also have receptors by which they obtain the cholesterol needed for building cell membranes and synthesizing hormones. These cells can regulate their cholesterol intake by adding or removing LDL receptors.

Approximately two thirds of the LDL cholesterol is removed from the bloodstream by the receptor-dependent mechanism. The number of LDL receptors on cell membranes determines the amount of LDL degradation (i.e., the more receptors on cells, the more LDL is broken down). Conditions that decrease the number or function of receptors (e.g., high dietary intake of cholesterol, saturated fat, or calories), increase blood levels of LDL.

The remaining one third is removed by mechanisms that do not involve receptors. Nonreceptor uptake occurs in various cells, especially when levels of circulating LDL cholesterol are high. For example, macrophage cells in arterial walls can attach LDL, thereby promoting accumulation of cholesterol and the development of atherosclerosis. The amount of LDL cholesterol removed by nonreceptor mechanisms is increased with inadequate numbers of receptors or excessive amounts of LDL cholesterol.

A high serum level of LDL cholesterol is atherogenic and a strong risk factor for coronary heart disease. The body normally attempts to compensate for high serum levels by inhibiting hepatic synthesis of cholesterol and cellular synthesis of new LDL receptors.

Very–low-density lipoprotein (VLDL) contains approximately 75% triglycerides and 25% cholesterol. It transports endogenous triglycerides (those synthesized in the liver and intestine, not those derived exogenously, from food) to fat and muscle cells. There, as with chylomicrons, lipoprotein lipase breaks down the molecule and releases fatty acids to be used for energy or stored as fat. The removal of triglycerides from VLDL leaves a cholesterol-rich remnant, which returns to the liver. Then the cholesterol is secreted into the intestine, mostly as bile acids, or it is used to form more VLDL and recirculated.

High-density lipoprotein (HDL) cholesterol, often referred to as "good cholesterol," is a small but very important lipoprotein. It is synthesized in the liver and intestine and some is derived from the enzymatic breakdown of chylomicrons and VLDL. It contains moderate amounts of cholesterol. However, this cholesterol is transported from blood vessel walls to the liver for catabolism and excretion. This reverse transport of cholesterol has protective effects against coronary heart disease.

The mechanisms by which HDL cholesterol exerts protective effects are unknown. Possible mechanisms include clearing cholesterol from atheromatous plaque; increasing excretion of cholesterol so less is available for reuse in the formation of LDL cholesterol; and inhibiting cellular uptake of LDL cholesterol. Regular exercise and moderate alcohol consumption are associated with increased levels of HDL cholesterol; obesity, diabetes mellitus, genetic factors, smoking, and some medications (e.g., steroids and beta blockers) are associated with decreased levels. HDL cholesterol levels are not directly affected by diet.

Box 55-2	Types of Dyslipidemias

Type I is characterized by elevated or normal serum cholesterol, elevated triglycerides, and chylomicronemia. This rare condition may occur in infancy and childhood.

Type IIa (familial hypercholesterolemia) is characterized by a high level of low-density lipoprotein (LDL) cholesterol, a normal level of very–low-density lipoprotein (VLDL), and a normal or slightly increased level of triglycerides. It occurs in children and is a definite risk factor for development of atherosclerosis and coronary artery disease.

Type IIb (combined familial hyperlipoproteinemia) is characterized by increased levels of LDL, VLDL, cholesterol, and triglycerides and lipid deposits (xanthomas) in the feet, knees, and elbows. It occurs in adults.

Type III is characterized by elevations of cholesterol and triglycerides plus abnormal levels of LDL and VLDL. This type usually occurs in middle-aged adults (40–60 years) and

is associated with accelerated coronary and peripheral vascular disease.

Type IV is characterized by normal or elevated cholesterol levels, elevated triglycerides, and increased levels of VLDL. This type usually occurs in adults and may be the most common form of hyperlipoproteinemia. Type IV is often secondary to obesity, excessive intake of alcohol, or other diseases. Ischemic heart disease may occur at 40 to 50 years of age.

Type V is characterized by elevated cholesterol and triglyceride levels with an increased level of VLDL and chylomicronemia. This uncommon type usually occurs in adults. Type V is not associated with ischemic heart disease. Instead, it is associated with fat and carbohydrate intolerance, abdominal pain, and pancreatitis, which are relieved by lowering triglyceride levels.

cerebrovascular, and peripheral vascular disease and are principal contributors to the significant morbidity and mortality of these conditions. Improvements in insulin resistance and lipid profiles are essential lifestyle modifications and constitute first-line treatment of metabolic syndrome. This chapter specifically addresses management of components of metabolic syndrome related to dyslipidemia; additional discussion of other factors is found in Chapters 26 and 50.

Dyslipidemia

Dyslipidemia (also called hyperlipidemia) is associated with atherosclerosis and its many pathophysiologic effects (e.g., myocardial ischemia and infarction, stroke, peripheral arterial occlusive disease). Ischemic heart disease has a high rate of morbidity and mortality. Elevated total cholesterol and LDL cholesterol and reduced HDL cholesterol are the abnormalities that are major risk factors for coronary artery disease. Elevated triglycerides also play a role in cardiovascular disease. For example, high blood levels reflect excessive caloric intake (excessive dietary fats are stored in adipose tissue; excessive proteins and carbohydrates are converted to triglycerides and also stored in adipose tissue) and obesity. High caloric intake also increases the conversion of VLDL to LDL cholesterol, and high dietary intake of triglycerides and saturated fat decreases the activity of LDL receptors and increases synthesis of cholesterol. Very high triglyceride levels are associated with acute pancreatitis.

Dyslipidemia may be primary (i.e., genetic or familial) or secondary to dietary habits, other diseases (e.g., diabetes mellitus, alcoholism, hypothyroidism, obesity, obstructive liver disease), and medications (e.g., beta blockers, cyclosporine, oral estrogens, glucocorticoids, sertraline, thiazide diuretics, anti–human immunodeficiency virus protease inhibitors). Types of dyslipidemia (also called *hyperlipoproteinemias* because increased blood levels of lipoproteins accompany increased

blood lipid levels) are described in Box 55-2. Although hypercholesterolemia is usually emphasized, hypertriglyceridemia is also associated with most types of hyperlipoproteinemia.

Initial Management of Dyslipidemia

Overall, the most effective blood lipid profile for prevention or management of metabolic syndrome and its sequelae is high HDL cholesterol, low LDL cholesterol, and low total cholesterol. A low triglyceride level is also desirable. NCEP III classified blood lipid levels and proposed the following guidelines as treatment goals for patients with lipid abnormalities:

Total serum cholesterol (mg/dL)

Normal or desirable = less than 200

Borderline high = 200 to 239

High = 240 or above

LDL cholesterol (mg/dL)

Optimal = less than 100

Near or above optimal = 100 to 129

Borderline high = 130 to 159

High = 160 to 189

Very high = 190 or above

HDL cholesterol (mg/dL)

High = more than 60

Low = less than 40

Triglycerides (mg/dL)

Normal or desirable = less than 150

Borderline high = 150 to 199

High = 200 to 499

Very high = 500 or above

For accurate interpretation of a patient's lipid profile, blood samples for laboratory testing of triglycerides should be drawn after the patient has fasted for 12 hours. Fasting is not required for cholesterol testing.

NCEP III recommends treatment of patients according to their blood levels of total and LDL cholesterol and their risk factors for cardiovascular disease (Table 55-1). Note that therapeutic lifestyle changes (TLC), including exercise, smoking cessation, changes in diet, and drug therapy, are recommended at lower serum cholesterol levels in patients who already have cardiovascular disease or diabetes mellitus. Also, the target LDL serum level is lower in these patients.

Guidelines include the following:

▪ Assess for, and treat, if present, conditions known to increase blood lipids (e.g., diabetes mellitus, hypothyroidism).

▪ Stop medications known to increase blood lipids, if possible.

▪ Start a low-fat diet. A Step I diet contains no more than 30% of calories from fat, less than 10% of calories from saturated fats (e.g., meat, dairy products), and less than 300 mg of cholesterol per day. A Step II diet contains no more than 30% of calories from fat, less than 7% of calories from saturated fat, and less than 200 mg of cholesterol per day. The Step II diet is more stringent and may be used initially in patients with more severe dyslipidemia, cardiovascular disease, or diabetes mellitus. It can decrease LDL cholesterol levels by 8% to 15%. Diets with more stringent fat restrictions than the Step II diet are not recommended because they produce little additional reduction in LDL cholesterol; raise serum triglyceride levels; and lower HDL cholesterol concentrations.

▪ Use the "Mediterranean diet," which includes moderate amounts of monounsaturated fats (e.g., canola, olive oils) and polyunsaturated fats (e.g., safflower, corn, cottonseed, sesame, soybean, sunflower oils) to also decrease risks of cardiovascular disease.

▪ Increase dietary intake of soluble fiber (e.g., psyllium preparations, oat bran, pectin, fruits and vegetables). This diet lowers serum LDL cholesterol by 5% to 10%.

▪ Dietary supplements (e.g., Cholestin) and cholesterol lowering margarines (e.g., Benecol, Take Control) can help reduce cholesterol levels. These products are considered to be foods, not drugs, and are costly.

▪ Start a weight-reduction diet if the patient is overweight or obese. Weight loss can increase HDL and decrease LDL.

▪ Emphasize regular aerobic exercise (usually 30 minutes at least three times weekly). This strategy increases blood levels of HDL.

▪ If the patient smokes, assist to develop a cessation plan. In addition to numerous other benefits, HDL levels are higher in nonsmokers.

▪ If the patient is postmenopausal, hormone replacement therapy can raise HDL and lower LDL.

▪ If the patient has elevated serum triglycerides, initial management includes efforts to achieve desirable body weight, ingest low amounts of saturated fat and cholesterol, exercise regularly, stop smoking, and reduce alcohol intake, if indicated. The goal is to reduce serum triglyceride levels to 200 mg/dL or less.

▪ Unless lipid levels are severely elevated, 6 months of intensive diet therapy and lifestyle modification may be undertaken before drug therapy is considered. It is essential that TLC continue during drug therapy because the benefits of diet, exercise, and drug therapy are additive.

Since the publication of the NCEP III in 2001, numerous clinical trials of statin therapy have been published. In 2004, more intensive treatment recommendations were established for those in the category of "very high" risk. Factors contributing to the increased risk include the presence of established cardiovascular disease or an acute coronary syndrome, with multiple major risk factors such as diabetes,

Table 55-1	National Cholesterol Education Program Recommendations for Treatment of Dyslipidemia		
Patient's Cardiovascular Disease Status	**THERAPEUTIC LIFESTYLE CHANGES (TLC)** LDL Cholesterol (mg/dL)	**DRUG THERAPY** LDL Cholesterol (mg/dL)	**GOAL OF THERAPY** LDL Cholesterol (mg/dL)
No or one risk factor	≥160	≥190	<160
More than two risk factors	≥130	≥160	<130
Has cardiovascular disease	≥100	≥130	<100

LDL, low-density lipoprotein.

obesity, hypertension (evidence of metabolic syndrome), high triglycerides, low HDL, and severe or poorly controlled risk factors such as continued cigarette smoking. These recommendations included consideration of treatment goals for LDL cholesterol to less than 70 milligrams per deciliter and earlier initiation of drug therapy in the presence of elevated triglyceride and low HDL levels. As current trials are continuing, the lower levels of LDL should be considered a therapeutic option for those at increased risk, with the goal of less than 100 milligrams per deciliter remaining as a strong recommendation for those not at high risk.

General Characteristics of Drugs Used for Management of Dyslipidemia

Dyslipidemic drugs are used to decrease blood lipids, prevent or delay the development of atherosclerotic plaque, promote the regression of existing atherosclerotic plaque, and reduce morbidity and mortality from cardiovascular disease. Clinical data

suggest that drug therapy may be efficacious even for those with mild to moderate elevations of LDL cholesterol. The drugs act by altering the production, absorption, metabolism, or removal of lipids and lipoproteins. Drug therapy is initiated when 6 months of dietary and other lifestyle changes fail to decrease dyslipidemia to an acceptable level. It is also recommended for patients with signs and symptoms of coronary heart disease, a strong family history of coronary heart disease or dyslipidemia, or other risk factors for atherosclerotic vascular disease (e.g., hypertension, diabetes mellitus, cigarette smoking). Although several dyslipidemic drugs are available, none is effective in all types of dyslipidemia.

Dyslipidemic Drugs: Classifications and Individual Drugs

Categories of drugs are described in this section; individual drugs are listed in Table 55-2. The sites of action of dyslipidemic drugs are found in Figure 55.1.

Table 55-2	Drugs at a Glance: Dyslipidemic Agents		
		ROUTES AND DOSAGE RANGES	
Generic/Trade Name	**Clinical Indications (Type of Dyslipidemia)**	**Adults**	**Children**
HMG-CoA Reductase Inhibitors (Statins)			
Atorvastatin (Lipitor)	Types IIa and IIb	PO 10–80 mg daily in a single dose	10–17y: 10 mg once daily to maximum of 20 mg/d
Fluvastatin (Lescol, Lescol XL)	Types IIa and IIb	PO 20–80 mg daily in 1 or 2 doses	10–16y: 20 mg once daily to maximum of 80 mg in 1 or 2 doses
Lovastatin (Mevacor, Altocor)	Types IIa and IIb	PO 20 mg daily with evening meal to 80 mg/d	10–17 y: 10–40 mg once daily with evening meal
Pravastatin (Pravachol)	Types IIa and IIb	PO 40–80 mg once daily; Elderly, PO 10 mg once daily initially	8–13 y: 20 mg/d; 14–18 y: 40 mg/d
Rosuvastatin (Crestor)	Types IIa and IIb, IV	PO 10–40 mg once daily	<18 y: not recommended
Simvastatin (Zocor)	Types 11a, 11b, IV, V	PO 5–80 mg once daily in the evening; Elderly, PO 5–20 mg once daily in the evening	10–17 y: 10 mg once daily in the evening to maximum of 40 mg/d
Fibrates			
Fenofibrate (TriCor)	Types IV, V (hypertriglyceridemia)	PO 48 mg once daily with meals increased if necessary to a maximum dose of 201 mg daily	

(continued on page 886)

Table 55-2	Drugs at a Glance: Dyslipidemic Agents (continued)		
		ROUTES AND DOSAGE RANGES	
Generic/Trade Name	**Clinical Indications (Type of Dyslipidemia)**	**Adults**	**Children**
Gemfibrozil (Lopid)	Types IV, V (hypertriglyceridemia)	PO 1200 mg daily, in 2 divided doses, 30 min before morning and evening meals	
Bile Acid Sequestrants			
Cholestyramine (Prevalite, Questran)	Type IIa	PO tablets, 4 g once or twice daily initially, gradually increased at monthly intervals to 8–16 g daily in 2 divided doses. Maximum daily dose, 24 g PO powder, 4 g 1–6 times daily	240 mg/kg/d in 3 divided doses
Colesevelam (WelChol)	Type IIa	PO 3.75 g daily in 1 or 2 doses with meals. Maximum daily dose, 4.375 g	
Colestipol (Colestid)	Type IIa	PO tablets, 2 g once or twice daily initially, gradually increased at 1- to 2-mo intervals, up to 16 g daily PO granules, 5 g daily initially, gradually increased at 1- to 2-mo intervals, up to 30 g daily in single or divided doses	
Cholesterol Absorption Inhibitor			
Ezetimibe (Zetia)	Types IIa and IIb	PO 10 mg once daily	<10 y: not recommended ≥10 y: PO 10 mg once daily
Miscellaneous			
Niacin (immediate-release)	Types II, III, IV, V	PO 2–6 g daily, in 3 or 4 divided doses, with or just after meals	PO 55–87 mg/kg/d, in 3 or 4 divided doses, with or just after meals
Niacin (extended-release)	Types IIa and IIb	PO 500–2000 mg daily	

HMG-CoA Reductase Inhibitors

The HMG-CoA reductase inhibitors or statins (e.g., **atorvastatin**) inhibit an enzyme (hydroxymethylglutaryl-coenzyme A reductase) required for hepatic synthesis of cholesterol. By decreasing production of cholesterol, these drugs decrease total serum cholesterol, LDL cholesterol, VLDL cholesterol, and triglycerides. They reduce LDL cholesterol within 2 weeks and reach maximal effects in approximately 4 to 6 weeks. HDL cholesterol levels remain unchanged or may increase.

These drugs are useful in treating most of the major types of dyslipidemia and are the most widely used dyslipidemic drugs. Studies indicate that these drugs can reduce the blood levels of C-reactive protein, which is associated with severe arterial inflammation that leads to heart attacks and strokes. The incidence of coronary artery disease is reduced by 25% to 60% and the risk of death from any cause by approxi-

mately 30%. Statins also reduce the risk of angina pectoris and peripheral arterial disease as well as the need for angioplasty and coronary artery grafting to increase or restore blood flow to the myocardium.

Applying Your Knowledge 55-1

You are counseling Mr. Watkins about his medication. He asks when he will need to have his laboratory work completed. How do you respond?

Atorvastatin is currently the most widely used statin and one of the most widely used drugs in the United States. There is indication that pravastatin may be preferred in patients who have had a transplant or who are receiving immunosuppres-

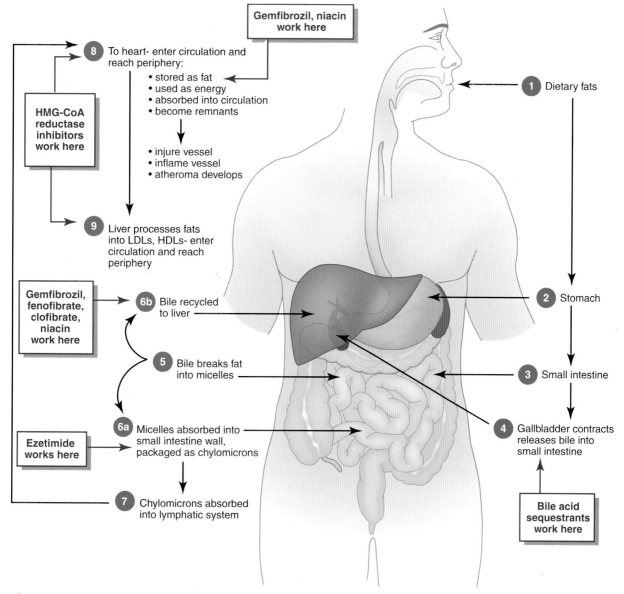

Figure 55-1 ■ Sites of dyslipidemic drugs.

sants, because it interacts less with immunosuppressant agents than other statins. There is controversy regarding clinical and subclinical effects of individual agents. Several studies have suggested that atorvastatin and **rosuvastatin** may possess some benefits that other statins do not. Multiple outcomes including intimal thickness, results of imaging studies, mortality, incidence of stroke, and progression of lesions have been studied, but there continue to be questions about the benefit profiles of individual drugs.

Absorption following oral administration varies by drug. **Lovastatin** and **pravastatin** are poorly absorbed; **fluvastatin** has the highest rate of absorption. Most of the statins undergo extensive first-past metabolism by the liver, which results in low levels of drug available for general circulation. Metabolism occurs in the liver, with 80% to 85% of drug metabolites excreted in feces and the remaining excreted in urine.

Statins are usually well tolerated; the most common adverse effects (nausea, constipation, diarrhea, abdominal cramps or pain, headache, skin rash) are usually mild and transient. More serious reactions include rare occurrences of hepatotoxicity and myopathy. Liver function studies should be monitored before onset of therapy, after 6 and 12 weeks of therapy, and intermittently during the course of therapy to detect any elevation or change. Statins can injure muscle tissue, resulting in muscle ache or weakness. Rarely is there progression to myositis and subsequent rhabdomyolysis, defined as muscle disintegration or dissociation. Factors that increase risk of myopathy include advanced age, frail or small body frame, high dosage of statins, concomitant use with fibrates, hypothyroidism, and multiple systemic diseases such as renal insufficiency secondary to diabetic nephropathy. Patients should be advised to notify their health care provider if unexplained muscle pain or tenderness occurs.

Statins are potentially teratogenic medications (pregnancy category D). Women of childbearing age should have contraceptive counseling to enhance awareness of the risks associated with statin use. Careful consideration should be given if potential benefits warrant use of the drug class in pregnant women despite potential risks.

Bile Acid Sequestrants

Bile acid sequestrants (e.g., **cholestyramine**) bind bile acids in the intestinal lumen. This causes the bile acids to be excreted in feces and prevents their being recirculated to the liver. Loss of bile acids stimulates hepatic synthesis of more bile acids from cholesterol. As more hepatic cholesterol is used to produce bile acids, more serum cholesterol moves into the liver to replenish the supply, thereby lowering serum cholesterol (primarily LDL). LDL cholesterol levels decrease within a week of starting these drugs and reach maximal reductions within a month. When the drugs are stopped, pretreatment LDL cholesterol levels return within a month.

These drugs are used mainly to reduce LDL cholesterol further in patients who are already taking a statin drug. The inhibition of cholesterol synthesis by a statin drug makes bile acid–binding drugs more effective. In addition, the combination increases HDL cholesterol and can further reduce the risk of cardiovascular disorders.

These drugs are not absorbed systemically, and their main adverse effects are abdominal fullness, flatulence, and constipation. They may decrease absorption of many oral medications (e.g., digoxin, folic acid, glipizide, propranolol, tetracyclines, thiazide diuretics, thyroid hormones, fat-soluble vitamins, warfarin). Other drugs should be taken at least 1 hour before or 4 hours after bile acid sequestrants. In addition, dosage of the interactive drug may need to be changed when a bile acid sequestrant is added or withdrawn.

Fibrates

Fibrates are derivatives of fibric acid (e.g., **gemfibrozil, fenofibrate**) and are similar to endogenous fatty acids. The drugs increase the oxidation of fatty acids in liver and muscle tissue and thereby decrease hepatic production of triglycerides, decrease VLDL cholesterol, and increase HDL cholesterol. These are the most effective drugs for reducing serum triglyceride levels, and their main indication for use is high serum triglyceride levels (>500 mg/dL). They are also useful for patients with low HDL cholesterol levels. In patients with coronary artery disease, management with gemfibrozil is associated with regression of atherosclerotic lesions on angiography.

These drugs are well absorbed following oral administration. Metabolism occurs in the liver and excretion is by urinary elimination. The main adverse effects are gastrointestinal discomfort and diarrhea, which may occur less often with fenofibrate than with gemfibrozil. The drugs may also increase cholesterol concentration in the biliary tract and formation of gallstones. For patients receiving warfarin, the warfarin dosage should be substantially decreased because fibrates displace warfarin from binding sites on serum albumin.

Niacin

Niacin (nicotinic acid) decreases both cholesterol and triglycerides. It inhibits mobilization of free fatty acids from peripheral tissues, thereby reducing hepatic synthesis of triglycerides and secretion of VLDL, which leads to decreased production of LDL cholesterol. Niacin is the most effective drug for increasing the concentration of HDL cholesterol. Disadvantages of niacin are the high doses required for dyslipidemic effects and the subsequent adverse effects. Niacin commonly causes skin flushing, pruritus, and gastric irritation and may cause hyperglycemia, hyperuricemia, elevated hepatic aminotransferase enzymes, and hepatitis. Flushing can be reduced by starting with small doses, gradually increasing doses, taking doses with meals, and taking 325 milligrams of aspirin about 30 minutes before niacin doses.

Niacin is rapidly absorbed from the gastrointestinal tract. Minimal metabolism occurs by the liver and the majority of the drug is excreted unchanged in the urine. Tablet strengths are not interchangeable; do not substitute immediate-release forms with long-acting ones.

Niacin is most effective in preventing heart disease when used in combination with another dyslipidemic drug such as a bile acid sequestrant or a fibrate. Its use with a statin lowers serum LDL cholesterol more than either drug alone, but the combination has not been studied in relation to preventing cardiovascular disease.

Cholesterol Absorption Inhibitor

The cholesterol absorption inhibitor (e.g., **ezetimibe**), the newest class of dyslipidemic drugs, acts in the small intestine to inhibit absorption of cholesterol and decrease the delivery of intestinal cholesterol to the liver, resulting in reduced hepatic cholesterol stores and increased clearance of cholesterol from the blood. This distinct mechanism is complementary to that of HMG-CoA reductase inhibitors.

This drug reduces total cholesterol and triglycerides and increases HDL. The drug is indicated as an adjunctive therapy to dietary management of hyperlipidemia. Administration may be with or without food, but it should be taken 2 hours before or 4 hours after a bile acid sequestrant. Therapeutic response is achieved within 2 weeks of initiation of therapy and maintained with continued use. The most common adverse effects include hypersensitivity reactions such as rash and nausea. This drug is contraindicated in pregnancy.

Nursing Process

Assessment

Assess the patient's status in relation to atherosclerotic vascular disease.

- Identify risk factors:
  - Hypertension
  - Diabetes mellitus
  - High intake of dietary fat and refined sugars
  - Obesity
  - Inadequate exercise
  - Cigarette smoking
  - Family history of atherosclerotic disorders
  - Dyslipidemia
- Signs and symptoms depend on the specific problem:
  - Dyslipidemia is manifested by elevated serum cholesterol (>200 mg/100 mL), triglycerides (>150 mg/100 mL), or both.
  - Coronary artery atherosclerosis is manifested by myocardial ischemia (angina pectoris, myocardial infarction).
  - Cerebrovascular insufficiency may be manifested by syncope, memory loss, transient ischemic attacks (TIAs), or strokes. Impairment of blood flow to the brain is caused primarily by atherosclerosis in the carotid, vertebral, or cerebral arteries.
  - Peripheral arterial insufficiency is manifested by impaired blood flow in the legs (weak or absent pulses; cool, pale extremities; intermittent claudication; leg pain at rest; and development of gangrene, usually in the toes because they are most distal to blood supply). This condition results from atherosclerosis in the distal abdominal aorta, the iliac arteries, and the femoral and smaller arteries in the legs.

Nursing Diagnoses

- Ineffective Tissue Perfusion related to interruption of arterial blood flow
- Imbalanced Nutrition: More Than Body Requirements of fats and calories
- Anxiety related to risks of atherosclerotic cardiovascular disease
- Disturbed Body Image related to the need for lifestyle changes
- Noncompliance related to dietary restrictions and adverse drug reactions
- Deficient Knowledge related to drug and diet therapy of dyslipidemia

Planning/Goals

The patient will

- Take lipid-lowering drugs as prescribed
- Decrease dietary intake of saturated fats and cholesterol
- Lose weight if obese and maintain the lower weight
- Have periodic measurements of blood lipids
- Avoid preventable adverse drug effects
- Receive positive reinforcement for efforts to lower blood lipid levels
- Feel less anxious and more in control as risks of atherosclerotic cardiovascular disease are decreased

Interventions

Use measures to prevent, delay, or minimize atherosclerosis.

- Help patients control risk factors. Ideally, primary prevention begins in childhood with healthful eating habits (e.g., avoiding excessive fats, meat, and dairy products; obtaining adequate amounts of all nutrients, including dietary fiber; avoiding obesity), exercise, and avoiding cigarette smoking. However, changing habits to a more healthful lifestyle is helpful at any time, before or after disease manifestations appear. Weight loss often reduces blood lipids and lipoproteins to a normal range. Changing habits is difficult for most people, even those with severe symptoms.
- Use measures to increase blood flow to tissues:
  - Exercise is helpful in developing collateral circulation in the heart and legs. Collateral circulation involves use of secondary vessels in response to tissue ischemia related to obstruction of the principal vessels. Patients with angina pectoris or previous myocardial infarction require a carefully planned and supervised program of progressive exercise. Those with peripheral arterial insufficiency usually can increase exercise tolerance by walking regularly. Distances should be determined by occurrence of pain and must be individualized.
  - Posture and position may be altered to increase blood flow to the legs in patients with peripheral arterial insufficiency. Elevating the head of the bed and having the legs horizontal or dependent may help. Elevating the feet is usually contraindicated unless edema is present or likely to develop.
- Although drug therapy is being increasingly used to prevent or manage atherosclerotic disorders, a major therapeutic option for management of occlusive vascular disease is surgical removal of atherosclerotic plaque or revascularization procedures. Thus, severe angina pectoris may be relieved by a coronary artery bypass procedure that detours blood flow around occluded vessels. This procedure also may be done after a myocardial infarction. The goal is to

Nursing Process continues on page 890

prevent infarction or reinfarction. TIAs may be relieved by carotid endarterectomy; the goal is to prevent a stroke. Peripheral arterial insufficiency may be relieved by aortofemoral, femoropopliteal, or other bypass grafts that detour around occluded vessels. Although these procedures increase blood flow to ischemic tissues, they do not halt progression of atherosclerosis.

The nursing role in relation to these procedures is to provide excellent preoperative and postoperative nursing care to promote healing, prevent infection, maintain patency of grafts, and help the patient to achieve optimum function.

■ Provide appropriate teaching related to drug therapy (see accompanying display).

■ Any dyslipidemic drug therapy must be accompanied by an appropriate diet; refer patients to a nutritionist. Overeating or gaining weight may decrease or cancel the lipid-lowering effects of the drugs.

■ Encourage adult patients to have their serum cholesterol level measured at least once every 5 years. Adults and children with a personal or family history of dyslipidemia or other risk factors should be tested more often.

■ The most effective measures for preventing dyslipidemia and atherosclerosis are those related to a healthful lifestyle (e.g., diet low in cholesterol and saturated fats, weight control, exercise).

■ Help patients and family members understand the desirability of lowering high blood lipid levels before serious cardiovascular diseases develop.

Evaluation

■ Observe for decreased blood levels of total and LDL cholesterol and triglycerides; observe for increased levels of HDL cholesterol.

■ Observe and interview regarding compliance with instructions for drug, diet, and other therapeutic measures.

■ Observe and interview regarding adverse drug effects.

■ Validate the patient's ability to identify foods high and low in cholesterol and saturated fats.

⊘ Applying Your Knowledge 55-3

How Can You Avoid This Medication Error?
You arrive at Mr. Watkins' home at 8:45 A.M. Mr. Watkins greets you and asks if you mind waiting a moment while he finishes his breakfast. While you are waiting, you prepare the correct doses of both his atorvastatin and gemfibrozil, which he receives routinely at 9:00 A.M. You then administer his medication.

Principles of Therapy

Drug Selection

Drug selection is based on the type of dyslipidemia and its severity. For single-drug therapy to lower cholesterol, a statin is preferred. To lower cholesterol and triglycerides, a statin, a cholesterol absorption inhibitor, gemfibrozil, or niacin may be used. To lower triglycerides, gemfibrozil, a cholesterol absorption inhibitor, or niacin may be used. Gemfibrozil, rather than niacin, is usually preferred for people with diabetes because niacin increases blood sugar.

When monotherapy is not effective, combination therapy is rational because the drugs act by different mechanisms. In general, a statin combined with a cholesterol absorption inhibitor or a bile acid sequestrant or niacin combined with a bile acid sequestrant are the most effective combinations in reducing total and LDL cholesterol. A fibrate, a cholesterol absorption inhibitor, or niacin may be used when a goal of therapy is to increase the level of HDL cholesterol. However, a fibrate–statin combination should be avoided because of increased risks of severe myopathy, and a niacin–statin combination increases the risks of hepatotoxicity. Adverse reactions from combination statin and cholesterol absorption inhibitor therapy are reported to be similar to those from statins alone.

Use in Special Populations

Use in Various Ethnic Groups

Little information has been reported on racial or ethnic differences for lipid-lowering drugs. Members of minority populations (e.g., African Americans, Mexican Americans) are less likely to be treated than Caucasians. Despite an increased prevalence of diabetes and obesity, Native Americans appear to have lower cholesterol levels than the United States population as a whole. This suggests that diet and exercises may be more useful than lipid-lowering drugs for this group.

Use in Children

Definitive evidence indicates that the development of atherosclerotic cardiovascular disease begins in early childhood and the rate of progression is greatly increased by lipid abnormalities. The frequency of dyslipidemia in children is on the rise, predominately associated with the concurrent epidemic of obesity and the metabolic syndrome. Therefore, a primary goal is to identify and manage dyslipidemia in at-risk children and adolescents to reduce the lipoprotein profile component on the risk burden of atherosclerosis. As with adults, initial management consists of diet therapy and management of any secondary causes, especially with younger children. Experts are calling for revisions of the existing 1992 guidelines for screening and managing dyslipidemia in children and adolescents. Since the initial publication of the guidelines, interventional studies in children with familial hyperlipidemia have shown statins to be the preferred pharmacological treatment in children and adolescents and supplementation with antioxidant vitamins and omega-3 fatty acids. Randomized clinical drug trials are ongoing in the pediatric age groups with primary high-risk lipid

Patient Teaching Guidelines | Dyslipidemic Drugs

General Considerations

▪ Heart and blood vessel disease causes a great deal of illness and many deaths. The basic problem is usually atherosclerosis, in which the arteries are partly blocked by cholesterol deposits. Cholesterol, a waxy substance made in the liver, is necessary for normal body functioning. However, excessive amounts in the blood increase the likelihood of having a heart attack, stroke, or leg pain from inadequate blood flow. One type of cholesterol (low-density lipoprotein [LDL] or "bad") attaches to artery walls, where it can enlarge over time and block blood flow. The other type (high-density lipoprotein [HDL] or "good") carries cholesterol away from the artery and back to the liver, where it can be broken down. Thus, the healthiest blood cholesterol levels are low total cholesterol (<200 mg/dL), low LDL (<130 mg/dL), and high HDL (>35 mg/dL). High levels of blood triglycerides, another type of fat, are also unhealthy.

▪ Dyslipidemic drugs are given to lower high concentrations of fats (total cholesterol, LDL cholesterol, and triglycerides) in your blood. The goal of management is to prevent heart attack, stroke, and peripheral arterial disease. If you already have heart and blood vessel disease, the drugs can improve your symptoms, activity level, and quality of life.

▪ A low-fat diet is needed. This is often the first step in treating high cholesterol or triglyceride levels, and may be prescribed for 6 months or longer before drug therapy is begun. When drug therapy is prescribed, the diet should be continued. An important part is reducing the amount of saturated fat (from meats, dairy products). In addition, eating a bowl of oat cereal daily can help lower cholesterol by 5% to 10%. Diet counseling by a dietitian or nutritionist can be helpful in developing guidelines that fit your needs and lifestyle. Overeating or gaining weight may decrease or cancel the lipid-lowering effects of the drugs.

▪ Other lifestyle changes that can help improve cholesterol levels include regular aerobic exercise (raises HDL); losing weight (raises HDL, lowers LDL, lowers triglycerides); and not smoking (HDL levels are higher in nonsmokers).

▪ Adults should have measurements of total cholesterol and HDL cholesterol at least once every 5 years. People with a personal or family history of dyslipidemia or other risk factors for cardiovascular disease should be tested more often.

▪ Techniques for home monitoring of cholesterol levels are improving and are more available for self-use. Patients may be instructed to perform self-monitoring and report their results to their health care provider. At present, equipment and supplies can be expensive, and most are not reimbursed by insurance companies.

▪ Atorvastatin and other statin-type dyslipidemic drugs may increase sensitivity to sunlight. Avoid prolonged exposure to the sun, use sunscreens, and wear protective clothing.

▪ Gemfibrozil may cause dizziness or blurred vision and should be used cautiously while driving or performing other tasks that require alertness, coordination, or physical dexterity. It also may cause abdominal pain, diarrhea, nausea, or vomiting. Notify a health care provider if these symptoms become severe.

▪ Skin flushing may occur with niacin. If it is distressing, taking one regular aspirin tablet (325 mg) 30 to 60 minutes before the niacin dose may decrease this reaction. Flushing usually decreases in a few days, but may recur when niacin dosage is increased. Ask your health care provider if there is any reason you should not take aspirin.

▪ Cholestyramine and colestipol can cause constipation. Increasing intake of dietary fiber can help prevent this adverse effect.

Self-Administration

▪ Take lovastatin with food; take fluvastatin, pravastatin, or simvastatin in the evening, with or without food. Food decreases stomach upset associated with lovastatin. All of these drugs may be more effective if taken in the evening or at bedtime, probably because more cholesterol is produced at nighttime and the drugs block cholesterol production.

▪ Take atorvastatin with or without food and without regard to time of day.

▪ Take fenofibrate with food; food increases drug absorption.

▪ Take gemfibrozil on an empty stomach, 30 minutes before morning and evening meals.

▪ Take immediate-release niacin with meals to decrease stomach upset; take timed-release niacin without regard to meals. Do not substitute immediate release forms with long-acting ones.

▪ Mix cholestyramine powder and colestipol granules with water or other fluids, soups, cereals, or fruits such as applesauce and follow with more fluid. These drug forms should not be taken dry.

▪ Do not take cholestyramine, coleseveiam, or colestipol with other drugs because they may prevent absorption of the other drugs. If taking other drugs, take them 1 hour before or 4 to 6 hours after cholestyramine or colestipol.

▪ Swallow colestipol tablets whole; do not cut, crush, or chew.

▪ Take ezetimibe with or without food at the same time each day. If taken in combination with a statin, take it at the same time (usually in the evening).

---

abnormalities to determine the safety and effectiveness of currently available lipid-lowering drugs. Recommended levels at which to initiate drug therapy for dyslipidemia have not been established in children.

Use in Older Adults

As with younger adults, diet, exercise, and weight control should be tried first. When drug therapy is required, statins are effective for lowering LDL cholesterol and usually are well tolerated by older adults. However, they are expensive. Niacin and bile acid sequestrants are effective, but older adults do not tolerate their adverse effects very well. In postmenopausal women, estrogen replacement therapy increases HDL cholesterol.

Older adults often have diabetes, impaired liver function, or other conditions that raise blood lipid levels. Thus, management of secondary causes is especially important. The older adult is also likely to have cardiovascular and other disorders that increase the adverse effects of dyslipidemic drugs. Overall, use of dyslipidemic drugs should be cautious, with close monitoring for therapeutic and adverse effects. Lower starting dosages are recommended for fenofibrate (67 mg/day), pravastatin (10 mg/day), and simvastatin (5 mg/day). Cholesterol absorption inhibitor as monotherapy (without statins) does not require dosage reduction in geriatric patients.

Use in Patients With Renal Impairment

Statins are metabolized by the liver and excreted partly through the kidneys (their main route of excretion is through bile). Drug plasma concentrations may be increased in patients with renal impairment and these drugs should be used cautiously; some need reduced dosage.

- With atorvastatin, plasma levels are not affected and dosage reductions are not needed.
- With fluvastatin, because it is cleared hepatically and less than 6% of the dose is excreted in urine, dosage reduction for mild to moderate renal impairment is unnecessary. Use caution with severe impairment. Recent randomized controlled clinical trials have demonstrated the drug's safety in kidney transplant recipients.
- With lovastatin, plasma concentrations are increased in patients with severe renal impairment (creatinine clearance < 30 mL/minute), and doses above 20 mg/day should be used with caution.
- With pravastatin, initiate therapy with 10 mg/day.
- With simvastatin, initiate therapy with 5 mg/day and monitor closely.
    Cholesterol absorption inhibitors as monotherapy (without statins) do not require dosage reduction in renal insufficiency.

Fibrates are excreted mainly by the kidneys and therefore accumulate in the serum of patients with renal impairment. With gemfibrozil, there have been reports of worsening renal impairment in patients whose baseline serum creatinine levels were higher than 2 milligrams per deciliter. A different type of dyslipidemic drug may be preferred in these patients. Fenofibrate is contraindicated in patients with severe renal impairment, and the recommended starting dose is 67 milligrams per day in patients with a creatinine clearance of less than 50 milliliters per minute. Drug and dose effects on renal function and triglyceride levels should be evaluated before dosage is increased.

Use in Patients With Hepatic Impairment

Statins are metabolized in the liver and may accumulate in patients with impaired hepatic function. They are contraindicated in patients with active liver disease or unexplained elevations of serum aspartate or alanine aminotransferase. They should be used cautiously, in reduced dosages, for patients who ingest substantial amounts of alcohol or who have a history of liver disease.

Liver function tests are recommended before starting a statin, at 6 and 12 weeks after starting the drug or increasing the dose, then every 6 months. Monitor patients who have increased serum aminotransferases until the abnormal values resolve. If the increases are more than three times the upper limit of normal levels and persist, the dose should be reduced or the drug discontinued.

Cholesterol absorption inhibitors as monotherapy (without statins) do not require dosage reduction in mild hepatic insufficiency. Fibrates may cause hepatotoxicity. Abnormal elevations of serum aminotransferases have occurred with both gemfibrozil and fenofibrate, but they usually subside when the drug is discontinued. Fenofibrate is contraindicated in severe hepatic impairment, including patients with primary biliary cirrhosis, pre-existing gallbladder disease, and persistent elevations in liver function test results. In addition, hepatitis (hepatocellular, chronic active, and cholestatic) has been reported after use of fenofibrate from a few weeks to several years. Liver function tests should be monitored during the first year of drug administration. The drug should be discontinued if elevated enzyme levels persist at more than three times the normal limit.

Niacin may cause hepatotoxicity, especially with doses above 2 grams daily, with timed-release preparations, and if given in combination with a statin or a fibrate.

Use in Home Care

For a patient with dyslipidemia, the home care nurse should reinforce teaching about the role of blood lipids in causing myocardial infarction, stroke, and peripheral arterial insufficiency; the prescribed management regimen and its goals; and the importance of improving dyslipidemia in preventing or improving cardiovascular disorders. In addition, the patient may need assistance in obtaining blood tests (e.g., lipids, liver function tests) and dietary counseling. Increasing availability of home cholesterol-monitoring devices will require additional patient teaching about technique and interpretation of the results.

Use of Herbal and Dietary Supplements

There is little evidence outlining the efficacy and safety of herbal and dietary supplements for reduction of cholesterol and the prevention of CAD. Concerns about drug interaction make the use of these agents potentially dangerous if taken in conjunction with standard lipid-lowering drug therapy. Therefore, a careful medication history should be taken on all patients, including over-the-counter, herbal, and supplemental medications.

Flax or flax seed is used internally as a laxative and a dyslipidemic agent. Absorption of all medications may be decreased when taken with flax, resulting in a less than therapeutic effect. Garlic is reportedly used as a dyslipidemic agent and as a possible antihypertensive, but there is little scientific support for such use. Bleeding may be increased when garlic is used with anticoagulants, and insulin doses may need to be decreased as a result of the hypoglycemic effect of garlic. Green tea is commonly used for its dyslipidemic effect and the caffeinated product can be a central nervous system stimulant. Soy is used as a food source and has been researched extensively. Use of soy to lower cholesterol (LDL and total cholesterol) has been documented. Significant interactions with other herbs or drugs have not been reported. Red yeast rice has been shown to lower cholesterol; however, dosage standardization is a concern.

Nursing Actions Drugs for Dyslipidemia

NURSING ACTIONS	RATIONALE/EXPLANATION
1. Administer accurately	
a. Give lovastatin with food; give fluvastatin on an empty stomach or at bedtime. Atorvastatin, pravastatin, or simvastatin may be given with or without food in the evening. Atorvastatin can be given without regard to time of day. Avoid giving with grapefruit juice.	Food decreases gastrointestinal (GI) upset associated with lovastatin. These drugs are more effective if taken in the evening or at bedtime, because more cholesterol is produced by the liver at night and the drugs block cholesterol production. Grapefruit juice increases serum drug levels.
b. Give fenofibrate with food.	Food increases drug absorption.
c. Give gemfibrozil on an empty stomach, about 30 minutes before morning and evening meals.	
d. Give immediate-release niacin with meals; give timed-release niacin without regard to meals.	The immediate-release formulation may cause gastric irritation.
e. Mix cholestyramine powder and colestipol granules with water or other fluids, soups, cereals, or fruits such as applesauce and follow with more fluid.	These drug forms should not be taken dry.
f. Do not give cholestyramine or colestipol with other drugs; give them 1 hour before or 4–6 hours after cholestyramine or colestipol.	Cholestyramine and colestipol prevent absorption of many drugs.
g. Instruct patients to swallow colestipol tablets whole; do not cut, crush, or chew.	
h. Give ezetimibe with or without food at the same time each day; give at night if used in combination with a statin.	Food does not affect absorption.
i. Give ezetimibe 2 hours before or 4 hours after bile sequestrants.	Cholestyramine and colestipol prevent absorption of many drugs.
2. Observe for therapeutic effects	
a. Decreased levels of total serum cholesterol, low-density lipoprotein cholesterol, and triglycerides, and increased levels of high-density lipoprotein cholesterol.	With statins, effects occur in 1–2 wk, with maximum effects in 4–6 wk. With fibrates and niacin, effects occur in approximately 1 mo. With cholestyramine and colestipol, maximum effects occur in approximately 1 mo.
3. Observe for adverse effects	
a. GI problems—nausea, vomiting, flatulence, constipation or diarrhea, abdominal discomfort	GI symptoms are the most common adverse effects of dyslipidemic drugs. Constipation is especially common with cholestyramine and colestipol.
b. With lovastatin and related drugs, observe for GI upset (see 2a), skin rash, pruritus, and myopathy.	Adverse effects are usually mild and of short duration. A less common but potentially serious effect is liver dysfunction, usually manifested by increased levels of serum aminotransferases. Serum aminotransferases (aspartate and alanine aminotransferase) should be measured before starting the drug, every 4–6 weeks during the first 3 months, then every 6–12 weeks or after dosage increases for 1 year, then every 6 months.
c. With niacin, flushing of the face and neck, pruritus, and skin rash may occur, as well as tachycardia, hypotension, and dizziness.	These symptoms may be prominent when nicotinic acid is used to lower blood lipids because relatively high doses are required. Aspirin 325 mg, 30 minutes before nicotinic acid, decreases the flushing reaction.
4. Observe for drug interactions	
a. Drugs that *increase* effects of lovastatin and related drugs:	
(1) Azole antifungals (e.g., fluconazole, itraconazole)	Risk of myopathy is increased. It is recommended that statin therapy be interrupted temporarily if systemic azole antifungals are needed.
(2) Cyclosporine	Risk of severe myopathy or rhabdomyolysis is increased.
(3) Erythromycin	Risk of severe myopathy or rhabdomyolysis is increased.

(continued on page 894)

Nursing Actions — Drugs for Dyslipidemia (continued)

NURSING ACTIONS	RATIONALE/EXPLANATION
(4) Fibrate dyslipidemics (e.g., fenofibrate, gemfibrozil)	Risk of severe myopathy or rhabdomyolysis is increased.
(5) Niacin	Risk of severe myopathy or rhabdomyolysis is increased.
(6) Drugs that *increase* effects of fluvastatin:	
(a) Alcohol, cimetidine, ranitidine, omeprazole	Increased blood levels
(7) Drugs that *increase* effects of ezetimibe:	
(a) Cyclosporine	Increased blood levels
b. Drugs that *decrease* effects of lovastatin and related drugs:	
(1) Bile acid sequestrant dyslipidemics	Decreased blood levels unless the drugs are taken 1–4 hours apart
(2) Antacids	Decrease absorption of atorvastatin
(3) Isradipine	This calcium channel blocker may decrease blood levels of lovastatin and its metabolites by increasing their hepatic metabolism.
(4) Rifampin	Decreases blood levels of fluvastatin
(5) St. John's wort	Decreases blood levels of atorvastatin
c. Drugs that *decrease* effects of fibrate dyslipidemic drugs:	
(1) Bile acid sequestrant dyslipidemic drugs	Decrease absorption unless the fibrate is taken about 1 hour before or 4–6 hours after the bile acid sequestrant

Key Concepts

- Unless a person has a genetic disorder of lipid metabolism, the amount of cholesterol in the blood is strongly related to dietary intake of saturated fat.

- For accurate interpretation of a patient's lipid profile, blood samples for laboratory testing of triglycerides should be drawn after the patient has fasted for 12 hours. Fasting is not required for cholesterol testing.

- Metabolic syndrome is a group of cardiovascular risk factors linked with obesity that include elevated waist circumference (central adiposity), elevated triglycerides, reduced high-density lipoprotein cholesterol, elevated blood pressure, and elevated fasting glucose.

- Lifestyle changes that can help improve cholesterol levels include a low-fat diet, regular aerobic exercise, losing weight, and not smoking.

- Take lovastatin with food; take fluvastatin, pravastatin, or simvastatin in the evening, with or without food; atorvastatin can be taken with or without food and without regard to time of day.

- Skin flushing may occur with niacin.

- Fibrates are the most effective drugs for reducing serum triglyceride levels.

Review and Application Exercises

Short Answer Exercises

1. How would you describe dyslipidemia to a patient?

2. What is the goal of management of dyslipidemia?

3. Differentiate lipid-lowering drugs according to their mechanisms of action.

4. What are the main nonpharmacologic measures to decrease total and LDL cholesterol and increase HDL cholesterol?

5. What are the main nonpharmacologic measures to decrease serum triglyceride levels?

NCLEX-Style Questions

6. The primary focus for prevention and management of metabolic syndrome and its sequelae is
   a. high HDL cholesterol, low LDL cholesterol, low total cholesterol
   b. low HDL cholesterol, low LDL cholesterol, low total cholesterol
   c. low triglycerides
   d. high HDL cholesterol, low LDL cholesterol, low triglycerides

7. Your patient, Mr. John Samuels, has not been able to decrease his LDL levels with lifestyle management, and his nurse practitioner has prescribed an HMG-CoA reductase inhibitor. You explain to him that these drugs, commonly called statins, are best administered
   a. with breakfast
   b. at noon
   c. with a snack in the early afternoon
   d. at night or bedtime

8. Your patient is on niacin (nicotinic acid) to decrease both her cholesterol and her triglycerides. In counseling her about taking this medication, you explain that flushing, a common adverse effect of niacin therapy, can be decreased by
   a. taking half the dose in the morning and half the dose at night
   b. taking 325 mg aspirin 30 minutes before the niacin
   c. taking the drug on an empty stomach
   d. taking niacin as monotherapy for dyslipidemia

9. A 48-year-old man visits the health care provider for his annual checkup. He is otherwise in good health, but assessment findings reveal a new onset of a slight increase in blood pressure and a total serum cholesterol of 240 mg/dL. What can the nurse anticipate as the preferred treatment for this patient?
   a. a low-lipid diet and an exercise program
   b. a low-lipid diet and a cholesterol synthesis inhibitor
   c. an exercise program and a fibrate
   d. a low-lipid diet, an exercise program, and niacin

10. A 36-year-old female patient has been taking lovastatin 40 mg PO daily for 6 months to treat mild dyslipidemia. At a clinic appointment, she tells the nurse she is 6 weeks' pregnant. The nurse counsels the patient to understand that it is likely that her midwife will counsel her
    a. to increase the dose of prenatal vitamins
    b. to reduce the dosage of her lovastatin to 20 mg PO daily
    c. to increase the dosage to 40 mg PO twice daily
    d. about discontinuing the drug during pregnancy

Selected References

American Academy of Pediatrics. (1992). National Cholesterol Education Program: Report of the Expert Panel on Blood Cholesterol Levels in Children and Adolescents. *Pediatrics, 89,* 525–584.

Drug facts and comparisons. (Updated monthly). St. Louis, MO: Facts and Comparisons.

Elesber, A. A. (2007). Coronary endothelial dysfunction and hyperlipidemia are independently associated with diastolic dysfunction in humans. *American Heart Journal, 153,* 1081–1087.

Fonseca, V. A. (2005). The metabolic syndrome, hyperlipidemia, and insulin resistance. *Clinical Cornerstone, 7,* 61–72.

Johnston, N. (2006). Improved identification of patients with coronary artery disease by the use of new lipid and lipoprotein biomarkers. *American Journal of Cardiology, 97,* 640–645.

Karch, A. M. (2007). *2008 Lippincott's nursing drug guide.* Philadelphia: Lippincott Williams & Wilkins.

Kasiske, B. L. (2006). An assessment of statin safety by nephrologists. *American Journal of Cardiology, 97,* 82C–85C.

Lacy, C. F., Armstrong, L. L., Goldman, M. P., & Lance, L. L. (2007). *Lexi-Comp's drug information handbook* (15th ed.). Hudson, OH: American Pharmaceutical Association.

Magnussen, C. G., Raitakari, O. T., Thomson, R., Juonala, M., Patel, D. A., Viikari, J. S. A., Marniemi, J., Srinivasan, S. R., Berenson, G. S., Dwyer, T., Venn, A. (2008). Utility of currently recommended pediatric dyslipidemia classifications in predicting dyslipidemia in adulthood: evidence from the Childhood Determinants of Adult Health (CDAH) Study, Cardiovascular Risk in Young Finns Study, and Bogalusa Heart Study. *Circulation, 117,* 32–42.

Matfin, G., & Porth, C. M. (2005). Alterations in cardiac function. In C. M. Porth (Ed.), *Pathophysiology: Concepts of altered health states* (7th ed., pp. 475–504). Philadelphia: Lippincott Williams & Wilkins.

McCrindle, B. W., Urbina, E. M., Dennison, B. A., et. al. (2007). Drug therapy of high-risk lipid abnormalities in children and adolescents: a scientific statement from the American Heart Association atherosclerosis, hypertension, and obesity in youth committee, council of cardiovascular disease in the young, with the council on cardiovascular nursing. *Circulation, 115,* 1948–1967.

McCrindle, B. W., Urbina, E. M., Dennison, B. A., Jacobson, M. S., Steinberger, J., Rocchini, A. P., Hayman, L. L., Daniels, S. R. (2007). Drug therapy of high-risk lipid abnormalities in children and adolescents: A scientific statement from the American Heart Association Atherosclerosis, Hypertension, and Obesity in Youth Committee, Council of Cardiovascular Disease in the Young, with the Council on Cardiovascular Nursing. *Circulation, 115,* 1948–1967.

McKenney, J. M. (2005). Pharmacologic options for aggressive low-density lipoprotein cholesterol lowering: Benefits versus risks. *American Journal of Cardiology, 96,* 60E–66E.

National Institutes of Health Expert Panel. (2001). *Third report of the National Cholesterol Education Program (NCEP) Expert Panel on Detection, Evaluation, and Treatment of High Blood Cholesterol in Adults (Adult Treatment Panel III)* (NIH Publication No. 01-3670). Bethesda, MD: National Institutes of Health.

Chapter Outline

Physiology of the Digestive System

KEY TERMS

- Alimentary canal
- Bile
- Digestion
- Elimination
- Esophagus
- Gallbladder
- Gastric juice
- Large intestine
- Liver
- Mucus
- Oral cavity
- Pancreas
- Pancreatic juices
- Peristalsis
- Saliva
- Small intestine
- Stomach

LEARNING OBJECTIVES

After studying this chapter, you will be able to:

1. Review roles of the main digestive tract structures.
2. List common signs and symptoms affecting gastrointestinal functions.
3. Identify general categories of drugs used to treat gastrointestinal disorders.
4. Discuss the effects of nongastrointestinal drugs on gastrointestinal functioning.

Introduction

The digestive system (Figure 56-1) consists of the *alimentary canal* (a tube extending from the *oral cavity* to the anus, approximately 25 to 30 feet [7.5–9 m] long) and the accessory organs (salivary glands, gallbladder, liver, and pancreas). The main function of the system is to provide the body with fluids, nutrients, and electrolytes in a form that can be used at the cellular level. The system also disposes of waste products that result from the digestive process (*elimination*).

The alimentary canal has the same basic structure throughout. The layers of the wall are mucosa, connective tissue, and muscle. *Peristalsis* propels food through the tract and mixes the food bolus with digestive juices. Stimulation of the parasympathetic nervous system (by vagus nerves) increases motility and secretions. Sympathetic stimulation promotes sphincter function and inhibits motility. The tract has an abundant blood supply, which increases cell regeneration and healing. Blood flow increases during *digestion* and absorption. Blood flow decreases with strenuous exercise, sympathetic nervous system stimulation (i.e., "fight or flight"), aging (secondary to decreased cardiac output and atherosclerosis), and conditions that shunt blood away from the digestive tract (e.g., heart failure, atherosclerosis).

Structures of the Digestive System

Oral Cavity

In the oral cavity, chewing mechanically breaks food into smaller particles, which can be swallowed more easily and provide a larger surface area for enzyme action. Food is also mixed with *saliva*, which lubricates the food bolus for swallowing and initiates the digestion of starch.

Esophagus

The *esophagus* is a musculofibrous tube about 10 inches (25 cm) long; its main function is to convey food from the pharynx to the stomach. It secretes a small amount of *mucus* and has some peristaltic movement. Each end of the esophagus functions as a sphincter. The upper esophageal sphincter prevents air from entering the esophagus during inspiration. The last 2 centimeters of the esophagus is the lower esophageal sphincter (LES). The function of the LES is to prevent reflux of acidic gastric contents into the esophagus.

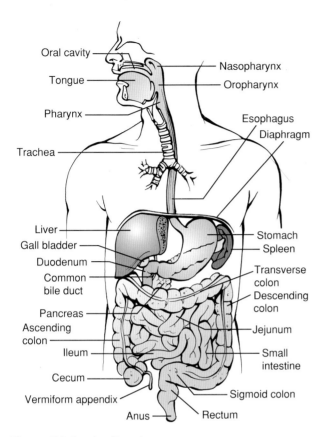

Oral cavity

Tongue

Pharynx

Trachea

Nasopharynx

Oropharynx

Esophagus

Diaphragm

Liver

Gall bladder

Duodenum

Common
bile duct

Pancreas

Ascending
colon

Ileum

Cecum

Vermiform appendix

Anus

Stomach

Spleen

Transverse
colon

Descending
colon

Jejunum

Small
intestine

Sigmoid colon

Rectum

Figure 56-1 ■ The digestive system.

Stomach

The *stomach* is a dilated area that serves as a reservoir. It churns and mixes the food with digestive juices; secretes mucus, hydrochloric acid, and enzymes; starts protein breakdown; and secretes intrinsic factor, which is necessary for absorption of vitamin B_{12} from the ileum. Although there is much diffusion of water and electrolytes through the gastric mucosa in both directions, there is little absorption of these substances. Carbohydrates and amino acids are also poorly absorbed. Only a few highly lipid-soluble substances, such as alcohol and some drugs, are absorbed in moderate quantities from the stomach.

The inlet of the stomach, the cardiac orifice, is at the terminal end of the esophagus. The stomach outlet is the pylorus, a ring-like muscle that opens into the beginning of the duodenum. The stomach normally holds about 1000 milliliters comfortably and empties in about 4 hours. Numerous factors influence the rate of gastric emptying, including the size of the pylorus, gastric motility, type of food, fluidity and composition of the chyme (the material produced by gastric digestion of food), and the state of the duodenum. Factors that cause rapid emptying include carbohydrate foods, increased motility, fluid chyme, and an empty duodenum. The stomach empties more slowly with decreased gastric tone and motility, fatty foods, and excessively acidic chyme. Cholecystokinin and gastric inhibitory peptide are released by the duodenum in response to an acidic pH, increased osmolality, or fatty acid composition of the chyme, delaying gastric emptying. When the chyme in the duodenum contains fats, the duodenal mucosa also produces a hormone, enterogastrone, which inhibits gastric secretion and motility. This allows a longer time for the digestion of fats in the small intestine.

Small Intestine

The *small intestine* consists of the duodenum, jejunum, and ileum and is approximately 20 feet (6 m) long. The duodenum makes up the first 10 to 12 inches (25–30 cm) of the small intestine. The pancreatic and bile ducts empty into the duodenum at the papilla of Vater. The small intestine contains numerous glands that secrete digestive enzymes, hormones, and mucus. For the most part, digestion and absorption occur in the small intestine, including absorption of most orally administered drugs.

Large Intestine

The *large intestine* consists of the cecum, colon, rectum, and anus. The ileum opens into the cecum. The colon secretes mucus and absorbs water.

Pancreas

The *pancreas* secretes enzymes required for the digestion of carbohydrates, proteins, and fats. It also secretes insulin, glucagon and somatostatin, hormones that regulate glucose metabolism and blood sugar levels.

Gallbladder

The *gallbladder* is a small pouch attached to the underside of the liver that stores and concentrates *bile*. It has a capacity of 50 to 60 milliliters. The gallbladder releases bile when fats are present in the duodenum.

Liver

The *liver* is a vital organ that performs numerous functions. It receives about 1500 milliliters per minute, or 25% to 30%, of the total cardiac output. About three fourths of the blood flow is venous blood from the stomach, intestines, spleen, and pancreas (portal circulation); the remainder is arterial blood through the hepatic artery. The hepatic artery carries blood to the connective tissue of the liver and bile ducts, then empties into the hepatic sinuses. Arterial blood mixes with blood from the portal circulation. Venous blood from the liver flows into the inferior vena cava for return to the systemic circulation. The ample blood flow facilitates the many functions of the liver, which are described below.

The liver serves as a blood reservoir for the body. The liver can eject 500 to 1000 milliliters of blood into the general circulation in response to stress, decreased blood volume, and sympathetic nervous system stimulation (e.g., hemorrhagic or hypovolemic shock).

The liver serves as a blood filter and detoxifier. Kupffer's cells in the liver phagocytize bacteria carried from the intestines by the portal vein. They also break down worn-out erythrocytes, saving iron for reuse in hemoglobin synthesis, and form bilirubin, a waste product excreted in bile. The liver metabolizes many body secretions and most drugs to prevent accumulation and harmful effects on body tissues.

Most drugs are active as the parent compound and are metabolized in the liver to an inactive metabolite, which is then excreted by the kidneys. However, some drugs become active only after formation of a metabolite in the liver.

The liver detoxifies or alters substances by oxidation, hydrolysis, or conjugation. Conjugation involves combining a chemical substance with an endogenous substance to produce an inactive or harmless compound. Essentially all steroid hormones, including adrenal corticosteroids and sex hormones, are at least partially conjugated in the liver and secreted into the bile. When the liver is damaged, these hormones may accumulate in body fluids and cause symptoms of hormone excess.

The liver plays a role in the metabolism of carbohydrate, fat, and protein. In carbohydrate metabolism, the liver converts glucose to glycogen for storage and reconverts glycogen to glucose when needed to maintain an adequate blood sugar concentration. Excess glucose that cannot be converted to glycogen is converted to fat. The liver also changes fructose and galactose, which cannot be used by body cells, to glucose, which provides energy for cellular metabolism. Fats are synthesized and catabolized by the liver. Amino acids from protein breakdown may be used to form glycogen, plasma proteins, and enzymes. In addition to glycogen, the liver also stores fat-soluble vitamins (i.e., vitamins A, D, E, K), vitamin B_{12}, iron, phospholipids, cholesterol, and small amounts of protein and fat.

The liver synthesizes bile; serum albumin and globulin; prothrombin; fibrinogen; blood coagulation factors V, VII, VIII, IX, XI, and XII; and urea. Formation of urea removes ammonia from body fluids. Large amounts of ammonia are formed by intestinal bacteria and absorbed into the blood. If the ammonia is not converted to urea by the liver, plasma ammonia concentrations rise to toxic levels and cause hepatic coma and death.

A final function of the liver is production of body heat by continuous cellular metabolism. The liver is the body organ with the highest rate of chemical activity during basal conditions, and it produces about 20% of total body heat.

Secretions of the Digestive System

Mucus

Mucus is secreted by mucous glands in every part of the gastrointestinal (GI) tract. The functions of mucus are to protect the lining of the tract from digestive juices, lubricate the food bolus for easier passage, promote adherence of the fecal mass, and neutralize acids and bases. Prostaglandins aid in protecting the gastrointestinal mucosa from injury.

Saliva

Saliva consists of mucus, ptyalin, and salivary amylase. It is produced by the salivary glands and totals about 1000 milliliters daily. Saliva has a slightly acidic to neutral pH (6–7); it lubricates the food bolus and begins starch digestion.

Gastric Juice

Gastric juice consists of mucus, digestive enzymes, hydrochloric acid, and electrolytes. The gastric glands secrete about 2000 milliliters of highly acidic (pH of 1–3) gastric juice daily. Secretion varies according to time of day, the time and type of food intake, psychological states, and other metabolic activities of the body. It is highest in the evening and lowest in the early morning. Secretion is stimulated by the parasympathetic nervous system (by the vagus nerve); the hormone gastrin; the presence of food in the mouth; and seeing, smelling, or thinking about food.

The major digestive enzyme in gastric juice is pepsin, a proteolytic enzyme (named before the "ase" system of naming enzymes) that functions best at a pH of 2 to 3. Hydrochloric acid provides the acid medium to promote pepsin activity. Gastrin, acetylcholine and histamine stimulate mechanisms that result in increased production of gastric acid from the gastric glands. The major function of gastric juice is to begin digestion of proteins. There is also a weak action on fats by gastric lipase and on carbohydrates by gastric amylase. A large amount of mucus is secreted in the stomach to protect the stomach wall from the proteolytic action of pepsin. When mucus is not secreted, gastric ulceration occurs within hours.

Pancreatic Juices

Pancreatic juices are alkaline (pH of 8 or above) secretions that contain amylase for carbohydrate digestion, lipase for fat digestion, and trypsin and chymotrypsin for protein digestion. They also contain large amounts of sodium bicarbonate, a base (alkali) that neutralizes the acid chyme from the stomach by reacting with hydrochloric acid. This protects the mucosa of the small intestine from the digestive properties of gastric juice. The daily amount of pancreatic secretion is about 1200 milliliters. The hormone cholecystokinin stimulates secretion of enzyme-rich pancreatic juices. Secretin stimulates increased production of bicarbonate-rich pancreatic juices.

Bile

Bile is an alkaline (pH of about 8) secretion that is formed continuously in the liver, carried to the gallbladder by the bile ducts, and stored there. The hormone cholecystokinin causes the gallbladder to contract and release bile into the small intestine when fats are present in intestinal contents. The liver secretes about 600 milliliters of bile daily. This amount is concentrated to the 50- to 60-milliliter capacity of the gallbladder. Bile contains bile salts, cholesterol, bilirubin, fatty acids, and electrolytes. Bile salts are required for digestion and absorption of fats, including fat-soluble vitamins. Most of the bile salts are reabsorbed and reused by the liver (enterohepatic recirculation); some are excreted in feces.

Effects of Drugs on the Digestive System

The digestive system and drug therapy have a reciprocal relationship. Many common symptoms (i.e., nausea, vomiting, constipation, diarrhea, abdominal pain) relate to GI dysfunction. These symptoms may result from a disorder in the digestive system, disorders in other body systems, or drug therapy. Many GI symptoms and disorders alter the ingestion, dissolution, absorption, and metabolism of drugs. Drugs may be administered to relieve these symptoms and disorders, but drugs administered for conditions unrelated to the digestive system may cause such symptoms and disorders. GI conditions may alter responses to drug therapy.

Drugs used in digestive disorders primarily alter GI secretion, absorption, or motility. They may act systemically or locally in the GI tract. The drug groups included in this section are laxatives, antidiarrheals, antiemetics, and drugs used for acid-peptic disorders. Other drug groups used in GI disorders include cholinergics (see Chap. 19), anticholinergics (see Chap. 20), corticosteroids (see Chap. 23), and anti-infective drugs (see Section 5).

Key Concepts

- The main functions of the digestive system are to provide the body with useable nutrition and dispose of waste products that result from the digestive process.
- Peristalsis propels food through the digestive tract and mixes the food bolus with digestive juices.
- Parasympathetic stimulation increases GI motility and secretions.
- Sympathetic stimulation promotes sphincter function and inhibits motility.
- Digestion begins in the oral cavity with mastication and digestion of starches.
- The esophagus is bordered by sphincters at each end and serves to convey food to the stomach.
- Failure of the lower esophageal sphincter results in reflux of gastric contents into the esophagus.
- Food is mixed with gastric juice, containing mucus, digestive enzymes such as pepsin, and hydrochloric acid in the stomach.

- Pepsin requires an acidic pH to effectively digest proteins.
- Gastrin, acetylcholine, and histamine stimulate secretion of gastric acid.
- Mucus and prostaglandins protect the stomach from the acidic pH of the gastric secretions
- Most nutrients and drugs are absorbed in the small intestine.
- Pancreatic juices are rich in bicarbonate and digestive enzymes.
- The gallbladder stores and releases bile into the small intestine when fats are present in the duodenum.
- The liver plays numerous roles in digestion, including metabolism of carbohydrates, fats, and proteins; storage of fat-soluble vitamins, vitamin B_{12}, iron, phospholipids, cholesterol, and a small amount of protein and fat; and synthesis of bile.

Review and Application Exercises

Short Answer Exercises

1. What is the main function of the GI system?
2. What is the role of the parasympathetic nervous system in GI function?
3. List factors affecting GI motility and secretions.

4. Describe important GI secretions and their functions.
5. What factors stimulate or inhibit GI secretions?
6. How does the GI tract affect oral medications?
7. How do oral medications affect the GI tract?

Selected References

Porth, C. M. (2005). Control of gastrointestinal function. In C. M. Porth (Ed.), *Pathophysiology: Concepts of altered health states* (7th ed., pp. 871–884). Philadelphia: Lippincott Williams & Wilkins.

Stanfield, C. (2008). Assessment of digestive and gastrointestinal function. In S. C. Smeltzer, B. G. Bare, J. L. Hinkle, & K. H. Cheever (Eds.), *Brunner & Suddarth's textbook of medical-surgical nursing* (11th ed., pp. 1120–1140). Philadelphia: Lippincott Williams & Wilkins.

LEARNING OBJECTIVES

After studying this chapter, you will be able to:

1. Assess patients for risk factors and manifestations of protein-calorie undernutrition.
2. Identify patients at risk for development of vitamin and/or mineral–electrolyte deficiency or excess.
3. Describe adverse effects associated with overdoses of vitamins.
4. Discuss the rationale for administering vitamin K to newborns.
5. Describe signs, symptoms, and treatment of sodium, potassium, magnesium, and chloride imbalances.
6. Describe signs, symptoms, and treatment of iron deficiency anemia.
7. Discuss the chelating agents used to remove excessive copper, iron, and lead from body tissues.
8. Apply nursing process skills to prevent, recognize, or treat nutritional imbalances.
9. Monitor laboratory reports that indicate nutritional status.

Applying Your Knowledge

Jane Farber is a 91-year-old woman who suffers from heart failure, osteoarthritis, and Parkinson's disease. Upon evaluation, you find that Mrs. Farber is undernourished and slightly dehydrated.

Introduction

Water, carbohydrates, proteins, fats, vitamins, and minerals are required to promote or maintain health, to prevent illness, and to promote recovery from illness or injury. Water is required for cellular metabolism and excretion of metabolic waste products; 2000 to 3000 milliliters are needed daily. Proteins are structural and functional components of all body tissues; the recommended amount for adults is 50 to 60 grams daily. Carbohydrates and fats mainly provide energy for cellular metabolism. Energy is measured in kilocalories (kcal) per gram of food oxidized in the body. Carbohydrates and proteins supply 4 kcal per gram; fats supply 9 kcal per gram.

Vitamins are required for normal body metabolism, growth, and development. They are components of enzyme systems that release energy from ingested carbohydrates, proteins, and fats. They also are required for formation of red blood cells, nerve cells, hormones, genetic material, and bone and other tissues. Minerals and electrolytes are essential constituents of bone, teeth, cell membranes, connective tissue, and many essential enzymes. They function to maintain fluid, electrolyte, and acid–base balance; maintain osmotic pressure; maintain nerve and muscle function; assist in transfer of compounds across cell membranes; and influence the growth process.

For all of these nutrients, patients' requirements vary widely, depending on age, sex, size, health or illness status, and other factors. This chapter discusses products to improve nutritional status in patients with deficiency states and excess states of selected vitamins and mineral–electrolytes.

Nutritional Deficiency States

Nurses encounter many patients who are unable to ingest, digest, absorb, or use sufficient nutrients to improve or maintain health. Debilitating illnesses such as cancer; acquired immunodeficiency syndrome; and chronic lung, kidney, or cardiovascular disorders often interfere with appetite and gastrointestinal (GI) function. Therapeutic drugs often cause anorexia, nausea, vomiting, diarrhea, or constipation. Nutritional deficiencies may impair the function of essentially every body organ. Signs and symptoms include unintended weight loss, increased susceptibility to infection, weakness and fatigability, impaired wound healing, impaired growth and development in children, edema, and decreased hemoglobin.

Nutritional Products

Various products are available to supplement or substitute for dietary intake. These may consist of liquid enteral formulas, intravenous (IV) fluids, pancreatic enzymes, vitamins, and minerals.

Liquid Enteral Products

Numerous liquid enteral formulas are available over-the-counter or in health care settings for oral or tube feedings. Many are nutritionally complete, except for water, when given in sufficient amounts (e.g., Ensure, Isocal, Sustacal, Resource).

Additional water must be given to meet fluid needs. Most oral products are available in a variety of flavors and contain 1 kcal per milliliter. Additional products are formulated for patients with special conditions (e.g., renal or hepatic failure, malabsorption syndromes) or needs (e.g., high protein, increased calories).

Intravenous Fluids

IV fluids are used when oral or tube feedings are contraindicated. Most are nutritionally incomplete and are used short term to supply fluids, electrolytes, and a few calories. Dextrose or dextrose and sodium chloride solutions are often used. When nutrients must be provided intravenously for more than a few days, a special *parenteral nutrition* formula can be designed to meet all nutritional needs or to supplement other feeding methods.

Pancreatic Enzymes

Pancreatic enzymes (amylase, protease, lipase) are required for absorption of carbohydrates, protein, and fat. Pancrelipase and others are commercial preparations used as replacement therapy in deficiency states, including cystic fibrosis, chronic pancreatitis, pancreatectomy, and pancreatic obstruction. Dosage is 1 to 3 capsules or tablets with each meal or snack.

Vitamins

Vitamins are obtained from foods or supplements. Although foods are considered the best source, studies indicate that most adults and children do not consume enough fruits, vegetables, cereal grains, dairy products, and other foods to consistently meet their vitamin requirements. In addition, some conditions increase requirements above the usual recommended amounts (e.g., pregnancy, lactation, various illnesses).

Historically, the major concern about vitamins was sufficient intake to promote health and prevent deficiency diseases. To this end, the Food and Nutrition Board of the National Academy of Sciences established recommendations for daily vitamin intake (Dietary Reference Intakes [DRIs]; see Box 57-1).

Box 57-1	Dietary Reference Intakes (DRIs)

Dietary Reference Intakes are the recommended amounts of vitamins (see Table 57-1) and some minerals (see Table 57-3). The current DRIs were established in 1997, 1998, and 2000 by the Food and Nutrition Board of the National Academy of Sciences and are intended to replace the Recommended Dietary Allowances (RDAs) used since 1989. DRIs consist of four subtypes of nutrient recommendations, as follows:
1. **Estimated Average Requirement** (EAR) is the amount estimated to provide adequate intake in 50% of healthy persons in a specific group.
2. **Recommended Dietary Allowance** (RDA) is the amount estimated to meet the needs of approximately 98% of

healthy children and adults in a specific age and gender group. The RDA is used to advise various groups about nutrient intake. It should be noted, however, that RDAs were established to prevent deficiencies and that they were extrapolated from studies of healthy adults. Thus, they may not be appropriate for all groups, such as young children and older adults.
3. **Adequate Intake (AI)** is the amount thought to be sufficient when there is not enough reliable, scientific information to estimate an average requirement. The AI is derived from data that show an average intake that appears to maintain health.

(continued on page 904)

Box 57-1	Dietary Reference Intakes (DRIs) (continued)

4. **Tolerable Upper Intake Level (UL)** is the maximum intake considered unlikely to pose a health risk in almost all healthy persons in a specified group; it is not intended to be a recommended level of intake.

With **vitamins,** the ULs for adults (19–70 years and older) are D, 50 mg; E, 1000 mg; C, 2000 mg; folate, 1000 mcg; niacin, 35 mg; and pyridoxine, 100 mg. With vitamins C and D and pyridoxine, the UL refers to the total intake from food, fortified food, and supplements. With niacin and folate, the UL applies to synthetic forms obtained from supplements, fortified foods, or a combination of the two. With vitamin E, the UL applies to any form of supplemental alpha-tocopherol. These ULs should not be exceeded.

There are inadequate data for establishing ULs for biotin, cyanocobalamin (B_{12}), pantothenic acid, riboflavin, and thiamine. As a result, consuming more than the recommended amounts of these vitamins should generally be avoided.

With **minerals,** ULs have been established for calcium (2.5 g), phosphorus (3–4 g), magnesium (350 mg), fluoride (10 mg), and selenium (400 mcg). The UL should not be exceeded for any mineral–electrolyte because all minerals are toxic in overdose. Except for magnesium, which is set for supplements only and excludes food and water sources, the stated UL amounts include those from both foods and supplements.

Currently, concern extends to excessive vitamin intake, which may also be detrimental to health. Vitamin supplements are widely promoted to increase health and prevent or treat illness. However, the supplements can be harmful if overused. As a result, the DRIs include the maximum Tolerable Upper Intake Levels (ULs) of some vitamins. **These amounts should not be exceeded.**

Vitamins are classified as fat soluble (A, D, E, K) and water soluble (B complex, C). *Fat-soluble vitamins* are absorbed from the intestine with dietary fat, and absorption requires the presence of bile salts and pancreatic lipase. Vitamin D is discussed mainly in Chapter 25 because of its major role in bone metabolism. Vitamin deficiencies occur with inadequate intake or disease processes that interfere with absorption or use of vitamins. Excess states occur with excessive intake of fat-soluble vitamins because these vitamins accumulate in the body. Excess states do not occur with dietary intake of water-soluble vitamins but may occur with vitamin supplements that exceed recommended amounts. Vitamins are described further in Table 57-1, and recommended dosages of vitamin preparations are listed in Table 57-2.

Vitamin Supplements

Vitamin supplements may be prescribed by health care providers, but most are self-prescribed. Because vitamins are essential nutrients, some people believe that large amounts (megadoses) promote health and provide other beneficial effects. However, excessive intake may cause harmful effects, and *megavitamins* should never be self-prescribed. Additional characteristics include the following:

- Vitamins from supplements exert the same physiologic effects as those obtained from foods.

- Vitamin supplements do not require a prescription.

- Vitamin products vary widely in number, type, and amount of specific ingredients.

- Preparations should not contain more than recommended amounts of vitamin D, folic acid, and vitamin A.

- Synthetic vitamins have the same structure and function as natural vitamins derived from plant and animal sources and are less expensive.

- Multivitamin preparations often contain minerals as well. **Large doses of all minerals are toxic.**

- Vitamins are often marketed in combination products with each other (e.g., antioxidant vitamins) and with herbal products (e.g., B-complex vitamins with ginseng, for "energy"). There is no reliable evidence to support the use of such products.

- Some vitamins (e.g., C; E; beta carotene, a precursor of vitamin A) have been thought to prevent heart disease, cancer, and other illnesses by their antioxidant effects. Antioxidants inactivate oxygen free radicals, potentially toxic substances formed during normal cell metabolism, and inhibit them from damaging body cells. However, the results of most research studies with antioxidant vitamin supplements have been disappointing and inconclusive. The consensus view seems to be that dietary vitamins from several daily servings of grains, fruits, and vegetables and a daily multivitamin supplement are beneficial for most children and adults, but vitamin supplements to prevent various chronic illnesses cannot be recommended with current evidence.

Mineral–Electrolytes

There are 22 minerals considered necessary for human nutrition. Some (calcium, phosphorus, sodium, potassium, magnesium, chlorine, sulfur) are required in relatively large amounts. Calcium and phosphorus are discussed mainly in Chapter 25 because of their major roles in bone metabolism. Sulfur is a component of cellular proteins, several amino acids, B vitamins, insulin, and other essential body substances. No recommended intake has been established; it is obtained from protein foods.

Other minerals are required in small amounts and are often called trace elements. Eight of these (chromium, cobalt,

Table 57-1	Vitamins			

VITAMIN/FUNCTION	RECOMMENDED DAILY INTAKE	FOOD SOURCES	SIGNS & SYMPTOMS OF DEFICIENCY	SIGNS & SYMPTOMS OF EXCESS
Fat-Soluble Vitamins				
Vitamin A (retinol) Required for normal vision, growth, bone development, skin, and mucous membranes	DRIs* *Females:* 14 y and older, 700 mcg; in pregnancy, 750–770 mcg; lactation, 1200–1300 mcg *Males:* 14 y and older, 900 mcg *Children:* 1–3 y, 300 mcg; 4–8 y, 400 mcg; 9–13 y, 600 mcg *Infants (AIs):* 0–6 mo, 400 mcg; 6–12 mo, 500 mcg	Preformed vitamin A: meat, butter and fortified margarine, egg yolk, whole milk, cheese made from whole milk Carotenoids: turnip and collard greens, carrots, sweet potatoes, squash, apricots, peaches, cantaloupe	Night blindness; xerophthalmia, which may progress to corneal ulceration and blindness; changes in skin and mucous membranes that lead to skin lesions and infections, respiratory tract infections, and urinary calculi	Anorexia, vomiting, irritability, skin changes (itching, desquamation, dermatitis); pain in muscles, bones, and joints; gingivitis; enlargement of spleen and liver; increased intracranial pressure; other neurologic signs. Congenital abnormalities in newborns whose mothers took excessive vitamin A during pregnancy. Acute toxicity, with increased intracranial pressure, bulging fontanels, and vomiting, may occur in infants who are given vitamin A.
Vitamin E Antioxidant in preventing destruction of certain fats, including the lipid portion of cell membranes; may increase absorption, hepatic storage, and use of vitamin A	RDAs† *Females:* 14 y and older, 15 mg; in pregnancy, 15 mg (22.5 IU); lactation, 19 mg (28.5 IU) *Males:* 14 y and older, 15 mg *Children:* 1–3 y, 6 mg; 4–8 y, 7 mg; 9–13 y, 11 mg *Infants (AIs):* 0–6 mo, 4 mg; 7–12 mo, 6 mg	Cereals, green leafy vegetables, egg yolk, milk fat, butter, meat, vegetable oils	Deficiency is rare.	Fatigue; nausea; headache; blurred vision; diarrhea
Vitamin K Essential for normal blood clotting. Activates precursor proteins, found in the liver, into clotting factors II, VII, IX, and X	1 mcg/kg	Green leafy vegetables (spinach, kale, cabbage, lettuce), cauliflower, tomatoes, wheat bran, cheese, egg yolk, liver	Abnormal bleeding (melena, hematemesis, hematuria, epistaxis, petechiae, ecchymoses, hypovolemic shock)	Clinical manifestations rarely occur. However, when vitamin K is given to someone who is receiving warfarin (Coumadin), the client can be made "warfarin-resistant" for 2–3 wk.
Vitamin D (see Chap. 25)				
Water-Soluble Vitamins				
B-Complex				
Biotin Essential in fat and carbohydrate metabolism	AIs *Females:* 14–18 y, 25 mcg; 19 y and older, 30 mcg; in pregnancy, 30 mcg; lactation, 35 mcg	Meat, egg yolk, nuts, cereals, most vegetables	Anorexia, nausea, depression, muscle pain, dermatitis	Not established

(continued on page 906)

| Table 57-1 | Vitamins (continued) | | | |

VITAMIN/FUNCTION	RECOMMENDED DAILY INTAKE	FOOD SOURCES	SIGNS & SYMPTOMS OF DEFICIENCY	SIGNS & SYMPTOMS OF EXCESS
	Males: 4–18 y, 25 mcg; 19 y and older, 30 mcg *Children:* 1–3 y, 8 mcg; 4–8 y, 12 mcg; 9–13 y, 20 mcg *Infants:* 0–6 mo, 5 mcg; 7–12 mo, 6 mcg			
Cyanocobalamin (B$_{12}$) Essential for normal metabolism of all body cells; normal red blood cells; normal nerve cells; growth; and metabolism of carbohydrate, protein, and fat	RDAs *Females:* 14 y and older, 2.4 mcg; in pregnancy, 2.6 mcg; lactation, 2.8 mcg *Males:* 14 y and older, 2.4 mcg *Children:* 1–3 y, 0.9 mcg; 4–8 y, 1.2 mcg; 9–13 y, 1.8 mcg *Infants (AIs):* 0–6 mo, 0.4 mcg; 7–12 mo, 0.5 mcg	Meat, eggs, fish, cheese	Pernicious anemia: decreased numbers of RBCs; large, immature RBCs; fatigue; dyspnea Severe deficiency: leukopenia, infection, thrombocytopenia, cardiac dysrhythmias, heart failure Neurologic signs and symptoms: paresthesias in hands and feet; unsteady gait; depressed deep-tendon reflexes; loss of memory; confusion; delusions; hallucinations; psychosis. Nerve damage may be irreversible.	Not established
Folic acid (folate) Essential for normal metabolism of all body cells; normal red blood cells; and growth	RDAs *Females:* 14 y and older, 400 mcg; in pregnancy, 600 mcg; lactation, 500 mcg *Males:* 14 y and older, 400 mcg *Children:* 1–3 y, 150 mcg; 4–8 y, 200 mcg; 9–13 y, 300 mcg *Infants (AIs):* 0–6 mo, 65 mcg; 7–12 mo, 80 mcg	Liver, kidney beans, fresh green vegetables (spinach, broccoli, asparagus), fortified grain products (e.g., breads, cereals, rice)	Megaloblastic anemia that cannot be distinguished from the anemia produced by B$_{12}$ deficiency; impaired growth in children; glossitis; GI problems	Not established
Niacin (B$_3$) Essential for glycolysis, fat synthesis, and tissue respiration. It functions as a coenzyme in many metabolic processes (after conversion to nicotinamide, the physiologically active form).	DRIs *Females:* 14 y and older, 14 mg; in pregnancy, 18 mg; lactation, 17 mg *Males:* 14 y and older, 16 mg *Children:* 1–3 y, 6 mg; 4–8 y, 8 mg; 9–13 y, 12 mg	Meat, poultry, fish, peanuts	Pellagra: erythematous skin lesions, GI problems (stomatitis, glossitis, enteritis, diarrhea), central nervous system problems (headache, dizziness, insomnia, depression, memory loss) Severe deficiency: delusions,	Flushing; pruritus; hyperglycemia; hyperuricemia; increased liver enzymes

VITAMIN/FUNCTION	RECOMMENDED DAILY INTAKE	FOOD SOURCES	SIGNS & SYMPTOMS OF DEFICIENCY	SIGNS & SYMPTOMS OF EXCESS
	Infants (AIs): 0–6 mo, 2 mg; 7–12 mo, 4 mg		hallucinations, impairment of peripheral motor and sensory nerves	
Pantothenic acid (B₅) Essential for metabolism of carbohydrate, fat, and protein (e.g., release of energy from carbohydrate; fatty acid metabolism; synthesis of cholesterol, steroid hormones, and phospholipids)	AIs *Females:* 14 y and older, 5 mg; in pregnancy, 6 mg; lactation, 7 mg *Males:* 14 y and older, 5 mg *Children:* 1–3 y, 2 mg; 4–8 y, 3 mg; 9–13 y, 4 mg *Infants:* 0–6 mo, 1.7 mg; 7–12 mo, 1.8 mg	Eggs, liver, salmon, yeast, cauliflower, broccoli, lean beef, potatoes, tomatoes	No deficiency state established	Not established
Pyridoxine (B₆) A coenzyme in metabolism of carbohydrate, protein, and fat; required for formation of tryptophan and conversion of tryptophan to niacin; helps release glycogen from the liver and muscle tissue; functions in metabolism of the central nervous system; helps maintain cellular immunity	DRIs *Females:* 14–18 y, 1.2 mg; 19–50 y, 1.3 mg; 51–70 and older, 1.5 mg; in pregnancy, 1.9 mg; lactation, 2.0 mg *Males:* 14–50 y, 1.3 mg; 51–70 y and older, 1.7 mg *Children:* 1–3 y, 0.5 mg; 4–8 y, 0.6 mg; 9–13 y, 1.0 mg *Infants (AIs):* 0–6 mo, 0.1 mg; 7–12 mo, 0.3 mg	Yeast, wheat germ, liver and other glandular meats, whole grain cereals, potatoes, legumes	Skin and mucous membrane lesions (seborrheic dermatitis, intertrigo, glossitis, stomatitis), neurologic problems (convulsions, peripheral neuritis, mental depression)	Not established
Riboflavin (B₂) A coenzyme in metabolism; necessary for growth; may function in production of corticosteroids and red blood cells and gluconeogenesis	DRIs *Females:* 14–18 y, 1.0 mg; 19 y and older, 1.1 mg; in pregnancy, 1.4 mg; lactation, 1.6 mg *Males:* 14 y and older, 1.3 mg *Children:* 1–3 y, 0.5 mg; 4–8 y, 0.6 mg; 9–13 y, 0.9 mg *Infants (AIs):* 0–6 mo, 0.3 mg; 7–12 mo, 0.4 mg	Milk, cheddar and cottage cheeses, meat, eggs, green leafy vegetables	Glossitis, stomatitis, seborrheic dermatitis, eye disorders (burning, itching, lacrimation, photophobia, vascularization of the cornea)	Not established
Thiamine (B₁) A coenzyme in carbohydrate metabolism; essential for energy production	DRIs *Females:* 14–18 y, 1.0 mg; 19 y and older, 1.1 mg; in pregnancy, 1.4 mg; lactation, 1.4 mg *Males:* 14 y and older, 1.2 mg	Meat, poultry, fish, egg yolk, dried beans, whole-grain cereal products, peanuts	Mild deficiency: fatigue, anorexia, retarded growth, mental depression, irritability, apathy, lethargy Severe deficiency (beriberi): peripheral neuritis; personality	Not established

(continued on page 908)

Table 57-1	Vitamins (continued)			

VITAMIN/FUNCTION	RECOMMENDED DAILY INTAKE	FOOD SOURCES	SIGNS & SYMPTOMS OF DEFICIENCY	SIGNS & SYMPTOMS OF EXCESS
	Children: 1–3 y, 0.5 mg; 4–8 y, 0.6 mg; 9–13 y, 0.9 mg *Infants (AIs):* 0–6 mo, 0.2 mg; 7–12 mo, 0.3 mg		disturbances; heart failure; edema; Wernicke-Korsakoff syndrome in alcoholics	
Vitamin C (ascorbic acid) Essential for formation of skin, ligaments, cartilage, bone, and teeth; required for wound healing and tissue repair, metabolism of iron and folic acid, synthesis of fats and proteins, preservation of blood vessel integrity, and resistance to infection	DRIs *Females:* 14–18 y, 65 mg; 19 y and older, 75 mg; in pregnancy, 80–85 mg; lactation, 115–120 mg *Males:* 14–18 y, 75 mg; 19 y and older, 90 mg *Children:* 1–3 y, 15 mg; 4–8 y, 25 mg; 9–13 y, 45 mg *Infants (AIs):* 0–6 mo, 40 mg; 7–12 mo, 50 mg	Fruits and vegetables, especially citrus fruits and juices	Mild deficiency: irritability, malaise, arthralgia, increased tendency to bleed Severe deficiency: scurvy and adverse effects on most body tissues (gingivitis; bleeding of gums, skin, joints, and other areas; disturbances of bone growth; anemia; and loosening of teeth). If not treated, coma and death may occur.	Renal calculi

*DRIs for vitamin A are expressed in retinol activity equivalents (RAEs), which include both preformed vitamin A and carotenoids. 1 RAE = 1 mcg retinol or 12 mcg beta carotene.

†Vitamin E activity is expressed in milligrams of alpha-tocopherol equivalents (alpha TE).

AIs, Adequate Intakes; DRIs, Dietary Reference Intakes; GI, gastrointestinal; RBCs, red blood cells; RDAs, Recommended Dietary Allowances.

Table 57-2	Drugs at a Glance: Vitamin Drug Preparations			

	ROUTES AND DOSAGE RANGES			
Generic/Trade Name	Adults	Children	Comments	
Fat-Soluble Vitamins				
Vitamin A (also called retinol)	*Deficiency,* PO, IM 100,000 IU daily for 3 d, then 50,000 IU daily for 2 wk, then 10,000–20,000 IU daily for another 2 mo	*Kwashiorkor,* Retinol 30 mg IM followed by intermittent oral therapy *Xerophthalmia (over 1 y old),* retinyl palmitate 110 mg PO or 55 mg IM plus another 110 mg PO at 1 and 3 or 4 d later	IM administration indicated when oral not feasible, as in anorexia, nausea, vomiting, preoperative and postoperative conditions, or malabsorption syndromes With xerophthalmia, vitamin E 40 IU should be coadministered to increase effectiveness of the retinol.	
Vitamin E	PO 100–400 IU daily	PO 15–30 IU daily	Should not be given IV because IV use has been associated with 38 infant deaths	

	ROUTES AND DOSAGE RANGES		
Generic/Trade Name	**Adults**	**Children**	**Comments**
Vitamin K Phytonadione (Mephyton)	Anticoagulant-induced pro-thrombin deficiency, PO, Sub-Q, IM 2.5–10 mg initially, repeat after 6–8 h (injected dose) or 12–48 h (oral dose) if needed (i.e., if prothrombin time still prolonged) Hypoprothrombinemia due to other causes, PO, Sub-Q, IM 2.5–25 mg	*Older children*, same as adults *Newborns*, prevention of hemorrhagic disease, IM 0.5–1 mg within 1 h after birth; may be repeated after 2–3 wk if mother received anticoagulant, anticonvulsant, antitubercular, or recent antibiotic drug therapy during pregnancy Treatment of hemorrhagic disease, Sub-Q, IM 1 mg	Do not give IV; unless necessary serious, ana-phylaxis-like reactions have occurred.
Water-Soluble Vitamins B-COMPLEX VITAMINS			
Calcium pantothenate (B$_5$)	Total parenteral nutrition, IV 15 mg daily	Total parenteral nutrition, over 11 y, IV 15 mg daily; 1–11 y, IV 5 mg daily	Deficiency states seen only with severe, multiple B-complex deficiency states
Cyanocobalamin (B$_{12}$)	PO 100–250 mcg daily IM 30 mcg daily for 5–10 d, then 100–200 mcg monthly	PO, IM, Sub-Q 10–100 mcg daily for 5–15 d, then 100–200 mcg monthly	Oral drug, alone or in multivitamin prepara-tions, is given for nutri-tional deficiencies.
Nascobal	Intranasal gel, 1 spray (500 mcg) in one nostril, once per wk		Parenteral B$_{12}$ should be given for pernicious anemia. Intranasal drug should not be used if rhinitis, nasal congestion, or upper respiratory infec-tion is present.
Folic acid	Deficiency, megaloblastic anemia, PO, Sub-Q, IM, IV up to 1 mg daily until symptoms decrease and blood tests are normal, then maintenance dose of 0.4 mg daily	PO, Sub-Q, IM, IV up to 1 mg daily until symptoms decrease and blood tests are normal, then a daily maintenance dose as fol-lows: infants, 0.1 mg; under 4 y, up to 0.3 mg; over 4 y, 0.4 mg	Oral administration preferred unless severe intestinal malabsorption is present
Niacin (nicotinic acid) Niacinamide (nicotinamide)	Deficiency, PO 50–100 mg daily Pellagra, PO Up to 500 mg daily Hyperlipidemia, PO 2–6 g daily (maximum dose, 6 g/d)	Safety and effectiveness not established for amounts exceeding the RDA	To reduce flushing with larger doses, start with smaller doses and gradu-ally increase them.
Pyridoxine (B$_6$)	Deficiency, PO, IM, IV 2–5 mg daily Anemia, peripheral neuritis, 50–200 mg daily	Safety and effectiveness not established for amounts exceeding the RDA	Usually given with isoniazid, an antituber-cular drug, to prevent peripheral neuropathy
Riboflavin	Deficiency, PO 5–10 mg daily In total parenteral nutrition, 3.6 mg/d	In total parenteral nutri-tion, IV over 11 y, 3.6 mg/d; 1–11 y, 1.4 mg/d	Deficiency rarely occurs alone; more likely with other vitamin deficiency states

(continued on page 910)

| Table 57-2 | Drugs at a Glance: Vitamin Drug Preparations (continued) | | |

| | ROUTES AND DOSAGE RANGES | | |
Generic/Trade Name	Adults	Children	Comments
Thiamine (B₁)	Deficiency, PO 10–30 mg daily; IM 10–20 mg 3 times daily for 2 wk, supplemented with 5–10 mg orally; IV 50–100 mg/d until able to take orally	Safety and effectiveness not established for amounts exceeding the RDA	Deficiency is common in alcoholics.
VITAMIN C Vitamin C (ascorbic acid)	Deficiency, PO, IM, IV 100–500 mg daily Urinary acidification, 2 g daily in divided doses Prophylaxis, 50–100 mg daily	Infants receiving formula, 35–50 mg daily for first few weeks of life	Excessive doses (e.g., 2000 mg or more daily) cause adverse effects and should be avoided.

IU, international units.

copper, fluoride, iodine, iron, selenium, and zinc) have relatively well-defined roles in human nutrition. Others (manganese, molybdenum, nickel, silicon, tin, and vanadium) are present in many body tissues and may be necessary for normal growth, structure, and function of connective tissue. However, requirements are unknown, and states of deficiency or excess have not been identified in humans.

Minerals occur in the body and foods mainly in ionic form. Ions are electrically charged particles. Metals (e.g., sodium, potassium, calcium, magnesium) form positive ions or cations; nonmetals (e.g., chlorine, phosphorus, sulfur) form negative ions or anions. These cations and anions combine to form compounds that are physiologically inactive and electrically neutral. When placed in solution, such as a body fluid, the components separate into electrically charged particles called *electrolytes*. At any given time, the body must maintain an equal number of positive and negative charges. Therefore, the ions are constantly combining and separating to maintain electrical neutrality or electrolyte balance.

These electrolytes also maintain the acid–base balance of body fluids. When foods are digested, they produce mineral residues that react chemically as acids or bases. Acids are usually anions (e.g., chloride, bicarbonate, sulfate, phosphate). Bases are usually cations (e.g., sodium, potassium, calcium, magnesium). If approximately equal amounts of cations and anions are present in the mineral residue, the residue is essentially neutral, and the pH of body fluids does not require adjustment. If there is an excess of cations (base), the body must draw on its anions (acid) to combine with the cations, render them physiologically inactive, and restore the normal pH of the blood. Excess cations combine with anions (e.g., phosphate) and are excreted in the urine; excess anions combine with hydrogen ions or other cations and are excreted in the urine.

Mineral–electrolytes are obtained from foods or supplements. Although most minerals are supplied by a well-

balanced diet, studies indicate that most adults and children do not ingest sufficient dietary calcium and that iron deficiency anemia is common in some populations. In addition, some conditions increase requirements (e.g., pregnancy, lactation, various illnesses), and some drug–drug interactions decrease absorption or use of minerals.

As with vitamins, goals for daily mineral intake have been established as DRIs. Thus far, DRIs and ULs have been established for calcium, phosphorus, magnesium, iron, fluoride, and selenium. **The UL should not be exceeded for any mineral–electrolyte.** Except for magnesium, which is set for supplements only and excludes food and water sources, the stated amounts include those from both foods and supplements. Mineral–electrolytes are described further in Table 57-3.

Mineral Supplements

Many people take mineral preparations as dietary supplements, usually in a multivitamin–mineral combination. Health care providers and patients should consider the following factors in relation to mineral supplements.

■ Nutritionists usually recommend dietary intake of nutrients rather than pharmaceutical supplements and emphasize that supplements do not compensate for an inadequate diet.

■ In general, **recommended daily doses should not be exceeded because all minerals are toxic at high doses.**

■ Multivitamin–mineral combinations recommended for age and gender groups contain different amounts of some minerals (e.g., postmenopausal women need less iron than younger women). This should be considered in choosing a product.

■ Iron supplements other than those in multivitamin–mineral combinations are usually intended for temporary use in the presence of deficiency or a period of increased need (e.g., pregnancy). They should not be taken otherwise because of the risk of accumulation and toxicity.

Table 57-3	Minerals and Electrolytes

MINERAL/FUNCTION	RECOMMENDED DAILY INTAKE	FOOD SOURCES	SIGNS & SYMPTOMS OF DEFICIENCY	SIGNS & SYMPTOMS OF EXCESS
Macro Minerals				
Sodium				
Assists in regulating osmotic pressure, water balance, conduction of electrical impulses in nerves and muscles, and electrolyte and acid–base balance Influences permeability of cell membranes and assists in movement of substances across cell membranes Participates in many intracellular chemical reactions	Approximately 2 g	In most foods. Proteins contain large amounts, vegetables and cereals contain moderate to small amounts, fruits contain little or no sodium. Major source in the diet is table salt added to food in cooking, processing, or seasoning. One teaspoon contains 2.3 g of sodium. Water in some areas may contain significant amounts of sodium.	Serum sodium less than 135 mEq/L; anorexia, nausea, and vomiting; ataxia; confusion; delirium; hypotension and tachycardia; muscle tremors; oliguria and increased BUN; seizures; weakness	Serum sodium greater than 145 mEq/L; disorientation; dry skin and mucous membranes; fever; hyperactive reflexes; hypotension; muscle rigidity; tremors and spasms; irritability; cerebral hemorrhage; coma; oliguria, concentrated urine, increased BUN
Potassium				
Within cells, helps maintain osmotic pressure, fluid and electrolyte balance, and acid–base balance In extracellular fluid, is required for conduction of nerve impulses and contraction of muscle Helps transport glucose into cells and is required for glycogen formation and storage Required for synthesis of muscle proteins	Approximately 40 mEq	Present in most foods, including meat, whole-grain breads or cereals, bananas, citrus fruits, tomatoes, and broccoli	Serum potassium less than 3.5 mEq/L; dysrhythmias and electrocardiographic changes; cardiac arrest; confusion; delirium; hyperglycemia; postural hypotension; muscle weakness; abdominal distention, constipation, paralytic ileus; polyuria, polydipsia, nocturia. Prolonged deficiency may increase serum creatinine and BUN.	Serum potassium greater than 5 mEq/L; muscle weakness; cardiotoxicity, with dysrhythmias or cardiac arrest Cardiac effects are not usually severe until serum levels are 7 mEq/L or above.
Magnesium				
Required for conduction of nerve impulses and contraction of muscle (especially important in functions of cardiac and skeletal muscles) Serves as a component of many enzymes Essential for metabolism of carbohydrate and protein	*Adults (DRIs):* Males 19–30 y, 400 mg; 31–70 y and older, 420 mg; females 19–30 y, 310 mg; 31–70 y and older, 320 mg; in pregnancy, 350–360 mg; lactation, 310–320 mg Upper Level (UL) or maximum intake from pharmaceutical preparations, 350 mg (does not include intake from food and water)	Present in many foods; diet that is adequate in other respects contains adequate magnesium. Good food sources include nuts, cereal grains, dark green vegetables, and seafoods.	Serum magnesium less than 1.5 mEq/L; ataxia; confusion; dizziness; irritability; muscle tremors, carpopedal spasm, nystagmus, generalized spasticity; seizures; tachycardia, hypotension, premature atrial and ventricular beats	Serum magnesium greater than 2.5 mEq/L; skeletal muscle weakness; cardiac dysrhythmias, hypotension; respiratory insufficiency; coma

(continued on page 912)

Table 57-3	Minerals and Electrolytes (continued)			

MINERAL/FUNCTION	RECOMMENDED DAILY INTAKE	FOOD SOURCES	SIGNS & SYMPTOMS OF DEFICIENCY	SIGNS & SYMPTOMS OF EXCESS
	Children (RDAs): 1–3 y, 80 mg; 4–8 y, 130 mg; 9–13 y, 240 mg; 14–18 y, 410 mg *Infants (AIs):* 0–6 mo, 30 mg; 7–12 mo, 75 mg			
Chloride Helps maintain osmotic pressure and electrolyte, acid–base, and water balance Forms hydrochloric acid (HCl) in gastric mucosal cells	80–110 mEq	Most dietary chloride is ingested as sodium chloride (NaCl), and foods high in sodium are also high in chloride.	Serum chloride less than 95 mEq/L; arterial blood pH greater than 7.45; dehydration; hypotension; low, shallow respirations; paresthesias of face and extremities; muscle spasms and tetany, which cannot be distinguished from the tetany produced by hypocalcemia	Serum chloride greater than 103 mEq/L; arterial blood pH less than 7.35; increased rate and depth of respiration; lethargy, stupor, disorientation, and coma if acidosis is not treated
Trace Elements **Chromium** Aids glucose use by increasing effectiveness of insulin and facilitating transport of glucose across cell membranes	Not established	Brewer's yeast and whole-wheat products.	Impaired glucose tolerance (hyperglycemia, glycosuria); impaired growth and reproduction; decreased life span	Not established
Cobalt A component of vitamin B_{12} that is required for normal function of all body cells and for maturation of red blood cells	Approximately 1 mg in the form of vitamin B_{12}	Animal foods, including liver, muscle meats, and shellfish. Fruits, vegetables, and cereals contain no cobalt as vitamin B_{12}.	Deficiency of vitamin B_{12} produces pernicious anemia.	Not established
Copper A component of many enzymes Essential for correct functioning of the central nervous, cardiovascular, and skeletal systems Important in formation of red blood cells, apparently by regulating storage and release of iron for hemoglobin	Approximately 2 mg	Many foods, including liver, shellfish, nuts, cereals, poultry, dried fruits	Decreased serum levels; decreased iron absorption; anemia from impaired erythropoiesis; leukopenia. Death can occur. In infants, anemia, chronic malnutrition and diarrhea, or Menke's syndrome (retarded growth and progressive mental deterioration) can occur.	Increased serum levels; Wilson's disease (a rare disorder characterized by accumulation of copper in brain, liver, and kidneys). Signs and symptoms vary according to affected organs.

MINERAL/FUNCTION	RECOMMENDED DAILY INTAKE	FOOD SOURCES	SIGNS & SYMPTOMS OF DEFICIENCY	SIGNS & SYMPTOMS OF EXCESS
Fluoride A component of tooth enamel Strengthens bones Adequate intake before ages 50–60 years may decrease osteoporosis and fractures during later years.	*Adults (AIs):* males 19–70 y and older, 4 mg; females 19–70 y and older, 3 mg; in pregnancy and lactation, 5 mg *Children (AIs):* 1–3 y, 0.7 mg; 4–8 y, 1 mg; 9–13 y, 2 mg; 14–18 y, 3 mg *Infants (AIs):* 0–6 mo, 0.01 mg; 7–12 mo, 0.5 mg	Beef, canned salmon, eggs. Very little in milk, cereal grains, fruits, and vegetables. Fluoride content of foods depends on fluoride content of soil where they are grown.	Dental caries and possibly a greater incidence of osteoporosis	Mottling of teeth and osteosclerosis.
Iodine Essential component of thyroid hormones	*Adults (RDAs):* males and females 19–51 y and older, 150 mcg; in pregnancy, 175 mcg; lactation, 200 mcg *Children:* 1–10 y, 10 mg; males 11–18 y, 12 mg; females 11–18 y, 15 mg *Infants:* 0–6 mo, 40 mcg; 6–12 mo, 50 mcg	Seafood is the best source. In vegetables, iodine content varies with the amount of iodine in soil where grown. In milk and eggs, content depends on the amount present in animal feed.	Thyroid gland enlargement; possible hypothyroidism	Iodism, with coryza, edema, fever, conjunctivitis, lymphadenopathy, stomatitis, vomiting
Iron Essential component of hemoglobin, myoglobin, and several enzymes: hemoglobin is required for transport and use of oxygen by body cells; myoglobin aids oxygen transport and use by muscle cells; enzymes are important for cellular metabolism.	*Adults (RDAs):* males 19–51 y and older, 10 mg; females 19–50, 15 mg; 51 y and older, 10 mg; in pregnancy, 30 mg; lactation, 15 mg *Children:* 1–10 y, 10 mg; males 11–18 y, 12 mg; females 11–18 y, 15 mg *Infants:* 0–6 mo, 6 mg; 6–12 mo, 10 mg	Liver and other organ meats, lean meat, shellfish, dried beans and vegetables, egg yolks, dried fruits, molasses, whole-grain and enriched breads. Milk and milk products contain essentially no iron.	Iron deficiency anemia: with gradual development of anemia, minimal symptoms occur; with rapid development or severe anemia, dyspnea, fatigue, tachycardia, malaise and drowsiness occur.	Acute iron intoxication: vomiting, diarrhea, melena, abdominal pain, shock, convulsions, and metabolic acidosis. Death may occur within 24 h if treatment is not prompt. Chronic iron overload (hemochromatosis): cardiac dysrhythmias, heart failure, diabetes mellitus, bronze pigmentation of skin, liver enlargement, arthropathy, and others
Selenium Important for function of myocardium and probably other muscles	*Adults (RDAs):* males and females 19–70 y and older, 55 mcg; in pregnancy, 60 mcg; lactation, 70 mcg *Children (RDAs):* 1–3 y, 20 mcg; 4–8 y, 30 mcg; 9–13 y, 40 mcg; 14–18 y, 55 mcg *Infants (AIs):* 0–6 mo, 15 mcg; 7–12 mo, 20 mcg	Fish, meat, breads, and cereals.	Deficiency most likely with long-term IV therapy. Signs and symptoms include myocardial abnormalities and other muscle discomfort and weakness.	Highly toxic in excessive amounts. Signs and symptoms include fatigue, peripheral neuropathy, nausea, diarrhea, and alopecia.

(continued on page 914)

Table 57-3	Minerals and Electrolytes (continued)			
MINERAL/FUNCTION	**RECOMMENDED DAILY INTAKE**	**FOOD SOURCES**	**SIGNS & SYMPTOMS OF DEFICIENCY**	**SIGNS & SYMPTOMS OF EXCESS**
Zinc A component of many enzymes that are essential for normal metabolism (e.g., carbonic anhydrase, lactic dehydrogenase, alkaline phosphatase) Necessary for normal cell growth, synthesis of nucleic acids (RNA and DNA), and synthesis of carbohydrates and proteins May be essential for use of vitamin A	*Adults (RDAs):* males 19–51 y and older, 15 mg; females, 19–51 y and older, 12 mg; in pregnancy, 15 mg; lactation, 16–19 mg *Children:* 1–10 y, 10 mg; males 11–18 y, 12 mg; females 11–18 y, 15 mg *Infants:* 0–6 mo, 40 mcg; 6–12 mo, 50 mcg	Animal proteins, such as meat, liver, eggs, and seafood. Wheat germ is also a good source.	Most evident in growing children and include impaired growth, hypogonadism in boys, anorexia, and sensory impairment (loss of taste and smell). Also, if the client has had surgery, wound healing may be delayed.	Unlikely with dietary intake but may develop with excessive ingestion or inhalation of zinc. Ingestion may cause nausea, vomiting, and diarrhea; inhalation may cause vomiting, headache, and fever.

AIs, Adequate Intakes; BUN, blood urea nitrogen; DRIs, Dietary Reference Intakes; RDAs, Recommended Dietary Allowances.

- Most adolescent and adult females probably benefit from a calcium supplement to achieve the recommended amount (1000–1300 mg daily). The amounts consumed in dairy products and other foods should be considered, and the UL of 2500 milligrams daily should not be exceeded.

- Although zinc is promoted for treatment of the common cold and to promote wound healing, there is insufficient evidence to support such uses. With colds, zinc reportedly helps some people and does not help others. With wounds, zinc is reportedly beneficial only if the patient has a zinc deficiency. More studies are needed before supplemental zinc can be recommended for general use.

Agents Used in Mineral–Electrolyte Imbalances

Mineral–electrolyte imbalances include both deficiency states and excess states. Most deficiency states occur with inadequate intake or excessive losses (e.g., vomiting, gastric suction, diarrhea, overuse of laxatives). Most excess states occur with excessive intake or impaired renal excretion.

Several pharmacologic agents are used to prevent or treat mineral–electrolyte imbalances. Usually, neutral salts of minerals (e.g., potassium chloride) are used in deficiency states, and nonmineral drug preparations are used in excess states. These agents are described below; routes and dosage ranges are listed in Table 57-4.

Cation Exchange Resin

Sodium polystyrene sulfonate (Kayexalate) is used to treat hyperkalemia. Given orally or rectally, the resin combines with potassium in the colon. Potassium is then eliminated from the body in the feces. Each gram of resin removes about 1 milliequivalent of potassium. Because the resin requires several hours to lower serum potassium levels, it may be used after other measures (e.g., IV insulin and glucose infusions) have lowered serum levels. Insulin and glucose lower serum potassium levels by driving potassium into the cells; they do not remove potassium from the body.

Chelating Agents (Metal Antagonists)

Deferasirox (Exjade) is an oral iron *chelating agent* (drug) that is used to treat chronic iron overload in children and adults who require frequent blood transfusions for severe, chronic anemia. Untreated iron accumulation from the transfusions can lead to heart and liver failure.

Deferasirox is absorbed with oral administration, with peak plasma levels in 1.5 to 4 hours. It is highly bound to serum albumin, metabolized by glucuronidation, and reabsorbed in the intestine or excreted in bile and feces. In clinical trials, the most common adverse effects were skin rash and gastrointestinal problems (e.g., abdominal pain, vomiting, diarrhea, and constipation).

Deferasirox was approved and marketed in 2005; in 2007, the U.S. Food and Drug Administration (FDA) issued warnings that acute renal failure, blood disorders (agranulocytosis, neutropenia, and thrombocytopenia), and a few deaths had been reported in patients taking the drug.

Deferoxamine (Desferal) is a parenteral drug used to remove excess iron from storage sites (e.g., ferritin, hemosiderin) in the body. It combines with the iron to produce a water-soluble compound that can be excreted by the kidneys.

Table 57-4 · **Drugs at a Glance:** Individual Agents Used in Mineral-Electrolyte and Acid-Base Imbalances

Drug	Indications for Use	ROUTES AND DOSAGE RANGES	
		Adults	**Children**
Cation Exchange Resin			
Sodium polystyrene sulfonate (Kayexalate)	Treatment of hyperkalemia	PO 15 g in 100–200 mL of water and 70% sorbitol, 1–4 times daily Rectally (retention enema) 30–50 g in 100–200 mL of water and 70% sorbitol q6h	
Chelating Agents (Metal Antagonists)			
Deferasirox (Exjade)	Chronic iron overload	PO 20 mg/kg initially, adjusted every 3–6 mo according to serum ferritin levels	Same as adults
Deferoxamine (Desferal)	Acute iron intoxication Hemochromatosis due to blood transfusions Hemosiderosis due to hemolytic anemia	IM 1 g initially, then 500 mg q4h for 2 doses, then 500 mg q4–12h if needed; maximum dose, 6 g/24 h IV infusion (for patients in shock) 1 g slowly (not to exceed 15 mg/kg/h), then 500 mg q4h for 2 doses, then 500 mg q4–12h if necessary; maximum dose, 6 g/24 h	Same as adults
Penicillamine (Cuprimine)	Wilson's disease Rheumatoid arthritis Cystinuria	Wilson's disease, PO 250 mg 4 times daily, increased gradually if necessary, up to 2 g daily Rheumatoid arthritis, PO 125–250 mg/d for 4 wk, increased by 125–250 mg/d at 1- to 3-mo intervals, if necessary usual maintenance dose, 500–750 mg/d; maximum dose, 1000–1500 mg/d	*Older children:* same as adults *Infants older than 6 mo and young children:* Wilson's disease, PO 250 mg daily, dissolved in fruit juice
Succimer (Chemet)	Lead poisoning		PO 10 mg/kg or 350 mg/m^2 q8h for 5 days, then q12h for 14 days (total of 19 days of drug administration) For young children who cannot swallow capsules, the capsule contents can be sprinkled on soft food or given with a spoon.
Iron Preparations			
Ferrous gluconate (Fergon)	Iron deficiency anemia	PO 320–640 mg (40–80 mg elemental iron) 3 times daily	PO 100–300 mg (12.5–37.5 mg elemental iron) 3 times daily *Infants:* PO 100 mg or 30 drops of elixir initially, gradually increased to 300 mg or 5 mL (15–37.5 mg elemental iron) of elixir daily, in divided doses

(continued on page 916)

Table 57-4 **Drugs at a Glance:** Individual Agents Used in Mineral-Electrolyte and Acid-Base Imbalances (continued)

Drug	Indications for Use	ROUTES AND DOSAGE RANGES Adults	Children
Ferrous sulfate (Feosol)	Iron deficiency anemia	PO 325 mg–1.2 g (60–240 mg elemental iron) daily in 3 or 4 divided doses	6–12 y: PO 120–600 mg (24–120 mg elemental iron) daily, in divided doses *Under 6 y:* 300 mg (60 mg elemental iron) daily, in divided doses
Iron dextran injection (InFeD)	Iron deficiency anemia	Dosage is calculated for individual clients according to hemoglobin and weight (see manufacturer's literature). A small test dose is required before therapeutic doses are given.	Dosage is calculated for individual patients according to hemoglobin and weight (see manufacturer's literature). A small test dose is required before therapeutic doses are given.
Magnesium Preparations **Magnesium oxide** **Magnesium hydroxide** **Magnesium sulfate**	Prevent or treat hypomagnesemia Treat hypertension or convulsions associated with toxemia of pregnancy or acute nephritis in children	Hypomagnesemia, PO magnesium oxide 250–500 mg 3–4 times daily, milk of magnesia 5 mL 4 times daily, or a magnesium-containing antacid 15 mL 3 times daily; IM (magnesium sulfate) 1–2 g (2–4 mL of 50% solution) 1–2 times daily based on serum magnesium levels Eclampsia, IM 1–2 g (2–4 mL of 50% solution) initially, then 1 g every 30 min until seizures stop Convulsive seizures, IM 1 g (2 mL of 50% solution) repeated PRN IV, do not exceed 150 mg/min (1.5 mL/min of a 10% solution, 3 mL/min of a 5% solution)	Convulsions, IM 20–40 mg/kg in a 20% solution; repeat as necessary
Potassium Preparation **Potassium chloride** (KCl)	Prevent or treat hypokalemia	PO 15–20 mEq 2–4 times daily IV 40–100 mEq/24 h, depending on serum potassium levels KCl **must** be diluted in dextrose or NaCl IV solution for IV use. **Maximum** *for serum K+ greater than 2.5 mEq:* diluted 40 mEq/L, infused 10 mEq/h to maximum dose of 200 mEq in 24 h **Maximum** *for serum K+ less than 2.5 mEq:* diluted 80 mEq/L, infused 40 mEq/h to maximum dose of 400 mEq in 24 h	IV infusion up to 3 mEq/kg or 40 mEq/m² daily Adjust amount of fluids to body size.

Drug	Indications for Use	ROUTES AND DOSAGE RANGES	
		Adults	**Children**
Sodium Preparation			
Sodium chloride (NaCl) injection	Hyponatremia	IV 1500–3000 mL of 0.22% or 0.45% solution/24 h depending on the patient's fluid needs; approximately 50 mL/h to keep IV lines open	
Zinc Preparation			
Zinc sulfate	Prevent or treat zinc deficiency	PO 25–50 mg elemental zinc (e.g., zinc sulfate 110–220 mg) daily	
Multiple Mineral–Electrolyte Preparations			
Oral solutions (e.g., Pedialyte) IV solutions (e.g., Normosol, Plasma-Lyte 148, Ringer's solution)	Prevent or treat fluid and electrolyte deficiencies	IV 2000–3000 mL/24 h, depending on individual fluid and electrolyte needs	IV, PO, amount individualized according to fluid and electrolyte needs (i.e., estimated fluid loss), age and weight (see manufacturer's literature)

The drug can remove 10 to 50 milligrams of iron per day. The urine becomes reddish brown from the iron content.

The major indication for use of deferoxamine is acute iron intoxication. The drug may also be used in chronic conditions characterized by accumulation of iron in tissues (e.g., hemochromatosis with blood transfusions, hemosiderosis due to certain hemolytic anemias).

Penicillamine (Cuprimine) chelates copper, zinc, mercury, and lead to form soluble complexes that are excreted in the urine. It is used mainly to remove excess copper in patients with Wilson's disease, a rare condition characterized by accumulation of copper in vital organs. It also can be used prophylactically, before clinical manifestations occur, in patients in whom this hereditary condition is likely to develop. Penicillamine may be used to treat cystinuria, a hereditary metabolic disorder characterized by large amounts of cystine in the urine and renal calculi. It may be used in lead poisoning and in severe rheumatoid arthritis that does not respond to conventional treatment measures.

Succimer (Chemet) chelates lead to form water-soluble complexes that are excreted in the urine. It is used to treat lead poisoning in children. After oral administration, peak blood levels are reached in 1 to 2 hours. The drug is metabolized in the liver and excreted in urine and feces, with a half-life of 2 days. The most common adverse effects are anorexia, nausea, vomiting, and diarrhea.

Iron Preparations

Iron preparations are used to prevent or treat iron deficiency anemia. For prevention, they are often given during periods of increased need (e.g., childhood, pregnancy). Oral ferrous salts (sulfate, gluconate, fumarate) are preferred, because they are well absorbed. Action starts in about 4 days, peaks in 7 to 10 days, and lasts 2 to 4 months. The drugs are not metabolized; a portion of a dose is lost daily in feces. Otherwise, the iron content is recycled and its half-life is unknown. Sustained-release or enteric-coated formulations are not as well absorbed as other preparations. Available ferrous salts differ in the amount of elemental iron they contain.

Adverse effects include nausea and other symptoms of GI irritation. Oral preparations also discolor feces, producing a black-green color that may be mistaken for blood in the stool. Iron preparations are contraindicated in patients with peptic ulcer disease, inflammatory intestinal disorders, anemias other than iron deficiency anemia, multiple blood transfusions, hemochromatosis, and hemosiderosis.

Ferrous sulfate P (Feosol), which contains 20% elemental iron (i.e., 65 mg per 325-mg tablet), is the prototype and often the preparation of choice. **Ferrous gluconate** (Fergon) may be less irritating to GI mucosa and therefore better tolerated than ferrous sulfate. It contains 12% elemental iron (i.e., 36 mg per 325-mg tablet). **Ferrous fumarate** (Feostat) contains 33% elemental iron (i.e., 33 mg per 100-mg tablet). As with dietary iron, only a portion is absorbed from pharmaceutical preparations and relatively large doses are needed to supply the 10 to 15 mg needed daily by most adults and children. Small amounts of iron are lost daily (about 0.5–1 mg) in urine, sweat, and sloughing of intestinal mucosal cells. Somewhat larger amounts (1–2 mg daily) are lost during menstruation. Thus, women of childbearing potential need larger amounts of iron than children, men, and postmenopausal women. Women who are pregnant have the greatest requirement and usually need an iron supplement. Although most iron products are available over-the-counter, their use should be discussed with a health care provider because of the toxicity that may occur with iron accumulation in body tissues.

Iron dextran injection (InFeD) is a parenteral form of iron useful in treating iron deficiency anemia when oral supplements cannot be used. One milliliter contains 50 milligrams of elemental iron. Indications for use include peptic ulcer or inflammatory bowel disease that may be aggravated by oral iron preparations, the patient's inability or unwillingness to take oral preparations, and a shortage of time for correcting the iron deficiency (e.g., late pregnancy or preoperative status). Contraindications include anemias not associated with iron deficiency and patients with hypersensitivity to the drug.

The drug is usually given IV. Drug action has a slow onset and peaks in 1 to 2 weeks. Dosage is calculated according to hemoglobin level and weight. A small IV test dose should be given before a therapeutic dose. The drug has a **BLACK BOX WARNING** about the risk of anaphylactic reactions and death.

Magnesium Preparations

Magnesium oxide or **hydroxide** may be given orally for mild hypomagnesemia in asymptomatic patients. **Magnesium sulfate** is given parenterally for moderate to severe hypomagnesemia, convulsions associated with pregnancy, and prevention of hypomagnesemia in total parenteral nutrition. Therapeutic effects in these conditions are attributed to the drug's depressant effects on the central nervous system and smooth, skeletal, and cardiac muscle. Oral magnesium salts may cause diarrhea; their uses as antacids and cathartics are discussed in Chapters 59 and 60, respectively.

Magnesium preparations are contraindicated in patients who have impaired renal function or who are comatose. Oral preparations of magnesium oxide or hydroxide act in 3 to 6 hours, are minimally absorbed systemically, and are excreted in urine. With parenteral magnesium sulfate, IM injections act in 1 hour and last 3 to 4 hours; IV administration produces immediate action that lasts about 30 minutes. The products are excreted in urine.

Potassium Preparation

Potassium chloride (KCl) is usually the drug of choice for preventing or treating hypokalemia because deficiencies of potassium and chloride often occur together. It may be prescribed for patients who are receiving potassium-losing diuretics (e.g., hydrochlorothiazide, furosemide), those who are receiving digoxin (hypokalemia increases risk of digoxin toxicity), and those who are receiving only IV fluids because of surgical procedures, GI disease, or other conditions. KCl also may be used to replace chloride in hypochloremic metabolic alkalosis

It is contraindicated in patients with renal failure and in those receiving potassium-saving diuretics, such as triamterene, spironolactone, or amiloride.

KCl can be given orally or IV; *dosage must be individualized according to serum potassium levels.* Oral preparations are available in flavored powders, liquids, effervescent tablets, and controlled- or extended-release tablets. These preparations act slowly and peak in 1 to 2 hours. IV preparations act rapidly; IV KCl **must** be well diluted (usually 20 mEq in 1 L of IV fluid)

and infused slowly (usually at a maximum rate of 10 mEq/h) to prevent hyperkalemia, cardiotoxicity, and severe pain at the injection site. With severe hypokalemia (e.g., serum potassium level below 2 mEq/L), a higher concentration and a faster infusion rate may be used with continuous monitoring of the electrocardiogram and frequent measurements of serum potassium levels.

Zinc Preparations

Zinc sulfate and **zinc gluconate** are available over-the-counter in various forms and strengths (e.g., tablets with 110 mg and capsules with 220 mg of zinc sulfate, equivalent to 25 or 50 mg of elemental zinc). Zinc is also an ingredient in several vitamin–mineral combination products. Zinc preparations are given orally as a dietary supplement to prevent or treat zinc deficiency. They have a slow onset of action and a delayed peak. They are metabolized in the liver and excreted in feces.

Multiple Mineral–Electrolyte Preparations

There are numerous electrolyte solutions for IV use to maintain or replace electrolytes when the patient is unable to eat and drink.

Oral electrolyte solutions (e.g., Pedialyte) contain several electrolytes and a small amount of dextrose. They are used to supply maintenance amounts of fluids and electrolytes when oral intake is restricted. They are especially useful in children for treatment of diarrhea and may prevent severe fluid and electrolyte depletion. The amount given must be carefully calculated, prescribed, and administered to avoid excessive intake. Oral solutions should not be used in severe circumstances in which IV fluid and electrolyte therapy is indicated, and they should not be mixed with other electrolyte-containing fluids, such as milk or fruit juices. In addition, they must be cautiously used in impaired renal function.

Nursing Process

Assessment

Assess each patient for current or potential nutritional deficiencies. Some specific assessment factors include the following:

- What are usual eating patterns?
- Does the patient appear underweight? If so, assess for contributing factors (e.g., appetite; ability to obtain, cook, or chew food). Calculate or estimate the body mass index (BMI); a BMI under 18.5 kg/m^2 indicates undernutrition.
- Does the patient have symptoms, disease processes, treatments, medications, or diagnostic tests that are likely to interfere with nutrition? For example, many illnesses and oral medications cause anorexia, nausea, vomiting, and diarrhea.

With vitamins, assessment factors include the following:

- Deficiency states are more common than excess states and people with other nutritional deficiencies are likely to have vitamin deficiencies as well.
- Deficiencies of water-soluble vitamins (B complex and C) are more common than those of fat-soluble vitamins.
- Vitamin deficiencies are usually multiple and signs and symptoms often overlap, especially with B-complex deficiencies.
- Vitamin requirements are increased during infancy, pregnancy, lactation, fever, hyperthyroidism, and many illnesses. Thus, a vitamin intake that is normally adequate may be inadequate in certain circumstances.
- Vitamin deficiencies are likely to occur in people who are poor, elderly, chronically or severely ill, or alcoholic.
- Vitamin excess states are rarely caused by excessive dietary intake but may occur with use of vitamin drug preparations, especially if megadoses are taken.

With mineral–electrolytes, assessment factors include the following:

- Deficiency states are more common than excess states unless a mineral–electrolyte supplement is being taken. However, deficiencies and excesses may be equally harmful, and both must be assessed.
- Patients with other nutritional deficiencies are likely to have mineral–electrolyte deficiencies as well. Moreover, deficiencies are likely to be multiple, with overlapping signs and symptoms.
- Many drugs influence gains and losses of minerals and electrolytes, including diuretics and laxatives.
- Minerals and electrolytes are lost with gastric suction, polyuria, diarrhea, excessive perspiration, and other conditions.

Assess laboratory reports when available:

- Check the complete blood count for decreased red blood cells, hemoglobin, and hematocrit. Reduced values may indicate iron deficiency anemia, and further assessment is needed.
- Check serum electrolyte reports for abnormal values. All major minerals can be measured in clinical laboratories. The ones usually measured are sodium, chloride, and potassium; carbon dioxide content, a measure of bicarbonate, is also assessed.

Nursing Diagnoses

- Imbalanced Nutrition: Less Than Body Requirements related to inadequate intake or impaired ability to digest nutrients
- Imbalanced Nutrition: More Than Body Requirements related to excessive intake of pharmaceutical preparations of vitamins and minerals

- Risk for Injury related to complications of tube or IV feedings
- Risk for Injury related to nutrient deficiency or overdose
- Deficient Knowledge: Nutritional needs and sources of nutrients

Planning/Goals

The patient will

- Improve nutritional status in relation to body needs
- Maintain fluid and electrolyte balance
- Ingest appropriate amounts of vitamins and mineral–electrolytes
- Avoid complications of enteral nutrition, including aspiration, diarrhea, and infection
- Avoid complications of parenteral nutrition
- Avoid overdoses and adverse effects of vitamins and minerals
- Avoid mineral–electrolyte supplements unless recommended by a health care provider
- Take mineral–electrolyte drugs as prescribed and have appropriate laboratory tests to monitor response

Interventions

- Promote a well-balanced diet for all patients. Five daily servings of fruits and vegetables provide adequate vitamins unless the patient has increased requirements or conditions that interfere with absorption or use of vitamins. An oral multivitamin may benefit most people, but it is not a substitute for an adequate diet. A diet that is adequate in protein and calories usually provides adequate minerals and electrolytes. Exceptions are calcium and iron, which are often needed as a dietary supplement in women and children.
- Treat symptoms or disorders that are likely to interfere with nutrition, such as pain, nausea, vomiting, or diarrhea.
- For patients who need increased protein-calorie intake, provide palatable supplements at appropriate times and encourage patients to take them.
- Promote exercise and activity. For undernourished patients, this may increase appetite, improve digestion, and aid bowel elimination.
- Minimize the use of sedative-type drugs when appropriate. Although no one should be denied pain relief, strong analgesics and other sedatives may cause drowsiness and decreased desire or ability to eat and drink as well as constipation and a feeling of fullness.
- Weigh patients at regular intervals. Calculate or estimate BMI when indicated.
- For patients receiving parenteral nutrition, monitor weight, fluid intake, urine output, vital signs, blood glucose, serum electrolytes, and complete blood count daily or weekly, according to the patient's status and whether he or she is hospitalized or at home.

Nursing Process continues on page 920

■ Mineral supplements are recommended only for current or potential deficiencies because all are toxic in excessive amounts.

■ For patients who have nasogastric tubes to suction, irrigate the tubes with isotonic sodium chloride solution. The use of tap water is contraindicated because it is hypotonic and would pull electrolytes into the stomach. Electrolytes are then lost in the aspirated and discarded stomach contents. For the same reason, only small amounts of ice chips or water are allowed per hour. Patients often request ice chips or water in larger amounts than desirable; the nurse must explain the reason for the restrictions.

Evaluation

■ Observe undernourished patients for quantity and quality of nutrient intake, weight gain, and improvement in laboratory tests of nutritional status (e.g., serum proteins, blood sugar, electrolytes).

■ Observe children for quantity and quality of food intake and appropriate increases in height and weight.

■ Interview and observe for signs and symptoms of complications of enteral and parenteral nutrition.

Principles of Therapy

Managing Nutritional Deficiencies

When possible, oral administration of liquid formulas, vitamins, and minerals is preferred. With vitamin and mineral supplements, larger doses are needed to treat deficiencies than are needed to prevent them. Treatment of deficiency states should be cautious, to avoid excess states.

Enteral Nutrition: Oral and Tube Feedings

When the GI tract is functional but the patient cannot ingest enough food and fluid, high-protein, high-calorie foods (e.g., milkshakes) or nutritionally complete supplements (e.g., Ensure) can be given with meals, between meals, and at bedtime. When oral feeding is contraindicated, tube feeding helps to maintain GI tract and immune system functioning. Guidelines for tube feedings include the following:

■ Several tubes and placement sites are available. For short-term use (about 4 weeks), a nasogastric tube may be used. For long-term feedings, a gastrostomy or jejunostomy tube may be inserted. Percutaneous endoscopic gastrostomy (PEG) tubes are often used. Nasointestinal tubes are recommended for patients at risk of aspiration from gastric feedings or with gastric disorders. Except for gastrostomy tubes, the tubes should be soft and small bore to decrease trauma.

■ When tube feedings are the patient's only source of nutrients, the feedings should be nutritionally complete and given in amounts calculated to provide adequate water, protein, calories, vitamins, and minerals.

■ For feedings that enter the stomach, intermittent administration is often used. For feedings that enter the duodenum or jejunum, a continuous drip method is required because the small bowel cannot tolerate the larger volumes of intermittent feedings. Continuous feedings require an infusion pump for accurate control of the flow rate. Water can be given with, after, or between regular feedings and with medications, according to the patient's fluid needs.

■ A potential complication of tube feeding is aspiration of the formula into the lungs. This is more likely to occur with unconscious patients. It can be prevented by correctly positioning patients, verifying tube placement, and giving feedings slowly.

 Patient Teaching Guidelines | **Nutritional Support Products, Vitamins, and Minerals**

General Considerations

■ Nutrition is extremely important in promoting health and recovery from illness. For people who are unable to take in enough nutrients because of poor appetite or illness, nutritional supplements can be very beneficial in improving nutritional status. For example, supplemental feedings can slow or stop weight loss; increase energy and feelings of well-being; and increase resistance to infection.

■ With oral or tube-feeding supplements, choose one or more that the patient is able and willing to take when possible.

■ With vitamins, supplements are often recommended because studies indicate that many adults and children do not ingest sufficient dietary vitamins. Supplements are also usually needed by pregnant women and by people who smoke, ingest large amounts of alcohol, have

impaired immune systems, or are elderly. When choosing a vitamin supplement, the following factors should be considered:

■ Avoid large doses of vitamins. They will not promote health, strength, or youth. In addition, excessive amounts of B vitamins and vitamin C are eliminated in urine and some can cause adverse effects (e.g., large doses of vitamin C can cause kidney stones; niacin [B_3] can cause stomach upset, flushing, skin rashes, itching, and aggravation of asthma and gout; pyridoxine [B_6] may cause numbness in limbs and difficulty in walking). Excessive amounts of vitamins A, D, E, and K are stored in the body and often lead to toxic effects. For example, high doses of vitamin A can result in headaches; diarrhea; nausea; loss of appetite; dry, itching skin; and elevated blood calcium. Excessive doses during pregnancy may cause birth defects.

- Although natural vitamins are advertised as being better than synthetic vitamins, there is no evidence to support this claim. The two types are chemically identical and used in the same way by the human body. Natural vitamins are more expensive.
- Sexually active women of childbearing potential need an adequate intake of folic acid to prevent severe birth defects in infants. To help prevent birth defects from folic acid deficiency, the Food and Drug Administration requires that folic acid be added to breads and cereal-grain products. This is estimated to add about 100 mcg of folic acid to the daily diet of most people. However, the recommended daily intake for adults is 400 mcg.
- Vitamins from supplements exert the same physiologic effects as those obtained from foods.
- Multivitamin preparations often contain minerals as well, usually in smaller amounts than those recommended for daily intake. Large doses of minerals are toxic.
- With minerals, a well-balanced diet contains all the minerals needed for health in most people. Exceptions are calcium and iron, which are often needed as a dietary supplement in women and children. Note that herbal preparations of chamomile, feverfew, and St. John's wort may inhibit iron absorption. The safest action is to take mineral supplements only on a health care provider's advice, in the amounts and for the length of time prescribed. All minerals are toxic when taken in excess. Additional considerations include:
  - Keep all mineral–electrolyte substances out of reach of children to prevent accidental overdose. Acute iron intoxication is a common problem among young children and can be fatal. Also, supervise children in using fluoride supplements (e.g., remind them to spit out oral rinses and gels rather than swallow them).
  - Keep appointments with health care providers for periodic blood tests and other follow-up procedures when mineral–electrolyte supplements are prescribed (e.g., potassium chloride). This helps prevent ingestion of excessive amounts.
  - Minerals are often contained in multivitamin preparations, with percentages of the recommended dietary allowances supplied. These amounts differ in various preparations and should be included in estimations of daily intake.

Self- or Caregiver Administration

- For oral supplemental feedings, take or give at the preferred time and temperature, when possible.
- For tube feedings:
  - Use or give with the patient in a sitting position, if possible, to decrease risks of strangling and pulling formula into the lungs.
  - Be sure the tube is placed correctly before each feeding. Ask a health care provider how to check placement with your type of tube.
  - Be sure the solution is room temperature. Cold formulas may cause abdominal cramping.
  - Do not take or give more than 1 pint (500 mL) per feeding, including 2 to 3 oz of water for rinsing the tube. This helps to avoid overfilling the stomach and possible vomiting.

- Take or give slowly, over approximately 30 to 60 minutes. Rapid administration may cause nausea and vomiting.
- With continuous feedings, change containers and tubing daily. With intermittent feedings, rinse all equipment after each use, and change at least every 24 hours. Most tube-feeding formulas are milk based and infection may occur if formulas become contaminated or equipment is not kept clean.
- Ask a health care provider about the amount of water to take or give. Most people receiving 1.5 to 2 quarts (1500–2000 mL) of tube feeding daily need approximately 1 quart (1000 mL) or more of water daily. However, patients' needs vary. Water can be mixed with the tube feeding formula, given after the tube feeding, or given between feedings. Be sure to include the amount of water used for rinsing the tube in the total daily amount.
- For giving medications by tube:
  - Give liquid preparations when available. When not available, some tablets may be crushed and some capsules may be emptied and mixed with 1 to 2 tablespoons of water. Ask a health care provider which medications can safely be crushed or altered, because some (e.g., long-acting or enteric-coated) can be harmful if crushed.
  - Do not mix medications with the tube-feeding formula because some medications may not be absorbed.
  - Do not mix medications; give each one separately.
  - Rinse the tube with water before and after each medication to get the medication through the tube and to keep the tube open.
- With supplementary vitamins, preparations differ widely in amounts and types of vitamin content. The product should not contain more than recommended amounts of vitamin D and vitamin A because of possible adverse effects.
- When choosing a vitamin supplement, compare ingredients and costs. Store brands are usually effective and less expensive than name brands.
- Vitamin C supplements are available in tablet and powder forms of various dosages, often in multivitamin and other preparations sold as antioxidants. In 2000, the recommended dietary allowance was increased from 60 mg daily to 75 mg for adult women and 90 mg for adult men. Large doses (e.g., 1000 mg or more daily) may cause adverse effects and should be avoided. An adequate amount of vitamin C can also be obtained by eating at least five servings of fruit and vegetables daily.
- Take oral niacin preparations, except for timed-release forms, with or after meals or at bedtime to decrease stomach irritation. In addition, sit or lie down for approximately 30 minutes after taking a dose. Niacin causes blood vessels to dilate and may cause facial flushing, dizziness, and falls. Facial flushing can be decreased by taking 325 mg of aspirin 30 to 60 minutes before a dose of niacin. Itching, tingling, and headache may also occur. These effects usually subside with continued use of niacin.
- Swallow extended-release products whole; do not break, crush, or chew them. Breaking the product delivers the entire dose at once and may cause adverse effects.
- Take prescribed vitamins as directed and for the appropriate time. In pernicious anemia, vitamin B_{12} injections

(continued on page 922)

Patient Teaching Guidelines | Nutritional Support Products, Vitamins, and Minerals (continued)

must be taken for the remainder of life. In pregnancy and lactation, vitamin supplements are usually taken only during this period of increased need.

- Take iron preparations with or after meals, with approximately 8 oz of fluid, to prevent stomach upset. Do not take iron with coffee or other caffeine-containing beverages, because caffeine decreases absorption (take iron and caffeine preparations at least 2 hours apart). Do not crush or chew slow-release tablets or capsules. With liquid preparations, dilute with water, drink through a straw, and rinse the mouth afterward to avoid staining the teeth. Expect that stools will be dark green or black.

- With potassium preparations, mix oral solutions or effervescent tablets with at least 4 oz of water or juice

to improve the taste, dilute the drug, and decrease gastric irritation. Do not crush or chew slow-release preparations. Take after meals initially to decrease gastric irritation. If no nausea, vomiting, or other problems occur, the drug can be tried before meals because it is better absorbed from an empty stomach. Do *not* stop taking the medication without notifying the health care provider who prescribed it, especially if also taking digoxin or diuretics. Excessive amounts should also be avoided. Do not use salt substitutes unless they are recommended by a health care provider; they contain potassium chloride and may result in excessive intake. Serious problems may develop from either high or low levels of potassium in the blood.

Parenteral Nutrition: IV Feedings

Parenteral feedings are indicated when the GI tract is non-functional, when nutritional needs cannot be met by enteral feedings, or when enteral feedings would aggravate conditions such as inflammatory bowel diseases or pancreatitis.

Short-Term IV Nutrition

For short-term use (e.g., 3–5 days), the goal is to provide adequate amounts of fluids and electrolytes and enough carbohydrate to minimize oxidation of body protein and fat for energy. The choice of specific solution depends on individual needs, but it should contain at least 5% dextrose. A frequently used solution is 5% dextrose in 0.22% sodium chloride, 2000 to 3000 mL in 24 hours (provides approximately 170 kcal/L, water, sodium, and chloride). KCl is often added, and vitamins may be added. These solutions are nutritionally inadequate.

Long-Term IV Nutrition

For long-term use (weeks to months), the goal is to provide all nutrients required for normal body functioning, including tissue repair. Basic solutions provide water, carbohydrate, protein, vitamins, and minerals; fat emulsions (e.g., Intralipid) are usually given separately to provide additional calories and essential fatty acids (500 mL of 10% emulsion provides 550 kcal). Guidelines include the following:

- Parenteral nutritional solutions can be administered through central or peripheral IV lines. Some solutions are hypertonic (from high concentrations of glucose) and must be given in a central vein so they can be diluted rapidly. Solutions that contain 5% or 10% dextrose are less hypertonic and can be given in a peripheral vein. However, they are nutritionally incomplete and used for a limited time (about 5–7 days).

- Fat emulsions are isotonic and may be given centrally or peripherally. When given peripherally, they are coinfused with dextrose–protein solution to help protect the vein from phlebitis.

- Dextrose–protein solutions are given through an in-line filter. Fat emulsions should not be filtered; they are "piggy-backed" into the IV line beyond the filter.

- Solutions should be administered with an infusion pump to maintain a steady and accurate flow rate.

- Sterile technique should be used in all aspects of preparation, administration, and site care. Most agencies have specific protocols for changing solution containers, administration sets, and dressings at the venipuncture site.

Managing Vitamin Disorders

Early recognition and treatment of vitamin disorders can prevent a mild deficiency or excess from becoming severe. For deficiency states, oral vitamin preparations are preferred when possible. Multiple deficiencies are common, and a multivitamin preparation used to treat them usually contains more than the recommended daily amount. These products should be used for limited periods. When fat-soluble vitamins are given to correct a deficiency, there is a risk of producing excess states. When water-soluble vitamins are given, excesses are less likely but may occur with large doses. For excess states, the usual treatment is to stop administration of the vitamin preparation. There are no specific antidotes or antagonists.

Vitamin A Disorders

With vitamin A deficiency, assist patients to increase intake of foods containing preformed vitamin A (e.g., meat, egg yolk, whole milk) or beta carotene (e.g., yellow fruits and vegetables such as cantaloupe, peaches, carrots, sweet potatoes) when feasible. If a supplement is required, vitamin A alone may be preferred over a multivitamin unless multiple deficiencies are present. Daily doses should not exceed 25,000 international units (approximately 7500 mcg RE; 1 mcg RE = 3.3 IU) daily unless a severe deficiency is present.

Vitamin A may be given IM if GI absorption is severely impaired or ocular symptoms are severe. With vitamin A excess, immediately stop known sources of the vitamin.

Vitamin K Disorders

With vitamin K deficiency, bleeding may occur spontaneously or in response to trauma. Thus, administration of vitamin K and measures to prevent bleeding are indicated. If the deficiency is not severe, oral vitamin K may be given for a few days until serum prothrombin activity returns to a normal range. In obstructive jaundice, bile salts must be given at the same time as oral vitamin K, or vitamin K must be given parenterally. In malabsorption syndromes or diarrhea, parenteral administration is probably necessary. A single dose of vitamin K may be sufficient.

There is a **BLACK BOX WARNING** that IV administration of vitamin K may result in an anaphylactic type of reaction with risks of shock, cardiorespiratory arrest, and death, even with drug dilution and slow administration. Therefore, the IV route should be used only if other routes cannot be used and the drug is deemed necessary. With severe bleeding, transfusions of plasma or whole blood may be preferred over IV vitamin K.

B-Complex Disorders

With B-complex vitamins, most deficiencies are multiple rather than single and treatment consists of increasing intake of foods containing B-complex vitamins (many foods, including meat, vegetables, and cereal grains) or giving multivitamin preparations. If a single deficiency seems predominant, that vitamin may be given alone or in addition to a multivitamin preparation. For example, folic acid deficiency may occur with inadequate dietary intake and intestinal disorders that inhibit absorption. In addition, folic acid is depleted by alcohol and several medications, including antibiotics containing trimethoprim (e.g., Bactrim), phenytoin, methotrexate, and oral contraceptives. Thiamine deficiency is common in alcoholics because of inadequate dietary intake and the use of large amounts of thiamine to metabolize ethanol.

Anemias Associated With B-Complex Vitamin Deficiencies

One type of anemia occurs with pyridoxine deficiency and is relieved by administration of pyridoxine. Another type, called *megaloblastic anemia* (because it is characterized by abnormally large, immature red blood cells), occurs with deficiency of folic acid or vitamin B_{12}. If megaloblastic anemia is severe, treatment is usually instituted with both folic acid and vitamin B_{12}.

In pernicious anemia, vitamin B_{12} must be given by injection because oral forms are not absorbed from the GI tract. The injections must be continued for life. Vitamin B_{12} is also given to prevent pernicious anemia in patients who are strict vegetarians, who have had gastrectomy, or who have chronic small bowel disease. Although folic acid relieves hematologic disorders of pernicious anemia, giving folic acid alone allows continued neurologic deterioration. Thus, an accurate diagnosis is required.

In other megaloblastic anemias, vitamin B_{12} or folic acid is indicated. Although both of these are included in many mul-

tivitamin preparations, they usually must be given separately for therapeutic purposes. With vitamin B_{12}, doses in excess of 100 micrograms are rapidly excreted in urine. With folic acid, doses in excess of 1 milligram are excreted in the urine.

Vitamin C Disorders

Treatment of vitamin C deficiency involves increased intake of vitamin C from dietary (e.g., fruits and vegetables) or pharmaceutical sources. Vitamin C is available alone for oral, IM, or IV administration. It is also an ingredient in most multivitamin preparations for oral or parenteral use.

In 2000, the DRI for vitamin C was increased from 60 milligrams daily to 75 milligrams for most adult women and 90 milligrams for most adult men. Some nutritionists recommend 120 milligrams per day; others recommend approximately 200 milligrams per day from five servings of fruits and vegetables or 100 milligrams per day of a vitamin C supplement. An additional recommendation is to avoid large doses (i.e., more than 1 g/day). With excessive intake of vitamin C supplements, the main concern is formation of calcium oxalate kidney stones and potential obstruction or other renal damage. There is no known benefit of such large amounts, and their use should be discouraged.

Managing Mineral–Electrolyte Disorders

When a mineral is given to correct a deficiency state, there is a risk of producing an excess state. Because both deficiencies and excesses may be harmful, the amount of mineral supplement should be titrated closely to the amount needed by the body. Larger doses are needed to treat deficiency states than are needed to prevent deficiencies from developing. When mineral–electrolyte drug preparations are needed, oral products are preferred when possible. They are safer, less likely to produce toxicity, more convenient to administer, and less expensive than parenteral preparations.

Potassium Disorders

Hypokalemia

- Assess for conditions contributing to *hypokalemia*, and attempt to eliminate them or reduce their impact.

- Assess severity by checking serum potassium levels and clinical manifestations. Serum potassium levels alone are inadequate because they may not accurately reflect depletion of body potassium or shifts of potassium into cells.

- In general, potassium supplements are indicated when serum potassium is below 3 milliequivalents per liter, when symptoms or electrocardiographic (ECG) changes indicate hypokalemia, and when patients are receiving digoxin, if necessary to maintain serum potassium above 3.5 milliequivalents per liter.

- KCl is the drug of choice in most instances. Controlled-release tablets or capsules with KCl in a wax matrix or microencapsulated form are preferred over liquids by most patients.

■ IV KCl is indicated when a patient cannot take an oral preparation or has severe hypokalemia. The serum potassium level should be measured and adequate urine output established before IV potassium therapy is started.

■ IV KCl must be well diluted to prevent sudden hyperkalemia, cardiotoxic effects, and phlebitis at the venipuncture site. The usual dilution is KCl 20 to 40 milliequivalents per 1000 milliliters of IV fluid.

■ Dosage must be individualized. Patients receiving IV fluids only are usually given 40 to 60 milliequivalents of KCl daily (e.g., 20 mEq KCl per 1000 mL of fluids at a flow rate of 100 to 125 mL/h). An infusion pump should be used to control flow rate accurately. Also, serum potassium levels must be checked frequently and dosage adjusted if indicated.

Hyperkalemia

■ Eliminate any exogenous sources of potassium, such as potassium supplements, penicillin G potassium, salt substitutes, and blood transfusion with old blood.

■ Treat acidosis, if present, because potassium leaves cells and enters the serum with acidosis.

■ Use measures that antagonize the effects of potassium, that cause potassium to leave the serum and re-enter cells, and that remove potassium from the body. Appropriate measures are determined mainly by serum potassium levels and ECG changes. Continuous cardiac monitoring is required. If the following measures fail to reduce hyperkalemia, peritoneal dialysis or hemodialysis may be used.
With severe *hyperkalemia* (serum potassium above 7 mEq/L and ECG changes indicating hyperkalemia), urgent treatment is required. IV **sodium bicarbonate** 45 milliequivalents, over a 5-minute period, causes rapid movement of potassium into cells. This can be repeated in a few minutes if ECG changes persist. **Calcium gluconate** 10%, 5 to 10 milliliters IV, is also given early in treatment to decrease the cardiotoxic effects of hyperkalemia. It is contraindicated if the patient is receiving digoxin, and it cannot be added to fluids containing sodium bicarbonate because insoluble precipitates are formed. IV **glucose and insulin** may also be infused. This causes potassium to move into cells, though not as quickly as administration of sodium bicarbonate.

With less severe hyperkalemia (or when serum potassium levels have been reduced by other measures), **sodium polystyrene sulfonate**, a cation exchange resin, can be given orally or rectally to remove potassium from the body. Each gram of the resin combines with 1 milliequivalent of potassium, and both are excreted in feces. The resin is usually mixed with water and sorbitol, a poorly absorbed, osmotically active alcohol that has a laxative effect. The sorbitol offsets the constipating effect of the resin and aids in its expulsion. Oral administration is preferred, and several doses daily may be given until serum potassium is normal. When given as an enema, the solution must be retained from 1 to several hours, or repeated enemas must be given for therapeutic effect.

Magnesium Disorders
Hypomagnesemia

For mild hypomagnesemia, oral magnesium preparations may be given. For moderate to severe and symptomatic hypomagnesemia, parenteral (IV or IM) magnesium sulfate may be given daily as long as hypomagnesemia persists or continuing losses occur. Initial dosage may be larger, but the usual maintenance dose is approximately 8 milliequivalents daily. A 10% solution is available in 10-milliliter vials that contain 8 milliequivalents of magnesium sulfate for adding to IV solutions. A 50% solution is available in 2-milliliter vials (8 mEq) for IM administration. Serum magnesium levels should be measured daily during treatment with a magnesium preparation.

Hypermagnesemia

■ Stop any source of exogenous magnesium, such as magnesium sulfate or magnesium-containing antacids and cathartics.

■ Have calcium gluconate available for IV administration. It is an antidote for the sedative effects of magnesium excess.

■ Increase urine output by increasing fluid intake, if feasible. This increases removal of magnesium from the body in urine.

■ Patients with chronic renal failure are the most likely to become hypermagnesemic. They may require peritoneal dialysis or hemodialysis to lower serum magnesium levels.

Iron Deficiency and Excess
Iron Deficiency Anemia

■ Anemia is a symptom, not a disease. Therefore, the underlying cause must be identified and eliminated, if possible.

■ Encourage increased dietary intake of foods with high iron content.

■ Ferrous sulfate is usually the drug of choice for oral iron therapy. Slow-release or enteric-coated products decrease absorption of iron but may cause less gastric irritation.

■ Dosage is calculated in terms of elemental iron. Iron preparations vary in the amount of elemental iron they contain. Ferrous sulfate, for example, contains 20% iron; thus, each 325-milligram tablet furnishes about 65 milligrams of elemental iron. With the usual regimen of one tablet three times daily, a daily dose of 195 milligrams of elemental iron is given. For most patients, probably half that amount would correct the deficiency. However, tablets are not manufactured in sizes to allow this regimen, and liquid preparations are not popular with patients. Thus, large doses are usually given, but smaller doses may be effective, especially if GI symptoms become a problem with higher dosages. Whatever the dose, only about 10% to 15% of the iron is absorbed. Most of the remainder is excreted in feces, which turn dark green or black.

■ Oral iron preparations are better absorbed if taken on an empty stomach. However, because gastric irritation is a common adverse reaction, they are more often given with or immediately after meals.

▪ Although normal hemoglobin levels return after approximately 2 months of oral iron therapy, an additional 6-month period of drug therapy is recommended to replenish the body's iron stores.

▪ Reasons for failure to respond to iron therapy include continued blood loss, failure to take the drug as prescribed, or defective iron absorption. These factors must be re-evaluated if no therapeutic response is evident within 3 to 4 weeks after drug therapy is begun.

▪ Parenteral iron is indicated when oral preparations may further irritate a diseased GI tract, when the patient is unable or unwilling to take the oral drugs, or when the anemia must be corrected rapidly.

▪ For severe iron deficiency anemia, blood transfusions may be most effective.

Iron Excess

Acute iron overdosage requires treatment as soon as possible, even if overdosage is only suspected and the amount taken is unknown. It is unnecessary to wait until the serum iron level is measured.

If treatment is begun shortly after oral ingestion of iron, aspiration of stomach contents by nasogastric tube or whole bowel irrigation with a polyethylene glycol solution (e.g., CoLyte) may be performed. Gastric lavage can be followed by instillation of 1% sodium bicarbonate solution, to form insoluble iron carbonate compounds, or 5 to 8 grams of deferoxamine (Desferal) dissolved in 50 milliliters of distilled water, to bind the iron remaining in the GI tract and prevent its absorption. Deferoxamine may also be given IM or IV to bind with iron in tissues and allow its excretion in the urine. Throughout the treatment period, supportive measures may be needed for GI hemorrhage, acidosis, and shock.

For chronic iron overload or hemochromatosis, the first step in treatment is to stop the source of iron, if possible. Phlebotomy is the treatment of choice for most patients because withdrawal of 500 milliliters of blood removes about 250 milligrams of iron. Phlebotomy may be needed as often as weekly and for as long as 2 to 3 years. For patients resistant to or intolerant of phlebotomy, deferoxamine can be given. Ten to 50 milligrams of iron are excreted daily in the urine with deferoxamine administration.

Effects of Vitamins and Minerals on Other Drugs

Folic acid decreases effects of phenytoin and may decrease absorption and effects of zinc. Niacin may increase the risk of rhabdomyolysis (a life-threatening breakdown of skeletal muscle) with statin cholesterol-lowering drugs (e.g., atorvastatin [Lipitor]). Vitamin A in large doses and vitamin E may increase the anticoagulant effect of warfarin. Vitamin C, 1000 milligrams daily or more, may decrease metabolism and increase the effects of estrogens and oral contraceptives.

Iron salts may decrease absorption of levodopa, levothyroxine, methyldopa, penicillamine, fluoroquinolones, and tetracyclines. Magnesium salts may decrease absorption and therapeutic effects of digoxin, fluoroquinolones, nitrofurantoin, penicillamine, and tetracyclines. Zinc salts may decrease absorption of fluoroquinolones and most tetracyclines (doxycycline is apparently not affected).

Use in Special Populations

Nutritional Support in Children

Children usually need sufficient water, protein, carbohydrate, and fat in proportion to their size to support growth and increased physical activity. However, reports of childhood obesity and inadequate exercise are steadily increasing. Therefore, the goal of nutritional support is to meet needs without promoting obesity.

For children with special needs in relation to nutrients, various enteral formulations are available for use. Some examples include Lofenalac for children with phenylketonuria (a disorder in which the amino acid phenylalanine cannot be metabolized normally); Nursoy and Soyalac, which contain soy protein, for children who are allergic to cow's milk; and Nutramigen and Pregestimil, which contain easily-digested nutrients for children with *malabsorption* or other GI problems.

With tube feedings, to prevent nausea and regurgitation, the recommended rate of administration is no more than 5 milliliters every 5 to 10 minutes for premature and small infants and 10 milliliters per minute for older infants and children. Preparation of formulas, positioning of children, and administration are the same as for adults to prevent aspiration and infection.

Parenteral nutrition may be indicated in infants and children who cannot eat or be fed enterally (e.g., during medical illnesses or perioperative states) to improve or maintain nutritional status. Overall, benefits include weight gain, increased height, increased liver synthesis of plasma proteins, and improved healing and recovery.

With **vitamins,** children need sufficient amounts to support growth and normal body functioning. If supplements are given, considerations include the following:

▪ Dosages should not exceed recommended amounts. There is a risk of overdosage by children and their parents. Because of manufacturers' marketing strategies, many supplements are available in flavors and shapes (e.g., animals, cartoon characters) designed to appeal to children. Because younger children may think of these supplements as candy and take more than recommended, they should be stored out of reach and dispensed by an adult. Because parents' desires to promote health may lead them to give unneeded supplements or to give more than recommended amounts, parents may need information about the potential hazards of vitamin overdoses.

▪ The content of supplements for infants and children younger than 4 years of age is regulated by the FDA; the content of preparations for older children is not regulated.

▪ Supplements given to children and adolescents should provide recommended amounts of vitamins. Except for single supplements of vitamin K and vitamin E in infants, multivitamin products are commonly used. For infants, liquid formulations usually include vitamins A, D, C, and B complex. Folic acid is not included because it is unstable in liquid form. For older children, chewable tablets usually contain vitamins A, D, C, and B complex, including folic acid.

■ A single IM dose of vitamin K is given to newborn infants to prevent hemorrhagic disease of newborns.

■ Preterm infants need proportionately more vitamins than term infants because their growth rate is faster and their absorption of vitamins from the intestine is less complete. A multivitamin product containing the equivalent of DRIs for term infants is recommended.

■ ULs have been established for some vitamins, and **these maximum daily amounts should not be exceeded.** For infants (birth to 12 months), the only UL is for vitamin D (25 mcg). For other children, ULs vary according to age, as listed in Table 57-5.

With **mineral–electrolytes,** children need sufficient amounts to support growth and normal body functioning. However, iron deficiency is common in young children and adolescent girls, and an iron supplement is often needed. Guidelines include the following:

■ A combined vitamin–mineral supplement every other day may be reasonable, especially for children who eat poorly.

■ If supplements are given, dosages should be discussed with a health care provider and usually should not exceed recommended amounts for particular age groups. ULs for children have been established for some minerals, and **these maximum daily amounts should not be exceeded.** They are listed in Table 57-6. The ULs for magnesium indicate maximum intake from pharmaceutical preparations; they do not include intake from food and water.

■ All minerals and electrolytes are toxic in overdose and may cause life-threatening adverse effects. All such drugs should be kept out of reach of young children and should never be referred to as "candy."

■ In areas where water is not fluoridated, a vitamin–mineral supplement containing fluoride may be indicated for infants and children. Many preparations of fluoride supplements are available for oral (tablets, chewable tablets, solutions) or topical (liquid rinse solutions or gels) use. Before using a pharmaceutical supplement, though, most dental professionals recommend that a patient's water supply be tested for fluoride. With numerous sources of fluoride available (e.g., infant formula, fruit juice, toothpaste, municipal water supplies, and supplements), however, children must also be guarded against excessive fluoride ingestion. To prevent excessive intake, all sources of fluoride should be considered, supplements used by children or adults should be kept out of the reach of children, supplements prescribed for children should be used only with adult supervision, and children using topical preparations should be reminded to spit them out and not to swallow them.

■ If KCl and other electrolyte preparations are used to treat deficiency states in children, serum electrolyte levels must be monitored. In addition, doses must be carefully measured and given no more often than prescribed to avoid toxicity.

■ Accidental ingestion of iron-containing medications and dietary supplements is a common cause of poisoning death in children younger than 6 years of age. To help prevent poisoning, products containing iron must be labeled with a warning and products with 30 milligrams or more of iron (e.g., prenatal products) must be packaged as individual doses. All iron-containing preparations should be stored in places that are inaccessible to young children.

Nutritional Support in Older Adults

Older adults are at risk of under nutrition with all nutrients. Inadequate intake may result from the inability to obtain and prepare food, disease processes that interfere with the ability to digest and use nutrients, and the use of drugs that decrease absorption of nutrients. When alternative feeding methods (tube feedings, IV fluids) are used, careful assessment of nutritional status is required to avoid deficits or excesses. With the high incidence of atherosclerosis, cardiovascular disease, and

Table 57-5	Vitamins: Tolerable Upper Intake Levels for Children			
VITAMIN	**1–3 YEARS**	**4–8 YEARS**	**9–13 YEARS**	**14–18 YEARS**
D	50 mg	50 mg	50 mg	50 mg
E	200 mg	300 mg	600 mg	800 mg
C	400 mg	650 mg	1200 mg	1800 mg
Folate	300 mcg	400 mcg	600 mcg	800 mcg
Niacin	10 mg	15 mg	20 mg	30 mg
Pyridoxine	30 mg	40 mg	60 mg	80 mg

Table 57-6	Minerals: Tolerable Upper Intake Levels for Children					
MINERAL	**BIRTH–6 MONTHS**	**7–12 MONTHS**	**1–3 YEARS**	**4–8 YEARS**	**9–13 YEARS**	**14–18 YEARS**
Calcium	No data	No data	2.5 g	2.5 g	2.5 g	2.5 g
Phosphorus	No data	No data	3 g	3 g	4 g	4 g
Fluoride	0.7 mg	0.9 mg	1.3 mg	2.2 mg	10 mg	10 mg
Magnesium	No data	No data	65 mg	110 mg	350 mg	350 mg
Selenium	45 mcg	60 mcg	90 mcg	150 mcg	280 mcg	400 mcg

diabetes mellitus in older adults, it is especially important that intake of animal fats and high-calorie sweets be reduced.

Vitamin requirements are the same as for younger adults, but deficiencies are common, especially of vitamins A and D, cyanocobalamin (B_{12}), folic acid, riboflavin, and thiamine. With vitamin B_{12}, for example, it is estimated that older adults only absorb 10% to 30% of the amount found in food. Every older adult should be assessed regarding vitamin intake (from foods and supplements) and use of drugs that interact with dietary nutrients. For most older adults, a daily multivitamin is probably desirable, even for those who seem healthy and able to eat a well-balanced diet. In addition, requirements may be increased during illnesses, especially those affecting GI function. Overdoses, especially of the fat-soluble vitamins A and D, may cause toxicity and should be avoided. ULs for older adults have been established for some vitamins (D, 50 mg; E, 1000 mg; C, 2000 mg; folate, 1000 mcg; niacin, 35 mg; pyridoxine, 100 mg), and **these amounts should not be exceeded**.

Applying Your Knowledge 57-1

You recognize that along with being undernourished, Mrs. Farber is also most likely deficient in vitamins. You confer with the physician. What will be the likely recommendation for Mrs. Farber?

Mineral–electrolyte requirements are also the same as for younger adults, but deficiencies of calcium and iron are common. Excess states also may occur in older adults. For example, decreased renal function promotes retention of magnesium and potassium. Hyperkalemia also may occur with the use of potassium supplements or salt substitutes. All minerals and electrolytes are toxic in overdose. ULs for older adults (over 65 years of age) have been established for calcium (2.5 g), phosphorus (3–4 g), fluoride (10 mg), magnesium (350 mg), and selenium (400 mcg), and **these maximum daily amounts should not be exceeded**. In general, serum levels of minerals and electrolytes should be monitored carefully during illness and measures taken to prevent either deficiency or excess states.

Applying Your Knowledge 57-2

It is important to assess patients for individual risk factors related to gender, health status, and age. For Mrs. Farber, what particular mineral–electrolyte deficiencies would you consider/explore?

Nutritional Support in Patients With Renal Impairment

Patients with impaired renal function usually have multiple metabolic disorders such as hyperglycemia, accumulation of urea nitrogen (the end product of protein metabolism), and increased serum triglyceride levels from disordered fat metabolism. With *enteral nutrition*, Amin-Aid may be given to provide amino acids, carbohydrates, and a few electrolytes for patients with renal failure. With parenteral nutrition, several amino acid solutions are formulated for patients with renal failure (e.g., Aminosyn-RF). In addition, patients with acute renal failure (ARF) often have hyperkalemia, hyperphosphatemia, and hypermagnesemia, so that potassium, phosphorus, and magnesium should be omitted until serum levels return to normal. IV fat emulsions should not be given to patients with ARF if serum triglyceride levels exceed 300 milligrams per deciliter. With chronic renal failure (CRF), high-calorie, low-electrolyte enteral formulations are usually indicated. Nepro is a formulation for patients receiving dialysis; Suplena, which is lower in protein and some electrolytes than Nepro, may be used in patients who are not receiving dialysis. Serum triglyceride levels should be measured before IV fat emulsions are given. Many patients with CRF have hypertriglyceridemia, which is worsened by fat emulsions and may cause pancreatitis.

With vitamins, patients with ARF who are unable to eat an adequate diet need a vitamin supplement to meet DRIs. Large doses of vitamin C should be avoided because urinary excretion is impaired. In addition, oxalate (a product of vitamin C catabolism) may precipitate in renal tubules or form calcium oxalate stones, obstruct urine flow, and worsen renal function. Patients with CRF often have deficiencies of water-soluble vitamins because many foods that contain these vitamins are restricted due to their potassium content. In addition, vitamin C is reabsorbed from renal tubules by a specific transport protein. When the transport protein becomes saturated, remaining vitamin C is excreted in urine. Vitamin C is removed by dialysis and patients receiving dialysis require vitamin C replacement. The optimal replacement dose is unknown but probably should not exceed 200 milligrams per day (to avoid increased oxalate and possible stones). Overall, a multivitamin with essential vitamins, including vitamin C 70 to 100 milligrams, pyridoxine 5 to 10 milligrams, and folic acid 1 milligram, is recommended for daily use.

With mineral–electrolyte products, several are contraindicated in patients with renal impairment, including magnesium and KCl, because of potential accumulation and toxicity. Frequent measurements of serum electrolyte levels may be indicated. In patients with CRF who are on hemodialysis and receiving supplemental erythropoietin therapy, sodium ferric gluconate complex (Ferrlecit) may be given IV during dialysis to treat iron deficiency anemia.

Nutritional Support in Patients With Hepatic Impairment

The liver is extremely important in digestion and metabolism of carbohydrate, protein, and fat as well as storage of nutrients. Thus, patients with impaired hepatic function are often undernourished, with impaired metabolism of foodstuffs, vitamin deficiencies, and fluid and electrolyte imbalances. Depending on the disease process and the extent of liver impairment, these patients have special needs in relation to nutritional support.

Patients with alcoholic hepatitis or cirrhosis have a high rate of metabolism and therefore need foods to supply extra energy. However, metabolic disorders interfere with the liver's ability to process and use foodstuffs. Patients with cirrhosis often have hyperglycemia. Patients with severe hepatitis often have hypoglycemia because of impaired hepatic production of glucose and possibly impaired hepatic metabolism of insulin.

Protein restriction is usually needed in patients with cirrhosis to prevent or treat hepatic encephalopathy, which is caused by excessive protein or excessive production of ammonia (from protein breakdown in the GI tract). For patients able to tolerate enteral feedings (usually by GI tube), Hepatic Aid II is formulated for patients with liver failure. When parenteral nutrition is necessary for patients with hepatic failure and hepatic encephalopathy, HepatAmine, a special formulation of amino acids, may be used. Other amino acid preparations are contraindicated in patients with hepatic encephalopathy and coma.

Enteral and parenteral fat preparations must be used very cautiously. Medium-chain triglycerides (e.g., MCT oil), which are used to provide calories in other malnourished patients, may lead to coma in patients with advanced cirrhosis. Patients who require parenteral nutrition may develop high serum triglyceride levels and pancreatitis if given usual amounts of IV fat emulsions. Sodium and fluid restrictions are often needed to decrease edema.

Vitamin deficiencies commonly occur in patients with chronic liver disease, because of poor intake and malabsorption. With hepatic failure, hepatic stores of vitamin A, pyridoxine, folic acid, riboflavin, pantothenic acid, vitamin B_{12}, and thiamine are depleted. Folic acid deficiency may lead to megaloblastic anemia. Thiamine deficiency may lead to Wernicke's encephalopathy. Therapeutic doses of vitamins should be given for documented deficiency states.

Niacin is contraindicated in liver disease because it may increase liver enzymes (alanine and aspartate aminotransferases, alkaline phosphatase) and bilirubin and cause further liver damage. Long-acting dosage forms may be more hepatotoxic than the fast-acting forms.

Iron dextran must be used with extreme caution in patients with impaired hepatic function. Also, overdoses of chromium and copper are hepatotoxic and should be avoided.

Nutritional Support in Patients With Critical Illness

Critically ill patients often have organ failures that alter their ability to ingest and use essential nutrients. Thus, they may be undernourished in relation to protein-calorie, vitamin, and mineral–electrolyte needs. Some considerations include the following:

■ With enteral nutrition, adequate calories and DRI-equivalent amounts of all vitamins are usually needed. Patients with respiratory impairment may need a formula that contains less carbohydrate and more fat than other products and produces less carbon dioxide (e.g., Pulmocare). Patients with cardiac or renal impairment who require fluid restriction may benefit from a more concentrated formula (e.g., 1.5 kcal/mL).

■ With parenteral nutrition, adequate types and amounts of nutrients are needed. When IV fat emulsions are given, they should be infused slowly, over 24 hours. With vitamins, the Nutrition Advisory Group of the American Medical Association (NAG-AMA) has established guidelines for daily intake, and parenteral multivitamin formulations are available for adults and children. Those for adults do not contain vitamin K, which is usually injected weekly. The usual dose is 2 to 4 milligrams. Vitamin K is included in pediatric parenteral nutrition solutions.

■ Electrolyte and acid–base imbalances often occur in critically ill patients and are usually treated as in other patients, with very close monitoring of serum electrolyte levels and avoiding excessive amounts of replacement products.

Nutritional Support in Home Care

The home care nurse is involved with nutritional matters in almost any home care setting. Because nutrition is so important to health, the home care nurse should take advantage of any opportunity for health promotion in this area. Health promotion may involve assessing the nutritional status of all members of the household, especially children, older adults, and those with obvious deficiencies, and providing assistance to improve nutritional status.

For patients receiving tube feedings at home, the home care nurse may teach about the goals of treatment, administration, preparation or storage of solutions, equipment (e.g., obtaining, cleaning), and monitoring responses (e.g., weight, urine output).

For patients receiving parenteral nutrition at home, solutions, infusion pumps, and other equipment are obtained from a pharmacy, home health agency, or independent company. The home care nurse may not be involved in the initial setup but is likely to participate in ongoing patient care, monitoring of patient responses, and supporting caregivers. In addition, the home care nurse may need to coordinate activities among prescribers, IV therapy personnel, and other health care providers.

With vitamins, the home care nurse needs to assess for indications of vitamin deficiencies or use of supplements, especially megadoses. If difficulties are found, the nurse may need to counsel household members about dietary sources of vitamins and adverse effects of excessive vitamin intake.

With mineral–electrolytes, the home care nurse needs to assess for indications of mineral–electrolyte deficiency or excess. Depending on assessment data, teaching may be needed about dietary sources of these nutrients, when mineral supplements are indicated or should be avoided, and safety factors related to iron supplements or exposure to lead in homes with small children.

⊘ Applying Your Knowledge 57-3

How Can You Avoid This Medication Error?
Mrs. Farber is taking an iron supplement. You tell the family to give her the iron supplement with her coffee.

Nursing Actions — Nutritional Products, Vitamins, and Mineral–Electrolytes

NURSING ACTIONS	RATIONALE/EXPLANATION
1. Administer accurately a. For **oral supplemental feedings,** chill liquids or pour over ice and give through a straw, from a closed container, between meals.	Chilling (or freezing) may improve formula taste and decrease formula odor. A straw directs the formula toward the back of the throat and decreases its contact with taste buds. A closed container also decreases odor. Giving between meals may have less effect on appetite at mealtimes.
b. For **tube feedings:** (1) Have the patient sitting, if possible. (2) Check tube placement before each feeding.	To decrease risks of aspirating formula into lungs To prevent aspiration or accidental instillation of feedings into lungs
(3) Give the solution at room temperature.	Cold formulas may cause abdominal cramping.
(4) If giving by intermittent instillation, do not give more than 500 mL per feeding, including water for rinsing the tube.	To avoid gastric distention, possible vomiting, and aspiration into lungs
(5) Give by gravity flow (over 30–60 minutes) or infusion pump.	Rapid administration may cause nausea, vomiting, and other symptoms.
(6) With continuous feedings, change containers and tubing daily. With intermittent bolus feedings, rinse all equipment after each use, and change at least every 24 hours.	Most tube-feeding formulas are milk based and provide a good culture medium for bacterial growth. Clean technique, not sterile technique, is required.
(7) Give additional water with, after, or between feedings.	To avoid dehydration and promote fluid balance. Most patients receiving 1500 to 2000 mL of tube-feeding formula daily will need 1000 mL or more of water daily.
(8) Rinse nasogastric tubes with at least 50–100 mL water after each bolus feeding or administration of medications through the tube.	To keep the tube patent and functioning. This water is included in calculation of fluid intake.
(9) When medications are ordered by tube, liquid preparations are preferred over crushed tablets or powders emptied from capsules.	Tablets or powders may stick in the tube lumen. This may mean the full dose of the medication does not reach the stomach. Also, the tube is likely to become obstructed.
c. With **pancreatic enzymes,** give before or with meals or food.	To be effective, these agents must be in the small intestine when food is present.
d. With **fat-soluble vitamins:** (1) Do not give oral preparations at the same time as mineral oil.	Mineral oil absorbs the vitamins and thus prevents their systemic absorption.
(2) For subcutaneous (Sub-Q) or intramuscular (IM) administration of vitamin K, aspirate carefully to avoid intravenous (IV) injection, apply gentle pressure to the injection site, and inspect the site frequently.	Vitamin K is given to patients with hypoprothrombinemia, which causes bleeding tendencies. Thus, any injection may cause trauma and bleeding at the injection site. IV phytonadione may cause hypotension and shock from an anaphylactic type of reaction. IV administration is not recommended.

(continued on page 930)

Nursing Actions — **Nutritional Products, Vitamins, and Mineral–Electrolytes** (continued)

NURSING ACTIONS	RATIONALE/EXPLANATION
e. With **B-complex vitamins:** (1) Give parenteral cyanocobalamin (vitamin B_{12}) IM or deep Sub-Q. (2) Give oral niacin, except for timed-release forms, with or after meals or at bedtime. Have the patient sit or lie down for about 30 minutes after administration. (3) Give IM thiamine deeply into a large muscle mass. Avoid the IV route.	To decrease anorexia, nausea, vomiting, diarrhea, and flatulence. Niacin causes vasodilation, which may result in dizziness, hypotension, and injury from falls. Vasodilation occurs within a few minutes and may last 1 hour. To decrease pain at the injection site. Hypotension and anaphylactic shock have occurred with rapid IV administration and large doses.
f. With **mineral–electrolyte preparations,** give oral drugs with food or immediately after meals; give IV preparations slowly, do not mix with any other drug in a syringe, and dilute as directed with compatible IV solutions.	Giving oral drugs with or after food decreases gastric irritation. Rapid IV administration may cause cardiac dysrhythmias or other serious problems. Mixing the drugs may cause drug inactivation or precipitation.
g. For **potassium supplements:** (1) For oral preparations, give with or after meals; do not crush controlled- or extended-release tablets; mix oral liquids, powders, and effervescent tablets in at least 4 oz of juice, water, or carbonated beverage. (2) For IV potassium chloride (KCl), **never** give undiluted drug IV; dilute 20–40 mEq in 1000 ml of IV solution, such as dextrose in water; be sure that KCl is mixed well with the IV solution; as a general rule, give potassium-containing IV solutions at a maximum rate of 10 mEq/h, for life-threatening dysrhythmias caused by hypokalemia, potassium can be replaced with 20–40 mEq/h with constant electrocardiogram (ECG) monitoring. Use an infusion pump and do not give potassium-containing IV solutions into a central venous catheter.	Giving with food decreases gastric irritation; crushing extended-release tablets causes the drug to be absorbed immediately rather than over several hours, as intended; mixing dilutes, disguises the taste, and decreases gastric irritation. Concentrated drug and transient hyperkalemia may cause life-threatening cardiotoxicity, severe pain, and vein sclerosis; adequate dilution decreases risks of hyperkalemia and cardiotoxicity and prevents or decreases pain at the infusion site; 10 mEq or less per hour is the safest amount and rate of potassium administration and it is usually effective; risks of hyperkalemia and life-threatening cardiotoxicity are greatly increased with high concentrations or rapid flow rates. Constant ECG monitoring can detect hyperkalemia. Infusion pumps can regulate the flow rate accurately. Administration through a central IV line can cause hyperkalemia and cardiac dysrhythmias or arrest.
h. For parenteral **magnesium sulfate** (1) Read the drug label carefully to be sure you have the correct preparation for the intended use. (2) For IM use, small amounts of 50% solution are usually given (1 g magnesium sulfate = 2 mL of 50% solution). (3) For IV use, a 5% or 10% solution is used for direct injection, intermittent infusion, or continuous infusion. Whatever concentration is used, administer no more than 150 mg/min (1.5 mL/min of 10% solution; 3 mL/min of 5% solution).	Magnesium sulfate is available in concentrations of 10%, 25%, and 50% and in sizes of 2-, 10-, and 20-mL ampules, as well as a 30-mL multidose vial.
i. For **iron preparations:** (1) Give tablets or capsules before meals, with 8 oz of water or juice, if tolerated. If gastric upset occurs, give with or after meals. Instruct patients not to crush or chew sustained-release preparations. (2) Dilute liquid iron preparations, give with a straw, and have the patient rinse the mouth afterward. (3) To give iron dextran IM, use a 2- to 3-inch needle and Z-track technique to inject the drug into the upper outer quadrant of the buttock. (4) To give iron dextran IV (either directly or diluted in sodium chloride solution and given over several hours), do not use the multidose vial.	Iron preparations are absorbed better if taken on an empty stomach. If taken with meals, note that bran, eggs, tea, coffee, and dairy products decrease iron absorption. Crushing or chewing releases all the medication at once, rather than over several hours, as intended. To prevent temporary staining of teeth To prevent discomfort and staining of Sub-Q tissue and skin The multidose vial contains phenol as a preservative and is not suitable for IV use. Ampules of 2 mL or 5 mL are available without preservative.

NURSING ACTIONS	RATIONALE/EXPLANATION
j. Refer to the individual drugs or package literature for instructions regarding administration of deferoxamine, penicillamine, IV sodium bicarbonate, and multiple electrolyte solutions.	
2. Observe for therapeutic effects	
a. With nutritional formulas given orally or by tube feeding, observe for weight gain and increased serum albumin. For infants and children receiving milk substitutes, observe for decreased diarrhea and weight gain.	Therapeutic effects depend on the reason for use (i.e. prevention or treatment of undernutrition).
b. With pancreatic enzymes, observe for decreased diarrhea and steatorrhea.	The pancreatic enzymes function the same way as endogenous enzymes to aid digestion of carbohydrate, protein, and fat.
c. With vitamins, observe for decreased signs and symptoms of deficiency:	
(1) With vitamin A, observe for improved vision, especially in dim light or at night, less dryness in eyes and conjunctiva (xerophthalmia), and improvement in skin lesions.	Night blindness is usually relieved within a few days. Skin lesions may not disappear for several weeks.
(2) With vitamin K, observe for decreased bleeding and more nearly normal blood coagulation tests (e.g., prothrombin time).	Blood coagulation tests usually improve within 4–12 hours.
(3) With B-complex vitamins, observe for decreased or absent stomatitis, glossitis, seborrheic dermatitis, neurologic problems (neuritis, convulsions, mental deterioration, psychotic symptoms), cardiovascular problems (edema, heart failure), and eye problems (itching, burning, photophobia).	Deficiencies of B-complex vitamins commonly occur together and produce many similar manifestations.
(4) With vitamin B_{12} and folic acid, observe for increased appetite, strength and feeling of well-being, increased reticulocyte counts, and increased numbers of normal red blood cells, hemoglobin, and hematocrit.	Therapeutic effects may be rapid and dramatic. The patient usually feels better within 24–48 hours, and normal red blood cells begin to appear. Anemia is decreased within approximately 2 weeks, but 4–8 weeks may be needed for complete blood count to return to normal.
(5) With vitamin C, observe for decreased or absent malaise, irritability, and bleeding tendencies (easy bruising of skin, bleeding gums, nosebleeds, and so forth).	
d. With mineral–electrolyte preparations, observe for decreased signs of deficiency.	
(1) With KCl or other potassium preparations, observe for decreased signs of hypokalemia and increased serum potassium levels.	
(2) With magnesium sulfate, observe for decreased signs of hypomagnesemia, increased serum magnesium levels, or control of convulsions.	
(3) With zinc sulfate, observe for improved wound healing.	
(4) With iron preparations, observe for increased vigor and feeling of well-being, improved appetite, less fatigue, and increased red blood cells, hemoglobin, and hematocrit. With parenteral iron, observe for an average increase in hemoglobin of 1 g/wk.	Therapeutic effects are usually evident within a month unless other problems are also present (e.g., vitamin deficiency, achlorhydria, infection, malabsorption).
3. Observe for adverse effects	
a. With commercial nutritional formulas (except Osmolite and Isocal), observe for hypotension, tachycardia, increased urine output, dehydration, nausea, vomiting, or diarrhea.	These adverse reactions are usually attributed to the hypertonicity of the preparations. They can be prevented or minimized by starting with small amounts of formula, given slowly.
b. With vitamin A, observe for signs of hypervitaminosis A (anorexia; vomiting; irritability; headache; skin disorders; pain in muscles, bones, and joints; other clinical manifestations; and serum levels of vitamin A above 1200 IV/dL).	Severity of manifestations depends largely on dose and duration of excess vitamin A intake. Very severe states produce additional clinical signs, including enlargement of liver and spleen, altered liver function, increased intracranial pressure, and other neurologic manifestations.
c. With Sub-Q or IM vitamin K, adverse effects rarely occur.	Vitamin K rarely produces adverse reactions. Giving IV phytonadione slowly may prevent adverse reactions.

(continued on page 932)

Nursing Actions Nutritional Products, Vitamins, and Mineral–Electrolytes (continued)

NURSING ACTIONS	RATIONALE/EXPLANATION
d. With B-complex vitamins, observe for hypotension and anaphylactic shock with parenteral niacin, thiamine, cyanocobalamin, and folic acid; anorexia, nausea, vomiting and diarrhea, and postural hypotension with oral niacin.	Adverse reactions are generally rare. They are unlikely with B-complex multivitamin preparations. They are most likely to occur with large IV doses and rapid administration.
e. With vitamin C megadoses, observe for diarrhea and rebound deficiency if stopped abruptly.	Adverse reactions are rare with usual doses and methods of administration.
f. With mineral–electrolytes, observe for excess states.	These are likely to occur with excessive dosages of supplements. They can usually be prevented by using relatively low doses in nonemergency situations and by frequent monitoring of serum levels of electrolytes and iron.
g. With potassium preparations, observe for hyperkalemia.	This is most likely to occur with rapid IV administration, high dosages or concentrations, or in the presence of renal insufficiency and decreased urine output.
h. With magnesium preparations, observe for hypermagnesemia.	See potassium preparations, above.
i. Gastrointestinal (GI) symptoms—anorexia, nausea, vomiting, diarrhea, and abdominal discomfort from gastric irritation	Most oral preparations of minerals and electrolytes are likely to cause gastric irritation. Taking the drugs with food or 8 oz of fluid may decrease symptoms.
j. Cardiovascular symptoms—cardiac dysrhythmias, hypotension, tachycardia, other symptoms of shock	Potentially fatal dysrhythmias may occur with hyperkalemia or hypermagnesemia; shock may occur with deferoxamine and iron dextran injections.
k. With Kayexalate, observe for hypokalemia, hypocalcemia, hypomagnesemia, and edema.	Although this drug is used to treat hyperkalemia, it removes calcium and magnesium ions as well as potassium ions. Because it acts by trading sodium for potassium, the sodium retention may lead to edema.
4. Observe for drug interactions	
a. With fat-soluble vitamins:	
(1) Bile salts *increase* effects.	Increase intestinal absorption
(2) Laxatives, especially mineral oil, *decrease* effects.	Mineral oil combines with fat-soluble vitamins and prevents their absorption if both are taken at the same time. Excessive or chronic laxative use decreases intestinal absorption.
(3) Antibiotics may *decrease* effects.	With vitamin K, antibiotics decrease production by decreasing intestinal bacteria. With others, antibiotics may cause diarrhea and subsequent malabsorption.
b. With B-complex vitamins:	
(1) Isoniazid (INH) *decreases* effect.	INH has an antipyridoxine effect. When INH is given for prevention or treatment of tuberculosis, pyridoxine is usually given also.
(2) With folic acid: alcohol, cholestyramine, methotrexate, oral contraceptives, phenytoin, sulfasalazine, and triamterene *decrease* effects.	Alcohol alters liver function and leads to poor hepatic storage of folic acid. Methotrexate and phenytoin act as antagonists to folic acid and may cause folic acid deficiency. Cholestyramine, oral contraceptives, and sulfasalazine decrease absorption of folic acid.
(3) With vitamin B_{12}, omeprazole (Prilosec) *decreases* effects.	Decreases absorption of B_{12} from foods
c. Drugs that *increase* effects of minerals and electrolytes and related drugs:	
(1) Cation exchange resin (Kayexalate): diuretics *increase* potassium loss; other sources of sodium *increase* the likelihood of edema.	Additive effects
(2) With iron salts:	
(a) Allopurinol (Zyloprim)	This drug may increase the concentration of iron in the liver. It should not be given concurrently with any iron preparation.
(b) Ascorbic acid (vitamin C)	Increases absorption of iron by acidifying secretions
(3) With potassium salts:	
(a) Angiotensin-converting enzyme (ACE) inhibitors (e.g., captopril)	May increase risks of hyperkalemia

NURSING ACTIONS	RATIONALE/EXPLANATION
(b) Diuretics, potassium-saving (spironolactone, triamterene, amiloride)	These drugs should not be given with a potassium supplement because of additive risks of producing life-threatening hyperkalemia.
(c) Salt substitutes	These contain potassium rather than sodium and may cause hyperkalemia if given with potassium supplements.
(d) Penicillin G potassium	This potassium salt of penicillin contains 1.7 mEq of potassium per 1 million units and increases risks of hyperkalemia.
d. Drugs that *decrease* effects of minerals and electrolytes and related drugs:	
(1) With oral iron salts:	
(a) Antacids	Decrease absorption. Iron is best absorbed in an acidic environment and antacids increase alkalinity.
(b) Caffeine	Decreases absorption. An iron preparation and a caffeine-containing substance (e.g., coffee) should be separated by at least 2 hours.
(c) Cimetidine (Tagamet)	Decreases absorption
(d) Pancreatic extracts	Decrease absorption
(2) With potassium salts:	
(a) Calcium gluconate	Decreases cardiotoxic effects of hyperkalemia and is therefore useful in the treatment of hyperkalemia
(b) Sodium polystyrene sulfonate (Kayexalate)	Used in treatment of hyperkalemia because it removes potassium from the body

Key Concepts

▪ Human nutrition for health requires sufficient water, carbohydrates, proteins, fats, vitamins, and minerals.

▪ Patients with other health problems often have nutritional deficiencies, such as protein-calorie undernutrition and vitamin deficiencies.

▪ All patients need to be assessed in terms of nutritional status. When problems are assessed, interventions to maintain or improve nutritional status are needed.

▪ Fat-soluble vitamins are A, D, E, and K; water-soluble vitamins are B complex and C.

▪ Nutrients are best obtained from foods; when they cannot be obtained from foods, they can be provided by oral, enteral (via GI tubes), or parenteral (IV) feedings to meet a patient's nutritional needs.

▪ Techniques for safe administration of oral, enteral, and parenteral feedings must be consistently followed because complications and harm to patients may occur with all methods.

▪ Adverse effects may occur with large doses of vitamin and mineral supplements; the maximum recommended amounts should not be exceeded.

▪ Although most adults and children probably benefit from a daily multivitamin, large doses of single vitamins do not prevent cancer or cardiovascular disease and should be avoided.

Review and Application Exercises

Short Answer Exercises

1. For patients who are unable to ingest food, which nutrients can be provided with enteral or IV nutritional formulas?

2. What is the role of lipid emulsions in parenteral nutrition?

3. What roles do vitamins play in normal body functioning?

4. Identify patient populations who are at risk for vitamin deficiencies and excesses.

5. Are fat-soluble or water-soluble vitamins more toxic in overdoses? Why?

6. For a patient who asks your advice about taking a multivitamin supplement daily, how would you reply? Justify your answer.

7. How do the vitamin requirements of children, older adults, and critically ill patients differ from those of healthy young and middle-aged adults?

8. What are the major roles of minerals and electrolytes in normal body functioning?

9. When a patient is given potassium supplements for hypokalemia, how do you monitor for therapeutic and adverse drug effects?

10. List the main steps in treatment of hyperkalemia. Identify patient populations at risk for development of hyperkalemia.

11. What are advantages and disadvantages of iron supplements?

12. List measures an adult can take to prevent accidental iron poisoning in small children.

NCLEX-Style Questions

13. Mr. H develops respiratory distress while receiving continuous tube feeding. After notifying the physician and stopping the feeding, the nurse should first
    a. Assess bowel sounds to determine if he has a paralytic ileus.
    b. Assess breath sounds to determine if he has aspirated tube-feeding formula.
    c. Perform nasal or tracheal suctioning.
    d. Aspirate stomach contents.

14. Which of the following statements by Mr. H's daughter who will care for him at home, leads you to believe that she has understood your teaching regarding tube feeding?
    a. "I will store unopened cans of formula in the refrigerator."
    b. "I will stop the feedings if he has more than two stools per day."
    c. "I will place him in a sitting position for his feedings."
    d. "I will give no more than 50 mL per hour."

15. Which of the following is a fat-soluble vitamin that is toxic in overdose?
    a. vitamin A
    b. vitamin B_1
    c. vitamin C
    d. folic acid

16. Teaching for a patient who is being started on an iron supplement should include information that the preparation
    a. may cause diarrhea
    b. may cause stools to be dark green or black
    c. should be taken with an antacid
    d. should not be taken with fruit juice

17. Which of the following IV electrolytes should be well diluted and never given as a bolus injection ("IV push") because it can cause fatal cardiac dysrhythmias?
    a. sodium bicarbonate
    b. magnesium sulfate
    c. sodium chloride
    d. potassium chloride

Selected References

Baron, R. B. (2007). Nutrition. In S. J. McPhee, M. A. Papadakis, & L. M. Tierney, Jr. (Eds.), *Current medical diagnosis and treatment 2007* (46th ed., pp. 1279–1310). New York: McGraw-Hill.

Brophy, D. F., & Gehr, T. W. B. (2005). Disorders of potassium and magnesium homeostasis. In J. T. DiPiro, R. L. Talbert, G. C. Yee, G. R. Matzke, B. G. Wells, & L. M. Posey (Eds.), *Pharmacotherapy: A pathophysiologic approach* (5th ed., pp. 967–981). New York: McGraw-Hill.

DeHart, R. M., & Yocom, S. J. (2005). Nutritional considerations in major organ failure. In J. T. DiPiro, R. L. Talbert, G. C. Yee, G. R. Matzke, B. G. Wells, & L. M. Posey (Eds.), *Pharmacotherapy: A pathophysiologic approach* (6th ed., pp. 2635–2658). New York: McGraw-Hill.

Drug facts and comparisons. (Updated monthly). St. Louis, MO: Facts and Comparisons.

Guyton, A. C., & Hall, J. E. (2006). *Textbook of medical physiology* (11th ed., pp. 865–880). Philadelphia: Elsevier Saunders.

Kumpf, V. J., & Chessman, K. H. (2005). Enteral nutrition. In J. T. DiPiro, R. L. Talbert, G. C. Yee, G. R. Matzke, B. G. Wells, & L. M. Posey (Eds.), *Pharmacotherapy: A pathophysiologic approach* (6th ed., pp. 2615–2634). New York: McGraw-Hill.

Linden, C. H., Rippe, J. M., & Irwin, R. S. (Eds.). (2006). *Manual of overdoses and poisonings.* Philadelphia: Lippincott Williams & Wilkins.

Lonn, E., Bosch, J., & Yusuf, S. (2005). Effects of long-term vitamin E supplementation on cardiovascular events and cancer: A randomized controlled trial. *Journal of the American Medical Association, 293,* 1338–1347.

Pleuss, J. (2005). Alterations in nutritional status. In C. M. Porth (Ed.), *Pathophysiology: Concepts of altered health states* (7th ed., pp. 217–238). Philadelphia: Lippincott Williams & Wilkins.

Smeltzer, S. C., Bare, B. G., Hinkle, J. L., & Cheever, K. H. (2008). *Brunner & Suddarth's textbook of medical-surgical nursing* (11th ed.). Philadelphia: Lippincott Williams & Wilkins.

Drugs to Aid Weight Management

LEARNING OBJECTIVES

After studying this chapter, you will be able to:

1. Promote healthful lifestyle measures to maintain body weight within a desirable range and avoid obesity.
2. Assess patients for risk factors and manifestations of obesity.
3. Calculate body mass index (BMI).
4. Counsel patients about the health consequences of obesity.
5. Assist overweight patients to develop and maintain a safe and realistic weight-loss program.
6. Identify reliable sources for information about nutrition, weight loss, and weight maintenance.
7. Assist patients with effective use of approved weight-loss drugs, when indicated.

Applying Your Knowledge

Halli Vargas is a 31-year-old woman who has had a weight problem all her life. She has been on any number of diets with a yo-yo effect of weight loss followed by weight gain. She is 5 feet 5 inches tall and weighs 265 pounds. Her adult nurse practitioner starts her on orlistat and prescribes a consultation with a dietitian.

Introduction

Carbohydrates, proteins, and fats are required for human nutrition. Either deficiencies or excesses impair health, cause illness, and impair recovery from illness or injury. Proteins are basic structural and functional components of all body cells and tissues; carbohydrates and fats serve primarily as sources of energy for cellular metabolism. Energy is measured in kilocalories (kcal, commonly called calories) per gram of food oxidized in the body. Carbohydrates and proteins supply 4 kcal per gram; fats supply 9 kcal per gram. Excessive amounts of any of these nutrients are converted to fat and stored in the body, resulting in excess weight and *obesity*. This chapter discusses obesity and treatment strategies, including drugs to aid weight loss and weight maintenance.

Overweight and Obese Adults

Being *overweight* and obese are widespread problems and are increasing in the United States, in both children and adults. They are considered major public health problems because of their association with high rates of morbidity and mortality. Overweight is defined as a *body mass index* (BMI) of 25 to 29.9 kilograms per square meter; obese is defined as a BMI of 30 or more kilograms per square meter. The BMI reflects weight in relation to height and is a better indicator than weight alone. The desirable range for BMI is 18.5 to 24.9 kilograms per square meter, with any values below

935

Box 58-1	Calculation of Body Mass Index (BMI) and Height and Weight Indicators for Overweight and Obese

BMI

Body mass index can be calculated as weight in kilograms divided by height in meters, squared; or as weight in pounds divided by height in inches, squared, multiplied by a conversion factor of 704.5 (listed as 703 in some sources), as follows:

$$BMI = \frac{Weight\ (pounds)}{Height\ (inches)^2} \times 704.5$$

Example: A person who weighs 150 lb and is 5'5" (65 in) tall

$$BMI = \frac{150\ lb}{65\ in \times 65\ in} \times 704.5 = \frac{105,675}{422.5} = 25$$

Weight Compared With Height as an Indicator for Being Overweight or Obese

Height (ft/in)	Weight (lb) Indicating Overweight (BMI 25)	Weight (lb) Indicating Obesity (BMI 30)
5'2" (62 inches)	135	165
5'3"	140	170
5'4"	145	175
5'5"	150	180
5'6"	155	185
5'7"	160	190
5'8"	165	195
5'9"	170	200
5'10"	175	205
5'11"	180	210
6'0"	185	220
6'1"	190	225
6'2" (74 inches)	195	230

18.5 indicating underweight and any values of 25 or above indicating excessive weight (Box 58-1). A large waist circumference (above 35 inches for women, above 40 inches for men) is another risk factor for overweight and obesity.

Obesity may occur in anyone but is more likely to occur in women, minority groups, and poor people. It results from consistent ingestion of more calories than are used for energy, and it substantially increases risks for development of numerous health problems (Box 58-2). Most obesity-related disorders are attributed mainly to the multiple metabolic abnormalities associated with obesity. Abdominal fat out of proportion to total body fat (also called central or visceral obesity), which often occurs in men and postmenopausal women, is considered a greater risk factor for disease and death than lower body obesity. In addition to the many health problems associated with

obesity, obesity is increasingly being considered a chronic disease in its own right. Although it has been the focus of much research in recent years, no current theory adequately explains the disorder and its resistance to treatment.

Prevalence

The prevalence of overweight people and obesity has dramatically increased during the past 25 years. Some authorities estimate that 60% of American adults are overweight or obese. There are differences in prevalence by gender, ethnicity, and socioeconomic status. In general, more women than men are obese, whereas more men than women are overweight; African-American women and Mexican Americans of both sexes have the highest rates of overweight and obesity in the United States; and women in lower socioeconomic classes are more likely to be obese than those in higher socioeconomic classes.

Etiology

The etiology of excessive weight is thought to involve complex and often overlapping interactions among physiologic, genetic, environmental, psychosocial, and other factors.

Physiologic Factors

In general, increased weight is related to an energy imbalance in which energy intake (food/calorie consumption) exceeds energy expenditure. Total energy expenditure represents the energy expended at rest (i.e., the basal or resting metabolic rate), during physical activity, and during food consumption. When a person ingests food, about 10% of the energy content of that food is expended in the digestion, absorption, and metabolism of nutrients. Foods that contain carbohydrates and proteins stimulate energy expenditure; high-fat foods have little stimulatory effect. The energy required to metabolize and to use food reaches a maximum level about 1 hour after the food is ingested. In addition, men tend to expend more energy than women because they have proportionally more muscle mass. Energy expenditure usually decreases in older men and women of all ages because these groups have less muscle tissue and more adipose tissue. Muscle is more metabolically active (i.e., has higher energy needs and burns more calories) than adipose tissue.

Excessive weight can result from eating more calories, exercising less, or a combination of the two factors. Consuming an extra 500 calories each day for a week results in 3500 excess calories or one pound of fat. Excess calories are converted to triglycerides and stored in fat cells (adipocytes). With continued intake of excessive calories, fat cells increase in both size and number.

Genetic Factors

Various studies indicate that a significant portion of weight variation within a given environment is genetic in origin. For example, identical twins raised in separate environments often have similar body types. Most cases of human obesity are attributed mainly to the combination of genetic susceptibility and environmental conditions.

Box 58-2	Health Risks of Obesity

Obesity is associated with serious health risks. Several disease states and chronic health problems are more prevalent in obese patients, as well as increased mortality. Studies indicate that a high body mass index (BMI) is associated with an increased risk of death from all causes, among both men and women, and in all age groups. In addition, a higher death rate occurs in people who gain weight of 10 kg or more after 18 years of age. Some of the major health risks include the disorders listed below. In general, these conditions tend to worsen as the degree of obesity increases and improve with weight loss.

Cancer

Obesity is associated with a higher prevalence of breast, colon, and endometrial cancers. With breast cancer, risks increase in postmenopausal women with increasing body weight. Women who gain more than 20 lb from age 18 to midlife have double the risk of breast cancer compared with women who maintain a stable weight during this period of their life. In addition, central obesity apparently increases the risk of breast cancer independent of overall obesity. In women with central obesity, this additional risk factor may be related to an excess of estrogen (from conversion of androstenedione to estradiol in peripheral fatty tissue) and a deficiency of sex hormone–binding globulin to combine with the estrogen.

Colon cancer seems to be more common in obese men and women. In addition, a high BMI may be a risk factor for a higher mortality rate with colon cancer. Endometrial cancer is clearly more common in obese women, with adult weight gain again increasing risk.

Cardiovascular Disorders

Obesity is a major risk factor for cardiovascular disorders and increased mortality from cardiovascular disease. Studies have confirmed the relationship between obesity and increased risk of coronary heart disease (CHD) and stroke in both men and women. In addition, obesity during adolescence is associated with higher rates and greater severity of cardiovascular disease as adults.

Obesity increases risks by aggravating other risk factors such as hypertension, insulin resistance, low HDL cholesterol, and hypertriglyceridemia. In addition, obesity seems to be an independent risk factor for cardiovascular disorders, and central obesity may be more important than BMI as a risk factor for death from cardiovascular disease. The increased mortality rate is seen even with modest excess body weight.

Hypertension, dyslipidemia, insulin resistance, and glucose intolerance are known cardiac risk factors that tend to cluster in obese individuals. Hypertension often occurs in obese persons and is thought to play a major role in the increased incidence of cardiovascular disease and stroke observed in patients with obesity. Metabolic abnormalities that occur with obesity and type 2 diabetes mellitus (e.g., insulin resistance and the resultant hyperinsulinemia) aggravate hypertension and increase cardiovascular risks. The combination of obesity and

hypertension is associated with cardiac changes (e.g., thickening of the ventricular wall, ischemia, and increased heart volume) that lead to heart failure more rapidly. Weight loss of as little as 4.5 kg (10 lb) can decrease blood pressure and cardiovascular risk in many people with obesity and hypertension.

Diabetes Mellitus

Obesity is strongly associated with impaired glucose tolerance, insulin resistance, and diabetes mellitus. In addition, obesity during adolescence is associated with higher rates of diabetes as adults as well as more severe complications of diabetes at younger ages.

The cellular effects by which obesity causes insulin resistance are unknown. Proposed mechanisms include down-regulation of insulin receptors, abnormal postreceptor signals, and others. Whatever the mechanism, the impaired insulin response stimulates the pancreatic beta cells to increase insulin secretion, resulting in a relative excess of insulin called hyperinsulinemia, and causes impaired lipid metabolism (increased low-density lipoprotein [LDL] cholesterol and triglycerides and decreased high-density lipoprotein [HDL] cholesterol). These metabolic changes increase hypertension and other risk factors for cardiovascular disease. As with cardiovascular disease and diabetes in general, central obesity seems to increase the likelihood of serious disease. The abdominal fat of central obesity seems to be more insulin resistant than peripheral fat deposited over the buttocks and legs. Intentional weight loss significantly reduces mortality in obese individuals with diabetes.

Dyslipidemias

Obesity strongly contributes to abnormal and undesirable changes in lipid metabolism (e.g., increased triglycerides and LDL cholesterol; decreased HDL cholesterol) that increase risks of cardiovascular disease and other health problems.

Gallstones

Obesity apparently increases the risk for developing gallstones by altering production and metabolism of cholesterol and bile. The risk is higher in women, especially those who have had multiple pregnancies or who are taking oral contraceptives. However, rapid weight loss with very–low-calorie diets is also associated with gallstones.

Metabolic Syndrome

Metabolic syndrome is a group of risk factors and chronic conditions that occur together and greatly increase the risks of diabetes mellitus, serious cardiovascular disease, and death. The syndrome is thought to be highly prevalent in the United States. Major characteristics include many of the health problems associated with obesity (e.g., dyslipidemias, hypertension, impaired glucose tolerance, insulin resistance, central obesity). More specifically, metabolic syndrome includes three or more of the following abnormalities:

(continued on page 938)

Box 58-2	Health Risks of Obesity (continued)

- Central obesity (waist circumference over 40 inches for men and over 35 inches for women)
- Serum triglycerides of 150 mg/dL or more
- HDL cholesterol below 40 mg/dL in men and below 50 mg/dL in women
- Blood pressure of 135/85 mm Hg or higher
- Serum glucose of 110 mg/dL or higher

Osteoarthritis

Obesity is associated with osteoarthritis (OA) of both weight-bearing joints, such as the hip and knee, and non–weight-bearing joints. Extra weight can stress affected bones and joints, contract muscles that normally stabilize joints, and may alter the metabolism of cartilage, collagen, and bone. In general, obese people develop OA of the knees at an earlier age and are more likely than nonobese people to require knee replacement surgery.

The important role of obesity in OA is supported by the observation that weight loss delays onset and reduces symptoms and disability. Weight reduction may also decrease infection, wound complications, and blood loss if surgery is required. Despite the benefits of weight loss, however, persons with OA have difficulty losing weight because painful joints limit exercise and activity.

Sleep Apnea

Sleep apnea commonly occurs in obese persons. A possible explanation is enlargement of soft tissue in the upper airways that leads to collapse of the upper airways with inspiration during sleep. The obstructed breathing leads to apnea with hypoxemia, hypercarbia, and a stress response. Sleep apnea is associated with increased risks of hypertension, possible right heart failure, and sudden death. Weight loss leads to improvement in sleep apnea.

Miscellaneous Effects

Obesity is associated with numerous difficulties in addition to those described above. These may include

- Nonalcoholic fatty liver disease, which is being increasingly recognized and which may lead to liver failure
- Poor wound healing
- Poor antibody response to hepatitis B vaccine
- A negative perception of people who are obese that affects their education, socioeconomic, and employment status
- High costs associated with treatment of the medical conditions caused or aggravated by obesity as well as the costs associated with weight-loss efforts
- In women, obesity is associated with menstrual irregularities, difficulty in becoming pregnant, and increased complications of pregnancy (e.g., gestational diabetes, higher rates of labor induction and cesarean section, and increased risk of neural tube and other congenital defects in offspring of obese women).
- In men, obesity is associated with infertility.
- In children and adolescents, obesity increases risk of bone fractures and muscle and joint pain. Knee pain is commonly reported, and changes in the knee joint make movement and exercise more difficult.

Environmental Factors

Environmental factors contributing to the greater number of overweight and obese individuals include increased food consumption and decreased physical activity. The ready availability and relatively low cost of a wide variety of foods, in addition to large portion sizes and high-calorie foods, promote overeating. In addition, many social gatherings are associated with eating or overeating.

In relation to physical activity, usual activities of daily living for many people, including work-related activities, require relatively little energy expenditure. In addition, few Americans are thought to exercise in the optimal frequency, intensity, or duration to maintain health and prevent excessive weight gain. For both adults and children, increased time watching television, playing video or computer games, and working on computers contribute to less physical activity and are thought to promote weight gain and obesity. In general, though, it is still unknown whether less physical activity leads to obesity or the physical effects of obesity lead to minimal physical activity.

Psychosocial Factors

Psychosocial disorders may be either a cause or an effect of obesity. Although much is still unknown about the psychological aspects of obesity development, depression and/or abuse may play a role. Obese people often report symptoms of depression, and some people overeat and gain weight during depressive episodes. It may be that obesity and depression commonly occur together and reinforce each other. A depressed person is less likely to take the active measures in diet and exercise that are required to lose weight, even if obesity is a prominent factor in the development of depression. In women, sexual, physical, and emotional abuse can result in obesity. Abuse during childhood and adolescence tends to produce more severe effects.

Other Factors

Diseases are rarely a major cause of obesity development. However, numerous disease processes may limit a person's ability to engage in calorie-burning physical activity. In addition, numerous prescription medications reportedly cause weight gain in some or most of the patients who take them (Box 58-3).

Overweight and Obese Children

Being overweight and obesity are common and increasing among children and adolescents, to the point of being called an "epidemic." Some studies estimate that 15% of children in the United States are overweight and that another 15% are

Box 58-3	Effects of Selected Medications on Weight

Antidepressants

Selective serotonin reuptake inhibitors (SSRIs), such as fluoxetine (Prozac, Sarafem) and related drugs, may promote weight loss with short-term use. However, with long-term use, they reportedly may cause as much weight gain as tricyclic antidepressants (TCAs) such as amitriptyline (Elavil). TCAs have long been associated with excessive appetite and weight gain. Mirtazapine (Remeron) and phenelzine (Nardil) are also associated with weight gain. The effects of bupropion (Wellbutrin, Zyban) on weight are unclear from clinical trials. Gain was reported when bupropion was used as a smoking deterrent, but both gain and loss occurred when used as an antidepressant. However, anorexia and weight loss occurred at a higher percentage rate than increased appetite and weight gain.

Antidiabetic Drugs

Although little attention is paid to the topic in most literature about diabetic drugs, weight gain apparently occurs with insulin, sulfonylureas, and the glitazones (but not with metformin, acarbose, or miglitol). Almost all patients with type 2 diabetes eventually require insulin; those who are failing on oral agents generally gain a large amount of body fat when switched to insulin therapy. Although the mechanism of weight gain is unknown, it may be related to the chronic hyperinsulinism induced by long-acting insulins and the sulfonylureas (which increase insulin secretion). Less weight is gained when oral drugs are given during the day and an intermediate- or long-acting insulin is injected at bedtime. This strategy is thought to cause less daytime hyperinsulinemia than the more traditional insulin strategies.

For near–normal-weight diabetic patients who require drug therapy, a sulfonylurea may be given. However, for obese patients, metformin is usually the initial drug of choice because it does not promote weight gain. Metformin may also be used to treat obese diabetic children, aged 10 to 16 years, who require drug therapy.

Antiepileptic Drugs

Weight gain commonly occurs with the use of antiepileptic drugs (AEDs). This has been observed for many years with older drugs (e.g., phenytoin, valproic acid, carbamazepine) and with newer AEDs (e.g., gabapentin, lamotrigine, tiagabine). Mechanisms by which the drugs promote weight gain are unclear but may involve stimulation of appetite and/or a slowed metabolic rate. Consequences of weight gain may include increased risks of diabetes mellitus, hypertension, and other physical health problems as well as psychological distress over appearance, especially in children and adolescents.

Antihistamines

Histamine$_1$ (H$_1$) antagonists (e.g., diphenhydramine, loratadine) reportedly increase appetite and cause weight gain.

Antihypertensives

The main antihypertensive drugs reported to cause weight gain are the beta blockers. The drugs can cause fatigue and decrease exercise tolerance and metabolic rate, all of which may contribute to weight gain. Other mechanisms may also be involved. As a result, some clinicians question the use of beta blockers in overweight or obese patients with uncomplicated hypertension. Alpha blockers may also cause weight gain, but apparently at a low incidence. Angiotensin-converting enzyme (ACE) inhibitors and calcium channel blockers are not reported to promote weight gain.

Antipsychotics

Weight gain is often reported and extensively documented with antipsychotic drugs. Although the exact mechanism is unknown, weight gain has been associated with antihistaminic effects, anticholinergic effects, and blockade of serotonin receptors. In addition, dietary factors and activity levels may also play significant roles.

Clozapine and olanzapine reportedly cause significant weight gain in 40% or more of patients. Compared with clozapine and olanzapine, risperidone causes less weight gain, and quetiapine and ziprasidone cause the least weight gain. Weight gain may lead to noncompliance with drug therapy. In addition to weight gain, clozapine and olanzapine adversely affect glucose regulation and can aggravate pre-existing diabetes or cause new-onset diabetes. The extent to which these effects are related to weight gain is unknown. For patients who are obese, diabetic, or at risk of developing diabetes, an antipsychotic drug that causes less weight gain would seem the better choice.

Cholesterol-Lowering Agents

Weight gain has been reported with the statin group of drugs; mechanisms and extent are unknown.

Corticosteroids

Systemic corticosteroids may cause increased appetite, weight gain, central obesity, and retention of sodium and fluid. Inhaled and intranasal corticosteroids have little effect on weight.

Gastrointestinal Drugs

Increased appetite and weight gain have been reported with the proton pump inhibitors (PPIs) such as omeprazole and others. The mechanisms and extent are unknown.

Hormonal Contraceptives

The weight gain associated with using hormonal contraceptives may be related more to retention of fluid and sodium than to increased body fat.

Mood Stabilizing Agent

Weight gain has been reported with long-term use of lithium, with approximately 20% of patients gaining 10 kg (22 lb) or more. This increased weight is attributed to fluid retention, consumption of high-calorie beverages as a result of increased thirst, or a decreased metabolic rate. Weight gain is a common reason for noncompliance with lithium therapy, and weight gain may be more common in women with lithium-induced hypothyroidism and in those who are already overweight.

at risk for becoming overweight, especially those with overweight parents. Overweight is defined as a BMI above the 85th percentile for the age group and obesity as a BMI above the 95th percentile.

Childhood obesity is a major public health concern because these children have or are at risk of developing hypertension, dyslipidemias, type 2 diabetes, and other disorders that may lead to major disability and death at younger adult ages than nonobese children. Obesity, type 2 diabetes, and other health problems are mainly attributed to poor eating habits and too little exercise. In addition, the child who is obese after 6 years of age is highly likely to be obese as an adult, especially if a parent is obese. Obesity in adults that began in childhood tends to be more severe.

In addition to major health problems, reduced energy, and less physical agility, obese children are often ridiculed or bullied by other children and may be discriminated against by adults in schools and workplaces.

General Characteristics of Drugs for Obesity

The National Heart, Lung, and Blood Institute (NHLBI) of the National Institutes of Health and most other organizations generally recommend reserving drug therapy for those with a BMI of 30 kilograms per square meter or greater and health problems (e.g., hypertension, dyslipidemia, coronary heart disease, type 2 diabetes, sleep apnea) that are likely to improve with weight loss. These organizations emphasize that drug therapy for obesity should be used as part of a weight-management program that also includes a sensible diet, physical activity, and behavioral modification. Guidelines also emphasize that drug therapy should be used to decrease medical risk and improve health rather than promote cosmetic weight loss.

Drug therapy for obesity has a problematic history, mainly because of serious adverse effects and rapid weight regain when the drugs were stopped. Some drugs (fenfluramine, dexfenfluramine, phenylpropanolamine) and a component of many over-the-counter and herbal weight-loss products (ephedra, ma huang) have been taken off the market because of their adverse effects.

Older drugs include amphetamines and similar drugs. Amphetamines (see Chap. 15) are not recommended because they are controlled substances (Schedule II) with a high potential for abuse and dependence. Benzphetamine, diethylpropion, phendimetrazine, and phentermine are adrenergic drugs (see Chap. 17) that stimulate the release of norepinephrine and dopamine in the brain. This action in nerve terminals of the hypothalamic feeding center suppresses appetite. These drugs, called appetite suppressants or *anorexiants*, are central nervous system (CNS) and cardiovascular stimulants and are contraindicated in cardiovascular disease, hyperthyroidism, glaucoma, and agitated states.

Of the adrenergic anorexiant drugs, only phentermine is commonly used. Sibutramine and orlistat are also commonly used and are the only weight-loss drugs approved for long-term use. According to some clinicians, sibutramine and orlistat may be continued as long as they are effective and adverse effects are tolerable. The drugs are described below; dosage ranges are listed in Table 58-1.

Individual Drugs

Phentermine

Phentermine (Adipex-P) is the most frequently prescribed adrenergic anorexiant. It is a Schedule IV drug and recommended only for short-term use (3 months or less). Its use is contraindicated in patients with hypertension or other cardiovascular disease and in those with a history of drug abuse. Because it increases blood pressure, phentermine should be used with caution even in patients with mild hypertension. The drug should also be used cautiously in patients with anxiety or agitation because of CNS stimulant effects. The most commonly reported adverse effects are nervousness, dry mouth, constipation, and hypertension.

Sibutramine

Sibutramine (Meridia) is a Schedule IV drug and the most commonly prescribed anti-obesity drug. It inhibits the reuptake of serotonin and norepinephrine in the brain, thereby increasing the amounts of these neurotransmitters. Clinical effects include increased satiety, decreased food intake, and a

Table 58-1	Drugs at a Glance: Drugs for Obesity

GENERIC/TRADE NAME	ROUTE AND DOSAGE RANGES
Appetite Suppressants	
Phentermine hydrochloride (Adipex-P, Ionamin, Pro-Fast)	PO 8 mg 3 times daily, 30 min before meals, or 15–37.5 mg daily in the morning
Sibutramine (Meridia)	PO 10–15 mg once daily, in the morning, with or without food
Fat Blocker	
Orlistat (Xenical, Alli)	PO 120 mg with each main meal, up to 3 capsules daily

faster metabolism rate. Sibutramine is approved by the U.S. Food and Drug Administration (FDA) for long-term use, but effects are mostly unknown beyond 1 to 2 years. The drug increases blood pressure and heart rate and is contraindicated in patients with cardiovascular disorders (e.g., coronary heart disease, dysrhythmias, heart failure, hypertension). It should be used cautiously in patients who take other medications that increase blood pressure and heart rate. It should also be used cautiously in patients with impaired hepatic function, narrow-angle glaucoma (may cause mydriasis), or a history of substance abuse or dependency. Sibutramine is not approved for use in children less than 16 years of age and is not recommended for women who are pregnant or lactating. The drug is contraindicated in people with severe renal or hepatic dysfunction.

Oral sibutramine is rapidly absorbed from the intestine and undergoes first-pass metabolism, during which time active metabolites are formed. Peak plasma levels of the active metabolites occur within 3 to 4 hours, and drug half-life is 14 to 16 hours. The long half-lives of the active metabolites allow for once-daily dosing. The drug is highly bound to plasma proteins and rapidly distributed to most body tissues, with the highest concentrations in the liver and kidneys. It is metabolized in the liver, mainly by the cytochrome P450 3A4 enzymes. The active metabolites produced by first-pass metabolism are further metabolized to inactive metabolites, which are then excreted in urine and feces.

Common adverse effects of sibutramine include dry mouth, headache, insomnia, nervousness, and constipation; cardiovascular effects include hypertension, tachycardia, and palpitations. Potentially serious drug interactions may occur if sibutramine is taken with other cardiovascular stimulants (increased risk of hypertension and dysrhythmias), CNS stimulants (increased anxiety and insomnia), and serotonergic drugs (serotonin syndrome). Other drugs that increase serotonin include the selective serotonin reuptake inhibitors (e.g., fluoxetine [Prozac] and related drugs), the triptan antimigraine drugs (e.g., sumatriptan [Imitrex]), dextromethorphan (a common ingredient in cough syrups), and lithium. The combination of sibutramine with any of these drugs may cause serotonin syndrome, a condition characterized by agitation, confusion, hypomania, impaired coordination, loss of consciousness, nausea, tachycardia, and other symptoms.

In clinical trials, people lost the most weight during the first 6 months of sibutramine therapy. However, continued drug therapy helped to maintain weight loss for 12 to 24 months. Most of the clinical trials included diet and behavioral modification techniques in addition to sibutramine therapy. As with other weight-loss drugs, studies indicate that sibutramine therapy is more effective when it is combined with lifestyle modification and diet than when used alone.

Orlistat

Orlistat (Xenical, Alli) differs from phentermine and sibutramine because it decreases absorption of dietary fat from the intestine (by binding to gastric and pancreatic lipases in the gastrointestinal [GI] tract lumen and making them unavailable to break down dietary fats into absorbable free fatty acids and monoglycerides). The drug blocks absorption of approximately 30% of the fat ingested in a meal; increasing dosage does not increase this percentage. Decreased fat absorption leads to decreased caloric intake, resulting in weight loss and improved serum cholesterol values (e.g., decreased total and low-density lipoprotein [LDL] cholesterol levels). The improvement in cholesterol levels is thought to be independent of weight-loss effects.

Orlistat is not absorbed systemically, and its action occurs in the GI tract. Consequently, it does not cause systemic adverse effects or drug interactions as phentermine and sibutramine do. Its main disadvantages are frequent administration (3 times daily) and GI symptoms (abdominal pain, oily spotting, fecal urgency, flatulence with discharge, fatty stools, fecal incontinence, and increased defecation). Adverse GI effects occur in almost all orlistat users but usually subside after a few weeks of continued drug usage. The drug also prevents absorption of the fat-soluble vitamins, A, D, E, and K. As a result, people taking orlistat should also take a multivitamin containing these vitamins daily. The multivitamin should be taken 2 hours before or after the orlistat dose. If taken at the same time, the orlistat prevents absorption of the fat-soluble vitamins.

Orlistat is intended for people who are clinically obese, not those wanting to lose a few pounds. In addition, high-fat foods still need to be decreased because total caloric intake is a major determinant of weight, and adverse effects (e.g., diarrhea; fatty, malodorous stools) worsen with high fat consumption. Long-term effects of orlistat are unknown. In addition to weight loss and reduced cholesterol levels, clinical trials found reduced severity and improved management of other health problems associated with obesity, such as diabetes and hypertension. In general, the addition of orlistat therapy to diet and other lifestyle changes produced greater weight loss than addition of a placebo. In some patients with impaired glucose tolerance, weight loss with orlistat and lifestyle changes prevented or delayed the occurrence of diabetes mellitus. After the medication was stopped, most patients regained weight.

Applying Your Knowledge 58-1

Ms. Vargas asks how orlistat will help her when nothing else in the past has been successful. How would you respond?

Herbal and Dietary Supplements

Many people use herbal or dietary supplements for weight loss, even though reliable evidence of safety and effectiveness are lacking. Some herbal products claim to decrease appetite and increase the rate at which the body burns calories. However, in most cases, there is no scientific evidence that they work at all. Some supplements for weight loss contain cardiovascular and

CNS stimulants that may cause serious, even life-threatening, adverse effects.

In general, many consumers do not seem to appreciate the benefits of proven weight-management techniques (e.g., appropriate diet and exercise) or the potential risks of taking unproven weight-loss products. Selected products are described below.

Glucomannan expands on contact with body fluids. It is included in weight-loss regimens because of its supposed ability to produce feelings of stomach fullness, thereby causing a person to eat less. It also has a laxative effect. There is little evidence to support its use as a weight-loss aid. Products containing glucomannan should not be used by people with diabetes; glucomannan may cause hypoglycemia alone and increases hypoglycemic effects of antidiabetic medications.

Guarana, a major source of commercial caffeine, is found in weight-loss products as well as caffeine-containing soft drinks, "energy" drinks, bodybuilding supplements, smoking-cessation products, vitamin supplements, candies, and chewing gums. Caffeine is the active ingredient; the amount varies among products, and caffeine content of any particular product cannot be accurately predicted. Guarana is promoted to decrease appetite and increase energy and mental alertness. It is contraindicated in patients with dysrhythmias and may aggravate gastroesophageal reflux disease (GERD) and peptic ulcer disease.

Adverse effects include diuresis, cardiovascular symptoms (premature ventricular contractions, tachycardia), CNS symptoms (agitation, anxiety, insomnia, seizures, tremors), and GI symptoms (nausea, vomiting, diarrhea). Such effects are more likely to occur with higher doses or concomitant use of guarana and other sources of caffeine. Adverse drug–drug interactions include additive CNS and cardiovascular stimulation with beta-adrenergic agonists (e.g., epinephrine, albuterol and related drugs, pseudoephedrine) and theophylline. In addition, concurrent use of cimetidine, fluoroquinolones, or oral contraceptives may increase or prolong serum caffeine levels and subsequent adverse effects.

Guar gum is a dietary fiber included in weight-loss products because it is bulk forming and produces feelings of fullness. Several small studies indicated it is no more effective than placebo for weight loss. It may cause esophageal or intestinal obstruction if not taken with an adequate amount of water and may interfere with the absorption of other drugs if taken at the same time. Adverse effects include nausea, diarrhea, flatulence, and abdominal discomfort.

Hydroxycitric acid (in Citrimax and other supplements) apparently suppresses appetite in animals, but there are no reliable studies that indicate its effectiveness in humans. One 12-week study did not show weight loss.

Laxative and diuretic herbs (e.g., aloe, rhubarb root, buckthorn, cascara, senna, parsley, juniper, dandelion leaves) are found in several products such as Super Dieter's Tea, Trim-Maxx Tea, and Water Pill. These products cause a significant loss of body fluids and electrolytes, not fat. Adverse effects may include low serum potassium levels, with subsequent cardiac dysrhythmias and other heart problems. In addition, long-term use of laxatives may lead to loss of normal bowel function and the necessity for continued use (i.e., laxative dependency).

Nursing Process

Assessment

Assess each overweight or obese patient for factors contributing to overweight and health risks related to excess weight, regardless of the reason for the contact. Some specific assessment factors include the following:

- Assess usual drinking and eating patterns, including healthful (e.g., whole-grain breads and cereals, fruits, vegetables, low-fat dairy products) and unhealthful (e.g., sugar-containing beverages and desserts, fried foods, saturated fat, fast foods, high-calorie snack foods) intake. The best way is to ask the patient to keep a food diary for 2 or 3 days. If food intake is not written down, people tend to underestimate the amount and caloric content. (If available, consult a nutritionist to assess a patient's diet and work with the patient to improve health and weight status.)

- Assess any obviously overweight person for health problems caused or aggravated by excessive weight (e.g., elevated blood pressure, other cardiovascular problems, diabetes mellitus, sleep apnea, osteoarthritis and other musculoskeletal disorders).

- Calculate the body mass index (see Box 58-1) and measure waist circumference.

- Check available reports of laboratory tests. Overweight patients may have abnormally high values for total and LDL cholesterol, triglycerides, and blood sugar and low values for high-density lipoprotein (HDL) cholesterol. If no laboratory reports are available, ask patients if a health care provider has ever told them they have high cholesterol or blood sugar.

- List all prescription and nonprescription medications being taken and ask about vitamins, herbals, and other dietary supplements. Review the list for drugs used to treat health problems associated with obesity, drugs that may promote weight gain, and any products that may be used to promote weight loss.

- Assess usual patterns of physical activity and exercise, including work and recreational activities.

- Assess motivation to develop and adhere to a weight-management plan. Ask if there are concerns about weight; if there is interest in a weight-management program to improve health; and what methods, over-the-counter products, or herbal or dietary supplements have been previously used to reduce weight, if any. The nurse must be very tactful in eliciting information and assessing whether a patient would like assistance with weight management. If the nurse–patient contact stems from a health problem caused or aggravated by excessive weight, the nurse may use this information to help motivate the patient to lose weight and improve health.

Nursing Diagnoses

- Imbalanced Nutrition: More Than Body Requirements related to excessive caloric intake
- Disturbed Body Image related to excessive weight gain
- Deficient Knowledge: Weight management

Planning/Goals

The patient will

- Reduce the impact of excessive weight on chronic health problems
- Modify lifestyle behaviors toward weight loss and weight maintenance at a more healthful level
- Avoid overuse of anorexiant drugs
- Avoid unproven weight-loss dietary supplements

Interventions

- Support programs/efforts to help promote a healthful lifestyle and prevent obesity (e.g., in families and schools).
- Serve as a role model by maintaining a healthful lifestyle and weight.
- Serve as a reliable source of information about weight loss and weight-loss products and programs.
- For an obese patient who reports interest and motivation in losing weight, assist to formulate realistic goals. Patients often expect to rapidly lose large amounts of weight with little or no effort. Most treatment programs result in a weight loss of 10% of body weight or less.
- Discuss health risks of obesity and anticipated benefits of achieving and maintaining a healthier weight. Emphasize that losing 5% to 10% of body weight is a reasonable goal and can significantly reduce the medical problems associated with being overweight.
- Assist patients to identify factors that support weight-loss efforts (e.g., family and friend encouragement) and factors that sabotage weight-loss efforts (e.g., having high-calorie foods readily available, frequently eating at fast-food restaurants).
- Promote exercise and activity. For overweight and obese patients, exercise may decrease appetite and distract from eating behaviors as well as increase calorie expenditure. For very sedentary, physically unfit patients, emphasize that any exercise can be beneficial and to start slowly, increasing the amount and intensity as physical condition improves.
- Encourage any efforts toward improving diet and increasing exercise to improve health.

- Weigh patients at regular intervals and measure waist circumference periodically.
- Refer patients to a nutritionist when indicated.
- Be alert for the psychological consequences of obesity and refer patients for counseling if indicated.
- Refer overweight and obese children to pediatric obesity specialists when possible.

Evaluation

- Observe overweight or obese patients for food intake, weight loss, decreased waist circumference, and appropriate use of exercise and anorexiant drugs.

Applying Your Knowledge 58-2

In addition to proper administration of her medication, what strategies should you review with Ms. Vargas to assist her in being successful with weight loss?

Principles of Therapy

Strategies to Prevent Becoming Overweight and Obese

Preventing excessive weight gain is a major struggle for many Americans as they fight the "battle of the bulge" daily. Many people want to lose weight, often more for appearance than for health. However, many are also unwilling or unable to adapt their lifestyles toward more healthful eating, exercising, and weight-controlling habits. As a result, millions of dollars are spent annually on weight-loss diets, products, and programs in an effort to find an easy way to lose weight. Health care providers need to promote efforts to prevent overweight and obesity when possible. When prevention is not possible, efforts should be aimed toward early recognition and treatment, before obesity and major health problems develop. Some strategies include the following:

- Personally practice a healthful lifestyle, primarily for one's own health and well-being, but also to serve as a role model and proponent for healthful practices in daily life.
- Provide or assist others to obtain reliable information about healthful lifestyle habits. For example, the U.S. Department of Health and Human Services and the Department of Agriculture publish *Dietary Guidelines for Americans* every 5 years. The 2005 update is available online at www.health-ierus.gov/dietaryguidelines. Selected recommendations are listed in Patient Teaching Guidelines.
- Use reliable resources for information about nutrition and weight management (Box 58-4).
- Read labels on food products and minimize the use of high-calorie products.
- Reduce fat, sugar, and salt when preparing meals.

Patient Teaching Guidelines — Weight Management and Drugs That Aid Weight Loss

General Considerations

- Because of the extensive health problems associated with overweight and obesity, individuals whose weight is within a normal range should try to prevent excessive weight gain by practicing a healthful lifestyle in terms of diet and exercise. Following are selected recommendations from the *Dietary Guidelines for Americans 2005*, published by the U.S. Department of Health and Human Services and the Department of Agriculture in January 2005 (updated every 5 years; available online at www.healthierus.gov/dietaryguidelines).
  1. Eat a variety of foods daily (e.g., 6–11 servings of whole-grain bread and cereals, 2 cups of fruit, 2 1/2 cups of vegetables, three or more servings of low-fat milk or other dairy products). Also limit intake of saturated fat (e.g., in meats and whole-milk dairy products), trans fats (e.g., hydrogenated oils in many commercial baked goods and other products), cholesterol, added sugars, salt, and alcohol. With trans fats, the amount in commercial products must be listed on the Nutrition Facts label. In addition, many restaurants have reduced or eliminated trans fats in their cooking oils. Canola oil and olive oil are healthy fats, but they have a high calorie content (120 calories per tablespoon), which must be considered in weight control efforts.
  2. To maintain body weight in a healthy range, balance diet (i.e., calories gained) with exercise (i.e., calories used). To prevent gradual weight gain over time, make small decreases in food and beverage calories and increase physical activity. Engage in regular physical activity and reduce sedentary activities to promote health, psychological well-being, and a healthy body weight. To reduce the risk of chronic disease, engage in at least 30 to 60 minutes of moderate-intensity physical activity, above usual activity, at work or home on most days of the week. For most people, greater health benefits can be obtained by engaging in physical activity of more vigorous intensity or longer duration.
  3. Physical fitness can be developed or improved by including cardiovascular conditioning, stretching exercises for flexibility, and resistance exercises or calisthenics for muscle strength and endurance.
- Individuals who are already overweight or obese should try to lose weight and maintain a lower weight because the likelihood of serious health problems and early death increases as weight increases. However, try to emphasize goals for improvement in health status rather than losing a large amount of weight. Remember that even a modest weight loss of 10 to 30 lbs can benefit your health. Most people are unlikely to achieve their "ideal" weight, and having unrealistic expectations sets one up for failure in any weight-loss program.
- Obesity is considered a chronic disease that requires long-term treatment, much like the treatment of diabetes and hypertension. Weight loss can be induced by severe calorie restriction, but without lifestyle changes (e.g., in eating and activity behavior), body fat is invariably regained. The safest and most effective way to lose weight and keep it off is permanent lifestyle changes that involve eating less and exercising more. Reducing caloric intake by 500 to

1000 calories per day allows the loss of 1 to 2 lb of fat per week, respectively. Higher levels of physical activity can help with weight loss and prevent weight regain. Additional health benefits include lower rates of cardiovascular disease and death.

- Use available resources. For example, if unable to implement needed changes alone, consult a nutritionist, qualified obesity expert, or behavioral therapist. Such clinicians can help modify the eating, activity, and thinking habits that predispose to obesity.
- In addition to feeling better, health benefits of weight loss may include reduced blood pressure, reduced blood fats, less likelihood of having a heart attack or stroke, and less risk for development of diabetes mellitus.
- Any weight loss program should include a nutritionally adequate diet with decreased calories and increased exercise.
- Regular physical examinations and follow-up care are needed during weight loss programs.
- Although many weight-loss supplements are available and heavily advertised in newspapers, magazines, and television, none is considered safe and effective and none is recommended for use. If you do choose to use any of these products, notify your primary health care provider. Depending on your condition (i.e., whether you have chronic health problems such as diabetes mellitus, hypertension, or others), the medications you take, and so forth, some weight-loss supplements can be harmful to your health.
- Diet and exercise are recommended for people who want to lose a few pounds. Medications to aid weight loss are usually recommended only for people whose health is endangered (i.e., those who are overweight and have other risk factors for heart disease, and those who are obese).
- Read package inserts and other available information about the drug being taken, who should not take the drug, instructions and precautions for safe usage, and so forth. Keep the material for later reference if questions arise. If unclear about any aspect of the information, consult a health care provider before taking the drug.
- Appetite-suppressant drugs must be used correctly to avoid potentially serious adverse effects. Because most of these drugs stimulate the heart and the brain, adverse effects may include increased blood pressure, fast heartbeat, irregular heartbeat, heart attack, stroke, dizziness, nervousness, insomnia (if taken late in the day), and mental confusion. In addition, prolonged use of prescription drugs may lead to psychological dependence.
- Avoid over-the-counter decongestants and allergy, asthma, cold remedies, and weight-loss herbal or dietary supplements when taking a prescription appetite suppressant. The combination can cause serious adverse effects from excessive heart and brain stimulation.
- Inform health care providers when taking an appetite suppressant, mainly to avoid other drugs with similar effects.
- Orlistat (Xenical) is not an appetite suppressant and does not cause heart or brain stimulation. It works in the intestines to keep fats in foods from being absorbed. It should be taken with a low-fat diet. Adverse effects include fatty stools and bloating. It is available over-

the-counter as Alli, with the recommended dosage one-half that of prescription Xenical.

Self-Administration

■ Take appetite suppressants in the morning to decrease appetite during the day and avoid interference with sleep at night.
■ Do not crush or chew sustained-release products.
■ With sibutramine (Meridia):
  ■ Take once daily, with or without food.
  ■ Have blood pressure and heart rate checked at regular intervals (the drug increases them).

■ Notify a health care provider if a skin rash, hives, or other allergic reaction occurs.
■ With orlistat (Xenical, Alli):
  ■ Take one capsule with each main meal or up to 1 hour after a meal, up to three capsules daily. If you miss a meal or eat a meal with no fat, you may omit a dose of orlistat.
  ■ Take a multivitamin containing fat-soluble vitamins (A, D, E, and K) daily, at least 2 hours before or after taking orlistat. Orlistat prevents absorption of fat-soluble vitamins from food or multivitamin preparations if taken at the same time.

Box 58-4	**Web Sites for Information on Nutrition and Weight Loss**

Aim for a Healthy Weight (www.nhlbi.nih.gov/health/public/heart/obesity/lose_wt/index.htm)
American Dietetic Association (www.eatright.org)
American Institute for Cancer Research (AICR) (www.aicr.org)
Centers for Disease Control and Prevention (CDC) (www.cdc.gov)
ConsumerLab (www.consumerlab.com)
National Center for Complementary and Alternative Medicine (NCCAM) (www.nccam.nih.gov)
National Institutes of Health, National Institute of Diabetes and Digestive and Kidney Disease: Weight Control Network (www.niddk.nih.gov/HealthEducation/HealthNutrit)
Natural Medicines Comprehensive Database (www.naturaldatabase.com)
ShapeUp America (www.shapeup.org)
The Obesity Society (www.obesity.org)
Weight Watchers (www.weightwatchers.com)

Management of Overweight and Obese Patients

Treatment options for obesity include diet, exercise, behavioral modification, drug therapy, and, if these options fail, possibly referring a patient for bariatric (weight-loss) surgery. The safest and most effective treatment for most people usually includes a combination of diet, exercise, and behavioral modification. Drug therapy and bariatric surgery are recommended only for seriously overweight people with major medical problems that can be improved by weight loss. In addition, neither of these treatments is a substitute for the necessary changes in eating and physical activity patterns.

The NHLBI issued a report entitled "Clinical Guidelines on the Identification, Evaluation and Treatment of Over-weight and Obesity in Adults," which is available at www.nhlbi.nih.gov/guidelines/obesity/ob_gdlns.htm; its recommendations are summarized in Box 58-5.

In addition to the NHLBI guidelines, additional recommendations and comments include the following:

■ Emphasize health benefits of weight reduction. There is strong evidence that weight loss reduces risk factors for cardiovascular disease, including blood pressure, serum triglycerides, and total and LDL cholesterol. It also increases HDL cholesterol. In addition, in overweight and obese people without diabetes, weight loss reduces blood glucose levels and the risk for development of type 2 diabetes.

■ For people who already have type 2 diabetes, weight loss reduces blood levels of glucose and glycosylated (A_{1c}) hemoglobin. These effects make the diabetes easier to manage, reduce complications of diabetes, and may allow smaller doses of antidiabetic medications. For people who already have hypertension, losing excess weight reduces blood pressure and may reduce the number or amount of antihypertensive drugs. For people who already have dyslipidemias, blood lipid profiles improve with weight loss.

■ Weight-loss diets wax and wane in popularity with the American public (Box 58-6). Although all of them can lead to weight loss if adhered to long enough, some are healthier than others and most are discarded before significant weight loss is achieved. Actually, any diet that reduces caloric intake in relation to caloric expenditure can lead to weight loss, and adherence is probably more important than the particular diet. Regardless of what some diet gurus and others say, total caloric intake must be considered because it is a major determinant of weight loss, gain, or maintenance.

■ Various formula diets or meal-replacement programs are available. The good ones contain high-quality protein, sugar as fructose, and a moderate amount of monounsaturated fat. The usual recommendation is to replace two meals daily for weight loss and one meal for weight maintenance. They can also be used as single meal replacements.

■ Although both calorie-reduced diets and sufficient exercise can lead to weight loss and maintenance, the NHLBI guide-

Box 58-5	NHLBI Report: "Clinical Guidelines on the Identification, Evaluation and Treatment of Overweight and Obesity in Adults"

■ Weight loss reduces health problems of individuals: decrease blood pressure if hypertensive; lower elevated levels of total cholesterol, LDL cholesterol, and triglycerides and raise low levels of HDL cholesterol if dyslipidemic; lower elevated blood glucose levels in persons with type 2 diabetes.

■ BMI is used to assess overweight and obesity and to estimate disease risks. Measure waist circumference initially and periodically to assess abdominal fat content. Weigh regularly to monitor body weight for gain, loss, or maintenance.

■ The initial goal of weight-loss therapy should be to reduce body weight by about 10% from baseline, at a rate of 1 to 2 pounds per week for a period of 6 months. Steady weight loss over a longer period reduces fat stores in the body, limits the loss of vital protein tissues, and avoids the sharp decline in metabolic rate that accompanies rapid weight loss. After weight loss, weight maintenance should be the priority goal, because weight regain is a problem with all weight-loss programs. In some cases, after a period of weight maintenance, additional losses may be desirable.

■ Dietary recommendations include low-calorie diets for weight loss, mainly reducing caloric intake by 500 to 1000 calories daily. Reducing dietary fat can reduce calories. However, reducing dietary fat without reducing total caloric intake does not produce weight loss. Vitamin and mineral supplements that meet age-related requirements are usually recommended with weight-loss programs that provide less than 1200 kcal for women or 1800 kcal for men.

■ Physical activity recommendations should be part of any weight-management program because physical activity contributes to weight loss, may decrease abdominal fat, increases cardiorespiratory fitness, and helps with weight maintenance. Initially, physical activity for 30 to 45 minutes, 3 to 5 days a week, is encouraged. Long-term, adults should try to accumulate at least 30 minutes or more of moderate-intensity physical activity on most days of the week.

■ In general, weight-loss and weight-maintenance programs should combine reduced-calorie diets, increased physical activity, and behavior therapy. After weight loss, weight-loss maintenance with dietary therapy, physical activity, and behavior therapy should be continued indefinitely. Drug therapy can also be used. However, drug safety and efficacy beyond 1 to 2 years of total treatment have not been established.

■ Behavioral modification can be helpful in a weight-loss program. The goals are to help patients modify their eating, activity, and thinking habits that predispose to obesity. Techniques include identifying triggers that promote overeating and barriers that keep one from adopting a more healthful lifestyle. One strategy is keeping an accurate record of food/calorie intake and physical activity (most people tend to underestimate food intake and overestimate activity). In addition, stress management, stimulus control, and social support are helpful. Patients who eat more when stressed can learn to manage stress more healthfully. Counseling by a behavioral therapist may be needed. Stimulus control has to do with avoiding or minimizing circumstances that promote overeating (e.g., cooking calorie-dense foods; having high-calorie snacks and "junk food" readily available; eating high-fat, high-calorie foods at fast-food restaurants). Social support involves family, friends, co-workers, and fellow dieters who encourage weight-loss efforts rather than sabotage them by urging one to eat high-calorie foods. In general, weight-loss regimens that use several of these strategies are more effective.

lines are based on studies indicating that a combination of the two strategies is more effective than either alone. However, many overweight and obese people may be physically unfit and unable or unwilling to increase activity. Thus, activity should be started slowly and gradually increased, with the goal of exercise becoming part of the daily routine. Aerobic exercise increases the metabolic rate during and for approximately 1 hour after activity. Consistent adherence to a reduced-calorie diet and exercise routine is a major factor in achieving weight control and health benefits.

■ For any patients following a weight-loss regimen, provide psychological support and positive reinforcement for efforts toward weight management. Programs or support groups involving supervision or regular participation within a social group appear to be more successful over time.

However, a systematic review that evaluated major commercial weight-loss programs found few high-quality studies. In general, there was more evidence of success with the Weight Watchers program than with Health Management Resources, OPTIFAST, Jenny Craig, or L.A. Weight Loss.

■ There seems to be increasing support for the long-term use of weight-loss medications in treatment of obesity. When drug therapy is indicated, a single drug in the lowest effective dose is recommended. As with most other drugs, low doses decrease risks of adverse drug effects. In addition, the National Institutes of Health do not recommend combining weight-loss medications except in the context of clinical trials. Thus far, studies indicate that combining sibutramine and orlistat has no additional benefit over using one of the drugs alone.

Box 58-6	Characteristics of Selected Diets

Various diets all work if total caloric intake is less than energy expenditure. Many diets are quite restrictive, however, and most people soon drop out and rapidly regain the weight they lost. As a result, the best "diet" is nutritionally adequate except for calories and is one the person can follow long term.

Low calorie. These diets provide 1200 to 1600 kcal per day. The usual recommendation is to reduce caloric intake by 500 to 1000 calories daily, to allow weight loss of 1 to 2 lb weekly. This rate of loss is likely to be more successful in terms of weight loss, and continuing a reduced-calorie diet promotes weight maintenance rather than weight regain. *Note that losing weight through diet alone, without increased physical activity, is unlikely to improve cardiovascular health.*

Very-low calorie. These diets usually consist of 800 calories or fewer per day. Numerous commercial products that promise "magical" results have been marketed. These diets result in rapid initial weight losses due mainly to diuresis and loss of sodium and water. Multiple health risks accompany such diets, including abnormalities in electrolytes, trace elements, and vitamins; gout; gallstones; cold intolerance; fatigue; lightheadedness; anemia; menstrual irregularities; and other problems.

The National Institutes of Health (NIH) recommends against using diets that provide fewer than 800 calories daily. If used at all, very–low-calorie diets should be used intermittently, for short periods, with a diet that maintains weight and is more nutritionally adequate.

Low fat. These diets do not cause significant weight loss unless caloric intake is reduced. Because fats are energy dense (9 cal/g), reducing fat is a practical way to reduce caloric intake. For both health and weight loss, current recommendations emphasize reducing intake of "bad" fats (e.g., saturated and trans fats) but including healthy mono- and polyunsaturated fats (e.g., olive and canola oil) within the caloric allotment.

Low carbohydrate. The weight loss that occurs with these diets (e.g., Atkins and South Beach) is attributed to caloric reduction or water loss rather than to the carbohydrate restriction. There have been no studies evaluating the long-term safety of these diets. In addition, numerous adverse effects may occur (e.g., constipation, dehydration, dyslipidemia, electrolyte imbalance, headache, aggravation of renal impairment, and hyperuricemia leading to gout).

Applying Your Knowledge 58-3

Ms. Vargas says she needs to lose 140 pounds and would like to accomplish this by her next birthday. How should you respond?

Management of Obesity in Special Populations

Managing Obesity in Children

Children in general need increased amounts of protein, carbohydrate, and fat in proportion to their size to support growth and increased physical activity. However, reports of childhood obesity have greatly increased over recent years, and childhood obesity has become a major public health concern. Therefore, the goal of nutrition is to meet needs without promoting obesity. When possible, specialists in childhood obesity should design and supervise treatment programs.

Efforts are needed toward both prevention and treatment of childhood obesity. Prevention should focus on identifying at-risk and overweight children and adolescents at an early stage, educating families about the health consequences of being overweight, and encouraging weight-control measures (e.g., a more active lifestyle, a low-fat diet, regular meals, avoidance of high-calorie snacks, drinking water instead of calorie-containing beverages, decreasing the time spent watch-

ing television and playing computer games). These measures are implemented successfully mainly within a family unit, and family support is needed to assist the child in weight control and a more healthful lifestyle. In addition, schools should teach children the basic principles of good nutrition and why eating a balanced diet is important to health.

Pediatric clinicians recommend treatment for children and adolescents who are overweight and have complications of obesity and for all children who are obese. Treatment of childhood obesity should focus on healthy eating and increasing physical activity. In general, children should not be put on "diets." For a child who is overweight, the recommended goal is to maintain weight or slow the rate of weight gain so that weight and BMI gradually decline as the child grows in height. If the child has already reached his or her anticipated adult weight, maintenance of that weight and prevention of additional gain should be the long-term treatment goal. If the child already exceeds the optimal adult weight, the goal of treatment should be a slow weight loss of 10 to 12 pounds per year until the optimal adult weight is reached. As with adults, increased activity is required for successful weight loss or management in children.

Family involvement and support are vital to children's weight management. Actually, the goal beyond weight control for a child is to develop healthier eating and exercise habits for long-term health benefits for the entire family. Studies indicate that children who eat adequate amounts of fruits, vegetables, and dairy products tend to continue these healthy eating habits. In general, young children who learn to eat a healthy diet are likely to reap the benefits throughout their lives. Improved diets and increased activity are unlikely to occur without active participation of parents and other caregivers.

Although drug therapy has not been generally recommended for treatment of childhood obesity, orlistat is approved for use in children aged 12 to 16 years and is considered safe and effective for weight reduction in overweight adolescents. As with adults, common adverse effects in clinical trials were gastrointestinal (e.g., diarrhea, flatulence) and reduced concentrations of fat-soluble vitamins. Sibutramine has not been studied in children under 16 years of age but is effective in reducing weight in adolescents. However, the drug may cause severe adverse effects (e.g., elevated blood pressure, tachycardia, depression, and suicidal ideations) and must be used cautiously. Metformin is undergoing investigation as a weight-loss drug in obese adolescents, both in nondiabetics and in those who have developed insulin resistance or type 2 diabetes.

Managing Obesity in Older Adults

Overweight and obesity are common among older adults. Although caloric needs are usually decreased, primarily because of slowed metabolism and decreased physical activity, most people continue usual eating patterns. With the high incidence of atherosclerosis and cardiovascular disease in older adults, it is especially important that intake of saturated and trans fats be reduced. Anorexiant drugs should be used very cautiously, if at all, because older adults often have cardiovascular, renal, or hepatic impairments that increase risks of adverse drug effects. With orlistat, the manufacturer recommends conservative use and dosage because older adults often have decreased renal, cardiac, and hepatic function.

Managing Obesity in Patients With Renal Impairment

In relation to drugs for obesity, little information is available about their use in patients with renal impairment. With sibutramine, dosage reductions are not recommended with mild to moderate impairment because the drug and its active metabolites are eliminated by the liver. However, some inactive metabolites are also formed and these are excreted renally. The drug is contraindicated in patients with severe renal impairment.

Managing Obesity in Patients With Hepatic Impairment

In relation to drugs for obesity, little information is available about their use in patients with hepatic impairment. Because sibutramine is metabolized in the liver, it is contraindicated in patients with severe hepatic impairment.

Managing Obesity in Home Care

The home care nurse may be involved with weight-management issues in almost any home care setting. Because nutrition, exercise, and weight control are so important to health, the home care nurse should take advantage of any opportunity for health promotion in this area. Health promotion may involve assessing the nutritional and fitness status of all members of the household and providing counseling or other assistance to improve health status. Those who are obviously overweight or who have obesity-related health problems must be approached with diplomacy and tact; they have probably tried repeatedly to lose weight and been told by previous health care providers that they need to lose weight. The home care nurse should be able to provide accurate information about realistic and successful techniques for losing weight and keeping it off; health benefits of even modest weight loss; and reasons to avoid "fad" diets, weight-loss herbal and dietary supplements, and programs that promise rapid and easy weight loss with little effort.

 Applying Your Knowledge 58-4

How Can You Avoid This Medication Error?

Ms. Vargas' prescription is for orlistat three times a day. She takes the dose with breakfast, lunch, and dinner. She has a meeting today that runs through lunch and so she skips lunch but takes her pill on time.

Nursing Actions | **Drugs for Weight Loss and Maintenance**

NURSING ACTIONS	RATIONALE/EXPLANATION
1. Administer accurately	
a. With phentermine:	
(1) Give single-dose drugs in the early morning.	For maximum appetite-suppressant effects during the day
(2) Give multiple-dose preparations 30 minutes before meals and the last dose of the day about 6 hours before bedtime.	For maximum appetite-suppressant effects at mealtime and to avoid interference with sleep from the drug's stimulating effects on the central nervous system (CNS)
b. With sibutramine, give once daily, in the morning.	
c. With orlistat, give one capsule with each main meal or up to 1 hour after a meal, up to three capsules daily. If a meal is missed or contains no fat, the dose can be omitted.	The drug needs to be in the gastrointestinal tract when fat-containing foods are eaten, to prevent fat absorption.

NURSING ACTIONS	RATIONALE/EXPLANATION
2. Observe for therapeutic effects a. With phentermine and sibutramine, observe for decreased caloric intake and weight loss.	The recommended rate of weight loss is 1–2 lb weekly.
b. With orlistat, observe for weight loss and improvements in health status (e.g., reduced LDL cholesterol, elevated HDL cholesterol, improved glycemic control, and reduced blood pressure).	Most weight loss occurs in the first 6 months of therapy, but the reduced weight can be maintained as long as orlistat is continued. The metabolic improvements are very beneficial for people with obesity-related health problems such as diabetes, dyslipidemia, hypertension, and metabolic syndrome.

3. Observe for adverse effects
  a. With phentermine and sibutramine, observe for:
    (1) Nervousness, insomnia, hyperactivity
	These effects result from excessive stimulation of the CNS. They are more likely to occur with large doses or too-frequent administration.

(2) Hypertension	Anorexiant drugs stimulate the sympathetic nervous system and may cause or aggravate hypertension.
(3) Development of tolerance to appetite-suppressant effects	This usually occurs within 4–6 weeks and is an indication for discontinuing drug administration. Continued administration and/or large doses do not maintain appetite-suppressant effects. Instead, they increase the incidence of adverse effects.
b. With orlistat, observe for abdominal cramping, gas pains, diarrhea, and fatty stools.	These effects commonly occur. They usually improve within a few weeks of continued drug use, but worsen with a high intake of dietary fat, which should be avoided.
4. Observe for drug interactions a. Drugs that *increase* effects of phentermine and sibutramine:	
(1) Antidepressants, tricyclic	May increase hypertensive effects
(2) Other CNS stimulants	Additive stimulant effects
(3) Other sympathomimetic drugs (e.g., epinephrine)	Additive hypertensive and other cardiovascular effects
b. Drugs that *decrease* effects of phentermine and sibutramine:	
(1) Antihypertensive drugs	Decrease blood pressure–raising effects of anorexiants
(2) CNS depressants (e.g., alcohol)	Antagonize or decrease effects
c. Drugs that *increase* effects of sibutramine:	
(1) Adrenergics (e.g., epinephrine, pseudoephedrine)	Additive increases in blood pressure
(2) Antidepressants (tricyclic antidepressants [TCAs; e.g., amitriptyline], selective serotonin reuptake inhibitors [SSRIs; e.g., fluoxetine])	TCAs and sibutramine increase levels of norepinephrine and serotonin in the brain; SSRIs increase serotonin levels. Concurrent use of these drugs may cause excessive CNS stimulation, hypertension, and serotonin syndrome and should be avoided.
(3) Antifungals (e.g., itraconazole and related azoles)	Decrease metabolism and may increase adverse effects and toxicity of sibutramine
(4) Antimigraine triptans (e.g., sumatriptan)	Additive serotonin effects
(5) Lithium	Additive serotonin effect

Key Concepts

- Overweight and obesity are major concerns because of their association with numerous health problems, including diabetes, hypertension, other cardiovascular disorders, and muscle and joint disorders.

- Ingesting 500 calories more per day than those used in exercise and physical activity leads to a weight gain of one pound in 1 week; decreasing caloric intake or increasing caloric output of 500 calories per day for 1 week leads to a weight loss of one pound.

- Reducing caloric intake and increasing caloric expenditure are part of any successful weight-loss program.

■ Weight-loss drugs are generally recommended only for people who are seriously overweight or have health problems associated with or aggravated by obesity.

■ Many people lose weight but regain it within a few months if they do not change their lifestyle habits toward eating more healthfully and exercising more.

Review and Application Exercises

Short Answer Exercises

1. Calculate the BMI for yourself, one or more members of your family, or a patient.

2. Assess eating and physical activity habits of yourself, one or more members of your family, or a patient. In general, do these habits promote health or obesity?

3. If you, the family member, or the patient has health problems related to overweight and obesity, list at least three things that can be done to improve health.

4. Debate whether or not it is important that health care providers demonstrate healthful practices in diet, exercise, and weight control to the general public.

5. With an overweight or obese patient who wants to lose weight, what are some nursing interventions to assist and support the patient?

6. List advantages and disadvantages of drug therapy for weight loss or maintenance.

NCLEX-Style Questions

7. In counseling a patient about weight loss diets, the nurse knows that a recommended low-calorie or reduced-calorie diet
   a. provides about 500 to 800 kcal per day.
   b. reduces daily intake to about 1800 kcal per day.
   c. is required for weight loss.
   d. focuses on high-fat, high-carbohydrate foods

8. Drug therapy for weight management may be prescribed for patients with which of the following?
   a. BMI of 22 and a desire to lose 10 pounds
   b. BMI of 24.5 and physically fit
   c. BMI of 27 or more with weight-related health problems
   d. BMI of 25–29 and healthy

9. Sibutramine (Meridia) may be contraindicated for patients with which of the following disorders?
   a. cardiovascular disease
   b. diabetes mellitus
   c. chronic fatigue syndrome
   d. gastroesophageal reflux disease

10. Orlistat (Xenical) aids weight loss by
    a. decreasing appetite
    b. increasing satiety and feelings of fullness
    c. increasing metabolism
    d. decreasing absorption of dietary fat

11. To decrease diarrhea with orlistat (Xenical), a patient should be instructed to
    a. avoid large amounts of fatty foods.
    b. drink eight glasses of water daily.
    c. avoid caffeine-containing beverages.
    d. increase physical activity.

Selected References

Baker, B. (2006). Weight loss and diet plans. *American Journal of Nursing, 106*, 52–59.

Baron, R. B. (2007). Nutrition. In S. J. McPhee, M. A. Papadakis, & L. M. Tierney, Jr. (Eds.), *Current medical diagnosis and treatment 2007* (46th ed., pp. 1279–1310). New York: McGraw-Hill.

Berkowitz, R. I., Fujioka, K., Daniels, S. R., Hoppin, A. G., Owen, S., Perry, A. C., et al. (2006). Effects of sibutramine treatment in obese adolescents. *Annals of Internal Medicine, 45*, 81–90.

Chanoine, J. P., Hampl, S., Jensen, C., Boldrin, M., & Hauptman, J. (2005). Effect of orlistat on weight and body composition in obese adolescents: A randomized controlled trial. *Journal of the American Medical Association, 293*, 2873–2883.

Daniels, J. (2006). Obesity: America's epidemic. *American Journal of Nursing, 106*, 40–49.

Drug facts and comparisons. (Updated monthly). St. Louis, MO: Facts and Comparisons.

Dunican, K. C., Desilets, A. R., & Montalbano, J. K. (2007). Pharmacotherapeutic options for overweight adolescents. *Annals of Pharmacotherapy, 41*, 1445–1455.

Expert Panel. (1998). Clinical guidelines on the identification, evaluation, and treatment of overweight and obesity in adults: Executive summary. *American Journal of Clinical Nutrition, 68*, 899–917.

Guyton, A. C., & Hall, J. E. (2006). *Textbook of medical physiology* (11th ed., pp. 865–880). Philadelphia: Elsevier Saunders.

Pereira, M., Kartashov, A. I., Ebbeling, C. B., et al. (2005). Fast-food habits, weight gain, and insulin resistance (the CARDIA study): 15-Year prospective analysis. *Lancet, 365*, 36–42.

Pleuss, J. (2005). Alterations in nutritional status. In C. M. Porth (Ed.), *Pathophysiology: Concepts of altered health states* (7th ed., pp. 217–238). Philadelphia: Lippincott Williams & Wilkins.

Raykowski, L. K. (2006). Popular diets: What practitioners should know. *Nurse Practitioner, 31*, 55–57.

Rosenbaum, M. (2007). Epidemiology of pediatric obesity. *Pediatric Annals, 36*, 89–94.

Sallmen, M., Sandler, D., Hoppin, J., Blair, A., & Baird, D. (2006). Reduced fertility among overweight and obese men. *Epidemiology, 17*, 520–523.

Small, L., Anderson, D., & Melnyk, B. M. (2007). Prevention and early treatment of overweight and obesity in young children: A critical review and appraisal of the evidence. *Pediatric Nursing, 33,* 149–161.

Smeltzer, S. C., Bare, B. G., Hinkle, J. L., & Cheever, K. H. (2008). *Brunner & Suddarth's textbook of medical-surgical nursing* (11th ed.). Philadelphia: Lippincott Williams & Wilkins.

St. Peter, J. V., & Khan, M. A. (2005). Obesity. In J. T. DiPiro, R. L. Talbert, G. C. Yee, G. R. Matzke, B. G. Wells, & L. M. Posey (Eds.), *Pharmacotherapy: A pathophysiologic approach* (6th ed., pp. 2659–2676). New York: McGraw-Hill.

Taylor, E. D., Theim, K. R., Mirch, M. C., Ghorbani, S., Tanofsky-Kraff, M., Adler-Wiles, D. C., et al. (2006). Orthopedic complications of overweight in children and adolescents. *Pediatrics, 117,* 2167–2174.

Tsai, A. G., & Wadden, T. A. (2005). Systematic review: An evaluation of major commercial weight loss programs in the United States. *Annals of Internal Medicine, 142,* 56–66.

Drugs Used for Peptic Ulcer and Acid Reflux Disorders

LEARNING OBJECTIVES

After studying this chapter, you will be able to:

1. Describe the main elements of peptic ulcer disease and gastroesophageal reflux disease (GERD).
2. Differentiate the types of drugs used to treat peptic ulcers and acid reflux disorders.
3. Discuss the advantages and disadvantages of proton pump inhibitors.
4. Differentiate between prescription and over-the-counter uses of histamine$_2$ receptor blocking agents.
5. Discuss significant drug–drug interactions with cimetidine.
6. Describe characteristics, uses, and effects of selected antacids.
7. Discuss the rationale for using combination antacid products.
8. Teach patients nonpharmacologic measures to manage peptic ulcers and GERD.

Apply Your Knowledge

Kathleen Daniels is a 54-year-old woman who has chronic GERD. She is prescribed rabeprazole 20 mg PO daily. She also takes OTC famotidine 10 mg twice a day as needed to control her heartburn. When needed, she also takes Mylanta 5 mL.

Introduction

Drugs to prevent or treat peptic ulcer and acid reflux disorders consist of several groups of drugs, most of which alter gastric acid and its effects on the mucosa of the upper gastrointestinal (UGI) tract. To aid understanding of drug effects, peptic ulcer disease and gastroesophageal reflux disease (GERD) are described below; related UGI disorders are described in Box 59-1.

Peptic Ulcer Disease

Peptic ulcer disease is characterized by ulcer formation in the esophagus, stomach, or duodenum, areas of the gastrointestinal (GI) mucosa that are exposed to gastric acid and pepsin. *Gastric* and *duodenal ulcers* are more common then esophageal ulcers.

Peptic ulcers are attributed to an imbalance between cell-destructive and cell-protective effects (i.e., presence of increased destructive mechanisms or presence of decreased protective mechanisms). Cell-destructive effects include those of gastric acid (hydrochloric acid), pepsin, *Helicobacter pylori* (*H. pylori*) infection, and ingestion of *nonsteroidal anti-inflammatory drugs (NSAIDs)*. Gastric acid, a strong acid that can digest the stomach wall, is secreted by parietal cells in the mucosa of the stomach antrum, near the pylorus. The parietal cells contain receptors for acetyl-

Box 59-1	Selected Upper Gastrointestinal Disorders

Gastritis

Gastritis, a common disorder, is an acute or chronic inflammatory reaction of gastric mucosa. Patients with gastric or duodenal ulcers usually also have gastritis. *Acute gastritis* (also called *gastropathy*) usually results from irritation of the gastric mucosa by such substances as alcohol, aspirin or other nonsteroidal anti-inflammatory drugs (NSAIDs), and others. *Chronic gastritis* is usually caused by *Helicobacter pylori* infection and it persists unless the infection is treated effectively. *H. pylori* organisms may cause gastritis and ulceration by producing enzymes (e.g., urease, others) that break down mucosa; they also alter secretion of gastric acid.

Nonsteroidal Anti-Inflammatory Drug Gastropathy

NSAID gastropathy indicates damage to gastroduodenal mucosa by aspirin and other NSAIDs. The damage may range from minor superficial erosions to ulceration and bleeding. NSAID gastropathy is one of the most common causes of gastric ulcers, and it may cause duodenal ulcers as well. Many people take NSAIDs daily for pain, arthritis, and other conditions. Chronic ingestion of NSAIDs causes local irritation of gastroduodenal mucosa; inhibits the synthesis of prostaglandins (which normally protect gastric mucosa by inhibiting acid secretion, stimulating secretion of bicarbonate and mucus, and maintaining mucosal blood flow); and increases the synthesis of leukotrienes and possibly other inflammatory substances that may contribute to mucosal injury.

Stress Ulcers

Stress ulcers indicate gastric mucosal lesions that develop in patients who are critically ill from trauma, shock, hemorrhage,

sepsis, burns, acute respiratory distress syndrome, major surgical procedures, or other severe illnesses. The lesions may be single or multiple ulcers or erosions. Stress ulcers are usually manifested by painless upper gastrointestinal (GI) bleeding. The frequency of occurrence has decreased, possibly because of improved management of sepsis, hypovolemia, and other disorders associated with critical illness and the prophylactic use of antiulcer drugs. However there is concern about inappropriate use of stress ulcer prophylaxis (See Evidence Based Practice Box).

Although the exact mechanisms of stress ulcer formation are unknown, several factors are thought to play a role, including mucosal ischemia, reflux of bile salts into the stomach, reduced GI-tract motility, and systemic acidosis. Acidosis increases severity of lesions, and correction of acidosis decreases their formation. In addition, lesions do not form if the pH of gastric fluids is kept at about 3.5 or above and lesions apparently form only when mucosal blood flow is diminished.

Zollinger-Ellison Syndrome

Zollinger-Ellison syndrome is a rare condition characterized by excessive secretion of gastric acid and a high incidence of ulcers. It is caused by gastrin-secreting tumors in the pancreas, stomach, or duodenum. Approximately two thirds of the gastrinomas are malignant. Symptoms are those of peptic ulcer disease, and diagnosis is based on high levels of serum gastrin and gastric acid. Treatment may involve long-term use of a proton pump inhibitor to diminish gastric acid, or surgical excision.

---

choline, gastrin, and histamine, substances that stimulate gastric acid production. Acetylcholine is released by vagus nerve endings in response to stimuli, such as thinking about or ingesting food. Gastrin is a hormone released by cells in the stomach and duodenum in response to food ingestion and stretching of the stomach wall. It is secreted into the bloodstream and eventually circulated to the parietal cells. Histamine is released from cells in the gastric mucosa and diffuses into nearby parietal cells. An enzyme system (*hydrogen, potassium adenosine triphosphatase*, or H^+, K^+-ATPase) catalyzes the production of gastric acid and acts as a gastric acid (proton) pump to move gastric acid from parietal cells in the mucosal lining of the stomach into the stomach lumen.

Pepsin is a proteolytic enzyme that helps digest protein foods and also can digest the stomach wall. Pepsin is derived from a precursor called pepsinogen, which is secreted by chief cells in the gastric mucosa. Pepsinogen is converted to pepsin only in a highly acidic environment (i.e., when the pH of gastric juices is 3 or less).

H. pylori is a gram-negative bacterium found in the gastric mucosa of most patients with chronic *gastritis*, about 75% of patients with gastric ulcers, and more than 90% of patients with duodenal ulcers. It is spread mainly by the fecal–oral route. However, iatrogenic spread by contaminated endoscopes, biopsy forceps, and nasogastric tubes has also occurred. After it moves into the body, the organism colonizes the mucus-secreting epithelial cells of the stomach mucosa and is thought to produce gastritis and ulceration by impairing mucosal function. Eradication of the organism accelerates ulcer healing and significantly decreases the rate of ulcer recurrence.

Cell-protective effects (e.g., secretion of mucus and bicarbonate, dilution of gastric acid by food and secretions, prevention of diffusion of hydrochloric acid from the stomach lumen back into the gastric mucosal lining, the presence of prostaglandin E, alkalinization of gastric secretions by pancreatic juices and bile, perhaps other mechanisms) normally prevent autodigestion of stomach and duodenal tissues and ulcer formation.

A gastric or duodenal ulcer may penetrate only the mucosal surface or it may extend into the smooth muscle layers. When superficial lesions heal, no defects remain. When smooth muscle heals, however, scar tissue remains and the mucosa that regenerates to cover the scarred muscle tissue may be defective. These defects contribute to repeated episodes of ulceration.

Although there is considerable overlap in etiology, clinical manifestations, and treatment of gastric and duodenal ulcers, there are differences as well. Gastric ulcers (which may be preceded by less severe mucosal defects such as erosions or gastritis) are often associated with stress (e.g., major trauma, severe medical illness), NSAID ingestion, or *H. pylori* infection of the stomach. They are often manifested by painless bleeding and take longer to heal than duodenal ulcers. Gastric ulcers associated with stress may occur in any age group and are usually acute in nature; those associated with *H. pylori* infection or NSAID ingestion are more likely to occur in older adults, especially in the sixth and seventh decades, and to be chronic in nature. Duodenal ulcers are strongly associated with *H. pylori* infection and NSAID ingestion, may occur at any age, occur about equally in men and women, are often manifested by abdominal pain, and are usually chronic in nature. They are also associated with cigarette smoking. Compared with nonsmokers, smokers are more likely to develop duodenal ulcers, their ulcers heal more slowly with treatment, and the ulcers recur more rapidly.

Gastroesophageal Reflux Disease

Gastroesophageal reflux disease (GERD), the most common disorder of the esophagus, is characterized by regurgitation of gastric contents into the esophagus and exposure of esophageal mucosa to gastric acid and pepsin. The same amount of acid-pepsin exposure may lead to different amounts of mucosal damage, possibly related to individual variations in esophageal mucosal resistance.

Acid reflux often occurs after the evening meal and decreases during sleep. The main symptom is heartburn (pyrosis), which increases with a recumbent position or bending over. Effortless regurgitation of acidic fluid into the mouth, especially after a meal and at night, is often indicative of GERD. Depending on the frequency and extent of acid-pepsin reflux, GERD may result in mild to severe esophagitis or esophageal ulceration. Pain on swallowing usually means erosive or ulcerative esophagitis.

The main cause of GERD is thought to be an incompetent lower esophageal sphincter (LES). Normally, the LES is contracted or closed and prevents the reflux of gastric contents. It opens or relaxes on swallowing to allow passage of food or fluid, then contracts again. Several circumstances contribute to impaired contraction of the LES and the resulting reflux, including foods (e.g., fats, chocolate), fluids (e.g., alcohol, caffeinated beverages), medications (e.g., beta adrenergics, calcium channel blockers, nitrates), gastric distention, cigarette smoking, and recumbent posture.

GERD occurs in men, women, and children but is especially common during pregnancy and after 40 years of age.

Classifications and Individual Drugs

Drugs used in the treatment of acid-peptic disorders promote healing of lesions and prevent recurrence of lesions by decreasing cell-destructive effects or increasing cell-protective effects. Several types of drugs are used, alone and in various combinations. *Antacids* neutralize gastric acid and decrease pepsin production, antimicrobials and bismuth can eliminate *H. pylori* infection, *histamine$_2$ receptor antagonists (H$_2$RAs)* and *proton pump inhibitors (PPIs)* decrease gastric acid secretion, sucralfate provides a barrier between mucosal erosions or ulcers and gastric secretions, and misoprostol restores prostaglandin activity. Types of drugs and individual agents are described in the following sections; dosages are listed in the Drugs at a Glance tables.

Antacids

Antacids are alkaline substances that neutralize acids. They react with hydrochloric acid in the stomach to produce neutral, less acidic, or poorly absorbed salts and to raise the pH (alkalinity) of gastric secretions. Raising the pH to approximately 3.5 neutralizes more than 90% of gastric acid and inhibits conversion of pepsinogen to pepsin. Commonly used antacids are aluminum, magnesium, and calcium compounds. Table 59-1 provides information for representative antacid products.

Antacids differ in the amounts needed to neutralize gastric acid (50–80 mEq of acid is produced hourly), in onset of action, and in adverse effects. Aluminum compounds have a low neutralizing capacity (i.e., relatively large doses are required) and a slow onset of action. They can cause constipation. In people who ingest large amounts of aluminum-based antacids over a long period, hypophosphatemia and osteomalacia may develop because aluminum combines with phosphates in the GI tract and prevents phosphate absorption. Aluminum compounds are rarely used alone for acid-peptic disorders. Magnesium-based antacids have a high neutralizing capacity and a rapid onset of action. They may cause diarrhea and hypermagnesemia. Calcium compounds have a rapid onset of action but may cause hypercalcemia and hypersecretion of gastric acid ("acid rebound") due to stimulation of gastrin release, if large doses are used. Consequently, calcium compounds are rarely used in peptic ulcer disease.

Commonly used antacids are mixtures of aluminum hydroxide and magnesium hydroxide (e.g., Gelusil, Mylanta, Maalox). Some antacid mixtures contain other ingredients, such as simethicone (contained in Mylanta) or alginic acid. **Simethicone** is an antiflatulent drug available alone as Mylicon. When added to antacids, simethicone does not affect gastric acidity. It reportedly decreases gas bubbles, thereby reducing GI distention and abdominal discomfort. Alginic acid (e.g., in Gaviscon) produces a foamy, viscous layer on top of gastric acid and thereby decreases backflow of gastric acid onto esophageal mucosa while the person is in an upright position.

Table 59-1	Drugs at a Glance: Representative Antacid Products				

| | **COMPONENTS** | | | | |
Trade Name	**Magnesium Oxide or Hydroxide**	**Aluminum Hydroxide**	**Calcium Carbonate**	**Other**	**Route and Dosage Ranges (Adults)**
Amphojel		300 or 600 mg/tab			PO 600 mg 5 or 6 times daily
Gelusil	200 mg/tab	200 mg/tab		Simethicone 25 mg/tab	PO 10 or more mL or 2 or more tablets after meals and at bedtime or as directed by physician to a maximum of 12 tablets or tsp/24 h
Maalox suspension	200 mg/5 mL	225 mg/5 mL			PO 30 mL 4 times daily, after meals and at bedtime or as directed by physician; maximal dose, 16 tsp/24 h
Mylanta	200 mg/tab, 200 mg/5 mL	200 mg/tab, 200 mg/5 mL		Simethicone 25 mg/tab, 20 mg/5 mL	PO 5–10 mL or 1–2 tablets q2–4h, between meals and at bedtime or as directed by physician.
Mylanta Double strength	400 mg/tab, 400 mg/5 mL	400 mg/tab, 400 mg/5 mL		Simethicone 30 mg/tab, 30 mg/5 mL	Same as Mylanta
Titralac			420 mg/tab, 1 g/5 mL	Glycine 180 mg/tab, 300 mg/5 mL	PO 1 tsp or 2 tablets, after meals or as directed by physician, to maximal dose of 19 tablets or 8 tsp/24 h

Antacids act primarily in the stomach and are used to prevent or treat peptic ulcer disease, GERD, esophagitis, heartburn, gastritis, GI bleeding, and *stress ulcers*. Aluminum-based antacids also are given to patients with chronic renal failure and hyperphosphatemia to decrease absorption of phosphates in food.

Magnesium-based antacids are contraindicated in patients with renal failure.

Helicobacter pylori Agents

Multiple drugs are required to eradicate *H. pylori* organisms and heal related ulcers. Effective combinations include two antimicrobials and a PPI or an H₂RA. For the antimicrobial component, two of the following drugs—**amoxicillin, clarithromycin, metronidazole,** or **tetracycline**—are used. A single antimicrobial agent is not used because of concern about emergence of drug-resistant *H. pylori* organisms. For patients with an active ulcer, adding an antisecretory drug (e.g., H₂RA or PPI) to an antimicrobial regimen accelerates symptom relief and ulcer healing. In addition, antimicrobial–antisecretory combinations are associated with low ulcer-recurrence rates.

A bismuth preparation is added to some regimens. Bismuth exerts antibacterial effects against *H. pylori* by disrupting bacterial cell walls, preventing the organism from adhering to gastric epithelium, and inhibiting bacterial enzymatic and proteolytic activity. It also increases secretion of mucus and bicarbonate, inhibits pepsin activity, and accumulates in ulcer craters.

Although several regimens are effective in *H. pylori* infection, a recent international consensus conference recommended a three-drug regimen with a PPI plus clarithromycin and either amoxicillin or metronidazole twice daily as the first treatment choice. An alternative regimen using metronidazole, a bismuth compound, tetracycline, and an antisecretory drug is very effective in healing ulcers. However, this regimen is not well tolerated, partly because of the multiple daily doses required. Because patient compliance is difficult with all the *H. pylori* eradication regimens, some drug combinations are packaged as individual doses to increase convenience. For example, Helidac contains bismuth subsalicylate, metronidazole, and tetracycline (taken with an H₂RA); Prevpac contains amoxicillin, clarithromycin, and lansoprazole. The newest combination product, Pylera, contains metronidazole, tetracycline, and bismuth subcitrate potassium. Bismuth subcitrate potassium has similar effects as bismuth subsalicylate without the risks associated with a salicylate. Table 59-2 provides further information.

Histamine₂ Receptor Antagonists (H₂RAs)

Histamine is a substance found in almost every body tissue and released in response to certain stimuli (e.g., allergic reactions,

Table 59-2	Drugs at a Glance: Drugs for Acid-Peptic Disorders	
GENERIC/TRADE NAME	**INDICATIONS FOR USE**	**ROUTES AND DOSAGE RANGES (ADULTS)**
Histamine$_2$ Receptor Antagonists	Treatment of peptic ulcers and GERD to promote healing, then maintenance to prevent recurrence Prevention of stress ulcers, GI bleeding, and aspiration pneumonitis Treatment of Zollinger-Ellison syndrome Treatment of heartburn	
Cimetidine (Tagamet)		*Duodenal or gastric ulcer*, PO 800 mg once daily at bedtime or 300 mg 4 times daily or 400 mg twice daily *Maintenance*, PO 400 mg at bedtime *IV injection*, 300 mg diluted in 20 mL of 0.9% NaCl solution q6–8h *IV intermittent infusion*, 300 mg diluted in 50 mL of dextrose or saline solution q6h Impaired renal function (creatinine clearance < 30ml/min). Give 25 mg/h IV for prevention of GI bleeding. PO or IV 300 mg q12h, may increase to every 8h if tolerated. IM 300 mg q6–8h *GERD*, PO 800 mg twice daily or 400 mg 4 times daily *Prevention of upper GI bleeding*, IV continuous infusion, 50 mg/h *Heartburn*, PO 200 mg once or twice daily as needed *Impaired renal function*, PO, IV 300 mg q8–12h
Famotidine (Pepcid, Pepcid RPD) **Famotidine 10 mg, calcium carbonate 800 mg, & magnesium hydroxide 165 mg** (Pepcid Complete)		*Duodenal or gastric ulcer*, PO or IV 40 mg once daily at bedtime or 20 mg twice daily for 4–8 wk; maintenance, PO or IV 20 mg once daily at bedtime *Zollinger-Ellison syndrome*, PO 20 mg q6h, increased if necessary *IV injection*, 20 mg q12h, diluted to 5 or 10 mL with 5% dextrose or 0.9% sodium chloride *IV infusion*, 20 mg q12h, diluted with 100 mL of 5% dextrose or 0.9% sodium chloride *Impaired renal function (creatinine clearance <50 mL/min)*, PO, IV 20 mg q24–48h *GERD*, PO 20 mg twice daily for 6–12 wk *Heartburn*, (Pepcid Complete) PO 1–2 tablets, chewed, daily as needed
Nizatidine (Axid)		*Duodenal or gastric ulcer*, PO 300 mg once daily at bedtime or 150 mg twice daily; maintenance, PO 150 mg once daily at bedtime *GERD*, PO 150 mg twice daily *Heartburn*, PO 75 mg 30–60 min before meals. *Impaired renal function (creatinine clearance [CrCl] 20–50 mL/min)*, PO 150 mg daily; CrCl <20 mL/min, PO 150 mg q48h

GENERIC/TRADE NAME	INDICATIONS FOR USE	ROUTES AND DOSAGE RANGES (ADULTS)
Ranitidine (Zantac)		*Duodenal ulcer,* PO 300 mg once daily at bedtime or 150 mg twice daily, maintenance 150 mg PO at bedtime. *IM* 50 mg q6–8h *IV injection,* 50 mg diluted to 100 mL in 5% dextrose or 0.9% sodium chloride solution q6–8h *IV intermittent infusion,* 50 mg diluted in 100 mL of 5% dextrose or 0.9% sodium chloride solution *Gastric ulcer or GERD,* PO 150 mg twice daily *Impaired renal function (CrCl <50 mL/min),* PO 150 mg q24h; IV, IM 50 mg q18–24h *Heartburn,* PO 75 mg as needed *H. Pyloric infection,* PO 400 mg twice daily for 4 weeks in combination with clarithromycin.
Proton Pump Inhibitors	Treatment of gastric and duodenal ulcers, for 4–8 wk Treatment of GERD with erosive esophagitis for 4–8 wk to promote healing, then maintenance to prevent recurrence Treatment of Zollinger-Ellison syndrome	
Esomeprazole (Nexium, Nexium IV, Nexium delayed-release capsules)		*GERD with erosive esophagitis,* PO 20–40 mg once daily for 4–8 wk; maintenance, 20 mg once daily, IV 20–40 mg daily up to 10 d
Lansoprazole (Prevacid, Prevacid IV)		*Duodenal ulcer,* PO 15 mg daily for healing and maintenance *Gastric ulcer,* PO 30 mg once daily, up to 8 wk *Erosive esophagitis,* PO 30 mg daily up to 8 wk; maintenance, 15 mg daily, IV 30 mg daily up to 7 d *H. pylori infection,* PO 30 mg (with amoxicillin and clarithromycin) twice daily for 14 d *Hypersecretory conditions,* PO 60–90 mg daily
Omeprazole (Prilosec, Prilosec OTC)		*Gastric ulcer,* PO 40 mg once daily for 4–8 wk *Duodenal ulcer,* PO 20 mg once daily for 4–8 wk *GERD,* with erosive esophagitis, PO 20 mg once daily *Zollinger-Ellison syndrome,* PO 60 mg once daily *Heartburn,* PO 20 mg for 14 days. May repeat treatment every 4 months if needed. *H. Pylori infection,* PO 40 mg daily for 14 days then 20 mg daily for 14 days, with clarithromycin.
Pantoprazole (Protonix, Protonix IV)		*GERD with erosive esophagitis,* PO, IV 40 mg once daily *Zollinger-Ellison syndrome,* PO, IV 40–80 mg q12h
Rabeprazole (Aciphex)		*Duodenal ulcer,* PO 20 mg once daily up to 4 wk *GERD,* PO 20 mg once daily for healing and maintenance *Zollinger-Ellison syndrome,* PO 60 mg once or twice daily
Miscellaneous Agents **Misoprostol** (Cytotec)	Prevention of aspirin and NSAID-induced gastric ulcers in selected clients	PO 100–200 mg 4 times daily with meals and at bedtime

(continued on page 958)

Table 59-2	Drugs at a Glance: Drugs for Acid-Peptic Disorders (continued)	
GENERIC/TRADE NAME	**INDICATIONS FOR USE**	**ROUTES AND DOSAGE RANGES (ADULTS)**
Sucralfate (Carafate)	Treatment of active duodenal ulcer to promote healing, then maintenance to prevent recurrence	*Treatment of active ulcer,* PO 1 g 4 times daily before meals and at bedtime *Maintenance therapy,* PO 1 g 2 times daily
Helicobacter pylori Agents **Antimicrobials** **Amoxicillin**	*H. pylori* infection causing gastric or duodenal ulcers	1g 2–3 times daily
Clarithromycin		PO 500 mg 3 times daily
Metronidazole		PO 250 mg 4 times daily
Tetracycline		PO 500 mg 4 times daily
Bismuth Subsalicylate	*H. pylori* eradication and GI upset (abdominal cramping, indigestion, nausea, diarrhea)	*Adults:* PO 525 mg (2 tabs or 30 mL) 4 times daily *Children:* 9–12 y, PO 1 tab or 15 mL; 6–9 y, PO 2/3 tab or 10 mL; 3–6 y, PO 1/3 tab or 5 mL; <3 y, consult physician. Dosage may be repeated every 30–60 min, if needed, up to 8 doses in 24 h.
Combination Regimens **Bisthmuth Subcitrate, metronidazole, tetracycline** (Pylera)		PO bisthmuth subcitrate 140 mg, metronidazole 125 mg, tetrayycline 125 mg. 3 caps 4 times daily with 8 oz water after meals and at bedtime for 10 days.
Bismuth Subsalicylate, metronidazole, and tetracycline (Helidac)		PO bismuth 525 mg (2 tabs), metronidazole 250 mg (1 tab), tetracycline 500 mg (1 capsule) 4 times daily for 14 d
Amoxicillin, clarithromycin, and lansoprazole (Prevpac)		PO amoxicillin 1 g, clarithromycin 500 mg, lansoprazole 30 mg twice daily, morning and evening, for 14 d

GERD, gastroesophageal reflux disease, including erosive esophagitis; GI, gastrointestinal; NSAID, nonsteroidal anti-inflammatory drug.

tissue injury). After it is released, histamine causes contraction of smooth muscle in the bronchi, GI tract, and uterus; dilation and increased permeability of capillaries; dilation of cerebral blood vessels; and stimulation of sensory nerve endings to produce pain and itching.

Histamine also causes strong stimulation of gastric acid secretion. Vagal stimulation causes release of histamine from cells in the gastric mucosa. The histamine then acts on receptors located on the parietal cells to increase production of hydrochloric acid. These receptors are called the H_2 receptors.

Traditional antihistamines or H_1 receptor antagonists prevent or reduce other effects of histamine but do not block histamine effects on gastric acid production. The H_2RAs inhibit both basal secretion of gastric acid and the secretion stimulated by histamine, acetylcholine, and gastrin. They decrease the amount, acidity, and pepsin content of gastric juices. A single dose of an H_2RA can inhibit acid secretion for 6 to 12 hours, and a continuous intravenous (IV) infusion can inhibit secretion for prolonged periods.

Clinical indications for use include prevention and treatment of peptic ulcer disease, GERD, esophagitis, GI bleeding due to acute stress ulcers, and *Zollinger-Ellison syndrome*. With gastric or duodenal ulcers, healing occurs within 6 to 8 weeks; with esophagitis, healing occurs in about 12 weeks. Over-the-counter (OTC) oral preparations, at lower dosage strengths, are approved for the treatment of heartburn.

There are no known contraindications, but the drugs should be used with caution in children, pregnant women, older adults, and patients with impaired renal or hepatic function. Dosage should be reduced in the presence of impaired renal function.

Adverse effects occur infrequently with usual doses and duration of treatment. They are more likely to occur with prolonged use of high doses and in older adults or those with impaired renal or hepatic function.

Cimetidine, ranitidine, famotidine, and nizatidine are the four available H_2RAs (see Table 59-2). **Cimetidine** was the first, and it is still widely used. It is well absorbed after oral administration. After a single dose, peak blood level is reached in 1 to 1.5 hours, and an effective concentration is maintained about 6 hours. The drug is distributed in almost all body tissues. Cimetidine should be used with caution during pregnancy because it crosses the placenta, and it should not be taken during lactation because it is excreted in breast milk. Most of an oral dose is excreted unchanged in the urine within 24 hours; some is excreted in bile and eliminated in feces. For acutely ill patients, cimetidine is given IV. A major disadvantage of cimetidine is that it inhibits the hepatic metabolism of numerous other drugs, thereby increasing blood levels and risks of toxicity with the inhibited drug.

Ranitidine is more potent than cimetidine on a weight basis, and smaller doses can be given less frequently. In addition, ranitidine causes fewer drug interactions than cimetidine. Oral ranitidine reaches peak blood levels 1 to 3 hours after administration and is metabolized in the liver; approximately 30% is excreted unchanged in the urine. Parenteral ranitidine reaches peak blood levels in about 15 minutes; 65% to 80% is excreted unchanged in the urine. **Famotidine** and **nizatidine** are similar to cimetidine and ranitidine.

Compared with cimetidine, the other drugs cause similar effects except they are less likely to cause mental confusion and gynecomastia (antiandrogenic effects). In addition, they do not affect the cytochrome P450 drug-metabolizing system in the liver and therefore do not interfere with the metabolism of other drugs.

Proton Pump Inhibitors (PPIs)

PPIs are strong inhibitors of gastric acid secretion. These drugs bind irreversibly to the gastric proton pump (e.g., the enzyme H^+, K^+-ATPase) to prevent the "pumping" or release of gastric acid from parietal cells into the stomach lumen, thereby blocking the final step of acid production. Inhibition of the proton pump suppresses gastric acid secretion in response to all primary stimuli, histamine, gastrin, and acetylcholine. Thus, the drugs inhibit both daytime (including meal-stimulated) and nocturnal (unstimulated) acid secretion.

Indications for use include treatment of peptic ulcer disease, erosive gastritis, GERD, and Zollinger-Ellison syndrome. PPIs are usually the drugs of choice for treatment of duodenal and gastric ulcers, GERD with erosive esophagitis, and Zollinger-Ellison syndrome. Compared with H₂RAs, PPIs suppress gastric acid more strongly and for a longer time. This effect provides faster symptom relief and faster healing in acid-related diseases. For example, healing of duodenal and gastric ulcers after 2 weeks is similar to the healing after 4 weeks of H₂RA therapy. The PPIs and H₂RAs are similarly effective in maintenance therapy of peptic ulcer disorders, with similar rates of ulcer recurrence. In patients with GERD, PPIs usually abolish symptoms within 1 to 2 weeks and heal esophagitis within 8 weeks. The drugs are also effective in maintenance therapy to prevent recurrence of esophagitis. In patients with *H. pylori*–associated ulcers, eradication of the organism with antimicrobial drugs is preferable to long-term maintenance therapy with antisecretory drugs.

The drugs usually are well tolerated; adverse effects are minimal with both short- and long-term use. Nausea, diarrhea, and headache are the most frequently reported adverse effects. However, long-term consequences of profound gastric acid suppression are unknown.

Omeprazole, esomeprazole, lansoprazole, pantoprazole, and **rabeprazole** are the available PPIs (see Table 59-2). Omeprazole was the first and is still widely used. It is well absorbed after oral administration, highly bound to plasma proteins (about 95%), metabolized in the liver, and excreted in the urine (about 75%) and bile or feces. Acid-inhibiting effects occur within 2 hours and last 72 hours or longer. When the drug is discontinued, effects persist for 48 to 72 hours or longer, until the gastric parietal cells can synthesize additional H^+, K^+-ATPase. The other drugs are very similar to omeprazole. Omeprazole (Prilosec OTC) has been approved for OTC sales for treating heartburn. If heartburn is not improved within 14 days of treatment, patients should be evaluated by their health care provider. A 2-week treatment with Prilosec OTC can be repeated every 4 months if needed to control heartburn.

Prostaglandin

Naturally occurring prostaglandin E, which is produced in mucosal cells of the stomach and duodenum, inhibits gastric acid secretion and increases mucus and bicarbonate secretion, mucosal blood flow, and perhaps mucosal repair. It also inhibits the mucosal damage produced by gastric acid, aspirin, and NSAIDs. When synthesis of prostaglandin E is inhibited, erosion and ulceration of gastric mucosa may occur. This is the mechanism by which aspirin and other NSAIDs are thought to cause gastric and duodenal ulcers (see Chap. 7).

Misoprostol (see Table 59-2) is a synthetic form of prostaglandin E approved for concurrent use with NSAIDs to protect gastric mucosa from NSAID-induced erosion and ulceration. It is indicated for patients at high risk of GI ulceration and bleeding, such as those taking high doses of NSAIDs for arthritis and older adults. The U.S. Food and Drug Administration (FDA) has issued a **BLACK BOX WARNING** to alert health care professionals that misoprostol is contraindicated in women of childbearing potential, unless effective contraceptive methods are being used, and during pregnancy, because it may induce abortion, premature birth, or birth defects. The most common adverse effects are diarrhea (occurs in 10%–40% of recipients) and abdominal cramping. Older adults may be unable to tolerate misoprostol-induced diarrhea and abdominal discomfort.

Sucralfate

Sucralfate is a preparation of sulfated sucrose and aluminum hydroxide that binds to normal and ulcerated mucosa. It is used to prevent and treat peptic ulcer disease. It is effective even though it does not inhibit secretion of gastric acid or pepsin, and it has little neutralizing effect on gastric acid. Its mechanism of action is unclear, but it is thought to act locally on the gastric and duodenal mucosa. Possible mechanisms include binding to the ulcer and forming a protective barrier between the mucosa and gastric acid, pepsin, and bile salts; neutralizing pepsin; stimulating prostaglandin synthesis in the mucosa; and exerting healing effects through the aluminum component. Sucralfate is effective in healing duodenal ulcers and in maintenance therapy to prevent ulcer recurrence. In general, the rates of ulcer healing with sucralfate are similar to the rates with H$_2$RAs.

Adverse effects are low in incidence and severity because sucralfate is not absorbed systemically. Constipation and dry mouth are most often reported. The main disadvantages of using sucralfate are that the tablet is large; it must be given at least twice daily; it requires an acid pH for activation and should not be given with an antacid, H$_2$RA, or PPI; and it may bind to other drugs and prevent their absorption. In general, sucralfate should be given 2 hours before or after other drugs.

Herbal and Dietary Supplements

Several herbal supplements are promoted as aiding heartburn, gastritis, and peptic ulcer disease. Most have not been studied in humans, and there is little, if any, evidence that they are either safe or effective for the proposed uses. Given the known safety and effectiveness of available drugs and the possible consequences of delaying effective treatment, the use of herbal supplements for any acid-peptic disorder should be discouraged.

Nursing Process

Assessment

Assess the patient's status in relation to peptic ulcer disease, GERD, and other conditions in which antiulcer drugs are used.

- Identify risk factors for peptic ulcer disease.
  - Cigarette smoking. Effects are thought to include stimulation of gastric acid secretion and decreased blood supply to gastric mucosa. (Nicotine constricts blood vessels.) Moreover, patients with peptic ulcers who continue to smoke heal more slowly and have more recurrent ulcers, despite usually adequate treatment, than those who stop smoking.
  - Stress, including physiologic stress (e.g., shock, sepsis, burns, surgery, head injury, severe trauma, medical illness) and psychological stress. One mechanism may be that stress activates the sympathetic nervous system, which then causes vasoconstriction in organs not needed for "fight or flight." Thus, stress may lead to ischemia in gastric mucosa, with ulceration if ischemia is severe or prolonged.
  - Drug therapy with aspirin and other NSAIDs, corticosteroids, and antineoplastics.

- Signs and symptoms depend on the type and location of the ulcer.
  - Periodic epigastric pain, which occurs 1 to 4 hours after eating or during the night and is often described as "burning" or "gnawing," is a symptom of a chronic duodenal ulcer.
  - GI bleeding occurs with acute or chronic ulcers when the ulcer erodes into a blood vessel. Clinical manifestations may range from mild (e.g., occult blood in feces, eventual anemia) to severe (e.g., hematemesis, melena, hypotension, shock).
  - GERD produces heartburn (a substernal burning sensation).

Nursing Diagnoses

- Pain related to effects of gastric acid on peptic ulcers or inflamed esophageal tissues
- Imbalanced Nutrition: Less Than Body Requirements related to anorexia and abdominal discomfort
- Constipation related to aluminum- or calcium-containing antacids and sucralfate
- Diarrhea related to magnesium-containing antacids and misoprostol
- Deficient Knowledge related to drug therapy and nonpharmacologic management of GERD and peptic ulcer disease

Planning/Goals

The patient will

- Take or receive antiulcer, anti-heartburn drugs accurately
- Experience relief of symptoms
- Avoid situations that cause or exacerbate symptoms, when possible
- Be observed for GI bleeding and other complications of peptic ulcer disease and GERD
- Maintain normal patterns of bowel function
- Avoid preventable adverse effects of drug therapy

Interventions

Use measures to prevent or minimize peptic ulcer disease and gastric acid–induced esophageal disorders.

- With peptic ulcer disease, helpful interventions may include the following:
  - General health measures such as a well-balanced diet, adequate rest, and regular exercise
  - Avoiding cigarette smoking and gastric irritants (e.g., alcohol, aspirin and NSAIDs, caffeine)
  - Reducing psychological stress (e.g., by changing environments) or learning healthful strategies of stress management (e.g., relaxation techniques, physical exercise). There is no practical way to avoid psychological stress because it is part of everyday life.

■ Long-term drug therapy with small doses of H$_2$RAs, antacids, or sucralfate. With "active" peptic ulcer disease, helping the patient follow the prescribed therapeutic regimen helps to promote healing and prevent complications (see accompanying Patient Teaching Guidelines).

■ Diet therapy is of minor importance in prevention or treatment of peptic ulcer disease. Some physicians prescribe no dietary restrictions, whereas others suggest avoiding or minimizing highly spiced foods, gas-forming foods, and caffeine-containing beverages.

■ With heartburn and esophagitis, helpful measures are those that prevent or decrease gastroesophageal reflux of gastric contents (e.g., avoiding irritant, highly spiced, or fatty foods; eating small meals; not lying down for 1 to 2 hours after eating; elevating the head of the bed; avoiding obesity, constipation, or other conditions that increase intra-abdominal pressure).

Evaluation

■ Observe and interview regarding drug use.

■ Observe and interview regarding relief of symptoms.

■ Observe for signs and symptoms of complications.

■ Observe and interview regarding adverse drug effects.

Applying Your Knowledge 59-1

In addition to taking her medication properly, you should instruct Ms. Daniels to take measures to avoid gastric irritation. What content would be included in this teaching plan?

Applying Your Knowledge 59-2

Ms. Daniels suffers from acid reflux. She should be taught measures that can help reduce the pain associated with heartburn. What should you teach her with regard to minimizing the symptoms of acid reflux?

Principles of Therapy

Drug Selection

All of the drugs used for acid-peptic disorders are effective for indicated uses; the choice of drugs may depend on etiology, acuity, severity of symptoms, cost, and convenience. General guidelines include the following:

Patient Teaching Guidelines ▪ Antiulcer and Anti-Heartburn Drugs

General Considerations

■ These drugs are commonly used to prevent and treat peptic ulcers and heartburn. Peptic ulcers usually form in the stomach or first part of the small bowel (duodenum), where tissues are exposed to stomach acid. Two common causes of peptic ulcer disease are stomach infection with a bacterium called *Helicobacter pylori* and taking nonsteroidal anti-inflammatory drugs (NSAIDs) such as ibuprofen and many others. Heartburn (also called gastroesophageal reflux disease) is caused by stomach acid splashing back onto the esophagus.

Peptic ulcer disease and heartburn are chronic conditions that are usually managed on an outpatient basis. Complications such as bleeding require hospitalization. Overall, these conditions can range from mild to serious, and it is important to seek information about the disease process, ways to prevent or minimize symptoms, and drug therapy.

■ With heartburn, try to minimize acid reflux by elevating the head of the bed; avoiding stomach distention by eating small meals; not lying down for 1 to 2 hours after eating; minimizing intake of fats, chocolate, citric juices, coffee, and alcohol; avoiding smoking (stimulates gastric acid production); and avoiding obesity, constipation, or other conditions that increase intra-abdominal pressure.

In addition, take tablets and capsules with 8 oz of water and do not take medications at bedtime unless instructed to do so. Some medications (e.g., tetracycline, potassium chloride tablets, iron supplements, nonsteroidal anti-inflammatory drugs [NSAIDS]) may cause "pill-induced" irritation of the esophagus (esophagitis) if not taken with enough liquid.

■ Most medications for peptic ulcer disease and heartburn decrease stomach acid. An exception is the antibiotics used to treat ulcers caused by *H. pylori* infection. The strongest acid reducers are omeprazole (Prilosec), esomeprazole (Nexium), lansoprazole (Prevacid), pantoprazole (Protonix), and rabeprazole (Aciphex). These are prescription drugs, except for omeprazole, which is approved for nonprescription use. Histamine-blocking drugs such as cimetidine (Tagamet), famotidine (Pepcid), and others are available as both prescription and over-the-counter (OTC) preparations. OTC products are indicated for heartburn, and smaller doses are taken than for peptic ulcer disease. These drugs usually should not be taken longer than 2 weeks without the advice of a health care provider. The concern is that OTC drugs may delay diagnosis and treatment of potentially serious illness. In addition, cimetidine can increase toxic effects of numerous drugs and should be avoided if you are taking other medications.

(continued on page 962)

Patient Teaching Guidelines — Antiulcer and Anti-Heartburn Drugs (cont'd)

Misoprostol (Cytotec) is given to prevent ulcers from NSAIDs, which are commonly used to relieve pain and inflammation with arthritis and other conditions. This drug should be taken only while taking a traditional NSAID such as ibuprofen. A related drug, celecoxib (Celebrex) is less likely to cause peptic ulcer disease. Do not take misoprostol if pregnant and do not become pregnant while taking the drug. If pregnancy occurs during misoprostol therapy, stop the drug and notify your health care provider immediately. Misoprostol can cause abdominal cramps and miscarriage.

Numerous antacid preparations are available, but they are not equally safe in all people and should be selected carefully. For example, products that contain magnesium have a laxative effect and may cause diarrhea; those that contain aluminum or calcium may cause constipation. Some commonly used antacids (e.g., Maalox, Mylanta) are a mixture of magnesium and aluminum preparations, an attempt to avoid both constipation and diarrhea. People with kidney disease should not take products that contain magnesium because magnesium can accumulate in the body and cause serious adverse effects. Thus, it is important to read product labels and, if you have a chronic illness or take other medications, ask your physician or pharmacist to help you select an antacid and an appropriate dose.

Self- or Caregiver Administration

■ Take antiulcer drugs as directed. Underuse decreases therapeutic effectiveness; overuse increases adverse effects. For acute peptic ulcer disease or esophagitis, drugs are given in relatively high doses for 4 to 8 weeks to promote

healing. For long-term maintenance therapy, dosage is reduced.

■ With Prilosec, Aciphex, Nexium, and Protonix, swallow the capsule whole; do not open, chew, or crush. With Prevacid, the capsule can be opened and the granules sprinkled on applesauce for patients who are unable to swallow capsules. Also, the granules are available in a packet for preparing a liquid suspension. Follow instructions for mixing the granules exactly. The granules should not be crushed or chewed.

■ Take cimetidine with meals or at bedtime. Take famotidine, nizatidine, and ranitidine with or without food. Do not take an antacid for 1 hour before or after taking one of these drugs.

■ Take sucralfate on an empty stomach at least 1 hour before meals and at bedtime. Also, do not take an antacid for 1 hour before or after taking sucralfate.

■ Take misoprostol with food.

■ For treatment of peptic ulcer disease, take antacids 1 and 3 hours after meals and at bedtime (4 to 7 doses daily), 1 to 2 hours before or after other medications. Antacids decrease absorption of many medications if taken at the same time. Also, chew chewable tablets thoroughly before swallowing, then drink a glass of water; allow effervescent tablets to dissolve completely and almost stop bubbling before drinking; and shake liquids well before measuring the dose.

■ Take Pepcid RPD orally disintegrating tablets by placing on tongue and allowing to dissolve with saliva. Taking with liquids not necessary.

■ PPIs are the drugs of first choice in most situations. They heal gastric and duodenal ulcers more rapidly and may be more effective in treating erosive esophagitis due to GERD, erosive gastritis, and Zollinger-Ellison syndrome than H_2RAs. They are also effective in eradicating *H. pylori* infection when combined with two antibacterial drugs. Omeprazole and rabeprazole are given only orally; esomeprazole, lansoprazole, and pantoprazole may be given orally or IV. PPIs are more expensive than H_2RAs. Many patients with GERD will experience a reoccurrence of symptoms when PPIs are discontinued; therefore, long-term maintenance therapy may be required.

■ *H. pylori* infection should be considered in most cases of peptic ulcer disease. If infection is confirmed by appropriate diagnostic tests, agents to eradicate the organisms should be drugs of first choice. The most-recommended drug regimen is a combination of a PPI and clarithromycin plus amoxicillin or metronidazole.

■ *H. pylori* eradication is helpful but insufficient as sole treatment to prevent NSAID-related ulcer disease in patients taking chronic NSAIDs. However, initial *H. pylori* eradication before beginning chronic NSAID therapy use may be helpful in preventing peptic ulcer formation. *H. pylori* infec-

tion should be considered in patients taking long-term aspirin or other NSAID therapy who experience bleeding. In patients on long-term NSAID therapy with peptic ulcers and bleeding ulcers, PPI treatment is more effective than *H. pylori* eradication in preventing reoccurrence of ulcers and bleeding.

■ H_2RAs have been replaced as first-choice drugs by the PPIs for most indications but are still widely used. Cimetidine may be less expensive, but it may cause confusion and antiandrogenic effects. It also increases the risks of toxicity with several commonly used drugs. Compared with cimetidine, other H_2RAs are more potent on a weight basis and have a longer duration of action, so they can be given in smaller, less frequent doses. In addition, they do not alter the hepatic metabolism of other drugs. OTC H_2RAs are indicated for the treatment of heartburn. In some cases, patients may depend on self-medication with OTC drugs and delay seeking treatment for peptic ulcer disease or GERD. For prescription or nonprescription uses, cimetidine is preferably taken by patients who are taking no other medications.

■ Antacids are often used as needed to relieve heartburn and abdominal discomfort. If used to treat acid-peptic disorders, they are more often used with other agents than alone and require a regular dosing schedule. The choice of antacid should be individualized to find a preparation that is acceptable to the patient in terms of taste, dosage, and convenience of administration. Some guidelines include the following:

■ Most commonly used antacids combine aluminum hydroxide and magnesium hydroxide. The combination decreases the adverse effects of diarrhea (with magnesium products) and constipation (with aluminum products). Calcium carbonate is effective in relieving heartburn, but it is infrequently used to treat peptic ulcers or GERD.

■ Antacids may be used more often now that low doses (e.g., two antacid tablets four times a day) have been shown to be effective in healing gastric and duodenal ulcers. All of the low-dose regimens contained aluminum, and the aluminum rather than acid neutralization may be the important therapeutic factor. Compared with other drugs for acid-peptic disorders, low-dose antacids are inexpensive and cause few adverse effects. In addition, tablets are as effective as liquids and usually more convenient to use.

■ Antacids with magnesium are contraindicated in renal disease because hypermagnesemia may result; those with high sugar content are contraindicated in diabetes mellitus.

■ Additional ingredients may be helpful to some patients. Simethicone has no effect on intragastric pH but may be useful in relieving flatulence or gastroesophageal reflux. Alginic acid may be useful in patients with daytime acid reflux and heartburn.

■ Sucralfate must be taken before meals, and this is inconvenient for some patients.

Ⓞ Applying Your Knowledge 59-3

How Can You Avoid This Medication Error?
Ms. Daniels finds that Maalox is less expensive than Mylanta so she switches her antacid brand. She complains that her heartburn is getting worse.

Guidelines for Therapy With Proton Pump Inhibitors

■ Recommended doses of PPIs heal most gastric and duodenal ulcers in about 4 weeks. Large gastric ulcers may require 8 weeks.

■ The drugs may be used to maintain healing of gastric and duodenal ulcers and decrease risks of ulcer recurrence.

■ A PPI and two antimicrobial drugs is the most effective regimen for eradication of H. pylori organisms.

■ With GERD, higher doses or longer therapy may be needed for severe disease and esophagitis. Lower doses can maintain symptom relief and esophageal healing.

Guidelines for Therapy With Histamine₂ Receptor Antagonists

■ For an acute ulcer, full dosage may be given up to 8 weeks. When the ulcer heals, dosage may be reduced by 50% for maintenance therapy to prevent recurrence.

■ For duodenal ulcers, a single evening or bedtime dose produces the same healing effects as multiple doses. Commonly used nocturnal doses are cimetidine 800 milligrams, ranitidine 300 milligrams, nizatidine 300 milligrams, or famotidine 40 milligrams.

■ For gastric ulcers, the optimal H_2RA dosage schedule has not been established. Gastric ulcers heal more slowly than duodenal ulcers and most authorities prescribe 6 to 8 weeks of drug therapy.

■ To maintain ulcer healing and prevent recurrence, long-term H_2RA therapy is often used. The drug is usually given as a single bedtime dose, but the amount is reduced by 50% (i.e., cimetidine 400 mg, ranitidine 150 mg, nizatidine 150 mg, or famotidine 20 mg).

■ For Zollinger-Ellison syndrome, high doses as often as every 4 hours may be required.

■ For severe reflux esophagitis, multiple daily doses may be required for adequate symptom control.

■ Dosage of all these drugs should be reduced in the presence of impaired renal function.

■ Antacids are often given concurrently with H_2RAs to relieve pain. They should not be given at the same time (except for Pepcid Complete) because the antacid reduces absorption of the other drug. H_2RAs usually relieve pain after 1 week of administration.

■ H_2RAs are available in a wide array of products. Precautions must be taken to ensure the correct formulation, dosage strength, and method of administration for the intended use. For example, cimetidine is available in tablets of 200, 300, 400, and 800 milligrams; an oral liquid with 300 milligrams per 5 milliliters; and injectable solutions. Ranitidine is available in tablets of 75 milligrams, capsules (Zantac GELdose) of 150 and 300 milligrams, liquid syrup with 15 milligrams per milliliter, effervescent granules of 150 milligrams, and injectable solutions of 1 milligrams per milliliter and 25 milligrams per milliliter. Nizatidine is available in tablets of 75 milligrams and capsules of 150 and 300 milligrams; famotidine is available in tablets of 10, 20, and 40 milligrams; chewable tablets of 10 milligrams; orally disintegrating tablets (Pepcid RPD) of 20 and 40 milligrams; a powder for oral suspension that contains 40 milligram per 5 milliliters when reconstituted; and injection solutions of 10 milligrams per milliliter and 20 milligrams per 50 milliliters.

■ All H₂RAs are available by prescription and OTC. When prescriptions are given, patients should be advised to avoid concomitant use of OTC versions of the same or similar drugs.

Guidelines for Therapy With Sucralfate

■ When sucralfate is used to treat an ulcer, it should be administered for 4 to 8 weeks unless healing is confirmed by radiologic or endoscopic examination.

■ When used long term to prevent ulcer recurrence, dosage should be reduced.

Guidelines for Therapy With Antacids

■ To prevent stress ulcers in critically ill patients and to treat acute GI bleeding, nearly continuous neutralization of gastric acid is desirable. Dose and frequency of administration must be sufficient to neutralize approximately 50 to 80 milliequivalents of gastric acid each hour. This can be accomplished by a continuous intragastric drip through a nasogastric tube or by hourly administration.

■ When a patient has a nasogastric tube in place, antacid dosage may be titrated by aspirating stomach contents, determining pH, and then basing the dose on the pH. (Most gastric acid is neutralized and most pepsin activity is eliminated at a pH above 3.5.)

■ When prescribing antacids to treat active ulcers, it has long been recommended to take them 1 hour and 3 hours after meals and at bedtime for greater acid neutralization. This schedule is effective but inconvenient for many patients. More recently, lower doses taken less often have been found effective in healing duodenal or gastric ulcers even though less acid neutralization occurs.

■ It was formerly thought that liquid antacid preparations were more effective. Now, tablets are considered as effective as liquids.

■ When antacids are used to relieve pain, they usually may be taken as needed. However, they should not be taken in high doses or for prolonged periods because of potential adverse effects.

Effects of Acid-Suppressant Drugs on Other Drugs

Antacids may prevent absorption of most drugs taken at the same time, including benzodiazepine antianxiety drugs, corticosteroids, digoxin, H₂RAs (e.g., cimetidine), iron supplements, phenothiazine antipsychotic drugs, phenytoin, fluoroquinolone antibacterials, and tetracyclines. Antacids increase absorption of a few drugs, including levodopa, quinidine, and valproic acid. These interactions can be avoided or minimized by separating administration times by 1 to 2 hours.

H₂RAs may alter the effects of several drugs. Most significant effects occur with cimetidine, which interferes with the metabolism of many commonly used drugs. Consequently, the affected drugs are eliminated more slowly, their serum levels are increased, and they are more likely to cause adverse effects and toxicity unless dosage is reduced.

Interacting drugs include antidysrhythmics (lidocaine, propafenone, quinidine), the anticoagulant warfarin, anticonvulsants (carbamazepine, phenytoin), benzodiazepine antianxiety or hypnotic agents (alprazolam, diazepam, flurazepam, triazolam), beta-adrenergic blocking agents (labetalol, metoprolol, propranolol), the bronchodilator theophylline, calcium channel blocking agents (e.g., verapamil), tricyclic antidepressants (e.g., amitriptyline), and sulfonylurea antidiabetic drugs. In addition, cimetidine may increase serum levels (e.g., fluorouracil, procainamide and its active metabolite) and pharmacologic effects of other drugs (e.g., respiratory depression with opioid analgesics) by unidentified mechanisms. Cimetidine also may decrease effects of several drugs, including drugs that require an acidic environment for absorption (e.g., iron salts, indomethacin, fluconazole, tetracyclines) and miscellaneous drugs (e.g., digoxin, tocainide) by unknown mechanisms.

Ranitidine, famotidine, and nizatidine do not inhibit the cytochrome P450 metabolizing enzymes. Ranitidine decreases absorption of diazepam if given at the same time and increases hypoglycemic effects of glipizide. Nizatidine increases serum salicylate levels in people taking high doses of aspirin.

PPIs have relatively few effects on other drugs. Omeprazole increases blood levels of some benzodiazepines (diazepam, flurazepam, triazolam), phenytoin, and warfarin, probably by inhibiting hepatic metabolism. These interactions have not been reported with the other PPIs.

Sucralfate decreases absorption of ciprofloxacin and other fluoroquinolones, digoxin, phenytoin, and warfarin. Sucralfate binds to these drugs when both are present in the GI tract. This interaction can be avoided or minimized by giving the interacting drug 2 hours before sucralfate.

Effects of Acid-Suppressant Drugs on Nutrients

Dietary folate, iron, and vitamin B₁₂ are better absorbed from an acidic environment. When gastric fluids are made less acidic by antacids, H₂RAs, or PPIs, deficiencies of these nutrients may occur. In addition, sucralfate interferes with absorption of fat-soluble vitamins, and magnesium-containing antacids interfere with absorption of vitamin A.

Use in Special Populations

Use in Children

Antacids may be given to ambulatory children in doses of 5 to 15 milliliters every 3 to 6 hours or after meals and at bedtime, as for adults with acid-peptic disorders. For prevention of GI bleeding in critically ill children, 2 to 5 milliliters may be given to infants and 5 to 15 milliliters to children every 1 to 2 hours. Safety and effectiveness of other antiulcer drugs have not been established for children.

Although most PPIs are not approved by the FDA for use in children, they are widely used in the treatment of peptic ulcer and gastroesophageal disease. They are also used to eradicate *H. pylori* organisms. Omeprazole is the only PPI approved by the FDA for children 2 years or older for the treatment of GERD or other acid related disorders. For children weighing less than 20 kilograms, the recommended dosage is 10 milligrams. For children weighing at least 20 kilograms, a dosage of 20 milligrams is recommended.

Use in Older Adults

All of the antiulcer, anti-heartburn drugs may be used in older adults. With antacids, smaller doses may be effective because older adults usually secrete less gastric acid than younger adults. Also, with decreased renal function, older adults are more likely to have adverse effects, such as neuromuscular effects with magnesium-containing antacids. Many physicians recommend calcium carbonate antacids (e.g., Tums) as a calcium supplement to prevent or treat osteoporosis in older women.

With H_2RAs, older adults are more likely to experience adverse effects, especially confusion, agitation, and disorientation with cimetidine. In addition, older adults often have decreased renal function, and doses need to be reduced.

Older adults often take large doses of NSAIDs for arthritis and therefore are at risk for development of acute gastric ulcers and GI bleeding. Thus, they may be candidates for treatment with misoprostol. Dosage of misoprostol may need to be reduced to prevent severe diarrhea and abdominal cramping.

Sucralfate is well tolerated by older adults. PPIs are also well tolerated; however, long-term use (>1 year) is associated with increased risk of hip fractures in adults older than 50 years. The risk of fractures increases the longer the medications are taken. This study also demonstrated that the risk of hip fractures is greater in those taking higher dosages of PPIs. The increased risk of fractures may be due to decreased calcium absorption due to achlorhydria resulting from PPI therapy. PPIs are probably the drug of choice for treating symptomatic GERD because evidence suggests that patients 60 years of age and older require stronger antisecretory effects than younger adults; however, appropriate dose and duration of therapy should be considered when treating GERD in older adults. H_2RAs are not associated with increased risk of hip fractures in older adult.

Use in Patients With Renal Impairment

Antacids containing magnesium are contraindicated in patients with impaired renal function (creatinine clearance < 30 mL/minute) because 5% to 10% of the magnesium may be absorbed and accumulate to cause hypermagnesemia. Antacids containing aluminum hydroxide have historically been used in patients with chronic renal failure because aluminum binds with phosphate in the GI tract, preventing phosphate absorption and hyperphosphatemia that commonly occurs in renal failure. However, aluminum may accumulate in patients with renal failure leading to encephalopathy, erythropoietin-resistant anemia, and osteomalacia. Antacids containing calcium carbonate are currently recommended for the purpose of controlling phosphate levels in patients with end-stage renal failure. Antacids with calcium carbonate can cause alkalosis and raise urine pH, and chronic use may cause renal stones and hypercalcemia.

With PPIs, no special precautions or dosage reductions are required in patients with renal impairment.

All of the available H_2RAs are eliminated through the kidneys, and dosage needs to be substantially reduced in patients with renal impairment to avoid adverse effects. Cimetidine may cause mental confusion in patients with renal impairment. It also blocks secretion of creatinine in renal tubules, thereby decreasing creatinine clearance and increasing serum creatinine level. With moderate to severe renal impairment, recommended dosages include cimetidine 300 milligrams every 12 hours, ranitidine 150 milligrams orally once daily or IV every 18 to 24 hours, and famotidine 20 milligrams at bedtime or every 36 to 48 hours if indicated. Dosage may be cautiously increased if necessary and if renal function is closely monitored. For patients on hemodialysis, an H_2RA should be given at the end of dialysis.

Use in Patients With Hepatic Impairment

PPIs are metabolized in the liver and may cause transient elevations in liver function tests. With omeprazole, bioavailability is increased because of decreased first-pass metabolism, and plasma half-life is increased. However, dosage adjustments are not recommended. Lansoprazole and rabeprazole should be used cautiously, and dosage should be reduced in patients with severe liver impairment.

H_2RAs are partly metabolized in the liver and may be eliminated more slowly in patients with impaired liver function. A major concern with cimetidine is that it can inhibit hepatic metabolism of many other drugs.

Use in Patients With Critical Illness

Gastric acid–suppressant drugs (e.g., PPIs, H_2RAs) and sucralfate are commonly used in critically ill patients. The PPIs are the strongest gastric acid suppressants and are usually well tolerated. For patients who cannot take drugs orally, a PPI can be given IV. The H_2RAs are used to prevent stress-induced gastric ulceration in adults and children. Except for patients with renal impairment, in whom dosage must be reduced, information about the pharmacokinetics of these drugs in critically ill patients is limited, and only cimetidine and ranitidine have been studied. Compared with healthy people, critically ill patients had a longer half-life and lower clearance rate for H₂RAs. The drugs are usually given by intermittent IV infusion. Ranitidine or famotidine is preferred because critically ill patients often require numerous other drugs with which cimetidine may interact and alter effects. Nizatidine is not available in a parenteral formulation.

Use in Home Care

All of the antiulcer, anti-heartburn drugs are commonly taken in the home setting, usually by self-administration. The home care nurse can assist patients by providing information about taking the drugs correctly and monitoring responses. If cimetidine is being taken, the home care nurse needs to assess for potential drug–drug interactions. With OTC H₂RAs, patients should be instructed to avoid daily use of maximum doses for longer than 2 weeks. If use of antacids or OTC H₂RAs seems to be excessive or prolonged, the patient should be assessed for peptic ulcer disease or GERD.

Evidence-Based Practice

59-1 Appropriate Use of Stress Ulcer Prophylaxis

PPIs or H₂RAs are often prescribed in both intensive care and nonintensive care settings in an effort to reduce the morbidity and mortality associated with gastrointestinal bleeding due to stress ulcers. It is estimated that between 27% and 50% of all hospitalized patients are prescribed medications for stress ulcer prophylaxis and about one-half of these patients are discharged with a prescription to continue taking these drugs. Although these medications have reduced the incidence of GI bleeding due to stress ulcers, several studies have examined the impact of inappropriate use of these medications. Increased health care costs and increased risk of adverse drug effects are the most commonly cited concerns. Guidelines for appropriate use of stress ulcer prophylaxis released by the American Society of Health Systems Pharmacists (1999) recommend preventative therapy in the presence of mechanical ventilation for more than 48 hours or when there is presence of coagulopathy (e.g., INR > 1.5, PTT > 2 times normal, or platelet count < 50,000). Research has shown that education regarding appropriate use of stress ulcer prophylaxis is effective in reducing the inappropriate use of these drugs.

Nursing Actions   Antiulcer Drugs

NURSING ACTIONS	RATIONALE/EXPLANATION
1. Administer accurately	
a. With proton pump inhibitors:	
(1) Give most of the drugs before food intake; give oral pantoprazole with or without food.	Manufacturer's recommendations
(2) Ask patients to swallow the tablets or capsules whole, without crushing or chewing.	Drug formulations are delayed-release and long-acting. Opening, crushing, or chewing destroys these effects. Manufacturer's recommendations. Enteric-coated, delayed-release granules are in oral capsules or separate packets. Chewing or crushing destroys the coating; mixing the granules with applesauce or other acidic substances preserves the coating of the granules, allowing them to remain intact until they reach the small intestine.
(3) For patients who are unable to swallow capsules, the lansoprazole capsule can be opened and the granules mixed with 60 mL of orange or tomato juice or sprinkled on 1 tablespoon of applesauce, Ensure pudding, cottage cheese, or yogurt, and swallowed immediately, without chewing. Esomeprazole capsules can be mixed with applesauce and swallowed without chewing.	
(4) To give lansoprazole granules as a liquid suspension, mix 1 packet with 30 mL of water (use no other liquids), stir well, and ask the patient to swallow immediately, without chewing the granules. Esomeprazole capsules can be opened, mixed with 50 mL of water, and swallowed or administered via nasogastric tube. Flush tube with water after administration.	
(5) With omeprazole, Do not substitute two 20-mg oral capsules or suspension packets for one 40-mg dose.	The 20-mg and 40-mg dosage contains the same amount of sodium bicarbonate. Substituting two 20-mg doses for one 40-mg dose results in administration of too much sodium bicarbonate.
(6) Give intravenous (IV) pantoprazole over 15 minutes, injected into a dedicated line or the Y-site of an IV infusion. Use the in-line filter provided; if injecting in a Y-site, the filter should be placed below the Y-site closest to the patient. Flush the IV line with 5% dextrose, 0.9% NaCl, or lactated Ringer's solution before and after pantoprazole administration. IV esomeprazole can be injected over no less than 3 minutes or infused over 10–30 minutes into a dedicated IV line. Flush the IV line with 5% dextrose or lactated Ringer's solution before and after esomeprazole administration.	

NURSING ACTIONS	RATIONALE/EXPLANATION
b. With histamine (H_2) blockers: (1) Give single oral doses at bedtime; give multiple oral doses of cimetidine with meals and at bedtime and other drugs without regard to food intake. (2) To give oral disintegrating tablets (Pepcid RPD), open blister package with dry hands immediately before use, place on tongue, and allow to dissolve with saliva to swallow. Administration with liquids not necessary. (3) To give cimetidine or ranitidine IV, dilute in 20 mL of 5% dextrose or normal saline solution, and inject over at least 2 minutes. For intermittent infusion, dilute in at least 50 mL of 5% dextrose or 0.9% sodium chloride solution, and infuse over 15–20 minutes. (4) To give famotidine IV, dilute with 5–10 mL of 0.9% sodium chloride injection, and inject over at least 2 minutes. For intermittent infusion, dilute in 100 mL of 5% dextrose or 0.9% sodium chloride, and infuse over 15–30 minutes.	The drugs are effective and convenient in a single oral dose at bedtime.
c. With antacids: (1) Do not give doses within approximately 1 hour of oral H_2 antagonists or sucralfate. (2) Shake liquids well before measuring the dose. (3) Instruct clients to chew antacid tablets thoroughly and follow with a glass of water. d. Give sucralfate 1 hour before meals and at bedtime. e. Give misoprostol with food. f. Follow package instructions for administering combination drug regimens for *Helicobacter pylori* infection (e.g., Prevpac, Helidac) and instruct patient to avoid alcohol during and 72 hours after therapy.	Antacids decrease absorption and therapeutic effectiveness of the other drugs. These preparations are suspensions and must be mixed thoroughly to give the correct dose. To increase the surface area of drug available to neutralize gastric acid To allow the drug to form its protective coating over the ulcer before high levels of gastric acidity. Sucralfate requires an acidic environment. After it has adhered to the ulcer, antacids and food do not affect drug action. Metronidazole may precipitate a disulfiram-like reaction if alcohol ingestion occurs with use.
2. Observe for therapeutic effects a. Decreased epigastric pain with gastric and duodenal ulcers; decreased heartburn with gastroesophageal reflux disorders b. Decreased gastrointestinal (GI) bleeding (e.g., absence of visible or occult blood in vomitus, gastric secretions, or feces) c. Higher pH of gastric contents d. Radiologic or endoscopic reports of ulcer healing	Therapeutic effects depend on the reason for use. Antacids should relieve pain within a few minutes. Proton pump inhibitors and H_2 antagonists relieve pain in 7–10 days by healing effects on peptic ulcers or esophagitis. The minimum acceptable pH with antacid therapy is 3.5. Healing usually occurs within 4 to 8 weeks.
3. Observe for adverse effects a. With proton pump inhibitors, observe for headache, diarrhea, abdominal pain, nausea, and vomiting. b. With H_2 antagonists, observe for diarrhea or constipation, headache, dizziness, muscle aches, fatigue, skin rashes, mental confusion, delirium, coma, depression, fever. c. With antacids containing magnesium, observe for diarrhea and hypermagnesemia. d. With antacids containing aluminum or calcium, observe for constipation.	These effects occur infrequently and are usually well tolerated. Adverse effects are uncommon and usually mild with recommended doses. Central nervous system effects have been associated with high doses in elderly patients or those with impaired renal function. With long-term administration of cimetidine, other adverse effects have been observed. These include decreased sperm count and gynecomastia in men, and galactorrhea in women. Diarrhea may be prevented by combining these antacids with other antacids containing aluminum or calcium. Hypermagnesemia may occur in patients with impaired renal function. These antacids should not be given to patients with renal failure. Constipation may be prevented by combining these antacids with other antacids containing magnesium. A high-fiber diet, adequate fluid intake (2000–3000 mL daily), and exercise also help prevent constipation.

(continued on page 968)

Nursing Actions Antiulcer Drugs (continued)

NURSING ACTIONS	RATIONALE/EXPLANATION
e. With sucralfate, observe for constipation.	The drug is not absorbed systemically and constipation is the most commonly reported adverse effect.
f. With misoprostol, observe for diarrhea, abdominal pain, nausea and vomiting, headache, uterine cramping, vaginal bleeding.	Diarrhea commonly occurs and may be severe enough to lead to dosage reduction or stopping the drug.
g. With bismuth, observe for black stools.	This is a harmless discoloration of feces; it does not indicate GI bleeding.
4. Observe for drug interactions	Most significant drug interactions alter the effect of the other drug rather than that of the antiulcer or anti–gastroesophageal reflux disease (GERD) drug.

a. Drugs that *alter* effects of proton pump inhibitors:
  (1) Clarithromycin *increases* effects of omeprazole.
  (2) Sucralfate *decreases* effects of lansoprazole.
	May increase blood levels
	Decreases absorption of lansoprazole, which should be given about 30 minutes before sucralfate if both are used.

b. Drugs that *decrease* effects of H$_2$ antagonists: (1) Antacids	Antacids decrease absorption of cimetidine and probably ranitidine. The drugs should not be given at the same time.

c. Drugs that *alter* effects of antacids:
  (1) Anticholinergic drugs (e.g., atropine) *increase* effects.
 	
  (2) Cholinergic drugs (e.g., dexpanthenol [Ilopan]) *decrease* effects.
d. Drugs that *decrease* effects of sucralfate:
  (1) Antacids
	May increase effects by delaying gastric emptying and by decreasing acid secretion themselves
	May decrease effects by increasing GI motility and rate of gastric emptying
	
	Antacids should not be given within 30 minutes before or after administration of sucralfate.

Key Concepts

- Peptic ulcers are attributed to an imbalance between cell-destructive and cell-protective effects. The most common location for a peptic ulcer is the duodenum followed by the stomach and esophagus.
- Cell-destructive effects include gastric acid (hydrochloric acid), pepsin, *Helicobacter pylori* infection, and ingestion of NSAIDs.
- Cell-protective effects include secretion of mucus and bicarbonate, dilution of hydrochloric acid by food and secretions, prevention of diffusion of hydrochloric acid from the stomach back into the gastric mucosal lining, the presence of prostaglandin E, and alkalinization of gastric secretions by pancreatic juices and bile.
- Gastroesophageal reflux disease (GERD) is characterized by regurgitation of acidic gastric contents into the esophagus, resulting in esophagitis or esophageal ulceration.
- Antacids are alkaline substances that neutralize acids.
- Aluminum antacids have low neutralizing capacity and often cause constipation.
- Magnesium antacids have high neutralizing capacity and may cause diarrhea and hypermagnesemia.

- Calcium antacids have high neutralizing capacity and rapid onset. They may cause rebound acidity and hypercalcemia.
- The treatment of choice for *Helicobacter pylori* infection is a PPI and clarithromycin plus either amoxicillin or metronidazole.
- The H$_2$RAs (e.g., cimetidine, famotidine, nizatidine, and ranitidine) inhibit secretion of gastric acid, decreasing the acidity of gastric juices. They are indicated for prevention and treatment of heartburn, peptic ulcer disease, GERD, esophagitis, GI bleeding due to stress ulcers, and hypersecretory syndromes such as Zollinger-Ellison syndrome.
- The PPIs (e.g., esomeprazole, lansoprazole, omeprazole, pantoprazole, rabeprazole) bind irreversibility to the gastric proton pump to prevent the release of gastric acid from parietal cels into the stomach lumen. They are considered drugs of choice for treatment of heartburn, gastric and duodenal ulcers, GERD, esophagitis, and hypersecretory syndromes such as Zollinger-Ellison syndrome.

■ Misoprostol is a synthetic form of prostaglandin E approved for concurrent use with NSAIDs to protect the gastric mucosa from NSAID-induced erosion and ulceration.

■ Sucralfate forms a protective barrier over mucosal ulcerations, protecting from exposure to gastric juices. It requires an acid pH to be effective.

Review and Application Exercises

Short Answer Exercises

1. What are risk factors for peptic ulcer disease?

2. What roles do gastric acid, pepsin, *H. pylori* organisms, prostaglandins, and mucus play in peptic ulcer occurrence?

3. How do the various drug groups heal ulcers or prevent their recurrence?

4. Compare H$_2$RAs and PPIs in indications for use and effectiveness.

5. What is the rationale for taking H$_2$ blockers at bedtime, sucralfate before meals, and antacids after meals?

6. Why are aluminum and magnesium salts often combined in antacid preparations?

7. For a patient who smokes cigarettes and is newly diagnosed with peptic ulcer disease, how would you explain that smoking cessation aids ulcer healing?

8. Compare and contrast peptic ulcer disease and GERD in terms of risk factors, drug therapy, and patient teaching needs.

NCLEX-Style Questions

9. When taking a patient's history, the nurse notes that the patient is taking warfarin and cimetidine, an H$_2$RA, concurrently. The nurse should anticipate that the
   a. warfarin effects would be increased
   b. cimetidine effects would be increased
   c. warfarin effects would be decreased
   d. cimetidine effects would be decreased

10. The nurse explains to the patient being discharged who is taking sucralfate that the medication should be administered
    a. at the same time as an antacid
    b. after meals
    c. with meals
    d. 2 hours before other drugs

11. A patient with *H. pylori* develops a related ulcer. He is placed on ranitidine and Helidac, a drug combination that contains bismuth, metronidazole, and tetracycline. The patient had been instructed not to consume alcohol, ignored the teaching, and drank beer. The patient presents to the emergency department with tachycardia, headache, diaphoresis, and nausea and vomiting. This disulfiram-like reaction occurred because of the interaction between the alcohol and which drug in the combination?
    a. ranitidine
    b. bismuth
    c. metronidazole
    d. tetracycline

12. A patient asks the nurse how sucralfate (Carafate) works. The nurse replies that sucralfate
    a. inhibits gastric acid secretion
    b. increases mucus and bicarbonate secretion
    c. binds to normal and ulcerated mucosa, creating a protective barrier
    d. enhances prostaglandin synthesis

13. One of the most common adverse effects of misoprostol that makes the drug difficult to tolerate in older adults is
    a. headache
    b. constipation
    c. hyperphosphatemia
    d. diarrhea

Selected References

American Society of Health System Pharmacists. (1999). ASHP therapeutic guidelines on stress ulcer prophylaxis. *American Journal of Health System Pharmacists, 56,* 347–379.

Berardi, R. R., & Welage, L. S. (2005). Peptic ulcer disease. In J. T. DiPiro, R. L. Talbert, G. C. Yee, G. R. Matzke, B. G. Wells, & L. M. Posey (Eds.), *Pharmacotherapy: A pathophysiologic approach* (6th ed., pp. 629–648). New York: McGraw-Hill.

Chicella, M. F., Batres, L. A., Heesters, M. S., & Dice, J. E. (2005). Prokinetic drug therapy in children: A review of current options. *Annals of Pharmacotherapy, 39,* 706–711.

Drug facts and comparisons. (Updated monthly). St. Louis, MO: Facts and Comparisons.

Go, M. F. (2005). Diagnosis and treatment of *Helicobacter pylori. Current Treatment Options in Gastroenterology, 8,* 163–174.

Hassall, E. (2005). Decisions in diagnosing and managing chronic gastroesophageal reflux in children. *Journal of Pediatrics, 146*(Suppl. 3), S3–S12.

Heidelbaugh, J. J., & Inadomi, J. M. (2006). Magnitude and economic impact of inappropriate use of stress ulcer prophylaxis in non-ICU hospitalized patients. *American Journal of Gastroenterology, 107,* 1–6.

Isselbacher, J. K. (2007, June 18). Hot topic: *Helicobacter pylori* infection: Latest concept in management. *Harrison's Online*. Retrieved July 5, 2007, from http://www.accessmedicine.com

Lam, N. P, Le, P. D., Crawford, S. Y., & Patel, S. (1999). National survey on stress ulcer prophylaxis. *Critical Care Medicine, 27*, 98–103.

Liberman, J. D., & Whelan, C. T. (2006). Brief report. Reducing inappropriate usage of stress ulcer prophylaxis among internal medicine residents: A practice-based educational intervention. *Journal of General Internal Medicine, 21*, 498–500.

Porth, C. M. (2005). *Pathophysiology: Concepts of altered health states* (7th ed.). Philadelphia: Lippincott Williams & Wilkins.

Smeltzer, S. C., Bare, B. G., Hinkle J. L., & Cheever, K. H. (2008). *Brunner & Suddarth's textbook of medical-surgical nursing* (11th ed., pp. 1209–1217). Philadelphia: Lippincott Williams & Wilkins.

Williams, D. B. & Schade, R. R. (2005). Gastroesophageal reflux disease. In J. T. DiPiro, R. L. Talbert, G. C. Yee, G. R. Matzke, B. G. Wells, & L. M. Posey (Eds.), *Pharmacotherapy: A pathophysiologic approach* (6th ed., pp. 613–628). New York: McGraw-Hill.

Yang, Y. X., Lewis, J. D., Epstein, S., & Metz, D. C. (2006). Long-term proton pump inhibitor therapy and risk of hip fracture. *Journal of the American Medical Association, 296*, 2947–2953.

Laxatives and Cathartics

LEARNING OBJECTIVES

After studying this chapter, you will be able to:

1. Differentiate the major types of laxatives according to effects on the gastrointestinal tract.
2. Differentiate the consequences of occasional use from those of chronic use.
3. Discuss rational choices of laxatives for selected patient populations or purposes.
4. Discuss bulk-forming laxatives as the most physiologic agents.
5. Discuss possible reasons for and hazards of overuse and abuse of laxatives.

Applying Your Knowledge

Mia Campbell is an 84-year-old woman. Her past health history includes arthritis, osteoporosis, hemorrhoids, and peptic ulcer disease. She is complaining about being constipated. You are her home care nurse.

Introduction

Laxatives and cathartics are drugs used to promote bowel elimination (*defecation*). The term *laxative* implies mild effects and elimination of soft, formed stool. The term *cathartic* implies strong effects and elimination of liquid or semiliquid stool. Because the different effects depend more on the dose than on the particular drug used, the terms often are used interchangeably.

Defecation

Defecation is normally stimulated by movements and reflexes in the gastrointestinal (GI) tract. When the stomach and duodenum are distended with food or fluids, gastrocolic and duodenocolic reflexes cause propulsive movements in the colon, which move feces into the rectum and arouse the urge to defecate. When sensory nerve fibers in the rectum are stimulated by the fecal mass, the defecation reflex causes strong peristalsis, deep breathing, closure of the glottis, contraction of abdominal muscles, contraction of the rectum, relaxation of anal sphincters, and expulsion of the fecal mass.

The cerebral cortex normally controls the defecation reflex so that defecation can occur at acceptable times and places. Voluntary control inhibits the external anal sphincter to allow defecation or contracts the sphincter to prevent defecation. When the external sphincter remains contracted, the defecation reflex dissipates, and the urge to defecate usually does not recur until additional feces enter the rectum or several hours later.

In people who often inhibit the defecation reflex or fail to respond to the urge to defecate, constipation develops as the reflex weakens. *Constipation* is the infrequent and painful expulsion of hard, dry stools. Although there is no "normal" number of stools because of variations in diet and other factors, most people report more than three bowel movements per week. Normal bowel elimination should produce a soft, formed stool without pain.

General Characteristics of Laxatives and Cathartics

Indications for Use

There are several rational indications for use:

- To relieve constipation in pregnant women, elderly patients whose abdominal and perineal muscles have become weak and atrophied, children with megacolon, and patients receiving drugs that decrease intestinal motility (e.g., opioid analgesics, drugs with anticholinergic effects)
- To prevent straining at stool in patients with coronary artery disease (e.g., post–myocardial infarction), hypertension, cerebrovascular disease, and hemorrhoids and other rectal conditions
- To empty the bowel in preparation for bowel surgery or diagnostic procedures (e.g., colonoscopy, barium enema)
- To accelerate elimination of potentially toxic substances from the GI tract (e.g., orally ingested drugs or toxic compounds)
- To prevent absorption of intestinal ammonia in patients with hepatic encephalopathy
- To obtain a stool specimen for parasitologic examination
- To accelerate excretion of parasites after anthelmintic drugs have been administered
- To reduce serum cholesterol levels (psyllium products)

Contraindications to Use

Laxatives and cathartics should not be used in the presence of undiagnosed abdominal pain. The danger is that the drugs may cause an inflamed organ (e.g., the appendix) to rupture and spill GI contents into the abdominal cavity with subsequent peritonitis, a life-threatening condition. Oral drugs also are contraindicated with intestinal obstruction and fecal *impaction*.

Classifications and Individual Drugs

Laxatives and cathartics are somewhat arbitrarily classified as bulk-forming laxatives, surfactant laxatives or stool softeners, saline cathartics, stimulant cathartics, lubricant or emollient laxatives, and miscellaneous. Individual drugs are listed in Table 60-1.

Bulk-Forming Laxatives

Bulk-forming laxatives (e.g., **polycarbophil, psyllium seed**) are substances that are largely unabsorbed from the intestine. When water is added, these substances swell and become gel-like. The added bulk or size of the fecal mass stimulates peristalsis and defecation. The substances also may act by pulling water into the intestinal lumen. Bulk-forming laxatives are the most physiologic laxatives because their effect is similar to that of increased intake of dietary fiber. They usually act within 12 to 24 hours but may take as long as 2 to 3 days to exert their full effects.

Surfactant Laxatives (Stool Softeners)

Surfactant laxatives (e.g., **docusate calcium, potassium, or sodium**) decrease the surface tension of the fecal mass to allow water to penetrate into the stool. They also act as a detergent to facilitate admixing of fat and water in the stool. As a result, stools are softer and easier to expel. These agents have little if any laxative effect. Their main value is to prevent straining while expelling stool. They usually act within 1 to 3 days and should be taken daily.

Saline Laxatives

Saline laxatives (e.g., **magnesium citrate, milk of magnesia**) are not well absorbed from the intestine. Consequently, they increase osmotic pressure in the intestinal lumen and cause water to be retained. Distention of the bowel leads to increased peristalsis and decreased intestinal transit time for the fecal mass. The resultant stool is semifluid. These laxatives are used when rapid bowel evacuation is needed. With oral magnesium preparations, effects occur within 0.5 to 6 hours; with sodium phosphate–containing rectal enemas, effects occur within 15 minutes.

Saline laxatives are generally useful and safe for short-term treatment of constipation, cleansing the bowel before endoscopic examinations, and treating fecal impaction. However, they are not safe for frequent or prolonged usage or for certain patients because they may produce fluid and electrolyte imbalances. For example, patients with impaired renal function are at risk of developing hypermagnesemia with magnesium-containing laxatives because some of the magnesium is absorbed systemically. Patients with congestive heart failure are at risk of fluid retention and edema with sodium-containing laxatives.

Polyethylene glycol–electrolyte solution (e.g., **NuLytely**) is a nonabsorbable oral solution that induces diarrhea within 30 to 60 minutes and rapidly evacuates the bowel, usually within 4 hours. It is a prescription drug used for bowel cleansing before GI examination (e.g., colonoscopy) and is contraindicated in patients with GI obstruction, gastric retention, colitis, or bowel perforation. Combination products such as **HalfLytely** combine polyethylene glycol with a stimulant cathartic, bisacodyl, to evacuate the colon in preparation for a colonoscopy. **Polyethylene glycol solution**

Table 60-1	**Drugs at a Glance:** Laxatives and Cathartics

	ROUTES AND DOSAGES RANGES	
Generic/Trade Name	**Adults**	**Children**
Bulk-Forming Laxatives		
Methylcellulose (Citrucel)	PO 1 heaping tbsp 1–3 times daily with water (8 oz or more)	*12 y and older:* PO same dosage as adults *6–11 y:* PO 1/2 the adult dosage in 8 oz water once daily
Polycarbophil (FiberCon, Mitrolan)	PO 1 g 1–4 times daily or PRN with 8 oz of fluid; maximum dose 4 g/24 h	*6–12 y:* PO 500 mg 1–3 times daily or PRN; maximum dose 2 g/24 h *2–6 y:* products vary, consult labels
Psyllium preparations (Metamucil, Effersyllium, Serutan, Perdiem Plain)	PO 1 rounded tsp 1–3 times daily, stirred in at least 8 oz water or other liquid	*12 y and older:* PO same dosage as adults *6–11 y:* PO 1/2 the adult dosage in 8 oz water once daily
Surfactant Laxatives (Stool Softeners)		
Docusate sodium (Colace)	PO 50–300 mg daily	*12 y and older:* PO same dosage as adults *6–11 y:* 100 mg daily *2–6 y:* products vary, consult labels
Docusate calcium (Surfak)	PO 240 mg daily	*12 y and older:* PO same dosage as adults
Saline Cathartics		
Magnesium citrate solution	PO 1/2–1 bottle at bedtime	*12 y and older:* PO same dosage as adults *6–11 y:* 1/2–1/4 bottle at bedtime
Magnesium hydroxide (milk of magnesia, magnesia magma)	Regular liquid: PO 30–60 mL at bedtime Concentrated liquid: PO 15–30 mL at bedtime	Regular liquid: *12 y and older:* PO same dosage as adults *6–11 y:* 15–30 mL at bedtime *2–5 y:* 5–15 mL at bedtime Concentrated liquid: *12 y and older:* PO same dosage as adults *6–11 y:* 7.5–15 mL at bedtime *2–5 y:* 2.5–7.5 mL at bedtime
Polyethylene glycol (PEG) solution (Miralax)	PO 17 g in 8 oz water	No pediatric dosage
Polyethylene glycol–electrolyte solution (PEG-ES) (CoLyte, GoLytely, NuLytely, OCL)	For bowel cleansing before GI examination: PO 240 mL every 10 min until 4 L is consumed	No recommended children's dose
Sodium phosphate and sodium biphosphate (Fleet Phosphosoda, Fleet Enema)	PO 20–40 mL in 8 oz water Rectal enema, 60–120 mL	*10 y and older:* PO 10–20 mL in 8 oz of water *5–10 y:* PO 5–10 mL in 8 oz of water Rectal enema, 60 mL
Stimulant Cathartics		
Bisacodyl (Dulcolax)	PO 10–15 mg Rectal suppository, 10 mg	*6 y and older:* PO 5 mg Rectal suppository, 5 mg
Cascara sagrada	PO tablets, 325 mg PO aromatic, 2.5–5 mL PO aromatic fluid extract, 2–6 mL	PO tablets and aromatic fluid extract: *12 y and older:* same dosage as adults PO aromatic: *2–12 y:* PO 1/5–1/2 tsp
Castor oil (Neoloid)	PO 15–60 mL	*5–15 y:* PO 5–30 mL depending on strength of emulsion *under 2 y:* PO 1.25–7.5 mL depending on strength of emulsion

(continued on page 974)

Table 60-1	Drugs at a Glance: Laxatives and Cathartics (continued)	
	ROUTES AND DOSAGES RANGES	
Generic/Trade Name	**Adults**	**Children**
Glycerin	Rectal suppository, 3 g	*under 6 y:* rectal suppository 1–1.5 g
Senna preparations (Senokot, Black Draught)	Granules, PO 1 level tsp once or twice daily Syrup, PO 2–3 tsp once or twice daily Tablets, PO 2 tablets once or twice daily For geriatric, obstetric, gynecologic patients, reduce all dosages by half	*Weight > 27 kg:* granules, syrup, and tablets, 1/2 the adult dosage
Combination Product HalfLytely and bisacodyl tablets Bowel Prep Kit	For bowel cleansing before colonoscopy: PO 4 bisacodyl tablets (5 mg each) with water. After bowel movement occurs, drink 8 oz of HalfLytely solution every 10 min until 2 L of solution is consumed.	Pediatric dosage not established
Lubricant Laxative Mineral oil (Agoral Plain, Milkinol, Fleet Mineral Oil Enema)	PO 15–30 mL at bedtime Rectal enema, 30–60 mL	*older than 6 y:* PO 5–15 mL at bedtime Rectal enema, 30–60 mL
Miscellaneous Medications Lactulose (Chronulac, Cephulac)	For constipation: PO 15–30 mL daily; maximum dose 60 mL daily Portal systemic encephalopathy: PO 30–45 mL 3 or 4 times daily, adjusted to produce two or three soft stools daily Rectally as retention enema, 300 mL with 700 mL water or normal saline, retained 30–60 min, every 4–6 h	*Infants:* PO 2.5–10 mL daily in divided doses *older children:* PO 40–90 mL daily in divided doses
Lubiprostone (Amitiza)	For chronic idiopathic constipation: PO 24 mcg twice daily with food	Pediatric dosage not established
Sorbitol	For hyperkalemia (with Kayexalate), PO 30–50 g daily	

(MiraLax) is an oral laxative that may be used to treat occasional constipation. Effects may require 2 to 4 days. It is a prescription drug and should not be taken longer than 2 weeks.

Stimulant Cathartics

The stimulant cathartics are the strongest and most abused laxative products. These drugs act by irritating the GI mucosa and pulling water into the bowel lumen. As a result, feces are moved through the bowel too rapidly to allow colonic absorption of fecal water, so a watery stool is eliminated. These drugs should not be used frequently or for longer than 1 week because they may produce serum electrolyte and acid–base imbalances (e.g., hypocalcemia, hypokalemia, metabolic acidosis or alkalosis).

Oral stimulant cathartics include **bisacodyl, cascara sagrada, castor oil, and senna products**. These products produce laxative effects in 6 to 12 hours. As a result, a single bedtime dose usually produces a morning bowel movement. Rectal suppository products include bisacodyl, which produces effects within 15 minutes to 2 hours, and **glycerin**. In addition to irritant, stimulant effects, glycerin exerts hyperosmotic effects in the colon. It usually acts within 30 minutes. Glycerin is not given orally for laxative effects.

Lubricant Laxative

Mineral oil is the only lubricant laxative used clinically. It lubricates the fecal mass and slows colonic absorption of water from the fecal mass, but the exact mechanism of action is unknown. Effects usually occur in 6 to 8 hours. Oral mineral oil may cause several adverse effects and is not recommended for long-term use. Mineral oil enemas are sometimes used to soften fecal impactions and aid their removal.

Miscellaneous Medications for Constipation

Lactulose is a disaccharide that is not absorbed from the GI tract. It exerts laxative effects by pulling water into the intestinal lumen. It is used to treat constipation and hepatic encephalopathy. The latter condition usually results from alcoholic liver disease in which ammonia accumulates and causes stupor or coma. Ammonia is produced by metabolism of dietary protein and intestinal bacteria. Lactulose decreases production of ammonia in the intestine. The goal of treatment is usually to maintain two to three soft stools daily; effects usually occur within 24 to 48 hours. The drug should be used cautiously because it may produce electrolyte imbalances and dehydration.

Lubiprostone (Amitiza) is indicated for the treatment of chronic idiopathic constipation in adults. Chronic idiopathic constipation, defined as the infrequent or difficult passage of stool, is characterized by abnormal GI motility, abdominal discomfort, bloating, and straining to pass hard, lumpy stools. Lubiprostone is poorly absorbed into the circulation and exerts its effect locally, activating chloride channels in the GI tract to increase the secretion of chloride rich fluids into the intestine. Increased intestinal fluid secretion stimulates intestinal motility, improving the passage of stool. Lubiprostone is metabolized by enzymes in the stomach and excreted in the urine and feces. Adverse effects include nausea and severe diarrhea. Taking lubiprostone with food may aid in decreasing nausea.

Sorbitol is a monosaccharide that pulls water into the intestinal lumen and has laxative effects. It is often given with sodium polystyrene sulfonate (Kayexalate), a potassium-removing resin used to treat hyperkalemia, to prevent constipation, and aid expulsion of the potassium–resin complex.

Herbal and Dietary Supplements

Many of the commonly used laxatives are plant based (e.g., cascara, psyllium, senna, castor oil). These have long been used and are safe and effective when used as directed.

Aloe is used most often as a topical remedy for burns and possibly other minor wounds. When used for this purpose, a gel-like liquid can be squeezed directly from a plant leaf onto the burned area. Oral aloe is sometimes used as a laxative. However, it is not recommended for this use because it is a strong stimulant laxative. With oral ingestion, aloe can cause

severe cramping and other potentially serious adverse effects, including hypokalemia and cardiac dysrhythmias.

Applying Your Knowledge 60-1

Based on Ms. Campbell's past health history, what is the most likely drug of choice?

Applying Your Knowledge 60-2

Given Ms. Campbell's complaint of constipation, what would you assess with regard to her bowel pattern and risk for constipation?

Nursing Process

Assessment

Assess patients for current or potential constipation.

- Identify risk factors.
- Diet with minimal fiber (e.g., small amounts of fruits, vegetables, and whole-grain products)
- Low fluid intake (e.g., <2000 mL daily)
- Immobility or limited activity
- Drugs that reduce intestinal function and motility (e.g., opioid analgesics, antacids containing aluminum or calcium, anticholinergics, calcium channel blockers, clozapine, diuretics, iron, phenothiazines, cholestyramine, colestipol, sucralfate, tricyclic antidepressants, vincristine). Overuse of antidiarrheal agents also may cause constipation.
- Conditions that may reduce intestinal function and motility (e.g., depression, eating disorders such as anorexia nervosa, hypothyroidism, hypercalcemia, multiple sclerosis, Parkinson's disease, spinal lesions)
- Hemorrhoids, anal fissures, or other conditions characterized by painful bowel elimination
- Elderly or debilitated patients
- Signs and symptoms include the following:
  - Decreased number and frequency of stools
  - Passage of dry, hard stools
  - Abdominal distention and discomfort
  - Flatulence

Nursing Diagnoses

- Constipation related to decreased activity; inadequate dietary fiber; inadequate fluid intake; drugs; or disease processes

Nursing Process continues on page 976

- Pain (abdominal cramping and distention) related to constipation or use of laxatives
- Noncompliance with recommendations for nondrug measures to prevent or treat constipation
- Risk for Deficient Fluid Volume related to diarrhea from frequent or large doses of laxatives
- Deficient Knowledge: Nondrug measures to prevent constipation and appropriate use of laxatives

Planning/Goals

The patient will

- Take laxative drugs appropriately
- Use nondrug measures to promote normal bowel function and prevent constipation
- Regain normal patterns of bowel elimination
- Avoid excessive losses of fluids and electrolytes from laxative use
- Be protected from excessive fluid loss, hypotension, and other adverse drug effects, when possible
- Be assisted to avoid constipation when at risk (eg, has illness or injury that prevents activity and food and fluid intake; takes medications that decrease GI function)

Interventions

- Assist patients with constipation and caregivers to
  - Understand the importance of diet, exercise, and fluid intake in promoting normal bowel function and preventing constipation
  - Increase activity and exercise
  - Increase intake of dietary fiber (e.g., vegetables, fruits, cereal grains)
  - Drink at least 2000 mL of fluid daily
  - Establish and maintain a routine for bowel elimination (e.g., going to the bathroom immediately after breakfast)
  - Understand and comply with drug therapy (see accompanying Patient Teaching Guidelines)
- Monitor client responses.
  - Record number, amount, and type of bowel movements.
  - Record vital signs. Hypotension and weak pulse may indicate deficient fluid volume.

Evaluation

- Observe and interview for improved patterns of bowel elimination.
- Observe for use of nondrug measures to promote bowel function.
- Observe for appropriate use of laxatives.
- Observe and interview regarding adverse effects of laxatives.

Principles of Therapy

Laxative Abuse

Laxatives and cathartics are widely available on a nonprescription basis and are among the most frequently abused drugs. One reason for overuse is the common misconception that a daily bowel movement is necessary for health and well-being, even with little intake of food or fluids. This notion may lead to a vicious cycle of events in which a person fails to have a bowel movement, takes a strong laxative, again fails to have a bowel movement, and takes another laxative before the fecal column has had time to become re-established (2–3 days with normal food intake). Thus, a pattern of laxative dependence and abuse is established.

Laxatives are also abused for weight control, probably most often by people with eating disorders and those who must meet strict weight requirements (e.g., some athletes). This is a very dangerous practice because it may lead to life-threatening fluid and electrolyte imbalances.

Drug Selection

In 2005, a review of published studies of efficacy and safety of medications for chronic constipation was completed to provide evidence-based recommendations for treatment. This review concluded that there was good evidence for the use of polyethylene glycol, lactulose, and psyllium to treat chronic constipation. There was minimal evidence in the published literature for many commonly used agents, including magnesium hydroxide, senna, bisacodyl, and stool softeners.

Clinically, the choice of a laxative or cathartic often depends on the reason for use and the patient's condition:

- For long-term use of laxatives or cathartics in patients who are older, unable or unwilling to eat an adequate diet, or debilitated, bulk-forming laxatives (e.g., Metamucil) usually are preferred. However, because obstruction may occur, these agents should not be given to patients with difficulty in swallowing or adhesions or strictures in the GI tract or to those who are unable or unwilling to drink adequate fluids.

- For patients in whom straining is potentially harmful or painful, stool softeners (e.g., docusate sodium) are the agents of choice.

- For occasional use to cleanse the bowel for endoscopic or radiologic examinations, saline or stimulant cathartics are acceptable (e.g., magnesium citrate, polyethylene glycol–electrolyte solution, bisacodyl). These drugs should not be used more than once per week. Frequent use is likely to produce laxative abuse.

- Oral use of mineral oil may cause potentially serious adverse effects (decreased absorption of fat-soluble vitamins and some drugs; lipid pneumonia if aspirated into the lungs). Thus, mineral oil is not an oral laxative of choice in any condition, although occasional use in the alert patient is unlikely to be harmful. It should not be used regularly.

Patient Teaching Guidelines | Laxatives

General Considerations

- Diet, exercise, and fluid intake are important in maintaining normal bowel function and preventing or treating constipation.
- Eat foods high in dietary fiber daily. Fiber is the portion of plant food that is not digested. It is contained in fruits, vegetables, and whole-grain cereals and breads. Bran, the outer coating of cereal grains such as wheat or oats, is an excellent source of dietary fiber and is available in numerous cereal products.
- Drink at least 6 to 10 glasses (8 oz each) of fluid daily if not contraindicated.
- Exercise regularly. Walking and other activities aid movement of feces through the bowel.
- Establish a regular time and place for bowel elimination. The defecation urge is usually strongest after eating and the defecation reflex is weakened or lost if repeatedly ignored.
- Laxative use should be temporary and not regular, as a general rule. Regular use may prevent normal bowel function, cause adverse drug reactions, and delay treatment for conditions that cause constipation.
- *Never* take laxatives when acute abdominal pain, nausea, or vomiting is present. Doing so may cause a ruptured appendix or other serious complication.
- After taking a strong laxative, it takes 2 to 3 days of normal eating to produce enough feces in the bowel for a bowel movement. Frequent use of a strong laxative promotes loss of normal bowel function, loss of fluids and electrolytes that your body needs, and laxative dependence.
- If you have chronic constipation and are unable or unwilling to eat enough fiber-containing foods in your diet, the next-best action is regular use of a bulk-forming laxative (e.g., Metamucil) as a dietary supplement. These laxatives act the same way as increasing fiber in the diet and are usually best for long-term use. When taken daily, they can prevent constipation. However, they may take 2 to 3 days to work and are not effective in relieving acute constipation.
- Your urine may be discolored if you take a laxative containing senna (e.g., Senokot) or cascara sagrada. The color change is not harmful.
- Some people use strong laxatives for weight control. This is an inappropriate use and a dangerous practice because it can lead to life-threatening fluid and electrolyte imbalances, including dehydration and cardiovascular problems.

Self- or Caregiver Administration

- Take all laxatives as directed and do not exceed recommended doses to avoid adverse effects.
- With bulk-forming laxatives, mix in 8 oz of fluid immediately before taking and follow with additional fluid, if able. *Never* take the drug dry. Adequate fluid intake is essential with these drugs.
- With bisacodyl tablets, swallow whole (do not crush or chew), and do not take within 1 hour of an antacid or milk. This helps prevent stomach irritation, abdominal cramping, and possible vomiting.
- Take magnesium citrate or milk of magnesia on an empty stomach with 8 oz of fluid to increase effectiveness.
- Refrigerate magnesium citrate before taking to improve taste and retain effectiveness.
- Mix lactulose with fruit juice, water, or milk, if desired, to improve taste.
- Take lubiprostone (Amitiza) with food.
- Notify your health care provider if severe diarrhea develops while taking lubiprostone.

Mineral oil is probably most useful as a retention enema to soften hard, dry feces and aid in their expulsion.

- In fecal impaction, a rectal suppository (e.g., bisacodyl) or an enema (e.g., oil retention or Fleet enema) is preferred. Oral laxatives are contraindicated when fecal impaction is present but may be given after the rectal mass is removed. After the impaction is relieved, measures should be taken to prevent recurrence. If dietary and other nonpharmacologic measures are ineffective or contraindicated, use of a bulk-forming agent daily or another laxative once or twice weekly may be necessary.

- Saline cathartics containing magnesium, phosphate, or potassium salts are contraindicated in patients with renal failure because hypermagnesemia, hyperphosphatemia, or hyperkalemia may occur.

- Saline cathartics containing sodium salts are contraindicated in patients with edema or congestive heart failure because enough sodium may be absorbed to cause further fluid retention and edema. They also should not be used in patients with impaired renal function or those following a sodium-restricted diet for hypertension.

- Polyethylene glycol–electrolyte solution is formulated for rapid and effective bowel cleansing without significant changes in water or electrolyte balance.

Use in Special Populations

Use in Children

Constipation is responsible for 3% of visits to pediatric clinics and up to 30% of visits to pediatric gastroenterologists. As in adults, increasing fluids, high-fiber foods, and exercise is preferred when possible.

Guidelines for treating constipation in infants and children developed by the North American Society for Pediatric Gastroenterology, Hepatology and Nutrition include the following recommendations:

- For infants:
  - Glycerin suppositories are often effective in infants and small children.
  - Lactulose or sorbitol can be used as stool softeners in infants.
  - Mineral oil or stimulant laxatives are not recommended for infants.

- For children:
  - Mineral oil, magnesium hydroxide, lactulose and sorbitol are effective for treating constipation in children.
  - Stimulant laxatives, such as senna or bisacodyl, can be used short-term as rescue therapy or in carefully selected patients with constipation that is difficult to treat. Polyethylene glycol–electrolyte solution in low dosages may be an effective long-term treatment for difficult to treat cases.

Parents should be advised not to give children any laxative more than once a week without consulting a health care provider. Polyethylene glycol–electrolyte solution is effective in treating acute iron overdose in children, although it is not approved by the U.S. Food and Drug Administration for this indication.

 Applying Your Knowledge 60-3

How Can You Avoid This Medication Error?

Ms. Campbell is concerned about not having a bowel movement. She takes a psyllium preparation at 8 A.M. She does not have a result by noon, so she takes milk of magnesia. She has not had a stool by supper, so she takes a glycerin suppository.

Use in Older Adults

As many as 15% to 20% of community-dwelling older adults and up to 50% of nursing home residents experience constipation. Laxatives are often used or overused. Nondrug measures to prevent constipation (e.g., increasing fluids and high-fiber foods, exercise) are much preferred to laxatives. If a laxative is required on a regular basis, a bulk-forming psyllium compound (e.g., Metamucil) is best because it is most physiologic in its action. If taken, it should be accompanied by a full glass of fluid. There have been reports of obstruction in the GI tract when a psyllium compound was taken with insufficient fluid. Regular use of stronger laxatives should be avoided; however, when necessary they should be taken infrequently at the lowest effective dose. Mineral oil should be avoided in bedfast elderly individuals due to the risks of lipid-aspiration pneumonia.

Use in Patients With Cancer

Many patients with cancer require moderate to large amounts of opioid analgesics for pain control. The analgesics slow GI motility and cause constipation. These patients often need a bowel-management program that includes routine laxative administration; however, a recent Cochrane review of research on laxatives for the management of constipation in palliative care found insufficient data to make a recommendation on the best laxative for these patients. Bulk-forming laxatives are not usually recommended for patients with cancer because they may not be able to drink adequate amounts of fluids required with these medications. One treatment option, stimulant laxatives (e.g., a senna preparation, bisacodyl) increase intestinal motility, which is the action that opiates suppress. These drugs may cause abdominal cramping, which may be lessened by giving small doses three or four times daily.

Use in Patients With Spinal Cord Injury

Spinal cord injury (SCI) impairs the ability of an individual to sense that a bowel movement is imminent and the ability to control the timing and place of bowel evacuation. Common problems that the individual with SCI must cope with include incontinence and fecal impaction, which if left untreated may result in perforation of the bowel.

SCIs above the twelfth thoracic vertebrae (T12) are referred to as upper motor neuron injuries. Individuals with this type of SCI are unable to sense when the bowel is full. The anal sphincter remains closed until the bowel becomes distended with stool, resulting in uncontrolled reflex emptying. Individuals with upper motor neuron injuries usually follow a bowel program that includes taking a daily stool softener such as docusate sodium and stimulating bowel movements at the desired time using digital stimulation and rectal suppositories such as bisacodyl or glycerin.

SCIs below T12 are referred to as lower motor neuron injuries. With this type of SCI, the muscles of the colon and anus remain relaxed or flaccid, resulting in constipation and incontinence. The bowel-control program for individuals with lower motor neuron injuries involves digital stimulation and manual removal of the stool. Initially, digital disimpaction should be done every other day. It may be necessary to increase the frequency of digital disimpaction to every day to avoid unplanned bowel movements or constipation and impaction.

With both types of SCIs the goal of the bowel program is to have regular bowel movements at a predictable time and place and to minimize "accidents." It is recommended to implement the bowel program at the same time each day, preferably after a meal. Factors that influence bowel activity must be considered in the bowel program. These factors include eating at regular intervals, including high-fiber foods in the diet, adequate intake of fluids in the diet, avoidance of medications and foods that may cause diarrhea or constipation, and an awareness of cues that a bowel movement may be imminent, such as sweating, restlessness, sensations of fullness in the lower abdomen, and piloerection or "goose bumps."

Use in Patients With Renal Impairment

Saline cathartics containing phosphate, sodium, magnesium, or potassium salts are usually contraindicated or must be used cautiously in the presence of impaired renal function. Ten percent or more of the magnesium in magnesium salts may be absorbed and cause hypermagnesemia; sodium phosphate and sodium biphosphate may cause hyperphosphatemia, hypernatremia, acidosis, and hypocalcemia; and potassium salts may cause hyperkalemia.

Use in Patients With Hepatic Impairment

Because most laxatives are not absorbed or metabolized extensively, they can usually be used without difficulty in patients with hepatic impairment. In fact, they are used therapeutically in patients with hepatic encephalopathy to decrease absorption of ammonia from dietary protein in the GI tract. Lactulose is usually given in dosages to produce two to three soft stools daily.

Use in Home Care

Laxatives are commonly self-prescribed and self-administered in the home setting. The home care nurse may become involved when visiting a patient for other purposes. The role of the home care nurse may include assessing usual patterns of bowel elimination, identifying patients at risk of developing constipation, promoting lifestyle interventions to prevent constipation, obtaining laxatives when indicated, and counseling about rational use of laxatives.

Nursing Actions   Laxatives and Cathartics

NURSING ACTIONS	RATIONALE/EXPLANATION
1. Administer accurately	
a. Give bulk-forming laxatives with at least 8 oz of water or other fluid. Mix with fluid immediately before administration.	To prevent thickening and expansion in the gastrointestinal (GI) tract with possible obstruction. These substances absorb water rapidly and solidify into a gelatinous mass.
b. With bisacodyl tablets, instruct the client to swallow the tablets without chewing and not to take them within an hour after ingesting milk or gastric antacids or while receiving cimetidine therapy.	The tablets have an enteric coating to delay dissolution until they reach the alkaline environment of the small intestine. Chewing or giving the tablets close to antacid substances or to cimetidine-treated clients causes premature dissolution and gastric irritation and results in abdominal cramping and vomiting.
c. Give saline cathartics on an empty stomach with 240 mL of fluid.	To increase effectiveness
d. Take lubiprostone with food.	Presence of food may help decrease nausea.
e. Refrigerate magnesium citrate and polyethylene glycol electrolyte solution before giving.	To increase palatability and retain potency
f. Castor oil may be chilled and followed by fruit juice or other beverage.	To increase palatability
g. Insert rectal suppositories to the length of the index finger, next to rectal mucosa.	These drugs are not effective unless they are in contact with intestinal mucosa.
2. Observe for therapeutic effects	
a. Soft to semiliquid stool	Therapeutic effects occur in approximately 1–3 days with bulk-forming laxatives and stool softeners; 6–8 hours with bisacodyl tablets, cascara sagrada, and senna products; 15–60 minutes with bisacodyl and glycerin suppositories.
b. Liquid to semiliquid stool	Effects occur in approximately 1–3 hours with saline cathartics and castor oil.
c. Decreased abdominal pain when used in clients with irritable bowel syndrome or diverticulosis	Pain results from straining to expel hard, dry feces.
d. Decreased rectal pain when used in clients with hemorrhoids or anal fissures	
3. Observe for adverse effects	
a. Diarrhea—several liquid stools, abdominal cramping. Severe, prolonged diarrhea may cause hyponatremia, hypokalemia, dehydration, and other problems.	Diarrhea is most likely to result from strong, stimulant cathartics (e.g., castor oil, bisacodyl, senna preparations), large doses of saline cathartics (e.g., milk of magnesia), or use of lubiprostone.
b. With bulk-forming agents, impaction or obstruction	Impaction or obstruction of the GI tract can be prevented by giving ample fluids with these agents and not giving the drugs to clients with known dysphagia or strictures anywhere in the alimentary canal.
c. With saline cathartics, hypermagnesemia, hyperkalemia, fluid retention, and edema	Hypermagnesemia and hyperkalemia are more likely to occur in patients with renal insufficiency because of impaired ability to excrete magnesium and potassium. Fluid retention and edema are more likely to occur in patients with congestive heart failure or other conditions characterized by edema. Polyethylene glycol–electrolyte solution produces the least change in water and electrolyte balance.
d. With mineral oil, lipid pneumonia and decreased absorption of vitamins A, D, E, and K	Lipid pneumonia can be prevented by not giving mineral oil to patients with dysphagia or impaired consciousness. Decreased absorption of fat-soluble vitamins can be prevented by not giving mineral oil with or shortly after meals or for longer than 2 weeks.

(continued on page 980)

Nursing Actions — Laxatives and Cathartics (continued)

NURSING ACTIONS	RATIONALE/EXPLANATION
4. Observe for drug interactions a. Drugs that *increase* effects of laxatives and cathartics: 　(1) GI stimulants (e.g., metoclopramide) b. Drugs that *decrease* effects of laxatives and cathartics: 　(1) Anticholinergic drugs (e.g., atropine) and other drugs 　with anticholinergic properties (e.g., phenothiazine 　antipsychotic drugs, tricyclic antidepressants, some 　antihistamines, and antiparkinson drugs) 　(2) Central nervous system depressants (e.g., opioid 　analgesics)	Additive stimulation of intestinal motility These drugs slow intestinal motility. Patients receiving these agents are at risk for development of constipation and requiring laxatives, perhaps on a long-term basis. Opioid analgesics commonly cause constipation.

Key Concepts

- Constipation is the infrequent and painful expulsion of hard, dry stools.
- Lifestyle modifications such as fluid and fiber intake and exercise are preferred to medications in the treatment of constipation.
- Laxatives and cathartics are drugs to promote bowel elimination.
- Common reasons for abuse of laxatives and cathartics include eating disorders, desire for strict weight control, or the belief that a daily bowel movement is necessary for health.
- Laxatives and cathartics should not be used in the presence of undiagnosed abdominal pain or other signs of intestinal obstruction due to the risks of perforation and peritonitis.
- Bulk-forming laxatives add mass to the feces, stimulating peristalsis and defecation. They must be taken with water to avoid obstruction. Generally, bulk-forming drugs are the most desirable laxative for long-term use.
- Surfactant laxatives decrease the surface tension of the fecal mass to allow water and fat to penetrate into the stool, making it softer and easier to expel. They have little true laxative effect.
- Saline laxatives increase the osmotic pressure in the intestinal lumen, resulting in the retention of water, which distends the bowel and stimulates peristalsis. They produce a

semifluid stool and may lead to fluid and electrolyte imbalances.
- Polyethylene glycol–electrolyte solution is a nonabsorbable oral solution that rapidly evacuates the bowel within 4 hours. It is useful for bowel cleansing before GI procedures.
- Stimulant cathartics are the strongest and most abused laxative products. They irritate the GI mucosa, pull water into the colon, and stimulate peristalsis. They produce a watery stool and may lead to fluid, electrolyte, and acid-base imbalances.
- Lubricant laxatives lubricate the fecal mass and slow colonic absorption of water from the fecal mass. These medications may interfere with the absorption of fat-soluble vitamins and if aspirated may result in a lipid aspiration pneumonia.
- Lactulose exerts an osmotic effect, pulling water into the colon and stimulating peristalsis. It is also useful in treating hepatic encephalopathy by decreasing the production of the waste product ammonia.
- Sorbitol is often given with sodium polystyrene sulfonate (Kayexalate) in the treatment of hyperkalemia to aid in the expulsion of the potassium-resin complex.
- Lubiprostone (Amitiza) aids in treating chronic idiopathic constipation by increasing intestinal fluid secretion, stimulating intestinal motility and defecation.

Review and Application Exercises

Short Answer Exercises

1. What are risk factors for development of constipation?
2. Describe nonpharmacologic strategies to prevent constipation.
3. Which type of laxative is, in general, the most desirable for long-term use? Which is the least desirable?
4. What are the most significant adverse effects of strong laxatives?

5. If an adult patient asked you to recommend an over-the-counter laxative, what information about the patient's condition would you need, and what would you recommend? Why?

NCLEX-Style Questions

6. Important points to include when teaching measures to promote healthy bowel function include all of the following except
   a. Increase activity.
   b. Eat a low-residue diet.
   c. Increase fluid intake.
   d. Establish regular bowel habits.

7. Which of the following oral medications is safe to use in a 60-year-old constipated patient with dysphagia?
   a. methylcellulose (Citrucel)
   b. psyllium (Metamucil)
   c. mineral oil (Agoral Plain)
   d. docusate sodium (Colace)

8. For which of the following patients is a laxative contraindicated?
   a. a patient with cancer taking daily narcotics for pain control
   b. a patient complaining of abdominal pain and distention
   c. a patient scheduled for a colonoscopy
   d. a patient with limited mobility due to Parkinson's disease

Selected References

Borowitz, S. M., Cox, D. J., Kovatchev, B., Ritterband, L. M., Sheen, J., & Sutphen, J. (2005). Treatment of childhood constipation by primary care physicians: Efficacy and predictors of outcome. *Pediatrics, 115,* 873–877.

Bosshard, W., Dreher, R., Schnegg, J. F., & Bula, C. J. (2004). The treatment of chronic constipation in elderly people: An update. *Drugs & Aging, 21,* 911–930.

Constipation Guideline Committee of the North American Society for Pediatric Gastroenterology. (2006, September). Evaluation and treatment of constipation in infants and children: Recommendations of the North American Society for Pediatric Gastroenterology. *Journal of Pediatric Gastroenterology and Nutrition, 43,* e1–e13. Retrieved July 16, 2007, from http://www.guideline.gov/summary/summary.aspx?doc_id=9792&nbr=005245&string=constipation+and+infants

Drug facts and comparisons. (Updated monthly). St. Louis, MO: Facts and Comparisons.

Loening-Bauche, V. (2005). Prevalence, symptoms and outcome of constipation in infants and toddlers. *Journal of Pediatrics, 146,* 359–363.

Miles, C. L., Fellowes, D., Goodman, M. L., & Wilkinson, S. (2007). Laxatives for the management of constipation in palliative care patients (Cochrane Review). *The Cochrane Library,* Issue 2.

Porth, C. M. (2005). Disorders of gastrointestinal function. In C. M. Porth (Ed.), *Pathophysiology: Concepts of altered health states* (7th ed., pp. 885–916). Philadelphia: Lippincott Williams & Wilkins.

Ramkumar, D., & Rao, S. (2005). Efficacy and safety of traditional medical therapies for chronic constipation: Systematic review. *American Journal of Gastroenterology, 100,* 936–971.

Smeltzer, S. C., Bare, B. G., Hinkle J. L., & Cheever, K. H. (2008). *Brunner & Suddarth's textbook of medical-surgical nursing* (11th ed., pp. 1232-1235). Philadelphia: Lippincott Williams & Wilkins.

Spruill, W. J., & Wade, W. E. (2005). Diarrhea, constipation, and irritable bowel syndrome. In J. T. DiPiro, R. L. Talbert, G. C. Yee, G. R. Matzke, B. G. Wells, & L. M. Posey (Eds.), *Pharmacotherapy: A pathophysiologic approach* (6th ed., pp. 677–692). New York: McGraw-Hill.

KEY TERMS

- Diarrhea
- Inflammatory bowel disorders
- Irritable bowel syndrome (IBS)
- Travelers' diarrhea

LEARNING OBJECTIVES

After studying this chapter, you will be able to:

1. Identify patients at risk for development of diarrhea.
2. Discuss guidelines for assessing diarrhea.
3. Describe types of diarrhea in which antidiarrheal drug therapy may be indicated.
4. Differentiate the major types of antidiarrheal drugs.
5. Discuss characteristics, effects, and nursing process implications of commonly used antidiarrheal agents.

Applying Your Knowledge

Frederico Mendoza is a 47-year-old salesman who travels extensively as part of his job. He recently returned from a trip to Mexico. He has been having diarrhea for the past 10 days and seeks advice on how to manage his symptoms.

Introduction

Antidiarrheal drugs are used to treat *diarrhea*, defined as the frequent expulsion of liquid or semi-liquid stools. Diarrhea is a symptom of numerous conditions that increase bowel motility, cause secretion or retention of fluids in the intestinal lumen, and cause inflammation or irritation of the gastrointestinal (GI) tract. As a result, bowel contents are rapidly propelled toward the rectum, and absorption of fluids and electrolytes is limited. Some causes of diarrhea include the following:

- Excessive use or abuse of laxatives. Laxative abuse may accompany eating disorders such as anorexia nervosa or bulimia.
- Intestinal infections with viruses, bacteria, or protozoa. A common source of infection is ingested food or fluid contaminated by a variety of organisms.
  - *Escherichia coli* O157:H7–related hemorrhagic colitis most commonly occurs with the ingestion of undercooked ground beef. A serious complication of *E. coli* O157:H7 colitis is hemolytic uremic syndrome (HUS), characterized by thrombocytopenia, microangiopathic hemolytic anemia, and renal failure. Children are especially susceptible to HUS, which is the leading cause of dialysis in pediatric patients. So-called *travelers' diarrhea* is usually caused by an enterotoxigenic strain of *E. coli* (ETEC). Fecal contamination of food or water is the most common source of ETEC-induced diarrhea.
  - Consumption of improperly prepared poultry may result in diarrhea due to infection with *Campylobacter jejuni*. In the United States, this is the most common bacterial organism identified in infectious diarrhea. In addition to diarrhea, vomiting, fever, and abdominal discom-

fort, *Campylobacter* bacteria produce neurotoxins, which may result in paralysis.

▪ *Salmonella* infections may occur when contaminated poultry and other meats, eggs, and dairy products are ingested. Elderly patients are especially susceptible to *Salmonella*-associated colitis.

▪ Several strains of *Shigella* may produce diarrhea. Infection most often results from direct person-to-person contact but may also occur via food or water contamination. Handwashing is especially important in preventing the spread of *Shigella* from person to person.

▪ Other diarrhea-producing organisms associated with contamination of specific foods include *Vibrio vulnificus* and *Vibrio parahaemolyticus* contamination of raw shellfish and oysters (particularly in the Gulf Coast states), *Clostridium perfringens* contamination of inadequately heated or reheated meats, *Staphylococcus aureus* contamination of processed meats and custard-filled pastries, *Bacillus cereus* contamination of rice and bean sprouts, and *Listeria monocytogenes* contamination of hot dogs and luncheon meats. Newborns, pregnant women, and older and immunocompromised individuals are especially susceptible to *L. monocytogenes* infection.

▪ Two of the most common viral organisms responsible for gastroenteritis and diarrhea are rotavirus or Norwalk-like virus (calicivirus). Vomiting is usually a prominent symptom accompanying virus-induced diarrhea.

▪ Undigested, coarse, or highly spiced food in the GI tract. The food acts as an irritant and attracts fluids in a defensive attempt to dilute the irritating agent. This may result from inadequate chewing of food or lack of digestive enzymes.

▪ Lack of digestive enzymes. Deficiency of pancreatic enzymes inhibits digestion and absorption of carbohydrates, proteins, and fats. Deficiency of lactase, which breaks down lactose to simple sugars (i.e., glucose and galactose) that can be absorbed by GI mucosa, inhibits digestion of milk and milk products. Lactase deficiency commonly occurs among people of African and Asian descent.

▪ *Inflammatory bowel disorders*, such as gastroenteritis, diverticulitis, ulcerative colitis, and Crohn's disease. In these disorders, the inflamed mucous membrane secretes large amounts of fluids into the intestinal lumen, along with mucus, proteins, and blood, and absorption of water and electrolytes is impaired. In addition, when the ileum is diseased or a portion is surgically excised, large amounts of bile salts reach the colon, where they act as cathartics and cause diarrhea. Bile salts are normally reabsorbed from the ileum.

▪ *Irritable bowel syndrome (IBS)* is a functional disorder of intestinal motility with no evidence of inflammation or tissue changes. It occurs more commonly in women than in men, affecting approximately 12% of adults in the United States. A change in bowel pattern (constipation, diarrhea, or a combination of both) accompanied by abdominal pain, bloating, and distention are the presenting symptoms. The

etiology is unknown; however, activation of 5-HT$_3$ (serotonin) receptors, which affect the regulation of visceral pain, colonic motility, and GI secretions, are thought to be involved in the pathophysiology of IBS.

▪ Drug therapy. Many oral drugs irritate the GI tract and may cause diarrhea, including acarbose, antacids that contain magnesium, antibacterials, antineoplastic agents, colchicine, laxatives, metformin, metoclopramide, misoprostol, selective serotonin reuptake inhibitors, tacrine, and tacrolimus. Antibacterial drugs are commonly used offenders that also may cause diarrhea by altering the normal bacterial flora in the intestine.

Antibiotic-associated colitis (also called pseudomembranous colitis) is a serious condition that results from oral or parenteral antibiotic therapy. By suppressing normal flora in the colon, antibiotics allow proliferation of other bacteria, especially gram-positive, anaerobic *Clostridium difficile* organisms. These organisms produce a toxin that causes fever, abdominal pain, inflammatory lesions of the colon, and severe diarrhea with stools containing mucus, pus, and sometimes blood. Symptoms may develop within a few days or several weeks after the causative antibiotic is discontinued. Other enteric pathogens that may overgrow in the presence of antibiotic therapy and result in colitis include *Salmonella, Clostridium perfringens* type A, *S. aureus*, and *Candida albicans*. Antibiotic-associated colitis is more often associated with ampicillin, cephalosporins, and clindamycin but may occur with any antibiotic or combination of antibiotics that alters intestinal microbial flora.

▪ Intestinal neoplasms. Tumors may increase intestinal motility by occupying space and stretching the intestinal wall. Diarrhea sometimes alternates with constipation in colon cancer.

▪ Functional disorders. Diarrhea may be a symptom of stress or anxiety in some patients. No organic disease process can be found in such circumstances.

▪ Hyperthyroidism. This condition increases bowel motility.

▪ Surgical excision of portions of the intestine, especially the small intestine. Such procedures decrease the absorptive area and increase fluidity of stools.

▪ Human immunodeficiency virus (HIV) infection/acquired immunodeficiency syndrome (AIDS). Diarrhea occurs in most patients with HIV infection, often as a chronic condition that contributes to malnutrition and weight loss. It may be caused by drug therapy, infection with a variety of microorganisms, or other factors.

Diarrhea may be acute or chronic and mild or severe. Most episodes of acute diarrhea are defensive mechanisms by which the body tries to rid itself of irritants, toxins, and infectious agents. These episodes are usually self-limiting and subside within 24 to 48 hours without serious consequences. If it is severe or prolonged, acute diarrhea may lead to serious fluid and electrolyte depletion, especially in young children and older adults. Chronic diarrhea may cause malnutrition and anemia and is often characterized by remissions and exacerbations.

Characteristics, Classifications, and Individual Antidiarrheal Drugs

Antidiarrheal drugs include a variety of agents, most of which are discussed in other chapters. When used for treatment of diarrhea, the drugs may be given to relieve the symptom (nonspecific therapy) or the underlying cause of the symptom (specific therapy). Individual drugs are listed in Table 61-1.

Nonspecific Therapy

A major element of nonspecific therapy is adequate fluid and electrolyte replacement. When drug therapy is required, nonprescription antidiarrheal drugs (e.g., loperamide) may be effective.

Overall, **opiates** and **opiate derivatives** (see Chap. 6) are the most effective agents for symptomatic treatment of diarrhea. These drugs decrease diarrhea by slowing propulsive movements in the small and large intestines. Morphine, codeine, and related drugs are effective in relieving diarrhea but are rarely used for this purpose because of their adverse effects. Opiates have largely been replaced by the synthetic drugs **diphenoxylate** and **loperamide**, which are used only for treatment of diarrhea and do not cause morphine-like adverse effects in recommended doses. Diphenoxylate requires a prescription.

Loperamide (Imodium) is a synthetic derivative of meperidine that decreases GI motility by its effect on intestinal muscles. Because loperamide does not penetrate the central nervous system (CNS) well, it does not cause the CNS effects associated with opioid use and lacks potential for abuse. Although adverse effects are generally few and mild, loperamide can cause abdominal pain, constipation, drowsiness, fatigue, nausea, and vomiting. For nonprescription use, dosages for adults should not exceed 8 milligrams per day; with supervision by a health care provider, maximum daily dosage is 16 milligrams per day. In general, loperamide should be discontinued after 48 hours if clinical improvement has not occurred.

Bismuth salts have antibacterial and antiviral activity; **bismuth subsalicylate** (Pepto-Bismol, a commonly used over-the-counter [OTC] drug) also has antisecretory and possibly anti-inflammatory effects because of its salicylate component.

Octreotide acetate is a synthetic form of somatostatin, a hormone produced in the anterior pituitary gland and in the pancreas. The drug may be effective in diarrhea because it decreases GI secretion and motility. It is used for diarrhea associated with carcinoid syndrome, intestinal tumors, HIV/AIDS, and diarrhea that does not respond to other antidiarrheal drugs.

Other nonspecific agents sometimes used in diarrhea are anticholinergics (see Chap. 20) and polycarbophil and psyllium preparations (see Chap. 60). Anticholinergic drugs, of which atropine is the prototype, are infrequently used because doses large enough to decrease intestinal motility and secretions cause intolerable adverse effects. The drugs are occasionally used to decrease abdominal cramping and pain (antispasmodic effects) associated with acute nonspecific diarrhea and chronic diarrhea associated with inflammatory bowel disease.

Polycarbophil (e.g., FiberCon) and psyllium are most often used as bulk-forming laxatives. They are occasionally used in diarrhea to adsorb toxins and water, decreasing the fluidity of stools. Polycarbophil is the only adsorbent drug evaluated to be effective by the U.S. Food and Drug Administration (FDA) over-the-counter review panel. Polycarbophil absorbs large amounts of water and produces stools of gelatin-like consistency. It may cause abdominal discomfort and bloating and may reduce the absorption of co-administered medications.

Specific Therapy

Specific drug therapy for diarrhea depends on the cause of the symptom and may include the use of enzymatic replacement therapy, bile salt–binding drugs, antibacterial agents, and 5-HT$_3$ serotonin receptor antagonists. Enzymatic replacement with **pancreatin** or **pancrelipase** is recommended when a deficiency of pancreatic enzymes results in malabsorption of nutrients and steatorrhea, which is a loose fatty stool. Bile-binding drugs such as **cholestyramine** or **colestipol** are useful in treating diarrhea due to bile salt accumulation in conditions such as Crohn's disease or surgical excision of the ileum. Antibacterial drugs are recommended for bacterial enteritis when diarrhea lasts longer than 48 hours, when the patient passes six or more loose stools in 24 hours, when diarrhea is associated with fever, or when blood or pus is seen in the stools. Although effective in preventing travelers' diarrhea, antibiotics usually are not recommended because their use may promote the emergence of drug-resistant microorganisms. Although effective in reducing diarrhea due to *Salmonella* and *E. coli* intestinal infections, antibiotics may induce a prolonged carrier state during which the infection can be transmitted to other people.

Rifaximin (Xifaxan) is a structural analog of the antimycobacterial drug, rifampin. It is a nonsystemic antibiotic that remains in the gut and is not absorbed into the bloodstream. It was specifically developed to treat travelers' diarrhea due to noninvasive strains of *E. coli* in patients older than 12 years of age. It should not be used for diarrhea in the presence of fever or bloody stools or for diarrhea due to pathogens other than *E. coli*. As with the use of other broad-spectrum antibiotics, superinfections may occur with rifaximin therapy, requiring termination of the medication and treatment.

Nitazoxanide (Alinia) is an antiprotozoal agent used specifically for treating diarrhea resulting from infection with *Giardia lamblia* or *Cryptosporidium parvum*. Caution should be used when administering Alinia concurrently with highly plasma-protein–bound medications such as warfarin, because the active metabolite of nitazoxanide is highly plasma-protein bound and such concurrent use may result in competitive drug interactions.

Table 61-1		**Drugs at a Glance:** Antidiarrheal Drugs		

			ROUTES AND DOSAGE RANGES	
Generic/Trade Name	**Characteristics**	**Clinical indications**	**Adults**	**Children**
Opiate-Related Drugs				
Paregoric	Morphine is the active ingredient. Paregoric contains 0.4 mg/mL of morphine. A Schedule III drug alone and a Schedule V in the small amounts combined with other drugs. Recommended doses and short-term use do not produce euphoria, analgesia, or dependence.	Symptomatic treatment of acute diarrhea	PO 5–10 mL 1–4 times daily (maximum of 4 doses) until diarrhea is controlled	PO 0.25–0.5 mL/kg 1–4 times daily (maximum of 4 doses) until diarrhea is controlled
Diphenoxylate with atropine sulfate (Lomotil)	A derivative of meperidine (Demerol) Commonly prescribed; decreases intestinal motility In recommended doses, does not produce euphoria, analgesia, or dependence. In high doses, produces morphine-like effects, including euphoria, dependence, and respiratory depression Naloxone (Narcan) is the antidote for overdose. Each tablet or 5 mL of liquid contains 2.5 mg of diphenoxylate and 0.025 mg of atropine. The atropine is added to discourage drug abuse. Contraindicated in patients with severe liver disease or glaucoma A Schedule V drug	Symptomatic treatment of acute or chronic diarrhea	PO 5 mg (2 tablets or 10 mL of liquid) 3 or 4 times daily; maximal daily dose, 20 mg	Liquid preparation (2.5 mg diphenoxylate and 0.025 mg atropine per 5 mL), PO 0.3–0.4 mg/kg/day in 4 divided doses. Contraindicated in children <2 y of age
Loperamide (Imodium)	A derivative of meperidine; decreases intestinal motility As effective as diphenoxylate, with fewer adverse effects in recommended doses. High doses may produce morphine-like effects. Naloxone (Narcan) is the antidote for overdose.	Symptomatic treatment of acute or chronic diarrhea	PO 4 mg initially, then 2 mg after each loose stool to a maximal daily dose of 16 mg. For chronic diarrhea, dosage should be reduced to the lowest effective amount (average 4–8 mg daily).	8–12 y, >30 kg: PO 2 mg 3 times daily 6–8 y, 20–30 kg: PO 2 mg twice daily 2–5 y, 13–20 kg: PO 1 mg 3 times daily Safety not established for children <2 y of age.

(continued on page 986)

Table 61-1 **Drugs at a Glance:** Antidiarrheal Drugs (continued)

Generic/Trade Name	Characteristics	Clinical indications	ROUTES AND DOSAGE RANGES Adults	Children
Antibacterial Agents				
Azithromycin	A macrolide (see Chap. 33)	Traveler's diarrhea acquired in SE Asia. Regardless of destination, may be preferred antibiotic for children and those unable to take quinolones.	PO 500 mg daily for 3 days.	PO 10 mg/kg on day 1, up to 500 mg; and 5 mg/kg on days 2 and 3, up to 250 mg.
Ciprofloxacin (Cipro)	A fluoroquinolone (See Chap. 31)	Diarrhea caused by susceptible strains of *Escherichia coli, Campylobacter jejuni, and Shigella* species	PO 500 mg q12h for 5–7 d	Not recommended for use
Erythromycin (E-Mycin)	A macrolide (see Chap. 33)	Intestinal amebiasis caused by *Entamoeba histolytica*	PO 250 mg 4 times daily for 10–14 d	PO 30–50 mg/kg/d, in divided doses, for 10–14 d
Metronidazole (Flagyl)	See Chap. 33	Diarrhea and colitis caused by *Clostridium difficile* organisms	*C. difficile* infection, PO 500 mg 3 times daily or 250 mg 4 times daily	Dosage not established for *C. difficile* infection
		Intestinal amebiasis	Intestinal amebiasis, PO 750 mg 3 times daily for 5–10 d	Intestinal amebiasis, PO 35–50 mg/kg/24 h (maximum 750 mg/dose), in 3 divided doses for 10 d
Nitazoxanide (Alinia)	Antiprotozoal agent	Diarrhea caused by *Giardia lamblia* or *Cryptosporidium parvum*	For *G. lamblia:* PO 500 mg tablet every 12 h with food or 25 mL (500 mg) oral suspension every 12 h with food for 3 d For *C. parvum:* adult dose not established	For *G. lamblia* and *C. parvum:* >12 y, same as adults 4–11 y, 10 mL (200 mg) oral suspension every 12 h with food for 3 d 1–3 y, 5 mL (100 mg) oral suspension every 12 h with food for 3 d
Rifaximin (Xifaxan)	Structural analog of rifampin; a broad-spectrum, nonspecific antibiotic that remains in the gut where it exerts its effects	Traveler's diarrhea caused by *E. coli*	PO 200 mg 3 times a day for 3 d	Dosage not established for children <12 y of age
Trimethoprim-sulfamethoxazole (TMP-SMX) (Bactrim, Septra)	See Chap. 32	Diarrhea caused by susceptible strains of *E. coli* or *Shigella* organisms Traveler's diarrhea	PO 160 mg of TMP and 800 mg of SMX q12h for 5 d or longer	PO 8 mg/kg of TMP and 40 mg/kg of SMX daily, in 2 divided doses, q12h, for 5 d or longer

ROUTES AND DOSAGE RANGES

Generic/Trade Name	Characteristics	Clinical indications	Adults	Children
Vancomycin	Cell wall synthesis inhibitor (see Chap. 33)	Diarrhea and colitis caused by *C. difficile* organism	PO 500 mg to 2 g per day in 3–4 divided doses for 7–10 d *or* PO 125 mg 3 or 4 times daily	PO 400 mg/kg/d in 4 divided doses for 7–10 d. Do not exceed 2 g/d.
Miscellaneous Drugs				
Alosetron (Lotronex)	A 5-HT$_3$ receptor antagonist	For women with diarrhea-predominant irritable bowel syndrome(IBS)	PO 0.5mg twice a day. May increase to 1mg after 4 weeks if needed	Not recommended
Bismuth subsalicylate (Pepto-Bismol)	Has antimicrobial, antisecretory, and possibly anti-inflammatory effects	Control of diarrhea, including traveler's diarrhea, and relief of abdominal cramping	PO 2 tablets or 30 mL every 30–60 min, if needed, up to 8 doses in 24 h	9–12 y, PO 1 tablet or 15 mL 6–9 y, PO 2/3 tablet or 10 mL 3–6 y, PO 1/3 tablet or 5 mL *Under 3 y*, consult pediatrician
Cholestyramine (Questran)	Binds and inactivates bile salts in the intestine (see chap. 55)	Diarrhea due to bile salts reaching the colon and causing a cathartic effect. "Bile salt diarrhea" is associated with Crohn's disease or surgical excision of the ileum.	PO 16–32 g/d in 120–180 mL of water, in 2–4 divided doses before or during meals and at bedtime	
Colestipol (Colestid)	Same as cholestyramine, above (see Chap. 55)	Same as cholestyramine	PO 15–30 g/d in 120–180 mL of water, in 2–4 divided doses before or during meals and at bedtime	
Octreotide (Sandostatin)	In GI tract, decreases secretions and motility (see Chap. 22)	Diarrhea associated with carcinoid tumors, HIV/AIDS, cancer chemotherapy or radiation, or diarrhea unresponsive to other drugs	Sub-Q IV 150–750/day divided over 2–4 doses. Start at 200-300 mcg/day divided over 2–4 doses for 2 weeks, then individualize dose to response.	Dosage not established
Pancreatin or pancrelipase (Viokase, Pancrease, Cotazym)	Pancreatic enzymes used only for replacement	Diarrhea and malabsorption due to deficiency of pancreatic enzymes	PO 1–3 tablets or capsules or 1–2 packets of powder with meals and snacks	PO 1–3 tablets or capsules or 1–2 packets of powder with each meal
Polycarbophil preparations (FiberCon)	Absorbs water and toxins and decreases fluidity of stools	Possibly effective for symptomatic treatment of diarrhea	PO 1g, 1–4 times daily. Do not exceed 4 g in 24 h. For severe diarrhea repeat dose every 30 min but do not exceed maximum dose.	6–12y: PO 500 mg 1–4 times daily. Do not exceed 2 g 124 h. *Under 6y:* products vary consist labels. For severediarrhea repeat dose every 30 min but do not exceed maximum dose.

AIDS, acquired immunodeficiency syndrome; GI, gastrointestinal; HIV, human immunodeficiency virus.

Alosetron (Lotronex) is a selective 5-HT$_3$ receptor antagonist indicated for treating women with chronic severe diarrhea-predominant IBS that has not responded to conventional therapy. Clinical studies have not demonstrated safety and efficacy of alosetron in men. Alosetron is rapidly absorbed orally with a bioavailability of 50% to 60%. It is moderately plasma protein bound (82%). Alosetron is extensively metabolized by the CYP 450 enzyme system (CYP 2C9, CYP 3A4, and CYP 1A2) with multiple metabolites produced that are excreted primarily in the urine. Caution must be used with concurrent administration with CYP1A2 and CYP3A4 inhibitors, and concurrent administration with fluvoxamine is contraindicated. Alosetron is also contraindicated in women with severe hepatic impairment. Reduced dosages may be needed in some women over 65 years of age to prevent drug accumulation and toxicity. A **BLACK BOX WARNING** alerts nurses to the serious GI adverse effects of alosetron. Severe constipation with possible obstruction, perforation, and hemorrhage is the most common problem. Ischemic colitis (reduced blood flow to the intestinal tract resulting in tissue damage) has also occurred. These serious conditions have resulted in hospitalizations, blood loss necessitating transfusion, surgery, and death in severe cases. Alosetron should not be given to patients with a history of GI disorders including chronic or severe constipation or sequelae of constipation, intestinal obstruction, stricture, toxic megacolon, GI perforation and/or adhesions, ischemic colitis, impaired intestinal circulation, thrombophlebitis or hypercoagulable state, Crohn's disease or ulcerative colitis, or diverticulitis.

To ensure safe and appropriate use of alosetron, the drug manufacturer has established a prescribing program, and only qualified health care providers enrolled in the program can prescribe this medication. Pharmacists must provide patients with a medication guide developed by the manufacturer at the time the medication is dispensed that includes the risks of taking alosetron and the situations under which the drug should be immediately discontinued. Each patient must sign a patient–physician agreement indicting that she (1) understands the risks of taking alosetron and agrees to take the medication, (2) will discontinue taking alosetron if constipation occurs, (3) will immediately notify the physician if constipation or signs of ischemic colitis occur, and (4) will stop taking alosetron and contact the physician after 4 weeks of therapy with alosetron if the symptoms of IBS are not controlled. The medication guide and patient–physician agreement are available at http://www.lotronex.com

Indications for Use

Despite the limitations of drug therapy in the prevention and treatment of diarrhea, antidiarrheal drugs are indicated in the following circumstances:

- Severe or prolonged diarrhea (>2–3 days), to prevent severe fluid and electrolyte loss
- Relatively severe diarrhea in young children and older adults. These groups are less able to adapt to fluid and electrolyte losses.

- In chronic inflammatory diseases of the bowel (ulcerative colitis and Crohn's disease), to allow a more nearly normal lifestyle
- In ileostomies or surgical excision of portions of the ileum, to decrease fluidity and volume of stool
- To reduce symptoms of diarrhea-predominant IBS
- HIV/AIDS–associated diarrhea
- When specific causes of diarrhea have been determined

Contraindications to Use

Contraindications to the use of antidiarrheal drugs include diarrhea caused by toxic materials, microorganisms that penetrate intestinal mucosa (e.g., pathogenic *E. coli*, *Salmonella*, *Shigella*), or antibiotic-associated colitis. In these circumstances, antidiarrheal agents that slow peristalsis may aggravate and prolong diarrhea. Opiates (morphine, codeine) usually are contraindicated in chronic diarrhea because of possible opiate dependence. Diphenoxylate and loperamide are contraindicated in children younger than 2 years of age.

Herbal and Dietary Supplements

Several herbal remedies are promoted for treatment of diarrhea. Most include tannins, substances with astringent properties that reduce intestinal inflammation and secretions. The leaves of edible berry plants (i.e., blackberry, blueberry, raspberry) are sometimes used in a "tea" made by pouring boiling water over 1 to 2 teaspoons of leaves, drunk up to six times daily. There is little objective evidence of effectiveness or toxicity.

Nursing Process

Assessment

Assess for acute or chronic diarrhea.

- Try to determine the duration of diarrhea; number of stools per day; amount, consistency, color, odor, and presence of abnormal components (e.g., undigested food, blood, pus, mucus) in each stool; precipitating factors; accompanying signs and symptoms (i.e, nausea, vomiting, fever, abdominal pain or cramping); and measures used to relieve diarrhea. When possible, look at stool specimens for possible clues to causation. Blood may indicate inflammation, infection, or neoplastic disease; pus or mucus may indicate inflammation or infection. Infections caused by *Shigella* organisms produce blood-tinged mucus. Infections caused by *Salmonella* or *E. coli* usually produce green, liquid or semiliquid stools. Inflammatory bowel disorders often produce non-bloody mucus.

- Try to determine the cause of the diarrhea. This includes questioning about such causes as chronic inflammatory diseases of the bowel, food intake, possible exposure to contaminated food, living or traveling in areas of poor sanitation, and use of laxatives or other drugs that may cause diarrhea. When available, check laboratory reports on stool specimens (e.g., culture reports).

- With severe or prolonged diarrhea, especially in young children and older adults, assess for dehydration, hypokalemia, and other fluid and electrolyte disorders.

Nursing Diagnoses

- Diarrhea related to GI infection or inflammatory disorders, other disease processes, dietary irritants, or overuse of laxatives

- Anxiety related to availability of bathroom facilities

- Deficient Fluid Volume related to excessive losses in liquid stools

- Pain (abdominal cramping) related to intestinal hyper-motility and spasm

- Deficient Knowledge: Factors that cause or aggravate diarrhea and appropriate use of antidiarrheal drugs

Planning/Goals

The patient will

- Take antidiarrheal drugs appropriately

- Obtain relief from acute diarrhea (reduced number of liquid stools, reduced abdominal discomfort)

- Maintain fluid and electrolyte balance

- Maintain adequate nutritional intake

- Avoid adverse effects of antidiarrheal medications

- Re-establish normal bowel patterns after an episode of acute diarrhea

- Have fewer liquid stools with chronic diarrhea

Interventions

Use measures to prevent diarrhea.

- Prepare and store food properly and avoid improperly stored foods and those prepared under unsanitary conditions. Dairy products, cream pies, and other foods may cause diarrhea ("food poisoning") if not refrigerated.

- Wash hands before handling any foods, after handling raw poultry or meat, and always before eating.

- Chew food well.

- Do not overuse laxatives (i.e., amount per dose or frequency of use). Many OTC products contain senna or other strong stimulant laxatives.

Provide education about drug therapy (see accompanying Patient Teaching Guidelines).

Regardless of whether antidiarrheal drugs are used, supportive therapy is required for the treatment of diarrhea. Elements of supportive care include the following:

- Replacement of fluids and electrolytes (2–3 quarts daily). Fluids such as weak tea; water; bouillon; clear soup; noncarbonated, caffeine-free beverages; and gelatin are usually tolerated and helpful. If the patient cannot tolerate adequate amounts of oral liquids or if diarrhea is severe or prolonged, intravenous fluids may be needed (i.e., solutions containing dextrose, sodium chloride, and potassium chloride).

- Avoid foods and fluids that may further irritate GI mucosa (e.g., highly spiced foods; "laxative" foods, such as raw fruits and vegetables).

- Increase frequency and length of rest periods, and decrease activity. Exercise and activity stimulate peristalsis.

- If perianal irritation occurs because of frequent liquid stools, cleanse the area with mild soap and water after each bowel movement, then apply an emollient, such as white petrolatum (Vaseline).

Evaluation

- Observe and interview for decreased number of liquid or loose stools.

- Observe for signs of adequate food and fluid intake (e.g., good skin turgor and urine output, stable weight).

- Observe for appropriate use of antidiarrheal drugs.

- Observe and interview for return of pre-diarrheal patterns of bowel elimination.

- Interview regarding knowledge and use of measures to prevent or minimize diarrhea.

Applying Your Knowledge 61-1

What factors would you include in your assessment of Mr. Mendoza?

Principles of Therapy

In most cases of acute, nonspecific diarrhea in adults, fluid losses are not severe and patients need only simple replacement of fluids and electrolytes lost in the stool. Acceptable replacement fluids during the first 24 hours include 2 to 3 liters of clear liquids (e.g., flat ginger ale, decaffeinated cola drinks or tea, broth, gelatin). Also, the diet should consist of bland foods (e.g., rice, soup, bread, salted crackers, cooked cereals, baked potatoes, eggs, applesauce). A regular diet may be resumed after 2 to 3 days.

Drug Selection

The choice of antidiarrheal agent depends largely on the cause, severity, and duration of diarrhea.

- For symptomatic treatment of diarrhea, diphenoxylate with atropine (Lomotil) or loperamide (Imodium) is probably the drug of choice for most people.

Patient Teaching Guidelines | Antidiarrheals

General Considerations

- Taking a medication to stop diarrhea is not always needed or desirable because diarrhea may mean the body is trying to rid itself of irritants or bacteria. Treatment is indicated if diarrhea is severe, prolonged, or occurs in young children or older adults, who are highly susceptible to excessive losses of body fluids and electrolytes.

- Try to drink 2 to 3 quarts of fluid daily. This helps prevent dehydration from fluid loss in stools. Water, clear broths, and noncarbonated, caffeine-free beverages are recommended because they are unlikely to cause further diarrhea.

- Avoid highly spiced or "laxative" foods, such as fresh fruits and vegetables, until diarrhea is controlled.

- Frequent and thorough handwashing and careful food storage and preparation can help prevent diarrhea.

- Consult a health care provider if diarrhea is accompanied by severe abdominal pain or fever, lasts longer than 3 days, or if stools contain blood or mucus. These signs and symptoms may indicate more serious disorders for which other treatment measures are needed.

- Stop antidiarrheal drugs when diarrhea is controlled to avoid adverse effects such as constipation.

- Bismuth subsalicylate (Pepto-Bismol) and loperamide (Imodium A-D) are available over the counter; diphenoxylate (Lomotil) is a prescription drug.

- Diphenoxylate and loperamide may cause dizziness or drowsiness and should be used with caution if driving or performing other tasks requiring alertness, coordination, or physical dexterity. In addition, alcohol and other drugs that cause drowsiness should be avoided.

- Pepto-Bismol may temporarily discolor bowel movements a grayish-black.

- Keep antidiarrheal drugs out of reach of children.

Self- or Caregiver Administration

- Take or give antidiarrheal drugs only as prescribed or directed on nonprescription drug labels.

- Do not exceed maximal daily doses of diphenoxylate (Lomotil), loperamide, or paregoric.

- With liquid diphenoxylate, use only the calibrated dropper furnished by the manufacturer for accurate measurement of dosages.

- With Pepto-Bismol liquid, shake the bottle well before measuring the dose; with tablets, chew them well or allow them to dissolve in the mouth.

- Add at least 30 mL of water to each dose of paregoric to help the drug dose reach the stomach. The mixture appears milky.

- Take cholestyramine or colestipol with at least 4 oz of water. These drugs should never be taken without fluids because they may block the gastrointestinal tract. Also, do not take within 4 hours of other drugs because they may combine with and inactivate other drugs.

- Take rifaximin with or without food for 3 days. Notify health care provider if your condition worsens or does not improve after 1 to 2 days.

- Use caution driving or operating machinery if experiencing dizziness while using rifaximin.

- Diabetic patients should be aware that Alinia oral suspension contains 1.48 g of sucrose per 5 mL.

- With Lotronex, if you become constipated, notice blood in your bowel movements, or experience a new worse or different pain in your stomach or abdomen, STOP taking Lotronex and notify your health care provider.

- In bacterial gastroenteritis or diarrhea, the choice of antibacterial drug depends on the causative microorganism and susceptibility tests.

- In ulcerative colitis, sulfonamides, adrenal corticosteroids, and other anti-inflammatory agents such as balsalazide (Colazal), mesalamine (Pentasa), and olsalazine (Dipentum) are the drugs of choice. The latter drugs are related to aspirin and nonsteroidal anti-inflammatory drugs (see Chap. 7 and Appendix A) and are contraindicated in patients with hypersensitivity to salicylates or any other product component. They are given orally or rectally and are thought to exert topical anti-inflammatory effects in ulcerative colitis.

- For treatment of women with diarrhea-predominant IBS that has not responded to conventional treatment, alosetron, a 5-HT$_3$ receptor antagonist may be prescribed.

- In antibiotic-associated colitis, stopping the causative drug is the initial treatment. If symptoms do not improve within 3 or 4 days, oral metronidazole or vancomycin is given for 7 to 10 days. Both are effective against *C. difficile*, but metronidazole is the drug of first choice and is much less expensive. Vancomycin may be given for severe disease or when metronidazole is ineffective. For approximately 6 weeks after recovery, relapse often occurs and requires re-treatment. Because relapse is not due to emergence of drug-resistant strains, the same drug used for the initial bout may be used to treat the relapse.

- In diarrhea caused by enzyme deficiency, pancreatic enzymes are given rather than antidiarrheal drugs.

- In bile-salt diarrhea, cholestyramine or colestipol may be effective.

- Although morphine and codeine are contraindicated in chronic diarrhea, they may occasionally be used in the treatment of acute, severe diarrhea. Dosages required for antidiarrheal effects are smaller than those required for analgesia. The following oral drugs and dosages are approximately equivalent in antidiarrheal effectiveness: 4 mg morphine, 30 mg codeine, 10 mL paregoric, 5 mg diphenoxylate, and 2 mg loperamide. A common and potentially fatal drug error is confusing paregoric (camphorated tincture of opium) with the much more potent drug Opium Tincture. Paregoric contains only 0.4 mg/mL of morphine, whereas Opium Tincture is much more concentrated, containing 10 mg/mL of morphine. Labels should be in place on Opium Tincture packaging identifying it as a poison, identifying the strength of morphine per mL as 10 mg/mL, and containing the statement, "Warning! DO NOT use Opium Tincture in place of paregoric."

Applying Your Knowledge 61-2

What is the most likely drug of choice for Mr. Mendoza?

Use in Special Populations

Use in Children

Antidiarrheal drugs, including antibiotics, are often used in children to prevent excessive losses of fluids and electrolytes. In small children, serious fluid volume deficit may rapidly develop with diarrhea. Worldwide, from 2000 to 2003, the World Health Organization estimated that diarrhea accounted for 18% of deaths in children less than 5 years of age during the first 28 days of life. Drug therapy should be accompanied by appropriate fluid replacement and efforts to decrease further stimuli. Oral rehydration solutions (e.g., Pedialyte solution and freezer popsicles) are commercially available in ready-to-use formulations in the United States. Packets of powder (containing glucose, sodium, potassium, chloride, and citrate), to be mixed with 1 liter of boiled or treated water, are available in developing countries and are usually provided by the World Health Organization.

Diphenoxylate contains atropine, and signs of atropine overdose may occur with usual doses. Diphenoxylate is contraindicated in children younger than 2 years of age; loperamide should not be used in children younger than 6 years, except with a pediatrician's supervision and should generally not be used for longer than 2 days in older children. Loperamide is a nonprescription drug.

Use in Older Adults

Diarrhea is less common than constipation in older adults, but it may occur from laxative abuse and bowel-cleansing procedures before GI surgery or diagnostic tests. Fluid volume deficits may rapidly develop in older adults with diarrhea. General principles of fluid and electrolyte replacement, measures to decrease GI irritants, and drug therapy apply as for younger adults. Most antidiarrheal drugs may be given to older adults, but cautious use is indicated to avoid inducing constipation.

Use in Patients With Renal Impairment

Diphenoxylate should be used with extreme caution in patients with severe hepatorenal disease because hepatic coma may be precipitated.

Use in Patients With Hepatic Impairment

Diphenoxylate should be used with extreme caution in patients with abnormal liver-function test results or severe hepatorenal disease because hepatic coma may be precipitated. With loperamide, monitor patients with hepatic impairment for signs of CNS toxicity. Loperamide normally undergoes extensive first-pass metabolism, which may be lessened by liver disease. As a result, a larger portion of a dose reaches the systemic circulation and may cause adverse effects. Dosage may need to be reduced. Alosetron is contraindicated in women with severe liver impairment.

Use in Immunocompromised Patients

Diarrhea often occurs in immunocompromised patients (e.g., those with AIDS, organ transplant, or anticancer chemotherapy) and may be difficult to treat with the usual antidiarrheal drugs. Octreotide may be effective, but it should be used only after other medications have failed because it is given by injection and is expensive.

Use in Home Care

Prescription and OTC antidiarrheal aids are often taken in the home setting. The role of the home care nurse may include advising patients and caregivers about appropriate use of the drugs, trying to identify the cause and severity of the diarrhea (i.e., risk of fluid and electrolyte deficit), and teaching strategies to manage the current episode and prevent future episodes. If octreotide is taken at home, the home care nurse may need to teach the patient or a caregiver how to administer subcutaneous injections.

Applying Your Knowledge 61-3

How Can You Avoid This Medication Error?
Mr. Mendoza is given loperamide for his diarrhea and sent home. He has a stool specimen examined for microorganisms. His report shows the presence of salmonella organisms. He continues to have diarrhea so you increase the dose of loperamide.

Nursing Actions   Antidiarrheals

NURSING ACTIONS	RATIONALE/EXPLANATION
1. Administer accurately	
a. WIth liquid diphenoxylate, use only the calibrated dropper furnished by the manufacturer for measuring dosage.	For accurate measurement
b. Add at least 30 mL of water to each dose of paregoric. The mixture appears milky.	To add sufficient volume for the drug to reach the stomach
c. Do not exceed maximal daily doses of diphenoxylate, loperamide, and paregoric. Also, stop the drugs when diarrhea is controlled.	To decrease risks of adverse reactions, including drug dependence
d. Give cholestyramine and colestipol with at least 120 mL of water. Also, do not give within approximately 4 hours of other drugs.	The drugs may cause obstruction of the gastrointestinal (GI) tract if swallowed in a dry state. They may combine with and inactivate other drugs.
2. Observe for therapeutic effects	
a. Decreased number, frequency, and fluidity of stools	Therapeutic effects are usually evident within 24–48 hours.
b. Decreased or absent abdominal cramping pains	
c. Signs of normal fluid and electrolyte balance (adequate hydration, urine output, and skin turgor)	
d. Resumption of usual activities of daily living	
3. Observe for adverse effects	
a. Constipation	Constipation is the most common adverse effect. It can be prevented by using antidiarrheal drugs only as prescribed and stopping the drugs when diarrhea is controlled. With Lotronex constipation may indicate a severe adverse effect and the health care provider should be notified.
b. Drug dependence	Dependence is unlikely with recommended doses but may occur with long-term use of large doses of paregoric, diphenoxylate, and difenoxin.
c. With diphenoxylate, anorexia, nausea, vomiting, dizziness, abdominal discomfort, paralytic ileus, toxic megacolon, hypersensitivity (pruritus, urticaria, angioneurotic edema), headache, and tachycardia With overdoses of a diphenoxylate–atropine or difenoxinatropine combination, respiratory depression and coma may result from diphenoxylate or difenoxin content and anticholinergic effects (eg, dry mouth, blurred vision, urinary retention) from atropine content.	Although numerous adverse reactions have been reported, their incidence and severity are low when diphenoxylate is used appropriately. Deliberate overdose and abuse are unlikely because of unpleasant anticholinergic effects. Overdose can be prevented by using the drug in recommended doses and only when required. Overdose can be treated with naloxone (Narcan) and supportive therapy.
d. With loperamide, abdominal cramps, dry mouth, dizziness, nausea, and vomiting	Abdominal cramps are the most common adverse effect. No serious adverse effects have been reported with recommended doses of loperamide. Overdose may be treated with naloxone, gastric lavage, and administration of activated charcoal.
e. With cholestyramine and colestipol, constipation, nausea, and abdominal distention	Adverse effects are usually minor and transient because these drugs are not absorbed from the GI tract.
f. With octreotide, diarrhea, headache, cardiac dysrhythmias, and injection-site pain	These are commonly reported adverse effects.
g. With rifaximin, flatulence, headache, stomach pain, urgent bowel movements, nausea, constipation, fever, vomiting, dizziness	These are commonly reported adverse effects.
h. With alosetron, constipation abdominal pain, abdominal distention, nausea, blood in bowel movements	These adverse effects indicate severe adverse GI effects including ischemic colitis and severe constipation. The medication should be discontinued and the health care provider notified.
4. Observe for drug interactions	Few clinically significant drug interactions have been reported with commonly used antidiarrheal agents.
a. Drugs that *increase* effects of antidiarrheal agents:	
(1) Central nervous system (CNS) depressants (alcohol, sedative-hypnotics, opioid analgesics, antianxiety agents, antipsychotic agents)	Additive CNS depression with opiate and related antidiarrheals. Opioid analgesics have additive constipating effects.

NURSING ACTIONS	RATIONALE/EXPLANATION
(2) Anticholinergic agents (atropine and synthetic anti-cholinergic antispasmodics; antihistamines and anti-depressants with anticholinergic effects)	Additive anticholinergic adverse effects (dry mouth, blurred vision, urinary retention) with diphenoxylate–atropine (Lomotil).
(3) With alosetron: CYPIA2 inhibitors (e.g., cimetidine, fluvoxamine, quinolone antibiotics) will *increase* the efects of alosetron.	CYPIA2 enzyme inhibition will reduce metabolism of alos-etron. Co-Administration with fluvoxamine is contraindicated.
(4) With Alosetron: CYP3A4 inhibitors (e.g., clar-ithromycin, ketaconazole, protease inhibitors) will *increase* the effects of alosetron.	CYP3A4 enzyme inhibition will reduce metabolism of alos-etron.
b. Nitazoxanide may *increase* the effect of highly protein-bound, narrow therapeutic-index drugs, such as warfarin, resulting in toxicity.	The active metabolite of nitazoxanide is 99.9% protein bound and may compete with other protein-bound medications at plasma protein binding sites.

Key Concepts

- Diarrhea is the frequent expulsion of liquid or semiliquid stools resulting from increased bowel motility, increased secretion or retention of fluids in the intestinal lumen, or inflammation/irritation of the GI tract.

- Overall, opiates and opiate derivatives are the most effec-tive nonspecific therapy for symptomatic treatment of diarrhea.

- Octreotide, a synthetic form of somatostatin, decreases GI secretion and motility. It is used for diarrhea associated with carcinoid syndrome, intestinal tumors, HIV/AIDS, and diarrhea that does not respond to other antidiarrheal drugs.

- Bismuth subsalicylate has antisecretory, antimicrobial, and possibly anti-inflammatory effects. It is used in the control of travelers' diarrhea and relief of abdominal cramping.

- Polycarbophil is used to treat diarrhea by adsorbing toxins and water, decreasing the fluidity of stools.

- Specific therapy for diarrhea is directed at the cause of the symptom and may include enzymatic replacement therapy, bile-salt binding drugs, antibacterial agents, and 5-HT$_3$ receptor antagonists.

- In bacterial gastroenteritis or diarrhea, the choice of anti-bacterial drug depends on the causative organism and sus-ceptibility tests.

- Because of the risk of severe GI adverse effects, use of alos-etron is subject to a mandated prescribing program. Only qualified health care providers enrolled in the program can prescribe this medication. Pharmacists are required to dis-tribute educational materials when dispensing alosetron. Patients must sign a patient–physician agreement before taking this medication.

Review and Application Exercises

Short Answer Exercises

1. What are some common causes of diarrhea?

2. In which populations is diarrhea most likely to cause seri-ous problems?

3. Which types of diarrhea do not require antidiarrheal drug therapy, and why?

4. How do antidiarrheal drugs decrease frequency or fluidity of stools?

5. What are adverse effects of commonly used antidiarrheal drugs?

6. If a patient asked you to recommend an OTC antidiarrheal agent, which would you recommend, and why?

7. Would your recommendation differ if the proposed recipi-ent were a child? Why or why not?

NCLEX-Style Questions

8. The nurse knows that an appropriate nursing measure when treating a 5-year-old child with a 1-day onset of mild diarrhea would be to
   a. Encourage a regular diet.
   b. Encourage intake of clear liquids.
   c. Encourage intake of milk products.
   d. Encourage no fluids for 24 hours.

9. A hospitalized patient on antibiotic therapy begins to experience fever, abdominal pain, and diarrhea containing

mucus, pus, and blood. The best nursing action in this situation is to

a. Continue the antibiotic because the patient has signs of a GI infection.

b. Monitor the patient's vital signs and notify the provider if there is further deterioration.

c. Withhold the antibiotic and notify the provider of the patient's condition.

d. Encourage fluid intake because fever is a sign of dehydration.

10. A patient with diarrhea begins to complain of eye pain after administration of diphenoxylate with atropine (Lomotil). The nurse should

a. Offer an OTC analgesic such as acetaminophen.

b. Discontinue the diphenoxylate with atropine and notify the provider.

c. Tell the patient this is a common side effect and will soon pass.

d. Apply a cool compress to the eyes for relief of the discomfort.

Selected References

Brye, J., Boschi-Pinto, C., Shibuya, K., Black, R. E., WHO Child Health Epidemiology Reference Group. (2005). WHO estimates of the causes of death in children. *Lancet, 365,* 1147–1152.

Drug facts and comparisons. (Updated monthly). St. Louis, MO: Facts and Comparisons.

Guerrant, R., Gilder, T., Steiner, T., Thielman, N., Slutsker, L., Tauxe, R., et al. (2001). Practice guidelines for the management of infectious diarrhea. *Clinical Infectious Diseases, 32,* 331–351.

Institute for Safe Medication Practices. (2002, February 20). *Hazard alert! Recurring confusion between tincture of opium and paregoric.* Retrieved August 22, 2005, from http://ismp.org/MSAarticles/recruitingPring/htm

Juckett, G. (2005). Travel medicine. *West Virginia Medical Journal, 100,* 222–225.

Porth, C. M. (2005). Disorders of gastrointestinal function. In C. M. Porth (Ed.), *Pathophysiology: Concepts of altered health states* (7th ed., pp. 885–916). Philadelphia: Lippincott Williams & Wilkins.

Schroeder, M. S. (2005). Clostridium difficile–associated diarrhea. *American Family Physician, 71,* 921–928.

Smeltzer, S. C., Bare, B. G., Hinkle, J. L., & Cheever, K. H. (2008). *Brunner & Suddarth's textbook of medical-surgical nursing* (11th ed., pp. 1237–1238). Philadelphia: Lippincott Williams & Wilkins.

Spruill, W. J., & Wade, W. E. (2005). Diarrhea, constipation, and irritable bowel syndrome. In J. T. DiPiro, R. L. Talbert, G. C. Yee, G. R. Matzke, B. G. Wells, & L. M. Posey (Eds.), *Pharmacotherapy: A pathophysiologic approach* (6th ed., pp. 677–692). New York: McGraw-Hill.

Antiemetics

LEARNING OBJECTIVES

After studying this chapter, you will be able to:

1. Identify patients at risk of developing nausea and vomiting.
2. Discuss guidelines for preventing, minimizing, or treating nausea and vomiting.
3. Differentiate the major types of antiemetic drugs.
4. Discuss characteristics, effects, and nursing process implications of selected antiemetic drugs.

Applying Your Knowledge

Nellie Snyder is a 38-year-old woman who has breast cancer. She is receiving radiation and chemotherapy. Ms. Snyder is experiencing significant nausea and vomiting. Her physician orders ondansetron 32 mg IV to be administered 30 minutes prior to her chemotherapy and 8 to 16 mg PO every 8 hours as needed. She also receives metoclopramide 10 mg PO four times a day: 30 minutes before meals and at bedtime.

Introduction

Antiemetic drugs are used to prevent or treat nausea and vomiting. *Nausea* is an unpleasant sensation of abdominal discomfort accompanied by a desire to vomit. *Vomiting* is the expulsion of stomach contents through the mouth. Nausea may occur without vomiting, and vomiting may occur without prior nausea, but the two symptoms often occur together.

Nausea and vomiting are common symptoms experienced by virtually everyone. These symptoms may accompany almost any illness or stress situation. Causes of nausea and vomiting include the following:

- Gastrointestinal (GI) disorders, including infection or inflammation in the GI tract, liver, gallbladder, or pancreas; impaired GI motility and muscle tone (e.g., gastroparesis); and overeating or ingestion of foods or fluids that irritate the GI mucosa
- Cardiovascular, infectious, neurologic, or metabolic disorders
- Drug therapy. Nausea and vomiting are the most common adverse effects of drug therapy. Although the symptoms may occur with most drugs, they are especially associated with alcohol, aspirin, digoxin, anticancer drugs, antimicrobials, estrogen preparations, and opioid analgesics.
- Pain and other noxious stimuli, such as unpleasant sights and odors
- Emotional disturbances; physical or mental stress
- Radiation therapy
- Motion sickness

■ Postoperative status, which may include pain, impaired GI motility, and receiving various medications

■ Pregnancy

Vomiting occurs when the *vomiting center* (a nucleus of cells in the medulla oblongata) is stimulated (Figure 62-1). Stimuli are relayed to the vomiting center by afferent signals from the *chemoreceptor trigger zone* (CTZ), the cerebral cortex, the sensory organs and the vestibular apparatus. The CTZ, composed of neurons in the fourth ventricle, can be activated by a variety of stimuli, including the presence of emetic substances (e.g., chemotherapy, opioids, ipecac) in the blood and cerebrospinal fluid and stimuli from the pharynx and gastrointestinal track. In cancer chemotherapy, *emetogenic* drugs are thought to stimulate the release of serotonin from the enterochromaffin cells of the small intestine; this released serotonin then activates 5-HT$_3$ receptors located on vagal afferent nerves in the CTZ to initiate the vomiting reflex. Activation of the CTZ is also thought to play a role in the nausea and vomiting associated with pregnancy. *Anticipatory nausea* triggered by memories and fear of nausea and vomiting is mediated by afferent signals from the higher centers of the cerebral cortex to the vomiting center. Noxious stimuli such as unpleasant odors or sights as well as pain are transmitted by afferent pathways from the sensory organs to the vomiting center. In *motion sickness*, rapid changes in body motion stimulate receptors in the inner ear (vestibular branch of the auditory nerve, which is concerned with equilibrium), and nerve impulses are transmitted to the vomiting center.

The vomiting center, CTZ, and GI tract contain benzodiazepine, cholinergic, dopamine, histamine, opiate, substance P/neurokinin, and serotonin receptors, which are stimulated by emetogenic drugs and toxins. When stimulated, the vomiting center initiates efferent impulses that stimulate the salivary center, cause closure of the glottis, contraction of abdominal muscles and the diaphragm, relaxation of the gastroesophageal sphincter, and reverse peristalsis, which moves stomach contents toward the mouth for ejection.

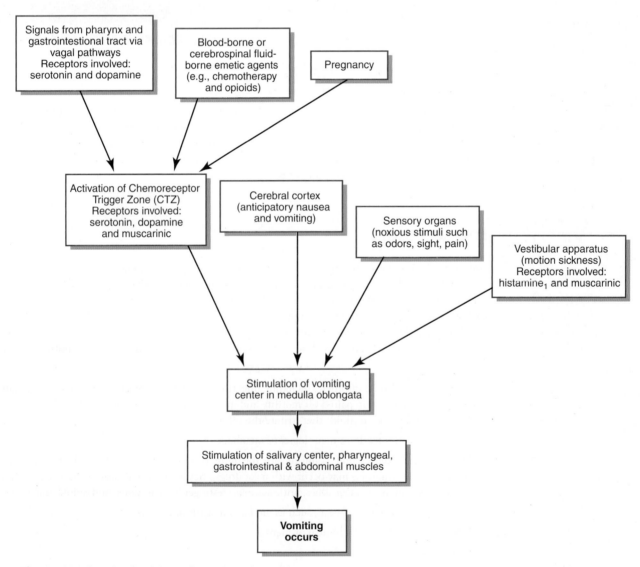

Figure 62-1 ■ Pathophysiology of nausea and vomiting.

General Characteristics of Antiemetic Drugs

Indications for Use

Antiemetic drugs are indicated to prevent and treat nausea and vomiting associated with surgery, pain, motion sickness, cancer chemotherapy, radiation therapy, and other causes.

Contraindications to Use

Antiemetic drugs are usually contraindicated when their use may prevent or delay diagnosis and when signs and symptoms of drug toxicity may be masked.

Classifications and Individual Drugs

Drugs used to prevent or treat nausea and vomiting belong to several different therapeutic classifications, and most have anticholinergic, antidopaminergic, antihistaminic, or antiserotonergic effects. In general, the drugs are more effective in prophylaxis than treatment. Most antiemetics prevent or relieve nausea and vomiting by acting on the vomiting center, CTZ, cerebral cortex, vestibular apparatus, or a combination of these. Major drugs are described in the following sections and in Table 62-1.

Table 62-1	Drugs at a Glance: Antiemetic Drugs

	ROUTES AND DOSAGE RANGES	
Generic/Trade Name	**Adults**	**Children**
Phenothiazines		
Prochlorperazine	PO 5–10 mg 3 or 4 times daily (sustained-release capsule, 10 mg twice daily) IM 5–10 mg q3–4h to a maximum of 40 mg daily Rectal suppository 25 mg twice daily	>10 kg, PO 0.4 mg/kg/d, in 3 or 4 divided doses IM 0.2 mg/kg as a single dose Rectal suppository 0.4 mg/kg/d, in 3 or 4 divided doses
Promethazine (Phenergan)	PO, IM, IV, rectal suppository 12.5–25 mg q4–6h (max dose PO, IM, rectal 50 mg. Max dose IV 25 mg	over 2 y, PO, IM, IV rectal suppository 0.25–0.5 mg/kg q4–6h (Max dose 25 mg) use lowest dose possible to prevent respiratory depression
Antihistamines		
Dimenhydrinate (Dramamine)	PO 50–100 mg q4–6h as needed (maximal dose, 400 mg in 24 h) IM 50 mg as needed IV 50 mg in 10 mL of sodium chloride injection, over 2 min	6–12 y, PO 25–50 mg q6–8h (maximal dose, 150 mg in 24 h) IM 1.25 mg/kg 4 times daily (maximal dose, 300 mg in 24 h)
Hydroxyzine (Vistaril) **Meclizine** (Antivert, Bonine)	IM 25–100 mg q4–6h as needed Motion sickness, PO 25–50 mg 1 h before travel Vertigo, PO 25–100 mg daily in divided doses	IM 0.5–1 mg/kg q4–6h Motion sickness, >12 y, PO 25–50 mg/d divided into 2 or 3 doses
Prokinetic Agent		
Metoclopramide (Reglan)	PO 10 mg 30 min before meals and at bedtime for 2–8 wk IV 2 mg/kg 30 min before injection of cisplatin and 2 h after injection of cisplatin, then 1–2 mg/kg q2–3h if needed, up to 4 doses	Dosage not established
5-HT$_3$ (Serotonin) Receptor Antagonists		
Dolasetron (Anzemet)	Prevention of PONV, PO 100 mg 2 h before surgery Prevention or treatment of PONV, IV 12.5 mg as a single dose, 15 min before cessation of anesthesia or as soon as nausea or vomiting develops	2–16 y, prevention of PONV, PO 1.2 mg/kg within 2 h before surgery. Maximum dose, 100 mg Prevention or treatment of PONV, IV 0.35 mg/kg as a single dose, 15 min before cessation of anesthesia or as soon as

(continued on page 998)

Table 62-1   Drugs at a Glance: Antiemetic Drugs (continued)

	ROUTES AND DOSAGE RANGES	
Generic/Trade Name	**Adults**	**Children**
	Prevention of chemotherapy-induced nausea and vomiting, PO 100 mg within 1 h before chemotherapy; IV 1.8 mg/kg as a single dose approximately 30 min before chemotherapy	nausea or vomiting develops. Maximum dose, 12.5 mg Prevention of chemotherapy-induced nausea and vomiting, PO 1.8 mg/kg within 1 h before chemotherapy, maximum dose 100 mg; IV 1.8 mg/kg as a single dose approximately 30 min before chemotherapy, maximum dose 100 mg
Granisetron (Kytril)	Cancer chemotherapy, PO 1 mg twice daily, first dose approximately 1 h before emetogenic drug, second dose 12 h later, only on days receiving chemotherapy; IV 10 mcg/kg infused over 5 min, 30 min before emetogenic drug, only on days receiving chemotherapy	2–16 y, IV 10 mcg/kg
Ondansetron (Zofran)	*Nausea and vomiting associated with highly emetogenic cancer chemotherapy:* PO 24 mg 30 min before start of single day chemotherapy	Pediatric dosage not established
	IV 0.15 mg/kg for 3 doses given 30 minutes before chemotherapy, repeat in 4 and 8 h; IV 32 mg as a single dose. Infuse over 15 min	6–18 mos, IV 0.15 mg/kg for 3 doses given 30 minutes before chemotherapy, repeat in 4 and 8 h. Infuse over 15 min.
	Nausea and vomiting associated with moderately emetogenic cancer chemotherapy: PO 8 mg for 2 doses given 30 min before chemotherapy, repeat in 8 h.	≥12 y, PO dosage same as adult 4–11 y, PO 4 mg given for 3 doses given 30 min before chemotherapy, repeat in 8 and 16 h.
	Post operative nausea and vomiting: PO 16 mg 1h before anesthesia IV 4 mg given over 2–5 min. IM 4 mg	PO dosage not established 1 mo–12 y, ≤40 kg: IV 0.1 mg/kg; ≥40 kg: IV 4 mg. Given over 2–5 min.
Palonosetron (Aloxi)	Cancer chemotherapy, IV 0.25 mg 30 min before emetogenic drug. Repeat dosing within a 7-day interval is not recommended.	Dosage not established
Substance P/Neurokinin 1 Receptor Antagonist		
Aprepitant (Emend)	Prevention of nausea and vomiting associated with highly emetic and moderately emetic chemotherapy: (administered as part of a 3-drug treatment that also includes a serotonin receptor antagonist and dexamethasone) Day 1: PO 125 mg 1 h before chemotherapy Day 2, 3: PO 80 mg in the morning	Pediatric dosage not established
Miscellaneous Agents		
Dronabinol (Marinol)	PO 5 mg/m² (square meter of body surface area) 1–3 h before chemotherapy, then q2–4h for a total of 4–6 doses daily. Dosage can be increased by 2.5 mg/m² increments to a maximal dose of 15 mg/m² if necessary.	Same as adults for treatment of chemotherapy-induced nausea and vomiting
Phosphorated carbohydrate solution (Emetrol)	PO 15–30 mL repeated at 15-min intervals until vomiting ceases	PO 5–10 mL repeated at 15-min intervals until vomiting ceases

Generic/Trade Name	ROUTES AND DOSAGE RANGES	
	Adults	**Children**
Scopolamine (Transderm Scop)	Motion sickness, PO IM, Sub-Q, 0.3–0.6 mg as a single dose. Transdermal disc (1.5 mg scopolamine) placed behind the ear every 3 d if needed	Motion sickness, PO, Sub-Q 0.006 mg as a single dose

PONV, postoperative nausea and vomiting.

Phenothiazines

Phenothiazines, of which **P** **chlorpromazine** (Thorazine) is the prototype, are central nervous system depressants used in the treatment of psychosis and psychotic symptoms in other disorders (see Chap. 9). These drugs have widespread effects on the body. Their therapeutic effects in nausea and vomiting (as in psychosis) are attributed to their ability to block dopamine from receptor sites in the brain and CTZ. When used as antiemetics, phenothiazines act on the CTZ and the vomiting center. Not all phenothiazines are effective antiemetics.

Phenothiazines are usually effective in preventing or treating nausea and vomiting induced by drugs, radiation therapy, surgery, and most other stimuli but are usually ineffective in motion sickness. These drugs cause sedation; **prochlorperazine** (Compazine) and **promethazine** (Phenergan) are commonly used. Because of their adverse effects (e.g., sedation, cognitive impairment, extrapyramidal reactions), phenothiazines are mainly indicated when other antiemetic drugs are ineffective or only a few doses are needed.

Antihistamines

Antihistamines are used primarily to prevent histamine from exerting its widespread effects on body tissues (see Chap. 45). Antihistamines used as antiemetic agents are the "classic" antihistamines or H_1 receptor blocking agents (as differentiated from cimetidine and related drugs, which are H_2 receptor blocking agents). The drugs are thought to relieve nausea and vomiting by blocking the action of acetylcholine in the brain. Antihistamines may be effective in preventing and treating motion sickness. Not all antihistamines are effective as antiemetic agents. Adverse anticholinergic effects include dizziness, confusion, dry mouth, thickened respiratory secretions, blurred vision, urinary retention, and tachycardia; therefore, patients with narrow-angle glaucoma, prostatic hyperplasia, and asthma are at greater risk for adverse effects.

Corticosteroids

Although corticosteroids are used mainly as antiallergic, anti-inflammatory, and antistress agents (see Chap. 23), they have antiemetic effects as well. The mechanism by which the drugs exert antiemetic effects is unknown; they may block prostaglandin activity in the cerebral cortex. **Dexamethasone** and **methylprednisolone** are commonly used in the management of chemotherapy-induced *emesis* and postoperative nausea and vomiting either alone or in combination with 5-HT_3 receptor antagonists and/or substance P/neurokinin 1 receptor antagonists. With short-term use, adverse effects associated with corticosteroids are mild (e.g., euphoria, insomnia, mild fluid retention).

Benzodiazepine Antianxiety Drugs

These drugs (see Chap. 8) are not antiemetics, but they are often used in multidrug regimens to prevent nausea and vomiting associated with cancer chemotherapy. The drugs produce relaxation, relieve anxiety, and inhibit cerebral cortex input to the vomiting center. They are often prescribed for patients who experience anticipatory nausea and vomiting before administration of anticancer drugs. *Lorazepam* (Ativan) is commonly used.

Prokinetic Agents

Metoclopramide (Reglan) is a *prokinetic* agent that increases GI motility and the rate of gastric emptying by increasing the release of acetylcholine from nerve endings in the GI tract (peripheral cholinergic effects). As a result, it can decrease nausea and vomiting associated with gastroparesis and other nonobstructive disorders characterized by gastric retention of food and fluids. Metoclopramide also has central antiemetic effects; it antagonizes the action of dopamine, a catecholamine neurotransmitter. Metoclopramide is given orally in diabetic gastroparesis and esophageal reflux. Historically, metoclopramide has been used IV during chemotherapy with cisplatin (Platinol) and other antineoplastic drugs to treat acute nausea and vomiting; however, 5-HT_3 receptor antagonists are now the preferred antiemetic for this indication. Metoclopramide is still used to prevent delayed nausea and vomiting associated with chemotherapy.

With oral administration of metoclopramide, action begins in 30 to 60 minutes and peaks in 60 to 90 minutes. With intramuscular (IM) use, action onset occurs in 10 to 15 minutes and peaks in 60 to 90 minutes. With IV use, action onset occurs in 1 to 3 minutes and peaks in 60 to 90 minutes. Adverse effects include sedation, restlessness, and extrapyramidal reactions (e.g., akathisia, dystonia, symptoms of Parkinson's disease).

Metoclopramide may increase the effects of alcohol and cyclosporine (by increasing their absorption) and decrease the effects of cimetidine and digoxin (by accelerating passage through the GI tract and decreasing time for absorption).

Metoclopramide is relatively contraindicated in Parkinson's disease because it further depletes dopamine and reduces the effectiveness of levodopa, a major antiparkinson drug.

5-Hydroxytryptamine$_3$ (5-HT$_3$ or Serotonin) Receptor Antagonists

Ondansetron (Zofran), **granisetron** (Kytril), **dolasetron** (Anzemet), and **palonosetron** (Aloxi) are used to prevent or treat moderate to severe nausea and vomiting associated with cancer chemotherapy, radiation therapy, and postoperative status. These drugs antagonize serotonin receptors, preventing their activation by the effects of emetogenic drugs and toxins.

Odansetron, granisetron, and dolasetron may be given intravenously (IV) or orally. Palonosetron is only given IV. All four of these drugs are metabolized in the liver. Adverse effects are usually mild to moderate, and common ones include diarrhea, headache, dizziness, constipation, muscle aches, and transient elevation of liver enzymes.

Ondansetron was the first drug of this group. Its half-life is 3 to 5.5 hours in most patients and 9 to 20 hours in patients with moderate or severe liver impairment. With oral drug, action begins in 30 to 60 minutes and peaks in about 2 hours. With IV drug, onset and peak of drug action are immediate.

Granisetron has a half-life of 6 hours with oral drug and 5 to 9 hours with IV drug; its half-life in patients with liver impairment is unknown. Action begins rapidly with IV injection and peaks in 30 to 45 minutes; action begins more slowly with oral drug and peaks in 60 to 90 minutes.

Dolasetron has a half-life of about 7 hours with both IV and oral drug, which is extended to 11 hours in patients with severe liver impairment. Action onset and peak occur rapidly with IV administration; with oral drug, onset is rapid and peak occurs in 1 to 2 hours.

Palonosetron is 62% plasma-protein bound and has a half-life of 40 hours. This prolonged half-life makes palonosetron effective for prevention of delayed emesis after chemotherapy. It is administered over 30 seconds and is given 30 minutes before chemotherapy via the same IV access. Drug action begins rapidly after IV administration.

Applying Your Knowledge 62-1

For what adverse effects would you assess Ms. Snyder, in relation to ondansetron?

Substance P/Neurokinin 1 Receptor Antagonists

Substance P is a peptide neurotransmitter in the neurokinin family. Substance P plays a role in mediating acute chemotherapy induced nausea and vomiting (along with serotonin) and is believed to be the primary mediator of delayed nausea and vomiting associated with chemotherapy. **Aprepitant** (Emend) is the first approved substance P/neurokinin 1 antagonist and

exerts its antiemetic effect by blockade of the NK$_1$ receptor. Aprepitant is often prescribed as part of combination therapy along with a 5-HT$_3$ receptor antagonist and corticosteroids to treat both acute and delayed nausea and vomiting associated with chemotherapy. Oral dosages of dexamethasone or methylprednisolone must be reduced by 50% and IV dosages of methylprednisolone must be reduced by 25% when co-administered with aprepitant due to CYP3A4 inhibition. Aprepitant is also indicated for prevention of postoperative nausea and vomiting.

Aprepitant is orally absorbed, reaching peak levels 4 hours after administration. It is highly protein bound. Aprepitant undergoes extensive hepatic metabolism by CYP450 enzyme systems. CYP3A4 is the primary enzyme of metabolism; however, CYP1A2 and CYP2C19 are also involved. Because aprepitant moderately inhibits as well as induces CYP3A4 enzymes and induces CYP2C9 enzymes, it has the potential for multiple drug interactions. Co-administration of aprepitant with pimozide (Orap), cisapride (Propulsid), terfenadine (Seldane), or astemizole (Hismanal) can produce life-threatening or fatal reactions and is contraindicated. (Terfenadine and astemizole are no longer available in the United States, and cisapride is only available through a limited access program to patients who have not responded to other treatments.) Aprepitant is eliminated primarily by hepatic metabolism. No dosage adjustments are required for renal impairment, mild to moderate hepatic impairment, or race, gender, or age. Aprepitant is not recommended for children.

Aprepitant reduces the effectiveness of oral contraceptive for up to 28 days after administration; therefore, alternate contraceptive methods are recommended during treatment and for 1 month following administration of aprepitant. Aprepitant induces the metabolism of warfarin. INR levels must be monitored for 2 weeks after treatment is initiated, especially during days 7 to 10 after treatment.

Miscellaneous Antiemetics

Dronabinol is a *cannabinoid* (derivative of marijuana) used in the management of nausea and vomiting associated with anticancer drugs and unrelieved by other drugs. Dronabinol causes the same adverse effects as marijuana, including psychiatric symptoms, has a high potential for abuse, and may cause a withdrawal syndrome when abruptly discontinued. As a result, it is a Schedule III drug under federal narcotic laws.

Withdrawal symptoms (e.g., insomnia, irritability, restlessness) may occur if dronabinol is abruptly stopped. Onset occurs within 12 hours, with peak intensity within 24 hours and dissipation within 96 hours. These symptoms are most likely to occur with high doses or prolonged use. Sleep disturbances may persist for several weeks.

Phosphorated carbohydrate solution (Emetrol) is a hyperosmolar solution with phosphoric acid. It is thought to reduce smooth muscle contraction in the GI tract and is available over the counter.

Scopolamine, an anticholinergic drug (see Chap. 20), is effective in relieving nausea and vomiting associated with motion sickness and radiation therapy for cancer. A transdermal patch is often used to prevent seasickness.

Herbal and Dietary Supplements

Ginger, commonly used in cooking, is promoted for use in preventing nausea and vomiting associated with motion sickness, pregnancy, postoperative status, and other conditions. A few studies have investigated its antiemetic activity in humans. In one randomized, double-blind study, 60 women undergoing gynecologic surgery were given either 1000 milligrams of powdered ginger root orally, 10 milligrams of metoclopramide (Reglan) IV, or a placebo, 1.5 hours before surgery. Results indicated that ginger was comparable with metoclopramide and that both treatments were more effective than placebo in preventing postoperative nausea and vomiting. Similar results were obtained in another study with 120 patients having gynecologic surgery; in this study, metoclopramide was given orally. Although these studies support the use of ginger, other studies do not. The general consensus seems to be that it is premature to recommend ginger for any therapeutic use until long-term, controlled studies are done.

Marijuana cigarettes, although illegal in most states and under federal law, have been used by some individuals to treat chemotherapy-induced nausea and vomiting. The National Cancer Institute Fact Sheet on Marijuana Use in Supportive Care for Cancer Patients points out concerns surrounding lack of consistent effect due to varying potency of marijuana, the need for additional research concerning the use of marijuana for supportive care, and the opinion that currently available antiemetic drugs are more effective for this purpose.

Nursing Process

Assessment

Assess for nausea and vomiting.

- Identify risk factors (e.g., digestive or other disorders in which nausea and vomiting are symptoms; drugs associated with nausea and vomiting).
- Interview regarding frequency, duration, and precipitating causes of nausea and vomiting. Also, question the patient about accompanying signs and symptoms, characteristics of vomitus (amount; color; odor; presence of abnormal components, such as blood), and any measures that relieve nausea and vomiting. When possible, observe and measure the vomitus.

Nursing Diagnoses

- Deficient Fluid Volume related to uncontrolled vomiting
- Imbalanced Nutrition: Less Than Body Requirements related to impaired ability to ingest and digest food

- Altered Tissue Perfusion: Hypotension related to fluid volume depletion or antiemetic drug effect
- Risk for Injury related to adverse drug effects
- Deficient Knowledge related to nondrug measures to reduce nausea and vomiting and appropriate use of antiemetic drugs

Planning/Goals

The patient will

- Receive antiemetic drugs at appropriate times, by indicated routes
- Take antiemetic drugs as prescribed for outpatient use
- Obtain relief of nausea and vomiting
- Eat and retain food and fluids
- Have increased comfort
- Maintain body weight
- Maintain normal bowel elimination patterns
- Have fewer vomiting episodes and less discomfort with cancer chemotherapy or surgical procedures

Interventions

Use measures to prevent or minimize nausea and vomiting.

- Assist patients to identify situations that cause or aggravate nausea and vomiting.
- Avoid exposure to stimuli when feasible (e.g., unpleasant sights and odors; excessive ingestion of food, alcohol, or nonsteroidal anti-inflammatory drugs).
- Because pain may cause nausea and vomiting, administration of analgesics before painful diagnostic tests and dressing changes or other therapeutic measures may be helpful.
- Administer antiemetic drugs 30 to 60 minutes before a nausea-producing event (e.g., radiation therapy, cancer chemotherapy, travel), when possible.
- Many oral drugs cause less gastric irritation, nausea, and vomiting if taken with or just after food. For any drug likely to cause nausea and vomiting, check reference sources to determine whether it can be given with food without altering beneficial effects.
- When nausea and vomiting occur, assess the patient's condition and report to the physician. In some instances, a drug (e.g., digoxin, an antibiotic) may need to be discontinued or reduced in dosage. In other instances (e.g., paralytic ileus, GI obstruction), preferred treatment is restriction of oral intake and nasogastric intubation.
- Eating dry crackers before rising in the morning and ingestion of small frequent protein meals may help prevent nausea and vomiting associated with pregnancy.
- Avoid oral intake of food, fluids, and drugs during acute episodes of nausea and vomiting. Oral intake may increase vomiting and risks of fluid and electrolyte imbalances.

Nursing Process continues on page 1002

■ Minimize activity during acute episodes of nausea and vomiting. Lying down and resting quietly are often helpful.

Give supportive care during vomiting episodes.

■ Give replacement fluids and electrolytes. Offer small amounts of food and fluids orally when tolerated and according to patient preference.

■ Record vital signs, intake and output, and body weight at regular intervals if nausea or vomiting occurs frequently.

■ Decrease environmental stimuli when possible (e.g., noise, odors). Allow the patient to lie quietly in bed when nauseated. Decreasing motion may decrease stimulation of the vomiting center in the brain.

■ Help the patient rinse his or her mouth after vomiting. Rinsing decreases the bad taste and corrosion of tooth enamel caused by gastric acid.

■ Provide requested home remedies when possible (e.g., a cool, wet washcloth to the face and neck).

Provide appropriate education for any drug therapy (see accompanying Patient Teaching Guidelines).

Evaluation

■ Observe and interview for decreased nausea and vomiting.

■ Observe and interview regarding ability to maintain adequate intake of food and fluids.

■ Compare current weight with baseline weight.

■ Observe and interview regarding appropriate use of antiemetic drugs.

Applying Your Knowledge 62-2

What nursing measures, in addition to the administration of medication, should you implement to reduce Ms. Snyder's nausea and vomiting?

Principles of Therapy

Drug Selection

Choice of an antiemetic drug depends largely on the cause of nausea and vomiting and the patient's condition.

■ To prevent chemotherapy-induced nausea and vomiting before receiving drugs with high emetic risk, the American Society of Clinical Oncology recommends a three-drug combination consisting of a 5-HT$_3$ receptor antagonist (ondansetron, granisetron, dolasetron, or palonosetron), dexamethasone, and aprepitant. For prevention of nausea and vomiting accompanying chemotherapy with moderate emetic risk, a 5-HT$_3$ receptor antagonist and dexamethasone are recommended. To prevent delayed emesis in patients receiving cisplatin and other high emetic risk chemotherapeutic agents, dexamethasone and aprepitant are recommended.

■ 5-HT$_3$ receptor antagonist s are usually considered drugs of first choice for postoperative nausea and vomiting.

■ Drugs with anticholinergic and antihistaminic properties are preferred for motion sickness. Antihistamines such as meclizine and dimenhydrinate are also useful for vomiting caused by labyrinthitis, uremia, or postoperative status.

■ For ambulatory patients, drugs causing minimal sedation are preferred. However, most antiemetic drugs cause some sedation in usual therapeutic doses.

■ Promethazine (Phenergan), a phenothiazine, is often used clinically for its antihistaminic, antiemetic, and sedative effects.

■ Although phenothiazines are effective antiemetic agents, they may cause serious adverse effects (e.g., hypotension, sedation, anticholinergic effects, extrapyramidal reactions that simulate signs and symptoms of Parkinson's disease). Consequently, phenothiazines other than promethazine usually should not be used, especially for pregnant, young, older, and postoperative patients, unless vomiting is severe and cannot be controlled by other measures.

■ Metoclopramide (Reglan) may be preferred when nausea and vomiting are associated with nonobstructive gastric retention.

■ When the nausea and vomiting associated with pregnancy are not controlled with lifestyle measures, some pharmacologic interventions may be appropriate (see Evidence-Based Practice Box: 62-1 Nausea and Vomiting During Pregnancy).

Drug Dosage and Administration

Dosage and route of administration depend primarily on the reason for use.

■ Doses of phenothiazines are much smaller for antiemetic effects than for antipsychotic effects.

■ Most antiemetic agents are available in oral, parenteral, and rectal dosage forms. As a general rule, oral dosage forms are preferred for prophylactic use and rectal or parenteral forms are preferred for therapeutic use.

■ Antiemetic drugs are often ordered PRN (as needed). As for any PRN drug, the patient's condition should be assessed before drug administration.

■ The use of antiemetic drugs is usually short term, from a single dose to a few days.

■ When nausea and vomiting are likely to occur because of travel, administration of emetogenic anticancer drugs, diagnostic tests, or therapeutic procedures, an antiemetic drug should be given before the emetogenic event. Pretreatment usually increases patient comfort and allows use of lower drug doses. It also may prevent aspiration and other potentially serious complications of vomiting.

Evidence-Based Practice

62-1 Nausea and Vomiting During Pregnancy

Seventy to eighty-five percent of pregnant women experience nausea and vomiting during pregnancy, also known as "morning sickness." The majority of these women experience mild to moderate symptoms, predominantly during the first 9 weeks of pregnancy. However, 0.5% to 2% of pregnant women will experience severe nausea and vomiting or hyperemesis gravidarum. Hyperemesis gravidarum is the second most common reason for hospitalization of pregnant women (after preterm labor) and is characterized by persistent vomiting, dehydration, ketonuria, electrolyte imbalances, and weight loss.

Practice guidelines from the American College of Obstetricians and Gynecologists (ACOG) include the following pharmacologic recommendations for treating nausea and vomiting during pregnancy:

■ Taking a multivitamin at the time of conception may be effective in decreasing the severity of morning sickness.
■ Treating nausea and vomiting early may aid in preventing progression to more severe symptoms.
■ There is consistent scientific evidence to support pyridoxine (vitamin B_6) 10 mg alone or with the antihistamine doxylamine 12.5 mg every 8 hours as needed.
■ Ginger 250 mg four times daily is a nonpharmacologic treatment supported by limited scientific evidence.
■ Antihistamine H_1-receptor blockers and phenothiazines have been shown to be safe and effective in treating nausea and vomiting that has not responded to other measures.
■ Although corticosteroids such as methylprednisolone may be effective in treating severe hyperemesis gravidarum, they should be reserved as a treatment of last resort due to the increased risk for fetal malformations such as cleft lip and cleft palate.

Use in Special Populations

Use in Patients Undergoing Chemotherapy

Several anticancer drugs may cause severe nausea and vomiting and much discomfort for patients. Cisplatin is one of the most emetogenic drugs. For this reason, new antiemetics are usually compared with older drugs in the treatment of cisplatin-induced nausea and vomiting. Some general management guidelines include the following:

■ Chemotherapy may be given during sleeping hours.
■ Some patients may experience less nausea and vomiting if they avoid or decrease food intake for a few hours before scheduled chemotherapy.
■ Antiemetic drugs should be given before the emetogenic drug to prevent nausea and vomiting when possible. Most often, they are given IV for rapid effects and continued for 2 to 3 days. Continuous IV infusion may be more effective than intermittent bolus injections.
■ The 5-HT_3 receptor antagonists (e.g., ondansetron) are usually considered the most effective antiemetics. They may be given in a single daily dose.
■ Metoclopramide, given IV in high doses, may be used alone or in combination with various other drugs. Diphenhydramine (Benadryl) may be given at the same time or PRN because high doses of metoclopramide often cause extrapyramidal effects (see Chap. 9).
■ Various combinations of antiemetic and sedative-type drugs are used, and research continues in this area. A commonly used regimen for prophylaxis when highly emetic chemotherapy is used is a corticosteroid (e.g., dexamethasone 12 mg PO on day 1 followed by 8 mg on days 2–4),

Patient Teaching Guidelines ▪ Antiemetic Drugs

General Considerations

■ Try to identify the circumstances that cause or aggravate nausea and vomiting and avoid them when possible.
■ Drugs are more effective in preventing nausea and vomiting than in stopping them. Thus, they should be taken before the causative event when possible.
■ Do not eat, drink, or take oral medications during acute vomiting episodes, to avoid aggravating the stomach upset.
■ Lying down may help nausea and vomiting to subside; activity tends to increase stomach upset.
■ After your stomach has settled down, try to take enough fluids to prevent dehydration and potentially serious problems. Tea, broth, and gelatins are usually tolerated.
■ Do not drive an automobile or operate dangerous machinery if drowsy from antiemetic drugs, to avoid injury.
■ If taking antiemetic drugs regularly, do not drink alcohol or take other drugs without consulting a health care provider. Several drugs interact with antiemetic agents, to increase adverse effects.
■ Dronabinol, which is derived from marijuana and recommended only for nausea and vomiting associated with cancer chemotherapy, can cause dizziness, drowsiness, mood changes, and other mind-altering effects. You

should avoid alcohol and other drugs that cause drowsiness. Also, do not drive or perform hazardous tasks requiring alertness, coordination, or physical dexterity, to decrease risks of injury.

Self- or Caregiver Administration

■ Take the drugs as prescribed: Do not increase dosage, take more often, or take when drowsy, dizzy, or unsteady on your feet. Several of the drugs cause sedation and other adverse effects, which are more severe if too much is taken.
■ To prevent motion sickness, take medication 30 minutes before travel and then every 4 to 6 hours, if necessary, to avoid or minimize adverse effects.
■ Take or give antiemetic drugs 30 to 60 minutes before a nausea-producing event, when possible. This includes cancer chemotherapy, radiation therapy, painful dressings, or other treatments.
■ Take dronabinol only when you can be supervised by a responsible adult because of its sedative and mind-altering effects.
■ Aprepitant (Emend) reduces the effectiveness of oral contraceptives; therefore, use an alternative form of birth control during therapy and for 1 month after therapy.

a 5-HT$_3$ receptor antagonist (e.g., ondansetron 32 mg IV on day 1), and aprepitant (125 mg PO day 1 and 80 mg PO on days 2–3).

Applying Your Knowledge 62-3

The physician orders Ms. Snyder to also receive diphenhydramine with her metoclopramide. What is the rationale for giving these two medications together?

Use in Children

Few studies of antiemetics have been done in children, and their usage is not clearly defined. Thus, antiemetic drug therapy should be cautious and limited to prolonged vomiting of known etiology.

- With the 5-HT$_3$ receptor antagonists, safety and efficacy of granisetron and dolasetron have not been established for children younger than 2 years of age, and there is little information available about the use of ondansetron in children 3 years of age and younger. Safety and efficacy of palonosetron has not been established in patients below the age of 18 years.

- The American Society of Clinical Oncology recommends the use of a 5-HT$_3$ receptor antagonist plus a corticosteroid before administering high-dose chemotherapy or chemotherapy with high to moderate emetic risk to pediatric oncology patients.

- Phenothiazines are more likely to cause dystonias and other neuromuscular reactions in children than in adults. Promethazine is the preferred phenothiazine, because its action is more like that of the antihistamines than the phenothiazines. However, promethazine should not be used in children with hepatic disease, Reye's syndrome, a history of sleep apnea, or a family history of sudden infant death syndrome. A **BLACK BOX WARNING** alerts nurses that promethazine is contraindicated in children less than 2 years of age due to the risk of potentially fatal respiratory depression. When using promethazine, the lowest effective dosage should be used and other drugs with respiratory depressant effects should not be given concurrently. Excessive doses may cause hallucinations, convulsions, and sudden death.

- Several antiemetics (e.g., cyclizine, scopolamine) are not recommended for use in children younger than 12 years of age.

- Metoclopramide often causes extrapyramidal reactions (e.g., dystonia) in children, even in small doses.

- Dronabinol may be used to prevent or treat chemotherapy-induced nausea and vomiting in children who do not respond to other antiemetic drugs. However, the drug should be used cautiously in children because of its psychoactive effects.

Use in Older Adults

Most antiemetic drugs cause drowsiness, especially in older adults, and therefore should be used cautiously. Efforts should be made to prevent nausea and vomiting when possible. Older adults are at risk of fluid volume depletion and electrolyte imbalances with vomiting.

Dronabinol should be used cautiously because older adults are usually more sensitive to the drug's psychoactive effects than young or middle-aged adults.

Use in Patients With Renal Impairment

Several drugs are commonly used for patients with renal impairment who have nausea and vomiting.

- Metoclopramide dosage should be reduced in patients with severe renal impairment to decrease drowsiness and extrapyramidal effects.

- Phenothiazines are metabolized primarily in the liver, and dosage reductions are not usually needed for patients with renal impairment. However, these drugs have anticholinergic effects and can cause urinary retention and orthostatic hypotension. They also can cause extrapyramidal symptoms and sedation in patients with end-stage renal disease (ESRD).

Use in Patients With Hepatic Impairment

Most antiemetic drugs are metabolized in the liver and should be used cautiously in patients with impaired hepatic function.

- With oral ondansetron, do not exceed an 8-mg dose; with IV use, a single, maximal daily dose of 8 mg is recommended.

- Phenothiazines are metabolized in the liver and eliminated in urine. In the presence of liver disease (e.g., cirrhosis, hepatitis), metabolism may be slowed and drug elimination half-lives prolonged, with resultant accumulation and increased risk of adverse effects. Thus, the drugs should be used cautiously in patients with hepatic impairment. Cholestatic jaundice has been reported with promethazine.

- Dronabinol normally undergoes extensive first-pass hepatic metabolism to active and inactive metabolites. Resultant plasma levels consist of approximately equal portions of the parent drug and the main active metabolite. In addition, the drug is eliminated mainly by biliary excretion, over several weeks. Thus, long-term use at recommended doses may lead to accumulation of toxic amounts of the drug and its metabolite, even in patients with normal liver function.

In patients with hepatic impairment, more of the parent drug and less of the active metabolite are likely to reach the bloodstream. Thus, therapeutic and adverse effects are less predictable. Also, impaired liver function can decrease metabolism and excretion in bile so that accumulation is likely and adverse effects may be increased and prolonged. The drug should be used very cautiously, if at all, in patients with moderate to severe hepatic impairment.

Use in Home Care

Antiemetics are usually given orally or by rectal suppository in the home setting. The home care nurse may need to assess patients for possible causes of nausea and vomiting and assist patients and caregivers with appropriate use of the drugs and other interventions to prevent fluid and electrolyte depletion. Teaching safety precautions with sedating drugs may also be needed.

Applying Your Knowledge 62-4

Ms. Snyder is concerned about the amount of medication she is receiving. She asks you to withhold her antiemetics until she actually vomits. You do as she requests.

Nursing Actions Antiemetics

NURSING ACTIONS	RATIONALE/EXPLANATION
1. Administer accurately	
a. For prevention of motion sickness, give antiemetics 30 minutes before travel and q4–6h, if necessary.	To allow time for drug dissolution and absorption
b. For prevention of vomiting with cancer chemotherapy and radiation therapy, give antiemetic drugs 30–60 minutes before treatment.	Drugs are more effective in preventing than in stopping nausea and vomiting.
c. Inject intramuscular antiemetics deeply into a large muscle mass (e.g., gluteal area).	To decrease tissue irritation
d. In general, do not mix parenteral antiemetics in a syringe with other drugs.	To avoid physical incompatibilities
e. Omit antiemetic agents and report to the physician if the patient appears excessively drowsy or is hypotensive.	To avoid potentiating adverse effects and central nervous system (CNS) depression
f. Mix intravenous (IV) ondansetron in 50 mL of 5% dextrose or 0.9% sodium chloride injection and infuse over 15 minutes.	
g. Mix granisetron in 20–50 mL of 5% dextrose or 0.9% sodium chloride injection and infuse over 5 minutes.	
h. With dolasetron:	
(1) Give oral drug 1–2 hours before chemotherapy; give IV drug about 30 minutes before chemotherapy.	For oral administration to patients who cannot swallow tablets, dolasetron injection can be mixed in apple or apple–grape juice. Specific instructions should be obtained from a pharmacy. When kept at room temperature, the diluted oral solution should be used within 2 hours.
(2) Give IV drug (up to 100-mg dose) by direct injection over 30 seconds or longer or dilute up to 50 mL with 0.9% sodium chloride, 5% dextrose, or 5% dextrose and 0.45% sodium chloride and infuse over 15 minutes.	
i. Infuse palonosetron IV over 30 seconds. Do not mix with other drugs. Flush the IV line with normal saline before and after administration of palonosetron.	Manufacturer's instructions
2. Observe for therapeutic effects	
a. Verbal reports of decreased nausea	
b. Decreased frequency or absence of vomiting	
3. Observe for adverse effects	
a. Excessive sedation and drowsiness	Excessive sedation may occur with usual doses of antiemetics and is more likely to occur with high doses. This may be minimized by avoiding high doses and assessing the patient's level of consciousness before each dose.
b. Anticholinergic effects—dry mouth, urinary retention	These effects are common to many antiemetic agents and are more likely to occur with large doses.
c. Hypotension, including orthostatic hypotension	Most likely to occur with phenothiazines; may also occur with 5-HT$_3$ antagonists
d. Extrapyramidal reactions—dyskinesia, dystonia, akathisia, parkinsonism	These disorders may occur with phenothiazines and metoclopramide.
e. With ondansetron and related drugs, observe for headache, diarrhea or constipation, dizziness, fatigue, and muscle aches. Bradycardia and hypotension may also occur.	These drugs are usually well tolerated, with mild to moderate adverse effects.

(continued on page 1006)

Nursing Actions   Antiemetics (continued)

NURSING ACTIONS	RATIONALE/EXPLANATION
f. With dronabinol, observe for alterations in mood, cognition, and perception of reality; dysphoria; drowsiness; dizziness; anxiety; tachycardia; and conjunctivitis. Dronabinol may also cause seizures or seizure-like activity. May lower the seizure threshold in those with pre-existing seizure disorders.	Tachycardia may be prevented with a beta-adrenergic blocking drug, such as propranolol (Inderal).
g. With aprepitant, observe for weakness, tiredness, dizziness, diarrhea or constipation, stomach pain, upset stomach, hiccups, and loss of appetite. Rare but serious adverse effects include hives, skin rashes, swelling of face, airways and extremities, hoarseness.	Notify provider if rare serious adverse effects occur.
4. Observe for drug interactions	
a. Drugs that *increase* effects of antiemetic agents:	
(1) CNS depressants (alcohol, sedative-hypnotics, antianxiety agents, other antihistamines or antipsychotic agents)	Additive CNS depression
(2) Anticholinergics (e.g., atropine)	Additive anticholinergic effects. Some phenothiazines and antiemetic antihistamines have strong anticholinergic properties.
(3) Antihypertensive agents	Additive hypotension
b. Drugs that *alter* effects of 5-HT$_3$ receptor antagonists:	
(1) Atenolol and cimetidine *increase* effects of dolasetron.	The drugs decrease dolasetron metabolism and clearance.
(2) Rifampin (and presumably other enzyme inducers) *decreases* effects of dolasetron and granisetron.	Enzyme inducers accelerate metabolism of affected drugs.
c. Drugs that *increase* effects of aprepitant:	
(1) CYP3A4 inhibitors (e.g., clarithromycin, diltiazem, ketaconazole, itraconazole, nelfinavir, ritonavir, troleandomycin)	These drugs drcrease the metabolism of aprepitant.
d. Drugs that *decrease* effects of aprepitant:	
(1) CYP3A4 inducers (e.g., carbmazepine, phenytoin, rifampin)	These drugs increase the metabolism of aprepitant.
(2) Paroxetine	

Key Concepts

- Antiemetic drugs are used to prevent or treat nausea and vomiting associated with surgery, pain, motion sickness, cancer chemotherapy, radiation therapy, and other causes.

- Antiemetic drugs are most effective when given before nausea and vomiting occurs.

- Nausea is an unpleasant sensation of abdominal discomfort accompanied by the desire to vomit.

- Vomiting is the expulsion of stomach contents through the mouth.

- The vomiting center, CTZ, and GI tract contain benzodiazepine, cholinergic (muscarinic), dopamine, histamine, opiate, substance P/neurokinin, and serotonin receptors that are stimulated by emetogenic drugs and toxins. Antiemetic drugs produce their effects by blockade of one or more of these receptors.

- The antiemetic effect of phenothiazines such as prochlorperazine and promethazine is due to blockade of dopamine receptors in the brain and CTZ. They are used to treat nausea induced by drugs, radiation therapy, surgery, and other stimuli but are considered ineffective in motion sickness.

- Classic H$_1$ blocking antihistamine drugs such as dimenhydrinate are thought to produce an antiemetic effect due to their anticholinergic properties. Antihistamines are used to prevent and treat nausea and vomiting due to motion sickness.

- The antiemetic mechanism of action of corticosteroids such as dexamethasone and methylprednisolone is unknown. These drugs are commonly used alone or in combination with 5-HT$_3$ serotonin receptor antagonists and/or substance P/neurokinin 1 receptor antagonists in the management of chemotherapy-induced emesis and postoperative nausea and vomiting.

- Benzodiazepines such as lorazepam produce relaxation, relieve anxiety, and inhibit cerebral cortex input to the vomiting center. They are prescribed for anticipatory nausea associated with cancer chemotherapy.

- Prokinetic agents such as metoclopramide increase the release of acetylcholine from nerve endings in the GI track, increasing GI motility and gastric emptying. It also antagonizes dopamine in the brain. Metoclopramide is prescribed to treat nausea and vomiting associated with gastroparesis and other nonobstructive disorders characterized by gastric retention of food and fluids and in the treatment of esophageal reflux. It is also useful in prevention of delayed nausea and vomiting associated with chemotherapy.

- 5-HT$_3$ serotonin receptor antagonists such as odansetron, granisetron, dolasetron, and palonosetron antagonize serotonin receptors, preventing their activation by emetogenic drugs and toxins. They are used to prevent and treat moderate to severe nausea associated with cancer chemotherapy, radiation therapy, and postoperative status.

- Substance P, a peptide neurotransmitter in the neurokinin family, plays a role in acute and delayed chemotherapy-induced nausea and vomiting. Aprepitant antagonizes the neurokinin 1 receptor, preventing activation by emetogenic chemotherapeutic drugs.

- Dronabinol is a cannabinoid used in the management of nausea and vomiting associated with chemotherapy unrelieved by other antiemetic drugs. It is a Schedule III drug under federal narcotic laws.

- Scopolamine is an anticholinergic drug effective in relieving nausea and vomiting associated with motion sickness and radiation therapy for cancer.

Review and Application Exercises

Short Answer Exercises

1. List common causes of nausea and vomiting or circumstances in which nausea and vomiting often occur.

2. How do antiemetic drugs prevent or relieve nausea and vomiting?

3. What are adverse effects of commonly used antiemetics?

4. Are antiemetics more effective if given before, during, or after nausea and vomiting?

5. Which antiemetics are usually given to control the nausea and vomiting that occur with certain antineoplastic drugs?

NCLEX-Style Questions

6. The nurse knows that antiemetics are most effective when administered
   a. before an emetogenic event occurs
   b. during an episode of nausea but before vomiting has occurred
   c. after the patient has experienced nausea and vomiting
   d. timing of administration has no impact on drug effectiveness

7. The nurse would question an order for which of the following antiemetics for treatment of motion sickness–induced nausea?
   a. prochlorperazine (Compazine)
   b. dimenhydrinate (Dramamine)
   c. meclizine (Antivert)
   d. scopolamine (Transderm Scop)

8. When administering 5-HT$_3$ receptor antagonists before cancer chemotherapy, the nurse should also be prepared to administer which of the following adjunctive medications?
   a. promethazine
   b. dexamethasone
   c. dronabinol
   d. hydroxyzine

Selected References

American College of Obstetricians and Gynecologists. (2004). ACOG Practice Bulletin. Clinical management guidelines for obstetrician-gynecologists: Nausea and vomiting of pregnancy. *Obstetrics and Gynecology, 103,* 803–811.

Davis, M. (2004). Nausea and vomiting of pregnancy: An evidence-based review. *Journal of Perinatal and Neonatal Nursing, 18,* 312–328.

DiPiro, C. V., & Taylor, A. T. (2005). Nausea and vomiting. In J. T. DiPiro, R. L. Talbert, G. C. Yee, G. R. Matzke, B. G. Wells, & L. M.

Posey (Eds.), *Pharmacotherapy: A Pathophysiologic Approach* (6th ed., pp. 665–676). New York: McGraw-Hill.

Drug facts and comparisons. (Updated monthly). St. Louis, MO: Facts and Comparisons.

Fetrow, C. W., & Avila, J. R. (2004). *Professional's handbook of complementary & alternative medicines* (3rd ed.). Springhouse, PA: Springhouse.

Kris, M. G., Hesketh, P. J., Somerfield, M. R., Feyer, P., Clark-Snow, R., Koeller, J. M., Morrow, G. R., Chinnery, L. W., Chesney, M. J.,

Gralla, R. J., & Grunberg, S. M. (2006). American Society of Clinical Oncology: Guideline for antiemetics in oncology. *Journal of Clinical Oncology, 24,* 1–16.

National Cancer Institute. *Fact Sheet. Marijuana use in supportive care for cancer patients.* Retrieved July 27, 2007, from http://www.cancer.gov/cancertopics/factsheet/Support/marijuana

Porth, C. M. (2005). Disorders of gastrointestinal function. In C. M. Porth (Ed.), *Pathophysiology: Concepts of Altered Health States* (7th ed., pp. 885–916). Philadelphia: Lippincott Williams & Wilkins.

SECTION 10

Drugs Used in Special Conditions

Chapter Outline

Drugs Used in Ophthalmic Conditions

KEY TERMS

- Conjunctiva
- Glaucoma
- Intraocular pressure (IOP)
- Keratitis
- Lacrimation
- Miosis
- Mydriasis
- Nasolacrimal occlusion
- Refraction
- Tonometry

LEARNING OBJECTIVES

After studying this chapter, you will be able to:

1. Review characteristics of ocular structures that influence drug therapy for eye disorders.
2. Discuss selected drugs in relation to their use in ocular disorders.
3. Use correct techniques to administer ophthalmic medications.
4. Assess for ocular effects of systemic drugs and systemic effects of ophthalmic drugs.
5. Teach patients, family members, or caregivers correct administration of eye medications.
6. For a patient with an eye disorder, teach about the importance of taking medications as prescribed to protect and preserve eyesight.

Applying Your Knowledge

Irene Molnar is a 75-year-old woman who has glaucoma. You are a home care nurse visiting Mrs. Molnar. Her physician has prescribed the following:

Acetazolamide (Diamox), 250 mg PO, every 6 hours
Timolol (Timoptic), one drop in each eye, twice daily
Pilocarpine (Isopto-Carpine), one drop of 2% solution in each eye, three times daily

Introduction

Basic Structure and Function of the Eye

The eye is the major sensory organ through which a person receives information about the external environment. Extensive discussion of vision and ocular anatomy is beyond the scope of this chapter, but some characteristics and functions are described to facilitate understanding of ocular drug therapy:

- The eyelids and lacrimal system function to protect the eye. The eyelid is a barrier to the entry of foreign bodies, strong light, dust, and other potential irritants. The *conjunctiva* is the mucous membrane lining of the eyelids. The canthi (singular, canthus) are the angles where the upper and lower eyelids meet. The lacrimal system produces a fluid that constantly moistens and cleanses the anterior surface of the eyeball. The fluid drains through two small openings in the inner canthus and flows through the nasolacrimal duct into the nasal cavity. When the conjunctiva is irritated or certain emotions are experienced (e.g., sadness), the lacrimal gland produces more fluid than the drainage system can accommodate. The excess fluid overflows the eyelids and becomes tears.

■ The eyeball is a spherical structure composed of the sclera, cornea, choroid, and retina, plus special refractive tissues. The sclera is a white, opaque, fibrous tissue that covers the posterior five sixths of the eyeball. The cornea is a transparent, special connective tissue that covers the anterior sixth of the eyeball. The cornea contains no blood vessels. The choroid, composed of blood vessels and connective tissue, continues forward to form the iris. The iris is composed of pigmented cells, the opening called the pupil, and muscles that control the size of the pupil by contracting or dilating in response to stimuli. Pupil constriction is called *miosis*; dilation is called *mydriasis*. The retina is the innermost layer of the eyeball.

■ For vision to occur, light rays must enter the eye through the cornea; travel through the pupil, lens, and vitreous body (discussed below); and be focused on the retina. Light rays do not travel directly to the retina. Instead, they are deflected in various directions according to the density of the ocular structures through which they pass. This process, called *refraction*, is controlled by the aqueous humor, lens, and vitreous body. The optic disk is the area of the retina where ophthalmic blood vessels and the optic nerve enter the eyeball.

■ The structure and function of the eyeball are further influenced by the lens, aqueous humor, and vitreous body. The lens is an elastic, transparent structure; its function is to focus light rays to form images on the retina. It is located behind the iris and is held in place by ligaments attached to the ciliary body. The aqueous humor is a clear fluid produced by capillaries in the ciliary body. Most of the fluid flows through the pupil into the anterior chamber (between the cornea and the lens and anterior to the iris). A small amount flows into a passage called Schlemm's canal, from which it enters the venous circulation. Normally, production and drainage of aqueous humor are approximately equal, and normal *intraocular pressure (IOP)* is maintained. Impaired drainage of aqueous humor causes increased IOP. The vitreous body is a transparent, jelly-like mass located in the posterior portion of the eyeball. It functions to refract light rays and maintain the normal shape of the eyeball.

Disorders of the Eye

The eye is subject to the development of many disorders that threaten its structure, function, or both. Some disorders in which ophthalmic drugs play a prominent role are discussed in the following sections.

Refractive Errors

Refractive errors include myopia (nearsightedness), hyperopia (farsightedness), presbyopia, and astigmatism. These conditions impair vision by interfering with the eye's ability to focus light rays on the retina. Ophthalmic drugs are used only in the diagnosis of the conditions; treatment involves prescription of eyeglasses or contact lenses.

Glaucoma

Glaucoma is one of the leading causes of blindness in the United States and the most common cause of blindness in African Americans. It is a group of diseases characterized by optic nerve damage and changes in visual fields. It is often characterized by increased IOP (above 22 mm Hg) but may also occur with normal IOP (below 21 mm Hg; average 15–16 mm Hg). Diagnostic tests for glaucoma include ophthalmoscopic examination of the optic disk, measurement of IOP (*tonometry*), and testing of visual fields.

The most common type of glaucoma is called primary open-angle glaucoma. Its etiology is unknown, but contributing factors include advanced age, a family history of glaucoma and elevated IOP, diabetes mellitus, hypertension, myopia, long-term use of corticosteroid drugs, and previous eye injury, inflammation, or infection. In addition, the incidence of glaucoma in African Americans is about three times higher than in non–African Americans. Closed-angle glaucoma is usually an acute situation requiring emergency surgery. It may occur when pupils are dilated and the outflow of aqueous humor is blocked. Darkness and drugs with anticholinergic effects (e.g., atropine, antihistamines, tricyclic antidepressants) may dilate the pupil, reduce outflow of aqueous humor, and precipitate acute glaucoma.

Inflammatory or Infectious Conditions

Inflammation may be caused by bacteria, viruses, allergic reactions, or irritating chemicals. Infections may result from foreign bodies, contaminated hands, contaminated eye medications, or infections in contiguous structures (e.g., nose, face, sinuses). Common inflammatory and infectious disorders include the following:

■ **Conjunctivitis** is a common eye disorder that may be caused by allergens (e.g., airborne pollens), bacterial or viral infections, or physical or chemical irritants. Symptoms include redness, tearing, itching, edema, and burning or gritty sensations. Bacterial conjunctivitis is often caused by *Staphylococcus aureus*, *Streptococcus pneumoniae*, or *Haemophilus influenzae* and produces mucopurulent drainage. Conjunctivitis with a purulent discharge is most often caused by the gonococcus; corneal ulcers and scarring may result.

■ **Blepharitis** is a chronic infection of glands and lash follicles on the margins of the eyelids, characterized by burning, redness, and itching. A hordeolum (commonly called a "stye") is often associated with blepharitis. The most common causes are seborrhea and staphylococcal infections.

■ *Keratitis* (inflammation of the cornea) may be caused by microorganisms, trauma, allergy, ischemia, and drying of the cornea (e.g., from inadequate *lacrimation*). The major symptom is pain, which ranges from mild to severe. Vision may not be affected initially. However, if not treated effectively, corneal ulceration, scarring, and impaired vision may result.

■ **Bacterial corneal ulcers** are most often caused by pneumococci and staphylococci. Pseudomonal ulcers are less common but may rapidly progress to perforation. Fungal ulcers may follow topical corticosteroid therapy or injury with plant matter, such as a tree branch. Viral ulcers are usually caused by the herpesvirus.

■ **Fungal infections** commonly occur and may often be attributed to frequent use of ophthalmic antibiotics and corticosteroids.

Ophthalmic Drug Therapy

Drug therapy of ophthalmic conditions is unique because of the location, structure, and function of the eye. Many systemic drugs are unable to cross the blood–eye barrier and achieve therapeutic concentrations in ocular structures. In general, penetration is greater if the drug achieves a high concentration in the blood, is fat soluble, is poorly bound to serum proteins, and if inflammation is present.

Because of the difficulties associated with systemic therapy, various methods of administering drugs locally have been developed. The most common and preferred method is topical application of ophthalmic solutions or suspensions (eye drops) to the conjunctiva. Drugs are distributed through the tear film covering the eye and may be used for superficial disorders (e.g., conjunctivitis) or for relatively deep ocular disorders (e.g., glaucoma). Topical ophthalmic ointments may also be used. In addition, ophthalmologists may inject medications (e.g., antibiotics, corticosteroids, local anesthetics) into or around various eye structures.

Classifications of Ophthalmic Drugs

Drugs used to diagnose or treat ophthalmic disorders represent numerous therapeutic classifications, most of which are discussed in other chapters. Major classes used in ophthalmology are described below.

Anesthetics (Local)

Topical ophthalmic anesthetics are used for various diagnostic and therapeutic procedures (e.g., tonometry, removal of foreign bodies or sutures, minor surgery on the cornea and conjunctivae). Proparacaine is a commonly used agent; after administration of one drop, anesthesia begins within 20 seconds and lasts 10 to 15 minutes. Injectable local anesthetics are administered by ophthalmologists, usually for eye surgery. Lidocaine is commonly used; it has a rapid onset and lasts 1 to 2 hours.

Antihistamines and Mast Cell Stabilizers

Antihistamines (H_1 receptor antagonists) and mast cell stabilizers (e.g., cromolyn) are used to decrease redness and itching associated with allergic conjunctivitis. Antihistamines inhibit the action of histamine, a substance produced by the body during an allergic reaction and which is the primary cause of itchy eyes. One antihistamine for allergic conjunctivitis, ketotifen (Zaditor), is available for over-the-counter purchase after several years of use as a prescription drug. Cromolyn acts by inhibiting the release of histamine and slow reacting substance of anaphylaxis (SRS-A) from mast cells. It is not useful in treatment of acute symptoms, and several days to weeks of use may be needed to elicit a therapeutic response.

Antimicrobials

Antimicrobials are used to treat bacterial, viral, and fungal infections of the external portion of the eye. Bacterial infections include conjunctivitis, keratitis, blepharitis, and corneal ulcers. The drugs are usually applied topically but may be given orally or intravenously. Sulfonamides (e.g., sulfacetamide) are commonly used to treat bacterial conjunctivitis. They have activity against both gram-positive and gram-negative organisms. Bacitracin, neomycin, polymyxin, erythromycin, tetracycline, gentamicin, tobramycin, and several fluoroquinolones (e.g., ciprofloxacin, ofloxacin) are also commonly used topical antibacterial drugs. Some clinicians recommend that the fluoroquinolones be reserved for bacterial keratitis and other serious infections. Natamycin is used to treat fungal infections; trifluridine is used for viral infections.

Autonomic Nervous System Drugs

These drugs are used for diagnostic and therapeutic purposes (see Chaps. 16 through 20). Phenylephrine is often used to dilate the pupil before ophthalmologic examinations or surgical procedures. Dosage is usually one drop initially and a second drop in 5 to 10 minutes. Dilation occurs within 30 minutes and lasts 2 to 3 hours. Numerous drugs are used to decrease IOP in glaucoma; they act by decreasing formation or increasing outflow of aqueous humor. Ophthalmic beta-adrenergic blocking agents (e.g., timolol) are most commonly used. Adrenergic vasoconstricting (decongestant) drugs are commonly used to decrease redness associated with allergic conjunctivitis.

Autonomic drugs indicated in one disorder may be contraindicated in another (e.g., anticholinergic drugs may be contraindicated in glaucoma). In addition, adrenergic mydriatics (e.g., phenylephrine) should be used cautiously in patients with hypertension, cardiac dysrhythmias, arteriosclerotic heart disease, and hyperthyroidism. Ophthalmic beta blockers usually have the same contraindications and precautions as oral or injected drugs (e.g., bradycardia, heart block, bronchospastic disorders).

Corticosteroids

Corticosteroids (see Chap. 23) are often used to treat inflammatory conditions of the eye (e.g., conjunctivitis, uveitis, keratitis) to reduce scarring and prevent loss of vision. The duration of treatment varies with the type of lesion and may range from a few days to several months. Corticosteroids are generally more effective in acute than chronic inflammatory conditions. Because these drugs are potentially toxic, they should not be used to treat minor disorders or disorders that can be effectively treated with safer drugs. When used, corticosteroids should be administered in the lowest effective dose and for the shortest effective time. Long-term use should be avoided when possible, because it may result in glaucoma, increased IOP, optic nerve damage, defects in visual acuity and fields of vision, cataracts, or secondary ocular infections.

Ophthalmologic corticosteroids may be administered topically, systemically, or both. They are contraindicated in eye infections caused by the herpesvirus because the drugs increase the severity of the infection. Ophthalmic preparations of corticosteroids combined with antimicrobial drugs are also available and commonly used for conditions in which both types of drugs are needed (e.g., keratoconjunctivitis, postoperatively).

Nonsteroidal Anti-inflammatory Drugs (NSAIDs)

NSAIDs, in ophthalmic formulations for topical use, may be used in eye disorders (see Table 63-3 and Chap. 7). As in other conditions, the drugs are thought to act by blocking the synthesis of inflammatory prostaglandins. Some clinicians use combinations of topical NSAIDs and corticosteroids to manage inflammatory disorders.

Prostaglandin Analogs

These are antiglaucoma drugs that reduce IOP by increasing the outflow of aqueous humor. The drugs may be used when a patient's IOP is not lowered adequately with a beta blocker or when a beta blocker is contraindicated for a patient. When compared with twice-daily ophthalmic timolol, the drugs were considered as effective as timolol. The drugs may be used in conjunction with other antiglaucoma medications (e.g., a beta blocker or carbonic anhydrase inhibitor [CAI]) if multiple drugs are required.

In clinical trials, the most common adverse effects were ocular burning, stinging, and itching. In addition, the drugs may cause a permanent darkening of eye color, especially in light-colored eyes, and alter eyelashes.

Nurses who are pregnant should handle prostaglandin analogs very carefully because the drugs may be absorbed through the skin. If accidental contact occurs, the exposed area should be washed immediately with soap and water.

Carbonic Anhydrase Inhibitors (CAIs) and Osmotic Agents

CAIs and osmotic agents are given to decrease IOP in glaucoma and before certain surgical procedures. CAIs lower IOP by decreasing production of aqueous humor. Oral CAIs are rarely used since the development of topical CAIs, beta blockers, and other newer glaucoma medications. Topical CAIs may be used alone but are most often used in combination with other glaucoma medications. With glycerin, a commonly used osmotic agent, maximum lowering of IOP occurs in 1 hour and lasts 4 to 5 hours.

Fluorescein

Fluorescein is a dye used in diagnosing lesions or foreign bodies in the cornea, fitting contact lenses, and studying the lacrimal system and flow of aqueous humor.

Individual Drugs

Individual drugs are described in Tables 63-1, 63-2, and 63-3.

| Table 63-1 | Drugs at a Glance: Drugs Used in Ocular Disorders* |

CLASSES OF DRUGS/ OCULAR EFFECTS	CLINICAL INDICATIONS	GENERIC/TRADE NAME	DOSAGE RANGES
Autonomic Nervous System Drugs			
Adrenergics			
Decreased production of aqueous humor Mydriasis Decreased IOP Vasoconstriction Photophobia	Glaucoma Ophthalmoscopic examination Reduction of adhesion formation with uveitis Preoperative and postoperative mydriasis Local hemostasis	**Phenylephrine (2.5% and 10% solutions)** (Neo-Synephrine)	Before ophthalmoscopy or refraction, 1 drop of 2.5% or 10% solution Preoperatively, 1 drop of 2.5% or 10% solution 30–60 min before surgery Postoperatively, 1 drop of 10% solution once or twice daily *Children:* Refraction, 1 drop of 2.5% solution
Alpha2 Adrenergic Agonists			
Decreased IOP	Glaucoma Prevention of increased IOP after ocular surgery	**Brimonidine** (Alphagan P)	1 drop in affected eye(s) 3 times daily, q8h
Beta Blockers			
Decreased production of aqueous humor Reduced IOP	Glaucoma	**Betaxolol** (Betoptic) **Carteolol**	1 or 2 drops in affected eye(s) twice daily 1 drop in affected eye(s) twice daily

(continued on page 1014)

Table 63-1		**Drugs at a Glance:** Drugs Used in Ocular Disorders* (continued)	
CLASSES OF DRUGS/ OCULAR EFFECTS	**CLINICAL INDICATIONS**	**GENERIC/TRADE NAME**	**DOSAGE RANGES**
		Levobunolol (Betagan)	1 or 2 drops in affected eye(s) once or twice daily
		Metipranolol (OptiPranolol)	1 drop in affected eye(s) twice daily
		Timolol maleate (Timoptic, Timoptic-XE)	1 drop in affected eye(s) twice daily; gel, 1 drop once daily
Cholinergics Increased outflow of aqueous humor Miosis	Glaucoma	**Pilocarpine (0.25%–10% solutions)** (Isopto Carpine, Pilocar)	Glaucoma, 1 drop of 1% or 2% solution in each eye 3 or 4 times daily
		Pilocarpine ocular system (Ocusert Pilo-20 or -40)	One system in conjunctival sac per wk
Anticholinergics Mydriasis Cycloplegia Photophobia	Mydriasis for refraction and other diagnostic purposes Before and after intraocular surgery Treatment of uveitis	**Atropine sulfate** (0.5%–3% solutions)	Before intraocular surgery, 1 drop After intraocular surgery, 1 drop once daily
		Cyclopentolate hydrochloride (Cyclogyl)	For refraction, 1 drop of 0.5% or 2% solution Before ophthalmoscopy, 1 drop of 0.5% solution *Children:* For refraction, 1 drop of 0.5%, 1%, or 2% solution, repeated in 10 min
		Homatropine hydrobromide (2% and 5% solutions)	Refraction, 1 drop of 5% solution every 5 min for 2 or 3 doses or 1 or 2 drops of 2% solution every 10–15 min for 5 doses Uveitis, 1 drop of 2% or 5% solution 2 or 3 times daily
		Tropicamide (0.5% and 1% solutions) (Mydriacyl)	Before refraction or ophthalmoscopy, 1 drop, repeated in 5 min, then every 20–30 min as needed to maintain mydriasis
Diuretics **Carbonic Anhydrase Inhibitors** Decreased production of aqueous humor Decreased IOP	Glaucoma Preoperatively in intraocular surgery	**Acetazolamide** (Diamox)	PO 250 mg q6h; sustained-release capsules, PO 500 mg q12h IV, IM 5–10 mg/kg/d in divided doses, q6h *Children:* PO 10–15 mg/kg/d in divided doses, q6–8h IV, IM 5–10 mg/kg q6h
		Brinzolamide (Azopt)	1 drop 3 times daily
		Dorzolamide (Trusopt)	1 drop 3 times daily
Osmotic Agents Reduced volume of vitreous humor Decreased IOP	Before intraocular surgery Treatment of acute glaucoma	**Glycerin** (Osmoglyn)	PO 1–1.5 g/kg, usually as a 50% or 75% solution 1–1½ h before surgery *Children:* Same as adults

CLASSES OF DRUGS/ OCULAR EFFECTS	CLINICAL INDICATIONS	GENERIC/TRADE NAME	DOSAGE RANGES
		Isosorbide (Ismotic)	Emergency reduction of IOP, PO 1.5 g/kg up to 4 times daily
		Mannitol (Osmitrol)	IV 1.5–2 g/kg as a 20% solution over 30–60 min *Children:* Same as adults
Prostaglandin Analogs Decreased IOP	Glaucoma	**Bimatoprost** (Lumigan)	1 drop once daily in the evening
		Latanoprost (Xalatan)	1 drop once daily in the evening
		Travoprost (Travatan)	1 drop once daily in the evening
Miscellaneous Agents **Anesthetics, Local** Surface anesthesia of conjunctiva and cornea	Tonometry Removal of foreign bodies Removal of sutures	**Proparacaine** (Alcaine)	Minor procedures, 1 or 2 drops of 0.5% solution
		Tetracaine (Pontocaine)	Minor procedures, 1 or 2 drops of 0.5% solution
Lubricants Serve as "artificial tears"	Protect the cornea during keratitis or diagnostic procedures Moisten contact lenses	**Methylcellulose** (Methulose) **Polyvinyl alcohol** (Liquifilm)	1 or 2 drops as needed 1 or 2 drops as needed

Antimicrobial agents are listed in Table 63-2; anti-allergic and anti-inflammatory agents are listed in Table 63-3.

IOP, intraocular pressure.

Table 63-2   **Drugs at a Glance:** Ophthalmic Antimicrobial Agents

	DOSAGE RANGES	
Generic/Trade Name	Adults	Children
Antibacterial Agents **Ciprofloxacin 3.5 mg/mL solution** (Ciloxan)	Corneal ulcer: Day 1, 2 drops q15min for 6 h, then q30min for rest of day; day 2, 2 drops q1h; days 3–14, 2 drops q4h Conjunctivitis: 1 or 2 drops q2h while awake for 2 d, then 1 or 2 drops q4h while awake for 5 d	Safety and efficacy not established in infants <1 y
Erythromycin 5% ointment (Ilotycin)		Prevention of neonatal gonococcal or chlamydial conjunctivitis, 0.5–1 cm in each eye
Gatifloxacin (Zymar)	1 drop in affected eye(s) every 2 h while awake, up to 8 times daily, for 2 d, then 1 drop up to 4 times daily while awake, for 5 d	Dosage not established
Gentamicin 3 mg/mL solution or 3 mg/g ointment (Garamycin)	1 drop q1–4h; ointment, apply 2 or 3 times daily	Same as adults
Levofloxacin 5 mg/mL solution (Quixin)	1 or 2 drops q2h up to 8 doses/d for 1 or 2 d, then q4h up to 4 doses/d for 5 d	Dosage not established

(continued on page 1016)

Table 63-2 Drugs at a Glance: Ophthalmic Antimicrobial Agents (continued)

| Generic/Trade Name | DOSAGE RANGES | |
	Adults	Children
Moxifloxacin (Vigamox)	1 drop in affected eye(s) 3 times daily for 7 d	Same as adults for children 1 y and older
Ofloxacin 3 mg/mL solution (Ocuflox)	Conjunctivitis: 1 or 2 drops q2–4h while awake for 2 d, then 4 times daily for 3–5 d	Same as adults for children 1 y and older
	Corneal ulcer: 1 or 2 drops q30min while awake, q4–6h during sleep, for 1–2 d, then q1h while awake for 4–6 d, then q4h while awake until healed	Dosage not established
Sulfacetamide 10% solution or ointment (Bleph-10), **15% solution** (Isopto Cetamide), **10% and 30% solution, 10% ointment** (Sodium Sulamyd)	Conjunctivitis, corneal ulcers, or other superficial infections caused by susceptible organisms: 1 or 2 drops q4h or 0.5 inch ointment 3 or 4 times daily, for 7–10 days	Safety and efficacy not established. Contraindicated in infants <2 mo of age
Sulfisoxazole 4% solution (Gantrisin)	1 or 2 drops 3 or more times daily	Safety and efficacy not established. Contraindicated in infants <2 mo of age
Tobramycin (0.3% solution and 3 mg/g ointment) (Tobrex)	1 or 2 drops 2–6 times daily or ointment 2 or 3 times daily	See manufacturer's instructions
Antiviral Agent		
Trifluridine 1% solution (Viroptic)	Keratoconjunctivitis or corneal ulcers caused by herpes simplex virus: 1 drop q2h while awake (maximum, 9 drops/d) until corneal ulcer heals, then 1 drop q4h (minimum, 5 drops/d), for 7 d	*older than 6 y:* Same as adults
Antifungal Agent		
Natamycin 5% suspension (Natacyn)	1 drop q1–2h for 3–4 d, then q3–4h for 14–21 d	Safety and efficacy not established

Table 63-3 Drugs at a Glance: Topical Ophthalmic Antiallergic and Anti-Inflammatory Agents

GENERIC/TRADE NAME	INDICATIONS FOR USE	ROUTES AND DOSAGE RANGES
Antiallergic Agents		
Azelastine (Optivar)	Allergic conjunctivitis	1 drop in affected eye(s) twice daily
Cromolyn (Crolom, Opticrom)	Treatment of seasonal allergic conjunctivitis, keratitis, and keratoconjunctivitis	1 or 2 drops in each eye 4–6 times daily at regular intervals
Emedastine (Emadine)	Allergic conjunctivitis	1 or 2 drops twice daily
Epinastine (Elestat)	Allergic conjunctivitis	1 drop in each eye twice daily
Ketotifen (Zaditor)	Allergic conjunctivitis	1 drop in affected eye(s) q8–12h
Lodoxamide (Alomide)	Conjunctivitis Keratitis	1 or 2 drops in affected eye(s) 4 times daily, for up to 3 mo
Olopatadine (Patanol)	Allergic conjunctivitis	1 or 2 drops twice daily

GENERIC/TRADE NAME	INDICATIONS FOR USE	ROUTES AND DOSAGE RANGES
Corticosteroids		
Dexamethasone (Decadron, Maxidex)	Inflammatory disorders of the conjunctiva, cornea, eyelid, and anterior eyeball (e.g., conjunctivitis, keratitis)	Solution or suspension 1 or 2 drops q1h daytime, q2h nighttime until response; then 1 drop q4h
	Corneal injury from chemical, radiation, or thermal burns, or penetration of foreign bodies	Postoperative inflammation, 1 or 2 drops 4 times daily, starting 24 h after surgery, for 2 wk
	Prevention of graft rejection after corneal transplant	Ointment thin strip 3 or 4 times daily until response, then once or twice daily
Fluorometholone (FML)	Inflammatory disorders	Solution 1 drop q1–2h until response, then less often
		Ointment thin strip 3 or 4 times daily until response, then once or twice daily
Loteprednol (Lotemax, Alrex)	Allergic conjunctivitis	Allergic conjunctivitis, 0.2%, 1 drop in affected eye(s) 4 times daily
	Keratitis	Keratitis, 0.5%, 1 or 2 drops in affected eye(s) 4 times daily
	Treatment of inflammation after ocular surgery	Postoperative inflammation, 0.5%, 1 or 2 drops in affected eye(s) 4 times daily starting 24 h after surgery and continuing for 2 wk
Prednisolone (Econopred, others)	Inflammatory disorders	Solution or suspension 1 or 2 drops q1–2h until response, then 1 drop q4h, then less frequently
		Ointment thin strip 3 or 4 times daily until response, then once or twice daily
Rimexolone (Vexol)	Treatment of anterior uveitis	Uveitis, 1 or 2 drops in affected eye q1h during waking hours for 1 wk, then 1 drop q2h for 1 wk, then taper until uveitis resolved
	Treatment of inflammation after ocular surgery	Postoperative inflammation, 1 or 2 drops in affected eye(s) 4 times daily starting 24 h after surgery and continuing for 2 wk
Nonsteroidal Anti-Inflammatory Drugs		
Diclofenac (Voltaren)	Treatment of inflammation after cataract surgery	1 drop to affected eye 4 times daily, starting 24 h after surgery, for 2 wk
Flurbiprofen (Ocufen)	Inhibition of pupil constriction during eye surgery	1 drop q30min for 4 doses, starting 2 h before surgery
Ketorolac (Acular)	Treatment of ocular itching due to seasonal allergic conjunctivitis	1 drop 4 times daily for approximately 1 wk

Nursing Process

Assessment

Assess the patient's condition in relation to ophthalmic disorders.

■ Determine whether the patient has impaired vision and, if so, the extent of the impairment. Minimal assessment includes the vision-impaired patient's ability to participate in activities of daily living, including safe ambulation. Maximal assessment depends on the nurse's ability and working situation. Some nurses do vision testing and ophthalmoscopic examinations.

■ Identify risk factors for eye disorders. These include trauma, allergies, infection in one eye (a risk factor for

Nursing Process continues on page 1018

infection in the other eye), use of contact lenses, infections of facial structures or skin, and occupational exposure to chemical irritants or foreign bodies.

▪ Signs and symptoms vary with particular disorders:

▪ Pain is usually associated with corneal abrasions or inflammation. Sudden, severe pain may indicate acute glaucoma, which requires immediate treatment to lower IOP and minimize damage to the optic nerve.

▪ Signs of inflammation (redness, edema, heat, tenderness) are especially evident with infection or inflammation of external ocular structures, such as the eyelids and conjunctiva. A watery or mucoid discharge also often occurs.

▪ Pruritus is most often associated with allergic conjunctivitis.

▪ Photosensitivity commonly occurs with keratitis.

Nursing Diagnoses

▪ Disturbed Sensory Perception: Visual, related to eye disorders

▪ Risk for Injury: Blindness related to inadequately treated glaucoma or ophthalmic infections

▪ Deficient Knowledge related to prevention and treatment of ocular disorders

Planning/Goals

The patient will

▪ Take ophthalmic medications as prescribed

▪ Follow safety precautions to protect eyes from trauma and disease

▪ Experience improvement in signs and symptoms (e.g., decreased drainage with infections, decreased eye pain with glaucoma)

▪ Avoid injury from impaired vision (e.g., falls)

▪ Avoid systemic effects of ophthalmic drugs

▪ Have regular eye examinations to monitor effects of antiglaucoma drugs

Interventions

Use measures to minimize ocular disorders.

▪ Promote regular eye examinations. This is especially important among middle-aged and older adults, who are more likely to have several types of ocular disorders. These patients are also more likely to experience ocular disorders as adverse effects of drugs taken for nonocular disorders.

▪ Assist patients at risk of eye damage from IOP (e.g., those with glaucoma; those who have had intraocular surgery, such as cataract removal) to avoid straining at stool (use laxatives or stool softeners if needed), heavy lifting, bending over, coughing, and vomiting when possible.

▪ Promote hand washing and keeping hands away from eyes to prevent eye infections.

▪ Cleanse contact lenses or assist patients in lens care, when needed.

▪ Treat eye injuries appropriately:

▪ For chemical burns, irrigate the eyes with copious amounts of water as soon as possible (i.e., near the area where the injury occurred). Do not wait for transport to a first-aid station, hospital, or other health care facility. Damage continues as long as the chemical is in contact with the eye.

▪ For thermal burns, apply cold compresses to the area.

▪ Superficial foreign bodies may be removed by irrigation with water. Foreign bodies embedded in ocular structures must be removed by a health care provider.

▪ Warm, wet compresses are often useful in ophthalmic inflammation or infections. They relieve pain and promote healing by increasing the blood supply to the affected area.

Evaluation

▪ Observe and interview for compliance with instructions regarding drug therapy and follow-up care.

▪ Observe and interview for relief of symptoms.

▪ Observe for systemic adverse effects of ophthalmic drugs (e.g., tachycardia and dysrhythmias with adrenergics; bradycardia or bronchoconstriction with beta blockers).

Applying Your Knowledge 63-1

When you arrive at Mrs. Molnar's house, she is in the middle of brushing her hair. She drops her hair brush and bends over to pick it up. This provides an opportunity to provide what patient teaching?

··

Principles of Therapy

General Guidelines for Ophthalmic Drug Therapy

▪ Topical application is the most common route of administration for ophthalmic drugs, and correct administration is essential for optimal therapeutic effects.

▪ Systemic absorption of eye drops can be decreased by closing the eye and applying pressure over the tear duct (*nasolacrimal occlusion*) for 3 to 5 minutes after instillation.

▪ When multiple eye drops are required, there should be an interval of 5 to 10 minutes between drops because of limited eye capacity and rapid drainage into tear ducts.

■ Absorption of eye medications is increased in eye disorders associated with hyperemia and inflammation.

■ Many ophthalmic drugs are available as eye drops (solutions or suspensions) and ointments. Ointments are administered less frequently than drops and often produce higher concentrations of drug in target tissues. However, they also cause blurred vision, which limits their daytime use, at least for ambulatory patients. For some patients, drops may be used during waking hours and ointments at bedtime.

■ Topical ophthalmic medications should not be used after the expiration date; cloudy, discolored solutions should be discarded.

■ Topical eye medications contain a number of inactive ingredients, such as preservatives, buffers, tonicity agents, antioxidants, and so forth. Some contain sulfites, to which some people may have an allergic reaction.

■ Some eye drops contain benzalkonium hydrochloride, a preservative, which is absorbed by soft contact lenses. The medications should not be applied while wearing soft contacts and should be instilled 15 minutes or longer before inserting soft contacts.

■ To increase safety and accuracy of ophthalmic drug therapy, the labels and caps of eye medications are color coded.

Patient Teaching Guidelines | Topical Eye Medications

General Considerations

■ Prevent eye disorders, when possible. For example, try to avoid long periods of reading and computer work; minimize exposure to dust, smog, cigarette smoke, and other eye irritants; wash hands often and avoid touching the eyes to decrease risks of infection. Use protective eyewear when indicated.

■ Do not use nonprescription eye drops (e.g., Murine, Visine) on a regular basis for longer than 48 to 72 hours. Persistent eye irritation and redness should be reported to a health care provider.

■ Have regular eye examinations and testing for glaucoma after 40 years of age.

■ Eye-drop preparations often contain sulfites, which can cause allergic reactions in some people.

■ If you have glaucoma, do not take any drugs without the ophthalmologist's knowledge and consent. Many drugs given for purposes other than eye disorders may cause or aggravate glaucoma. Also, wear a medical alert bracelet or carry identification that states you have glaucoma. This helps to avoid administration of drugs that aggravate glaucoma or to maintain treatment of glaucoma, in emergencies.

■ If you have an eye infection, wash hands before and after contact with the infected eye to avoid spreading the infection to the unaffected eye or to other people. Also, avoid touching the unaffected eye.

■ If you wear contact lenses, wash your hands before inserting them and follow instructions for care (e.g., cleaning, inserting or removing, and duration of wear). Improper or infrequent cleaning may lead to infection. Overwearing is a common cause of corneal abrasion and may cause corneal ulceration. The lens wearer should consult an ophthalmologist when eye pain occurs. Antibiotics are often prescribed for corneal abrasions to prevent development of ulcers.

■ If you wear soft contact lenses, do not use any eye medication without consulting a specialist in eye care. Some eye drops contain benzalkonium hydrochloride, a preservative, which is absorbed by soft contacts. The medication should not be applied while wearing soft contacts and should be instilled 15 minutes or longer before inserting soft contacts.

■ Never use eye medications used by someone else and never allow your eye medications to be used by anyone

else. These preparations should be used by one person only and they are dispensed in small amounts for this purpose. Single-person use minimizes cross-contamination and risks of infection.

■ Many eye drops and ointments cause temporary blurring of vision. Do not use such medications just before driving or operating potentially hazardous machinery.

■ Avoid straining at stool (use laxatives or stool softeners if necessary), heavy lifting, bending over, coughing, and vomiting when possible. These activities increase intraocular pressure, which may cause eye damage in glaucoma and after eye surgery.

Self-Administration

■ If using more than one eye medication, be sure to administer the correct one at the correct time. Benefits depend on accurate administration.

■ Check expiration dates; do not use any eye medication after the expiration date and do not use any liquid medications that have changed color or contain particles.

■ Shake the container if instructed to do so on the label. Solutions do not need to be shaken; suspensions should be shaken well to ensure the drug is evenly dispersed in the liquid and not settled in the bottom of the container.

■ Wash hands thoroughly.

■ Tilt head back or lie down and look up.

■ Pull the lower eyelid down to expose the conjunctiva (mucous membrane).

■ Place the dropper directly over the eye. Avoid contact of the dropper with the eye, finger, or any other surface. Such contact contaminates the solution and may cause eye infections and serious damage to the eye, with possible loss of vision.

■ Look up just before applying a drop; look down for several seconds after applying a drop.

■ Release the eyelid, close the eyes, and press on the inside corner of the eye with a finger for 3 to 5 minutes. Closing the eyes and blocking the tear duct helps the medication be more effective by slowing its drainage out of the eye.

■ Do not rub the eye; do not rinse the dropper.

■ If more than one eye drop is ordered, wait 5–10 minutes before instilling the second medication.

■ Use the same basic procedure to insert eye ointments.

You are teaching Mrs. Molnar how to administer her medication. What do you teach her about administering eye drops?

Ocular Infections

Guidelines for drug therapy of ocular infections include the following:

- Drug therapy is usually initiated as soon as culture material (eye secretions) has been obtained, often with a broad-spectrum antibacterial agent or a combination of two or more antibiotics.

- Topical administration is used most often, and recommended drugs include bacitracin, polymyxin B, and sulfacetamide. These agents are rarely given systemically. They do not cause sensitization to commonly used systemic antibiotics and do not promote growth of drug-resistant microorganisms. Other antibacterial drugs available in ophthalmic formulations include erythromycin, gentamicin, tobramycin, several fluoroquinolones (ciprofloxacin, gatifloxacin, moxifloxacin, ofloxacin), and combination products.

- In severe infections, antibacterial drugs may be given both topically and systemically. Because systemic antibiotics penetrate the eye poorly, large doses are required to attain therapeutic drug concentrations in ocular structures. Drugs that reach therapeutic levels in the eye when given in proper dosage include ampicillin and dicloxacillin. Gentamicin and other antibiotics penetrate the eye when inflammation is present.

- Combination products containing two or more antibacterials are available for topical treatment of external ocular infections. These products are most useful when therapy must be initiated before the infecting microorganism is identified. Mixtures (e.g., polymyxin B and bacitracin) provide a broader spectrum of antibacterial activity than a single drug.

- Fixed-dose combinations of an antibacterial agent and a corticosteroid (e.g., Blephamide, Maxitrol, NeoDecadron, Poly-Pred) are available for topical use in selected conditions (e.g., staphylococcal keratitis, blepharoconjunctivitis, bacterial conjunctivitis, some postoperative inflammatory reactions).

- Trifluridine (Viroptic) is the drug of choice in eye infections caused by the herpes simplex virus. Ganciclovir is available for treatment of cytomegalovirus (CMV) retinitis in patients with acquired immunodeficiency syndrome (AIDS).

- Natamycin (Natacyn) is the drug of choice in fungal eye infections. It has a broad spectrum of antifungal activity and is nonirritating and nontoxic.

Corneal Abrasions

Injuries to the cornea cause pain, tearing, photophobia, and a foreign-body or gritty feeling in the eye. These symptoms can be worsened by exposure to light, blinking, and rubbing the injured surface against the inside of the eyelid. Initial management involves removal of foreign bodies and analgesia with topical NSAIDs or oral analgesics. Topical antibiotics also may be used. Most corneal abrasions heal in 24 to 72 hours.

Patients who wear contact lenses are at higher risk of developing abrasions that become infected and ulcerate. For these patients, an antipseudomonal antibiotic (e.g., gentamicin or a fluoroquinolone) should be used. In addition, the patient should avoid wearing contact lenses until the abrasion is healed and antibiotic therapy completed.

Glaucoma

For chronic glaucoma, the goal of drug therapy is to slow disease progression by reducing IOP. Topical beta blockers are first-line drugs and commonly used. They may be used alone or in combination with other antiglaucoma drugs. Several are available for ophthalmic use. Most adverse effects of systemic beta blockers may also occur with ophthalmic preparations and their use may be restricted in patients with respiratory or cardiac disease.

Other first-line drugs, which may be used with or instead of beta blockers, include brimonidine, prostaglandin analogs, and topical CAIs.

Use in Special Populations

Use in Children

Topical ophthalmic drug therapy in children differs little from that in adults. Few studies of ophthalmic drug therapy in children have been reported, and many conditions for which adults need therapy (e.g., cataract, glaucoma) rarely occur in children. A major use of topical ophthalmic drugs in children is to dilate the pupil and paralyze accommodation for ophthalmoscopic examination. As a general rule, the short-acting mydriatics and cycloplegics (e.g., cyclopentolate, tropicamide) are preferred because they cause fewer systemic adverse effects than atropine and scopolamine. In addition, lower drug concentrations are usually given empirically because of the smaller size of children and the potential risk of systemic adverse effects.

Use in Older Adults

Older adults are at risk for development of ocular disorders, especially glaucoma and cataracts. General principles of ophthalmic drug therapy are the same as for younger adults. In addition, older adults are likely to have cardiovascular disorders that may be aggravated by systemic absorption of topical eye medication. Thus, accurate dosage and occlusion of the nasolacrimal duct in the inner canthus of the eye are needed to prevent adverse drug effects (e.g., hypertension, tachycardia, or dysrhythmias with adrenergic drugs; bradycardia, heart block, or bronchoconstriction with beta blockers).

For what are possible systemic effects of Mrs. Molnar's eye drops the nurse should monitor?

Use in Home Care

The home care nurse may be involved in the care of patients with acute or chronic eye disorders. As with other drug therapy, the nurse may need to teach patients and caregivers reasons for use, accurate administration, and assessment of therapeutic and adverse responses to eye medications. The nurse may also need to encourage periodic eye examinations and measurements of IOP to promote optimal vision and prevent blindness.

Nursing Actions   Ophthalmic Drugs

NURSING ACTIONS	RATIONALE/EXPLANATION
1. Administer accurately	
a. Read labels of ophthalmic medications carefully.	To avoid error, because many drugs are available in several concentrations
b. Read medication orders carefully and accurately.	To avoid error. Avoid abbreviations (e.g., OS, OD, OU) .
c. For hospitalized patients, keep eye medications at the bedside.	Eye medications should be used by one person only. They are dispensed in small amounts for this purpose. This minimizes cross-contamination and risk of infection.
d. Wash hands before approaching the patient for instillation of eye medications.	To reduce risks of infection
e. To administer eye drops, have the client lie down or tilt the head backward and look upward. Then, pull down the lower lid to expose the conjunctival sac, and drop the medication into the sac. After instillation, have the patient close the eyes gently, and apply pressure to the inner canthus.	Drug absorption and concentration in ocular tissues depend partly on the length of time the medication is in contact with ocular tissues. Contact time is increased by closing the eyes (delays outflow into the nasolacrimal duct) and by placing pressure on the inner canthus (delays outflow and decreases side effects resulting from systemic absorption).
f. When instilling ophthalmic ointments, position the patient as above, and apply a ¼-inch to ¼-inch strip of ointment to the conjunctiva.	
g. Do not touch the dropper tip or ointment top to the eye or anything else.	To avoid contamination of the medication and infection
h. When crusts or secretions are present, cleanse the eye before administering medication.	If the eye is not cleansed, the drug may not be absorbed.
i. When two or more eye drops are scheduled for the same time, they should be instilled at least 5 minutes apart.	To avoid drug loss by dilution and outflow into the nasolacrimal duct
2. Observe for therapeutic effects	Therapeutic effects depend on the reason for use.
a. With beta-blocking agents, observe for decreased intraocular pressure (IOP).	Lowering of IOP usually occurs within a month; periodic measurements should be done.
b. With mydriatics, observe for dilation of the pupil.	Mydriasis begins within 5–15 minutes after instillation.
c. With miotics, observe for constriction of the pupil.	
d. With antimicrobial drugs, observe for decreased redness, edema, and drainage.	
e. With osmotic agents, observe for decreased IOP.	With oral glycerin, maximal decrease in IOP occurs approximately 1 hour after administration, and effects persist for about 5 hours. With intravenous mannitol, maximal decreased IOP occurs within 30–60 minutes and lasts 6–8 hours.
3. Observe for adverse effects	
a. Local effects:	
(1) Irritation, burning, stinging, blurred vision, discomfort, redness, itching, tearing, conjunctivitis, keratitis, allergic reactions	These effects may occur with any topical ophthalmic agent. Burning and stinging occur with instillation and are usually transient. Allergic reactions may occur with the active ingredient, preservatives, or other components.
(2) With prostaglandin analogs—permanent darkening of eye color may occur, especially in light-colored eyes. Changes in the length and thickness of eyelashes may also occur.	Changes in eye color and eyelashes may not be noticeable for months to years after starting drug use. These effects are most problematic in clients receiving treatment in one eye.
(3) With antibacterial agents—superinfection or sensitization	Superinfection caused by drug-resistant organisms may occur. Sensitization means that topical application induces antibody formation. Therefore, if the same or a related drug is subsequently administered systemically, an allergic reaction may occur. Sensitization can be prevented or minimized by avoiding topical administration of antibacterial agents that are commonly given systemically.

(continued on page 1022)

Nursing Actions **Ophthalmic Drugs** (continued)

NURSING ACTIONS	RATIONALE/EXPLANATION
(4) With anticholinergics, adrenergics, corticosteroids—glaucoma or increased IOP	Mydriatic drugs (anticholinergics and adrenergics) may cause an acute attack of angle closure in patients with closed-angle glaucoma by blocking outflow of aqueous humor. Topical corticosteroids raise IOP in some patients. The "glaucomatous" response occurs most often in patients with chronic, primary open-angle glaucoma and their relatives. It also may occur in clients with myopia or diabetes mellitus. The magnitude of increased IOP depends on the concentration, frequency of administration, duration of therapy, and anti-inflammatory potency of the corticosteroid. This effect can be minimized by checking IOP every 2 months in patients receiving long-term therapy with topical corticosteroids.
(5) With miotic drugs—decreased vision in dim light	These agents prevent pupil dilation, which normally occurs in dim light or darkness.
b. Systemic effects:	Systemic absorption and adverse effects of eye drops can be prevented or minimized by closing the eyes or applying pressure to the inner canthus (nasolacrimal occlusion) after instillation of the medications. Pressure may be applied by the nurse or the patient.
(1) With beta-blocking agents—bradycardia, bronchospasm, and others (see Chap. 18)	These agents may be absorbed systematically and cause all the adverse effects associated with oral or injected drugs.
(2) With miotics—sweating, nausea, vomiting, diarrhea, abdominal pain, bradycardia, hypotension, bronchoconstriction. Toxic doses produce ataxia, confusion, convulsions, coma, respiratory failure, and death.	These cholinergic or parasympathomimetic effects occur rarely with pilocarpine. Acute toxicity may be reversed by an anticholinergic agent, atropine, given IV.
(3) With anticholinergic mydriatics—dryness of the mouth and skin, fever, rash, tachycardia, confusion, hallucinations, delirium	These effects are most likely to occur with atropine and in children and older adults. Tropicamide (Mydriacyl) rarely causes systemic reactions.
(4) With adrenergic mydriatics—tachycardia, hypertension, premature ventricular contractions, tremors, headache	Systemic effects are uncommon. They are more likely to occur with repeated instillations of high drug concentrations (e.g., phenylephrine [Neo-Synephrine] 10%).
(5) With carbonic anhydrase inhibitors—anorexia, nausea, vomiting, diarrhea, paresthesias, weakness, lethargy	Nausea, malaise, and paresthesias (numbness and tingling of extremities) commonly occur with oral drugs, which are given only when topical drugs are not effective.
(6) With osmotic diuretics—dehydration, nausea, vomiting, headache, hyperglycemia and glycosuria with glycerin (Osmoglyn)	These agents may produce profound diuresis and dehydration. Oral agents (e.g., glycerin) are less likely to cause severe systemic effects than IV agents (e.g., mannitol). These agents are usually given in a single dose, which decreases the risks of serious adverse reactions unless large doses are given.
(7) With corticosteroids, see Chapter 23.	Serious adverse effects may occur with long-term use of corticosteroids.
(8) With antibacterial agents, see Chapter 29 and the chapter on the individual drug group.	Adverse effects may occur with all antibacterial agents.
(9) With ophthalmic nonsteroidal anti-inflammatory drugs—potential for increased bleeding	Systemic absorption may interfere with platelet function and increase risks of bleeding with surgery or anticoagulant therapy.
(10) With prostaglandin analogs—headache, cold/flu/upper respiratory infection, bronchitis, sinusitis, muscle and joint pain, chest pain	These were the most commonly reported systemic adverse effects in clinical trials, similar in incidence to placebo.
4. Observe for drug interactions	
a. Drugs that *increase* effects of antiglaucoma drugs:	
(1) Other antiglaucoma drugs	Antiglaucoma drugs may be used in various combinations for additive effects when a single drug does not decrease IOP sufficiently.
b. Drugs that *increase* effects of adrenergic (sympathomimetic) ophthalmic drugs:	
(1) Anticholinergic ophthalmic drugs	The combination (e.g., atropine and phenylephrine) produces additive mydriasis.
(2) Systemic adrenergic drugs	Additive risks of adverse effects (e.g., tachycardia, cardiac dysrhythmias, hypertension)

NURSING ACTIONS	RATIONALE/EXPLANATION
c. Drugs that *decrease* effects of adrenergic ophthalmic preparations:	
(1) Cholinergic ophthalmic drugs	Antagonize mydriatic effects of adrenergic drugs
d. Drugs that *increase* effects of antiadrenergic ophthalmic preparations:	
(1) Systemic antiadrenergics (e.g., propranolol, atenolol, metoprolol, nadolol, timolol)	When the patient is receiving a topical beta blocker in ocular disorders, administration of systemic beta-blocking agents in cardiovascular disorders may cause additive systemic toxicity.
e. Drugs that *increase* effects of anticholinergic ophthalmic drugs:	
(1) Adrenergic ophthalmic agents	Additive mydriasis
(2) Systemic anticholinergic drugs (e.g., atropine) and other drugs with anticholinergic effects (e.g., some antihistamines, antipsychotic agents, and tricyclic antidepressants)	Additive anticholinergic effects (mydriasis, blurred vision, tachycardia). These drugs are hazardous in narrow-angle glaucoma.
f. Drugs that *decrease* effects of cholinergic ophthalmic drugs:	
(1) Anticholinergics and drugs with anticholinergic effects (e.g., atropine, antipsychotic agents, tricyclic antidepressants, some antihistamines)	Antagonize antiglaucoma (miotic) effects of cholinergic drugs
(2) Corticosteroids	Long-term use of corticosteroids, topically or systemically, raises IOP and may cause glaucoma. Therefore, corticosteroids decrease effects of all drugs used for glaucoma.
(3) Sympathomimetic drugs	Antagonize miotic (antiglaucoma) effect

Key Concepts

- Drug therapy of eye disorders is unique because of the location, structure, and function of the eye.
- Eye medications represent several different drug classes.
- Most eye medications are given as eye drops.
- Therapeutic effects of eye drops depend on accurate administration.
- Eye medications should be kept sterile to avoid infection.
- Local eye medications may cause systemic effects; systemic drugs may affect eye function.

Review and Application Exercises

Short Answer Exercises

1. List common disorders of the eye for which drug therapy is indicated.
2. Do ophthalmic medications need to be sterile? Why or why not?
3. What are important principles and techniques related to the nurse's administration of ophthalmic drugs?
4. For a patient with newly prescribed eye drops, how would you teach self-administration principles and techniques?

NCLEX-Style Questions

5. What is a major purpose of occluding tear ducts for 3 to 5 minutes after administering eye drops?
   a. to prevent eye infections
   b. to prevent systemic absorption of the drug
   c. to make self-administration easier
   d. to use a smaller drug dosage

6. When a patient has two different eye drops ordered at the same time, how should the nurse administer them?
   a. The drops should be given one immediately after the other.
   b. Wait 5 to 10 minutes between drops.
   c. Wait 30 seconds between drops.
   d. Reschedule the medications to be given 1 hour apart.

7. For a patient receiving an ophthalmic beta blocker and a systemic beta blocker, the nurse is alerted that which of the following effects is likely to occur?
   a. increased bradycardia
   b. increased nausea
   c. increased antiglaucoma effect
   d. increased blood pressure

8. People who wear contact lenses should be educated by the nurse that they are at high risk of developing which of the following eye disorders?
   a. cataract
   b. glaucoma
   c. corneal abrasion
   d. allergic conjunctivitis

9. A patient with an inflammatory eye disorder has been prescribed corticosteroid eye drops and asks the nurse why this has been prescribed. The nurse is correct in telling the patient that these drops are used to
   a. dilate pupils prior to surgery
   b. constrict pupils in glaucoma
   c. prevent cataract development
   d. prevent scarring and loss of vision

Selected References

Carroll, E. W., Porth, C. M., & Curtis, R. L. (2005). Alterations in vision. In C. M. Porth (Ed.), *Pathophysiology: Concepts of altered health states* (7th ed., pp. 1291–1327). Philadelphia: Lippincott Williams & Wilkins.

Drug facts and comparisons. (Updated monthly). St. Louis, MO: Facts and Comparisons.

Lacy, C. F., Armstrong, L. L., Goldman, M. P., & Lance, L. L. (2006). *Drug information handbook* (14th ed.). Hudson, OH: Lexi-Comp, Inc.

Lesar, T. S., Fiscella, R. G., & Edward, D. (2005). Glaucoma. In J. T. DiPiro, R. L. Talbert, G. C. Yee, G. R. Matzke, B. G. Wells, & L. M.

Posey (Eds.), *Pharmacotherapy: A pathophysiologic approach* (6th ed., pp. 1713–1727). New York: McGraw-Hill.

Navarro, V. (2008). Assessment and management of patients with eye and vision disorders. In S. C. Smeltzer, B. G. Bare, J. L. Hinkle, & K. H. Cheever (Eds.), *Brunner & Suddarth's textbook of medical-surgical nursing* (11th ed., pp. 2042–2091). Philadelphia: Lippincott Williams & Wilkins.

Riordan-Eva, P. (2007). Eye. In S. J. McPhee, M. A. Papadakis, & L. M. Tierney, Jr. (Eds.), *Current medical diagnosis and treatment 2007* (46th ed., pp. 151–181). New York: McGraw-Hill.

Drugs Used in Dermatologic Conditions

KEY TERMS

- Acne
- Candidiasis
- Dermatitis
- Emollient
- Erythema
- Keratin
- Melanocytes
- Pruritus
- Psoriasis
- Rosacea
- Tinea pedis
- Urticaria

LEARNING OBJECTIVES

After studying this chapter, you will be able to:

1. Review characteristics of skin structures that influence drug therapy of dermatologic disorders.
2. Discuss antimicrobial, anti-inflammatory, and selected miscellaneous drugs in relation to their use in dermatologic disorders.
3. Use correct techniques to administer dermatologic medications.
4. Teach patients, family members, or caregivers correct administration of dermatologic medications.
5. For patients with "open lesion" skin disorders, teach about the importance and techniques of preventing infection.
6. Practice and teach measures to protect the skin from the damaging effects of sun exposure.

Applying Your Knowledge

Ginger Hertzfeld is a 15-year-old female student at the high school where you are the school nurse. She tells you that she has a red and itchy rash. Ginger is very modest and shy and will not show you the rash but wants advice on an over-the-counter preparation she can use to treat it.

Introduction

Basic Structure and Function of the Skin

The skin is the largest body organ and the interface between the internal and external environments. It is composed of the epidermis and dermis. Epidermal or epithelial cells begin in the basal layer of the epidermis and migrate outward, undergoing degenerative changes in each layer. The outer layer, called the stratum corneum, is composed of dead cells and keratin. The dead cells are constantly being shed (desquamated) and replaced by newer cells. Normally, approximately 1 month is required for cell formation, migration, and desquamation. When dead cells are discarded, keratin remains on the skin. *Keratin* is a tough protein substance that is insoluble in water, weak acids, and weak bases. Hair and nails, which are composed of keratin, are referred to as appendages of the skin.

Melanocytes are pigment-producing cells located at the junction of the epidermis and the dermis. These cells produce yellow, brown, or black skin coloring in response to genetic influences, melanocyte-stimulating hormone released from the anterior pituitary gland, and exposure to ultraviolet (UV) light (e.g., sunlight).

The dermis is composed of elastic and fibrous connective tissue. Dermal structures include blood vessels, lymphatic channels, nerves and nerve endings, sweat glands, sebaceous glands, and hair follicles. The dermis is supported underneath by subcutaneous tissue, which is composed primarily of fat cells.

The skin has numerous functions, most of which are protective, including the following:

- Serves as a physical barrier against loss of fluids and electrolytes and against entry of microorganisms, foreign bodies, and other potentially harmful substances
- Detects sensations of pain, pressure, touch, and temperature through sensory nerve endings
- Assists in regulating body temperature through production and elimination of sweat
- Serves as a source of vitamin D when exposed to sunlight or other sources of UV light. Skin contains a precursor for vitamin D.
- Excretes water, sodium, chloride, lactate, and urea in sweat
- Inhibits growth of many microorganisms by its acidic pH (4.5–6.5)

Mucous membranes are composed of a surface layer of epithelial cells, a basement membrane, and a layer of connective tissue. They line body cavities that communicate with the external environment (e.g., mouth, vagina, anus). Mucous membranes receive an abundant blood supply because capillaries lie just beneath the epithelial cells.

Disorders of the Skin

Dermatologic disorders may be primary (i.e., originate in the skin or mucous membranes) or secondary (i.e., result from a systemic condition, such as measles or adverse drug reactions). This chapter emphasizes selected primary skin disorders and the medications used to prevent or treat them.

Inflammatory Disorders

Dermatitis

Dermatitis, also called eczema, is a general term denoting an inflammatory response of the skin to injuries from irritants, allergens, or trauma. Whatever the cause, dermatitis is usually characterized by *erythema* (redness), *pruritus* (itching), and skin lesions. It may be acute or chronic.

- **Atopic dermatitis** is a common disorder characterized by dry skin, pruritus, and lesions that vary according to the extent of inflammation, stages of healing, and scratching. Scratching damages the skin and increases the risks of secondary infection. Acute lesions are reddened skin areas containing papules and vesicles; chronic lesions are often thick, fibrotic, and nodular.

  The cause is uncertain but may involve allergic, hereditary, or psychological elements. Approximately 50% to 80% of patients have asthma or allergic rhinitis; some have a family history of these disorders. Thus, exposure to possible causes or exacerbating factors such as allergens, irritating chemicals, foods, and emotional stress should be considered. The condition may occur in all age groups but is more common in children.

- **Contact dermatitis** results from direct contact with irritants (e.g., soaps, detergents) or allergens (e.g., clothing materials or dyes, jewelry, cosmetics) that stimulate inflammation. Irritants cause tissue damage and dermatitis in anyone with sufficient contact or exposure. Allergens cause dermatitis only in sensitized or hypersensitive people. The location of the dermatitis may indicate the cause (e.g., facial dermatitis may indicate an allergy to cosmetics).

- **Seborrheic dermatitis** is a disease of the sebaceous glands characterized by excessive production of sebum. It may occur on the scalp, face, or trunk. A simple form involving the scalp is dandruff, which is characterized by flaking and itching of the skin. More severe forms are characterized by greasy, yellow scales or crusts with variable amounts of erythema and itching.

- **Urticaria** ("hives") is an inflammatory response characterized by a skin lesion called a wheal, a raised edematous area with a pale center and red border, which itches intensely. Histamine is the most common mediator of urticaria and it causes vasodilation, increased vascular permeability, and pruritus.

  Histamine is released from mast cells and basophils by both allergic (e.g., insect bites, foods, drugs) and nonallergic (e.g., radiocontrast media, opiates, heat, cold, pressure, UV light) stimuli. An important difference between allergic and nonallergic reactions is that many allergic reactions require prior exposure to the stimulus, whereas nonallergic reactions can occur with the first exposure.

- **Drug-induced skin reactions** can occur with virtually any drug and can resemble the signs and symptoms of virtually any skin disorder. Topical drugs usually cause a localized, contact-dermatitis type of reaction and systemic drugs cause generalized skin lesions. Skin manifestations of serious drug reactions include erythema, facial edema, pain, blisters, necrosis, and urticaria. Systemic manifestations may include fever, enlarged lymph nodes, joint pain or inflammation, shortness of breath, hypotension, and leukocytosis. Drug-related reactions usually occur within the first or second week of drug administration and subside when the drug is discontinued.

Psoriasis

Psoriasis is a chronic, inflammatory disorder attributed to activated T lymphocytes, which produce cytokines that stimulate abnormal growth of affected skin cells and blood vessels. The abnormal growth results in excessively rapid turnover of epidermal cells. Instead of 30 days from formation to elimination of normal epidermal cells, epidermal cells involved in psoriasis are abnormal in structure and have a lifespan of about 4 days. Skin lesions of psoriasis are erythematous, dry, and scaling. The lesions may occur anywhere on the body but commonly involve the skin covering bony prominences, such as the elbows and knees. Skin lesions may be tender, but they do not usually cause severe pain or itching. However, the lesions are unsightly and usually cause embarrassment and mental distress.

The disease is characterized by remissions and exacerbations. Exacerbating factors include infections, winter weather, some drugs (e.g., beta blockers, lithium), and possibly stress, obesity, and alcoholism.

Rosacea

Rosacea is a chronic disease characterized by erythema, telangiectases (fine, red, superficial blood vessels), and acne-like lesions of facial skin. Hyperplasia of the nose (rhinophyma) eventually develops. The etiology is thought to be excessive production of certain inflammatory proteins. Rosacea usually occurs in middle-aged and older people, more often in men than women. Spicy foods, heat, alcohol, and embarrassment can worsen the condition.

Dermatologic Infections

Bacterial Infections

Bacterial infections of the skin are common; they are most often caused by streptococci or staphylococci.

- **Cellulitis** is characterized by erythema, tenderness, and edema, which may spread to subcutaneous tissue. Generalized malaise, chills, and fever may occur.
- **Folliculitis** is an infection of the hair follicles that most often occurs on the scalp or bearded areas of the face.
- **Furuncles** and **carbuncles** are infections usually caused by staphylococci. Furuncles (boils) may result from folliculitis. They usually occur in the neck, face, axillae, buttocks, thighs, and perineum. Furuncles tend to recur. Carbuncles involve many hair follicles and include multiple pustules. Carbuncles may cause fever, malaise, leukocytosis, and bacteremia. Healing of carbuncles often produces scar tissue.
- **Impetigo** is a superficial skin infection caused by streptococci or staphylococci. An especially contagious form is caused by group A beta-hemolytic streptococci. This form occurs most often in children.

Fungal Infections

Fungal infections of the skin and mucous membranes are most often caused by *Candida albicans*.

- **Oral *candidiasis*** (thrush) involves mucous membranes of the mouth. It often occurs as a superinfection after the use of broad-spectrum systemic antibiotics.
- **Candidiasis of the vagina and vulva** occurs with systemic antibiotic therapy and in women with diabetes mellitus.
- **Intertrigo** involves skin folds or areas where two skin surfaces are in contact (e.g., groin, pendulous breasts).
- **Tinea infections** (ringworm) are caused by fungi (dermatophytes). These infections may involve the scalp (tinea capitis), the body (tinea corporis), the foot (tinea pedis), and other areas of the body. *Tinea pedis*, commonly called athlete's foot, is a common type of ringworm infection.

Viral Infections

Viral infections of the skin include verrucal (warts) and herpes infections. There are two types of herpes simplex infections: type 1 usually involves the face or neck (e.g., fever blisters or cold sores on the lips), and type 2 involves the genitalia. Other herpes infections include varicella (chickenpox) and herpes zoster (shingles).

Trauma

Trauma refers to a physical injury that disrupts the skin. When the skin is broken, it may not be able to function properly. The major problem associated with skin wounds is infection. Common wounds include lacerations (cuts or tears), abrasions (shearing or scraping of the skin), puncture wounds, surgical incisions, and burn wounds.

Ulcerations

Cutaneous ulcerations are usually caused by trauma and impaired circulation. They may become inflamed or infected.

- **Pressure ulcers** (also called decubitus ulcers) may occur anywhere on the body when external pressure decreases blood flow. They are most likely to develop in patients who are immobilized, incontinent, malnourished, and debilitated. Common sites include the sacrum, trochanters, ankles, and heels. In addition, abraded skin is susceptible to infection and ulcer formation.
- **Venous stasis ulcers**, which usually occur on the legs, result from impaired venous circulation. Other signs of venous insufficiency include edema, varicose veins, stasis dermatitis, and brown skin pigmentation. Bacterial infection may occur in the ulcer.

Acne

Acne is a common disorder characterized by excessive production of sebum and obstruction of hair follicles, which normally carry sebum to the skin surface. As a result, hair follicles expand and form comedones (blackheads and whiteheads). Acne lesions vary from small comedones to acne vulgaris, the most severe form, in which follicles become infected and irritating secretions leak into surrounding tissues to form inflammatory pustules, cysts, and abscesses. Most patients have a variety of lesion types at one time. At least four pathologic events take place within acne-infected hair follicles: (1) androgen-mediated stimulation of sebaceous gland activity, (2) abnormal keratinization leading to follicular plugging (comedone formation), (3) proliferation of the bacterium *Propionibacterium acnes* within the follicle, and (4) inflammation.

Acne occurs most often on the face, upper back, and chest because large numbers of sebaceous glands are located in these areas. One etiologic factor is increased secretion of male hormones (androgens), which occurs at puberty in both sexes. This leads to increased production of sebum and proliferation of *P. acnes* bacteria, which depend on sebum for survival. The *P. acnes* organisms contain lipase enzymes that break down free fatty acids and produce inflammation in acne lesions. Other causative factors may include medications (e.g., phenytoin, corticosteroids) and stress (i.e., the stress mechanism may involve stimulation of androgen secretion). There is no evidence that certain foods (e.g., chocolate) or lack of cleanliness cause acne.

External Otitis

External otitis is an infection of the external ear characterized by pain, itching, and drainage. The external ear is lined with epidermal tissue, which is susceptible to the same skin disorders that affect other parts of the body. External otitis is most often caused by *Pseudomonas aeruginosa* and *Staphylococcus aureus* organisms and may be treated with antimicrobial ear drops for 7 to 10 days.

Anorectal Disorders

Hemorrhoids and anal fissures are common anorectal disorders characterized by pruritus, bleeding, and pain. Inflammation and infection may occur.

Dermatologic Drug Therapy

Many dermatologic medications are applied topically to skin and mucous membranes. The drugs may improve barrier function, soften and remove scaly lesions, alter inflammation in the skin, alter blood flow, exert antimicrobial effects, or affect proliferating cells. Components of topical medications include an active drug and additives that facilitate application to skin and mucous membranes. Numerous dosage forms have been developed for topical application to various parts of the body and for various therapeutic purposes (see Box 64-1). Many topical drugs are available in several dosage forms.

Topical medications are used primarily for local effects and systemic absorption is undesirable. Major factors that increase systemic absorption of topical agents include damaged or inflamed skin, high concentrations of drug, and application of drug to the face or mucous membranes, to large areas of the body, or for prolonged periods.

Types of Dermatologic Drugs

Many different drugs are used to prevent or treat dermatologic disorders; most fit into one or more of the following categories:

■ **Antimicrobials** are used to treat infections caused by bacteria, fungi, and viruses (see Chaps. 29–36). When used in dermatologic infections, antimicrobials may be administered locally (topically) or systemically (orally or parenterally). Topical antibacterials (Table 64-1) are used to treat superficial skin disorders such as acne and skin infections. Systemic antibacterials (e.g., cephalosporins) are used for soft-tissue infections such as cellulitis and postoperative wound infections. Tetracyclines are used for acne and rosacea; fluoroquinolones (e.g., ciprofloxacin) may be used to treat soft-tissue infections caused by gram-negative organisms.

■ **Antiseptics** kill or inhibit the growth of bacteria, viruses, or fungi. They are used primarily to prevent infection. Skin surfaces should be clean before application of antiseptics.

■ **Corticosteroids** (see Chap. 23) are used to treat the inflammation present in many dermatologic conditions. They are most often applied topically (Table 64-2) but also may be given orally or parenterally.

Box 64-1	Dosage Forms of Topical Medications

Medications for application to skin and mucous membranes mix an active drug with preservatives, emulsifying agents, and an appropriate base or vehicle. Numerous dosage forms are available for various conditions and therapeutic uses, as follows.

■ **Creams** are emulsions of oil in water that may be greasy or nongreasy. They leave a thin coating of oil on the skin as the water evaporates. Creams retain moisture in the skin and are cosmetically acceptable for use on the face and other visible areas of the body. They also may be used in hairy, moist, intertriginous areas. Creams are especially useful in subacute dermatologic disorders.

■ **Gels** are transparent colloids, which are solid at room temperature but melt on contact with the skin. They dry and leave a film over the area that helps retain moisture in the skin. They are especially useful in subacute dermatologic disorders.

■ **Lotions** are suspensions of insoluble substances in water. They cool, dry, and protect the skin. They are most useful in subacute dermatologic disorders.

■ **Ointments** are oil-based substances that usually contain a medication in an emollient vehicle, such as petrolatum or lanolin. Ointments occlude the skin and promote retention of moisture. Thus, they are especially useful in chronic skin disorders characterized by dry lesions. Ointments should usually be avoided in hairy, moist, and intertriginous areas of the body because of potential maceration, irritation, and secondary infection.

■ **Pastes** are a mixture of powder and ointment.

■ **Powders** have absorbent, cooling, and protective effects. Powders usually should not be applied in acute exudative disorders or on denuded areas because they tend to cake, occlude the lesions, and retard healing. Also, some powders (e.g., cornstarch) may lead to secondary infections by promoting growth of bacteria and fungi.

■ **Solutions** include water, alcohol, and propylene glycol, but not oil.

■ **Sprays** and **aerosols** are similar to lotions.

■ **Topical otic medications** are usually liquids. However, creams or ointments may be used for dry, crusted lesions, and powders may be used for drying effects.

■ **Topical vaginal medications** may be applied as douche solutions, vaginal tablets, or vaginal creams used with an applicator.

■ **Anorectal medications** may be applied as ointments, creams, foams, and rectal suppositories.

■ **Emollients** and **moisturizers** (e.g., lanolin) are used to relieve dry skin and pruritus.

■ **Enzymes** may be used to débride burn wounds, decubitus ulcers, and venous stasis ulcers. They promote healing by removing necrotic tissue.

■ **Immunosuppressants** (see Chap. 41) may be used to treat inflammatory skin disorders. Two topical agents, tacrolimus

(Protopic) ointment and pimecrolimus (Elidel) cream, are used for moderate to severe atopic dermatitis. However, the drugs have **BLACK BOX WARNINGS** about a possible increased risk of skin cancer and lymphoma. Precautions include using the drugs only when other drugs are ineffective and avoiding long-term use. Several systemic biologic agents, including alefacept (Amevive), efalizumab (Raptiva), etanercept (Enbrel), and infliximab (Remicade), are used for the treatment of severe psoriasis. These agents have **BLACK BOX WARNINGS** about increased risks for developing infections and their long-term effects are unknown.

▪ **Keratolytics** are used to treat keratin-containing skin conditions. Alpha hydroxy acids (e.g., glycolic acid) are used to treat wrinkles and sun-damaged skin. These acids are a component of many "antiaging" cosmetics and other products. Salicylic acid is used to remove warts, corns, and calluses.

▪ **Retinoids** are vitamin A derivatives that are active in proliferation and differentiation of skin cells. These agents are commonly used to treat acne, psoriasis, aging and wrinkling of skin from sunlight exposure, and skin cancers. Retinoids are contraindicated in women of childbearing potential unless the women have negative pregnancy tests; agree to use effective contraception before, during, and after drug therapy; and agree to take the drugs as prescribed. These drugs have been associated with severe fetal abnor-

malities and have **BLACK BOX WARNINGS** about the risks and precautions for safe use. With isotretinoin (Accutane), for example, manufacturers are required to maintain records of doctors who prescribe the drug, pharmacies that distribute it, and patients who take it. Prescribers and pharmacies must inform patients about the risks of taking the drug, have them sign informed-consent documents, and obtain proof of negative pregnancy tests (two tests before starting isotretinoin and a monthly test during therapy).

▪ **Sunscreens** are used to protect the skin from the damaging effects of UV radiation, thereby decreasing skin cancer and signs of aging, including wrinkles. Dermatologists recommend sunscreen preparations that block both UVA and UVB and have a "sun protection factor" (SPF) value of 30 or higher. The SPF is determined by the ratio of sunlight exposure needed to cause erythema in users of a sunscreen versus the exposure needed to cause erythema in nonusers. These highly protective sunscreens are especially needed by people who are fair skinned, allergic to sunlight, or using medications that increase skin sensitivity to sunlight (e.g., estrogens, tetracyclines).

Individual Drugs

Individual Drugs are described in Tables 64-1, 64-2, and 64-3.

| Table 64-1 | **Drugs at a Glance:** Topical Antimicrobial Agents |

GENERIC/TRADE NAME	INDICATIONS FOR USE	APPLICATION
Antibacterial Agents		
Azelaic acid (Azelex, Finacea)	Acne Rosacea	To lesions, twice daily
Bacitracin	Bacterial skin infections	To affected area, 1–3 times daily
Benzoyl peroxide	Acne	To affected areas, once or twice daily
Clindamycin (Cleocin T)	Acne	To affected areas, twice daily
Erythromycin (Akne-Mycin)	Acne	To affected areas, twice daily
Gentamicin (Garamycin)	Skin infections caused by susceptible organisms	To infected areas, 3–4 times daily
Metronidazole (MetroGel, Noritate)	Rosacea	To affected area, once or twice daily
Mupirocin (Bactroban)	Impetigo caused by *Staphylococcus aureus*, beta-hemolytic streptococci, or *Streptococcus pyogenes* Eradication of nasal colonization with methicillin-resistant S. *aureus*	Impetigo: Ointment, to affected areas, 3 times daily. Other skin lesions: Cream, 3 times daily for 10 d Eradication of nasal colonization: Ointment from single-use tube, one half in each nostril, morning and evening for 5 d
Retaptamulin (Altabax)	Impetigo	To affected area, twice daily for 5 d
Silver sulfadiazine (Silvadene)	Prevent or treat infection in burn wounds caused by *Pseudomonas* and many other organisms	To affected area, once or twice daily, using sterile technique

(continued on page 1030)

| Table 64-1 | | **Drugs at a Glance:** Topical Antimicrobial Agents (continued) | |

GENERIC/TRADE NAME	INDICATIONS FOR USE	APPLICATION
Combination Products		
Bacitracin and polymyxin B (Polysporin)	Bacterial skin infections	To lesions, 1–3 times daily
Erythromycin/benzoyl peroxide (Benzamycin)	Acne	To affected areas, twice daily
Neomycin, polymyxin B, and bacitracin (Neosporin)	Bacterial skin infections	To lesions, 2 or 3 times daily
Antifungal Agents		
Butenafine (Mentax)	Tinea pedis	To affected area, once daily for 2–4 wk
Ciclopirox (Loprox)	Tinea infections Cutaneous candidiasis	To affected area, twice daily for 2–4 wk
Clotrimazole (Lotrimin)	Tinea infections Cutaneous candidiasis	To affected areas, twice daily for 2–4 wk
Econazole (Spectazole)	Tinea infections Cutaneous candidiasis	To affected areas, once daily for tinea infections, twice daily for candidiasis
Ketoconazole (Nizoral)	Tinea infections Cutaneous candidiasis Seborrheic dermatitis	Tinea infections and candidiasis, to affected areas once daily for 2–4 wk Seborrheic dermatitis, twice daily for 4 wk
Miconazole (Micatin)	Tinea infections Cutaneous candidiasis	To affected area, once daily for 2–4 wk
Naftifine (Naftin)	Tinea infections	To affected areas, once daily with cream, twice daily with gel
Nystatin (Mycostatin)	Candidiasis of skin and mucous membranes	To affected areas, 2 or 3 times daily until healed
Oxiconazole (Oxistat)	Tinea infections	To affected areas, once or twice daily for 2–4 wk
Terbinafine (Lamisil)	Tinea infections	To affected areas, twice daily for 1–4 wk
Tolnaftate (Tinactin)	Tinea infections	To affected areas, twice daily for 2–4 wk
Antiviral Agents		
Acyclovir (Zovirax)	Herpes genitalis Herpes labialis in immunosuppressed patients	To lesions, q3h 6 times daily for 7 d
Penciclovir (Denavir)	Herpes labialis	To lesions, q2h while awake for 4 d

| Table 64-2 | | **Drugs at a Glance:** Topical Corticosteroids | |

GENERIC/TRADE NAME	DOSAGE FORMS	POTENCY
Alclometasone (Aclovate)	Cream, ointment	Low
Augmented betamethasone dipropionate (Diprolene)	Cream, gel, lotion, ointment	Ointment, very high; cream, high
Betamethasone dipropionate (Alphatrex, others)	Aerosol, cream, lotion, ointment	Cream and ointment, high; lotion, medium
Betamethasone valerate (Valisone, others)	Cream, foam, lotion, ointment	Ointment, high; cream, medium

GENERIC/TRADE NAME	DOSAGE FORMS	POTENCY
Clobetasol (Temovate)	Cream, gel, ointment, scalp application	Very high
Desonide (Tridesilon)	Cream, lotion, ointment	Low
Desoximetasone (Topicort)	Cream, gel, ointment	Medium
Dexamethasone (Decadron)	Aerosol, cream	Low
Fluocinolone (Synalar, others)	Cream, oil, ointment, shampoo, solution	High
Fluocinonide (Lidex)	Cream, gel, ointment, solution	High
Flurandrenolide (Cordran)	Cream, lotion, ointment, tape	Medium
Fluticasone (Cutivate)	Cream, ointment	Medium
Halobetasol (Ultravate)	Cream, ointment	Very high
Hydrocortisone (Cortaid, others)	Cream, lotion, ointment, solution, spray, roll-on stick	Medium or low
Mometasone (Elocon)	Cream, lotion, ointment	Medium
Triamcinolone acetonide (Aristocort, Kenalog, others)	Aerosol, cream, lotion, ointment	0.5% cream and ointment, high; lower concentrations, medium

| **Table 64-3** | **Drugs at a Glance:** Miscellaneous Dermatologic Agents |

GENERIC/ TRADE NAME	DERMATOLOGIC EFFECTS	CLINICAL INDICATIONS	METHOD OF ADMINISTRATION
Enzyme			
Trypsin (Granulex)	Débriding effects	Débridement of infected wounds (e.g., decubitus and varicose ulcers)	Topically by spray twice daily
Immunomodulators			
Pimecrolimus (Elidel)	Anti-inflammatory	Atopic dermatitis	Topically to affected skin, twice daily
Tacrolimus (Protopic)	Anti-inflammatory	Atopic dermatitis	Topically to affected skin, twice daily
Retinoids			
Acitretin (Soriatane)	Related to vitamin A	Severe psoriasis	PO 25–50 mg/d
Adapalene (Differin)	Reportedly causes less burning, itching, redness, and dryness than tretinoin	Acne vulgaris	Topically to skin lesions once daily
Isotretinoin (Accutane)	Inhibits sebum production and keratinization	Severe cystic acne Disorders characterized by excessive keratinization (e.g., pityriasis, ichthyosis) *Mycosis fungoides*	PO 1–2 mg/kg/d, in 2 divided doses, for 15–20 wk
Tazarotene (Tazorac)	A prodrug; mechanism of action is unknown	Acne Psoriasis	Topically to skin, after cleansing, once daily in the evening
Tretinoin (Retin-A)	Irritant	Acne vulgaris	Topically to skin lesions once daily
Other Agents			
Becaplermin (Regranex)	A recombinant human platelet-derived growth factor	Diabetic skin ulcers	Topically to ulcer; amount calculated according to size of the ulcer
Calcipotriene (Dovonex)	Synthetic analog of vitamin D that helps to regulate skin-cell production and development	Psoriasis	Topically to skin lesions twice daily

(continued on page 1032)

Table 64-3	**Drugs at a Glance:** Miscellaneous Dermatologic Agents (continued)		
GENERIC/ TRADE NAME	**DERMATOLOGIC EFFECTS**	**CLINICAL INDICATIONS**	**METHOD OF ADMINISTRATION**
Capsaicin (Zostrix)	Depletes substance P (which transmits pain impulses) in sensory nerves of the skin	Relief of pain associated with rheumatoid arthritis, osteoarthritis, and neuralgias	Topically to affected area, up to 3 or 4 times daily
Coal tar (Balnetar, Zetar, others)	Irritant	Psoriasis Dermatitis	Topically to skin, in various concentrations and preparations (e.g., creams, lotions, shampoos, bath emulsion). Also available in combination with hydrocortisone and other substances
Colloidal oatmeal (Aveeno)	Antipruritic	Pruritus	Topically as a bath solution (1 cup in bathtub of water)
Dextranomer (Debrisan)	Absorbs exudates from wound surfaces	Cleansing of ulcers (e.g., venous stasis, decubitus) and wounds (e.g., burn, surgical, traumatic)	Apply to a clean, moist wound surface q12h initially, then less often as exudate decreases
Fluorouracil (Efudex)	Antineoplastic	Actinic keratoses Superficial basal cell carcinomas	Topically to skin lesions twice daily for 2–6 wk
Masoprocol (Actinex)	Inhibits proliferation of keratin-containing cells	Actinic keratoses	Topically to skin lesions morning and evening for 28 d
Salicylic acid	Keratolytic, antifungal	Removal of warts, corns, calluses Superficial fungal infections Seborrheic dermatitis Acne Psoriasis	Topically to skin lesions
Selenium sulfide (Selsun)	Antifungal, antidandruff	Dandruff Tinea versicolor	Topically to scalp as shampoo once or twice weekly

Applying Your Knowledge 64-1

You ask Ginger to describe her rash. She says that it is red and very itchy. Upon further questioning, she tells you that she has had it before but cannot remember what it is called. She also has a history of seasonal allergies. Ginger agrees to let you look at the rash. Her history and the appearance of the rash suggest dermatitis. What can Ginger use to help relieve the itching and inflammation?

Herbal Preparations

Many supplements are promoted for use in skin conditions. Most have not been tested adequately to ensure effectiveness. At the same time, however, topical use rarely causes serious adverse effects or drug interactions. Two topical agents for which there is some support of safety and effectiveness are aloe and oat preparations.

Aloe is often used as a topical remedy for minor burns and wounds (e.g., sunburn, cuts, abrasions) to decrease pain, itching, and inflammation and to promote healing. Its active ingredients are unknown. Wound healing is attributed to moisturizing effects and increased blood flow to the area. Reduced inflammation and pain may result from inhibition of arachidonic acid metabolism and formation of inflammatory prostaglandins. Reduced itching may result from inhibition of histamine production.

Commercial products are available for topical use, but fresh gel from the plant may be preferred. When used for this purpose, a clear, thin, gel-like liquid can be squeezed directly from a plant leaf onto the burned or injured area several times daily if needed.

Aside from oral use as a cereal, a good source of dietary fiber, and a well-documented cholesterol-lowering product, **oat** preparations are used topically to treat minor skin irritation and pruritus associated with common skin disorders. Oats contain gluten, which forms a sticky mass that has emollient effects and holds moisture in the skin when it is mixed with a liquid. For topical use, oats are contained in bath products, cleansing bars, and lotions (e.g., Aveeno products) that can be used once or twice daily. They should not be used near the eyes or on inflamed skin. After use, bath products should be washed off with water.

Nursing Process

Assessment

Assess the patient's skin for characteristics or lesions that may indicate current or potential dermatologic disorders.

- When a skin rash is present, interview the patient and inspect the area to determine the following:
  - **Appearance of individual lesions.** Lesions should be described as specifically as possible so that changes can be identified. Terms commonly used in dermatology include *macule* (flat spot), *papule* (raised spot), *nodule* (small, solid swelling), *vesicle* (blister), *pustule* (pus-containing lesion), *petechia* (flat, round, purplish-red spot the size of a pinpoint, caused by intradermal or submucosal bleeding), and *erythema* (redness). Lesions also may be described as weeping, dry and scaly, or crusty.
  - **Location or distribution.** Some skin rashes occur exclusively or primarily on certain parts of the body (e.g., face, extremities, trunk), and this distribution may indicate the cause.
  - **Accompanying symptoms.** Pruritus occurs with most dermatologic conditions. Fever, malaise, and other symptoms may occur as well.
  - **Historic development.** Appropriate questions include
    - When and where did the skin rash appear?
    - How long has it been present?
    - Has it changed in appearance or location?
    - Has it occurred previously?
  - **Etiologic factors.** In many instances, appropriate treatment is determined by the cause. Some etiologic factors include the following:
    - **Drug therapy.** Many commonly used drugs may cause skin lesions, including antibiotics (e.g., penicillins, sulfonamides, tetracyclines), narcotic analgesics, and thiazide diuretics. Skin rashes due to drug therapy are usually generalized and appear abruptly.
    - **Irritants or allergens** may cause contact dermatitis. For example, dermatitis involving the hands may be caused by soaps, detergents, or various other cleansing agents. Dermatitis involving the trunk may result from allergic reactions to clothing.
    - **Communicable diseases** (e.g., measles, chickenpox) cause characteristic skin rashes and systemic signs and symptoms.

- When skin lesions other than rashes are present, assess appearance, size or extent, amount and character of any drainage, and whether the lesion appears infected or contains necrotic material. Bleeding into the skin is usually described as *petechiae* (pinpoint hemorrhages) or *ecchymoses* (bruises). Burn wounds are usually described in terms of depth (partial or full thickness of skin) and percentage of body surface area. Burn wounds with extensive skin damage are rapidly colonized with potentially pathogenic microorganisms. Venous stasis, pressure, and other cutaneous ulcers are usually described in terms of diameter and depth.

- When assessing the skin, consider the age of the patient. Infants are likely to have "diaper" dermatitis, miliaria (heat rash), and tinea capitis (ringworm infection of the scalp). School-aged children have a relatively high incidence of measles, chickenpox, and tinea infections. Adolescents often have acne. Older adults are more likely to have dry skin, actinic keratoses (lesions on sun-exposed skin formerly thought to be premalignant but now considered early-stage squamous cell cancer), and skin cancer.

- Assess for skin neoplasms. Basal cell carcinoma, the most common type, may initially appear as a pale nodule, most often on the head and neck. Squamous cell carcinomas may appear as actinic keratoses or ulcerated areas. These lesions may occur anywhere on the body but are more common on sun-exposed parts, such as the face and hands. Malignant melanoma is the most serious skin cancer. It involves melanocytes, the pigment-producing cells of the skin. Malignant melanoma may occur in pigmented nevi (moles) or previously normal skin. In nevi, malignant melanoma may be manifested by enlargement and ulceration. In previously normal skin, lesions appear as irregularly shaped pigmented areas. Although it can occur in almost any area, malignant melanoma is most likely to be located on the back in Caucasians and in toe webs and on soles of the feet in African Americans or Asians.

- Color changes and skin rashes are more difficult to detect when assessing dark-skinned patients. Some guidelines include the following:
  - Adequate lighting is required; nonglare daylight is best. The illumination provided by overhead lights is inadequate for most purposes.
  - Some skin rashes may be visible on oral mucous membranes.
  - Petechiae are not visible on dark-brown or black skin, but they may be visible on oral mucous membranes or the conjunctiva.

Nursing Process continues on page 1034)

■ When skin disorders are present, assess the patient's psychological response to the condition. Many patients, especially those with chronic disorders, feel self-conscious and depressed.

Nursing Diagnoses

■ Disturbed Body Image related to visible skin lesions

■ Anxiety related to potential for permanent scarring or disfigurement

■ Pain related to skin lesions and pruritus

■ Risk for Injury: Infection related to entry of microbes through damaged skin

Planning/Goals

The patient will

■ Apply topical drugs correctly

■ Experience relief of symptoms

■ Use techniques to prevent or minimize skin damage and disorders

■ Avoid scarring and disfigurement when possible

■ Be encouraged to express concerns about acute and chronic body-image changes

Interventions

Use measures to prevent or minimize skin disorders.

■ Use general measures to promote health and increase resistance to disease (i.e., maintain nutrition, rest, and exercise).

■ Practice good personal hygiene, with at least once-daily cleansing of skin areas with high bacterial counts, such as underarms and perineum.

■ Practice safety measures to avoid injury to the skin. Any injury, especially one that disrupts the integrity of the skin (e.g., lacerations, puncture wounds, scratching of skin lesions) increases the likelihood of skin infections.

■ Avoid known irritants or allergens. Have the patient substitute nonirritating soaps or cleaning supplies for irritating ones; use hypoallergenic jewelry and cosmetics if indicated; wear cotton clothing if indicated.

■ Use measures to relieve dry skin and pruritus. Dry skin causes itching, and itching promotes scratching. Scratching relieves itching only if it is strong enough to damage the skin and serve as a counterirritant. Skin damaged or disrupted by scratching is susceptible to invasion by pathogenic microorganisms. Thus, dry skin may lead to serious skin disorders. Older adults are especially likely to have dry, flaky skin. Measures to decrease skin dryness include the following:

■ Alternating complete and partial baths. For example, the patient may alternate a shower or tub bath with a sponge bath (of face, hands, underarms, and perineal areas). Warm water, mild soaps, and patting dry are recommended because hot water, harsh soaps, and rubbing with a towel have drying effects on the skin.

■ Liberal use of lubricating creams, lotions, and oils. Bath oils, which usually contain mineral oil or lanolin oil and a perfume, are widely available. If bath oils are used, precautions against falls are necessary because the oils make bathtubs and shower floors slippery. Creams and lotions may be applied several times daily.

■ Prevent pressure ulcers by avoiding trauma to the skin and prolonged pressure on any part of the body. In patients at high risk for development of pressure ulcers, major preventive measures include frequent changes of position and correct lifting techniques. Various pressure-relieving devices (e.g., special beds and mattresses) also are useful. Daily inspection of the skin is needed for early detection and treatment of beginning pressure ulcers.

■ Avoid excessive exposure to sunlight and other sources of UV light. Although controlled amounts of UV light are beneficial in some dermatologic disorders (e.g., acne, psoriasis), excessive amounts cause wrinkling, dryness, and malignancies. If prolonged exposure is necessary, protective clothing and sunscreen lotions decrease skin damage.

■ When skin rashes are present, cool, wet compresses or baths are often effective in relieving pruritus. Water or normal saline may be used alone or with additives, such as colloidal oatmeal (e.g., Aveeno) or baking soda. A cool environment also tends to decrease pruritus. The patient's fingernails should be cut short and kept clean to avoid skin damage and infection from scratching.

■ For severe itching, a systemic antihistamine may be needed.

Evaluation

■ Observe and interview regarding use of dermatologic drugs.

■ Observe for improvement in skin lesions and symptoms.

■ Interview regarding use of measures to promote healthy skin and prevent skin disorders.

Applying Your Knowledge 64-2

What nonpharmacologic measures would you recommend for Ginger?

Principles of Therapy

Goals of Therapy

General treatment goals for many skin disorders are to relieve symptoms (e.g., dryness, pruritus, inflammation, infection), eradicate or improve lesions, promote healing and repair, restore skin integrity, and prevent recurrence. Specific goals often depend on the condition being treated. With acne, for example, goals are to reduce the number of lesions.

General Guidelines for Dermatologic Drug Therapy

- Pharmacologic therapy may include a single drug or multiple agents used concurrently or sequentially.

- For severe skin conditions, a dermatologist is best qualified to prescribe medications and other treatments. Because many skin conditions are so visible, early and aggressive treatment may be needed to prevent additional tissue damage, repeated infections, scarring, and mental anguish.

- Topical medications are preferred, when effective, and many preparations are available. Astringents and lotions are usually used as drying agents for "wet," oozing lesions, and ointments and creams are used as "wetting" agents for dry, scaling lesions.

- To relieve pruritus, skin lubricants, systemic antihistamines, and topical corticosteroids are important elements.

- Topical corticosteroids are used for both acute and chronic inflammatory and pruritic lesions. However, when acute lesions involve extensive areas or chronic lesions are resistant to topical drugs, systemic corticosteroid therapy may be needed. Prednisone 0.5 to 1 mg/kg/day is often used for 1 to 3 weeks.

Patient Teaching Guidelines — Topical Medications for Skin Disorders

General Considerations

- Severe dermatologic disorders should be treated by a dermatologist.
- Promote healthy skin by a balanced diet, personal hygiene measures, avoiding excessive exposure to sunlight, avoiding skin injuries, and lubricating dry skin. Healthy skin is less susceptible to inflammation, infections, and other disorders. It also heals more rapidly when disorders or injuries occur.
- Prevent actinic keratosis and skin cancer by minimizing sun exposure, wearing sun-protective clothing, and using sunscreen. Such measures should begin in early childhood.
- Common symptoms of skin disorders are inflammation, infection, and itching and the goal of most drug therapy is to relieve these symptoms and promote healing. Systemic medications (e.g., oral antihistamines, antibiotics and corticosteroids) may be used for severe disorders, at least initially, but most medications are applied directly to the skin. There is a wide array of topical products, both prescription and over-the-counter.
- It is important to use the correct topical medication and the correct amount for the condition being treated. Topical corticosteroids, for example, come in many vehicles (e.g., creams, lotions, ointments) that cannot be used interchangeably. In addition, they should not be covered with occlusive dressings unless instructed to do so
- Adverse effects of topical medications may involve the skin (e.g., irritation, infection) where the drug is applied or the entire body, when the drug is absorbed into the bloodstream. Systemic absorption is increased when the drug is highly potent; applied to inflamed skin, over a large surface area, or frequently; or covered with an occlusive dressing (e.g., plastic wrap). Systemic absorption is of most concern with corticosteroid preparations.
- Some ways to prevent or decrease skin disorders include
  - Identifying and avoiding, when possible, substances that cause skin irritation and inflammation (e.g.,

harsh cleaning products, latex gloves, cosmetics, pet dander)
  - Bathing in warm water with a mild cleanser (e.g., Cetaphil), patting skin dry, and applying lotions or oils (e.g., Eucerin, mineral oil) to lubricate skin and decrease dryness
  - Avoiding scratching, squeezing, or rubbing skin lesions. These behaviors cause additional skin damage and increase risks of infection. Fingernails should be cut short; cotton gloves can be worn at night.
  - Maintaining a cool environment; preventing sweating
  - Applying cold compresses to inflamed, itchy skin
  - Using baking soda or colloidal oatmeal (Aveeno) in bath water to relieve itching
- If you are taking an oral antihistamine to relieve itching, it should be taken on a regular schedule, around the clock, for greater effectiveness.
- Misinformation about acne is common. Acne is not caused by dirt, washing does not improve acne, and vigorous scrubbing may worsen acne lesions. There is also no evidence that acne is caused by eating chocolate or other foods. Recommendations for managing acne include using non–acne-producing cosmetics, moisturizers, and sunscreens; washing and bathing with lukewarm water and a gentle cleanser (e.g., Dove); and avoiding sun exposure if taking a tetracycline or retinoid anti-acne medication. (The drugs increase risks of sunburn.) After treatment is started, improvement may take several weeks.
- People with psoriasis can obtain information and support from
National Psoriasis Foundation (NPF)
6600 SW 92nd Avenue, Suite 30
Portland, OR 97223
Telephone: 1-800-723-9166
E-mail: getinfo@npfusa.org
Web site: http//www.psoriasis.org
- Unavoidable skin lesions or scars can often be hidden or rendered less noticeable with makeup or clothing.

(continued on page 1036)

Patient Teaching Guidelines | Topical Medications for Skin Disorders (continued)

- Women can wear cosmetics over most topical medications. If unclear, ask a health care provider whether makeup is permissible. With acne, use noncomedogenic make-up, moisturizers, and sunscreens.
- If taking an oral retinoid (e.g., Accutane), avoid vitamin supplements containing vitamin A and excessive exposure to sunlight to decrease risks of excessive vitamin A intake and photosensitivity.
- Because adult household contacts of children with ringworm of the scalp may be asymptomatic carriers, they should use a shampoo containing ketoconazole daily until the infected child is clear of signs and symptoms.

Self-Administration

- Use topical medications only as prescribed or according to the manufacturer's instructions (for over-the-counter products). Use the correct preparation for the intended area of application (i.e., skin, ear, vagina).
- For topical application to skin lesions, cleanse the skin and remove previously applied medication to promote drug contact with the affected area of the skin.
  - Wash the skin and pat it dry.
  - Apply a small amount of the drug preparation and rub it in well. A thin layer of medication is effective and decreases the incidence and severity of adverse effects. With acne and rosacea, preventing skin lesions is easier than eliminating lesions that are already present. As a result, topical medications should be applied to the general area of involvement rather than individual lesions.
  - For burn wounds, broken skin, or open lesions, apply the drug with sterile gloves or sterile cotton-tipped applicators to prevent infection.

- Wash hands before and after application. Wash before to avoid infection; wash afterward to avoid transferring the drug to the face or eyes and causing adverse reactions.
- For minor wounds and abrasions, cleansing with soap and water is usually adequate. If an antiseptic is used, an iodine preparation (e.g., aqueous iodine solution 1%) is preferred. Alcohol should not be applied to open wounds. Hydrogen peroxide may help with cleansing but it is a weak antiseptic.
- With azelaic acid (Azelex) for acne, use for the full prescribed period, do not use occlusive dressings or wrappings, and keep away from mouth, eyes, and other mucous membranes (if it gets into eyes, wash eyes with a large amount of water).
- With benzoyl peroxide for acne:
  - With cleansing solutions, wash affected areas once or twice daily. Wet skin areas to be treated before applying the cleanser. Rinse thoroughly and pat dry. Reduce use if excessive drying or peeling occurs.
  - With other dosage forms, apply once daily initially and gradually increase to two or three times daily if needed. Cleanse skin, let dry completely, and apply a small amount over the affected area. Reduce dosage if excessive drying, redness, or discomfort occurs. If excessive stinging or burning occurs after any single application, remove with mild soap and water and resume use the next day. Keep away from eyes, mouth, and inside of nose. Rinse with water if contact occurs with these areas. Avoid other sources of skin irritation (e.g., sunlight, sunlamps, other topical acne medications).

Applying Your Knowledge 64–3

Ginger requires teaching about applying the hydrocortisone. What points should you cover?

Use of Topical Corticosteroids

Because of the extensive use of topical corticosteroids and the risks of potentially serious adverse effects, numerous precautions, guidelines, and recommendations have evolved to increase safety and effectiveness of these drugs.

Drug Selection

Choice of drug depends mainly on the acuity, severity, location, and extent of the condition being treated. For acute lesions, a more potent corticosteroid may be needed, at least initially; for chronic lesions, the least-potent preparation that is effective is indicated (see Table 64-2).

- Low-potency drugs (e.g., hydrocortisone) are preferred when likely to be effective. They are especially recommended for use in children, on large areas, and on body sites especially prone to corticosteroid damage (e.g., face, scrotum, axillae, flexures, skin folds).
- Mid-potency drugs (e.g., flurandrenolide) are usually effective in nonintertriginous areas in children and adults.
- High-potency drugs (e.g., fluocinolone) are used for acute or severe disorders and areas resistant to lower-potency agents. Short-term or intermittent use (e.g., every other day, 3 or 4 consecutive days per week, once per week) may be more effective and cause fewer adverse effects than continuous use of lower-potency products. These drugs may also be alternated with lower-potency agents.
- Very–high-potency drugs (e.g., clobetasol, halobetasol) usually are used for less absorptive areas such as soles of feet, palms of hands, and thick skin plaques. Usage should not exceed 2 consecutive weeks and total dosage should not exceed 50 g/week because of the potential for these drugs to suppress the hypothalamic–pituitary–adrenal (HPA) axis. Clobetasol suppresses the HPA axis at doses as low as 2 g/day. These drugs should not be used with occlusive dressings or for children younger than 12 years of age.

■ Drug potency and clinical use vary with the dosage form, and many topical corticosteroids are available in creams, ointments, and other preparations. Creams are usually the most acceptable to patients; ointments penetrate the epidermis better and are often used for chronic dry or scaly lesions; lotions are recommended for intertriginous areas and the scalp. Some preparations are available in aerosol sprays, gels, and other dosage forms.

Drug Dosage

Dosage depends on the drug concentration, the area of application, and the method of application.

■ The skin covering the face, scalp, scrotum, and axillae is more permeable to corticosteroids than other skin surfaces, and these areas can usually be treated with less potent formulations, smaller amounts, or less frequent applications.

■ Drug absorption and risks of systemic toxicity are significantly increased when the drug is applied to inflamed skin or covered by an occlusive dressing. Application should be less frequent and limited to isolated, resistant areas when occlusive dressings are used.

■ The drug should be applied sparingly. Some clinicians recommend twice-daily applications until a clinical response is obtained, then decreasing to the least-frequent schedule needed to control the condition.

■ With continuous use, one or two applications daily may be as effective as three or four applications, because the drugs have a repository effect.

■ If an occlusive dressing is applied, leave it on overnight or for at least 6 hours. However, do not leave it in place for more than 12 hours in a 24-hour period.

■ After long-term use or after using a potent drug, taper dosage by switching to a less potent agent or applying the drug less frequently. Discontinuing the drug abruptly can cause a rebound effect, in which the skin condition worsens.

Drug Therapy in Selected Skin Conditions

The choice of topical dermatologic agents depends primarily on the reason for use and patient response.

Acne

Numerous prescription and nonprescription anti-acne products are available.

Antimicrobial drugs include both topical and systemic agents. Topical drugs are indicated for mild to moderate acne, often in combination with a topical retinoid to maximize reduction in severity and number of lesions. Azelaic acid (Azelex) has antibacterial activity against *P. acnes* and is reportedly as effective as benzoyl peroxide or topical erythromycin. Benzoyl peroxide is an effective topical agent that is available in numerous preparations (e.g., gel, lotion, cream, wash) and concentrations (e.g., 2.5%–10%). Lotion and cream preparations are the least irritating. Clindamycin and erythromycin are also available in topical dosage forms. These drugs reduce *P. acnes* bacteria and are equally effective. Combination products of topical clindamycin or erythromycin and benzoyl peroxide are more effective than antibiotics alone. Best results require 8 to 12 weeks of therapy, and maintenance therapy is usually required. Adverse effects of topical antibiotics include erythema, peeling, dryness, and burning as well as development of resistant strains of *P. acnes*. Recommendations for reducing drug resistance include using topical retinoids or benzoyl peroxide or both when using topical antibiotics and avoiding long-term use of topical or oral antibiotics when feasible. Benzoyl peroxide can also cause an irritant dermatitis and bleach hair, clothes, and bed linens.

Oral antimicrobials are first-line treatment for patients with moderate to severe inflammatory acne. These drugs have both antimicrobial and anti-inflammatory effects. They reduce *P. acnes* organisms and thereby inhibit production of *P. acnes*–induced inflammatory cytokines. Commonly used oral antibiotics include tetracycline, doxycycline, minocycline, and erythromycin. Tetracycline and erythromycin suppress leukocyte chemotaxis and bacterial lipase activity; minocycline and doxycycline inhibit cytokines and proteinase enzymes that contribute to inflammation and tissue breakdown. Resistance to the tetracyclines is less common than to erythromycin and is least with minocycline. All oral antibiotics require at least 6 to 8 weeks of use. Although there are no established guidelines for duration of use, some clinicians encourage using the drugs for shorter periods and avoiding long-term use as maintenance therapy, to decrease the development of resistant *P. acnes* organisms.

Retinoids, in both systemic and topical forms, may be used for moderate to severe acne. All topical retinoids (tretinoin, adapalene, tazarotene) reduce acne lesions, usually within 12 weeks. Tretinoin is often used with other products because it may require several months to decrease acne lesions if used alone. Adapalene gel causes less skin irritation and is better tolerated than tretinoin and tazarotene, but tazarotene may be more effective. Topical retinoids should be applied to the entire area of involvement, starting with about 30 seconds' duration and building up to an hour or more. Maintenance therapy is usually required.

Oral isotretinoin (Accutane) may be used for patients with severe acne who do not respond to safer drugs. Its anti-acne effects include suppression of sebum production, inhibition of comedone formation, and inhibition of inflammation. Approximately 70% to 80% of patients have a long-term remission. Major drawbacks are teratogenic and other adverse effects. This drug must never be given to a woman of childbearing potential unless she agrees to baseline and monthly pregnancy tests and to practice adequate contraceptive measures during and for 6 months after the drug is discontinued. In addition, baseline and 1-month measurements of cholesterol, fasting triglycerides, and liver function are recommended because the drug may increase these values.

Oral antiandrogens may be given to female patients with high blood levels of androgens (e.g., testosterone). Combination oral contraceptive pills decrease the amount of free testosterone circulating in the bloodstream and therefore may improve acne. Norgestimate/ethinyl estradiol (Ortho Tri-Cyclen) and norethindrone acetate/ethinyl estradiol (Estrostep) are FDA-approved for treatment of acne.

Anorectal Disorders

In anorectal disorders, most preparations contain a local anesthetic, emollients, and perhaps a corticosteroid. These preparations relieve pruritus and pain but do not cure the underlying condition. Some preparations contain ingredients of questionable value, such as vasoconstrictors, astringents, and weak antiseptics. No particular mixture is clearly superior.

Dermatitis

Both systemic and topical agents are usually needed. Sedating, systemic antihistamines such as diphenhydramine or hydroxyzine are often used to relieve itching and promote rest and sleep. An oral antibiotic such as clindamycin, dicloxacillin, a cephalosporin, or a macrolide may be given for a week to treat secondary infections. An oral corticosteroid such as prednisone may be needed initially for severe inflammation, but topical corticosteroids are most often used.

Coal-tar preparations have anti-inflammatory and antipruritic actions and can be used alone or with topical corticosteroids. However, these agents have an unpleasant odor and they stain clothing. They are usually applied at bedtime.

Additional preparations include moisturizers and lubricants (e.g., Aquaphor) for dry skin and itching, mild skin cleansers (e.g., Basis, Cetaphil) to avoid further skin irritation, and baking soda or colloidal oatmeal (e.g., Aveeno) in baths or soaks for pruritus.

External Otitis

Otic preparations of various dermatologic medications are used. Hydrocortisone is the corticosteroid most often included in topical otic preparations. It relieves pruritus and inflammation in chronic external otitis. Systemic analgesics are usually required.

Pressure Ulcers

In pressure ulcers, the only clear-cut guideline for treatment is avoiding further pressure on the affected area. Many topical agents are used, most often with specific procedures for dressing changes, skin cleansing, and so on. No one agent or procedure is clearly superior. Consistent implementation of a protocol (e.g., position changes; inspection of current or potential pressure areas; dressing changes; use of alternating, pressure-relieving mattresses) may be more effective than drug therapy.

Psoriasis

Localized lesions are usually treated by a combination of topical agents, such as a corticosteroid during daytime hours and a coal-tar ointment at night. Coal-tar preparations work slowly but produce longer remissions. Newer antipsoriasis drugs such as calcipotriene (Dovonex) or tazarotene (Tazorac) may also be used. Calcipotriene is reportedly as effective as topical fluocinonide. However, its onset of action is slower than that of a topical corticosteroid. A combination of calcipotriene and

a topical corticosteroid may be used initially for rapid improvement, after which the calcipotriene can be continued as monotherapy. Tazarotene is a topical retinoid that may cause cutaneous irritation.

Generalized psoriasis, which requires systemic treatment or body phototherapy, should be managed by dermatologists. Systemic therapy may involve oral retinoids, methotrexate, or biologic immunosuppressants. Acitretin is the oral retinoid of choice for treatment of severe psoriasis. Like other oral retinoids, acitretin is teratogenic. Thus, women of childbearing potential who take acitretin should be instructed to avoid ingesting alcohol and to use adequate contraception while taking the drug and for at least 3 years thereafter. Methotrexate is an antineoplastic drug that has long been used to treat psoriasis because it suppresses inflammation and proliferation of T lymphocytes. It may cause significant adverse effects. Biologic immunosuppressants (e.g., alefacept, efalizumab, etanercept, infliximab) reduce the activity of T lymphocytes and the inflammation of skin lesions. They are used to treat moderate to severe psoriasis and all have potentially serious adverse effects.

Phototherapy can involve natural sunlight, which is highly effective. Most patients with psoriasis notice some remission during summer months. Office phototherapy treatments are usually performed three to five times weekly.

Rosacea

Mild skin cleansers (e.g., Cetaphil), oral tetracycline, and topical metronidazole are commonly used; oral isotretinoin and topical metronidazole are also effective. These medications prevent or treat acneiform lesions; they have little to no effect on other aspects (e.g., erythema, telangiectasia, hyperplasia of connective tissue and sebaceous glands).

Urticaria

Systemic drug therapy with antihistamines (H_1 receptor antagonists) is the major element of drug therapy. In addition, an epinephrine injection may be used initially, and topical medications may be applied to relieve itching. With chronic *urticaria*, the goal of treatment is symptom relief. Antihistamines are most effective when given before histamine-induced urticaria occurs and should be given around the clock, not just when lesions appear.

Use in Special Populations

Use in Children

Children and adolescents may develop a wide range of dermatologic disorders, including acne, atopic dermatitis, skin rashes, and skin and skin structure infections. Few guidelines have been developed for drug therapy of most skin disorders in this group; some precautions with topical and systemic drugs are described below.

With topical agents, cautious use is recommended. Infants, and perhaps older children, have more permeable skin and are more likely to absorb topical drugs than adults. In addition, absorption is increased in the presence of broken or damaged skin. With topical corticosteroids, which are often used to treat atopic dermatitis, suppression of the HPA axis (see Chap. 23), Cushing's disease, and intracranial hypertension have been reported in children. Signs of impaired adrenal function may include delayed growth and low plasma cortisol levels. Signs of intracranial hypertension may include headaches and swelling of the optic nerve (papilledema) on ophthalmoscopic examination. The latter may lead to blindness if pressure on the optic nerve is not relieved. Because children are at high risk for development of systemic adverse effects with topical corticosteroids, these drugs should be used only if clearly indicated, in the smallest effective dose, for the shortest effective time, and usually without occlusive dressings. In addition, a low-potency agent should be used initially in infants and in intertriginous areas of older children. If a more potent drug is required for severe dermatitis, the child should be examined often and the strength of the drug reduced as skin lesions improve.

With systemic drugs, an oral antibiotic is often needed to treat skin and skin structure infections. Most of these infections are caused by *Staphylococcus aureus* and *Streptococcus pyogenes*. However, the prevalence of infections caused by methicillin-resistant *S. aureus* continues to increase, and the choice of drug should be based on culture and sensitivity tests. In areas with high resistance rates, the commonly prescribed cephalosporin antibiotics may not be effective. Further, if an oral retinoid (e.g., isotretinoin) is prescribed for adolescent females with severe acne, all precautions regarding negative pregnancy tests and thorough counseling must be followed.

Use in Older Adults

Older adults often have thin, dry skin and are at risk of pressure ulcers if mobility, nutrition, or elimination is impaired. Principles of topical drug therapy are generally the same as for younger adults. In addition, topical corticosteroids should be used with caution on thinned or atrophic skin.

Use in Home Care

Skin disorders are commonly treated at home by patients or caregivers. When a home care nurse is involved, responsibilities may include assessing patients, other members of the household, and the home environment for risks of skin disorders; teaching preventive or treatment measures; assisting with treatment; and assessing response to treatment.

Applying Your Knowledge 64–4

Ginger's rash has spread to her face. As a teenager, she thinks it looks horrible. What would be an appropriate nursing diagnosis?

Nursing Actions | Dermatologic Drugs

NURSING ACTIONS	RATIONALE/EXPLANATION
1. Administer accurately	
a. Use the correct preparation for the intended use (i.e., dermatologic, otic, vaginal, anorectal)	Preparations may differ in drug contents and concentrations.
b. For topical application to skin lesions:	
(1) Wash the skin, and pat it dry.	To cleanse the skin and remove previously applied medication. This facilitates drug contact with the affected area of the skin.
(2) Apply a small amount of the drug preparation, and rub it in well.	A thin layer of medication is effective and decreases the incidence and severity of adverse effects.
(3) For burn wounds, broken skin, or open lesions, apply the drug with sterile gloves or sterile cotton-tipped applicators.	To prevent infection
(4) Use the drug only for the individual patient.	To avoid bacterial cross-contamination between patients
(5) Wash hands before and after application.	Wash hands before to avoid exposing the patient to infection; wash hands afterward to avoid transferring the drug to your own face or eyes and causing adverse reactions.
2. Observe for therapeutic effects	Therapeutic effects depend on the medication being used and the disorder being treated.
a. With dermatologic conditions, observe for healing of skin lesions.	With acne and rosacea, improvement may require 6–12 weeks of therapy.
b. With external otitis, observe for decreased pain and pruritus.	
c. With vaginal disorders, observe for decreased vaginal discharge and pruritus.	
d. With anorectal disorders, observe for decreased pain and pruritus.	

(continued on page 1040)

Nursing Actions Dermatologic Drugs (continued)

NURSING ACTIONS	RATIONALE/EXPLANATION
3. Observe for adverse effects a. Local irritation or inflammation—burning on application, erythema, skin rash, pruritus	Incidence of adverse effects is low with topical agents. Local effects may occur with most topical agents but may be more likely with antiseptics, local anesthetics, and antimicrobials.
b. With topical corticosteroids, observe for local and systemic effects. (1) Local effects include skin atrophy, striae, telangiectasia, hypopigmentation, rosacea, dermatitis, acne, and allergic and irritant reactions.	These effects commonly occur with prolonged use, frequent application, and higher-potency drugs. Atrophy or thinning of skin is more likely in the face, groin, and axillae. Allergic and irritant reactions to preservatives, fragrances, and other ingredients may prevent healing or worsen dermatitis.
(2) Systemic effects include suppression of adrenal function, hypertension, hyperglycemia, muscle weakness, osteoporosis, cataracts, glaucoma, and growth retardation in children.	Systemic effects are more likely with more potent agents (e.g., clobetasol can cause suppression of the hypothalamic–pituitary–adrenal axis with as little as 2 g daily); application over large areas of skin; prolonged use; and the use of occlusive dressings. In addition, children are at higher risk because they may absorb proportionally larger amounts and be more sensitive to systemic toxicity. Little adrenal suppression is likely to occur with doses less than 50 grams weekly for an adult and 15 grams weekly for a small child, unless occlusive dressings are used.
c. With topical antibiotics, superinfection and sensitization may occur.	Superinfection with drug-resistant organisms may occur with any antibacterial agent; diarrhea and pseudomembranous colitis may occur with topical clindamycin. Sensitization may cause serious allergic reactions if the same drug is given systemically at a later time.
d. With oral retinoids, observe for hypervitaminosis A (nausea, vomiting, headache, blurred vision, eye irritation, conjunctivitis, skin disorders, abnormal liver function, musculoskeletal pain, increased plasma triglycerides, depression, and suicidal ideation).	Adverse effects commonly occur with usual doses but are more severe with higher doses.
4. Observe for drug interactions	Clinically significant drug interactions rarely occur with topical agents.

Key Concepts

■ Staphylococci and streptococci are the most common bacterial causes of skin infection, and methicillin-resistant *S. aureus* (MRSA) infections are increasing.

■ Careful assessment of types and locations of lesions can aid diagnosis and treatment of many skin disorders.

■ Topical drugs are used to treat most skin disorders; accurate application is essential to maximize therapeutic effects.

■ Special precautions are needed for safe use of topical corticosteroids, especially in children.

■ Special precautions are needed for safe use of oral retinoids in female patients of childbearing potential.

■ Systemic adverse effects may occur with topical drug therapy; skin disorders may occur with systemic drugs.

Review and Application Exercises

Short Answer Exercises

1. What are the main functions of the skin?

2. Describe interventions to promote skin health and integrity.

3. During initial assessment of a patient, what signs and symptoms may indicate common skin disorders?

4. Which patient groups are at risk for development of common skin disorders (e.g., skin infections, pressure ulcers)?

5. Compare topical and systemic corticosteroids in terms of adverse effects.

6. If an adolescent patient with acne asks your advice about over-the-counter topical drugs, which would you recommend, and why?

7. List general principles of using topical agents for common skin disorders.

NCLEX-Style Questions

8. Neosporin topical ointment has been ordered for a teenaged outpatient being seen for follow-up care for several healing lesions following a bicycle accident. The nurse knows that topical medications are usually applied for what kinds of effects?
   a. rapid
   b. slow
   c. local
   d. systemic

9. Systemic absorption of topical medications is greatest in
   a. damaged skin
   b. intact skin
   c. soles of the feet
   d. skin of the elbows and knees

10. Your teenaged client is using tretinoin (Retin-A). Which of the following statements indicates that he understands the teaching you have done?
    a. "I will apply the medication three times daily for 6 weeks."
    b. "My skin may become red and irritated from the medication."
    c. "I am excited that my acne should be mostly gone by next week."
    d. "This medication will increase my tolerance to sunlight."

11. Over-the-counter benzoyl peroxide is an effective treatment for many cases of
    a. acne
    b. psoriasis
    c. tinea infections
    d. dermatitis

12. In general, a licensed health care provider with prescriptive authority should prescribe the use of all topical
    a. antifungal drugs
    b. anti-acne drugs
    c. antibacterial drugs
    d. high-potency corticosteroids

Selected References

Berger, T. G. (2007). Skin, hair, and nails. In S. J. McPhee, M. A. Papadakis, & L. M. Tierney, Jr. (Eds.), *Current medical diagnosis and treatment 2007* (46th ed., pp. 87–150). New York: McGraw-Hill.

Buys, L. M. (2007). Treatment options for atopic dermatitis. *American Family Physician, 75,* 523–528.

Cheigh, N. H. (2005). Atopic dermatitis. In J. T. DiPiro, R. L. Talbert, G. C. Yee, G. R. Matzke, B. G. Wells, & L. M. Posey (Eds.), *Pharmacotherapy: A pathophysiologic approach* (6th ed., pp. 1785–1792). New York: McGraw-Hill.

Roebuck, H. L. (2006). Acne: Intervene early. *The Nurse Practitioner, 31,* 25–43.

Simandl, G. (2005). Alterations in skin function and integrity. In C. M. Porth (Ed.), *Pathophysiology: Concepts of altered health states* (7th ed., pp. 1449–1493). Philadelphia: Lippincott Williams & Wilkins.

West, D. P., West, L. E., Musumeci, M. L., & Micali, G. (2005). Acne vulgaris. In J. T. DiPiro, R. L. Talbert, G. C. Yee, G. R. Matzke, B. G. Wells, & L. M. Posey (Eds.), *Pharmacotherapy: A pathophysiologic approach* (6th ed., pp. 1755–1768). New York: McGraw-Hill.

West, D. P., West, L. E., Scuderi, L.. & Micali, G. (2005). Psoriasis. In J. T. DiPiro, R. L. Talbert, G. C. Yee, G. R. Matzke, B. G. Wells, & L. M. Posey (Eds.), *Pharmacotherapy: A pathophysiologic approach* (6th ed., pp. 1769–1783). New York: McGraw-Hill.

Drug Use During Pregnancy and Lactation

KEY TERMS

- Abortifacients
- Eclampsia
- Fetotoxic
- Organogenesis
- Oxytocic
- Preeclampsia
- Preterm labor
- Prostaglandins
- Teratogenic
- Tocolytics

LEARNING OBJECTIVES

After studying this chapter, you will be able to:

1. Discuss reasons for minimizing drug use during pregnancy and lactation.
2. Describe selected fetotoxic and teratogenic drugs.
3. Discuss guidelines for drug therapy of pregnancy-associated signs and symptoms.
4. Discuss guidelines for drug therapy of selected chronic disorders during pregnancy and lactation.
5. Discuss which immunizations are considered safe for use during pregnancy and which are contraindicated.
6. Teach females of childbearing potential to avoid prescribed and over-the-counter drugs when possible and to inform all health care providers if there is a possibility of pregnancy.
7. Discuss the role of the home care nurse working with the pregnant woman.
8. Discuss drugs used during pregnancy complications and normal labor and delivery in terms of their effects on the mother and newborn infant.
9. Describe abortifacients in terms of characteristics and nursing process implications.

Applying Your Knowledge

Annie Blevins is a 30-year-old woman who comes to the primary care facility where you work to receive her annual checkup. She was recently married and both she and her husband want to start trying to get pregnant. Before her marriage, Mrs. Blevins took Ortho Tri-Cyclen to prevent pregnancy. She has since discontinued taking the oral contraceptive.

Introduction

Drug use before and during pregnancy and during lactation requires special consideration and, in general, should be avoided or minimized when possible. In sexually active women of reproductive age and ability who may become pregnant (i.e., are not consistently using effective contraception), the concern is that the woman may ingest drugs that are potentially harmful to the fetus (*fetotoxic*) before she knows she is pregnant. *Organogenesis* (formation of fetal organs) occurs during the first 2 to 8 weeks after conception. During pregnancy, any drugs ingested by the mother may affect the fetus. Drug effects on the fetus are often unknown, especially with newer drugs, and few drugs are considered completely safe. During lactation, many drugs are excreted in breast milk and reach the nursing infant in varying amounts. Some drugs should be avoided during lactation; some can be continued with precautions to decrease infant exposure.

Despite these concerns, however, many pre-pregnant, pregnant, and lactating women take drugs for various reasons, including acute disorders that may or may not be associated with pregnancy, chronic disorders that require continued treatment during pregnancy or lactation, and habitual use of non-therapeutic drugs (e.g., alcohol, tobacco, others). Many of the drugs in this chapter are described elsewhere; they are discussed here in relation to pregnancy and lactation. Other drugs that are used mainly during pregnancy are discussed in greater detail, including those used to terminate pregnancy (*abortifacients*), drugs used to stop preterm labor (*tocolytics*), and drugs used during labor and delivery.

Pregnancy

During pregnancy, mother and fetus undergo physiologic changes that influence drug effects. In pregnant women, physiologic changes alter drug pharmacokinetics (Table 65-1). In general, drug effects are less predictable because plasma volume expansion decreases plasma drug concentrations, and increased metabolism by the liver and increased elimination by the kidneys shorten the duration of drug actions and effects.

Maternal–Placental–Fetal Circulation

Drugs ingested by the pregnant woman reach the fetus through the maternal–placental–fetal circulation, which is completed about the third week after conception. On the maternal side, arterial blood pressure carries blood and drugs to the placenta. In the placenta, maternal and fetal blood are separated by a few thin layers of tissue, which drugs can readily cross. Placental transfer begins the fifth week after conception. After drugs enter the fetal circulation, relatively large amounts are pharmacologically active because the fetus has low levels of serum albumin and thus low levels of drug binding. Most drug molecules are transported to the liver, where they are metabolized. Metabolism occurs slowly because the fetal liver is immature in quantity and quality of drug-metabolizing enzymes. Drugs metabolized by the fetal liver are excreted by fetal kidneys into amniotic fluid. Excretion also is slow and inefficient due to immature development of fetal kidneys. Other drug molecules are transported directly to the heart, which then distributes them to the brain and coronary arteries. Drugs enter the brain easily because the blood–brain barrier is poorly developed in the fetus. Approximately half of the drug-containing blood is then transported through the umbilical arteries to the placenta, where it re-enters the maternal circulation. Thus, the mother can metabolize and excrete some drug molecules for the fetus.

Drug Effects on the Fetus

Drug effects are determined mainly by the type and amount of drugs, the duration of exposure, and the level of fetal growth and development when exposed to the drugs. The fetus is sensitive to drug effects because it is small, has few plasma

Table 65-1	Pregnancy: Physiologic and Pharmacokinetic Changes
PHYSIOLOGIC CHANGE	**PHARMACOKINETIC CHANGE**
Increased plasma volume and body water, approximately 50% in a normal pregnancy Increased cardiac output (30%–50%) and increased blood flow to the uterus, kidneys, skin, and breasts	After it is absorbed into the bloodstream, a drug (especially if water soluble) is distributed and "diluted" more than in the nonpregnant state. Drug dosage requirements may increase. However, this effect may be offset by other pharmacokinetic changes of pregnancy.
Increased weight (average 25 lb) and body fat	Drugs (especially fat-soluble ones) are distributed more widely. Drugs that are distributed to fatty tissues stay in the body longer because they are slowly released from storage sites into the bloodstream.
Decreased serum albumin. The rate of albumin production is increased. However, serum levels fall because of plasma volume expansion. Also, many plasma-protein binding sites are occupied by hormones and other endogenous substances that increase during pregnancy.	The decreased capacity for drug binding leaves more free drug available for therapeutic or adverse effects on the mother and for placental transfer to the fetus. Thus, a given dose of a drug may produce greater effects than it would in the nonpregnant state.
During most of a pregnancy, increased renal blood flow and glomerular filtration rate secondary to increased cardiac output	Increased excretion of drugs by the kidneys, especially those excreted primarily unchanged in the urine (e.g., lithium, penicillins)
In late pregnancy, renal blood flow may decrease when the woman assumes a supine position, secondary to the increased size and weight of the uterus.	Decreased renal blood flow may result in delayed excretion and prolonged effects of renally excreted drugs.
Increased hormones (e.g., estrogen, progesterone) induce drug-metabolizing enzymes in the liver.	Increased metabolism and clearance of many drugs

proteins that can bind drug molecules, and has a weak capacity for metabolizing and excreting drugs. In addition, the fetus is exposed to any drugs circulating in maternal blood. When drugs are taken on a regular schedule, fetal blood usually contains 50% to 100% of the amount in maternal blood. This means that *any drug that stimulates or depresses the central nervous, cardiovascular, respiratory, or other body system in the mother has the potential to stimulate or depress those systems in the fetus.* In some cases, fetotoxicity occurs.

A major concern about drug effects on the fetus is teratogenicity (anatomic malformations or birth defects). Drug-induced teratogenicity is most likely to occur when drugs are taken during the first trimester of pregnancy (Fig. 65-1). For drugs taken during the second and third trimesters, adverse effects are usually manifested in the neonate (birth to 1 month) or infant (1 month to 1 year) as growth retardation, respiratory problems, infection, or bleeding. It should be emphasized, however, that *drugs taken at any time during pregnancy can affect the baby's brain because brain development continues throughout pregnancy and after birth.*

The incidence of drug-induced teratogenicity is unknown. The U.S. Food and Drug Administration (FDA) requires manufacturers to assign a pregnancy risk category to new drugs to indicate their potential for causing birth defects (Box 65-1). Relatively few therapeutic drugs are considered fetotoxic or *teratogenic* (Box 65-2), and these can usually be avoided during pregnancy. In contrast, nontherapeutic drugs (e.g., alcohol, cocaine, heroin, marijuana, methamphetamine,

nicotine) are fetotoxic or teratogenic and should be avoided during pregnancy. Caffeine has not been associated with birth defects, but high amounts (more than 400 mg/day) have been associated with preterm births and other complications of pregnancy and should also be avoided.

Fetal Therapeutics

Although the major concern about drugs ingested during pregnancy is adverse effects on the fetus, a few drugs are given to the mother for therapeutic effects on the fetus. These include digoxin for fetal tachycardia or heart failure, levothyroxine for hypothyroidism, penicillin for exposure to maternal syphilis, and prenatal corticosteroids to promote surfactant production to improve lung function and decrease respiratory distress syndrome in preterm infants.

Maternal Therapeutics

Thus far, the main emphasis on drug use during pregnancy has related to actual or potential adverse effects on the fetus. Despite the general principle that drug use should be avoided when possible, pregnant women may require drug therapy for various illnesses, increased nutritional needs, pregnancy-associated problems, chronic disease processes, treatment of preterm labor, induction of labor, and pain management during labor.

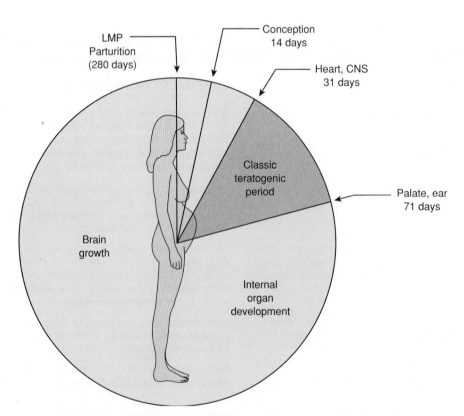

Figure 65-1 ■ The gestational clock showing the classic teratogenic risk assessment. (Adapted from Niebyl, J. [1999]. Drugs and related areas in pregnancy. In J. Sciarra [Ed.], *Obstetrics and gynecology.* Philadelphia: Lippincott Williams & Wilkins.)

Box 65-1	FDA Pregnancy Categories

A. Adequate studies in pregnant women demonstrate no risk to the fetus.

B. Animal studies indicate no risk to the fetus, but there are no adequate studies in pregnant women, or animal studies show adverse effects, but adequate studies in pregnant women have not demonstrated a risk.

C. Risk is unknown and cannot be ruled out. Animal studies demonstrate fetotoxicity, but the drugs have not been adequately studied in humans. However, potential benefits may justify the potential risks.

D. Positive evidence of harm to human fetuses. If needed in a life-threatening situation or a serious disease, the drug may be acceptable if safer drugs cannot be used or are ineffective.

X. Contraindicated in pregnancy. Studies in animals or humans, or postmarketing adverse reaction reports, or both, have demonstrated fetal abnormalities. The risk of use in a pregnant woman clearly outweighs potential benefit.

Herbal and Dietary Supplements

Pregnancy increases nutritional needs, and vitamin and mineral supplements are commonly used. **Folic acid** supplementation is especially important to prevent neural-tube birth defects (e.g., spina bifida). Such defects occur early in pregnancy, often before the woman realizes she is pregnant. For this reason, it is recommended that all women of childbearing potential ingest 400 or 600 micrograms of folic acid daily from food and/or a supplement. In addition, pregnancy increases folic acid requirements and deficiencies are common. A supplement is usually needed to supply adequate amounts.

Herbal supplements are not recommended during pregnancy. **Ginger** has been used to relieve nausea and vomiting during pregnancy, with a few studies supporting its use. Overall, it has not been proven effective but is probably safe for use.

Applying Your Knowledge 65-1

What nutritional advice should you give to Mrs. Blevins?

Pregnancy-Associated Symptoms and Their Management

Anemias

Three types of anemia are common during pregnancy. One is physiologic anemia (often defined as a hemoglobin below 10 g/dL or hematocrit below 30%), which results from

Box 65-2	Selected Drugs That Are Fetotoxic or Teratogenic

Risk Category D

*Angiotensin-converting enzyme (ACE) inhibitors (e.g., captopril and others)

*Angiotensin II receptor blockers (ARBs; e.g., losartan and others)

Antibacterials (aminoglycosides, tetracyclines, tigecycline, trimethoprim in third trimester)

Antidepressants (imipramine, nortriptyline, paroxetine)

Antiepileptics (carbamazepine, phenytoin, valproic acid)

Antifungals (voriconazole)

Antimanic agent (lithium)

Antineoplastics (ibritumab, idarubicin, ifosfamide, imatinib, irinotecan)

Antithyroid agents (e.g., propylthiouracil)

Antivirals (efavirenz)

Benzodiazepine antianxiety agents (e.g., alprazolam, diazepam, lorazepam)

Beta blockers (atenolol; acebutolol, betaxolol, esmolol, metoprolol, propranolol, timolol, second and third trimesters, by experts, category B or C by manufacturer)

Bisphosphonates (pamidronate, zoledronic acid)

Diuretic (hydrochlorothiazide, by expert, category B by manufacturer)

Nicotine replacement products (oral inhaler, nasal spray, transdermal patch)

Nonsteroidal anti-inflammatory drugs (e.g., ibuprofen, naproxen; during third trimester)

Opioid analgesics (with prolonged use or high doses at term)

Risk Category X

Anticoagulant (warfarin)

Antineoplastics (e.g., cyclophosphamide, methotrexate)

Antirheumatoid arthritis drug (leflunomide)

Antiviral (ribavirin)

Benzodiazepine sedative/hypnotics (e.g., flurazepam)

Female sex hormones (estrogens, progestins, oral contraceptives)

Male sex hormones (androgens, anabolic steroids)

Nicotine replacement product, chewing gum

Retinoids (e.g., acitretin, isotretinoin, and several topical preparations)

Statin cholesterol-lowering drugs (e.g., atorvastatin, others)

*ACE inhibitors and ARBs were formerly considered category C during the first trimester and category D during the second and third trimesters. Recent evidence indicates that the drugs are fetotoxic if taken at any time during pregnancy.

Sources: Drug Facts and Comparisons; Drug Information Handbook.

expanded blood volume. A second is iron-deficiency anemia, which is often related to long-term nutritional deficiencies. A third type is folic acid–deficiency anemia. The recommended daily intake of folic acid doubles during pregnancy, from 400 to 800 micrograms, and a folic acid supplement is often prescribed.

For many years, it was considered "best practice" to routinely prescribe daily iron supplements for pregnant women to prevent or treat iron-deficiency anemia. More recently, studies indicate that use of the supplements in women who are not anemic may lead to excessive levels of hemoglobin, iron overload, and hypertension in the mother and premature birth or low birth weight (for gestational age) in the infant.

Constipation

Constipation often occurs during pregnancy, probably from decreased peristalsis. Preferred treatment, if effective, is to increase exercise and intake of fluids and high-fiber foods. If a laxative is required, a bulk-producing agent (e.g., Metamucil) is the most physiologic for the mother and safest for the fetus because it is not absorbed systemically. A stool softener (e.g., docusate) or an occasional saline laxative (e.g., milk of magnesia) may also be used. Mineral oil should be avoided because it interferes with absorption of fat-soluble vitamins. Reduced absorption of vitamin K can lead to bleeding in newborns. Castor oil, all strong laxatives, and excessive amounts of any laxative should be avoided because they can cause uterine contractions and initiate labor.

Gastroesophageal Reflux Disease

Gastroesophageal reflux disease (GERD), of which heartburn (pyrosis) is the main symptom, occurs in one third or more of pregnant women. Hormonal changes relax the lower esophageal sphincter, and the growing fetus increases abdominal pressure. These developments allow gastric acid to splash into the esophagus and cause discomfort and esophagitis. In addition, GERD may trigger asthma attacks in pregnant women with asthma.

Nonpharmacologic interventions include eating small meals; not eating for 2 to 3 hours before bedtime; avoiding caffeine, gas-producing foods, and constipation; and sitting in an upright position. For patients who do not obtain adequate relief with these measures, drug therapy may be needed. Antacids may be used if necessary. Because little systemic absorption occurs, the drugs are unlikely to harm the fetus if used in recommended doses. A histamine$_2$ (H$_2$) receptor antagonist such as ranitidine (Zantac) may also be used. Proton pump inhibitors such as esomeprazole (Nexium) are thought to be safe, but some clinicians reserve them for patients for whom H$_2$ blockers are ineffective.

Gestational Diabetes

Gestational diabetes is glucose intolerance first found during pregnancy. Women with risk factors (e.g., obesity; age older than 35 years; family history of diabetes; being Hispanic, Native American, Asian, or African American; previous pregnancy with stillbirth, spontaneous abortion, fetal anomalies, or large baby) should be screened at the first prenatal visit. Most women without risk factors, or whose initial test was normal, should be tested between 24 and 28 weeks of gestation. The criterion for a diagnosis of diabetes is a fasting plasma glucose level of more than 126 milligrams per deciliter or a nonfasting glucose level of more than 200 milligrams per deciliter. Women with gestational diabetes are at higher risk for complications of pregnancy.

The goal of treatment is to keep blood glucose levels as nearly normal as possible because even mild hyperglycemia is detrimental to the fetus. Initial management includes diet, moderate exercise, and frequent self-monitoring of blood glucose levels. For women who are obese, mild calorie restriction may be indicated (severe calorie restriction is harmful to the developing fetus and should be avoided). If these interventions are inadequate, drug therapy may be needed. Insulin is usually the drug of choice for treatment of diabetes during pregnancy because it does not cross the placenta and has a long history of safe usage. Oral antidiabetic drugs have generally been contraindicated. However, several studies indicate that glyburide is safe to use and acarbose, metformin, and miglitol seem to cause minimal fetal risk.

When the pregnancy ends, blood glucose levels usually return to a normal range within a few weeks. However, two thirds of these women will have gestational diabetes in subsequent pregnancies and up to half will develop overt diabetes within 15 years.

Nausea and Vomiting

Nausea and vomiting often occur, especially during early pregnancy. Dietary management (e.g., eating small, frequent meals, limiting or avoiding high fat and high fiber foods) is recommended. Antiemetic drugs should be given only if nausea and vomiting are severe enough to threaten the mother's nutritional or metabolic status. No antiemetic medications are FDA-approved for use during pregnancy, although some have been used without apparent teratogenic effects.

Pregnancy-Induced Hypertension

Pregnancy-induced hypertension includes preeclampsia and eclampsia, conditions that endanger the lives of mother and fetus. *Preeclampsia* is manifested by hypertension and proteinuria (blood pressure with systolic above 140 mm Hg or diastolic above 90 mm Hg and proteinuria above 300 mg in 24 hours). It may occur after 20 weeks of gestation and up to 6 weeks postpartum.

Preeclampsia most often occurs during a first pregnancy, but it may occur in women with chronic hypertension, diabetes mellitus, or multiple fetuses. Some women can be observed on an outpatient basis, with frequent monitoring of mother and fetus. Women who are noncompliant with follow-up care or who have severe preeclampsia should be hospitalized. Drug therapy for severe preeclampsia includes intravenous hydralazine or labetalol (see Chap. 52) for blood pressure control, and magnesium sulfate (see Chap. 57 and "Tocolytics," below) for prevention or treatment of seizures. Drug therapy reduces perinatal deaths and severe maternal hypertension. If not effectively treated, preeclampsia may progress to *eclampsia*, which is characterized by potentially fatal seizures. The only cure is delivery of the baby; cesarean section is needed in some cases.

Selected Infections

Group B streptococcal infections may affect the pregnant woman and the neonate. Women colonized with group B streptococci (estimated at 10%–30% of pregnant women) have increased risks of adverse fetal outcomes (e.g., transmitting the bacteria to the infant during delivery, resulting in potential bacteremia, meningitis, or pneumonia) and maternal outcomes (urinary tract infection, preterm delivery, postpartum endometritis). Because of the potentially serious consequences of infection with group B streptococci, pregnant women should have a vaginal culture performed at 35 to 37 weeks of gestation. A positive culture indicates infection that should be treated. In addition, an IV antibiotic that is effective against group B streptococci should be started at the onset of labor or with rupture of membranes and continued until delivery.

Human immunodeficiency virus (HIV) infection in pregnant women requires antiretroviral drug therapy for the mother and to prevent transmission to the infant. In general, highly active antiretroviral therapy (HAART) is recommended as for nonpregnant women. The goal of treatment is to achieve an HIV plasma RNA load of less than 400 copies per milliliter.

For young children, almost all HIV infections are transmitted perinatally, either in utero, during labor and delivery, or in breast milk. Antiretroviral drug therapy for the pregnant woman reduces perinatal transmission by about two thirds. During labor, IV zidovudine is given until delivery. After delivery, the infant should be given zidovudine for 6 weeks, with or without other antiretroviral drugs.

Children with HIV infection have failure to thrive, central nervous system abnormalities, and developmental delays as major manifestations. *Pneumocystis jiroveci* pneumonia (PCP) is an opportunistic infection that may occur in infants, most often between 3 and 6 months of age, and is a major cause of early mortality in HIV-infected children. Trimethoprim-sulfamethoxazole (TMP-SMZ; Bactrim) is recommended for prophylaxis and should be started by 4 to 6 weeks of age for all infants born to HIV-infected mothers. Because of the potentially serious consequences for infants born to HIV-infected mothers, it is recommended that all pregnant women be tested for HIV infection.

Urinary tract infections (UTIs) commonly occur during pregnancy and may include asymptomatic bacteriuria, cystitis, and pyelonephritis. Asymptomatic bacteriuria should be treated in pregnant women because of its association with cystitis and pyelonephritis. If untreated, symptomatic cystitis occurs in approximately 30% of pregnant women. Asymptomatic bacteriuria and UTIs are also associated with increased preterm deliveries and low birth weights. Hospitalization and IV antibiotics may be needed for management of pyelonephritis.

Applying Your Knowledge 65-2

Mrs. Blevins becomes pregnant. She calls the office complaining of constipation. What do you recommend?

Management of Chronic Diseases During Pregnancy

Asthma

Asthma is one of the most common, potentially serious medical conditions to complicate pregnancy. It is associated with increased risk of infant death, preeclampsia, preterm birth, low birth weight, and congenital malformations. These risks are higher with severe asthma and lower with well-controlled asthma. Asthma attacks, which are usually accompanied by hypoxia, hypocapnia, and alkalemia, should be treated promptly, with hospitalization if indicated. Respiratory infections are common triggers for acute asthma exacerbations.

Because asthma is unpredictable during pregnancy (i.e., symptoms may improve, worsen, or stay about the same), all women with asthma should be monitored closely when pregnant and treated when indicated. Some women with asthma do not require drug therapy during pregnancy. For those who need drug therapy, treatment is considered safer for the fetus than poor asthma control. In general, drug therapy during pregnancy is similar to that in nonpregnant women. Commonly used drugs include orally inhaled beta$_2$ agonists (e.g., albuterol), inhaled cromolyn, and inhaled and systemic corticosteroids (e.g., budesonide, beclomethasone, prednisone). The regular use of inhaled corticosteroids decreases the number of asthma exacerbations during pregnancy, and systemic corticosteroids are used for severe exacerbations. Women taking an oral corticosteroid near term require "stress doses" at the time of delivery. Oral theophylline may also be used. Serum theophylline levels should be monitored, and values of 5 to 12 micrograms per milliliter are recommended during pregnancy.

The National Asthma Education and Prevention Program (NAEPP) publishes recommendations for drug therapy and other aspects of managing asthma during pregnancy. These recommendations, which were updated in 2007 and continued previous drug therapy guidelines, are summarized in Box 65-3.

Antiasthma drug therapy is continued during lactation for mothers breast-feeding their baby. The amount of medication reaching the infant through breast milk is less than the amount received in utero through the placenta.

Diabetes Mellitus

Diabetes increases the risks of pregnancy for both mother and fetus, and the hormonal changes of pregnancy have diabetogenic effects that may cause or aggravate diabetes. Maternal risks include retinopathy, preeclampsia, and pyelonephritis; fetal risks include congenital malformations and perinatal death. Because diabetic retinopathy progresses in many pregnant women, patients should be examined by an ophthalmologist each trimester.

The goal of treatment is to maintain a near-normal blood glucose level, because even mild hyperglycemia may be harmful to the fetus. In general, pregnancy makes diabetes more

Box 65-3	National Asthma Education and Prevention Program (NAEPP) Expert Panel Report: Managing Asthma During Pregnancy: Recommendations for Pharmacologic Treatment—2007 Update

General Recommendations

- Controlling asthma during pregnancy is important because poorly controlled asthma can lead to serious medical problems for pregnant women and their fetus(es).
- Because asthma severity changes during pregnancy for most women, pregnant patients with persistent asthma should have their asthma checked at least monthly by a health care provider (e.g., clinicians providing obstetric care should monitor asthma severity during each prenatal visit).
- Assist patients to identify and avoid or limit exposure to triggers that precipitate or worsen acute asthma symptoms (e.g., tobacco smoke, allergens such as dust mites).
- Women with other conditions that can worsen asthma (e.g., allergic rhinitis, sinusitis, gastroesophageal reflux) should have those conditions treated as well.

Drug Therapy Recommendations

- Evidence indicates that it is safer to take medications than to have asthma exacerbations.
- A stepwise approach to asthma care similar to that used in the NAEPP general asthma treatment guidelines for children and nonpregnant adults is recommended (see Chap. 44). Under this approach, medication is stepped up in intensity if needed and stepped down when possible, depending on asthma severity.
- For quick relief of acute asthma symptoms, albuterol, a short-acting, inhaled beta$_2$ agonist, should be used, and pregnant women with asthma should have this medication available at all times.
- For treatment of persistent asthma (e.g., women who have symptoms at least 2 days a week or 2 nights a month), asthma medication is needed daily to prevent exacerbations. Inhaled corticosteroids are preferred to control the underlying inflammation. Budesonide (Pulmicort) is often used because there are more data on its safety during pregnancy than for other inhaled corticosteroids. However, there are no data indicating that other inhaled corticosteroids are unsafe during pregnancy, and other inhaled corticosteroids may be continued if they effectively control a patient's asthma. Alternative daily medications are leukotriene receptor antagonists such as montelukast (Singulair) or zafirlukast (Accolate), cromolyn (Intal), or theophylline.
- For patients whose persistent asthma is not well controlled on low doses of inhaled corticosteroids alone, the guidelines recommend either increasing the dose of inhaled corticosteroid or adding another medication (e.g., a long-acting beta agonist such as salmeterol [Serevent]).
- Oral corticosteroids may be required for the treatment of severe asthma. The guidelines note that there are conflicting data regarding the safety of oral corticosteroids during pregnancy. However, severe, uncontrolled asthma poses a definite risk to the mother and fetus and use of oral corticosteroids may be warranted.

---

difficult to manage effectively. Some women who were previously able to control diabetes with diet may require insulin during pregnancy. Women who already take insulin usually need larger doses as pregnancy advances. Recommendations for management include the following:

- For a planned pregnancy, women with diabetes can have a better outcome if they can maintain normal or near-normal blood glucose levels and normal glycosylated hemoglobin (A$_{1c}$) levels for at least 2 months prior to conception. Previously, it was recommended that women taking oral antidiabetic drugs should be switched to insulin prior to pregnancy. Although insulin is still the drug of choice during pregnancy, several studies indicate that oral glyburide is safe and effective. In addition, acarbose, miglitol, and metformin are thought to have little risk for the fetus.
- Tight blood glucose control is needed throughout pregnancy. It is especially important early in the first trimester, when fetal organs are being formed, because poor glycemic control increases the risks of birth defects. The usual goals for tight glucose control are fasting and preprandial capillary blood glucose levels of approximately 65 mg/dL (equivalent to a plasma concentration of 75 mg/dL) and 1-hour postprandial levels of less than 120 mg/dL (plasma value less than 140 mg/dL). During this time, it is recommended that women monitor their blood glucose levels at least daily and sometimes more often.

- Insulin is the antidiabetic drug of choice during pregnancy. Human insulin should be used because it is least likely to cause an allergic response. Because insulin requirements vary according to the stage of pregnancy, the diabetic patient's blood glucose levels must be monitored closely and insulin therapy individualized. It is especially important that sufficient insulin is given to prevent maternal acidosis. Uncontrolled acidosis is likely to interfere with neurologic development of the fetus. Careful dietary control and other treatment measures are also necessary throughout pregnancy.
- Insulin requirements usually decrease during the first trimester and increase during the second and third trimesters. During the ninth month, insulin needs are approximately 50% greater than at preconception and the increase is greater among women with type 2 diabetes. Obese women with type 2 diabetes may need much higher insulin doses because of the additional insulin resistance of pregnancy.

■ During labor and delivery, short-acting insulin and frequent blood glucose tests are used to control diabetes, as during other acute situations.

■ During the postpartum period, insulin requirements fluctuate because stress, trauma, infection, surgery, or other factors associated with delivery tend to increase blood glucose levels and insulin requirements. At the same time, termination of the pregnancy reverses the diabetogenic hormonal changes and decreases insulin requirements. Short-acting insulin is given, and dosage is based on frequent measurements of blood glucose. After the insulin requirement is stabilized, the patient may be able to return to the prepregnancy treatment program.

Epilepsy

Although antiepileptic drugs (AEDs) are generally considered fetotoxic or teratogenic, they must often be taken during pregnancy because seizures may also be harmful to mother and fetus. Fortunately, most pregnancies (more than 90%) result in normal infants. Despite the usually good outcomes, women with epilepsy have higher risks of preeclampsia, preterm labor, and stillborn births. In addition, the incidence of birth defects is two to three times higher in fetuses exposed to AEDs than in those not exposed. If an AED is required, one drug (monotherapy) should be used because the rate of major birth defects (e.g., cardiac defects, neural tube defects) in infants exposed to one AED is higher than those not exposed and even higher in infants exposed to two or more AEDs. The lowest dose that controls seizures is also recommended. Infants whose mothers took AEDs for bipolar disorder rather than for epilepsy also have higher rates of birth defects. The effects of newer AEDs during pregnancy are largely unknown.

Plasma drug levels should be checked monthly during pregnancy. Approximately one third of women with epilepsy have an increased number of seizures during pregnancy. This is attributed to physiologic changes of pregnancy (e.g., increased blood volume) that lower plasma levels of AEDs.

Women with epilepsy should take a folic acid supplement (at least 400 mcg daily) all the time and 800 micrograms or more during pregnancy to prevent or reduce neural tube defects (e.g., spina bifida). Supplemental vitamin K (e.g., 10 mg/day) is also recommended during the last month of pregnancy to prevent bleeding in neonates. AEDs are associated with a neonatal bleeding disorder characterized by decreased levels of vitamin K–dependent clotting factors. The prenatal vitamin K supplement is in addition to the injection of vitamin K usually given to all neonates immediately after birth.

Hypertension

Chronic hypertension is defined as blood pressure above 140/90 mm Hg that begins before conception or in the first 20 weeks of pregnancy and persists after delivery. Hypertension that is initially diagnosed during pregnancy and does not resolve after pregnancy also is classified as chronic. Whenever it occurs, chronic hypertension is associated with increased maternal and fetal risks (e.g., preeclampsia, abruptio placentae, intrauterine growth restriction, preterm delivery, perinatal death). In women with chronic hypertension, blood pressure often decreases during the first and second trimesters and increases during the third trimester.

Management of chronic hypertension during pregnancy consists of nonpharmacologic and pharmacologic therapies. Nonpharmacologic interventions (e.g., avoiding excessive weight gain, sodium restriction, increased rest) should be emphasized. If drug therapy is required, methyldopa has not been associated with adverse effects on the fetus or neonate. Beta blockers and calcium channel blockers may also be used. With beta blockers, fetal and neonatal bradycardia, hypotension, hypoglycemia, and respiratory depression have been reported. As a result, some authorities recommend avoiding the drugs during the first trimester and stopping them 2 to 3 days before delivery. *Angiotensin-converting enzyme (ACE) inhibitors and angiotensin II receptor blockers (ARBs), which are commonly used in other populations, are contraindicated during pregnancy.*

Drugs That Alter Uterine Motility

Abortifacients

Abortion is the termination of pregnancy before 20 weeks. It may occur spontaneously or be intentionally induced. Medical abortion may be induced by prostaglandins and an antiprogestin (Table 65-2). *Prostaglandins* may be used to terminate pregnancy during the second trimester. In the female reproductive system, prostaglandins E and F are found in the ovaries, myometrium, and menstrual fluid. They stimulate uterine contraction and probably help initiate and maintain the normal birth process. Drug preparations of prostaglandins are capable of inducing labor at any time during pregnancy. **Misoprostol** (Cytotec), a prostaglandin developed to prevent gastric ulcers associated with nonsteroidal anti-inflammatory drugs (NSAIDs) (see Chap. 59), is being given orally or intravaginally for first- or second-trimester termination. It is not FDA approved for this use.

Tocolytics

Drugs given to inhibit labor and maintain the pregnancy are called tocolytics. Uterine contractions with cervical changes before 37 weeks of gestation are considered *preterm labor*. Preterm labor may occur spontaneously or be precipitated by premature rupture of membranes or other factors. Drug therapy is most effective when the cervix is minimally dilated and membranes are intact. Tocolytic drugs do not reduce the number of preterm births, but they may prolong pregnancy from 2 to 7 days. The goal of tocolytic treatment is to postpone birth long enough to reduce problems associated with prematurity (e.g., respiratory distress, bleeding in the brain, infant death). For example, the delay may allow antenatal administration of a corticosteroid (e.g., betamethasone) to the mother to

Table 65-2   Drugs at a Glance: Abortifacients, Prostaglandins, Tocolytics, and Oxytocics

GENERIC/TRADE NAME	ROUTES AND DOSAGE RANGES
Prostaglandins	
Carboprost tromethamine (Hemabate)	IM 250 mcg q1.5–3.5h, depending on uterine response, up to 48 hours. Maximum total dose, 12 mg.
Dinoprostone (Prostin E$_2$ vaginal suppository)	Intravaginally 20 mg, repeated q3–5h until abortion occurs. Maximum dose, 240 mg.
Misoprostol (Cytotec)	PO 200–400 mcg q12h; termination usually complete within 48 h Intravaginally 25 mcg (1/4 of a 100-mcg tablet) q3–6h
Tocolytics	
Magnesium sulfate	IV infusion, loading dose 3–4 g mixed in 5% dextrose injection and administered over 15–20 min Maintenance dose 1–2 g/h, according to serum magnesium levels and deep-tendon reflexes PO 250–450 mg q3h, to maintain a serum level of 2.0–2.5 mEq/L
Nifedipine (Procardia)	PO 10 mg every 20 min for 3 or 4 doses; maximum dose 40 mg in 1 h; then 10–20 mg q4–6h
Terbutaline (Brethine)	IV infusion 10 mcg/min, titrated up to a maximum dose of 80 mcg/min until contractions cease PO 2.5 mg q4–6h as maintenance therapy
Oxytocic	
Oxytocin (Pitocin)	During labor and delivery, IV by infusion pump, 2 milli units/min, gradually increased to 10 milli units/min, if necessary, to produce 3 or 4 contractions within 10-min periods. Prepare a solution of 10 mU/mL by adding 10 units (1 mL) of oxytocin to 1000 mL of 0.9% sodium chloride. To control postpartum hemorrhage, IV 10–40 units added to 1000 mL of 0.9% sodium chloride, infused at a rate to control bleeding To prevent postpartum bleeding, IM 3–10 units (0.3–1 mL) as a single dose

improve pulmonary maturity and function in the infant when it is born. In addition, the mother may need to be transported to a facility equipped to deal with high-risk deliveries. Magnesium sulfate, nifedipine, some NSAIDs, and terbutaline are used as tocolytics. They are described below and in Table 65-2.

Magnesium sulfate has long been given IV as a first-line agent. However, studies indicate that the drug is ineffective as a tocolytic, and some clinicians recommend stopping usage for this purpose. In addition, if used, the drug requires special precautions for administration and monitoring because of potentially severe adverse effects. Safety measures include a unit protocol that standardizes drug concentration, flow rate, type of infusion pump, and frequency and type of assessment data to be documented (e.g., serum magnesium levels, respiratory status, reflexes, uterine activity, urine output). The antidote, calcium gluconate, should be readily available for use if hypermagnesemia occurs.

These safety measures are needed because hypotension, muscle paralysis, respiratory depression, and cardiac arrest can occur with overdoses of magnesium sulfate. Close monitoring of serum levels and signs of hypermagnesemia is required. In addition, infants born to mothers who recently received magnesium sulfate should be assessed for hypermagnesemia and respiratory depression.

Nifedipine is a calcium channel blocking drug that decreases uterine contractions. Its use is associated with fewer adverse effects than magnesium sulfate or terbutaline. However, a common adverse effect is maternal hypotension, which may reduce blood flow between the placenta and the uterus.

NSAIDs, such as **indomethacin**, inhibit uterine prostaglandins that help to initiate the uterine contractions of normal labor. Maternal adverse effects include nausea, heartburn, dizziness, and GI bleeding. In addition, a few instances of serious neonatal complications, including patent ductus arteriosus, have been reported.

Terbutaline is a beta-adrenergic agent that inhibits uterine contractions by reducing intracellular calcium levels. Adverse effects may include hyperkalemia, hyperglycemia, cardiac dysrhythmias, hypotension, and pulmonary edema.

Drugs Used During Labor and Delivery at Term

At the end of gestation, labor usually begins spontaneously and proceeds through delivery of the neonate. If labor does not occur spontaneously, it may be induced by a drug that stimulates uterine contraction. Drugs often used during labor, delivery, and the immediate postpartum period include an oxytocic, analgesics, and anesthetics.

Labor Induction

Prostaglandin preparations (e.g., Prepidil or Cervidil formulations of **dinoprostone**) may be administered to promote cervical ripening (i.e., the cervix becomes softer and thinner, to facilitate labor) or induce labor at or near full-term gestation. Prostaglandins F_{2alpha} and E_2 stimulate uterine contractions by increasing intracellular calcium concentrations and activating the actin–myosin contractile units of uterine muscle. About 13% of pregnancies end in labor induction. Reasons for induction include gestation longer than 42 weeks, suspected fetal growth retardation, maternal hypertension, and premature rupture of membranes.

Oxytocics

The most commonly used *oxytocic* drug is **Pitocin**, a synthetic form of oxytocin (a hormone produced in the hypothalamus and released by the posterior pituitary gland; see Chap. 22). Pitocin may be used to induce labor or to strengthen weak uterine contractions during labor. Physiologic doses produce a rhythmic uterine contraction–relaxation pattern that approximates the normal labor process. An IV solution of 10 milliunits per milliliter is used for infusion, and dosage (flow rate) is titrated according to frequency and strength of contractions. Pitocin is contraindicated for antepartum use in the presence of fetal distress, preterm labor, previous uterine surgery, and severe preeclampsia. Maternal condition and fetal heart rate must be closely monitored during Pitocin administration. Maternal adverse effects include hypotension, excessive uterine stimulation, and uterine rupture.

After delivery, Pitocin is the drug of choice for prevention or control of postpartum uterine bleeding. The drug reduces uterine bleeding by contracting uterine muscle. It also plays a role in letdown of breast milk to the nipples during lactation.

Analgesics

During early labor, pain occurs with uterine contractions; during later stages, pain occurs with perineal stretching. Parenteral opioid analgesics (e.g., IV or IM **meperidine, morphine,** or **fentanyl**) are commonly used to control pain during labor and delivery. They may prolong labor and cause sedation and respiratory depression in the mother and neonate. Meperidine may cause less neonatal depression than other opioid analgesics. **Butorphanol** is also widely used. If neonatal respiratory depression occurs, it can be reversed by **naloxone** (Narcan).

Regional analgesia may also be used and may be more effective than IV analgesics. Epidural analgesia involves administration of an opioid (e.g., fentanyl, morphine) through a catheter placed in the epidural space for that purpose. Following a cesarean section, a long-acting form of morphine (e.g., Duramorph) can be injected into the epidural catheter to provide analgesia up to 24 hours. Possible adverse effects include maternal urinary retention, but no significant effects on the fetus have been noted.

Anesthetics

Local anesthetics also are used to control discomfort and pain. They are injected by physicians for regional anesthesia in the pelvic area. Epidural blocks involve injection into the epidural space of the spinal cord. **Bupivacaine** is commonly used. With regional anesthesia, the mother is usually conscious and comfortable, and the neonate is rarely depressed. **Fentanyl** may be combined with a small amount of a local anesthetic for both analgesia and anesthesia.

Neonatal Therapeutics

In the neonate, any drug must be used cautiously. Drugs are usually given less often because they are metabolized and excreted slowly. Immature liver and kidney function prolongs drug action and increases risks of toxicity. Also, drug therapy should be initiated with low doses, especially with drugs that are highly bound to plasma proteins. Neonates have few binding proteins, which leads to increased amounts of free, active drug and increased risk of toxicity. When a health care provider is assessing the neonate, drugs received by the mother during pregnancy, labor and delivery, and lactation must be considered.

At birth, some drugs are routinely administered to prevent hemorrhagic disease of the newborn and ophthalmia neonatorum. Hemorrhagic disease of the newborn occurs because the intestinal tract lacks the bacteria that normally synthesize vitamin K and there is little if any dietary intake of vitamin K. Vitamin K is required for liver production of several clotting factors, including prothrombin. Thus, the neonate is at increased risk of bleeding during the first week of life. One dose of phytonadione 0.5 to 1 milligram is injected at delivery or on admission to the nursery.

Ophthalmia neonatorum is a form of bacterial conjunctivitis that may cause ulceration and blindness. It may be caused by several bacteria, most commonly *Chlamydia trachomatis*, a sexually transmitted organism. Erythromycin ointment 0.5% is applied to each eye at delivery. It is effective against both chlamydial and gonococcal infections.

Nursing Process

Assessment

Assess each female patient of reproductive age for possible pregnancy. If the patient is known to be pregnant, assess status in relation to pregnancy, as follows:

- Length of gestation
- Use of prescription, over-the-counter, herbal, nontherapeutic, and illegal drugs. If used, assess specifically for those drugs known to be fetotoxic or teratogenic.
- Acute and chronic health problems that may influence the pregnancy or require drug therapy

Nursing Process continues on page 1052

■ With preterm labor, assess length of gestation, the frequency and quality of uterine contractions, the amount of vaginal bleeding or discharge, and the length of labor. Also determine whether any tissue has been expelled from the vagina. When abortion is inevitable, an oxytocic drug may be given. When stopping labor is possible or desired, a tocolytic drug may be given.

■ When spontaneous labor occurs in normal, full-term pregnancy, assess frequency and quality of uterine contractions, amount of cervical dilatation, fetal heart rate and quality, and maternal blood pressure.

■ Assess antepartum women for intention to breast-feed.

Nursing Diagnoses

■ Risk for Injury: Damage to mother, fetus, or neonate from maternal ingestion of drugs

■ Noncompliance related to ingestion of nonessential drugs during pregnancy

■ Risk for Injury related to possible damage to mother or infant during the birth process

■ Deficient Knowledge: Drug effects during pregnancy and lactation

Planning/Goals

The patient will

■ Avoid unnecessary drug ingestion when pregnant or likely to become pregnant

■ Use nonpharmacologic measures to relieve symptoms associated with pregnancy or other health problems when possible

■ Obtain optimal care during pregnancy, labor and delivery, and the postpartum period

■ Avoid behaviors that may lead to complications of pregnancy and labor and delivery

■ Breast-feed safely and successfully if desired

Interventions

■ Use nondrug measures to prevent or minimize the need for drug therapy during pregnancy.

■ Promote or provide optimal prenatal care to promote a healthy pregnancy (e.g., regular monitoring of blood pressure, weight, blood sugar, urine protein; counseling about nutrition and other healthful activities).

■ Assist women with chronic health problems (e.g., asthma, diabetes, hypertension) to manage the disorders effectively and decrease risks of harm to themselves and their babies.

■ Help patients and families cope with complications of pregnancy.

■ Counsel candidates for therapeutic abortion about methods and expected outcomes; counsel abortion patients about contraceptive techniques.

Evaluation

■ Observe and interview regarding actions taken to promote reproductive and general health.

■ Observe and interview regarding compliance with instructions for promoting and maintaining a healthy pregnancy.

■ Interview regarding ingestion of therapeutic and nontherapeutic drugs during pre-pregnant, pregnant, and lactating states.

■ Observe and interview regarding the health status of the mother and neonate.

Principles of Therapy

General Guidelines: Pregnancy

■ Regardless of the designated pregnancy risk category or presumed safety, no drug should be used during pregnancy unless it is clearly needed and potential benefit to the mother outweighs the risk of potential harm to the fetus.

■ Although the teratogenicity of many drugs is unknown, most medications required by pregnant women can be used safely and most children are born healthy.

■ When drug therapy is required, the choice of drug should be based on the stage of pregnancy and available drug information. During the first trimester, for example, an older drug that has not been associated with fetotoxic or teratogenic effects is usually preferred over a newer drug of unknown fetotoxicity or teratogenicity.

■ Any drugs used during pregnancy should be given in the lowest effective doses and for the shortest effective time.

■ Counsel pregnant women about the use of immunizations during pregnancy. Live-virus vaccines (e.g., measles, mumps, rubella) should be avoided because of possible harmful effects to the fetus. Vaccines against pneumococcal pneumonia, meningococcal meningitis, and hepatitis A can be used if indicated. Influenza vaccine is indicated in all women who are pregnant during influenza season. (However, FluMist, a live virus vaccine given by nasal spray, should *not* be given to pregnant women.) In addition, hepatitis B vaccine (if the mother is high risk and negative for hepatitis B antigen) and toxoids (e.g., diphtheria, tetanus) are considered safe for use. Hyperimmune globulins can be given to pregnant women who are exposed to hepatitis B, tetanus, or varicella (chickenpox).

Applying Your Knowledge 65-3

Mrs. Blevins asks you about over-the-counter and prescription drug use during her pregnancy. What do you tell her?

General Guidelines: Lactation

- The American Academy of Pediatrics (AAP) supports breast-feeding as optimal nutrition for infants during the first year of life and does not recommend stopping maternal drug therapy unless necessary. In some instances, mothers may pump and discard breast milk while receiving therapeutic drugs to maintain lactation.

- Most systemic drugs taken by the mother reach the infant in breast milk. For some, the amount of drug is too small to cause significant effects; for others, effects on the nursing infant are unknown or potentially adverse. Drugs that are generally contraindicated are listed in Box 65-4.

- Give medications only when clearly indicated, weighing potential benefit to the mother against possible harm to the nursing infant. For contraindicated drugs, it is usually recommended that the mother stop the drug or stop breast-feeding.

- Any drugs used during lactation should be given in the lowest effective dose for the shortest effective time.

- Most over-the-counter and prescription drugs, taken in moderation and only when needed, are thought to be safe.

- Women with HIV infection should not breast-feed. The virus can be transmitted to the nursing infant.

Patient Teaching Guidelines — Drug Use During Pregnancy and Lactation

- Any systemic drug ingested by a pregnant woman reaches the fetus and may interfere with fetal growth and development. For most drugs, safety during pregnancy has not been established, and all drugs are relatively contraindicated. Therefore, any drug use must be cautious and minimal to avoid potential damage to the fetus.

- Avoid drugs when possible and use them very cautiously when necessary. If women who are sexually active and not using effective contraception take any drugs, there is a high risk that potentially harmful agents may be ingested before pregnancy is suspected or confirmed. It is estimated that 50% or more of pregnancies are unplanned.

- Lifestyle or nontherapeutic drugs associated with problems during pregnancy include alcohol, caffeine, and cigarette smoking. Women should completely avoid alcohol when trying to conceive and throughout pregnancy; no amount is considered safe. Caffeine intake should be limited to about three caffeinated beverages per day; excessive intake should be avoided. Women who smoke should quit if possible during pregnancy to avoid the effects of nicotine, carbon monoxide, and other chemicals on the fetus. However, the use of nicotine replacement products during pregnancy is not recommended.

- Herbal supplements are not recommended; their effects during pregnancy are largely unknown.

- Measures to prevent the need for drug therapy include a healthful lifestyle (adequate nutrition, exercise, rest, and sleep; avoiding alcohol and cigarette smoking) and avoiding infection (personal hygiene, avoiding contact with people known to have infections, maintaining indicated immunizations).

- Nondrug measures to relieve common health problems include positioning, adequate food and fluid intake, and deep breathing.

- See a health care provider as soon as pregnancy is suspected.

- Inform any health care provider from whom treatment is sought if there is a possibility of pregnancy.

- Many drugs are excreted in breast milk to some extent and reach the nursing infant. The infant's health care provider should be informed about medications taken by the nursing mother and consulted about potential drug effects on the infant. Before taking over-the-counter medications, consult a health care provider. In regard to nontherapeutic drugs, recommendations include the following:
  - Alcohol should be used in moderation and nursing should be withheld temporarily after alcohol consumption (1–2 hours per drink). Alcohol reaches the baby through breast milk, with the highest concentration about 30 to 60 minutes after drinking (60–90 minutes if taken with food). The effects of alcohol on the baby are directly related to the amount of alcohol the mother consumes. Moderate to heavy drinking (two or more drinks per day) can interfere with the ability to breast-feed, harm the baby's motor development, and slow the baby's weight gain. If you plan to drink (e.g., wine with dinner), you can avoid breast-feeding for a few hours (until the alcohol has time to leave your system) or you can pump your milk before drinking alcohol and give it to the baby after you have had the alcohol. You can also pump and discard the milk that is most affected by the ingested alcohol.
  - Caffeine is considered compatible with breast-feeding. However, large amounts should be avoided because infants may be jittery and have difficulty sleeping.
  - Cigarette smoking is contraindicated. Nicotine and an active metabolite are concentrated in milk and the amounts reaching the infant are proportional to the number of cigarettes smoked by the mother. Ideally, the mother who smokes would stop. If unable or unwilling to stop, she should decrease the number of cigarettes as much as possible, avoid smoking before nursing, and avoid smoking (or allowing other people to smoke) in the same room with the infant. The risk for sudden infant death syndrome (SIDS) is greater when a mother smokes or when the baby is around secondhand (passive) smoke. Maternal smoking and passive smoke may also increase respiratory and ear infections in infants.
  - All drugs of abuse (e.g., cocaine, heroin, marijuana, methamphetamine, phencyclidine) are contraindicated.

How Can You Avoid This Medication Error?

Mrs. Blevins delivers a healthy baby and is breast-feeding. At her 6-week checkup, she is told she can resume normal sexual relations. Mrs. Blevins does not want to have another child for a while, so she resumes taking the birth control pills that she took prior to becoming pregnant.

Home Care

Many obstetric patients with conditions such as preterm labor, hyperemesis, and elevated blood pressure are managed in the home. The home care nurse who assists in managing these patients should be an obstetric specialist who is knowledgeable about normal pregnancy and potential complications. The nurse should be aware of the drugs being used to treat the complicated obstetric patient as well as maternal use of any nonprescription and nontherapeutic drugs. A systematic assessment of maternal and fetal responses should be made on each visit.

Home care visits also allow for assessment of compliance with the proposed management plan. Understanding of previous teaching should be evaluated on each visit. It is especially important for the patient to know the danger signs and symptoms that may necessitate notifying a health care provider.

The overall goal of home care is to maintain the pregnancy to the most advanced gestational age possible. Home care follow-up by a nurse has been demonstrated to positively affect the outcome of a high-risk pregnancy.

Box 65-4	Selected Drugs That Are Contraindicated or Not Recommended During Lactation

Angiotensin converting enzyme (ACE) inhibitors (e.g., captopril, others)

Angiotensin receptor blockers (ARBs; e.g., losartan, others)

Antibacterials (aminoglycosides, fluoroquinolones, tetracyclines, sulfamethoxazole/trimethoprim)

Antidepressants (e.g., amitriptyline, bupropion, citalopram, fluoxetine, venlafaxine, others)

Antidiabetic drugs (oral) (e.g., glimepiride, glipizide, metformin, pioglitazone, rosiglitazone)

Antiepileptics (carbamazepine, lamotrigine, levetiracetam, phenytoin, tiagabine, topiramate, zonisamide)

Antifungals (e.g., itraconazole, terbinafine)

Antihistamines (cetirizine, clemastine, desloratadine, diphenhydramine, loratadine)

Antimanic agent (lithium)

Antipsychotics (e.g., clozapine, olanzapine, risperidone, others)

Antirheumatic immunosuppressant drugs (e.g., etanercept, infliximab)

Antivirals (e.g., famciclovir)

Benzodiazepine antianxiety and sedative/hypnotic drugs (e.g., alprazolam, diazepam, triazolam, others)

Beta blockers (e.g., metoprolol, others)

Calcium channel blockers (e.g., amlodipine, diltiazem, others)

Diuretics (e.g., hydrochlorothiazide)

Histamine$_2$ receptor antagonists (e.g., cimetidine, ranitidine)

Nonbenzodiazepine sedative/hypnotics (e.g., ramelteon, zolpidem)

Nonsteroidal anti-inflammatory drugs (e.g., naproxen, tolmetin)

Opioid analgesics (codeine, hydromorphone, methadone)

Proton pump inhibitors (e.g., esomeprazole, omeprazole, others)

Retinoids (e.g., isotretinoin)

Statin cholesterol-lowering drugs (e.g., atorvastatin, simvastatin, others)

Sources: Drug Facts and Comparisons; Drug Information Handbook

Nursing Actions | Abortifacients, Prostaglandins, Tocolytics, and Oxytocics

NURSING ACTIONS	RATIONALE/EXPLANATION
1. Administer accurately a. With prostaglandin abortifacients (e.g., Hemabate, Prostin E$_2$) and prostaglandin cervical ripening agents (e.g., Cervidil), consult manufacturers' instructions.	These drugs are given according to specific protocols and should be administered only by nurses experienced in their use and aftercare of patients.
b. Give intravenous magnesium sulfate via an infusion pump; read the drug label carefully to be sure of using the correct preparation for the intended use; when available, use premixed IV bags of 20 g magnesium sulfate in 500 mL of IV fluid; clearly label IV bags; use a	Magnesium sulfate is a high-risk drug and should be given only by experienced labor and delivery nurses who are knowledgeable about safe administration and monitoring patients. The nurse should assess and document maternal status and fetal status before starting the drug infusion, remain at the

NURSING ACTIONS	RATIONALE/EXPLANATION
separate 100-mL (4 g) or 150-mL (6 g) IV piggyback solution for the initial bolus dose; give the initial bolus over 20–30 minutes; titrate the maintenance dose (1–2 g/hour) according to serum magnesium levels; have a second nurse check all IV bags containing magnesium sulfate and all infusion pump settings; have IV calcium gluconate readily available.	bedside during bolus infusions, and monitor the patient frequently throughout drug administration. Magnesium sulfate is available in different concentrations and sizes as well as a multidose vial. Calcium gluconate is an antidote for an overdose of magnesium sulfate. One ampule of 1 g (10 mL of a 10% solution) can be given IV over 3 minutes to relieve signs and symptoms of hypermagnesemia.
c. Give terbutaline IV initially, via an infusion pump, then by mouth (PO).	Although not FDA-approved for tocolysis, there is extensive clinical experience with the drug.
d. For IV oxytocin, dilute the drug in an IV sodium chloride solution, and piggyback the solution into a primary IV line. Use an infusion pump to administer.	Oxytocin may cause water intoxication, which is less likely to occur if the drug is given in a saline solution. Piggybacking allows regulation of the oxytocin drip without interrupting the main IV line.
e. Give intramuscular oxytocin immediately after delivery of the placenta.	To prevent excessive postpartum bleeding
2. Observe for therapeutic effects	
a. When an abortifacient is given, observe for the onset of uterine bleeding and the expulsion of the fetus and placenta.	Abortion usually occurs within 24 hours after a prostaglandin is administered.
b. When a tocolytic drug is given in threatened abortion or preterm labor, observe for absent or decreased uterine contractions.	The goal of drug therapy is to stop the labor process. Uterine activity may be assessed by maternal self-report, palpation, or electronic fetal monitoring. Tocolytic blood levels of magnesium sulfate range from 4.8–9.6 mg/dL.
c. When magnesium sulfate is given in preeclampsia, observe for an absence or decrease of seizures.	Blood levels of 3–6 mg/dL are considered optimal for anti-seizure effects.
d. When oxytocin is given to induce or augment labor, observe for firm uterine contractions at a rate of three to four per 10 minutes. Each contraction should be followed by a palpable relaxation period. Examine periodically for cervical dilatation and effacement.	Uterine contractions should become regular and increase in duration and intensity.
e. When oxytocin is given to prevent or control postpartum bleeding, observe for a small, firm uterus and minimal vaginal bleeding.	These agents control bleeding by causing strong uterine contractions. The uterus can be palpated in the lower abdomen.
3. Observe for adverse effects	
a. With prostaglandins, observe for:	
(1) Nausea, vomiting, diarrhea	These are the most common adverse effects; they result from stimulation of gastrointestinal smooth muscle.
(2) Fever, cardiac dysrhythmias, bronchospasm, convulsions, chest pain, muscle aches	These effects occur less often. Bronchospasm is more likely to occur in patients with asthma; seizures are more likely in patients with known epilepsy.
b. With magnesium sulfate, observe for:	
(1) Hypermagnesemia—respiratory depression and failure, depressed deep-tendon reflexes, muscle weakness, hypotension, cardiac dysrhythmias, cardiac arrest	Hypermagnesemia is most likely to occur with rapid IV administration, high dosages or concentrations, and decreased urine output.
(2) Headache, vomiting, nausea, chest pain, lethargy, visual disturbances, weakness	
(3) Change in fetal heart rate	
c. With oxytocin, observe for:	
(1) Excessive stimulation of uterine contractility (hypertonicity; rupture; cervical and perineal lacerations; fetal hypoxia; dysrhythmias; death or damage from rapid, forceful propulsion through the birth canal)	Most likely to occur when excessive doses are given to initiate or augment labor.
(2) Hypotension or hypertension	Usual doses cause little change in blood pressure; large doses may cause an initial drop, followed by sustained elevation.
(3) Water intoxication (convulsions, coma)	
4. Observe for drug interactions	
a. Drugs that *alter* effects of prostaglandins:	
(1) Aspirin and other nonsteroidal anti-inflammatory agents, such as ibuprofen	These drugs inhibit effects of prostaglandins. When given concurrently with abortifacient prostaglandins, the abortive process is prolonged.

(continued on page 1056)

Nursing Actions — Abortifacients, Prostaglandins, Tocolytics, and Oxytocics (continued)

NURSING ACTIONS	RATIONALE/EXPLANATION
b. Drug that *alters* effects of magnesium sulfate: (1) Calcium gluconate	Calcium gluconate is an antidote for magnesium sulfate overdose.
c. Drugs that *alter* effects of oxytocin: (1) Vasoconstrictors, such as epinephrine and other adrenergic drugs	Additive vasoconstriction with risks of severe, persistent hypertension and intracranial hemorrhage

Key Concepts

■ Major concerns with drug use during pregnancy are feto-toxicity and teratogenicity. A developing fetus is exposed to any drugs circulating in the mother's bloodstream.

■ Fetal organs are formed during the first trimester of pregnancy, possibly before a woman knows she is pregnant. The fetus' brain continues to develop throughout pregnancy and after birth.

■ A folic acid supplement is recommended for women who may become pregnant and during pregnancy to prevent neural tube defects.

■ Drugs should be avoided during pregnancy when possible and used cautiously when required.

■ Some drugs should be avoided during lactation; all drugs should be used cautiously.

Review and Application Exercises

Short Answer Exercises

1. Why should drugs be avoided during pregnancy and lactation when possible?

2. How does insulin therapy for diabetes mellitus differ during pregnancy?

3. What is the rationale for using methyldopa to treat hypertension during pregnancy?

4. How are asthma and seizure disorders managed during pregnancy?

5. In a patient receiving a tocolytic drug to inhibit uterine contractions, how would you assess the patient for adverse drug effects?

6. In a patient receiving an oxytocin infusion to induce or augment labor, what interventions are needed to increase safety and decrease adverse drug effects?

7. Which immunizations are safe to be administered during pregnancy? Which are contraindicated?

8. A pregnant patient asks you about using herbal supplements. What would you tell her? Why?

NCLEX-Style Questions

9. A daily vitamin K supplement is recommended during the last month of pregnancy for women receiving long-term drug therapy for which of the following conditions?
   a. asthma
   b. diabetes mellitus
   c. hypertension
   d. seizure disorders

10. For a patient receiving a continuous IV magnesium sulfate infusion for tocolysis, which of the following medications should the nurse have readily available?
    a. diazepam (Valium)
    b. methyldopa
    c. calcium gluconate
    d. phenytoin (Dilantin)

11. Betamethasone (Celestone) is ordered for a patient experiencing preterm labor at 34 weeks gestation. The nurse explains to the patient that the drug is being given to
    a. enhance fetal lung maturity
    b. counteract the effects of tocolytic therapy
    c. treat intrauterine infection
    d. decrease need for a cesarean section

12. A drug of choice for treating group B streptococcal infection in a pregnant woman is
    a. penicillin
    b. fluoroquinolone
    c. aminoglycoside
    d. tetracycline

13. Which of the following drugs is used after delivery to prevent or control postpartum uterine bleeding?
    a. vitamin K
    b. oxytocin
    c. magnesium sulfate
    d. betamethasone

Selected References

American Diabetes Association. (2006). Position statement: Gestational diabetes mellitus. *Diabetes Care, 29*(Suppl. 1, 543–548).

Born, D., & Barron, M. L. (2005). Herb use in pregnancy: What nurses should know. MCN: *Journal of Maternal/Child Nursing, 30*, 201–206.

Cooper, W. O., Hernandez-Diaz, S., Arbogast, P. G., Dudley, J. A., Dyer, S., Gideon, P. S., et al. (2006). Major congenital malformations after first-trimester exposure to ACE inhibitors. *New England Journal of Medicine, 354*, 2443–2451.

Crombleholme, W. R. (2007). Obstetrics. In S. J. McPhee, M. A. Papadakis, & L. M. Tierney, Jr. (Eds), *Current medical diagnosis and treatment 2007* (46th ed., pp. 782–806). New York: McGraw-Hill.

Drug facts and comparisons. (Updated monthly). St. Louis, MO: Facts and Comparisons.

Guyton, A. C., & Hall, J. E. (2006). *Textbook of medical physiology* (11th ed.). Philadelphia: Elsevier Saunders.

Lacy, C. F., Armstrong, L. L., Goldman, M. P., & Lance, L. L. (2006). *Drug information handbook* (14th ed.). Hudson, OH: Lexi-Comp.

Langer, O., Yogev, Y., Xenakis, E. M. J., & Rosenn, B. (2005). Insulin and glyburide therapy: Dosage, severity level of gestational diabetes, and pregnancy outcome. *American Journal of Obstetrics and Gynecology, 192*, 134–139.

Louik, C., Lin, A. E., Werler, M. M., Hernandez-Diaz, S., & Mitchell, A. A. (2007). First-trimester use of selective serotonin-reuptake inhibitors and the risk of birth defects. *New England Journal of Medicine, 356*, 2675–2683.

McCarter-Spaulding, D. E. (2005). Medications in pregnancy and lactation. MCN: *Journal of Maternal/Child Nursing, 30*, 10–17.

National Asthma Education and Prevention Program (NAEPP) Expert Panel. *Managing asthma during pregnancy: Recommendations for pharmacologic treatment—2007 update.* National Institutes of Health,

item 08-4051 (prepublication copy). Retrieved September 21, 2007, from http://www.nhlbi.nih.gov/guidelines/asthma/asthgdln.htm

Patka, J. H., Lodolce, A. E., & Johnston, A. K. (2005). High-versus low-dose oxytocin for augmentation or induction of labor. *Annals of Pharmacotherapy, 39*, 95–101.

Pigarelli, D. L., Kraus, C. K., & Potter, B.E. (2005). Pregnancy and lactation: Therapeutic considerations. In J. T. DiPiro, R. L. Talbert, G. C. Yee, G. R. Matzke, B. G. Wells, & L. M. Posey (Eds.), *Pharmacotherapy: A pathophysiologic approach* (6th ed., pp. 1425–1442). New York: McGraw-Hill.

Porth, C. M. (2005). *Pathophysiology: Concepts of altered health states* (7th ed.). Philadelphia: Lippincott Williams & Wilkins.

Scollan-Koliopoulos, M., Guadagno, S., & Walker, E. A. (2006). Gestational diabetes management: Guidelines to a healthy pregnancy. *Nurse Practitioner, 31*, 14–18.

Simhan, H. N., & Caritis, S. N. (2007). Prevention of preterm delivery. *New England Journal of Medicine, 357*, 477–487.

Simpson, K. R., & Creehan, P. A. (2007). *Perinatal nursing* (3rd ed.). Philadelphia: Wolters Kluwer Health/Lippincott Williams & Wilkins.

Spencer, A. P., & Wingate, S. (2005). Cardiovascular drug therapy in women. *Journal of Cardiovascular Nursing, 20*, 410–419.

Young, V. S. L. (2005). Teratogenicity and drugs in breast milk. In M. A. Koda-Kimble, L. Y. Young, W. A. Kradjan, et al. (Eds.), *Applied therapeutics: The clinical use of drugs* (8th ed., pp. 47-1–47-32). Philadelphia: Lippincott Williams & Wilkins.

Ziaei, S., Norrozi, M., Faghihzadeh, S., & Jafarbegloo, E. (2007). A randomised placebo-controlled trial to determine the effect of iron supplementation on pregnancy outcome in pregnant women with haemoglobin under 13.2 g/dl. *BJOG: An International Journal of Obstetrics and Gynaecology, 114*, 684–688.

The International System of Units

The International System of Units (Système International d'Unites or SI units), which is based on the metric system, has been adopted by many countries in an attempt to standardize reports of clinical laboratory data among nations and disciplines. A major reason for using SI units is that biologic substances react in the human body on a molar basis.

The International System, like the conventional or traditional system, uses the kilogram for measurement of mass or weight and the meter for measurement of length. The major difference is that the International System uses the mole for measurement of amounts per volume of a substance. A mole is the amount of a chemical compound of which its weight in grams equals its molecular weight. Thus, the concentrations of solutions are expressed in moles, millimoles, or micromoles per liter (mol/L, mmol/L, micromol/L) rather than the conventional measurement of mass per volume, such as grams or milligrams per 100 mL or dL. A few laboratory values are the same in conventional and SI units, but many differ dramatically. Moreover, "normal values" in both systems often vary, depending on laboratory methodologies and reference sources. Thus, *laboratory data should be interpreted in light of the patient's clinical status and with knowledge of the "normal values" of the laboratory performing the test.*

Serum Drug Concentrations

Measuring the amount of a drug in blood plasma or serum is often useful in the clinical management of various disorders. For example, serum drug levels may be used to guide drug dosage (e.g., with aminoglycoside antibiotics such as gentamicin); to evaluate an inadequate therapeutic response; and to diagnose or manage drug toxicity. Listed below are generally accepted therapeutic serum drug concentrations, in conventional and SI units, for some commonly used drugs. In addition, toxic concentrations are listed for acetaminophen and salicylate. Note that SI units have not been established for some drugs.

DRUG	CONVENTIONAL UNITS	SI UNITS
Acetaminophen	0.2–0.6 mg/dL Toxic >5 mg/dL	13–40 μmol/L >300 μmol/L
Amikacin	(Peak) 16–32 mcg/mL (Trough) ≤8 mcg/mL	20–30 mg/L
Amitriptyline	110–250 ng/mL	375–900 nmol/L
Carbamazepine	4–12 mcg/mL	17–50 μmol/L
Desipramine	125–300 ng/mL	470–825 nmol/L
Digoxin	0.5–2.2 ng/mL	1–2.6 nmol/L
Disopyramide	2–8 mcg/mL	6–18 μmol/L
Ethosuximide	40–110 mcg/mL	280–780 μmol/L
Gentamicin	(Peak) 4–8 mcg/mL (Trough) ≤2 mcg/mL	5–10 mg/L
Imipramine	200–350 ng/mL	530–950 nmol/L
Lidocaine	1.5–6 mcg/mL	6–21 μmol/L
Lithium	0.5–1.5 mEq/L	0.5–1.5 mmol/L
Maprotiline	50–200 ng/mL	180–270 nmol/L
Nortriptyline	50–150 ng/mL	190–570 nmol/L
Phenobarbital	15–50 mcg/mL	65–170 μmol/L
Phenytoin	10–20 mcg/mL	40–80 μmol/L
Primidone	5–12 mcg/mL	25–45 μmol/L
Procainamide	4–8 mcg/mL	17–40 μmol/L
Propranolol	50–200 ng/mL	190–770 nmol/L
Protriptyline	100–300 ng/mL	380–1140 nmol/L
Quinidine	2–6 mcg/mL	4.6–9.2 μmol/L
Salicylate	100–200 mg/L Toxic >200 mg/L	724–1448 μmol/L >1450 μmol/L
Theophylline	10–20 mcg/mL	55–110 μmol/L

(continued on page 1060)

(Continued)

DRUG	CONVENTIONAL UNITS	SI UNITS
Tobramycin	(Peak) 4–8 mcg/mL (Trough) ≤2 mcg/mL	5–10 mg/L
Valproic acid	50–100 mcg/mL	350–700 μmol/L
Vancomycin	(Peak) 30–40 mg/mL (Trough) 5–10 mg/mL	(Peak) 20–40 mg/L (Trough) 5–10 mg/L

dL, deciliter; mcg, microgram; mEq, milliequivalent; mmol, millimole; ng, nanogram; nmol, nanomole; μmol, micromole.

Anesthetics, Adjunctive Drugs, and Nursing Considerations

Anesthetics interrupt the conduction of painful nerve impulses from a site of injury to the brain. They are given to prevent pain and promote relaxation during surgery, childbirth, and some diagnostic tests and treatments.

General Anesthetics

General anesthetics produce profound central nervous system (CNS) depression, during which there is complete loss of sensation, consciousness, pain perception, and memory. The drugs include inhalation and intravenous (IV) agents and can be used for almost any surgical, diagnostic, or therapeutic procedure. General anesthesia is often started with a fast-acting IV drug (e.g., propofol, thiopental) then maintained with a mixture of an anesthetic gas and oxygen given by inhalation. The IV agent produces rapid loss of consciousness and provides a pleasant induction and recovery. An anesthetic barbiturate or propofol may be used alone for anesthesia during brief diagnostic tests or surgical procedures. Selected agents and their characteristics and uses are listed in Table C-1.

General Anesthetic Adjunctive Drugs

Several drugs are used along with general anesthetics. *Antianxiety agents* and *sedative-hypnotics* are given to decrease anxiety, promote rest, allow easier induction of anesthesia, and allow smaller doses of anesthetics. These drugs may be given the night before to aid sleep and 1 or 2 hours before the scheduled procedure. In addition, midazolam (Versed) is often used in ambulatory surgical or invasive diagnostic procedures and for regional anesthesia. It has a rapid onset and short duration of action, causes amnesia, produces minimal cardiovascular adverse effects, and reduces the dose of opioid analgesics required during surgery. *Anticholinergic drugs* are given to prevent vagal effects (e.g., bradycardia, hypotension) associated with general anesthesia and surgery. Vagal stimulation occurs with some inhalation anesthetics and with surgical procedures in which there is manipulation of the pharynx, trachea, peritoneum, stomach, intestine, or other viscera, and procedures in which pressure is exerted on the eyeball.

Neuromuscular blocking agents (see Table C-1) cause muscle relaxation, an important component of general anesthesia, and allow the use of smaller amounts of anesthetic agents. They are also used to facilitate mechanical ventilation, control increased intracranial pressure, and treat status epilepticus. Artificial ventilation is necessary because these drugs paralyze muscles of respiration as well as other skeletal muscles. The drugs do not cause sedation; therefore, unless recipients are unconscious, they can see and hear environmental activities and conversations. These commonly used drugs prevent acetylcholine from acting at neuromuscular junctions. As a result, the nerve cell membrane is not depolarized, the muscle fibers are not stimulated, and skeletal muscle contraction does not occur. The drugs should be used very cautiously in patients with renal or hepatic impairment because the drug or its metabolites may accumulate and cause prolonged paralysis.

Nursing Considerations With General Anesthetics and Neuromuscular Blocking Agents

- General anesthetics should be administered *only* by anesthesiologists or nurse anesthetists and *only* in locations where staff, equipment, and drugs are available for emergency use or cardiopulmonary resuscitation. Most nurses care for patients before and after administration of general anesthetics.

| Table C-1 | General Anesthetics and Neuromuscular Blocking Agents |

GENERIC/TRADE NAME	CHARACTERISTICS
General Inhalation Anesthetics	
Desflurane (Suprane), **enflurane** (Ethrane), **isoflurane** (Forane), **sevoflurane** (Ultane)	These drugs are similar volatile liquids used for induction and maintenance of general anesthesia. They are given by anesthesiologists or nurse anesthetists.
Nitrous oxide	One of the oldest and safest anesthetics; given with oxygen to prevent hypoxia; has rapid induction and recovery; used for anesthesia with IV barbiturates, neuromuscular blocking agents, opioid analgesics, and stronger inhalation anesthetics; used alone for analgesia in dentistry, obstetrics, and brief surgical procedures
General Intravenous Anesthetics	
Alfentanil (Alfenta), **remifentanil** (Ultiva), **sufentanil** (Sufenta)	These drugs are rapid-acting opioid-analgesic anesthetics used as a primary anesthetic or as an analgesic adjunct with other general anesthetics.
Etomidate (Amidate)	A nonanalgesic hypnotic used for induction and maintenance of general anesthesia; may be used with nitrous oxide for short operative procedures
Methohexital (Brevital), **thiopental** (Pentothal)	Ultra–short-acting barbiturates used to induce general anesthesia. For major surgery, the drugs are used with inhalation anesthetics and muscle relaxants.
Midazolam (Versed)	A short-acting benzodiazepine. Given IV or IM for preoperative sedation. Given IV for conscious sedation during short endoscopic or other diagnostic procedures; induction of general anesthesia; and maintenance of general anesthesia with nitrous oxide and oxygen for short surgical procedures. Adverse effects of IV drug include respiratory depression, apnea, and death.
Propofol (Diprivan)	A rapid-acting hypnotic used for induction or maintenance of general anesthesia, with other agents. Also used alone for sedation in critical care units. Recovery occurs a few minutes after the drug is stopped. Adverse effects include hypotension, apnea, and other signs of central nervous system depression.
Neuromuscular Blocking Agents	
Atracurium (Tracium), **Cisatracurium** (Nimbex), **Rocuronium** (Zemuron), **Vecuronium** (Norcuron)	These are intermediate-acting, nondepolarizing skeletal muscle relaxants used with general anesthesia for surgical procedures and to facilitate endotracheal intubation and mechanical ventilation. They may cause hypotension and their effects can be reversed by neostigmine (Prostigmin).
Pancuronium	An older, long-acting drug used during surgery after general anesthesia has been induced or to aid endotracheal intubation or mechanical ventilation. It may cause hypotension, and effects can be reversed by neostigmine (Prostigmin).
Succinylcholine	A depolarizing, short-acting drug that may be used during surgery and brief procedures, such as endoscopy and endotracheal intubation. It is used less often than the nondepolarizing agents described above. Adverse effects include malignant hyperthermia, a life-threatening condition.

■ If a medical disorder of a vital organ system (cardiovascular, respiratory, renal) is present, it should be corrected before anesthesia is given, when possible. Such disorders increase the risks of complications with anesthesia and surgery. Additional risk factors include cigarette smoking, obesity, and limited exercise or activity.

■ Compared with adults, children are at greater risk of complications (e.g., laryngospasm, bronchospasm, aspiration, postoperative nausea and vomiting) and death from general anesthetics and adjunctive drugs.

■ Compared with younger adults, older adults often have physiologic changes and pathologic conditions that make them more susceptible to adverse effects of anesthetics, neuromuscular blocking agents, and adjunctive medications. Thus, lower doses of these agents are usually needed.

■ During preanesthetic nursing assessments, patients should be asked about drug allergies and the use of prescription drugs, nonprescription drugs, and herbal or dietary supplements. With herbal products, the American Society of Anesthesiologists recommends that all herbals be stopped 2 or 3 weeks before any surgical procedure because some (e.g., feverfew, garlic, ginkgo biloba, ginseng) can increase risks of bleeding and some (e.g., kava, valerian) can increase effects of sedatives.

■ Effects of anesthetics wear off gradually and the nurse must observe and safeguard patients during this recovery period. With general anesthetics and neuromuscular blocking agents, frequent (e.g., every 5–15 minutes) assessment of cardiovascular and respiratory function is needed until the client wakes up and is breathing well. This is usually done in a postanesthesia recovery (PAR) area. Observe for adverse effects, including excessive sedation (e.g., delayed awakening, failure to respond to verbal or tactile stimuli); respiratory problems (e.g., laryngospasm, hypoxia, hypercarbia); cardiovascular problems (e.g., hypotension, tachycardia and other cardiac dysrhythmias, fluid and electrolyte imbalances); and other problems (e.g., restlessness, nausea, vomiting).

■ Propofol and neuromuscular blocking agents are commonly used in critical care units, usually for patients who are intubated and mechanically ventilated. These drugs should be administered and monitored only by health care personnel who are skilled in the management of critically ill patients, including cardiopulmonary resuscitation and airway management. Critical care nurses must often care for patients receiving IV infusions of the drugs and titrate dosage and flow rate to achieve desired effects and minimize adverse effects. Consult drug literature regarding accurate administration and monitoring of these drugs.

Local Anesthetics

Local anesthetics, given to produce loss of sensation and motor activity, are applied to or injected into localized areas of the body. The drugs decrease the permeability of nerve cell membranes to ions, especially sodium. This action reduces excitability of cell membranes; when excitability falls low enough, nerve impulses cannot be initiated or conducted by the anesthetized nerves. As a result, the drugs prevent the cells from responding to pain impulses and other sensory stimuli.

Anesthetic effects dwindle as drug molecules diffuse out of neurons into the bloodstream. The drugs are then transported to the liver for metabolism, mainly to inactive metabolites. The metabolites are excreted in the urine, along with a small amount of unchanged drug. Commonly used local anesthetics are listed in Table C-2.

Selected Types of Local Anesthesia

■ *Spinal* anesthesia involves injecting the anesthetic agent into the cerebrospinal fluid, usually in the lumbar spine. The anesthetic blocks sensory impulses at the root of peripheral nerves as they enter the spinal cord. Spinal anesthesia is especially useful for surgery involving the lower abdomen and legs.

■ *Epidural* anesthesia, which involves injecting the anesthetic into the epidural space, is used most often in obstetrics during labor and delivery. This route is also used to provide analgesia (often with a combination of a local anesthetic and an opioid) for patients with postoperative or other pain.

When the combination is used, the dosage of both drugs must be reduced to avoid respiratory depression and other adverse effects.

■ *Topical* anesthesia involves application of a local anesthetic to skin and mucous membranes. The anesthetic is usually an ingredient in ointments, solutions, or lotions designed for use at particular sites. For example, preparations are available for use on eyes, ears, nose, oral mucosa, perineum, hemorrhoids, and skin. These preparations are used to relieve pain and itching of dermatoses, sunburn, minor skin wounds, hemorrhoids, sore throat, and other conditions. The main adverse effect is allergic reactions.

Nursing Considerations With Local Anesthetics

■ Some local anesthetic is absorbed into the bloodstream and circulated through the body, especially when injected or applied to mucous membrane. *Systemic absorption accounts for most of the potentially serious adverse effects of local anesthetics.* These adverse effects include CNS stimulation (e.g., hyperactivity, excitement, seizure activity) followed by CNS depression; cardiovascular depression (e.g., hypotension, dysrhythmias); and allergic reactions (e.g., hives and other skin lesions; itching; edema; possible anaphylactoid symptoms, including severe hypotension). Serious adverse effects are more likely to occur with large doses, high concentrations, injections into highly vascular areas, or accidental injection into a blood vessel.

■ Except with IV lidocaine for cardiac dysrhythmias, local anesthetic solutions must not be injected into blood vessels because of the high risk of serious adverse reactions involving the cardiovascular system and CNS.

■ Local anesthetics given during labor cross the placenta and may depress muscle strength, muscle tone, and rooting behavior in newborns. In addition, if a local anesthetic (e.g., bupivacaine) is infused epidurally with an opioid analgesic (e.g., fentanyl), dosage of both agents must be reduced to decrease risks of respiratory arrest.

■ Epinephrine, a vasoconstrictor, is often added to a local anesthetic to slow systemic absorption, prolong anesthetic effects, and control bleeding. This combination should *not* be given IV or in excessive dosage because the drugs can cause serious systemic toxicity, including cardiac dysrhythmias. In addition, the combination should *not* be used for nerve blocks in areas supplied by end arteries (fingers, ears, nose, toes, penis) because it may produce ischemia and gangrene.

■ For topical anesthesia, use the local anesthetic only on the body part and condition for which it was prescribed. Most preparations are specifically made to apply on certain areas, and they cannot be used effectively and safely on other body parts. Also, teach patients to cleanse the site before application, if needed, so that the drug has direct contact

Table C-2	Local Anesthetics

GENERIC/TRADE NAME	CHARACTERISTICS
Injectable Drugs	
Articaine (Septodont)	Used for local infiltration (injection) and nerve block for dental and periodontal procedures or oral surgery. Effects occur in 1–6 min and last 1 h.
Bupivacaine (Marcaine)	Used for infiltration, nerve block, and epidural anesthesia during childbirth. With injection, effects occur in 5 min and last 2–4 h. With epidural administration, effects occur in 10–20 min and last 3–5 h. May cause systemic toxicity (e.g., decreased cardiac output, dysrhythmias, CNS stimulation possibly proceeding to seizures).
Chloroprocaine (Nesacaine)	Used for infiltration, nerve block, and epidural anesthesia. Effects occur in 6–12 min and last 30 min. Rapidly metabolized and less likely to cause systemic toxicity than other local anesthetics
Lidocaine (Xylocaine)	Used for local infiltration, nerve block, and spinal and epidural anesthesia. With injection, effects occur in less than 2 min and last 30–60 min. With epidural use, effects occur in 5–15 min and last 1–3 h. Lidocaine is also given IV to prevent or treat cardiac dysrhythmias. (Warning: Do not use preparations containing epinephrine for dysrhythmias.)
Mepivacaine (Carbocaine)	Used for infiltration, nerve block, and epidural anesthesia. With injection, effects occur in 3–5 min and last 0.75–1.5 h. With epidural use, effects occur in 5–15 min and last 1–3 h.
Prilocaine (Citanest)	Used for infiltration, nerve block, and epidural anesthesia. With injection, effects occur in less than 2 min and last 60 min. With epidural use, effects occur in 5–15 min and last 1–3 h.
Ropivacaine (Naropin)	Used for local or regional surgical anesthesia and obstetric or postoperative analgesia. Given by injection or epidural infusion. With epidural use, effects occur in 10–30 min and last up to 6 h.
Topical Drugs	
Benzocaine (Americaine, Lanacane, Solarcaine, others)	Used on skin and mucous membranes to relieve pain and itching of sunburn, other minor burns and wounds, skin abrasions, earache, hemorrhoids, sore throat, and other conditions. Available over-the-counter in aerosol sprays, throat lozenges, rectal suppositories, lotions, and ointments. May cause allergic reactions.
Dibucaine (Nupercainal)	Used on skin and mucous membranes. Anesthetic effects occur in less than 15 min and last 3–4 h. May cause local allergic reactions
Dyclonine (Dyclone)	Used to relieve pain of mouth or anogenital lesions and to anesthetize mucous membranes of throat and gastrointestinal tract for endoscopic procedures. Effects occur in less than 10 min and last less than 60 min.
Lidocaine (Xylocaine, Dentipatch, others)	One of the most commonly used local anesthetics. Available in several preparations, including lidocaine viscous, which is used orally for numbing of the mouth and throat, and topical patches for relief of painful conditions such as postherpetic neuralgia and to provide oral anesthesia for superficial dental procedures. With topical use, effects occur in 2–5 min and last 15–45 min.
Pramoxine (Tronothane)	Used for skin wounds, dermatoses, hemorrhoids, endotracheal intubation, and sigmoidoscopy
Proparacaine (Alcaine)	Used to anesthetize the eye for tonometry and for removal of sutures, foreign bodies, and cataracts
Tetracaine (Pontocaine)	Used for topical anesthesia

with the affected area; and to avoid using the product longer or applying more often than directed because skin irritation, rash, and hives can develop.

■ When used to anesthetize nasal, oral, pharyngeal, laryngeal, tracheal, bronchial, or urethral mucosa, local anesthetics should be given in low concentrations and at the lowest effective dosages. The drugs are well absorbed through mucous membranes and may cause systemic adverse reactions.

■ A mixture of lidocaine and prilocaine (Eutectic Mixture of Local Anesthetics [EMLA]) was formulated to penetrate intact skin, provide local anesthesia, and decrease pain of vaccinations and venipuncture, especially in children. The cream is applied at the injection site with an occlusive dressing at least 60 minutes before vaccination or venipuncture. It should not be used on abraded skin or mucous membranes.

Drugs For Erectile Dysfunction

DRUG CATEGORY	CHARACTERISTICS
Phosphodiesterase Type 5 Inhibitors	**Mechanism of Action:** Improves erectile function by inhibiting the enzyme responsible for the breakdown of cyclic guanosine monophosphate (cGMP), a vasodilatory neurotransmitter in corporal tissues of the penis. **Indications:** Treatment of erectile dysfunction in men who are healthy enough for sexual activity. Sildenafil is also approved for the treatment of pulmonary arterial hypertension. **Contraindications/Cautions:** Contraindicated in patients taking organic nitrates due to risk of severe hypotension resulting in dizziness, syncope, heart attack or stroke. Use with caution in patients taking alpha blockers due to risk of hypotension. Vardenafil prolongs the QT interval and should not be used with other drugs with similar effect particularly Class I and II antiarrrythmics (see Ch. 50). Concurrent use of substantial amounts of alcohol can increase the risk of orthostatic hypotension, tachycardia, dizziness and headache. **Adverse Effects:** Common adverse reactions include: headache, facial flushing, dyspepsia, nasal congestion and dizziness. Sildenafil and vardenafil reduce blood pressure. Sildenafil (and to a lesser degree vardenafil) increases the risk of light sensitivity, blurred vision and loss of blue-green color discrimination. Tadalafil is associated with back and muscle pain. Rarely, adverse effects associated with phosphodiesterase inhibitors include development of nonarteritic ischemic optic neuropathy due to obstruction of blood flow to the optic nerve, resulting in irreversible loss of vision; and sudden permanent hearing loss accompanied by dizziness and tinnitus. Priapism is rare and usually associated with excessive dosing or concurrent use with another erectogenic drug. Persistent priapism requires prompt medical treatment to avoid permanent penile damage. Persistent erections are treated by aspiration of blood from the corpus cavernosum, followed by irrigation with a vasoconstrictor such as epinephrine.

GENERIC (TRADE NAME)	INDIVIDUAL CHARACTERISTICS	ROUTES AND DOSAGE RANGES
Sildenafil (Viagra)	Time to peak effect: 1 h Duration: 4 h High fat meals will delay absorption and reduce peak levels.	PO 25-100 mg 1 h before sexual activity. Reduced dose with age over 65 years, concurrent use of CYP 3A4 inhibitors*, and renal or hepatic impairment.
Tadalafil (Cialis)	Time to peak effect: 2 h Duration: 24-36 h Meals do not impact absorption rate or peak levels.	PO 5-20 mg 2 h or more before anticipated sexual activity. Reduced dose with age over 65 years, renal or hepatic impairment and concurrent use of CYP3A4 inhibitors*.
Vardenafil (Levitra)	Time to peak effect: 1 h Duration: 4 h High fat meals will delay absorption and reduce peak levels.	PO 5-20 mg 1 h before sexual activity. Reduced dose with age over 65, hepatic impairment and concurrent use of CYP 3A4 inhibitors.*

*CYP3A4 inhibitors include azole antifungals, erythromycin, and saquinavir.

DRUG CATEGORY	CHARACTERISTICS
Prostaglandin E₁	**Mechanism of Action:** Relaxes trabecular smooth muscle and dilates cavernosal arteries, resulting in penile engorgement and reduced venous outflow. **Indications:** Treatment of erectile dysfunction in men who are healthy enough for sexual activity. **Contraindications/Cautions:** Not for use in patients at risk for priapism (e.g., sickle cell anemia or trait, multiple myeloma, leukemia). Use intracavernosal injections with caution in patients concurrently receiving anticoagulants due to risk of bleeding. Not recommended for concurrent use with other vasoactive agents. Alprostadil is pregnancy category C. Do not use intraurethral alprostadil if the partner is pregnant unless a condom barrier is used. **Adverse Effects:** Intracavernosal injection is associated with burning sensations, prolonged erection and priapism. Long term use is associated with penile fibrosis. Intraurethral administration is associated with penile pain.

GENERIC (TRADE NAME)	INDIVIDUAL CHARACTERISTICS	ROUTES AND DOSAGE RANGES
Intracavernosal Injection: Alprostadil (Caverject aqueous, Caverject powder, Edex powder)	Onset: following injection Duration: With proper dose, erection should not last longer than 1 hour Comes in an aqueous preparation and a power preparation that must be reconstituted prior to single use. Aqueous injection may be stored frozen up to 3 months and may be moved to the refrigerator for up to 7 days prior to use. Do not refreeze. Remove foil covering and allow to reach room temperature immediately prior to use. Store Caverject powder at or below 77 ° F for up to 3 months. Reconstituted solution must be used within 24 hours. Edex powder can be stored at controlled room temperature.	Intracavernosal injection: Inject along the dorsolateral aspect of the proximal third of the penis, avoiding visible veins. Rotate injection sites from one side of the penis to the other and change injection site with each dose. Injection may be used no more than 3 times per week and only once in 24 hours. Initial injection done in physician's office to determine dose adequate to achieve satisfactory erection without causing priapism.
Intraurethral Administration: Alprostadil (Muse)	Onset: 5-10 minutes Duration: 30-60 minutes Store unopened foil pouches in refrigerator. May be kept at controlled room temperature up to 14 days prior to use.	Intraurethral: Prior to introducing pellet into urethra, the patient should void. Residual urine in urethra aids in dispersing the medication. Intraurethral administration may be used no more than two times in 24 hours. Adequate dosage to produce satisfactory erection is determined in physician's office.

CYP3A4 inhibitors include azole antifungals, erythromycin, and saquinavir.

Glossary

Abortifacient: drug used to terminate pregnancy.

Absorption: the process that occurs from the time a drug enters the body to the time it enters the bloodstream to be circulated.

Acetylcholine: a neurotransmitter in the cholinergic system located in many areas of the brain, with high concentrations in the motor cortex and basal ganglia; also a neurotransmitter in the autonomic nervous system and at peripheral neuromuscular junctions; exerts excitatory effects at synapses and nerve–muscle junctions and inhibitory effects at some peripheral sites, such as organs supplied by the vagus nerve.

Acetylcholinesterase: enzyme responsible for the immediate breakdown of acetylcholine when released from the nerve ending.

Acne: a common disorder characterized by excessive production of sebum and obstruction of hair follicles, which normally carry sebum to the skin surface.

Acromegaly: a chronic disease, resulting from excessive secretion of growth hormone (GH), characterized by an abnormal pattern of bone and connective-tissue growth associated with an increased incidence of diabetes mellitus and hypertension.

Addison's disease: primary adrenocortical insufficiency; inadequate production of both cortisol and aldosterone.

Addisonian crisis: also known as adrenocortical insufficiency; mimics hypovolemic and septic shock.

Adrenocortical insufficiency: See addisonian crisis.

Adrenocorticotropic hormone (ACTH): also referred to as corticotropin-releasing hormone or factor (CRH or CRF); causes release of corticotropin in response to stress and threatening stimuli; most often secreted during sleep.

Adrenergic drugs: produce effects similar to those produced by stimulation of the sympathetic nervous system and therefore have widespread effects on body tissues.

Aldosterone: the main mineralocorticoid and is responsible for approximately 90% of mineralocorticoid activity; sodium resorption by the kidneys, potassium is lost in the urine.

Alopecia: temporary hair loss; commonly occurs during chemotherapy.

Agranulocytosis: an acute condition caused by loss or absence of granulocyte white blood cells.

Akathisia: manifested by motor restlessness and inability to be still, usually occurs in the first few months of treatment with antipsychotics.

Akinesia: inability to move.

Agonists: drugs that produce effects similar to those produced by naturally occurring hormones, neurotransmitters, and other substances.

Alcohol abuse: acute or chronic consumption of alcohol in excess of the limits accepted by the person's culture; may not necessarily be dependent on alcohol.

Alpha-adrenergic blocking drugs: act primarily in the skin, mucosa, intestines, lungs, and kidneys to block or prevent alpha-mediated vasoconstriction.

Alpha$_1$ receptors: receptors on surface membranes of target tissues and organs; mainly postsynaptic.

Alpha$_2$ receptors: receptors on surface membranes of target tissues and organs; mainly presynaptic.

Alzheimer's disease: the most common type of dementia in adults; is characterized by abnormalities in the cholinergic, serotonergic, noradrenergic, and glutamatergic neurotransmission systems.

Anabolic steroids: synthetic drugs with increased anabolic activity and decreased androgenic activity compared with testosterone.

Analgesia: loss of pain sensation.

Anaphylactic shock: characterized by hypotension due to massive vasodilation and acute airway obstruction due to bronchoconstriction caused by release of histamine and other chemical mediators in response to a severe allergic reaction.

Anaphylaxis: a type I immunoglobulin E-mediated allergic reaction to a foreign substance (antigen) that has entered the body; occurs on second or subsequent exposure to an antigen. Symptoms develop rapidly; typical symptom onset ranges from 30 minutes to 2 hours after exposure to the antigen.

Androgens: male sex hormones, primarily testosterone, secreted by the testes in men, the ovaries in women, and the adrenal cortex of both sexes.

Angina pectoris: chest pain that results from a deficit in myocardial oxygen supply (myocardial ischemia) in relation to myocardial oxygen demand, most often caused by atherosclerotic plaque in the coronary arteries.

Angiogenesis: the process of forming new blood vessels.

Angiotensin converting enzyme (ACE) inhibitor: drug that decreases activation of the renin-angiotensin-aldosterone system; specifically, the drug prevents inactive angiotensin I from being converted to angiotensin II.

Angiotensin II receptor blocker (ARB): similar to ACE inhibitor, although the mechanism of action is blockade of the angiotensin II receptor site.

Anhedonia: lack of pleasure.

Anorexiant: drug that suppresses the appetite.

Anticipatory nausea: triggered by fears of nausea and vomiting; conditioned response to either chemotherapy or nausea in pregnancy.

Antagonist: drug that inhibits cell function by occupying receptor sites.

Antiadrenergic drug: decreases or blocks the effects of sympathetic nerve stimulation.

Antibacterial: drug used to treat bacterial infections; used interchangeably with antibiotic.

Antibiotic: drug used to treat bacterial infections.

Antibiotic resistance: bacteria resistant to the effects of antibiotic drugs; occurs in most human pathogens.

Anticholinesterase: indirect-acting cholinergic drug that decreases the inactivation of acetylcholine in the synapse by the enzyme acetylcholinesterase.

Anticoagulants: drugs that prevent formation of new clots and extension of clots already present; they do not dissolve formed clots.

Anticonvulsant: an antiseizure drug; also referred to as antiepileptic drug (AED).

Antidepressant discontinuation syndrome: occurs with sudden termination of most antidepressant drugs; symptoms occur more rapidly and may be more intense with drugs that have a short half-life and/or with long-term antidepressant therapy.

Antidiuretic hormone (ADH): functions to regulate water balance; is secreted when body fluids become concentrated and when blood volume is low.

Antiemetic: drug that is used to prevent or treat nausea and vomiting.

Antigen: foreign substance.

Anti-inflammatory: drug that is indicated when the inflammatory response is inappropriate, abnormal, or persistent, or destroys tissue.

Anti-microbial: drug used to prevent or treat infections caused by pathogenic microorganisms.

Antimuscarinic drug: drug that interacts with muscarinic cholinergic receptors in the brain, secretory glands, heart, and smooth muscle to produce an anticholinergic response.

Anterograde amnesia: short-term memory loss.

Anticholinergic drug: blocks the action of acetylcholine on the parasympathetic nervous system.

Antigen: a foreign substance that initiates immune responses; antigens have specific sites that interact with immune cells to induce the immune response; when discussing hypersensitivity conditions they are referred to as allergens.

Anti-infective: drug used to treat infection.

Anti-oncogene: a tumor suppressor gene that normally functions to inhibit inappropriate cellular growth and proliferation.

Antiplatelet drug: drug that prevents one or more steps in the prothrombotic activity of platelets.

Antipyretics: drugs that have the ability to relieve pain, fever, and/or inflammation, symptoms associated with many injuries and illnesses.

Antiprostaglandin drugs: drugs such as aspirin, NSAIDs, and acetaminophen that inhibit the synthesis of prostaglandins.

Antiretroviral drugs: Antiviral medications used in the treatment of retroviral infections such as HIV.

Antiretroviral therapy (ART): used in treatment of HIV infection; newer drugs and drug combinations that are more effective in viral suppression, cause fewer serious adverse effects, and are more convenient for patients to take.

Antitussives: drugs that suppress cough by depressing the cough center in the medulla oblongata or the cough receptors in the throat, trachea, or lungs.

Anxiety: a common disorder that may be referred to as nervousness, tension, worry, or other terms that denote an unpleasant feeling.

Anxiety disorder: severe anxiety that is prolonged and impairs the ability to function in usual activities of daily living.

Anxiolytics: anti-anxiety drugs.

Arachidonic acid: a fatty acid present in cell membranes that is metabolized by cyclooxygenase (COX) enzymes to produce prostaglandins.

Atherosclerosis: disease process that often leads to pathologic thrombosis; begins with accumulation of lipid-filled macrophages (i.e., foam cells) on the inner lining of arteries. Foam cells develop in response to elevated blood lipid levels and eventually become fibrous plaques, often in arteries supplying the heart, brain, and legs.

Attention-deficit hyperactivity disorder (ADHD): most common psychiatric or neurobehavioral disorder in children; it is characterized by persistent hyperactivity, a short attention span, difficulty completing assigned tasks or schoolwork, restlessness, and impulsiveness.

Autonomic nervous system (ANS): controls involuntary activities in smooth muscle, secretory glands, and in the visceral organs of the body such as the heart.

Autoregulation: the ability of body tissues to regulate their own blood flow.

Bacteria: unicellular microorganisms sub-classified according to whether they are aerobic (require oxygen) or anaerobic (cannot live in the presence of oxygen), their reaction to Gram's stain (gram positive or gram negative), and their shape (e.g., cocci, bacilli).

Bactericidal: the action of an antibacterial drug that kills the microorganism.

Bacteriostatic: the action of an antibacterial drug that inhibits growth of the microorganism.

Basal ganglia: the area in the midbrain that controls smooth voluntary movement.

Bioavailability: the portion of a drug dose that reaches the systemic circulation and is available to act on body cells.

Biotechnology: the process of manipulating deoxyribonucleic acid (DNA) and ribonucleic acid (RNA) and recombining genes into hybrid molecules that can be inserted into living organisms (*Escherichia coli* bacteria are often used) and repeatedly reproduced.

Biotransformation: also referred to as metabolism; when drugs are altered from their original form into a new form by the body.

Bipolar disorder: mood disorder characterized by episodes of depression alternating with episodes of mania.

Bisphosphonates: drugs that bind to bone and inhibit calcium resorption from bone; used mainly in the treatment of hypercalcemia and osteoporosis.

Blood glucose level: blood sugar level in the body.

Blood glucose meter: device that measures how much glucose is in the blood.

Bradykinesia: slow movement.

Body mass index(BMI): reflects weight in relation to height and is a better indicator than weight alone when determining the fitness level of a person.

Bradykinin: a peptide that causes vasodilation and lowers blood pressure.

Brand or trade name: name given to a drug designated and patented by the manufacturer.

Breakthrough pain: acute pain in people who have been receiving opioids for chronic pain.

Broad spectrum antibacterials: drugs that are effective against several groups of microorganisms, including gram positive and gram negative microoganisms.

Calcitonin: used in the treatment of hypercalcemia and osteoporosis.

Cannabinoid: derivative of marijuana.

Cancer: used to describe many disease processes with the common characteristics of uncontrolled cell growth, invasiveness, and metastasis.

Candidiasis: infection either containing or caused by *Candida* fungi.

Carcinomas: the most common type of malignant cancer; derived from epithelial tissues (skin, mucous membrane, linings and coverings of viscera).

Cardiogenic shock: occurs when the myocardium has lost its ability to contract efficiently and maintain an adequate cardiac output.

Cardioselective beta blockers: drugs that have more effect on beta$_1$ receptors than on beta$_2$ receptors; may cause less bronchospasm, less impairment of glucose metabolism, and less peripheral vascular insufficiency, than non-selective beta blockers.

Catechol-O-methyltransferase (COMT): an enzyme that degrades and inactivates catecholamines such a dopamine, epinephrine, norepinephrine.

Cathartics: drugs with strong laxative effects and elimination of liquid or semiliquid stool.

Ceiling drug: an opioid whose dosage cannot be increased above a certain amount without causing severe adverse effects.

Cell cycle: the interval between the "birth" of a cell and its division into two daughter cells.

Central adiposity: elevated waist circumference.

Chemoreceptor trigger zone (CTZ): one of the central sites that relays stimuli to the vomiting center.

Chemotherapy: treatment of disease with drugs that kill cells, usually indicates treatment for cancer or infection.

Cholesterol: component of cell membrane that is produced and processed in the liver; a fat that is essential for the formation of steroid hormones; it is produced in cells and taken in by dietary sources.

Cholinergic drugs: stimulate the parasympathetic nervous system in the same manner as acetylcholine.

Choreoathetoid: twisting, worm-like movements of the face and tongue

Chronotropy: affects the rate of occurrence; such as heart rates.

Clinical pathways: guidelines for the care of patients with particular conditions.

Clonic: spasms that alternate between contraction and relaxation.

Colonization: the presence of normal microbial flora or transient environmental organisms that do not harm the host.

Community-acquired infections: are usually acquired outside of the hospital.

Conjunctiva: the mucous membrane lining of the eyelids.

Constipation: the infrequent and painful expulsion of hard, dry stools.

Controlled substances: drugs that are categorized by federal law according to therapeutic usefulness and potential for abuse.

Convoluted tubules: along with glomerul; comprise the nephrons; referred to as convoluted because the tubules contain many twists and turns.

Convulsion: a tonic-clonic type of seizure characterized by spasmodic contractions of involuntary muscles.

Coronary artery disease (CAD): the development and progression of atherosclerotic plaque; results in impaired blood flow to the myocardium.

Corticosteroids: steroid hormones produced by the adrenal cortex; include androgens, glucocorticoids, and mineralocorticoids.

Corticotropin: an anterior pituitary hormone obtained from animal pituitary glands; may be used as a diagnostic test to differentiate primary adrenal insufficiency from secondary adrenal insufficiency caused by inadequate pituitary secretion of corticotropin.

Cortisol: the main glucocorticoid secreted as part of the body's response to stress.

Cretinism: congenital hypothyroidism; occurs when a child is born with a poorly functioning or absent thyroid gland.

Crystalluria: presence of crystals in the urine.

Cyclooxygenase (COX): enzyme required for prostaglandin formation; there are two forms: Cox-1 and Cox-2.

Cyclothymia: a mild type of bipolar disorder that involves periods of hypomania and depression that do not meet the criteria for mania and major depression.

Cushing's disease: adrenocortical hyperfunction; may result from excessive corticotropin or a primary adrenal tumor

Cycloplegia: paralysis in the ciliary muscle of the eye.

Decongestants: drugs that decrease the blood flow to the upper respiratory tract and decrease the overproduction of secretions.

Defecation: bowel elimination that is normally stimulated by movements and reflexes in the gastrointestinal (GI) tract.

Delusions: false beliefs that persist in the absence of reason or evidence.

Depression: the most common mental illness, is characterized by depressed mood, feelings of sadness or emotional upset, and it occurs in all age groups.

Dermatitis: a general term denoting an inflammatory response of the skin to injuries from irritants, allergens, or trauma; also referred to as eczema.

Detection of antigens: technique to identify pathogens that uses features of culture and serology but reduces the time required for diagnosis.

Diabetes mellitus: a chronic disease characterized by disordered metabolism of carbohydrates, fats, and protein, and hyperglycemia, due to a deficiency in the amount on action of insulin. There are 3 main forms of diabetes: Type 1, Type 2, and gestational diabetes.

Diarrhea: a symptom of numerous conditions that increase bowel motility; cause secretion or retention of fluids in the intestinal lumen; and cause inflammation or irritation of the gastrointestinal (GI) tract.

Diuretics: drugs that increase renal excretion of water, sodium, and other electrolytes – increasing urine formation and output; useful in preventing renal failure by their ability to sustain urine flow.

Directly observed therapy (DOT): a health care provider (or other responsible adult) observes the patient taking each dose of antiTB drugs; recommended for all drug regimens and considered mandatory in intermittent schedules and regimens for MDR-TB.

Disease modifying antirheumatic drugs (DMARDs): include a variety of medications used to relieve symptoms and slow joint destruction (so-called disease-modifying effects); the drugs of choice to treat active rheumatoid arthritis (Level B-C).

Distributive shock: characterized by massive vasodilation, which results in a relative hypovolemia; further divided into anaphylactic, neurogenic, and septic shock.

Distribution: transport of drug molecules within the body; after a drug is injected or absorbed into the bloodstream, it is carried by the blood and tissue fluids to its sites of action, metabolism, and excretion.

Dopamine: a neurotransmitter in the dopaminergic system; is inhibitory in the basal ganglia but may be excitatory in other areas. Repeated stimulation of dopamine receptors decreases their numbers (down-regulation) and their sensitivity to dopamine (desensitization).

Dopaminergic drugs: increase the amount of dopamine in the brain by various mechanisms.

Dosage forms: forms in which drugs are manufactured; vary according to the drugs' chemical characteristics, reason for use and route of administration; some available in one dosage form and others in multiple forms; forms include: liquids, tablets, capsules, suppositories, and transdermal and pump delivery systems.

Down regulation: decrease in receptor number or responsiveness.

Dromotropy: influencing conduction of electrical impulses in cardiac muscles and nerves.

Drug classifications: Drugs are classified according to their effects on particular body systems, their therapeutic uses, and their chemical characteristics.

Drug withdrawal reactions: signs and symptoms that occur when some drugs are abruptly discontinued or their dosage is decreased; occur with ethanol dependence, opioids, benzodiazepines, and antidepressants.

Dwarfism: a condition marked by severely decreased linear growth and, frequently, severely delayed mental, emotional, dental, and sexual growth as well; caused by a lack of growth hormone (GH).

Dyskinesia: difficulty in performing voluntary movements.

Dyslipidemia: abnormal lipid levels in the blood, associated with atherosclerosis and its many pathophysiologic effects (e.g., myocardial ischemia and infarction, stroke, peripheral arterial occlusive disease).

Dysmenorrhea: pain associated with menstruation

Dysthymia: involves a chronically depressed mood and at least two other symptoms of depression for 2 years.

Dystonia: uncoordinated, twisting and repetitive movements of the neck, face, eyes, tongue, trunk, or extremities.

Edema: the excessive accumulation of fluid in body tissues.

Effector organ: target organ containing receptors for a neurotransmitter, hormone or other chemical; stimulation of receptors on an effector organ produces a response.

Embolus: an object that migrates through the circulation until it lodges in a blood vessel, causing occlusion; may be a thrombus, fat, air, amniotic fluid, a bit of tissue, or bacterial debris.

Emesis: the act of vomiting.

Emetogenic: drugs that cause vomiting.

Emollient: lubricants used to relieve pruritus and dryness of the skin.

Endogenous analgesia system: body system for relieving pain by suppressing the transmission of pain signals from peripheral nerves; may also inhibit pain signals at other points in the pain pathway.

Endorphins: peptides found in the brain that interact with opioid receptors to inhibit perception and transmission of pain signals.

Epinephrine: the drug of choice for the treatment of anaphylaxis. It relieves bronchospasm, laryngeal edema, and hypotension; a catecholamine.

Ergogenic: an increase in muscular work capacity caused by drugs that enhance athletic performance.

Erythema: redness of the skin.

Excretion: elimination of a drug from the body; effective excretion requires adequate functioning of the circulatory system and of the organs of excretion (kidneys, bowel, lungs, and skin).

Expectorants: drugs given orally to liquefy respiratory secretions and allow for ease of removal.

Extrapyramidal reaction: movement disorders such as tardive dyskinesia, akathesia, dystonia, and drug-induced parkinsonism that may occur with usage of antipsychotic drugs.

Extravasation: leaking of medication into soft tissues around the venipuncture site.

Enteric-coated: tablets and capsules that are coated with a substance that is insoluble in stomach acid.

Enterohepatic recirculation: drugs or metabolites that are excreted in bile, reabsorbed from the small intestine, returned to the liver, metabolized, and eventually excreted in urine.

Enzyme inducting drugs: stimulate liver cells to produce larger amounts of drug-metabolizing enzymes; accelerate drug metabolism because larger amounts of the enzymes (and more binding sites) allow larger amounts of a drug to be metabolized during a given time.

Enzyme inhibiting drugs: inhibit production of drug-metabolizing enzymes and often occurs with concurrent administration of two or more drugs that compete for the same metabolizing enzymes; occurs within hours or days of starting an inhibiting agent.

Epilepsy: seizures that occur in a chronic, recurrent pattern.

Estrogen: produced primarily by the ovaries and secondarily by the adrenal cortex; promotes growth of specific body cells and development of most female secondary sexual characteristics.

Extensively drug-resistant tuberculosis (XDR-TB): indicates resistance to the second-line drugs used to treat multidrug-resistant tuberculosis (MDR-TB).

Euthyroid: normal thyroid gland functioning.

Evidence-based practice: a conscientious and continuing effort to provide high-quality care to patients by obtaining and analyzing the best available scientific evidence from research; the scientific evidence is integrated with the nurse's clinical expertise and the patient's preferences and values to yield "best practices" for a patient with a particular disease process or health problem.

Extrapyramidal effects: neuromuscular symptoms (i.e., abnormal movements) brought on by usage of antipsychotic drugs.

Fetotoxic: drugs harmful to the fetus

Fibrinolysin: see plasmin.

First messenger: the ligand that binds the receptor on target tissues.

First-pass effect: initial metabolism of some oral drugs as they are carried from the intestine to the liver by the portal circulatory system prior to reaching the systemic circulation for distribution to site of action.

"Five rights": the basic requirements for accurate drug administration; require knowledge of the drugs to be given and the patients who are to receive them as well as specific nursing skills and interventions.

Floppy iris syndrome: possible surgical complication of cataract surgery for patients taking alpha$_1$-blockers. The drugs may cause the pupil to constrict and the iris to relax.

Fungi: plant-like organisms that live as parasites on living tissue or as saprophytes on decaying organic matter.

Gamma amino butyric acid (GABA): abundant in the brain and spinal cord; the major inhibitory neurotransmitter in the CNS, with a role in many neuronal circuits.

Generic name: is related to the chemical or official name of the drug; independent of the manufacturer and often indicates the drug group.

Genital herpes: an infection caused by the herpes simplex virus (HSV) and produces recurrent, painful, blister-like lesions on skin and mucous membranes.

Gingival hyperplasia: an overgrowth of gum tissue, common in children.

Glaucoma: group of diseases characterized by optic nerve damage and changes in visual fields; characterized by increased IOP (above 22 mm Hg) but may also occur with normal IOP (below 21 mm Hg); average 15–16 mm Hg; one of the leading causes of blindness in the United Statues.

Glucagon: a pancreatic hormone that raises blood glucose levels by stimulating the liver to convert glycogen into glucose. Opposes insulin.

Gluconeogenesis: the formation of glucose from non-carbohydrate sources such as fats and amino acids.

Glucose: sugar in the blood; major stimulus of insulin secretion.

Glucocorticoid: includes cortisol, corticosterone, and cortisone; secreted cyclically, with the largest amount being produced in the early morning and the smallest amount produced during evening hours.

Glutamate: the most important excitatory neurotransmitter, occurs in high concentrations in most areas of the CNS.

Glycylcycline: a new class of antibiotics that are structurally related to tetracyclines, and share many of their properties; used for the treatment of complicated skin and skin structure infections caused by methicillin-resistant *Staphylococcus aureus* (MRSA) and vancomycin-sensisitive *Enterococcus faecalis*, as well as treatment of complicated intra-abdominal infections.

Goiter: visible enlargement of the thyroid gland.

Gonadotropin-releasing hormone (GnRH): causes release of follicle-stimulating hormone (FSH) and luteinizing hormone (LH).

Graves' disease: antibody-mediated autoimmune disease resulting in hyperthyroidism. Most common cause of hyperthyroidism.

Gray syndrome: a dangerous condition that occurs in newborns who are given chloramphenicol; may lead to fatalities.

Growth hormone: stimulates growth of body tissues; regulates cell division and protein synthesis required for normal growth and promotes an increase in cell size and number, including growth of muscle cells and lengthening of bone.

Hallucinations: sensory perceptions of people or objects that are not present in the external environment.

Hallucinogen: a substance that produces hallucinations.

Hemostasis: the prevention or stoppage of blood loss from an injured blood vessel and is the process that maintains the integrity of the vascular compartment.

Hepatitis: inflammation of the liver usually caused by a viral infection.

Herpesvirus: any virus belonging to the family Herpesviridae.

Highly active antiretroviral therapy (HAART): several combinations of antiretroviral drugs used at one time to treat HIV/AIDS.

Histamine: found mainly in mast cells surrounding blood vessels and is released when these tissues are injured.

Hormones: chemical messengers to transmit information between body cells and organs.

Human immunodeficiency virus (HIV): an infection caused by a retrovirus that infects the immune system; there are two types of HIV virus identified, HIV-1 and HIV-2; most infections in U.S. are caused by HIV-1; HIV-2 infection occur mainly in Africa; virus is most commonly spread by sexual intercourse; injection of intravenous drugs with contaminated needles; and mucous membrane contact with infected blood or body fluids.

Hypnotic: a drug that produces sleep.

Hypersensitivity: or allergy; may occur with almost any drug; it is unpredictable and unrelated to dose; occurs in patients who have been previously exposed to the drug or a similar substance and who have developed antibodies; drugs react with antibodies to cause cell damage and the release of histamine and other intracellular substances; subsequently producing reactions ranging from mild skin rashes to anaphylactic shock.

Hypercalcemia: abnormally high blood calcium level.

Hyperkalemia: greater than normal concentration of potassium in the blood.

Hyperlipoproteinemias: types of dyslipidemias; increased blood levels of lipoproteins.

Hyperparathyroidism: excessive production of parathyroid hormone (PTH); caused by a tumor or hyperplasia of a parathyroid gland.

Hypertensive crisis: extreme elevations in blood pressure which may result in acute organ damage such as a stroke or MI.

Hyperuricemia: elevated levels of uric acid in the blood resulting from accelerated generation of uric acid through purine metabolism or impaired renal excretion of uric acid.

Hypocalcemia: abnormally low blood calcium level; may be caused by inadequate intake of calcium and Vitamin D.

Hypokalemia: abnormally small amount of potassium in the blood.

Hypomania: persistent irritable mood but absence of psychotic symptoms characteristic of true mania.

Hypoparathyroidism: insufficient production of parathyroid hormone.

Hypothalamus: the link between the nervous and endocrine systems; controls secretions of almost all hormones from the pituitary gland; secretes hormones called releasing and inhibitory factors, which regulate functions of the anterior pituitary.

Hypothalamic-pituitary-adrenocortical (HPA) axis: a negative feed back mechanism by which the body controls cortisol secretion.

Hyperthyroidism: excessive secretion of thyroid hormone; usually involves an enlarged thyroid gland that has an increased number of cells and an increased rate of secretion.

Hypothyroidism: occurs when disease or destruction of thyroid gland tissue causes inadequate production of thyroid hormones.

Hypovolemic shock: a loss of intravascular fluid volume that may be due to actual blood loss or relative loss from fluid shifts within the body.

Immunocompetent: a normal immune response

Immunocompromise: an impaired or weakened immune system.

Immunosuppression: suppression of immune system

Impaction: a mass of hard, dry stool in the rectum; caused by chronic constipation.

Impaired fasting glucose (IFG): an individual with a fasting blood glucose level between 100 mg/dL to 125 mg/dL; also referred to as prediabetes.

Inflammatory bowel disorder: disease characterized by inflammation of the intestines (e.g., ulcerative colitis, Crohn's disease).

Inhibiting hormone: produced by the hypothalamus; decreases hormone secretion that corresponds to each of the major hormones of the anterior pituitary gland.

Inotropy: changes in the force of myocardial contraction.

Insulin: a protein hormone secreted by beta cells in the pancreas; facilitates glucose utilization by cells; absence of insulin results in diabetes mellitus.

Insulin pump: a wearable delivery system for continuous Sub-Q insulin infusion; the insulin dosage is programmed into the pump and the appropriate amount of insulin is injected into the adipose tissue through a needle inserted into the Sub-Q area.

Intraocular pressure (IOP): the pressure inside the eye.

Intrinsic sympathetic activity (ISA): partial agonist activity at adrenergic receptors exerted by beta blockers with ISA properties, due to structural similarity with catecholamines.

Irritable bowel syndrome: a functional disorder of intestinal motility characterized by absence of inflammation or tissue changes; a change in bowel pattern (constipation, diarrhea, or a combination of both); and abdominal pain, bloating, and distention.

Jaundice: yellow discoloration of the skin due to excessive levels of bilirubin in the blood.

Keratin: a tough protein substance that is insoluble in water, weak acids, and weak bases.

Keratitis: inflammation of the cornea.

Ketoacidosis: a metabolic acidosis due to accumulation of ketone bodies formed by the breakdown of fatty acids and amino acids for energy in the absence of insulin.

Ketolides: newer class of antibiotics that belong to the macrolide group; have a more broad spectrum effect compared to macrolides, especially in *Streptococcus pneumoniae infections*.

Lancet: sharp instrument used to prick the finger for blood test.

Lacrimation: production of tears

Laxatives: drugs with mild effects and elimination of soft, formed stool.

Leukemias: cancers of the bone marrow characterized by overproduction of abnormal white blood cells; there are four main types: acute lymphocytic; acute myelogenous; chronic lymphocytic; and chronic myelogenous.

Leukopenia: abnormally low white blood cell count.

Ligands: neurotransmitters as well as medications and hormones that can bind to receptors in the ANS.

Lincosamide: similar to macrolides in its mechanism of action and antimicrobial spectrum.

Lipopeptide: a new class of antibiotics that kills gram positive bacteria by inhibiting synthesis of bacterial proteins, DNA and RNA.

Lipoproteins: specific proteins in plasma that transport blood lipids; each contains cholesterol, phospholipid, and triglyceride bound to protein; vary in density and amounts of lipid and protein.

Loop diuretics: inhibit sodium and chloride reabsorption in the ascending limb of the loop of Henle, where reabsorption of most filtered sodium occurs; diuretics of choice when rapid effects are required and when renal function is impaired.

Macrolides: may be bacteriostatic or bactericidal, depending on drug concentration in infected tissues; widely used for treatment of respiratory tract and skin/soft tissue infections caused by streptococci and staphylococci.

Malignant: cells that grow in an uncontrolled fashion and avoid the restraints (e.g., contact with other cells) that stop the growth of normal cells.

Malignant hyperthermia: a rare but life-threatening complication of anesthesia characterized by hypercarbia, metabolic acidosis, skeletal muscle rigidity, fever, and cyanosis.

Mania: an emotional disorder characterized by euphoria or irritability; usually occurs in bipolar disorder.

Medication history: information about a patient's use of prescription and non-prescription drugs.

Melanocytes: pigment-producing cells located at the junction of the epidermis and the dermis; produce yellow, brown, or black skin coloring in response to genetic influences, melanocyte-stimulating hormone released from the anterior pituitary gland, and exposure to ultraviolet light.

Membrane-stabilizing effect: beta blockers that produce myocardial depression.

Menopause: permanent end of the menstrual cycle; usually occurs in women aged 48-55.

Metabolism: the rate at which cells burn energy.

Metabolic syndrome: a cluster of several cardiovascular risk factors linked with obesity, elevated waist circumference, elevated triglycerides, reduced high-density lipoprotein cholesterol, elevated blood pressure, and elevated fasting glucose.

Metastasis: the spread of malignant cells from one part of the body to another.

Methicillin-resistant _Staphylococcus aureus_ (MRSA): microorganisms resistant to broad-spectrum antibiotics such as penicillin, erythromycin; frequently colonizes nasal passages of health care workers and is increasing as a cause of infection in critical care units.

Methicillin-resistant staphylococcal species non-aureus (SSNA): other strains of antibiotic-resistant staphylococci.

Mineralocorticoid: steroid hormones released by the adrenal cortex; they cause sodium and water retention and potassium excretion.

Miosis: pupil constriction

Monoamine oxidase inhibitors (MAOIs): class of antidepressants used to treat depressive disorders; considered third line medications in the treatment of depression because of a high incidence of food and drug interactions which potentially lead to hypertensive crisis.

Monotherapy: the use of a single drug in drug therapy; has the advantages of fewer adverse drug effects, fewer drug–drug interactions, lower cost, and usually greater patient compliance.

Motion sickness: rapid changes in body motion stimulate receptors in the inner ear (vestibular branch of the auditory nerve, which is concerned with equilibrium), and nerve impulses are transmitted to the vomiting center.

Mottling: permanent discoloration of skin or teeth.

Mucolytics: administered by inhalation to liquefy mucus in the respiratory tract; solutions of mucolytic drugs may be nebulized into a face mask or mouthpiece or instilled directly into the respiratory tract through a tracheostomy.

Mucositis: inflammation and erosion of oral mucous membrane.

Multidrug-resistant tuberculosis (MDR-TB): indicates organisms that are resistant to isoniazid (INH) and rifampin, the most effective drugs available, with or without resistance to other antitubercular drugs; 24 months of drug therapy is often recommended; cure rate is 50%.

Muscarinic receptors: located in most internal organs, including the cardiovascular, respiratory, gastrointestinal, and genitourinary systems. When activated by acetylcholine, the affected cells may be excited or inhibited in their functions.

Muscle spasm: a sudden, involuntary, painful muscle contraction that occurs with musculoskeletal trauma or inflammation.

Mutation: abnormal structural change in the genetic material of a cell.

Myasthenia gravis: an autoimmune disorder in which autoantibodies are thought to destroy nicotinic receptors for acetylcholine on skeletal muscle. As a result, acetylcholine is less able to stimulate muscle contraction, and muscle weakness occurs.

Mycobacterium avium complex (MAC) disease: caused by atypical mycobacteria; occurs mainly in people with advanced human immunodeficiency virus (HIV) infection.

Myelosuppression: bone marrow depression.

Myocardial infarction: interruption in blood supply to a portion of the heart; most commonly due to thrombus formation at the site of a ruptured atherosclerotic plague in the coronary artery. If untreated, infarction or death of myocardium occurs.

Mydriasis: pupil dilation.

Myxedema: adult hypothyroidism; occurs more often in women than in men.

Narcolepsy: sleep disorder that is characterized by daytime "sleep attacks" in which the person goes to sleep at any place or at any time.

Nasolacrimal occlusion: applying pressure on the tear duct.

Nausea: an unpleasant sensation of abdominal discomfort accompanied by a desire to vomit.

Negative feedback: the influence of the output of a system affects the stimulus for the system (e.g., hormone secretion produces an effect that shuts off the stimulus for further hormone secretion).

Neonatal withdrawal syndrome: Occurs in newborns who were exposed to CNS depressants during the third trimester.

Common symptoms include irritability, prolonged crying, respiratory distress, rigidity and possibly seizures.

Nephron: the functional unit of the kidney; each kidney contains approximately 1 million nephrons.

Nephropathy: any disease of the kidney.

Nephrotoxicity: toxic or damaging effect of a substance on the kidney; potentially serious because renal damage interferes with drug excretion, causing drug accumulation and increased adverse effects.

Neuron: structural unit of the nervous system.

Neurogenic shock: due to massive vasodilation caused by suppression of the sympathetic nervous system.

Neuroleptic: antipsychotic drug used to treat disorders that involve thought processes.

Neuroleptic malignant syndrome: a rare but potentially fatal adverse effect; characterized by rigidity, severe hyperthermia, agitation, confusion, delirium, dyspnea, tachycardia, respiratory failure and acute renal failure.

Neuropathic: pain that is caused by lesions or physiologic changes that injure peripheral pain receptors, nerves, or the CNS.

Neurotransmission: neurotransmitters, synapses, and receptors work together to produce communication networks; the interactions between and among these systems promote order or disorder in the body's physical and mental processes.

Neutropenia: low neutrophil count.

Neurotransmitters: chemical substances that carry messages from one neuron to another, or from a neuron to other body tissues, such as cardiac or skeletal muscle.

Nicotinic receptors: located in motor nerves and skeletal muscle; when activated by acetylcholine, the cell membrane depolarizes and produces muscle contraction.

Nitrous oxide: a nonflammable, nonexplosive gas that supports combustion; widely used as a rapidly acting, reversible, nondepressant to supplement other anesthetics.

Nociceptors: pain receptors that are abundant in arterial walls, joint surfaces, muscle fascia, periosteum, skin and soft tissues; they are scarce in most internal organs.

Non-ceiling opioid: opioid with no upper limit to the dosage that can be given to patients who have developed tolerance to previous dosages.

Nonsteroidal anti-inflammatory drugs (NSAIDs): inhibit the synthesis of prostaglandins; used to prevent and treat mild to moderate pain and inflammation.

Norepinephrine: mainly an excitatory neurotransmitter that stimulates the brain to generalized increased activity.

Nosocomial infections: hospital-acquired; may be more severe and difficult to manage because they often result from drug-resistant microorganisms and occur in people whose immunity is impaired.

Nursing process: systematic way of gathering and using information to plan and provide individualized patient care and to evaluate the outcomes of care through use of assessment, nursing diagnosis, planning/goals, interventions, and evaluation.

Obesity: defined as a body mass index (BMI) of 30 or more kg/m^2

Oncogenes: abnormal genes that are mutations of normal growth-regulating genes referred to as proto-oncogenes.

Opioid receptors: delta, kappa, and mu receptors located in the brain and spinal cord; endogenous opioids as well as opioid medications serve as ligands.

Opportunistic: microorganisms that are usually normal endogenous or environmental flora and nonpathogenic; they produce disease in hosts whose defense mechanisms are impaired.

Oral glucose tolerance test (OGTT): test used to determine how the body handles sugar; indicates if a patient has prediabetes or diabetes; test consists of drinking a liquid containing glucose, followed by a blood test 1 hour after consumption.

Organogenesis: formation of fetal organs

Osmotic diuretics: produce rapid diuresis by increasing the osmolarity of plasma and pulling water out of tissues into the bloodstream.

Osteoporosis: decreased bone density and weak, fragile bones that often lead to fractures, pain, and disability.

Ototoxic: adverse effects on the structures of the ear, especially the cochlea and auditory nerve.

Over-the-counter (OTC) drugs: drugs that are available without a prescription.

Overweight: defined as a body mass index (BMI) of 25 to 29.9 kilograms per square meter (kg/m^2)

Oxazolidinones: a newer class of antibiotics; active against aerobic gram-positive bacteria, in which it acts by inhibiting protein synthesis.

Oxytocin: posterior pituitary hormone; it initiates uterine contractions at the end of gestation to induce childbirth, and it causes milk to move from breast glands to nipples.

Paget's disease: an inflammatory skeletal disease that affects older people; characterized by a high rate of bone turnover, bone deformity and pain.

Pain: unpleasant, uncomfortable sensation that usually indicates tissue damage and impels a person to remove the cause of the damage or seek relief from the pain.

Paranoia: the belief that other people control their thoughts, feelings, and behaviors or seek to harm them.

Parasympathetic nervous system: a division of the autonomic nervous system that regulates the routine activities of digestion and elimination; functions stimulated by the parasympathetic nervous system are often described as resting, reparative, or vegetative functions. They include digestion, excretion, cardiac deceleration, anabolism, and near vision.

Parathyroid hormone (PTH): helps regulate calcium and bone metabolism; stimulated by low serum calcium levels

Parkinson's disease: a chronic, progressive, degenerative disorder of the central nervous system (CNS) characterized by resting tremor, bradykinesia, rigidity, and postural instability; also called parkinsonism.

Patient-controlled analgesia: allows the patient to self-administer pain medication through the push of a button on an infusion pump; the amount of drug in each dose delivered is preset and limited.

Penicillin-binding proteins: the binding site within the bacterial cell wall for penicillins; binding disrupts the bacterial cell wall, resulting in bacterial cell lysis.

Parenteral: route of drug administration; injected.

Pharmacoeconomics: involves the costs of drug therapy, including costs of purchasing; dispensing; storage; administration; laboratory and other tests used to monitor patient responses; and losses due to expiration.

Pharmacodynamics: reactions between living systems and drugs; drug actions on target cells and the resulting alterations in cellular biochemical reactions and functions

Pharmacogenetics: study of genetic variations that result in interindividual differences in drug response.

Pharmacotherapy: the use of drugs to prevent, diagnose, or treat signs, symptoms and disease processes.

Pharmacokinetics: drug movement through the body to reach sites of action, metabolism, and excretion.

Phospholipids: major components of the cell membrane portion of all body cells.

Plasmin: an enzyme that breaks down the fibrin meshwork that stabilizes blood clots; also referred to as fibrinolysin.

Plasminogen: an inactive protein found in many body tissues and fluids

Post antibiotic effect: a persistent effect of an antimicrobial on bacterial growth after brief exposure of the organisms to a drug.

Post-ganglionic: nerve fibers from the ganglia to target or effector tissues of the heart, blood vessels, glands, other visceral organs, and smooth muscle.

Pre-ganglionic: nerve fibers from the CNS along the presynaptic nerves to ganglia.

Postsynaptic: occurring after a synapse

Physical dependence: involves physiologic adaptation to chronic use of a drug so that unpleasant symptoms occur when the drug is stopped, when its action is antagonized by another drug, or when its dosage is decreased.

Psychological dependence: involves feelings of satisfaction and pleasure from taking the drug.

Placebo: an inactive substance similar in appearance to the actual drug

Postnatal depression: a major depressive episode occurring after the birth of a child

Potassium-sparing diuretics: act at the distal tubule to decrease sodium reabsorption and potassium excretion; often given in combination with potassium losing diuretics.

Prediabetes: see Impaired fasting glucose.

Preeclampsia/eclampsia: pregnancy induced hypertension that endangers the lives of mother and fetus; preeclampsia is manifested by hypertension and proteinuria; if not effectively treated it may lead to eclampsia, which is characterized by potentially fatal seizures.

Prescription drugs: one of two routes of access to therapeutic drugs; order for medication is written by a licensed health care provider.

Pressor drug: raises blood pressure; maintains tissue perfusion and a mean arterial pressure of at least 80 to 100 mm Hg by producing vasoconstriction and increased blood pressure.

Presynaptic: occurring before a synapse.

Preterm labor: uterine contractions with cervical changes before 37 weeks of gestation; may occur spontaneously or be precipitated by premature rupture of membranes or other factorss.

Prodrugs: drugs initially inactive and exert no pharmacologic effects until they are metabolized.

Progestin: female sex hormone produced along with estrogen by the ovaries and adrenal cortex; most often used in combination with an estrogen in contraceptive products.

Prokinetics: increase the release of acetylcholine from nerve endings in the GI tract, increasing GI motility and gastric emptying; also antagonize dopamine in the brain; useful in prevention of delayed nausea and vomiting associated with chemotherapy.

Prostaglandins: chemical mediators found in most body tissues; they help regulate many cell functions and participate in the inflammatory response; help initiate uterine contractions in labor.

Protein binding: many drugs form a compound with plasma proteins, mainly albumin, which act as carriers; allows part of a drug dose to be stored and released as needed.

Proto-oncogenes: normal growth-regulating genes; present in all body cells; when exposed to carcinogens and genetically altered to oncogenes, they may operate continuously and cause abnormal, disordered, and unregulated cell growth.

Prototype: an example of a group of drugs, often the first one of the group to be developed.

Pruritus: itching.

Psoriasis: a chronic, inflammatory disorder attributed to activated T lymphocytes which produce cytokines that stimulate abnormal growth of affected skin cells and blood vessels; results in excessively rapid turnover of epidermal cells; skin lesions may occur anywhere but typically occur on the elbows and knees.

Psychosis: a severe mental disorder characterized by disorganized thought processes, hallucinations, and delusions.

Pyrogen: fever producing agent.

Quaternary amines: anticholinergic drugs that carry a positive charge and are lipid insoluble; they do not readily cross cell membranes; are poorly absorbed from the GI tract and do not cross the blood–brain barrier.

Receptors: proteins that are embedded in cell membranes of body tissues.

Red man syndrome: an adverse reaction when vancomycin is administered too quickly; hypotension, flushing, and skin rash may occur.

Refraction: light rays deflected in various directions according to the density of the ocular structures through which they pass.

Releasing hormones: produced by the hypothalamus; accelerate the secretion of anterior pituitary hormones.

Remission: the symptom free period in disease; particularly cancer.

Retrovirus: virus with an RNA genome that relies on reverse transcriptase to transform its genome from RNA to DNA. HIV is a retrovirus.

Reye's syndrome: a potentially fatal disease characterized by encephalopathy and fatty liver accumulations. It is associated with the use of aspirin and NSAIDs after viral infections such as chickenpox or influenza in children and adolescents.

Rhinitis: inflammation and congestion of nasal mucosa; most common cause of sinusitis.

Rhinorrhea: secretions discharged from the nose.

Rosacea: a chronic disease characterized by erythema, telangiectases (fine, red, superficial blood vessels) and acne-like lesions of facial skin; usually occurs in middle-aged and older people and more commonly in men then women.

Salicylism: may occur with an acute overdose of a salicylate drug or with chronic use of therapeutic doses, especially the higher doses taken for anti-inflammatory effects.

Sarcomas: malignant tumors that develop from connective tissue (muscle, bone, cartilage, fibrous tissue, fat, blood vessels).

Schizophrenia: a variety of related psychotic disorders; symptoms include: agitation, behavioral disturbances, delusions, disorganized speech, hallucinations, insomnia, and paranoia.

Sedative: drug that produces CNS depression.

Second messenger: a signaling molecule that activates proteins inside cells to exert a cellular response.

Seizure: involves a brief episode of abnormal electrical activity in nerve cells of the brain that may or may not be accompanied by visible changes in appearance or behavior.

Seizure threshold: the amount of stimulation required to produce a seizure.

Selective serotonin reuptake inhibitors (SSRIs): first line medications in the treatment of depression.

Septic shock: due to massive vasodilation in response to overwhelming infection.

Serology: identifies infectious agents indirectly by measuring the antibody level (titer) in the serum of a diseased host.

Serotonin: a major neurotransmitter in the CNS; thought to produce sleep by inhibiting CNS activity and arousal; serotonin receptors are associated with mood, anxiety, and temperature regulation.

Serotonin syndrome: a serious and sometimes fatal reaction characterized by hypertensive crisis, hyperpyrexia, extreme agitation progressing to delirium and coma, muscle rigidity, and seizures; may occur due to combined therapy with an SSRI and an MAO inhibitor or other drugs that potentiate serotonin neurotransmission.

Serum drug level: a laboratory measurement of the amount of a drug in the blood at a particular time.

Serum half-life: also called elimination half-life, is the time required for the serum concentration of a drug to decrease by 50%.

Signal transduction: movement of signals from outside the cell to inside the cell.

Sinusitis: inflammation of the paranasal sinuses, air cells that connect with the nasal cavity and are lined with similar mucosa.

Somatotropin: see growth hormone.

Spasticity: caused by nerve damage in the brain and spinal cord, it is a permanent condition that may be painful and disabling; involves increased muscle tone or contraction and stiff, awkward movements.

Status epilepticus: repeated seizures or a seizure that lasts for at least 30 minutes; may be convulsive, nonconvulsive, or partial.

Steroids: lipid soluble hormones produced by the gonadal organs or the adrenal cortex.

Stomatitis: see mucositis.

Streptogramins: class of antibacterial drugs; produced by a bacterium of the genus *Streptomyces* (*S. graminofaciens*).

Substance abuse: self-administration of a drug for prolonged periods or in excessive amounts to the point of producing physical or psychological dependence; impairing functions of body organs; reducing the ability to function in usual activities of daily living; and decreasing the ability and motivation to function as a productive member of society; excessive use of drugs or alcohol.

Substance P: a peptide neurotransmitter in the neurokinin family; plays a role in neurotransmission of pain impulses.

Substantia nigra: dopamine producing nerve cells; site of origination for Parkinson's disease.

Sulfonamides: bacteriostatic against a wide range of gram-positive and gram-negative bacteria, although increasing resistance is making them less useful.

Susceptibility: tests that determine which drugs are likely to be effective against the organism causing an infection.

Sustained-release: controlled release oral tablets or capsules; slowly absorbed medication; effects prolonged, usually 12-24 hours; contain relatively large amounts of active drug.

Sympathetic nervous system: a branch of the autonomic nervous system responsible for a basal level of activity (sympathetic tone). Becomes more active during stress and its action during the stress response is termed the fight-or-flight reaction.

Synapse: a microscopic gap that separates neurons in a chain.

Systemic effects: drugs that are absorbed by the body, circulated through the bloodstream to their sites of action in various body tissues, and eventually eliminated from the body.

Tardive dyskinesia: an irreversible late extrapyramidal effect of some antipsychotic drugs.

Teratogenic: having adverse effects on the fetus.

Tertiary amines: anticholinergic drugs that are uncharged lipid-soluble molecules; able to cross cell membranes readily; are well absorbed from the gastrointestinal (GI) tract and conjunctiva, and they cross the blood–brain barrier.

Testosterone: male sex hormone; secreted by the Leydig's cells in the testes.

Tetany: prolonged and painful spasms of the voluntary muscles, associated with hypocalcemia.

Tetracyclines: antibacterials effective against a wide range of gram-positive and gram-negative organisms, although they are usually not drugs of choice.

Thiazides: diuretic drugs that are chemically related to the sulfonamides; often prescribed for the management of hypertension and heart failure; they act to decrease reabsorption of sodium, water, chloride, and bicarbonate in the distal convoluted tubule of the kidney.

Thrombocytopenia: low platelet count.

Thrombogenesis: formation of a blood clot.

Thrombolysis: the break down or dissolution of blood clots.

Thrombolytic: a drug that dissolves blood clots.

Thrombus: presence of a blood clot.

Thyroiditis: a common cause of primary hypothyroidism; it is an autoimmune disorder characterized by inflammation of the thyroid gland.

Thyroid-stimulating hormone (TSH): regulates secretion of thyroid hormones.

Thyroid storm: a rare but severe complication characterized by extreme symptoms of hyperthyroidism; most likely to occur in patients with hyperthyroidism that has been inadequately treated, especially when stressful situations occur; also known as thryotoxic crisis.

Thyroxine: one of three hormones produced by the thyroid gland.

Tinea pedis: a common type of ringworm infection; also called athlete's foot.

Tocolytics: drugs used to stop preterm labor

Tolerance: patients who have developed drug tolerance through long-term use of lesser doses.

Tonic: muscle spasms with sustained contraction.

Tonic-clonic: most common type of seizure; often referred to as a major motor seizure. The tonic phase involves sustained contraction of skeletal muscles; abnormal postures, such as opisthotonos; and absence of respiration, during which the person becomes cyanotic. The clonic phase is characterized by rapid rhythmic and symmetric jerking movements of the body.

Tonometry: diagnostic test to measure the pressure inside the eye (IOP) to determine if glaucoma is present.

Tophi: deposits of uric acid crystals in the joints, kidneys, and soft tissues.

Topical: application of drug to skin or mucus membrane.

Transdermal: absorption of drug through the skin.

Travelers' diarrhea: occurs during or shortly after travel; usually caused by fecal contamination of food and/or water.

Up-regulation: the increase in receptor responsiveness when they are chronically exposed to substances that block their function.

Uricosuric: drug that increases urinary excretion of uric acid.

Urinary antiseptics: used only to treat urinary tract infections; may be bactericidal for sensitive organisms in the urinary tract.

Urticaria: an inflammatory response characterized by a skin lesion called a wheal, a raised edematous area with a pale center and red border, which itches intensely; also known as hives.

Vancomycin-resistant enterococci (VRE): pathogenic bacteria that are resistant to vancomycin.

Vasodilators: a drug that causes dilation of the blood vessels.

Vasogenic shock: see distributive shock.

Vasopressor: a substance that constricts blood vessels and raises blood pressure.

Viral hepatitis: liver inflammation due to a virus; there are five different viruses that cause viral hepatitis: Hepatitis A, B, C, D, and G.

Viral load: a measure of the number of HIV RNA particles within the blood; it does not measure viral levels in tissues, where viral reproduction may be continuing.

Virus(es): intracellular parasites that survive only in living tissues; they are officially classified according to their structure, but are more commonly described according to origin and the disorders or symptoms they produce.

Vitamin D (calciferol): a fat-soluble vitamin that includes both ergocalciferol (obtained from foods) and cholecalciferol (formed by exposure of skin to sunlight); functions as a hormone and plays an important role in calcium and bone metabolism; main action of vitamin D is to raise serum calcium levels by increasing intestinal absorption of calcium and mobilizing calcium from bone.

Vomiting: the expulsion of stomach contents through the mouth.

Vomiting center: a nucleus of cells in the medulla oblongata.

Chapter 2

2-1   Mrs. Green is elderly and has a failing memory. Instead of a calendar, a pill tray or box with divided sections for each day and each time of day might work more effectively. The pill box should be filled by the nurse on her weekly visits and Mrs. Green should be instructed on the proper use of the pill container. The family or some other close support person should also be instructed regarding Mrs. Green's medication schedule and if a family member is available between visits, oversight of her medication should help prevent overdosage.

Chapter 3

3-1   This medication error occurred because the medication was given to the wrong patient. You did not check the patient's name band and relied on the patient to respond to your calling his name. In this situation, the patient had been asleep and may have been responding simply to being awakened. Also, Mr. Sanchez's memory deficits and altered mental status may have contributed. Accurate identification of the patient is imperative, especially when the patient may be confused or unable to respond appropriately.

Chapter 4

4-1   Ibuprofen is used to manage Mr. Walker's arthritis. Hypertension is an indication for both furosemide and captopril. Most likely, Mr. Walker takes famotidine to treat heartburn. The dosages are all within the normal range and are on the lower end of the dosage range, which is appropriate for the elderly.

4-2   Potential nursing diagnoses for Mr. Walker might include Noncompliance to appropriate drug therapy, Risk for Injury related to Adverse Drug Effects, Risk for Injury related to Overdose, Risk for Loneliness, and Deficient Knowledge related to Drug Administration.

4-3   Mr. Walker takes several medications in various amounts at several times during the day. Older adults often have trouble administering more than three or four drugs. Mr. Walker is currently taking four different medications. Implement strategies to make sure Mr. Walker is taking the right drug, in the right dose, at the right time. Make sure that Mr. Walker's drugs are clearly labeled. Create a chart clearly depicting his medication regimen, or use/prepare a special drug container with prepared doses labeled with the correct time. Enlist his daughter's help.

Chapter 6

6-1   4 mg of morphine. Because this is the initial 24 hours after surgery and the pain is severe, morphine is the drug of choice. Start with the lowest effective dose and increase as needed. Larger doses have an increased risk of causing adverse effects. Also recognize that Mr. Harris has used pain medication for a long time and may require a higher dose of medication to control his pain.

6-2   Prepare to administer naloxone (Narcan) and assist with ventilation as needed. Naloxone is the drug of choice for opioid overdose.

6-3   Lortab is 5 mg of hydrocodone and 500 mg of acetaminophen. What is ordered is oxycodone. Roxicet 5/500 is 5 mg of oxycodone and 500 mg of acetaminophen. The nurse must recognize the difference between oral pain medications and these two different opioids.

Chapter 7

7-1   GI bleeding. Taking ASA, caffeine, and naproxen sodium may lead to GI irritation and bleeding.

7-2   It is necessary to recognize that cold and flu medication frequently has acetaminophen added for analgesic effect. The cumulative effects of multiple medications with acetaminophen may lead to hepatic failure.

7-3   The patient needs to increase fluid intake to 2 to 3 liters of fluid a day and take drugs with food. This will decrease gastric irritation and help maintain kidney function.

7-4   The total amount of acetaminophen may approach or exceed 9000 milligrams (9 g) in a 24-hour period, and this may lead to hepatic damage. The maximum recommended daily dose of acetaminophen should not exceed 4 grams in 24 hours.

Chapter 8

8-1   Help Mrs. Portman's daughter understand how the drugs help to manage her mother's anxiety and symptoms of agitation. The concern for the patient's safety needs to be emphasized. Perhaps a team meeting of the health care professionals involved in her mother's care would help her to accept the plan to care for her mother.

8-2   Prepare to administer alprazolam 0.25 mg, the smallest ordered dose. Daytime drowsiness or impaired mobility are signs of too much medication. Also, Mrs. Portman is elderly, so one half of the adult dose is recommended.

8-3   These symptoms are typical for withdrawal of benzodiazepines. Tapering the drug may reduce the likelihood of withdrawal symptoms or Mrs. Portman may need to continue on the medication for a longer period of time.

Chapter 9

9-1   Parkinsonism is a common side effect of antipsychotic medication. Notify the physician; antiparkinson drugs may be given along with the antipsychotic drugs.

9-2   The dizziness is most likely due to orthostatic hypotension as a side effect of the risperidone. Have Ms. Jones change position gradually, lie down for an hour after taking her medication, elevate her legs when in a sitting position, and avoid hot baths.

9-3   These symptoms are typical of neuroleptic malignant syndrome. This is a rare but potentially fatal reaction that requires rapid treatment.

Chapter 10

10-1   The nurse should never leave an antidepressant at the bedside. Charting the medication as given when it has not yet been taken by the patient is not truthful, and the patient may forget to take the medication or may hold the medication for a later time and save up multiple doses. This is especially problematic with a patient suffering from depression because he or she may have suicidal ideations.

10-2   Some antidepressant medications, such as sertraline, are in the class of selective serotonin reuptake inhibitors (SSRIs), which may not reach a therapeutic effect for up to 2 to 4 weeks. Provide appropriate teaching for both the patient and his wife regarding therapeutic effect. Check to make sure that Mr. Mehring is taking the right dosage. Encourage him to continue taking the medication.

10-3   Check with the physician to see if Mr. Mehring's dose can be taken once a day in the morning. If this is not possible, then check to see if a different SSRI can be given that has once-a-day dosing. Taking the dose in the morning may solve Mr. Mehring's sleeping difficulty if the problem is due to the drug and not due to the depression.

Chapter 11

11-1   Monitor the phenytoin level. The normal free phenytoin level is 0.8 to 2 mcg/mL. Adequate serum levels are needed for seizure control.

11-2   Ask if Frank is taking a monoamine oxidase (MAO) inhibitor, which may be used to treat depression. Carbamazepine should not be taken within 14 days of an MAO inhibitor.

11-3   The patient must always taper the dosage of an AED gradually, or the seizures may exacerbate.

Chapter 12

12-1   Provide patient teaching and inform Mrs. Sung that the drug she is taking acts quickly and must be taken several times a day in order to provide relief of her symptoms. The half-life of levodopa/carbidopa is only 1 to 3 hours. Her friend is most likely taking a different medication.

12-2   A referral for physical therapy is most appropriate. Gait training and a widened stance will provide Mrs. Sung with increased balance and a better base of support.

12-3   The pharmacy provided the correct drug and the correct strength; however, it provided the extended-release form of the drug when the immediate-release form was ordered. In addition to checking the drug name and strength, you must check the dosage form.

Chapter 13

13-1   Patients with MS should be encouraged to avoid emotional stress; exposure to extremes in environmental temperature; infection; and excessive fatigue

13-2   Baclofen should not be given if it causes excessive muscle weakness and impairs rather than facilitates mobility and function. Contact Mrs. Milweski's physician.

13-3   Provide patient/caregiver teaching. Baclofen should be given with milk or food to reduce gastrointestinal irritation.

Chapter 14

14-1   The first step is for Mr. Wilson to realize he is abusing alcohol and other drugs. His cooperation in the treatment program is critical to his success. The program should consist of psychological counseling, referral to a self-help group, and drug therapy.

14-2   A benzodiazepine antianxiety agent is the drug of choice. This drug will help Mr. Wilson participate in his rehabilitation program and can be gradually reduced in dosage. Taking a benzodiazepine will provide Mr. Wilson with adequate sedation and will also have a significant anticonvulsant effect.

14-3   Antabuse is a drug that interferes with the metabolism of alcohol. If Mr. Wilson drinks alcohol while on Antabuse, he will experience hypotension, tachycardia, syncope, blurred vision, headache, and confusion. Mr. Wilson must know what he is taking and cooperate with the treatment plan.

14-4   Mr. Wilson needs further instruction regarding his medication. He can stop taking Zyban when he no longer craves nicotine; however, he must continue to take the Antabuse.

Chapter 15

15-1   Inform the teacher that there is no legitimate use of this drug by athletes. Kevin, his parents, and the principal of the school should be informed of the behavior. There is no need to disclose any of Kevin's personal health information.

15-2 Kevin is most likely having a toxicity reaction. Place him in a cool room that has minimal external stimulation. Monitor Kevin's heart rate, blood pressure, and temperature.

15-3 Losing weight is a common adverse effect of methylphenidate. Evaluate how well Kevin is eating. Provide tips on taking drugs safely and accurately. Instruct Kevin to take his medication 30 to 45 minutes before meals and to take his last dose of the day before 6 pm. Taking the drugs before meals will minimize the drug's appetite-suppressing effects, and taking this medication before 6 pm will avoid interference with sleep.

Chapter 17

17-1 Epinephrine is not given orally because the enzymes in the GI tract and liver destroy it.

17-2 Epinephrine 1:1000 has a 1 mg/1 mL concentration. To yield a 1:10,000 solution, 10 mL of normal saline should have been used. Read drug-mixing instructions carefully.

17-3 Mr. Sobechenko has had an anaphylactic reaction to an antibiotic. Make sure to advise Mr. Sobechenko of his allergy and note it on his chart. Observe the patient for increased blood pressure, tachycardia, and hyperglycemia (adverse effects of epinephrine).

Chapter 18

18-1 Lopressor will act as an antianginal and antihypertensive drug for Mr. Jones. It also may protect the heart from reinfarction.

18-2 Clonidine is effective in reducing blood pressure. Clonidine exerts its effect by reducing central nervous system outflow, a physiologic effect that raises blood pressure.

18-3 Beta-blocking medication should be discontinued slowly, over 1 to 3 weeks. Notify the physician and pharmacy if the patient cannot/will not take the substituted drug; do not stop the beta-blocker drugs abruptly.

18-4 Diabetic patients are prone to hypoglycemia as an adverse effect of their antidiabetic medication. Mr. Jones is at risk for more severe and prolonged hypoglycemia because he is taking Lopressor (metoprolol). The nurse should assess the blood sugar in a diabetic patient more carefully.

Chapter 19

19-1 The nurse should follow the patient request. Most patients with myasthenia gravis require a higher dose of medication with increased physical activity. Ms. Humbarger is probably not as active in the hospital and will require less medication.

19-2 Betty Humbarger is experiencing a myasthenic crisis. Signs and symptoms having an onset within approximately 1 hour after a dose of an anticholinesterase drug are more likely to be caused by a cholinergic crisis or too much drug. Signs and symptoms beginning 3 hours or more after an anticholinesterase drug are more likely to be caused by a myasthenic crisis or too little drug. The nurse should respond to a myasthenic crisis by the administration of more anticholineserase drug.

Chapter 20

20-1 The nurse should expect to see an increase in the heart rate. Atropine is an anticholinergic drug that blocks the parasympathetic vagus nerve, thereby preventing slowing.

20-2 Encourage the patient to increase the fiber in his diet and to drink 2-3 quarts of fluid a day, unless otherwise contraindicated, to help with the constipation. Notify the physician of Mr. Smoot's urinary retention and constipation.

20-3 Mr. Bing has a history of glaucoma. Scopolamine is an anticholinergic medication and is contraindicated for a patient with glaucoma.

Chapter 22

22-1 The ordered dose is to be given in two divided doses. The nurse should have administered 0.1 mL in the first dose and the other 0.1 mL in the second dose.

22-2 Monitor Mr. Rojas's daily weight, intake and output, and when available, the urine specific gravity. A patient with diabetes insipidus will lose 8 to 10 L of urine a day or more. The nurse must monitor the fluid status of the patient.

22-3 Mr. Rojas is most likely having a serious adverse reaction to the desmopressin. Hyponatremia and water retention should be reported to the physician and you should continue to monitor the patient.

22-4 The nurse has a professional responsibility to discuss the situation with the boys' mother. Excessive hormone increases the risk of health problems for Miguel and Juan needs an adequate dose to be therapeutic.

Chapter 23

23-1 Notify Ms. Hubble's physician. This is a sign of thrush or oral candidiasis, a fungal infection. The patient requires immediate treatment and may not be able to continue on the prednisone if the infection becomes systemic. Systemic fungal infections are a contraindication to the administration of corticosteroids.

23-2 Prednisone is a drug that will treat the symptoms of COPD, but it is not designed to cure the underlying disease process. Because the drug reduces respiratory inflammation, Ms. Hubble will have less difficulty with breathing.

23-3   Prednisone causes hyperglycemia in many patients and especially in patients with diabetes mellitus. The physician should be notified for a change in Ms. Hubble's diabetic medication. Also, the nurse should review Ms. Hubble's diet.

23-4   The teaching plan should include taking the drug as ordered, carrying medical alert identification that includes the drugs taken, taking measures to avoid infection, and observing for any signs of infection or delayed wound healing. The nurse should encourage activity as tolerated to prevent osteoporosis, and teach the patient when to seek medical attention.

Chapter 24

24-1   Change the medication time to 7:30 a.m. to assure that Synthroid is given on an empty stomach. Taking the drug on an empty stomach will increase its absorption.

24-2   Teach Ms. Zalewski to maintain a diet that is low in fat and calories and high in fiber, and to monitor for variations in weight.

24-3   Evaluate Ms. Zalewski's TSH level. The normal range is 0.5–4.2 microunits/L. Her symptoms are typical of a patient with hyperthyroidism. Notify the prescriber of these symptoms.

24-4   Synthroid should not be given with an antacid, iron preparation, or sucralfate. These drugs decrease the absorption of Synthroid. If the patient requires an antacid, the antacid should be given 2 hours before or 4 to 6 hours after the dose of Synthroid.

Chapter 25

25-1   Alendronate must be taken 30 minutes prior to any intake of food, fluid, or other medication. Alendronate is very poorly absorbed from the gastrointestinal tract and any other substance will diminish the absorption of this medication.

25-2   For most individuals, a daily intake of between 1000 to 1500 mg of calcium is recommended. Milk and dairy products contain high levels of calcium. Two 8-oz glasses of milk provide one half of the daily calcium requirement (600 mg). Postmenopausal women should increase their calcium intake to 1500 mg per day. Weight-bearing exercise and adequate vitamin D intake are also important teaching points.

25-3   Any patient taking alendronate needs to be instructed to remain in an upright position for at least 30 minutes after taking this medication. Avoiding the supine position reduces the risk of esophageal irritation.

Chapter 26

26-1   This insulin is a mixed type composed of both regular and NPH insulins. The peak times for both of these insulins would be when Mr. Coulter is most likely to experience hypoglycemia. The nurse should be especially watchful for the signs and symptoms of hypoglycemia at 2 to 3 hours after insulin administration and again at 8 to 12 hours after administration.

26-2   Measure Mr. Coulter's blood glucose level if possible. Also, give the patient 15 grams of carbohydrate. This would include sugar, candy, fruit juice, or 4 ounces of regular soda.

26-3   Deficient Knowledge: Antidiabetic drugs and administration, diet and management of hypoglycemia and other complications. Based on assessment data, this is a priority diagnosis and nursing interventions are necessary.

26-4   You should hold the metformin for 48 hours prior to any diagnostic test involving radiographic contrast media. Mr. Coulter will be NPO the morning of the test and should not take his medication until the test is over and he is able to eat. The metformin will continue on hold for 48 hours after the test. The combination of metformin and contrast media containing iodine may lead to renal failure and/or lactic acidosis.

Chapter 27

27-1   Explain to Vickie that her color-coded tablets have different amounts of medication in them, making them more closely resemble the normal variations in hormones in the body. Emphasize the need to take the tablets in the correct sequence.

27-2   Vickie should stop taking the oral contraceptives and her pregnancy state should be evaluated. Pregnancy is a contraindication for continuation of the hormones. Damage may occur to the fetus if oral contraceptives are taken during pregnancy.

27-3   Instruct Vickie to take her pills with food or at bedtime to reduce nausea. If the nausea continues and she cannot take the pills in continued sequence, perhaps considering another form of contraception would be appropriate.

27-4   Vickie should have been instructed to use an alternate method of birth control while she is on antibiotics. Antibiotics decrease the effectiveness of oral contraceptives

Chapter 28

28-1   Teach Ms. Watson to weigh herself and to have her blood pressure assessed regularly. She should call her physician immediately if she becomes pregnant.

28-2   Assess for hirsutism, deepening of the voice, and menstrual irregularities.

28-3   You have an obligation to explain the health risks of untreated hypertension. Patient teaching guidelines would include discussing health habits that may be contributing to the problem.

Chapter 29

29-1 Teach all patients to take all of the prescribed doses and not to stop when their symptoms are relieved. Failure to take all of the medication may lead to an increased risk for a drug-resistant infection. Additionally, teach all patients not to take antibiotics left over from a previous illness. The likelihood of having the right drug in the right amount to adequately treat the infection is extremely small. This practice of taking leftover medication may also lead to an increased risk of developing a drug-resistant infection.

29-2 Collect specimens for culture before the first dose of an antibiotic is given, unless a life-threatening infection is present. Practice impeccable infection-control principles, including frequent and thorough hand hygiene, proper use of gloves, and proper handling and disposal of body fluids. Schedule antibiotics at evenly spaced intervals around the clock, to maintain therapeutic blood levels. Check specific recommendations with regard to the administration of the antibiotic with food and other medication to decrease binding to food and drugs and prevent inactivation. Follow all instructions for mixing and storing medication and check expiration dates. Give parenteral antibiotics alone; do not mix with any other drug, to avoid chemical and physical incompatibilities that may cause drug precipitation or inactivation. Flush the IV tubing after each dose to ensure the entire dose is administered.

Chapter 30

30-1 First-generation cephalosporins are the drug of choice for surgical prophylaxis. They are active against a large number of bacteria and have a low incidence of adverse effects.

30-2 The physician, pharmacist, and nurse should ask Ms. Jang if she has ever taken penicillin and if she has ever had an allergic reaction. Penicillin is the most common cause of drug-induced anaphylaxis.

30-3 Tell Ms. Jang to call 911. She should be transported to the nearest emergency facility immediately. This is most likely a severe reaction to the penicillin.

30-4 The nurse should recognize that piperacillin-tazobactam (Zosyn) is a combination of a penicillin and a beta-lactamase inhibitor. An allergy to any penicillin means that Ms. Jang cannot receive any other penicillin-containing drug.

Chapter 31

31-1 Mr. Dallas should wait for 2 hours before or after he has taken the Cipro before taking an antacid for his indigestion. Antacids interfere with the absorption of fluoroquinolones from the GI tract.

31-2 Assess Mr. Dallas's hearing and his renal function because gentamicin is ototoxic and nephrotoxic.

31-3 The patient should be encouraged to take 2 to 3 liters of fluid a day unless contraindicated. The intake of fluid will help prevent nephrotoxicity.

Chapter 32

32-1 Sharon needs fluid intake of at least 2 to 3 liters daily. The fluid will keep her urine diluted and reduce the multiplication of bacteria.

32-2 The Bactrim will increase the skin's sensitivity to sunlight and sunburn. Sharon is already at risk due to the tetracycline. Advise her to wear sunscreen and protective clothing.

32-3 Tetracyclines should not be taken within 2 hours of food that contains dairy products; antacids; or iron supplements. The combination of a tetracycline with calcium, iron, aluminum, or magnesium results in an insoluble compound that prevents the absorption of tetracycline.

Chapter 33

33-1 Azithromycin should be taken on an empty stomach with 6 to 8 ounces of water. Do not take any antacid products for 2 hours before or 2 hours after a dose of azithromycin. Take the medication at the same time each day until all of the pills are gone. Adequate water intake aids absorption. Taking the drug at regular intervals helps to maintain a therapeutic blood level. Finishing the drug will help decrease the risks of inadequate treatment and drug resistance.

33-2 Assess for the occurrence of adverse GI effects such as nausea, vomiting, or continued diarrhea. Mr. Nikki should be aware that he may have a metallic taste in his mouth due to the metronidazole. Also observe for CNS adverse effects, such as seizures or peripheral neuropathy.

33-3 Teach Mr. Nikki to monitor himself for abdominal pain, nausea, vomiting, diarrhea, and/or yellow discoloration of the eyes or skin.

Chapter 34

34-1 The primary reason for MDR-TB is a failure to take the medication as prescribed.

34-2 Assess for the occurrence of hepatotoxicity. The signs and symptoms might include anorexia, nausea, fatigue, malaise, and/or jaundice. You would also want to monitor the liver enzymes ALT and AST for an increase.

34-3 Rifampin may cause a red-orange coloration to the urine and other body fluids. Although it will permanently stain clothing and other objects, it is not harmful to the patient.

Chapter 35

35-1 The nurse should look at the results of the CBC, HIV-RNA and the CD4+ cell count to measure Tony's response to his drug therapy.

35-2   He may take his Combivir with food to decrease the GI upset; however, he should take the Efavirenez on an empty stomach.

35-3   Filgrastim is given because zidovudine in the Combivir depresses the bone marrow and causes neutropenia. Filgrastim should increase the white cell count.

Chapter 36

36-1   Charlotte should be assessed for pregnancy before taking fluconazole. Azole drugs are contraindicated in pregnancy.

36-2   Assess for nausea, vomiting, diarrhea, abdominal pain, headache, or skin rash, although these symptoms only occur in about 3% of patients. You should also be aware of the risk of liver dysfunction

36-3   Patients who receive IV amphotericin B should be assessed for fever, chills, and tachypnea. Infusion reactions from IV amphotericin B should be reported. Charlotte should be premedicated with acetaminophen, diphenhydramine, and a corticosteroid.

Chapter 37

37-1   Metronidazole is contraindicated in the first trimester of pregnancy. Also, the patient should avoid all forms of alcohol while taking this medication.

37-2   Teach Ms. Michelson to use proper hand and other personal hygiene techniques. She should avoid raw fish and undercooked meat. Encourage Ms. Michelsen to take all of her medication and to have follow-up care.

37-3   Chlorquine should be taken with meals to decrease GI irritation.

Chapter 39

39-1.   Assess for the presence of fever, immunosuppressive drug therapy, immunodeficiency states, leukemia, lymphoma or generalized malignancy and pregnancy. The administration of vaccines and toxoids is usually contraindicated with these conditions.

39-2.   The best source for current immunization information is the CDC Web site (www.cdc.gov). Health care providers should update their knowledge at least annually.

39-3.   Do not use any vaccine that has been stored at room temperature. To maintain effectiveness of the vaccine, MMR requires refrigeration and protection from light.

Chapter 40

40-1   Teach Mrs. Paul to get adequate rest and sleep, to eat a nutritious diet and to practice meticulous personal hygiene.

40-2   Pegfilgrastim should not be administered for 14 days before the next dose of chemotherapy or within 24 hours following a treatment.

40-3   An adequate intake of iron is needed for epoetin alfa to be effective. A nutritional supplement of iron is usually necessary in addition to dietary sources.

Chapter 41

41-1   Monitor Mr. Kinney's WBC and platelet counts. The adverse reactions to mycophenolate are neutropenia and thrombocytopenia.

41-2   Cyclosporine and sirolimus should not be given at the same time. The drugs should be taken 4 hours apart. The concomitant administration of cyclosporine and sirolimus can increase the blood level of sirolimus to possible toxic levels.

41-3   The following teaching points are appropriate: Do not substitute brands of cyclosporine, and report to the primary care provider if a decreased urinary output is observed. Take mycophenolate on an empty stomach. Take sirolimus 4 hours after the dose of cyclosporine and do not take it with grapefruit juice. All of these drugs should be taken at the same time each day and you should report to the primary care provider if you cannot take the medication as ordered for any reason. Take no other drugs without medical supervision. Take precautions to prevent infection.

41-4   Mr. Kinney is at a greatly increased risk of a serious infection and perhaps a life-threatening complication. In addition to the immunosuppressed state putting Mr. Kinney at risk for infection, the immunosuppressant drugs slow the proliferation of lymphocytes and damage rapidly dividing nonimmune cells.

Chapter 42

42-1   The most common adverse effects are bone marrow depression, mucositis, alopecia, and GI ulceration. Julia will need periodic blood tests to determine the degree of bone marrow depression. Nutrition will be important. Julia should have a plan for the alopecia (perhaps including purchasing a wig prior to her hair loss). Be sure to review medications to prevent and treat the adverse effects with Julia.

42-2   Although there is some risk, the benefit is that Herceptin will bind with a substance called *human epidermal growth factor receptor(2)*, which is present in excess in 25%- 30% of women with breast cancer.

42-3   Tell Julia that every precaution is taken when administering this medication and that she will be medicated before the infusion to reduce the occurrence of a serious allergic reaction.

42-4   Ensure that the orders are appropriate; do not accept verbal or telephone orders.

Chapter 44

44-1　The salmeterol in the Advair is long acting and only for prophylaxis of acute bronchoconstriction. The appropriate medication for acute asthma attacks is the albuterol.

44-2　Explain to Lynne that she is receiving the same type of medication in her inhaled Advair (contains fluticasone). An inhaled corticosteroid will minimize systemic absorption and adverse effects. Topical application will reduce the inflammation.

44-3　Respiratory assessment should consist of observation of the patient's breathing pattern. Observe for a respiratory rate less than 12 or above 24 breaths per minute, dyspnea, cough, or wheezing respirations. Indications of severe respiratory distress include tachypnea, the use of accessory muscles, and hypoxia.

Chapter 45

45-1　Loratadine should be taken on an empty stomach. Do not take both loratadine and diphenhydramine. Wear sunscreen if exposed to sunlight. Inform your physician if you become pregnant, and do not consume alcohol.

45-2　First-generation antihistamines such as diphenhydramine are less costly and may provide an alternative to the higher cost of the second-generation antihistamines. Caution Ms. Fisher that if she switches drugs, the first-generation drugs cause more drowsiness.

45-3　Since the nurse is unlikely to have an opportunity to teach about individual OTC medications, it is important to advise. Ms. Fisher to read the medication label on all OTC medication. She needs to be especially careful when medicating a small child. Loratadine is only approved for use in children 2 years and older.

Chapter 46

46-1　Remind everyone of the need for frequent and thorough hand hygiene. Infected people with viruses on their hands touch objects that uninfected people will touch, thereby transferring the viruses.

46-2　Appropriate patient teaching with regard to nasal sprays should include not using a nasal spray for more than 7 days. Rebound nasal swelling can occur with excessive or extended use.

46-3　Nonpharmacologic measures would be most appropriate to consider. Intake of adequate fluids, frequent and thorough hand hygiene, and proper disposal of soiled tissues should be reinforced. Chlorpheniramine is an antihistamine. Mr. Hobbs should avoid using an antihistamine; it will dry nasal secretions but it will also dry lower respiratory secretions and may worsen secretion retention and cough. The use of expectorants, such as guaifenesin, has not clearly been supported by research, and many authorities do not support its use.

Chapter 48

48-1　Digitalization in adults is accomplished by the administration of a total dose of 0.75 to 1.0 mg of digoxin in divided doses over a 24-hour period. Although digitalization engenders a higher risk of toxicity, the maximum drug effect will be reached more rapidly.

48-2　The normal digoxin level is 0.5 to 2.0 ng/mL. Toxic serum levels are greater than 2 ng/mL; however, toxicity may occur at any serum level.

48-3　When taken orally, the absorption of digoxin depends on the preparation. Capsules have better absorption than the tablets and should not be substituted equally.

Chapter 49

49-1　The normal therapeutic serum level of lidocaine is 2 to 5 mcg/mL. The risk of adverse effects is reduced when the drug is administered within the therapeutic range. Lidocaine will also not decrease AV conduction or myocardial contractility with therapeutic doses.

49-2　The amiodarone is given to prevent the recurrence of AF and at this low dose it has less toxicity. You should monitor for thyroid dysfunction, pulmonary fibrosis, myocardial depression, hypotension, bradycardia, hepatic dysfunction, CNS disturbances, peripheral neuropathy, bluish discoloration of the skin, and reduced visual acuity.

49-3　Bradycardia may indicate impending heart block or cardiovascular collapse. You should stop the IV infusion and report to the physician if there are marked changes in the rate, rhythm, or quality of the pulse.

Chapter 50

50-1　Mr. Gerald should be taught to never take sildenafil or other drugs in this class while on nitroglycerin. The combination can produce life-threatening hypotension.

50-2　Beta blockers are used in the treatment of CAD for a number of reasons. They reduce the frequency and severity of anginal attacks. Beta blockers also decrease exercise-induced tachycardia. They additionally are more effective at decreasing the likelihood of silent ischemia and improve the mortality rate after an MI.

50-3　Diltiazem is a calcium channel blocker. The drug will improve blood supply to the myocardium and decrease the workload on the heart. In addition, the diltiazem will reduce coronary artery vasospasm, which is most likely the cause of the pain that Mr. Gerald experiences at rest.

Chapter 51

51-1 The nurse needs to monitor the BP and pulse every 5-15 min. until Mr. Alrashed has a sufficient BP and his BP stabilizes. The nurse needs to also assess the IV site frequently, monitor mental status, distal pulses, urine output and skin temperature closely.

51-2 Phentolamine is administered to prevent tissue necrosis in the tissue surrounding the area of infiltration.

51-3 All solutions should be clear in color. The brown discoloration indicates the solution is decomposed and no longer safe to use. The solution should be discarded and new solution obtained.

Chapter 52

52-1 Be aware that compliance is a common problem with patients who have hypertension. Explore the reasons for the noncompliance, such as: is the patient unable to make lifestyle changes; is the patient experiencing adverse effects from the medication; is the patient able to afford the cost of the medication; and does the patient understand this asymptomatic disorder and the many complications that hypertension can cause? As always, provide appropriate teaching.

52-2 Encourage the patient to reduce weight and sodium intake, to get regular physical activity, to stop smoking, and to moderate alcohol intake. These measures can prevent prehypertension and reduce blood pressure in patients with elevated blood pressure. The patient should also understand antihypertensive drug therapy. Always review other behaviors that may decrease the therapeutic response, such as taking over-the-counter medication.

52-3 Due to their efficacy, calcium channel blockers are the drugs of first choice for the treatment of hypertension in African Americans, according to the JNC 7.

Chapter 53

53-1 This provides an opportunity to teach Ms. Bass that avoiding foods high in sodium will help her diuretic to work more effectively. Table salt is an obvious food to avoid, but she should also read the sodium content of food containers and avoid those high in sodium, such as potato chips and other salty snacks.

53-2 Spironolactone is a potassium-sparing diuretic. This diuretic will enhance diuresis without depleting potassium like furosemide would. You should observe for hyperkalemia with patients taking a potassium-sparing diuretic.

53-3 IV-push furosemide should be given over 1 to 2 minutes, up to a 40-milligram dose. Too-rapid administration may lead to increased ototoxicity.

Chapter 54

54-1 The main reason anticoagulants are used is to prevent the formation of new clots and the extension of clots that are already present. Heparin does not dissolve a clot that is already formed. The main adverse effect is bleeding.

54-2 The goal of therapy with heparin is to maintain the aPTT at 1.5 to 2.5 times the baseline value. In most patients, the goal will be 45 to 70 seconds.

54-3 Have the blood work evaluated before any warfarin is given. Subsequent assessment of PT/INR should be performed before the second dose of warfarin is given.

54-4 Aspirin is used in long-term therapy for the prevention of clot formation in atrial fibrillation and to prevent a future myocardial infarction.

Chapter 55

55-1 Inform Mr. Watkins that he will need to have blood analysis performed in 4 to 6 weeks. He will need to be without food for the triglyceride level. In addition to lipid levels, the physician will check liver function.

55-2 Although this group of drugs is usually well tolerated, potential adverse effects include nausea, constipation, diarrhea, abdominal cramps or pain, headache, and skin rash. Tell Mr. Watkins to notify his health care provider if he notices **unexplained muscle pain or tenderness:** This can be a warning sign of rhabdomyolysis, a destruction of the muscle. Patients at higher risk are the elderly; those on a high dose of a statin; those with a small body frame; and those concurrently taking gemfibrozil, such as Mr. Watkins.

55-3 Gemfibrozil must be administered at least 30 minutes before food and on an empty stomach.

Chapter 57

57-1 Include the administration of a multivitamin with her daily nourishment. The undernourished frequently have deficiencies in vitamins A, D, B_{12}, folic acid, riboflavin, and thiamine.

57-2 In the elderly, the most common mineral-electrolyte deficiencies are of calcium and iron. Excess states are also possible. Serum levels of minerals and electrolytes should be monitored carefully and measures taken to prevent both deficiency and excess.

57-3 Iron preparations are to be administered before meals for best absorption. When given with coffee, tea, or dairy products, absorption is decreased.

Chapter 58

58-1 Orlistat works by blocking the fat absorbed from the intestine. This drug will block approximately 30% of the fat ingested in a meal. It is important to teach that increasing the dose will not increase the percentage of fat blocked. This drug also blocks the absorption of fat-soluble vitamins, so you should advise Ms. Vargas to take a multivitamin at a different time than the orlistat.

58-2 Strategies should include the practice of a healthy lifestyle by eating a variety of foods daily and by eating a diet rich in whole grains, vegetables, and low-fat dairy products. Limit the intake of saturated fat, trans fat, cholesterol, added sugars, salt, and alcohol. Ms. Vargas must also include some regular physical activity.

58-3 The initial goal of weight-loss therapy should be to reduce body weight by about 10 percent from baseline weight at a rate of one to two pounds per week for the first 6 months. Assist Ms. Vargas to set a realistic and healthy goal.

58-4 The dose of orlistat should not be taken if the patient misses a meal. Teach Ms. Vargas to omit the dose if a meal is missed.

Chapter 59

59-1 Teach Ms. Daniels to avoid cigarette smoking, alcohol, caffeine, aspirin, and NSAIDs.

59-2 Acid reflux can be reduced by avoiding stomach distention. Eating small meals will reduce gastric distention. Teach Ms. Daniels not to lie down for at least 1 to 2 hours after eating. Foods and drinks that can increase acid reflux include fats, chocolate, citric juices, coffee, and alcohol. Take medication with 8 oz of water. Control obesity, constipation, or other causes of increased intra-abdominal pressure. It may also be helpful to elevate the head of the bed to reduce acid reflux.

59-3 When providing patient teaching about drug therapy, include the reasons why each medication has been selected. Make sure to encourage the patient to ask questions. Teach Ms. Daniels that the reason she is to take Mylanta is because it contains simethicone; Maalox does not. Although simethicone will not reduce gastric acid, it does relieve gas and reflux.

Chapter 60

60-1 Ms. Campbell is elderly, has hemorrhoids and has chronic disease and should not strain when having a bowel movement. Docusate sodium is most likely the drug of choice. This drug has little laxative effect. Docusate sodium will work by decreasing the surface tension of the fecal mass, thereby allowing water to enter the stool. It will also act as a detergent to facilitate the addition of fat and water to the stool, thereby making it easier to expel.

60-2 Assess for the number of stools, the appearance of the fecal mass, any abdominal distention or discomfort, or flatulence. Evaluate the drugs Ms. Campbell is taking because they may reduce intestinal function. Also, assess risk factors such as decreased activity and a diet with minimal fiber intake and low fluid intake.

60-3 Ms. Campbell has taken much more medication than needed. The psyllium preparation will usually act in 12 to 24 hours but may take as long as 2 to 3 days to exert the full effect. Milk of magnesia is a saline cathartic that will usually have an effect in 0.5 to 6 hours. Ms. Campbell did not allow either of these medications enough time to work. She also administered a stimulant cathartic that should not be used in older patients. Teach Ms. Campbell about drug actions, including how long before each drug takes effect. Also, provide guidance on appropriate drug selection.

Chapter 61

61-1 Determine the number of stools each day and the amount, consistency, color, odor, and presence of abnormal components in each stool. Ask Mr. Mendoza what measures he has initiated to relieve the diarrhea and if he has any other symptoms, such as nausea and vomiting or fever. The most obvious cause of Mr. Mendoza's diarrhea is his recent trip to Mexico; however, also consider chronic inflammatory diseases of the bowel, use of laxative or other drugs, and food intake.

61-2 The drug of choice to treat diarrhea is loperamide. Mr. Mendoza should be instructed to take no more than 8 mg per day: 4 mg initially then 2 mg after each loose stool. If his symptoms persist for more than 48 hours, Mr. Mendoza should consult his physician.

61-3 Mr. Mendoza should discontinue the use of loperamide. Antidiarrheal agents are contraindicated in diarrhea caused by microorganisms. In these circumstances, antidiarrheal agents that slow peristalsis may aggravate and prolong diarrhea.

Chapter 62

62-1 Assess for headache, diarrhea or constipation, dizziness, fatigue, and muscle aches.

62-2 Encourage Ms. Snyder to minimize activity during acute nausea and vomiting. Avoid oral intake of food, fluids, and drugs, because this may increase vomiting. Encourage Ms. Snyder to take antiemetics 30 to 60 minutes before meals or a nausea-producing event such as radiation or chemotherapy. Avoid exposure to stimuli as much as possible; this includes unpleasant sights and odors, alcohol, and excessive ingestion of food or drugs that irritate the gastric mucosa.

62-3 Diphenhydramine is given with metoclopramide to decrease metoclopramide's extrapyramidal effects.

62-4 You should follow the patient's wishes whenever possible; however, Ms. Snyder needs to understand that the antiemetic medication will work much better when given to prevent nausea and vomiting rather than to treat it. Convey to her that the pretreatment approach will increase her comfort and allow the use of lower doses of the drugs.

Chapter 63

63-1 Instruct Mrs. Molnar to avoid activities that increase IOP. She should avoid straining at stool, heavy lifting, bending over, coughing, and vomiting when possible.

63-2 Wash hands before applying the medications. To decrease the systemic absorption of eye drops, instruct Mrs. Molnar to close the eye and apply pressure to the tear duct for 3 to 5 minutes after instillation. When multiple eye drops are prescribed, there should be an interval of 5 to 10 minutes between the medications.

63-3 The nurse should observe for bradycardia, arrhythmias and bronchoconstriction.

Chapter 64

64-1 The drug of choice for Ginger is most likely a low-potency, topical hydrocortisone.

64-2 Teach Ginger that dry skin and pruritus are aggravated by hot water and harsh soap, so she should take warm baths and use a gentle cleanser. Patting the skin dry with a towel and using a lotion will reduce the irritation. She may also take a colloidal-oatmeal bath to help relieve the pruritus.

64-3 Apply hydrocortisone sparingly, in a thin layer. Ginger may apply it twice daily until the itch and redness are resolved. If she experiences relief with less frequent application, she should use the drug less often.

64-4 The most appropriate nursing diagnosis based on these data is Disturbed Body Image related to visible skin lesions.

Chapter 65

65-1 Instruct Mrs. Blevins to begin to take 400 to 600 micrograms of folic acid daily. Folic acid supplementation can prevent neural-tube birth defects.

65-2 Tell Mrs. Blevins that constipation is a common occurrence during pregnancy. The best treatment is to increase amount of exercise and intake of fluids and high-fiber foods. If a laxative is needed, a bulk-producing agent is recommended because it is safest for both mother and fetus.

65-3 All systemically absorbed drugs in the mother's blood-stream will reach the fetus. Drugs are listed with an FDA pregnancy risk category based on the amount of risk to the fetus. Drugs categorized as risk category X should not be used at all during pregnancy. Most drugs are risk category C and should be discussed with the physician. These drugs should only be used when the potential benefit to the mother outweighs the risk to the fetus.

65-4 Mrs. Blevins needs a new prescription for birth control without estrogen. Ortho Tri-Cyclen contains estrogen; estrogen is contraindicated while she is breast-feeding.

Index

Page numbers followed by f indicate figures; t, tables; b, boxes

A

abacavir (Ziagen), 565t, 574
abatacept (Orencia), 656t, 664
abbreviations, 32, 33t
abciximab (ReoPro), 866t, 869
Abelcet (amphotericin B lipid complex), 585t, 593–594, 596–597
Abilify (aripiprazole), 156t, 160t, 162, 169, 171, 181t
abortifacients, 1049, 1050t, 1054–1055
absence seizure, 197
absolute refractory period, 780
absorption, 11–12
acarbose (Precose), 420t, 440
Accolate (zafirlukast), 720–721, 723, 727
AccuNeb (albuterol), 715, 715t–716t
Accupril (quinapril), 829t
Accutane (isotretinoin), 1031t, 1037
acebutolol (Sectral), 299t, 784t, 787, 830t
Aceon (perindopril), 829t
acetaminophen (Tylenol)
    antidote for, 23t, 121
    in children, 123
    patient teaching about, 119–120
    dosage of, 107t, 121
    in hepatic-impaired patients, 124
    in home care, 124
    indications for, 104–105, 105, 121
    metabolism of, 112
    in older adults, 123–124
    opioid/acetaminophen products, 88t
    pharmacokinetics of, 112
    in renal-impaired patients, 124
    toxicity, 121
acetazolamide (Diamox), 1014t
acetic acid derivatives, 111
acetylcholine
    cholinergic receptor stimulation by, 314
    description of, 75, 271
    dopamine and, 218
    functions of, 313–314
acetylcysteine (Mucomyst)
    antidote uses of, 23t
    description of, 121
    mucolytic uses of, 749t
acetylsalicylic acid. See aspirin
achlorhydria, 965
acid reflux, 954
acid-base balance, 910
acidosis, 431
Aciphex (rabeprazole), 957t, 959
acitretin (Soriatane), 1031t
Aclovate (alclometasone), 1030t
acne, 1027, 1037–1038

acquired immunodeficiency syndrome
    description of, 373
    human immunodeficiency virus progression to, 561b
ACTH (corticotropin), 347, 349t, 351
Acthar Gel (corticotropin), 349t, 351
ActHIB (*Haemophilus influenzae* b conjugate vaccine), 629t
Actifed Cold & Allergy, 749t
Actimmune (interferon gamma-1b), 645t
Actinex (masoprocol), 1032t
Actinomycin D (dactinomycin), 680t
Actiq (fentanyl), 83, 84t
Activase (alteplase), 867t, 870
activated charcoal, 22b–23b, 263
activated partial thromboplastin time, 873–874
active immunity, 616, 626
active transport, 12b
active tuberculosis, 543
Activella, 449t
Acto Plus Met (pioglitazone/metformin), 421t
Actonel (risedronate), 398, 399t, 407
Actos (pioglitazone), 420t, 439, 440
Acular (ketorolac), 1017t
acute ingestion, 244
acute pain
    description of, 80b, 91
    opioid analgesics for, 91–92, 95
acute renal failure, 64, 927
acyclovir (Zovirax), 563t, 567, 575, 576, 1030t
Adalat (nifedipine), 802t, 804, 831t
adalizumab (Humira), 656t, 663
adapalene (Differin), 1031t
adaptive immunity, 616
Adderall, 258
Addison's disease, 360, 362
additive effects, 17
adefovir (Hepsera), 564t
A-delta fibers, 80
Adenocard (adenosine), 785t–786t, 788
adenosine (Adenocard), 785t–786t, 788
adenosine diphosphate receptor antagonists, 869
adequate intake, 903b
Adipex-P (phentermine hydrochloride), 940, 940t, 948–949
adjuvant chemotherapy, 695
administration of drugs
    abbreviations commonly used in, 32, 33t
    in critical-illness patients, 66
    dosages. See drug dosages
    drug preparations for, 68
    ear medications, 46
    ear solutions, 35t
    eye solutions, 35t, 46
    gastrointestinal, 37t